Pathophysiology

Concepts of Altered Health States

Carol Mattson Porth
R.N., M.S.N., Ph.D. (Physiology)
Associate Professor, School of Nursing
University of Wisconsin-Milwaukee
Adjunct Assistant Professor
Department of Physiology
Medical College of Wisconsin
Milwaukee, Wisconsin

Pathophysiology
Concepts of Altered Health States

THIRD EDITION

With 18 contributors
Illustrated by Carole Russell Hilmer and others

J.B. Lippincott Company   Philadelphia

Grand Rapids   London
New York   Sydney
St. Louis   Tokyo
San Francisco

Acquisitions Editor: David P. Carroll
Project Editor: Dina Kamilatos
Manuscript Editors: Mary Frawley, Patrick O'Kane
Indexer: Nancy Weaver
Art Director: Susan Hess Blaker
Design Coordinator: Ellen C. Dawson
Interior and Cover Designer: Ellen C. Dawson
Production Manager: Carol A. Florence
Production Coordinator: Caren Erlichman
Compositor: Tapsco
Printer/Binder: Murray Printing Company

Cover photographs (left to right): Diabetic retinopathy *(Courtesy National Eye Institute);* Retinoblastoma; Healthy red blood cells *(Courtesy of S.T.E.M. Laboratories and Fisher Scientific);* Sickle cells *(Brunner LS, Suddarth DS: Textbook of Medical–Surgical Nursing, 3rd ed);* Healthy lung tissue *(Courtesy of Kenneth Siegesmund, Ph.D., Anatomy Department, The Medical College of Wisconsin);* Emphysematous lung tissue *(Courtesy of Kenneth Siegesmund, Ph.D., Anatomy Department, The Medical College of Wisconsin)*

3rd Edition

3 5 6 4

Library of Congress Cataloging-in-Publication Data

Porth, Carol.
  Pathophysiology: concepts of altered health states / Carol
Mattson Porth; with contributors; illustrated by Carole Russell
Hilmer and others.—3rd ed.
      p. cm.
  Includes bibliographies and index.
  ISBN 0-397-54723-4
  1. Physiology, Pathological. 2. Nursing. I. Title.
  [DNLM: 1. Disease—nurses' instruction. 2. Pathology—nurses'
instruction. 3. Physiology—nurses' instruction.   QZ 4 P851p]
RB113.P67   1990
616.07—dc20
DNLM/DLC
for Library of Congress   89-12503
                                                        CIP

Any procedure or practice described in this book should be applied by the health-care practitioner under appropriate supervision in accordance with professional standards of care used with regard to the unique circumstances that apply in each practice situation. Care has been taken to confirm the accuracy of information presented and to describe generally accepted practices. However, the authors, editors, and publisher cannot accept any responsibility for errors or omissions or for any consequences from application of the information in this book and make no warranty, express or implied, with respect to the contents of the book.

Every effort has been made to ensure drug selections and dosages are in accordance with current recommendations and practice. Because of ongoing research, changes in government regulations and the constant flow of information on drug therapy, reactions and interactions, the reader is cautioned to check the package insert for each drug for indications, dosages, warnings and precautions, particularly if the drug is new or infrequently used.

Contributors

Laura J. Burke, R.N., M.S.N.
  Cardiovascular Clinical Specialist
  Sinai Samaritan Medical Center
  Milwaukee, Wisconsin

Robin L. Curtis, Ph.D.
  Associate Professor
  Department of Anatomy and Cellular Science and
    Department of Physical Medicine Rehabilitation
  Medical College of Wisconsin
  Milwaukee, Wisconsin

Sheila M. Curtis, R.N., M.S.
  Lecturer, University of Wisconsin-Milwaukee
    School of Nursing
  Doctoral Student
  Marquette University
  Milwaukee, Wisconsin

Susan E. Dietz, R.N., M.S.M.
  Health Education Specialist
  Division of Sexually Transmitted Diseases
  Center for Prevention Services
  Centers for Disease Control
  Atlanta, Georgia

W. Michael Dunne, Jr., Ph.D.
  Assistant Professor of Pathology and Pediatrics
  Medical College of Wisconsin
  Milwaukee, Wisconsin

Sylvia Eichner, R.N., M.S.N.
  Clinical Nurse Specialist, Spinal Cord Injury
  Froedtert Memorial Lutheran Hospital
  Milwaukee, Wisconsin

Susan Gallagher-Lepak, R.N., M.S.N.
  Transplant Clinical Nurse Specialist
  Froedtert Memorial Lutheran Hospital
  Milwaukee, Wisconsin

Kathryn J. Gaspard, Ph.D.
  Education Supervisor
  The Blood Center of Southeastern Wisconsin
  Milwaukee, Wisconsin

Kathleen E. Gunta, R.N., M.S.N.
  Clinical Nurse Specialist
  Sinai Samaritan Medical Center
  Milwaukee, Wisconsin

Linda S. Hurwitz, R.N., M.S.N.
  Director of Nursing
  Pediatrics, Obstetrics, and Gynecology
  The Presbyterian Hospital of the City of New York
  Columbia-Presbyterian Medical Center
  New York, New York

Patricia McCowen Mehring, R.N., M.S.N.
  Obstetrical-Gynecological Nurse Practitioner
  Women's Care
  Waukesha, Wisconsin

Janice Smith Pigg, R.N., M.S.N.
  Nurse Consultant, Rheumatology
  Midwest Arthritis Treatment Center
  Director, Musculoskeletal Services
  Columbia Hospital
  Milwaukee, Wisconsin

Joan Pleuss, R.D., M.S., C.D.E.
  Senior Research Dietician
  Clinical Research Center
  Medical College of Wisconsin at Froedtert
    Memorial Lutheran Hospital
  Milwaukee, Wisconsin

Eileen Sherburne, R.N., M.S.N.
  Certified Neurological Nurse
  Neurology and Pulmonary Rehabilitation Clinic
  Children's Hospital of Wisconsin
  Milwaukee, Wisconsin

Gladys Simandl, R.N.
  Doctoral Candidate
  University of Wisconsin-Milwaukee School of
    Nursing
  Milwaukee, Wisconsin

Stephanie M. Stewart, R.N., M.S.N.
  Doctoral Candidate and Associate Professor
  Bellin College of Nursing
  Green Bay, Wisconsin

Darlene G. Thornhill, R.N., M.S.N.
  Formerly Patient Care Director
  Medical College of Wisconsin
  Clinical Research Center
  Milwaukee, Wisconsin

Nancie Urban, R.N., M.S.N., C.C.R.N.
  Director of Critical Care Services
  Sinai Samaritan Medical Center
  Milwaukee, Wisconsin

Preface

The meaning of pathophysiology, or physiology of altered health, reflects not so much the pathologic processes that take place but the physiologic changes and responses that produce signs and symptoms. These changes determine, to a large extent, whether a disease will be disabling, and are thus of concern to most health-care professionals.

As a nurse-physiologist, my major aim in writing *Pathophysiology: Concepts of Altered Health States* was to relate normal body functioning to the physiologic changes that occur as a result of illness, as well as the body's remarkable ability to compensate for these changes. A conceptual model that integrates developmental and preventive aspects of health was used. Selection of content was based on common health problems, including the special health needs of children and elderly persons. The book provides the rationale, but not the "how to's" of health care, the specifics of drug therapy, or the particulars of diagnostic methods. It is assumed that the reader will have access to more complete reference sources in these areas than this book could provide.

My second aim was to present the content in an easily understood manner. Concepts from physiology, biochemistry, physics, and other sciences are reviewed as deemed appropriate. Diagrams to aid in visualizing the content and tables to aid in identifying and summarizing essential information have been included throughout the text. Objectives appear at the beginning of each chapter. A comprehensive bibliography is provided in many chapters.

The book is organized into units: the first deals with the cellular aspects of disease, the second with body defenses, and the others with alterations in organ and system function. The content of the book has been organized into three areas of focus based on the health–illness continuum: (1) control of normal body function; (2) pathophysiology, or alterations in body function; and (3) system or organ failure, regardless of pathologic state (*e.g.*, heart failure and renal failure). In some sections, separate chapters have been devoted to each of these areas, while in others, the content has been integrated within a single chapter.

This third edition has been greatly expanded and reorganized. An entire new chapter has been devoted to acquired immunodeficiency syndrome (AIDS); two other new chapters, one on alterations in thermal regulation and another on alterations in nutrition, have been added; and the entire unit on alterations in neuromuscular function has been reorganized. These additions and changes reflect the newer concerns in health care as well as the expressed needs of my colleagues and students.

As with previous editions, every effort was made to make the text as accurate and as up-to-date as possible. This was accomplished through an extensive review of the literature and through the use of critiques provided by students, faculty, and content specialists. As this vast amount of information was processed, inaccuracies or omissions may have occurred. Readers are encouraged to contact me about such errors. Such feedback is essential to the continued development of the book.

Carol Mattson Porth, R.N., M.S.N., Ph.D.

Acknowledgments

As with previous editions, many persons contributed to the development of this edition.

Carole Russell Hilmer, medical illustrator, deserves a special commendation for her tireless effort in creating the illustrations for this edition as well as previous editions of the book. She has been able to take ordinary ideas and develop them into both attractive and instructive figures.

The students in my classes deserve a special commendation, because their questions, comments, and enthusiasm provided the motivation needed for a task such as this.

A number of people were kind enough to review parts of the text and make helpful suggestions: John E. Ridely III, M.D., Elizabeth Boldt, R.N., Elias A. Lianos, M.D., Betty Pearson, R.N., Ph.D., and John Kosko, M.D. In addition, there are a number of persons who reviewed the text for the publisher, but who are unknown to the author. These persons made valuable comments and are to be commended.

The contributing authors deserve a special mention, for they worked long hours to supply essential content. Mary Rice, Pharm.D., read the pharmacology content to ensure its accuracy.

Several previous contributing authors were not able to participate in this edition: Debbie L. Cook, R.N., M.S.N., C.N.M., Pamela M. Schroeder, R.N., M.S.N., Mary Wierenga, R.N., Ph.D., and E. Ronald Wright, Ph.D. Their contributions to previous editions greatly facilitated the preparation of this edition.

Several other persons deserve special recognition. Georgianne Heymann, R.N., B.S.N., served as my local editor for the book. As with the previous edition, she provided not only excellent editorial services, but encouragement and support when the tasks associated with manuscript preparation became most dismal. Jill A. Barney, M.S, also edited sections of the book and provided helpful input. Heidi Habel, nursing student, conducted library searches, typed manuscripts, made copies, and read manuscripts. I also want to thank Michelle Heeg and Heather Robison, B.S.N., for their help in copying and conducting library searches.

Contents

UNIT III: ALTERATIONS IN OXYGENATION OF TISSUES

UNIT IV: ALTERATIONS IN BODY FLUIDS

UNIT V: ALTERATIONS IN GENITOURINARY FUNCTION

UNIT VI: ALTERATIONS IN METABOLISM, ENDOCRINE FUNCTION, AND NUTRITION

UNIT VII: ALTERATIONS IN NEUROMUSCULAR FUNCTION

Pathophysiology

Concepts of Altered Health States

Alterations in Cell Function and Growth

CHAPTER 1

Carol Mattson Porth
Robin L. Curtis

Cell and Tissue Characteristics

Functional components of the cell
Nucleus
Cytoplasm and its organelles
  Ribosomes
  Endoplasmic reticulum
  Golgi complex
  Mitochondria
  Lysosomes
  Microtubules and
    microfilaments

Cell membrane
  Membrane junctions
  Membrane transport
  Membrane potentials
Cellular energy metabolism
Anaerobic metabolism
Aerobic metabolism
  Citric acid cycle
  Oxidative phosphorylation

Tissue types
  Cell differentiation
  Embryonic origin of tissue types
  Epithelial tissue
  Connective tissue
  Muscle tissue
  Nervous tissue

Objectives

After you have studied this chapter, you should be able to meet the following objectives:

_____ List the components of the cell nucleus and the function of each.

_____ State the composition of the ribosomes.

_____ Differentiate rough ER and smooth ER according to function.

_____ State the function of the Golgi complex.

_____ State the composition of the cytoplasm.

_____ Explain why the mitochondria are described as the power plants of the cell.

_____ State a possible role of the lysosomes in irreversible shock.

_____ Define *microtubule, microfilament,* and *centriole* on the basis of function.

_____ State four functions of the cell membrane.

_____ State the mechanisms of membrane transport.

_____ Explain the function of the intercellular junctions.

_____ Describe the process of cell differentiation.

_____ Use the equilibrium (Nernst) equation to explain how an increase or decrease in serum potassium affects the resting membrane potential.

_____ Describe the movement of charge and the changes in membrane potential that occur during an action potential.

_____ Explain why the basic tissue types are described in terms of their embryonic origin.

_____ Characterize the three types of epithelium.

_____ State the function of each of the three types of connective tissue.

_____ Describe the properties of muscle tissue.

_____ State the general function of nervous tissue.

In order to understand the functioning of the human body in health and disease, it is necessary to understand how the individual cells of the body are structured and how they function. The cell is the smallest functional unit that an organism can be divided into and still retain the characteristics necessary for life. Cells, in turn, are organized into larger functional units called *tissue,* and it is the tissues that form body structures and organs. Although the cells of different tissues and organs vary in structure and function, there are certain characteristics that are common to all cells. Cells are remarkably similar in their ability to exchange materials with their immediate environment, in obtaining energy from organic nutrients, in synthesizing complex molecules, and in duplicating themselves. It is at the level of the cell that most disease processes exert their effects. Some diseases affect the cells of a single organ, others affect the cells of a particular tissue type, and still others affect the cells of the entire organism.

The substances that make up the cells of living organisms are collectively referred to as *protoplasm.* Protoplasm is composed of water, proteins, lipids, carbohydrates, and electrolytes. Water makes up 70% to 85% of the cell's protoplasm. The second most abundant constituent (10–20%) of protoplasm is the cell proteins, which form cell structures and the enzymes necessary for cellular reactions. Lipids constitute 2% to 3% of most cells and are insoluble in water. They serve as a cellular storage form for nutrients and combine with proteins to form the membranes that separate the various compartments of the cell. Only small amounts of carbohydrates are found in the cell, and these are used primarily for fuel. The major intracellular electrolytes are potassium, magnesium, phosphate, sulfate, and bicarbonate. There are also smaller quantities of sodium, chloride, and calcium. These electrolytes facilitate the generation and transmission of electrochemical impulses in nerve and muscle cells. Intracellular electrolytes participate in reactions that are necessary for cellular metabolism. In this chapter, we discuss the functional components of the cell, cellular energy metabolism, tissue types, and membrane potentials.

Functional components of the cell

Although diverse in their organization, all cells have common structures that perform unique and special functions. When seen under a light microscope, three major components of the cell become evident: the nucleus, the cytoplasm, and the cell membrane (Figure 1-1).

The nucleus

The nucleus is the control center for the cell. It contains the individual units of heredity—*the genes*—which are strung along the chromosomes. In a resting cell the chromosomes appear as darkly stained granules known as *chromatin material.* Chemically, each gene consists of deoxyribonucleic acid (DNA). Genes control cellular activity by determining the type of proteins, enzymes, and other substances that are made by the cell. The nucleus is also the site of ribonucleic acid (RNA) synthesis. There are three kinds of RNA: messenger RNA (mRNA), which carries the

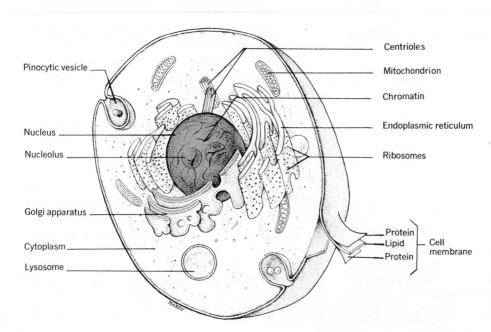

Figure 1-1 A composite cell designed to show, in one cell, all of the various components of the nucleus and cytoplasm. (*Chaffee EE, Greisheimer EM: Basic Physiology and Anatomy, 3rd ed. Philadelphia, JB Lippincott, 1974*)

Pinocytic vesicle

Nucleus

Nucleolus

Golgi apparatus

Cytoplasm

Lysosome

Centrioles

Mitochondrion

Chromatin

Endoplasmic reticulum

Ribosomes

Protein
Lipid — Cell membrane
Protein

instructions from DNA for protein synthesis to the cytoplasm; ribosomal RNA (rRNA), which moves to the cytoplasm where it becomes the site of protein synthesis, and transfer RNA (tRNA), which serves as an amino acid transport system for protein synthesis. In addition to the chromatin, the nucleus contains one or two rounded bodies called *nucleoli.* It is here that rRNA is synthesized. The nuclear contents are surrounded by a double-walled nuclear membrane. The pores present in this membrane allow fluids, electrolytes, RNA, and other materials to move between the nuclear and cytoplasmic compartments.

The cytoplasm and its organelles

The cytoplasm surrounds the nucleus, and it is here that the work of the cell takes place. The cytoplasm is essentially a colloidal solution that contains water, electrolytes, suspended proteins, neutral fats, and glycogen molecules. Although they do not contribute to the cell's function, pigments may also accumulate in the cytoplasm. Some pigments, such as melanin, which gives skin its color, are normal constituents of the cell. Others, such as carbon and coal dust, which are commonly found in the lungs of coal miners and persons living in polluted environments, are abnormal.

Embedded within the cytoplasm are the *organelles,* or inner organs of the cell. These include the ribosomes, endoplasmic reticulum, Golgi complex, mitochondria, lysosomes, microtubules, and microfilaments.

Ribosomes

The ribosomes serve as sites of protein synthesis in the cell. They are small particles of nucleoproteins (rRNA and proteins) that can be found attached to the wall of endoplasmic reticulum or as free ribosomes (Figure 1-2). The free ribosomes are scattered singly in the cytoplasm or joined to form functional units called *polyribosomes.* The free ribosomes are involved in the synthesis of proteins, such as intracellular enzymes, that are used within the cell. The ribosomes that are attached to the endoplasmic reticulum synthesize proteins that are exported from the cell.

Endoplasmic reticulum

The endoplasmic reticulum (ER) is an extensive system of paired parallel membranes that connects various parts of the inner cell (see Figure 1-2). The space between the paired ER membrane layers is connected with the space between the two membranes of the double-layered nuclear membrane, allowing for

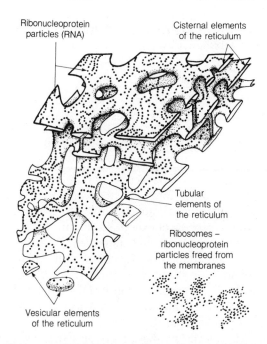

Figure 1-2 Three-dimensional view of the granular endoplasmic reticulum with ribosomal RNA. (*Modified from Bloom W, Faucett DW: Histology, 10th ed. Philadelphia, WB Saunders, 1975*)

transport between the nucleus and the cytoplasm. There are two types of ER—rough and smooth. The rough ER is studded with ribosomes. The function of the rough ER is to segregate proteins that are being exported from the cell from other components of the cytoplasm and modify their structure. Hormone synthesis by glandular cells and plasma protein production by liver cells take place in the rough ER. The smooth ER is free of ribosomes but is often attached to the rough ER. The functions of the smooth ER vary in different cells. The sarcoplasmic reticulum of skeletal and cardiac muscle cells is a form of smooth ER. Calcium ions needed for muscle contraction are stored and released from cisterns located in the sarcoplasmic reticulum of these cells.

In the liver, the smooth ER is involved in glycogen storage and drug metabolism. An interesting form of adaptation occurs in the smooth ER of the liver cells responsible for metabolizing certain drugs such as phenobarbital. It is known that repeated administration of phenobarbital leads to a state of increased tolerance to the drug, such that the same dose of drug no longer produces the same degree of sedation. This response has been traced to increased drug metabolism due to increased synthesis of drug-metabolizing enzymes by the ER membrane. This system is sometimes called the *microsomal system* because the ER can be fragmented in the laboratory, and when this is done, small vesicles called *microsomes* are formed. The microsomal system responsible for metabolizing phenobarbital has a crossover effect that influences the metabolism of other drugs that use the same metabolic pathway.

Golgi complex

The Golgi complex (or apparatus) consists of flattened membranous saccules and cisterns that communicate with the ER and acts as a receptacle for hormones and other substances that the ER produces. It then modifies and packages these substances into secretory granules. The secretory granules move out of the Golgi complex into the cytoplasm and, following an appropriate signal, are then released from the cell through the process of exocytosis. Figure 1-3 is a diagram of the synthesis and movement of a hormone through the endoplasmic reticulum and Golgi complex. In addition to secreting proteins, the Golgi complex is thought to produce some of the large carbohydrate molecules that are needed to combine with proteins produced in the rough ER to form glycoproteins. Many cells synthesize proteins that are larger than the active product. Insulin, for example, is synthesized as a larger inactive proinsulin molecule that is cut apart and reassembled into a smaller active insulin molecule in the Golgi complex of the beta cells of the pancreas.

Mitochondria

The mitochondria are literally the "power plants" of the cell, for it is here that the energy-rich compound adenosine triphosphate (ATP), which powers the various cellular activities, is generated. The mitochondria require oxygen to capture energy contained in foodstuffs and convert it into the high-energy bonds of ATP. The enzymes involved in oxidative metabolism are present only in the mitochondria.

The mitochondria are encased in a double membrane. An outer membrane encloses the periphery of the mitochondria and an inner membrane is enfolded to form the cristae, which aid in the production and temporary storage of ATP (Figure 1-4). The mitochondria are located close to the site of energy consumption in the cell: for example, near the myofibrils in muscle cells. The number of mitochondria in a given cell type is largely determined by the type of activity that the cell performs and the amount of energy that is needed to perform this activity.

Lysosomes

The lysosomes essentially form the digestive system of the cell. They consist of small membrane-enclosed vesicles or sacs that contain hydrolytic enzymes capable of breaking down worn-out cell parts so that they can be recycled. They also envelope or destroy foreign material that enters the cell. The enzymes contained in the lysosomes are so powerful that they are often called "suicide bags," because under abnormal conditions their contents can be released, causing lysis and the destruction of cellular contents. Under other conditions their contents can be released into the extracellular spaces, destroying the surrounding cells. One theory of irreversible shock suggests that this stage of shock is caused, at least in part, by widespread release of lysosomal enzymes from cells that have been damaged by lack of oxygen.

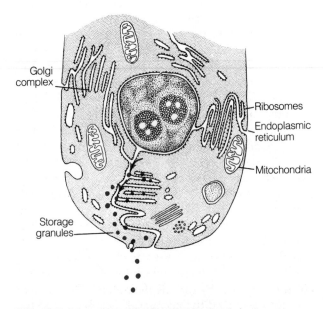

Figure 1-3 Hormone synthesis and secretion. In hormone secretion, the hormone is synthesized by the ribosomes that are attached to the rough endoplasmic reticulum (ER). It moves from the rough ER to the Golgi complex where it is stored in the form of secretory granules. These leave the Golgi complex and are stored within the cytoplasm until released from the cell in response to an appropriate signal.

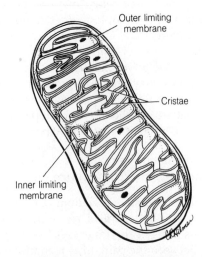

Figure 1-4 Mitochondrion. The inner membrane forms transverse folds called cristae. It is here that the enzymes needed for the final step in adenosine triphosphate (ATP) production (oxidative phosphorylation) are located.

Microtubules and microfilaments

The *microtubules* are long, rigid, threadlike structures dispersed throughout the cytoplasm.

Microtubules function in a number of ways. They (1) maintain the shape of cells—long cell processes like the axons of nerve cells exist only because they are reinforced by numerous microtubules; (2) serve as a transport system for the movement of compounds and organelles within the cell; (3) construct the mitotic spindle; and (4) provide for the support and movement of cilia and flagella. Because they control cell shape and movement, the microtubules and microfilaments are often called the *cytoskeletal* system.

In cilia and sperm, the microtubules occur in doublets. The centrioles, which will be discussed next, contain microtubules arranged in triplets. It appears that microtubules can be rapidly assembled and disassembled according to the needs of the cell. The assembly of microtubules is halted by the action of the plant alkaloid colchicine. In the laboratory this compound is used to halt cell mitosis. It is also used in the treatment of gout. It is thought that the drug's ability to reduce the inflammatory reaction associated with this condition stems from its ability to interfere with microtubular function and leukocyte motility.

The *microfilaments* occur in association with the microtubules. The contractile muscle proteins—actin, myosin, and troponin—are examples of microfilaments found in muscle cells. Microfilaments are also found in the microvilli of the intestinal brush border surface.

Abnormalities of the cytoskeletal system may constitute important causes of alterations in cellular function. For example, proper functioning of the microfilaments and microtubules is essential for various stages of leukocyte migration. In certain disease conditions, such as diabetes mellitus, alterations in leukocyte mobility and migration may interfere with the chemotaxis and phagocytosis of the inflammatory response and predispose to the development of bacterial infection.[1]

The *centrioles* are cylindrical structures composed of highly organized microtubules. A centriole is composed of nine bundles, each containing three microtubules that are arranged in a pinwheel configuration. The centrioles serve as a template for microtubule formation and organization. In dividing cells, they form the mitotic spindle that aids in the separation and movement of the chromosomes during cell division.

The cell membrane

The cell is enclosed in a thin membrane that separates the intracellular contents from the extracellular environment. To distinguish it from the other cell membranes, such as the mitochondrial or nuclear membranes, the cell membrane is often called the *plasma membrane*. In many respects, the plasma membrane is one of the most important parts of the cell. The functions of the cell membrane include (1) acting as a semipermeable membrane that separates the intracellular and extracellular environments; (2) providing receptors for hormones and other biologically active substances; (3) participating in the electrical events that occur in nerve and muscle cells; and (4) aiding in the regulation of growth and proliferation. It is also thought that the cell membrane may play an important role in the behavior of cancer cells,[2] which will be discussed in Chapter 5.

The cell membrane consists of an organized arrangement of lipids, carbohydrates, and proteins (Figure 1-5). According to current theories, the lipids form a bilayer structure that is essentially impermeable to all but the lipid-soluble substances. It is believed that globular proteins are embedded in this lipid bilayer and that these proteins participate in the transport of lipid-insoluble particles through the plasma membrane. According to this schema, some of the globular proteins move within the membrane structure acting as carriers, some are attached to either side of the membrane, and others pass directly through the membrane and communicate with both the inside and the outside of the cell. It is probable that these latter proteins form channels that permit passage of substances such as water and ions such as sodium, hydrogen, and chloride. There are different membrane channels for different ions. For example, one set of pores, called the *sodium channels,* are selectively permeable to sodium.

The cell surface has been observed, under the electron microscope, to be surrounded by a fuzzy-looking layer called the *cell coat,* or *glycocalyx.* This layer is made up of glycolipid and glycoprotein molecules that participate in cell membrane interactions. The cell coat contains the sites for hormone recognition, the ABO blood group antigens and other tissue antigens.

Microvilli are elongated protrusions of the cell membrane that are arranged as a series of tubular extensions. These extensions greatly increase the surface area of the cell membrane. This specialized cell membrane arrangement facilitates the absorption of fluids and other materials. Microvilli are found in the lumen of the small intestine and renal tubules.

Cilia are long protuberances of the cell membrane with the tapered ends that are characteristic of many cell types, particularly the epithelium. They are anchored in the cytoplasm by a structure similar to the centriole, and extending from this structure is a series of microtubules that are surrounded by the cell membrane. By sliding the microfilaments on each other, the cilia are capable of a sweeping type of movement.

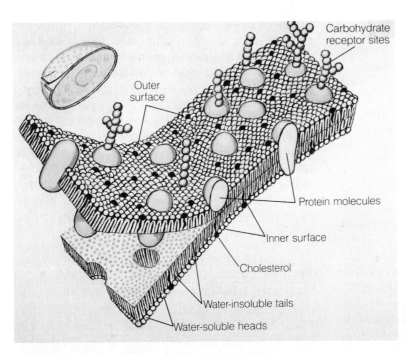

Carbohydrate receptor sites

Outer surface

Protein molecules

Inner surface

Cholesterol

Water-insoluble tails

Water-soluble heads

Figure 1-5 Cell membrane. The right end is intact, but the left end has been split along the plane of the lipid tails. (*Chaffee EE, Lytle IM: Basic Physiology and Anatomy, 4th ed. Philadelphia, JB Lippincott, 1980*)

Longer cilia are called *flagella*. The cilia provide a mechanism for cell movement or, if the location of the cell is fixed, as in the respiratory tract, for the movement of adjacent fluids.

Membrane junctions

With the exception of blood cells, most cells are organized into tissues and organs. In these tissues or organs, cells are held together by the intercellular adhesions that connect the membranes of adjacent cells.

There are at least three types of intercellular junctions that join the cell membranes of adjacent cells to form a unit. One type of intercellular junction, known as a *desmosome*, is disk-shaped and can be likened to a rivet. A second type, the *zona occludens* or *tight junction*, actually fuses the membranes of adjacent cells together. This type of intercellular connection is found in tissues such as the skin that are subject to considerable stretching and in epithelial tissues that separate two compartments with different chemical compositions (*e.g.*, bladder and gastrointestinal tract lining). A third and less common form of intercellular junction involves the close approximation of the cell membranes with the formation of apparent pores between the cytoplasms of the two cells. These *nexus*, or *gap junctions*, possess low electrical-resistance properties and permit electrical communication between cells. The type of cell junction varies with the function of the tissue type. Tissues that facilitate the absorption of fluid usually have cells that are connected by tight junctions. The intercalated disks that join the myocardial fibers of the heart muscle are nexus with low-resistance electrical properties.

Membrane transport

There is a constant movement of molecules and ions across the cell membrane. This movement is facilitated by diffusion, osmosis, facilitated diffusion, active transport, pinocytosis, phagocytosis, and exocytosis (Figure 1-6).

Diffusion. Diffusion refers to the process whereby molecules of gases and other substances move from an area of higher concentration to an area of lower concentration and become equally distributed across the cell membrane. Lipid-soluble molecules such as oxygen, carbon dioxide, alcohol, and fatty acids become dissolved in the lipid matrix of the cell membrane and diffuse through the membrane in the same manner that diffusion occurs in water. Other substances diffuse through minute pores in the cell membrane.

Osmosis. Osmosis is concerned with the passage of water across a semipermeable membrane. It is regulated by the concentration of osmotically active particles present on either side of the membrane. For example, when a greater number of osmotically active particles is present on one side of a semipermeable membrane, water will move down its concentration gradient from the side that has the lesser number of particles to the side with the greater number of particles. This movement of water will continue until the solute particles on both sides of the membrane are equally diluted or until the hydrostatic pressure created by the movement of water opposes its flow.

Facilitated diffusion. Facilitated diffusion involves a carrier system. Some substances, such as glucose, cannot pass through the cell membrane be-

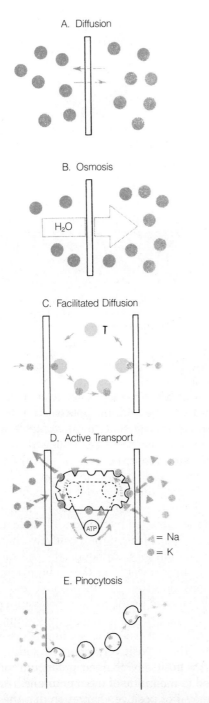

A. Diffusion

B. Osmosis

H₂O

C. Facilitated Diffusion

T

D. Active Transport

ATP

• = Na
• = K

E. Pinocytosis

Figure 1-6 Mechanisms of membrane transport. *A* represents diffusion, in which particles move to become equally distributed across the membrane. In *B* the osmotically active particles regulate the flow of water. In *C*, facilitated diffusion uses a carrier system. *D* represents active transport, in which selected molecules are transported across the membrane using the energy-driven (ATP) pump. The membrane forms a vesicle in *E* that engulfs the particle and then transports it across the membrane, where it is released. This is called pinocytosis.

cause they are not lipid soluble or they are too large to pass through the membrane's pores. These substances combine with a special lipid-soluble carrier at the membrane's outer surface, are carried across the membrane attached to the carrier, and are then re-

leased at the inner surface of the membrane. In facilitated diffusion a substance can move only from an area of higher concentration to an area of lower concentration. The rate at which a substance moves across the membrane through the process of facilitated diffusion depends on the difference in concentration between the two sides of the membrane, the amount of carrier that is available for transport, and the rapidity with which the carrier binds and releases the substances that are being transported.[2] It is thought that insulin, which increases glucose transport, may increase either the amount of carrier that is present or the rate at which the reactions between glucose and the carrier take place.

Active transport. Whereas diffusion and facilitated diffusion move substances from an area of higher concentration to one of lower concentration, active transport can move substances across the cell membrane against a concentration gradient, from a lower to a higher concentration. Active transport requires expenditure of energy from the hydrolysis of adenosine triphosphate (ATP). The sodium and potassium membrane transport system, sometimes called the *sodium-potassium pump,* is an example of active transport. The sodium-potassium pump moves sodium from the inside to the outside of the cell, where its concentration is about 14 times greater than inside, and then returns potassium to the inside, where its concentration is about 35 times greater than it is outside the cell. Were it not for the activity of the sodium-potassium pump, sodium would accumulate within the cell, causing cellular swelling because water would move into the cell along an osmotic gradient (see Chapter 2).

Pinocytosis. Pinocytosis is a mechanism by which the cell membrane engulfs particles and forms a membrane-covered vesicle. The vesicle then breaks away from the inner surface of the cell membrane and moves into the cytoplasm, where its contents are eventually freed by the action of lysosomes or other cytoplasmic enzymes. Pinocytosis refers to the ingestion of small amounts of extracellular fluid and dissolved particles; it is important in the transport of proteins and strong solutions of electrolytes.

Phagocytosis. Phagocytosis is a mechanism similar to pinocytosis, except that larger indentations occur in the cell membrane. Phagocytosis involves the attachment of the particle to the phagocytic cell, engulfment, and killing or degradation of the microorganism or particle. This mechanism allows the cell to ingest large particles such as bacteria and cell debris. Blood neutrophils and macrophages (see Chapter 10) are phagocytic cells.

Exocytosis. Exocytosis is the mechanism for the secretion of intracellular substances into the extracellular spaces. It is the reverse of pinocytosis in that a fluid-filled vacuole fuses to the inner side of the cell membrane and an opening occurs to the outside of the cell surface. This opening allows the contents of the vacuole to be released into the extracellular fluid. Exocytosis is important in removing cellular debris from the cell and releasing substances such as hormones, which have been synthesized within the cell.

Membrane potentials

Electrical potentials exist across the membranes of most, if not all, cells in the body. In excitable tissues, such as nerve or muscle cells, changes in the membrane potential are necessary for generation and conduction of impulses. In other types of cells, such as glandular cells, changes in the membrane potential contribute to other functions.

An electrical potential describes the ability of separated electrical charges of opposite polarity (+ and −) to do work; it is measured in volts (V). The terms *potential difference* and *voltage* are synonymous. Voltage is always measured with respect to two points in a system. For example, the potential difference between the two terminals in a car battery is 6 V or 12 V. Since the total amount of charge that can be separated by a biological membrane is very small, the potential differences are very small. Membrane potentials are measured in millivolts. (A *millivolt* is 1/1000 of a volt.) The voltage or potential difference between the inside and the outside of a cell can be measured in the laboratory by inserting a very fine electrode into the cell and another into the extracellular fluid surrounding the cell and connecting the two electrodes to a voltmeter (Figure 1-7). The movement of charge between two points is called *current;* it occurs when a potential difference has been established and the charged particles are able to move between the two points.

Both extracellular and intracellular fluids are electrolyte solutions containing about 150 mEq to 160 mEq of positively charged ions and an equal concentration of negatively charged ions; these are the *current-carrying ions* responsible for generating and conducting the electrical potentials of the cell. Generally, there is a minute excess of positive ions outside the cell membrane and an equal excess of negative ions inside the cell membrane. Because of the extreme thinness of the cell membrane, these charges accumulate on either side of the membrane, contributing to the establishment of a membrane potential.

Origin of the membrane potential. The uneven distribution of the various ions in the extracellular and intracellular fluids is required for the existence of a membrane potential. Three factors contribute to the origin of the resting membrane potential: (1) the presence of large numbers of nondiffusible intracellu-

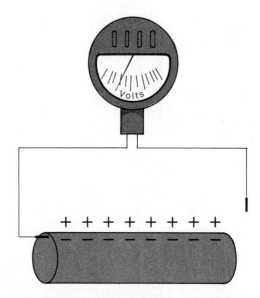

Figure 1-7 Alignment of charge along the cell membrane. The electrical potential is negative on the inside of the cell membrane in relation to the outside.

lar anions, such as protein ions, sulfate ions, and phosphate ions; (2) the selective permeability of the resting membrane to the positively charged potassium ion; and (3) the sodium-potassium pump (Figure 1-8). In the resting state, most excitable membranes are 50 to 100 times more permeable to potassium ions than to sodium ions; because of this, there is limited movement of sodium ions to the inside of the membrane. Despite this enhanced permeability, the positively charged potassium ions remain inside the membrane, attracted by the nondiffusible intracellular anions and repelled by the positively charged extracellular sodium ions. Although the cell membrane is relatively impermeable to the sodium ion, some sodium ions do cross the membrane and are subsequently extruded by the sodium-potassium membrane pump. In the process of removing sodium ions from inside the membrane, the sodium-potassium pump extrudes three positively charged sodium ions for every two positively charged potassium ions that are returned to the inside of the membrane, resulting in a net removal of positive charges so that the inside becomes more negative than the outside.

There is no pump for the chloride ion. Although the membrane is permeable to the ion, it remains on the outside of the membrane because it is attracted by the positively charged sodium ions and repelled from moving to the inside of the membrane by the nondiffusible intracellular anions.

Diffusion potentials. The effects of the major electrolytes (sodium and potassium) on body membrane potentials are determined by the electrolyte concentrations on the inside and outside of the membrane and by the membrane's permeability to the electrolytes. A membrane potential produced by dif-

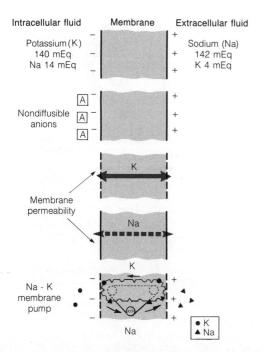

Intracellular fluid — Membrane — Extracellular fluid

Potassium (K) 140 mEq
Na 14 mEq

Sodium (Na) 142 mEq
K 4 mEq

Nondiffusible anions

Membrane permeability

Na - K membrane pump

● K
▲ Na

Figure 1-8 Mechanisms in the development of membrane potentials. Three factors contribute to the difference in electrical potential (negative on the inside and positive on the outside) and Na$^+$ and K$^+$ concentration across the cell membrane: (1) the presence of nondiffusible anions on the inside of the membrane, which attract the positively charged K$^+$ ions; (2) selective permeability of the resting membrane to Na$^+$ and K$^+$ (the resting membrane is 100 times more permeable to K$^+$ than to Na$^+$) so that K$^+$ diffuses and remains inside the membrane and Na$^+$ remains outside; and (3) the Na$^+$-K$^+$ membrane pump, which extrudes three Na$^+$ ions for every two K$^+$ ions admitted, resulting in a net removal of positive charge from inside the membrane.

fusion of an ion reflects the driving force of the ion's concentration gradient across the membrane and the electrical forces that oppose its movement. In the resting or unexcited state, the concentration of potassium ions inside of the cell is about 35 times that on the outside of the cell. The diffusion gradient caused by this concentration difference would cause potassium ions to move out of the cell were it not for the opposing force provided by the positively charged sodium ions on the outside of the membrane. An *equilibrium potential* is one in which there is no net movement of ions because the diffusion and electrical forces are exactly balanced. The equilibrium potentials for sodium and potassium can be calculated using the following equation:

$$E \text{ (millivolts)} = -61 \times \log \frac{\text{ion concentration inside}}{\text{ion concentration outside*}}$$

where E is the equilibrium potential for the ion and −61 is a constant derived from the gas constant, the absolute temperature, the valence of the ion, and a

* Known as the Nernst equation

term for converting natural logarithms to base 10. For example, if the concentration of an ion inside the membrane is 100 millimolar (mM) and the concentration outside is 10 mM, the equilibrium potential for that ion would be −61 (100/10 = 10 and the log of 10 is 1). That is, it would take 61 mV of charge on the inside of the membrane to balance the diffusion potential created by the concentration difference across the membrane for this ion. Two conditions are necessary for a membrane potential to occur as a result of diffusion: (1) the membrane must be selectively permeable, allowing a single type of ion to diffuse through membrane pores, and (2) the concentration of the diffusible ion must be greater on one side of the membrane than on the other.

If the membrane were permeable only to potassium and there were no pumping of ions across the membrane, the equilibrium potential for the potassium ion, using normal intracellular and extracellular ion concentrations, would be −94 mV (−61 × log 140 mM/4 mM). This value approximates the −70 mV to −90 mV resting membrane potential that has been reported for nerve fibers. Likewise, the equilibrium potential for sodium would be about +61 mV (−61 × log 14 mM/140 mM). This value approaches the +45 mV reported for the fraction of a second that occurs at the peak of the action potential overshoot when the membrane is much more permeable to the sodium ion than to the potassium ion.

When the membrane is permeable to several different ions, the diffusion potential that develops depends on the concentration difference for each of the ions, their charges, and the permeability of the membrane to each of these ions.

Action potentials. Action potentials are abrupt, pulselike changes in the membrane potential that last a few ten-thousandths to a few thousandths of a second. In a nerve fiber an action potential can be elicited by any factor that suddenly increases the permeability of the membrane to the sodium ion. It is thought that there are pores or channels in the cell membrane through which the current-carrying ions flow. The sodium and potassium ions use different channels as they move through the membrane, allowing the membrane to change its permeability during different phases of the action potential. It is also thought that these channels are guarded by electrically charged "gates" that open and close with changes in the membrane potential (Figure 1-9). There are similar channels for the calcium ion in the membrane, and it is these channels that are blocked by the calcium channel-blocking drugs used in treatment of cardiovascular disease.

When charges of opposite polarity (+ and −) are aligned across the membrane, it is said to be polarized. The changes that occur in excitable tissue

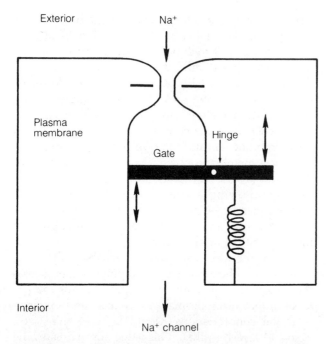

Figure 1-9 A hypothetical model of a sodium channel through the plasma membrane of an axon. A narrow pore (0.3 × 0.5 nm) with a negatively charged wall provides selectivity to hydrated sodium ions. When the gate is opened during the initial stage of depolarization, the flow of sodium is greatly increased.

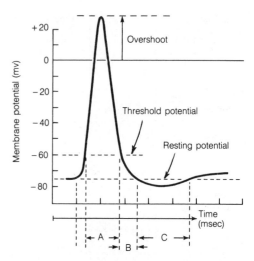

A = Absolute refractory period (active potential and partial recovery)
B = Relative refractory period
C = Positive relative refractory period

Figure 1-10 The time course of the action potential recorded at one point of an axon with one electrode inside and one on the outside of the plasma membrane. The rising part of the action potential is called the spike. The rising phase plus approximately the first half of the repolarization phase is equal to the absolute refractory period (*A*). The portion of the repolarization phase that extends from the threshold to the resting membrane potential represents the relative refractory period (*B*). The remaining portion of the repolarization phase to the resting membrane potential is equal to the negative after potential (*C*). Hyperpolarization is equal to the positive relative refractory period.

during an action potential can be divided into three phases—the resting or polarized state, depolarization, and repolarization (Figure 1-10).

The *resting membrane potential* is characterized by the relatively low permeability of the membrane to the rapid flow of charged ions. During this phase, there is about 70 mV less charge on the inside of the membrane (−70 mV) than on the outside. This difference in concentration of charge is necessary for the establishment of current flow once the membrane becomes permeable to the flow of charged ions.

The *threshold potential* (about −60 mV) represents the membrane potential at which neurons or other excitable tissue are stimulated to fire. Stimuli that excite a neuron produce marked increases in membrane permeability and an increased flow of sodium ions across the membrane, causing it to become less negative and moving it toward the threshold potential. When the threshold potential is reached, the sodium gates swing open and there is a rapid inflow of positively charged sodium ions across the membrane. Once a neuron reaches the minimal threshold for excitation, it is committed to fire and its response will be maximal. This is called the *all-or-none law.*

Depolarization represents the phase of the action potential during which the membrane is highly permeable to sodium ions. During this phase, the sodium gates are open and there is reversal of the membrane potential; the inside of the membrane be-

comes positive (about +30 mV). In neurons the sodium ion gate remains open for only about a quarter of a millisecond, and then closes quickly.

The third phase of the action potential is called *repolarization*. During this phase, the polarity of the resting membrane potential is reestablished. This is accomplished as sodium channels close and sodium permeability decreases while potassium permeability increases. The outflow of positively charged potassium ions returns the membrane potential toward negativity. The sodium-potassium pump gradually reestablishes the resting ionic concentrations on each side of the membrane.

The membrane of an excitable cell must be sufficiently repolarized before it can be reexcited. In the process of repolarization, the membrane remains refractory (will not fire) until the repolarization is about one-third complete. This period, which lasts about half a millisecond, is called the *absolute refractory period*. There is an additional portion of the recovery period during which the membrane can be excited, but only by a stronger-than-normal stimulus. This period is called the *relative refractory period*.

The excitability of a neuron or muscle fiber depends on the amount of change in membrane potential that is needed to initiate an action potential. When the resting membrane potential becomes extremely negative, the membrane is said to be *hyperpolarized.* When this happens, reexcitation becomes more difficult or does not occur. *Hypopolarization,* on the other hand, represents the situation in which the resting membrane potential *becomes less negative.* When the resting membrane potential approaches the threshold potential, the membrane becomes extremely excitable and may undergo spontaneous depolarization.

Alterations in membrane excitability. There are a number of factors that alter membrane excitability. Among these are (1) changes in the resting membrane potential and (2) changes in the permeability of the membrane.

Serum levels of potassium exert a strong influence on the repolarization (and resting membrane potential) of excitable tissue. When serum levels of potassium decrease, the resting membrane potential becomes more negative, and nerve and muscle fibers become hyperpolarized, sometimes to the extent that they cannot be reexcited. *Familial periodic paralysis* is a hereditary condition in which extracellular potassium levels periodically fall to low levels, causing muscle paralysis (see Chapter 27). An increase in serum potassium, on the other hand, interferes with the repolarization of the membrane; it causes hypopolarization, and the resting membrane potential moves closer to threshold levels and then to zero. When this happens, the strength of the action potential is decreased. This is because there is a decrease in the difference in charge between the two sides of the membrane, and consequently less charge is available to move through the membrane during each action potential. Should the resting potential be reduced so that it approaches zero, the membrane will remain depolarized. This situation is similar to what happens when the car battery goes dead and needs to be recharged. Elevations in serum potassium exert their greatest effect on the conduction system of the heart. The force of cardiac contractions becomes weaker until eventually repolarization is inadequate to maintain excitability, and the heart stops beating.

Neural excitability is markedly altered by changes in membrane permeability. Calcium ions decrease membrane permeability to sodium ions. If there are not enough calcium ions available, the permeability of the membrane increases and, as a result, membrane excitability increases—sometimes to the extent that spontaneous muscle movements (tetany) occur. *Local anesthetic agents* (such as procaine or cocaine) act directly on neural membranes to decrease their permeability to sodium.

In summary, the cell is a remarkably autonomous structure that functions in a manner strikingly similar to that of the total organism. The cell nucleus controls cell function and is the mastermind of the cell, whereas the cytoplasm contains the cell's inner organs and is the cell's work site. Cells contain other structures such as microtubules and microfilaments, which are needed for the special functions that they perform. Cells are separated from their external environment by a semipermeable cell membrane that aids in regulating the osmotic and ionic homeostasis of the cell's interior. Semipermeability to Na^+ and K^+, impermeability to larger negative cytoplasmic ions, and the action of a Na^+–K^+ pumping mechanism results in a net electrical charge differential (negative inside) across the cell membrane. Electrical potentials (negative on the inside and positive on the outside) exist across the membranes of most, if not all, cells in the body. These electrical potentials result from the selective permeability of the cell membrane to Na^+ and K^+, the presence of nondiffusible anions inside the cell membrane, and the activity of the Na^+–K^+ membrane pump, which extrudes Na^+ from the inside of the membrane and returns K^+ to the inside. In the resting state, excitable tissues such as neurons and muscle cells are impermeable to the flow of electrically charged ions. An action potential is an abrupt, pulselike change in the membrane potential. It consists of a depolarization phase during which the membrane is permeable to the rapid inflow of charged ions, causing the reversal (positive on the inside and negative on the outside) of the membrane potential, and a repolarization phase during which the resting membrane potential is reestablished. The threshold potential is the change in membrane potential that is sufficient to produce an action potential.

Cellular energy metabolism

Energy is defined as the ability to do work. Cells utilize oxygen and the breakdown products of the foods we eat to produce the energy needed for muscle contraction, transport of ions and molecules, and synthesis of enzymes, hormones, and other macromolecules. *Energy metabolism* refers to the processes by which fats, proteins, and carbohydrates from the foods we eat are converted into energy or complex energy sources in the cell. There are two phases of metabolism, *catabolism* and *anabolism.* Catabolism consists of the breaking down of substances, particularly the breaking down of food and body tissues with the resultant liberation of energy. Anabolism is a building-up process in which more complex molecules are formed from simpler ones.

The special carrier for cellular energy is *adenosine triphosphate* (ATP). The ATP molecule consists of adenosine, a nitrogenous base; ribose, a five-carbon sugar; and three phosphate groups (Figure 1-11). The phosphate groups contain two high-energy bonds that store seven calories each; free energy from foodstuffs is transformed into energy that is stored in these bonds. ATP is often referred to as the "energy currency" of the cell; energy can be "saved or spent" using ATP as an exchange currency.

There are two sites of energy production in the cell: (1) the anaerobic (without oxygen) glycolytic pathway, which is located in the cytoplasm, and (2) the aerobic (with oxygen) pathways in the mitochondria.

Anaerobic metabolism

Glycolysis is the process by which energy is liberated from glucose. It occurs in the cytoplasm of the cell and can proceed anaerobically, or without the presence of oxygen. Glycolysis is an important energy provider for cells that lack mitochondria, the cell structure in which aerobic metabolism occurs (Figure 1-12). The process also provides energy in situations when delivery of oxygen to the cell is either delayed or impaired. The process involves a sequence of reactions that converts glucose to pyruvate with the concomitant production of ATP from adenosine diphosphate (ADP). The net gain of energy from the glycolysis of one molecule of glucose is two ATP molecules and two molecules of pyruvate.

Glycolysis requires the presence of an oxidative-reduction enzyme called nicotinamide-adenine dinucleotide (NAD^+) as a hydrogen acceptor. Oxygen, which combines with the hydrogen from NADH in an energy-producing reaction, is needed to maintain NAD^+ levels for glycolysis.

If oxygen is present, the two molecules of pyruvate move into the mitochondria, where they enter the citric acid cycle. When oxygen is lacking, pyruvate is converted to lactic acid and released into the extracellular fluid as a means of restoring NAD^+ levels so that glycolysis can proceed. Indeed, glycolysis

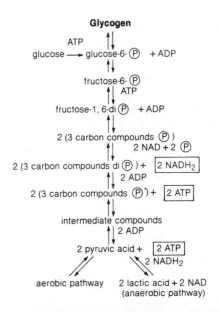

Figure 1-12 The glycolytic pathway. ℗ = phosphate.

could proceed for only a few seconds if pyruvic acid were not removed from the cytoplasm. The conversion of pyruvate to lactic acid is reversible, so that once the oxygen supply has been restored, lactic acid is converted back either to pyruvic acid or to glucose. Heart cells are particularly efficient in converting lactic acid to pyruvic acid and then using this as a fuel source. While relatively inefficient in terms of energy yield, the glycolytic pathway is important during periods of decreased oxygen delivery, such as occurs in skeletal muscle during the first few minutes of exercise.

Aerobic metabolism

Aerobic metabolism occurs in the cell's mitochondria. The mitochondria are oval organelles located in the cell's cytoplasm (see Figure 1-4). The oxidative processes responsible for the production of energy occur in the mitochondria, and it is here that hydrogen and carbon molecules from the fats, proteins, and carbohydrates in our diet are broken down and combined with molecular oxygen to form carbon dioxide and water as energy is released. Unlike lactic acid, which is an end product of anaerobic metabolism, carbon dioxide and water are relatively harmless and easily eliminated from the body. The mitochondria have two membrane systems: an outer membrane and an inner membrane with a series of ridges called the *cristae*. Hence, the mitochondria have two compartments: an intermembrane space between the inner and outer membrane and an internal matrix, which is bounded by the inner membrane. The reactions of the citric acid cycle and fatty acid oxidation occur in the internal matrix, whereas the respiratory

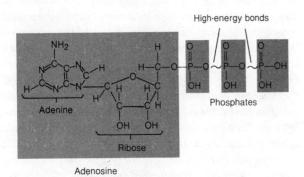

Figure 1-11 Structure of the adenosine triphosphate (ATP) molecule.

assembly for oxidative phosphorylation is an integral part of the inner membrane.

The citric acid cycle

The citric acid cycle, sometimes called the *tricarboxylic acid* or *Kreb's cycle,* provides the final common pathway for the metabolism of nutrients (Figure 1-13). In the citric acid cycle, an activated two-carbon molecule of acetyl-coenzyme A (acetyl-CoA) condenses with a four-carbon molecule of oxaloacetic acid and then moves through a series of enzyme-mediated steps in which hydrogen and carbon dioxide are formed. The hydrogen atoms become attached to one of two special carriers, NAD^+ or flavin adenine dinucleotide (FAD), for transfer to the electron transport system. The carbon dioxide molecules are carried to the lungs and then exhaled. Two carbon atoms are lost in one turn of the cycle, neither from the original acetyl-CoA; these two are then lost as carbon dioxide in the second revolution of the cycle. In the citric acid cycle each of the two pyruvate molecules that were formed in the cytoplasm from one molecule of glucose yields another molecule of ATP along with two molecules of carbon dioxide and eight hydrogen atoms. These hydrogen molecules are transferred to the electron transport system on the inner mitochondrial membrane for oxidation. In addition to pyruvate from the glycolysis of glucose, products of amino acid and fatty acid degradation enter the citric acid cycle.

Oxidative phosphorylation

Oxidative metabolism, which supplies 90% of the body's energy needs, is the process in which inorganic phosphate is coupled with adenosine diphosphate (ADP) to form ATP as hydrogen electrons are transferred from $FADH_2$ and NADH to molecular oxygen by a series of electron carriers that are present in the inner mitochondrial membrane. As molecular oxygen combines with the electrons from the hydrogen atom, water is formed. In a 24-hour period of time, oxidative metabolism supplies the body with 300 ml to 500 ml of water.

Cyanide causes death by poisoning the enzymes needed for one of the final steps in the oxidative phosphorylation sequence.

In summary, cellular energy metabolism is the process whereby the carbohydrates, fats, and proteins from the foods we eat are broken down and converted into energy that is stored in the form of ATP's high-energy bonds. There are two sites of energy metabolism in cells: the mitochondria and the cytoplasmic matrix. The most efficient of these pathways are the aerobic pathways that are located in the mitochondria. These pathways require oxygen and produce carbon dioxide and water as end products. The glycolytic pathway, which is located in the cytoplasm, involves the breakdown of glucose to form ATP. The formation of lactic acid allows this process to proceed in the absence of oxygen.

Tissue types

In the preceding sections we discussed the individual cell and its metabolic processes. Although cells are similar, their structure and function vary according to the needs of the tissues. There are four categories of specialized tissue: epithelium, connective tissue, muscle, and nerve. This section provides a brief overview of these tissue types as preparation for understanding the subsequent chapters in this and other units.

Cell differentiation

The formation of different types of cells and the disposition of these cells into tissue types is called *cell differentiation.* Following conception, the fertilized ovum divides and subdivides and ultimately forms over a hundred different cell types. The process of cell differentiation normally moves forward and is irreversible, producing cells that are more specialized than their predecessors. This means that once differentiation has occurred, the tissue type does not move backward to an earlier stage of differentiation. Usually, a highly differentiated cell loses its ability to undergo cell division.

Although most cells proceed through differentiation into specialized cell types, many tissues contain a few cells that apparently are only partially dif-

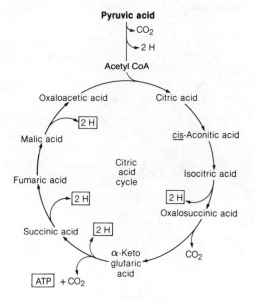

Figure 1-13 The citric acid cycle.

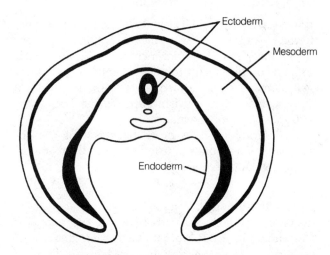

Figure 1-14 The embryonic tissue layers.

ferentiated. These cells are still capable of cell division and serve as a stem cell, or reserve source, for continued production of specialized cells throughout the life of the organism. This is one of the major processes that make regeneration possible in some (but not all) tissues. Skeletal muscle, for example, has relatively few undifferentiated cells to serve as a reserve supply. Cancer cells are thought to originate from undifferentiated stem cells (see Chapter 5 for further discussion).

Embryonic origin of tissue types

The four basic tissue types are often described in terms of embryonic origin. The very young embryo is essentially a three-layered tubular structure (Figure

Table 1–1. Classification of tissue types

Tissue type	Location*
Epithelial	
Covering and lining of body surfaces	
Simple epithelium	
Squamous	Lining of blood vessels and body cavities
Cuboidal	Covering of ovaries and thyroid gland
Columnar	Lining of intestine and gallbladder
Pseudostratified epithelium	Trachea and respiratory passages
Stratified epithelium	
Squamous keratinized	Skin
Squamous nonkeratinized	Mucous membranes of mouth, esophagus, and vagina
Transitional	Bladder
Glandular	
Endocrine	Pituitary, thyroid, adrenal, others
Exocrine	Sweat glands and glands in gastrointestinal tract
Connective	
Loose	Fibroblasts, adipose tissue, endothelial vessel lining
Hematopoietic	Blood cells, myeloid tissue (bone marrow), lymphoid tissue
Supporting tissues	Connective tissue and cartilage, bone and joint structures
Muscle	
Skeletal	Skeletal muscles
Cardiac	Myocardium
Smooth	Gastrointestinal tract, blood vessels, bronchi, bladder, others
Nervous	
Neurons	Central and peripheral neurons and nerve fibers
Supporting cells	Glial and ependymal cells in central nervous system, Schwann and satellite cells in peripheral nervous system

* Not inclusive.

1-14). The outer layer of the tube is called the *ecto-derm;* the middle layer, the *mesoderm;* and the inner layer, the *endoderm.* All of the adult body tissues origi-nate from these three cellular layers. Epithelium has its origin in all three embryonic layers, connective tissue and muscle develop from the mesoderm, and nervous tissue develops from the ectoderm. Mesen-chymal tissue is a precursor to connective tissue and has its origin in the mesoderm. The epithelial lining of the gut, the respiratory tract, and much of the urinary system is derived from the endoderm.

All of the more than 100 different types of body cells can be classified under four basic or pri-mary tissue types: epithelial, connective, muscle, and nervous. Each of the primary tissue types has various subdivisions. The four tissue types and the major subdivisions are summarized in Table 1-1.

—— Epithelial tissue

Epithelial tissue covers the body's outer sur-face, lines the internal surface, and forms the glandu-lar tissue. The epithelium protects (skin and mucous membranes), secretes (glandular tissue and goblet cells), absorbs (intestinal mucosa), and filters (renal glomeruli). The epithelial cells are avascular—that is, they have no blood vessels of their own and must receive oxygen and nutrients from the capillaries of the connective tissue on which the epithelium rests (Figure 1-15). To survive, the epithelial cells must be kept moist. Even the seemingly dry skin epithelium is kept moist by a nonvitalized waterproof layer of kera-tin that prevents evaporation of moisture from the deeper living cells. Epithelium is able to regenerate quickly when injured.

Epithelial cells that cover the body or line body cavities are classified into three types according to the shape of the cells and the number of layers that are present: *simple, stratified,* and *pseudostratified.* The terms *squamous* (thin and flat), *cuboidal* (cube-shaped), and *columnar* (resembling a column) refer to the cell shapes (Figure 1-16).

Simple epithelium contains a single layer of cells. Simple squamous epithelium is adapted for fil-tration; it is found lining the blood vessels, lymph nodes, and alveoli of the lungs. The single layer of squamous epithelium that lines the inside of the heart and blood vessels is known as the *endothelium.* A simi-lar type of layer, called the *mesothelium,* is found in the serous membranes that line the pleura and the peri-cardial and peritoneal cavities. *Simple cuboidal epithe-lium* is found on the surface of the ovary and in the thyroid. *Simple columnar epithelium* lines the intestine. One form of simple columnar epithelium has hairlike

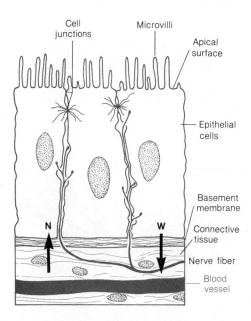

Figure 1-15 Typical arrangement of epithelial cells in relation to underlying tissues and blood supply. Epithelial tissue has no blood supply of its own, but relies on the blood vessels in the underlying connective tissue for nutrition (*N*) and elimination of wastes (*W*).

projections called *cilia,* and another produces mucous and is called a *goblet* cell.

Pseudostratified columnar epithelium is a mix-ture of columnar cell types. Because some of these cells do not reach the surface of the tissue, it gives the appearance of stratified epithelium. Pseudostratified columnar ciliated epithelium with goblet cells forms the lining of most of the upper respiratory tract.

Stratified epithelium contains more than one layer of cells and is designed to protect the body sur-face. *Keratin* is a tough, fibrous protein that is formed from flattened dead cells. Stratified squamous kera-tinized epithelium makes up the epidermis of the skin, and nonkeratinized cells are found on wet surfaces such as the mouth and tongue.

Transitional epithelium is similar to stratified keratinized epithelium with the exception that its su-perficial cells can change shape and become thinner when the tissue is stretched. Such tissue can be stretched without pulling the superficial cells apart. Transitional epithelium is well adapted for the lining of organs, such as the bladder, that are constantly changing their volume.

Glandular epithelium can be divided into two types: exocrine and endocrine. The *exocrine glands* have ducts and discharge their secretions directly onto the epithelial surface where they are located. Sweat glands and alveolar glands are examples of exocrine glands. The *endocrine glands* produce secretions that move directly into the bloodstream.

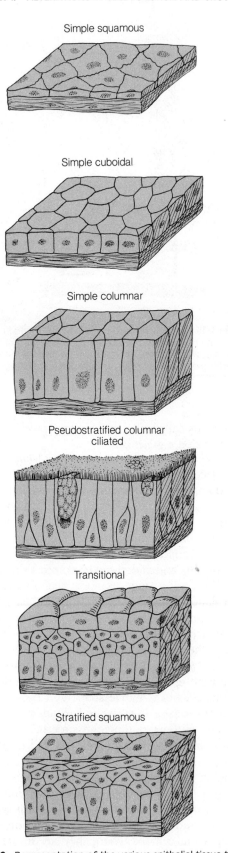

Simple squamous

Simple cuboidal

Simple columnar

Pseudostratified columnar ciliated

Transitional

Stratified squamous

Figure 1-16 Representation of the various epithelial tissue types.

Connective tissue

Connective tissue is the most abundant tissue in the body. As its name indicates, it connects and holds tissues together. Connective tissue is unique in that it includes nonliving forms of intracellular substances, such as collagen fibers and the tissue gel that fills the intercellular spaces. Connective tissue can be divided into three types: *loose connective tissue, hematopoietic* types of connective tissue, and *strong supporting* types of tissue.

Loose connective tissue. The loose connective tissue is soft and pliable and contains large amounts of intercellular substance (Figure 1-17). Loose connective tissue supports the epithelial tissues and provides the means by which these tissues are nourished. In an organ containing both functioning epithelial tissue and supporting connective tissue, the term *parenchymal tissue* is used to describe the functioning epithelium in contradistinction to the connective tissue framework. Cells of loose connective tissue include fibroblasts; mast cells; adipose or fat cells; and the endothelial cells that line blood vessels.

The fibroblasts secrete substances that form the intercellular matrix that supports and connects body cells. These intercellular substances are of two types: the fibrous type (collagen, elastin, and reticular fibers), which holds cells together, and the amorphous type, which fills the tissue spaces. *Collagen* is the most common protein in the body; it is a tough, nonliving white fiber that serves as the structural framework for skin, ligaments, tendons, and numerous other structures. *Elastin* acts like a rubber band, for it can be stretched and then return to its original form. Elastin fibers are abundant in structures, such as the aorta, that are subjected to frequent stretching. Reticular fibers are extremely thin fibers that create a flexible network in organs that are subjected to changes in form or volume, such as the spleen, liver, uterus, or intestinal muscle layer. The amorphous (nonliving) intercellular ground substance that fills the tissue spaces has a gel-like consistency and is sometimes referred to as tissue gel. Hyaluronic acid, which is one of the main components of tissue gel, has the ability to hold vast amounts of water; it facilitates the even dispersion of intercellular fluids and aids in the exchange of cellular nutrients and metabolites. In certain physiological or pathological conditions, a condition called *edema* develops in which there is an excess accumulation of water in the tissue gel of the intercellular matrix (see Chapter 28).

The *basement membrane* or basal lamina is a special type of intercellular matrix that is present where connective tissue comes in contact with the tissue it supports. A basement membrane is found along the interface between connective tissue and

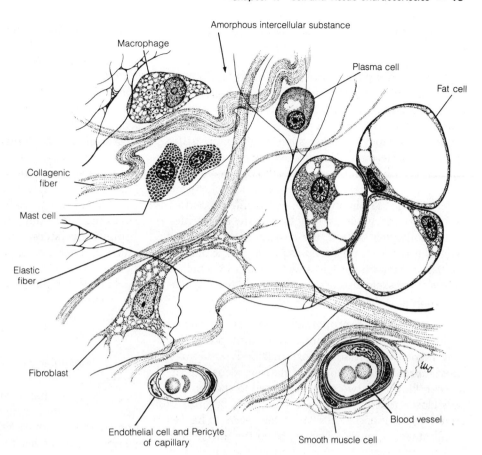

Macrophage

Amorphous intercellular substance

Plasma cell

Fat cell

Collagenic
fiber

Mast cell

Elastic
fiber

Fibroblast

Figure 1-17 Diagrammatic
representation of cells that may
be seen in loose connective
tissue. The cells lie in an
intercellular matrix that is bathed
in tissue fluid that originates in
capillaries. (*Cormack DH: Ham's
Histology, 9th ed, p 170.
Philadelphia, JB Lippincott, 1987*)

Endothelial cell and Pericyte
of capillary

Smooth muscle cell

Blood vessel

muscle fibers, Schwann cells of the peripheral nervous system, the basal surface of endothelial cells, and fat cells. These basement membranes bond cells to the underlying or surrounding connective tissues, serve as selective filters for particles that pass between connective tissue and other cells, and contribute to cell regeneration and repair.[3] The presence of the basement membrane around the muscle cell is necessary for establishment of a new myoneural junction and reinnervation of a denervated muscle cell.

Hematopoietic tissue.   The hematopoietic types of connective tissue include the blood cells, bone marrow, and lymphatic tissue. The role of the hematopoietic system in inflammation and immunity is discussed in Chapters 10 and 11; the reticulocyte, or red blood cell, is discussed in Chapter 16.

Strong supporting connective tissue.   The third form of connective tissue—the strong supporting form—consists of dense connective tissue, cartilage, and bone. The dense connective tissues are rich in collagen and form the tendons and ligaments that join muscle to bones and bones to bones. A layer of dense connective tissue also forms a capsule for many organs and body structures such as the kidney and heart. Dense connective tissue does not require many capillaries because it is composed largely of nonliving col-

lagen fibers. Cartilage and bone are discussed in Chapter 54.

Muscle tissue

There are three types of muscle tissue: *skeletal, cardiac,* and *smooth.* Skeletal and cardiac muscles are striated muscles. The actin and myosin filaments in these muscle types are arranged in striations, giving the muscle fibers a striped appearance.

Skeletal muscle is the largest tissue in the body, accounting for 40% to 45% of the total body weight. Most skeletal muscle is attached to bones, and its contraction is responsible for movement of the skeleton. It differs from cardiac and smooth muscle in that it is under voluntary control and is innervated by the somatic nervous system.

Cardiac muscle is found in the myocardium. Myocardial muscle is designed to pump blood continuously. It has inherent properties of automaticity, rhythmicity, and conductivity. The pumping action of the heart is controlled by impulses originating in the cardiac conduction system and is modified by blood-borne neural mediators and impulses from the autonomic nervous system.

Smooth muscle is found in many organs, including the blood vessels, the iris of the eye, and tubes such as the ureters and bile ducts that connect many internal organs.

Neither skeletal nor cardiac muscle is able to undergo the mitotic activity needed to replace injured cells. Smooth muscle, however, may proliferate and undergo mitotic activity. Some increases in smooth muscle are physiologic, such as occurs in the uterus during pregnancy. Others, such as the increase in smooth muscle that occurs in the arteries of persons with chronic hypertension, are pathologic.

Although the three types of muscle tissue differ significantly in structure, contractile properties, and control mechanisms, they have many similarities. In the following section, the structural properties of skeletal muscle are presented as the prototype of muscle tissue. Smooth muscle and the ways in which it differs from skeletal muscle are then discussed. Cardiac muscle is described in Chapter 20.

Structural properties. Muscle tissue is highly specialized for contractility and producing movement of internal and external body structures. Most muscle cells are long and narrow, a characteristic that allows the two ends of the cell to shorten and pull closer together during contraction. Because of their length, muscle cells are called *fibers*. The cell membrane of a muscle fiber is called the *sarcolemma*, and the cytoplasm is referred to as the *sarcoplasm*. Embedded in the sarcoplasmic reticulum are the contractile elements, *actin* and *myosin* (Figure 1-18). The sarcoplasmic reticulum, which is comparable to the endoplasmic reticulum, is composed of longitudinal

tubules that run parallel to the muscle fiber and surround the actin and myosin filaments. The sarcoplasmic reticulum ends in enlarged, saclike regions called the *lateral sacs*, or *terminal cisternae*. The lateral sacs store calcium to be released during muscle contraction. A second system of tubules consists of the *transverse*, or *T-tubules*, which run perpendicular to the muscle fiber. The lumen of the transverse tubule is continuous with the extracellular fluid compartment; and the membrane of the T-tubule is able to propagate action potentials, which are rapidly conducted over the surface of the muscle fiber and into the sarcoplasmic reticulum. As the action potential moves through the lateral sacs, the sacs release calcium, which initiates muscle contraction. The membrane of the sarcoplasmic reticulum also has an active transport mechanism for pumping the calcium ions back into the reticulum as a means of removing them from the vicinity of the actin and myosin cross-bridges on termination of muscle contraction.

Molecular mechanisms of contraction. In striated muscle the thin, lighter filaments and the thick, darker filaments are arranged in striations that give the muscle a striped appearance. Although the striated pattern appears to be continuous across a single fiber, the fiber is actually composed of a number of independent cylindrical elements called *myofibrils*. The myofibril, in turn, consists of smaller filaments that form a regular repeating pattern along the length of the myofibril; each of these units is called a *sarcomere*. The sarcomeres, which contain the thin actin and thick myosin filaments, are the functional units of the contractile system in muscle. A sarcomere extends from one Z line to another Z line. The dark A bands contain the thick myosin filaments and the lighter I bands contain the thin actin filaments. The Z lines consist of short elements that interconnect and provide the thin filaments from two adjoining sarcomeres with an anchoring point. The H zone in the center of the sarcomere corresponds to the space between the thin filaments; only thick filaments are found in this area. In the center of the H zone is a thin, dark band known as the *M line;* it is produced by linkages between the thick filaments.

During muscle contraction, the thick myosin and the thin actin filaments slide past each other, causing shortening of the muscle fiber while the length of the individual thick and thin filaments remains unchanged. The structures that produce the sliding of the filaments are the myosin heads that form cross-bridges with the thin actin filaments (Figure 1-19). When activated by ATP, the cross-bridges swivel in a fixed arc, much like the oars of a boat, as they become attached to the actin filament. During contraction, each cross-bridge undergoes its own cycle

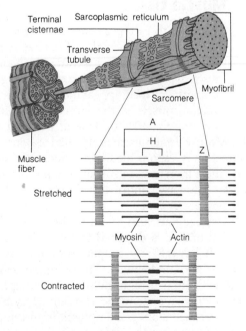

Figure 1-18 Muscle fiber, structures of the myofibril, and the relationship between actin and myosin filaments when the muscle is stretched or contracted.

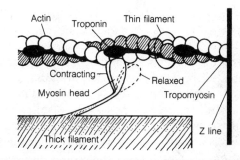

Figure 1-19 Molecular structure of the thin actin filament and the thicker myosin filament of striated muscle. The thin filament is a double-stranded helix of actin molecules with tropomyosin and troponin molecules lying along the grooves of the actin strands. During muscle contraction, the ATP-activated heads of the thick myosin filament swivel into position, much like the oars on a boat, form a cross-bridge with a reactive site on tropomyosin and then pull the actin filament foreward. During muscle relaxation the troponin molecules cover the reactive sites on tropomyosin.

of movement, forming a bridge attachment and releasing it, and then moving to another site where the same sequence of movement occurs. This has the effect of pulling the thin and thick filaments past each other.

Myosin is the chief constituent of the thick filament; it consists of a thin tail, which provides the structural backbone for the filament, and a globular head. Each globular head contains a binding site able to bind to a complementary site on the actin molecule. In addition to the binding site for actin, each myosin head has a separate active site that catalyzes the breakdown of ATP to provide the energy needed to activate the myosin head so that it can form a cross-bridge with actin. Following contraction, myosin also binds ATP as a means of breaking the linkage between actin and myosin. The myosin molecules are bundled together side by side in the thick filaments so that half have their heads toward one end of the filament and their tails toward the other end, while the other half are arranged in the opposite manner.

The thin filaments are composed mainly of actin, a globular protein that is lined up in two rows that coil around each other to form a long helical strand. Associated with each actin filament are two regulatory proteins, tropomyosin and troponin (see Figure 1-19). *Tropomyosin,* which lies in grooves of the actin strand, provides the site for attachment of the globular heads of the myosin filament. In the noncontractile state, *troponin* covers the tropomyosin binding sites and prevents formation of cross-bridges between the actin and myosin. The binding of calcium to troponin during an action potential uncovers the actin binding sites for formation of cross-bridges with the myosin molecule. Following breaking of the linkage between actin and myosin, the concentration of cal-

cium around the myofibrils decreases as calcium is actively transported into the sarcoplasmic reticulum by a membrane pump that uses energy derived from ATP.

Smooth muscle. Smooth muscle is often called *involuntary muscle* because its activity arises either spontaneously or through activity of the autonomic nervous system. On the whole, smooth muscle contraction tends to be slower and more sustained than skeletal or cardiac muscle contraction. Smooth muscle cells are spindle-shaped and considerably smaller than skeletal muscle fibers. There are no Z or M lines in smooth muscle fibers, and the cross-striations are absent. The contractile filaments of actin and myosin are scattered throughout the cytoplasm. The lack of Z lines and regular overlapping of the contractile elements provide for a greater range of tension development. This is important in hollow organs that undergo changes in volume, with consequent changes in the length of the smooth muscle fibers in their walls. Even at large increases in volume, the smooth muscle fiber retains some ability to develop tension, whereas such distention would have stretched skeletal muscle beyond the area where the thick and thin filaments overlap. Smooth muscle is generally arranged in sheets or bundles. In hollow organs, such as the intestines, the bundles are organized into two layers —an outer, longitudinal layer and an inner, circular layer. In blood vessels, the bundles are arranged in a circular or helical manner around the vessel wall.

Smooth muscle differs from skeletal muscle in the way its cross-bridges are formed. In smooth muscle, calcium binds to a smooth muscle cytoplasmic protein, *calmodulin;* the calcium–calmodulin complex binds to and activates the myosin-containing thick filaments, which then interact with actin. The sarcoplasmic reticulum is less well developed in smooth muscle than in skeletal muscle, and there are no transverse tubules connected to the cell membrane. Thus, smooth muscle relies on the entrance of extracellular calcium across the cell membrane as well as the release of calcium from the sarcoplasmic reticulum for muscle contraction. This dependence on movement of extracellular calcium across the cell membrane during muscle contraction contributes to the effectiveness of calcium-blocking drugs that are used in treatment of cardiovascular disease.

Smooth muscle may be divided into two broad categories according to the mode of activation: multiunit and single-unit, or visceral, smooth muscle. *Multiunit* smooth muscle has no inherent activity, but depends on the autonomic nervous system for its activation. Smooth muscle of this type is found in the iris, in the walls of the vas deferens, and attached to hairs in the skin. *Single-unit* smooth muscle is able to contract spontaneously in the absence of either nerve or hormonal stimulation. Normally, a large number of muscle fibers contract synchronously, hence the term *single-unit*. The action potentials originating from pacemaker cells show regular slow waves of depolarization and are transmitted from cell to cell by nexus formed by the fusion of adjacent cell membranes. The intensity of contraction increases with the frequency of the action potential. Certain hormones, other agents, and local factors can modify smooth muscle activity by either depolarizing or hyperpolarizing the membrane. The smooth muscle of the intestinal tract, the uterus, and small-diameter blood vessels is single-unit smooth muscle.

Nervous tissue

Nervous tissue is a specialized form of tissue designed for communication purposes. The nervous tissue develops from the ectoderm of the embryo and includes the neurons, the supporting cells of the nervous system, and the ependymal cells that line the ventricular system. The structure and organization of the nervous system are discussed in Chapter 46.

In summary, body cells are organized into four basic tissue types: epithelial, connective, muscle, and nervous. The epithelium covers the body surfaces and forms the functional components of the glandular structures. Connective tissue supports and connects body structures; it forms the bones and skeletal system, the joint structures, the blood cells, and the intercellular substances. Muscle tissue is a specialized tissue that is designed for contractility. There are three types of muscle tissue: skeletal, cardiac, and smooth. Nervous tissue is designed for communication purposes and includes the neurons, the supporting neural structures, and the ependymal cells that line the ventricles of the brain and the spinal canal.

References

1. Robbins SL, Cotran RS: Pathologic Basis of Disease, 2nd ed, p 11. Philadelphia, WB Saunders, 1979
2. Guyton A: Medical Physiology, 7th ed, p 92. Philadelphia, WB Saunders, 1986
3. Cormack DH: Ham's Histology, 9th ed, pp 165–168. Philadelphia, JB Lippincott, 1987

CHAPTER 2

Cellular Adaptation and Injury

Objectives

After you have studied this chapter, you should be able to meet the following objectives:

_____ State the general purpose of changes in cell structure and function that occur as the result of normal adaptive processes.

_____ State the relationship between changes in cell structure and function that occur as a result of normal adaptive processes and the stimuli producing these changes.

_____ Describe cell changes that occur with atrophy, hypertrophy, hyperplasia, metaplasia, and dysplasia.

_____ State the general conditions under which atrophy, hypertrophy, hyperplasia, metaplasia, and dysplasia occur.

_____ Describe three types of reversible cell changes that can occur with cell injury.

_____ State the difference in outcome between intracellular accumulations due to systemic disorders and those due to inborn errors of metabolism.

_____ Cite the reasons for the changes that occur with the wet and dry forms of gangrene.

_____ Describe cell changes that occur with hypoxia, electrical injury, and thermal injury.

_____ Define the term *free radical*.

_____ Relate free-radical formation to cell injury and death.

_____ Explain how injurious effects of biologic agents differ from those produced by physical and chemical agents.

_____ Differentiate between the effects of ionizing and nonionizing radiation in terms of their ability to cause cell injury.

_____ State how nutritional imbalances contribute to cell injury.

When confronted with stresses that tend to disrupt its normal structure and function, the cell undergoes adaptive changes that permit survival and maintenance of function. This chapter addresses cellular responses to stress, injury, and death.

Cellular adaptation

Cells adapt to changes in the internal environment just as the total organism adapts to changes in the external environment. Cells may adapt by undergoing changes in size, number, and type. These changes, occurring singly or in combination, may lead to atrophy, hypertrophy, hyperplasia, metaplasia, and dysplasia. In contrast to abnormal adaptive responses, normal adaptive responses occur in response to need and an appropriate stimulus. Once the need has been removed, the adaptive response ceases.

Atrophy

Atrophy refers to a decrease in the size of a body part brought about by loss of cell substance resulting in a shrinkage in cell size. When confronted with a decrease in work demands or adverse environmental conditions, most cells are able to revert to a smaller size and a lower and more efficient level of functioning that is compatible with survival. The size of all the structural components of the cell usually decreases as the cell atrophies.

The general causes of atrophy can be grouped into the following categories: (1) disuse, (2) denervation, (3) lack of endocrine stimulation, (4) decreased nutrition, and (5) ischemia. Cell size, particularly in muscle tissue, is related to work load. As the work load of a cell diminishes, there is a general decrease in oxygen consumption and protein synthesis. The cell conserves energy by decreasing the number and size of its organelles and other structures. Disuse atrophy is seen in the muscles of extremities that have been encased in plaster casts. Denervation atrophy is a form of disuse atrophy that occurs in the muscles of paralyzed limbs. Lack of endocrine stimulation causes the atrophic involutional changes that occur in the reproductive structures during menopause. During prolonged periods of interference with general nutrition, such as occurs during starvation or other disease conditions, the body often undergoes a generalized wasting of tissue mass. Ischemia results from localized lack of blood flow and delivery of oxygen and nutrients to the affected tissues. In peripheral vascular disease there is often atrophy of the muscles and skin in the affected extremities due to ischemia.

In some situations, a collection of yellow-brown pigment called *lipofuscin* accompanies the retrogressive changes that occur with atrophy. This form of atrophy is referred to as *brown atrophy*. The discoloration is thought to represent an accumulation of indigestible residues from within the cell. It is seen more commonly in heart, nerve, and liver cells than in other types of tissue. Lipofuscin itself is not injurious to cell structure or function.[1] The accumulation of lipofuscin increases with age, and it is sometimes referred to as the wear-and-tear pigment.

Hypertrophy

Hypertrophy is an increase in the amount of functioning tissue mass of an organ or part caused by an increase in cell size. It results from increased functional demands or specific hormonal stimulation. It is most commonly seen in cardiac and skeletal muscle tissue. These types of tissue cannot adapt to an increase in work load by mitotic division and formation of more cells. The pregnant uterus undergoes both hypertrophy and hyperplasia as the result of estrogen stimulation.

In hypertrophy there is an increase in the functional components of the cell that allows it to achieve an equilibrium between demand and functional capacity. For example, as muscle cells hypertrophy, additional microfilaments, cell enzymes, and ATP are synthesized. The mechanism underlying the increase in cell components is not completely understood. It is thought to be related to a decreased rate of protein degradation with a slightly increased rate of protein synthesis.[1] Whatever the mechanism, a limit is eventually reached beyond which further enlargement of the tissue mass is no longer able to compensate for the increased work demands. The limiting factors for continued hypertrophy may be related to limitations in blood flow.[1]

Hypertrophy may occur as the result of either normal physiologic or pathologic conditions. The increase in muscle mass associated with exercise is an example of physiologic hypertrophy. Pathologic hypertrophy may be adaptive or compensatory. Examples of adaptive hypertrophy are the thickening of the urinary bladder due to long-continued obstruction of urinary outflow and the myocardial hypertrophy that results from valvular heart disease or hypertension. Compensatory hypertrophy is the enlargement of a remaining organ or tissue after a portion has been surgically removed or rendered inactive. For instance, if one kidney is removed, the remaining kidney enlarges to compensate for the loss.

Hyperplasia

Hyperplasia is an increase in the number of cells of a tissue or organ. Hyperplasia occurs in tissues with cells that are capable of mitotic division, such as the epidermis, intestinal epithelium, and glandular tissue. Nerve cells and skeletal and cardiac muscle do not divide and therefore have no capacity for hyperplastic growth. As with other normal adaptive cellular responses, hyperplasia is a controlled process that occurs in response to an appropriate stimulus and ceases once the stimulus has been removed. There are two types of stimuli that are generally associated with hyperplasia—physiologic and nonphysiologic. Breast and uterine enlargement during pregnancy are examples of a physiologic hyperplasia that is hormonally regulated. An example of a nonphysiologic form of hyperplasia occurs in response to abnormal hormonal stimulation of target cells. Hyperplasia of target cells in the endometrium occurs with excessive estrogen production; the abnormally thickened uterine layer may bleed excessively and frequently.

Metaplasia

Metaplasia is the conversion from one adult cell type to another adult cell type. It allows for substitution of cells that are better able to tolerate environmental stresses. The conversion of cell types never oversteps the boundaries of the primary groups of tissue (epithelial or connective). In metaplasia, one type of epithelial cell may be converted to another type of epithelial cell but not to a connective tissue cell. An example of metaplasia is the adaptive substitution of stratified squamous epithelial cells for the ciliated columnar epithelial cells in the trachea and large airways in the person who is a habitual cigarette smoker. Metaplasia of epithelial tissue occurs in chronic irritation and inflammation. For unknown reasons, a vitamin A deficiency tends to cause squamous metaplasia of the respiratory tract. Metaplasia occurs in response to a stimulus and is potentially reversible.

Dysplasia

Dysplasia is deranged cell growth of a specific tissue that results in cells that vary in size, shape, and appearance. Minor degrees of dysplasia occur in association with chronic irritation or inflammation.

Dysplasia classically occurs in the uterine cervix, oral cavity, gallbladder, and respiratory passages. Habitual cigarette smokers often have dysplastic changes in their airways. Although dysplasia is abnormal, it is adaptive in that it is potentially reversible once the irritating cause has been found and removed. Dysplastic tissue changes may progress to neoplastic disease, a feature that makes dysplasia a phenomenon of great importance.

In summary, cells adapt to changes in their environment and in their work demands by changing size, number, and character. Changes include atrophy—a shrinking of tissue due to a decrease in cell size and functional components within the cell; hypertrophy—an increase in tissue size brought about by an increase in cell size and functional components within the cell; hyperplasia—an increase in cell number; metaplasia—the conversion of one adult cell type to another adult cell type; and dysplasia—disordered cell growth resulting in altered cell structure. Normal adaptive changes are consistent with the needs of the cell and occur in response to an appropriate stimulus. The changes are reversed once the stimulus has been withdrawn.

Cell injury

The extent to which any injurious agent can cause cell injury and death depends, in large measure, on the intensity and duration of the injury and the type of cell that is involved. When cells are injured or the need to adapt becomes overwhelming, degenerative changes begin to appear. Degeneration is a retrogressive process in which there is a cellular deterioration along with changes in both the chemical structure and microscopic appearance of the cell. Degeneration can follow many paths that eventually lead to cell changes, which may be reversible or irreversible. Irreversible changes consist of necrosis (cell death) and tissue dissolution. Frequently, however, the final outcome is not reached because somewhere along the way the process is reversed, allowing cells and tissues to return to their normal state.

Reversible cell injury

The manifestations of reversible cell injury fall into three main categories: cellular swelling, fatty changes, and intracellular accumulations.

Cellular swelling

An accumulation of water within the cell is an early manifestation of almost all types of cell injury. When this happens, the cytoplasm of the cell develops a cloudy appearance (cloudy swelling). It has been postulated that the swelling is caused by a decrease in adenosine triphosphate (ATP) and impaired function of the sodium pump. This leads to an accumulation of intracellular sodium and subsequent waterlogging of the cell, with the appearance of vacuoles if water continues to accumulate. These vacuoles probably represent the collection of water in the endoplasmic reticulum.

Fatty changes

Fatty cellular changes are linked to intracellular accumulation of fat. When fatty changes occur, small vacuoles of fat disperse throughout the cytoplasm. The process is usually more ominous than cloudy swelling, and although it is reversible, its presence usually indicates severe injury. These fatty changes may occur because normal cells are presented with an increased fat load or because injured cells are unable to metabolize the fat properly. In obesity, fatty infiltrates often occur within and between the cells of the liver and heart because of an increased fat load. Pathways for fat metabolism may be impaired during cell injury and fat may accumulate within the cell as production exceeds use and export. The liver, where most fats are synthesized and metabolized, is particularly susceptible to fatty change, but fatty change may also occur in the kidney, the heart, and other organs.

Intracellular accumulations

Under certain conditions, various substances may accumulate in both normal and abnormal cells. Robbins has grouped these substances into three categories: (1) normal cellular constituents, such as lipids, proteins, and carbohydrates, which are present in large amounts; (2) abnormal substances, such as those resulting from inborn errors of metabolism; and (3) products of excessive intracellular synthesis.[1] The previously described fatty changes are an example of intracellular accumulation of a normal cell constituent.

There are a number of genetic disorders that disrupt the metabolism of selected substances. A normal enzyme may be replaced with an abnormal one, resulting in the formation of a substance that cannot be utilized or eliminated from the cell; or an enzyme may be missing, so that an intermediate product accumulates within the cell. For example, there are at least ten inborn errors of glycogen metabolism, most of which lead to the accumulation of intracellular glycogen stores. In the most common form of this disorder, von Gierke's disease, large amounts of glycogen accumulate in the liver and kidneys because of a deficiency of the enzyme glucose-6-phosphatase. Without this enzyme, glucose-6-phosphate, stored in the form of glycogen, cannot be broken down to form glucose. In a similar manner, other enzyme defects lead to the accumulation of other substances.

Pigments are colored substances that may accumulate within cells. They can be either endogenous (arising from within the body) or exogenous (arising from outside the body) in origin. Icterus, or jaundice, is a yellow discoloration of tissue caused by the retention of endogenous bile pigments. This condition may result from increased bilirubin production due to red blood cell destruction, obstruction of bile passage into the intestine, or toxic diseases that affect the liver's ability to remove bilirubins from the blood. One of the most common exogenous pigments is carbon in the form of coal dust. In coal miners or individuals ex-

posed to heavily polluted environments, the accumulation of carbon or other environmental dusts may cause serious lung disease. Lung disease associated with coal dust is termed *anthracosis* and that associated with silica (sand dust) is called *silicosis*. The formation of a blue lead line along the margins of the gum is one of the diagnostic features of lead poisoning.

Whatever the nature or cause of the abnormal accumulation, it implies storage of some substance by a cell. If the accumulation is due to a correctable systemic disorder such as hyperbilirubinemia, which causes jaundice, the accumulation is reversible. If the disorder cannot be corrected, as often occurs in many inborn errors of metabolism, the cells become overloaded, causing cell injury and death.

Irreversible cell injury and death

Necrosis means death of a cell, organ, or tissue that is still a part of the body. Widespread necrosis can occur without somatic (body) death. With cell death there are marked changes in the appearance of both the cytoplasmic contents and the nucleus. These changes are often not visible, even under the microscope, for hours following cell death. The dissolution of the necrotic cell or tissue can follow several paths: the cell can undergo liquefaction (liquefaction necrosis); it can be transformed to a gray, firm mass (coagulation necrosis); or it can be converted to a cheesy material by infiltration of fatlike substances (caseous necrosis). *Liquefaction necrosis* occurs when some of the cells die but their catalytic enzymes are not destroyed. An example of liquefaction necrosis is the softening of the center of an abscess with discharge of its contents. During *coagulation necrosis,* acidosis denatures the enzymatic and structural proteins of the cell. This type of necrosis is characteristic of hypoxic injury and is seen in infarcted areas. An infarction occurs when an artery supplying an organ or part of the body becomes occluded and no other source of blood supply exists. As a rule, the infarct is conical in shape and corresponds to the distribution of the artery and its branches. An artery may be occluded by an embolus, a thrombus, disease of the arterial wall, or pressure on the vessel from without. *Caseous necrosis,* or cheesy necrosis, is associated with tubercular lesions.

Gangrene

The term *gangrene* is applied when a considerable mass of tissue undergoes necrosis (Figure 2-1). Gangrene may be classified as either dry or moist. Dry gangrene is usually due to interference with arterial blood supply to a part without interference with venous return. Strictly speaking, it is a form of coagu-

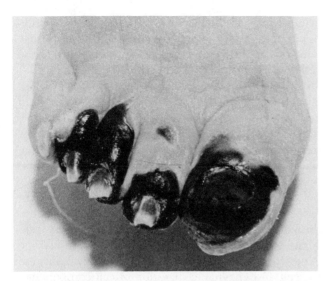

Figure 2-1 Photograph of a foot with dry gangrene of the first four toes. Note the sharp line of demarcation between the normal and necrotic tissue. *(Courtesy of M. Wagner, M.D. The Anatomy Department, Medical College of Wisconsin)*

lation necrosis. Moist, or wet, gangrene is primarily due to interference with the venous return from the part. Bacterial invasion plays an important role in the development of wet gangrene and is responsible for many of its prominent symptoms. Dry gangrene is confined almost exclusively to the extremities, whereas moist gangrene may affect either the internal organs or the extremities.

In dry gangrene, the part becomes dry and shrinks; the skin wrinkles, and its color changes to dark brown or black. The spread of dry gangrene is slow, and its symptoms are not as marked as those of wet gangrene. The irritation caused by the dead tissue produces a line of inflammatory reaction (line of demarcation) between the dead tissue of the gangrenous area and the healthy tissue. If bacteria invade the necrotic tissue, dry gangrene is converted to wet gangrene.

In moist gangrene, the area is cold, swollen, and pulseless. The skin is moist, black, and under tension. Blebs form on the surface, liquefaction occurs, and a foul odor (due to bacterial action) is present. There is no line of demarcation between the normal and diseased tissues and the spread of tissue damage is rapid. Systemic symptoms are usually severe, and death may occur unless the condition can be arrested.

Gas gangrene is a special type of gangrene that is due to infection of devitalized tissues by one of several clostridial bacteria. These anaerobic bacteria produce toxins that cause shock, hemolysis, and death of muscle cells. Characteristic of this disorder are the bubbles of gas that form in the muscle. Gas gangrene is a serious and potentially fatal disease. Treatment includes administration of gas gangrene antitoxin.

Because the organism is anaerobic, oxygen is sometimes administered in a hyperbaric chamber.

In summary, cell injury can be caused by a number of agents. The injury may produce sublethal and reversible cellular damage or may lead to irreversible cell injury and death. Necrosis refers to cell death. There are three forms of cell necrosis: (1) liquefaction necrosis, which occurs when cell death does not result in inactivation of intracellular enzymes; (2) coagulation necrosis, which occurs with ischemia; and (3) caseous necrosis, which is associated with tubercular lesions. Necrosis of large areas of tissue leads to gangrene. Gangrene can be classified as dry or wet gangrene. Dry gangrene is essentially a form of coagulation necrosis, and wet gangrene is due to bacterial invasion of the necrotic area.

Types of cell injury

There are many ways in which cell damage can occur. The common forms of injury tend to fall into several categories: (1) hypoxic cell injury, (2) cell injury due to physical agents, (3) radiation injury, (4) chemical injury, (5) injury due to biologic agents, and (6) injury associated with nutritional imbalances. Some agents, such as heat, produce direct cell injury; other factors, such as genetic derangements, produce their effects indirectly by predisposing to cell injury, inflammation, and immune responses. Although these mechanisms are normally protective in nature, they can cause cell injury and death.

Many injurious agents exert their damaging effects through a reactive chemical species called a *free radical.*[2-4] In most atoms, the outer electron orbitals are filled with paired electrons moving in opposite directions to balance their spin. A free radical is a highly reactive chemical species that contains a single unpaired electron that is highly unstable and will combine with almost any cell component. Oxygen with its two unpaired outer electrons, is the most frequent source of free radicals. During the course of normal cell metabolism, cells process energy-producing oxygen into water; in some reactions, a free superoxide radical is formed. Uncontrolled radical production causes damage to cell membranes, cross-linking of cell proteins, inactivation of cell enzyme systems, and nucleic acid interactions that induce mutations in the genetic code. Under normal conditions, most cells have chemical mechanisms that protect them from the injurious effects of free radicals. These protective mechanisms commonly break down when the cell is deprived of oxygen or exposed to certain chemical agents, radiation, or other injurious agents.

Free-radical formation is a particular threat to

tissues in which the blood flow has been interrupted and then restored. During the period of interrupted flow, the intracellular mechanisms that control free radicals are inactivated or damaged. When blood flow is restored, the cell is suddenly confronted with an excess of free radicals that it cannot control. Scientists are currently investigating the use of free-radical scavengers that would protect against cell injury during periods when protective cellular mechanisms are impaired.

Hypoxic injury

One of the most common causes of tissue injury is hypoxia. Hypoxia deprives the cell of oxygen and interrupts oxidative metabolism and the generation of ATP. The actual time necessary to produce irreversible cell damage depends on the degree of oxygen deprivation and the metabolic needs of the cell. Well-differentiated cells such as those in the heart, brain, and kidney require large amounts of oxygen to provide energy for their special functions. Brain cells, for example, begin to undergo permanent damage following 4 to 6 minutes of oxygen deprivation. Furthermore, there is often a fine margin between the time involved in reversible and irreversible cell damage. In one study it was found that the epithelial cells of the proximal tubule of the kidney in the rat could survive 20 but not 30 minutes of ischemia.[5]

Hypoxia can result from an inadequate amount of oxygen in the air, respiratory disease, decreased blood flow due to circulatory disease (ischemia), anemia, or inability of the cells to utilize oxygen. In edema, the distance for diffusion of oxygen may become a limiting factor. In hypermetabolic states the cells may require more oxygen than can be supplied by normal respiratory function and oxygen transport. Hypoxia also serves as the ultimate cause of cell death in other injuries. For example, toxins from certain microorganisms interfere with cellular utilization of oxygen, and a physical agent such as cold causes severe vasoconstriction and impairs blood flow.

Hypoxia literally causes a power failure within the cell with widespread effects on the cell's functional and structural components. As oxygen tension within the cell falls, oxidative metabolism ceases and the cell reverts to anaerobic metabolism, using the cell's limited glycogen stores in an attempt to maintain vital cell functions. Cellular pH falls as lactic acid and inorganic phosphates resulting from hydrolysis of ATP accumulate within the cell. This reduction in pH can have profound effects on intracellular structures. Clumping of the nuclear chromatin occurs, and myelin figures, which derive from destructive changes in cell membranes and intracellular structures, are seen within the cytoplasm and extracellular spaces.

One of the earliest effects of reduced ATP is

acute cellular swelling caused by failure of the energy-dependent sodium-potassium membrane pump, which extrudes sodium and returns potassium to the cell. With impaired function of this pump, intracellular potassium levels decrease, and sodium and water accumulate within the cell. The movement of fluid and ions into the cell is associated with dilatation of the endoplasmic reticulum, increased membrane permeability, and decreased mitochondrial function.[1]

To this point, the cellular changes are reversible if oxygenation is restored. If the oxygen supply is not restored, however, there is a continued loss of essential enzymes, proteins, and ribonucleic acid through the hyperpermeable membrane of the cell. Injury to the lysosomal membranes results in leakage of destructive lysosomal enzymes into the cytoplasm of the cell and enzymatic digestion of cell components. The leakage of intracellular enzymes through the permeable cell membrane into the extracellular fluid is used as an important clinical indicator of cell injury and death. These enzymes enter the blood and can be measured by laboratory tests. For example, heart muscle liberates glutamic-oxaloacetic transaminase (GOT), creatine phosphokinase (CPK), and lactate dehydrogenase (LDH) when injured. Because different types of tissue have different enzymes, the presence of elevated levels of specific enzymes provides information about the location of tissue injury due to hypoxia.

Injury due to physical agents

Physical agents responsible for cell and tissue injury include mechanical forces, extremes of temperature, and electrical forces. Injury due to mechanical forces occurs as the result of body impact with another object. Either the body or the mass can be in motion, or, as sometimes happens, both can be in motion at the time of impact. These types of injuries split and tear tissue, fracture bones, injure blood vessels, and disrupt blood flow.

Extremes of heat and cold cause damage to the cell, its organelles, and its enzyme systems. Exposure to low-intensity heat (43° to 46°C), such as occurs with partial-thickness burns and severe heat stroke, causes cell injury by inducing vascular injury, accelerating cell metabolism, inactivating temperature-sensitive enzymes, and disrupting the cell membrane.[1] With more intense heat, coagulation of blood vessels and tissue proteins occurs.

Exposure to cold induces vasoconstriction by direct action on blood vessels and also by reflex activity of the sympathetic nervous system. The resultant decrease in blood flow may lead to hypoxic tissue injury, depending on the degree and duration of cold exposure. Injury due to freezing is probably a combination of ice-crystal formation and vasoconstriction.

The decreased blood flow leads to capillary stasis and arteriolar and capillary thrombosis. Edema results from increased capillary permeability.

Electrical injuries can affect the body in two ways—through extensive tissue injury and disruption of neural and cardiac impulses. The effect of electricity on the body is mainly determined by (1) the type of circuit (direct or alternating), (2) its voltage, (3) its amperage, (4) the resistance of the intervening tissue, (5) the pathway of the current, and (6) the duration of exposure.[1]

Alternating current (AC) is usually more dangerous than direct current (DC) because it causes violent muscle contractions, preventing release of the electrical source and sometimes resulting in fractures and dislocations. In electrical injuries, the body acts as a conductor of the electrical current; that is, the current enters the body from an electrical source such as an exposed wire and then passes through the body and exits to another conductor, such as the moisture on the ground or a piece of metal the person is holding. The pathway that a current takes is of critical importance because the electrical energy disrupts impulses in excitable tissues. Current flow through the brain may interrupt respiratory impulses from medullary centers, and current flow through the chest may cause fatal cardiac arrhythmias.

In electrical circuits, resistance to the flow of current transforms electrical energy into heat. This is why the elements in electrical heating devices are made of highly resistive metals. Much of the tissue damage produced by electrical injuries is due to heat production in tissues that have the highest electrical resistance. Resistance to electrical current varies from the greatest to the least as follows: bone, fat, tendons, skin, muscles, blood, and nerves. The most severe tissue injury usually occurs at the skin sites where the current enters and leaves the body. After electricity has penetrated the skin, it passes rapidly through the body along the lines of least resistance—through body fluids and nerves. Degeneration of vessel walls may occur and thrombi may form as current flows along the blood vessels. This can cause extensive muscle and deep tissue injury. Thick, dry skin is more resistant to the flow of electricity than thin, wet skin. It is generally believed that the greater the skin resistance, the greater the amount of local skin burn; the less the resistance, the greater the deep and systemic effects.

——— Radiation injury

Electromagnetic radiation comprises a wide spectrum of wave-propagated energy ranging from ionizing gamma rays to radio-frequency waves (Figure 2-2). A photon is a particle of radiation energy. Radiation energy above the visible ultraviolet range is called *ionizing radiation* because the photons have

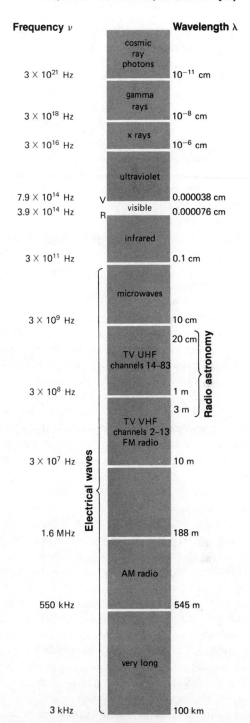

Figure 2-2 The electromagnetic spectrum. The frequencies are shown on the left side of the diagram, and the corresponding wavelengths appear on the right. The frequencies and wavelengths are related by $C = \nu\lambda$, where C = the speed of light in free space (3×10^8 m/sec) and is the same for all wavelengths of the electromagnetic spectrum. (*Hooper HO, Gwynne P: Physics and the Physical Perspectives. New York, Harper & Row, 1980*)

enough energy to knock electrons off atoms and molecules. Radiation energy at frequencies below that of visible light is often referred to as *nonionizing* radiation. Ultraviolet radiation represents the portion of the spectrum of electromagnetic radiation just above the visible range. It contains increasingly energetic rays that are powerful enough to disrupt intracellular bonds and cause sunburn.

Ionizing radiation

The spectrum of ionizing radiation includes two distinct forms of energy propagation: electromagnetic waves and fast-moving particles. Gamma waves and x-rays are similar in their interaction with body tissues but differ in their origin; x-rays are machine-generated, and gamma rays are emitted from the spontaneous decay of radioactive materials. Both of these forms of radiation are very energetic and extremely penetrating, and they assume characteristics of both waves and particles.

Particulate radiation involves particles of definite mass and charge given off by both naturally occurring and artificially produced radioactive elements, processes of fission (atomic reactors), and particle accelerators. Naturally occurring radioactive substances (*e.g.,* radium) and artificially produced radioisotopes undergo spontaneous decay, during which they emit radiant energy. This rate of decay varies greatly and is expressed in terms of the half-life of the product, or the time necessary to reduce its radioactivity to one-half its initial value. The half-life of a radioisotope may be as short as a fraction of a second, or it may be as long as 1638 years (radium).[6]

Ionizing radiation affects cells by causing ionization of molecules and atoms within the cells either by directly hitting the target molecules or by producing free radicals that interact with critical cell components. It can immediately kill cells, interrupt cell replication, or cause a variety of mutations, which may or may not be lethal. The cell's initial response to radiation exposure is characterized by swelling, disruption of the mitochondria and other organelles, alterations in the cell membrane, and marked changes in the nucleus. Because of inhibition of DNA synthesis and interference with the mitotic process, rapidly dividing cells such as those of the bone marrow and gastrointestinal epithelium are more susceptible to radiation injury than nondividing cells. Cancer cells are rapidly proliferating cells; therefore, radiation therapy is often used in treating cancer.

Dose-dependent vascular changes occur in all irradiated tissues. During the immediate postirradiation period, only vessel dilatation takes place (*e.g.,* the initial erythema of the skin after radiotherapy). Later, or with higher levels of radiation, destructive changes occur in small blood vessels such as the capillaries and venules.

At relatively low doses, both normal cells and cancer cells are able to repair radiation damage. If, however, cell recovery is not complete at the time of the next exposure, there may be additional damage. The importance of cell repair in protecting against radiation injury is evidenced by the vulnerability of persons who lack repair enzymes to ultraviolet-induced skin cancer. In a disease called *xeroderma pigmentosum,* an enzyme needed for DNA replication to repair sunlight-induced defects is lacking, and this results in the development of a mutant cancer cell line.

Nonionizing radiation

Nonionizing radiation includes infrared light, ultrasound, microwaves, and laser energy. Unlike ionizing radiation, which can directly break chemical bonds, nonionizing radiation exerts its effects by causing vibrations and rotations of atoms and molecules. Essentially, all of this vibrational and rotational energy is eventually converted to thermal energy. Because all of these types of radiation are finding increasing usage for industrial, domestic, and medical purposes, there is increasing concern about the safety, dosimetry, and long-term effects of exposure to these types of radiation. In laboratory animals, for example, cataracts and lymphocyte dysfunction have been associated with exposure to microwave radiation.[7] Unquestionably, much of this damage was due to local and general hyperthermia.[8] A number of epidemiologic studies on the ocular effects of occupational exposure have not found an increase in lens opacity in humans.[4]

Ultrasound, too, has been shown to alter nerve transmission in lower animals; but, again, this was related to the thermal effects.[1] Questions regarding the safety of ultrasound during pregnancy as a routine screening method have prompted the National Institutes of Health and the Federal Drug Administration to sponsor a consensus development conference on diagnostic ultrasound in pregnancy. The group advised that "data on the clinical efficacy and safety do not allow a recommendation for routine screening of the fetus at this time." They further cautioned that "ultrasound examinations performed solely to satisfy the family's desire to know fetal sex, or obtain a picture of the fetus, should be discouraged."[9]

Chemical injury

Chemical agents can injure the cell membrane and other cell structures, block enzymatic pathways, coagulate cell proteins, and disrupt the osmotic and ionic balance of the cell. There are many injurious chemicals—even excessive amounts of simple table salt (sodium chloride) can cause cell damage by disrupting the cell's osmotic and ionic homeostasis. Chemicals can destroy cells at the site of contact. Corrosive substances such as strong acids and bases destroy cells as they come into contact with the body. Other chemicals may injure cells in the process of metabolism or elimination. Carbon tetrachloride (CCl_4), for example, causes little damage until it is metabolized by liver enzymes to a highly reactive free radical ($CCl_3 \cdot$). Carbon tetrachloride is extremely toxic to liver cells. Still other types of chemicals are selective in their sites of action. Carbon monoxide has a special affinity for the hemoglobin molecule.

Injury due to biologic agents

Biologic agents differ from other injurious agents in that they are able to replicate and thus can continue to produce their injurious effects. These agents range from submicroscopic viruses to the larger parasites. Biologic agents cause cell injury by a number of diverse mechanisms: viruses enter the cell and become incorporated into its synthetic machinery. Certain bacteria elaborate exotoxins that interfere with cellular production of ATP. Other bacteria, such as the gram-negative bacilli, release endotoxins that cause cell injury and increased capillary permeability. Still other microorganisms produce their effects through inflammatory or immune mechanisms. Infectious processes are discussed in Chapter 9.

Injury associated with nutritional imbalances

Both nutritional excesses and nutritional deficiencies predispose to cell injury. Obesity and diets high in saturated fats are thought to predispose to atherosclerosis. The body requires more than 60 organic and inorganic substances, in amounts ranging from micrograms to grams. These nutrients include minerals, vitamins, certain fatty acids, and specific amino acids. Dietary deficiencies can occur in the form of starvation, in which there is a deficiency of all nutrients and vitamins, or because of a selective deficiency of a single nutrient or vitamin. Iron-deficiency anemia, scurvy, beriberi, and pellagra are examples of injury caused by the lack of specific vitamins or minerals. The protein and calorie deficiencies that occur with starvation cause widespread tissue damage.

In summary, the causes of cell injury are many and diverse. One common cause is hypoxia. This can result from inadequate oxygen in the air, cardiorespiratory disease, anemia, or the inability of the cells to use oxygen. The impairment of blood flow to an area of the body is called *ischemia*. It produces a state of localized hypoxia. Among the physical agents that produce cell injury are mechanical forces that produce tissue trauma, extremes of temperature, electricity, and radiation. Free-radical formation is an important cause of cell injury in hypoxia and following exposure to radiation and certain chemical agents. Chemical agents can cause cell injury through several mechanisms; they can block enzymatic pathways, cause coagulation of tissues, or disrupt the osmotic or ionic balance of the cell. Biologic agents differ from other injurious agents in that they are able to replicate and continue to produce injury. Among the nutritional factors that contribute to cell injury are excesses and deficiencies of nutrients, vitamins, and minerals.

References

1. Robbins SL, Cotran RS, Kumar V: Pathologic Basis of Disease, 3rd ed, pp 23, 31, 31, 17, 6, 462, 464, 470. Philadelphia, WB Saunders, 1984
2. American Heart Association: Oxygen free radicals: When a good element goes bad. Cardiovascular Research Report. Summer:12, 1987
3. Dart RC, Sanders AB: Oxygen free radicals and myocardial reperfusion injury. Ann Emerg Med 17:53, 1988
4. McCord JM: Oxygen-derived free radicals in postischemic tissue injury. N Engl J Med 312, No. 3:159, 1985
5. Vogt MT, Farber E: On the molecular pathology of ischemic renal cell death: Reversible and irreversible cellular and mitochondrial metabolic alterations. Am J Pathol 53: 1, 1968
6. Robbins SL, Cotran RS, Kumar V: Pathologic Basis of Disease, 2nd ed, p 551. Philadelphia, WB Saunders, 1979
7. Erwin DN: An overview of the biological effects of radiofrequency radiation. Milit Med 148, No. 2: 113–117, 1983
8. Djordjevic Z, Kolak A, Djokovic V et al: Results of our 15-year study on biological effects of microwave exposure. Aviat Space Environ Med 54, No. 6:539–542, 1983
9. Ultrasound use in pregnancy. FDA Drug Bull 14, No. 1:6, 1984

CHAPTER 3

Genetic Control of Cell Function and Inheritance

Genetic control of cell function
  Gene structure
  Genetic code
  Protein synthesis
    Messenger RNA
    Transfer RNA
    Ribosomal RNA

Regulation of gene expression
  Gene mutations
Chromosomes
  Autosomes
  Sex chromosomes
  Chromosome studies

Patterns of inheritance
  Definitions
  Mendel's law
  Pedigree
Gene technology
  Gene mapping
  Recombinant DNA technology

Objectives

After you have studied this chapter, you should be able to meet the following objectives:

_____ State the definition of a gene.

_____ Describe the structure of a gene.

_____ Explain the mechanisms whereby genes control cell function.

_____ Explain how genetic information is transferred from one generation to another generation.

_____ Compare the functions of messenger RNA, transfer RNA, and ribosomal RNA.

_____ Describe the concept of induction and repression in terms of gene function.

_____ Describe the pathogenesis of gene mutation.

_____ Construct a hypothetical pedigree according to Mendel's law.

_____ Contrast genotype and phenotype.

_____ Define *gene mapping*.

_____ List the steps in constructing a karyotype using cytogenetic studies.

_____ List the steps in developing a gene product such as human insulin using recombinant DNA technology.

The word *gene* is defined somewhat differently by the various scientific disciplines. There are breeding genetic units, cellular chromosomal or cytogenetic genes, functional polypeptide genes, and nucleoprotein structural unit genes, as well as others. In all of these terms, the word gene stands for the *fundamental unit of information storage*. This information is stored in the structure of an extremely stable macromolecule within the nucleus of each cell. Because of this stable structure, the genetic information survives the many processes of reduction division of the gametes (ovum and sperm), fertilization, and the many cell divisions involved in the formation of a new organism from the single-celled zygote formed by the union of an ovum and sperm.

Genes determine the types of proteins and enzymes that are made by the cell, and hence control not only inheritance but the day-to-day function of all the cells in the body. For example, genes control the type and quantity of hormones that a cell produces, the antigens and receptors that are present on the cell membrane, and the synthesis of enzymes needed for metabolism. More than 3000 genes have been identified. With few exceptions, each gene provides the instructions for the synthesis of a single protein. This chapter includes discussions of genetic regulation of cell function, chromosomal structure, patterns of inheritance, and gene technology.

Genetic control of cell function

The genetic information needed for protein synthesis is inscribed on *deoxyribonucleic acid (DNA)* contained in the cell nucleus. A second type of nucleic acid, *ribonucleic acid (RNA)*, is involved in the actual synthesis of cellular enzymes and proteins. *Messenger RNA* transcribes the instructions for protein synthesis from the DNA molecule and carries them into the cytoplasm, whereas *ribosomal RNA* translates the message into production language that can be used by the cell's polypeptide-building machinery. *Transfer RNA* delivers the appropriate amino acids to the ribosome, where they are incorporated into the protein being synthesized. This process for the control of cell function is illustrated in Figure 3-1.

The nuclei of all the cells in an organism each contain the same accumulation of genes derived from the gametes of the two parents. This means that liver cells contain the same genetic information as skin and muscle cells. For this to be true, the molecular code must be duplicated prior to each succeeding cell division, or mitosis. Theoretically, although not yet achieved in humans, any of the highly differentiated cells of an organism could be used to produce a com-

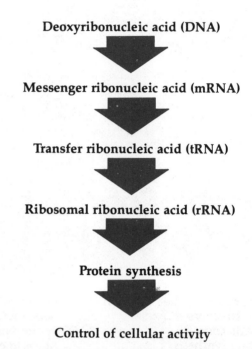

Figure 3-1 DNA-directed control of cellular activity through synthesis of cellular proteins. Messenger RNA carries the transcribed message, which directs protein synthesis, from the nucleus to the cytoplasm. Transfer RNA selects the appropriate amino acids and carries them to ribosomal RNA, where assembly of the proteins takes place.

plete, genetically identical organism, or clone. From this it becomes evident that each particular tissue uses only some of the information stored in the genetic code. Although information required for the function of other types of tissues is still present, it is repressed.

── Gene structure

The stable structure that stores the genetic information within the nucleus is a very long, double-stranded, chainlike molecule of DNA in which the two strands coil around a common axis to form a double helix. The DNA molecule is composed of nucleotides, which consist of (1) phosphoric acid, (2) a five-carbon sugar called deoxyribose, and (3) one of four nitrogenous bases. The four bases can be divided into two groups: the purine bases adenine and guanine, which have two nitrogen ring structures, and the pyrimidine bases thymine and cytosine, which have one ring. Alternating groups of sugar and phosphoric acid form the backbone of the molecule, whereas the paired bases project inward from the sides of the sugar molecule. The entire chain is like a spiral staircase, with the paired bases representing the steps (Figure 3-2C).

There is a precise pairing of the nucleotides in the double-stranded DNA molecule. The nucleotides exist in complementary pairs of a purine and pyrimidine base: adenine is paired with thymine and gua-

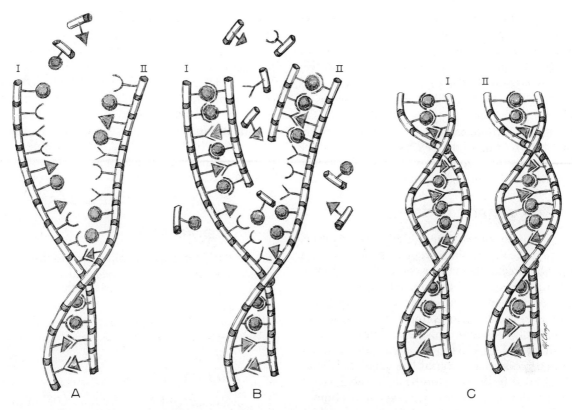

Figure 3-2 Schematic representation of the replication of DNA. (**A**) Prior to cell division, the bonds between the nitrogenous bases are broken, the two strands separate, and each strand takes with it the bases attached to its side. (**B**) The bases attached to each single strand attract free-floating nucleotide units and pair off in the usual way: adenine with thymine, guanine with cytosine. (**C**) The end result is two exact replicas of the original DNA molecule, and the cell is ready to undergo division. (*Chaffee EE, Lytle IM: Basic Physiology and Anatomy, 4th ed. Philadelphia, JB Lippincott, 1980*)

nine with cytosine (Figure 3-3). Each nucleotide in a pair is on one strand of the DNA molecule, with the bases of the pair loosely bound by a hydrogen bond. Because of the looseness of the bond, the two strands can pull apart with ease so that the genetic information can be duplicated or transcribed (Figure 3-2**A**).

A gene can be regarded as being represented by several hundred to a thousand base pairs. Of the two DNA strands, only one is used in transcribing the information for the cell's polypeptide-building machinery. If the genetic information of one strand is meaningful, then the complementary code of the other strand will not make sense and will therefore be ignored. Both strands, however, are involved in DNA duplication. Prior to cell division, the two strands of the helix separate and a complementary molecule is organized next to each original strand. Thus, two strands make four strands, with each strand joined to a new complementary strand (Figure 3-2**B**). During cell division, the newly duplicated double-helix molecules are separated and placed in each daughter cell by the mechanics of mitosis. As a result, each of the daughter cells again contains the meaningful strand and the complementary strand joined in the form of a

double helix. Replication of DNA has been termed *semiconservative* because each new daughter molecule contains one parental strand.

The very long DNA molecule is combined with several types of protein and small amounts of

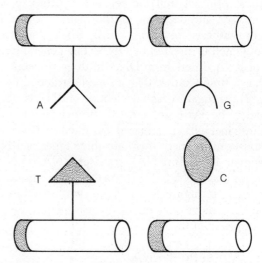

Figure 3-3 Pairing of the nucleotides in DNA. Thymine pairs with adenine and cytosine with guanine.

RNA into a complex known as *chromatin.* Chromatin is the more readily stainable portion of the cell nucleus. Some of these proteins form binding sites for repressor molecules and hormones that regulate genetic transcription. Other proteins may themselves block genetic transcription by preventing access of nucleotides to the surface of the DNA molecule. A specific group of proteins, called *histones,* are thought to control the folding of the DNA strands. As will be discussed later, the chromatin coils and folds over to form chromosomes during cell division.

The genetic code

The four bases guanine, adenine, cytosine, and uracil make up the alphabet of the genetic code. A sequence of three of these bases constitutes the fundamental triplet code used in transmitting the genetic information needed for protein synthesis; this triplet code is called a *codon.* An example is the nucleotide sequence GCU (guanine, cytosine, and uracil), which is the triplet RNA code for the amino acid alanine. The genetic code is a universal language used by all living cells: that is, the code for the amino acid tryptophan is the same in a bacterium, a plant, and a human being. There are also start and stop codes, which signal the beginning and end of a protein molecule. Mathematically, the 4 bases can be arranged in 64 different combinations ($4 \times 4 \times 4 = 64$). This means 64 combinations can be used to specify amino acids. Because there are 20 amino acids that can be used in protein synthesis, there must be several codes for the same amino acid. It has been discovered that 18 of the amino acids have more than one code word.

Protein synthesis

Although DNA determines the type of biochemical product that the cell will synthesize, the transmission and decoding of information needed for protein synthesis are carried out by RNA, the formation of which is directed by DNA. The general structure of RNA differs from DNA in three respects: (1) RNA is a single- rather than a double-stranded molecule; (2) the sugar in each nucleotide of RNA is ribose instead of deoxyribose; and (3) the pyridimine base thymine, in DNA, is replaced by uracil in RNA. As previously mentioned, there are three types of RNA: messenger RNA (mRNA), transfer RNA (tRNA), and ribosomal RNA (rRNA). As the name implies, all three forms of ribonucleic acid are synthesized in the nucleus and move through the nuclear membrane into the cytoplasm of the cell.

Messenger RNA

Messenger RNA is a long molecule containing several hundred to several thousand nucleotides, which are codons that are exactly complementary to code words on the genes. Messenger RNA is formed by a process called *transcription,* in which the weak hydrogen bonds of the DNA are broken so that free RNA nucleotides can pair with their exposed DNA counterparts on the meaningful strand of the DNA molecule. As with the base pairing of the DNA strands, complementary RNA bases will pair with the DNA bases (uracil, which replaces thymine in RNA, pairs with adenine). The joining together of the RNA molecule is catalyzed by the transcriptase enzyme, which is active only in the presence of DNA.

Transfer RNA

Transfer RNA transfers amino acids to protein molecules being synthesized by ribosomal structures; it has two recognition sites: one for the mRNA codon for the amino acid and a second for the amino acid itself. There are different types of tRNA, and each type recognizes and binds only one type of amino acid.

Ribosomal RNA

Ribosomal RNA constitutes 60% of the ribosome in which protein synthesis occurs. The remainder of the ribosome is structural proteins and enzymes needed for protein synthesis. Ribosomal RNA uses the "blueprint" transcribed on mRNA in assembling proteins. This process is called *translation.* There is no specificity of ribosomes for synthesis of a particular protein; a particular mRNA can direct protein synthesis in any ribosome. During protein synthesis most ribosomes become attached to the endoplasmic reticulum. This attachment facilitates transport of the protein end product and is particularly important in cells that produce substances, such as hormones, that are released from the cell.

Proteins are made from a standard set of 20 amino acids, which are joined end to end to form the long polypeptide chains of protein molecules. Each polypeptide may have as many as 100 to more than 300 amino acids in it. During protein synthesis, mRNA comes in contact with and then passes through the ribosome—much in the same manner that a tape moves through a tape player. As mRNA passes through the ribosome, rRNA translates the message into assembly language, and tRNA delivers the appropriate amino acids for attachment to the growing polypeptide chain. The long mRNA molecule usually travels through and directs protein synthesis in more than one ribosome at a time. As the first part of the mRNA is read by the first ribosome, it moves on to a second, and then a third; as a result, ribosomes that are actively involved in protein synthesis are often found in clusters called *polyribosomes.* The process of protein synthesis is depicted in Figure 3-4.

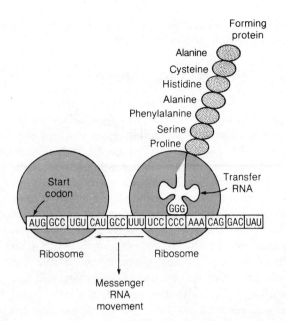

Figure 3-4 Postulated mechanism by which a protein molecule is formed in ribosomes in association with messenger RNA and ribosomal RNA. (Guyton A: Medical Physiology, 7th ed. Philadelphia, WB Saunders, 1986)

Regulation of gene expression

Although all cells contain the same genes, not all genes are active all of the time, nor are the same genes active in all cell types. On the contrary, only a small, select group of genes is active in directing protein synthesis in the cell, and this group varies from one cell type to another. In order for different types of cells to develop in the body as a result of cell differentiation, the protein synthesis in some cells must be different from that in others. Furthermore, in order to adapt to an ever-changing environment, certain cells may need to produce varying amounts and types of proteins. In addition, there are certain enzymes, such as carbonic anhydrase, that all cells must synthesize for the fundamental metabolic process on which life depends.

At present there are believed to be at least two types of genes that control protein synthesis: (1) structural genes that specify the amino acid sequence of a polypeptide chain and (2) genes that serve a regulatory function without stipulating the structure of protein molecules. The degree to which a gene or particular group of genes is active is referred to as *gene expression*. A phenomenon termed *induction* is an important process whereby gene expression is increased. Except in early embryonic development, induction is produced by some external influence. A *repressor* is a substance produced by a regulatory gene that acts to prevent protein synthesis. Some genes are normally dormant and can be activated by inducer substances, and other genes are naturally active and can be inhibited by repressor substances.

Genetic mechanisms for the control of protein synthesis are much better understood in microorganisms than in humans. It can be assumed, however, that many of the same principles apply. The mechanism that has been most extensively studied is the one by which the synthesis of particular proteins can be turned on and off. In *Escherichia coli (E. coli)* grown in a nutrient medium containing the disaccharide lactose, an enzyme (galactosidase) can be isolated that catalyzes the splitting of lactose into a molecule of glucose and a molecule of galactose; this is necessary if lactose is to be metabolized by *E. coli*. On the other hand, if the *E. coli* is grown in a medium that does not contain lactose, very little of the enzyme is produced. From these and other studies, it is theorized that the synthesis of a particular protein, such as galactosidase, requires a series of reactions, each of which is catalyzed by a specific enzyme. The formation of all of the enzymes needed for the synthetic process is controlled by a sequence of genes that are located on adjacent sites on the same chromosome. This area of the DNA strand is called an *operon*. The rate at which the operon functions to transcribe RNA, and therefore sets into motion the enzymatic system for the synthetic process, is controlled by a small adjacent segment of the DNA molecule. This small segment functions as a control unit for the operon; it can activate or repress the function of the operon. The control unit for the operon often monitors levels of the synthesized product and regulates the activity of the operon in a negative feedback manner; whenever there is enough of the required product, the operon becomes inactive. The operon can also be activated by an inducer substance: some of the steroid hormones, for example, perform their hormonal action by activating operons in this manner. Regulatory genes located elsewhere in the genetic complex can exert control over an operon through activator or repressor substances, as can the availability of the transcriptase enzyme needed for transcription of RNA. Not all genes are subject to induction and repression; many appear to lack control genes and are continually active.

Gene mutations

Rarely, accidental errors in duplication or destruction of parts of the genetic code occur. Such changes are called *mutations*. Many of these mutations are caused by environmental agents, chemicals, and radiation. If the duplicating cell line that contains such a change forms gametes, or germ cells, then the mutation can be transmitted to the offspring. Much more frequently, the affected cell line differentiates into one or more of the many tissues of the body and thus is not transmissible to the next generation. These are *somatic mutations* and they result in genetic differences between the cells and tissues of the same organism, producing what is called a *genetic mosaic*. Occasionally, a person is born with one brown eye and one blue eye as a result of a somatic mutation. The change or loss of gene information is just as likely to affect the fundamental processes of cell function or organ differentiation. Such somatic mutations in the early embryonic period can result in embryonic death or congenital malformations. Somatic mutations are important causes of cancer and other tumors in which cell differentiation and growth get out of hand. Fishermen, farmers, and others who are excessively exposed to the ultraviolet radiation of sunlight have an increased risk of developing skin cancer resulting from potential radiation damage to the genetic structure of the skin-forming cells.

In summary, genes are the fundamental unit of information storage in the cell. They determine the types of proteins and enzymes that are made by the cell and therefore control not only inheritance but day-to-day cell function. Genes store information in the form of a very stable macromolecule called DNA. Genes transmit information in the form of a triplet code, which uses the nitrogenous bases of the four nucleotides (adenine, guanine, thymine, and cytosine) of which the DNA molecule is composed. The transfer of stored information into production of cell products is accomplished through a second type of macromolecule called RNA. Messenger RNA transcribes the instructions for product synthesis from the DNA molecule and carries it into the cell's cytoplasm, where ribosomal RNA utilizes the information to direct product synthesis. Transfer RNA acts as a carrier system for delivering the appropriate amino acids to the ribosomes, where the synthesis of cell products occurs. Although all cells contain the same genes, only a small, select group of genes is active in a given cell type. In all cells some genetic information is repressed while other information is expressed. Gene mutations represent accidental errors in duplication or destruction of parts of the genetic code.

Chromosomes

The genetic information of a cell is organized, stored, and retrieved in the form of small cellular structures called *chromosomes*. There are 46 human chromosomes—22 pairs of autosomes and 1 pair of sex chromosomes.

Autosomes

Each of the autosomes appears to be identical to its partner, but each pair is different in genetic content and appearance from the other pairs. These 22 pairs have the same appearance in all individuals, and each has been given a numerical designation for classification purposes.

Sex chromosomes

The sex chromosomes constitute the 23rd pair of chromosomes (Figure 3-5). They determine the sex of an individual. There are two sex chromosomes: the Y in the male coming from the father and the X from the mother. All normal females have two X chromosomes, one from each parent. It is believed that of the two X chromosomes in the female only one is active in controlling the expression of genetic traits. Both X chromosomes are involved, however, in transmission to the offspring. In the female the active X chromosome is invisible, whereas the inactive X chromosome can be demonstrated, on appropriate nuclear staining, as the *chromatin mass* or *Barr body*. Thus the genetic sex of a child can be determined by microscopic study of cell or tissue samples. The total number of X chromosomes is equal to the number of Barr bodies (inactive X chromosomes) plus one (active X chromosome). For example, the cells of a normal female will have one Barr body, and therefore a total of two X chromosomes. A male will have no Barr bodies. In the female, whether the X chromosome derived from the mother or that derived from the father is active is determined within a few days after conception; the selection is random for each postmitotic cell line. This is called the Lyon principle (after Mary Lyon, the British geneticist who developed it).

Chromosome studies

Cytogenetics is the study of the structure and numerical characteristics of the cell's chromosomes. Chromosome studies can be done on any tissue or cell

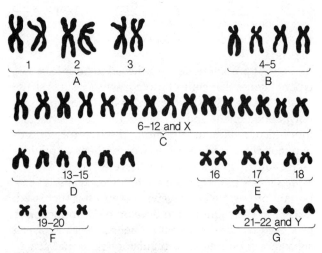

Figure 3-5 Normal male karyotype. The first 22 pairs of chromosomes are the autosomes and the last 2 chromosomes are the sex chromosomes, in this case an X and Y chromosome. (*Singer S: Human Genetics. San Francisco, WH Freeman and Co., Copyright © 1978*)

that will grow and divide in culture. The lymphocytes from venous blood are frequently used for this purpose. Once the cultured cells have been fixed and spread on a slide, they are stained to demonstrate chromosomal banding patterns so that they can be identified. The chromosomes are then photographed, and each chromosome is cut from the photograph and arranged according to the standard set by the 1971 Paris Chromosome Conference to form the *karyotype* (or chromosome picture) of the individual.[1] This arrangement is called an *idiogram*.

In summary, the genetic information in a cell is organized, stored, and retrieved in the form of small cellular structures called chromosomes. There are 46 chromosomes arranged in 23 pairs. Twenty-two of these pairs are autosomes. The 23rd pair contains the sex chromosomes, which determine the sex of an individual. A karyotype is a photograph of an individual's chromosomes. It is prepared by special laboratory techniques in which body cells are cultured, fixed, stained to demonstrate identifiable banding patterns, and photographed.

Patterns of inheritance

At a particular point on the DNA molecule, the genetic code may be capable of controlling the production of an observable trait. Such a segment of the DNA molecule is called a *gene locus*. Alternative forms of the gene code are possible (one inherited from the mother and the other from the father), and each form may produce a different aspect of the trait. Alternative forms of a gene at the same locus are called *alleles*.

Definitions

Genetics has its own set of definitions. The *genotype* of an individual is a term for the genetic information stored in the base sequence triplet code. The *phenotype* refers to the recognizable traits, physical or biochemical, that are associated with a specific genotype. There are many instances in which the genotype is not evident by available detection methods. Thus, more than one genotype may have the same phenotype. Some brown-eyed people are carriers of the code for blue eyes and other brown-eyed persons are not. Phenotypically, these two types of brown-eyed people are the same, but genotypically they are different.

When it comes to a genetic disorder, not all individuals with a mutant gene are affected to the same extent. *Expressivity* refers to the expression of the gene in the phenotype, which can range from mild to severe. *Penetrance* means the ability of a gene to express its function. Seventy-five percent penetrance means that only 75% of the individuals of a particular genotype will demonstrate a recognizable phenotype.

A locus is the location or site on a chromosome (*i.e.*, along the DNA molecule) where a gene pair is located. When only one pair of genes is involved in the transmission of information, the term *single-gene* is used. Single-gene traits follow the mendelian laws of inheritance. *Polygenic* inheritance involves multiple genes at different loci, each gene exerting a small additive effect in determining a trait. Most human traits are determined by multiple pairs of genes, many with alternate codes, accounting for some of the dissimilar forms that occur with certain genetic disorders. Polygenic traits are predictable, but less so than single-gene traits.

Mendel's law

The main feature of inheritance is predictability: given certain conditions, the likelihood of the occurrence or recurrence of a specific trait is remarkably predictable. The units of inheritance are the genes, and the pattern of single-gene expression can be predicted using Mendel's law, with some modification as the result of knowledge accumulated since 1865, the date of Mendel's publication.

It was Mendel who discovered the basic pattern of inheritance by conducting carefully planned experiments with simple garden peas. From his experiments with wrinkled and round peas, Mendel proposed that inherited traits are transmitted from parents to offspring by means of independently inherited factors—now known as genes—and that these factors are transmitted as recessive and dominant traits. Mendel labeled dominant factors (his round peas) "A" and recessive (his wrinkled peas) "a." Geneticists continue to use capital letters to designate dominant traits and lower-case letters to identify recessive traits. The possible combinations that can occur with transmission of single-gene dominant and recessive traits can be described by constructing a figure using capital and lower-case letters.

The observable traits are inherited from one's parents. During maturation, the germ cells (sperm and ovum) of both parents undergo meiosis, or reduction division, in which the number of chromosomes is divided in half (from 46 to 23). At this time, the two alleles from a gene locus separate so that each germ cell gets only one allele from each pair. According to Mendel's law, the alleles from the different gene loci segregate independently and then recombine in a random fashion in the zygote that is formed by the union of the two germ cells. Individuals in whom the two alleles of a given pair are the same (AA or aa) are called *homozygotes*. *Heterozygotes* have different (Aa) alleles at a gene locus.

A *recessive trait* is one that is expressed only in a homozygous pairing; a *dominant trait* is one that is expressed in either a homozygous or a heterozygous pairing. All persons with a dominant allele inherit that trait. A *carrier* is a person who is heterozygous for a recessive trait and does not manifest the trait. For example, if the genes for blond hair were determined to be recessive and those for brunet hair dominant, then only persons with a genotype with two alleles for blond hair would be blond, and all persons with either one or two brunet alleles would have dark hair.

── Pedigree

A pedigree is a graphic method for portraying a family history of an inherited trait. It is constructed from a carefully obtained family history and is useful for tracing the pattern of inheritance for a particular trait.

In summary, inheritance represents the likelihood of the occurrence or recurrence of a specific genetic trait. The genotype refers to information that is stored in the genetic code of an individual. The phenotype represents the recognizable traits, physical and biochemical, that are associated with the genotype. Expressivity refers to the expression of a gene in the phenotype, and penetrance is the ability of a gene to express its function. The point on the DNA molecule that controls the inheritance of a particular trait is called a gene locus. Alternate codes at one gene locus are called alleles. According to Mendel's law, the two alleles at a gene locus can transmit recessive or dominant traits. A recessive trait is one that is expressed only when there is homozygous pairing of the alleles. A dominant trait is expressed with either homozygous or heterozygous pairing of the alleles. A pedigree is a graphic method for portraying a family history of an inherited trait.

Gene technology

── Gene mapping

Gene mapping is the assignment of genes to specific chromosomes or parts of the chromosome. The initial assignment of a gene to a particular chromosome was made in 1911 for the color blindness gene that was inherited from the mother—that is, followed the X-linked pattern of inheritance.[2] In 1968 the specific location of the Duffy blood group on the long arm of chromosome 1 was determined.[3] At pres-

ent the locations of more than 1300 expressed human genes have been mapped to a specific chromosome and most of them to a specific region on the chromosome.[4]

A number of methods have been used for gene mapping. The most important ones currently used are family linkage studies, gene dosage methods, in situ hybridization, and somatic cell hybridization. Often the specific assignment of a gene is made possible by the use of information from several mapping techniques.

Linkage studies assume that genes occur in a linear array along the chromosomes. During meiosis, the paired chromosomes of the diploid germ cell exchange genetic material in a phenomenon called *crossing over*. This exchange involves not individual, but large blocks of genes, each accounting for a sizable fraction of the chromosome. Although the point at which one block separates from another occurs in a random fashion, the closer together two genes are on the same chromosome the greater the chance they will be passed on together to the offspring. When two inherited traits occur together at a rate significantly greater than would occur by chance, they are said to be linked.

There are several methods of using the crossing over and recombination of genes to map a particular gene. In one method, any gene that is already assigned to a chromosome can be used as a marker to assign other linked genes. For example, it was found that both an extra-long 1 chromosome and the Duffy blood group were inherited as a dominant trait, placing the position of the blood group gene close to the extra material on the 1 chromosome. Color blindness has been linked to hemophilia A in some pedigrees, hemophilia to glucose-6-phosphatase deficiency in others, and color blindness and glucose-6-phosphatase deficiency in still others. Therefore, all three genes must be located in a small section of the X chromosome. Linkage analysis can be used clinically to identify affected persons in a family with a known genetic defect. Two autosomal recessive disorders successfully diagnosed prenatally (using amniocentesis) by linkage studies are congenital adrenal hyperplasia (due to 21-hydroxylase deficiency and linked to an HLA type) and hemophilia A (which is linked to glucose-6-phosphatase deficiency in some families). Postnatally, linkage studies have been used in diagnosing hemochromatosis, which is closely linked to another immune response gene or human leukocyte antigen (HLA) type (see discussion in Chapter 11). Persons with this disorder are unable to metabolize iron, and it accumulates in the liver and other organs. It cannot be diagnosed by conventional means until irreversible damage has been done. Given a family history of the disorder, HLA typing can determine if the gene is present; if present, dietary restriction of iron intake may be used to prevent organ damage.

Dosage studies involve measuring enzyme activity. Autosomal genes are normally arranged in pairs, and normally both are expressed. If both alleles are present and both are expressed, then the activity of the enzyme should be 100%. If one member of the gene pair is missing, only 50% of the enzyme activity will be present, reflecting the activity of the remaining normal allele.

In situ hybridization involves the use of a recombinant DNA probe to locate genes that do not express themselves in cell culture. It begins with the extraction of mRNA that is specific for a particular protein. The mRNA is then used as a template for synthesis of the complementary DNA strand. The complementary DNA, labeled with a radioisotope, binds to the gene to which it is complementary and serves as a probe for gene location. For example, mRNA for two components of the hemoglobin A molecule (Hb a and Hb b) were extracted from the red blood cell, and through this method it was found that the gene for Hb a was located on chromosome 16 and the gene for Hb b on chromosome 11.

Somatic cell hybridization involves the fusion of a mouse or Chinese hamster cell line with human leukocytes or fibroblasts to produce a rodent–human somatic cell. These hybrids preferentially lose human chromosomes in a random manner during cell mitosis, so it is possible to obtain cells with different partial combinations of human chromosomes. In this way the correlation of the expression of human gene markers, such as production of a specific enzyme, can be linked to a particular chromosome.

—— Recombinant DNA technology

During the course of the past several decades, genetic engineering has provided the methods for manipulating nucleic acids and recombining genes (recombinant DNA) into hybrid molecules that can be inserted into unicellular organisms and reproduced many times over. Each hybrid molecule gives rise to a genetically identical population, called a *clone,* that reflects its common ancestor.

The techniques of gene isolation and cloning are based on the fact that the genes of all organisms, from bacteria through mammals, have a similar molecular organization. Gene cloning requires cutting a DNA molecule apart, modifying and reassembling its fragments, and producing copies of the modified DNA, its mRNA, and its gene product. Cutting apart the DNA molecule is accomplished through the use of a bacterial enzyme, called a *restriction enzyme,* that binds to DNA wherever a particular short sequence of base pairs is found and then cleaves the molecule at a specific nucleotide site. In this way, a long DNA molecule can be broken down into smaller discrete fragments with the intent that one of the fragments will contain the gene of interest. At present, there are more than 100 restriction enzymes commercially available that will cut DNA at different recognition sites.

Replication of the selected gene fragment is accomplished through insertion of the DNA fragments into a unicellular organism such as a bacterium. To do this, a cloning vector such as a bacterial virus or a small DNA circle that is found in most bacteria, called a *plasmid,* is used. Both viral and plasmid vectors replicate autonomously in the host bacterial cell. In the process of gene cloning, a bacterial vector and the fragments from a DNA molecule are mixed together and joined by a special enzyme called a *DNA ligase.* The recombinant vectors are then introduced into a suitable culture of bacteria and the bacteria allowed to replicate and express the recombinant vector gene. Sometimes mRNA that is taken from a tissue that expresses a high level of the gene is used to produce a complementary DNA molecule that can be used in the cloning process. Because the fragments of the entire DNA molecule are used in the cloning process, additional steps are taken to identify and separate the clone that contains the gene of interest.

In terms of biological research and technology, cloning makes it possible to identify the DNA sequence in a gene and produce the protein product encoded by a gene. The specific nucleotide sequence of a cloned DNA fragment can often be identified by analyzing the amino acid sequence and mRNA codons of its protein product. It is also possible to synthesize short sequences of base pairs that can be radioactively labeled and used to identify their complementary sequence. In this way, it is possible to identify normal and abnormal gene structures.

Proteins that formerly were only available in small amounts can now be made in large quantities once their respective genes have been isolated. For example, genes encoding for insulin and growth hormone have been cloned as a means of producing these hormones for pharmacological use. Although quite different from inserting genetic material into a unicellular organism such as a bacteria, techniques are now available for inserting genes into the genome of intact multicellular plants and animals. However, the introduction of the cloned gene into the multicellular organism can only influence the few cells that acquire the gene. An answer to this problem would be the insertion of the gene into a germ cell (sperm or ovum) in which the gene would be replicated in all of the differentiating cell types. Even so, techniques for cell insertion are very limited. Not only are moral and ethical issues involved, but these techniques cannot direct the inserted DNA to attach to a particular chromosome nor can they supplant an existing gene by knocking it out of its place.

In summary, gene mapping is a method used to assign genes to particular chromosomes or parts of the chromosome. Methods currently used in gene mapping are somatic cell hybridization and use of recombinant DNA. Somatic cell hybridization is a method used to obtain cells with partial combinations of human chromosomes and involves fusion of mouse or Chinese hamster cell lines with human leukocytes or fibroblasts. It is used in linkage studies, which assign a chromosomal location to genes based on their close association with other genes of known location. Recombinant DNA studies involve the extraction of specific types of messenger RNA that are used in synthesis of complementary DNA strands. The complementary DNA strands, labeled with a radioisotope, bind with the genes for which they are complementary and are used as gene probes.

References

1. ISCN (1981): An International System for Human Cytogenetic Nomenclature—High Resolution Banding (1981). Birth Defects, 17, No. 5, New York: March of Dimes Foundation, 1981
2. Wilson EB: The sex chromosomes. Arch Mikrosc Anat. 77:249, 1911
3. McKusick VA: The anatomy of the human genome. Hosp Pract 16, No. 4: 82, 1981
4. McKusick VA: The new genetics and clinical medicine: A summing up. Hosp Pract 23, No. 7:178, 1988

CHAPTER 4

Genetic and Congenital Disorders

Genetic and chromosomal disorders
  Single-gene disorders
    Disorders of autosomal inheritance
    Disorders of sex-linked inheritance
    Manifestations of single-gene disorders
  Polygenic disorders
  Chromosome disorders
    Alterations in chromosome duplication
    Alterations in chromosome number
    Alterations in chromosome structure

Disorders due to environmental influences
  Period of vulnerability
  Teratogenic agents
    Irradiation
    Chemicals and drugs
    Infectious agents

Diagnosis and counseling
  Genetic assessment
  Prenatal diagnosis
    Ultrasound
    Amniocentesis
    Chorionic villus sampling
    Cytogenic and biochemical analyses

Objectives

After you have studied this chapter, you should be able to meet the following objectives:

_____ Define the term *congenital defect.*

_____ Describe three types of single-gene disorders.

_____ Contrast polygenic disorders with single-gene disorders.

_____ Describe two chromosomal abnormalities that demonstrate aneuploidy.

_____ Describe three patterns of chromosomal breakage and rearrangement.

_____ Relate maternal age and occurrence of Down's syndrome.

_____ Cite the most susceptible period of intrauterine life for development of defects due to environmental agents.

_____ State the cautions that should be observed when considering use of drugs during pregnancy.

_____ List four infectious agents that cause congenital defects.

_____ List types of information that are usually considered when doing an assessment of genetic risk.

_____ Cite examples of fetal information that can be obtained with use of amniocentesis, chorionic villus sampling, and ultrasound.

Genetic and congenital disorders are important at all levels of health care because they affect all age groups and can involve any of the body organs and tissues. A congenital defect has been described as any structural, functional, or biochemical abnormality in development that originates before or shortly after birth and causes an immediate or a delayed abnormality in the structure and function of an organ.[1] There are two general categories of congenital defects: (1) those that have a hereditary basis, such as single-gene and polygenic abnormalities or chromosomal aberrations, and (2) abnormalities that are caused by environmental agents such as maternal disease, radiation, or drugs. One-quarter million infants are born with physical or mental damage in the United States each year.[2] More than 60,000 Americans die of birth defects annually. It has been estimated that 80% of birth defects arise as the result of genetic disorders, and the remaining 20% represent the effects of agents such as infection, drugs, and physical injury to the fetus.[3]

This chapter is designed to provide an overview of genetic and congenital disorders and is divided into three parts: (1) genetic and chromosomal disorders, (2) disorders due to environmental agents, and (3) diagnosis and counseling.

Genetic and chromosomal disorders

A mutant gene is implied by the sudden appearance of a genotype in a demonstrably noncarrier pedigree. Genetic disorders represent changes (or mutations) in gene function or changes in chromosomal structure. A genetic disorder can involve a single-gene trait or it can involve a polygenic trait. Polygenic traits are observable characteristics that result from the additive interactions of more than one, and sometimes many, gene loci. The shape of the nose, body height, native intelligence, and other characteristics involve polygenic inheritance. Almost all of the hereditary traits that are of importance in most individuals result from the interaction between many independently associated gene loci and the environment.

The effects of an abnormal genetic trait may be present at birth or may not become apparent until later in life. Huntington's chorea, for example, usually has its onset between 20 and 30 years of age. Some diseases tend to run in families, and it is thought that the combined effects of genetic predisposition and environmental factors influence the development of these diseases. This is true of some types of diabetes mellitus, hypertension, and cancer.

Every individual probably has five to eight recessive genes that would cause defects if present in the homozygous state.[4] About 80% to 85% of these abnormal genes are from the pedigree (inherited) and the remainder represent new mutations.

── Single-gene disorders

At last count there were more than 3000 single-gene disorders; although individually rare, they collectively account for approximately 1% of all adult and 5% of all pediatric hospital admissions.[5] Single-gene disorders may be dominant or recessive, and genes located on the nonsex chromosomes (autosomal genes) or those located on the sex chromosomes may be affected. Disorders of the Y, or male, chromosome are extremely rare. Chart 4-1 lists some of the common defects in each of these categories.

── Disorders of autosomal inheritance

The autosomes are represented on 22 homologous pairs of chromosomes. The autosomes on each chromosome are arranged in strict order, with each gene occupying a specific location or locus, and in pairs, with one maternal and one paternal member. The two members of a gene pair are called alleles. If both members of a gene pair are identical then the

---

Chart 4-1: Some disorders of Mendelian or single-gene inheritance

Autosomal dominant

Achondroplasia (short-limb dwarfism)
Adult polycystic kidney disease
Huntington's chorea
Hypercholesterolemia
Marfan's syndrome
Multiple neurofibromatosis (von Recklinghausen's disease)
Osteogenesis imperfecta
Spherocytosis
von Willebrand's disease (bleeding diathesis)

Autosomal recessive

Color blindness
Cystic fibrosis
Glycogen storage diseases
Oculocutaneous albinism
Phenylketonuria (PKU)
Renal glycosuria
Sickle cell disease
Tay-Sachs disease
Wilson's disease

X-linked recessive

Bruton-type agammaglobulinemia
Classic hemophilia
Duchenne-type muscular dystrophy

person is *homozygous* for the locus; if both members are different, then the person is *heterozygous*. Any gene-determined characteristic is a trait. If the trait is only expressed in the heterozygote, it is said to be *dominant;* and if it is only expressed in the homozygote, it is *recessive.*

Although gene expression usually follows a dominant or recessive pattern, it is possible for both alleles (members) of a gene pair to be fully expressed in the heterozygote, a condition called *codominance.* The term *polymorphism* describes the condition in which there are multiple allelic forms of the same gene. Histocompatibility and blood group inheritance are examples of both codominance and polymorphism.

A single mutant gene may be expressed in many different parts of the body. Marfan's syndrome is a defect in connective tissue that has widespread effects involving skeletal, eye, and cardiovascular structures. In other single-gene disorders, the same defect can be caused by mutations at several different loci. Childhood deafness can result from 16 different types of autosomal recessive mutations.

In autosomal dominant disorders, a single mutant allele from an affected parent is transmitted to an offspring regardless of sex. The unaffected relatives of the parent or unaffected siblings of the offspring do not transmit the disorder. The affected individual has a 50% chance of transmitting the disorder to each offspring (Figure 4-1). Autosomal dominant disorders are characterized by reduced penetrance and variable expressivity, an age of onset that is later in life (*e.g.,* Huntington's chorea), and a mutant gene that tends to involve a structural or a regulatory protein. Although there is a 50% chance of inheriting a dominant genetic disorder, there can be wide variation in gene expression. When a person inherits a dominant mutant gene but fails to express it, the trait is described as having *reduced penetrance.* Penetrance is expressed in mathematical terms; a 50% penetrance indicates that a per-

son who inherits the defective gene has a 50% chance of expressing the disorder. The person who has a mutant gene but does not express it is an important exception to the rule that unaffected persons do not transmit an autosomal dominant trait. These persons can transmit the gene to their descendants and so produce a skipped generation. Autosomal dominant disorders can also display variable expressivity, meaning that they can be expressed differently among individuals. Polydactyly or supernumerary digits, for example, may be expressed in either the fingers or the toes.

Autosomal recessive disorders are manifested only when both members of the gene pair are mutant alleles. In this case, both parents may be unaffected but are carriers of the defective gene. Autosomal recessive disorders affect both sexes. The occurrence risk in each pregnancy is one in four for an affected child, two in four for a carrier child, and one in four for a normal (noncarrier, unaffected) homozygous child (Figure 4-2). With autosomal recessive disorders, the expression of the gene tends to be more uniform than with autosomal dominant disorders; the age of onset is frequently early in life; and in many cases enzyme proteins are affected by the mutation.

Disorders of sex-linked inheritance

Sex-linked inheritance is almost always associated with the X, or female, chromosome and is predominantly recessive. The common pattern of inheritance is one in which an unaffected mother carries one normal and one mutant allele on the X chromosome. This means that she will have a 50% chance of transmitting the defect to her sons and that her female children will have a 50% chance of being carriers of the mutant gene. When the affected male procreates, he will transmit the defect to all of his daughters, who

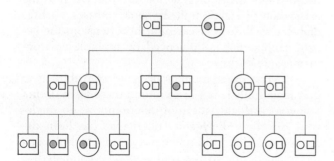

Figure 4-1 Simple pedigree for inheritance of an autosomal dominant trait. The colored circle represents the mutant gene. An affected parent with an autosomal dominant trait has a 50% chance of passing the mutant gene on to each child regardless of sex.

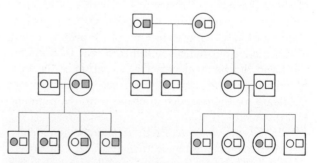

Figure 4-2 Simple pedigree for inheritance of an autosomal recessive trait. The colored circle and square represent a mutant gene. When both parents are carriers of a mutant gene there is a 25% chance of an affected child, a 50% chance of a carrier child, and a 25% chance of a nonaffected/noncarrier child regardless of sex. All children (100%) of an affected parent will be carriers.

will then become carriers of the mutant gene. Since the genes of the Y chromosome are unaffected, the affected male will not transmit the defect to any of his sons and they will not be carriers or transmit the disorder to their children.

Manifestations of single-gene disorders

Many single-gene disorders result in inborn errors of metabolism. These biochemical defects involve the formation of abnormal structural proteins, abnormal biochemical mediators or enzymes, or abnormal membrane-bound transport systems or receptor proteins.

Structural protein defects are usually manifested as autosomal dominant disorders. An example is *Marfan's syndrome,* described previously as a disorder of the connective tissues that is manifested by changes in the skeleton, the eyes, and the cardiovascular system. Characteristics of the skeletal defects are a long thin body, hyperextensive joints, arachnodactyly (spider fingers), and scoliosis. Defects of the eye include the upward displacement of the lens and the potential for retinal detachment. Involvement of connective tissue in the cardiovascular system may lead to mitral valve disease and a tendency for development of a dissecting aortic aneurysm. Abraham Lincoln's extremely long legs and the unequal lengths of his thumbs suggest that he may have been mildly affected by Marfan's syndrome. Both Abraham Lincoln and a distant male cousin, who was diagnosed as having Marfan's syndrome, are descendants of Mordecai Lincoln II. Although Mordecai almost certainly had the gene for Marfan's syndrome, he showed no signs of the disorder, probably because in him the gene had low expressivity.[6]

Primary enzyme defects are usually autosomal recessive. These enzyme defects may result in any of the following: (1) deficiency of a metabolic end-product, (2) production of harmful intermediates or toxic by-products of metabolism, or (3) accumulation of destructive substances within the cell. In *albinism,* the basic biochemical defect is the absence or nonfunctioning of the enzyme tyrosinase. This enzyme is necessary for the production of melanin, the pigment that gives skin its color.

Phenylketonuria (PKU) is another genetically inherited primary enzyme defect. In this disorder, there is a deficiency of phenylalanine hydroxylase, the enzyme needed for conversion of phenylalanine to tyrosine, and as a result of this deficiency, toxic levels of phenylalanine accumulate in the blood. Like other inborn errors of metabolism, PKU is inherited as a recessive trait and is manifested only in the homozygote. It is possible to identify carriers of the trait by subjecting them to a phenylalanine test in which a large dose of phenylalanine is administered orally and the rate at which it disappears from the bloodstream is measured. PKU occurs once in approximately 10,000 births, and damage to the developing brain almost always results when high concentrations of phenylalanine and other metabolites persist in the blood. Newborn infants are now routinely screened for abnormal levels of serum phenylalanine. Infants with the disorder are treated with a special diet that restricts phenylalanine intake. Dietary treatment must be started early in neonatal life because the untreated affected child may have evidence of arrested brain development by 4 months of age.[7]

Tay-Sachs disease is caused by an accumulation of ganglioside GM_2 (a glycolipid) in body tissues due to an enzyme deficiency (hexosaminidase A), resulting in gangliosidosis. It is inherited as an autosomal recessive disorder. The disease is particularly prevalent among eastern European (Ashkenazi) Jews. Infants with Tay-Sachs appear normal at birth but begin to manifest neurologic signs at about 6 months of age. These neurologic manifestations eventually lead to muscle flaccidity, dementia, and finally death at about 2 to 3 years of age. Although there is no cure for the disease, analysis of the blood serum for a deficiency of hexosaminidase A allows for accurate identification of the genetic carriers for the disease.

Membrane-associated transport defects can be either dominant or recessive. Hereditary *spherocytosis,* an autosomal dominant trait, is a form of hemolytic anemia that is caused by a defect in sodium transport in the red cell. *Renal glycosuria,* on the other hand, is an autosomal recessive trait that involves glucose transport in the renal tubules.

Polygenic disorders

Polygenic disorders are conditions in which two or more genes or gene loci are influential in the expression of a gene trait. In some diseases, such as diabetes mellitus and essential hypertension, the genetic component is influenced by multiple environmental influences.

The exact number of genes contributing to polygenic traits is not known, and these traits do not follow a clear-cut pattern of inheritance as do single-gene disorders. Polygenic inheritance has been described as a threshold phenomenon in which the factors contributing to the trait might be compared to water filling a glass.[8] Using this analogy, one might say that expression of the disorder occurs when the glass overflows. Conditions that are thought to arise through polygenic inheritance include the following:

allergies, anencephaly, cleft lip or palate, clubfoot, congenital dislocation of the hip, congenital heart disease, diabetes mellitus, hydrocephalus, myelomeningocele, pyloric stenosis, and urinary tract malformation.

Although polygenic traits cannot be predicted with the same degree of accuracy as the mendelian single-gene mutations, characteristic patterns exist. First, polygenic congenital malformations involve a single organ or tissue that is derived from the same embryonic developmental field. Second, the risk of recurrence in future pregnancies is for the same or a similar defect. This means that parents of a child with polygenic cleft palate defect have an increased risk of having another child with a cleft palate, but not with spina bifida. Third, the increased risk (compared with the general population) among first-degree relatives of the affected person is 2% to 5%, and among second-degree relatives it is about one-half that amount.[8] Furthermore, the risk increases with increasing incidence of the defect among relatives. This means that the risk is greatly increased when a second child with the defect is born to a couple. The risk also increases with severity of the disorder and when the defect occurs in the sex not generally affected by the disorder.

Chromosome disorders

Chromosome disorders involve a change in chromosome number or structure that results in damage to sensitive genetic mechanisms or in reproductive disorders.[9] During cell division in nongerm cells (mitosis), the chromosomes replicate, so that each cell receives a full diploid number. During the process of germ-cell (sperm and ovum) formation, a special form of cell division called *meiosis* takes place. During this division, the double sets of 22 autosomes and the 2 sex chromosomes (normal diploid number) become reduced to single sets (haploid number) in each gamete. At the time of conception, the haploid number in the ovum and that in the sperm join and restore the diploid number of chromosomes. Chromosome defects usually develop because of defective movement during meiosis or breakage of a chromosome with loss or translocation of genetic material.

Alterations in chromosome duplication

Mosaicism. *Mosaicism* is the presence in one individual of two or more cell lines characterized by distinctive karyotypes. This defect results from an accident during chromosomal duplication. Sometimes mosaicism consists of an abnormal karyotype and a normal one, in which case the physical deformities caused by the abnormal cell line are usually less severe.

Alterations in chromosome number

A change in chromosome number is called *aneuploidy.* Among the causes of aneuploidy are failure of separation of the chromosomes during oogenesis or spermatogenesis. This can occur in either the autosomes or the sex chromosomes and is called *nondisjunction.* Nondisjunction gives rise to germ cells that have an even number of chromosomes (22 or 24). The products of conception that are formed from this even number of chromosomes will have an uneven number of chromosomes, either 45 or 47. *Monosomy* refers to the presence of only one member of a chromosome pair. The defects associated with monosomy of the autosomes are severe and usually cause abortion. Monosomy of the X chromosome (45, X/O), or Turner's syndrome, causes less severe defects. *Polysomy,* or the presence of more than two chromosomes to a set, occurs when a germ cell containing more than 23 chromosomes is involved in conception. This defect has been described for both the autosomes and the sex chromosomes. Trisomies of chromosomes 8, 13, 18, and 21 are the more common forms of polysomy of the autosomes. There are several forms of polysomy of the sex chromosomes in which one or more extra X or Y chromosomes are present.

Trisomy 21 (Down's syndrome). Trisomy 21, or Down's syndrome, is the most common form of chromosome disorder. It has an incidence of 1 in 800 births.[10] The condition is usually accompanied by moderately severe mental retardation.

The risk of having a baby with Down's syndrome is greater in women who are 35 years of age or older at the time of delivery (Table 4-1). The sharp

Table 4-1. The relationship between maternal age and the risk of Down's syndrome in a newborn child

Maternal age (years)	Approximate risk of occurrence
20–24	1 in 1350
25–29	1 in 1175
30–35	1 in 750
36–40	1 in 250
41–45	1 in 65
46–50	1 in 25(?)

(Wisniewski LP, Hirschhorn K: A Guide to Human Chromosome Defects, 2nd ed. White Plains, March of Dimes Birth Defects Foundation, BD: OAS XVI(6), 1980)

rise in incidence of Down's syndrome children born to older women may occur for several reasons. Although males continue to produce sperm throughout their reproductive life, females are born with all the oocytes they will ever have. These oocytes may change as a result of the aging process. Also with increasing age there is a greater chance of a woman having been exposed to damaging environmental agents such as drugs, chemicals, and radiation. However, recent evidence suggests that in 20% to 30% of trisomy 21 the extra chromosome is of paternal origin.[10]

The physical features of a child with Down's syndrome are distinctive, and therefore the condition is usually apparent at birth. These features include a small and rather square head. There is upward slanting of the eyes, small and malformed ears, an open mouth, and a large and protruding tongue. The child's hands are usually short and stubby with fingers that curl inward, and there is usually only a single palmar (simian) crease. There are often accompanying congenital heart defects. Of particular concern is the much greater risk that these children have for the development of acute leukemia—20 times greater than other children.[11]

Monosomy X (Turner's syndrome). Turner's syndrome describes a monosomy of the X chromosome (45,X/O) with gonadal agenesis, or absence of the ovaries. This disorder is present in about 1 out of every 2500 live births. There are variations in the syndrome, with abnormalities ranging from essentially none to webbing of the neck with redundant skin folds, nonpitting edema of the hands and feet, and congenital heart defects (particularly coarctation of the aorta). Characteristically, the female with Turner's syndrome is short in stature, but her body proportions are normal. She does not menstruate and shows no signs of secondary sex characteristics. Administration of the female sex hormones (estrogens) may cause the secondary sexual characteristics to develop and may produce additional skeletal growth. The infertility associated with Turner's syndrome cannot be reversed. When a mosaic cell line (45,X/O and 46,X/X or 45,X/O and 46,X/Y) is present, the manifestations associated with the chromosomal defect tend to be less severe.

Polysomy X (Klinefelter's syndrome). Klinefelter's syndrome is characterized by an X-chromatin–positive (47,X/X/Y) male and is associated with testicular dysgenesis. In rare cases, there may be more than one extra X chromosome: for example, 47,X/X/X/Y. The incidence of Klinefelter's syndrome is about 1 in 600. The condition may not be detected in the newborn. The infant usually has normal male genitalia, with a small penis and small, firm testicles. Hypogonadism during puberty usually leads to a tall stature

with abnormal body proportions in which the lower part of the body is longer than the upper part. Later in life, the body build may become heavy with a female distribution of subcutaneous fat and variable degrees of breast enlargement. There may be deficient secondary male sex characteristics, such as a voice that remains feminine in pitch and sparse beard and pubic hair. There may be sexual dysfunction, along with complete infertility and impotence. Personality problems may occur, but the intellect is usually normal. Replacement hormone therapy with testosterone is used to treat the disorder.

Alterations in chromosome structure

Aberrations in chromosome structure occur when there is a break in one or more of the chromosomes followed by rearrangement or deletion of the chromosome parts. Among the factors believed to cause chromosome breakage are the following: (1) exposure to radiation sources, such as x-rays; (2) influence of certain chemicals; (3) extreme changes in the cellular environment; and (4) viral infections.

A number of patterns of chromosome breakage and rearrangement can occur (Figure 4-3). There can be a *deletion* of the broken portion of the chromosome. When one chromosome is involved, the broken parts may be *inverted. Isochromosome formation* occurs when the centromere, or central portion, of the chromosome separates horizontally instead of vertically. *Ring formation* results when deletion is followed by uniting of the chromatids to form a ring. *Translocation* occurs when there are simultaneous breaks in two chromosomes from different pairs with exchange of chromosome parts. With a balanced reciprocal translocation, no genetic information is lost; therefore, persons with translocations are generally normal. These persons are, however, translocation carriers and may have both normal and abnormal children. A special form of translocation called a *centric fusion* or *Robertsonian translocation* involves two acrocentric chromosomes in which the centromere is near the end. Typically the break occurs near the centromere affecting the short arm in one chromosome and the long arm in the other. Transfer of chromosomes leads to one long and one extremely short chromosome (see Figure 4-3). Often the short fragments are lost. In this case, the person has only 45 chromosomes, but the amount of genetic material that is lost is so small that it often goes unnoticed. Difficulty, however, arises during meiosis; the result is gametes with an unbalanced number of chromosomes. A rare form of Down's syndrome can occur in the offspring of persons in whom there has been a translocation of the centric fusion type.

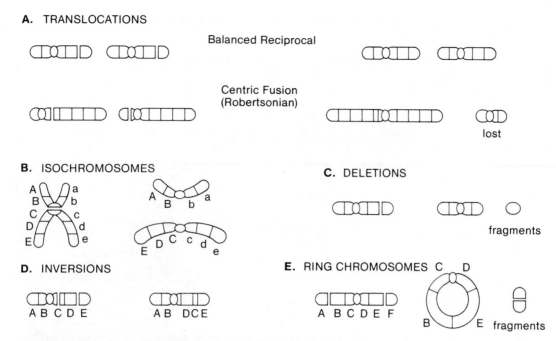

Figure 4-3 Rearrangement following breaks in chromosome structures. (*From Robbins SL, Kumar V: Basic Pathology, 4th ed, p 120. Philadelphia, WB Saunders, 1987*)

The manifestations of aberrations in chromosome structure will depend to a great extent on the amount of genetic material that is lost. Many cells suffering unrestituted breaks will be eliminated within the next few mitoses because of deficiencies that may in themselves be fatal. This is beneficial because it prevents the damaged cells from becoming a permanent part of the organism or, if it occurs in the gametes, from giving rise to grossly defective zygotes. Some altered chromosomes, such as those that occur with translocations, will be passed on to the next generation.

In summary, genetic and congenital disorders affect all age groups and all body structures. Genetic disorders can affect a single gene (mendelian inheritance) or several genes (polygenic inheritance). Chromosome disorders result from a change in chromosome number or structure. A change in chromosome number is called aneuploidy. Monosomy involves the presence of only one member of a chromosome pair; it is seen in Turner's syndrome, in which there is monosomy of the X chromosome. Polysomy refers to the presence of more than two chromosomes in a set. Klinefelter's syndrome involves polysomy of the X chromosome. Trisomy 21 (Down's syndrome) is the most common form of chromosome disorder. Alterations in chromosome structure involve either deletion or addition of genetic material, which may involve a translocation of genetic material from one chromosome pair to another.

Disorders due to environmental influences

The developing embryo is subject to many nongenetic influences. Following conception, development is influenced by the environmental factors that the embryo shares with the mother. The physiologic status of the mother—her hormone balance, her general state of health, her nutritional status, and the drugs she takes—undoubtedly influences the development of the unborn child. For example, diabetes mellitus is associated with increased risk of congenital anomalies. Smoking is associated with lower than normal neonatal weight. Alcohol, in the context of chronic alcoholism, is known to cause fetal abnormalities. Some agents cause early abortion. Measles and other infectious agents cause congenital malformations. Other agents, such as radiation, can cause chromosomal and genetic defects as well as developmental disorders.

Period of vulnerability

The embryo's development is most easily disturbed during the period when differentiation and development of the organs is taking place. This time interval is often referred to as the period of *organogenesis;* it extends from day 15 to day 60 after conception. Environmental influences during the first 2 weeks following fertilization may interfere with implantation

Highly Sensitive Periods of Development In Terms of Teratogenic Effects

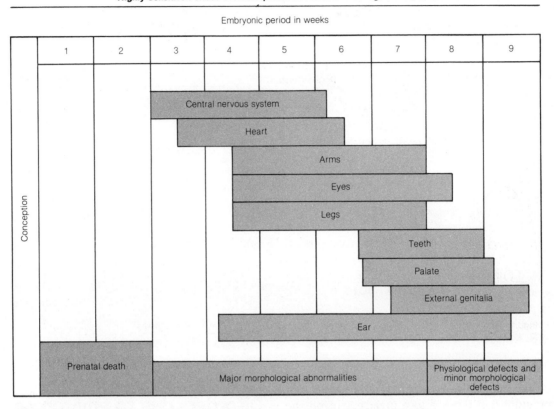

Embryonic period in weeks

Figure 4-4 Susceptible periods during embryologic development during which teratogenic agents are most likely to impair development of the various body structures. (*Developed from information included in Moore KL: The Developing Human, 2nd ed. Philadelphia, WB Saunders, 1977*)

and result in abortion or very early resorption of the products of conception. Each organ has a critical period during which it is highly susceptible to environmental derangements (Figure 4-4). Often the effect is expressed at the biochemical level just before the organ begins to develop. The same agent may affect different organ systems that are developing at the same time.

Teratogenic agents

A teratogenic agent is one that produces abnormalities during embryonic or fetal development. For discussion purposes, teratogenic agents have been divided into three groups: (1) irradiation, (2) drugs and chemical substances, and (3) infectious agents. Chart 4-2 lists commonly identified agents in each of these groups.

Irradiation

Heavy doses of ionizing radiation have been shown to cause microcephaly, skeletal malformations, and mental retardation. At present there is no evidence that diagnostic levels of radiation cause congenital abnormalities. Because the question of safety remains, however, many agencies require that the day of

Chart 4-2: Teratogenic agents

Irradiation

Drugs and chemical substances
Alcohol
Anticoagulants
    Warfarin
Anticonvulsants
    Paramethadione
    Phenytoin
    Trimethadione
Cancer drugs
    Aminopterin
    Methotrexate
    6-mercaptopurine
Progestins and oral contraceptive drugs
Propylthiouracil
Tetracycline
Thalidomide

Infectious agents
Viruses
    Cytomegalovirus
    Herpes simplex virus
    Measles (rubella)
    Mumps
    Chickenpox
Nonviral factors
    Syphilis
    Toxoplasmosis

a woman's last menstrual period be noted on all radiologic requisitions. Other institutions may require a pregnancy test before any extensive diagnostic x-ray studies are performed. Radiation is not only teratogenic but also mutagenic, and there is the possibility of effecting inheritable changes in genetic materials. Administration of therapeutic doses of radioactive iodine (^{131}I) during the 13th week of gestation, the time when the fetal thyroid is beginning to concentrate iodine, has been shown to interfere with thyroid development.

Chemicals and drugs

Some of the best-documented chemical teratogens are the organic mercurials, which cause neurologic deficits and blindness. Sources of exposure to mercury include contaminated food (fish) and water.

A number of drugs are suspected of being teratogens, but only a few have been identified with certainty. Perhaps the best known of these drugs is thalidomide, which has been shown to give rise to a full range of malformations, including phocomelia (short flipper-like appendages) of all four extremities. Other drugs known to cause fetal abnormalities are the antimetabolites used in the treatment of cancer, the anticoagulant drug warfarin, several of the anticonvulsant drugs, ethyl alcohol, and cocaine. Some drugs affect a single developing structure; for example, propylthiouracil can impair thyroid development and tetracycline can interfere with the mineralization phase of tooth development. The progestins, which are included in many birth control pills, can cause virilization of a female fetus depending on their dosage and timing.

Fetal alcohol syndrome. Only recently have the teratogenic effects of alcohol been described in the literature. Alcohol has widely variable effects on fetal development, ranging from minor abnormalities to a unique constellation of anomalies that has been termed the *fetal alcohol syndrome*.[12] One out of 750 infants born in the United States manifests some characteristics of the syndrome.[13]

The fetal alcohol syndrome is associated with several severe problems: (1) central nervous system dysfunction ranging from hypotonia and poor muscle coordination to moderate mental retardation, (2) craniofacial anomalies that can include microcephaly and a cluster of facial and eye defects, (3) deficient growth, and (4) other problems such as cardiovascular defects. Each of these defects can vary in severity, which probably reflects the amount of alcohol consumed as well as hereditary and environmental influences.

Evidence suggests that the consumption of 89 ml of alcohol per day—equivalent to six hard drinks —constitutes a major risk to the fetus.[12] Although clinical studies have focused on the consequences of chronic maternal alcoholism, there is inadequate information about the possible adverse effects of lower alcohol intake, including social drinking. In studies using pregnant monkeys, alcohol administration produced transient but marked collapse of the umbilical cord, causing severe hypoxia and acidosis in the fetus.[13] If this phenomenon occurs in humans, it could explain the teratogenicity of alcohol. Even in late gestation, the unborn child could be at risk for alcohol-induced hypoxia.

Because many drugs are suspected of causing fetal abnormalities, and even those that were once thought to be safe are now being viewed critically, it seems unwise for women in their childbearing years to use drugs unnecessarily. This pertains to nonpregnant women as well as pregnant ones because many developmental defects occur very early in pregnancy. As happened with thalidomide, the damage to the embryo often occurs before pregnancy is suspected or confirmed.

Cocaine babies. Of recent concern is the increasing use of cocaine by pregnant women. Among the effects of cocaine use during pregnancy is a decrease in uteroplacental blood flow, maternal hypertension, stimulation of uterine contractions, and fetal vasoconstriction. The decrease in uteroplacental blood flow is associated with an increase in preterm births, lower birth weight, and delivery of small for gestational age infants.[13a,b] Maternal hypertension may increase the risk of abruptio placentae, particularly if it is accompanied by a decrease in uteroplacental blood flow.[13a] Fetal vasoconstriction has been suggested as the cause of fetal anomalies, particularly limb reduction defects and urogenital tract defects such as hydronephrosis, hypospadias and undescended testicles, and ambiguous genitalia.[13b,c] Sudden infant death syndrome (SIDS) has also been more common in babies of mothers who have used cocaine during their pregnancy.[13d] Other reported effects of maternal cocaine use on the infant are small head size, altered neonatal behavior patterns, and impaired neonatal brainstem auditory system development.[13e] One study reported that 39% of 28 cocaine-exposed babies exhibited cerebral infarctions as documented on cranial ultrasound at birth.[13f] Although the immediate effects of maternal cocaine use on infant behavior are now being reported, the long-term effects are largely unknown.

Unfortunately cocaine addiction often impacts on the behavior of the pregnant woman to the extent that the need to procure larger amounts of the drug overwhelms all other considerations of maternal and fetal well-being; hence, other factors such as malnutrition, use of other drugs and teratogens, and lack of prenatal care may also contribute to fetal disorders.

—— **Infectious agents**

Many microorganisms cross the placenta and enter the fetal circulation, often producing multiple malformations. The acronym TORCH stands for *toxoplasmosis, other, rubella, cytomegalovirus,* and *herpes,* which are the agents most frequently implicated in fetal anomalies.[14] "Other" stands for type B hepatitis virus, coxsackie virus B, mumps, poliovirus, rubeola, varicella, listeria, gonorrhea, streptococcus, and treponema. Of these, hepatitis B poses the greatest threat to mother and infant. The TORCH screening test examines the infant's serum for the presence of antibodies to these agents. These infections tend to cause similar clinical manifestations, including microcephaly, hydrocephaly, defects of the eye, and hearing problems. Cytomegalovirus may cause mental retardation and rubella virus may cause congenital heart defects.

Toxoplasmosis is a protozoal infection that can be contracted by eating raw or poorly cooked meat. The domestic cat also seems to carry the organism, excreting the protozoa in its stools. It has been suggested that pregnant women should avoid contact with the excrement from the family cat. *Rubella* (German measles) is a commonly recognized viral teratogen. About 15% to 20% of babies born to women who have had rubella during the first trimester have abnormalities.[15] The epidemiology of the *cytomegalovirus* is largely unknown. Some babies are severely affected at birth and others, though having evidence of the infection, have no symptoms. In some symptom-free babies, brain damage becomes evident over a span of several years. There is also evidence that some babies contract the infection during the first year of life and in some of them the infection leads to retardation a year or two later. *Herpes simplex* 2 is considered to be a genital infection and is usually transmitted through sexual contact. The infant acquires this infection either *in utero* or in passage through the birth canal.

In summary, a teratogenic agent is one that produces abnormalities during embryonic or fetal life. It is during the early part of pregnancy (15 to 60 days after conception) that environmental agents are most apt to produce their deleterious effects on the developing embryo. A number of environmental agents can be damaging to the unborn child, including radiation, drugs and chemicals, and infectious agents. The fetal alcohol syndrome is a recently recognized risk for infants of women who regularly consume alcohol during pregnancy. Because many drugs have the potential for causing fetal abnormalities, often at a very early stage of pregnancy, it is recommended that women of childbearing age avoid unnecessary use of drugs.

Diagnosis and counseling

The birth of a defective child is a traumatic event in any parent's life. Usually two issues must be resolved. The first deals with the immediate and future care of the affected child and the second with the possibility of future children in the family having a similar defect. Genetic assessment and counseling can help to determine whether the defect was inherited as well as the risk of recurrence. Prenatal diagnosis provides a means of determining whether the unborn child has certain types of abnormalities.

—— **Genetic assessment**

Effective genetic counseling involves accurate diagnosis and communication of the findings and of the risks of recurrence, to the parents and other family members who need such information. Counseling may be provided following the birth of an affected child, or it may be offered to persons at risk for having defective children (siblings of persons with birth defects). A team of trained counselors can help the family to understand the problem and can support their decisions about having more children.

Assessment of genetic risk and prognosis is usually directed by a clinical geneticist, often with the aid of laboratory and clinical specialists. A detailed family history (pedigree), a pregnancy history, and detailed accounts of both the birth process and postnatal health and development are included. A careful physical examination of the affected child and often of the parents and siblings is usually needed. Laboratory work, including chromosomal analysis and biochemical studies, often precedes a definitive diagnosis.

The creases and dermal ridges on the palms and soles are examined in a genetic study called *dermatoglyphic analysis*. This is of value because the dermal ridges are formed by 16 weeks of gestation and any abnormalities will document the time during which the developmental defect occurred. Dermatoglyphic analysis includes examination of the patterns of the arches on the fingertips, the flexion creases of the fifth finger, and the arch pattern of the base of the great toe. One of the most readily identified creases is the palmar (simian) crease (Figure 4-5). For additional information on dermatoglyphic analysis, the reader is referred to other sources, including those listed in the reference section at the end of this chapter.

—— **Prenatal diagnosis**

Prenatal diagnosis is aimed at detecting fetal abnormalities. Among the methods used for fetal diagnosis are ultrasonography, amniocentesis, chori-

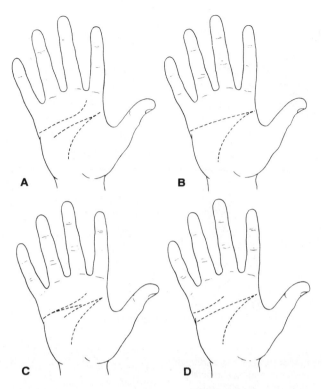

Figure 4-5 The transverse palmar crease. Hands **A** and **C** are normal. Hand **B** shows the typical transverse or simian crease. It is found in about 4% of the normal population and in about 50% of persons with Down's syndrome and certain other chromosomal defects. The sydney line **D** can be regarded as a variant of B and has the same significance. (*Valentine GH: The Chromosome Disorders, 3rd ed. Philadelphia, JB Lippincott, 1975*)

onic villus sampling, and laboratory methods to determine the biochemical and genetic makeup of the fetus. Alpha-fetoprotein screening is also used. Prenatal diagnosis is indicated in about 8% of pregnancies. Termination of pregnancy is only indicated in a small number of cases; in the rest, the fetus is normal and the procedure provides reassurance for the parents. Prenatal diagnosis can also provide the information needed for prescribing prenatal treatment for the fetus. For example, if congenital adrenal hyperplasia is diagnosed, the mother can be treated with adrenal cortical hormones to prevent masculinization of a female fetus.

Ultrasound

Ultrasound is a noninvasive diagnostic method that uses reflections of high-frequency sound waves to visualize soft tissue structures. Since its introduction in 1958, it has been used during pregnancy to determine fetal size, fetal position, and placental location. Improved resolution and real-time units have enhanced the ability of ultrasound scanners to detect congenital anomalies. With this more sophisticated equipment, it is now possible to obtain information such as measurements of hourly urine output in a high-risk fetus.[16] Ultrasound makes possible the *in utero* diagnosis of hydrocephalus, spina bifida, facial defects, congenital heart defects, congenital diaphragmatic hernias, disorders of the gastrointestinal tract, and skeletal anomalies. Intrauterine diagnosis of congenital abnormalities permits planning of surgical correction shortly after birth, preterm delivery for early correction, selection of cesarean section to reduce fetal injury, and in some cases *in utero* therapy. At present, 40% of obstetric practices in the United States have all of their patients undergo ultrasound scanning at least once during pregnancy.[16] When a congenital abnormality is suspected, a diagnosis made using ultrasound can generally be obtained by weeks 16 to 18 of gestation.

Amniocentesis

Amniocentesis involves the withdrawal of a sample of amniotic fluid from the pregnant uterus by means of a needle inserted through the abdominal wall (Figure 4-6). The procedure is useful in women over age 35, who have an increased risk of giving birth to a baby with Down's syndrome, in parents who have another child with chromosomal abnormalities, and in situations in which either parent is known to be a carrier of an inherited disease. Ultrasound is used to gain additional information and to guide the placement of the amniocentesis needle. Both the amniotic fluid and cells that have been shed by the fetus are studied. Usually a determination of fetal status can be made by the 16th to 17th week of pregnancy. For chromosomal analysis, the fetal cells are grown in culture and the result is available in 2 to 3 weeks. To test for inborn errors of metabolism such as Tay-Sachs disease, the amniotic fluid cells are grown in culture for 4 to 6 weeks in order to provide sufficient cells to assay for the appropriate enzyme. The amniotic fluid can also be tested using various biochemical tests.

Chorionic villus sampling

Sampling of the chorionic villi from the fetus is performed at 8 to 12 weeks of gestation. The biopsy is taken through the cervix using a catheter and gentle suctioning under ultrasound guidance. Sometimes an abdominal approach is needed if the transcervical approach is inadequate or if a sample is required after the 12th week of gestation. The tissue that is obtained can be used for fetal chromosome studies, DNA analysis, and biochemical studies. The fetal tissue does not have to be cultured, and fetal chromosome analysis can be made available in 24 hours. DNA analysis and biochemical tests can be completed in 1 to 2 weeks because the tissue does not have to be cultured.

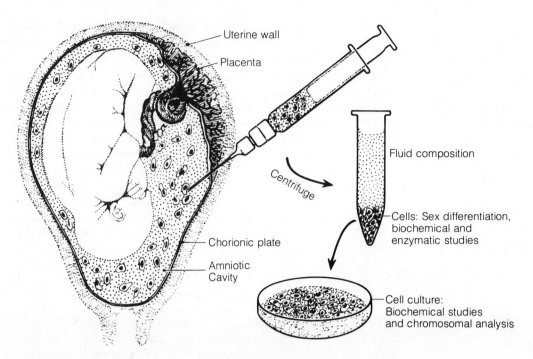

Figure 4-6 Amniocentesis. A needle is inserted into the uterus through the abdominal wall and a sample of amniotic fluid is withdrawn for chromosomal and biochemical studies. (*Department of Health, Education and Welfare: What Are the Facts About Genetic Disease? Washington, DC, 1977*)

Cytogenetic and biochemical analyses

Amniocentesis and chorionic villus sampling yield cells that can be used for cytogenetic and DNA analyses. Cytogenetic studies are used for fetal karyotyping to determine the chromosome makeup of the fetus. It is done to detect abnormalities of chromosome number and structure. Karyotyping also reveals the sex of the fetus. This may be useful when an inherited defect is known to affect only one sex.

DNA analysis is done on cells extracted from the amniotic fluid or obtained by chorionic villus sampling. It is done to detect genetic defects such as inborn errors of metabolism. The defect may be established through direct demonstration of the molecular defect or through methods that break the DNA into fragments so that the fragments may be studied to determine the presence of an abnormal gene. Direct demonstration of the molecular defect is done by growing the amniotic fluid cells in culture and measuring the enzymes that the cultured cells produce. Many of the enzymes are expressed in the chorionic villi; this permits earlier prenatal diagnosis because the cells do not need to be subjected to prior culture. DNA studies are used to detect genetic defects that cause inborn errors of metabolism such as Tay-Sachs disease, glycogen storage diseases, and familial hypercholesterolemia. Prenatal diagnoses are now possible for more than 70 inborn errors of metabolism.

Alpha-fetoprotein (AFP) is a major fetal plasma protein and has a structure similar to the albumin that is found in postnatal life. AFP is made initially by the yolk sac and later by the liver. It peaks at about 12 to 14 weeks in the fetus and falls thereafter.[17] AFP is found in the amniotic fluid at about one-hundredth the concentration found in fetal serum. AFP reaches the maternal bloodstream and can be measured by laboratory methods. The normal maternal serum AFP rises from 13 weeks and peaks at 32 weeks gestation. In pregnancies where the fetus has a neural tube defect (anencephaly and open spina bifida) or certain other malformations such as an anterior abdominal wall defect, maternal and amniotic levels of AFP are elevated. Screening of maternal blood samples is usually done between weeks 16 to 20 of gestation. If the AFP is elevated, a second serum sample is taken and ultrasound studies are advised to check for a missed abortion or multiple pregnancy, both of which produce elevated AFP levels. When a second maternal blood sample is found to contain elevated levels of AFP, more extensive ultrasound and amniocentesis are advised.

In summary, genetic and prenatal diagnosis and counseling are done in an effort to determine the risk of having a child with a genetic or chromosomal disorder. They often involve a detailed family history (pedigree), examination of any affected and other family members, and laboratory studies including chromosomal analysis and biochemical studies. They are usually done by a genetic counselor and a specially prepared team of health care professionals. Both ultrasound and amniocentesis can be used to screen for congenital defects. Ultrasound is used for determination of fetal size and position and for the presence of structural anomalies. Amniocentesis and chorionic villus sampling are used to obtain specimens for cytogenetic and biochemical studies. They are currently used in the prenatal diagnosis of over 60 genetic disorders.

References

1. Goldman AS (Key Consultant): Congenital Defects. Washington, DC, US Department of Health, Education and Welfare, Public Health Service, 1983
2. Facts/1984. White Plains, NY, March of Dimes, 1984
3. National Institutes of Health: What Are the Facts About Genetic Disease? Washington, DC, US Department of Health, Education and Welfare, Public Health Service, 1977
4. Erbe RW: Principles of medical genetics. N Engl J Med 294(6):381, 294(5):480, 1976
5. McKusick VA: Mendelian Inheritance in Man: Catalogs of Autosomal Dominant, Autosomal Recessive, and X-linked Phenotypes. Baltimore, Johns Hopkins University Press, 1983
6. Singer S: Human Genetics, p 13. San Francisco, WH Freeman and Co., 1978
7. Vaughn VC, McKay RJ, Nelson WE: Nelson Textbook of Pediatrics, 10th ed, p 132. Philadelphia, WB Saunders, 1975
8. Riccardi VM: The Genetic Approach to Human Disease, pp 92, 500. New York, Oxford University Press, 1977
9. A Guide to Chromosome Defects, 2nd ed, The National Foundation—March of Dimes Birth Defects 16, No. 6:5, 1980
10. De LaCruz D, Muller JZ: Facts about Down syndrome. Child Today 13, No.6:3, 1983
11. Hassold TJ, Jacobs PA: Trisomy in man. Ann Rev Genet 18:69, 1984
12. National Institute of Alcohol Abuse and Alcoholism: Critical Review of the Fetal Alcohol Syndrome. Rockville, MD, Alcohol, Drug Abuse, and Mental Health Administration, 1977
13. Mukherjee AB, Hodgen GD: Maternal alcohol exposure induces transient impairment of umbilical circulation and fetal hypoxia in monkeys. Science 218:700, 1982
13a. MacGregor SN, Keith LG, Chasnoff IJ, Rosner MA, Chisnum GM, Shaw P, Minogue JP: Cocaine use during pregnancy: Adverse outcome. Am J Obstet Gynecol 157(3):686, 1987
13b. Chasnoff IJ, Griffith DR: Cocaine: Clinical studies of pregnancy and the newborn. Annals New York Acad Sci 562:260, 1989
13c. Chasnoff IJ, Chisum GM, Kaplan WE: Maternal cocaine use and genitourinary malformations. Teratology 37:201, 1988
13d. Riley JB, Brodsky NL, Porat R: Risk of SIDS in infants with *in utero* cocaine exposure: A prospective study (Abstract). Pediatr Res 23, 454A, 1988
13e. Shih B, Cone-Wesson B, Reddix B, Wu PYK: Effects of maternal cocaine abuse on the neonatal auditory system (Abstract). Pediatr Res 23:264A, 1988
13f. Dixon SD, Bejar R: Brain lesions in cocaine- and methamphetamine-exposed neonates (Abstract). Pediatr Res 23:405A, 1988
14. DeVore NE, Jackson VM, Piening SL: TORCH infections. Am J Nurs 83:1660, 1983
15. Dudgeon JA: Infectious causes of human malformations. Br Med J 32:77, 1976
16. Hill LM, Breckle R, Gehrking RT: The prenatal detection of congenital malformations by ultrasonography. Mayo Clin Proc 58:805, 1983
17. Connor JM, Ferguson-Smith MA: Essential Medical Genetics, 2nd ed, p 191. London, Blackwell Scientific Publications, 1987

Bibliography

Annas GJ: Routine prenatal genetic screening. N Engl J Med 317, No. 22:1407, 1987

Casey CT: Genetic therapy: Somatic gene transplants. Hosp Pract 22, No. 8:181, 1987

Chervenak FA, Isaacson G, Mahoney MJ: Advances in the diagnosis of fetal defects. N Engl J Med 315, No. 5:305, 1986

Cline MJ: Gene therapy: Current status. Am J Med 83:291, 1987

Dabney BJ: The role of human genetic monitoring in the workplace. J Occup Med 23:626, 1981

Denniston C: Low level radiation and genetic risk estimation in man. Ann Rev Genet 16:329–355, 1982

Fabricant JD, Legator MS: Etiology, role and detection of chromosomal aberrations in man. J Occup Med 23, No.9:617, 1981

Fraser FC: Genetic counseling: Using the information wisely. Hosp Pract 23, No. 6:245, 1988

Gelehrter TD: The family history and genetic counseling: Tools for preventing and managing genetic disorders. Genetic Diseases 73, No. 6:119, 1983

German J: Embryonic stress hypothesis of teratogenesis. Am J Med 76:293, 1984

Golden NL et al: Maternal alcohol use and infant development. Pediatrics 70, No. 6:931, 1982

Hill LM: Effects of drugs and chemicals on the fetus and newborn. Mayo Clin Proc 59:707–716, 1984

Hill LM: Effects of drugs and chemicals on the fetus and newborn. (Part 2). Mayo Clin Proc 59:755–765, 1984

Hill LM et al: The prenatal detection of congenital malformations by ultrasonography. Mayo Clin Proc 58:805–826, 1983

Janerich DT, Polednak AP: Epidemiology of birth defects. Epidemiol Rev 5:16–37, 1983

Kalter H, Warkany J: Congenital malformations: Etiological factors and their role in prevention. N Eng J Med 308, No. 8:424–430, 1983

Kalter H, Warkany J: Congenital malformations: Etiological

factors and their role in prevention. (Part 2). N Eng J Med 308, No. 9:491–497, 1983

Marx JL: Cytomegalovirus: A major cause of birth defects. Science 190:1184, 1975

McKusick VA: The morbid anatomy of the human genome. (Parts 1, 2, 3, 4) Medicine 65: 1, 1966; 66:1, 237, 1987; 67:1, 1987

McKusick VA: The new genetics and clinical medicine: A summing up. Hosp Pract 23, No. 6:177, 1988

Mukherjee AB, Hodgen GD: Maternal ethanol exposure induces transient impairment of umbilical circulation and fetal hypoxia in monkeys. Science 218, No. 4573:700–702, 1982

Nitowsky HM: Fetal alcohol syndrome and alcohol-related birth defects. N Y State J Med 82, No. 7:1214–1217, 1982

Perejda AJ, Abraham PA, Carnes WH: Marfan's syndrome: Structural, biochemical, and mechanical studies of the aortic media. J Lab Clin Med 106:376, 1985

Prockop DJ, Kivirikko KI: Heritable diseases of collagen. N Eng J Med 311, No. 6:376–385, 1984

Shiono H, Kadowaki J: Dermatoglyphics of congenital abnormalities without chromosomal aberrations: A review of clinical applications. Clin Pediatr 14:1003, 1975

Tomasi TB: Structure and function of alpha-fetoprotein. Annu Rev Med 28:453, 1977

Valle D: Genetic disease: An overview of current therapy. Hosp Pract 22, No. 7:167, 1987

Wilson JG: Teratogenic effects of environmental chemicals. Fed Proc 36, No. 5:1698, 1977

CHAPTER 5

Alterations in Cell Differentiation: Neoplasia

Concepts of cell growth and differentiation
    The cell cycle
    Cell replication
    Cell differentiation
Neoplasia
    Characteristics of neoplasms
      Benign neoplasms
      Malignant neoplasms
    Cancer cell characteristics
      Anaplasia
      Cell surface and membrane changes
      Metabolic changes

Carcinogenesis
    Heredity
    Oncogenes and oncogenic viruses
    Carcinogens
    Immunologic defects
Tumor growth and spread
General effects
Diagnostic methods
    Staging and grading of tumors

Cancer treatment
    Surgery
    Radiation therapy
    Pharmacologic therapy

Objectives

After you have studied this chapter, you should be able to meet the following objectives:

_____ List the most common sites of cancer in men and women.

_____ Describe the five phases of the cell cycle.

_____ Cite the method used for naming benign and malignant neoplasms.

_____ Define the term *neoplasm* and explain how neoplastic growth differs from the normal adaptive changes seen in atrophy, hypertrophy, and hyperplasia.

_____ State at least six ways in which benign and malignant neoplasms differ.

_____ State the difference between solid and hematologic cancers.

_____ Relate the properties of cell differentiation to the development of a cancer cell line and the behavior of the tumor.

_____ Relate environmental factors to the development of cancer.

_____ State the purpose of the clinical staging of cancer.

_____ Use the concepts of growth fraction and doubling time to explain the growth of cancerous tissue.

_____ Explain the pathogenesis of metastasis.

_____ Describe the surveillance capacity of the immune system.

_____ Describe the general effects of cancer on body systems.

_____ Compare the methods used in obtaining a Pap smear and a tissue biopsy sample.

_____ Explain the rationale for use of radiation in the treatment of cancer.

_____ Cite the difference between external beam radiation therapy and radiation therapy using an internal radiation source.

_____ Describe the adverse effects of radiation therapy.

_____ Compare the action of cell-cycle-specific and cell-cycle-independent chemotherapeutic drugs.

Cancer is the second leading cause of death in the United States. The disease affects all age groups, causing more deaths in children 3 to 14 years of age than any other disease. The American Cancer Society has estimated that over 75 million Americans, or one out of every four alive today, will develop cancer during their lifetimes. In 1988, about 985,000 persons were diagnosed as having cancer.[1] It has been estimated that with present methods of treatment, 49% of persons who develop cancer each year will be alive 5 years later.

The term *neoplasm* comes from a Greek word meaning *new formation*. In contrast to the tissue growth that occurs with hypertrophy and hyperplasia, a neoplasm serves no useful purpose but tends to increase in size and persist at the expense of the rest of the body. Furthermore, neoplasms do not obey the laws of normal tissue growth. For example, they do not occur in response to an appropriate stimulus, and they continue to grow after the stimulus has ceased or the needs of the organism have been met.

Cancer is not a single disease; rather, the term describes almost all forms of malignant neoplasia. As shown in Figure 5-1, cancer can originate in almost any organ, with the lung being the most common site in men and the breast in women. Cancers vary greatly in curability. Cancers such as acute lymphocytic leukemia, Hodgkin's disease, testicular and ovarian cancers, and osteogenic sarcoma, which only a few decades ago had a poor prognosis, are today cured in many cases. This change is mainly due to advances in chemotherapy. On the other hand, lung cancer, which is the leading cause of death in the United States, is very resistant to therapy, and although some progress has been made in its treatment, mortality rates remain high. This chapter provides a general overview of cancer (malignant neoplasia) along with a brief discussion of benign neoplasia. Specific forms of cancer are discussed elsewhere in the book.

Concepts of cell growth and differentiation

Neoplasia is a disorder of cell growth and replication. Cell division and replication are inherent adaptive mechanisms for body cells, and in a single day many of these cells are replaced by new cells. Normally the new cells are identical in structure and function to the cells they replace. When abnormal or mutant cells do develop, usually either they are defective and incapable of survival or they are destroyed by the body's immune system.

The cell cycle

The life of a cell is called the *cell cycle*. It consists of the interval between the midpoint of mitosis in a cell and the subsequent midpoint of mitosis in one or both daughter cells. *Mitosis* is the period of time when cell division is actually taking place. The cell cycle is divided into five distinct phases, for which *gap* or *G* terminology is used (Figure 5-2). G_1 is the

CANCER INCIDENCE AND DEATHS BY SITE AND SEX — 1985 ESTIMATES

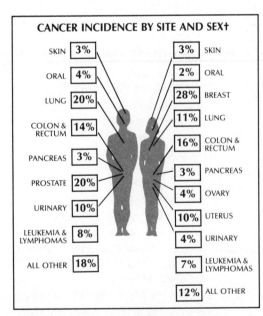

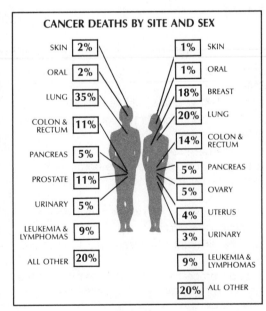

†Excluding non-melanoma skin cancer and carcinoma in situ.

Figure 5-1 Cancer Incidence and deaths (1988 estimates) by site and sex. (*Cancer Facts. New York, American Cancer Society: 1988*)

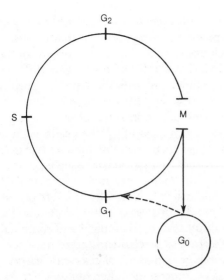

Figure 5-2 Phases of the cell cycle. The cycle represents the interval from the midpoint of mitosis to the subsequent end point in mitosis in a daughter cell. G_1 is the postmitotic phase during which RNA and protein synthesis is increased and cell growth occurs. G_0 is the resting or dormant phase of the cell cycle. The S phase represents synthesis of nucleic acids with chromosome replication in preparation for cell mitosis. During G_2, RNA and protein synthesis occurs as in G_1.

first gap, the postmitotic phase during which DNA synthesis ceases while RNA and protein synthesis and cell growth take place. Toward the end of G_1, some critical event occurs that commits the cell to continue through the phases of the gap cycle and enter mitosis.

G_0 is the resting or dormant phase in which the cell performs all activities except those related to proliferation. Cells can leave G_1 and enter G_0. The time spent in G_0 varies according to the cell type, and not all cells spend time in G_0. It is believed that some special growth signal is needed to move cells that have been dormant in G_0 back into the cell cycle.

During the S phase, or synthesis phase, DNA replication occurs, giving rise to two separate sets of chromosomes. G_2 is the premitotic phase. During this phase, as in G_1, DNA synthesis ceases while synthesis of RNA and protein continues.

The M phase represents mitosis. Mitosis is subdivided into four stages: prophase, metaphase, anaphase, and telophase (Figure 5-3). During *prophase,* the centrioles in the cytoplasm separate and move toward opposite sides of the cell, the chromosomes become shorter and thicker, and the nuclear membrane breaks up so that there is no longer a barrier between the chromosomes and the cytoplasm. *Metaphase* involves the organization of the chromosome pairs in the midline of the cell and the formation of a mitotic spindle composed of the microtubules. *Anaphase* is the period during which splitting of the chromosome pairs occurs, with the microtubules pulling each set of 46 chromosomes toward the opposite cell pole in preparation for cell separation. Cell division is completed during *telophase,* when the mitotic spindles vanish and a new nuclear membrane develops and encloses each of the sets of chromosomes.

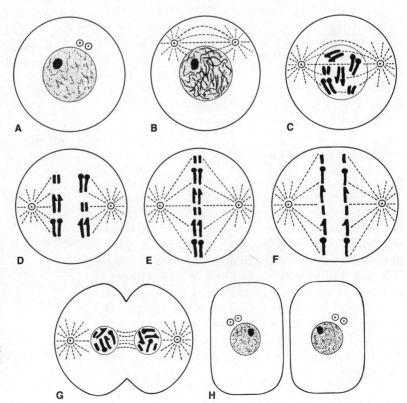

Figure 5-3 Cell mitosis. **A** and **H** represent the nondividing cell; **B, C,** and **D** represent prophase; **E** represents metaphase; **F** represents anaphase; and **G** represents telophase. (*Chaffee EE, Greisheimer EM: Basic Physiology and Anatomy, 3rd ed. Philadelphia, JB Lippincott, 1974*)

Cell replication

The term *proliferation* refers to the process by which cells multiply and bear offspring. In normal tissue, cell proliferation is regulated so that the number of cells actively dividing is equivalent to the number dying or being shed. In terms of cell proliferation, the 100 or more cell types of the body can be divided into three large groups: (1) the well-differentiated neurons and cells of skeletal and cardiac muscle that are unable to divide and reproduce; (2) the parent, or progenitor cells, that continue to divide and reproduce, such as blood cells, skin cells, and liver cells; (3) the undifferentiated stem cells that can be triggered to enter the cell cycle and produce large numbers of progenitor cells when the need arises. The rates of reproduction of these cells vary greatly. White blood cells and cells that line the gastrointestinal tract live several days and must be replaced constantly. In most tissues, the rate of cell reproduction is greatly increased when tissue is injured or lost. Bleeding, for example, stimulates the rapid reproduction of the blood-forming cells of the bone marrow. In highly specialized tissue the genetic program for cell replication is normally repressed, but it can be resumed under certain conditions. The liver, as an example, has extensive regenerative capabilities under certain conditions.

For very rapidly reproducing cells, the entire cell cycle occupies about 16 hours. For others, such as liver cells, the cycle takes about 10,000 hours.[2] The duration of the G_2 period (8 hours), S period (2 hours), and mitosis (0.07 hours) are almost identical for all cell types. It is the duration of G_1 and G_0 that determines the duration of the cell cycle.[2] When only a low rate of cell reproduction is needed to maintain health of tissues, the cells remain dormant in the G_0 phase of G_1; when a more rapid rate of reproduction is needed, the G_0 dormant period is shortened.

Cell differentiation

Cell differentiation is the process whereby cells are transformed into different and more specialized cell types as they proliferate. Cell differentiation determines what a cell will look like, how it will function, and how long it will live. For example, a red blood cell is programmed to develop into a concave disk that functions as a vehicle for oxygen transport and lives 120 days. Cancer cells have two important properties that underlie the nature of the disease: (1) they grow and divide with less restraint than normal cells and (2) they do not differentiate normally. Therefore, they do not function properly and do not die on time.

All of the different cell types of the body originate from a single cell—the fertilized ovum. As the embryonic cells increase in number, they engage in an orderly process of differentiation that is necessary for the development of all the various organs of the body. What makes the cells of one organ different from those of another organ is the type of genes that are expressed. Although all cells have the same complement of genes, only a small number of these genes are expressed in postnatal life. When cells, such as those of the developing embryo, differentiate and give rise to committed cells of a particular tissue type, the appropriate genes are maintained in an active state while the rest become inactive. Normally, the rate of cell reproduction and the process of cell differentiation are precisely controlled in both prenatal and postnatal life so that both of these mechanisms cease once the appropriate numbers and kinds of cells are formed.

The process of differentiation occurs in orderly steps; with each progressive step, increased specialization is exchanged for a loss of ability to develop different cell characteristics and different cell lines. The more highly specialized a cell becomes, the more likely it is to lose its ability to undergo mitosis. Neurons, which are the most highly specialized cells in the body, lose their ability to divide and reproduce once development of the nervous system is complete. More importantly, there are no reserve or parent cells to direct their replacement. In other, less specialized tissues, such as the skin and mucosal lining, cell renewal continues throughout life.

But even in the continuously renewing cell populations, there are highly specialized cells that are similarly unable to divide. An alternative mechanism provides for their replacement. In this case, there are progenitor cells of the same lineage that have not yet differentiated to the extent that they have lost their ability to divide. These cells are sufficiently differentiated that their daughter cells are limited to the same cell line, but they are insufficiently differentiated to preclude the potential for active proliferation. As a result these parent, or progenitor, cells are able to provide large numbers of end cells. The progenitor cells, however, have limited capacity for self-renewal and they become limited to producing a single type of end cell.

A third type of cell, called a *stem cell*, remains incompletely differentiated throughout life. Stem cells are reserve cells that remain quiescent until there is a need for end-cell replenishment, and then they divide to replenish or increase the progenitor cell population (Figure 5-4).

In summary, the term *neoplasm* refers to a new growth. In contrast to normal cellular adaptive processes such as hypertrophy and hyperplasia, neoplasms do not obey the laws of normal cell growth. They serve no useful purpose, they do not occur in

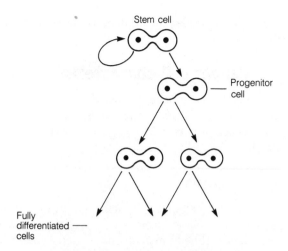

Figure 5-4 Mechanism of cell replacement.

response to an appropriate stimulus, and they continue to grow at the expense of the host. The life of a cell is called the cell cycle. It is divided into five phases: (1) G_1 represents the postmitotic phase, during which RNA and protein synthesis occurs; (2) G_0 is the resting or dormant phase of the cell cycle; (3) the S phase is the synthesis phase, during which DNA replication occurs; (4) G_2 is the premitotic phase and is similar to G_1 in terms of RNA and protein synthesis; (5) the M phase is the phase during which cell mitosis occurs. Cell proliferation is normally regulated so that the number of cells that are actively dividing is equal to the number dying or being shed. Differentiation is the process whereby these stem cells are transformed into a more specialized cell type. Differentiation determines the structure, function, and life span of a cell. As a cell line becomes more differentiated, it becomes more highly specialized in its function and less able to divide.

Neoplasia

Characteristics of neoplasms

Neoplasms are composed of two types of tissue: parenchymal tissue and supporting tissue. The functioning cells of a tumor are representative of parenchymal tissue. The supporting tissue consists of the connective tissue, blood vessels, and lymph structures. Most neoplasms involve the parenchymal tissue of an organ.

By definition, a tumor is a swelling that can be caused by a number of conditions, including inflammation and trauma. Although they are not synonymous, the terms *tumor* and *neoplasm* are often used interchangeably. The Latin word *malus* means bad; hence a *malignant* tumor is a bad tumor. It will usually cause suffering and death unless treated and controlled. A benign tumor is a *good tumor.* A benign tumor does not usually cause death unless by its location it interferes with vital functions.

Tumors are usually identified by the addition of the suffix *-oma* to the name of the parenchymal tissue type from which the growth originated. Thus, a benign tumor of glandular epithelial tissue is called an *adenoma,* and a benign tumor of bone tissue, an *osteoma.* The term *carcinoma* is used to designate a malignant tumor of epithelial tissue origin. In the case of a malignant adenoma, the term *adenocarcinoma* is used. Malignant tumors of mesenchymal origin are called *sarcomas:* for example, osteosarcoma. *Oncology* is the study of tumors and their treatment. Table 5-1 lists the names of selected benign and malignant tumors according to tissue types.

Benign and malignant neoplasms are generally differentiated by their (1) cell characteristics, (2) manner of growth, (3) rate of growth, (4) potential for metastasizing and spreading to other parts of the body, (5) ability to produce generalized effects, (6) tendency to cause tissue destruction, and (7) capacity to cause death. The characteristics of benign and malignant neoplasms are summarized in Table 5-2.

Benign neoplasms

Benign tumors are characterized by well-differentiated cells, a slow progressive rate of growth that may come to a standstill or regress, an expansive manner of growth, the presence of a well-defined fibrous capsule, and failure to metastasize to distant sites. Benign tumors are composed of well-differentiated cells that resemble their normal counterparts. For example, the cells of a uterine leiomyoma resemble uterine smooth muscle cells. For some unknown reason, benign tumors seem to have lost the ability to suppress the genetic program for cell replication, but retain the program for normal cell differentiation. Benign tumors grow by expansion and are enclosed in a fibrous capsule. This is in sharp contrast to malignant neoplasms, which grow by infiltrating the surrounding tissue (Figure 5-5). The presence of the capsule is responsible for a sharp line of demarcation between the benign tumor and the adjacent tissues, a factor that facilitates surgical removal. The formation of the capsule is thought to represent the reaction of the surrounding tissues to the tumor.

Benign tumors do not undergo degenerative changes as readily as malignant tumors, and they do not usually cause death unless by their location they interfere with vital functions. For instance, a benign tumor growing in the cranial cavity can eventually cause death by compressing brain structures. Benign tumors can also cause disturbances in the function of adjacent or distant structures by producing pressure on tissues, blood vessels, or nerves. Some benign tumors are also known for their ability to cause alterations in body function due to abnormal elaboration of hormones.

Malignant neoplasms

In contrast to benign tumors, malignant neoplasms tend to grow rapidly, spread widely, and kill regardless of their original location. The destructive nature of malignant tumors is related to the changes in their rate of growth, lack of cell differentiation, and ability to spread and metastasize. Their malignant potential usually depends on their degree of undifferentiation. Because of their rapid rate and manner of growth, malignant tumors compress blood vessels and outgrow their blood supply causing ischemia and tissue necrosis, rob normal tissues of amino acids and essential nutrients, and liberate enzymes and toxins that destroy both tumor tissue and normal tissue. The generalized effects of malignant tumor growth are discussed later in this chapter.

There are two categories of cancer—solid tumors and hematologic cancers. Solid tumors initially are confined to a specific tissue or organ. As the growth of a solid tumor progresses, cells are shed from the original tumor mass and travel through the blood and lymph streams to produce metastasis in distant sites. Hematologic cancers involve the blood and lymph systems and are disseminated diseases from the beginning.

Cancer cell characteristics

Cancer cells have distinct characteristics that differentiate them from normal cells. These include anaplasia, cell surface and membrane changes, antigenic changes, and metabolic changes.

Anaplasia

Cancer cells, as distinguished from normal cells, fail to undergo normal cell proliferation and differentiation. The term *anaplasia* is used to describe the lack of cell differentiation in cancerous tissue. Undifferentiated cancer cells are altered in appearance and nuclear size and shape from the cells in the tissue where the cancer originated. For example, when examined under the microscope, cancerous tissue that originated in the liver does not have the appearance of normal liver tissue. The degree of anaplasia that a tumor displays varies. Some cancers display only slight anaplasia and others display marked anaplasia. As a general rule, the more undifferentiated the tumor, the more frequent the mitoses and the more rapid the rate of growth. The degree of anaplasia can be determined by a pathologist during tissue studies and is used in the grading of tumors.

Table 5–1. Names of selected benign and malignant tumors according to tissue types

Tissue type	Benign	Malignant
Epithelial tumors		
Surface	Papilloma	Squamous cell carcinoma
Glandular	Adenoma	Adenocarcinoma
Connective tissue tumors		
Fibrous	Fibroma	Fibrosarcoma
Adipose	Lipoma	Liposarcoma
Cartilage	Chondroma	Chondrosarcoma
Bone	Osteoma	Osteosarcoma
Blood vessels	Hemangioma	Hemangiosarcoma
Lymph vessels	Lymphangioma	Lymphangiosarcoma
Muscle tumors		
Smooth	Leiomyoma	Leiomyosarcoma
Striated	Rhabdomyoma	Rhabdomyosarcoma
Nerve cell tumors		
Nerve cell	Neuroma	
Glial tissue		Glioma
Nerve sheaths	Neurilemoma	Neurilemic sarcoma
Hematologic tumors		
Granulocytic		Myelocytic leukemia
Erythrocytic		Erythroleukemia
Plasma cells		Multiple myeloma
Lymphoid		Lymphocytic leukemia

Because cancer cells lack differentiation, they do not function properly and do not die on time. In some types of leukemia, for example, the lymphocytes do not follow the normal developmental process: they do not differentiate fully, they do not acquire the ability to destroy bacteria, and they do not die on schedule. Instead, these long-lived defective cells tend to crowd out normal blood cells, leaving the body less able to defend itself during infection.

In tissues capable of regeneration, replacement cells usually derive from undifferentiated stem cells. When a stem cell divides, one daughter cell retains the stem cell characteristics, and the other becomes a progenitor daughter cell. The progeny of each progenitor cell continues along the same genetic program, with the differentiating cells undergoing multiple mitotic divisions in the process of becoming a mature cell type and with each generation of cells becoming more specialized. In this way a single stem cell can give rise to the many cells needed for normal tissue repair or blood cell responses. When the dividing cells become fully differentiated, they are no longer capable of mitosis. In the immune system, for example, appropriately stimulated B cells become progressively more differentiated as they undergo successive mitotic divisions until they become mature plasma cells that can no longer divide but are capable of producing large amounts of antibody. It is thought that cancer cells develop from mutations that occur during the differentiation process (Figure 5-6). When the mutation occurs early in the process, the resulting tumor is poorly differentiated and highly malignant; when it occurs later in the process, more fully differentiated and less malignant tumors result.

Poorly differentiated cancer cells often display changes in their karyotype, or organization of cell chromosomes. Mitosis, in normal cells, yields two identical cells, each with a normal arrangement of

Table 5-2. Characteristics of benign and malignant neoplasms

Characteristics	Benign	Malignant
Cell characteristics	Well differentiated cells that resemble normal cells of the tissue from which the tumor originated	Cells often bear little resemblance to the normal cells of the tissue from which they arose; there is both anaplasia and pleomorphism
Mode of growth	Tumor grows by expansion and does not infiltrate the surrounding tissues; usually encapsulated	Grows at the periphery and sends out processes that infiltrate and destroy the surrounding tissues
Rate of growth	Rate of growth is usually slow	Rate of growth is variable and is dependent on level of differentiation; the more anaplastic the tumor, the more rapid the rate of growth
Metastasis	Does not spread by metastasis	Gains access to the blood and lymph channels and metastasizes to other areas of the body
General effects	Is usually a localized phenomenon that does not cause generalized effects unless by its location it interferes with vital functions	Often causes generalized effects such as anemia, weakness, and weight loss
Destruction of tissue	Does not usually cause tissue damage unless its location interferes with blood flow	Often causes extensive tissue damage as the tumor outgrows its blood supply or encroaches on blood flow to the area; may also produce substances that cause cell damage
Ability to cause death	Does not usually cause death unless by its location it interferes with vital functions	Will usually cause death unless growth can be controlled

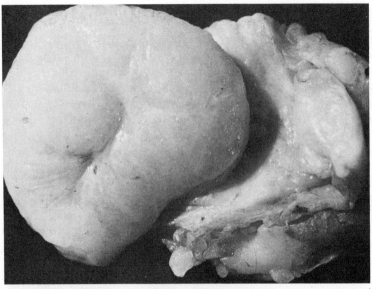

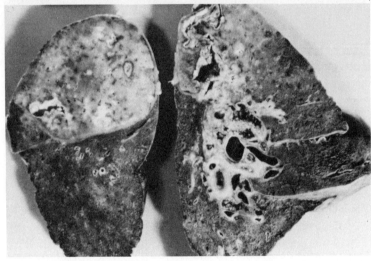

Figure 5-5 Photograph of a benign encapsulated fibroadenoma of the breast at the top and a bronchogenic carcinoma of the lung at the bottom. Note that the fibroadenoma has sharply defined edges, whereas the bronchogenic carcinoma is diffuse and infiltrates the surrounding tissues.

chromosomes. Normal diploid cells have a double set of chromosomes, and when they divide they form two identical cells. *Polyploidy* is cell division that results in a cell receiving more than two complete sets of chromosomes. *Aneuploidy* refers to abnormal cell division

in which daughter cells receive an uneven number of chromosomes; one cell may receive 47 chromosomes and another 45. Cancerous tumors often undergo abnormal mitosis and display polyploidy or aneuploidy. These cells often have multiple mitotic spindles that

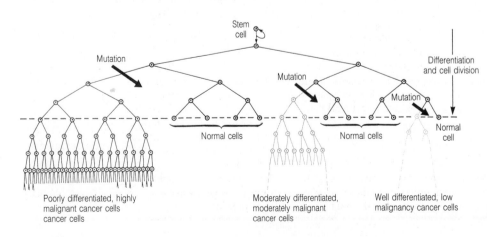

Figure 5-6 Mutation of a cancer cell line. (*Prescott DM, Flexer AS: Cancer, the misguided cell. Sunderland, Massachusetts, Sinauer Associates, 1986*)

result in uneven division of nuclear or cytoplasmic contents. The term *pleomorphism* refers to variations in size and shape of cells and cell nuclei.

Cell surface and membrane changes

In addition to changes in cell growth and differentiation, cancer cells display alterations in cell surface and membrane characteristics. These changes include alterations in contact inhibition; loss of cohesiveness and adhesion; impaired cell-to-cell communication; and elaboration of degradative enzymes that participate in invasion and metastatic spread. Contact inhibition is the cessation of growth once a cell comes in contact with another cell. Contact inhibition usually switches off cell growth by blocking the synthesis of DNA, RNA, and protein. In wound healing, contact inhibition causes fibrous tissue growth to cease at the point where the edges of the wound come together. Cancer cells, on the other hand, tend to grow rampant without regard for other tissue. Loss of cohesiveness and adhesiveness permits shedding of the tumor's surface cells; these cells appear in the surrounding body fluids or secretions and can be detected using the Papanicolaou (Pap) test. Although many of the membrane changes reported for cancer cells have only been observed with individual cancer cells in the laboratory, there is reason to believe that these same properties exist in cancer cells in the body; and these changes account for the invasive and destructive nature of cancer cell growth. Impaired cell-to-cell communication may interfere with formation of intercellular connections and responsiveness to membrane-derived signals. The production of degradative enzymes, such as fibrinolysins, contributes to the breakdown of the intercellular matrix and promotes cancer's invasive and metastatic properties.

Antigenic changes. Cell surface antigens are coded by the genes of a cell. Many transformed cancer cells produce antigens that are immunologically distinct from normal cell antigens. Possibly it is these antigens that are recognized as foreign by the body's immune system, contributing to the body's defense against the survival of abnormal cell types and the development of cancer.

There are fetal antigens, or neoantigens, expressed during intrauterine and early postnatal life that are completely repressed in the mature organism. Serum alpha-fetoprotein is one such antigen; it is a useful marker in persons with primary liver cell cancer or germ cell tumors of the ovary or testes. Carcinoembryonic antigen, another embryonic antigen not normally found in the adult, is present in approximately 75% of persons with colorectal cancer.[3] The reappearance of fetal antigens in certain types of cancers reflects the undifferentiated nature of these tumors

and is thought to result from expression or enhanced activation of genes coding for these antigens. The presence of these antigens, which can be detected through laboratory studies, is useful in diagnosis and follow-up treatment of these neoplasms.

Metabolic changes

Cancer cells often utilize markedly different biochemical and metabolic pathways than their normal cell counterparts. There are also changes in the membrane transport of sugars and amino acids by tumor cells. Cancer cells have been called *nitrogen traps* because they tend to rob normal cells of amino acids. There are a number of changes in biochemical behavior associated with cancer cells; many of the changes resemble those associated with rapid growth of fetal and immature cells. Most cancers elaborate enzymes (proteases and glycosidases) that break down proteins and contribute to the invasiveness of the tumor. Some tumors are transformed into cells that elaborate hormones. For example, some forms of bronchogenic carcinoma produce antidiuretic hormone (ADH) and adrenocorticotropic hormone (ACTH). As with neoantigens, the biochemical changes displayed by cancer cells are attributed to expression of genes that are normally repressed.

Carcinogenesis

The term *carcinogenesis* refers to the process by which a normal tissue type is transformed into cancerous tissue. There are many theories regarding the mechanisms and related risk factors of carcinogenesis; they include the role of heredity, oncogenes and oncogenic viruses, carcinogenic agents, and immunologic defects.

Heredity

Certain types of cancers seem to run in families. Breast cancer, for example, occurs more frequently in women whose grandmothers, mothers, aunts, and sisters also have had a cancerous disease. Cancer is found in approximately 10% of persons having one affected first-degree relative, in approximately 15% of persons having two affected family members, and in 30% of persons having three affected family members.[4]

The genetic predisposition for development of cancer has been documented for a number of cancerous and precancerous lesions that follow mendelian inheritance patterns (Table 5-3). Fortunately, most of these neoplasms are extremely rare—probably accounting for less than 5% of all cancers in the general population.[3]

Table 5–3. Some cancers and cancer-predisposing diseases with Mendelian inheritance patterns

Dominant (autosomal)	Recessive (autosomal)
Adenocarcinoma (primarily colon and endometrium)	Albinism
Familial polyposis of colon	Ataxia telangiectasia
Gardner's syndrome (predisposes to colonic cancer)	Bloom's syndrome
	Franconi's aplastic anemia
Melanocarcinoma	Xeroderma pigmentosum
Multiple endocrine adenomatosis (MEA)	
Neurofibromatosis (von Recklinghausen's disease)	
Retinoblastoma	

(Modified from Robbins SL, Cotran RS: Pathologic Basis of Disease, 2nd ed. Philadelphia, WB Saunders, 1979. Fagan-Dubin L: Causes of cancer. Cancer Nurs 2(6):436, 1979. Copyright © by Masson Publishing USA, Inc., New York.)

Among the inherited forms of cancer are retinoblastoma and multiple polyposis of the colon. In about 40% of cases, retinoblastoma (a form of eye cancer that occurs most frequently in small children) is inherited as an autosomal dominant trait; the remainder are nonhereditary. The penetrance of the genetic trait is high; in carriers of the dominant retinoblastoma gene, the penetrance for this gene is 95% for at least one tumor, and the affected person may be unilaterally or bilaterally affected.[5] Familial polyposis of the colon also follows an autosomal dominant inheritance pattern. Individuals who inherit the gene develop polypoid adenomas of the colon, and almost all are fated to develop cancer by age 50.[3]

Oncogenes and oncogenic viruses

Recently, it has been found that many cancer cells contain specific genes, the *oncogenes,* that are responsible for the many malignant traits of these cells.[6–9] To date some 30 or more oncogenes have been identified that can, when appropriately activated, produce cancer in animals and cause cancerous transformation of laboratory cultured cells.

The oncogene theory dates back to 1911 when Francis Peyton Rous discovered a virus that causes sarcomas in chickens. Over the years various oncogenic viruses have been identified that can produce cancerous transformations in laboratory cell cultures and animals. As the research with virus-induced cell transformation progressed, it was discovered that normal cells contain DNA sequences very similar to the viral genes that cause cancerous transformation of laboratory cells. These DNA sequences, called proto-oncogenes, appear to have essential roles in the nor-

mal growth and proliferation of cells. The involvement of these genes in the cancer process probably involves a somatic mutation that takes place in a specific target tissue, converting its proto-oncogenes into oncogenes. It has been suggested that cancer-predisposing genes may act in several ways—they may affect the rate at which carcinogens are metabolized to the active forms that damage cell genes; they may affect the ability to repair consequent DNA damage; they may alter immune surveillance function, affecting the body's ability to recognize and destroy tumor cells; or they may affect gene functions controlling normal cell growth and proliferation.[4] Significantly, it appears the acquisition of a single oncogene is not sufficient to convert cells into full-blown tumor cells. Instead, cancerous transformation appears to require the action of many independently activated genes. A recent discovery is that a very different class of genes, tumor-suppressing or anti-oncogenic genes, may be involved in some forms of cancerous transformation. These tumor-suppressing genes seem to be involved in controlling cellular growth. When this type of gene is inactivated, a block to proliferation is removed and the cells begin a program of unregulated growth.

An oncogenic virus is a virus that can induce cancer. Viruses, which are small particles containing genetic (DNA or RNA) material, enter a host cell and become incorporated into its chromosomal DNA or take control of the cell's machinery for the purpose of producing viral proteins. The extent to which viruses contribute to human cancers is unknown. A retrovirus contains RNA that is copied in reverse direction into the genome of the host cell. Retroviruses have been shown to induce leukemias, sarcomas, and lymphomas in a wide variety of fowl and animals. On occasion, genital warts (condyloma acuminatum) which are caused by the human papilloma DNA virus, can progress to squamous cell carcinoma. Herpes simplex virus type II, which is also a DNA virus, has been associated with uterine cervical cancer.

Carcinogens

A carcinogen is an agent capable of causing cancer. The role of environmental agents in causation of cancer was first noted in 1775 by Sir Percivall Pott, who related the high incidence of scrotal cancer in chimney sweeps to their exposure to coal soot. In 1915, Yamagiwa and Ichikawa conducted the first experiments in which a chemical agent was used to produce cancer. These investigators found that a cancerous growth developed when they painted a rabbit's ear with coal tar. Coal tar has since been found to contain potent polycyclic aromatic hydrocarbons. Since then, literally hundreds of carcinogenic agents have been identified. In fact, it has been estimated that 80% to 85% of human cancers are associated with exposure to environmental or chemical agents (Chart 5-1).[10]

Chemical carcinogens. Literally hundreds of chemical carcinogenic agents exist; some have been found to cause cancers in animals and others are known to cause cancers in humans. These agents include both natural (*e.g.*, aflatoxin B_1) and manmade products (*e.g.*, vinyl chloride). Usually, carcinogenic agents can be divided into two categories: (1) direct-acting agents and (2) procarcinogens, which are metabolized and converted into carcinogenic agents in the body. Direct-acting agents do not require activation in the body to become carcinogenic. Among these agents are the alkylating drugs used in the treatment of cancer (to be discussed). Procarcinogens, which include the polycyclic hydrocarbons and the azo dyes, are the most potent carcinogens known.[3] With the procarcinogens, cancer usually develops in the organ where the agent is metabolized or stored for elimination: for example, in the bladder in persons exposed to aniline dyes.

Chemical carcinogens form highly reactive ions (electrophiles) that bind with the nucleophilic residues on DNA, RNA, or cellular proteins. The action of these ions tends to cause cell mutation or alteration in synthesis of cell enzymes and structural proteins in a manner that alters cell replication and interferes with cell regulatory controls.

The effects of carcinogenic agents are usually dose dependent—the larger the dose or the longer the

---

Chart 5-1: Some chemical and environmental agents known to be carcinogenic in humans

Polycyclic hydrocarbons
 Soots, tars, and oils
 Cigarette smoke

Industrial agents
 Asbestos
 Vinyl chloride
 Arsenic compounds
 Aniline and azo dyes
 Nickel and chromium compounds
 Acrylonitrile
 a-Naphthylamine
 b-Naphthylamine
 Benzene
 Carbon tetrachloride

Food and drugs
 Smoked foods
 Nitrosamines (used in preservation of meats)
 Aflatoxin B_1 (mold that grows in nuts and grains)
 Phenacetin
 Diethylstilbestrol
 Estrogens

---

duration of exposure, the greater the risk that cancer will develop. There is usually a time delay ranging from 5 to 30 years from the time of exposure to the development of cancer. This is unfortunate, because many persons may have been exposed to the agent and its carcinogenic effects before the association is recognized. This occurred, for example, with the use of diethylstilbestrol, which was widely used in the United States from the mid-1940s to 1970 to prevent miscarriages. But it was not until the late 1960s that many cases of vaginal adenosis and adenocarcinoma in young women were found to be a result of their exposure *in utero* to diethylstilbestrol.[11]

Two occupational carcinogens of particular interest are *asbestos* and *vinyl chloride*.[12] Although the history of asbestos disease dates back to the early 1900s, it was not until the late 1960s that the full spectrum of the problem became evident. Exposure to asbestos is associated with cancer of the lung, cancer of the stomach, and a rare form of malignancy (mesothelioma) that affects the pleura and peritoneum. The population groups at increased risk of developing cancer due to asbestos exposure include not only those persons who work directly with the mineral, but also those who live in the vicinity of industrial installations where asbestos is used in one way or another and persons who live in the same household as the asbestos worker. The risk of cancer in these groups is increased even further if they also smoke cigarettes, which points to an additive effect. Until 1973 (when its use was banned), asbestos was frequently used as a fireproofing spray in many high-rise buildings. There is now concern that the air circulating through some buildings in which a dry type of asbestos fireproofing was applied may be contaminated with asbestos fibers. There is also concern about how exposure to asbestos can be controlled when these buildings need to be demolished.

Vinyl chloride, which is used in the rubber industry, is associated with hemangiosarcoma of the liver. As with many other carcinogenic agents, the relationship between vinyl chloride exposure and the development of cancer was not discovered until a large number of workers had been exposed to the chemical. In 1974, the U.S. Department of Labor established regulations for vinyl chloride exposure in industry.

Radiation. Among the well-documented causes of cancer is radiation, including ultraviolet rays from sunlight, x-rays, radioactive chemicals, and other forms of radiation. As with other carcinogens, the effects of radiation are usually additive, and there is usually a long delay between the time of exposure and the time that cancer can be detected. This is true of skin cancer, which is caused by overexposure to the sun and is many years in the making. Skin cancer is an occupational hazard of farmers and sailors, particularly those who work in the southwest United States. Equally hazardous is the practice of sun-bathing to achieve a suntan.

Another example of the ultimate consequences of radiation exposure is the therapeutic radiation of the head and neck—particularly in infants and small children—in which there may be a time lag as long as 35 years before thyroid cancer is detected.[13] Even more dramatic are the long-term effects of radiation on the survivors of the atomic blasts in Hiroshima and Nagasaki: between 1950 and 1970, the death rate from leukemia alone in the most heavily exposed population groups in Hiroshima was 147 per 100,000, or 30 times the expected rate.[14]

Immunologic defects

One characteristic of mutant and cancer cells is that they develop neoantigens that attach to the surface of the cell. *Immune surveillance* is a term often used to describe the mechanism by which an organism develops an immune response against the antigens expressed by a tumor.[15] The role of the immune system in the destruction of a cancer cell is depicted in Figure 5-7.

It has been suggested that the development of cancer might be associated with impairment or decline in the surveillance capacity of the immune system. For example, increases in cancer incidence have been observed in persons with immunodeficiency diseases and in persons with renal transplants who are

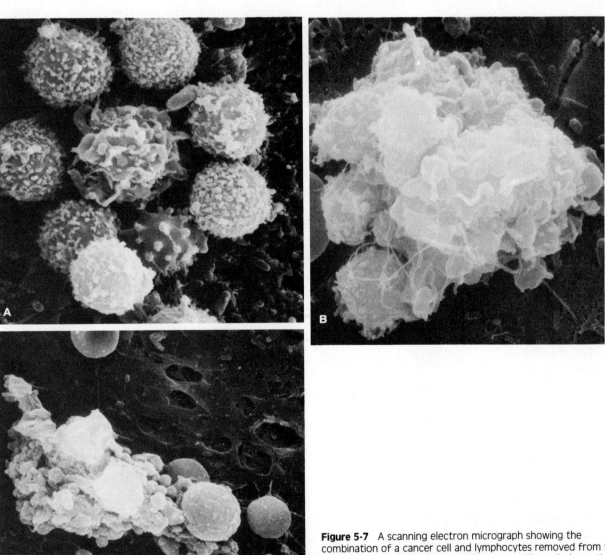

Figure 5-7 A scanning electron micrograph showing the combination of a cancer cell and lymphocytes removed from the same patient and studied in the laboratory. Photo **A** shows the lymphocytes surrounding the cancer cell (60 min). Photo **B** shows the lymphocytes attacking the cancer cell (150 min). In Photo **C,** the integrity of the cancer cell has been destroyed (240 min). *(Courtesy of Kenneth Siegesmund, Ph.D., and Burton A. Waisbren Sr., M.D. The Anatomy Department, The Medical College of Wisconsin.)*

receiving immunosuppressant drugs. The incidence of cancer is also increased in the elderly, in whom there is a known decrease in immune activity. The recent association of Kaposi's sarcoma with acquired immunodeficiency syndrome (AIDS) further emphasizes the role of the immune system in preventing malignant cell proliferation. Although seemingly simple, the role of immunity in the development of cancer is still largely uncertain. At present it cannot be said with any certainty that the immune system is able to protect against all forms of cancer. Many growing tumors appear to suppress the immune response. Furthermore, it is well recognized that some conventional types of cancer treatment—chemotherapy and radiation—tend to suppress the immune response. *Immunotherapy,* which will be discussed later in this chapter, is a cancer treatment modality designed to heighten the patient's general immune responses so as to increase tumor destruction.

—— Tumor growth and spread

The rate of tissue growth in both normal and cancerous tissue depends on three factors: (1) the number of cells that are actively dividing or moving through the cell cycle, (2) the cell-cycle time, and (3) the number of cells that are being lost. One of the reasons cancerous tumors often seem to grow so rapidly relates to the size of the cell pool that is actively engaged in cycling. It has been shown that the cell-cycle time of cancerous tissue cells is not necessarily

shorter than that of normal cells; rather, cancer cells do not die on schedule. In addition, the growth factors that allow cells to enter G_0 when they are not needed for cell replacement is lacking; therefore a greater percentage of cells are actively engaged in cycling than occurs in normal tissue.[16]

The ratio of dividing cells to resting cells in a tissue mass is called the *growth fraction.* The *doubling time* is the length of time it takes for the total mass of cells in a tumor to double. As the growth fraction increases, the doubling time decreases. When normal tissues reach their adult size, an equilibrium between cell birth and cell death is reached. Cancer cells, however, continue to divide and multiply until limitations in blood supply and nutrients retard their growth.

Experimentally it is possible to measure the cell-cycle time and the percentage of cells that are cycling during a given period of time and then to estimate the doubling time. From this information, it is possible to estimate the rate of cell increase per hour for the different types of tumors. Knowledge of cell-cycle time and the rate of cell increase is used in planning cancer therapy.

A tumor is generally undetectable until it has doubled 30 times and contains more than a billion (1 $\times 10^9$) cells. At this point it is about 1 cm in size (Figure 5-8). After 35 doublings the mass contains more than a trillion (1×10^{12}) cells, which is sufficient to kill the host.

Cancer in situ is a localized preinvasive lesion. Depending on its location, this type of lesion can

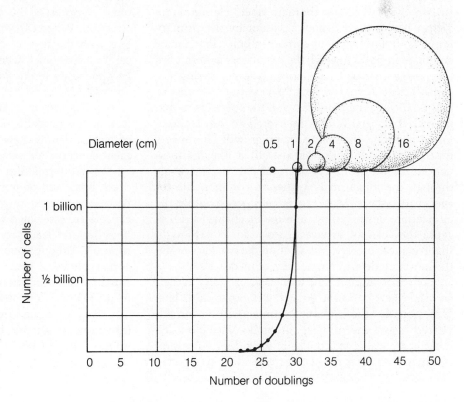

Figure 5-8 Growth curve of a hypothetical tumor on arithmetic coordinates. Note the number of doubling times before the tumor reaches an appreciable size. *(Adapted from Collins VP et al: Observations of growth rates of human tumors. Am J Roent Rad Ther Nuclear Med 76:988, 1956. Charles C Thomas, Publisher)*

usually be removed surgically or treated so that the chances of recurrence are small. For example, cancer in situ of the cervix is essentially 100% curable.

The spread of cancer can take many forms: direct extension, seeding of cancer cells within body cavities, or metastatic spread through the blood or lymph pathways. Cancers grow by infiltration, direct extension, or invasion of the surrounding tissues. The word *cancer* is derived from the Latin word meaning crablike, because cancerous growth spreads by sending crablike projections into the surrounding tissues. Unlike benign tumors, which are encapsulated, malignant tumors have no sharp line of demarcation separating them from the surrounding tissue, and this often makes complete surgical removal of the tumor difficult. *Seeding* of cancer cells into body cavities occurs when a tumor erodes into these spaces and tumor cells drop onto the serosal surface. For example, a tumor may penetrate the wall of the stomach and its cells implant on the surfaces of the peritoneal cavity.

Metastatic spread occurs when a malignant tumor invades the vascular or lymphatic channels and parts of the tumor break loose and travel to distant parts of the body, where implantation occurs. Lymphatic spread is more typical of carcinomas, whereas sarcomas usually spread through the vascular channels. When metastasis occurs by way of the lymphatic channels, the tumor cells lodge first in the regional lymph nodes that receive drainage from the tumor site. The regional lymph nodes may contain the tumor cells for a time, but eventually the cells break loose and gain access to more distant nodes and to the bloodstream by way of the thoracic duct. Hematologic spread begins with venous invasion by the primary tumor and formation of tumor emboli. The tumor emboli then travel through the circulatory system until they lodge in small capillaries. Before entering the general circulation, the venous blood from the gastrointestinal tract, the pancreas, and the spleen is routed through the portal vein to the liver. The liver is therefore a common site of metastatic growth for cancers that originate in these organs. In a like manner, venous blood from all parts of the body travels through the lungs, making these a common site for cancer metastasis. Most cancer cells perish within the circulation, destroyed by immune mechanisms or because they cannot survive in isolation. It is thought that receptors on cancer cells or on the capillary endothelium may determine the sites of metastasis.

Some tumors tend to metastasize early in their course, whereas others do not metatasize until late. Occasionally, the metastatic tumor will be far advanced before the primary tumor becomes clinically detectable. Malignant tumors of the kidney, for example, may go completely undetected and be asymptomatic even when a metastatic lesion is found in the lung. To a great extent, metastatic tumors retain many of the characteristics of the primary tumor from which they had their origin. Because of this, it is usually possible to determine the site of the primary tumor from the cellular characteristics of the metastatic tumor.

General effects

There is probably not a single body function left unaffected by the presence of cancer (Table 5-4). Because tumor cells replace normal functioning parenchymal tissue, the initial manifestations of cancer usually reflect the primary site of involvement. For example, cancer of the lung initially produces impairment of respiratory function; then as the tumor grows and metastasizes, other body structures become affected.

Cancer disrupts tissue integrity. As cancers grow, they compress and erode blood vessels, causing ulceration and necrosis along with frank bleeding and sometimes hemorrhage. One of the early warning signals of colorectal cancer is blood in the stool. Cancer cells may also produce enzymes and metabolic toxins that are destructive to the surrounding tissues. Usually, tissue damaged by cancerous growth does not heal normally. Instead, the damaged area persists and often continues to grow; hence a second warning signal of cancer—a sore that does not heal.

Cancer has no regard for normal anatomic boundaries—as it grows, it invades and compresses adjacent structures. Abdominal cancer, for example, often compresses the viscera and causes bowel obstruction. When cancer affects the brain, it may interfere with the flow of cerebral fluid as well as other cerebral functions. Cancer may obstruct lymph flow and penetrate serous cavities causing pleural effusion and ascites.

Cancer, in its late stages, often causes pain. In fact, pain is probably one of the most dreaded aspects of cancer. Pain management is one of the major treatment concerns for persons with incurable cancers.

Abnormalities in a person's energy, carbohydrate, lipid, and protein regulation are common manifestations during progressive tumor growth. Many cancers are associated with weight loss and wasting of body fat and lean protein, a condition called *cancer cachexia.* Although anorexia, reduced food intake, and abnormalities of taste are common in persons with cancer and are often accentuated by treatment methods, the extent of weight loss and protein wasting cannot be explained in terms of diminished food intake alone. It recently has been suggested that a hormone called cachectin, or tissue necrosis factor, is responsible for the tissue wasting.[17,18] Cachectin, which is produced by the macrophages in response to tumor growth or tissue destruction, has been credited with suppressing the enzymes needed for fat storage; hence, the loss of fat tissue. The hormone's capabilities range from eliciting fever and other inflammatory responses to mediating endotoxic shock secondary to trauma, burns, and sepsis. At this time the role of the tumor necrosis factor and its full impact on cancer cachexia is uncertain. It has been suggested by some that the hormone may be an endogenous antineoplastic agent.[18]

In addition to signs and symptoms at the sites of primary and metastatic disease, cancer can produce manifestations in sites that are not directly affected by the disease. Such manifestations are collectively referred to as *paraneoplastic syndromes.* Some of these manifestations are caused by the elaboration of hormones by cancer cells and others are due to the production of circulating factors that produce nonmetastatic hematopoietic, neurologic, and dermatologic syndromes. For example, cancers may produce procoagulation factors that contribute to an increased risk of venous thrombosis. It is estimated that about 7% of persons with cancer are affected by these syndromes.[19] The three most common endocrine syndromes associated with cancer are: (1) the syndrome of inappropriate antidiuretic hormone (ADH) secretion (Chapter 27), (2) Cushing's syndrome due to ectopic adrenocorticotropic hormone (ACTH) production (Chapter 44), (3) and hypercalcemia (Chapter 27). Hypercalcemia of malignancy does not appear to be

related to parathyroid hormone but to some other circulating factor or factors. The paraneoplastic syndromes may be the earliest indication that a person has cancer; and they may also signal early recurrence of the disease in previously treated persons. In some persons with cancer, a paraneoplastic syndrome such as hypercalcemia can be disabling and even life-threatening.

Diagnostic methods

The methods used in the diagnosis and staging of cancer are determined largely by the location and type of cancer suspected. There are a number of diagnostic procedures that are used in diagnosis of cancer, including x-ray studies; endoscopic examinations; urine and stool tests for blood; blood tests for tumor markers; bone marrow aspirations; ultrasound imaging; magnetic resonance imaging (MRI); and computed tomography (CT scan). Two diagnostic methods will be discussed in this chapter, the Pap smear and tissue biopsy.

The Pap smear is an example of the type of test called *exfoliative cytology.* It consists of microscopic examination of a properly prepared slide by a cytotechnologist or pathologist for the purpose of detecting the presence of abnormal cells. The usefulness of exfoliative cytology relies on the fact that the cancer cells lack the cohesive properties and intercellular junctions that are characteristic of normal tissue; without these characteristics, cancer cells tend to exfoliate and be-

Table 5–4. General effects on body function associated with cancer growth

Overall effect	Related tumor action
Altered function of the involved tissue	Destruction and replacement of parenchymal tissue by neoplastic growth
Bleeding and hemorrhage	Compression of blood vessels, with ischemia and necrosis of tissue; or tumor may outgrow its blood supply
Ulceration, necrosis, and infection of tumor area	Ischemia associated with rapid growth, with subsequent bacterial invasion
Obstruction of hollow viscera or communication pathways	Expansive growth of tumor with compression and invasion of tissues
Effusion in serous cavities	Impaired lymph flow from the serous cavity or erosion of tumor into the cavity
Increased risk of vascular thrombosis	Abnormal production of coagulation factors by the tumor, obstruction of venous channels, and immobility
Anemia	Bleeding and depression of red blood cell production
Bone destruction	Metastatic invasion of bony structures
Hypercalcemia	Destruction of bone due to metastasis and/or production by the tumor of parathyroid hormone or parathyroid-like hormone
Pain	Liberation of pain mediators by the tumor, compression, and/or ischemia of structures
Cachexia, weakness, wasting of tissues	Catabolic effect of the tumor on body metabolism along with selective trapping of nutrients by rapidly growing tumor cells
Inappropriate hormone production, *e.g.,* ADH or ACTH secretion by cancers such as bronchogenic carcinoma	Production by the tumor of hormones or hormone-like substances that are not regulated by normal feedback mechanisms

come mixed with secretions surrounding the tumor growth. The routine performance of a Pap smear (once every 3 years after two initial negative tests 1 year apart) in women over age 20 is recommended as a means of detecting in situ cervical cancer.[1] Exfoliative cytology can also be performed on other body secretions, including nipple drainage, pleural or peritoneal fluid, gastric washings, and others.

A *biopsy* is the removal of a tissue specimen for microscopic study. It can be obtained by needle aspiration (needle biopsy) or by endoscopic methods, such as bronchoscopy or cystoscopy, which involve the passage of a scope through an orifice and into the involved structure. In some instances a surgical incision is made. If the tumor is small, the entire tumor may be removed; or if the tumor is too large to be removed, a specimen may be excised for examination. Tissue diagnosis is of critical importance in designing the treatment plan should cancer cells be found.

Staging and grading of tumors

At present, there are two basic methods for classifying cancers: (1) grading according to the histologic or cellular characteristics of the tumor and (2) staging according to the spread of the disease. Both methods are used to prognosticate the course of the disease and to aid in selecting an appropriate treatment or management plan. Grading of tumors involves the microscopic examination of cancer cells to determine their level of differentiation and the number of mitoses. Cancers are classified as grade I, II, III, and IV with increasing anaplasia. Staging of cancers uses methods to determine the progress and spread of the disease. It may utilize surgery to determine tumor size and lymph node involvement.

The clinical staging of cancer is intended to provide a means by which information related to the progress of the disease, the methods and success of treatment modalities, and the prognosis can be communicated to others. The TNM system, which has evolved from the work of the International Union Against Cancer (IUAC) and the American Joint Committee on Cancer Staging and End Stage Reporting (AJCCS), is used by many cancer facilities. This system, which is briefly described in Chart 5-2, quantifies the disease into stages, using three tumor components: (1) *T* stands for the extent of the primary tumor, (2) *N* refers to the involvement of the regional lymph nodes, and (3) *M* describes the extent of the metastatic involvement. The time of staging is indicated as: cTNM, clinical-diagnostic staging; pTNM, postsurgical resection–pathologic staging; sTNM, surgical-evaluative staging; rTNM, retreatment staging; and aTNM, autopsy staging.[20] The TNM system further defines each specific type of cancer, such as breast cancer. The rationale for use of the system

---

Chart 5–2:   TNM classification system

T* subclasses

Tx—tumor cannot be adequately assessed

T0—no evidence of primary tumor

TIS—carcinoma *in situ*

T1, T2, T3, T4—progressive increase in tumor size and/or involvement

N†

Nx—regional lymph nodes cannot be assessed clinically

N0—no evidence of regional node metastasis

N1, N2, N3—increasing involvement of regional lymph nodes

M‡ subclasses

Mx—not assessed

M0—no distant metastasis

M1—distant metastasis present, specify site(s)

Histopathology

GX—grade cannot be assessed

G1—well differentiated grade

G2—moderately well differentiated grade

G3—poorly differentiated grade

G4—undifferentiated

* T = Primary tumor.
† N = Regional lymph nodes.
‡ M = Distant metastasis.
(Developed from: Beahrs OH, Myers MH (eds): Manual for Staging of Cancer, ed 3, p 7. Philadelphia, JB Lippincott, 1988)

---

encompasses the need to classify the disease at various time periods—initial diagnosis, presurgical treatment, postsurgical treatment, and so on.

Cancer treatment

The goals of current treatment methods fall into three categories: *curative, palliative,* and *adjunctive.* The most common modalities are surgery, radiation, chemotherapy, and endocrinotherapy. In recent years, immunotherapy has been added to the list of treatment modalities. Interferon and hyperthermia are being used on an experimental basis. A current practice in the treatment of cancer is the use of a carefully planned program that combines the benefits of multiple treatment modalities and the expertise of a team of medical specialists such as a medical oncologist, surgical oncologist, and radiologist.

Surgery

Surgery is used for diagnosis, the staging of cancer, the removal of the tumor, and palliation (relief of symptoms) when cure cannot be effected. The type of surgery to be used is determined by the extent of the disease and the structures involved. When the tumor is small, the entire lesion can often be removed; when the tumor is large or involves vital tissues, surgical removal may be impossible.

Surgical techniques have been expanded to

include electrosurgery, cryosurgery, chemosurgery, and laser surgery.[21] *Electrosurgery* uses the cutting and coagulating effects of high-frequency current applied by needle, blade, or electrodes. Once considered a palliative type of procedure, it is now being used as an alternative treatment for certain cancers of the skin, oral cavity, and rectum. *Cryosurgery* involves the instillation of liquid nitrogen into the tumor through a probe. It is used in treating cancers of the oral cavity, brain, and prostate. *Chemosurgery* is used in skin cancers. It involves the use of a corrosive paste in combination with multiple frozen sections to ensure complete removal of the tumor. *Laser surgery* uses a laser beam to resect a tumor. It has been used effectively in retinal and vocal cord surgery.

Cooperative efforts between cancer centers throughout the world have helped to standardize and improve surgical procedures, determine which cancers benefit from surgical intervention, and establish in what order surgical and other treatment modalities should be used. Increased emphasis has also been placed on the development of surgical techniques, such as limb salvage surgery, which is used in the treatment of osteogenic sarcoma to preserve functional abilities while permitting complete removal of the tumor.

Radiation therapy

About 50% of patients with cancer receive radiation therapy, either alone or in combination with other forms of treatment.[22] Radiation can be used singly as the primary method of treatment, as presurgical or postsurgical therapy, with chemotherapy, or with chemotherapy and surgery. Survival rates approaching 90% have been reported with early detection and the use of radiation therapy for seminoma of the testes, Hodgkin's disease, and cancers of the larynx and cervix.[22]

Ionizing radiation was discovered by Marie and Pierre Curie and Wilhelm Conrad Roentgen just before the turn of the century. Development of the first sealed vacuum x-ray tube followed, during the 1920s, along with quantitative methods for measuring radiation dosage. During this same period, Claude Regaud (Foundation Curie in Paris) was able to show that fractionated—small, sublethal—doses of radiation could permanently halt spermatogenesis, whereas no single lethal dose could do so without causing severe damage to the surrounding tissues. It was this observation that linked radiation to the treatment of cancer. Another advance in radiation therapy followed the atomic bomb, with the development of radioactive cobalt. Since then, advances in technology have resulted in the development of sophisticated equipment that produces high-voltage x-ray and electronic beams capable of delivering a therapeutic dose

of radiation to the tumor without causing lethal damage to surrounding tissues.

Radiation acts at the cellular level, causing cell death as particles of radioactive energy break chemical bonds, disrupting DNA and interfering with cell activity and mitosis. Radiation exerts its greatest effect during certain phases of the cell cycle, particularly during early DNA synthesis of the S phase and in the mitotic or M phase of the cycle. To some extent, radiation is injurious to all cells, but most of all to the poorly differentiated and rapidly proliferating cells of cancer tissue. Radiation also injures such rapidly proliferating cells as those of the bone marrow and the mucosal lining of the gastrointestinal tract. Recovery from sublethal doses of radiation occurs in the interval between the first dose of radiation and subsequent doses. Normal tissue appears to be able to recover from radiation damage more readily than cancerous tissue.

The term *radiosensitivity* describes the sensitivity of cells to radiation, and it varies widely. For example, lymphomas are highly radiosensitive, whereas rhabdomyosarcomas are much less so. The radiation dose that is chosen for treatment of a particular cancer is determined by factors such as the radiosensitivity of the tumor type and the size of the tumor. The *lethal tumor dose* is defined as the dose that achieves 95% tumor control.[23] With external radiation sources, this dose is divided into a series of smaller, fractionated doses. With the use of fractionated doses, it is more likely that the cancer cells will be dividing and in the vulnerable period of the cell cycle. This dose also allows time for normal tissues to repair the radiation damage. Selecting alternative entrance sites for radiation also helps to spare normal tissue. For example, radiation can be directed at an internal tumor from various points marked off on the front, back, and sides of the body, so that the maximum radiation is directed at the tumor, while the rest of the body receives only minimal radiation.

Administration. Radiation can be administered by using an external machine or an internal source. The machines used to deliver *external radiation* are categorized into the kilovoltage (1000 eV) and megavoltage (1 million eV) range. The early x-ray machines that were used for radiation therapy delivered low-penetrance rays in the *kilovoltage* (KeV) range. These rays exert their maximum tumor dose within 1 cm to 2 cm of the skin surface and are now used only in superficial skin lesions or tumors located near the skin surface. *Megavoltage* (MeV) machines include the cobalt machines, betatrons, and linear accelerators. The MeV machines produce rays that are more penetrating and have more sharply defined edges then the KeV machines; this allows for the delivery of curative doses of radiation without causing damage to skin or other tissues. The rays from the MeV machines also spare bone structures. With KeV beams, absorption was markedly higher in bone than in soft tissues, but with the MeV machines this difference does not exist; soft tissue and bone have the same absorption rate—a factor that has allowed delivery of a cancericidal dose of radiation in the vicinity of bone without extensive damage to the bone structures.

Internal radiation therapy involves the insertion of radioactive sources within a body cavity, body tissues, or close to the surface being treated. The radioisotopes most commonly used for this purpose are cobalt-60, iridium-192, iodine-125, iodine-131, phosphorus-32, cesium-137, gold-198, and radium-226. Internal radiation can be administered in the form of either sealed or unsealed radiation sources. *Sealed radiation sources* are packed within applicators that can be formed into almost any size or shape. Most commonly they are packed into needles, beads, seeds, ribbons, or catheters, which are then implanted directly into the tumor. Both removable and permanent implants are used. Removable devices make it possible to insert a radioactive material into a tumor area for a period of time (1 or 2 days to a week) and then remove it. The radioactive sources that are used most commonly for this purpose are radium-226, cesium-137, and iridium-192. Cancer of the cervix and uterus is often treated with removable radium implants. Radioactive materials with a relatively short half-life, such as gold-198, radon, or iodine-125, are commonly encapsulated and used in permanent implants. This type of treatment is used for oral, bladder, and prostate cancers. *Unsealed internal radiation sources* are either injected intravenously, administered by mouth, or instilled into a body cavity. Iodine-131, which is given by mouth, is used in the treatment of thyroid cancer. Gold-198 and phosphorus-32 are instilled directly into body cavities to control effusions (collections of fluid within a serous cavity).

Internal radiation sources are a source of radiation exposure as long as a sealed implant remains in the body or an unsealed implant or injected radioisotope emanates rays of radiant energy. It is essential that the type of ray that is being emitted and the half-life of the radioisotope be considered when care is provided for a person receiving internal radiation. Some radioisotopes such as phosphorus-32 produce only beta rays, which do not create a radiation hazard because of the limited range of beta radiation. Others, such as radium implants, pose a radiation hazard because they emit gamma rays. Institutions that practice nuclear medicine must be licensed by the Atomic Energy Commission and have a radiation protection supervisor, who has the responsibility of establishing policies and maintaining radiation safety within the institution.

Radiation responsiveness. *Radiation responsiveness* refers to the manner in which a tumor responds to irradiation. Several factors may alter the tumor's response to irradiation. One of these is tumor oxygenation. Many rapidly growing tumors outgrow their blood supply and become deprived of oxygen. It is now recognized that the hypoxic cells of these tumors are more resistant to radiation than normal or well-oxygenated tumor cells. Ways of increasing oxygen delivery to these tumors during radiation therapy are being investigated, as are agents that act as oxygen substitutes. These agents increase the production of free radicals during radiation in a manner similar to oxygen. Another factor is radiosensitivity. Studies are being conducted in hopes of finding ways to increase the radiosensitivity of tumors by altering their DNA in a manner that either makes it more sensitive to radiation or less able to repair radiation damage.

Radioprotectors are substances that selectively protect normal tissue such as bone marrow, salivary glands, and the gastrointestinal mucosa from the effects of radiation without interfering with its effects on cancer tissue. These substances are also being studied.[24]

Adverse effects. Because radiation affects all rapidly proliferating cells, it usually causes some adverse effects. Tissues that are most frequently affected are the skin, the mucosal lining of the gastrointestinal tract, and the bone marrow. Radiation effects are dose dependent: with moderate doses of radiation to the skin, the hair falls out either spontaneously or when being combed, by about the 10th to the 14th day; with larger doses, erythema develops (much like a sunburn) and may turn brown; and at very high doses, the skin is denuded. Fortunately, epithelialization takes place after the treatments have been stopped. The effects of irradiation on the oral and pharyngeal mucous membranes are similar to those that occur on the skin. Radiation-induced bone marrow depression leads to a decrease in white blood cell and platelet production and thus to an increased risk of infection and bleeding tendencies. Other systemic signs associated with irradiation include anorexia, nausea, vomiting, fatigue, profuse perspiration, and even chills. These effects are temporary and reversible.

Protection from radiation. Protection from radiation is a concern of persons who are in contact with radiation. The three basic considerations in protection are shielding, time, and distance. *Shielding* is practiced by persons who are in contact with radiation for long periods, such as radiologists and radiologic technicians; they are shielded by special walls or body coverings such as lead aprons, gloves, and throat collars. Increased *time* spent in contact with a radiation source increases exposure. Finally, *distance* must be considered. According to the *inverse square law* that applies to radiation exposure, one can reduce exposure from x-ray or gamma radiation to one-fourth simply by doubling the distance from the radiation source. At a distance of 2 feet from the radiation source, a person receives one-fourth the exposure that he or she would receive at a distance of 1 foot from the source; at a distance of 4 feet, the exposure is one-fourth that received at a distance of 2 feet.

Pharmacologic therapy

Chemotherapy. In the past three decades, cancer chemotherapy has evolved as a major treatment modality. Drugs may be the chief form of treatment or they may be used adjunctively to other treatments. Chemotherapy is now the primary treatment for most hematologic and some solid tumors, including choriocarcinoma, acute and chronic leukemia, Burkitt's lymphoma, and multiple myeloma.

Cancer chemotherapeutic drugs exert their effects through several mechanisms. At the cellular level, they exert their lethal action by creating adverse conditions that prevent cell growth and replication. These mechanisms include disrupting production of essential enzymes; inhibiting DNA, RNA, and protein synthesis; and preventing cell mitosis. These agents act by first-order kinetics: that is, they kill a percentage rather than a constant number of cells. They are most effective in treating tumors that have a high growth fraction because of their ability to kill rapidly dividing cells.

The anticancer drugs may be classified as either cell-cycle specific or cell-cycle nonspecific. Drugs are cell-cycle specific if they exert their action during a specific phase of the cell cycle. For example, methotrexate, an antimetabolite, acts by interfering with DNA synthesis and thereby interrupts the S phase of the cell cycle. Drugs that are cell-cycle nonspecific affect cancer cells through all the phases of the cell cycle. The alkylating agents, which are cell-cycle nonspecific, act by disrupting DNA when the cells are in the resting state as well as when they are dividing. Chemotherapeutic drugs that have similar structures and effects on cell function are generally grouped together, and these drugs usually have similar toxic effects and side effects (Table 5-5). Because they differ in their mechanisms of action, combinations of cell-cycle-specific and cell-cycle-nonspecific agents are often used to treat cancer.

Combination chemotherapy has been found to be more effective than treatment with a single drug. With this method, several drugs with different mechanisms of action, metabolic pathways, times of onset of action and recovery, side effects, and onsets of side effects are used. The regimens for combination therapy are often referred to by acronyms. Two well-known combinations are MOPP (nitrogen mustard, vincristine [Oncovin], procarbazine, and prednisone), used in the treatment of Hodgkin's disease, and CMF (cyclophosphamide, methotrexate, and 5-fluorouracil), used in the treatment of breast cancer. The maximum possible drug doses are usually used to ensure the maximum cell-kill. The routes of administration and dosage schedules are carefully designed to ensure optimal delivery of the active forms of the drugs to a tumor during the sensitive phase of the cell cycle.[25]

Adverse effects. Because cancer cells derive from normal cells, they retain many of the latter's properties; thus, chemotherapeutic drugs will affect both the neoplastic cells and the rapidly proliferating cells of normal tissue. The *nadir* (lowest point) is the point of maximal toxicity for a given adverse effect of a drug and is stated in the time it takes to reach that point. The nadir for leukopenia with thiotepa occurs at 14 days after initiation of treatment. Since many toxic effects of chemotherapeutic drugs persist for some time after the drug is discontinued, the nadir times and recovery rates are useful guides in evaluating the effects of cancer therapy.

Anorexia, nausea, vomiting, and diarrhea are common problems associated with cancer chemotherapy. They occur within minutes or hours of drug administration and are thought to be due to stimulation of the chemoreceptor trigger zone (vomiting center) in the medulla or the autonomic nervous system. The symptoms usually subside within 24 to 48 hours and often can be relieved by antiemetics. Some drugs cause stomatitis and damage to the rapidly proliferating cells of the gastrointestinal tract mucosal lining. Most chemotherapeutic drugs suppress bone marrow function and formation of blood cells, leading to anemia, leukopenia, and thrombocytopenia. With severe granulocytopenia there is risk of developing serious infections. Hair loss results from impaired proliferation of the hair follicles and is a side effect of a number of cancer drugs; it is usually temporary and the hair tends to regrow when treatment is stopped. The rapidly proliferating structures of the reproductive system are particularly sensitive to the action of the cancer drugs. Women may experience changes in menstrual flow or amenorrhea. Men may develop oligospermia and azoospermia. Many of these agents may also have teratogenic or mutagenic effects leading to fetal abnormalities.

Recent epidemiological studies have shown an increased risk of second malignancies such as acute nonlymphocytic leukemia following long-term use of alkylating agents,[26,27] and semustine[28] for treatment of various forms of cancer. These second malignancies

Table 5–5. Agents used in treatment of cancer

Agent	Mechanism of action	Major toxic manifestations
Alkylating agents		
Chlorambucil (Leukeran) Busulfan (Myleran) Cyclophosphamide (Cytoxan) Ifosfamide (Ifex) Mechlorethamine (HN_2, Mustargen) Melphalan (Alkeran L-Pam) Thiotepa	Interfere with DNA replication by attacking DNA synthesis throughout the cell cycle	Bone marrow depression with leukopenia, thrombocytopenia, and bleeding; cyclophosphamide may cause alopecia and hemorrhagic cystitis
Antimetabolites		
Methotrexate (Methotrexate) 6-mercaptopurine (6-MP, Purinethol) 6-thioguanine (6-TG, Thioguan) 5-fluorouracil (5-FU, Fluorouracil) Cytarabine (Ara-C, Cytosar) 5-fluorodeoxyridine (FUDR, Floxidine)	Structural analogs of essential metabolites; therefore, interfere with synthesis of these metabolites	Bone marrow depression, oral and gastrointestinal ulceration
Antibiotics		
Doxorubicin (Adriamycin) Bleomycin (Blenoxane) Dactinomycin (Cosmegen) Daunorubicin (Daunomycin, Cerubidin) Mitoxantrone (Novantrone) Plicamycin (Mithramycin, Mithracin) Mitomycin C (Mutamycin)	Interfere with DNA or RNA synthesis, varying with the drug	Stomatitis, gastrointestinal tract disturbances, and bone marrow depression Doxorubicin and daunorubicin cause cardiac toxicity at cumulative doses over 500 mg/m² (mitoxantrone may be less cardiotoxic) Bleomycin can cause alopecia and pulmonary fibrosis, but only minimal bone marrow depression
Plant alkaloids		
Etoposide (VePesid)	Interferes with DNA synthesis.	Etoposide: bone marrow depression, alopecia
Vinblastine (Velban) Vincristine (Oncovin)	Interfere with cell mitosis	Vinblastine: alopecia, areflexia and bone marrow depression Vincristine: neurotoxicity with ataxia and impaired fine motor skills, constipation, and paralytic ileus
Steroid hormones and antagonists		
Androgens Estrogens Progestins Adrenal cortical hormones	Cell-cycle nonspecific Influence cell membrane receptors	Specific to action of the hormone
Tamoxifen (Nolvadex)	Antiestrogen	Retinopathy (rare), hot flashes, nausea, and vomiting
Leuprolide (Lupron)	Inhibits gonadotropin secretion	Hot flashes, gynecomastia; increased bone pain and difficulty urinating during first few weeks of therapy
Flutamide (Eulexin)	Antiandrogen	Diarrhea
Others		
Asparaginase (Elspar)	Inhibits protein synthesis	Fever, hypersensitivity
Carmustine (BICNU)	Antimetabolite and alkylating agent	Bone marrow depression
Carboplatin (Paraplatin)	Inhibits DNA, RNA, protein synthesis	Bone marrow depression
Cisplatin (Cis-Platinum, Platinol)		Renal damage
Dacarbazine (DTIC-Dome)	Interferes with DNA, RNA synthesis, antimetabolite	Bone marrow depression
Hydroxyrurea (Hydrea)	DNA selective antimetabolite	Bone marrow reaction Allergic reactions to tartrazine dye
Lomustine (CCNu, CeeNu)	Interferes with DNA, RNA synthesis	Bone marrow depression
Procarbazine (Matulane)	Inhibits DNA, RNA, protein synthesis	CNS depression

are thought to result from direct cellular changes that are produced by the drug or from suppression of the immune response.

Endocrine therapy. Endocrine therapy consists of the administration of exogenous hormones in large, nonphysiologic doses or the ablation of organs (ovaries, testes, or adrenal glands) responsible for hormone production. This treatment is used in cancers that are responsive to or dependent on hormones for growth. Among the tumors known to be responsive to hormonal manipulations are those of the breast, prostate, thyroid gland, and uterine endometrium. Hormone therapy also involves use of the adrenal corticosteroid hormones. These compounds inhibit mitosis and are cytotoxic to cells of lymphocytic origin. Hormones are cell-cycle nonspecific and are thought to alter the synthesis of RNA and proteins by binding to receptor sites. Unresponsiveness to hormonal manipulation is thought to be related to the absence of specific receptors for the hormone on the tumor.

Light-activated drugs (photophoresis). One of the goals of cancer therapy is the development of treatment methods that affect the cancer cells while sparing normal body tissues. One strategy is to use light-activated drugs that are inert unless they are exposed to the correct wavelength of light. In this way only those tissues that are exposed to both the drug and light become the target for the drug's action. One such drug, 8-methyoxypsoralen (8-MOP) is used in the treatment of cutaneous T-cell lymphoma.[29] The treatment is accomplished by giving the 8-MOP, removing blood from the body and exposing the white blood cells and plasma that have been separated from the whole blood to ultraviolet rays, and then returning the blood to the body.

Immunotherapy. Immunotherapy remains largely investigational and is usually used in conjunction with other forms of treatment. Immunotherapeutic methods fall into three categories. The first is *active nonspecific immune therapy,* whose purpose is to stimulate the immune response. One such agent is BCG (bacillus Calmette-Guérin), an attenuated strain of the bacterium that causes bovine tuberculosis. The second method is *specific immune therapy,* a method that is somewhat similar to immunization in that it involves the use of antigens, from either the patient's tumor or an antigenically similar tumor from another patient, as a challenge to the patient's immune system to produce immune cells against the tumor antigen. The third method is *transfer of passive tumor immunity,* which is accomplished through the administration of antisera or effector substances. Transfer factor is an extract of stimulated lymphocytes that are capable of transferring specific delayed hypersensitivity to other lymphocytes.

Interferons. Interferons are a group of glycoproteins that are synthesized by a number of cells in response to a variety of stimuli including viral infections (see Chapter 11). The interferons belong to a class of compounds called the *biologic response modifiers,* which fight cancer by stimulating the body's immune system. At present 20 interferons have been identified in humans. There are three broad groups of interferons: alpha, beta, and gamma. Most of the subtypes belong to the alpha group. The exact physiological roles of each of the interferons remain unclear. They appear to inhibit viral replication and may also be involved in inhibiting tumor protein synthesis and in prolongating the cell cycle and increasing the percentage of cells in the G_0 phase.[30] In addition interferons stimulate natural killer cells and T-lymphocyte killer cells.

Although until recently the availability of interferon was limited because it could only be obtained from white blood cells and fibroblasts, large amounts can now be produced using techniques of recombinant DNA synthesis. Interferon is used in combination with other forms of cancer treatment and as a single-agent treatment. The best responses to interferon have occurred in hairy cell leukemia, cutaneous T-cell lymphoma, nodular lymphoma, and chronic myeloid leukemia.[31] There has been some success in treatment of melanoma and renal carcinoma. Interferon has proved useful in treating papillomas and condylomas, and its role as a local agent will probably expand. Future research is expected to focus on combining interferons with other forms of cancer therapy and establishing optimal doses and treatment protocols.

In summary, neoplasms may be either benign or malignant. The growth of a benign tumor is restricted to the site of origin, and the tumor will not cause death unless it interferes with vital functions. Cancer or malignant neoplasms, on the other hand, grow wildly and without organization, spread to distant parts of the body, and cause death unless checked. Tumors are named by the addition of the suffix *-oma* to the name of the tissue type. The term carcinoma refers to a malignant tumor of epithelial cell origin and the term sarcoma to a malignant tumor of mesenchymal cell origin. Benign and malignant tumors differ in terms of: (1) cell characteristics, (2) manner of growth, (3) rate of growth, (4) potential for metastasis, (5) ability to produce generalized effects, (6) tendency to cause tissue destruction, and (7) capacity to cause death. Cancer cells are often poorly differentiated in comparison to normal cells; they display abnormal membrane characteristics, they have abnormal antigens, they produce abnormal biochemical products, and they have abnormal karyotypes. Carcinogenesis is the process of cancer formation. The mechanisms involved in cancer development are many and complex. It is likely that cancer occurs because of interactions among many risk factors, including heredity, oncogenes and oncoviruses, chemical and environmental carcinogenic agents, cancer-causing viruses, immunologic defects, and precancerous lesions. It has been estimated that carcinogenic agents are involved in 80% to 85% of cancers, probably in association with other risk factors.

The methods used in diagnosis of cancer vary with the type of cancer that is present and its location. Since many cancers are curable if diagnosed early, health care practices designed to promote early detection are important. These practices include breast self-exam in the female, testicular self-exam in the male, and consulting of a physician when any of the early warning signals of cancer are present. The pap smear and tissue biopsy are used to detect the presence of cancer cells and in diagnosis. There are two basic methods of classifying tumors: (1) grading according to the histologic or tissue characteristics and (2) clinical staging according to spread of the disease. Histologic studies are done in the laboratory using cells or tissue specimens. The TNM system for clinical staging of cancer uses tumor size, lymph node involvement, and presence of metastasis.

Treatment plans that use more than one type of therapy, often in combination, are now providing cures for a number of cancers that a few decades ago had a poor prognosis and are increasing the life-expectancy in other types of cancer. Surgical procedures are now more precise as a result of improved diagnostic equipment and new techniques such as laser surgery. Radiation equipment and radioactive sources permit greater and more controlled destruction of cancer cells while causing less damage to normal tissues. Combination chemotherapy regimes have provided cures for cancers that were previously viewed as uncurable. Successes with use of immunotherapy and interferon offer hope that the body's own defenses can be used in fighting cancer.

References

1. Cancer Facts 1988: New York, American Cancer Society, 1988
2. Prescott DM, Flexer AS: Cancer: The Misguided Cell, p 61. Sunderland MA, Sinauer Assoc., 1986
3. Robbins SL, Cotran RS, Kumar V: Pathologic Basis of Disease, 3rd ed, pp 268, 255, 264, 268. Philadelphia, WB Saunders, 1984
4. Lynch HT: Familial risk and cancer control. J Am Med Assoc 236, No. 6:585, 1976
5. Knudson AG: Heredity and human cancer. Am J Path 77, No.1:77, 1974
6. Friend SH, Dryja TP, Weinberg RA: Oncogenes and tumor suppressing genes. N Engl J Med 318:618, 1988
7. Marx JL: What do oncogenes do? Science 223:673, 1984
8. Gordon H: Oncogenes. Mayo Clin Proc 60:696, 1985
9. Sibbitt WL: Oncogenes, normal cell growth, and connective tissue disease. Ann Rev Med 39:123, 1988
10. Farber E: Chemical carcinogenesis. N Engl J Med 305:1378, 1981
11. Poskanzer DC, Herbst A: Epidemiology of vaginal adenosis and adenocarcinoma associated with exposure to stilbesterol in utero. Cancer 39, No. 4:1792, 1977
12. Nicholson WJ: Cancer following occupational exposure to asbestos and vinyl chloride. Cancer 39, No. 4: 1972, 1977
13. Favus MJ, Schneider AB, Stachura ME, et al: Thyroid cancer occurring as a late consequence of head and neck irradiation: Evaluation of 1056 patients. N Engl J Med 294:1019, 1976
14. Jablon S, Kato H: Studies of the mortality of A-bomb survivors: 5. Radiation dose and mortality, 1950–1970. Radiat Res 50:649, 1972
15. Burnett FM: Immunologic aspects of malignant disease. Lancet 1:1171, 1967
16. Baserga R: The cell cycle. N Engl J Med 304:453, 1981
17. Beutler B, Cerami A: Cachectin: More than a tumor necrosis factor. N Engl J Med 316:379, 1987
18. Rothstein JL, et al: Tumor necrosis factor: A potent effector molecule for tumor cell killing by activated macrophages. Proc Natl Acad Sci USA 83:8318, 1986
19. Ihde DC: Paraneoplastic syndromes. Hosp Pract 22 (Aug 15):105, 1987
20. Beahrs OH, Myers MH (eds): Manual for Staging of Cancer, 2nd ed, p 6. Philadelphia, JB Lippincott, 1983
21. Patterson WB: Principles of surgical oncology. In Rubin P (ed): Clinical Oncology ed. 6, p 35. American Cancer Society, 1983
22. Bloomer WD, Hellman S: Normal tissue responses to radiation therapy. N Engl J Med 293:80, 1975
23. Rubin P, Poulter C: Principles of radiation and cancer radiotherapy. In Rubin P(ed): Clinical Oncology, 5th ed, p 33. New York. American Cancer Society, 1978
24. Phillips TL, Wasserman TH: Promise of radiosensitizers and radioprotectors in treatment of human cancers. Cancer Treat Rep 68:291, 1984
25. Krakoff IRL: Cancer chemotherapeutic agents. CA: A Cancer J for Clinicians 31, No. 3:4, 1981
26. Pederson-Bjergaard J, Larsen SO: Incidence of acute nonlymphocytic leukemia, preleukemia and acute myeloproliferative syndrome up to 10 years after treatment of Hodgkin's disease. N Engl J Med 307:964, 1982
27. Coltman CA Jr, Dixon DO: Second malignancies complicating Hodgkin's disease: A Southwest Oncology Group 10 year followup. Cancer Treat Rep 66:1023, 1982
28. Boise JD, Greene MH, Killen JY, et al: Leukemia and

preleukemia after adjuvant treatment of gastrointestinal cancer with Semustine. N Engl J Med 309:1079, 1983

29. Edelson RL: Light-activated drugs. Sci Am 259, No. 2:68, 1988

30. Goldstein D, Laszio J: The role of interferon in cancer therapy: A current perspective. CA: A Cancer J for Clinicians 38, No. 5:258, 1988

Bibliography

Bailar JC, Smith EM: Progress against cancer. N Engl J Med 314:1226, 1986

Bingham CA: The cell cycle and cancer chemotherapy. Am J Nurs 78, No.7:1201, 1978

Bishop JM: The molecular genetics of cancer. Science 235:305, 1987

Brodt P: Tumor immunology—Three decades in review. Ann Rev Med 37:447, 1983

Buckley I: Oncogenes and the nature of malignancy. Adv Cancer Res 50:71, 1988

Burnett FM: Immunological aspects of malignant disease. Lancet 1:1171, 1967

Cohen LA: Diet and cancer. Sci American 257, No. 5:42, 1987

Cooper GM: Activation of transforming genes in neoplasms. Br J Cancer 50:137, 1984

Dvorak HF: Tumors: Wounds that do not heal. N Engl J Med 315:1650, 1986

Ensminger WD, Gyves JW: Regional cancer chemotherapy. Cancer Treatment Reports 68, No. 1:101, 1984

Farber E: Chemical carcinogenesis. N Eng J Med 305, No. 23:1379, 1981

Fenoglio CM, Lefkowitch JH: Viruses and cancer. Med Clin N Amer 67, No. 5:1105, 1983

Frye RJM, Aninsworth EJ: Radiation injury: Some aspects of the oncogenic effects. Fed Proc 36, No. 5:1703, 1977

Gallo RC: The virus-cancer story. Hosp Pract 18, No. 6:79, 1983

Gilbert F: Retinoblastoma and cancer genetics. N Engl J Med 314:1248, 1986

Heidelberger C: Chemical carcinogenesis. Annu Rev Biochem 44:79, 1975

Insogna KL, Broadus AE: Hypercalcemia of malignancy. Ann Rev Med 38:241, 1987

Knudson AG: Genetics of human cancer. Ann Rev Med 20:231, 1986

Krontiris TG: The emerging genetics of human cancer. N Eng J Med 309, No. 7:404, 1983

Lyon JL: Radiation exposure and cancer. Hosp Pract 19 (7):159, 1984

McIntire KR: Tumor Markers: How useful are they? Hosp Pract 19 (12):55, 1984

Miller EC, Miller JA: Mechanisms of chemical carcinogenesis. Cancer 47:1055, 1981

Moldawer NP, Murray JL: The clinical uses of monoclonal antibodies in cancer research. Cancer Nurs (8):207, 1985

Moldawert LL, Georgieff M, Lundholm K: Interleukin I, tumor necrosis factor-alpha (cachectin) and the pathogenesis of cancer cachexia. Clin Physiol 7:263, 1987

Moskowitz M: Cost-benefit of determinations of screening mammography. Radiologic Clin North Am 25:1680, 1987

Mundy GR: Ectopic hormonal syndromes in neoplastic disease. Hosp Pract 22 (4):179, 1987

Old LJ: Tumor necrosis factor. Scientific Am 258, No. 5:59, 1988

Purtilo DT: Defective immune surveillance in viral carcinogenesis. Lab Invest 51, No. 4:373, 1984

Richter MP, Kligerman MM: Particle-beam radiation therapy 1983: Evaluation and recommendations. Cancer Treatment Reports 68, No. 1:303, 1984

Schmaier AH: Oncologic emergencies. Med Times 111, No. 2:87, 1983

Scott RE, Wille JJ: Mechanisms for the initiation and promotion of carcinogenesis: A review and a new concept. Mayo Clin Proc 59:107, 1984

Sibbit WL: Oncogenes, normal cell growth, and connective tissue disease. Ann Rev Med 39:123, 1988

Winters WD: Viruses and cancer. Am J Nurs 78, No. 2:249, 1978.

Alterations in Body Defenses

CHAPTER 6

Stress and Adaptation

Objectives

After you have studied this chapter, you should be able to meet the following objectives:

_____ State Selye's definition of stress.

_____ Define the term *stressor*.

_____ Cite two factors that influence the nature of the stress response.

_____ Compare specific and nonspecific stress responses.

_____ Explain the interactions of the nervous system in mediating the stress response.

_____ Describe the stress responses of the autonomic nervous system, the hypothalamus-pituitary-adrenal axis, the immune system, and the musculoskeletal system.

_____ Explain the purpose of adaptation.

_____ Describe the components of a simple control system.

_____ Describe the function of a negative feedback system.

_____ Cite Cannon's four features of homeostasis.

_____ List at least six factors that influence an individual's adaptive capacity.

_____ Relate experience and previous learning to the process of adaptation.

_____ Contrast anatomic and physiologic reserve.

_____ Describe the circadian rhythms for body temperature and cortisol.

_____ Relate the concept of entrainment to hunger.

_____ Relate the effect of social cues on the sleep–wakefulness cycle in third shift workers.

_____ Explain the methods used in biofeedback training.

_____ Describe the four factors that are involved in various relaxation techniques.

_____ Contrast relaxation exercises with the methods used in imagery.

Health is a dynamic state in which energy must be expended continuously in order to adapt to life stresses. Much of this energy is used to recruit physiologic and psychologic behaviors that oppose or compensate for perceived threats to the integrity of the internal environment. In this respect, the human body is truly an amazing structure. It is able to withstand exposure to environmental stresses while maintaining its internal environment within the very narrow confines of what is termed *normal*. From astronauts who have traveled to the moon and from explorers of the ocean's depths, we have learned that vital physiologic functions such as heart rate, blood pH, and body temperature remain remarkably similar to those observed under normal environmental conditions. Even in advanced disease states, the body maintains much of its adaptive capacity and is able to compensate and maintain the internal environment within relatively normal limits.

Stress

In recent years, interest in the roles that stress and altered adaptive processes play in the development of disease has increased. Hypertension, heart disease, and peptic ulcer are but a few of the diseases that have been associated with stress. Stress may contribute directly to the production of disease or it may contribute to the development of behaviors such as smoking, overeating, and drug abuse, which increase the risk of disease.

Stress has been defined in many ways. To the physicist, the term refers to a force, strain, or pressure applied to a system. To the lay person, stress frequently implies exposure to excessive demands or environmental conditions that cause emotional upset and tension. To the psychologist, stress can be anything that alters the psychologic homeostatic processes.[1] To the anthropologist, stress is adversity: coercion between people or between the environment and humans, or between history and humankind.[2] Hans Selye, the world-renowned endocrinologist and pioneer in the field of stress research, has described stress as the nonspecific response of the body to any demand made on it.[3] Because the primary focus of this book is on physiology, Selye's theory of stress is used here.

—— Stressors

The events or environmental agents responsible for initiating the stress response are called *stressors*. According to Selye, stressors may be endogenous, arising from within the body, or exogenous, arising from outside the body.[3] Stressors can be physical, psychologic, or sociologic. They include mental and physical effort, extremes of temperature, hunger, thirst, and fatigue, and other everyday experiences. Mason has suggested that emotional reactions to the stressor serve as the final common pathway for the stress response, emphasizing the need to consider the impact that learning and emotion have on the response.[4]

Of particular interest are the differences in the body's response to stressors that threaten the integrity of the body's physiologic environment and those that threaten the integrity of the individual's psychosocial environment. Many of the body's responses to physiologic stressors are controlled on a moment-by-moment basis by feedback mechanisms that limit their utilization and duration of action. For example, the baroreflex-mediated rise in heart rate that occurs when one moves from the recumbent to the standing position is almost instantaneous and subsides within seconds. Furthermore, the response to physiologic stressors that threaten the integrity of the internal environment is specific to the stress—the body does not usually raise the body temperature when a rise in heart rate is needed. In contrast, the response to psychologic stressors is not regulated with the same degree of specificity and feedback control—instead, the effect may be inappropriate and sustained.

Stressors can assume a number of patterns in relation to time. They may also be classified as follows: (1) acute time-limiting, (2) event-sequencing, (3) chronic intermittent, or (4) chronic sustained stressors.[5] An acute time-limiting stressor is any event that occurs within a short period and does not usually recur. Event-sequencing stressors are situations in which a stressor initiates a series of stress-producing events (*e.g.*, being fired from a job). Chronic intermittent stress occurs in response to discrete, intermittent stimuli to which a person is habitually exposed. Chronic sustained stressors are those to which a person is continuously exposed. The frequency or chronicity of circumstances in which the body is asked to respond to a stressor often determines the availability and efficiency of stress responses. The response of the immune system, for example, is more rapid and more efficient on second exposure to a pathogen than it is on first exposure. On the other hand, chronic exposure to a stressor can fatigue the stress response system and impair its effectiveness.

—— The stress response

In explaining the stress response, Selye proposed that two factors determine the nature of the stress response: (1) the properties of the stressor and (2) the conditioning of the individual being stressed.[3]

Most stressors produce both specific and nonspecific responses. For example, the joy of becoming a new parent and the sorrow of losing a parent are completely different experiences, yet their stressor effect —the nonspecific demand for adjustment to a new situation—can be quite similar. The specific stress responses alert an individual to the presence of the stressor, whereas the nonspecific effects, which involve neuroendocrine responses such as increased autonomic nervous system activity, are designed to maintain or reestablish normality and are independent of specific responses. The ability of the same stressor to produce different responses and disorders in different individuals indicates the adaptive capacity of the individual, or what Selye termed *conditioning factors*. These conditioning factors may be internal (genetic predisposition, age, sex, or others) or external (exposure to environmental agents, treatment with certain drugs, or dietary factors).[3]

Manifestations of the stress response

The manifestations of the stress response—a pounding headache, cold moist hands, a stiff neck, and increased incidence of infections—reflect, for the most part, the nonspecific aspects of the stress response. They include responses of the autonomic nervous system, the endocrine system, the musculoskeletal system, and the immune system. The integration of these responses, which occurs at the level of the central nervous system, is elusive and complex. It relies on communication between the cerebral cortex, the limbic system, the thalamus, the hypothalamus, and the reticular formation and reticular activating system (Figure 6-1). The thalamus functions as a relay center for incoming impulses from all parts of the body and is important in sorting out and distributing sensory input. The reticular formation modulates mental alertness, autonomic nervous system activity, and skeletal muscle tone; but it does this using input and output from other neural structures. Likewise, the hypothalamus modulates the functioning of both the endocrine and the autonomic nervous system (see Figure 6-1). The limbic system is involved with the emotional components (fear, excitement, rage, anger) of the stress response.

Musculoskeletal responses

The musculoskeletal tension that occurs during the stress response reflects the increased activity of the reticular formation and its influence on the muscle spindles and the gamma loop (descending neural pathways, gamma motor neurons, spindle muscle fibers, afferent neurons, and alpha motor neurons), which control muscle tone. Muscle tension can remain as a prolonged manifestation of the stress response and can cause stiffness of the neck, backache, headaches, and other complaints.

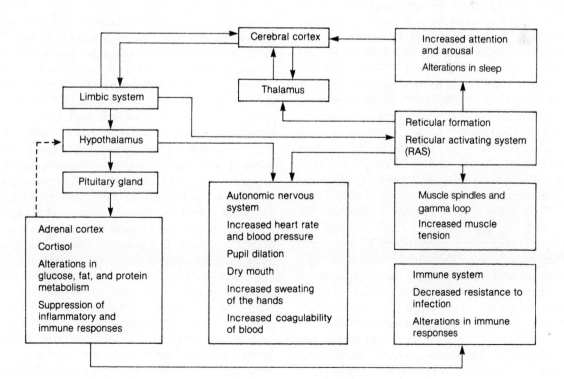

Figure 6-1 Stress pathways. The broken line represents negative feedback.

Autonomic nervous system responses

The autonomic nervous system manifestation of the stress reaction has been termed the *fight-or-flight response*. This is the most rapid of the stress responses and represents the basic survival response of our primitive ancestors when confronted with the perils of the wilderness and its inhabitants. In the presence of danger, the alternatives were clear—run away or stand up and fight. The heart and respiratory rates increase, the hands and feet become moist, the pupils dilate, the mouth becomes dry, and the activity of the gastrointestinal tract decreases. The autonomic nervous system is also involved in less-threatening situations. For example, it is the autonomic nervous system that controls the circulatory responses to activities of daily living such as moving from the seated or lying to the standing position.

Hypothalamic-pituitary-adrenal responses

The hypothalamic-pituitary-adrenal response is the mechanism that regulates body levels of adrenocortical hormones (mainly cortisol). The production of cortisol by the adrenal gland is controlled by the adrenocorticotropic hormone (ACTH) from the anterior pituitary. ACTH, in turn, is controlled by the corticotropin-releasing factor from the hypothalamus. The influence of emotion and stress on cortisol production is largely through the central nervous system by means of the hypothalamus. Cortisol is involved in maintaining blood glucose levels, facilitating fat metabolism, supporting vascular responsiveness, and modulating central nervous system (CNS) function.[6] In addition, cortisol affects mineral turnover in bone, hematopoiesis, muscle function, immune responses, and renal function. The adrenocortical hormones are discussed in Chapter 44. Other hormones (growth hormone, thyroid hormone, vasopressin, the sex hormones, and others) are also involved in the stress response. These hormones are discussed in other sections of this text.

As a young medical student, Selye noted that patients suffering from diverse disease conditions had many signs and symptoms in common. He noted that "whether a man suffers from a loss of blood, an infectious disease, or advanced cancer, he loses his appetite, his muscular strength, and his ambition to accomplish anything; usually the patient also loses weight and even his facial expression betrays that he is ill."[3] Selye referred to this as the "syndrome of just being sick." To Selye, the response to stress was a process that enabled the body to resist the stressor in the best possible way by enhancing the function of the

system best able to respond to it. He termed this response the *general adaptation syndrome (GAS)*. The GAS involves three stages: (1) the alarm stage, (2) the stage of resistance, and (3) the stage of exhaustion. The hypothalamic-pituitary-adrenal axis assumes a pivotal role in stress homeostasis during the alarm stage. Selye observed a triad of adrenal enlargement, thymus atrophy, and gastric ulcers in the rats used in his original studies. During the alarm stage no one organ system is predominantly active. The most appropriate channels of defense are recruited during the stage of resistance. During this second stage, the increased cortisol levels that were present during the first stage drop, because they are no longer needed. During the third stage—the stage of exhaustion—the reaction spreads because of wear and tear on the most appropriate channel of adaptation.[7]

Selye contended that many ailments, such as various emotional disturbances, mildly annoying headaches, insomnia, upset stomach, gastric and duodenal ulcers, and certain types of rheumatic disorders, as well as cardiovascular and kidney diseases, appear to be initiated or encouraged by the "body itself because of its faulty adaptive reactions to potentially injurious agents."[3]

Immunologic responses

There is increasing interest in the effect that stress has on the immunologic responses. The occurrence of the oral disease acute necrotizing gingivitis, in which the normal bacterial flora of the mouth becomes invasive, is well known by dentists to be associated with acute stress, such as final exams.[8] Similarly, herpes simplex I (cold sores) often develops during periods of inadequate rest, fever, ultraviolet radiation, and emotional upset. In this case, the resident herpes virus is kept in check by body defenses, most likely by T-lymphocytes, until a stressful event occurs and causes suppression of the immune system.

The exact mechanism by which stress produces its effect on the immune response is unknown and probably varies from individual to individual, depending on genetic endowment and environmental factors. It is known, however, that the stress response induces changes in a number of hormonal factors that affect the immune response. The hallmark of the stress response, as first described by Selye, is the presence of conditions (increased corticosteroid production and atrophy of the thymus) known to suppress the immune response. This process can be utilized clinically, as in the administration of pharmacologic preparations of the corticosteroid hormones to suppress the inflammatory and immune response. The existence of a feedback loop between the immune system and the hypothalamic-pituitary-adrenal system suggests the intriguing possibility that there may be interaction between the two systems in decreasing resistance to infection and in the surveillance function of the immune system in preventing neoplastic cell development (see Chapter 5). The receptors for a number of CNS-controlled hormones and neuromediators reportedly have been found on lymphocytes. Among these are receptors for glucocorticoids, insulin, testosterone, catecholamines, estrogens, histamine, acetylcholine, and growth hormone.[9] The presence of a hormone receptor on a cell suggests that the cell's function is influenced by the hormone.

In summary, stress is defined in many ways. Hans Selye, the world-renowned endocrinologist and pioneer in the field of stress research, defines stress as the nonspecific response of the body to any demands made on it. The event or environmental agent that produces the stress is called a stressor. Stressors may be physical, psychologic, or social. They include mental and physical effort, extremes of temperature, hunger, thirst, fatigue, and other everyday experiences. Most stressors produce both specific and nonspecific responses. The specific responses alert the individual to the nature of the stressor and assist in establishing definitive measures to deal with it. The nonspecific responses are designed to maintain or reestablish normality.

Adaptation

The ability to adapt to a wide range of environments and stressors is not peculiar to humans. According to René Dubos (a microbiologist noted for his study of human response to the total environment), "adaptability is found throughout life and is perhaps the one attribute that distinguishes most clearly the world of life from the world of inanimate matter."[10] Living organisms, no matter how primitive, do not submit passively to the impact of environmental forces. They attempt to respond adaptively, each in its own unique and most suitable manner. The higher the organism on the evolutionary scale, the larger its repertoire of adaptive mechanisms and its ability to select and limit aspects of the environment to which it will respond. The most fully evolved mechanisms are the social responses through which individuals or groups modify their environments, their habits, or both, in order to achieve a way of life that is suited to their needs.[10]

Human beings, because of their highly developed nervous system and intellect, usually have alternative mechanisms for adapting and have the ability to control many aspects of the environment. Air conditioning and central heating limit the need to adapt to extreme changes in environmental temperature. The control of microbial growth, immunization, and the availability of antibiotics eliminates the need to respond to common infectious agents. On the other hand, modern technology creates new challenges for adaptation and provides new sources of stress, such as increased noise, air pollution, exposure to chemicals that reduce the microbial agents in the environment and increase the shelf life of the foods we eat, and changes in the biologic rhythms imposed by shift work and transcontinental flights.

── Constancy of the internal environment

The environment in which the cells live is not the external environment that surrounds the organism, but a local fluid environment that surrounds each cell. It is from this internal environment that cells receive their nourishment and it is into this fluid that they secrete their wastes. Even the contents of the gastrointestinal tract and lungs do not become part of the internal environment until they have been absorbed into the extracellular fluid. A multicellular organism is able to survive only as long as the composition of the internal environment is compatible with the survival needs of the individual cells. Even a small change in the pH of the body fluids can disrupt the metabolic processes of individual cells. Claude Bernard, a nineteenth-century physiologist, was the first to clearly describe the central importance of a stable internal environment (*milieu interne*). Bernard recognized that body fluids that surround the cells and the various organ systems provide the means for exchange between the external and the internal environments.

── Homeostasis

The concept of a stable internal environment was supported by Walter B. Cannon, who emphasized that this kind of stability, which he termed *homeostasis*, was achieved through a system of carefully coordinated physiologic processes that oppose change. He pointed out that these processes were largely automatic.

Cannon emphasized that homeostasis involves not only resistance to external disturbances, but also resistance to disturbances from within. In his book *Wisdom of the Body*, published in 1939, Cannon presented four tentative propositions to describe the general features of homeostasis:

1. Constancy in an open system, such as our bodies represent, requires mechanisms that act to maintain this constancy. Cannon based this proposition on insights into the ways by which steady

states such as glucose concentrations, body temperature, and acid–base balance were regulated.

2. Steady-state conditions require that any tendency toward change be automatically met with factors that resist change. An increase in blood sugar results in thirst as the body attempts to dilute the concentration of sugar in the extracellular fluid.

3. The regulating system that determines the homeostatic state consists of a number of cooperating mechanisms acting simultaneously or successively. Blood sugar is regulated by insulin, glucagon, and other hormones that control its release from the liver or its uptake by the tissues.

4. Homeostasis does not occur by accident, but is the result of organized self-government. With this postulate, Cannon emphasized that when a factor is known to shift homeostasis in one direction, it is reasonable to expect mechanisms that have the opposite effect. In the homeostatic regulation of blood sugar, one would expect to find mechanisms that both raise and lower blood sugar.[11]

Control systems

The ability of the body to function under conditions of change in the internal and external environment depends on the thousands of control systems that serve to regulate body function. The body's control systems regulate cellular function, control the life processes, and integrate the interrelated functions of the different organ systems.

The most intricate of these control systems is the genetic control system that regulates cellular function, including cell structure and replication (see Chapter 3). Other control systems regulate function within organs and systems, whereas still others operate throughout the body to integrate the functions of the different organ systems. The concentration of carbon dioxide in the extracellular spaces is regulated by the respiratory and nervous systems, and the blood sugar concentration is controlled mainly by the liver and pancreas.

A homeostatic control system is a collection of interconnected components that function to keep a physical or chemical parameter of the body relatively constant. At least three essential components exist in a control system: (1) a *sensor,* which detects changes in product or function, (2) a *comparator,* which compares the sensed value with an acceptable range, and (3) an *effector system,* which returns the function or product to the acceptable range (Figure 6-2).

System efficiency

The effectiveness of a system is determined by the amount of change (amplification or gain) that occurs within the system in response to changes in external chemical or physical parameters. In his textbook of physiology, Guyton uses the example of a 1-degree Fahrenheit change in body temperature (from 98°F to 99°F) that occurs when environmental temperature is increased from 60°F to 110°F.[12] As body temperature rises because of the change in external temperature, sensors in the system detect the error, and sufficient compensation, in terms of radiation and evaporative heat losses from the skin, returns the temperature to within 1 degree Fahrenheit of the set point of the system. Were it not for the efficiency of the control system, the body temperature would have risen 50 degrees Fahrenheit instead of 1 degree Fahrenheit (Figure 6-3).

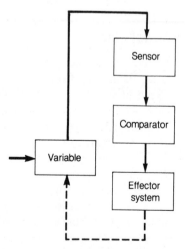

Figure 6-2 A simple control system consisting of a sensor that monitors a physiological variable, a comparator that compares the actual value of the monitored variable with the set-point of the system, and an effector system that functions to correct the disturbance (*solid line*). The broken line represents feedback control.

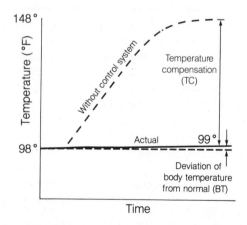

Figure 6-3 Effects on body temperature of suddenly increasing the air temperature 50° F, showing the hypothetical effect without a control system and the actual effect with a normal control system. (*Guyton A: Textbook of Medical Physiology,* 7th ed. Philadelphia, WB Saunders, 1986)

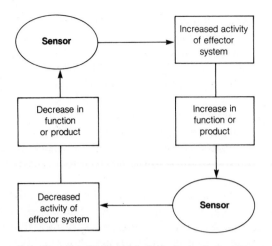

Figure 6-4 Negative feedback control of a body function, hormone level, or biochemical product.

Feedback systems

Most control systems in the body operate by *negative feedback mechanisms,* which function in a manner similar to the thermostat on a heating system. When the monitored function decreases below the set point of the system, the feedback mechanism causes the function to increase, and when the function is increased above the set point, the feedback mechanism causes it to decrease (Figure 6-4). For example, in the negative feedback mechanism that controls blood glucose levels, an increase in blood glucose stimulates an increase in insulin which enhances the removal of glucose from the blood. When sufficient glucose has left the bloodstream to cause blood glucose levels to fall, the release of glucose from the liver and the recruitment of other counterregulatory mechanisms cause the blood glucose to rise.

The reader is likely to ask why most physiologic control systems function under negative rather than *positive feedback mechanisms.* * The answer is that a positive feedback mechanism interjects instability rather than stability into a system. It produces a vicious circle in which the initiating stimulus produces more of the same. In a positive feedback system, exposure to an increase in environmental temperature would invoke compensatory mechanisms designed to increase rather than decrease body temperature.

Factors affecting adaptation to stress

Adaptation and homeostasis are idealized concepts. In practice, the body has available to it a wide variety and range of responses for adjusting to

* Some of the amplifying circuits in the nervous system function through positive feedback mechanisms.

the external and internal environments, and conditions do not always return to their original state.

Generally speaking, adaptation affects the whole person. When adapting to stress, the body uses those behaviors that are most efficient and effective—the body will not "use a baseball bat to kill a mosquito." Nor will the body use long-term mechanisms when short-term adaptation mechanisms are sufficient. The increase in heart rate that accompanies a febrile illness is a temporary response designed to deliver additional oxygen to the tissues during the short period when the elevated temperature increases the metabolic needs of the tissues (the increase in heart rate also expedites delivery of heat-carrying blood to the skin surface, where the heat can be lost to the external environment). On the other hand, adaptive responses such as hypertrophy of the left ventricle in persons with systemic hypertension are long-term responses.

Adaptation is affected by a number of factors, including previous experience and learning, physiologic reserve, rapidity of onset, genetic endowment and age, health status, nutrition, circadian rhythms, and psychosocial factors (Figure 6-5).

Previous experience and learning

Dubos cites the case of an old Chinese fisherman (the type depicted on the scrolls of the Sung era) as an example of the effect that experience and learning have on adaptation:

> The fisherman appears fully at ease and relaxed in his primitive boat, floating on a misty lake, or even a

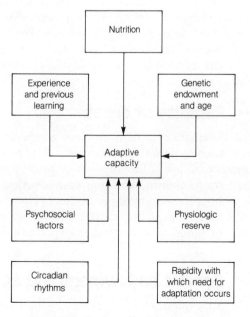

Figure 6-5 Factors affecting adaptation.

polluted and crowded harbor. He has probably experienced many tribulations in the course of his years of struggle and poverty, but has survived by becoming almost totally identified with his environment. In fact he is so well adapted to it that he will probably live for many more years, without modern comfort, sanitation, or medical care, just by letting his existence be ruled by what he considers to be the inalterable laws of the seasons and nature. . . . In the course of his life, he developed different protective mechanisms that increased his immunologic, physiologic, and psychic resistance to the physico-chemical hardships, the parasites, and the social conflicts which threatened him every day. Finally, he has elected to spend the rest of his life in the environment in which he has evolved and to which he has become adapted. Robust though he appears and really is, he probably would soon become sick if he moved into an area where the parasites, physiologic stresses, and social customs differ from the ones among which he has spent his early life.[10]

Physiologic reserve

The trained athlete is able to increase cardiac output 6- to 7-fold during exercise. The safety margin for adaptation of most body systems is considerably greater than that needed for normal activities. The red blood cells carry more oxygen than the tissues can use, the liver and fat cells store excess nutrients, and bone tissue has a storage of calcium in excess of that needed for normal neuromuscular function. The ability of body systems to increase their function given the need to adapt is known as the *physiologic reserve*. It is noteworthy that many of the body organs such as the lungs, kidneys, and adrenal glands are paired to provide not only a physiologic but an *anatomic reserve* as well. Both organs are not needed to ensure the continued existence and maintenance of the internal environment. Many individuals function normally with only one lung or one kidney. In kidney disease, for example, signs of renal failure do not occur until about 90% of the functioning nephrons have been destroyed.

Rapidity of onset

Adaptation is most efficient when changes occur gradually rather than suddenly. It is possible, for instance, to lose a liter or more of blood through chronic gastrointestinal bleeding over a period of a week without developing signs of shock. However, a sudden hemorrhage that causes loss of an equal amount of blood is apt to cause hypotension and shock.

Genetic endowment and age

Adaptation is further affected by the availability of adaptive responses and flexibility in selecting the most appropriate and economical response. The greater the number of available responses, the more effective the capacity to adapt.

Genetic endowment can ensure that the systems that are essential to adaptation—the immune system, the metabolism and waste elimination systems, and so on—function adequately. Even a gene that has deleterious effects may prove adaptive in some environments. In Africa, the gene for sickle cell anemia persists in some populations because it provides some resistance to the parasite that causes malaria.[10]

The capacity to adapt is decreased at the extremes of age. The ability to adapt is impaired by the immaturity of an infant as it is by the decline in functional reserve that occurs with age. For example, the infant has difficulty concentrating urine because of immature renal structures and is therefore less able than an adult to cope with decreased water intake or exaggerated water losses. A similar situation exists in the elderly due to age-related changes in renal function.

Health status

Health status, both physical and mental, determines physiologic and psychologic reserves and is a strong determinant of the ability to adapt. For example, persons with heart disease are less able to adjust to stresses that require the recruitment of cardiovascular responses. Likewise, severe emotional stress often produces disruption of physiologic function and limits the ability to make appropriate choices related to long-term adaptive needs. Those who have worked with acutely ill persons know that the will to live often has a profound influence on survival during life-threatening illnesses.

Nutrition

There are 50 to 60 essential nutrients, including minerals, lipids, certain fatty acids, vitamins, and specific amino acids. Deficiencies or excesses of any of these nutrients can alter one's health status and impair the ability to adapt. The importance of nutrition to enzyme function, immune response, and wound healing are well known. On a worldwide basis, malnutrition may be one of the most common causes of immunodeficiency. Among the problems associated with dietary excess are obesity and alcohol abuse. Obesity is a common problem. It predisposes to a number of health problems, including atherosclerosis and hypertension. Alcohol is a well-known nutrient that is often used in excess. It acutely affects the brain function and, with long-term use, can seriously impair the function of the liver, brain, and other vital structures.

— Circadian rhythms

Time and rhythms are fundamental properties of life. In the past 20 to 30 years it has become increasingly evident that biologic rhythms play an important role in adaptation to stress, the development of illness, and response to medical treatment.

Although the previously discussed concepts of homeostasis and the constancy of the internal environment hold true, most of the bodily functions are continuously changing, many with a regular oscillatory rhythm. The frequencies of bodily rhythms cover almost every dimension of time (*e.g.*, some brain waves have a rhythm that oscillates once per fraction of a second, respiration has a rhythm of several seconds, and the menstrual cycle a monthly rhythm). Many rhythms such as sleep, rest and activity, work and leisure, and eating and drinking oscillate with a frequency similar to that of the 24-hour light–dark solar day. The term *circadian*, from the Latin *circa* (about) and *dies* (day) is used to describe these 24-hour diurnal rhythms.

The first studies of endogenous circadian rhythms in human subjects isolated from time cues were conducted in cellars or caves in which time, light, temperature, noise, and social cues could be controlled or eliminated.[13,14] Subsequent studies have been done in specially constructed isolation rooms. Under these conditions, the fundamental properties of human circadian rhythms have been more thoroughly defined. When a biologic rhythm persists in the absence of any environmental periodicity it is said to be free-running. It has been found that human beings have a free-running period of about 25 hours; therefore, if their circadian pacemakers were not reset (exposed to environmental cues), they would lose about 1 hour out of the 24-hour clock each day.

Circadian rhythms can arise from within the organism or they can develop as the result of environmental influences. Geographic events such as temperature, light and dark, and seasonal cycles, which occur periodically, serve as regular, predictable environmental synchronizers for circadian rhythms. The process of synchronization of the biologic clock by environmental influences is termed *entrainment*. Hunger can be entrained by meal schedules. The external influences that are capable of entraining the biologic clock have been given the name *zeitgebers* from the German word meaning time-giver or synchronizer. Endogenous circadian rhythms arise from within the individual.

Figure 6-6 shows the normal circadian rhythms for sleep stages, body temperature, plasma concentrations of growth hormone and cortisol, and urinary excretion of potassium. The body temperature is highest in the evening and lowest at the end of sleep time. Adrenocorticotropic hormone (ACTH) and

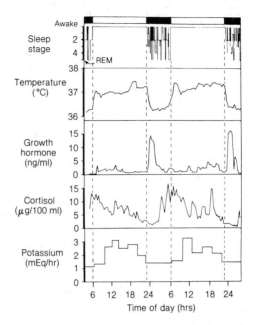

Figure 6-6 Circadian rhythms in sleep, body temperature, plasma concentration of growth hormone and plasma cortisol, and urinary excretion of potassium measured over 48 hr in a normal human subject. Sleep stages include rapid-eye-movement (REM) sleep and non-REM sleep, stages 1 through 4. Body temperature was measured rectally. The light–dark cycle is indicated by the horizontal bar at top. (*Moore-Ede MC, Czeisler CA, Richardson GS: Circadian timekeeping in health and disease. N Engl J Med 309[9]:330, 1983*)

cortisol are secreted in tandem. In persons with a normal sleep-wake cycle, serum cortisol levels reach their peak shortly after rising, at about 8 A.M. or 9 A.M. Growth hormone is secreted at the onset of sleep. Evidence suggests that endogenous control of circadian rhythms is vested in neurons that are located in the suprachiasmatic nucleus of the hypothalamus.[15]

As was mentioned previously, endogenous circadian rhythms adopt a longer, 25-hour day when studied under free-running conditions. The circadian rhythms for body temperature, urine elimination, and cortisol secretion maintain a free-running rhythm when an individual becomes desynchronized from the environment. This has been shown to be true in blind persons who are not exposed to the usual light-dark stimuli. The sleep–wakefulness cycle has been shown to be weakly entrained. For 20% to 30% of subjects under free-running conditions in one study, the period between awakenings became longer than 25 hours, lengthening to 30 to 33 hours in some subjects.[16] In these individuals the vegetative functions of temperature control, urine elimination, and cortisol secretion remained on a 25-hour rhythm.

Like any physiologic regulatory system, the circadian system occasionally misfunctions. In some disease states, such as Cushing's disease, there is a loss of circadian rhythms for cortisol. Periodic mood swings from mania to hypomania to depression in manic-depressive patients have been linked to changes in phase relationships of circadian rhythms.[16] Internal desynchronization of rhythms may explain some sleep disorders. Aschoff suggests that some of the sleep problems in the elderly may arise from loss of entrainment of the circadian system.[13]

Important questions related to circadian rhythms are whether or not certain pharmacologic agents have different effects when given at different times of the day or night and whether or not the degree of their effectiveness depends on the time of administration. Halberg, using laboratory mice, has shown that the sensitivity of the organism to many stimuli, including ethanol, barbiturates, and exposure to carcinogens, is quite different at different times of the day or night and depends on the phase of the circadian rhythm. In the human, it has been shown that administration of corticosteroid drugs produces less suppression of the hypothalamic-hypophyseal-adrenal axis when synchronized with the normal circadian peaks in cortisol levels.[14]

Shift changes and the time-zone changes associated with transcontinental flights are external influences that affect circadian rhythms. Shift changes usually involve a conflict situation in which the sleep–wakefulness cycle is reversed while social contacts keep the night worker entrained to a day-active cycle. With transcontinental flight, there is a complete phase shift in circadian rhythms. For a time change of 5 to 6 hours it takes several days to become entrained to local time. Less time is usually required to adjust after westward flights than after eastward flights, probably because the endogenous clock adjust more readily to a longer day than to a shorter day.[17]

Psychosocial factors

A number of studies relate social factors and life events to illness. Scientific interest in the social environment as a cause of stress has gradually broadened to include the social environment as a resource that modulates the relationship between stress and health. For example, married persons have consistently been found to be mentally and physically healthier than unmarried persons, these differences being more pronounced among men than among women.[18,19]

Social networks contribute in a number of ways to an individual's psychosocial and physical integrity. The configuration of significant others that constitutes this network functions to mobilize the resources of the individual; these people share the individual's tasks and provide monetary support, materials and tools, and guidance in improving problem-solving capabilities.[20] There is evidence that persons who have social supports or social assets may live longer and have a lower incidence of somatic illness.[21,22] Social support has been viewed in terms of both the number of relationships a person has and the person's perception of these relationships. Thus, close relations with others can involve not only positive effects but also the potential for conflict and may, in some situations, leave the individual less able to cope with life stressors. There is also the belief that social supports are likely to be protective only in the presence of stressful circumstances.[23]

Holmes and Rahe (1967) defined *social stressors* as any set of circumstances the advent of which signifies or requires changes in an individual's ongoing life pattern.[24] According to this definition, exposure to social stresses does not cause disease but may alter the individual's susceptibility at a particular time and may therefore serve as a precipitating factor. A Schedule of Recent Experiences, developed by Holmes and Rahe, is an instrument used to measure recent life experiences. The scale lists 43 life changes (*e.g.*, promotion, divorce, being fired) to which subjects respond by indicating how many times in the preceding year each event has occurred. Each event is rated with a score, and the sum of these scores is used to determine the amount of stress associated with recent life change events.

In summary, physiologic adaptation involves the ability to maintain the constancy of the internal environment in the face of a wide range of changes in the internal and external environments. It involves control systems that regulate cellular function, control life's processes, and integrate the function of the different body systems. Adaptation is affected by a number of factors, including experience and previous learning, the rapidity with which the need to adapt occurs, genetic endowment and age, health status, nutrition, circadian rhythms, and psychosocial factors.

Treatment of stress

Stress is a normal part of everyday life. However, excessive or inappropriate stress responses can disrupt normal functioning and contribute to the production of disease. Among the nonpharmacologic methods used to assist individuals in controlling the manifestations of the stress response are biofeedback, relaxation, and imagery.

Biofeedback

Biofeedback is a technique in which an individual learns to control physiologic functioning. It involves electronic monitoring of one or more physiologic responses to stress with immediate feedback of the specific response to the person undergoing treatment. Basmajian defined biofeedback as "the technique for using equipment (usually electronic) to reveal to human beings some of their internal physiological events, normal and abnormal, in the form of visual and auditory signals in order to teach them to manipulate these otherwise involuntary or unfelt events by manipulating the displayed signal."[25]

Several types of responses are currently used: electromyographic (EMG), electrothermal, and electrodermal (EDR). The EMG response involves the measurement of electrical potentials from muscles, usually the forearm extensor or frontalis. This is used to gain control over the contraction of striated skeletal muscles that occurs with anxiety and tension. The electrothermal sensors monitor the skin temperature of the fingers or toes. The sympathetic nervous system exerts significant control over blood flow to the distal parts of the body such as the digits of the hands and feet. Consequently, anxiety is often manifested by a decrease in the skin temperature of the digits of the hands and feet. The EDR sensors measure tonic or phasic changes in the electrical activity or conductivity of the skin (usually the hands) in response to anxiety. Fearful and anxious persons often have cold and clammy hands, which leads to an increase in conductivity.

Biofeedback is used to treat anxiety and tension in conditions such as vascular and tension headaches, Raynaud's disease, and low back pain.

── Relaxation

Practices for evoking the relaxation response are numerous. They are found in virtually every culture, and are credited with a generalized decrease in sympathetic nervous system activity and in musculoskeletal tension. According to Benson, four elements are integral to the various relaxation techniques: (1) a repetitive mental device, (2) a passive attitude, (3) decreased muscle tonus, and (4) a quiet environment. Benson developed a simple noncultural method that is commonly used for achieving relaxation. The instructions for this technique are as follows:

> Sit quietly in a comfortable position. Close your eyes. Deeply relax all your muscles, beginning at your feet and progressing up to your face. Keep them deeply relaxed.
>
> Breathe through your nose. Become aware of your breathing. As you breathe out, say the word "one" silently to yourself. Continue for 20 minutes. You may open your eyes to check the time, but do not use an alarm. When you are finished, sit quietly for several minutes, at first with closed eyes and later with open eyes.
>
> Do not worry about whether you are successful in achieving a deep level of relaxation. Maintain a positive attitude and permit relaxation to occur at its own pace. Expect distracting thoughts, ignore them, and continue repeating "one."

> Practice the technique once or twice daily, but not within two hours after a meal, since the digestive processes seem to interfere with elicitation of the anticipated changes.[26]

Progressive muscle relaxation, originally developed by Edmund Jacobson, is another method of relieving tension.[27] His procedure consisted of approximately 50 training sessions. Jacobson's methods have been modified by a number of therapists in an effort to increase their efficiency and practicality.[28,29] Progressive muscle relaxation involves the systematic contraction and relaxation of major muscle groups (typically, 15 groups are used initially). As the person learns to relax, the various muscle groups are combined. Eventually, the person learns to relax individual muscle groups without first contracting them.[30]

── Imagery

Imagery is another technique that can be used to achieve relaxation. One method is scene visualization, in which the person is asked to sit back, close the eyes, and concentrate on a scene narrated by the therapist. Whenever possible all five senses are involved; the person is asked to see, feel, smell, hear, and taste aspects of the visual experience. Other types of imagery involve imaging the appearance of each of the major muscle groups and how they feel during tension.

In summary, stress is a normal part of everyday living. However, when the stress response is excessive or inappropriate, it can disrupt body function and contribute to disease production. Nonpharmacologic methods used in the treatment of stress include biofeedback, relaxation, and imagery. Biofeedback involves the electronic monitoring of one or more physiological responses with immediate feedback of the response to the person undergoing treatment. Relaxation involves physical and mental exercises to achieve mental relaxation and a decrease in muscle tension. Imagery uses scene visualization as a means of controlling the stress response.

References

1. Burchfield SR: The stress response: A new perspective. Psychosom Med 41:661, 1979
2. Hartmann F: An anthropological consideration of the stress response. Contrib Nephrol 30:7, 1982
3. Selye H: The evolution of the stress concept. Am Sci 61:692, 1973
4. Mason JW: The re-evaluation of the concept of nonspecificity in stress theory. J Psychiatr Res 7:323, 1971
5. Cohen F: Stress and bodily illness. Psychiatr Clin North Am 4, No. 2:269, 1981

6. Berne RM, Levy MN: Physiology. St. Louis, CV Mosby, 1983

7. Selye H: Stress Without Distress, p 6. New York, New American Library, 1974

8. Dworkin SF: Psychosomatic concepts and dentistry: Some perspectives. J Peridontol 40:647, 1969

9. Solomon GF, Amkraut GF: Psychoneuroendocrinological effects on the immune response. Annu Rev Microbiol 35:155–184, 1981

10. Dubos R: Man Adapting, pp 256, 258, 261, 264. New Haven, Yale University Press, 1965

11. Cannon WB: The Wisdom of the Body, pp 299–300. New York: WW Norton, 1932

12. Guyton AC: Textbook of Medical Physiology, 7th ed, p 8. Philadelphia, WB Saunders, 1986

13. Aschoff J: Circadian systems in man and their implications. Hosp Pract 11, No. 5:51, 1976

14. Halberg F: Implications of biological rhythms for clinical practice. Hosp Pract 12, No. 1:139, 1977

15. Wagner DR, Weitzman ED: Neuroendocrine secretion and biological rhythms in man. Psychiatr Clin North Am 3, No. 2:223, 1980

16. Wehr TA, Muscettola G, Goodwin FK et al: Phase advance of the circadian sleep-wake cycle as an antidepressant. Science 206:710, 1979

17. Arendt J, Marks V: Physiological changes underlying jet lag. Br Med J 284:144, 1982

18. Ortmeyer CF: Variations in mortality, morbidity, and health care by marital status. In Erhardt CE, Berlin JE (eds): Mortality and Morbidity in the United States. Cambridge, Harvard University Press, 1974

19. Gove WR: Sex, marital status, and mortality. Am J Sociol 79:45, 1973

20. Greenblatt M, Becerra RM, Serafetinides EA: Social networks and mental health: An overview. Am J Psychiatr 139, No. 8:977, 1982

21. Berkman LF, Syme S: Social networks, host resistance, and mortality: A nine-year follow-up study of Alameda County residents. Am J Epidemiol 109:186, 1979

22. House JS, Robbins C, Metzner HL: The association of social relationships and activities with mortality: Prospective evidence from the Tecumseh Community Health Study. Am J Epidemiol 116:123, 1982

23. Kaplan BH, Cassel J, Gore S: Social support and health. Med Care 15, No. 5 (Suppl):48, 1977

24. Holmes TH, Rahe RH: The social readjustment rate scale. J Psychosom Res 11:213, 1967

25. Basmajian J: Biofeedback—Principles and Practice for Clinicians. Baltimore, Williams & Wilkins, 1979

26. Benson H: Systemic hypertension and the relaxation response. N Engl J Med 296, No. 20:1152, 1977

27. Jacobson E: Progressive Relaxation. Chicago, University of Chicago Press, 1958

28. Wolpe J: The Practice of Behavior Therapy. New York, Pergamon, 1973

29. Nigl A, Fischer-Williams M: Treatment of musculo-ligamentous low back strain with electromyographic biofeedback and relaxation training. Psychosomatics 21:495, 1980

30. Fischer-Williams M, Nigl AF, Sovine DL: A Textbook of Biological Feedback. New York, Human Science Press, 1981

Bibliography

—— Circadian rhythms

Bassler SF: The origins and development of biological rhythms. Nurs Clin N Am 11:575, 1976

Minors DS, Waterhouse JM: Circadian Rhythms and the Human. Boston, Wright PSG, 1981

Moore-Ede MC, Czeisler CA, Richardson GS: Circadian timekeeping in health and disease: Basic properties of circadian pacemakers. N Engl J Med 309:469, 1983

Moore-Ede MC, Czeisler CA, Richardson GS: Circadian timekeeping in health and disease: Clinical implications of circadian rhythmicity. N Engl J Med 309:530, 1983

Reisne T: Neurohumoral aspects of ACTH release. Hosp Pract 23 (3):77, 1988

Smolensky MH, Reinberg A: The chronotherapy of corticosteroids: practical application of chronobiologic findings to nursing. Nurs Clin N Am 11:609, 1976

Stephens GJ: Periodicity in mood, affect, and instinctual behavior. Nurs Clin N Am 11:595, 1976

Takahashi JS, Zatz M: Regulation of circadian rhythmicity. Science 217:1104, 1982

Tom CK: Nursing assessment of biological rhythms. Nurs Clin N Am 11:621, 1976

Weitzman ED: Biologic rhythms and hormone secretion patterns. Hosp Prac 8:79, 1976

Zucker I: Light, behavior, and biologic rhythms. Hosp Prac 10:83, 1976

—— Stress

Brown GM, Seggie J: Neuroendocrine mechanisms and their implications for psychiatric research. Psych Clin N Am 3:205, 1980

Ganong WF: The stress response—A dynamic overview. Hosp Pract 23 (6):155, 1988

Davenport HW: Signs of anxiety, rage or distress. Physiologist 24:1, 1981

Haggerty RJ: Breaking the link between stress and illness in children. Postgrad Med 74:287, 1983

Haskett RF, Rose RM: Neuroendocrine disorders and psychopathology. Psych Clin N Am 4:239, 1981

McEwen BS: Glucocorticoid receptors in the brain. Hosp Pract 23 (8):107, 1988

Mills FJ: The endocrinology of stress. Aviat Space Environ Med 56:642, 1985

Rose RM: Endocrine responses to stressful psychological events. Psych Clin N Am 3:251, 1980

Sachar EJ, Asni G, Halbreich U, Nathan RS, Halpern F: Recent studies in the neuroendocrinology of major depressive disorders. Psych Clin N Am 3:313, 1980

Selye H: Confusion and controversy in the stress field. J Human Stress 6:37, 1975

Stein M: A biophysical approach to immune function and medical disorders. Psych Clin N Am 4:203, 1981

Strain GW: Nutrition, brain function and behavior. Psych Clin N Am 4:253, 1981

Timmreck TC, Braza GF, Mitchell JH: Stress and aging. Geriatrics 6:113, 1980

Winogrod IR: Health, stress, and coping in the elderly. Wis Med J 81:27, 1982

CHAPTER 7

Alterations in Temperature Regulation

Objectives

After you have studied this chapter, you should be able to meet the following objectives:

_____ Differentiate between body core temperature and skin temperature and relate the differences to methods used for measuring body temperature.

_____ Describe the mechanisms of heat production in the body.

_____ Define the terms _conduction, radiation, convection,_ and _evaporation_ and relate them to the mechanisms for heat loss from the body.

_____ Name the stimulus for changing the set point of the thermoregulatory center in fever.

_____ Describe the four stages of fever.

_____ Cite the possible purposes of fever.

_____ Explain what is meant by intermittent, remittent, sustained, and relapsing fevers.

_____ State the relationship between body temperature and heart rate.

_____ List the five goals of fever treatment and provide at least one example of treatment for each goal.

_____ Explain the action of aspirin and acetaminophen in reducing body temperature during fever.

_____ Explain the mechanism of fever reduction through the use of tepid sponge baths and a cooling mattress.

_____ Differentiate between the physiological mechanisms involved in fever and hyperthermia.

_____ List the possible mechanisms of drug-related fevers.

_____ Compare the mechanisms of malignant hyperthermia and neuroleptic malignant syndrome.

_____ State the definition of hypothermia.

_____ Explain the reason that children can sometimes survive asphyxia and submersion hypothermia.

_____ Describe special precautions that are needed when monitoring body temperature in a person with hypothermia.

_____ Compare the manifestations of mild, moderate, and severe hypothermia and relate to changes in physiologic functioning that occur with decreased body temperature.

_____ Describe methods for achieving passive, active total, and active core rewarming.

Virtually all biochemical processes in the body are affected by changes in temperature. Metabolic processes speed up or slow down depending on whether body temperature is rising or falling. Body temperature is normally maintained within a range of 35.8°C to 37.4°C (96.6–99.3°F). Within this range there are individual differences and diurnal variations; internal core temperatures reach their highest point in late afternoon and evening and their lowest point in the early morning hours (Figure 7-1). The content in this chapter is organized into three sections: regulation of body temperature, fever and hyperthermia, and hypothermia.

Body temperature regulation

Body temperature reflects the difference between heat production and heat loss and varies with exercise and extremes of temperature. Properly protected, the body can function in environmental conditions that range from −50°C (−58°F) to +50°C (122°F). Individual body cells, however, cannot tolerate such a wide range of temperatures—at −1°C (30.2°F), ice crystals form; and at +45°C (113°F), cell proteins coagulate. It is only for short periods of time that cells can tolerate an internal body temperature of +41°C.[1]

Most of the body's heat is produced by the deeper core tissues (muscles and viscera) of the body, which are insulated from the environment and protected against heat loss by the subcutaneous tissues and skin (Figure 7-2). Adipose tissue is a particularly good insulator, conducting heat only one-third as effectively as other tissues. Heat loss occurs when the heat from the body's inner core is transferred to the skin surface by the circulating blood. If no heat were lost by the body at rest, the temperature of the body would rise 1°C (1.8°F)/hr; with light work, the temperature would rise 2°C/hr.

Temperatures differ in various parts of the body, core temperatures being higher than those at the skin surface. Generally the rectal temperature is used as a measure of core temperature. Core temperatures may also be obtained from the esophagus using a flexible thermosensor. The oral temperature, taken sublingually, is usually 0.2°C (0.36°F) to 0.51°C (0.9°F) lower than the rectal temperature. Rectal temperature probably provides a more accurate estimate of core temperature during exercise involving the legs, since the blood from the exercising muscles returns to the circulation by way of the abdominal veins. Because of location, esophageal temperatures closely reflect the temperature of the heart and thoracic organs. The axillary temperature can also be used as an estimate of core temperature. However, the parts of the body shell must be pressed closely together because this method requires considerable heat to accumulate before the final temperature is reached.

Body temperature is regulated by the thermoregulatory center in the hypothalamus. This center integrates input from various thermal receptors located throughout the body with output responses that either conserve body heat or increase its dissipation. It is the temperature of the body core rather than surface temperature that is regulated. The thermostatic set point of the thermoregulatory center is set so that the temperature of the body is regulated within the previously mentioned normal range of 35.8°C to 37.4°C. When body temperature begins to rise above the normal range, heat-dissipating behaviors are initiated; when the temperature falls below the normal range, heat production is increased. Core temperatures above 41°C (105.8°F) or below 34°C (93.2°F) usually mean that thermoregulation is impaired (Figure 7-3). Body responses that produce, conserve, and dissipate heat are described in Table 7-1. Spinal cord injuries

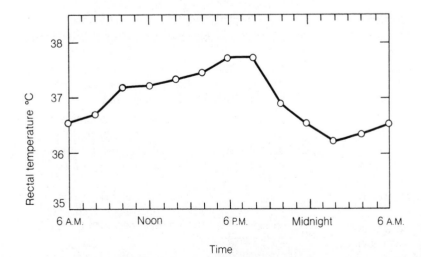

Figure 7-1 Normal diurnal variations in body temperature.

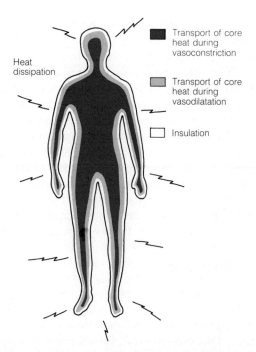

Figure 7-2 Control of heat loss. Body heat is produced in the deeper core tissues of the body, which is insulated by the subcutaneous tissues and skin to protect against heat loss. During vasodilatation, circulating blood transports heat to the skin surface, where it dissipates into the surrounding environment. Vasoconstriction decreases the transport of core heat to the skin surface and vasodilatation increases transport.

Legend:
- Transport of core heat during vasoconstriction
- Transport of core heat during vasodilatation
- Insulation

Heat dissipation

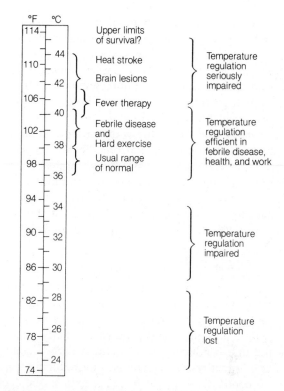

Figure 7-3 Body temperatures under different conditions. (*Dubois EF: Fever and the Regulation of Body Temperature. Springfield, IL, Charles C Thomas, 1948*)

that transect the cord at the cervical level can seriously impair temperature regulation. This is because the hypothalamus can no longer control skin blood flow or sweating.

Aside from the thermostatic mechanisms of temperature regulation, persons engage in other behaviors to regulate body temperature. These behaviors include the selection of proper clothing and regulation of environmental temperature through heating systems and air-conditioning. Body positions that hold the extremities close to the body prevent heat loss and are commonly assumed in cold weather.

Mechanisms of heat production

The body's main source of heat production is metabolism. There is a 1° Fahrenheit (0.56°C) increase in body temperature for every 7% increase in metabolism. The sympathetic neurotransmitters, epinephrine and norepinephrine, which are released when an increase in body temperature is needed, act at the cellular level to shift metabolism so that energy production (ATP) is reduced and heat production is increased. This may be one of the reasons that fever tends to produce feelings of weakness and fatigue. Thyroid hormone increases cellular metabolism, but this response usually requires several weeks to reach maximal effectiveness.

Fine involuntary actions such as shivering and chattering of the teeth can produce a three- to five-fold increase in body temperature. Shivering is initiated by impulses from the hypothalamus. The first muscle change that occurs with shivering is a general increase in muscle tone followed by an oscillating rhythmic tremor involving the spinal-level reflex that controls muscle tone. Because no external work is performed, all the energy liberated by the metabolic processes from shivering is in the form of heat.

Physical exertion increases body temperature. With strenuous exercise, more than three-quarters of the increased metabolism resulting from muscle activity appears as heat within the body and the remainder appears as external work.

Mechanisms of heat loss

Most of the body's heat losses occur at the skin surface as heat from the blood moves to the skin and from there into the environment. There are numerous arteriovenous (A-V) shunts under the skin surface that allow blood to move directly from the arterial to the venous system. These A-V shunts are much like the radiators in a heating system. When the shunts are open, body heat is freely dissipated to the skin and surrounding environment; when the shunts are closed, heat is retained in the body. The blood flow in the A-V shunts is controlled almost exclusively by the sympathetic nervous system in response to changes in core temperature and environmental temperature. Contraction of the pilomotor muscles of the skin, which produces goose bumps, reduces the surface area available for heat loss.

Heat is lost from the body through radiation, conduction, and convection from the skin surface; through the evaporation of sweat and insensible perspiration; through the warming and humidifying of inspired air; and through urine and feces. Of these mechanisms, only heat losses that occur at the skin surface are directly under hypothalamic control.

Conduction

Conduction is the direct transfer of heat from one molecule to another. Blood carries, or conducts, heat from the inner core of the body to the skin surface. Normally only a small amount of body heat is lost through conduction to a cooler surface. Cooling blankets or mattresses that are used for reducing fever rely on conduction of heat from the skin to the cool surface of the mattress. Heat can also be conducted in the opposite direction—from the external environment to the body surface. For instance, body temperature may rise slightly after a hot bath.

Water has a specific heat several times greater than air, so water absorbs far greater amounts of heat than air. Hence, the loss of body heat can be excessive and life-threatening in situations of cold water immersion or cold exposure in damp or wet clothing.

The conduction of heat to the body's surface is influenced by blood volume. In hot weather, the body compensates by increasing blood volume as a means of dissipating heat. Persons who are not acclimated to a hot environment can increase their total blood volume by 10% within 2 to 4 hours of heat exposure. A mild swelling of the ankles during hot weather provides evidence of blood volume expansion. Exposure to cold produces a cold diuresis and a reduction in blood volume as a means of controlling the transfer of heat to the body's surface.

Radiation

Radiation is the transfer of heat through the air or a vacuum. Heat from the sun is carried by radiation. Heat loss by radiation varies with the temperature of the environment. Environmental temperature must be less than that of the body for heat loss to occur. Normally about 60% to 70% of body heat is dissipated by radiation.

Convection

Convection refers to heat transfer through the circulation of air currents. Normally a layer of warm air tends to remain near the body's surface; convection

Table 7–1. Heat loss and heat gain responses used in regulation of body temperature

Heat gain		Heat loss	
Body response	Mechanism of action	Body response	Mechanism of action
Vasoconstriction of the superficial blood vessels	Confines blood flow to the inner core of the body, with the skin and subcutaneous tissues acting as insulation to prevent loss of core heat	Dilatation of the superficial blood vessels	Delivers blood containing core heat to the periphery where it is dissipated through: Radiation Conduction Convection
Contraction of the pilomotor muscles that surround the hairs on the skin	Reduces the heat loss surface of the skin	Sweating	Increases heat loss through evaporation
Assumption of the huddle position with the extremities held close to the body	Reduces the area for heat loss		
Shivering	Increases heat production by the muscles		
Increased production of epinephrine	Increases the heat production associated with metabolism		
Increased production of thyroid hormone	Is a long-term mechanism that increases metabolism and heat production		

causes continual removal of the warm layer and replacement with air from the surrounding environment. The wind-chill factor that is often included in the weather report combines the effect of convection due to wind with the actual still-air temperature.

Evaporation

Evaporation involves the use of body heat to convert water on the skin to water vapor. Water that diffuses through the skin independent of sweating is called insensible perspiration. Insensible water losses are greatest in a dry environment. Sweating occurs through the sweat glands and is controlled by the sympathetic nervous system. Unlike other sympathetically mediated functions, in which the catecholamines serve as neuromediators, sweating is mediated by acetylcholine. This means that anticholinergic drugs, such as atropine, can interfere with heat loss by interrupting sweating.

Evaporative heat losses involve both insensible perspiration and sweating, with 0.58 calories being lost for each gram of water that is evaporated.[2] As long as body temperature is greater than the atmospheric temperature, heat is lost through radiation. However, when the temperature of the surrounding environment becomes greater than skin temperature, evaporation is the only way the body can rid itself of heat. Any condition that prevents evaporative heat losses will cause the body temperature to rise.

In summary, body temperature is normally maintained within a range of 35.9°C to 37.4°C (96.6°F to 99.3°F). Most of the body's heat is produced by metabolic processes that occur within deeper core structures (muscles and viscera) of the body. Heat loss occurs at the body's surface when heat from core structures is transported to the skin by the circulating blood. Heat is lost from the body through radiation, conduction, convection, and evaporation. The thermoregulatory center in the hypothalamus functions to modify heat production and heat losses as a means of regulating body temperature.

Increased body temperature

Fever and hyperthermia describe an increase in body temperature that is outside the normal range. True fever is a disorder of thermoregulation in which there is upward displacement of the hypothalamic set point for temperature control. In hyperthermia the set point is unchanged, but the mechanisms that control body temperature are ineffective in meeting the challenge of maintaining body temperature during exposure to high ambient temperature or the excess heat production that occurs with strenuous exertion.

Fever

The literature on fever dates back to the writings of Hippocrates, which contain many descriptions of the febrile-course diseases, such as typhoid fever.[3] However, it was not until the development of the thermometer that actual measurements of body temperature became possible. One of the first studies of body temperature was conducted by the German physician Carl Wunderlich, who in 1868 studied the body temperature of 25,000 of his patients with observations made twice daily with a foot-long thermometer held in the axilla for a period of 20 minutes. From his observations, Wunderlich observed that the thermometer was a useful instrument for providing insight into the condition of the sick. Today temperature is one of the most frequent physiological responses to be monitored during illness.

Mechanisms

Fever, or pyrexia, describes an elevation in body temperature that is caused by an upward displacement of the set point of the hypothalamic thermoregulatory center. When the fever has broken, the set point returns to its prefever setting. Fevers that are regulated by the hypothalamus usually do not rise above 41°C (105.8°F), suggesting a built-in thermostatic safety mechanism. Temperatures above that level are usually the result of superimposed activity, such as convulsions, hyperthermic states, or direct involvement of the temperature control center.[4] The mechanisms for controlling temperature are not well developed in the infant. Hence, in infants under 3 months, a mild elevation in temperature (i.e., rectal temperature of 38°C [100.4°F]) can indicate serious infection and requires immediate medical attention.[5] The presence of fever in elderly persons is also more likely to indicate serious infection or disease.[6]

Fever can be caused by a number of substances that collectively incite the production of a fever-producing mediator called pyrogen. Pyrogen-producing substances include viruses, bacteria, and other microorganisms, products of inflammation, antigen-antibody complexes, drugs, and chemicals. These substances are ingested by macrophages that become activated and then release a substance that was formerly called endogenous pyrogen. Recently, endogenous pyrogen was found to be the same as interleukin-1, an inflammatory mediator that produces other signs of inflammation such as leukocytosis, anorexia, and malaise (see Chapter 10). Interleukin-1 produces fever by increasing the set point of the hypothalamic thermoregulatory center, probably through the action of prostaglandin E.

Many noninfectious disorders, such as myocardial infarction, pulmonary emboli, and neoplasms, produce fever. In these conditions the injured or abnormal cells incite the production of endogenous pyrogen (interleukin-1). For example, trauma and surgery can be associated with up to 3 days of fever.[7,8] Some malignant cells, such as those of leukemia and Hodgkin's disease, secrete endogenous pyrogen.

A fever that has its origin in the central nervous system is sometimes referred to as a *neurogenic fever*. It is usually caused by central nervous system trauma, intracerebral bleeding, or an increase in intracranial pressure. Neurogenic fevers are characterized by a high temperature that is resistant to antipyretic therapy and is not associated with sweating.

Purpose

The purpose of fever is not completely understood. However, from a purely practical standpoint, fever is a valuable index to health status. For many persons, fever signals the presence of an infection and may legitimize the need for treatment. In ancient times, fever was thought to "cook" the poisons that caused the illness. With the availability of antipyretic drugs in the late 19th century, the belief that fever was useful began to wane, probably because most antipyretic drugs also had analgesic effects. There is little research to support the belief that fever is harmful unless the temperature rises above 40°C (104°F). Animal studies have demonstrated a clear survival advantage in infected members with fever as compared with animals that were unable to develop a fever. It has been shown that small elevations in temperature like those that occur with fever enhance immune function. There is increased motility and activity of the white blood cells, stimulation of interferon production, and activation of T-cells.[9,10] Many of the microbial agents that cause infection grow best at normal body temperatures and their growth is inhibited by temperatures within the fever range. For example, the rhinoviruses responsible for the common cold are cultured best at 33°C (91.4°F), which is close to the temperature in the nasopharynx; temperature-sensitive mutants of virus that cannot grow at temperatures above 37.5°C (99.5°F) produce fewer signs and symptoms.[11]

Patterns

The patterns of temperature change in persons with fever vary and may provide information about the nature of the causative agent.[12,13] These patterns can be described as intermittent, remittent, sustained, or relapsing. An *intermittent* fever is one in which temperature returns to normal at least once every 24 hours. In a *remittent* fever, by contrast, the temperature does not return to normal and varies a few degrees in either direction. In a *sustained*, or *continuous*, fever the temperature remains above normal with minimal variations. A *recurrent* or *relapsing* fever is one in which there is one or more episodes of fever, each as long as several days, with one or more days of normal temperature between episodes.

Critical to the analysis of a fever pattern is the relationship of heart rate to the level of temperature elevation. Normally a 1°C rise in temperature produces a 15 beat/minute increase in heart rate (1°F, 10 beats/minute).[12] Most people respond to an increase in temperature with an appropriate increase in heart rate. The observation that a rise in temperature is not accompanied by the anticipated change in heart rate can provide useful information about the cause of the fever. For example, a heart rate that is slower than would be anticipated can occur with legionnaires' disease and drug fever, and a heart rate that is more rapid than anticipated can be symptomatic of hyperthyroidism and pulmonary emboli.

Manifestations

The reactions that occur in body temperature during fever usually consist of four stages: (1) a prodrome, (2) a chill during which the temperature rises, (3) a flush, and (4) defervescence.[14] During the first or prodromal period, there are nonspecific complaints such as mild headache and fatigue, general malaise, and fleeting aches and pains. Vasoconstriction and piloerection usually precede the onset of shivering. At this point the skin is pale and covered with goose flesh. There is a feeling of being cold and an urgency to put on more clothing or covering and to curl up in a position that conserves body heat. The prodromal stage is followed by the second stage—the onset of a generalized shaking chill; and even as the temperature rises, there is the uncomfortable sensation of being chilled. When the shivering has caused the body temperature to reach the new set point of the temperature control center, the shivering ceases and a sensation of warmth develops. At this point, the third stage begins, during which cutaneous vasodilation occurs and the skin becomes warm and flushed. The fourth, or defervescence, stage of the febrile response is marked by the initiation of sweating. Not all persons proceed through the four stages of fever development. Sweating may be absent and fever may develop gradually with no indication of a chill or shivering.

Common manifestations of fever are anorexia, myalgia, arthralgia, and fatigue. These discomforts are worse when the temperature rises rapidly or exceeds 39.5°C (103.1°F). Respiration is increased and the heart rate is usually elevated. The occurrence of chills commonly coincides with the introduction of pyrogen into the circulation. Many of the manifestations of fever are related to the increases in the metabolic rate, increased need for oxygen, and use of body proteins as an energy source. Dehydration occurs because of sweating and the rapid respiratory rate that results in increased vapor losses. With prolonged fever, there is increased breakdown of endogenous fat stores. If fat catabolism is rapid, metabolic acidosis may result.

Headache is a common accompaniment to fever and is thought to result from the vasodilation of cerebral vessels occurring with fever. Delirium is possible when the temperature in fever exceeds 40°C (104°F). In the elderly, confusion and delirium may follow moderate elevations in temperature. Due to increasingly poor oxygen uptake by the aging lung, pulmonary function may prove to be a limiting factor in the hypermetabolism that accompanies fever in older individuals. Confusion, incoordination, and agitation commonly reflect cerebral hypoxemia. Febrile convulsions can occur in some children. They usually occur with rapidly rising temperatures or at a threshold temperature that differs with each child.

Herpetic lesions, or fever blisters, that develop in some persons during fever are due to a separate infection by the type I herpes simplex virus that is activated by a rise in body temperature.

Treatment

The methods of fever treatment focus on (1) modification of the external environment as a means of increasing heat transfer from the internal to the external environment, (2) support of the hypermetabolic state that accompanies fever, (3) protection of vulnerable body organs and systems, and (4) treatment of the infection or condition causing the fever. Since fever is a disease symptom, its manifestation suggests the need for treatment of the primary cause.

Modification of the environment ensures that the environmental temperature facilitates heat transfer away from the body. Sponge baths (with cool water or an alcohol solution) can be used to increase evaporative heat losses. More profound cooling can be accomplished through the use of a cooling mattress, which facilitates the conduction of heat from the body into the coolant solution that circulates through the mattress. Care must be taken so that cooling methods do not produce vasoconstriction and shivering that decrease heat loss and increase heat production.

Adequate fluids and sufficient amounts of simple carbohydrates are needed to support the hypermetabolic state and to prevent the tissue break-

down that is characteristic of fever. Additional fluids are needed for sweating and to balance the insensible water losses from the lungs that accompany an increase in respiratory rate. Fluids are also needed to maintain an adequate vascular volume for heat transport to the skin surface.

Antipyretic drugs, such as aspirin and acetaminophen, are often used to alleviate the discomforts of fever and protect vulnerable organs, such as the brain, from extreme elevations in body temperature. These drugs act by inhibiting prostaglandin synthesis and thereby resetting the hypothalamic temperature control center to a lower level.

Hyperthermia

Hyperthermia describes an increase in body temperature that occurs without a change in the set point of the hypothalamic thermoregulatory center. It includes (in order of increasing severity) heat syncope, heat cramps, heat exhaustion, and heatstroke. Malignant hyperthermia describes a rare genetic disorder of anesthetic-related hyperthermia. Fever and hyperthermia may also occur as the result of a drug reaction.

A number of factors predispose to hyperthermia. If muscle exertion is continued for long periods in warm weather, as often happens with athletes, military recruits, and laborers, excessive heat loads are generated.[15] Adequate circulatory function is essential for heat dissipation. Elderly persons and persons with cardiovascular disease are at increased risk. Drugs that increase muscle tone and metabolism or reduce heat loss can impair thermoregulation. Infants and small children who are left in a closed car for even short periods of time in hot weather are potential victims of hyperthermia. Florence Nightingale in *Notes on Nursing* observed that an excess of blankets is the commonest cause of fever in the hospital.[16]

Heat syncope

Heat syncope is characterized by a sudden episode of unconsciousness resulting from cutaneous vasodilation and subsequent hypotension. Usually the episode follows vigorous exercise. The systolic blood pressure is usually less than 100 mmHg, the pulse is weak, and the skin is cool and moist. The treatment consists of recumbency and rest in a cool place and administration of fluids by mouth or intravenously.

Heat cramps

Heat cramps are slow, painful, skeletal muscle cramps and spasms, usually in the muscles that are most heavily used, that last for 1 to 3 minutes. Cramping results from salt depletion that occurs when fluid losses due to heavy sweating are replaced by water alone. The muscles are tender, and the skin is usually moist. Body temperature may be normal or slightly elevated. There is almost always a history of vigorous activity preceding the onset of symptoms.

Treatment consists of drinking an oral saline solution and resting in a cool environment. Because their absorption is slow and unpredictable, salt tablets are not recommended. Salt tablets can also cause gastric irritation, vomiting, and cerebral edema. Strenuous physical activity should be avoided for several days, while dietary sodium replacement is continued.

Heat exhaustion

Heat exhaustion is related to a gradual loss of salt and water, usually following prolonged and heavy exertion in a hot environment. The symptoms include thirst, fatigue, nausea, oliguria, giddiness, and finally delirium. Gastrointestinal flu-like symptoms are common. Hyperventilation in association with heat exhaustion may contribute to heat cramps and tetany by causing respiratory alkalosis. The skin is moist, the rectal temperature is usually over 37.8°C (100°F), and the heart rate is elevated (usually more than half again the normal resting rate). Signs of heat syncope and heat cramps may accompany heat exhaustion.

Like heat cramps, heat exhaustion is treated by rest in a cool environment, the provision of adequate hydration, and salt replacement. Intravenous fluids are administered when adequate oral intake cannot be achieved.

Heatstroke

Heatstroke is a severe, life-threatening failure of thermoregulatory mechanisms resulting in an excessive rise in body temperature—a core temperature greater than 40°C (104°F), absence of sweating, and loss of consciousness. Evaporation serves as the major mechanism for heat dissipation in a warm environment, and conditions that interrupt this mechanism predispose to increased body temperature and heatstroke.

Heatstroke is seen most commonly in the elderly and disabled. Mortality may be as high as 80% in persons over 65 years of age. In the United States, approximately 5000 deaths occur each year from heatstroke, two-thirds of these in persons over age 60 years.[17] In the elderly, the problem is often one of impaired heat loss and failure of homeostatic mechanisms, so body temperature rises with any increase in environmental temperature. Elderly persons with decreased perception of environmental temperature changes and decreased mobility are at particular risk, since they may also be unable to take appropriate measures such as removing clothing, moving to a

cooler environment, and increasing fluid intake. This is particularly true of elderly individuals who live alone in small and poorly ventilated housing units and who may be too confused or weak to complain or seek help at the onset of symptoms.

The symptoms of heatstroke include dizziness, weakness, emotional lability, nausea and vomiting, confusion, delirium, blurred vision, convulsions, collapse, and coma. The skin is hot and usually dry, and the pulse is typically strong initially. The blood pressure may be elevated at first, but hypotension develops as the condition progresses. As vascular collapse occurs, the skin becomes cool.

Associated abnormalities include electrocardiograph changes consistent with heart damage, blood coagulation disorders, potassium and sodium depletion, and signs of liver damage.

Treatment consists of rapidly reducing the core temperature. Care must be taken that the cooling methods used do not produce vasoconstriction or shivering and thereby decrease the cooling rate or induce heat production. Two general methods of cooling are used. One method involves submersion in cold water or application of ice packs, and the other, spraying the body with tepid water while a fan is used to enhance heat dissipation through convection. Whatever method is used, it is important that the temperature of vital structures, such as the brain, heart, and liver be reduced rapidly since tissue damage ensues when core temperatures rise above 43°C (109.4°F). Selective brain cooling has been reported by fanning the face during hyperthermia.[18,19] Blood flows from the emissary venous pathways of the skin on the head through the bones of the skull to the brain. In hyperthermia, face fanning is thought to cool the venous blood that flows through these emissary veins and thereby produce brain cooling by enhancing heat exchange between the hot arterial blood and the surface-cooled venous blood within the intracranial venous spaces.

Malignant hyperthermia

Malignant hyperthermia is an autosomal dominant metabolic disorder in which heat generated by uncontrolled skeletal muscle contraction can produce severe and potentially fatal hyperthermia. The muscle contraction is caused by an abnormal release of intracellular calcium from the mitochondria and sarcoplasmic reticulum (see Chapter 1).

In affected persons an episode of malignant hyperthermia is triggered by exposure to certain stresses or general anesthetic agents. The incidence of malignant hyperthermia from anesthetic agents is 1 in 15,000 in children and 1 in 50,000 to 100,000 in adults.[20] The syndrome is most frequently associated with the halogenated anesthetic agents and the depolarizing muscle relaxant succinylcholine.[21] There are also various nonoperative precipitating factors, including trauma, exercise, environmental heat stress, and infection. The condition is particularly dangerous in a young person who has a large muscle mass to generate heat.

During malignant hyperthermia the body temperature rises as high as 43°C (109.4°F) at a rate of 1°C every five minutes. An initial sign of the disorder, when the condition occurs during anesthesia, is skeletal-muscle rigidity. Cardiac arrhythmias and a hypermetabolic state follow in rapid sequence unless the triggering event is immediately discontinued. In addition to discontinuing the triggering agents, treatment includes measures to cool the body and the administration of dantrolene, a muscle relaxant drug. At present there is no accurate screening test for the condition. A family history of malignant hyperthermia should be considered when general anesthesia is needed, since there are agents available that do not trigger the hyperthermic response.

Drug fever and neuroleptic malignant syndrome

Drug fever has been defined as fever coinciding with the administration of a drug and disappearing once the drug has been discontinued.[22–24] Drugs can induce fever by several mechanisms: they can interfere with heat dissipation; they can alter temperature regulation by the hypothalamic centers; they can act as direct pyrogens; they can injure tissues directly; or they can induce an immune response.[21] Peripheral heat dissipation can be impaired by atropine, antihistamines, and tricyclic antidepressants, which decrease sweating, or by sympathomimetic drugs, which produce peripheral vasoconstriction. Thyroid hormone can increase heat production. Bleomycin (an anticancer drug), amphotericin B (an antifungal drug), and allergic extracts and vaccines that contain bacterial and viral products can all act to induce the release of pyrogens. Intravenously administered drugs can lead to infusion-related phlebitis with production of cellular pyrogens that produce fever. Treatment with anticancer drugs can cause the release of endogenous pyrogen from the cancer cells that are destroyed. Administration of certain anesthetic agents can cause life-threatening malignant hyperthermia in genetically predisposed individuals. Antipsychotic drugs have been shown to produce a similar syndrome called the neuroleptic malignant syndrome.

Hypersensitivity reactions. The most common cause of drug fever is a hypersensitivity reaction. Hypersensitivity drug fevers develop after several weeks of exposure to the drug, cannot be explained in terms of the drug's pharmacologic action, are not related to dose, disappear when the drug is stopped, and reappear when the drug is readministered. The fever pattern is typically spiking in nature and exhibits a normal diurnal rhythm.[25] In addition, persons with drug fevers often experience other signs of hypersensitivity reactions, such as arthralgias, urticaria, myalgias, gastrointestinal discomfort, and rashes. The person may be unaware of the fever and appear to be well for the degree of fever that is present. Often a fever precedes other more serious effects of a drug reaction, and for this reason, the early recognition of drug fever is important. In a study of 68 cases of drug fever, of which 31 were fatal, an early fever was present in 30% of the cases.[26] Some of the most commonly cited causes of drug fever are aminosalicylic acid (an antituberculosis drug), amphotericin B, antihistamines, barbiturates, cocaine derivatives, methyldopa (an antihypertensive drug), novobiocin (an antibiotic), penicillin, and quinidine sulfate (a cardiac dysrhythmic drug).[24] This list is not inclusive; many other drugs can induce drug fever. Drug fever should be suspected whenever the temperature elevation is unexpected and occurs despite improvement in the condition for which the drug was prescribed.

Neuroleptic malignant syndrome. Neuroleptic malignant syndrome, which is usually explosive in onset, consists of hyperthermia, muscle rigidity, alterations in consciousness, and autonomic nervous system dysfunction. The hyperthermia is accompanied by tachycardia (120 to 180 beats/min) and cardiac dysrhythmias, labile blood pressure (70/50 mm Hg to 180/130 mm Hg), postural instability, dyspnea, and tachypnea (18 to 40 breaths/min).[27] Permanent brain damage may result, and the mortality rate is nearly 30%.[28]

The disorder is associated with neuroleptic medications and may occur in up to 1% of persons taking such drugs.[28] Some of the most commonly implicated drugs are haloperidol, chlorpromazine, thioridazine, and thiothixene. All of these drugs block dopamine receptors in the basal ganglia and hypothalamus. Hyperthermia is thought to result either from alterations in the function of the hypothalamic thermoregulatory center caused by decreased dopamine levels or from uncontrolled muscle contraction like that occurring with anesthetic-induced malignant hyperthermia. Many of the neuroleptic drugs increase muscle contraction, suggesting that this mechanism might contribute to the neuroleptic malignant syndrome.

Treatment for neuroleptic malignant syndrome includes the immediate discontinuance of the neuroleptic drug, measures to decrease body temperature, and treatment of dysrhythmias and other complications of the disorder. Bromocriptine (a dopamine agonist) and dantrolene (a muscle relaxant) may be used as part of the treatment regimen.

In summary, fever and hyperthermia refer to an increase in body temperature outside the normal range. True fever is a disorder of thermoregulation in which there is an upward displacement of the set point for temperature control. In hyperthermia, the set point is unchanged but the challenge to temperature regulation exceeds the thermoregulatory center's ability to control body temperature. Fever can be caused by a number of factors, including microorganisms, trauma, and drugs or chemicals, all of which incite the release of interleukin-1 (formerly called endogenous pyrogen). The reactions that occur during fever consist of four stages: (1) a prodrome, (2) a chill, (3) a flush, and (4) defervescence. A fever can follow an intermittent, remittent, sustained, or recurrent pattern. The manifestations of fever are largely related to dehydration and an increased metabolic rate. The treatment of fever focuses on (1) modifying the external environment as a means of increasing heat transfer to the external environment; (2) supporting the hypermetabolic state that accompanies fever; (3) protecting vulnerable body tissues; and (4) treating the infection or condition causing the fever. Hyperthermia includes heat syncope, heat cramps, heat exhaustion, and heatstroke. Among the factors that contribute to the development of hyperthermia are prolonged muscular exertion in a hot environment, disorders that compromise heat dissipation, and hypersensitivity drug reactions. Malignant hyperthermia is an autosomal dominant disorder that can produce a severe and potentially fatal increase in body temperature. Heat production results from uncontrolled muscle contraction that is caused by an abnormal release of intracellular calcium. The condition is commonly triggered by general anesthetic agents and muscle relaxants used during surgery. The neuroleptic malignant syndrome is associated with neuroleptic drug therapy and is thought to result from alterations in the function of the thermoregulatory center or from uncontrolled muscle contraction.

Decreased body temperature

—— Hypothermia

Hypothermia is defined as a core (rectal, esophageal, or tympanic) temperature less than 35°C.[29–31] Core body temperatures in the range of 34°C to 35°C (93.2°F to 95°F) are considered mildly hypothermic; 30°C to 34°C (86°F to 93.2°F), mod-

erately hypothermic; and less than 30°C (86°F), severely hypothermic.[32,33] Accidental hypothermia may be defined as a spontaneous decrease in core temperature, usually in a cold environment and associated with an acute problem but without primary pathology of the temperature regulating center. The term *submersion hypothermia* is used when cooling follows acute asphyxia such as occurs in drowning.[34] In children the rapid cooling process, in addition to the diving reflex which triggers apnea and circulatory shunting to establish a heart-brain circulation (see Chapter 20), may account for the surprisingly high survival rate following submersion. The diving reflex is greatly diminished in adults. Children have been reported to survive 10 to 40 minutes of submersion asphyxia.[35,36] Controlled hypothermia may be used during certain types of surgeries to decrease brain metabolism.

Oral temperatures are markedly inaccurate during hypothermia because of severe vasoconstriction and sluggish blood flow. Although esophageal temperatures or temperatures measured near the tympanic membrane provide the most exact estimate of core temperature during hypothermia, these methods are often impractical; therefore, rectal temperatures are usually used. Most clinical thermometers only measure temperature in the range of 35°C to 42°C (95°F to 107.6°F); so a special thermometer that registers as low as 25°C (77°F) or an electrical thermistor probe is needed for monitoring temperatures in persons with hypothermia.[33]

Systemic hypothermia may result from exposure to prolonged cold (atmospheric or submersion). The condition may develop in otherwise healthy persons in the course of accidental exposure. Because water conducts heat more readily than air, body temperature drops rapidly when the body is submerged in cold water or when clothing becomes wet. In persons with altered homeostasis due to debility or disease, hypothermia may follow exposure to relatively small decreases in atmospheric temperature. Elderly and inactive persons living in inadequately heated quarters are particularly vulnerable to hypothermia. Acute alcoholism is a common predisposing factor. Persons with cardiovascular disease, cerebrovascular disease, malnutrition, and hypothyroidism are also predisposed to hypothermia. The use of sedatives and tranquilizing drugs may be a contributing factor.

—— Manifestations

With mild hypothermia, intense shivering generates heat and sympathetic nervous system activity is raised to resist lowering of temperature. Vasoconstriction can be profound, heart rate is accelerated, and stroke volume is increased. Blood pressure increases slightly, and hyperventilation is common. Exposure to cold augments urinary flow (cold diuresis) before there is any fall in temperature. Dehydration and increased hematocrit may develop within a few hours of even mild hypothermia, augmented by an extracellular-to-intracellular water shift.

With moderate hypothermia, shivering gradually decreases and the muscles become rigid. Shivering usually ceases at 27°C (80.6°F). Consciousness is usually lost at 30°C (86°F). Heart rate and stroke volume are reduced, and blood pressure falls. The greatest effect of hypothermia is exerted through a decrease in the metabolic rate, which falls to 50% of normal at 28°C (82.4°F).[37] Associated with this decrease in metabolic rate is a decrease in oxygen consumption and carbon dioxide production. There is roughly a 6% decrease in oxygen consumption per degree Celsius decrease in temperature. A decrease in carbon dioxide production leads to a decrease in respiratory rate. Respirations decrease as temperatures drop below 32.2°C (90°F). Decreases in mentation, the cough reflex, and respiratory tract secretions, may lead to difficulty in clearing secretions and aspiration.

In terms of cardiovascular function, there is a gradual decline in heart rate and cardiac output that occurs as hypothermia progresses. Blood pressure initially rises, and then gradually falls. There is increased risk of dysrhythmia developing, probably from myocardial hypoxia and autonomic nervous system imbalance. Ventricular fibrillation is a major cause of death in hypothermia.

Carbohydrate metabolism and insulin activity is decreased, resulting in a hyperglycemia that is proportional to the level of cooling. A cold-induced loss of cell membrane integrity allows intravascular fluids to move into the skin, giving the skin a puffy appearance. Acid–base disorders occur with increased frequency at temperatures below 25°C (77°F) unless adequate ventilation is maintained. Extracellular sodium and potassium concentrations decrease and chloride levels increase. There is a temporary loss of plasma from the circulation along with sludging of red blood cells and increased blood viscosity as the result of trapping in the small vessels and skin.

The signs and symptoms of hypothermia include poor coordination, stumbling, slurred speech, irrationality and poor judgment, amnesia, hallucinations, blueness and puffiness of the skin, dilation of the pupils, decreased respiratory rate, weak and irregular pulse, and stupor.

——— Treatment

The treatment of hypothermia consists of rewarming, support of vital functions, and the prevention and treatment of complications. There are three methods of rewarming: passive rewarming, active total rewarming, and active core rewarming. Passive rewarming is done by removing the person from the cold environment, covering with a blanket, supplying warm fluids (oral or intravenous), and allowing rewarming to occur at the person's own pace. Active total rewarming involves immersing the person in warm water or placing heating pads or hot water bottles on the surface of the body, including the extremities. Active core rewarming places major emphasis on rewarming the trunk, leaving the extremities, containing the major metabolic mass, cold until the heart rewarms.[30] Active rewarming can be done by instilling warmed fluids into the gastrointestinal tract, peritoneal dialysis, extracorporeal blood warming, in which blood is removed from the body and passed through a heat exchanger and then returned to the body, or warming by inhalation of oxygen warmed to 42°C to 46°C (107.6°F to 114.8°F).

Persons with mild hypothermia usually respond well to passive rewarming in a warm bed. Persons with moderate or severe hypothermia do not have the thermoregulatory shivering mechanism and require active rewarming. During rewarming, the cold acidotic blood from the peripheral tissues is returned to the heart and central circulation. If this is done too rapidly or before cardiopulmonary function has been adequately reestablished, the hypothermic heart cannot respond to the increased metabolic demands of warm peripheral tissues.

In summary, hypothermia is a potentially life-threatening disorder in which the body's core temperature drops below 35°C (95°F). Accidental hypothermia can develop in otherwise healthy persons in the course of accidental exposure and in elderly or disabled persons with impaired perception or response to cold. Alcoholism, cardiovascular disease, malnutrition, and hypothyroidism contribute to the risk of hypothermia. The greatest effect of hypothermia is a decrease in the metabolic rate, leading to a decrease in carbon dioxide production and respiratory rate. The signs and symptoms of hypothermia include poor coordination, stumbling, slurred speech, irrationality, poor judgment, amnesia, hallucinations, blueness and puffiness of the skin, dilation of the pupils, decreased respiratory rate, weak and irregular pulse, stupor, and coma. The treatment for moderate and severe hypothermia includes active rewarming.

References

1.   Vick R: Contemporary Medical Physiology, p 886. Menlo Park CA, Addison Wesley, 1984
2.   Guyton A: Textbook of Medical Physiology, 7th ed, p 851. Philadelphia, WB Saunders, 1986

3. Atkins L: Fever: The old and new. J Infect Dis 149:339, 1984
4. Bernheim HA, Block LH, Atkins E: Fever: Pathogenesis, pathophysiology, and purpose. Ann Intern Med 91:262, 1979
5. Kruse J: Fever in children. Am Family Pract 37(2):127, 1988
6. Keating HJ, Klimek JJ, Levine DS, et al: Effect of age on the clinical significance of fever in ambulatory adult patients. J Am Geriatric Soc 32:282, 1984
7. Fraser I, Johnstone M: Significance of early postoperative fever in children. Br Med J 282:1299, 1981
8. Pien FD, Ho PWL, Fergusson DJG: Fever and infection after cardiac operation. Ann Thorac Surg 33:382, 1982
9. Kluger MJ: Fever: A hot topic. News Physiol Sci 1:25, 1986
10. Roberts NJ: Temperature and host responses. Microbiol Rev 43:241, 1979
11. Rodbard D: The role of regional temperature in the pathogenesis of disease. N Engl J Med 305:808, 1981
12. McGee ZA, Gorby GL: The diagnostic value of fever patterns. Hosp Pract 22 (10):103, 1987
13. Cunha BA: Implications of fever in the critical care setting. Heart Lung 13:460, 1984
14. Sodeman WA, Sodeman TM: Pathologic Physiology: Mechanisms of Disease, 6th ed, p 546. Philadelphia, WB Saunders, 1979
15. Danzl DF: Hyperthermic syndromes. Am Family Pract 37(6):157, 1988
16. Florence Nightingale: Notes on Nursing, p 45. London, Brandon/Systems Press Inc, 1970
17. Halle A, Repasy A: Classic heatstroke: A serious challenge for the elderly. Hosp Pract 22 (5): 26, 1987
18. Brinnel H, Nagasaka T, Cabanac M: Enhanced brain protection during passive hyperthermia in humans. Eur J Appl Physiol 56:540, 1987
19. Cabanac M: Keeping a cool head. News Physiol Sci 1 (Apr):41, 1986
20. Britt BA, Kalow W: Malignant hyperthermia: A statistical review. Can Anaesth Soc J 17:293, 1970
21. Nelson TE, Flewellen EH: The malignant hyperthermia syndrome. N Engl J Med 309:416, 1983
22. Tabor PA: Drug-induced fever. Drug Intell Clin Pharm 20:413, 1986
23. Mackowiak PA, LeMaistre CF: Drug fever: A critical appraisal of conventional concepts. Ann Intern Med 106:728, 1986
24. Hofland SL: Drug fever: Is your patient's fever drug-related. Crit Care Nurs 5:29,1985
25. Musher DM, Fainstein V, Young EJ, et al: Fever patterns: Their lack of clinical significance. Arch Intern Med 139:1225, 1979
26. Cluff LE, Johnson JE: Drug fever. Prog Allergy 8:149, 1964
27. Parker WA: Neuroleptic malignant syndrome. Crit Care Nurse 7:40, 1987
28. Goldwasser HD, Hooper JF: Neuroleptic malignant syndrome. Am Family Pract 38(5):211, 1988
29. Reuler JB: Hypothermia: Pathophysiology, clinical settings, and management. Ann Intern Med 89:519, 1978
30. Fitzgerald FT, Jessop C: Accidental hypothermia: A report of 22 cases and review of the literature. Ann Rev Med :127, 1982
31. Celestina FS, Van Noord GR, Miraglia CP: Accidental hypothermia in the elderly. J Family Pract 26:259, 1988
32. Lonning PE, Skulberg A, Abyholm F: Accidental hypothermia. Acta Anaethesiol Scand 30:601, 1986
33. Division of Environmental Hazards and Health Effects: Hypothermia-associated death—United States, 1968–1980. MMWR 34, No 48, Atlanta, Centers for Disease Control, 1985
34. Conn AW: Near drowning and hypothermia. Can Med Assoc J 120:397, 1979
35. Siebke H, Beivik H, Rod T: Survival after 40 minutes submersion with cerebral sequelae. Lancet 1:1275, 1975
36. Moss JF: The management of accidental severe hypothermia. New York J Med 88:411, 1988
37. Wong KC: Physiology and pharmacology of hypothermia. West J Med 138:227, 1983

Bibliography

Donaldson JF: Therapy of acute fever: A comparative approach. Hosp Pract 16 (Sept):125, 1981

Done AK: Treatment of fever in 1982: A review. Am J Med (746B):27, 1983

Gutierrez-Nuñez JJ, Ibañez AR, Stevens MB, et al: Fever without focus. Am Fam Pract 32:138, 1985

Harrison MH: Effects of thermal stress and exercise on blood volume in humans. Physiol Rev 65:149, 1985

Hubbard RW, Matthew CB, Durkot MJ, et al: Novel approaches to the pathophysiology of heatstroke: The energy depletion model. Ann Emerg Med 16:1066, 1987

Jafek BW, Solomons CC, Masson NC, et al: Current concepts of malignant hyperthermia. Otolaryngol Head Neck Surg 89:891, 1981

Kimmel S, Gemmill DW: The young child with fever. Am Fam Pract 37:196, 1988

McAlpin CH, Martin BJ, Lennox LM, et al: Pyrexia in infection in the elderly. Age Ageing 15:230, 1986

McCarron K: Fever—The cardinal sign. Crit Care Quart 9 (June):15, 1986

Nadel ER: Recent advances in temperature regulation during exercise in humans. Fed Proc 44:2286, 1985

Newman J: Evaluation of sponging to reduce body temperature in febrile children. Can Med Assoc J 132:641, 1985

Orlowski JP: Drowning, near-drowning, and ice-water submersions. Ped Clin North Am 34:75, 1987

Rosendorff C: Neurochemistry of fever. South Afr J Med Sci 41:23, 1976

Samples JF, Van Cott ML, Long C, et al: Circadian rhythms: Basis for screening for fever. Nurs Res 34:377, 1985

Simon HE: Extreme pyrexia. Hosp Pract 21 (5A):123, 1986

Steele RW, Tanaka PT, Lara RP: Evaluation of sponging and of oral antipyretic therapy to reduce fever. J Pediatr 77:824, 1970

Stern RC: Pathophysiologic basis for symptomatic treatment of fever. Pediatrics 59:92, 1978

CHAPTER 8

Gladys Simandl

Alterations in Skin Function and Integrity

Structure of the skin
  Epidermis
  Basement membrane zone
  Dermis
  Subcutaneous tissue
  Skin appendages
    Hair
    Sebaceous glands
    Sweat glands
    Nail
Manifestations of skin disorders
  Lesions and rashes
  Pruritus
Developmental skin problems
  Infancy and childhood
    Rashes associated with
      childhood disorders
  Adolescence and young
    adulthood
  Old age
    Common skin problems

Primary disorders of the skin
  Mechanical processes
  Infectious processes
    Fungal infections
    Bacterial infections
    Viral infections
  Inflammatory skin disorders
    Acne
    Lichen planus
    Psoriasis
    Pityriasis rosea
  Allergic skin responses
    Contact dermatitis
    Eczema
    Drug-induced skin eruptions

**Insect bites, vectors, ticks,
  and parasites**
  Scabies
  Pediculosis
  Bedbugs
  Ticks
  Mosquitoes
  Chiggers
  Fleas
Photosensitivity and sunburn
Neoplasms
  Nevi
  Basal cell carcinoma
  Squamous cell carcinoma
  Malignant melanoma
Black skin
  Vitiligo

Objectives

After you have studied this chapter, you should be able to meet the following objectives:

_____ List five functions of the skin.

_____ Explain the development of the keratin layer of the epidermis.

_____ Describe the function of the melanocytes.

_____ List the structures of the dermis and state their function.

_____ Describe the innervation of the sweat glands and the arrector pili (pilomotor) muscles.

_____ Compare the distribution and secretory activity of the eccrine and apocrine sweat glands.

_____ State the location and function of the sebaceous glands.

_____ Describe the following skin rashes and lesions: macule, patch, papule, plaque, nodule, tumor, wheal, vesicle, bulla, pustule, erosion, crust, ulcer, scale, fissure, lichenification, petechiae, ecchymosis.

_____ Cite two theories used to explain the physiology of pruritus.

_____ Differentiate between a strawberry hemangioma and a port-wine stain hemangioma in terms of appearance and outcome.

_____ Describe the distinguishing features of rashes associated with roseola infantum, rubeola, rubella, chickenpox, and scarlet fever.

(continued)

_____ Define the term *keratosis* and compare the seborrheic and actinic keratoses.

_____ Relate the behavior of fungi to the production of superficial skin lesions associated with tinea or ringworm.

_____ Explain the dermatomal distribution of herpes zoster lesions.

_____ Compare acne vulgaris, acne conglobata, and acne rosacea in terms of appearance and location of lesions.

_____ State three contributing factors in acne vulgaris.

_____ Cite three goals of acne treatment and one example of a treatment method for each goal.

_____ Describe the appearance of psoriasis lesions.

_____ Explain the action of the drug methoxsalen that is used in the PUVA treatment for psoriasis.

_____ Differentiate between lesions seen in infantile and adult forms of eczema.

_____ Relate the life cycle of the *Sarcoptes scabiei* to the skin lesions seen in scabies.

_____ Utilize knowledge of the life cycles of *Pediculus humanus corporis* and *P. humanus capitis* to explain the lesions associated with body and head lice.

_____ Explain methods used in treating pediculosis and eradicating lice and their nits from bedding and clothing.

_____ Compare the life cycles of bedbugs and ticks.

_____ List three drugs that produce photosensitivity.

_____ State the relationship between sun exposure and skin cancer.

_____ Compare the appearance of basal cell carcinoma, squamous cell carcinoma, and malignant melanoma.

_____ Cite changes in a mole that are suggestive of cancerous transformation.

_____ Provide a physiologic explanation for the red, white, and blue mottled appearance of malignant melanoma.

_____ Compare the appearance of atopic dermatitis, pityriasis rosea, psoriasis, tinea versicolor, and lichen planus in white and black skin.

The skin is primarily an organ of protection. It is the largest organ of the body and forms the major barrier between the internal organs and the external environment. The skin of an average-sized adult covers approximately 18 square feet and weighs 6 pounds to 9 pounds.[1,2] As the body's first line of defense, the skin is continuously subjected to potentially harmful environmental agents, including solid matter, liquids, gases, sunlight, and microorganisms. Although the skin may become bruised, lacerated, burned, or infected, it has remarkable properties that allow for a continuous cycle of healing, shedding, and cell regeneration.

In addition to protection, the skin serves several other important functions. The skin is richly innervated with pain, temperature, and touch receptors. Skin receptors relay the numerous qualities of touch, such as pressure, sharpness, dullness, and pleasure to the central nervous system (CNS) for localization and fine discrimination. Further, the skin is important in regulating body temperature (see Chapter 7). Through CNS control, blood vessels in the skin are dilated or constricted to maintain thermoregulation and to regulate sweat production. The skin also plays an essential role in vitamin D synthesis and fluid and electrolyte balance. Finally, a less well known property of the skin is its ability to store glycogen and contribute to glucose metabolism.[3]

Importantly, skin may demonstrate outwardly what occurs in the body systemically. A number of systemic diseases are manifested by skin disorders: for example, systemic lupus erythematous, several forms of cancer, and Kaposi's sarcoma associated with AIDS. This means that although skin eruptions frequently represent primary disease of the skin, they may also be a manifestation of systemic disease. Hence, careful attention to the history and the assessment of the client's concerns is imperative.

The skin also has an elusive quality of reflecting emotional states regardless of disease. It is through the skin that warmth and human affection are given and received. The skin conveys notions of health, beauty, integrity, and love. Society emphasizes the body and, in particular, the skin to the degree that even slight imperfections may evoke a wide variety of human responses. As more is learned about the skin through scientific investigations, the importance of considering mind-body connectedness when working with people who have skin disorders is becoming increasingly apparent. Sensitivity to these concerns is of extreme importance in helping persons deal with their skin problems.

Structure of the skin

Because of the great variations in structure in different parts of the body, normal skin is difficult to describe.[4] Corresponding variations are found in the properties of the skin, such as the thickness of skin layers, the distribution of sweat glands, and the number and size of hair follicles. For example, the skin is thicker on the palms and soles of the feet, hair follicles are densely distributed in the scalp, and apocrine sweat glands are confined to the axillae and the anogenital area. Nevertheless, certain structural properties are common to all skin in all areas of the body. The skin is composed of two layers: the epidermis (outer layer) and the dermis (inner layer). A basement membrane zone (BMZ) divides the two layers. The subcutaneous tissue, a layer of loose connective and fatty tissues, binds the dermis to the underlying tissues of the body (Figure 8-1).

Epidermis

The functions of the skin depend on the properties of its outermost layer, the epidermis. The epidermis not only covers the body, but is also special-

ized to form the various skin appendages: hair, nails, and glandular structures. Its cells produce a fibrous protein called *keratin,* which is essential to the protective function of skin, and a pigment called *melanin,* which protects against ultraviolet radiation. The epidermis contains openings for two types of glands: sweat glands, which produce watery secretions, and sebaceous glands, which produce an oily secretion called *sebum.* The epidermis is composed of stratified squamous epithelium, which when viewed under the microscope is seen to consist of five distinct layers, or strata, that represent a progressive differentiation of epidermal cells: stratum germinativum, or basal layer; stratum spinosum; stratum granulosum; stratum lucidum; and stratum corneum (see Figure 8-1).

The first layer, the stratum corneum, consists of dead, keratinized cells. This layer contains the most cell layers and the largest cells of any zone of the

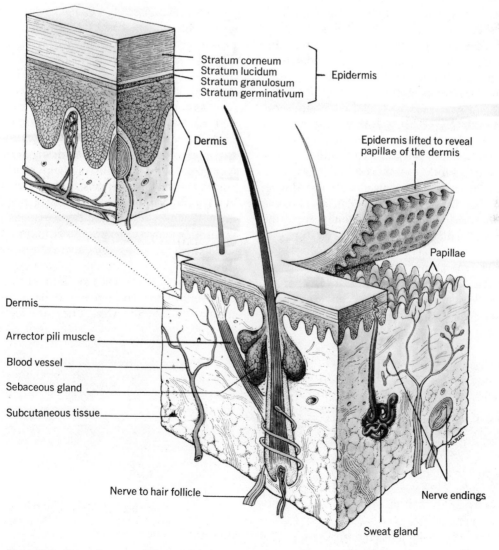

Figure 8-1 Three-dimensional view of the skin. (*Chaffee EE, Lytle IM: Basic Anatomy and Physiology, 4th ed. Philadelphia, JB Lippincott, 1980*)

epidermis. It ranges from 15 layers thick in areas such as the face to 25 layers or more on the arm.[5] In specialized areas, such as the palms of the hands or soles of the feet, 100 or more layers are present.[5]

The stratum lucidum, or second layer, is thin and transparent. It consists of transitional cells that retain some of the functions of living skin cells from the layers below and resemble the cells of the stratum corneum. This layer can be seen on the palms of the hands and soles of the feet.

The stratum granulosum, the third layer of the epidermis, consists of granular cells that are the most differentiated cells of the living skin. The cells in this layer are unique in that two polar functions are occurring simultaneously. While some cells are losing cytoplasm and DNA structures, others continue to synthesize keratin.

The fourth layer, the stratum spinosum, is formed as the progeny of the basal cell layer move upward. This layer is two to four layers thick, and its cells become differentiated as they migrate outward, toward the skin surface (Figure 8-2). Keratinocytes, Langerhans' cells, and melanocytes are present in this layer. The cells of this layer are commonly referred to as prickle cells because they develop a spiny appearance as their cell borders interact.

The stratum germinativum, or stratum basale, is the deepest layer of the epidermis. It consists of a single layer of basal cells that are attached to the basement membrane. The basal cells, which are columnar in shape, produce new skin cells that move toward the skin surface to replace cells lost during normal skin shedding. Unlike the other layers of the epidermis, the basal cells do not migrate toward the skin surface, but remain stationary in the stratum germinativum.

Besides the layers, the epidermis houses four major cell types: keratinocytes, melanocytes, Langerhans' cells, and Merkel's cells. These cells are derived from the basal layer of the epidermis—that is, new cells of the epidermis are produced from the basal cells. Each cell type is discussed in the following paragraphs.

The keratinocyte is the major cell of the epidermis. It is able to synthesize DNA and produce keratin. The keratinocyte changes morphologically as it is pushed toward the outer layer of the epidermis. For example, in the basal layer, the keratinocyte is round. As it is pushed into the stratum spinosum, the keratinocyte becomes multisided; it becomes flatter in the granular layer and is flattened and elongated in the stratum corneum (see Figure 8-2). Keratinocytes also change cytoplasmic structure and composition as they are pushed outward. This transformation from viable cells to the dead cells of the stratum corneum is called *keratinization.*

Melanocytes are pigment-synthesizing cells. They are almost always located in the basal layer. They function to produce pigment granules called melanosomes, which contain melanin, the brown substance that gives skin its color. Although melanocytes remain in the basal layer, the melanosomes are transferred to the keratinocytes through a dendritic process. During this transfer, the normally round melanocytes become dendritic in shape. The dendrite tip of the melanocyte is engulfed by a nearby keratinocyte, and the melanosomes are transferred (Figure 8-3). Each melanocyte is capable of supplying several keratinocytes with melanin. It is the amount of melanin in the keratinocytes that determines a person's skin color. The melanin pigment protects the skin from the ultraviolet sun rays, and exposure to ultraviolet rays increases the production of melanin. Black-skinned and white-skinned people have the same amount of melanocytes; however, the number of melanosomes produced differs greatly among individuals.

Langerhans' cells are located in the suprabasal layers of the epidermis and become established among the keratinocytes. They are few in number

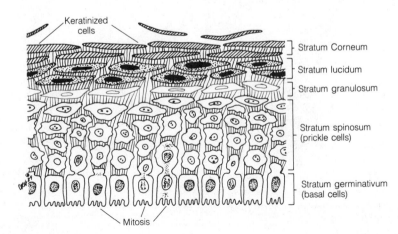

Keratinized cells

Stratum Corneum

Stratum lucidum

Stratum granulosum

Stratum spinosum (prickle cells)

Stratum germinativum (basal cells)

Mitosis

Figure 8-2 Epidermal cells. The basal cells undergo mitosis and then change their size and shape as they move upward to produce new skin cells which replace cells that are lost during normal cell shedding.

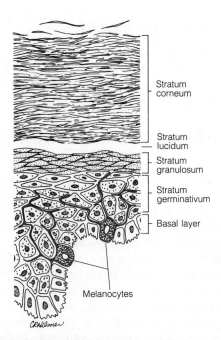

Figure 8-3 Melanocytes. The melanocytes, which are located in the basal layer of the skin, produce melanin pigment granules that give skin its color. The melanocytes have threadlike cytoplasmic-filled extensions that are used in passing the pigment granules to the keratinocytes.

compared with the keratinocytes. They are derived from precursor cells originating in the bone marrow and continuously repopulate the epidermis.[6] Like melanocytes, they are dendritic in shape and have clear cytoplasms. Microscopically, they resemble a tennis racquet and are therefore easy to differentiate from other skin cell types. The exact origin of these cells remains unknown, as does their function. Research has indicated that they may play a role in the cutaneous immune response and serve as a possible source of prostaglandins[7,8]

Merkel's cells consist of free nerve endings attached to modified epidermal cells. Their origin remains unknown, and they are the least densely populated cell of the epidermis. Merkel's cells are found on the skin of the fingers, toes, lips, oral cavity, and outermost sheath of hair follicles (the touch areas). Merkel's cells function as mechanoreceptors, or touch receptors.[9]

The movement of the cells to the surface of the skin can best be described as random or nonsynchronized. Keratinocytes pass other keratinocytes, melanocytes, and Langerhans' cells as they migrate in a seemingly random fashion. However, the cells are connected with minute points of attachment called *desmosomes*. Desmosomes keep the cells from detaching and provide some structure to the skin while it is in perpetual motion. The basal layer, however, provides the underlying structure and stability for the epidermis.

Basement membrane zone

The BMZ is a layer of tissue that connects the epidermis to the dermis, both structures contributing to its formation. Characteristics of the BMZ have become more defined over the past few years. Essentially, the BMZ contains collagen fibers and glycoproteins and consists of four distinct layers, all contributing to the adhesion and elasticity of the skin. The collagen fibers provide the skin with tensile strength, anchorage, and elasticity. The glycoproteins are believed to be associated with cohesion. The function of the BMZ as a barrier remains debatable, as many substances are able to penetrate it. Lymphocytes, neutrophils, and Langerhans' cells easily penetrate the BMZ; however, the BMZ has been found to bar larger molecules.

Dermis

The dermis is the connective tissue layer that separates the epidermis from the subcutaneous fat layer. It supports the epidermis and serves as its primary source of nutrition. The two layers of the dermis, the papillary dermis and the reticular dermis, are composed of cells, fibers, and ground substances as well as nerves and blood vessels. The pilar (hair) structures and glandular structures are embedded in this layer and elaborated upon in the epidermis.

The papillary dermis (pars papillaris) is a thin superficial layer that lies adjacent to the epidermis. It consists of collagen fibers and ground substance. The basal cells of the epidermis project into the papillary dermis, forming dermal papillae (see Figure 8-1). Dermal papillae contain capillary venules, which serve to nourish the epidermal layers of the skin. This layer of the dermis is well vascularized. Lymph vessels and nerve tissue are also found in this layer.

The reticular dermis (pars reticularis) is the thicker area of the dermis and forms the bulk of the dermis. This is the layer from which the tough leather hides of animals are made. The reticular dermis is characterized by a mesh of three-dimensional collagen bundles interconnected with large elastic fibers and ground substance.

The ground substance is a viscid gel, rich in mucopolysaccharides. The collagen fibers are oriented parallel to the body's surface in any given area. These collagen bundles may be organized lengthwise, as on the abdomen, or in round blocks, as in the heel. The direction of surgical incisions is often determined by this organizational pattern. The epidermis extends deep into the reticular dermis and either terminates there or extends into the subcutaneous layer. Blood vessels, lymph vessels, and nerve fibers are found in this area. Extremely small nerve endings extend into the papillary dermis.

Cells found in the dermis include fibroblasts, macrophages, and mast cells. Limited numbers of lymphocytes are found around dermal blood vessels. Fibroblasts synthesize the connective tissue matrix. They also secrete enzymes needed to break down and thereby remodel the matrix. Macrophages are abundant in the dermis and serve to synthesize certain enzymes that enhance or suppress lymphocyte activity, certain prostaglandins, and interferon. Mast cells are also abundant, but their exact function remains unknown.

The microvasculature of the dermal papillae is linked to the larger vessels that exist between the dermal papillae. These vessels transport epidermal nutrients and waste products and also function in thermoregulation. The lymphatic system of the skin, which combats certain infectious skin invasions, is also limited to the dermis.

The innervation of the skin is complex. The skin, with its accessory structures, serves as an organ for receiving sensory information from the environment. Accordingly, it is well supplied with sensory nerves. In addition, it contains nerves that supply the blood vessels, sweat glands, and arrector pili muscles. The receptors for touch, pressure, heat, cold, and pain are widely distributed in the skin. Because of the variation in function among the different types of nerve endings, it is generally agreed that sensory modalities are not associated with a particular type of receptor. For example, the sensations of pain, touch, and pressure probably result from multiple stimuli. The final sensation may be the result of central summation in the CNS, which mediates patterned responses.

Most of the skin's blood vessels are under sympathetic nervous system control. The sweat glands are innervated by cholinergic fibers but controlled by the sympathetic nervous system. Likewise, the sympathetic nervous system controls the arrector pili (pilomotor) muscles that cause hairs on the skin to stand up. Contraction of these muscles tends to cause the skin to dimple, producing "goose pimples."

Subcutaneous tissue

The subcutaneous tissue layer consists primarily of fat and connective tissues that lend support to the vascular and neural structures supplying the outer layers of the skin. There is controversy about whether or not the subcutaneous tissue should be considered an actual layer of the skin. However, the eccrine glands and deep hair follicles extend to this layer, and several skin diseases involve the subcutaneous tissue.

Skin appendages

The skin houses a variety of appendages including hair, nails, and sebaceous and sweat glands. The distribution as well as the function of the appendages varies.

Hair

Hair is a structure that originates from hair follicles in the dermis. Most hair follicles are associated with sebaceous glands, and these structures combine to form the pilosebaceous apparatus. The entire hair structure consists of the hair follicle, sebaceous gland, hair muscle (arrector pili), and, in some instances, the apocrine gland (Figure 8-4). Hair is a keratinized structure that is pushed upward from the hair follicle. Growth of the hair is centered in the bulb (base) of the hair follicle and the hair undergoes changes as it is pushed outward. Hair has been found to go through cyclic phases identified as anagen (the growth phase), catagen (the atrophy phase), and telogen (the resting phase). A vascular network at the site of the follicular bulb nourishes and maintains the hair follicle. Melanocytes are found in the bulb and are responsible for the color of the hair. The arrector pili muscle, located under the sebaceous gland, provides a thermoregulation function by contracting and reducing the skin surface area that is available for the dissipation of body heat.

Sebaceous glands

The sebaceous glands (see Figure 8-4) secrete a fatty material called sebum, which lubricates hair and skin. Sebum prevents undue evaporation of moisture from the stratum corneum during cold weather and helps to conserve body heat. It is also thought to possess some bactericidal and fungicidal properties. It is the sebaceous glands that are most involved in the development of acne (discussed later in this chapter).

Sweat glands

There are two types of sweat glands: eccrine and apocrine (see Figure 8-4). Eccrine sweat glands are simple tubular structures that originate in the dermis and open directly to the skin surface. They vary in density and are located over the entire body surface. Their purpose is to transport sweat to the outer skin surface to regulate body temperature.

Apocrine sweat glands are fewer in number than eccrine sweat glands. They are larger and located deep in the dermal layer. They open through a hair follicle, even though a hair may not be present, and are found primarily in the axillae and groin. The

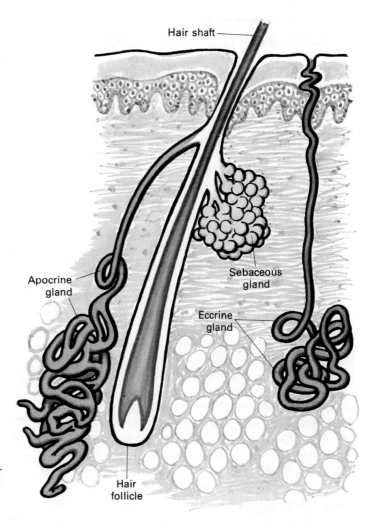

Figure 8-4 The glandular structures of the skin. Note that the apocrine and sebaceous glands open into the hair follicle, whereas the eccrine gland opens directly onto the surface of the skin. (*Chaffee EE, Lytle IM: Basic Anatomy and Physiology, 4th ed. Philadelphia, JB Lippincott, 1980*)

major difference between these glands and the eccrine glands is that they secrete an oily substance. In animals, apocrine secretions give rise to distinctive odors that enable animals to recognize the presence of others. In humans, apocrine secretions are sterile until mixed with the bacteria on the skin surface and then they produce what is commonly known as body odor.

Nail

The nail is a hardened keratinized plate that protects the fingers and toes and enhances dexterity. The nail is the end product of dead matrix cells that grow from the nail plate. Unlike hair, nails grow continuously unless permanently damaged or diseased.

In summary, the skin is primarily an organ of protection. It is the largest organ of the body and forms the major barrier between the internal organs and the external environment. In addition, the skin is richly innervated with pain, temperature, and touch receptors; it synthesizes vitamin D and plays an es-

sential role in fluid and electrolyte balance. It contributes to glucose metabolism through its glycogen stores. The skin is composed of two layers, the epidermis and the dermis, separated by a basement membrane zone. A layer of subcutaneous tissue binds the dermis to the underlying organs and tissues of the body. The epidermis contains five layers, or strata, and is the outermost layer of the skin. The major cells of the epidermis are the keratinocytes, melanocytes, Langerhans' cells, and Merkel's cells. These cells, which remain in the stratum germinativum (or basal layer) of the epidermis, are the source of the cells in all five layers of the epidermis. The keratinocytes, which are the major cells of the epidermis, are transformed from viable keratinocytes to dead keratin as they move from the innermost layer of the epidermis (stratum germinativum) to the outermost layer (stratum corneum). The melanocytes are pigment-synthesizing cells that give skin its color. The dermis provides the epidermis with support and nutrition and is the source of blood vessels, nerves, and skin appendages (hair follicles and sebaceous glands, nails, and sweat glands).

Manifestations of skin disorders

The skin is a unique organ in which numerous signs are immediately observable. These signs contribute to accurate diagnosis and treatment. In many cases, the skin may relay signs of other organic dysfunction. The most common manifestations of skin disorders are rashes, lesions, and pruritus.

Lesions and rashes

Rashes are temporary eruptions of the skin, such as those associated with childhood diseases, heat rash, diaper rash, or drug-induced eruptions. The term *lesion* usually refers to a traumatic or pathologic loss of normal tissue continuity, structure, or function. Sometimes the components of a rash are referred to as lesions. The various types of lesions are described in Tables 8-1, 8-2, and 8-3. Rashes and lesions may range in size from a fraction of a millimeter (as in petechiae) to many centimeters (as in a decubitus ulcer, or pressure sore). They may be blanched (white), reddened (erythematous), hemorrhagic or purpuric (containing blood), or pigmented. Skin lesions may be vascular in origin (Table 8-1); they may occur as primary lesions arising in previously normal skin (Table 8-2); or they may develop as secondary lesions resulting from primary lesions (Table 8-3).

Pruritus

Pruritus, or itching, is a symptom common to many skin disorders. Pruritus may be present with dry skin and often accompanies major skin disorders. Itching may also be symptomatic of other organ disorders, such as diabetes or biliary disease, when no skin anomaly exists. Physiologically, two theories exist regarding itch. The first is that an anatomically distinct itch receptor exists, although none has been found to date, perhaps because of their scarcity and small size.[10] The second theory is that itching is the sensation experienced by an individual when multiple nerve fibers in the skin are stimulated (e.g., pain and touch). The CNS interprets these sensations as itch through central summation.

The latter theory, that pain and itch are transmitted through the same nerve pathways, is generally more accepted. However, the sensations are perceived as quite distinct from each other. Whether there are two receptors or one, the mediator of the itch response remains unknown. Several substances, such as histamine and morphine, are known to increase itching. Prostaglandins and warmth can also trigger the itch phenomenon.

The well-known response to an itch is scratching; this can cause skin excoriations. Excoriated skin is much more susceptible to infectious processes, and measures to reduce pruritus and prevent scratching should therefore be taken. Because vasodilatation increases itching, a common method of reducing pruritus is the use of cold applications. Application of topical corticosteroids may be helpful in some situations. Administration of systemic antihistamines and corticosteroids may be indicated in severe pruritus. Phototherapy may be used with the chronic forms of itching associated with internal organic disease processes.

In summary, skin lesions, rashes, and pruritus are common manifestations of skin disorders. Rashes are temporary skin eruptions. Lesions result from traumatic or pathologic loss of the normal continuity, structure, or function of the skin. Lesions may be vascular in origin; they may occur as primary lesions in previously normal skin; or they may develop as secondary lesions resulting from primary lesions. Pruritus, or itching, is a symptom common to many skin disorders. Scratching because of pruritus can lead to excoriation, infection, and other complications.

Developmental skin problems

Many skin problems occur more commonly in certain age groups. Because of aging changes, infants, adolescents, and elderly persons tend to have different skin problems.

Infancy and childhood

Infancy connotes the image of perfect, unblemished skin. For the most part, this is true; however, several congenital skin lesions, such as mongolian spots, hemangiomas, and nevi are associated with the early neonatal period. *Mongolian spots* are caused by selective pigmentation. They usually occur on the buttocks or sacral area and are commonly seen in the yellow or black race. *Hemangiomas* are vascular disorders of the skin. Two types of hemangiomas are commonly seen in infants and small children: bright-red, raised strawberry hemangiomas and flat, reddish-purple port-wine stain hemangiomas. The strawberry hemangiomas begin as small red lesions that are noted shortly after birth. They may remain as small superficial lesions or extend to involve the subcutaneous tissue. Strawberry hemangiomas usually disappear before 5 to 7 years of age without leaving an appreciable scar. Port-wine stain hemangiomas are rare, usually occur on the face, and are disfiguring. They do not disappear with age, and there is no satisfactory treatment. Usually cover-up cosmetics are used in an attempt to conceal their disfiguring effects.

The term *nevus,* discussed later in this chapter, is used to denote any congenital colored lesion.[11] Nevi may vary in shape or size and they may be present at birth or develop later in life.

Because of its newness, infant skin is also sensitive to irritation, injury, and extremes of temperature. Prolonged exposure to a warm humid environment can lead to prickly heat, and too-frequent bathing can cause dryness and lead to skin problems. The contents of soiled diapers, if not changed frequently, can lead to contact dermatitis and bacterial infections. Cradle cap is usually attributed to infrequent and in-

Table 8–1. Vascular and purpuric lesions of the skin

	Vascular			Purpuric	
	Cherry angioma	Spider angioma	Venous star	Petechia	Ecchymosis
Color	Bright or ruby red; may become brownish with age	Fiery red	Bluish	Deep red or reddish purple	Purple or purplish blue, fading to green, yellow, and brown with time
Size	1–3 mm	Very small up to 2 cm	Variable, from very small to several inches	Usually 1–3 mm	Variable, larger than petechiae
Shape	Round, flat, or sometimes raised, may be surrounded by a pale halo	Central body, sometimes raised, surrounded by erythema and radiating legs	Variable. May resemble a spider or be linear, irregular, cascading	Round, flat	Round, oval, or irregular; may have a central subcutaneous flat nodule
Pulsatility	Absent	Often demonstrable in the body of the spider, when pressure is applied with a glass slide	Absent	Absent	Absent
Effect of pressure	May show partial blanching, especially if pressure is applied with the edge of a pinpoint	Pressure over the body causes blanching of the spider	Pressure over center does not cause blanching	None	None
Distribution	Trunk, also extremities	Face, neck, arms, and upper trunk; almost never below the waist	Most often on the legs, near veins; also anterior chest	Variable	Variable
Significance	None; increase in size and numbers with aging	Liver disease, pregnancy, vitamin B deficiency; also occurs in some normal people	Often accompanies increased pressure in the superficial veins, as in varicose veins	Blood extravasated outside the vessels; may suggest increased bleeding tendency or emboli to skin	Blood extravasated outside the vessels; often secondary to trauma; also seen in bleeding disorders

(Bates B: A Guide to Physical Examination and History Taking, 4th ed. Philadelphia, JB Lippincott, 1987)

adequate washing of the scalp. Table 8-4 summarizes common skin problems of the infant and small child.

The primary factor in preventing infant skin disorders is careful attention to the skin. Baby lotions are helpful in maintaining skin moisture, while baby powder acts as a drying agent. Both are useful aids when used selectively and according to the nature of the skin problem (excessive moisture or dryness). Baby powders containing talc can cause serious respiratory problems if inhaled; therefore, containers should be kept out of the reach of small children. Cornstarch works well for this purpose, and baby powders containing cornstarch are available on the market. Unnecessary bathing should be avoided, and clothing appropriate to the environment should be worn.

Diaper rash results from a combination of ammonia and other breakdown products of urine. The treatment includes frequent change of diapers with careful cleansing of the irritated area to remove the waste products. This is important particularly in hot weather. Exposing the irritated area to air is helpful. Use of plastic pants should be discouraged. Diapers washed in gentle detergent and thoroughly rinsed to remove all traces of waste products help to reduce the risk of diaper rash. Although disposable diapers may help in some cases, their plastic backing may further augment the problem unless they are changed frequently.

Prickly heat results from constant maceration of the skin because of prolonged exposure to a warm and humid environment; this leads to midepidermal obstruction and rupture of the sweat glands. The treatment includes the removal of excessive clothing, cooling the skin with warm water baths, drying the skin with powders, and avoiding hot humid environments.

Cradle cap is usually treated by mild shampooing and gentle combing to remove the scales. Application of oil is no longer recommended, as this can compound the problem.

As children become mobile and interact with

Table 8–2. Primary lesions (may arise from previously normal skin)

Circumscribed, flat, nonpalpable changes in skin color	Palpable elevated solid masses	Circumscribed superficial elevations of the skin formed by free fluid in a cavity within the skin layers
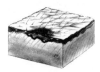	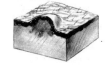	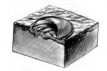
Macule—Small, up to 1 cm.* Example: freckle, petechia	*Papule*—Up to 0.5 cm. Example: an elevated nevus	*Vesicle*—Up to 0.5 cm; filled with serous fluid. Example: herpes simplex
Patch—Larger than 1 cm. Example: vitiligo	*Plaque*—A flat, elevated surface larger than 0.5 cm, often formed by the coalescence of papules	*Bulla*—Greater than 0.5 cm; filled with serous fluid. Example: 2nd degree burn
	Nodule—0.5 cm to 1–2 cm; often deeper and firmer than a papule	*Pustule*—Filled with pus. Examples: acne, impetigo
	Tumor—Larger than 1–2 cm	
	Wheal—A somewhat irregular, relatively transient, superficial area of localized skin edema. Example: mosquito bite, hive	

* Authorities vary somewhat in their definitions of skin lesions by size. Dimensions given in this table should be considered approximate, not rigid.

(Bates B: A Guide to Physical Examination and History Taking, 4th ed. Philadelphia, JB Lippincott, 1987)

Table 8–3. Secondary lesions (result from changes in primary lesions)

Loss of skin surface

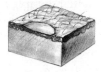

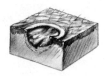

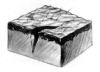

Erosion—Loss of the superficial epidermis; surface is moist but does not bleed. Example: moist area after the rupture of a vesicle, as in chickenpox

Ulcer—A deeper loss of skin surface; may bleed and scar. Examples: stasis ulcer of venous insufficiency, syphilitic chancre

Fissure—A linear crack in the skin. Example: athlete's foot

Material on the skin surface

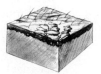

Crust—The dried residue of serum, pus, or blood. Example: impetigo

Scale—A thin flake of exfoliated epidermis. Examples: dandruff, dry skin, psoriasis

Miscellaneous

Lichenification—Thickening and roughening of the skin and increased visibility of the normal skin furrows. Example: atopic dermatitis

Atrophy—Thinning of the skin with loss of the normal skin furrows; the skin looks shinier and more translucent than normal. Example: arterial insufficiency

Excoriation—A scratch mark

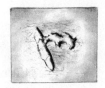

Scar—Replacement of destroyed tissue by fibrous tissue

Keloid—A hypertrophied scar

* Authorities vary somewhat in their definitions of skin lesions by size. The dimensions given in this table should be considered approximate, not rigid.

(Bates B: A Guide to Physical Examination and History Taking, 4th ed. Philadelphia, JB Lippincott, 1987)

Table 8–4. Common skin lesions of infants and small children

Lesion	Appearance
Congenital dermatoses	
Hemangiomas	
Strawberry	Bright-red raised and rounded lesions; may enlarge with growth of infant and then regress; usually disappear by 5 to 7 years of age
Port-wine stain	Flat reddish-purple disfiguring lesion; usually found on the face; does not disappear with age
Mongolian spot	Light blue, gray-green to slate gray macule; commonly located in the lumbosacral area; usually disappears with age
Nevi (moles)	Vary in size, shape, and location; usually brown-black, flat or raised macules or papules; borders are usually well defined and rounded
Irritative and inflammatory dermatoses	
Cradle cap	Yellowish, greasy, and crusted collection of vernix and shedding skin on scalp
Prickly heat	Tiny vesicles usually located on the neck, back, chest, trunk, abdomen, and folds of skin; pruritus is common
Diaper rash	Erythematous macular rash; blister formation, excoriation, and infection may develop

the environment, they become susceptible to the myriad skin disorders affecting people of all age groups. Children, because of their cognitive and physiological development, are also more prone to accidents that may result in major skin trauma, such as lacerations and burns. Careful activity supervision consistent with the developmental needs of children is the prime factor in preventing these traumas. Besides interacting with the environment, children are frequently in close contact with other children. As a result, conditions such as head lice, tinea capitis, and impetigo are more frequently seen in children. Epidemiologically, the incidence of roseola, rubeola, rubella, and chickenpox is also highest in this age group; hence, these diseases have become known as the childhood diseases.

Rashes associated with childhood disorders

Roseola infantum. Roseola infantum is a contagious viral disease that generally affects children under 4 and usually children about 1 year of age. It produces a characteristic maculopapular rash covering the trunk and spreading to the appendages. A rapid rise in temperature to 105°F and coldlike symptoms accompany the disease. Unlike rubella, no cervical or postauricular lymph node adenopathy occurs. The symptoms usually subside within 3 to 5 days. Roseola infantum is frequently mistaken for rubella. Rubella can usually be ruled out by the age of the child as well as the absence of lymph node adenopathy. Generally, children under 6 to 9 months do not develop rubella because they retain some maternal antibodies. Blood antibody titers may be taken to determine the actual diagnosis. In most cases, there are no long-term effects from this disease.

Treatment for roseola infantum is palliative; there is no vaccine for prevention. Antipyretic drugs such as acetaminophen (Datril or Tylenol) and cooling baths are used to reduce the fever. Rest and fluids are recommended for recuperation and body rehydration. Pruritus may accompany the other symptoms, but this is rare. If severe, pruritus can be treated with topical lotions such as Caladryl.

Rubeola. Rubeola (hard measles, 7-day measles) is a communicable viral disease caused by morbillivirus. The characteristic rash is macular and blotchy; sometimes the macules become confluent. The rubeola rash usually begins on the face and spreads to the appendages. There are several accompanying symptoms: a fever of 100°F or greater, Kopliks spots (small, irregular red spots with a bluish white speck in the center) on the buccal mucosa, and mild to severe photosensitivity. Coldlike symptoms and general malaise and myalgia are often present. In severe cases, the macule may hemorrhage into the skin tissue or onto the outer body surface. This is called hemorrhagic measles. Measles is more severe in malnourished children. Complications include otitis media, pneumonia, and encephalitis.

Rubeola is a disease preventable by vaccine, and immunization is required by law in most states. Immunization is accomplished by injection of a live-virus vaccine. A single injection after 15 months of age is sufficient to produce immunity. For a positive diagnosis of rubeola, most states require antibody titers. Blood titers are usually drawn during the disease process and 6 weeks after the symptoms have resided.

The treatment for rubeola is symptomatic. Children are kept in darkened rooms; antipyretic medications are given to reduce the fever; and rest and fluids are encouraged. If marked dehydration exists or the symptoms are severe, the physician should be consulted.

Rubella. Rubella (3-day measles, German measles) is a childhood disease caused by the rubella virus. It is characterized by a diffuse, punctate, macular rash that begins on the trunk and spreads to the arms and legs. Mild febrile states occur; generally the fever is less than 100°F. Postauricular, suboccipital, and cervical lymph node adenopathy are common. Coldlike symptoms usually accompany the disease in the form of cough, congestion, and coryza.

Rubella generally has no long-lasting sequelae; however, the transmission of the disease to pregnant women early in the gestation period may result in severe teratogenic effects in the unborn fetus. Among the teratogenic effects are cataracts, microcephaly, mental retardation, deafness, patent ductus arteriosus, glaucoma, purpura, and bone defects. Most states have laws requiring immunization to prevent the transmission of rubella to pregnant women. Immunization is accomplished by live-virus injection. A single injection after 15 months of age is considered adequate in the prevention of rubella. Cases of rubella in unimmunized children are rare provided the level of immunization in the general population remains high. As with rubeola, the treatment is symptomatic.

Chickenpox. Chickenpox is a common communicable childhood disease. It is caused by the herpes zoster virus, which is also the agent in shingles. The characteristic skin lesion occurs in three stages: macule, vesicle, and granular scab. The macular stage is characterized by rapid development (within hours) of macules over the trunk of the body, spreading to the limbs, buccal mucosa, scalp, axillae, upper respiratory tract, and conjunctiva. During the second stage, the macules vesiculate (become filled with water, or blister) and may become depressed or umbilicated (raised blisters with depressed centers). The vesicles break open, and a scab forms during the third stage. Crops of lesions occur successively, so that all three forms of the lesion are usually visible by the third day of the illness. Mild to extreme pruritus accompanies these lesions and can be a complicating factor by leading to scratching and subsequent development of secondary bacterial infections. Chickenpox is also accompanied by coldlike symptoms, including cough, coryza, and sometimes photosensitivity. Mild febrile states usually occur. Side effects, such as pneumonia, septic complications, and encephalitis, are rare.

The treatment, as in most of the other childhood diseases, is palliative. To date, no vaccine is available to prevent chickenpox. Antipyretic drugs such as acetaminophen are given to reduce fever; they may also relieve local discomfort. Pruritus is relieved with lukewarm baths and applications of topical antipruritics such as Caladryl lotion. Home remedies, such as baking soda baths, also relieve itching. The physician should be notified in cases of severe pruritus. Oral administration of diphenhydramine (Benadryl) or other antihistamines may be prescribed. Rest and fluids are important in recuperation and rehydration.

Scarlet fever. Scarlet fever is a systemic reaction to the toxins produced by the group A beta-hemolytic streptococci. It occurs when the person is sensitized to the toxin-producing variants of streptococci. It frequently occurs in association with streptococcal sore throat (strep throat); but it may also be associated with a wound, skin infection, or puerperal infection. Scarlet fever is characterized by a pink punctate skin rash on the neck, chest, axillae, groin, and thighs. When palpated, the rash feels like fine sandpaper. There is flushing of the face with circumoral pallor. Other symptoms include high fever, nausea and vomiting, strawberry tongue, raspberry tongue, and skin desquamation. Complications of scarlet fever include otitis media, peritonsillar abscess, rheumatic fever, acute glomerulonephritis, and cholera. Penicillin is the drug of choice for treatment.

Adolescence and young adulthood

The most common disorder of adolescence and young adulthood is acne vulgaris (discussed later in this chapter). The increased production of sex hormones and oils contribute to this problem. The problem associated with childhood diseases are less common in this age group; however, diseases such as pityriasis rosea are more commonly seen. Also, chronic skin diseases may exacerbate or change with the aging process.

Old age*

The elderly person may experience a variety of skin disorders as well as exacerbation of earlier skin problems because of the aging process. Physiologically, in the skin of the elderly person the dermal-epidermal junction is flattened; dermal and subcutaneous mass is lost; the capillary loops are shortened; and the number of melanocytes, Langerhans' cells, and Merkel's cells is reduced. This results in less padding, thinning of the skin, and changes in color and elasticity. The skin is much less resilient to environmental and mechanical trauma, and tissue repair takes longer. Similarly, there is less hair and nail growth, and the hair loses pigment.

Dry skin and pruritus associated with dry skin are common in the elderly. Reduced activity of the sebaceous glands and sweat glands contributes to this problem. For some elderly persons, these changes may be a great help in clearing a lifelong struggle with acne.

* This section is reprinted from Porth C, Kapke K: Aging and the skin. Geriatric Nursing 3:160–161, 1983. Copyright American Journal of Nursing Company. Reprinted by permission.

Common skin problems

The most common skin problems in the elderly are skin tags, keratoses, lentigines, and vascular lesions (Table 8-5). Many of these problems reflect continued exposure to sun and weather over the years.

Skin tags. Skin tags are soft, pedunculated, brown or flesh-colored papules appearing on the front or side of the neck or in the axilla. Ranging in size from a pinhead to the size of a pea, the tags have the normal color and texture of the skin.

Keratoses. A keratosis is a horny growth or a condition characterized by an abnormal growth of the keratinizing cells of the epidermis. *Seborrheic keratoses* are sharply circumscribed, wartlike lesions that seem to rest on top of the skin. They usually begin as yellow-to-brown flat lesions of less than 1 cm and may become larger, dark-brown to coal-black lesions with a greasy appearance.

Table 8–5. Skin lesions common among elders

Lesion	Appearance
Skin tags	Small protrusions (pinhead to size of pea), color and texture of normal skin
Seborrheic keratoses	Raised, sharply circumscribed, wartlike growths, yellow-brown to brown-black color, often multiple, usually on face or trunk
Actinic keratoses	Premalignant, slightly raised, light-to-dark-brown, scaly lesions on "weathered" areas, scale is adherent and returns each time it is removed
Senile lentigines	Flat, tan-to-brown macules, usually on face or hands, often called liver spots
Malignant lentigines	Premalignant lesions; slow growing, flat, light-to-dark-brown mottled "freckles"; usually larger than senile lentigines
Senile angiomas	Small ruby red or purplish vascular tumors; usually on the trunk
Telangiectases	Dilatations of capillaries or terminal arteries; located on the skin surface, often on face, particularly around the nose
Venous lakes	Flat, small, bluish blood vessels, frequently seen on the back of hands, ears, and lips

(From Porth C, Kapke K: Aging and the skin. Geriatr Nurs (May/June) 3:161, 1983. Copyright American Journal of Nursing Company. Reprinted by permission.)

Keratoses are usually found on the face or trunk, sometimes in the form of a solitary lesion and in other cases as literally hundreds of lesions. Although seborrheic keratoses are benign, they must be differentiated from nevi, or moles, which are formed from clusters of melanocytes, because a change in the color, texture, or size of a nevus may indicate malignant transformation to a melanoma.

Actinic (solar) keratoses are premalignant skin lesions that develop on sun-exposed areas. The lesions, ranging in size from 0.1 to 1 cm or larger, usually appear as dry, brown, and scaly areas, although some may have a shiny surface. A slight erythematous area often encircles the lesion.

Actinic lesions are often multiple and more easily felt than seen. When scale is present, it is extremely adherent, and efforts at removal often cause capillary bleeding. The scale tends to recur when it is removed. Characteristic of actinic keratoses is the "weathered" appearance of the surrounding skin. Enlargement, induration, or ulceration of the lesions suggests malignant transformation.

Lentigines. Senile lentigines are the brown, so-called liver spots often seen on sun-exposed areas. Over-the-counter (OTC) creams and lotions containing hydroquinone (Eldoquin, Solaquin, and others) may be used to temporarily bleach these spots. This agent interferes with the synthesis of new pigment but does not destroy existing pigment.

In the concentration approved for OTC preparations, however, hydroquinone has limited usefulness. In the higher concentrations available in prescription preparations, hydroquinone may cause inflammation with burning, tingling, and stinging. Despite the limited usefulness of OTC preparations, their effects may make some people feel less self-conscious about skin discoloration. The success of treatment depends on avoiding sunlight completely or consistently applying a high-potency sunscreen.

Malignant lentigines, sometimes referred to as Hutchinson's melanotic freckles, begin as premalignant lesions arising from the melanocytes and are usually larger than the senile lentigines. They start as a small, light- to dark-brown mottled area that is flat with the surface of the skin and grows laterally. Growth may continue at a variable rate over many years. As malignant changes occur, the area grows vertically and becomes elevated.

Vascular lesions. Vascular lesions consist of vascular tumors and chronically dilated blood vessels. *Senile angiomas* are small, ruby-red or purplish vascular tumors, usually compressible and found mainly on the trunk. *Senile ectasia* refers to a slightly raised erythematous papule that is composed of dilated capillaries. They are usually 2 mm to 5 mm in diameter and located on the trunk. *Telangiectases* are single dilated blood vessels (capillaries or terminal arteries) that appear most frequently on the cheeks and the nose—areas long exposed to excessive sunlight and harsh weather.

Venous lakes are usually seen on the exposed body parts, particularly the backs of the hands, ears, and lips. They consist of small, flat, bluish blood vessels that have a lakelike appearance. The color of the lesion can usually be blanched when sustained pressure is applied to one side. Senile angiomas and venous lakes can be removed by fulguration if a person desires.

In summary, many skin problems occur in specific age groups. Common in infants are diaper rash, prickly heat, and cradle cap. Rashes associated with such childhood diseases as roseola, rubeola, rubella, and chickenpox are seen in young children afflicted with these diseases. Acne vulgaris is a common disorder of adolescence and young adulthood. Skin changes that occur as a part of the aging process predispose the elderly to dry skin, keratosis, lentigines, and vascular skin lesions.

Primary disorders of the skin

Primary skin disorders are those originating in the skin. They include infectious processes, inflammatory conditions, allergic reactions, parasitic infestations, overexposure or hypersensitivity to sunlight, and neoplasms. Although most of these disorders are not life-threatening, they can affect the quality of life.

Mechanical processes

Areas of skin that are rubbed repeatedly may result in necrosis of the stratum spinosum. This can cause blisters, calluses, or corns.

A *blister* is a vesicle or fluid-filled papule. Blisters of mechanical origin form from the repeated friction caused by repeated rubbing on a single area of the skin. Histologically, there is degeneration of epidermal cells and a disruption of intercellular junctions that causes the layers of the skin to separate. As a result, fluid accumulates and a noticeable bleb forms on the skin surface. Blisters are best protected by adding layers of padding (such as adhesive bandages or gauze) to prevent further blister formation. Breaking the skin on a blister to remove the fluid is inadvisable because of the risk of secondary infections.

Prolonged repeated rubbing can produce a *callus* or area of increased skin production (hyperker-

atosis). Increased cohesion between cells results in both hyperkeratosis and decreased skin shedding.

Corns are small, well-circumscribed conical keratinous thickenings of the skin. They usually appear on the toes from rubbing or ill-fitting shoes. The actual corn is a small encapsulated body of hardened keratinous material. Pain often accompanies corns. Corns may be surgically removed, but they will recur if the causative agent is not removed.

Infectious processes

The skin is subject to attack by a number of microorganisms. Normally the skin flora, sebum, immune responses, and other protective mechanisms guard the skin against infection. Depending on the virulence of the infecting agent and the competence of the host's resistance, infections may result.

Fungal infections

Fungal infections of the skin are classified as superficial and deep types. The superficial infections are called dermatophytoses; they are commonly known as *tinea*, or *ringworm*. Different forms of tinea affect different body areas. Tinea can affect the body (tinea corporis), scalp (tinea capitis), beard (tinea barbae), hands (tinea manus), feet (tinea pedis), nails (tinea unguium), or groin and upper aspects of the thigh (tinea cruris; see jock itch, Chapter 35). Deep fungal infections involve the epidermis, dermis, and subcutis. Infections that are typically superficial may exhibit deep involvement in immunosuppressed individuals.

A fungus is a free-living saprophytic plantlike organism (see Chapter 9). Certain strains of fungi are considered normal flora. Fungi causing superficial skin infections live on the dead, keratinized cells of the epidermis. They emit an enzyme that enables them to digest keratin, which results in superficial skin scaling, nail disintegration, and hair structure breakage. An exception to this is the invading fungus of tinea versicolor, which does not produce a keratolytic enzyme. Individual species of three genera have been identified as the invading fungi in most forms of tinea: *Microsporum, Epidermophyton,* and *Trichophyton.*

Diagnosis of fungal infections is primarily done by microscopic examination of skin scrapings. Hyphae are threadlike filaments that grow from spores and are visible microscopically. Mycelia are macroscopic aggregations of hyphae. The fungal spores, the reproducing bodies of fungi, are rarely seen on skin scrapings. Potassium hydroxide (KOH) preparations are used to prepare slides of skin scrapings. The KOH disintegrates human tissue and leaves behind the hyphae for examination. With another method of diag-

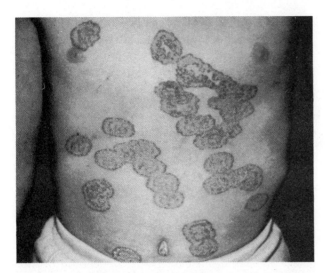

Figure 8-5 Tinea corporis. *(Sauer GC: Manual of Skin Diseases, 4th ed. Philadelphia, JB Lippincott, 1980)*

nosis, a Wood's light (ultraviolet light) is directed onto the affected area; under the light, many fungi will fluoresce a green to yellow-green color.

Tinea corporis. Tinea corporis (ringworm of the body) can be caused by any of the fungal agents. Usually, it is caused by *Microsporum canis* or *M. audouini*; less frequently it is caused by *Trichophyton rubrum* or *T. mentagrophytes*.

The lesions vary depending on the fungal agent. However, the most common types of lesions are round, oval, or circular patches (Figure 8-5).

There is central clearing of the patches with raised red borders consisting of vesicles, papules, or pustules. The lesion begins as a red papule and enlarges with central healing. The borders are sharply defined; lesions may coalesce. Pruritus, a mild burning sensation, and erythema frequently accompany the skin lesion.

Tinea corporis affects all ages; however, children seem most prone to infection. Transmission is most commonly from kittens, puppies, and other children who have infections. Less common forms are from foot and groin infections.

Treatment of mild cases is generally with over-the-counter antifungal preparations containing tolnaftate or undecylenic acid. Tinactin contains a 1% tolnaftate base, whereas Desenex and other name brands contain undecylenic acid. Both of these topical agents are effective if used correctly. Griseofulvin, an oral prescription antifungal agent, is warranted in severe cases.

Tinea capitis. Tinea capitis (ringworm of the scalp) is separated into two types: primary (noninflammatory) and secondary (inflammatory). Primary lesions characteristically present as grayish round hairless patches, or balding spots, on the head. The lesion varies in size and is most commonly seen on the back of the head (Figure 8-6). Mild erythema, crust, or scale may be present. The child is usually symptomless, although occasionally pruritus may exist. The primary form of tinea capitis is caused by *M. audouini* and *M. canis* transferred from kittens, puppies, and other humans. Epidemics have occurred from *Trichophyton tonsurans* and *M. audouini* and represent human-to-human transmission.

Children aged 3 to 8 are primarily affected. Tinea capitis seldom occurs in an adult; this has been partially attributed to the higher content of fatty acids in the sebum after puberty, a finding that has generated the development of several antifungal agents with fatty acid bases. These antifungal agents revolutionized treatment, replacing the old remedies in which children were often subjected to head shavings and use of harsh shampoos and salves.

The inflammatory type of tinea capitis is caused by a virulent strain of *T. mentagrophytes, T.*

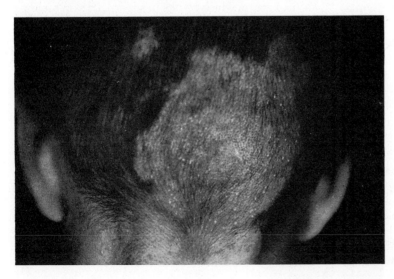

Figure 8-6 Tinea capitis. *(Sauer GC: Manual of Skin Diseases, 4th ed. Philadelphia, JB Lippincott, 1980)*

verrucosum, and *Microsporum gypseum*. The onset is acute, and lesions are usually localized to one area. The initial lesion consists of a pustular scaly round patch with broken hairs. A secondary bacterial infection is common and may lead to a painful circumscribed, boggy, and indurated lesion called a *kerion*. The highest incidence is in children and in farmers who work with infected animals.

The treatment for both forms of tinea capitis is primarily griseofulvin, an oral antifungal agent. Topical ointments are sometimes indicated in addition. Wet packs and medicated shampoos, along with antibiotics, may be prescribed for the secondary types of infection.

Tinea pedis. Tinea pedis (athlete's foot, ringworm of the feet) is a common skin disorder primarily affecting the spaces between the toes, the soles of the feet, or the sides of the feet. It is caused by *T. mentagrophytes* and *T. rubrum*. The lesions vary from a mild scaling lesion to a painful exudative, erosive, inflamed lesion with fissuring. Lesions are often accompanied by pruritus and foul odor.

Evidence suggests that athlete's foot occurs in two forms, simple and complex. Simple forms of tinea pedis have high fungal populations and low bacterial growths. They are characterized by mild to moderate skin peeling and are largely asymptomatic. Complex tinea pedis has a higher bacterial count (*Proteus* and *Pseudomonas*) with a receding fungal count. Complex forms involve maceration of tissue, inflammation, and fissuring. Pruritus and pain are often present.[12]

Some people are prone to chronic tinea pedis. Mild forms are more common during dry environmental conditions. Exacerbations in the mild form occur as a result of hot weather, sweating, and exercise, or when the feet are exposed to moisture or occlusive shoes. Tinea pedis may occur alone or in combination with other infections such as tinea corporis or tinea cruris. Patches may occur on the hands; this is known as the intradermal, or dermatophytid, reaction.

Simple forms of tinea pedis are treated with topical application of antifungals such as tolnaftate. In the past, complex forms have been treated with oral griseofulvin and topical antifungal agents. Based on their study, Klingman and Leyden[12] now suggest the combination of antibiotics (neomycin sulfate) and tolnaftate in the treatment of complex forms. Other treatment and preventive modalities include scrupulous cleansing and drying of affected areas, clean dry socks, and changing of socks daily. When bathed, the feet should be dried after other parts of the body to prevent spread of the disease.

Tinea unguium. Tinea unguium, or ringworm of the nails (onchomycosis), is a chronic fungal infection of the nails of the hands or feet. Tinea of the toenails is common; tinea of the fingernails is less common. Toenail infection is common in people prone to chronic infections of tinea pedis. Often, the infection in the toenails becomes a ready source for future infections of the foot. It may begin from a crushing injury to a toenail or from the spread of tinea pedis. Usually tinea unguium is caused by *T. rubrum* or *T. mentagrophytes*. The infection usually begins at the tip of the nail, where the fungus digests the keratin of the nail. Initially, the nail appears opaque, white, or silvery. The nail then turns yellow or brown. This condition remains unchanged for years and may involve only one or two nails. Generally, there is no discomfort. Gradually, the nail thickens and becomes frail as the infection spreads to the entire nail and nail plate. The nail cracks and thickens, and the nail plate separates from the nail bed as the nail becomes permanently discolored and distorted. Spreading to other nails may occur.

The prognosis for fungal infections of the toenail is poor. The treatment usually involves oral griseofulvin for up to 1 year. It rarely produces a cure, and some authorities recommend not using griseofulvin or only using the drug with removal of the infected toenails. Even with this therapy, recurrence is frequent. Fingernail infections are more easily treated. Oral griseofulvin therapy for 6 months to 1 year has been successful but is dependent on the persistence of both the therapist and the patient.

Tinea manus. Tinea manus (ringworm of the hands) is rarely a primary infection. The primary site of infection is usually tinea pedis with tinea manus occurring as a secondary infection. A diagnostic differentiation among hand diseases is that tinea manus usually occurs only on one hand, whereas other infectious processes, such as contact dermatitis and psoriasis, affect both hands.

The same fungal agents responsible for tinea pedis are found active in tinea manus, *T. rubrum* and *T. mentagrophytes*. The characteristic lesion is a blister on the palm or finger surrounded by erythema. Chronic lesions are scaly and dry. Cracking and fissuring may occur. The lesions may spread to the plantar surfaces of the hand; if chronic, tinea manus may lead to tinea of the fingernails. The treatment of choice is oral griseofulvin therapy for approximately 3 months.

Tinea barbae. Tinea barbae (ringworm of the beard) is rare. It occurs primarily in farmers, who contract it from infected cattle. It is usually caused by *T. verrucosum*, found in cattle, or *T. mentagrophytes*, found in dogs and horses. Historically, the name had its origin during the time when tinea barbae was transmitted person-to-person by contaminated barbers' razors and combs.

The milder form of tinea barbae involves lesions similar to those found in tinea corporis or tinea capitis. A macule spreads into a patch with raised borders and central clearing. Vesicles and papules may be found. Alopecia accompanies involved areas. Severe forms include pustule formation with bacterial infection. The beard hairs break off close to the skin surface and are easily pulled out.

The usual mode of treatment is oral griseofulvin therapy with or without topical antifungal applications. Boric acid wet packs are sometimes indicated. The benefits of antibiotic therapy are limited to secondary bacterial infections.

Tinea versicolor. Tinea versicolor is a fungal infection involving the upper chest, the back, and sometimes the arms. The causative agent is *Malassezia furfur*. The infection occurs primarily in young adults in tropic and temperate regions; however, cases have been reported in the northern states.

The characteristic lesion is a yellow, pink, or brown sheet of scaling skin. The name *versicolor* is derived from the multicolored variations of the lesion. The patches are depigmented and do not tan when exposed to ultraviolet light, and the skin has an overall appearance of being "dirty." These cosmetic defects often bring the patient to the physician in the summer months. The theory is that the fungus filters the ultraviolet light, thus preventing tanning. In darker-skinned persons, the depigmented areas are more apparent.

Although there is no specific drug that will prevent the recurrence of tinea versicolor, selenium sulfide, found in several shampoo preparations, has been a most effective treatment measure. Boiling or steam-pressing clothes may prevent recurrence.

Dermatophytid reaction. A secondary skin eruption may occur in persons allergic to one of the dermatophytes, and this is called a dermatophytid, or intradermal (ID), reaction. It may occur during an acute episode of a fungal infection. The most common reaction occurs on the hands, in response to tinea pedis. The lesions are vesicles with erythema extending over the palms and fingers of the hand; extension to other areas may occur. Less commonly, there can be a more generalized reaction in which papules or vesicles erupt on the trunk or extremities. These eruptions may resemble tinea corporis and may become excoriated and infected with bacteria. Treatment revolves around treating the primary site of infection. The ID reaction will resolve in most cases without intervention if the primary site is cleared.

Candidal (monilial) infections. Candidiasis (moniliasis) is a fungal infection caused by *Candida albicans*. This yeastlike fungus is a normal inhabitant of the gastrointestinal tract, mouth, and vagina (see genital *C. albicans,* Chapter 38). The skin problems that result are due to the release of irritating toxins on the skin surface. Some conditions predispose a person to candidal infections, such as diabetes mellitus, antibiotic therapy, pregnancy, use of birth control pills, poor nutrition, and immunosuppressed diseases.

C. albicans thrives in warm, moist intertriginous areas of the body. The rash is red with well-defined borders. Patches erode the epidermis, and there is scaling (Figure 8-7). Severe forms of infection may involve pustules or vesiculopustules. A differential diagnostic feature of candidal in comparison with tinea infection is the presence of satellite lesions. These satellite lesions are maculopapular and are found outside the clearly demarcated borders of the candidal infection. The appearance of candidal infections varies according to the site; Table 8-6 summarizes site characteristics.

Treatment measures vary according to the location. Preventive measures, such as wearing rubber gloves, are encouraged for people with infections of the hands. Intertriginous areas are often separated with clean cotton cloth. Nystatin (Mycostatin), an antibiotic available in tablets, powder, or vaginal suppositories, is effective in control of infection.

Bacterial infections

Bacteria are considered normal flora of the skin. Most bacteria are not pathogenic; however, when pathogenic bacteria invade the skin, superficial or systemic infections may develop. Bacterial infections are classified as primary, or superficial, and secondary, or deep. Impetigo is an example of a primary bacterial infection, and infected ulcers are an example of a secondary bacterial infection.

Bacterial infections are usually cultured for diagnosis. In addition to antibiotic therapy, the treatment of bacterial infections often includes hygiene

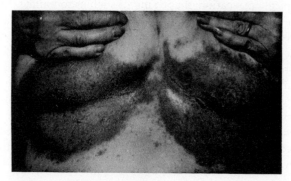

Figure 8-7 Submammary candidiasis. Note the satellite lesions beyond the border of the eruption. (*Demis DJ [ed]: Clinical Dermatology. Philadelphia, Harper & Row, 1985*)

Table 8–6. Candidal infections: location and appearance of lesions

Location	Appearance
Breasts, groin, axillae, anus, umbilicus, toe or fingerwebs	Red lesions with well-defined borders and presence of satellite lesions; lesions may be dry or moist
Vagina	Red, oozing lesions with sharply defined borders and inflamed vagina; cervix may be covered with moist, white plaque; cheesy, foul-smelling discharge; presence of pruritus and burning
Glans penis (balanitis)	Red lesions with sharply defined borders; penis may be covered with white plaque; presence of pruritus and burning
Mouth (thrush)	Creamy white flakes on a red, inflamed mucous membrane; papillae on tongue may be enlarged
Nails	Red, painful swelling around nail bed; common in people who often have their hands in water

education, general isolation procedures, and dietary management.

Impetigo. Impetigo is a common superficial bacterial infection caused by staphylococci or beta-hemolytic streptococci. It is most common among young infants and children, although older children and adults occasionally contract the disease. It is highly communicable in the younger population.

Initially, impetigo appears as a small vesicle or pustule, or a large bulla. The primary lesion ruptures, leaving a denuded area that discharges a honey-colored serous liquid; the liquid hardens on the skin surface and deposits a honey-colored crust with a stuck-on appearance (Figure 8-8). New vesicles erupt within hours. Pruritus often accompanies the disease, and the skin excoriations that result from scratching multiply the infection sites. Lesions are most often found on the face, but they can occur anywhere on the body. Untreated, impetigo can last for weeks and may continue to spread and become a deeper bacterial infection requiring emergency medical attention. A possible complication of untreated impetigo is post-streptococcal acute glomerulonephritis.

Treatment measures vary among physicians. Some physicians treat the lesions locally: crusts are removed with soaks, infected areas are washed with bacteriostatic soaps, and topical antibiotics are applied. Other physicians believe that impetigo should be treated systemically with antibiotics to prevent glomerulonephritis.

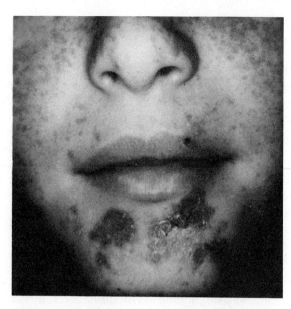

Figure 8-8 The crusted lesions of impetigo. (*Demis DJ [ed]: Clinical Dermatology. Philadelphia, Harper & Row, 1985*)

Ecthyma. Ecthyma is an ulcerative form of impetigo, usually secondary to minor trauma. It frequently occurs on the buttocks and thighs of children. The lesions are similar to those of impetigo. A vesicle or pustule ruptures, leaving a skin erosion or ulcer that weeps and dries to a crusted patch, often resulting in scar formation. With extensive ecthyma, there is a low-grade fever and extension of the infection to other organs. The treatment is the same as for impetigo. When other organs are involved, oral or intramuscular penicillin is indicated.

Viral infections

Viruses are intracellular pathogens. They have no organized cell structure but consist of a DNA or RNA core surrounded by a protein coat. Viruses rely completely on live cells for reproduction. The viruses seen in skin lesion disorders tend to be DNA-containing viruses. Viruses invade the keratinocyte, begin to reproduce, and cause cellular proliferation or cellular death. The rapid increase in viral skin diseases has been attributed to the use of birth control medication and corticosteroid drugs, which have immunosuppressive qualities, and the use of antibiotics, which alter the bacterial flora of the skin.[13] As the number of bacterial infections has decreased, there has been a proportional rise in viral skin diseases.

Verrucae. Verrucae, or warts, are common benign papillomas caused by DNA-containing papovaviruses. Although warts vary in gross appearance depending on their location, they all have a similar histologic appearance (Table 8-7). The wart is not a mass of uniform tumor cells but, like other skin diseases, is an exaggeration of the normal skin composition. There is an irregular thickening of the stratum spinosum and greatly increased thickening of the stratum corneum. The human papilloma viruses (HPVs), the subgroup of the papovaviruses that cause human warts, are not found in animals and invade only the skin and mucous membrane of humans.

Warts resolve spontaneously when immunity to the virus develops. The immune response may be delayed for years; after 5 years, 95% of warts left untreated will have disappeared. In earlier years, treatment measures were directed at eradicating all wart tissue, primarily by excision. Since this frequently left scars, current treatment is directed at irritation of the wart with liquid nitrogen or acid chemicals. Cryotherapy and salicylic acid paint or plasters have also been effective.

Herpes simplex (cold sore, fever blister). Herpes simplex virus (HSV) infections of the skin and mucous membrane are common (Figure 8-9). Two types of herpesvirus infect humans, type I and type II. Most of the HSV I infections occur above the waist. HSV I may result when external infection is spread to other parts of the body through the occupational hazards that exist in professions such as dentistry and medicine, and some athletics. Type II is responsible for most infections in the genital region (see Chapter 38).

Herpesvirus lesions usually begin with a burning or tingling sensation. Vesicles and erythema follow and progress to pustules, ulcers, and crusts before healing. The lesion is most common on the lips, face, and mouth. Pain is common, and healing takes place within 10 to 14 days.

Herpes simplex viral infections are of two types: primary and secondary. The primary infection usually consists of a high fever, sore throat, painful vesicles, and ulcers of the tongue, palate, gingiva, buccal mucosa, and lips. The primary infection results in the development of antibodies to the virus so that recurrences (secondary infections) are more localized and less severe. Following an initial infection, the herpesvirus persists in the trigeminal and other ganglia in the latent state. Recurrent lesions are common in a small percentage of people; precipitating factors may be stress, sunlight exposure, menses, or injury.

There is no cure for herpes simplex; most treatment measures are palliative. Lidocaine (Xylocaine) or diphenhydramine (Benadryl) application and aspirin help relieve pain. Cold compresses help in the acute stages. Severe forms have been treated with idoxuridine (IDI, Stoxil), which prevents certain aspects of DNA synthesis and thereby inhibits viral reproduction without causing cell injury. To date, the most effective treatment has been the drug acyclovir. Acyclovir is an antimetabolite that inhibits herpesvirus replication. It is the prototype of all the antiviral drugs and is most effective in topical solutions and creams.

Herpes zoster. Herpes zoster (shingles) is an acute localized inflammatory disease of a dermatome segment of the skin. It is caused by the same herpesvirus that causes chickenpox—varicella-zoster. It is believed to be the result of reactivation of a latent

Table 8-7. Types and characteristics of verrucae (warts)

Type	Location	Appearance
Verruca vulgaris (common warts)	Anywhere on the skin, usually on the hands	Ragged dome-shape with growth above the skin surface
Verruca filiformis	Eyelids, face, neck	Long finger-like projections
Verruca plana (flat wart)	Forehead, dorsum of hand	Small flat tumors, may be barely visible
Verruca plantaris (plantar wart)	Sole of foot	Flat to slightly raised growth extending deep into skin; painful; bleeding occurs with superficial trimming; coalesced plantar warts are referred to as mosaic warts
Condyloma acuminata	Mucous membrane of the penis, female genitalia, perianal areas, and rectum	Large moist projections with rough surfaces; usually pink or purple in color

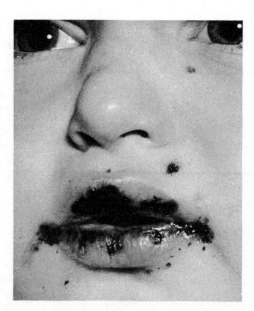

Figure 8-9 Primary herpes simplex in a two-year-old child. (*Sauer GC: Manual of Skin Diseases, 4th ed. Philadelphia, JB Lippincott, 1980*)

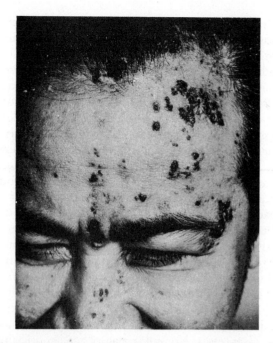

Figure 8-10 Herpes zoster involving the ophthalmic branch of the trigeminal nerve. (*Sauer GC: Manual of Skin Disease, 5th ed. Philadelphia, JB Lippincott, 1985*)

varicella-zoster virus that has been present in the sensory dorsal ganglia since childhood infection. During an attack of shingles, the reactivated virus travels from the ganglia to the skin of the corresponding dermatome.

The clinical picture of herpes zoster is the eruption of vesicles with erythematous bases that are restricted to skin areas supplied by sensory neurons of a single or associated group of dorsal root ganglia. Eruptions are generally unilateral in the thoracic region, trunk, and face. In immunosuppressed persons, the lesions may extend beyond the dermatome. New crops of vesicles erupt for 3 to 5 days along the nerve pathway. The lesions are deeper and more confluent than those of chickenpox. The vesicles dry, form crusts, and eventually fall off. The lesions usually clear in 2 to 3 weeks. Severe pain and paresthesia are common. In the elderly, herpes zoster is a particularly serious condition that may be long-lasting and eventually lead to death. Pain reports from elderly individuals indicate an increased severity and lengthy episodes of up to 1 year. Postherpetic neuralgia is the most important complication occurring in people over the age of 50. Eye involvement can result in permanent blindness and occurs in 50% of the cases involving the ophthalmic division of the trigeminal nerve (Figure 8-10).

Treatment is primarily palliative except when complications occur. Topical agents used are Burow's compresses or aqueous alcohol lotions. Pain medication is indicated in severe cases. Systemic corticosteroids have been effective in healthy patients over 50

years old with severe pain. High doses of interferon, an antiviral glycoprotein, have been effective in people with cancer when the lesions are limited to the dermatome. The drug acyclovir has proved effective in treating some cases of herpes zoster, but it remains under investigation.

Inflammatory skin disorders

The inflammatory skin diseases listed here are generally of unknown cause or etiology. They are usually localized to the skin and are rarely associated with a specific internal disease. They produce marked variations in normal skin, usually papulosquamous in nature. Inflammation and erythema are common. These disorders, which include acne, lichen planus, psoriasis, and pityriasis rosea, are among the most common skin disorders.

Acne

Acne is commonly referred to as a disorder of the pilosebaceous (hair and sebaceous gland) unit. The sebaceous glands empty into the hair follicle and the pilosebaceous unit opens to the skin surface by means of a widely dilated opening called a *pore* (see Figure 8-4). The sebaceous glands are largest on the face, scalp, scrotum, but are present in all areas of the skin except for the soles of the feet and palms of the hands. The sebaceous cells are derived from the epidermal keratin cell and have a structure similar to epidermal cells except that they accumulate lipid droplets. The sebaceous glands produce a complex lipid mixture called *sebum,* from the Latin word meaning tallow or grease. Sebum consists of a mixture of free fatty acids, triglycerides, diglycerides, monoglycerides, sterol esters, wax esters, and squalene. Sebum production occurs as a holocrine process in which the sebaceous cells are completely broken down and their lipid contents emptied through the sebaceous duct into the hair follicle. The amount of sebum produced depends on two factors: (1) the size of the sebaceous gland, and (2) the rate of cellular growth. Sebaceous cell proliferation and sebum production are uniquely responsive to direct hormonal stimulation by androgen. In men, testicular androgens are the main stimulus for sebaceous activity; in women, adrenal and ovarian androgens maintain sebaceous activity.

Acne lesions consist of comedones (whiteheads and blackheads), papules, pustules, and in severe cases, cysts. Noninflammatory acne consists primarily of comedones, whereas inflammatory acne consists of erythematous-based pustules and cysts. Blackheads are plugs of material that accumulate in sebaceous glands that open to the skin surface. The color of blackheads results from melanin that has moved into the sebaceous glands from adjoining epidermal cells. Whiteheads are pale, slightly elevated papules with no visible orifice. The inflammatory lesions are believed to develop from the escape of sebum into the dermis and the irritating effects of the fatty acids that are contained in the sebum.

There are several forms of acne. Three types of acne occur during different stages of the life cycle: acne vulgaris is the most common form among adolescents and young adults; acne conglobata develops later in life, and acne rosacea occurs in older adults. There are numerous other types of acne with varying etiologic agents and influences.

Acne vulgaris. Acne vulgaris develops in about 80% to 90% of all people during adolescence or young adulthood and accounts for about 25% of all visits to the dermatologist. In women, acne may persist up to 30 years of age; however, the overall incidence is higher in men.

Acne vulgaris lesions form primarily on the face and neck and, to a lesser extent, on the back, chest, and shoulders (Figure 8-11). The lesions are thought to result from increased activity of the sebaceous glands and plugging of the pilosebaceous ducts.

The cause of acne vulgaris is unknown, but is probably multifactorial. Several contributing factors have been determined: (1) the influence of androgens on sebaceous cell activity; (2) increased proliferation

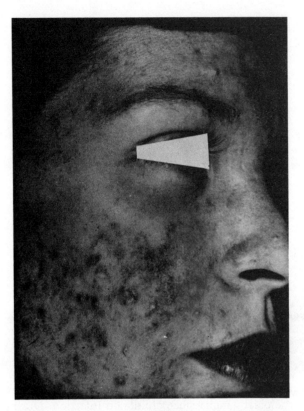

Figure 8-11 Acne vulgaris. (*Demis DJ [ed]: Clinical Dermatology. Philadelphia, Harper & Row, 1985*)

of the keratinizing epidermal cells that form the sebaceous cells; (3) increased sebum production in relation to the severity of the disease; (4) decreased amounts of linoleic acid in the sebum; and (5) presence of the *Propionibacterium acnes* organism. The *P. acnes* organism contains lipases, and these enzymes can result in lipolysis and production of the free fatty acids which produce inflammation.[14]

The importance of preventive measures as a child nears puberty cannot be overstated. These include frequent washing of the involved areas, avoiding touching the face with the hands, shampooing hair and scalp regularly, keeping hair away from the face, avoiding use of creams and moisturizers, and using water-based, rather than oil-based, makeup. Exposure to sunlight is often helpful. Squeezing, rubbing, or picking of comedones should be avoided. A balanced diet is recommended, and stressful or fatigue-producing activities should be minimized. Although there is little empirical evidence to support these measures, therapists recommend them depending on their views on acne and the person's symptoms.

Preventive measures are also used to treat acne. Mild forms of acne respond well to stringent hygiene measures in addition to the topical application of acne creams, ointments, and lotions. Numerous commercial products are available that contain peeling, drying, and antibiotic agents. Products with resorcinol, salicylic acid, or sulfur bases are helpful in drying and peeling the skin. Oil-based preparations should be avoided, because they contribute to the problem.

Treatment of severe acne is based upon four objectives supported by current knowledge of the condition: (1) correction of the defect in epidermal cell proliferation, (2) lessening of sebaceous gland activity, (3) reduction of the *P. acnes* population, and (4) reduction of the inflammatory process. Many of the treatment modalities may be used alone or in combination with other treatments.

Acne creams and lotions contain keratolytic agents such as sulfur, salicylic acid, and resorcinol that act as chemically abrasive agents to loosen comedones and exert a peeling effect on the skin. Tretinoin (Retin-A), an acid derivative of vitamin A, is a stronger keratolytic agent, but it is irritating. It helps remove comedones by increasing mitotic activity at the base of the follicle. Comedones are then pushed out from below. Because tretinoin is applied topically, it remains chiefly on the epidermis with minimal absorption into the circulation.

Oral low-dose tetracycline has been used effectively for years. Tetracycline has no effect on sebum production, but it does decrease the amount of free fatty acids. Tetracycline requires a sufficient treatment period to establish effective blood levels. Side effects are minimal, which is why the drug has remained so useful. However, it does have teratogenic effects and should not be given to pregnant women. Erythromycin, another antibiotic, also has been effective in acne treatment. Of the sulfonamides, dapsone (diaminodeniphylsulfone) has been effective in severe cystic acnes. However, the side effects are many and the drug should be used with caution and close monitoring. Tetracycline, erythromycin, and clindamycin are now available for topical application.

Estrogens decrease sebum production; however, because of the high dosages required, they are contraindicated in men. In women, estrogen therapy is administered in 2-week or 3-week treatment periods and regulated with the menstrual cycle. Side effects are those associated with any estrogen therapy, such as nausea, weight gain, spotting, breast tenderness, amenorrhea, thromboembolic disorders, and a possible increased risk of cancer.

Glucocorticoid therapy has been limited primarily to severe resistive cases. The therapy results in remarkable healing, yet acne usually returns after the therapy has been terminated.

Isotretinoin (Accutane), an orally administered synthetic retinoid or acid form of vitamin A, reduces sebum secretion and has been proven useful in the treatment of cystic acne. Its effects are thought to be related more to hormonal activity rather than the vitamin activity its origin would indicate.[15] In carefully planned dosages, oral isotretinoin has cleared major cases of acne and initiated long-term remissions of the disease. It is administered for 3-month to 4-month treatment periods. Because of its many side effects, it should only be used in persons with severe acne. Common side effects are dryness of the mouth and other mucous membranes, conjunctivitis, and pruritus. Although the exact mode of action is not known, it decreases sebaceous gland activity, reduces the *P. acnes* count, and has an anti-inflammatory effect.

Other treatment measures for acne include surgery, ultraviolet irradiation, x-ray irradiation, cryotherapy, and intralesional glucocorticosteroid injection. Acne surgery involves the aspiration of comedones with small-bore needles or devices designed to extract comedone contents. Scarring is a common sequela if done improperly. The use of ultraviolet irradiation, which involves exposure to either hot or cold quartz lights for specified periods, remains controversial, but continues to be used in treatment of some forms of acne. X-ray therapy reduces the size of the sebaceous glands for brief periods; its use has decreased over time because of the risk of thyroid cancer in persons exposed to the treatment. Cryotherapy (freezing with carbon dioxide slushes, liquid nitrogen, dry ice, or acetone) has been effective in promoting healing of lesions by removing the outer layers of skin. Injection of glucocorticosteroids using a syringe or needleless injector is limited to severe nodulocystic forms of acne. It has been effective in promoting cyst healing, but usually has to be repeated frequently.

Acne conglobata. Acne conglobata occurs later in life and is a chronic form of acne. Comedones, papules, pustules, nodules, abscesses, cysts, and scars occur on the back, buttocks, and chest, and to a lesser extent on the abdomen, shoulders, neck, face, upper arms, and thighs. The comedones have multiple openings and their discharge is odoriferous, serous, and purulent or mucoid. Healing leaves deep keloidal lesions. Afflicted persons have anemia and increased white blood cell counts, sedimentation rates, and neutrophil counts. The treatment is difficult and stringent. It often includes debridement, systemic corticosteroid therapy, oral retinoids, and systemic antibiotics.

Acne rosacea. Acne rosacea is a chronic acne that occurs in middle-aged and older adults. The characteristic lesion is an erythema or telangiectasia with or without acneiform components (comedones, pustules, nodules). The cause is unknown, and the onset is insidious. It begins with redness over the nose and cheeks and may extend to the chin and forehead. After years of affliction, acne rosacea may develop into an irregular, bullous hyperplasia (thickening) of the nose, known as *rhinophyma*. The sebaceous follicles and openings enlarge, while the skin color changes to a purple red. Treatment measures are similar to those for acne vulgaris; there is no specific treatment. Patients are told to avoid vascular-stimulating agents such as heat, cold, sunlight, hot liquids, highly seasoned foods, and alcohol. Rhinophyma can be treated surgically.

Other acnes. There are numerous other forms of acne. The symptoms vary depending on the source or age of onset. Treatment measures for these acnes vary depending on the precipitating agent and the extent of the lesions. Many of the previously discussed treatment measures have been used with varying degrees of success.

Acne fulminans is manifested by a sudden eruption of large, inflamed, tender lesions on the back and chest that ulcerate, heal, and scar. Teenage boys are most affected by this type of acne. *Steatocystoma multiplex* consists of an eruption of many cystic lesions of various sizes on the trunk of men and women of young adult age. *Neonatal acne* occurs on the newborn infant, typically on the nose and cheeks; it usually clears without treatment. *Drug acnes* occur as an untoward reaction to certain pharmacologic agents, most commonly steroids, iodides (in cough mixtures), and bromides (in sedatives). *Tropical acne* consists of deep, large inflammatory lesions on the trunk and buttocks. This acne is usually the result of living in tropical climates and is therefore seen most often on men who serve in the armed forces.

Acne that results from the exposure to occupational compounds or chemicals is called *occupational acne*. Many of the precipitating agents are the same as those that may cause allergic responses, cutting oils being the most offensive. *Acne aestivalis* is a form of acne that results from sun exposure. Lesions are commonly found on the shoulders, arms, neck, and chest of young adult women. *Acne cosmetica* is believed to be caused by cosmetics. The exact etiologies are unknown because of the variety of cosmetic agents used by women. Even after cosmetic use has been discontinued, this acne usually persists and is difficult to heal. *Acne detergicans* is believed to be caused by compulsive washing of the face with soaps, while *acne mechanica* develops from repeated trauma to the skin. A common form of acne mechanica is seen on football players from the rubbing of their helmets. *Pomade acne* follows the hairline and is most commonly seen on black males. *Acne excoriée des jeunes filles* is a mild form of acne seen in adolescent girls.

The lesions spread from scratching and picking that are believed to be of emotional origin.

Lichen planus

The term *lichen* is of Greek origin and means *tree-moss*. The term is applied to skin disorders characterized by small, firm, papular lesions that are set very close together. Lichen planus is a relatively common chronic, pruritic disease involving inflammation and papular eruption of the skin and mucous membranes. Idiopathic lichen planus is of unknown etiology; but, like other diseases, it is associated with a variety of drugs and chemicals in susceptible persons. Lichen planus may involve a cell-mediated immune response that occurs in the basal cells. There is basal cell degeneration with reduced cell mitosis. There are variations in the pattern of lesions (annular, linear) as well as differences in the sites (mucous membranes, genitalia, nails, scalp). The characteristic lesion is a shiny white-topped, purple, polygonal papule. These lesions appear on the wrist, ankles, and trunk of the body (Figure 8-12).

In the majority of people, lichen planus is a self-limiting disease. Treatment measures include discontinuation of all medications, followed by treatment with topical corticosteroids and occlusive dressings. Systemic corticosteroids may be indicated in severe cases. Antipruritic agents are helpful in reducing itch.

Psoriasis

Psoriasis is a common, papulosquamous disease characterized by white, scaling patches of various sizes. Psoriasis occurs worldwide, although the incidence is lower in warmer, sunnier climates. In the United States it affects 1% of the population. The average age of onset is in the third decade.

The disease, which can persist throughout life

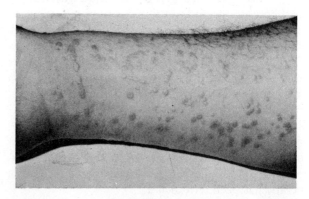

Figure 8-12 Lichen planus. Note the discrete papules on the forearm. On the wrist, the papules have a linear configuration. *(Demis DJ [ed]: Clinical Dermatology. Philadelphia, Harper & Row, 1985)*

and exacerbate at unpredictable times, is classified as a chronic ailment. A few cases, though, have been known to clear and not recur. The cause of psoriasis is unknown. There is often a background of psoriasis in the family, indicating a hereditary factor—approximately one-third of the cases have a genetic history. Skin trauma is a common precipitating factor in persons predisposed to the disease (prepsoriasis). This reaction of the skin to the original trauma, which can be of any type, is called the Koebner reaction. There appears to be an association between psoriasis and arthritis. Psoriatic arthritis occurs in 5% to 7% of persons with psoriasis.

Histologically, the migration time of the keratinocyte from the basal cell layer of the stratum corneum decreases from the normal 14 days to approximately 4 to 7 days. This process is *hyperkeratosis*. In psoriasis there is thinning of the suprapapillary plate and clubbing of the dermal papillae. Capillary beds show permanent damage even when the disease is in remission or has resolved.

There are various forms of psoriasis. A chronic stationary form called *psoriasis vulgaris* is the most common form. The lesions may occur anywhere on the skin, but most often involve the elbows, knees, and scalp (Figure 8-13). The primary lesions are papules that vary in shape. The papules form into plaques with thick and silvery scales. A differential diagnostic finding is that the plaques bleed from minute points when removed, which is known as *Auspitz* sign. Secondary lesions are uncommon, but there may be excoriation, thickening, or oozing. In the black person the plaques may turn purple.

Another form of psoriasis, called *eruptive (guttata)* psoriasis is more common as an early onset form of the disease. Its lesions are smaller and usually limited to the upper trunk and extremities. Generalized pustular psoriasis is a distinct form of the disease that is distinguished by a fever that lasts for several days following eruptions of small pustules. The pustules occur over the trunk and extremities and may include nail beds, palms of the hands, and soles of the feet. Psoriatic erythroderma affects all body surfaces including the hands, feet, nails, trunk, and extremities. *Psoriasis annularis* is a rare form of the disease, and as its name implies, the lesions are annular in shape.

There are a variety of treatment regimes for psoriasis. Anthralin applied topically has been effective in resolving lesions in approximately 2 weeks. A variation of the treatment, called the Ingram method, involves coal tar applications, ultraviolet-B radiation, followed by anthralin paste application. Coal or wood tar (crude tar or wood extract) is one of the oldest and yet one of the most effective forms of treatment. The skin is covered with a film of coal tar for a period of up to several weeks. The exact mechanism of action of the tar products is unknown, but the side effects of the treatment are few. Coal tar preparations may contain other compounds. The Goeckerman regimen consists of combining the therapeutic effects of coal tar and ultraviolet light.

Topical, systemic, and intralesionally applied corticosteroids are useful in the treatment of psoriasis. Topical corticosteroids are most effective if they are potent and used under occlusive dressings. Severe cases or acute exacerbations of the disease may warrant the use of systemic corticosteroid therapy. Intralesional injections of the corticosteroid drug triamcinolone are effective in resistant lesions.

Another treatment modality is photochemotherapy using a light-activated form of the drug

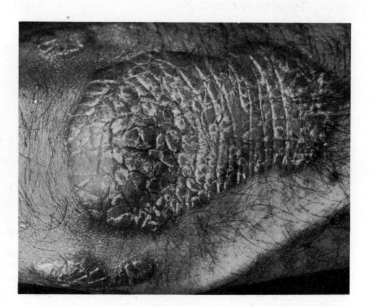

Figure 8-13 Psoriasis on the elbow. (*Sauer GC: Manual of Skin Diseases, 5th ed. Philadelphia, JB Lippincott, 1985*)

methotrexate—methoxsalen (8-MOP). Methoxsalen is a psoralen, a light-activated drug that exerts its actions when exposed to ultraviolet-A rays in the 320-nm to 400-nm wavelength range. The combination treatment regimen of psoralen (P) and ultraviolet light (UVA) is known by the acronym PUVA. Methotrexate, which is also used in cancer treatment, is an antimetabolite that inhibits DNA synthesis and thus prevents cell mitosis. Methotrexate has been effective in treating psoriasis when given without phototherapy, but the drug has many side effects, including nausea, malaise, leukopenia, thrombocytopenia, and liver function abnormalities. Because methoxsalen is inert until it is exposed to UVA light, its effects are limited to the skin cells that are exposed to both the drug and the UVA light. Methoxsalen is given orally prior to UVA exposure. Activated by UVA, methoxsalen inhibits DNA synthesis and thus prevents cell mitosis, thereby decreasing the hyperkeratosis that occurs with psoriasis. The treatment produces a remission, but not a cure. Even though there has been a high success rate with PUVA treatment, it must be used cautiously, since it can induce accelerated aging of exposed skin, skin cancer, development of cataracts, and alterations in immune function. In addition, the skin remains sensitive to sunlight until the methoxsalen is excreted, so that persons receiving PUVA treatment should be cautioned to avoid sun exposure for 8 hours following treatment.

Retinoids are currently under investigation for the treatment of psoriasis. Climatotherapy (moving to a warm climate with saltwater baths for 4 weeks to 6 weeks) has also been an effective treatment. All treatments are palliative, as a cure for psoriasis has not yet been developed.

Pityriasis rosea

Pityriasis rosea is a skin rash of unknown origin that primarily affects young adults. The incidence is highest in spring and fall. The belief is that it could be viral, but to date no virus has been isolated. Cases occur in clusters and among people who are in close contact with each other, indicating an infectious spread; however, there are no data to support communicability.

The characteristic lesion is a macule or papule with surrounding erythema. The lesion spreads with central clearing much like tinea corporis. This initial lesion is a solitary lesion called the herald patch and is usually on the trunk or neck. As the lesion enlarges and begins to fade away (2–10 days), successive crops of lesions appear on the trunk and neck. The extremities, face, and scalp may be involved, and mild to severe pruritus may occur. The disease is self-limiting and usually disappears within 6 to 8 weeks. Treatment measures are palliative and include topical steroids, antihistamines, and colloid baths. Systemic corticosteroids may be indicated in severe cases.

Allergic skin responses

Allergic skin responses involve the body's immune system and are caused by hypersensitivity reactions (see Chapter 12). They include contact dermatitis, atopic and nummular eczema, and drug reactions.

Contact dermatitis

Contact dermatitis is a common inflammation of the skin. There are two types of contact dermatitis —irritant and allergic. Irritant contact dermatitis occurs in people who are in contact with a sufficient amount of the irritant to cause a reaction (Figure 8-14). It can occur from mechanical means such as rubbing (wool, fiberglass), chemical irritants (those found in common household cleaning products), or environmental irritants (plants, urine). Allergic contact dermatitis is the cell-mediated allergy response brought about by sensitization to an allergen. It is a type IV sensitivity (see Chapter 12). This type is dependent on hapten migration into the skin to produce an immune reaction. Many contact allergens are capable of producing the inflammatory skin response (Table 8-8). The crude forms of many naturally occurring substances are rarely allergenic. It is the additives in the form of dyes and perfumes that account for the major sources of known allergens. Additional examples are poison ivy, chemicals, and metal sources such as jewelry.

The initial contact dermatitis lesion ranges from a mild erythema with edema to vesicles or large

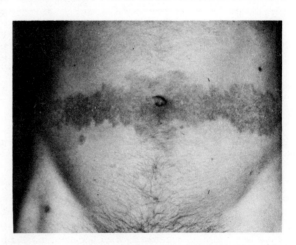

Figure 8-14 Contact dermatitis resulting from a component of rubber. (Demis DJ [ed]: Clinical Dermatology. Philadelphia, Harper & Row, 1985)

bullae. Secondary lesions from bacterial infection may occur. Lesions can occur almost anywhere on the body. The typical poison ivy lesion consists of vesicles or bullae in a linear pattern. The vesicles and bullae break and weep, leaving an excoriated area.

Treatment measures are aimed at removing the source of the irritant. In some cases, this may mean that the person needs to modify his or her behavior in the home or workplace to avoid the irritant. The actual treatment regimen differs according to the type of irritant and the severity of the reaction. Minor cases are treated by washing the affected areas to remove further sources of irritation; by applying antipruritic creams and lotions; and by bandaging the exposed areas. More extreme cases are treated with wet dressings, systemic corticosteroids, and oral antihistamines.

—— Eczema

There are two forms of eczema, atopic and nummular. Atopic eczema (also called atopic dermatitis) is a common skin disorder that occurs in two clinical forms, infantile and adult. It is associated with a type I hypersensitivity reaction (see Chapter 12). There is usually a family history of asthma, hay fever, or atopic dermatitis. The infantile form is characterized by vesicle formation, oozing, and crusting with excoriations. It usually begins in the cheeks and may progress to involve the scalp, arms, trunk, and legs (Figure 8-15). The infantile form usually becomes milder and often disappears after the age of 3 or 4 years. Adolescents and adults generally have dry, leathery, and hyperpigmented or hypopigmented lesions located in the antecubital and popliteal areas that may spread to the neck, hands, feet, or eyelids, and behind the ears. Itching may be severe with both forms, and secondary infections are common.

Although the cause of atopic eczema or dermatitis is largely unknown, several mechanisms have been proposed. The first is the role of allergens in eliciting pruritus by interacting with IgE on mast cells and macrophages in a manner similar to that which produces bronchospasm in persons with extrinsic bronchial asthma. The second, which involves an imbalance between cholinergic- and adrenergic-receptor responses, is similar to the nonallergic reaction that occurs in intrinsic asthma. A third mechanism proposes a beta-adrenergic blockade caused by histamine, prostaglandins, and other inflammatory mediators. As with the hyperreactive response of the bronchial smooth muscle that is seen in asthma, these mechanisms propose a hyperreactive skin response with a lowered itch threshold and proliferation of T-lymphocytes and macrophages. This response promotes collagen deposition and epidermal hyperplasia with subsequent thickening of the skin.

The treatment measures for eczema are designed around the chronic nature of the disease. Exposure to environmental irritants and foods that cause exacerbation of the symptoms is avoided. Wool and lanolin (wool fat) often aggravate the condition. Dryness of the skin often causes the condition to become worse. For this reason, bathing and the use of soap and water should be reduced. Avoidance of temperature changes and stress helps to minimize abnormal and cutaneous vascular and sweat responses. Acute weeping lesions are treated with soothing lotions, soaps, baths, or wet dressings. Subacute or subsiding lesions may be treated with lotions containing mild

---

Table 8–8. Sources of contact dermatitis allergens

Sources	Possible allergens
Clothing	Raw material such as wool, polyester, cotton; dyes and sizers in new fabrics and clothing; detergents used to wash clothing
Cosmetics	Dyes, perfumes, oils (*e.g.,* lanolin, coconut oil, olive oil, palm oil)
Cleaning products (soaps, detergents)	Fats, alkali, perfumes, dyes, formaldehyde, hydrochloric acid, sodium carbonate, ammonium hydroxide, and germicidal agents
Occupational exposure	Metals, metal salts, and alloys (nickel); resin, natural and synthetic; tung oil, linseed oil, turpentine; usually the allergens are from the processing of rubber rather than crude rubber (acids, alkalies, solvents, soaps, dust, heat) and are more common from rubber products (gloves, footwear, condoms)
Plants and woods	Ragweed; lichens; poison ivy, oak, and sumac; pine (more from resin and turpentine); caterpillars; and growth on trees and plants
Soap ingredients	
Fats	Coconut oil, olive oil, palm oil, rosin, and fish or whale oil
Alkali	Sodium hydroxide, potassium hydroxide, sodium carbonate, trisodium phosphate, sodium tripolyphosphate, pyrophosphate, sodium silicate
Perfumes	Seed oil, oil of bergamot, bitter almond oil, eucalyptus oil, geranium oil, lavender oil, peppermint oil, rosemary oil, musk
Coloring agents	D&C yellow No. 11, eosin, rhodamine, fuchsin, ultramarine green

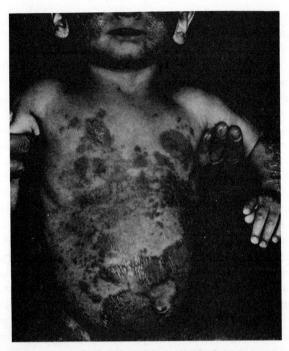

Figure 8-15 Severe infantile atopic dermatitis. (*Demis DJ [ed]: Clinical Dermatology. Philadelphia, Harper & Row, 1985*)

Table 8–9. Types of rashes associated with drug-induced skin eruptions

Drugs	Type of rash
Barbiturates, arsenic, sulfonamides, quinine	Resembles measles
Barbiturates, arsenic, codeine, morphine	Resembles scarlet fever
Bismuth, gold, barbiturates	Resembles pityriasis rosea
Quinine, procaine, antihistamines	Eczematous
Isoniazid, para-aminosalicylic acid combinations	Resembles nummular eczema
Penicillin, salicylates, opium	Urticaria
Bromides, iodides, testosterone, ACTH	Pustular (acne)
Sulfonamides, penicillin, phenylbutazone	Vesicular, bullous
Quinacrine, arsenic, gold	Lichen planus
Contraceptive drugs, quinacrine	Pigment changes
Arsenic, mercury	Keratosis and epitheliomas

antipruritic agents. Chronic dry lesions are treated with ointments and creams containing lubricating, keratolytic, and antipruritic agents as indicated. Topical or systemic corticosteroid therapy may be indicated for severe cases.

The exact etiology of nummular eczema is unknown. There is usually a history of asthma, hay fever, or atopic dermatitis. Lesions consist of coin-shaped (nummular) papulovesicular patches mainly involving the arms and legs. The disease is chronic and most often occurs in elderly men. Lichenification and secondary bacterial infections are common. Ingestion of iodides and bromides usually aggravates the condition. The treatment is palliative. Frequent bathing and foods rich in iodides and bromides should be avoided. Topical corticosteroids and antibiotics are prescribed as necessary.

Drug-induced skin eruptions

Without exception, any drug can cause a localized or generalized skin eruption. Generally, topical drugs are responsible for a localized contact dermatitis type of rash, whereas systemic drugs cause generalized skin lesions. Table 8-9 describes the characteristics of selected drug-induced skin eruptions.

The diagnosis of a drug sensitivity depends almost entirely on accurate reporting by the patient, because the lesions from drug sensitization differ greatly. Drug reactions mimic almost all other skin lesions described in this chapter. The treatment is aimed at eliminating the offending drug. Mild skin eruptions are treated symptomatically, whereas severe systemic drug eruptions often require systemic corticosteroid therapy and antihistamines.

Insect bites, vectors, ticks, and parasites

The skin is susceptible to a variety of disorders as a result of an invasion or infestation by bugs, ticks, or parasites. The rash, or sometimes singular lesion, differs depending on the causative agent.

Scabies

Scabies is caused by a mite (*Sarcoptes scabiei*) that burrows into the epidermis. After a female mite is impregnated, she burrows into the skin and lays two to three eggs each day for 4 or 5 weeks. Three to 5 days later, the eggs hatch and the larvae migrate to the skin surface. At this point, they burrow into the skin only for food or for protection. The larvae molt and become nymphs; they molt once more to become adults. Once they are impregnated, the cycle is repeated.

The characteristic lesion is a small burrow, approximately 2 mm long, that may be red to red-brown in color. Small vesicles may cover the burrows. The areas most commonly affected are the interdigital web of the finger, flexor surface of the wrist, inner surface of the elbow, axilla, female nipple, penis, belt line, and gluteal crease (Figure 8-16). Pruritus is common and may result from the burrows, the fecal material of the mite, or both. Excoriations may develop from scratching, and secondary bacterial infec-

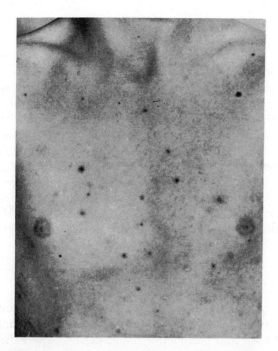

Figure 8-16 Scabies on the chest (K.C.G.H.). (*Sauer GC: Manual of Skin Diseases, 5th ed. Philadelphia, JB Lippincott, 1985*)

tions and severe skin lesions may occur if the condition is untreated.

Scabies affects all people in all socioeconomic classes. Usually more prevalent in times of war and famine, it reached pandemic proportions in the 1970s, perhaps as a result of poverty, sexual promiscuity, and worldwide travel.

Diagnosis is done by skin scrapings. Mineral oil is applied to the skin and a scraping is obtained. A positive diagnosis relies on the presence of the mite or its feces. The treatment is simple and curative. Lindane lotion or cream (Kwell) is applied over the entire skin surface for 12 hours. Repeat applications may be recommended in certain cases, but one treatment is usually sufficient. Controversy exists over bathing before the treatment. Some physicians no longer recommend bathing before the treatment, perhaps to enhance full drug effectiveness.[16] Clothes and towels are disinfected with hot water and detergent. Treatment of outer clothing and furniture is unnecessary because the mite cannot live away from the body for more than a few hours. If symptoms persist following treatment, the patient should be advised not to retreat the condition without consulting the physician. A red-brown nodule, thought to be an allergic response from the mite parts left on the skin, may form after treatment.

Pediculosis

Pediculosis is the term for infestation with lice (genus *Pediculus*). Lice are gray, gray-brown, or red-brown, oval, wingless insects that live off the blood of humans and animals. Lice are host-specific; lice that live on animals do not transfer to humans, and vice versa. Lice are also host-dependent; they cannot live apart from the host beyond a few hours. As with scabies, the incidence of pediculosis increased in the 1970s to pandemic levels, probably because of increases in poverty, sexual experiences, and worldwide travel.

Three types of lice affect humans: *Pediculus humanus corporis* (body lice), *Pediculus pubis* (pubic lice), and *Pediculus humanus capitis* (head lice). Although these three types differ biologically, they have similar life cycles. The life cycle of a louse consists of an unhatched egg or "nit," three molt stages, an adult reproductive stage, and death. Before adulthood, lice live off the host and are incapable of reproduction. After fertilization, the egg is laid by the female louse along a hair shaft. These nits appear pearl-gray to brown. Depending on the site, a female louse can lay anywhere between 150 and 300 nits in her life. The life span of a feeding louse is 30 to 50 days. Lice are equipped with stylets that pierce the skin. Their saliva contains an anticoagulant that prevents host blood from clotting while the louse is feeding. A louse takes up to 1 mg of blood during a feeding.

Pediculosis corporis. Pediculosis corporis is infestation with *Pediculus humanus corporis,* or body lice, which are chiefly transferred through contact with infested clothing and bedding. The lice live in the clothes fibers, coming out only to feed. Unlike the pubic louse and the head louse, the body louse can survive 10 to 14 days without the host. The typical lesion is a macule at the site of the bite. Papules and wheals may develop. The infestation is pruritic and evokes scratching that brings about a characteristic linear excoriation. Eczematous patches are frequently found. Secondary lesions may become scaly and hyperpigmented and leave scars. Areas typically affected are the shoulders, trunk, and buttocks. The presence of nits in the seams of clothes confirms a diagnosis of body lice. Treatment measures consist of eradicating the louse and nits both on the body and on clothing. Washing clothes in hot water and steam pressing or dry-cleaning them is recommended. Special attention is given to the seams. Merely storing clothing in plastic bags for 2 weeks will rid clothes of lice. Many physicians prefer not to treat the body unless nits are in evidence on hair shafts. If treatment is indicated, lindane shampoo or topical preparations containing gamma benzene hexachloride, pyrethrum, or malathion are recommended.

Pediculosis pubis. Pediculosis pubis (the infestation known as crabs, or pubic lice) is a nuisance disease that is uncomfortable and embarrassing. The disease is spread by intimate contact with someone harboring *Phthirus pubis*. Lice and nits are located in the pubic area of males and females. Occasionally they may be found in secondary sex sites such as the beard in males or the axilla in males and females. Symptoms include intense itching and irritation of the skin. Diagnosis is made on the basis of symptoms and microscopic examination. The treatment is the same as that used for head lice.

Pediculosis capitis. Pediculosis capitis, or infestation with head lice, primarily affects white-skinned people; it is relatively unknown in darker-skinned persons. In addition, the incidence is higher in female children, although hair length has not been indicated as a contributing factor. Infestations of head lice are usually confined to the nape of the neck and behind the ears. Less frequently, head lice are found on the beard, pubic areas, eyebrows, and body hairs.

Head lice are primarily transmitted by human-to-human contact. A positive diagnosis depends on the presence of firmly attached nits on hair shafts. Crawling adults are rarely seen. Pruritus and scratching of the head are the primary indicators that head lice may be present. The scalp may appear red and excoriated from scratching. In severe cases, the hair becomes matted together in a crusty foul-smelling "cap." An occasional morbilliform rash, which may be misdiagnosed as rubella, may occur with lymphadenopathy.

Head lice are treated with gamma benzene hexachloride preparations (Kwell). The medicated shampoo is applied to dry hair in sufficient quantity to wet the hair and skin. After the hair and head are massaged, small amounts of water are added to produce a lather. The head is scrubbed for 4 minutes, rinsed, and dried. The treatment may be repeated after 1 week to eliminate the hatching nits. Dead nits may be removed with a finetoothed comb.

Bedbugs

The common bedbug, *Cimex lectularius,* is a reddish-brown insect, 3 mm to 6 mm long, that turns purple after feeding. Like lice, bedbugs feed on human blood. Unlike lice, bedbugs can alternate hosts from human to animal, and they live up to and sometimes beyond 1 year. When not feeding, bedbugs stay hidden in the cracks and crevices of furniture, mattresses, wallpaper, picture frames, baseboards, flooring, door locks, or any darkened area. They are nocturnal feeders, and when squashed, they emit a foul odor.

The *Cimex* bite is painless. The characteristic lesion is a pruritic oval or oblong wheal with a small hemorrhagic punctum at the center. Bullous lesions are not uncommon. Usually, lesions are multiple and arranged in rows or clusters on the face, neck, hands, and arms. No area is exempt. The wheal is probably a type I sensitivity reaction to the anticoagulant saliva of the bedbug. Secondary excoriation and bacterial infections may occur.

Differential diagnosis is made by taking an accurate history as to the time of day during which the lesions occur. Because of the painless bite, it is not uncommon for the victim to awake with one or several pruritic papules. Topical antipruritics are used in the treatment. The source of the bedbug must be eliminated or recurrence is inevitable. Professional extermination is advised because of the many hiding places of *Cimex*. Bedbugs have been known to feed from animal populations when forced from their living quarters. Upon rehabitation in the same quarters, the bedbug will once again find the unsuspecting human host.

Ticks

Ticks are insects that live in woods and underbrush. They attach themselves to human and animal hosts and burrow into the epidermis, where they feed on blood. The tick bite itself is not problematic; the dangers stem rather from the infectious bacteria or viruses that they carry to human hosts. There are many tick-borne illnesses, including Central European encephalitis, Q fever, babesiasis, and relapsing fever. The most common tick-borne disease in the United States is Rocky Mountain spotted fever (RMSF), which is caused by a tick that carries *Rickettsia rickettsii*. RMSF used to be localized to the Rocky Mountain area, but by 1982 most states had reported a case of RMSF.

The initial tick bite appears as a papule or macule with or without a central punctum. The tick burrows in and enlarges as it feeds. The tick must be attached to the human host for 4 to 6 hours before the rickettsiae are activated by the blood. Rickettsiae are found in the tick feces and body parts. The rickettsiae then enter the bloodstream and multiply in the body tissues. Within 4 to 8 days the patient experiences fever, headache, muscle aches, nausea, and vomiting. A rash that starts on the wrist or ankle follows. The characteristic rash is a macular or maculopapular rash that spreads to the rest of the body. Other symptoms include generalized edema, conjunctivitis, petechial lesions, photophobia, lethargy, confusion, and cranial nerve deficits.

The treatment for RMSF requires hospitalization and antibiotic therapy. The most important measure is to prevent tick bites by using insect repellents while engaged in activities in the woods. Once a tick has attached itself, it is important to remove all the body parts to limit the possibility of infection. Ticks may be removed by slowly pulling them, dousing them with mineral oil or alcohol before removing them with a tweezers, or applying a hot match to the end of the tick. The latter method is not the most effective, as the tick may regurgitate into the open wound.

Lyme disease is a tick-borne disease characterized by a distinctive skin lesion, erythema chronicum migrans (ECM). ECM is a red macule or papule that extends in an annular fashion with a central clearing, which has been called the *bull's eye*. The disease is caused by a spirochete, *Borrelia burgdorferi,* and occurs in three stages: (1) appearance of the ECM, (2) cardiac and neurologic manifestations that present weeks to months later, and (3) arthritis, which develops weeks to years later in about 60% of cases. The disease was named Lyme disease after the town in Connecticut where the disease was discovered due to the efforts of a mother who reported eight cases of juvenile arthritis. Although incidence rates are highest along the coasts and in the Midwest, cases have occurred across the United States and in several other countries. Treatment consists of tetracycline and penicillin therapy and is most effective if initiated during the ECM stage.

Mosquitoes

Most people are aware of the bite of the mosquito. The typical lesion is a raised wheal on an erythematous base accompanied by pruritus that occurs within 45 minutes of the bite. A second type of reaction is the delayed response. Eight to 12 hours after the bite, the lesion becomes raised, erythematous, and indurated, with extensive pruritus or pain. This reaction peaks 24 hours to 72 hours after the bite. The saliva of the mosquito is believed to be the source of the skin reaction. Although severe skin reactions are possible, they are rare. Insect repellents are encouraged for prevention; local antipruritics are used for treatment.

Chiggers

Chiggers are common in the southern United States but can be found as far north as Canada. The chigger resides in grasses and bushes. The mite attaches to legs and thighs and punctures the skin to obtain food. Chigger bites are pruritic papules seen wherever the chigger encounters resistance, such as the top of socks, at the beltline, or around the neckband area. Secondary lesions are excoriations from scratching that have become infected by bacteria. The treatment is palliative, and insect repellent is encouraged for prevention.

Fleas

The sources for human fleas are usually dogs and cats. Geographically, specific fleas have been identified that seem to pester newcomers rather than natives of an area. The characteristic lesion is a highly pruritic papule with a central punctum and is generally seen on covered parts of the body. The treatment measures are symptomatic; insect repellents are advised.

Photosensitivity and sunburn

Physical and mechanical stimuli such as fire, electromagnetic radiation, and ionizing radiation can cause skin burns (see Chapter 2). Many of these burns occur accidentally in the home or workplace. Ultraviolet light, or sunlight, also causes skin changes. The obvious and desired skin change is tanning; yet most forms of skin cancer are directly related to sun exposure. Besides cancerous lesions, several skin alterations, such as senile lentigines, have been linked to sun exposure. Exposure to the sun, as well as harsh weather, has also been linked to early wrinkling and aging of the skin. Some drugs are classified as photosensitive drugs because they produce an exaggerated response to ultraviolet light when the drug is taken in combination with sun exposure (Chart 8-1).

The skin, as an organ, is the protective shield against harmful ultraviolet rays from the sun. Living epidermal cells are damaged when 280-nm to 310-nm wavelengths penetrate the skin.

The wavelength of sunlight in an area is determined by the ozone layer. Ozone absorbs wavelengths shorter than 320 nm; the shortest wavelength of sunlight reaching the earth is about 290 nm. Smoke and fog may play a part in reducing the intensity of ultraviolet radiation.[17]

Human cells release vasoactive and injurious chemicals, resulting in vasodilation and sunburn. The melanin in the stratum corneum protects the skin by absorbing the ultraviolet rays and the skin responds to sunlight exposure by increasing its melanin content as a means of preventing destruction of the lower skin layers.

Sunburn ranges from mild to severe. A mild sunburn consists of varying degrees of redness 2 to 12 hours after exposure to the sun. Varying degrees of inflammation, vesicle eruption, weakness, chills, fever, malaise, and pain accompany more severe forms of sunburn. Scaling and peeling follow any overexposure to sunlight. Black skin also burns and may appear grayish or gray-black.

Chart 8-1: Drugs that induce photosensitivity

Sulfonamides
Thiazide diuretics
Furosemide
Sulfonylurea hypoglycemia agents
Tetracycline (particularly demeclocycline)
Phenothiazine, antipsychotic drugs
Nalidixic acid

If the desired outcome of sun exposure is a good suntan, prevention of excessive exposure to harmful ultraviolet rays is the best policy. Early morning and late afternoon sun exposures are less harmful because the ultraviolet rays are longer. Although longer-wavelength rays are less apt to cause severe sunburn, they, too, have been implicated in the development of skin cancers. The FDA now requires a rating on all commercial suntan preparations based on their ability to occlude ultraviolet light.

The ratings are generally on a scale of 1 to 15, with 1 being least occlusive to sunlight. Some commercial products have ratings of 22 or higher. Para-aminobenzoic acid (PABA) is the most effective blocking ingredient in many of these suntan creams. Suntan creams should be used diligently and according to the individual's tendency to burn rather than tan. Another preventive measure includes knowing about sunlight and how to protect the skin. Shade does not necessarily protect people from the sun's rays, because ultraviolet rays are reflected from many surfaces. Sand is a good reflector of sunlight and, therefore, a person can get sunburned even sitting under an umbrella on a sandy beach. Water absorbs ultraviolet light, and does not reflect it, as is commonly thought.[17]

Severe sunburns are treated with boric acid soaks and topical creams to limit pain and maintain skin moisture. Extensive second- and third-degree burns require hospitalization and specialized burn care techniques.

Neoplasms

There are a number of premalignant and malignant skin lesions. Most of these are found on the skin surfaces exposed to sun and harsh weather. Nevi are common benign tumors of the skin. Cancer of the skin is the most common of all cancers. With the exception of malignant melanoma, the overall cure rate for skin cancer is higher than 90%.[18]

Nevi

Nevi, or moles, are common congenital or acquired tumors of the skin. Almost all adults have nevi, some in greater numbers than others. Nevi can be pigmented or nonpigmented, flat or elevated, and hairy or nonhairy. Pigmented nevi are derived from neural crest-derived cells (nevocellular nevi) that include modified melanocytes of various shapes. Histologically, most nevi begin as aggregates of well-defined cells located within the lower epidermal layer that lies adjacent to the dermis. These nevi are called *junctional nevi*. Eventually, nevus cells begin to grow into the dermis. *Compound nevi* contain both epider-

mal and dermal components. *Dermal nevi* are located within the dermis.

Generally, nevocellular nevi are tan to deep brown, uniformly pigmented, small papules with well-defined and rounded borders. Blue nevi have a blue-black color. Moles are important because of their capacity for transformation to malignant melanomas. The relationship between preexisting benign nevi and malignant melanoma is unclear. Although the average person has about 20 moles, only 4 people out of 100,000 develop a malignant melanoma.[16] It is known that two types of pigmented nevus are associated with malignant transformation; these are the congenital melanocytic nevi and the large atypical or dysplastic nevi (discussed later in this chapter). Because of the possibility of malignant transformation, any mole that undergoes a change in size, thickness, or color, causes itching, or bleeds, warrants immediate medical attention.

Basal cell carcinoma

Basal cell carcinoma is the most common form of skin cancer (Figure 8-17). Light-skinned people are more susceptible; blacks and Orientals are rarely affected. It is a nonmetastasizing tumor that will extend wide and deep if left untreated. These tumors are most frequently seen on the head and neck and, less commonly, on the skin surfaces unexposed to the sun. Basal cell carcinoma usually occurs in people who are exposed to great amounts of sun.

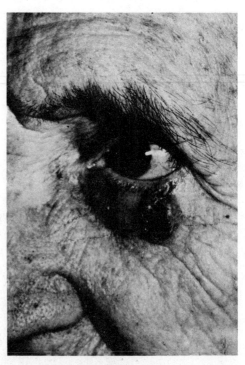

Figure 8-17 Nodular basal cell carcinoma with central ulceration. (*Demis DJ* [ed]: *Clinical Dermatology. Philadelphia, Harper & Row, 1985*)

The most common type of basal cell carcinoma is the noduloulcerative basal cell epithelioma. It begins as a small, smooth shiny nodule that enlarges over time. Telangiectatic vessels are frequently seen beneath the surface. Over the years, a central depression forms that progresses to an ulcer surrounded by the original shiny, waxy border.

The second most common basal cell carcinoma is the superficial form, which is most often seen on the chest or back. It begins as a flat, nonpalpable erythematous plaque. The red scaly areas slowly enlarge with nodular borders and telangiectatic bases. This type of skin cancer is difficult to diagnose because it mimics other dermatologic problems.

In both cases, tumors are biopsied for diagnosis. The treatment depends on the site and extent of the lesion. Curettage with electrodesiccation, surgical excision, irradiation, and chemosurgery are effective in removing all cancerous cells. Patients should be checked at regular intervals for recurrence.

Squamous cell carcinoma

Squamous cell carcinomas are malignant tumors of the outer epidermis. There are two types of squamous cell carcinoma: intraepidermal squamous cell carcinoma and invasive squamous cell carcinoma. Intraepidermal squamous cell carcinoma remains confined to the epidermis for a long time, but may at some unpredictable time penetrate the basement membrane to the dermis and then metastasize to the regional lymph nodes. Invasive squamous cell carcinoma can develop from intraepidermal carcinoma or from a premalignant lesion. It may be slow or fast growing with metastasis.

Squamous cell carcinoma is a scaly, keratotic slightly elevated lesion with an irregular border,

usually with a shallow chronic ulcer. Later lesions grow outward, show large ulcerations, and have persistent crusts and raised, erythematous borders. These lesions occur on sun-exposed areas of the skin, particularly the nose, forehead, helixes of the ears, lower lip, and back of the hands (Figure 8-18).

The mechanisms of squamous cell carcinoma development are unclear. The effects of sunlight are uncertain; however, most squamous cell cancers occur in sun-exposed areas of the skin. Outdoor people are more affected, and there is less incidence in dark-skinned people. Other suspected causes include exposure to arsenic, gamma radiation, tars, and oils.

Treatment measures are aimed at the removal of all cancerous tissue using methods such as electro-surgery, excision surgery, chemosurgery, or radiation therapy. Following removal, the area is observed closely for signs of recurrence.

Malignant melanoma

Malignant melanoma is a malignant tumor of the melanocytes. It is a rapidly progressing, metastatic form of cancer that accounts for 1% to 3% of all cancers.[11] It is the primary cause of death of all skin diseases. Early diagnosis and knowledge of precursor lesions have led to earlier intervention and to increased survival of people who have malignant melanoma.

Malignant melanomas differ in size and shape (Figure 8-19). The vast majority seem to arise from preexisting benign nevi or as new molelike growths.[19] Usually they are slightly raised and black or

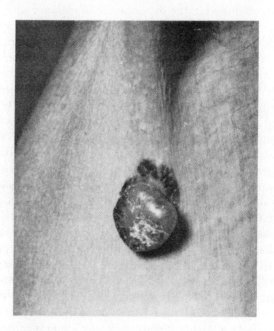

Figure 8-19 Malignant melanoma. On posterior axillary fold (K.C.G.H.). (*Sauer GC: Manual of Skin Diseases, 4th ed. Philadelphia, JB Lippincott, 1980*)

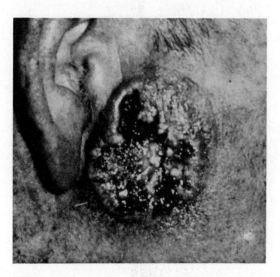

Figure 8-18 Squamous cell carcinoma. (*Demis DJ [ed]: Clinical Dermatology. Philadelphia, Harper & Row, 1985*)

brown. Borders are irregular and surfaces are uneven. Periodically, melanomas ulcerate and bleed; there may be surrounding erythema, inflammation, and tenderness. Dark melanomas are often mottled with red, blue, and white shades. These three colors represent three concurrent processes: melanoma growth (blue), inflammation and the body's attempt to localize and destroy the tumor (red), and scar tissue formation (white). Malignant melanomas can appear anywhere on the body. They are frequently found on sun-exposed areas, but sun exposure alone does not account for the development of melanomas. In men, they are frequently found on the trunk, head, neck, and arms; in women, they are found on the legs, arms, trunk, head, and neck.

Four types of melanomas have been identified. Lentigo maligna melanoma is a slow-growing flat nevus and occurs primarily on sun-exposed areas. Superficial spreading melanoma is characterized by a raised-edged nevus with lateral growth. It has a disorderly appearance in color and outline and tends to have a biphasic growth, horizontally and vertically. It typically ulcerates and bleeds with growth. This type of lesion accounts for 70% of all melanomas. Nodular melanoma is raised and initially grows vertically, is of a uniform blue-black color, and is sharply delineated. These lesions tend to look like blood blisters. Acral-lentiginous melanoma occurs primarily in blacks and Orientals on the palms of the hands, soles of the feet, nail beds, and mucous membranes. It has the appearance of lentigo maligna.

Most melanomas arise as new lesions, but some appear to develop in association with other preexisting benign nevi. Three precursor lesions have been identified in the development of melanoma: lentigo maligna, congenital melanocytic nevi, and dysplastic nevi. Recognition of these precursors is important to the early diagnosis and treatment of melanoma. Lentigo maligna is a flat lesion that looks like an irregular freckle. The lesion is tan-brown to black with irregular pigmentation and borders; it spreads and may look like a stain. Lentigo malignas frequently occur in elderly patients on sun-exposed areas. Congenital melanocytic nevi are large, brown to black hyperpigmented nevi that are present at birth. Generally, they are found on the hands, shoulders, buttocks, entire arm, or trunk of the body. Some involve large areas of the body in garment-like fashion. These nevi darken with age, and hairs that are present in the lesion become coarser. Malignant changes often occur at an early age (generally by age 10).[11] Dysplastic nevi are flat to slightly raised lesions consisting of neural crest-derived cells (nevocellular nevi) and often have a diameter greater than 1 cm. A person may have hundreds of these lesions; typically, they occur on both sun-exposed and covered areas of the body.

They vary in shade from brown and red to flesh tones with irregular borders. There is some familial tendency to develop dysplastic nevi.

The prognosis of malignant melanoma depends on the depth of the lesion and the extent of the disease process. Stage I patients have no evidence of tumor growth in regional lymph nodes, and the disease process is limited to the localized lesion area. Survival rates for these people, with surgical intervention, is uncertain but is longer than for either of the other two stages. Stage II melanomas have metastasized to the regional lymph nodes. Five-year to 10-year survival rates have been reported for people in this stage of the disease process. Stage III malignant melanoma involves metastasis to distant organs in the body. The prognosis is poor, with survival ranging up to 16 months.[20]

The best treatment is early detection. Patients should be taught to watch for changes in existing nevi or the development of new nevi. Color changes (variegation), irregular borders, bleeding, and growth of nevi should be brought to the attention of a dermatologist. Treatment measures vary depending on the severity. Deep and wide excisions with skin grafts are used. Systemic immunotherapy, chemotherapy, and

Table 8–10. Common normal variations in black skin

Variation	Appearance
Futcher (Voigt's) Line	Demarcation between darkly pigmented and lightly pigmented skin in upper arm; follows spinal nerve distribution; common in black and Japanese populations
Midline hypopigmentation	Line or band of hypopigmentation over the sternum, dark or faint, lessens with age; common in Latin American and black populations
Nail pigmentation	Linear dark bands down nails or diffuse nail pigmentation, brown, blue, or blue-black
Oral pigmentation	Blue to blue-gray pigmentation of oral mucosa; gingivae also affected
Palmar changes	Hyperpigmented creases, small hyperkeratotic papules, and tiny pits in creases
Plantar changes	Hyperpigmented macules, can be multiple with patchy distribution, irregular borders, and variance in color

(Developed from information in Rosen T, Martin S: Atlas of Black Dermatology. Boston, Little, Brown, 1981)

radiation therapy are indicated when the disease becomes systemic.

In summary, primary disorders of the skin include infectious processes, inflammatory conditions, allergic reactions, parasitic infestations, skin reactions to sunlight, and neoplasms. Superficial fungal infections are called dermatophytoses and are commonly known as tinea, or ringworm; they include tinea corporis, tinea capitis, tinea barbae, tinea manus, tinea pedis, tinea unguium, and tinea versicolor. Impetigo, which is caused by staphylococci or beta-hemolytic streptococci, is the most common superficial bacterial infection. Viruses are responsible for verrucae (warts), herpes simplex I lesions (cold sores or fever blisters), and herpes zoster (shingles). Noninfectious inflammatory skin conditions such as acne, lichen planus, psoriasis, and pityriasis rosea are generally of unknown etiology. They are usually localized to the skin and are rarely associated with specific internal disease. Allergic skin responses involve the body's immune system and are caused by hypersensitivity reactions to allergens, environmental agents, drugs, and other substances. The skin is sensitive to a number of disorders resulting from invasion or infestation by bugs, ticks, or parasites. The rash or bite from such invasion is usually singular and varies with the agent. Neoplasms of the skin include basal cell carcinoma, squamous cell carcinoma, and melanoma, with basal cell carcinoma being the most common form. Repeated exposure to the ultraviolet rays of the sun is the principal cause of skin cancer.

Black skin

There are several skin disorders common to blacks that are not commonly found in whites. Similarly, many skin disorders that affect white-skinned peoples do not affect darker-skinned persons, such as skin cancers. Literature related specifically to black skin disorders is rare; frequently, common occurrences in black skin are mistaken for anomalies.

The greater number of melanosomes produced and transferred to the keratinocyte is responsible for the darker pigmentation in blacks. In other words, blacks do not have more melanocytes than whites, but the production of pigment is increased. Skin pallor, cyanosis, and erythema are more difficult to see in black people. Also, normal variations in skin structure and skin tones make evaluation of black skin difficult (Table 8-10). Often, verbal histories must be relied on to indicate skin changes. Hypopigmentation refers to a loss of pigmentation, and hyperpigmentation refers to excessive melanin production. Often these signs accompany black skin disorders and are important to accurate diagnosis. The appearances of skin disorders listed in Table 8-11 are common to the American black who represents a blend of African Negro, European Caucasian, and Native American.

Table 8–11. Appearance of common disorders of black skin

Disorder	Appearance
Hot-comb alopecia	Well-defined patches of scalp alopecia on crown; extends down; decreased number of follicular orifices; hair loss irreversible; due to use of hot comb with petroleum, more common with Afro hairstyles
Infantile acropustulosis	Crops of vesicopustules for 7 to 10 days, followed by a 2 to 3 week remission before recurrence; pruritus; affects palms and soles of feet in children 2 to 10 months of age; resolves by 3 years of age
Keloids	Firm, smooth, shiny hairless elevated scars, sometimes hyperpigmented; often with symptomatic pruritus, tenderness, or pain; extremely common even with simple wounds on ears, neck, jaw, cheeks, upper chest, shoulders, and back
Mongolian spot	Very common; ill-defined light blue to slate gray macule in lumbosacral area; usually disappears, but may persist through adulthood
Atopic dermatitis	Follicular lesion development that progresses to a lichenification stage; hyperpigmented lichenifications are interspersed with excoriated pink patches; common in blacks
Pityriasis rosea	Lesions are salmon-pink, dull-red, or dark-brown; profuse fine scales, not commonly seen in white skin; postinflammatory pigmentary changes are more common in blacks
Psoriasis	Does not commonly occur in blacks; distribution is similar, but the plaques are bright-red, violet, or blue-black; pigment changes may persist after treatment
Tinea versicolor	Common in blacks, increased incidence in tropical climates; hypopigmented or extremely hyperpigmented patches, gray to dark brown; occurs more often on the face in blacks than in whites
Lichen planus	Papules are deep purple from pigmentary leakage; oral lesions are uncommon; hypertrophic lesions are more common in blacks than in whites

(Developed from information in Rosen T, Martin S: Atlas of Black Dermatology. Boston, Little, Brown, 1981)

Vitiligo

Vitiligo is a pigmentary problem of concern to darkly pigmented people of all races. It also affects whites, but not as often. The lesion is a macular depigmentation with definite borders on the face, axillae, neck, or extremities. The borders are smooth. The patches vary in size from small to large macules involving great skin surfaces. The large macular type is much more common. Depigmented areas, which burn in sunlight, appear white or flesh-colored or sometimes grayish-blue. Vitiligo appears at any age, in men and women alike, and usually occurs before the age of 21 years. It has been on the rise in India, Pakistan, and Far Eastern countries. Although the cause is unknown, inheritance and autoimmune factors have been implicated. Vitiligo also seems to be implicated as a cutaneous expression of a systemic disorder, especially thyroid disease.[21] The areas affected enlarge over time.

Treatment regimens for vitiligo remain experimental. Psoralen administration in conjunction with ultraviolet radiation (PUVA) has been successful in patients who have involvement of 40% or more of the skin surface. Cosmetics and sunscreens are used for camouflage.

In summary, black skin has an increased number of melanosomes. Thus, skin pallor, cyanosis, and erythema are more difficult to evaluate. Some skin disorders that are common in blacks are not common in whites, and vice versa. The manifestations of common skin disorders are also different. Vitiligo, a condition of depigmentation, is a problem of concern to darkly pigmented people of all races.

References

1. Arey LB: Human Histology, p 186. Philadelphia, WB Saunders, 1974
2. Jacob SW, Fracone CA, Lossow WJ: Structure and Function in Man, 4th ed, p 75. Philadelphia, WB Saunders, 1978
3. Arndt KA, Jick H: Rates of cutaneous reactions to drugs. JAMA 235:918, 1976
4. Pinkus H, Mehregan AH: A Guide to Dermatohistopathology, 3rd ed, p 5. New York, Appleton-Century-Crofts, 1981
5. Holbrook KA, Odland GF: Regional differences in the thickness (cell layers) of the human stratum corneum: An ultrastructural analysis. J Invest Dermatol 62:415, 1974
6. Katz SI, Tamaki K, Sachs DH: Epidermal Langerhans cells are derived from cells originating in the bone marrow. Nature 282:324, 1979
7. Silberberg-Sinakin I, Baer RL, Thorbekke G: Langerhans cells: A review of their nature with emphasis on their immunologic functions. Prog Allergy 24:268, 1978
8. Tamaki K, Stingl G, Katz SJ: The origin of Langerhans cells. J Invest Dermatol 74:309, 1980
9. Hartschuh W, Grube D: The Merkel cell—A member of the APUD cell system: Fluorescence and electron microscopic contribution to the neurotransmitter function of the Merkel cell granules. Arch Dermatol Res 265:115, 1979
10. Herndon JH: Pruritus. In Moschella SL (ed): Dermatology Update, pp 185–196. New York, Elsevier Biomedical, 1982
11. Robbins SL, Cotran RS, Kumar V: Pathologic Basis of Disease, 3rd ed, pp 1275, 1279, 1298. Philadelphia, WB Saunders, 1984
12. Klingman AM, Leyden J: The interaction of fungi and bacteria in the pathogenesis of athlete's foot. In Maibach HI, Aly R (eds): Skin Microbiology: Relevance to Clinical Infection, pp 203–219. New York, Springer-Verlag, 1981
13. Nasemann T: Viral diseases of the skin, mucous membrane and genitalia. Philadelphia, WB Saunders, 1977
14. Strauss JS: Biology of the sebaceous gland and the pathophysiology of acne vulgaris. In Soter NA, Baden HP (eds): Pathophysiology of Dermatologic Diseases, pp 159–173, 1984
15. Dicken CH: Retinoids: A review. J Am Acad Dermatol 11(4): 541–552, 1984
16. Parish LC, Witkowski JA, Cohen HB: Clinical picture of scabies. In Parish LC, Nutting WB, Schwartzman RM (eds): Cutaneous Infestations of Man and Animal, pp 70–78. New York, Praeger, 1983
17. Pathak MA, Fitzpatrick TB, Greiter F, Kraus EW: Preventive treatment of sunburn, dermatoheliosis, and skin cancer with sun protective agents. In Fitzpatrick TB, Eisen AZ, Wolf K, Austen KF (eds): Dermatology in Medicine: Textbook and Atlas, pp 1507–1522. New York: McGraw-Hill, 1987
18. Facts on Skin Cancer. New York, American Cancer Society, 1978
19. Sherman CD, McCune CS, Rubin P: Malignant melanoma. In Rubin P (ed): Clinical Oncology, 6th ed, p 190. New York, American Cancer Society, 1983
20. Sober AJ, Rhodes AR, Day CL, Fitzpatrick TB, Mihm MC: Primary melanoma of the skin: Recognition of precursor lesions and estimation of prognosis in Stage I. In Fitzpatrick TB, Eisen AZ, Wolff K, Freedburg IM, Austen KF (eds): Update: Dermatology in General Medicine. New York, McGraw-Hill, 1983
21. Mosher DB, Pathak MA, Fitzpatrick TB: Vitiligo: Etiology, pathogenesis, diagnosis, and treatment. In Fitzpatrick TB, Eisen AZ, Wolff K, Freedburg IM, Austen KF (eds): Update: Dermatology in General Medicine. New York, McGraw-Hill, 1983

Bibliography

Abel E: Psoriasis: Problems with PUVA therapy. Cutis 33:255, 1984
Adams RM: Occupational Skin Disease. New York, Grune & Stratton, 1983

Benenson AS (ed): Control of Communicable Diseases in Man. Washington, DC, American Public Health Association, 1981

Bruno NP, Beacham BE, Burnett, JW: Adverse effects of isotretinoin therapy. Cutis 33:484, 1984

Burton JL: Essentials of Dermatology. New York, Churchill Livingstone, 1985

Callen JP, Dahl MV, Golitz LE, Rasmussen JE, Stegman SJ (eds): Current Issues in Dermatology, vol 1. Boston, G. K. Hall Medical, 1984

Cohen S: Skin rashes in infants and children. Am J Nurs 78:1, 1978

Connolly SM: Allergic contact dermatitis: When to suspect it and what to do. Postgrad Med 74:227, 1983

De Launey WE, Land WA: Principles and practice of dermatology, 2nd ed. Sydney, Butterworths, 1984

Dilaimy MS, Owen WR, Sima B: Keratosis punctata of the palmar creases. Cutis 33:394, 1984

DiLorenzo PA: The clinical approach to pruritus. Cutis 3:1087, 1967

Domonkos AN, Arnold HL, Odom RB: Andrew's Diseases of the Skin: Clinical Dermatology, 7th ed. Philadelphia, WB Saunders, 1982

Epstein E, Epstein E (eds): Skin Surgery, 5th ed. Springfield, IL, Charles C Thomas, 1982

Farber EM, Cox AJ (eds): Psoriasis: Proceedings of the Third International Symposium. New York, Grune & Stratton, 1981

Fitzpatrick TB, Eisen AZ, Wolff K, Freedberg IM, Austen KF (eds): Update: Dermatology in Medicine. New York, McGraw-Hill, 1983

Fitzpatrick TB, Eisen AZ, Wolf K, Austen KF (eds): Dermatology in Medicine: Textbook and Atlas. New York, McGraw-Hill, 1987

Fraser MC, McGuire DB: Skin cancer's early warning system. Am J Nurs 84:1232, 1984

Greer KE: Common Problems in Dermatology. Chicago, Year Book Medical, 1987

Gunnoe RE: Diseases of the nails: How to recognize and treat them. Postgrad Med 74:357, 1983

Halder RM: Hair and scalp disorders in blacks. Cutis 32:378, 1983

Halder RM, Grimes PE, McLaurin CI, Kress MA, Kenny JA: Incidence of common dermatoses in a predominantly black dermatologic practice. Cutis 32:388, 1983

Hanifin JM: Atopic dermatitis. Postgrad Med 74:188, 1983

Henderson AL: Skin variations in blacks. Cutis 32:376, 1983

Kaplan AP: Chronic urticaria. Postgrad Med 74:209, 1983

Knopf AW, Bart RS, Rodriguez-Sains RS, Ackerman AB: Malignant Melanoma. New York, Masson Publishing, 1979

Lynch PJ: Sunlight and aging of the skin. Cutis 18:451, 1976

McLaurin CI: Unusual patterns of common dermatoses in blacks. Cutis 32:352, 1983

Miller LH: Herpes zoster in the elderly. Cutis 18:427, 1976

Orkin M, Maibach HI: Current views of scabies and pediculosis pubis. Cutis 33:85, 1984

Orkin M, Maibach HI: Scabies, a current pandemic. Postgrad Med 66:53, 1979

Ragozzino MW, Melton LJ, Kurland LT, Chu CP, Perry HO: Population-based study of herpes zoster and its sequelae. Med 61:310, 1982

Rosen T, Martin S: Atlas of Black Dermatology. Boston, Little, Brown, 1981

Waisman M: A clinical look at the aging skin. Postgrad Med 66:87, 1979

Weller TH: Varicella and herpes zoster: Changing concepts of the natural history, control, and importance of a not-so-benign virus. N Engl J Med 309:1362, 1983

Wilson BL: Skin problems common to blacks: A nursing perspective. In Gorline LL, Stegbauer CC (eds): Common Problems in Primary Care. St Louis, CV Mosby, 1982

Zugerman C: Dermatology in the workplace. Am Fam Pract 26:103, 1982

CHAPTER 9

W. Michael Dunne, Jr.

Mechanisms of Infectious Disease

Terminology
Agents of infectious disease
  Viruses
  Bacteria
    Spirocetes
    Mycoplasmas
  Rickettsiae and chlamydiae
  Fungi
  Parasites
Mechanisms of infection
  Epidemiology of infectious
    diseases

Portal of entry
  Penetration
  Direct contact
  Ingestion
  Inhalation
Source
Symptomatology
Disease course
  Incubation period
  Prodromal stage
  Acute stage
  Convalescent stage
  Resolution

Site of infection
Virulence factors
  Toxins
  Adherence factors
  Evasive factors
  Invasive factors
Diagnosis of infectious diseases
Therapy of infectious diseases
  Antimicrobial agents
  Immunotherapy
  Surgical intervention

Objectives

After you have studied this chapter, you should be able to meet the following objectives:

_____ Define the terms: *host, infectious disease, colonization, microflora, commensalism, mutualism, parasitic relationship, virulence, pathogen, saprophyte.*

_____ Describe the structure, host–microorganism interaction, and mechanisms of reproduction for viruses, bacteria, rickettsiae, and chlamydiae, fungi, and parasites.

_____ Use the concepts of incidence, portal of entry, source of infection, symptomatology, disease course, site of infection, agent, and host characteristics to explain the mechanisms of infectious diseases.

_____ Differentiate between incidence and prevalence and among endemic, epidemic, and panepidemic.

_____ Describe the stages of an infectious disease following the point at which the potential pathogen enters the body.

_____ List the systemic manifestations of infectious disease.

_____ State the two criteria used in the diagnosis of an infectious disease.

_____ Explain the difference between culture, serology, and antigen or metabolite detection methods for diagnosis of infectious disease.

_____ Cite three general intervention methods that can be used in treatment of infectious illnesses.

_____ State four basic mechanisms whereby antibiotics exert their action.

_____ Differentiate between the terms *bactericidal* and *bacteriostatic.*

_____ Explain the actions of IGIV and cytokines in treatment of infectious illnesses.

All living creatures share two basic purposes of life—survival and reproduction. This tenet applies equally to humans and to members of the microbial world including bacteria, viruses, fungi, and protozoa. To satisfy these goals, organisms must extract nutrients essential for growth and proliferation from the environment; for countless organisms, that environment is the human body. Normally, the contact between humans and microorganisms is incidental and in certain situations may actually benefit both organisms. Under extraordinary circumstances, however, the invasion of the human body by microorganisms can produce harmful and potentially lethal consequences. These consequences are collectively termed *infectious diseases.*

Terminology

All scientific disciplines evolve with a distinct vocabulary, and the study of infectious diseases is no exception. Therefore, the most appropriate way to approach this subject is with a brief discussion of the terminology used to characterize interactions between humans and microbes.

Any organism capable of supporting the nutritional and physical growth requirements of another is called a *host.* Throughout this chapter, the term *host* will most often refer to humans supporting the growth of microorganisms. The term *infection* describes the presence and multiplication of a living organism on or within the host. Occasionally, the terms infection and *colonization* are used interchangeably.

One common misconception should be dispelled early on; not all contacts between microorganisms and humans are injurious. The exposed surfaces of the human body (internal and external) are normally and harmlessly inhabited by a multitude of bacteria collectively referred to as the *normal microflora* (Table 9-1). Although the colonizing bacteria acquire nutritional needs and shelter, the host is not adversely affected by the relationship. An interaction such as this is called *commensalism.* The term *mutualism* is applied to an infection in which the microorganism and the host derive benefits from the interaction. For example, certain inhabitants of the human intestinal tract extract nutrients from the host and, in turn, secrete essential vitamin by-products of metabolism (*e.g.,* vitamin K), which are absorbed and used by the host. A *parasitic relationship* is one in which only the

Table 9-1. Location and variety of nonpathogenic normal human microflora

Area	Site(s)	Bacteria Gram-positive	Gram-negative	Myco-bacteria	Parasites	Myco-plasmas	Fungi	Chlamydia/ Rickettsia	Spiro-chetes
Upper respiratory tract	Mouth, nose	+++	+++	+	+	+	+	0	+
	Nasopharynx	(Aerobes and	(Aerobes and	0	(Protozoans)	0	(Yeast)	0	0
	Throat	anaerobes	anaerobes)						
Lower respiratory tract	Larynx	0	0	0	0	0	0	0	0
	Trachea	0	0	0	0	0	0	0	0
	Lungs	0	0	0	0	0	0	0	0
External surfaces	Skin	++++	+	+	0	0	+	0	0
	Outer ear	(Aerobes and	(Transient)	0	0	0	(Yeast)	0	0
	Eyes	anaerobes)	0	0	0	0	0	0	0
Upper gastro-intestinal tract	Stomach	+	+	+	0	0	0	0	0
	Duodenum	(Transient)	(Transient)	(Transient)					
	Esophagus	0	0	0	0	0	0	0	0
	Jejunum	0	0	0					
Lower gastro-intestinal tract	Ileum	+++	++++	+	+	0	+	0	+
	Colon	(Predominantly anaerobes)	(Predominantly anaerobes)	0	(Protozoans)	0	(Yeast)		0
External genito-urinary tract	Vagina	++	++	0	0	+	+	0	+
	Anterior urethra	0	0	0	0	0	(Yeast)	0	0
Internal genito-urinary tract	Cervix, ovaries	0	0	0	0	0	0	0	0
	Fallopian tubes	0	0	0	0	0	0	0	0
	Uterus, prostate	0	0	0	0	0	0	0	0
	Bladder, kidney	0	0	0	0	0	0	0	0
	Testes, epididymis	0	0	0	0	0	0	0	0
Body fluids	Blood, urine	0	0	0	0	0	0	0	0
	Spinal fluid	0	0	0	0	0	0	0	0
	Synovial fluid	0	0	0	0	0	0	0	0
	Peritoneal fluid	0	0	0	0	0	0	0	0

Key: 0 = none; + = rare; ++ = few; +++ = moderate; ++++ = many.

infecting organism benefits from the relationship. If the host sustains injury or pathologic changes in response to a parasitic infection, the process is called an *infectious disease.*

The severity of an infectious disease can range from mild to life-threatening depending on many variables including the health of the host at the time of infection and the *virulence* (disease-producing potential) of the microorganism. A select group of microorganisms called *pathogens* are so virulent that they are rarely found in the absence of disease. Fortunately, there are very few human pathogens among the microbial world. Most microorganisms are harmless *saprophytes,* (*i.e.,* free living organisms obtaining their growth from dead or decaying organic material from the environment). However, it is important to remember that all microorganisms, even saprophytes and members of the normal flora, can be *opportunistic pathogens,* capable of producing an infectious disease when the health and immunity of the host has been severely weakened by illness, famine, or medical therapy.

In summary, throughout life, humans are continuously and harmlessly colonized by a multitude of microscopic organisms. This relationship is kept in check by the intact defense mechanisms of the host (mucosal and cutaneous barriers, normal immune function) and the innocuous nature of most environmental microorganisms. Those factors that either weaken the resistance of the host or increase the virulence of colonizing microorganisms can disturb the equilibrium of the relationship and cause disease. The degree to which the balance is shifted in favor of the microorganism determines the severity of illness.

Agents of infectious disease

The agents of infectious disease include viruses, bacteria, rickettsiae, and chlamydiae, fungi, and parasites.

Viruses

Viruses are the smallest obligate intracellular pathogens. They are incapable of replication outside of a living cell. They have no organized cellular structures but simply consist of a protein coat (capsid) surrounding a nucleic acid core (genome) of either RNA or DNA—never both (Figure 9-1). Some viruses are enclosed within a lipoprotein envelope derived from the cytoplasmic membrane of the parasitized host cell. Certain viruses are continuously shed from the infected cell surface enveloped in buds

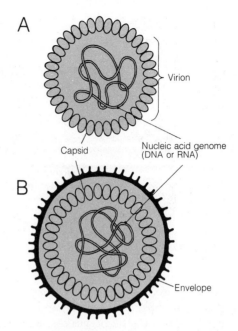

Figure 9-1 The structure of viruses. The basic structure of a virus includes a protein coat surrounding an inner core of nucleic acid (either DNA or RNA). Some viruses may also be enclosed in a lipoprotein outer envelope.

pinched from the cytoplasmic membrane. Enveloped viruses include members of the herpesvirus group and paramyxoviruses such as influenza.

Viruses must penetrate a susceptible living cell and use the biosynthetic machinery of the cell to produce viral progeny. The process of viral replication is shown in Figure 9-2. Not all viral agents cause the lysis and death of the host cell during the course of replication. Still other viruses enter the host cell and insert their genetic material (genome) into the host cell chromosome where the genome remains in a latent, nonreplicating state for long periods of time without causing disease. Under the appropriate stimulation, the virus will undergo active replication and produce symptoms of disease months to years later. Members of the herpesvirus group and adenovirus are the best examples of latent viruses. Herpesviruses include the viral agents of chickenpox and zoster (shingles), genital herpes, cytomegalovirus infections, infectious mononucleosis, and fever blisters. In each of these, the resumption of the latent viral replication may produce symptoms of primary disease (*e.g.,* genital herpes) or cause an entirely different symptomatology (*e.g.,* shingles instead of chickenpox).

Within the past decade, members of the retrovirus group have received considerable attention following identification of the human immunodeficiency viruses (HIV) as the causative agent of AIDS. The retroviruses have a unique mechanism of replication; after entry into the host cell, the viral RNA genome is first translated into DNA by a viral enzyme called

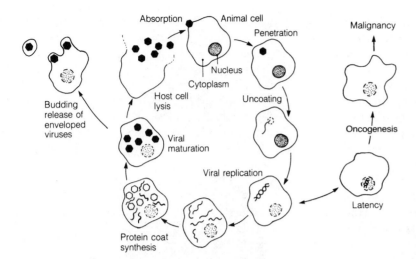

Figure 9-2 Schematic representation of the many possible consequences of viral infection of host cells including cell lysis (poliovirus), continuous release of budding viral particles or latency (herpesviruses) and oncogenesis (papovaviruses).

reverse transcriptase. The viral DNA copy is then integrated into the host chromosome and exists in a latent state similar to the herpesviruses. Reactivation and replication require a reversal of the entire process. Some retroviruses lyse the host cell during the process of replication. In the case of HIV, the infected cells regulate the immunologic defense system of the host and their lysis leads to a permanent suppression of the the immune response. In addition to causing infectious diseases, certain viruses also have the ability to transform normal host cells into malignant cells during the replication cycle. This group of viruses is referred to as *oncogenic* and includes certain retroviruses and DNA viruses such as the herpesviruses, adenoviruses, papovaviruses.

The viruses of humans and animals have been categorized somewhat arbitrarily according to various characteristics including the type of viral genome, the mechanism of replication (the retroviruses), the mode of transmission (anthropod-borne viruses or enteroviruses), and the type of disease produced (hepatitis A and B viruses) just to name a few.

—— Bacteria

Bacteria are autonomously replicating unicellular organisms known as *prokaryotes* because they lack an organized nucleus. Compared to nucleated eukaryotic cells (see Chapter 1), the structure of the bacterial cell is small and relatively primitive (Figure 9-3). Bacteria approximate the size of the eukaryotic mitochondria (about 1 micron in diameter) and may in fact be the evolutionary ancestors of mitochondria.

Bacteria contain no organized intracellular organelles and only a single chromosome (genome) of DNA. Many bacteria transiently harbor smaller extrachromosomal pieces of circular DNA called plasmids. Occasionally, plasmids will contain genetic information that increases the virulence of the organism. Simi-

lar to eukaryotic cells, but unlike viruses, bacteria contain both DNA and RNA.

The prokaryotic cell is organized into an internal compartment called the *cytoplasm,* which contains the reproductive and metabolic machinery of the cell. The cytoplasm is surrounded by a flexible lipid membrane (cytoplasmic membrane), which, in turn, is enclosed within a rigid cell wall. The structure and synthesis of the cell wall determine whether the microscopic shape of the bacterium is spherical (*cocci*), helical (*spirilla*), or elongate (*bacilli*). Most bacteria produce a cell wall composed of a distinctive polymer known as *peptidoglycan.* This polymer is only produced by prokaryotes—not eukaryotes—and, therefore, is an ideal target for antibacterial therapy. Several bacteria synthesize an extracellular capsule composed of protein or carbohydrate. The capsule protects the organism from environmental hazards such as the immunologic defenses of the host.

Certain bacteria are motile as the result of external whiplike appendages called *flagella*. The rotary action of the flagella transports the organism through a liquid environment like a propeller. Bacteria can also produce hairlike structures projecting from the cell surface called *pili* or *fimbrae,* which enable the organism to adhere to surfaces such as mucous membranes or other bacteria.

Most prokaryotes reproduce asexually by simple cellular division. The number of planes in which an organism divides can influence the microscopic morphology. For instance, when the cocci divide in chains they are called *streptococci;* in pairs, *diplococci;* and in clusters, *staphylococci.* The growth rate of bacteria varies significantly among different species and depends to a great deal on physical growth conditions and the availability of nutrients. In the laboratory, a single bacterium placed in a suitable growth environment such as an agar plate will reproduce to the extent that it will form a visible colony composed of millions of bacteria within a few hours. The physical appearance of the colony can be quite distinctive for each type of bacteria. Some bacteria produce highly resistant *spores* when faced with an unfavorable environment. The spores exist in a quiescent state almost indefinitely until suitable growth conditions are encountered. The spores then germinate, and the organism resumes normal metabolism and replication.

Bacteria are extremely adaptable life forms. They inhabit almost every environmental extreme on earth including humans. However, each individual bacterial species has a well-defined set of growth parameters including nutrition, temperature, light, humidity, and atmosphere. Bacteria with extremely strict growth requirements are called *fastidious*. For example, *Neisseria gonorrhoeae*, the bacterium that causes gonorrhea, cannot live for extended periods of time outside the human body. Some bacteria require oxygen for growth and metabolism and are called *aerobes;* others cannot survive in an oxygen-containing environment and are called *anaerobes*. An organism capable of adapting its metabolism to aerobic or anaerobic conditions is termed *facultatively anaerobic*.

In the laboratory, bacteria are generally classified according to the microscopic appearance and staining properties of the cell. The gram-stain, originally developed in 1884 by the Danish bacteriologist Christian Gram, is still the most widely used staining procedure today. Bacteria are designated *gram-positive* if they are stained purple by a primary basic dye (usually crystal violet); organisms that are not stained by the crystal violet but are counterstained a red color by a second dye (safranine) are called *gram-negative*. The staining characteristics and microscopic morphology are used in combination to describe bacteria. For example, *Streptococcus pyogenes*, the agent of scarlet fever and rheumatic fever, is a gram-positive streptococcus that is spherical, grows in chains, and stains purple by gram-stain. *Legionella pneumophila*, the bacterium responsible for Legionnaire's disease, is a gram-negative rod. For purposes of identification and classification, each member of the bacterial kingdom is categorized into a small group of biochemically and genetically related organisms called the *genus* and further subdivided into distinct individuals with the genus called *species*. The genus and species assignment of the organism is reflected in its name (*e.g.,* *Staphylococcus* [genus] *aureus* [species]).

Spirochetes

The spirochetes are an eccentric category of bacteria that are mentioned separately because of their unusual cellular morphology and mechanism of motility. Technically, the spirochetes are gram-negative rods but are distinctive in that the cell is helical in shape and the length of the organism is many times its width. A series of filaments are wound about the cell wall and extend the entire length of the cell. These filaments propel the organism through an aqueous environment in a corkscrew motion. Spirochetes are anaerobic or facultatively anaerobic organisms and contain three genera: *Leptospira, Borrelia,* and *Treponema.* Each genus has both saprophytic and pathogenic strains. The pathogenic leptospires infect a wide variety of wild and domestic animals. Infected animals shed the organisms into the environment through the urinary tract. Transmission to humans occurs by contact with infected animals or urine-contaminated surroundings. Leptospires gain access to the host directly through mucous membranes or breaks in the skin. In contrast, the borreliae are transmitted from infected animals to humans through the bite of an arthropod vector such as lice or ticks. Included among the genus *Borrelia* are the agents of relapsing fever (*B. recurrentis*) and Lyme disease (*B. burgdorferi*). Pathogenic *Treponema* species require no intermediates and are spread from person to person by direct contact. The most important member of the genus is *T. pallidum,* the cause of syphilis.

Mycoplasmas

The mycoplasmas are unicellular prokaryotes capable of independent replication. These organisms are less than one-third the size of bacteria and contain a small DNA genome approximately one-half the size of the bacterial chromosome. The cell is composed of cytoplasm surrounded by a membrane, but, unlike bacteria, the mycoplasmas do not produce a rigid peptidoglycan cell wall. As a consequence, the microscopic appearance of the cell is highly variable, ranging from coccoid forms to filaments, and the mycoplasmas are resistant to cell wall inhibiting antibiotics (*e.g.,* penicillins and cephalosporins). The mycoplasmas of humans are divided into three genera: *Mycoplasma, Ureaplasma,* and *Acholeplasma.* The first two of these require cholesterol from the environment to produce the cell membrane; the *Acholeplasma* do not. In the human host, mycoplasmas are commensals, but a number of species are capable of producing serious diseases in humans including pneumonia (*M. pneumoniae*), genital infections (*M. hominis* and *U. urealyticum*), and maternally transmitted respiratory infections to low birth weight infants (*U. urealyticum*).

Rickettsiae and chlamydiae

The rickettsiae and chlamydiae combine the characteristics of both viral and bacterial agents to produce disease in humans. Both are obligate intracellular pathogens like the viruses and yet both syn-

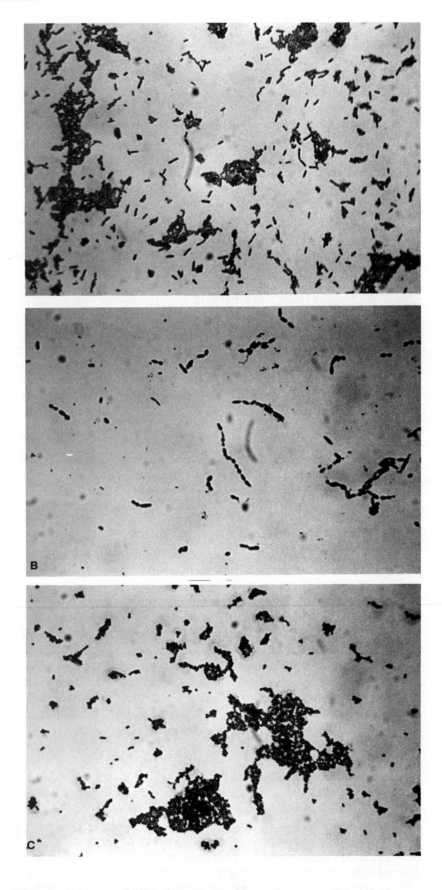

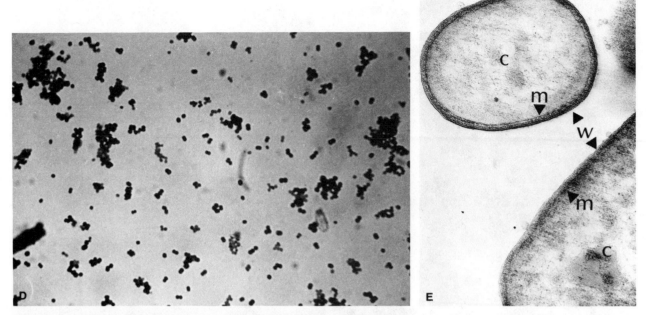

Figure 9-3 A sampling of the microscopic morphology of bacteria demonstrating the variability of size and shape including streptococci (**A**), bacilli (**B**), staphylococci (**C**), and diplococci (**D**). Also shown (**E**) is an electron micrograph of a cross-sectioned gram-negative bacterium showing the simple procaryotic cell structure including the cytoplasm (*c*), cytoplasmic membrane (*m*), and the bacterial cell wall (*w*).

thesize a rigid peptidoglycan cell wall, reproduce asexually by cellular division, and contain both RNA and DNA similar to the bacteria.

The rickettsiae depend on the host cell for essential vitamins and nutrients, while the chlamydiae appear to scavenge intermediates of energy metabolism such as ATP. The rickettsiae infect but do not produce disease in the cells of certain arthropods such as fleas, ticks, and lice. The organisms are accidentally transmitted to humans through the bite of the arthropod (vector) and produce a number of potentially lethal diseases including Rocky Mountain spotted fever and epidemic typhus.

The chlamydiae are slightly smaller than the rickettsiae but are structurally similar. Unlike the rickettsiae, chlamydiae are transmitted directly between susceptible vertebrates without an intermediate arthropod host. Transmission and replication of chlamydiae occur through a defined life cycle. The infectious form, called an *elementary body,* attaches to and enters the host cell where it transforms into a larger *reticulate body.* The latter undergoes active replication into multiple elementary bodies, which are shed into the extracellular environment to initiate another infectious cycle. Chlamydial diseases of humans include sexually transmitted genital infections (see Chapter 38), ocular infections, and pneumonia of the newborn (*Chlamydia trachomatis*), as well as respiratory disease acquired from infected birds (*C. psittaci*).

Fungi

The fungi are free-living, eukaryotic saprophytes found in every habitat on earth. Some are members of the normal human microflora. Fortunately, very few fungi are capable of causing diseases in humans, and most of these are incidental self-limited infections of skin and subcutaneous tissue. Serious fungal infections are rare and usually initiated through puncture wounds or inhalation. Despite their normally harmless nature, fungi can cause serious life-threatening opportunistic diseases when host defense capabilities have been disabled.

The fungi can be separated into two groups, yeasts and molds, based on rudimentary differences in their morphology (Figure 9-4). The yeasts are single-celled organisms, approximately the size of a red blood cell, that reproduce by a budding process. The buds separate from the parent cell and mature into an identical daughter cell. Molds, on the other hand, produce long, hollow, branching filaments called *hyphae.* Some molds produce cross walls, which segregate the hyphae into compartments—others do not. A limited number of fungi are capable of growing as yeasts at one temperature and as molds at another. These organisms are called dimorphic fungi and include a number of human pathogens such as the agents of blastomycosis, histoplasmosis, and coccidioidomycosis (San Joaquin Valley fever).

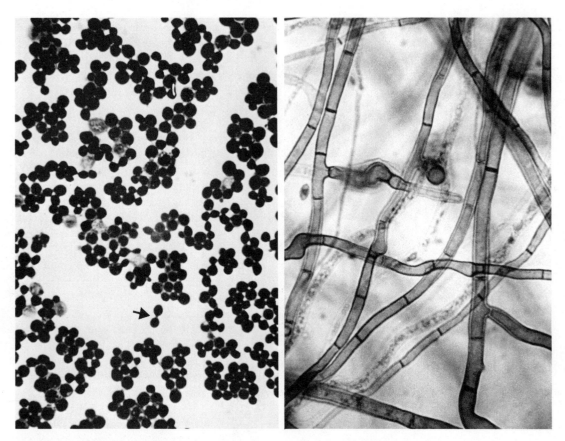

Figure 9-4 The microscopic morphology of the fungal pathogens of humans. The yeasts (*left*) are single-celled organisms that reproduce by a budding process (*arrow*). The molds (*right*) produce long branched or unbranched filaments called *hyphae*. A number of fungal pathogens called *dimorphic fungi* can exist either as yeasts or molds depending on the temperature of the environment.

The visual appearance of a fungal colony tends to reflect its cellular composition. Colonies of yeast are generally smooth with a waxy or creamy texture. Molds tend to produce cottony or powdery colonies composed of mats of hyphae collectively called a *mycelium*. The mycelium can penetrate the growth surface or project above the colony like the roots and branches of a tree. Both yeasts and molds produce a rigid cell wall layer that is chemically unrelated to the peptidoglycan of bacteria, and, therefore, is not susceptible to the effects of penicillin-like antibiotics.

Most fungi are capable of either sexual or asexual reproduction. The former process involves the fusion of zygotes with the production of a recombinant zygospore. Asexual reproduction involves the formation of highly resistant spores called *conidia* or *sporangiospores,* which are borne by specialized structures that arise from the hyphae. Molds are identified in the laboratory by the characteristic microscopic appearance of the asexual fruiting structures and spores. Just like the bacterial pathogens of humans, fungi can only produce disease in the human host if they can grow at the temperature of the infected body site. For example, a number of fungal pathogens called the *dermatophytes* are incapable of growing at core body temperature (37°C) and the infection is limited to the cooler cutaneous surfaces. Diseases caused by these organisms (ringworm, athlete's foot, jock itch) are collectively called superficial mycoses. Systemic mycoses are serious fungal infections of deep tissues and, by definition, are caused by organisms capable of growth at 37°C. Yeasts such as *Candida albicans* are commensals of the skin, mucous membranes, and gastrointestinal tract and are capable of growth at a wider range of temperatures. Intact immune mechanisms and competition for nutrients provided by the bacterial flora normally keep colonizing fungi in check. Alterations in either of these components by disease states or antibiotic therapy can upset the balance permitting fungal overgrowth and setting the stage for opportunistic infections.

Parasites

In a strict sense, any organism that derives benefits from its biologic relationship with another organism is a parasite. In the study of microbiology, however, the term *parasite* has evolved to designate members of the animal kingdom that infect and cause disease in other animals and includes protozoa, helminths, and arthropods.

The protozoa are unicellular animals with a complete complement of eukaryotic cellular machinery including a well-defined nucleus and organelles. Reproduction may be sexual or asexual and life cycles may be simple or complicated with several maturation stages requiring more than one host for completion. Most are saprophytes, but a few have adapted to the accommodations of the human environment and produce a variety of diseases including malaria, amebic dysentery, and giardiasis. Protozoan infections can be passed directly from host to host (*e.g.*, sexual contact), indirectly through contaminated water or food, or via an arthropod vector. Direct or indirect transmission results from the ingestion of highly resistant cysts or spores that are shed in the feces of an infected host. When the cysts reach the intestine, they mature into vegetative forms called trophozoites which, in turn, are capable of asexual reproduction or cyst formation. Most trophozoites are motile by means of flagella, cilia, or ameboid motion.

The helminths are a collection of wormlike parasites, which include the roundworms (nematodes), tapeworms (cestodes), and flukes (trematodes). The helminths reproduce sexually within the definitive host, and some require an intermediate host for the development and maturation of offspring. Humans can serve as the definitive or intermediate host and in certain diseases (*e.g.*, trichinosis) as both. Transmission of helminth diseases occurs primarily through the ingestion of fertilized eggs (ova) or the penetration of infectious larval stages through the skin—either directly or with the aid of an arthropod vector. Helminth infections can involve many organ systems and sites including the liver and lung, urinary and intestinal tracts, circulatory and central nervous systems, and muscle. Although most helminth diseases have been eradicated from the United States, they are still a major health concern of developing nations.

The parasitic arthropods of humans and animals include the vectors of infectious diseases (*i.e.*, ticks, mosquitoes, and biting flies) and the ectoparasites. The ectoparasites infest external body surfaces and cause localized tissue damage or inflammation secondary to the bite or burrowing action of the arthropod. The most prominent human ectoparasites are mites (scabies), chiggers, lice (head, body, and pubic), and fleas. Transmission of ectoparasites occurs directly by contact with immature or mature forms of the arthropod or its eggs found on the infested host or the host's clothing, bedding, or grooming articles (*e.g.*, combs and brushes). Many of the ectoparasites are vectors of other infectious diseases including endemic typhus and bubonic plague (fleas) and epidemic typhus (lice). A summary of the salient characteristics of human microbial pathogens is presented in Table 9-2.

In summary, this section of the chapter underscores the extreme diversity of procaryotic and eucaryotic microorganisms capable of causing infectious diseases in humans. With the advent of immunosuppressive medical therapy and immunosuppressive diseases such as AIDS, the number and type of potential microbic pathogens, the so-called opportunistic pathogens, have increased dramatically. However, the majority of infectious illnesses in humans will continue to be caused by only a small fraction of the organisms that comprise the microscopic world.

Table 9-2. Comparison of characteristics of human microbial pathogens

Organism	Defined nucleus	Genomic material	Size*	Intracellular/ extracellular	Motility
Virus	No	DNA or RNA	0.02–0.3	I	–
Bacteria	No	DNA	0.5–15	I/E	±
Mycoplasmas	No	DNA	0.2–0.3	E	–
Spirochetes	No	DNA	6–15	E	+
Rickettsias	No	DNA	0.2–2	I	–
Chlamydia	No	DNA	0.3–1	I	–
Yeasts	Yes	DNA	2–60	I/E	–
Molds	Yes	DNA	2–15 (hyphal width)	E	–
Protozoans	Yes	DNA	1–60	I/E	+
Helminths	Yes	DNA	2 mm–>1 m	E	+

* Micrometers unless indicated.

Mechanisms of infection

Epidemiology of infectious diseases

Epidemiology, in the context of this chapter, is the study of factors, events, and circumstances that influence the transmission of infectious diseases among humans. The ultimate goal of the epidemiologist is to devise strategies that interrupt or eliminate the spread of an infectious agent. To accomplish this, infectious diseases must be classified according to incidence, portal of entry, source, symptomatology, disease course, site of infection, agent, and host characteristics so that potential outbreaks may be predicted and averted or appropriately treated. Each of these categories will be discussed in detail with the exception of agents and host, which have already been reviewed.

Epidemiology is a science of rates. The expected frequency of any infectious disease must be calculated so that gradual or abrupt changes in frequency can be observed. The term *incidence* is used to describe the number of new cases of an infectious disease that occur within a defined population (*e.g.,* per 100,000 people) over an established period of time (monthly, quarterly, yearly). Disease prevalence indicates the number of active cases at any given time. A disease is considered endemic in a particular geographic region if the incidence and prevalence are expected and relatively stable. An epidemic describes an abrupt and unexpected increase in the incidence of disease over endemic rates. A pandemic refers to the spread of disease beyond continental boundaries. The advent of rapid, worldwide travel has increased the likelihood of pandemic transmission of pathogenic microorganisms.

Portal of entry

The portal of entry refers to the process by which a pathogen enters the body, gains access to susceptible tissues, and causes disease. Among the potential modes of transmission are penetration, direct contact, ingestion, and inhalation.

Penetration

Any disruption in the integrity of the surface barriers such as the skin or mucous membranes is a potential site for invasion of microorganisms. The break may be the result of accidental injury (abrasions, burns, wounds), medical procedures (surgery, catheterization), another infection (chickenpox), or inoculation (intravenous drug abuse, animal or arthropod bites). The latter mode of transmission can be extremely injurious because large numbers of microorganisms can be introduced directly into potentially vital sites relatively unscathed by the host's primary defenses.

Direct contact

Some pathogens are transmitted directly from infected tissue or secretions to exposed, intact mucous membranes without a prerequisite for damaged mucosal barriers. This is especially true of certain sexually transmitted diseases such as gonorrhea, syphilis, chlamydial infections, and herpes where exposure of uninfected membranes to pathogens occurs during intimate contact.

However, the transmission of these agents is not limited to sexual contact and can also occur during birth when the mucous membranes of the child come in contact with infected vaginal secretions of the mother.

Ingestion

The entry of pathogenic microorganisms through the oral cavity and gastrointestinal tract represents one of the more efficient means of disease transmission in humans. Many bacterial, viral, and parasitic infections, including cholera, typhoid fever, dysentery (amebic and bacillary), traveler's diarrhea, and hepatitis A, are initiated through the ingestion of contaminated food and water. This mechanism of transmission necessitates that an infectious agent survives the low *p*H and enzyme activity of gastric secretions and the peristaltic action of the intestines in numbers sufficient to establish infection (infectious dose). Ingested pathogens also must compete successfully with the normal bacterial flora of the bowel for nutritional needs. Persons with reduced gastric acidity (achlorhydria) due to disease or medication are more susceptible to infection by this route because the number of ingested microorganisms surviving the gastric environment is greater.

Inhalation

The respiratory tract of healthy individuals is equipped with a multitiered defense system to prevent potential pathogens from entering the lungs. The surface of the respiratory tree is coated with a layer of mucous that is continuously swept away from the lungs and toward the mouth by the beating motion of ciliated epithelial cells. Humidification of inspired air increases the size of aerosolized particles, which then are effectively filtered by the mucous membranes of the upper respiratory tract. Coughing also aids in the removal of particulate matter from the lower respiratory tract. Respiratory secretions contain antibodies and enzymes capable of inactivating infectious agents. Particulate matter and microorganisms that ultimately reach the lung are cleared by phagocytic cells. Despite this impressive array of protective mechanisms, a number of pathogens can invade the human body through the respiratory tract, including agents of bacterial pneumonia (*Streptococcus pneumoniae, Legionella pneumophila*), meningitis (*Neisseria meningitidis*), tuberculosis, and the viruses responsible for measles, mumps, rubella, and chickenpox. Defective pulmonary function or mucociliary clearance caused by noninfectious processes (*e.g.,* cystic fibrosis, or emphysema) or smoking can increase the risk of inhalation-acquired diseases.

It is important to remember that the portal of entry does not dictate the site of infection. Ingested pathogens may penetrate the intestinal mucosa, disseminate through the circulatory system and cause diseases in other organs such as the lung or liver. Whatever the mechanisms of entry, the transmission of infectious agents is directly related to the number of infectious agents absorbed by the host.

Source

The source of an infectious disease refers to the location, host, object, or substance from which the infectious agent was acquired: essentially the who, what, where, and when of disease transmission. The source may be endogenous (*i.e.,* acquired from the host's own microbial flora as would be the case in an opportunistic infection) or exogenous (*i.e.,* acquired from sources in the external environment such as the water, soil, air, or food). The infectious agent can originate from another human being, as from mother to child during gestation (congenital infections) or birth (perinatal infections). Zoonoses are a category of infectious diseases passed to humans from another animal species. The spread of infectious diseases through biting arthropods (vectors) has already been mentioned.

Source can denote a place—infections that develop in patients while they are hospitalized are termed *nosocomial,* and those that are acquired outside of health-care facilities are called *community acquired.*

The source may also pertain to the body substance that is the most likely vehicle for transmission, such as feces, blood, body fluids, respiratory secretions, and urine. Infections can be transmitted from person to person through shared inanimate objects (fomites) contaminated with infected body fluids. An example of this mechanism of transmission would include the spread of the AIDS virus through the use of shared syringes by intravenous drug abusers.

Symptomatology

The term *symptomatology* refers to the collection of signs and symptoms expressed by the host during the disease course. This is also known as the *clinical picture* or disease presentation and can be quite characteristic of any given infectious agent. In terms of pathophysiology, symptoms are the outward expression of the struggle between invading organisms and the retaliatory inflammatory and immune responses of the host (see Chapters 10 and 11). The symptoms of an infectious disease may be quite specific and reflect the site of infection (*e.g.,* diarrhea, rash, convulsions, hemorrhage). Conversely, symptoms such as fever, myalgia, headache, and lethargy are relatively nonspecific and can be shared by a number of diverse infectious diseases. The symptoms of a diseased host might be obvious, as in the cases of chickenpox or measles. Other covert symptoms, such as hepatitis or an increased white blood cell count, may require laboratory testing to detect. Accurate recognition and documentation of symptomatology can aid in the diagnosis of an infectious disease.

Disease course

The course of any infectious disease can be divided into several distinguishable stages following the point of time in which the potential pathogen enters the host. These stages are: the incubation period, the prodromal stage, the acute stage, the convalescent stage, and the resolution stage (Figure 9-5). These stages are based on the progression and intensity of the host's symptoms over time. The duration of each phase and the pattern of the overall process can be quite specific for different pathogens, thereby aiding in the diagnosis of an infectious disease.

Incubation period

The incubation period is the phase during which the pathogen begins active replication without producing recognizable symptoms in the host. The incubation period may be short, as in the case of salmonellosis (6–24 hours) or prolonged such as hepatitis B (50–180 days). The duration of the incubation period can be influenced by additional factors including the general health of the host, the portal of entry, and the infectious dose of the pathogen.

Prodromal stage

The hallmark of the prodromal stage is the initial appearance of symptoms in the host, although the clinical picture during this time may be only a vague sense of not feeling well. The host may experience mild fever, myalgia, headache, and malaise. These are constitutional changes shared by a great number of disease processes. Once again, the duration of the prodromal stage can vary considerably from host to host.

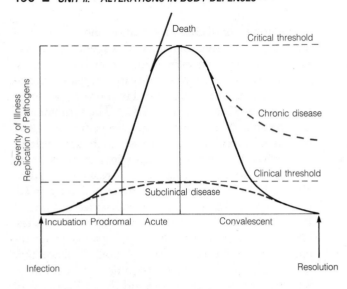

Figure 9-5 The stages of a primary infectious disease as they appear in relation to the severity of symptoms and the numbers of infectious agents. The clinical threshold corresponds with the initial expression of recognizable symptoms while the critical threshold represents the peak of disease intensity.

Acute stage

The acute stage consists of the period during which the host experiences the maximum impact of the infectious process corresponding to rapid proliferation and dissemination of the pathogen. During this phase, toxic by-products of microbial metabolism, cell lysis, and the immune response mounted by the host combine to produce tissue damage and inflammation. The symptoms of the host are pronounced and more specific than the prodromal stage, usually typifying the pathogen and site(s) of involvement.

Convalescent stage

The convalescent period is characterized by the containment of infection, progressive elimination of the pathogen, repair of damaged tissue, and resolution of associated symptoms. Similar to the incubation period, the time required for complete convalescence may be days, weeks, or months depending on the type of pathogen and the voracity of the host's immune response.

Resolution

The resolution is the total elimination of a pathogen from the body without residual signs or symptoms of disease. Several notable exceptions of the classic presentations of an infectious process have been recognized. *Chronic* infectious diseases have a markedly protracted and sometimes irregular course. The host may experience symptoms of the infectious process continuously or sporadically for months or years without a convalescent phase. In contrast, *subclinical* or *subacute* illness progresses from infection to resolution without clinically apparent symptoms. A disease is termed *insidious* if the prodromal phase is protracted; a *fulminant* illness is characterized by abrupt onset of symptoms with little or no prodrome.

Obviously, fatal infections are variants of the typical disease course.

Site of infection

The anatomical location of an infectious process is usually designated by adding the suffix *-itis* (Gr., inflammation) to the name of the involved tissue (*e.g.*, bronchitis, infection of the bronchi and bronchioles; encephalitis, brain infection; carditis, infection of the heart). These are general terms, however, and they apply equally to inflammation due to infectious and noninfectious causes (see Chapter 10). The suffix *-emia* is used to designate the presence of a substance in the blood; hence the terms *bacteremia, viremia,* and *fungemia* describe the presence of these infectious agents in the bloodstream. The term sepsis, or septicemia, refers to the presence of microbial toxins in the blood.

The site of an infectious disease is determined ultimately by the type of pathogen, the portal of entry, and competence of the host's immunologic defense system. Many pathogenic microorganisms are very restricted in their capacity to invade the human body. *Mycoplasma pneumoniae,* influenza viruses, and *Legionella pneumophila* rarely cause disease outside the respiratory tract; infections caused by *Neisseria gonorrhoeae* are generally confined to the genitourinary tract; and shigellosis and giardiasis seldom extend beyond the gastrointestinal tract. These are considered localized infectious diseases. The newly recognized bacterium *Campylobacter pylori* is an extreme example of a site-specific pathogen. *C. pylori* is considered a probable agent of gastric ulcers and has not been implicated in disease processes elsewhere in the human body. Bacteria such as *Hemophilus influenzae* type b, a prominent pathogen of young children and *Borrelia burgdorferi,* the agent of Lyme disease, tend to disseminate from the primary site of infection to involve other locations and organ systems. These are examples of systemic pathogens. Most systemic infections disseminate throughout the body by way of the circulatory system.

An abscess is a localized pocket of infection composed of devitalized tissue, microorganisms, and the host's phagocytic white blood cells—in essence a stalemate in the infectious process. The spread of the pathogen has been contained by the host, but white cell function within the toxic environment of the abscess is hampered, and the elimination of microorganisms is retarded. Abscesses, in general, must be surgically drained to effect a complete cure.

Virulence factors

Virulence factors are substances or products generated by infectious agents that enhance their ability to cause disease. Although number and type of microbial products that fit this description are numerous, they can generally be grouped into four categories: (1) toxins, (2) adherence factors, (3) evasive factors, and (4) invasive factors (Table 9-3).

Toxins

Toxins are substances that alter or destroy the normal function of the host or host's cells. Toxin production is a trait chiefly monopolized by bacterial pathogens, although certain fungal and protozoan pathogens also elaborate substances toxic to humans. Bacterial toxins have a diverse spectrum of activity and exert their effects on a wide variety of host target cells. For classification purposes, however, the bacterial toxins can be divided into two main types: *exotoxins* and *endotoxins*.

Exotoxins are proteins released from the bacterial cell during growth. Bacterial exotoxins enzymatically inactivate or modify key cellular constituents leading to cell death or dysfunction. Diphtheria toxin,

for example, inhibits cellular protein synthesis; botulism toxin decreases the release of neurotransmitter from cholinergic neurons, causing flaccid paralysis; tetanus toxin decreases the release of neurotransmitter from inhibitory neurons, producing spastic paralysis; and cholera toxin induces fluid secretion into the lumen of the intestine, causing diarrhea. Other examples of exotoxin-induced diseases include pertussis (whooping cough), anthrax, traveler's diarrhea, toxic shock syndrome, and a host of food-borne illnesses (food poisoning). Bacterial exotoxins that produce vomiting and diarrhea are sometimes referred to as *enterotoxins*.

By comparison, endotoxins do not contain protein, are not actively released from the bacterium during growth, and have no enzymatic activity. Rather, endotoxins are complex molecules composed of lipid and polysaccharides found in the cell wall of gram-negative bacteria. Studies of different endotoxins have indicated that the lipid portion of the endotoxin confers the toxic properties of the molecule. Endotoxins are potent activators of a number of regulatory systems in humans. A small amount of endotoxin in the circulatory system (endotoxemia) can induce clotting, bleeding, inflammation, hypotension, and fever. The sum of the physiologic reactions to endotoxins is sometimes called *endotoxic shock*.

Adherence factors

No interaction between microorganisms and humans can progress to infection or disease if the pathogen is unable to attach to and colonize the host. The process of microbial attachment may be site specific (mucous membranes or skin surfaces), cell specific (T-lymphocytes, respiratory epithelium), or nonspecific (moist or charged surfaces). In any of these cases, adherence requires a positive interaction between the surfaces of host cells and the infectious agent. The site to which microorganisms adhere is

---

Table 9–3. **Examples of virulence factors produced by pathogenic microorganisms**

Factor	Category	Organism	Effect on host
Cholera toxin	Exotoxin	*Vibrio cholerae* (bacterium)	Secretory diarrhea
Diphtheria toxin	Exotoxin	*Corynebacterium diphtheriae* (bacterium)	Inhibits protein synthesis
Lipopolysaccharide	Endotoxin	Many gram-negative bacteria	Fever, hypotension, shock
Toxic shock toxin	Enterotoxin	*Staphylococcus aureus* (bacterium)	Rash, diarrhea, vomiting, hepatitis
Hemagglutinin	Adherence	Influenzae virus	Establishment of infection
Pili	Adherence	*Neisseria gonorrhoeae* (bacterium)	Establishment of infection
Leukocidin	Evasive	*Staphylococcus aureus*	Kills phagocytes
IgA protease	Evasive	*Hemophilus influenzae* (bacterium)	Inactivates antibody
Capsule	Evasive	*Cryptococcus neoformans* (yeast)	Prevents phagocytosis
Collagenase	Invasive	*Pseudomonas aeruginosa* (bacterium)	Penetration of tissue
Protease	Invasive	*Aspergillus* (mold)	Penetration of tissue
Phospholipase	Invasive	*Clostridium perfringens* (bacterium)	Penetration of tissue

called a *receptor,* and the reciprocal molecule or substance that binds to the receptor is called a *ligand* or *adhesin.* Receptors may be proteins, carbohydrates, lipids, or complex molecules composed of all three. Similarly, ligands may be simple or complex molecules, and in some cases, highly specific structures. Ligands that bind to specific carbohydrates are called *lectins.* Certain bacteria produce hairlike structures protruding from the cell surface called *pili* or *fimbriae,* which anchor the organism to receptors on host cell membranes to establish an infection. Many viral agents including influenza, mumps, measles, and adenovirus produce filamentous appendages or spikes called *hemagglutinins,* which recognize carbohydrate receptors on the surfaces of specific cells in the upper respiratory tract of the host. After initial attachment, a number of bacterial agents become embedded in a gelatinous matrix of polysaccharides called a slime or mucous layer. The slime layer serves two purposes: it anchors the agent firmly to host tissue surfaces and it protects the agent from the immunologic defenses of the host.

Evasive factors

A number of factors produced by microorganisms enhance virulence by evading various components of the host's immune system. Extracellular polysaccharides (capsules, slime, or mucous layers) discourage engulfment and killing of pathogens by the phagocytic white blood cells (neutrophils and macrophages) of the host. Certain bacterial, fungal, and parasitic pathogens avoid phagocytosis by excreting leukocidins—toxins that deplete the host of neutrophils and macrophages by causing specific and lethal damage to the cytoplasmic membrane of white blood cells. Other pathogens, such as the bacterial agents of listeriosis and Legionnaires' disease are adapted to survive and reproduce within phagocytic white blood cells after ingestion, avoiding or neutralizing the usually lethal products contained within the lysosomes of the cell. Other unique strategies employed by pathogenic microbes to evade immunologic surveillance have evolved solely to avoid recognition by host antibodies. Strains of *Staphylococcus aureus* produce a surface protein (protein A), which immobilizes immunoglobulin G, holding the antigen-binding region harmlessly away from the organisms. This pathogen also secretes a unique enzyme called coagulase. Coagulase converts soluble human coagulation factors into a solid clot, which envelops and protects the organism from phagocytic host cells and antibody. *Hemophilus influenzae* and *Neisseria gonorrhoeae* secrete enzymes that cleave and inactivate secretory immunoglobulin A, thus neutralizing the primary defense of the respiratory and genital tracts at the site of infection.

Borrelia species, including the agents of Lyme disease and relapsing fever, alter surface antigens during the disease course to avoid immunologic detection. So it appears that the ingenuity to devise strategic defense systems and stealth technologies are not limited to humans. Viruses such as HIV cause impaired function of immunoregulatory cells. Although this property certainly increases the virulence of these agents, it is not considered a virulence factor in the true sense of the definition.

Invasive factors

Simply defined, invasive factors are products produced by infectious agents that facilitate the penetration of anatomical barriers and host tissue. In general, most invasive factors are enzymes capable of destroying cellular membranes (phospholipases), connective tissue (elastases, collagenases), intercellular matrices (hyaluronidase), and structural protein complexes (proteases). It is the combined effects of invasive factors, toxins, and antimicrobial and inflammatory substances released by host cells to counter infection that mediate the tissue damage and pathophysiology of infectious diseases.

Diagnosis of infectious diseases

The diagnosis of an infectious disease requires two criteria: the recovery of a probable pathogen or evidence of its presence from the infected site(s) of a diseased host and accurate documentation of clinical signs and symptoms (symptomatology) compatible with an infectious process. In the laboratory, the diagnosis of an infectious agent is accomplished using three basic techniques: (1) culture, (2) serology, or (3) the detection of characteristic antigens or metabolites produced by the pathogen.

Culture refers to the propagation of a microorganism outside of the body usually on or in artificial growth media such as agar plates or broth (Figure 9-6). The specimen from the diseased host is inoculated into broth or on to the surface of an agar plate, and the culture is placed in a controlled environment (incubator) until the growth of microorganisms becomes detectable. In the case of a bacterial pathogen, identification is based on microscopic appearance and Gram's stain reaction, shape, texture, and color (morphology) of the colonies, and by a panel of reactions that "fingerprint" salient biochemical characteristics of the organism. Certain bacteria such as *Mycobacterium leprae,* the agent of leprosy, and *Treponema pallidum,* the syphilis spirochete, will not grow on artificial media and require additional methods of identification. Fungi and mycoplasmas are cultured in much the same way as bacteria but with more reliance on microscopic and colonial morphology for identification. Chlamydia, rickettsia, and all human viruses are

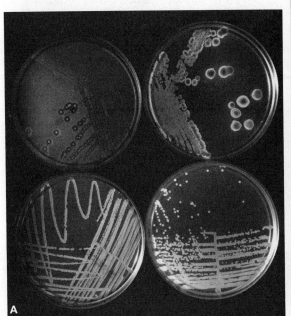
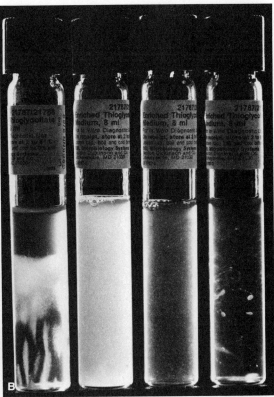

Figure 9-6 Variability of the macroscopic appearance of bacteria cultured on solid, agar-containing medium (**A**) or liquid broth medium (**B**). On solid surfaces, bacteria form distinct colonies, which increase in size and cell density with time until nutrients are depleted. Bacteria cultured in broth form a variety of growth patterns ranging from particulate to homogenous, turbid suspensions. Anaerobic bacteria cultured in liquid medium tend to grow best at the bottom of the tube where the concentration of molecular oxygen is lowest.

obligate intracellular pathogens. As a result, the propagation of these agents in the laboratory requires the inoculation of eukaryotic cells grown in culture (cell cultures). A cell culture consists of a flask containing a single layer, or monolayer, of eukaryotic cells covering the bottom and overlaid with broth containing essential nutrients and growth factors. When a virus infects and replicates within cultured eukaryotic cells, it produces pathologic changes in the appearance of the cell called cytopathic effect or CPE (Figure 9-7). CPE can be detected microscopically, and the pattern and extent of cellular destruction is often characteristic of a particular virus. Although culture media have been developed for the growth of certain human protozoa and helminths in the laboratory, the diagnosis of parasitic infectious diseases has traditionally relied on microscopic, or in the case of worms, visible identification of organisms, cysts, or ova directly from infected patient specimens.

Serology, the study of serum, is an indirect means of identifying infectious agents by measuring serum antibodies in the diseased host. A tentative diagnosis can be made if the antibody level, also called *antibody titer,* against a specific pathogen rises during the acute phase of the disease and falls during convalescence. Serologic identification of an infectious agent is not as accurate as culture, but it may be a useful adjunct, especially for the diagnosis of diseases caused by pathogens that cannot be cultured (*e.g.,* hepatitis B virus). The measurement of antibody titers has another advantage in that specific antibody types such as IgM and IgG are produced by the host during different phases of an infectious process; IgM-specific antibodies generally rise and fall during the acute phase, while the synthesis of the IgG class of antibodies increases during the acute phase and remains elevated until or beyond resolution. Measurements of class-specific antibodies are also useful in the diagnosis of congenital infections. IgM antibodies do not cross the placenta, while certain IgG antibodies are transferred passively from mother to child during the final trimester of gestation. Consequently, an elevation of pathogen-specific IgM antibodies found in the serum of a neonate must have originated from the child and, therefore, indicates congenital infection. A similarly increased IgG titer in the neonate does not distinguish congenital from maternal infection.

The technology of *direct antigen detection* has

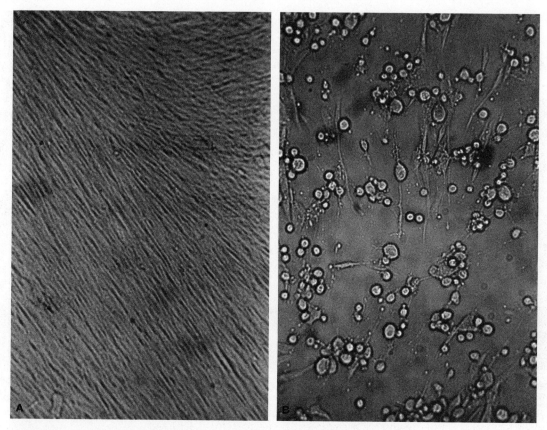

Figure 9-7 The microscopic appearance of a monolayer of uninfected human fibroblasts grown in cell culture (**A**) and the same cells following infection with herpes simplex virus (**B**) demonstrating the cytopathic effect (CPE) caused by viral replication and concomitant cell lysis.

evolved rapidly over the past decade and in the process has revolutionized the diagnosis of infectious diseases. Antigen detection incorporates features of culture and serology but reduces by a fraction the time required for diagnosis. In principle, this method relies on purified antibodies to detect antigens of infectious agents in specimens obtained from the diseased host. The source of antibodies used for antigen detection can be animals immunized against a particular pathogen or *hybridomas*. Hybridomas are created by fusing normal antibody-producing spleen cells from an immunized animal with malignant myeloma cells, which synthesize large quantities of antibody. The result is a cell that produces an antibody called a *monoclonal antibody*, which is highly specific for a single antigen and a single pathogen. Regardless of the source, the antibodies are labeled with a substance that allows microscopic or overt detection when bound to the pathogen or its products. Generally, the three types of labels used for this purpose are fluorescent dyes, enzymes, and particles such as latex beads. Fluorescent antibodies allow visualization of an infectious agent with the aid of a fluorescent microscope. Depending on the type of fluorescent dye used, the organism may appear a bright green or orange color against a black background, making detection extremely easy. En-

zyme-labeled antibodies function in a similar manner. The enzyme is capable of converting a colorless compound into a colored substance, thereby permitting detection of antibody bound to an infectious agent without the use of a fluorescent microscope. Finally, particles coated with antibodies will clump together, or agglutinate, when the appropriate antigen is present in a specimen. Particle agglutination is especially useful when examining infected body fluids such as urine, serum, or spinal fluid.

Very recently, an exciting method of detecting infectious agents in host specimens has been developed called *DNA probe hybridization*. Small fragments of DNA are cut from the genome of a specific pathogen and labeled with compounds that allow detection. The labeled DNA "probes" are then added to specimens from an infected host. If the pathogen is present, the probe will attach to the corresponding piece of DNA on the genome of the infectious agent permitting rapid diagnosis.

Therapy of infectious diseases

The goal of treatment for an infectious disease is complete removal of the pathogen from the host and the restoration of normal physiologic function to damaged tissues. Most infectious diseases of humans are self-limiting, that is, they require little or no medical therapy for a complete cure. When an infectious process gains the upper hand and therapeutic intervention is essential, the choice of treatment may be medicinal through the use of antimicrobial agents; immunologic with antibody preparations, vaccines, or substances that stimulate and improve the host's immune function; or surgical by removing infected tissues. The decision of which therapeutic modality or combination of therapies is based on the extent, urgency, and location of the disease process, the pathogen, and the availability of effective antimicrobial agents.

Antimicrobial agents

The use of chemicals, potions, and elixirs in the treatment of infectious diseases dates back to the earliest records of human medicine. Well over 2000 years ago Greek and Chinese physicians recognized that certain substances were useful for preventing or curing wound infections. Although the biologic activity of these compounds was not understood, some may have inadvertently contained by-products of molds that resemble modern antibiotics. From that time until the late 1800s when the relationship between infection and microorganisms was finally accepted, the evolution of anti-infective therapy was less than explosive. It was not until the advent of World War II, following the introduction of sulfonamides and penicillin, that the development of antimicrobial compounds matured into a science of great consequence. Today the comprehensive list of effective anti-infective agents is burgeoning. Most antimicrobial compounds can be categorized roughly according to mechanism of anti-infective activity, chemical structure, and target pathogen (e.g., antibacterial, antiviral, antifungal, or antiparasitic agents).

Antibacterial agents. Antibacterial agents are generally called antibiotics. Most antibiotics are actually produced by other microorganisms—primarily bacteria and fungi—as by-products of metabolism and, in general, are only effective against other prokaryotic organisms. An antibiotic is considered *bactericidal* if it causes irreversible and lethal damage to the bacterial pathogen and *bacteriostatic* if its inhibitory effects on bacterial growth are reversed when the agent is eliminated. Antibiotics can be classified into families of compounds with related chemical structure and activity (Table 9-4).

Not all antibiotics are effective against all pathogenic bacteria. Some agents are only effective against gram-negative bacteria, others are specific for gram-positive organisms. The so-called broad-spectrum antibiotics, such as the newest class of cephalosporins, are active against a wide variety of gram-positive and gram-negative bacteria. Members of the *Mycobacterium* genus, including *M. tuberculosis*, are extremely resistant to the effects of the major classes of antibiotics and require an entirely different spectrum

Table 9-4. Classification and activity of the antibacterial agents (antibiotics)

Family	Example	Target site	Side-effects
Penicillins	Ampicillin	Cell wall	Allergic reactions
Cephalosporins	Cephalexin	Cell wall	Allergic reactions
Monobactams	Aztreonam	Cell wall	Skin rash
Aminoglycosides	Tobramycin	Ribosomes (protein synthesis)	Hearing loss Nephrotoxicity
Tetracyclines	Doxycycline	Ribosomes (protein synthesis)	Gastrointestinal irritation Allergic reactions Teeth and bone dysplasia
Macrolides	Clindamycin	Ribosomes (protein synthesis)	Colitis Allergic reactions
Sulfonamides	Sulfadiazine	Folic acid synthesis	Allergic reactions Anemia Gastrointestinal irritation
Glycopeptides	Vancomycin	Ribosomes (protein synthesis)	Allergic reactions Hearing loss Nephrotoxicity
Quinolones	Ciprofloxacin	DNA synthesis	Gastrointestinal irritation
Miscellaneous	Chloramphenicol	Ribosomes (protein synthesis)	Anemia Hepatotoxicity
	Rifampin	Ribosomes (protein synthesis)	Allergic reactions
	Trimethoprim	Folic acid synthesis	Same as sulfonamides

of agents for therapy. The four basic mechanisms of the antibiotics are: (1) inhibition of bacterial peptidoglycan synthesis (penicillins, cephalosporins, glycopeptides); (2) inhibition of bacterial protein synthesis (aminoglycosides, macrolides, tetracyclines, chloramphenicol, and rifampin); (3) interruption of nucleic acid synthesis (fluoroquinolones, nalidixic acid); and (4) interference with normal metabolism (sulfonamides and trimethoprim).

Despite lack of antibiotic activity against eukaryotic cells, many cause unwanted or toxic side-effects in humans including allergic responses (penicillins, cephalosporins, sulfonamides, and glycopeptides), hearing and kidney impairment (aminoglycosides), and liver or bone marrow toxicity (chloramphenicol). Of greater concern is the increasing prevalence of bacteria resistant to the effects of antibiotics. The ways in which bacteria acquire resistance to antibiotics are becoming as numerous as the number of antibiotics. Bacterial resistance mechanisms include the production of enzymes that inactivate antibiotics, genetic mutations that alter antibiotic binding sites, alternative metabolic pathways that bypass antibiotic activity, and changes in the filtration qualities of the bacterial cell wall that prevent access of antibiotics to the target site within the organism. It is the continuous search for a better mousetrap that makes anti-infective therapy such a fascinating aspect of infectious diseases.

Antiviral agents. Unlike antibiotics, the list of effective antiviral agents, although increasing, is relatively small. The reason for this is host toxicity—viral replication requires the use of eukaryotic host cell enzymes and the drugs that effectively interrupt viral replication are likely to interfere with host cell reproduction as well. Almost all antiviral compounds are man-made and, with very few exceptions, the primary target of antiviral compounds is viral RNA or DNA synthesis. Agents such as acyclovir, vidarabine, and ribavirin mimic the nucleoside building blocks of RNA and DNA. During active viral replication, the nucleoside counterfeits inhibit the host or viral enzymes required to duplicate the viral genome, thus preventing the spread of infectious viral progeny to other susceptible host cells. Similar to the specificity of antibiotics, antiviral agents may be active against RNA viruses only, DNA viruses only, or occasionally both. Antiviral agents such as zidovudine, which are under evaluation in the treatment of AIDS, have targeted the HIV-specific enzyme reverse transcriptase for inhibition. This key enzyme is essential for viral replication and has no counterpart in the infected eukaryotic host cells. Experimental approaches to antiviral therapy include compounds that inhibit viral attachment to susceptible host cells and drugs that prevent uncoating of the viral genome once inside the host cell. Although the treatment of viral infections with antimicrobial agents is a relatively recent endeavor, reports of viral mutations resulting in resistant strains have already appeared in medical journals.

Antifungal agents. The target site of the two most important families of antifungal agents is the cytoplasmic membranes of yeasts or molds. Fungal membranes differ from human cell membranes in that they contain the sterol ergosterol instead of cholesterol. The polyene family of antifungal compounds (amphotericin B, nystatin) preferentially bind to ergosterol and form holes in the cytoplasmic membrane causing leakage of the fungal cell contents and, eventually, lysis of the cell. The imidazole class of drugs (miconazole, ketoconazole) inhibit the synthesis of ergosterol, thereby damaging the integrity of the fungal cytoplasmic membrane. Both types of drugs bind, to a certain extent, to the cholesterol component of host cell membranes and elicit a variety of toxic side-effects in treated patients. The nucleoside analogue 5-fluorocytosine (5-FC) disrupts fungal RNA and DNA synthesis but without the toxicity associated with the polyene and imidazole drugs. Unfortunately, 5-FC demonstrates little or no antifungal activity against molds or dimorphic fungi and is primarily reserved for infections caused by yeasts.

Antiparasitic agents. Because of the extreme diversity of human parasites and their growth cycles, a review of current antiparasitic therapies and agents would be highly impractical and lengthy. Similar to other infectious disease caused by eukaryotic microorganisms, treatment of parasitic illnesses is based on exploiting essential components of the parasite's metabolism or cellular anatomy that are not shared by the host. Any relatedness between the target site of the parasite and the cells of the host increases the likelihood of toxic reactions in the host. Continued development of improved antiparasitic agents suffers greatly from economic considerations as well. Parasitic diseases of humans are primarily the scourge of poor, underdeveloped, third-world nations. As a result, the financial incentives to produce more effective therapies are nonexistent. Resistance among human parasites to standard, effective therapy is also a major concern. In Africa, Asia, and South America the incidence of chloroquine-resistant malaria (*Plasmodium falciparum*) is on the rise. Resistant strains require more complicated, expensive, and potentially toxic therapy with a combination of agents.

Immunotherapy

One of the most recent and exciting approaches to the treatment of infectious diseases is immunotherapy. This strategy involves supplementing or stimulating the host's immune response so that the spread of a pathogen is limited or reversed. Several products are available for this purpose including intravenous immune globulin (IVIG) and cytokines. IVIG is a pooled preparation of antibodies obtained from normal, healthy immune human donors that is infused as an intravenous solution. In theory, pathogen-specific antibodies present in the infusion will facilitate neutralization, phagocytosis, and clearance of infectious agents above and beyond the capabilities of the diseased host. Hyperimmune immunoglobulin preparations, which are also commercially available, contain high titers of antibodies against specific pathogens including hepatitis B virus, cytomegalovirus, rabies, and varicella-zoster (chickenpox) virus. Cytokines are substances produced by human white blood cells that, in very small quantities, stimulate white cell replication, phagocytosis, antibody production, and the induction of fever, inflammation, and tissue repair—all of which counteract infectious agents and hasten recovery. With the advent of genetic engineering and cloning, many cytokines, including interferon and interleukins, have been produced in the laboratory and are currently being evaluated experimentally as anti-infective agents. One of the most efficient (and often overlooked) means of preventing infectious diseases is immunization. Proper and timely adherence to recommended vaccination schedules in children and boosters in adults effectively reduces the senseless spread of vaccine-preventable illnesses such as measles, mumps, pertussis, and rubella, which still occur in the United States with alarming frequency.

Surgical intervention

Prior to the discovery of antimicrobial agents, surgical removal of infected tissues, organs, or limbs was occasionally the only option available to prevent the demise of the infected host. Today, medicinal therapy with antibiotics and other anti-infective agents is an effective solution for a great majority of infectious diseases. However, surgical intervention is still an important option for cases in which (1) the pathogen is resistant to currently available treatments, (2) containment of rapidly progressing infectious process is the only means of saving the patient (gas gangrene), or (3) access to an infected site by antimicrobial agents is limited and surgical drainage (abscesses), cleaning of the site (debridement), or removal of organs or necrotic tissue (*e.g.*, appendectomy) will hasten the recovery process. In certain situations, surgery may be the only means of effecting a complete cure as in the case of endocarditis (infected

heart valves) in which the diseased valve must be replaced with a mechanical or biologic valve to restore normal function.

In summary, the ultimate outcome of any interaction between microorganisms and the human host is decided by a complex and ever-changing set of variables that take into account the overall health and physiologic function of the host, and the virulence and infectious dose of the microbe. In many instances, disease is an inevitable consequence, but with continued advancement of science and technology, the vast number of cases can either be eliminated or rapidly cured with appropriate therapy. It is the intent of those who study infectious diseases to understand thoroughly the pathogen, the disease course, the mechanisms of transmission, and the host response to infection. This knowledge will lead to development of improved diagnostic techniques, revolutionary approaches to anti-infective therapy, and hopefully, the eradication or control of those microscopic agents that cause frightening devastation and loss of life throughout the world.

Bibliography

Beachey EH: Bacterial adherence: Adhesin-receptor interactions mediating the attachment of bacteria to mucosal surfaces. J Infect Dis 143:325, 1981

Donowitz GR, Mandell GL: Beta-lactam antibiotics (parts 1 and 2). N Engl J Med 318:419, 490, 1988

Flier JS, Underhill LH: Medical consequences of persistent viral infections. N Engl J Med 314(6):359, 1986

Jones JE: Pinworms. Am J Fam Pract 38(3):159, 1988

Lennette EH, Balows A, Hausler WJ Jr et al (eds): Manual of Clinical Microbiology. Washington DC, American Society for Microbiology, 1985

Musher DM: The gram-positive cocci: I. Streptococci. Hosp Pract 23(3):63, 1988

Musher DM: The gram-positive cocci: II. Staphylococci. Hosp Pract 23(4):179, 1988

Musher DM: The gram-positive cocci: III. Resistance to antibiotics. Hosp Pract 23(5):105, 1988

Petri WA: Tick-borne diseases. Am Fam Pract 37(6):95, 1988

Sharp AH, Fields BN: Pathogenesis of viral infections. N Engl J Med 312(8):486, 1985

Sheagren JN: *Staphlococcus aureus*. N Engl J Med 3109(21,22):1437, 1984

Stechenberg BW: Lyme disease: The latest great imitator. Pediatr Infect Dis 7:402, 1988

Treadwell TL: Gram-negative bacteremia. Hosp Pract 23(7):117, 1988

Wright SW, Trott AT: North American tick-borne diseases. Ann Emerg Med 17(9):964, 1988

CHAPTER 10

Inflammation and Repair

The inflammatory response
  Acute inflammation
    Vascular response
    Cellular response
    Inflammatory mediators
    Inflammatory exudates
    Resolution of acute
      inflammation
    The acute-phase response

Chronic inflammation
  Nonspecific chronic
    inflammation
  Granulomatous inflammation

Tissue healing and repair
  Regeneration
  Connective tissue repair
    Healing by first or second
      intention
    Keloid formation
    Factors that affect wound
      healing

Objectives

After you have studied this chapter, you should be able to meet the following objectives:

_____ Define *inflammation*.

_____ Explain why the inflammatory response is beneficial to the body.

_____ List at least five general causes of inflammation.

_____ Cite one universal characteristic of the inflammatory response.

_____ State the five cardinal signs of inflammation and describe the physiologic mechanisms involved in production of each of these signs.

_____ Describe the early hemodynamic changes that occur in acute inflammation.

_____ State the three patterns of the hemodynamic response that occur with an inflammatory reaction.

_____ Describe the four stages of the cellular phase of the acute inflammatory response.

_____ State the function of granular leukocytes.

_____ Define *diapedesis*.

_____ Relate chemotaxis to leukocyte activity.

_____ Describe the process of phagocytosis.

_____ List the components of the reticuloendothelial system.

_____ State one distinctive characteristic of chemical inflammatory mediators.

_____ Contrast the five types of inflammatory exudates.

_____ Describe three patterns of resolution of acute inflammation.

_____ State the mediator of the acute-phase response and list the manifestations of the response.

_____ State the characteristics of chronic inflammation.

_____ Relate the sequence of events in soft tissue repair.

_____ Describe the process of scar tissue development.

_____ Define *first intention* and *second intention* in relation to wound healing.

_____ Relate the influence of local and systemic factors on wound healing.

The ability of the body to sustain injury, resist attack by microbial agents, and repair damaged tissue is dependent on the inflammatory reaction, the immune response, tissue regeneration, and fibrous tissue replacement. This chapter focuses on the local manifestations of acute and chronic inflammation, the repair process, systemic signs of inflammation, and selected disease states that affect the inflammatory cells. Chapter 11 discusses the immune response.

Inflammation is the local reaction of vascularized tissue to injury.[1] Although the effects of inflammation are often viewed as undesirable because they are unpleasant and cause discomfort, the process is essentially a beneficial one that allows a person to live with the effects of everyday stress. Without the inflammatory response, wounds would not heal and minor infections would become overwhelming.

On the other hand, inflammation also produces undesirable effects. The crippling effects of rheumatoid arthritis, for example, have their origin in the inflammatory response.

The inflammatory response

The inflammatory response is closely intermeshed with wound healing and reparative processes. It acts to neutralize or destroy the offending agent, to restrict the tissue damage to the smallest possible area, to alert the individual to the impending threat of tissue injury, and to prepare the injured area for healing. Wound healing and tissue repair begin during the active stages of inflammation and serve to repair the damage caused by the injurious agent.

The causes of inflammation are many and varied. Although it is quite common to equate inflammation with infection, it is important to recognize that almost all types of injury are capable of inciting the response and that only a small number of inflammatory responses are related to infections. The injurious agents that cause inflammation can arise from outside the body (*exogenous*) or from within the body (*endogenous*). Common causes of inflammation are trauma, surgery, infection, caustic chemicals, extremes of heat and cold, immune responses, and ischemic damage to body tissues.

Although the inflammatory response can be initiated by a wide variety of injurious agents, the sequence of physiologic events that follow is remarkably similar. The inflammatory response involves *a sequence of specific physiologic behaviors that occur in response to injury by a nonspecific agent.* An acute inflammatory response will follow the same course, whether the injury is caused by a streptococcal infection or by tissue necrosis associated with myocardial

infarction. The extent of the injury will vary and the site of inflammation will be different, but the tissue response and systemic manifestations will be similar. The body will, however, *use only those behaviors in the sequence that are needed to minimize tissue damage.* A small area of local swelling and redness may be sufficient to prevent injury from a mosquito bite, whereas other, more serious conditions, such as appendicitis, may incite leukocytosis, fever, and formation of an exudate.

Inflammation can be acute or chronic. Acute inflammation is the typical short-term response associated with all types of tissue injury. It involves hemodynamic changes, formation of an exudate, and the presence of granular leukocytes. Chronic inflammation follows a less uniform and more persistent pattern. It involves the presence of nongranular leukocytes and usually results in more extensive formation of scar tissue and deformities.

Inflammatory conditions are named by adding the suffix -*itis* to the affected organ or system. For instance, neuritis refers to inflammation of a nerve, pericarditis to inflammation of the pericardium, and appendicitis to inflammation of the appendix. A further description of the inflammatory process might indicate whether the process was acute or chronic and what type of exudate was formed, for example, acute fibrinous pericarditis.

Acute inflammation

The classic description of acute inflammation has been handed down through the ages. In the first century A.D., the Roman physician Celsus described the local reaction to injury in terms of what has come to be known as the cardinal signs of inflammation. These signs are *rubor* (redness), *tumor* (swelling), *calor* (heat), and *dolor* (pain). In the second century A.D., Galen added a fifth cardinal sign, *functio laesa* or loss of function.

The manifestations of acute inflammation can be divided into two categories, *hemodynamic* and *white blood cell responses*. At the biochemical level, many of the responses that occur during acute inflammation are associated with the release of chemical mediators. Both the hemodynamic responses and white blood cell responses contribute to the *inflammatory exudates* that characterize the acute inflammatory response. Each of these aspects of acute inflammation is discussed separately.

Vascular response

The hemodynamic, or vascular, changes that occur with inflammation begin almost immediately following injury and are initiated by a momentary constriction of small vessels in the area. This momentary period of vasoconstriction is followed immediately by vasodilation of the arterioles and venules that supply the area. As a result, the area becomes congested and warm—the *redness* and *warmth* are characteristic of acute inflammation. Accompanying this hyperemic response is an increase in capillary permeability, which allows fluid to escape into the tissue and to cause *swelling*. *Pain* and *impaired function* follow as the result of tissue swelling and release of chemical mediators. The reader can simulate the hemodynamic responses that occur with acute inflammation by running the sharp edge of a fingernail along the inner aspect of the arm. The response has been termed the *triple response.*[2] Within seconds, the line will redden as the first response takes place. The second response is a red flare that develops on both sides of the line, which represents the hyperemic phase of the inflammatory response. Within several minutes, the third response occurs as the line becomes slightly raised due to swelling resulting from an increase in capillary permeability. The flare response that occurs with this type of stimulus is highly variable; some persons will have only a slight response while others will have an exaggerated one.

The hemodynamic changes that occur during the early stages of inflammation are beneficial in that they aid in controlling the effects of the injurious agent. During this stage, the exudation of fluid out of the capillary into the tissue spaces helps *dilute* the toxic and irritating agents. Sometime later, white blood cells accumulate in the area and leave the capillary as part of the exudate. As fluid moves out of the capillary, *stagnation* of flow and *clotting* of blood in the small capillaries that supply the inflamed area occur. This aids in *localizing* the effects of the injury.

Depending on the severity of injury, the hemodynamic changes that occur with the inflammatory reaction follow one of three patterns of response. The first is an immediate transient response, which occurs with minor injury. The second is an immediate sustained response, which occurs with more serious injury and continues for several days. With this response there is actual damage to the vessels in the area. The third type of response is a delayed response—the increase in capillary permeability is delayed for a period of 4 to 24 hours. A delayed response often accompanies radiation types of injuries, such as a sunburn.

Cellular response

The cellular stage of acute inflammation is marked by movement of white blood cells (leukocytes) into the area of injury. This stage includes (1) the margination or pavementing of white blood cells, (2)

emigration of white blood cells, (3) chemotaxis, and (4) phagocytosis. A description of white blood cells precedes the discussion of cellular events that occur in acute inflammation.

The leukocytes, or white blood cells, develop from the primordial stem cells located in the bone marrow and lymphoid tissue. The leukocytes are larger and less numerous than the red blood cells. There are two types of white blood cells, granular and nongranular leukocytes. The different types of leukocytes are illustrated in Figure 10-1.

Granular leukocytes. The granular leukocytes are identifiable because of their cytoplasmic granules and are commonly referred to as granulocytes. In addition to their cytoplasmic granules, these white blood cells have distinctive multilobar nuclei. The granulocytes are divided into three types (neutrophils, eosinophils, and basophils) according to the staining properties of the granules (Figure 10-1).

The *neutrophils*, which constitute 60% to 70% of the total number of white blood cells, have granules that are neutral and hence do not stain with either an acid or a basic dye. Because these white cells have nuclei that are divided into three to five lobes, they are often called *polymorphonuclear (PMN) leukocytes.* The neutrophils are the first cells to arrive at the site of inflammation, usually appearing within 90 minutes of injury. Neutrophils increase greatly during the inflam-

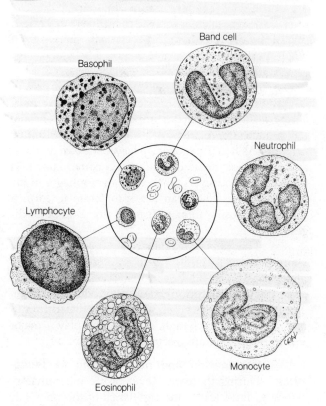

Basophil
Band cell
Neutrophil
Lymphocyte
Eosinophil
Monocyte

Figure 10-1 White blood cells involved in the inflammatory response.

matory process. When this happens, immature forms of neutrophils are released from the bone marrow. These immature cells are often called *bands* or *stabs* because of the horseshoe shape of their nuclei. The neutrophils have a life span of only about 10 hours and, therefore, must be constantly replaced if their numbers are to be adequate.

The cytoplasmic granules of the *eosinophils* stain red with the acid dye eosin. These leukocytes constitute 1% to 3% of the total number of white blood cells and increase during allergic reactions and parasitic infections. It is thought that they detoxify the agents or chemical mediators associated with allergic reactions and assist in terminating the response.

The granules of the *basophils* stain blue with a basic dye. These cells constitute only about 0.3% to 0.5% of the white blood cells. The granules in the basophils contain heparin and histamine and are similar to those of the mast cells. The basophils are thought to be involved in allergic and stress responses.

Nongranular leukocytes. There are two groups of nongranular leukocytes, the monocytes and the lymphocytes. The *monocytes* are the second order of cells to arrive at the inflammation site; their arrival usually requires 5 hours or more. Within 48 hours, however, the monocytes are usually the predominant cell type in the inflamed area. Monocytes are the largest of the white blood cells and constitute about 3% to 8% of the total leukocyte count. The circulating life span of the monocyte is three to four times longer than that of the granulocytes, and these cells survive for a longer period of time in the tissues. The monocytes, which are phagocytic cells, are often referred to as *macrophages*. The monocytes engulf larger and greater quantities of foreign material than the neutrophils. These leukocytes play an important role in chronic inflammation and are also involved in the immune response. When the monocyte leaves the vascular system and enters the tissue spaces, it becomes known as a *histiocyte*. Histiocytes function as macrophages in the inflamed area. They can also proliferate to form a capsule, enclosing foreign material that cannot be digested.

The *lymphocytes* constitute 20% to 30% of the white blood cell count. There are two types of lymphocytes, B cells and T cells. The B cells form plasma cells, and they are concerned with antibody formation. The T cells are concerned with cell-mediated immunity. Both types of lymphocytes, which play a major role in immunity, are discussed in Chapter 11.

Margination and pavementing of leukocytes. During the early stages of the inflammatory response, fluid leaves the capillaries of the microcirculation causing blood viscosity to increase. As this occurs, the leukocytes begin to *marginate*, or move to the periphery of the blood vessel. As the process continues, the marginated leukocytes begin to adhere to the vessel lining in preparation for emigration from the vessel. The cobblestone appearance of the vessel lining due to margination of leukocytes has led to the term *pavementing*.

Emigration of leukocytes. Emigration is a mechanism whereby the leukocytes extend *pseudopodia* (false feet), pass through the capillary walls by ameboid movement, and then migrate into the tissue spaces. The movement of white blood cells through the wall of the capillary occurs by means of a process called *diapedesis*. Along with the emigration of leukocytes, there is also an escape of red cells from the capillary. The red cells may escape singly or in small jets at points where the capillaries have become distended.

Chemotaxis. The leukocytes, after emigrating through the vessel wall, wander through the tissue space guided by the presence of bacteria and cellular debris. The process by which leukocytes are attracted to bacteria and cellular debris is called *chemotaxis*. Chemotaxis can be positive or negative, meaning that it can act either to attract or to repel the leukocytes. Many substances are capable of acting as chemotaxic agents, including infectious organisms, plasma-protein fractions (complement), and tissue debris.

Phagocytosis. In the final stage of the cellular response, the neutrophils and monocytes engulf and degrade the bacteria and cellular debris in a process called *phagocytosis* (Figure 10-2). The neutrophils are sometimes called *microphages* because they con-

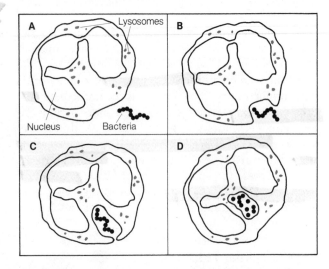

Figure 10-2 Phagocytosis by a neutrophil. In **A**, a neutrophil has emigrated from the capillary; in **B**, it is attracted to the bacteria through chemotaxis; and in **C**, it engulfs the bacteria. **D** shows the final stages of phagocytosis: the bacteria are degraded by the enzymes and digestive materials contained in the cytoplasmic granules of the neutrophil.

centrate on the phagocytosis of bacteria and small particles. The monocytes, or *macrophages,* remove tissue debris and larger particles from the area of inflammation.

Leukocytosis. Leukocytosis refers to an increase in white blood cell numbers. Acute inflammatory conditions, particularly those of bacterial origin, are accompanied by marked increases in white blood cell numbers with a disproportionate increase seen in the neutrophilic count. A differential blood count measures both the total number of white blood cells and the percentage of each type of blood cell. Table 10-1 compares the normal white blood cell count with that sometimes seen in an acute infection.

The reticuloendothelial system. In addition to the mobile white cells that circulate in the bloodstream, there are nonmobile phagocytic cells widely scattered throughout the body. These cells are collectively referred to as the reticuloendothelial system. There are the Kupffer's cells in the liver sinusoids, the alveolar macrophages, the microglia of the brain, and the macrophages located in the spleen, bone marrow, and lymphoid tissues. These cells ingest the debris of dead cells, bacteria, and inert foreign matter. The lymphoid organs (lymph nodes, spleen, and tonsils) are discussed in Chapter 11.

Inflammatory mediators

Although inflammation is precipitated by injury and cell death, its signs and symptoms are produced by chemical mediators such as histamine, the plasma proteases, prostaglandins, slow-reacting substance of anaphylaxis, and other neutrophil and lymphocyte factors. Other mediators have been identified, but their role in the inflammatory process is still unclear. The chemical mediators are stored in inactive form in various body cells such as neutrophils, basophils, mast cells, and platelets. The process of mediator activation requires a number of sequential steps

Table 10-1. Example of a normal white blood count (wbc) compared with white blood count during an acute infection

	Normal	Acute infection
Total WBC (cells per mm³)	5,000–10,000	16,000–18,000
Polymorphonuclear leukocytes (PMNs, %)	69	85
Stabs (% of PMNs)	—	12
Lymphocytes (%)	29	14
Monocytes (%)	2	1

Table 10-2. Signs of inflammation and corresponding chemical mediators

Inflammatory response	Chemical mediator
Swelling, redness, and tissue warmth (vasodilatation and capillary permeability)	Histamine Prostaglandins Bradykinin
Tissue damage	Neutrophil, macrophage, and lysosomal enzymes
Chemotaxis	Complement fractions
Pain	Prostaglandins Bradykinin
Fever	Prostaglandins Endogenous pyrogens
Leukocytosis	Leukocyte-stimulating factor

that control the reaction and prevent the process from occurring by chance. If this were not true, most of us would be constantly covered with swollen and reddened areas over much of our bodies. Table 10-2 describes the prominent manifestations of inflammation and the chemical substances that mediate their occurrence.

Histamine. Histamine is widely distributed throughout the body. It can be found in platelets, basophils, and mast cells. Histamine causes dilatation of arterioles and enhanced permeability of capillaries and venules. It is the first mediator in the initial inflammatory response. Antihistamine drugs suppress this immediate transient response induced by mild injury.

Plasma proteases. The plasma proteases consist of the kinins, complement and its fractional components, and clotting factors. One of the kinins, bradykinin, causes increased capillary permeability and pain. The complement system consists of a number of component proteins and their cleavage products. These substances interact with the antigen–antibody complexes and mediate immunologic injury and inflammation (see Chapter 11). The clotting system is discussed in Chapter 15.

Prostaglandins. The prostaglandins, so named because they were first identified in the prostate gland, are ubiquitous tissue proteins composed of lipid-soluble acids derived from arachidonic acid, which is stored in cell membrane phospholipids. The synthesis of prostaglandins occurs in two stages: (1) arachidonic acid is liberated from the phospholipids of the cell membrane and (2) then converted to prostaglandins. This second stage requires the enzyme cyclo-oxygenase. Prostaglandins contribute to vasodilation, capillary permeability, and the pain and fever that accompany inflammation. There are a number of prostaglandins. The stable prostaglandins (PGE₁ and PGE₂) induce inflammation and potentiate the effects of histamine and other inflammatory mediators. The prostaglandin thromboxane A₂ promotes platelet aggregation and vasoconstriction. Prostacycline (PGI₂) has the opposite effect. It relaxes vascular smooth muscle and inhibits platelet aggregation. Drugs such as aspirin and indomethacin (a nonsteroidal anti-inflammatory drug) inhibit prostaglandin synthesis by suppressing cyclo-oxygenase activity. The glucocorticoid hormones secreted from the adrenal cortex (or given as a drug) are known to curtail the availability of arachidonic acid for prostaglandin production.[3] The glucocorticoid drugs have come to be known as anti-inflammatory drugs because of their ability to suppress the inflammatory response.

Leukotrienes. The leukotrienes are a group of chemical mediators capable of inciting the inflammatory response. Their name was chosen because they were discovered on the leukocyte and they have a chemical triene structure. One of the leukotrienes, the slow-acting substance of anaphylaxis, causes slow and sustained constriction of the bronchioles and is an important inflammatory mediator in bronchial asthma and immediate hypersensitivity reactions (see Chapter 12). The leukotrienes have also been reported to have an effect on the permeability of the postcapillary venules; adhesion properties of the endothelial cells; extravasation of the white blood cells; and chemotaxis of polymorphonuclear cells, eosinophils, and monocytes.[4] Like the prostaglandins, the leukotrienes are formed from arachidonic acid but they use the lipoxygenase pathway, which involves the enzyme lipoxygenase. Thus, it now appears that prostaglandins and leukotrienes are part of a larger biologic control system based on arachidonic acid. Depending on the active enzymes in the stimulated cell, arachidonic acid can be converted to several biologically active compounds, which regulate various cellular responses to injury.

Neutrophil and lymphocyte products. The neutrophils and lymphocytes contribute a number of mediators to the inflammatory process. The neutrophils release mediators that increase vascular permeability, act as a chemotactic factor for monocytes, and cause tissue damage. Much of the tissue damage done during the acute inflammatory process is caused by the lysosomal enzymes of the neutrophil. The lymphocytes release mediators called lymphokines. These mediators have numerous actions including chemotaxis of macrophages, neutrophils, and basophils.

Inflammatory exudates

Characteristically the acute inflammatory response involves production of exudates. These exudates can vary in terms of fluid, plasma protein, and cell content. Acute inflammation can produce serous, fibrinous, membranous, purulent, and hemorrhagic exudates. Inflammatory exudates are often composed of a combination of these types.

Serous exudate. The initial exudate that enters the inflammatory site is largely plasma. Serous drainage is a watery exudate low in protein content. A blister contains serous fluid. A catarrhal inflammation is one that affects the mucous membranes and is associated with an increase in watery secretions and desquamation of the epithelial cells. Hay fever is an example of a catarrhal inflammatory response.

Fibrinous exudate. Fibrinous exudates contain large amounts of fibrinogen and form a thick and sticky meshwork, much like the fibers of a blood clot. Fibrinous exudates are frequently encountered in the serous cavities of the body. Acute rheumatic fever often causes development of a fibrinous pericarditis. A fibrinous exudate must be removed through fibrinolytic activity of enzymes before healing can take place. Failure to remove the exudate leads to ingrowth of fibroblasts and subsequent development of scar tissue and adhesions. A fibrinous exudate may be beneficial in that it tends to glue the inflamed structures together thereby preventing the spread of infection. In appendicitis, for example, the initial formation of a fibrinous exudate serves to localize the organisms in the region of the appendix and thus prevents the generalized spread of the infection to the peritoneal cavity.

Membranous exudate. Membranous or pseudomembranous exudates develop on mucous membrane surfaces. The development of a membranous exudate occurs as necrotic cells become enmeshed in a fibrinopurulent exudate that coats the mucosal surface. *Diphtheria* was known for its ability to produce a membranous exudate on the surface of the trachea and major bronchi. *Thrush* is a monilial infection of the oral cavity that produces patches of membranous inflammation. *Membranous enterocolitis* is a severe membranous inflammatory condition of the bowel mucosa related to a disturbance in the normal bowel flora due to treatment with a variety of broad-spectrum antibiotics.

Purulent exudate. A purulent (suppurative) exudate contains pus, which is composed of the remains of white blood cells, proteins, and tissue debris. Purulent infections are caused by a number of pyogenic or pus-forming bacteria. An *abscess* is a localized collection of pus. Abscesses may occur at the site of injury, or they may develop as the result of metastatic spread of infectious organisms and tissue debris through the bloodstream. An abscess is encapsulated in a so-called pyogenic membrane, which consists of layers of fibrin, inflammatory cells, and granulation tissue. An abscess may need to be incised and the pus removed before healing can occur.

Cellulitis, or phlegmonous inflammation, is a subgroup of suppurative infections that involve massive necrosis of tissue along with production of purulent infiltrates. Instead of producing small localized collections of pus, certain pyogenic organisms (usually the streptococci) elaborate a large amount of spreading factor, the hyaluronidases, which break down the fibrin meshwork and other barriers designed to localize the infection.

Hemorrhagic exudate. A hemorrhagic exudate occurs in situations in which severe tissue injury causes damage to blood vessels or when there is diapedesis of red blood cells from the capillaries. Often a hemorrhagic exudate accompanies other forms of exudate. A serosanguineous exudate describes a combination of serous and hemorrhagic exudates.

Resolution of acute inflammation

Acute inflammation can be resolved in one of three ways: (1) it can undergo resolution, with the injured area returning to normal or near-normal appearance and function; (2) it can progress, and suppurative processes may develop; or (3) it can proceed to the chronic phase. In the process of responding to injury, the body will use only those behaviors in the inflammatory sequence that are necessary to prevent or halt the destruction of tissue.

The acute-phase response

Infection, injury, and inflammatory processes produce a constellation of systemic effects that are often collectively referred to as the acute-phase response. The acute-phase response, which usually begins within hours or days of the onset of inflammation or infection, includes leukocytosis (discussed earlier in the chapter), fever and increased metabolism (see Chapter 7), increased erythrocyte sedimentation rate (ESR), decreased plasma iron levels and anemia, skeletal muscle catabolism and negative nitrogen balance, anorexia, and increases in lassitude and sleep.[5–7]

The manifestations of the acute-phase response, which has the characteristics of a generalized host response irrespective of the localized or systemic nature of the inciting agent, are associated with the production of a mediator molecule called interleukin-1. The term interleukin-1 was first proposed in 1979.[5] Until that time, the terms lymphocyte-activating factor, endogenous pyrogen (fever mediator), and leukocytic endogenous mediator (the inducer of leukocytosis) had been used to designate the macrophage products responsible for the systemic effects of inflammation. Considerable evidence supports the concept that these products are the same or are related, and

hence they are collectively referred to as interleukin-1. A second interleukin, interleukin-2 (formerly T-cell growth factor), stimulates T-cell growth (see Chapter 11). The sources of interleukin-1 are the phagocytic blood monocytes and tissue macrophages. In most cases, the mediator molecule enters the circulation and, much like a hormone, travels to distant target sites where it exerts its effects. An indication that interleukin-1 may have a role in normal physiology is its detection in the plasma of healthy women and observation that its level varies with the menstrual cycle.[8]

During the acute-phase response, the liver dramatically increases the synthesis of acute-phase proteins such as fibrinogen and the C-reactive protein, which may serve several different nonspecific host-defense functions.[6] These acute-phase proteins contribute to the increased sedimentation rate of the erythrocytes. There is evidence that decreased levels of serum iron have an important protective role in combating various bacteria.[5] Sequestering of iron in the liver during the acute-phase response causes a rapid drop in serum iron levels, contributing to the development of anemia in some persons. Other factors such as decreased red-cell survival also contribute to the anemia, but the role of interleukin-1 in this process is unclear.

The metabolic changes that occur with the acute-phase response include skeletal muscle catabolism and liberation of amino acids that are used in the synthesis of lymphokines, immunoglobulins, fibroblasts, and collagen needed for repair of injured tissue. Fat metabolism decreases during the acute-phase response and amino acids are also used for glucose production and energy. A common manifestation of infection and inflammation is a decrease in food appetite that occurs at a time during which metabolism and the need for energy substrates are often markedly increased. This acute-phase anorexia can be a major factor in the negative nitrogen balance and body weight loss that occurs with injury and infection.

Disorders of interleukin-1 production and its effects may contribute to the pathology of some chronic inflammatory conditions. Elevated levels have been reported in the serum of persons with fever, sepsis, and Crohn's disease. Interleukin-1 has also been detected in joint effusions of persons with rheumatoid arthritis and other joint disease.

The numerous effects of interleukin-1 in producing the acute-phase response can be used as a means for monitoring the inflammatory process. The measurement of fever, white blood cell count, and ESR are well-established procedures for monitoring many disease states. The ESR is a laboratory test that measures the speed at which erythrocytes settle when an anticoagulant is added to the blood. In this test, the blood to which the anticoagulant is added is placed in a long, narrow tube and the speed at which the cells settle is observed. Methods for measuring interleukin-1 have also been developed.[5] Although these methods are not well standardized at present, it seems likely that they will be refined and used to monitor the inflammatory response.

Chronic inflammation

To this point, we have discussed acute inflammation associated with a self-limiting stimulus, such as a burn or infection, that is rapidly controlled by host defenses. Chronic inflammation, on the other hand, is self-perpetuating and may last for weeks, months, or even years. It may develop in the course of a recurrent or progressive acute inflammatory process or as the result of a low-grade smoldering response that fails to evoke an acute response. Characteristic of chronic inflammation is an infiltration by mononuclear cells (macrophages, lymphocytes, and plasma cells) rather than neutrophils, such as occurs in acute inflammation. Chronic inflammation also involves the proliferation of fibroblasts rather than exudates. As a result, the risk of scarring and deformity developing is usually considerably greater than in acute inflammation.

In contrast to agents that provoke sufficient initial tissue injury to evoke the acute inflammatory response, agents that evoke chronic inflammation are typically low-grade persistent irritants that are unable to penetrate deeply or spread rapidly. Among the causes of chronic inflammation are foreign bodies such as talc, silica, asbestos, and certain surgical suture materials. Many viruses provoke a chronic inflammatory response, as do certain bacteria, fungi, and larger parasites of moderate to low virulence. Examples are the tubercle bacillus, the treponema of syphilis, and the actinomyces. The presence of injured or altered tissue, such as that surrounding a tumor or healing fracture, may also incite chronic inflammation. In many cases of chronic inflammation, such as sarcoidosis, the inciting agent is unknown. Little is known about the mediators of the chronic inflammatory response. Immunologic mechanisms are thought to play an important role in chronic inflammation.[9]

There are two patterns of chronic inflammation: (1) a nonspecific chronic inflammation and (2) granulomatous inflammation.

Nonspecific chronic inflammation

Nonspecific chronic inflammation involves a diffuse accumulation of macrophages and lymphocytes at the site of injury. Macrophages are accumulated from three sources: (1) continued recruitment of monocytes, the precursors of tissue macrophages, from the circulation in response to chemotaxic factors; (2) local proliferation of macrophages after they have left the bloodstream; (3) prolonged survival and immobilization of macrophages within the inflammatory site.[1] These mechanisms lead to fibroblast proliferation with subsequent scar formation that, in many cases, replaces normal supporting connective tissue elements or functional parenchymal tissue of the involved structure. For example, scar tissue resulting from chronic inflammation of the bowel causes narrowing of the bowel lumen, and in chronic glomerulonephritis there is a loss of functional nephrons.

Granulomatous inflammation

A granulomatous lesion is a form of chronic inflammation. A granuloma is typically a small, 1-mm to 2-mm lesion in which there is a massing of macrophages surrounded by lymphocytes. These modified macrophages resemble epithelial cells and are sometimes called *epithelioid cells*. Like other macrophages, the epithelioid cells that form a granuloma are derived from blood monocytes. Granulomatous inflammation is associated with foreign bodies such as splinters, sutures, silica, and talc particles, and with microorganisms such as those that cause tuberculosis, syphilis, sarcoidosis, deep fungal infections, and brucellosis. These types of agents have one thing in common—they are poorly digestible and are usually not easily controlled by other inflammatory mechanisms.

The epithelioid cells in granulomatous inflammation may either clump in a mass (granuloma) or coalesce, forming a large multinucleated giant cell that attempts to surround the foreign agent. Some giant cells may contain as many as 200 nuclei. A giant cell is usually surrounded by granuloma cells, and a dense membrane of connective tissue eventually encapsulates the lesion and isolates it. A tubercle is a granulomatous inflammatory response to the tubercle bacillus. Peculiar to the tuberculosis granuloma is the presence of a caseous (cheesy) necrotic center. In the past, surgical gloves were dusted with talc so they could be slipped on easily, but particles of talc frequently ended up in the surgical field and caused granulomatous lesions to develop. Surgical gloves are now dusted with an absorbable starch that does not cause this problem.

In summary, inflammation describes a local response to tissue injury and can present as an acute or chronic condition. Acute inflammation is the local response of tissue to a nonspecific form of injury. The classic signs of inflammation are redness, swelling, local heat, pain, and loss of function. Acute inflammation involves a hemodynamic phase in which blood flow and capillary permeability is increased and a cellular phase during which there is an increase in white cell movement in the area. Although acute inflammation is usually self-limiting, chronic inflammation is more prolonged and is usually caused by persistent irritants, most of which are insoluble and resistant to phagocytosis and other inflammatory mechanisms. Chronic inflammation usually involves the presence of lymphocytes, plasma cells, and macrophages.

Tissue healing and repair

The degree to which body structures return to their normal state following injury is largely dependent on the body's ability to replace the parenchymal cells and to arrange them as they were originally. Repair can assume one of two forms: regeneration or fibrous scar-tissue replacement. Regeneration describes the process by which cells are replaced with cells of a similar type and function so that there is little evidence that injury has occurred. Healing by fibrous replacement, on the other hand, involves the substitution of a fibrous–connective tissue scar for the original tissue.

Regeneration

The ability to regenerate varies with tissue types. Body cells are divided into three types according to their ability to undergo regeneration: (1) labile, (2) stable, or (3) permanent cell types.

Labile cells are those that continue to regenerate throughout life. These cells include the surface epithelial cells of the skin and mucous membranes of the gastrointestinal tract. A constant daily turnover of cells occurs with these tissue types.

Stable cells are those that normally stop dividing when growth ceases. These cells are capable, however, of undergoing regeneration when confronted with an appropriate stimulus. In order for stable cells to regenerate and restore tissues to their original state, the underlying structural framework must be present. When this framework has been destroyed, the replacement of tissues will be haphazard. The reader will recall that epithelial tissue relies on the blood supply from the underlying connective tissues for nourishment. The hepatocytes of the liver are one form of stable cell, and the importance of the structural framework to regeneration is evidenced by two forms of liver disease. In viral hepatitis, for example, there is selective destruction of the parenchymal liver cells while the structural cells remain unharmed. Consequently, once the disease has subsided, the injured cells regenerate and liver function returns to

normal. On the other hand, in cirrhosis of the liver, fibrous bands of tissue form and replace the normal structural framework of the liver, causing disordered replacement of liver cells and disturbance of liver function.

Permanent, or fixed cells, are those that cannot undergo mitotic division. The fixed cells include nerve cells, as well as skeletal and cardiac muscle cells. As will be discussed later, the nerve axon can regenerate under certain conditions in which the nerve cell body is uninjured.

Connective tissue repair

The sequence of events that occurs with laceration of the skin and underlying tissues is familiar to most readers. This type of injury is followed almost immediately by bleeding into the area and the development of a blood clot (Figure 10-3). Within several hours, the clot loses fluid and becomes a hard, dehydrated scab that serves to protect the area. At about the same time, phagocytic white blood cells begin to enter the injured area and break down and remove the inflammatory debris. Shortly thereafter, cells called fibroblasts arrive and begin to build scar tissue by synthesizing collagen fibers and other proteins. Meanwhile, the epithelial cells at the margin of the

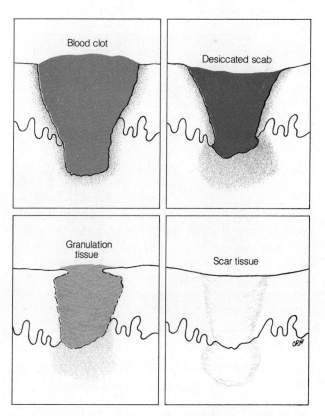

Figure 10-3 Events that follow skin and subcutaneous tissue injury.

wound begin to regenerate and move toward the center of the wound, forming a new surface layer that is similar to that destroyed by the injury. When healing is complete, the scab falls off. With the exception of the desiccated scab, repair of injury to internal structures follows a similar pattern.

The primary objective of the healing process is to fill the gap created by tissue destruction and to restore the structural continuity of the injured part. When regeneration cannot occur, healing by fibrous-tissue substitution provides the means for maintaining this continuity. Although scar tissue fills the gap created by tissue death, it does not repair the structure with functioning parenchymal cells.

Healing by fibrous substitution begins during the early stages of inflammation as macrophages invade the area and begin to digest the invading organisms and the cellular debris. The *fibroblasts* are connective-tissue cells that are responsible for the formation of *collagen* and other *intercellular elements* needed for wound healing.

As early as 24 hours following injury, fibroblasts and vascular endothelial cells begin to enter the area, and by the third to the fifth day proliferation of both fibroblasts and small blood vessels occurs (Figure 10-4). As this happens, the area becomes filled with a specialized form of soft, pink granular tissue called *granulation tissue*. This tissue is edematous and

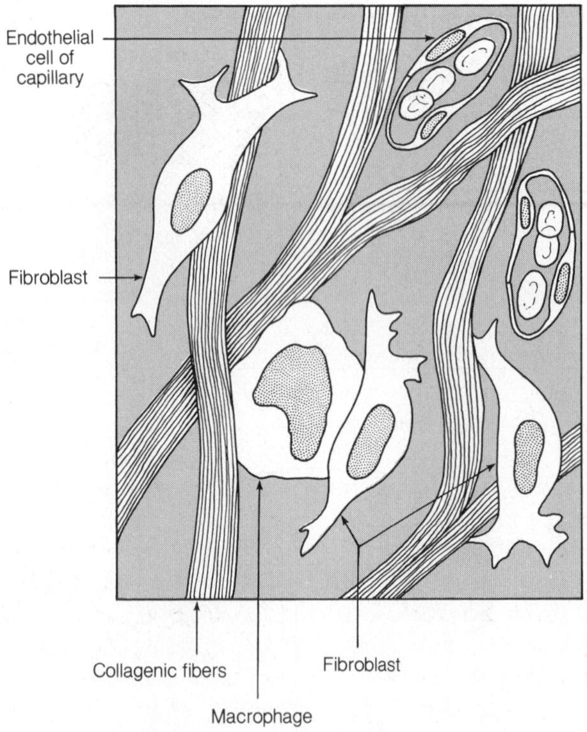

bleeds easily because of the numerous, newly developed, fragile and leaky capillary buds. At times excessive granulation tissue, sometimes referred to as "proud flesh," may form. This excess granulation tissue protrudes from the wound and prevents reepithelization from taking place. Surgical removal or chemical cauterization of the defect allows healing to proceed.

As the process of scar-tissue development progresses, there is a further increase in extracellular collagen and a decrease in active fibroblastic function. The small blood vessels become thrombosed and degenerate. As this happens the collagen fibers begin to mature and shorten, and a dense devascularized scar is formed. *Wound contraction* contributes heavily to the healing of surface wounds. As a result, the scar that is formed is considerably smaller than the original wound. Cosmetically, this may be desirable because it reduces the size of the visible defect. On the other hand, contraction of scar tissue over joints and other body structures tends to limit movement and to cause deformities.

As a result of loss of elasticity, scar tissue that is stretched fails to return to its original length. Most wounds do not regain their original tensile strength once healing has occurred. They usually begin to increase in strength between 10 and 14 days following injury; after this they rapidly increase in strength and, by the end of 3 months, reach a plateau at about 70% to 80% of their unwounded strength.[1]

Healing by first or second intention

Wounds can be divided into two types—those in which there is minimal tissue loss and that heal by first *intention* and those that have significant tissue loss and heal by *second intention* (Figure 10-5). Both visible skin wounds and invisible wounds of the internal organs heal by either first or second intention. A sutured surgical incision is an example of healing by first intention (healing directly, without granulations). Visible wounds that heal by second intention are burns and decubitus ulcers. When healing by second intention occurs, granulation tissue proliferates into the injured area. The granulation tissue fills the defect and allows reepithelization to occur, beginning at the wound edges and continuing to the center, until the entire wound is covered. Healing by second intention is slower than healing by first intention and results in the formation of more scar tissue. A wound that might otherwise have healed by first intention may become infected and then heal by second intention.

Keloid formation

An abnormality in healing by scar tissue repair is *keloid* formation. Keloids involve excessive production of bulging tumorlike scar-tissue masses. The

Endothelial cell of capillary

Fibroblast

Collagenic fibers

Fibroblast

Macrophage

Figure 10-4 Cells involved in the development of granulation tissue. Collagen fibers and vascular endothelial cells usually begin to enter the wound area around the third to sixth day following injury.

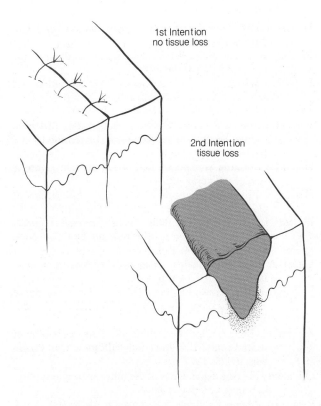

1st Intention
no tissue loss

2nd Intention
tissue loss

Figure 10-5 Healing by first and second intention.

tendency to develop keloids is more common in blacks and seems to have a genetic basis.

Factors that affect wound healing

Many factors, both local and systemic, influence wound healing. Science has not found any way to hasten the normal process of wound repair, but there are many factors that impair healing.

Age. The rate of skin replacement slows with aging. Healing of open wounds and epithelization of skin takes longer in the elderly.

Nutrition. Adequate nutrition that includes essential amino acids, vitamins A and C, and zinc is essential for normal wound repairs. Cystine, an amino acid, is needed for synthesis of the mucopolysaccharides by the fibroblast. Vitamin C aids in collagen formation and capillary development. Zinc is thought to be an enzyme cofactor. In animal studies, zinc has been found to aid in re-epithelization. It is of interest that although a zinc deficiency tends to impair healing, zinc therapy does not seem to improve healing.[10]

Infection. Infection tends to impair wound healing. Both wound contamination and host factors that increase susceptibility to infection predispose to wound infection. Increased susceptibility to infection is associated with conditions that lead to a deficiency in leukocytes or impaired leukocyte function. Neutro-

phils in the diabetic, for example, have diminished chemotaxic and phagocytic ability. This may explain why diabetics are highly vulnerable to bacterial wound invasion.

Hormonal influences. The therapeutic administration of adrenal corticosteroids is known to influence the inflammatory process and to delay healing. These hormones decrease capillary permeability during the early stages of inflammation, impair the phagocytic property of the leukocytes, and inhibit fibroblast proliferation and function.

Blood supply. In order for healing to occur, wounds must have adequate blood flow to supply the necessary nutrients and to remove the resulting waste, local toxins, bacteria, and other debris. Impaired wound healing due to poor blood flow may occur as a result of wound conditions, such as swelling, or may be caused by preexisting conditions. Arterial disease and venous pathology are well-documented causes of impaired wound healing.

Wound separation. Approximation of the wound edges, that is, suturing of an incision type of wound, greatly enhances healing and prevents infection. Epithelization of a wound with closely approximated edges occurs within 1 to 2 days. Large gaping wounds tend to heal more slowly because it is often impossible to effect wound closure with these types of wounds.

Presence of foreign bodies. Foreign bodies tend to invite bacterial contamination and delay healing. Fragments of wood, steel, glass, and the like may have entered the wound at the site of injury and can be difficult to locate when the wound is treated. Sutures are also foreign bodies and, although needed for the closure of surgical wounds, they are an impediment to healing. This is why sutures are removed as soon as possible after surgery.

In summary, the ability of tissues to repair damage due to injury is dependent on the body's ability to replace the parenchymal cells and to organize them as they were originally. Regeneration describes the process by which tissue is replaced with cells of a similar type and function. Healing by regeneration is limited to tissue with cells that are able to divide and to replace the injured cells. Body cells are divided into types according to their ability to regenerate: (1) labile cells, such as the epithelial cells of the skin and gastrointestinal tract, which continue to regenerate throughout life; (2) stable cells, such as those in the liver, which normally do not divide but which are capable of regeneration when confronted with an appropriate stimulus; and (3) permanent or fixed cells, such as nerve cells, which are unable to regenerate. Scar-tissue repair involves the substitution of fibrous connective tissue for injured tissue that cannot be repaired by regeneration.

References

1. Robbins SL, Cotran RS, Kumar V: Pathologic Basis of Disease, 3rd ed, pp 40, 62, 79. Philadelphia, WB Saunders, 1984
2. Lewis T: Blood Vessels of the Human Skin and Their Responses. London, Shaw, 1927
3. Claman HN: Glucocorticoids I: Anti-inflammatory mechanisms. Hosp Pract 18, 7:123, 1983
4. Samuelsson B: Leukotrienes: Mediators of immediate hypersensitivity reactions and inflammation. Science 220:568, 1983
5. Dinarello CA: Interleukin-1 and the pathogenesis of the acute-phase response. N Engl J Med 311:1413, 1984.
6. Dinarello C: Interleukins. Ann Rev Med 37:173, 1986
7. Duff G: Many roles for interleukin-1. Nature 313:353, 1985.
8. Cannon JG, Dinarello CA: Increased plasma interleukin-1 activity in women after ovulation. Science 227:1277, 1985.
9. Houck JC: Inflammation: A quarter century of progress. J Invest Dermatol 67:124, 1976
10. Neldner KH, Hambridge KM: Zinc therapy. N Engl J Med 292:879, 1975

Bibliography

Allison AC: Role of macrophage activation in the pathogenesis of chronic inflammation and its pharmacologic control. Adv Inflam Res 1:201, 1984

Bruno P: The nature of wound healing. Nurs Clinic North Am 14:667, 1979

Demmers LM: Prostaglandins in human disease. Clin Lab Med 4:889, 1984

Feuerstein G, Hallenbeck JM: Leukotrienes in health and disease. FASEB J 1:186, 1987

Ford-Hutchinson AW: Leukotrienes: Their formation and role as inflammatory mediators. Federation Proc 44:25, 1985

Ford-Hutchinson A, Letts G: Biological actions of leukotrienes: State of the art lecture. Hypertension (Suppl II):44, 1986

Holt PG: Immune and inflammatory function in cigarette smokers. Thorax 42:241, 1987

Hotter A: Physiologic aspects and clinical implications of wound healing. Heart Lung 11:522, 1982

Jett MF, Lancaster LE: The inflammatory-immune response: The body's defense against invasion. Crit Care Nurs 5 (Sept/Oct)B:64, 1983

Lasser A: The mononuclear phagocytic system: A review. Human Pathol 14:108, 1983

Lichtenstein IL, Herzikoff S, Shore JM, et al: The dynamics of wound healing. Surg Gynecol Obstet April: 686, 1970

Montandon D, D'Andiran G, Gabbiani G: The mechanism of wound contraction and epithelialization. Clin Plastic Surg 4:325, 1977

O'Flaherty JT: Age dependency of the inflammatory response. Lab Invest 56:600, 1986

Ryan GB, Majno G: Acute inflammation: A review. Am J Pathol 86:185, 1977

Solomkin JS, Simmons RL: Cellular and subcellular mediators of acute inflammation. Surg Clin N Am 62:225, 1983

Vane J, Botting R: Inflammation and the mechanism of action of anti-inflammatory drugs. FASEB J 1:89, 1987

Wade BH, Mandell GL: Polymorphonuclear leukocytes: Dedicated professional phagocytes. Am J Med 74:686, 1983

Weismann G, Smolen JE, Korchak HM: Release of inflammatory mediators from stimulated neutrophils. N Engl J Med 303:27, 1980

CHAPTER 11

The Immune Response

Immune system
   Self versus nonself: the role of the major histocompatibility complex antigens
   Immune cells
      T-lymphocytes
      B-lymphocytes
      Macrophages
      Natural killer cells

Lymphoid organs
   Thymus
   Lymph nodes
   Spleen
   Other lymphoid tissues

Immunity and immune mechanisms
Antigens
Immune mechanisms
   Humoral immunity
   Cell-mediated immunity
   Complement system
   Lymphokines
   Phagocytosis
Aging and the immune response

Objectives

After you have studied this chapter, you should be able to meet the following objectives:

_____ State the functions of the immune system.

_____ Briefly describe the source of monoclonal antibodies and cite their contribution to the understanding of the immune system.

_____ Explain the significance of the major histocompatibility complex (MHC) and the human leukocyte antigen (HLA).

_____ Differentiate between the central and peripheral lymphoid structures.

_____ Trace the differentiation of the T-lymphocytes from bone marrow stem cells to mature regulatory and effector cells.

_____ Trace the differentiation of a B-lymphocyte from a bone marrow stem cell to a mature plasma cell or memory cell.

_____ State the function of the five classes of immunoglobulins.

_____ Describe the function of the macrophage.

_____ Define *immune response*.

_____ Differentiate between specific and nonspecific immune mechanisms.

_____ Describe the characteristics of an antigen.

_____ Differentiate between passive and active immunity.

_____ Contrast humoral and cell-mediated immunity.

_____ Differentiate between primary and secondary immune responses.

_____ Relate the complement system to the immune response.

_____ Describe the four stages of phagocytosis.

_____ Describe the actions of the lymphokines: interleukin-2 and interferons.

_____ Characterize the changes in the immune response that occur in the elderly.

The immune system is a complex network of specialized organs and cells that protects the body from destruction by foreign agents and microbial pathogens, degrades and removes damaged or dead cells, and exerts a surveillance function to prevent the development and growth of malignant cells. The immune system consists of the immune cells and the lymphoid organs and tissues. In many respects, the complexity of the immune system parallels that of the nervous system. It is able to distinguish self from nonself, remember previous experiences, and react accordingly.[1] Once an individual has the mumps, the immune system remembers the experience and protects against getting the disease again. Not only is the immune system capable of memory, it is also able to respond with great diversity and specificity. It can recognize many millions of nonself molecules and produce specific molecules that match up with and counteract each of them. This chapter is divided into two parts: the first focuses on the immune system and the second on immunity and immune mechanisms.

The immune system

The immune system consists of the immune cells and the central and peripheral lymphoid structures. The central immune organs, the bone marrow and the thymus, are the sites of immune cell production. The peripheral lymphoid structures consist of lymph nodes, spleen, tonsils, intestinal lymphoid tissue, and aggregates of lymphoid tissue occurring in nonlymphoid organs. The immune cells interact with antigens in the peripheral lymphoid structures. The lymphoid organs are connected by networks of lymph channels and blood vessels. The immune cells travel throughout the body and into and out of the lymphoid tissue. As they move throughout the body, the immune cells selectively seek out and destroy foreign antigens and materials, while recognizing and sparing the host cells that are identified as self.

Within the last two decades, major scientific advances have enhanced the understanding of the immune system. To a great extent these advances have resulted from several new technologies including methods for developing monoclonal antibodies and advances in molecular biology used to determine the genetic basis for antigen recognition.

Monoclonal antibodies are produced in a laborious process that fuses an antibody-producing spleen cell from an animal (usually a mouse) with a malignant myeloma cell.[2,3] The fusion of the two cells results in a singe fused cell, or clone, capable of producing a highly specific antibody (see Chapter 9). The precision of the monoclonal antibody is such that it recognizes a single antigenic site, such as one of those located on the cell surface of hematopoietic or tumor cells.

The stages in the life history of an immune cell are marked by expression of a changing variety of membrane-bound antigen markers. These antigens are not present on bone marrow stem cells but develop as an expression of the differentiation process. For example, membrane-bound antigens differ among T cells according to their level of maturation and among subsets of mature T cells such as T4 and T8 cells. Thus, monoclonal antibodies can be used for distinguishing among cells of mononuclear phagocytic lineage, in delineating between B cells and T cells, and in differentiating between subsets of T cells. It was through the use of monoclonal antibodies that the pathogenesis of acquired immune deficiency syndrome (AIDS) was made possible.

Self versus nonself: the role of the major histocompatibility complex antigens

The ability of the immune system to distinguish self from nonself resides in cell surface antigens that are unique to each person. These antigens are coded by a large cluster of genes called the *major histocompatibility complex* (MHC) located on the short arm of chromosome 6. In humans, the histocompatibility antigens are called the *human leukocyte antigens* (HLA) because they were first detected on the leukocyte. The histocompatibility antigens are similar in many respects to the ABO antigens found on red blood cells, which are matched for transfusion purposes.

The histocompatibility antigens are inherited as part of the genetic makeup of an individual. Seven closely linked gene loci—HLA-A, HLA-B, HLA-C, HLA-D, HLA-DR, HLA-DQ, and HLA-DP—have been identified. Each of the seven gene loci is occupied by multiple alleles, or alternate genes, that code for the development of each cell surface antigen. There are at least 23 possible gene products or antigens for the A loci and 47 antigens for the B loci. Each of the antigens is numbered, HLA-A1, HLA-A2, and so on. An international workshop meets every 2 to 3 years to update the nomenclature of the HLA complex.

An individual's HLA type is inherited. Because of their close linkage, the combination of HLA genes at each locus is usually inherited as a unit. This unit is called a *haplotype*. Each person inherits a chromosome from each parent and, therefore, has two HLA haplotypes for each gene locus. By simple mendelian inheritance, there is a 25% chance that two siblings will share the same haplotype, a 50% chance that they will share one haplotype, and a 25% chance that they will share no haplotype. Unlike blood types, common HLA types are highly unlikely. When one considers that there are at least 23 gene products for the HLA-A locus and 47 gene products for the HLA-B gene locus, the diversity of HLA types among the general population becomes tremendous. With the exception of identical twins, the chances of two persons having exactly the same HLA type are very unlikely. The typing of histocompatibility antigens is important in tissue grafting and organ tranplantation. The closer the matching of HLA types, the less the chance of rejection.

Based on their tissue distribution and structure, HLA antigens have been subdivided into two classes: Class I MHC antigens—also called the classic histocompatibility antigens—include the HLA-A, HLA-B, and HLA-C antigens, and class II MHC antigens—also called immune antigens (Ia)—include the HLA-D, HLA-DR, HLA-DQ, and HLA-DP antigens. Class I MHC proteins are found on the surface of nucleated cells, and class II MHC proteins appear on only a few types of cells that are part of the immune system, such as B-lymphocytes and macrophages.

The immune cells

The primary cells of the immune system are the small white blood cells called *lymphocytes*. Lymphocytes represent 20% to 30% of the leukocytes (Figure 11-1). Like other blood cells, they are derived from stem cells in the bone marrow (Figure 11-2). One class of lymphocytes, the B-lymphocytes (B cells), undergoes maturation in the bone marrow. The other class of lymphocytes, the T-lymphocytes (T cells), completes maturation in the thymus. About 60% to 70% of the lymphocytes are T cells, and 10% to 20% are B cells.[4] Most of the remaining lymphocytes are not identified as either T cells or B cells, but as a null cell population called natural killer cells. Under the microscope, both T-lymphocytes and B-lymphocytes have similar appearances. However, both types of lymphocytes express different surface antigens and both have functional properties that distinguish them. Within both lymphocyte populations are subsets of cells with their own special properties. In addition to lymphocytes, cells of the mononuclear phagocytic system, monocytes and macrophages, serve as accessory cells for the immune system. The macrophages capture the antigen, process it, and present it to the lymphocytes.

Both B-lymphocytes and T-lymphocytes manifest immunologic specificity, that is, they are programmed to respond to a specific antigen. B-cell specificity is expressed as antibody receptor proteins and

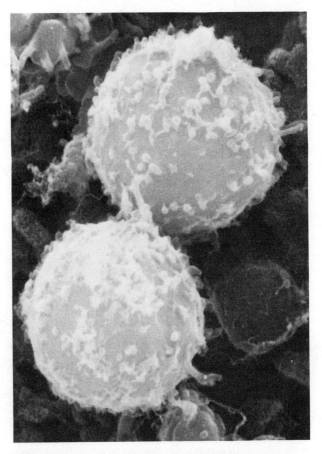

Figure 11-1 A scanning micrograph of two lymphocytes. (*Courtesy of Kenneth Siegesmund, Ph.D., Anatomy Department, Medical College of Wisconsin*)

T-cell specificity is expressed as cell surface receptors. Within the T-cell and B-cell populations are both effector cells and memory cells. Effector cells (activated T cells and antibody-producing plasma cells of the B-cell population) are instrumental in causing destruction of the antigen. Effector cell specificity is accomplished through an antigen-stimulated gene reshuffling process, resulting in a clone of cytotoxic T cells or plasma cells with receptors that exactly match those of the stimulating antigen. In the case of the plasma cells, the antigen receptors are expressed on the antibody (immunoglobulin) that is produced. Memory cells are formed following initial exposure to the antigen. They revert to an inactive state, but are able to rapidly proliferate and increase the intensity of the immune response with subsequent exposure to the specific antigen of which they have a memory. There is considerable interaction among immune cells. Only certain antigens will stimulate B cells. With most immune responses that elicit a humoral (antibody) response, T-lymphocytes interact with B-lymphocytes, facilitating their activation and regulating their differentiation. The functions of the macrophage are essential to both T-cell and B-cell function.

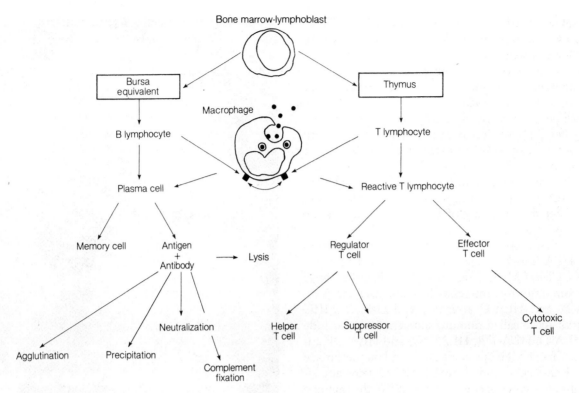

Figure 11-2 The development of cellular and humoral immunity.

T-lymphocytes

The T-lymphocytes function in the activation of other T cells and B cells, in the control of viral infections, in the rejection of grafts of foreign tissues, and in delayed hypersensitivity reactions (see Chapter 12). Collectively these immune responses are referred to as cell-mediated or cellular immunity. The T cells take the lead in the immune response when they recognize antigen presented on the surface of macrophages. Activated in this way, T cells produce soluble factors that recruit other T cells and B cells. T-lymphocytes can only recognize antigen when it is associated with MHC membrane-bound products. This dual recognition of both nonself antigen and the self MHC gene products is important for activation of both cytotoxic effector cells and immunoregulatory cells.[5]

The T-lymphocytes arise from precursors in the bone marrow, travel to the thymus where they are programmed to differentiate into T cells. T cells have a life span of years; they leave the thymus and circulate throughout the body in the bloodstream. Selected subpopulations of T cells transiently seed the lymph nodes, spleen, or other peripheral immune tissues and then reenter the circulation in a lymphaticovenous communication system.

There are two populations of T cells: regulatory T cells and effector T cells. Both regulatory and effector T cells synthesize and release soluble immune mediators called lymphokines (to be discussed). The T-cell regulatory functions involve amplification of cell-mediated cytotoxicity by other T cells and immunoglobulin production by B cells. Regulatory T cells act by either enhancing or suppressing the action of the B-lymphocytes. These cells are called the helper and suppressor T cells. The helper T cells may be the switch to the immune system. B cells can recognize antigen independent of T-cell stimulation, but their proliferation and terminal differentiation require activation by helper T cells. The suppressor T cells seem to be equally important in regulating the immune response by providing negative feedback; they make the immune response self-limiting. The cytotoxic or killer T cells serve as effector cells. The cytotoxic T cell destroys by binding to cell surface antigens on the target cell and releasing lymphokines that destroy the cell membrane on the target cell. The close contact between the cytotoxic T cell and the target cell ensures that neighboring cells are not indiscriminately destroyed.

The mature T cells contain surface markers, which can be used to define T-cell subsets. Two subsets of T cells, T4 and T8, are distinguished by their surface antigens. About 70% of mature T cells carry the T4 antigen and 30% carry the T8 antigen. The T4 cells, the helper and inducer T cells, possess CD4 antigens; they recognize antigen in association with class II MHC products. The T8 cells, suppressor and cytotoxic T cells, possess CD8 antigens; they recognize antigen in association with class I MHC gene products. A T3 or CD3 antigen is present on all peripheral T cells. The CD3 antigen is associated with the T-cell receptor that recognizes and binds foreign antigens.

B-lymphocytes

The B-lymphocytes are responsible for humoral immunity. Humoral immunity provides for elimination of bacterial invaders, neutralization of bacterial toxins, prevention of viral reinfection, and immediate allergic responses (see Chapter 12).

The B-lymphocytes can be identified by the presence of B-cell antigens, immunoglobulin and complement receptors, and class II MHC antigens on their surface. They are called *B-lymphocytes* because in fowl, B-cell precursors migrate from the bone marrow to a hindgut structure, the bursa of Fabricius, where they differentiate and mature. Because mammals do not have a bursa of Fabricius, the differentiation of B cells is thought to occur in the bone marrow.

Soon after their formation in the bone marrow, B cells enter the circulation and migrate to the spleen or other peripheral lymphoid structures. The migration of the B cells from the bone marrow to the spleen is an antigen-independent process. In the absence of antigen stimulation, the life of a B cell ends after this process. Most B cells reaching the spleen die within a few days.[6] B cells that encounter antigens complementary to their surface immunoglobulin receptor and receiving T-cell help undergo a series of changes that transform them into either memory cells or into immunoglobulin (antibody)-secreting plasma cells. The antigen molecules that bind to immunoglobulin receptors are taken into the B cell, partially digested, and the antigen fragments are recycled to the B-cell surface and expressed in association with the class II MHC antigens. The combination of antigen fragments and the MHC molecules are recognized by helper T cells. In this way, B cells can present antigen to helper T cells and stimulate the production of T-cell factors that stimulate the antigen-presenting B cell to divide and undergo terminal differentiation into mature plasma cells, which produce thousands of antibody molecules per second before their death a day or so later.[6]

The immunoglobulins have been divided into five classes: IgG, IgA, IgM, IgD, and IgE (Table 11-1). Each of the immunoglobulins is composed of two heavy (H) chains and two light (L) chains (Figure 11-3). The heavy chains in each of the classes of immunoglobulins are antigenically distinctive, and it is this distinction that permits division of the immunoglobulins into classes through the use of immunoelectrophoresis. The amino acid sequence of each of the heavy chains and each of the light chains has a con-

Table 11–1. Classes of immunoglobulins

Class	Percent of total	Characteristics
IgG	75.0	Present in majority of B cells; contains antiviral, antitoxin, and antibacterial antibodies; only immunoglobulin that crosses the placenta; responsible for protection of newborn; activates complement and binds to macrophages
IgA	15.0	Predominant immunoglobulin in body secretions, such as saliva, nasal and respiratory secretions, breast milk; protects mucous membranes
IgM	10.0	Forms the natural antibodies such as those for ABO blood antigens; prominent in early immune responses; activates complement
IgD	0.2	Action is not known; may affect B-cell maturation
IgE	0.004	Binds to mast cells and basophils; involved in allergic and hypersensitivity reactions

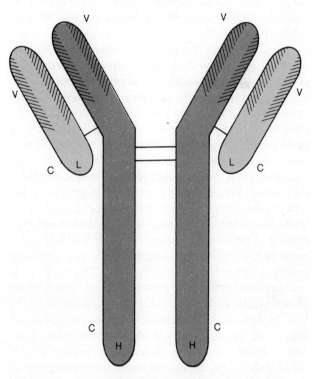

Figure 11-3 Basic immunoglobulin structure formed from four polypeptide chains bound together. Light chains (*L*), heavy chains (*H*), constant amino acid region (*C*), and variable amino acid region (*V*). Antigens bind to the variable region of the immunoglobulin.

stant (C) region and a variable (V) region. An antigen reacts with the variable region. Each different type of immunoglobulin is produced by a separate clone of B cells and has a different amino acid sequence in the variable region, which provides it with the specificity needed to react with a single antigen. Clonal diversity is generated during the early stages of B-cell differentiation—a process that involves a series of immunoglobulin-gene rearrangements. As the immature B cell achieves a functional gene arrangement for immunoglobulin production, it begins to express membrane-bound IgM molecules. Over the next couple of days most B cells also begin to produce IgD. Within each B-cell clone, some members switch from the expression of IgM and IgD to the expression of IgG, IgA, or IgE.[7]

IgG (gamma globulin) is the most abundant of the immunoglobulins. It circulates in body fluids and is the only immunoglobulin that crosses the placenta. In the past several years it has been found that there are four subsets of IgG (IgG1, IgG2, IgG3, and IgG4). IgG1 is the predominant subclass (58%–71% of the total IgG), IgG2 (19%–31%), IgG3 (5%–8%), and IgG4 (1%–5%).[8] IgG subclass restrictions have been reported for antibodies against many bacterial and viral antigens. For example, tetanus toxoid antibody is found predominantly with the IgG1 subclass and IgG2 appears to be specific for bacteria that are encapsulated with a polysaccharide covering such as pneumococcus, *Hemophilus influenzae,* and *Neisseria meningitides.*

IgA, the second most abundant of the immunoglobulins, is found in saliva, tears, and bronchial, gastrointestinal, prostatic, and vaginal secretions. It is a secretory immunoglobulin and is considered to be a primary defense against local infections. The difference in protection afforded by the IgG and the IgA immunoglobulins can be illustrated using the two types of polio vaccine—Salk and Sabin. With some viral infections, such as poliovirus, systemic infection follows an initial mucosal phase during which the virus replicates in the mucosa of the portal of entry. In these infections, circulating IgG antibodies are important in preventing systemic disease. The Salk polio vaccine (killed virus administered by injection) prompts the production of systemic IgG antibodies and protects against the systemic effects of the virus. However, the Salk vaccine does not stimulate production of IgA secretory antibodies, and there can be growth of the organisms in the gastrointestinal tract and establishment of a carrier state. With the oral Sabin polio vaccine, IgA secretory antibody production is induced and virus replication and subsequent mucosal penetration are prevented as is systemic dissemination of the virus and development of the carrier state.

IgE is involved in allergic and hypersensitivity reactions. It binds to mast cells and causes release of histamine and other mediators of allergic reactions.

Macrophages

The monocytes and tissue macrophages are a part of the mononuclear phagocyte system, formerly called the *reticuloendothelial system.* All of the cells of the mononuclear phagocytic system arise from a common precursor in the bone marrow that gives rise to the blood monocytes, which migrate to the various tissues where they are transformed into macrophages.[9] The tissue macrophages are scattered in connective tissue or clustered in organs such as the lung (alveolar macrophages), liver (Kupffer's cells), spleen sinusoids, lymph nodes, peritoneum, central nervous system (microglial cells), and other areas. Langerhans cells are macrophages that are located in the skin; they are involved in cell-mediated immune reactions of the skin such as delayed contact hypersensitivity and they play an important role in induction of contact sensitivity (see Chapter 12).[10] The cells of the mononuclear phagocyte system, also called *accessory cells,* are antigen-capturing cells. They participate in the immune response by capturing and breaking down microorganisms and antigen-containing substances and presenting the antigen to the lymphocytes in a form that increases its immunogenicity (Figure 11-4). In the process of phagocytosis, the macrophage ingests the foreign substance, digests it, and then moves the antigen fragments to the cell surface along with class II

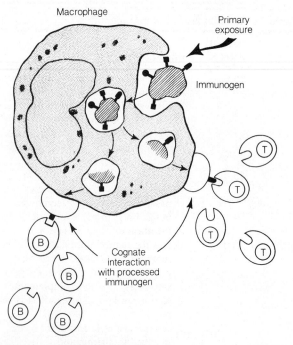

Figure 11-4 The interaction between the immunogen (antigen), macrophage, and lymphocytes.

MHC gene products. It is the combined antigen fragments and class II MHC gene products that are recognized by T cells. The interaction between the modified antigen particles on the macrophage receptors and the lymphocyte stimulates lymphocyte differentiation and proliferation. These receptor-site interactions also appear to provide the stage for T-cell and B-cell interactions; they facilitate the helper role of the T-lymphocytes in terms of B-cell function. The interaction between antigen-presenting macrophages and T cells appears to be limited to helper T cells that bear the CD4 protein on their membrane. Because the helper T cell cannot be triggered by free antigens, presentation of antigen by macrophages or other accessory cells is essential for induction of cell-mediated immunity.[11] Macrophages also produce interleukin-1, which is a mediator for the inflammatory process (see Chapter 10), and they can act under T-cell influence to destroy bacteria and tumor cells. Lymphokines produced by the effector T cells cause migration or activation of the macrophages.

Although macrophages can ingest microorganisms and other foreign antigens prior to the development of specific antibodies, the process is accelerated when antibodies are present. Frequently, soluble proteins that are injected in deaggregated form as vaccine antigens are not attracted to accessory cells and do not provoke antibody formation. For this reason, immunization vaccines are often developed by creating particulate immunogens (alum precipitation or formation of oily droplets), which incite antibody formation and carry the antigen to the accessory cell.[12] As soon as antibody is formed, any remaining soluble antigen is rapidly taken into accessory cells within hours.

Natural killer cells

Natural killer cells are a distinct population of non-B and non-T cells characterized by their ability to identify quickly and lyse a variety of tumor cells, virus-infected cells, and fungi.[13] Unlike cytotoxic T cells, natural killer cells function without prior sensitization. The activity of natural killer cells is augmented by interferons and interleukin-2. Although, the primary physiologic role of the natural killer cells is unclear, natural killer cells appear to play a role in tumor rejection (immune surveillance) and in resistance to infection.

Lymphoid organs

Thymus

The thymus is an elongated flat bilobed structure that is located in the neck below the thyroid gland and extends into the upper part of the thorax behind the top of the sternum. The thymus is a fully developed organ at birth and weighs about 15 to 20 g.[14] After birth, the thymus grows slowly, reaching a maximum size of about 40 g at puberty. It then regresses in size, its lymphoid tissue being replaced by adipose tissue so that in the adult its substance is difficult to distinguish from the adipose tissue in which it is embedded. Nevertheless, some thymus tissue persists into old age.

The function of the thymus is central to the development of the immune system. During embryonic development, the thymus is the first organ to begin the manufacture of lymphocytes. There is evidence that precursor cells of some of the nonthymic lymphoid tissues (e.g., lymph nodes and spleen) originate in the thymus and migrate at various times before and after birth to sites where they establish germinal centers for maintaining the body's immunologic defenses. Impaired thymus function has been associated with immunologic deficiency disorders. If the thymus is removed from certain animals at birth or it is congenitally absent, as it is in certain human conditions, there is a decrease of lymphocytes in the blood, a marked depletion or absence of T-lymphocytes, and an absence of thymus-dependent lymphocytes in the peripheral lymphoid tissues.[15]

Thymic epithelial cells produce soluble factors that influence the growth and maturation of T cells. Maturation of the lymphocytes in the thymus takes about 2 to 3 days, after which the mature lymphocytes migrate from the thymus gland into the bloodstream. From the bloodstream they enter the inner cortex of the lymph nodes, the periarterial sheaths of the spleen, and other thymus-dependent regions of the peripheral lymphoid tissue.[15] In addition to lymphocytes that arise from resident cells within the thymus, certain hematopoietic cells from the bone marrow are capable of migrating to the thymus where they are somehow instructed to become mature lymphocytes. Before birth, the thymus is the major source of lymphocytes; in later life, the precursor cells migrate to the thymus.

Lymph nodes

The lymph nodes serve two functions: (1) they remove foreign materials from lymph before it enters the bloodstream and (2) they are centers for proliferation of immune cells. They are located along the lymph ducts, which lead from the tissues to the thoracic duct. Each lymph node processes lymph from a discrete, adjacent anatomical site (see Chapter 14, Figure 14-3). Many lymph nodes are situated in the axillae, groin, and along the great vessels of the neck, thorax, and abdomen.[16] A lymph node consists of outer cortex and inner medulla and is surrounded by a connective tissue capsule (Figure 11-5). Lymph enters the node through afferent channels that penetrate the capsule and leaves through the deep indentation in the hilus. Because of the lymph nodes' spongelike structure, the macrophages, lymphocytes, and granulocytes flow slowly through them. The reticular meshwork serves as a surface on which macrophages attach and phagocytose antigens. The T-lymphocytes are more abundant in the medullary portion of the node, and the B-lymphocytes are more abundant in the cortex. The T-lymphocytes proliferate on antigenic stimulation and create germinal centers in the medullary region after stimulation. These centers contain macrophages, growing T-lymphocytes, and smaller adult cells. The cortical germinal centers contain mainly B-lymphocytes and appear to be concerned with antibody production.

Spleen

The spleen, which is roughly the size of a clenched fist, is located in the abdomen at the level of the 9th, 10th, and 11th ribs. The spleen is composed of red and white pulp. The red pulp is well supplied with arteries and is the area where senescent and injured red blood cells are destroyed. The white pulp contains concentrated areas of lymphocytes called periarterial lymphoid sheaths, which surround the central arterioles. Although T-lymphocytes are found in the spleen, it is primarily a B-lymphocyte-containing organ.

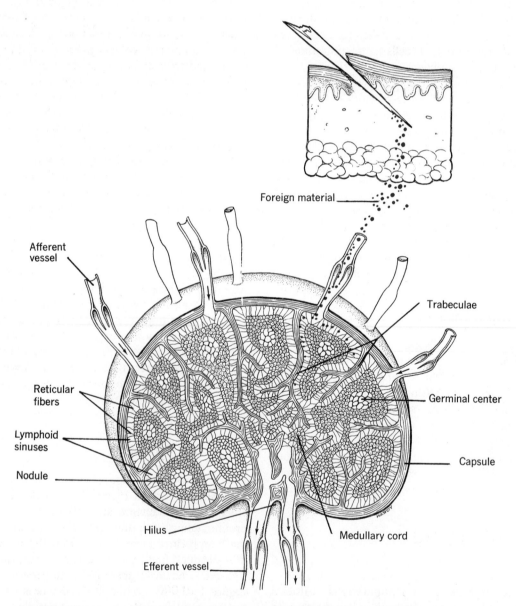

Figure 11-5 Structural features of a lymph node. Bacteria that gain entry to the body are filtered out of the lymph as it flows through the node. (*Chaffee EE, Lytle IM: Basic Physiology and Anatomy, 4th ed. Philadelphia, JB Lippincott, 1980*)

Other lymphoid tissues

The tonsils have a structure similar to the lymph, thymus, and lymph nodes. Like the thymus, the tonsils are rather large during childhood and regress in size with age. Other important collections of lymphoid tissue exist in the appendix and Peyer's patches in the intestine.

In summary, the immune system is a complex network of organs and cells that serve to protect the body against invasion by foreign agents and proliferation of abnormal and malignant cells. The immune system is able to distinguish self from nonself through cell surface antigens coded by the MHC genes on the sixth chromosome. There are two classes of MHC antigens: Class I gene products found on most nucleated body cells and class II products found on selected immune cells. The immune system includes the immune cells and the central and peripheral lymphoid organs. The primary cells of the immune system are the B- and T-lymphocytes. The B-lymphocytes are the source of antibody, and the T-lymphocytes are the source of cell-mediated immunity. The helper T cells, a subset of T cells, act as a switch for the immune response. They are necessary for B-cell proliferation and differentiation. The macrophages of the mononuclear phagocytic system are antigen-capturing cells. They capture, modify, and present antigen to the lymphocytes in a form that increases its antigenicity. The central lymphoid structures consist of the bone marrow and thymus gland where blood cells are produced. The bone marrow is the source of both lymphocytes and mononuclear phagocytic cells. The T-lymphocytes travel from the bone marrow to the thymus where they are programmed to differentiate into mature and functional T cells. The proliferation and maturation of B-lymphocytes occur in the bone marrow. When fully differentiated, the B-lymphocyte becomes an antibody-producing plasma cell. The peripheral lymphoid structures consist of the lymph nodes, spleen, tonsils, intestinal lymphoid tissue, and aggregates of other lymphoid tissue. The interaction between antigens and immune cells occurs in the peripheral lymphoid structures.

Immunity and immune mechanisms

Immunity is a normal adaptive response designed to protect the body against potentially harmful foreign substances, infections, and other sources of nonself antigens. Immunity can be either natural or acquired. *Natural immunity* is species specific. It is the reason that humans do not contract certain animal diseases, such as feline distemper. *Innate immunity* is the immunity one is born with. It is genetically controlled and involves natural immunity, heredity, race, and sex. *Acquired immunity* is that protection which an individual gains through active or passive means.

The *immune response* describes the interaction between an antigen (immunogen) and an antibody (immunoglobulin) or reactive T-lymphocyte. The process of acquiring the ability to respond to an antigen is known as immunization.

Active immunity is acquired through immunization or actually having a disease. It is long-lived immunity developed by the body's own immune system. Active immunity does not provide immediate protection upon first exposure to an invading agent or vaccine. It takes a few days to weeks before the immune response is sufficiently developed to contribute to the destruction of the pathogen. With subsequent exposure to the same agent, however, the immune system is usually able to react within minutes to hours.

Passive immunity is temporary immunity transmitted or borrowed from another source. An infant receives passive immunity from its mother *in utero* and from antibodies that it receives from its mother's breast milk. Passive immunity can also be transferred through injection of antiserum, which contains the antibodies for a specific disease, or through the use of pooled gamma globulin, which contains antibodies for a number of diseases. Both antiserum and gamma globulin are obtained from blood plasma.

Antigens

An antigen is any substance recognized as foreign (nonself) by the immune system. An antigen can be a microorganism, such as a virus or a bacterium, or it can be a foreign protein or polysaccharide. Tissues or cells from another individual, unless it is an identical twin, can also act as antigens. Antigens have specific *antigenic determinant sites*, or *epitopes*, which interact with immune cells to induce the immune response.[17] All antigens carry different epitopes, allowing the immune system to recognize the antigen as nonself and as different from other antigens. The number of antigenic determinant sites on a molecule is roughly proportional to its molecular weight, with one site existing for each 10,000 or so units of molecular weight.[17] A complete antigen has two or more sites. Large protein and polysaccharide molecules make good antigens because of their complex chemical structure and multiple antigenic determinant sites. Smaller molecules (those with a molecular weight of less than 10,000) usually make poor antigens. There are some substances that cannot act as antigens by themselves, but have antigenic determinant sites can combine with carrier substances and then ac antigens. These substances, which usually have a low molecular weight, are called *haptens*. House dust, animal danders, and plant pollens are haptens.

The site of access to the body may influence the antigenic strength of a substance. For example, the digestive enzymes often hydrolyze and destroy the antigenic quality of otherwise fully antigenic materials. When these same substances are given parenterally (injected), greater amounts of the antigen are available for interacting with the antigen-processing cells. The oral polio vaccine is one exception; when taken into the gastrointestinal tract, it invades the lining of the intestine and reproduces itself.[14]

Immune mechanisms

Immune mechanisms are of two types: specific and nonspecific. There are two types of specific immunologic responses, humoral and cell-mediated, that not only recognize self from nonself, but also distinguish between antigens (Figure 11-2). Nonspecific immunologic defense mechanisms such as the complement system, lymphokines, and phagocytosis can recognize self from nonself, but cannot distinguish between agents or pathogens.

Humoral immunity

Humoral immunity depends on B-lymphocytes and plasma cell production of immunoglobulins. Antigen–antibody reactions can take several forms. Combination of antigen with antibody can result in precipitation of antigen–antibody complexes, agglutination or clumping of cells, neutralization of bacterial toxins, lysis and destruction of pathogens or cells, adherence of antigen to immune cells, facilitation of phagocytosis through opsonization, and complement activation. Some of these reactions, such as opsonization, occur because of complement activation.

Two types of responses occur in the development of humoral immunity (Figure 11-6). A primary immune response occurs when the antigen is first introduced into the body. During this primary response, there is a latent period before the antibody can be detected in the serum. This latent period involves the recognition of antigen by the B cells and the development of a clone of plasma cells that will produce the antibody. This period usually takes from 48 to 72 hours, after which the detectable antibody titer continues to rise for a period of 10 days to 2 weeks. Recovery from many infectious diseases occurs at about the time during the primary response when the antibody titer is reaching its peak. The secondary response occurs on second or subsequent exposures to the antigen. During the secondary response, the rise in antibody titer occurs sooner and reaches a higher

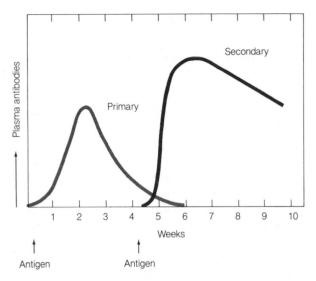

Figure 11-6 Primary and secondary responses of the humoral immune system to the same antigen.

level. There are two forms of plasma cells that develop during the primary response: one produces the antibody and the other becomes a memory cell, which records the information needed for antibody production. During the secondary response, the memory cells recognize the antigen and stimulate production of plasma cells, which produce the specific antibody. The booster immunization given for some infectious diseases, such as tetanus, makes use of the secondary response. For a person who has been previously immunized, administration of a booster shot causes an almost immediate rise in antibody titer to a level sufficient to prevent development of the disease.

Cell-mediated immunity

In cell-mediated immunity, the action of the T-lymphocytes and the macrophages predominates. The most aggressive phagocyte, the activated macrophage, becomes so only after exposure to a T-cell lymphokine.[14] Cell-mediated immunity provides protection against viruses and cancer cells. In addition to its protective effects, cell-mediated immunity is responsible for delayed hypersensitivity and transplant reactions.

The antigen recognition receptor sites on the T cell are similar to those that are expressed by the immunoglobulins. A T cell receptor site has a variable region that is modified to match the particular antigen that a particular clone of T cells has been programmed to defend against. Activated T cells exert their effect through the synthesis of lymphokines and transfer factor. Once T cells have been activated by signals required for antigen-specific activation, they release lymphokines, which then act in an antigen-nonspecific manner on other populations of inflammatory cells, irrespective of their antigen specificity.

Some subsets of effector T cells produce an intracellular RNA-type macromolecule called *transfer factor*. Its function is similar to that of RNA in that it provides the pattern for production of lymphokines. Immediately after a T cell responds to an antigen, it begins to produce transfer factor. Transfer factor then converts other T-lymphocytes into lymphokine-producing cells. It has been shown that transfer factor can be used to transfer passive cell-mediated immunity from one animal to another. In humans, transfer factor has been used experimentally for treatment of resistant infections, such as mucocutaneous candidiasis, and as an adjuvant therapy for certain types of cancer.

Cytotoxic T cells play an important role in host defense against viral infections. In order for the T8 population of cells to exert their cytotoxic effects, they must first recognize viral determinants in conjunction with class I MHC molecules displayed on the cell surface. In this way, cytotoxic T cells can selectively destroy viral infected cells, while sparing noninfected cells.

The complement system

The complement system is the primary mediator of the humoral immune response that enables the body to produce inflammation and facilitate the localization of an infective agent. The complement system, like the blood coagulation system, consists of a group of proteins that are normally present in the circulation as functionally inactive precursor components of the system. These proteins constitute 10% to 15% of the plasma-protein fraction. In order for a complement reaction to occur, each of the complement components must be activated in the proper sequence. Uncontrolled activation of the complement system is prevented by the instability of the activated combining sites at each sequence of the process. In addition, several serum proteins have been identified that serve to modulate and limit activation of the complement system. There are two parallel but independent mechanisms for activation of the complement system: the classic and alternate pathways.

The classic complement pathway is activated when target cells are able to evoke a complement-fixing antigen–antibody response (Figure 11-7). Only immune responses involving immunoglobulins IgG (IgG1, IgG2, and IgG3) and IgM activate complement, and it is probable that complement is bound in all antigen–antibody reactions that involve these two classes of immunoglobulins. In addition the classic complement pathway can be activated by a group of chemically diverse substances, including DNA, C-reactive protein, and certain cellular membranes and trypsin-like enzymes.[17] Table 11-2 lists immune responses that occur as the result of complement fixation.

The alternate (properdin) pathway is activated by complex polysaccharides or enzymes. This system bypasses the first two steps of the classic complement pathway, but requires the presence of C3b.

Following activation of the complement system, interactions ranging from lysis of a spectrum of different kinds of cells, bacteria, and viruses to direct mediation of the inflammatory process occur. First, complement has been shown to mediate the lytic destruction of many kinds of cells including red blood cells, platelets, bacteria, viruses, and lymphocytes. Ei-

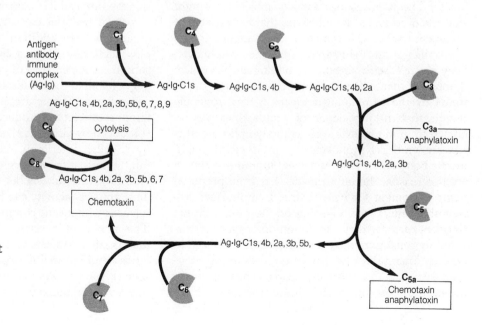

Figure 11-7 Classic complement pathway and major biologic activities (*in blocks*). (*Adapted from Barrett JT: Textbook of Immunology, 4th ed. St. Louis, CV Mosby, 1983*)

Table 11–2. Complement-mediated immune responses

Response	Effect
Cytolysis	Destruction of cell membrane of body cells or pathogens
Adherence of immune cells	Adhesion of antigen–antibody complexes to the inert surfaces of cells or tissues such as the reticuloendothelial cells that line the blood vessels and have the capacity for phagocytosis
Chemotaxis	Chemical attraction of phagocytic cells to foreign agents
Anaphylaxis	Degranulation of mast cells with release of histamine and other inflammatory mediators
Opsonization	Modification of the antigen so that it can be easily digested by a phagocytic cell

ther complement pathway may induce cytolysis. Second, a major biologic function of complement activation is opsonization—the coating of antigen–antibody complexes that facilitates clearance of these complexes by the fixed macrophage system. Third, chemotactic complement products can trigger an influx of leukocytes that remain fixed in the area of complement activation through attachment to specific sites on C3b and C4b molecules. Fourth, production of anaphylatoxin and kinin products can lead to contraction of smooth muscle, increased vascular permeability, and edema. Fifth, complement mediated phagocytosis facilitates the destruction of an infectious agent.

—— Lymphokines

The lymphokines are low molecular weight products of activated lymphocytes that are capable of influencing other inflammatory cells, including the macrophages, the neutrophil, and the lymphocyte. They are released in response to antigen, but unlike antibodies, their chemical composition is not determined by the stimulating antigen. It was originally thought that the production of lymphokines was restricted to immune cells such as the lymphocyte. It is now known that lymphokines are produced throughout the body and are not restricted to immune cells.[17] For this reason, the term *cytokine* has been proposed as a replacement for lymphokine. Lymphokines can exert their effect locally, acting on the same cell that produces them or they can act on other types of surrounding cells. Lymphokines can also be produced in sufficient quantities that they gain access to the circulatory system and act hormonally to produce profound systemic effects. Several lymphokines have been named according to their biologic effect (*e.g.,* B-cell differentiating factor and T-cell growth factor). Because most lymphokines have more than one function, names that indicate biologic activity are often misleading. For example, interleukin-1 is a mediator of many of the inflammatory responses including fever, and interleukin-2 acts as a growth factor for activated T cells, induces the synthesis of other lymphokines, and activates cytotoxic lymphocytes. Therefore, at the Sixth International Congress of Immunology in 1986, it was agreed that all new lymphokines would be named first according to their biologic properties and then assigned an interleukin number.[18] However, some of the lymphokines such as interferon have retained their original names. Table 11-3 describes the prominent biologic properties of human lymphokines.

Interleukin-2. The term *interleukin* is used to describe substances produced by and acted on by leukocytes. The presence of interleukin-2, also known as T-cell growth factor, is necessary for proliferation and function of helper, suppressor, and cytotoxic T-lymphocytes. Interleukin-2 interacts with T-lymphocytes by binding to specific membrane receptors that are present on activated T-cells but not on resting T-cells.[18] The expression of interleukin-2 receptors can be triggered by the binding of a specific antigen to the cell surface. Sustained T-cell proliferation relies on the presence of both interleukin-2 and interleukin-2 receptors—if either is missing, cell proliferation will cease and the cell will die.[19] Cyclosporin, a drug used to prevent rejection of heart, kidney, and liver transplants, functions primarily by inhibiting the synthesis of interleukin-2.[19]

Interferons. The interferons are a family of lymphokines that protect neighboring cells from invasion by intracellular parasites. This includes viruses, rickettsia, malarial parasites, and other intracellular organisms.[14] In addition, bacterial toxins, complex polysaccharides, and a number of other chemical substances are capable of inducing interferon production. Not all of these substances that induce interferon are antigenic. There are at least three types of interferon: α interferon (produced by T cells), β interferon (produced by fibroblasts), and γ interferon (produced by T cells). Interferon interacts at the gene level to inhibit translation of messenger RNAs, which regulate viral protein synthesis but not host protein synthesis. This antiviral activity can be transferred to neighboring cells without the continued presence of interferon. The actions of interferon are pathogen nonspecific, that is, they are effective against different types of viruses and intracellular parasites. They are, however, species specific. Animal interferons will not provide protection in humans. Of recent interest is the cell growth-regulating action of interferons. The ability of interferon to slow growth of cancer cells has prompted investigation into its use in treatment of cancer (see Chapter 5).

Phagocytosis

Phagocytosis is a nonspecific response in which injured cells and antigens are ingested by phagocytic cells. Phagocytosis is mainly the function of two types of cells: the neutrophils and the monocytes or macrophages. Phagocytosis involves four distinct but interrelated steps: (1) chemotaxis, (2) opsonization, (3) engulfment, and (4) intracellular killing. Although structurally different, both the neutrophils and the macrophages approach phagocytosis in a similar manner.

Chemotaxis involves the chemical attraction of phagocytic cells to foreign agents or pathogens. Granulocyte and macrophage chemotaxis can be stimulated by many factors including fragments of the fifth complement factor, chemotaxic factors produced by lymphocytes, and compounds elaborated by bacteria.

Defects in chemotaxis result in a decreased ability to respond to infections and overcome injury.

Opsonization renders pathogens more susceptible to ingestion by phagocytic cells. The virulence of many organisms, such as *Streptococcus pneumoniae*, *Klebsiella pneumoniae*, and *Hemophilus influenzae*, results from surface factors that inhibit attachment of the phagocytic cells. Opsonins provide binding sites for attachment of the phagocyte to the pathogen. Two opsonins are immunoglobulin (IgG) and the C_{3b} fragment of the complement system.

Engulfment occurs once the phagocyte recognizes the agent as foreign. Cytoplasm-filled extensions of the cell membrane surround and enclose the agent, forming a membrane-enclosed phagocytic vesicle or phagosome. Interiorization occurs as the phagosome breaks away from the cell membrane and moves into the cell. Once inside the cell, the phagosome merges with a lysosome and lysosomal enzymes digest the agent.

Intracellular killing of pathogens is accomplished through a number of mechanisms in association with an acid pH environment, enzymes, and oxy-

Table 11–3. Prominent biologic properties of human lymphokines

Lymphokine	Biologic properties
Interleukin-1 (alpha and beta)	Activates resting T cells; is cofactor for hematopoietic growth factors; induces fever, sleep, ACTH release, neutrophilia, and other systemic acute-phase responses; stimulates synthesis of lymphokines, collagen, and collagenases; activates endothelial and macrophagic cells; mediates inflammation, catabolic processes, and nonspecific resistance to infection.
Interleukin-2	Is growth factor for activated T cells; induces the synthesis of other lymphokines; activates cytotoxic lymphocytes.
Interleukin-3	Supports the growth of pluripotent (multilineage) bone-marrow stem cells; is growth factor for mast cells.
Colony-stimulating factor (CSF)	
Granulocyte-macrophage CSF	Promotes neutrophilic, eosinophilic, and macrophagic bone-marrow colonies; activates mature granulocytes.
Granulocyte CSF	Promotes neutrophilic colonies.
Macrophage CSF	Promotes macrophagic colonies.
Interleukin-4 (B-cell stimulating factor-1)	Is growth factor for activated B cells; induces DR expression on B cells; is growth factor for resting T cells; enhances cytolytic activity of cytotoxic T cells; is mast-cell growth factor.
B-cell stimulating 2 (B-cell differentiating factor)	Induces the differentiation of activated B cells into immunoglobulin-secreting plasma cells; is identical with beta$_2$-interferon, plasmacytoma growth factor, and hepatocyte-stimulating factor.
Gamma-interferon	Induces class I, class II (DR), and other surface antigens on a variety of cells; activates macrophages and endothelial cells; augments or inhibits other lymphokine activities; augments natural killer cell activity; exerts antiviral activity.
Interferon (alpha and beta)	Exerts antiviral activity; induces class I antigen expression; augments natural killer cell activity; has fever-inducing and antiproliferative properties.
Tumor necrosis factor (alpha and beta)	Is direct cytotoxin for some tumor cells; induces fever, sleep, and other systemic acute-phase responses; stimulates the synthesis of lymphokines, collagen, and collagenases; activates endothelial and macrophagic cells; mediates inflammation, catabolic processes, and septic shock.

(Dinarello CA, Mier JW: Lymphokines. N Engl J Med 317(15):941, 1987)

gen-dependent myeloperoxidases and peroxides. Neutrophils contain granules that participate in destruction of the agent. Neutrophils are generally concerned with the phagocytosis of bacteria and organisms that rely on evading phagocytosis for survival.

Aging and the immune response

Aging is characterized by a declining ability to adapt to environmental stresses. One of the factors thought to contribute to this problem is a decline in immune responsiveness. This includes changes in both cell-mediated and antibody-mediated immune responses. Elderly persons tend to be more susceptible to infections, they have more evidence of autoimmune and immune complex disorders than younger persons, and they have a higher incidence of cancer.

The alterations in immune function that occur with advanced age are not fully understood. There is a decrease in the size of the thymus gland, which is thought to affect T-cell function. The size of the gland begins to decline shortly after sexual maturity, and by age 50 it has usually diminished to 15% or less of its maximum size.[20] There is also a progressive decrease in absolute numbers of lymphocytes, which begins during middle life; during the sixth decade this number has decreased to 70% of the value seen in younger persons.[21] This mainly represents a decrease in T cells, especially helper T cells. As a result, delayed hypersensitivity responses, which are mediated by helper T cells, are diminished in the elderly. Likewise, there is impairment of antibody responses. This impairment is also thought to result from changes in the T-cell rather than the B-cell population. In addition to a decrease in helper T-cell function, there is evidence that suppressor functions of the immune system are altered as a result of the aging process. Impairment of suppressor function is thought to contribute to the increase in autoantibodies and autoimmune disorders in the elderly.

In summary, immunity is the resistance to a disease that is provided by the immune system. An immune response involves an antigen an antibody or effector T cell. It can be acquired actively (through immunization or actually having a disease) or passively (by receiving antibodies or immune cells from another source). Antigens have antigenic determinant sites, which the immune system uses to recognize the antigen as nonself and to distinguish it from other antigens. Immune mechanisms can be classified into two types: specific and nonspecific. Specific immunity involves humoral and cellular mechanisms; it can recognize self from nonself and can distinguish between antigens. Nonspecific immune mechanisms can distinguish between self and nonself but cannot differentiate between antigens. It includes the complement system, the lymhokines, and phagocytic functions of the neutrophils and macrophages. The effectiveness of the immune response decreases with aging.

References

1. National Institutes of Health: Understanding the Immune System, No.84-529. Washington, DC, US Dept of Health and Human Services, 1983
2. Diamond BA, Yelton DE, Scharff MD: Monoclonal antibodies. N Engl J Med 304:1344, 1981
3. Keller RH, Milson TJ, Janicek KM et al: Monoclonal antibodies: Clinical utility and the misunderstood epitope. Lab Med 15:795, 1984
4. Robbins SL, Kumar V: Basic Pathology, 4th ed, p 129. Philadelphia, WB Saunders, 1987
5. Royer HD, Rienherz EL: T lymphocyte ontogeny, function, and relevance to clinical disorders. N Engl J Med 317:1136, 1987
6. Cooper MD: B lymphocytes. N Engl J Med 317:1452, 1987
7. Rosen FS, Cooper MD, Wedgewood RJP: The primary immunodeficiencies (first of two parts). N Engl J Med 311:235, 1984
8. Ochs HD, Wedgwood RJ: IgG subclass deficiencies. Annu Rev Med 38:325, 1987
9. Johnson RB: Monocytes and macrophages. N Engl J Med 318:747, 1988
10. Lasser A: The mononuclear phagocytic system: A review. Hum Pathol 14:108, 1983
11. Unanue ER, Allen PM: The immunoregulatory role of the macrophage. Hosp Pract 22(4):87, 1987
12. Nossal GJV: The basic components of the immune system. N Engl J Med 316:1320, 1987
13. Herberman RB: Natural killer cells. Hosp Pract 17(4):93, 1982
14. Barrett JT: Textbook of Immunology, 4th ed, pp 79, 215–216, 212. Philadelphia, WB Saunders, 1983
15. Smith LH, Their SO: Pathophysiology, p 167. Philadelphia, WB Saunders, 1981
16. Cormack DH: Ham's Histology, 9th ed, p 249. Philadelphia, JB Lippincott, 1987
17. Stites DP, Stobo JD, Wells JV: Basic & Clinical Immunology, 6th ed, pp 20, 134, 114. Los Altos, CA, Lange Medical Publications, 1987
18. Dinarello CA, Mier JW: Lymphokines. N Engl J Med 317:940, 1987
19. Dinarello CA, Mier JW: Interleukins. Annu Rev Med 37:173, 1986
20. Weksler ME: The senescence of the immune response. Hosp Pract 16(10):55, 1981
21. Fundenberg HH, Stites DP, Caldwell JL et al: Clinical Immunology, 3rd ed, p 329. Los Altos, CA, Lange Medical Publications, 1980

Bibliography

Acuto O, Reinherz EL: The human T-cell receptor. N Engl Med 312:1100, 1985

Davis MM: Molecular genetics of T-cell antigen receptors. Hosp Pract 23(5):157, 1988

Desforges JF: T-cell receptors. N Engl J Med 313:576, 1985

Dinone MA, Young JD: How lymphocytes kill tumor and other cellular targets. Hosp Pract 22(5a):59, 1987

Fearon DT: Complement, C receptors, and immune complex disease. Hosp Pract 23(8):63, 1988

Fitch FW: T-cell clones and T-cell receptor. Microbiol Rev 50:50, 1986

Haddy RI: Aging, infections, and the immune system. J Family Pract 27:409, 1988

Kimber I. Natural killer cells. Med Lab Sci 42:60, 1985

Marrack P, Kappla J: The T cell and its receptor. Sci Am 254(2):36, 1986

Muller HJ: The membrane attack complex of complement. Annu Rev Immunol 4:503, 1986

Naughton JL, Creasey AA: Advances in interferon research. West J Med 136:227, 1982

Schattner A, Duggan DB: Natural killer cells—Toward clinical application. Am J Hematol 18:435, 1985

Schifferli JA, Yin CN, Peters DK: The role of complement and its receptor in the elimination of immune complexes. N Engl J Med 315:488, 1986

Schumaker VN: Activation of the first component of complement. Annu Rev Immunol 5:21, 1987

Tonegawa S: The molecules of the immune response. Sci Am 122, 1986

Waldman TA, Tsudd M: Interleukin-2 receptors: Biology and therapeutic potential. Hosp Pract 22(1):77, 1987

Young JD, Cohn ZA: How killer cells kill. Sci Am 258(1):38, 1988

CHAPTER 12

Alterations in the Immune Response

Immunodeficiency disease
   Antibody (B-cell)
      immunodeficiency
   Cellular (T-cell)
      immunodeficiency
   Combined antibody (B-cell)
      and cellular (T-cell)
      immunodeficiency
   Disorders of the complement
      system
   Disorders of phagocytosis

Allergy and hypersensitivity
   Type I allergic responses
      Seasonal pollen allergy and
         allergic rhinitis
      Food allergies
      Atopic dermatitis
   Type II cytotoxic reactions
   Type III immune complex
      reactions

Type IV cell-mediated
   hypersensitivity
   Transplant rejection
   Autoimmune disease
      Probable mechanisms
      Systemic lupus erythematosus

Objectives

After you have studied this chapter, you should be able to meet the following objectives:

_____ List the most important categories of immunodeficiency disease and state one example of each category.

_____ Relate the function of the complement system to the manifestations of hereditary angioneurotic edema.

_____ State the proposed mechanisms of dysfunction in primary disorders of phagocytosis.

_____ List the manifestations of primary disorders of phagocytosis.

_____ Compare the immune mechanisms involved in type I, type II, type III, and type IV hypersensitivity immune reactions.

_____ List the goals for treatment of seasonal pollen allergy and allergic bronchitis.

_____ Compare the hypersensitivity reactions associated with serum sickness and the Arthus reaction.

_____ Explain the implications of a positive tuberculin test.

_____ Discuss the rationale for matching of HLA and MHC types in organ transplantation.

_____ Compare the immune mechanisms involved in transplant rejection and graft-versus-host disease.

_____ Discuss the role of the suppressor and helper T cells in the regulation of self-tolerance.

_____ Describe three or more postulated mechanisms underlying autoimmune disease.

_____ State the significance of the LE factor in systemic lupus erythematosus.

Although the immune response is a normal protective mechanism, it can cause disease when the response is deficient (immunodeficiency disease), inappropriate (allergy and hypersensitivity), or misdirected (autoimmune disease). All of these alterations in the immune response are discussed in this chapter.

Immunodeficiency disease

Immunodeficiency can be defined as an abnormality of the immune system that inhibits normal immune responsiveness. There are four major types of immune mechanisms that defend the body against assault by viral, bacterial, fungal, and other agents: (1) antibody-mediated (B-cell) immunity, (2) cell-mediated (T-cell) immunity, (3) complement factors, and (4) phagocytosis. The immunodeficiency state may be primary (hereditary or congenital) or secondary (acquired after birth), and it may involve one or more of these immune mechanisms. Both primary and secondary deficiencies lead to the same spectrum of disease.[1] The severity and manifestations of the disorder depend on the type and degree of deficiency that is present.[2] The major categories of immunodeficiency are summarized in Chart 12-1. The acquired im-

---

Chart 12–1: Immunodeficiency states*

Antibody (B-Cell) immunodeficiency

Primary
  Transient hypogammaglobulinemia of infancy
  Common variable immunodeficiency
  X-linked hypogammaglobulinemia
  Selective deficiency of IgG, IgA, IgM
Secondary
  Decreased synthesis of immunoglobulins (lymphomas)
  Increased loss of immunoglobulins (nephrotic syndrome)
  Production of defective immunoglobulins (multiple myeloma)

Cellular (T-Cell) immunodeficiency

Primary
  Congenital thymic aplasia (DiGeorge's syndrome)
  Abnormal T-cell production (Nezelof's syndrome)
Secondary
  Malignant disease (Hodgkin's disease and others)
  Transient suppression of T-cell production and function due to an acute viral
    infection such as measles
  AIDS

Combined antibody (B-Cell) and cellular (T-Cell) immunodeficiency

Primary
  Severe combined immunodeficiency (autosomal or sex-linked recessive)
  Wiskott–Aldrich syndrome (immunodeficiency, thrombocytopenia, and eczema)
  Immunodeficiency with ataxia and telangiectasia
Secondary
  X-radiation
  Immune suppressant and cytotoxic drugs
  Aging

Complement abnormality

Primary
  Selective deficiency in a complement component
  Angioneurotic edema (complement 1 inactivator deficiency)
Secondary
  Acquired disorders in which complement is used

Phagocytic dysfunction

Primary
  Chronic granulomatous disease
  Glucose-6-phosphate dehydrogenase deficiency
  Job's syndrome
Secondary
  Drug induced (*e.g.,* corticosteroid and immunosuppressive therapy)
  Diabetes

* Examples are not inclusive.

munodeficiency syndrome (AIDS) is discussed in Chapter 13.

Antibody (B-cell) immunodeficiency

At birth a baby is partially protected by maternal IgG antibodies. During the first 4 to 5 months of life there is a gradual decline in serum IgG levels as these antibodies are destroyed; the IgG level reaches its lowest point at about 5 to 6 months. At about this time, the infant's immune system begins to function and the antibody level begins to rise, reaching adult levels when the infant is about 12 to 16 months of age. Some babies may, however, experience a delay in onset of gamma globulin production that could last until 2 to 3 years of age—transient hypogammaglobulinemia. These babies are particularly susceptible to bacterial and respiratory infections and to bronchitis. Usually, the condition is self-limiting and immunoglobulin production becomes normal sometime between the second and third years of life.

A much more serious disorder of immunoglobulin deficiency is a sex-linked inherited condition that is usually restricted to males and has an incidence of 1 in 100,000 live births.[3] This form of X-linked hypogammaglobulinemia was first described by Bruton in 1952 and is sometimes called Bruton's disease. It is thought that in these infants the pre-B cells fail to develop and as a result there is a deficiency in both B cells and plasma cells. Symptoms of the disorder usually begin to develop at about the time that maternal antibodies have been depleted (age 5 to 6 months). Children with this disorder are particularly prone to develop severe recurrent episodes of pharyngitis, otitis media, skin infections, and respiratory tract infections from exposure to common pathogens. Diagnosis is based on demonstration of low levels of immunoglobulins in the serum. Treatment for the condition consists of injections of gamma globulin and treatment of the infections with antibiotics.

Common variable immunodeficiency (acquired hypogammaglobulinemia) consists of a group of clinical syndromes characterized by reduced levels of serum immunoglobulins, impaired ability to produce immunoglobulins following antigen exposure, and increased incidence of pyogenic (pus-forming) infections. The symptoms are similar to those of X-linked hypogammaglobulinemia but do not appear until later in life (usually between ages 15 and 35 years), and both males and females are affected equally. Affected individuals fail to produce significant levels of immunoglobulins secondary to a lack of plasma cells. Characteristically, there is a lack of germinal centers and plasma cells in the lymph nodes and spleen. These individuals have a high incidence of autoimmune disease and higher than normal incidence of abnormalities in T-cell immunity. A rheumatoid-like disorder develops in 30% of these individuals.[1] The cause of the disorder is unknown. Of interest is the greater than average incidence of autoimmune disease among first-degree relatives, which suggests a genetic basis. Treatment includes replacement therapy with human immune globulins.

A selective deficiency of IgA is the most common form of primary immunodeficiency state known. It occurs in 1 out of every 500 individuals and consists of a virtual lack of both serum and secretory IgA.[3] Most individuals with the disorder are asymptomatic, although some may have repeated respiratory infections, diarrhea, and increased incidence of asthma and other allergies. The disorder is thought to consist of a defect in the terminal stage of B-cell development. Patients with IgA deficiencies may experience an anaphylactic reaction when given a blood transfusion because the IgA in the donor blood is often recognized as a foreign agent.[4]

Cellular (T-cell) immunodeficiency

There are very few primary forms of T-cell deficiency. One such condition is a congenital failure of thymus gland development (*DiGeorge's syndrome*). The condition occurs as a defect associated with embryonic development of the third and fourth pharyngeal pouches. These embryonic structures are also involved in development of other parts of the head and neck, and babies born with this disorder also fail to develop the parathyroid gland and have congenital defects of the face and heart. Another condition, *Nezelof's syndrome,* is a genetically (autosomal recessive) determined disorder in which there is faulty development of the thymus gland and T-cell production, but lack of other developmental defects.

Temporary suppression of T-cell function has been reported following acute viral infections, such as measles. Viruses may actually damage the lymphocytes or mononuclear phagocytes, or they may inhibit their function. Some viruses have been found to damage cells in the thymus and thymus-dependent areas of the spleen and lymph nodes. Secondary forms of cellular immunodeficiency occur with some diseases of the lymphoid tissue, including Hodgkin's disease, a neoplastic disease of lymphoid tissue. Persons with Hodgkin's disease have impaired T-cell function and what is called *anergy,* or the failure to respond to a variety of skin antigens, including the tuberculin test. In terms of the protective function of the T cells, persons with Hodgkin's disease have a well-defined predisposition to develop tuberculosis, fungal and yeast infections, and herpes zoster varicella. The immunodeficiency observed with Hodgkin's disease and other neoplasms may be due to a number of factors including the effects of the tumor, depression of the immune system associated with irradiation and drugs used in treatment of cancer, and malnutrition.

Combined antibody (B-cell) and cellular (T-cell) immunodeficiency

A complete lack of both humoral and cellular immunity causes early susceptibility to infection. The deficiency state can be sex-linked or autosomal recessive. Infants with the disorder seldom survive beyond the first year of life because of poor resistance to infection unless confined to a sterile environment. Of recent interest was the boy from Houston, Texas, who was able to survive for more than 12 years in a sterile plastic bubble environment.[5] A histocompatible bone-marrow transplant is the treatment of choice.

There are several other combined forms of humoral and cellular immunodeficiency. These conditions are accompanied by other abnormalities. One of these is the *Wiskott-Aldrich syndrome,* which is accompanied by thrombocytopenia and eczema. Another is *ataxia-telangiectasia,* in which loss of muscle coordination and blood vessel dilatation are combined with deficits in IgA and IgE production and T-lymphocyte function.

Disorders of the complement system

Complement plays a critical role in both specific and nonspecific immune responses. It is necessary for normal chemotaxis and killing of bacteria (see Chapter 11). Alterations in the complement system can consist of a deficiency of one or more of its components or acquired disorders in which complement is involved in the pathogenesis of the condition.

There are several known abnormalities of the complement system. One of the better-known defects is a condition called *hereditary angioneurotic edema,* which is caused by a congenital deficiency of complement 1 inactivator. The uncontrolled activation of this component of the complement system leads to sporadic attacks of subcutaneous edema, which are associated with minor trauma to the affected part. In extensive reactions, edema of the face, neck, and joints may occur. Edema of the throat may make breathing difficult, and edema of the abdominal organs may produce intense abdominal pain.

Other deficiencies of the complement system have been described, and many are associated with recurrent infections. A decrease in complement levels has also been observed in a number of autoimmune disorders such as lupus erthymatosus, poststreptococcal glomerulonephritis, and autoimmune hemolytic anemia. The reason for this deficiency is unknown. Many of the actions of complement are essential for phagocytosis and clearing the body of immune complexes. It has been suggested that a deficiency in classic complement components may lead to inadequate solubility and clearance of immune complexes.[6]

Disorders of phagocytosis

Phagocytosis is an important defense mechanism in terms of removal of bacteria and foreign agents from the body. As with other alterations in immune function, defects in phagocytosis may occur as a primary genetic or congenital defect or secondary to drug therapy or disease states. Primary disorders of phagocytosis are usually caused by enzyme deficiencies within the metabolic pathways used by the phagocytes for killing bacteria or destroying other agents. *Chronic granulomatous disease* is inherited as an X-linked disorder of phagocytosis. The metabolic pathways of both neutrophils and monocytes are abnormal, and susceptibility to organisms that usually are of low virulence, such as *Staphylococcus epidermidis, Candida,* and *Aspergillus,* increases. The disorder usually becomes apparent during the first year of life. Manifestations include marked lymphadenopathy and hepatosplenomegaly associated with impaired phagocytic function of cells within these structures. Infections of the lymph nodes, skin, lungs, gastrointestinal tract, liver, and bone are common. Treatment includes use of antibiotics, and, in some cases, white cell infusions. *Job's syndrome* results in eczematoid skin lesions, otitis media, and chronic nasal discharge. It is thought to be a variant of chronic granulomatous disease. Deficiency of leukocyte glucose-6-phosphate-dehydrogenase is associated with a form of hemolytic anemia (see Chapter 16). When this deficiency is present, there is impairment of glucose metabolism by the leukocytes, which are unable to destroy certain organisms.

Secondary disorders of phagocytosis can occur in a number of conditions. Opsonins are substances that alter an agent so that it can undergo phagocytosis. Antibodies and complement are the two main opsonins. Thus, deficiencies of either antibodies or complement cause impairment of phagocyte function. Immunosuppressive and corticosteroid drugs decrease the number of phagocytic cells and impair phagocytosis. Impaired phagocytic function is thought to contribute to the high incidence of infections that occur in persons with poorly controlled diabetes. The defect appears to involve a reduction in opsonic activity and a decrease in intracellular killing of organisms, probably related to altered glucose metabolism of the phagocytes.[7]

In summary, immunodeficiency states describe an absolute or relative lack (or dysfunction) of immune cells or other factors, such as complement, which defend the body from invasion by foreign agents or the growth of malignant cells. There are four types of immunodeficiency states: (1) antibody (B-cell) immunodeficiency, (2) cellular (T-cell) immunodeficiency, (3) disorders of the complement system, and (4) impairment of phagocytosis. These immunodeficiency states can be primary (hereditary or congenital) or secondary (acquired after birth) and may involve one or more immune mechanisms. The severity of immunodeficiency states is dependent on the type and degree of deficiency present.

Allergy and hypersensitivity

Allergy and hypersensitivity are immune responses in which the antigen is an environmental agent, food, or drug that is not intrinsically harmful. Gell, Coombs, and Lachman have divided allergic responses into four categories:[8]

I. *Type I* is an IgE-mediated response that causes release of histamine and slow-reacting substance of anaphylaxis (SRS-A) from mast cells. The types of reactions seen in this category are anaphylaxis and atopic allergies such as hay fever, asthma, and urticaria (hives).
II. *Type II* is an IgG- or IgM-mediated response. It is a cytotoxic reaction that most often involves complement, but this is not a requirement. Certain drug reactions fit into this category.
III. *Type III* is an IgG- or IgM-mediated antigen–antibody complex reaction. Serum sickness is a type III response.
IV. *Type IV* is a cell-mediated response in which sensitized T-lymphocytes react with an antigen to cause inflammation. Contact dermatitis is a type IV response, as is the tuberculin reaction.

—— Type I allergic responses

The term *atopy* is used to describe allergic conditions that have a familial predisposition. About 1 out of every 10 persons in the United States suffers from symptomatic allergies of this type.

Atopic immune responses result from immunoglobulin IgE activity. These immunoglobulins are sometimes called *reagins*. Reagins function only when they are attached to mast cells or basophils. Atopic reactions include anaphylaxis, seasonal pollen allergy (hay fever), allergic rhinitis, and atopic skin reactions. This discussion focuses on general concepts of atopy and seasonal pollen allergy, allergic rhinitis, food allergies, and atopic dermatitis. Anaphylactic shock is discussed in Chapter 23, and bronchial asthma is discussed in Chapter 25.

Mast cells (tissue cells) and basophils (blood cells) have granules that contain mediators involved in allergic reactions. In predisposed individuals, allergen stimulation causes IgE to bind to mast cells. On subsequent exposure, the allergen binds to the IgE on the sensitized mast cells, and this results in a series of reactions that culminate in the release of histamine and vasoactive substances from the mast cell (Figure 12-1). Three primary mediators are released from mast cells during an allergen-IgE-mediated response: (1) *histamine,* which causes increased vascular permeability; (2) *eosinophil chemotactic factor,* which attracts eosinophils and neutrophils; and (3) *neutral proteases,* which cleave complement and protein products to generate other inflammatory mediators such as prostaglandin, leukotrienes, and platelet-activating factor.

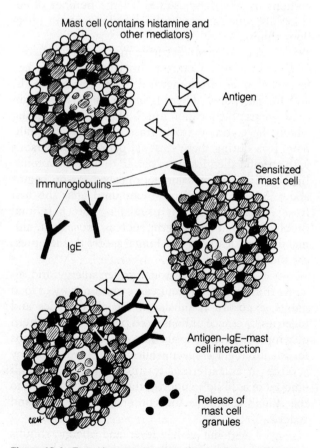

Figure 12-1 Type I immune response that involves an allergen (antigen), immunoglobulin (IgE), and mast cell. Exposure to the allergen causes sensitization of the mast cell with subsequent binding of the allergen, which causes release of mast cell granules containing inflammatory mediators such as histamine and SRS-A.

Prostaglandins can cause smooth muscle contraction. Leukotrienes are potent vasoactive and spasmogenic agents and are important in type I hypersensitivity reactions. On a molar basis, they are several thousand times more active than histamine in causing vascular permeability and bronchospasm.[9] Because their release is slower than histamine, these leukotrienes are referred to as slow-reacting substance of anaphylaxis (SRS-A). Platelet-activating factor causes platelet aggregation and histamine release.

Seasonal pollen allergy and allergic rhinitis

Seasonal pollen allergy (hay fever) is associated with sneezing, itching, and watery drainage from the eyes and nose. The conjunctiva is usually reddened and swollen and there is often an accompanying irritation and itching of the pharynx and outer ear canal. The nasal mucosa is usually pale and boggy. Nasal polyps are grapelike cystic masses commonly associated with allergic rhinitis. Microscopic examination of a properly stained smear of nasal secretions usually demonstrates a large number of eosinophils, whereas neutrophils predominate in infectious rhinitis.

A person with hay fever may be allergic to one or more inhalants. Common inhalants that cause hay fever are pollens from ragweed, trees, grasses, weeds, and fungal spores. There is usually a season within each geographic location in the United States during which the common trees, grasses, and weeds pollinate. It is during these seasonal periods that persons with specific allergies are expected to have symptoms. In the Midwest, for example, ragweed season begins about August 15 and continues until after the first frost. Allergic rhinitis is usually a more perennial problem, caused by allergens such as house dust, animal danders, feathers, and fungal spores that are present the year round.

Diagnosis of seasonal pollen allergy and allergic rhinitis usually requires a careful history of food habits, exposure to inhalants, use of cosmetics and toiletries, presence of household pets, seasonal pattern of symptoms, and so forth. Skin tests provide a means for identifying the specific allergies. This is done by scratch or intradermal testing in which a small amount of a dilute solution of the antigen is applied to the skin; the area is then observed for edema and redness.

Treatment of hay fever and allergic rhinitis consists of avoiding the allergen when possible, treating the symptoms, and desensitizing for the antigen. When an individual responds to a single allergen, such as feathers in a bed pillow, it is often possible to eliminate the allergen. Antihistamine drugs usually provide symptomatic relief at the onset of the season, but their effectiveness often wanes as the season continues. Nasal decongestants of the sympathomimetic type are effective by themselves or with antihistamines. The anti-inflammatory steroid drugs are usually reserved for severe hay fever that cannot be controlled by other methods. Desensitization involves frequent (usually weekly) injections of the offending antigen(s). The antigens, which are given in increasing doses, stimulate production of high levels of IgG, which acts as a blocking antibody by combining with the antigen before it can combine with the cell-bound IgE antibodies.

Food allergies

Food allergies can occur at any age, although they are usually more common in children. They are usually type I allergic responses and frequently accompany other manifestations of atopic allergy. The reaction occurs when IgE antibodies in the intestinal mucosa react with the food allergen, causing release of mediators of the immune response. Systemic manifestations result from absorption of these mediators into the bloodstream. Allergens are usually food proteins or partially digested food products. Carbohydrates, fats, and food additives such as flavoring, preservatives, and food colorings are also potential allergens. Closely related foods can contain common or cross-reacting antigens. For example, some individuals may be allergic to all legumes (beans, peas, and peanuts). Some allergens are heat labile and are destroyed by cooking. Diagnosis of food allergies is usually based on history rather than skin tests, which are often inaccurate. Avoidance of the food rather than desensitization is recommended.

Atopic dermatitis

Another form of type I hypersensitivity reaction is atopic dermatitis. The disorder is usually associated with a family history of atopy and a history of other allergies. Up to 70% of persons with atopic dermatitis have some type of allergic respiratory disorder and 70% have a family history of atopy.[10] This disorder typically appears in early childhood and either disappears or becomes less severe with age. Onset is in the first year of life in 60% of cases and within the first 5 years of life in 90%.[10] In infants the lesions are usually oozing, weeping, and eczematous. Consequently, the condition is often referred to as eczema in this age group. The lesions usually affect the forehead, cheeks, and extensor surfaces of the extremities in infants and small children. At later ages, the neck and antecubital and popliteal spaces are more commonly affected. The skin is dry, erythematous, and pruritic (itchy). This leads to excoriations, papules, and scaling. The disease usually improves spontaneously during the summer months.

The cause of atopic dermatitis is uncertain. IgE levels are elevated, and histamine release seems important. It does not seem to be related to exposure to specific allergens, although food allergies may be demonstrated in children. Milk, wheat, eggs, corn, fish, and legumes are common food allergens. Recent studies suggest a partial defect in cell-mediated immunity.

Treatment includes the application of nonirritating lubricants to decrease the dryness of the skin. If a sensitivity to foods is noted, these foods are eliminated from the diet. Because foods have been implicated as a cause of eczema in infants, only one new solid food is usually added to an infant's diet at a time. Topical corticosteroid may be used to reduce the inflammatory response. The most common complication is secondary infection.

Type II cytotoxic reactions

In type II reactions, IgM or IgG immunoglobulins react with cell-surface antigens to activate the complement system and produce direct damage to the cell surface (Figure 12-2). The cytotoxic reactions include transfusion reactions, hemolytic disease of the newborn, autoimmune hemolytic anemia, and certain drug reactions in which antibodies are formed to react with the drug that is complexed to the red-cell antigens.

Type III immune complex reactions

Type III reactions involve the complement-activating IgG and IgM immunoglobulins and the classic complement pathway. This type of reaction is characterized by the formation of an immune complex that initiates an acute inflammatory reaction in the tissues. The immune complexes become attached to walls of blood vessels where they cause tissue damage by activating the complement system. Two of the more common immune complex disorders are serum sickness and the Arthus reaction (Figure 12-3).

Serum sickness develops in about 50% of persons receiving bovine or horse antitoxin against tetanus, gas gangrene, and other infections.[11] Fortunately, antitoxin therapy is infrequently used today because most individuals have been actively immunized for tetanus and human antisera are available. At present the most common cause of serum sickness is an adverse reaction to drugs such as penicillin. The symptoms of serum sickness usually appear at about 7 to 10 days following exposure to the offending antigen. The signs and symptoms that occur at this time include urticaria, patchy or generalized rash, extensive edema (usually of the face, neck, and joints), and fever. In previously sensitized individuals, severe and even fatal forms of serum sickness may occur either immediately or within several days after the sensitizing drug or serum is administered.

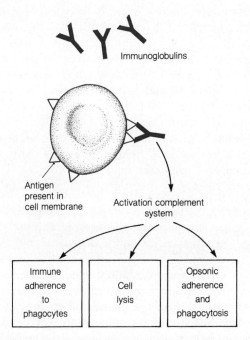

Figure 12-2 Type II cytotoxic immune reactions that involve immunoglobulins (IgG and IgM) and cell-surface antigens with activation of the complement system.

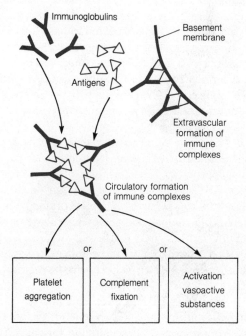

Figure 12-3 Type III immune complex reactions that involve complement-activating IgG and IgM immunoglobulins with formation of blood-borne or extravascular immune complexes and their effects.

The Arthus reaction is a local reaction to the immune complex. It consists of vasculitis and tissue necrosis at the site of antigen exposure. The reaction causes erythema and swelling, which begins within several hours and progresses to form a central area of cellular necrosis. Usually the area dries and heals within a week. The Arthus reaction is involved in hypersensitivity pneumonitis and extrinsic alveolitis (see Chapter 25). These disorders include farmer's lung, caused by breathing dust from moldy hay; pigeon breeder's disease, caused by exposure to pigeon droppings and danders; and humidifier lung, caused by inhalation of fungal spores that grow in humidifiers. Allergic pneumonitis is characterized by a dry cough, shortness of breath, fever, and general malaise that appears about 6 to 8 hours after exposure to the antigen. The symptoms subside within a few days, but reappear with each subsequent exposure to the agent.

Type IV cell-mediated hypersensitivity

Cell-mediated hypersensitivity reactions involve T-lymphocytes that have been sensitized to locally deposited antigens. The reaction is mediated by release of lymphokines, direct cytotoxicity, or both (Figure 12-4). Cell-mediated immunity is also called *delayed hypersensitivity*, compared with immediate hypersensitivity, which is caused by immunoglobulins such as IgE. Two of the more common types of cell-mediated immunity are the tuberculin test and contact dermatitis.

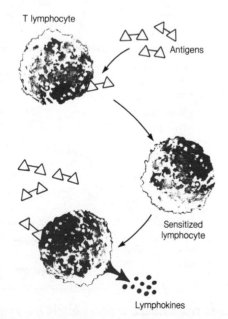

T lymphocyte

Antigens

Sensitized lymphocyte

Lymphokines

Figure 12-4 Type IV immune response that involves an antigen, sensitized T-lymphocyte, and lymphokines. Exposure to the antigen causes sensitization of the lymphocyte with release of lymphokines on subsequent exposures.

The tuberculin test, in which a purified component of the tubercle bacillus is injected intradermally, produces a delayed type of hypersensitivity reaction. In a previously sensitized individual, there is redness and swelling at the site of injection as the sensitized T-type lymphocytes interact with the tuberculin antigen. The reaction usually develops gradually over a period of 48 to 72 hours. As a point of clarification, it is important to recognize that the tuberculin test merely indicates that an individual has been sensitized to the tuberculosis bacillus through a previous exposure—it does not mean that the person has the disease.

Contact dermatitis is an acute or chronic dermatitis that results from direct contact with different chemical agents or other irritants, such as cosmetics, hair dyes, metals, and drugs applied to the skin. Two of the best known types of contact dermatitis are due to poison ivy and poison oak. When the sap from these plants comes in contact with the skin, neoantigens are formed, and sensitization to these new antigens develops. Contact dermatitis lesions usually consist of erythematous macules, papules, and vesicles (blisters). The affected area often becomes swollen and warm, with exudation, crusting, and development of a secondary infection. The location of the lesions often provides a clue as to the nature of the antigen causing the disorder.

In summary, hypersensitivity and allergic reactions are immune responses in which the antigen is an environmental agent, food, or drug usually considered harmless. There are four basic types of hypersensitivity responses: (1) type I responses, which are mediated by the IgE immunoglobulins and include anaphylactic shock, hay fever, and bronchial asthma; (2) type II cytotoxic reactions, which are caused by IgG- or IgM-activated complement and include hemolytic responses due to blood transfusion reactions; (3) type III hypersensitivity reactions in which IgG or IgM reacts with an antigen to form an immune complex that causes local tissue injury; and (4) type IV cell-mediated responses in which sensitized T-lymphocytes react with an antigen to cause inflammation and tissue injury.

Transplant rejection

Organ transplantation, once considered only life-saving, has now been transformed into a life-enhancing and technologically advanced form of therapy. The success of transplantation can be greatly enhanced by appropriate matching of the major histocompatibility complex (MHC) antigens (see Chapter 11) and the use of immunosuppression drugs.

Organ transplantation involves a donor and a

recipient. The donor can be living related as in kidney transplantation, living unrelated as in a human leukocyte antigen (HLA) compatible bone marrow transplantation, or an unrelated brain-dead donor (cadaver). With kidney transplants using living related donors there is a 90% 1-year graft survival when the donor and recipient are identical twins as compared with a 56% 1-year graft survival when the donor and recipient do not share either HLA haplotype.[9] With cadaver transplants, matching of class II MHC antigens produces a marked improvement in graft success. This is probably because the class II antigens trigger T-cell responses, which are believed to be important in graft rejection. On the other hand, there is only minimal to moderate improvement in graft survival when only MHC I antigens match.[9]

Transplant rejection usually involves both cellular and humoral immunity and is a complex process. There are three basic patterns of transplant rejection: hyperacute, acute, and chronic. In bone marrow transplantation, which is used increasingly for hematologic malignancies and certain immune deficiency diseases, there is a threat of both transplant rejection and graft-versus-host disease.

A hyperacute response occurs almost immediately following the transplant; in kidney transplants, it can often be noted at the time of surgery. As soon as blood flow from the recipient to the donor kidney has been established, the kidney, instead of becoming pink and viable-looking, becomes cyanotic, mottled, and flaccid in appearance. Sometimes the onset of the reaction is not so sudden, but develops over a period of hours or several days. The hyperacute transplant rejection is caused by the presence of existing recipient antibodies to the graft that act at the level of the vascular epithelium to incite an Arthus type of reaction. These antibodies have usually developed in response to previous blood transfusions, pregnancies in which the mother develops antibodies to fetal antigens that have been inherited from the father, or infections with HLA cross-reacting bacteria or viruses.

Acute rejection is seen in the first months following transplant. In the patient with a kidney transplant, acute rejection is evidenced by signs of renal failure. Acute rejection often involves both humoral and cell-mediated immune responses.

Chronic rejection occurs over a period of months following transplant and is largely caused by cell-mediated immune responses. In renal transplant patients this rejection pattern causes a gradual rise in serum creatinine over a period of 4 to 6 months.[12]

Graft-versus-host disease occurs when immunologically competent bone marrow cells and their precursors recognize the recipient's tissue as foreign, a condition that is potentially lethal. HLA matching helps to prevent graft-versus-host disease but does not prevent it because the donor T cells can react against minor histocompatibility antigens. As a precaution, the donor T cells may be depleted with anti-T$_3$ antibodies and complement.[9]

Previous blood transfusions have proven to be beneficial in cadaver renal transplant survival. The mechanisms for the transfusion benefit are thought to be through the development of specific and nonspecific suppressor T cells and through the generation of blocking antibodies against recipient antibodies that would reject the donor graft.

Immunosuppression is a necessity in almost all organ transplantation except in the case of identical twins. Two drugs that are used to provide immunosuppression are the corticosteroids and cyclosporin. Cyclosporin, which acts by suppressing interleukin-2–mediated lymphocyte activation, has definitely improved the long-term success of cadaver and some living related transplants.

Autoimmune disease

Inherent in the normal immune response is the ability of the immune system to recognize body cells as self and to distinguish them from nonself. There is a normal immunologic tolerance to self-antigens, which prevents damage to body tissues by the immune system. Autoimmune disease can be viewed as a disruption in immunologic tolerance, which results in damage to body tissues or cells normally recognized as self. It should be remembered that antibody can be formed in response to injured, antigenically changed tissue. Also, autoantibodies can be demonstrated in a number of persons who do not have autoimmune disease. Robbins and Kumar suggest that the designation of autoimmune disease should be based on: (1) evidence of an autoimmune reaction, (2) the judgment that the immunologic findings are not secondary to another condition, and (3) the lack of other identified causes for the disorder.[9]

Autoimmune diseases can affect almost any cell or tissue in the body. There are known or suspected autoimmune disorders of blood cells and various body tissues and disorders that affect multiple organs and systems. Chart 12-2 describes some of the probable autoimmune diseases. Systemic lupus erythematosus is presented in this chapter as an example of an autoimmune disease. Many of the other autoimmune disorders are discussed in other sections of the book.

Probable mechanisms

The ability to recognize self from nonself resides in the human leukocyte antigen (HLA), which is coded by the major histocompatibility complex (MHC) genes (see Chapter 11). Autoimmunity can

Chart 12–2: Probable autoimmune diseases

Systemic

Systemic lupus erythematosus
Rheumatoid arthritis
Dermatomyositis
Scleroderma
Sjögren's syndrome
Mixed connective-tissue disease

Blood

Autoimmune hemolytic anemia
Idiopathic thrombocytopenic purpura
Neutropenia and lymphopenia

Other organs

Hashimoto's thyroiditis
Thyrotoxicosis
Goodpasture's syndrome
Pernicious anemia
Myasthenia gravis
Primary biliary cirrhosis
Chronic active hepatitis
Ulcerative colitis
Autoimmune adrenalitis
Juvenile autoimmune diabetes
Premature gonadal failure
Sympathetic ophthalmia
Temporal arteritis
Acute idiopathic polyneuritis
Insulin-resistant diabetes

(Adapted from Robbins SL, Cotran RS: Pathologic Basis of Disease, p 293. Philadelphia, WB Saunders, 1979)

involve abnormal T-cell or B-cell reactivity. One of the differences between the two types of immune cells is that B cells can recognize an isolated antigen in and apart from the rest of the immune system, whereas peripheral T cells cannot. For normal T-cell response, the antigen must be presented on the surface of a cell such as a macrophage that also displays proteins of the MHC. This dual recognition requirement affects all three major T-cell populations: cytotoxic T cells, which damage target cells directly, and helper and suppressor T cells, which, respectively, stimulate or restrict B cells and other T cells. It has been proposed that the helper and suppressor T cells are the master switches to the immune system.

Self-tolerance is the lack of immune responsiveness to an individual's own tissue antigens. Most self-antigens can be visualized as hapten-carrier complexes. For self-antigens, T-cell self-tolerance is probably the rule. B cells, on the other hand, are capable of recognizing the haptenic determinants of self-antigens and form anti-hapten antibodies. This process can only occur, however, if helper T cells send appropriate activating signals to hapten-carrying B cells. Alternatively, the activity of hapten-carrying B cells can be inhibited by suppressor T cells. The absence or suppression of T helper cells probably keeps the B cells from secreting anti-self antibodies.

Multiple mechanisms may explain the loss of self-tolerance and susceptibility autoimmune disorders. Among the proposed mechanisms are: (1) genetic predisposition and influence of the human leukocyte antigens in rejection of a person's own tissues, (2) interactions with chemical, physical, or biologic agents that trigger an immune response involving self-antigens, and (3) abnormalities in immune cells that lead to an inappropriate immune response. Because of the complexity of the immune system, it seems unlikely that autoimmune disease results from a single mechanism.

Familial clustering of several autoimmune diseases suggests a genetic predisposition. The genetic predisposition may be linked to an inherited HLA type or to other factors. It has been observed that certain human leukocyte antigens occur more frequently in persons with certain disease conditions (Table 12-1). For example, it has been shown that 90% of persons with ankylosing spondylitis have HLA-B27 antigen; whereas only 7% of a control group without the disease have the antigen. Other HLA-associated diseases are Reiter's syndrome and HLA-B27, rheumatoid arthritis and HLA-DR4, and systemic lupus erythematosus and HLA-DR3. The basis for these associations is unclear. It may be that certain MHC immune response genes that code the human leukocyte antigens facilitate immune responses against self-antigens.

There are multiple ways in which exogenous chemicals and microbial agents can interact with the immune system to alter self-tolerance. Among these mechanisms are modification of the carrier determinant of the self-antigen, cross-reactions of external agents with human antigens, and by abnormal B-cell activation. Drugs and viruses may modify self-antigen carrier proteins and help bypass T-cell regulation. For example, the antihypertensive drug methyldopa can interact with intrinsic red blood cell proteins to produce an autoimmune hemolytic anemia. In this case the hemolytic anemia goes away once the drug has been discontinued. Cross-reactions can occur between human antigens and certain microbes if they share the same antigenic specificity. In rheumatic fever, for example, the streptococcus M protein cross-reacts with heart tissue. Several microorganisms and their products (particularly endotoxin) can bypass normal T-cell regulation of the immune response, directly stimulating B-cell proliferation and production of antibody. Such an effect can follow infection with gram-negative bacteria.

Because helper and suppressor T cells are pivotal to the immune response, any decline in suppressor T cells or increase in helper T cells affords the potential for the development of autoimmunity. For example, in multiple sclerosis, fluctuations in suppressor T cells parallels exacerbations and remissions of the disease.[13] It is not known, however, if the abnormality is a primary event or merely an accompanying phenomenon.

—— Systemic lupus erythematosus

Systemic lupus erythematosus (SLE) is a chronic autoimmune disease that affects multiple body systems. Recent studies indicate that the prevalence of the disease is about 1 in 2000.[14] The disease is seen most frequently in the 20- to 40-year-old age group, with about 85% of the affected persons being women. Blacks are affected more frequently than whites. There is a strong familial predisposition for development of the disease.

A lupus-like reaction that is indistinguishable both clinically and in the laboratory from spontaneously occurring SLE can also develop from the continual use of a number of drugs, especially the antihypertensive drug hydralazine and the antiarrhythmic drug procainamide. Drug-induced reactions usually disappear once the drug has been discontinued.

The immunologic abnormalites associated with SLE are uncertain. Evidence suggests a familial predisposition. There is a high incidence among identical twins, family members have an increased incidence of SLE, and there is a positive association in the North American Caucasian population between SLE and the HLA-DR2 and DR3 antigens coded by the MHC genes.[9] Persons with SLE have increased production of both self and nonself antigens suggesting B-cell hyperactivity. The basis for the B-cell hyperactivity could result from several mechanisms. In theory, excessive helper T-cell function or defective suppressor T-cell function could alter the B-cell response.

One of the first cellular changes to develop in SLE of immunologic origin is the presence of *LE cells* in the blood. The LE cells are neutrophils that contain a large LE body that has been engulfed. This LE body originates from the nucleus of certain white blood cells that have undergone nuclear changes and have been stripped of their cytoplasm by other phagocytic leukocytes. The LE factor responsible for this reaction has been identified as an antideoxyribonucleoprotein (anti-DNA) antibody of the IgG type. The relationship between the LE factor found in the serum and the development of the body changes that occur with SLE is still obscure. However, absence of the LE factor is a strong indication against a diagnosis of SLE.[1]

The disease affects many organs and body systems, including the skin, joints, kidneys, and serosal surfaces. The *skin* lesions include the classic "butterfly" rash that extends over the nose and cheeks—the sign of the red wolf for which the disease is named. There is extreme sensitivity to sunlight, and the rash

Table 12–1. HLA and disease associations

Disease	HLA antigen	Frequency In patients (%)	In controls (%)
Ankylosing spondylitis	B27	90	7
Reiter's disease	B27	76	6
Acute anterior uveitis	B27	55	8
Psoriasis	B13	18	4
	B17	29	8
	B16	15	5
Graves' disease	B8	47	21
Celiac disease (gluten-sensitive enteropathy)	D3	95	15
Dermatitis herpetiformis	B8	62	27
Myasthenia gravis	B8	52	24
Multiple sclerosis	D2	60	15
	B7	36	25
Acute lymphatic leukemia	A2	63	37
Hodgkin's disease	B5	25	16
	B1	39	32
	B8	26	22
Chronic hepatitis	B8	68	18
Ragweed hay fever			
Ra 5 sensitivity	B7	50	19
Allergen E sensitivity	Multiple (in family studies)		

(Krupp MA, Chatton MJ (eds): Current Medical Diagnosis and Treatment. Copyright 1981 by Lange Medical Publications, Los Altos, CA. Reproduced with permission.)

appears in areas of the body that are exposed to sunlight. Depending on the course of the disease, the rash may resolve without problems or it may progress to form scars, hypo- or hyperpigmentation, or discoid lesions. A *polyarthritis* occurs in about 90% of persons with SLE; it can affect any of the joints and is often the first manifestation of the disease. The arthritis seldom causes deformities, and erosive lesions usually are not observed on x-ray films. Involvement of the *serous cavities* can lead to pleural and pericardial effusion and pleurisy. *Renal* involvement is a common and serious complication of SLE. The most severe type of renal lesion observed in SLE is proliferative glomerulonephritis, which may be associated with nephrosis and renal failure. It is probably due to immune-complex deposition in the glomerular basement membrane. Among the other manifestations of SLE are *neurologic* disorders such as severe depression, psychosis, and convulsions. *Ocular* disturbances may also occur, including conjunctivitis. The disease is often called the great imitator because it affects so many body systems and can imitate so many different disease conditions.

The course of SLE is highly variable and unpredictable. Some persons have a benign form of the disease and require only supportive care; in others the disease presents with an acute onset and follows a progressive downhill trajectory. More often the disease is characterized by flare-ups and remissions spanning a period of years and even decades. The prognosis for persons with SLE seems to be better than older reports would indicate. Recent studies have shown 10-year survival rates exceeding 85%.[14]

Persons with photosensitivity should be cautioned against sun exposure and should apply a protective skin lotion when out of doors. Acute attacks of the disease are usually treated with adrenal corticosteroid drugs. Immunosuppressant drugs may be used to treat persons who are resistant to the corticosteroid drugs. The most frequently observed serious complication of SLE is renal disease followed by central nervous system involvement. Another important cause of sickness and death is infection, related in part to the use of corticosteroid drugs.

In summary, autoimmune diseases represent a disruption in self-tolerance that results in damage to body tissues by the immune system. Autoimmune diseases can affect almost any cell or tissue of the body. Normally self-tolerance is maintained by suppressor and helper T-cells that recognize self-antigens and regulate and protect the body from inappropriate immune responses. Among the proposed mechanisms to explain the loss of self-tolerance and susceptibility to autoimmune disorders are: (1) genetic predisposition and influence of the HLA antigens in rejection of a person's own tissue, (2) interactions with chemical, physical, and biologic agents that trigger an abnormal immune response, and (3) abnormalities in immune cells that lead to an inappropriate immune response directed against self-antigens. Systemic lupus erythematosus was presented as a chronic autoimmune disease that affects multiple body systems.

References

1. Stites DP, Stobo JD, Wells JV: Basic and Clinical Immunology, 6th ed, pp 317, 439, 359. Norwalk CO, Appleton Lange, 1987
2. Wedgewood RJ, Rosen FS, Paul NW (eds): Primary immunodeficiency disease: Report of the International Workshop held September 12–16, 1982, at Rosario Resort, Orcas Island, Washington. Birth Defects 19:345, 1983
3. Baradana EJ: A conceptual approach to immunodeficiency. Med Clin North Am 65(5):959, 1981
4. Sodeman WA, Sodeman TM: Pathologic Physiology: Mechanisms of Disease, p 125. Philadelphia, WB Saunders, 1979
5. Kangilas KJ (ed): Plastic bubble remains boy's home. JAMA 237:521, 1977
6. Smith LH, Their SO: Pathophysiology, p 234. Philadelphia, WB Saunders, 1981
7. Rayfield EJ, Ault MJ, Keutsch GT et al: Infection and diabetes: The case for glucose control. Am J Med 72:439, 1982
8. Gell RGH, Coombs RRA, Lachman PJ (eds): Clinical Aspects of Immunology, 3rd ed. Oxford, Blackwell Scientific, 1975
9. Robbins SL, Kumar V: Basic Pathology, 4th ed, pp 137, 148, 149, 154. Philadelphia, WB Saunders, 1987
10. Hanifin JM: Atopic dermatitis. Postgrad Med 74(3):188, 1983
11. Barrett JT: Textbook of Immunology, 4th ed, p 380. St Louis, CV Mosby, 1983
12. Robbins SL, Cotran RS, Kumar V: Pathologic Basis of Disease, 3rd ed, p 174. Philadelphia, WB Saunders, 1984
13. Huddlestone JR, Olstone MBA: T-suppressor (T$_G$) lymphocytes fluctuate in parallel with changes in the clinical course of patients with multiple sclerosis. J Immunol 123:1615, 1979
14. Shearn MA: Arthritis and musculoskeletal disorders. In Schroeder SA, Krupp MA, Tierney LM (eds): Current Medical Diagnosis and Treatment, p 503. Norwalk, CO, Appleton Lange, 1988

Bibliography

Bach FH, Sachs DH: Transplantation immunology. N Engl J Med 317:489, 1987
Becker MJ, Drucker I, Farkas R et al: Monocytemediated regulation of cellular immunity in humans: Loss of suppressor activity with ageing. Clin Exp Immunol 45:439, 1981

Buissert PD: Allergy. Sci Am 247(2):86, 1982

Clift RA, Rainer S: Histocompatible bone marrow transplants in humans. Annu Rev Med 5:43, 1987

Fauci AS (Moderator): Activation and regulation of human immune responses: Implications in normal and disease states (NIH Conference). Ann Intern Med 99:61, 1983

Geha RS: Regulation of IgE synthesis in atopic disease. Hosp Pract 23 (2):91, 1988

Gilliland BC: Serum sickness and immune complexes. N Engl J Med 311:1435, 1984

Goodwin JS, Searles RP, Tung SK: Immunological responses of a healthy elderly population. Clin Exp Immunol 48:403, 1982

Herberman RB: Natural killer cells. Hosp Pract 17(4):93, 1982

Jett MF, Lancaster LE: The inflammatory-immune response: The body's defense against invasion. Crit Care Nurse 5:64, 1983

Jones JV: Plasmapheresis: Current research and success. Heart Lung 9:671, 1980

Kantor FS: Autoimmunities: Disease of dysregulation. Hosp Pract 23 (7):75, 1988

Lippmann SM, Arnett FC, Conley CL et al: Genetic factors predisposing to autoimmune diseases. Am J Med 73:827, 1982

McChesney MB, Oldstone MBA: Viruses perturb lymphocyte functions: Selected principles characterizing virus-induced immunosuppression. Annu Rev Immunol 5:279, 1987

Hirschhorn R: Metabolic defects and immunodeficiency disorders. N Engl J Med 308:714, 1983

Rosen FS, Cooper MD, Wedgwood RJ: The primary immunodeficiencies (Parts I and II). N Engl J Med 311:300, 1984

Ruddy S: Hereditary angioedema: Undersuspected, underdiagnosed. Hosp Pract 23 (8):91, 1988

Schaller JG, Hansen JA: HLA relationships to disease. Hosp Pract 16(5):41, 1981

Schoenfeld Y, Schwartz RS: Immunologic and genetic factors in autoimmune disease. N Engl J Med 311:1019, 1984

Schumak KH: Therapeutic plasma exchange. N Engl J Med. 310:762, 1984

Serafin WE, Austin KF: Mediators of immediate hypersensitivity reactions. N Engl J Med 317:30, 1987

CHAPTER 13

Susan E. Dietz

Acquired Immunodeficiency Syndrome (AIDS)

Objectives

After you have studied this chapter, you should be able to meet the following objectives:

_____ Briefly trace the history of the AIDS epidemic.

_____ State the virus responsible for AIDS and explain how it differs from most other viruses.

_____ Describe the mechanisms of HIV transmission and relate them to the need for public awareness and concern regarding the spread of AIDS.

_____ Describe the alterations in immune function that occur in persons with AIDS.

_____ Explain the possible significance of a positive antibody test for HIV infection.

_____ Describe the universal precautions for HIV infection.

_____ Differentiate between the EIA and Western blot antibody detection tests for HIV infection.

_____ List the four stages of AIDS and describe the symptoms, psychosocial issues, and management concerns for each stage.

At the beginning of the AIDS epidemic many Americans had little sympathy for people with AIDS. The feeling was that somehow people from certain groups deserved their illness. Let us put those feelings behind us. We are fighting a disease, not people. Those who are already afflicted are sick people and need our care as do all the sick patients. The country must face this epidemic as a unified society. We must prevent the spread of AIDS while at the same time preserving humanity and intimacy.

C. Everett Koop, MD, ScD
Surgeon General[1]

The acquired immunodeficiency syndrome (AIDS) is a disease of the immune system. It is caused by a retrovirus that selectively attacks and destroys the immune system. The Centers for Disease Control (CDC) have estimated that the total number of persons infected with HIV in the United States is 1 million to 1.5 million.[2] The incidence and prevalence of HIV infection and AIDS in the United States have been highest in the East and West Coast regions and lowest in the northern Midwest and Mountain states. In addition, prevalence has been greater in urban than rural areas. HIV infection and AIDS have been concentrated among young and early middle-aged men (ages 20–39). It disproportionately affects blacks and Hispanics.[3]

Data from 1986 on heart disease, all cancers, and cerebrovascular diseases (including stroke) show that these conditions each killed 10 to 50 times as many Americans as AIDS.[2]

However, AIDS is the only major disease in the United States in which mortality is substantially increasing; it is the leading cause of death for men 25 years to 44 years of age in several large cities in the United States.[2] In years of potential life lost before age 65, AIDS increased in rank among diseases from 13th in 1984 to 8th in 1986.[2] This change reflects the young age of those who have died of AIDS and the increasing number of deaths.

The AIDS epidemic

The first recognized cases of AIDS occurred in the summer of 1981 as reports began to appear of *Pneumocystis carinii* pneumonia and Kaposi's sarcoma in previously healthy people.[4] Both of these conditions had previously occurred only in persons who were severely immunocompromised. The condition became known early on as the acquired immune deficiency syndrome, although its causes and modes of transmission were not immediately obvious.[4]

The virology of AIDS progressed with amazing efficiency; in 1983, within 3 years of the first recognized cases, the virus causing AIDS had been identified.[4] The virus was initially known by various names, including human T-lymphotropic virus type III (HTLV-III), lymphadenopathy-associated virus (LAV), and AIDS related/associated virus (ARV).[4] The internationally accepted term is now human immunodeficiency virus (HIV).[5]

First described among homosexual men in June 1981, AIDS was recognized among intravenous drug users and Haitians the following year and among recipients of blood or blood products, infants born to mothers at risk, heterosexual sexual partners of persons with AIDS, and Africans as early as 1983.[6] Studies of these diverse groups led to the conclusion that AIDS was an infectious disease spread by blood, sexual contact, and perinatally from mother to child. The cumulative world total of AIDS was 11,965 cases through 1984.[7] As of March 21, 1988, 136 countries or territories throughout the world had reported a total of 84,256 cases with 54,233 of the cases being reported in the United States.[7] Reporting of cases is not uniform throughout the world, so there may be countries not accurately represented in these figures.

The absence of a cure or preventive vaccine has led to broad and increasing public concern. In the year 1991, it is estimated that 25% to 50% of New York City's medical-surgical hospital beds will be constantly occupied by persons with AIDS.[8] Studies have also estimated that the average direct health-care cost for each person with AIDS is between $30,000 and $150,000. Of these costs, inpatient care accounted for approximately 90%. It is unclear if all HIV-infected individuals are moving toward AIDS at different rates or if some individuals will remain asymptomatic for the rest of their lives. Cohort studies show that 48% of infected persons will develop HIV-related illness within 10 years.[9] Extrapolations of current data have predicted a 65% to 100% progression to AIDS after 16 years of infection.[10] This variability in incubation period could be related to cofactors including the status of the immune system, genetic variation among infected individuals, or variable virulence among different strains of the virus. Some HIV-infected persons may experience the less severe symptoms of AIDS only.

In summary, acquired immunodeficiency syndrome (AIDS) is an infectious disease of the immune system caused by the human immunodeficiency virus (HIV). First described in June 1981, it has established worldwide prevalance and has since become the only major disease in the United States with a substantially increasing mortality rate. The efficient progression of the virus, along with the absence of a cure or preventive vaccine, has generated an ever-increasing public awareness and concern.

Transmission of HIV infection

HIV is transmitted from one individual to another through sexual contact, by blood exchange, or perinatally. HIV is not transmitted through casual contact.[6] It is not spread by mosquitoes or other insect vectors.[6] When infected blood, semen, or vaginal secretions from one person are deposited onto a mucous membrane or into the bloodstream of another person, it is possible for transmission to occur.

Blood, semen, and vaginal secretions contain HIV in sufficient concentrations to transmit the infection.[6] Contact with semen occurs during sexual intercourse (vaginal and anal), oral sex (fellatio), and donor insemination. Exposure to vaginal secretions occurs during vaginal intercourse and oral sex (cunnilingus). In most cities in the United States, HIV is transmitted primarily through sexual contact. Although 74% of the cases of AIDS in the United States have been among homosexual or bisexual men, in other parts of the world heterosexual transmission is the leading route of HIV infection.[6]

The sharing of unsterilized intravenous needles and syringes contaminated with blood containing HIV is a direct route for blood-to-blood transmission. Twenty-five percent of all the cases in the United States have occurred among persons who use intravenous drugs, and 17% have occurred among persons in whom intravenous drug use is the only risk factor.[6] This risk behavior has also created a route for heterosexual and perinatal transmission of HIV. Intravenous drug users who are infected with HIV can pass the virus on to sex partners and, in the case of pregnant women, to their offspring. It is estimated that 90% of intravenous drug users are heterosexual and 30% are women.[6] Of these women, 90% are in their childbearing years.[6]

Transfusions of whole blood, plasma, platelets, or red blood cells may transmit HIV.[6] However, blood transfusions have accounted for only a small percentage of AIDS in the United States (2% in adults and 12% in children).[6] All donations of blood in the United States have been screened for HIV since mid-1985. There will continue to be cases of AIDS identified as being transmitted by transfusions for some time due to the long incubation period of HIV. Factor VIII, the clotting factor used by persons with hemophilia, is derived from the pooled blood of many donors. Before HIV screening, the virus was transmitted to persons with hemophilia through infusions of factor VIII.[6] Although factor VIII is now heat-treated to kill HIV, 70% to 80% of persons with hemophilia have already become infected. Other blood products, such as gamma globulin or hepatitis B vaccine, have not been implicated in transmission of HIV.[6]

HIV may be transmitted from infected women to their offspring by three possible routes: *in utero* through the maternal–placental circulation, by inoculation or ingestion of blood and other infected fluids during labor and delivery, and through infected breast milk after birth.[6] The majority of documented cases of HIV infection and AIDS in infants and small children have occurred as a result of maternal-to-offspring transmission during pregnancy or in the perinatal period.[6] Although studies of pregnancy outcome have shown a wide range of infant infection rates, it has been estimated that the rate of perinatal transmission is 40% to 50%. This rate may increase as clinical disease appears and altered immune status worsens.

AIDS among health-care workers in the United States results primarily from infection that occurs outside the work setting. A small number of health-care workers have been infected with HIV through occupational exposure.[11] The CDC has recommended that "Universal Blood and Body Fluid Precautions" be used for all patients in the health-care setting (Chart 13-1).[11] Because health-care workers may be caring for persons whose HIV status is not known, this is the most prudent way to prevent occupational exposure. Studies have shown the occupational risk of acquiring HIV in the health-care setting to be low. It is most often associated with percutaneous inoculation (needlestick) of blood from a patient

---

Chart 13-1: General principles of universal precautions*

1. Take care to prevent injuries when using needles, scalpels, and other sharp instruments or devices. Do not recap used needles by hand, and do not bend, break, or otherwise manipulate used needles by hand. Place used disposable syringes and needles, scalpel blades, and other sharp items in puncture-resistant containers for disposal. Locate the puncture-resistant containers as close to the use area as possible.
2. Use protective barriers (*i.e.*, gloves, gowns, masks, protective eyewear) to prevent exposure to blood, body fluids containing visible blood, and other fluids to which universal precautions apply. The type of protective barrier(s) should be appropriate for the procedure being performed and the type of exposure anticipated.
3. Immediately and thoroughly wash hands and other skin surfaces that are contaminated with blood, body fluids containing visible blood, or other body fluids to which universal precautions apply.

* This list is abbreviated.
(Centers for Disease Control: Update: Universal precautions for prevention of transmission of human immunodeficiency virus, hepatitis B virus, and other blood-borne pathogens in health-care settings. MMWR 37:377, 1988)

with HIV.[12] The risk of seroconversion following needlestick exposure to the blood of an HIV-infected patient is estimated to be less than 0.5%.[11]

In summary, the transmission of HIV is from one individual to another through sexual contact, blood exchange, or perinatally. Transmission occurs when the infected blood, semen, or vaginal secretions of one person are deposited onto a mucous membrane or into the bloodstream of another person. The primary route of transmission is through intimate sexual contact. Although blood-exchange transmission may occur with intravenous drug use, blood transfusion, or occupational exposure in a health-care setting, only a small percentage of HIV transmission is attributable to blood transfusion or occupational exposure. Infected women may transmit the virus to their offspring *in utero,* during labor and delivery, or through breast milk. HIV infection is not transmitted through casual contact or by insect vectors.

Pathophysiology of AIDS

Since the first description of AIDS, considerable strides have been made in our understanding of the pathophysiology of the disease. The virus, its mechanism of action, HIV screening tests, and some treatment methods have all been discovered within a few years of the beginning of the epidemic.

The HIV belongs to a class of viruses called retroviruses, which carry their genetic information in RNA rather than DNA (see Chapter 9). The HIV infects a limited number of cell types in the body including a subset of T4-lymphocytes called helper T4 cells[6] and macrophages.[13] The HIV has also been found in brain tissue. In the bloodstream, HIV binds to specific receptors on the surface of the T4-lymphocytes. The virus then enters the lymphocyte and sheds its protein coat. Viral RNA is transcribed into DNA using a special enzyme called reverse transcriptase, and a portion of the viral DNA becomes integrated into the host cell DNA. The virus then enters a latent phase, which may last for several years. During this time, individuals remain asymptomatic although HIV infection can be documented through serologic tests that identify antibodies to viral proteins. These antibodies are usually detectable 1 to 3 months after infection. The presence of these antibodies does not convey any protection against the virus.

The T4 cells are a subset of lymphocytes that are necessary for normal immune function (see Chapter 11). Among other functions, the helper T4 cell recognizes foreign antigens, infected cells, and helps activate the antibody-producing B-lymphocytes.

The T4 cells also orchestrate cell-mediated immunity, which involves cytotoxic T8-lymphocytes and natural killer cells. Also influenced by T4 cells are the phagocytic monocytes and macrophages. In the process of infecting and selectively destroying the T4-lymphocytes, which are pivotal cells in the immune response, the HIV strips the individual with AIDS of protection against common environmental organisms and mutant (cancerous) cells that develop during normal cell division.

Clinical manifestations

Once infected with HIV, some individuals develop an acute mononucleosis-like syndrome soon after infection.[14] This acute phase may include fever, sweats, myalgia, arthralgias, malaise, sore throat, nausea, vomiting, and headache. Physical findings include generalized lymphadenopathy, hepatic and splenic enlargement, and transient macular erythematous rashes.[10]

The acute phase may be followed by a relatively latent period of years before many other symptoms occur. This period, previously referred to as the AIDS-related complex (ARC), is now considered part of the AIDS case definition. During this time persons with HIV infection present with lymphadenopathy. Persistent lymphadenopathy related to HIV is usually defined as lymph nodes that are chronically swollen for more than 3 months in at least two locations, not including the groin.[15] The lymph nodes may be sore or visible externally, but this is not always true. The lymphadenopathy may be accompanied by fatigue, fever, weight loss, night sweats, and diarrhea.

An abrupt onset of severe illness tends to be precipitated by an opportunistic infection. Opportunistic infections involve common organisms that normally do not produce infection unless there is impaired immune function. With immune system failure, these infections become progressively more severe and difficult to treat. The presence of an opportunistic infection or neoplasm is an essential feature in the diagnosis of AIDS (see Chart 13-2). The complications of AIDS include opportunistic infections of the respiratory and gastrointestinal tract, central nervous system involvement, Kaposi's sarcoma, and the wasting syndrome.

Respiratory manifestations

Pneumocystis carinii pneumonia (PCP) is the most common opportunistic disease in people with AIDS.[16] *Pneumocystis carinii* pneumonia is caused by a fungus that is common in soil, houses, and many other places in the environment. In people with healthy immune systems, its presence does not cause infection or disease. In people with AIDS, *Pneumocystis carinii* can multiply quickly in the lungs and cause pneumonia.[16] These symptoms may be acute or gradually progressive. Individuals may also complain of chest pain or sputum production. Physical examination may demonstrate only fever and tachypnea; rales may be absent and breath sounds normal. Chest x-ray may show interstitial infiltrates, but a normal chest film does not rule out *Pneumocystis carinii* pneumonia. The specific diagnosis can be made in some persons by examination of induced sputum, but most will require bronchoalveolar lavage or lung biopsy.

Other organisms that cause pulmonary infections in persons with AIDS include *Mycobacterium tuberculosis,* cytomegalovirus (CMV), *Mycobacterium avium*-intracellular (MAI), *Toxoplasma gondii,* and *Cryptococcus neoformans.*[15] Pneumonia may also occur due to the more common pulmonary pathogens, including *Streptococcus pneumoniae, Hemophilus influenzae,* and *Legionella pneumophila.* Some persons may be infected with multiple organisms. In persons with AIDS, tuberculosis is likely to be extrapulmonary and in two or more disease sites.[16]

Gastrointestinal manifestations

Esophageal candidiasis is another common opportunistic infection occurring among persons with AIDS.[16] Other opportunistic organisms causing esophagitis include CMV and herpes simplex virus (HSV).[16] Individuals experiencing these infections usually complain of painful swallowing or retrosternal pain. Endoscopy, with esophageal brushings or biopsy, is required for definitive diagnosis.

Diarrhea or gastroenteritis also occurs commonly in persons with AIDS. Symptoms may be the result of a protozoal infection by *Cryptosporidium.*[16] This watery diarrhea may produce gallons of stool per day and last for months. Symptoms this severe lead to weakness and potential death from fluid loss. Stool

---

Chart 13–2:   Case definition

A case of AIDS can be diagnosed under the following conditions:

I.   Without an HIV antibody test or one with inconclusive results, the absence of other causes of immunodeficiency and a definitive diagnosis of:
  ■ Candidiasis of the esophagus, trachea, bronchi, or lungs
  ■ Crypotococcosis, extrapulmonary
  ■ Cryptosporidiosis with diarrhea persisting over 1 month
  ■ Cytomegalovirus disease of an organ other than the liver, spleen, or lymph nodes in a patient over 1 month of age
  ■ Herpes simplex virus infection causing a mucocutaneous ulcer that persists longer than 1 month; or bronchitis, pneumonia, or esophagitis for any duration affecting a patient over 1 month of age
  ■ Kaposi's sarcoma affecting a patient under 60 years of age
  ■ Lymphoma of the brain (primary) affecting a patient under 60 years of age
  ■ Lymphoid interstitial pneumonia and/or pulmonary lymphoid hyperplasia affecting a child under 13 years of age
  ■ *Mycobacterium avium* complex or *M. kansasii* disease, disseminated (at other than or in addition to the lungs, skin, or cervical or hilar lymph nodes)
  ■ *Pneumocystis carinii* pneumonia
  ■ Progressive multifocal leukoencephalopathy
  ■ Toxoplasmosis of the brain affecting a patient over 1 month of age
II. With laboratory evidence of HIV infection and a definitive diagnosis of:
  ■ The combination of at least two bacterial infections within a 2-year period, multiple or recurrent, affecting a child under 13 years of age (septicemia, pneumonia, meningitis, bone or joint infection, or abscess of an internal organ or body cavity—excluding otitis media or superficial skin or mucosal abscesses, caused by *Hemophilus, Streptococcus,* or other pyogenic bacteria)
  ■ Coccidioidomycosis, disseminated
  ■ HIV encephalopathy (HIV infection or AIDS dementia)
  ■ Hystoplasmosis, disseminated
  ■ Isoporiasis with diarrhea persisting over 1 month
  ■ Kaposi's sarcoma
  ■ Lymphoma of the brain (primary)
  ■ Other non-Hodgkins lymphoma of B-cell or unknown immunogenic phenotype
  ■ Any mycobacterial disease caused by mycobacteria other than *M. tuberculosis,* disseminated
  ■ Disease caused by *M. tuberculosis,* extrapulmonary
  ■ HIV wasting syndrome (emaciation, "slim disease")
III. When laboratory test results are negative for HIV infection, and:
  ■ All other causes of immunodeficiency are excluded
  ■ The patient has had a definitively diagnosed case of any of the diseases in list II and a helper T-lymphocyte count under 400/mm.

(From Centers for Disease Control: Revision of the CDC Surveillance Case Definition for Acquired Immunodeficiency Syndrome. MMWR 36:35, 1987)

specimens are examined and cultured for identification of the organism.

Nervous system manifestations

Neurologic complications of HIV infections occur frequently and may affect either the peripheral or central nervous system.[17] These complications arise from the direct effects of the retrovirus in the CNS and from secondary opportunistic infections.[17] There may be neurologic symptoms in HIV-infected persons who are otherwise asymptomatic.[17] *T. gondii* is a common opportunistic pathogen infecting the CNS in persons with AIDS. The typical presentation includes fever, altered mental status, seizures, or motor deficits.[16] Computerized tomography (CT scans) may show lesions, but brain biopsy is necessary in many cases for definitive diagnosis.

Primary central nervous system (CNS) lymphoma and high-grade B-cell lymphoma have been diagnosed with increased frequency in persons with AIDS.[17] The latter tumors often present with extranodal involvement of the gastrointestinal tract, CNS, bone marrow, myocardium, or kidneys. The clinical course of these lymphomas is marked by rapid progression and death despite treatment.

A common neurologic syndrome attributed directly to HIV is called subacute encephalitis or AIDS dementia complex.[17] It occurs in more than 15% of persons with AIDS, but the prevalence in otherwise healthy seropositive individuals is not known.[17] It is marked by subtle cognitive or behavioral dysfunction occurring over weeks to months. Individuals may initially develop memory loss, difficulty in concentrating, euphoria, social withdrawal, or lethargy.[17] These early signs are easily confused with depression or drug abuse and may be ignored until they eventually progress to severe dementia with motor disturbances, ataxia, tremor, spasticity, and paraplegia. CT scans show a characteristic pattern of cerebral atrophy with prominent sulci and ventricles.[17] Examination of the cerebrospinal fluid typically shows a mild pleocytosis with an elevated protein or lowered glucose concentration.[17] AIDS dementia complex may initially occur without any other signs or symptoms of AIDS.

Cryptococcus neoformans is a yeast that typically causes meningitis with fever and headache. Disseminated disease may be found in persons with AIDS involving the lungs, kidneys, skin, and other organs.[15] Cryptococcal meningitis is diagnosed by laboratory testing of the cerebrospinal fluid.

In addition to disorders of the CNS, HIV causes abnormalities of the peripheral nervous system in some individuals. A painful sensory neuropathy occurs in 30% to 50% of persons with AIDS and an unknown percentage of other HIV-infected persons.[16] Painful dysesthesias, numbness, weakness, and those symptoms related to dysfunction of the autonomic nervous system may occur.

Kaposi's sarcoma

Kaposi's sarcoma (KS) is a cancer of the connective tissues that support blood vessels. This is an opportunistic cancer and occurs in immunosuppressed individuals (*i.e.,* transplant patients and persons with AIDS). There is a great diversity in the clinical manifestations of Kaposi's sarcoma. It usually begins as one or more macules, papules, or violet lesions, which enlarge and become darker. They may coalesce to form raised plaques or tumors. These irregular-shaped tumors can be anywhere from one-eighth of an inch to silver dollar size. Tumor nodules are frequently located on the trunk, neck, and head (especially the tip of the nose). They are usually painless in the early stages, but discomfort may develop as the tumor ages. Invasion of internal organs, including the lungs, gastrointestinal tract, and lymphatic system, occurs commonly. Here the tumors may obstruct organ function or rupture causing internal bleeding. The progression of Kaposi's sarcoma may be slow or rapid. Biopsy of suspicious lesions is needed to make a definitive diagnosis. Both chemotherapy and radiation therapy have been extensively used for palliative treatment of the tumors. Treatment of malignancy by itself is unlikely to improve survival, because most patients die of opportunistic infections rather than tumor effects.[16]

Wasting syndrome

HIV wasting syndrome is now formally considered in the case definition of AIDS.[15] It is so commonly found that it has characterized the person with AIDS. In Africa, AIDS has become known as "slim disease" due to this condition. With the wasting syndrome there is profound involuntary weight loss, which is over 10% of baseline body weight.[15] There is also severe diarrhea and chronic weakness with fever. This diagnosis is used when no other opportunistic infections or neoplasms can be identified as causing these symptoms.[15]

Diagnosis

The most accurate and cost-effective method for identifying HIV at this time is the utilization of antibody detection tests. The first commercial assays for HIV were introduced in 1985 to screen donated blood. Since then their use has been expanded to include evaluating individuals at increased risk of HIV infection and as a component of the case definition of

AIDS. The two assays currently in widespread use are the enzyme-linked immunoassay (EIA or ELISA) and the Western blot (WB) assay.[15] In light of the psychosocial issues related to HIV and AIDS, sensitivity and confidentiality must be maintained whenever testing is implemented. If testing is done, it must be carried out with pre- and post-test counseling and with expressed consent of the person being tested.

The EIA test detects antibodies produced in response to HIV infection. It is based on the light absorbance of antigen–antibody complexes in sample wells compared to control wells.[13] The test kit contains beads or microtiter wells coated with HIV antigens. When a serum sample is added, HIV antibodies in the serum bind to the antigen-coated surface. After additional washings and incubations, the amount of bound HIV antibody is measured indirectly with a spectrophotometer. The test is considered reactive if the measured light absorbance is greater than a cut-off value established from known positive and negative controls.[13] Samples that are initially reactive are retested and those that are repeatedly reactive are then tested by a supplemental test such as the Western blot.[15]

The Western blot assay is based on the identification of antibodies to specific viral antigens. Prior to the test, HIV antigens are separated by electrophoresis and transferred (blotted) to nitrocellulose paper.[13] The serum sample is then added, allowing specific HIV antibodies to bind with specific viral antigen bands. This technique permits the identification of antibodies to specific HIV core or envelope proteins and glycoproteins.[13] When certain combinations of the antibody bands are identified, the test is considered positive. In public health practice, the Western blot is run only on those samples that are initially reactive on the EIA.

The serologic tests for detecting HIV antibodies have proved to be extremely sensitive and specific. When serum tests are strongly reactive or borderline by EIA and also positive by Western blot, it is considered to have been infected by HIV.[15] It is important for both tests to be done because, in some situations, misinformation can be generated by EIA testing alone. The EIA test, when used in groups with a high prevalence of infection (*i.e.*, sexually active homosexual men), has a high predictive value.[18] However, when it is used in groups of low prevalence of infection, most of the positive results are low reactive and generally turn out to be false-positive tests.[18] As with other viral infections, it is possible for viral replication to occur before antibodies are detectable. For HIV this "window phase" occurs immediately after infection and appears to last for a few weeks in most individuals. It has been known to last up to 6 months.[18] Except during this window phase, current data indicate a serum repeatedly negative by EIA test result is not virtually infected with HIV in all instances.[18] For purposes of surveillance and monitoring of the course of the epidemic, the CDC has made a specific case for definition of AIDS (Chart 13-2).[15]

Prevention of HIV infection

Because there is currently no cure for AIDS, adopting risk-free or low-risk behavior is the best protection against the disease. Abstinence or mutually monogamous sexual relationships between two uninfected partners are ways to avoid HIV infection and other sexually transmitted diseases. Proper use of condoms may provide another form of protection from the disease by not allowing the exchange of semen or vaginal secretions during intercourse.

The use of recreational drugs provides another avenue for HIV transmission. Avoiding recreational drug use and particularly the practice of sharing needles is important to AIDS prevention. Individuals concerned about their risk should be encouraged to get information and counseling in regards to their infection status.

Universal precautions

Universal precautions are intended to prevent parenteral, mucous membrane, and nonintact skin exposures of health-care workers to blood-borne pathogens. These precautions apply to body fluids known to contain HIV.[11] Blood is the single most important source of HIV pathogens in the occupational setting.[11] Universal precautions also apply to semen and vaginal secretions. Although both of these fluids have been implicated in sexual transmission of HIV, they have not been implicated in occupational transmission from patient to health-care worker.[11] Because the associated risk of transmission is unknown, universal precautions should also be used with tissues and cerebrospinal, pleural, peritoneal, pericardial, and amniotic fluids.[11] Universal precautions do not apply to the following fluids unless they contain visible blood because the risk of transmission is extremely low or nonexistent: feces, nasal secretions, sputum, sweat, tears, urine, saliva, and vomitus. Epidemiologic studies have not shown HIV to be transmitted by any of these fluids in health-care or community settings.[11] General infection control practices should include the use of gloves for digital examinations of mucous membranes and endotracheal suctioning and handwashing after contact with body fluids. The general principles of universal precautions are listed in Chart 13-1.

Study results have indicated that HIV is very sensitive to chemical disinfectants. Commonly used germicides at recommended concentrations inactivated HIV within 2 minutes to 10 minutes. Sodium hypochlorite (household bleach) diluted 1:10 and 70% alcohol (ethyl, isopropyl) inactivated the virus within 1 minute of exposure.[19] The results of these studies do not necessitate any changes in currently recommended procedures for sterilization or disinfection in public, private, or health-care facilities.[20]

——— Management

There is currently no cure for AIDS. Opportunistic diseases are treated individually with standard and experimental protocols (such as antibiotics, antifungals, anticancer therapies). At the time of this writing, there is only one antiviral agent approved by the United States Food and Drug Administration for treatment of HIV. Azidothymidine (AZT or Zidovudine) is a competitive inhibitor of reverse transcrip-

tase, which inhibits viral replication.[21] Clinical trials showed that AZT increased survival of persons with AIDS. Investigations of other antiviral drugs and vaccines are currently underway.[21]

Theoretically, infection might increase disease progression through activation of the immune system.[22] Therefore, individuals with AIDS should be advised to avoid infections as much as possible and seek evaluation promptly whenever they occur. They should be encouraged to avoid alcohol, nonprescription drugs, and smoking. A balanced diet, moderate exercise, and stress management are all positive factors in maintaining a healthy life-style.

The care of persons with AIDS can be divided into four stages (Table 13-1). It is not known how many individuals will proceed from stage I to stage II. Once diagnosed with AIDS (stage II), the survival rate is approximately 50% at 1 year and 15% at 5 years.[23]

Table 13-1. Stages of AIDS, symptoms and management

Stage	Symptoms	Psychosocial issues	Management
I HIV infection (pre-AIDS)	Acute flulike symptoms: night sweats, weight loss, fatigue, fever	Depression, reduction in social activities due to fear or symptoms; absenteeism from work; confusion and fear regarding symptoms	Referral to community support agencies for counseling, education, support groups, and medical research programs
II Diagnosis of AIDS	First opportunistic infection or multisystem involvement	Symptoms may cause medical leaves from work, increased isolation, possible difficulty in activities of daily living. Fatigue may increase sleep needs. Increased financial outlay for medications to support symptom management.	Evaluation by appropriate health professionals to determine the ability to cope with diagnosis, treatment programs, availability of support systems, nutritional needs, drug interactions and compliance. Provide for in-home assistance, professional nursing, and physical therapy visits as needed. Arrange for professional counseling/therapy to facilitate coping with realities and effects of illness.
III Repetitive opportunistic infections, multisystem	Manifestations of total system failures (pulmonary, gastrointestinal, neurologic); malnutrition, loss of muscle mass, skin breakdown, loss of teeth	Acute disease processes may force person to remain homebound, unable to care for self, loss of outside social activities. Repeated acute episodes may require permanent medical leave and dependence on public or private medical benefits. Depression, rage, fear, dementia may be expressed.	Re-evaluation of medication and nutritional status. Increased attendant care needs; dependent on family/caregiver availability. Skilled nursing to manage care and administer intravenous fluids and medications.
IV Active dying	As dying begins, treatment modalities are less effective, increasing need for management, symptoms caused by multisystem failures	Probably bed-bound, requiring full care. Outside contacts limited to close friends, family, caregivers. Experiences confusion from isolation, drug side-effects, and disease effects.	Provide for hospice care (some patients may choose to continue treatment program). Continuous attendant care probably required. Skilled nursing visits needed for care plan management and support during dying process.

(Sedaka S, O'Reilly M: The financial implications of AIDS. Caring 5:38–46, 1986)

The prejudice toward people with AIDS has been widely publicized. There are numerous reports of persons with HIV infection or AIDS who have lost their jobs and have been abandoned by their families. A recent study of college students indicated that prejudice toward those dying from AIDS was greater than that felt for those dying of cancer.[24]

The psychologic effects of AIDS may be as devastating as the physical effects. When AIDS strikes, the dramatic impact of this catastrophic illness is compounded by complex reactions on the part of members of the health-care team, the individual, his or her partner, friends, and family.[25] These reactions may be influenced by inadequate information, fear of contagion, shame, prejudices, and condemnation of risk behaviors. In addition to the fear and grief associated with death, the person with AIDS may also experience guilt, anger, and uncertainty. Questioning and self-examination are common as the person attempts to understand what is happening. The person is confronted with questions—Why did I get this disease? Will the medical treatment help? Am I going to die? Did I give this disease to someone else? How can I protect myself and the people I love? Will someone take care of me when I am sick? What will happen to my family/partner when I die? Will my family, friends, and colleagues reject me? Will I lose my job, benefits, apartment, belongings?

The person with HIV infection and AIDS may feel helpless, hopeless, stigmatized, and out of control.[25] AIDS affects all spheres of life. Isolated from peers and with a weakened sense of identity, the person may be anxious, depressed, and miserable. Acknowledging a diagnosis of AIDS my be the first indication to family and colleagues of otherwise hidden life-styles of the individual (*i.e.,* homosexuality or drug use). This increases the strain on relationships with important support persons.

To deal with these complex issues, the health-care team must recognize and accept their fears, prejudices, and emotions concerning those with AIDS. Their feelings must not prevent caregivers from acknowledging the intrinsic human worth of all individuals and their right to be treated with dignity and care.[25] It is also important for members of the health-care team to have adequate support for their own emotional needs generated from working with persons with AIDS. Grief, anxiety, and concern over stigmatization are normal feelings. They should be acknowledged and dealt with through peer support or professional counseling in order to reduce burnout and further emotional strain. The emotional stress, feelings of isolation, and sadness experienced by the person with AIDS can be devastating. It is important for persons with the disease to have as much information and control over activities as possible.[25] They should be encouraged to direct their energies in a positive manner and continue with their social and group activities as tolerated. All appropriate social support systems (*e.g.,* AIDS service organizations, community groups, religious organizations) should be used whenever possible.

In summary, HIV, a retrovirus, infects the body's T4 lymphocytes and macrophages, becoming integrated into the host cell DNA. Manifestations of infection, such as acute mononucleosis-like symptoms, may occur immediately following transmission or appear after a relatively latent phase that may last several years. This period, previously referred to as the AIDS-related complex (ARC), is accompanied by lymphadenopathy. The end of the latent period is marked by the onset of severe illness brought about by opportunistic infection. The complications of these infections, which are manifested throughout the respiratory, gastrointestinal, and nervous systems, include pneumonia, esophagitis, diarrhea, gastroenteritis, tumor, wasting syndrome, altered mental states, seizures, and motor deficits. The diagnosis of HIV is made using the enzyme-linked immunoassay and the Western blot assay, antibody detection tests that have proven to be extremely sensitive and reliable. Risk-free or low-risk behavior is the best protection against HIV infection since there is currently no cure for AIDS. Abstinence or mutually monogamous sexual relationships between two uninfected partners, the use of condoms, avoiding drug use and the sharing of needles, and the practice of universal precautions by health-care workers is essential to stop the spread of HIV. At this time there is only one antiviral agent approved for treatment of HIV. Management of AIDS is divided into four stages that address the individual's physical and emotional well-being.

References

1. Koop CE: The Surgeon General's Report on Acquired Immune Deficiency Syndrome, p 6. US Department of Health and Human Services, 1986
2. Centers for Disease Control: Quarterly Report to the Domestic Policy Council on the Prevalence and Rate of Spread of HIV and AIDS in the United States. MMWR 37:224, 1988
3. Centers for Disease Control: Human immunodeficiency virus infection in the United States. MMWR 36:802, 1987
4. Curran JW, Morgan WM, Hardy AM et al: The epidemiology of AIDS: Current status and future prospects. Science 229:1352, 1985
5. Montagnier L, Alizon M: The human immune deficiency virus (HIV): An update. In Gluckman JC, Vilmer E (eds): Proceedings of the Second International Conference on AIDS, p 13. Paris, Elsevier, 1986

6. Friedland GH, Klein RS: Transmission of the human immunodeficiency virus. N Engl J Med 317:1125, 1987

7. Centers for Disease Control: Update: Acquired immune deficiency syndrome (AIDS)—Worldwide. MMWR 37:224, 1988

8. Weinberg DS, Murray HW: Coping with AIDS. N Engl J Med 317:1469, 1987

9. Hessol NA, Rutherford GW, Lifson A, et al: The natural history of HIV infection in a cohort of homosexual and bisexual men: A decade of follow-up. In the Proceedings of the IV International Conference on AIDS, p 4096. Stockholm, Sweden, 1988

10. Lemp GA, Hessol NA, Rutherford GW, et al: Projections of AIDS morbidity and mortality in San Francisco using epidemic models. In the Proceedings of the IV International Conference on AIDS, p 4682. Stockholm, Sweden, 1988

11. Centers for Disease Control: Update: Universal precautions for prevention of transmission of human immunodeficiency virus, hepatitis B virus, and other blood-borne pathogens in health-care settings. MMWR 37:377, 1988

12. Centers for Disease Control: Update: Acquired immunodeficiency syndrome and human immunodeficiency virus infection among health-care workers. MMWR 37:229, 1988

13. Levy JA. The human immunodeficiency virus (HIV) and its pathogenic properties. In Schinaz RF, Nahmias AJ (eds): AIDS in Children, Adolescents and Heterosexual Adults, pp 117–25. New York, Elsevier, 1988

14. Ho DD, Sarngadharan MG, Resnick L et al: Primary human T- lymphotropic virus type III infection. Ann Intern Med 103:880, 1985

15. Centers for Disease Control: Revision of the CDC Surveillance Case Definition for Acquired Immunodeficiency Syndrome. MMWR 36:3S, 1987

16. Sherertz RA: Acquired immune deficiency syndrome. Med Clin of North Am 69:637, 1985

17. Price RW, Brew B, Sidtis J et al: The brain in AIDS: Central nervous system HIV-1 infection and AIDS dementia complex. Science 239:586, 1988

18. Francis DP, Chin J: The prevention of acquired immunodeficiency syndrome in the United States. JAMA 257:1357, 1987

19. Resnick L, Veren K, Salhuddin SK et al: Stability and inactivation of HTLV-III/LAV under clinical and laboratory environments. JAMA 255:1887, 1986

20. Martin LS, McDougal JS, Loskoske SL: Disinfection and inactivation of the human T-lymphotropic virus type III/lymphadenopathy-associated virus. J Infect Dis 152:400, 1985

21. Fischl MA, Richman D, Grieco M, et al: The efficacy of azidothymidine (AZT) in the treatment of patients with AIDS and AIDS-related complex. A double-blind, placebo controlled trial. N Engl J Med 317(4):185, 1987

22. Quinn TC, Piot P, McCormick JB et al: Serologic and immunologic studies in patients with AIDS in North America and Africa. The potential role of infectious agents as cofactors in human immunodeficiency virus infection. JAMA 257:2617, 1987

23. Rothenberg R, Woelfel M, Stoneburner R et al: Survival with the acquired immunodeficiency syndrome. N Engl J Med 317:1297, 1987

24. Lester D: Prejudice toward AIDS patients versus other terminally ill patients. Am J Public Health 78:854, 1988

25. O'Brien AM, Oerlemans-Bunn M, Blachfield JC: Nursing the AIDS patient at home. AIDS Patient Care 1:21, 1987

Bibliography

Anders KH, Guerra WF, Tomiyasu U: The neurophysiology of AIDS. Am J Pathol 124:537, 1986

Fineberg HV: Education to prevent AIDS: Prospects and obstacles. Science 239:4840, 1988

Fineberg HV: The social dimensions of AIDS. Sci Am 259(10):128, 1988

Fishman JA: An approach to pulmonary infection in AIDS. Hosp Pract 23(4):196, 1988

Gallo RC: The first human retrovirus. Sci Am 255(6):88, 1986

Gallo RC: The AIDS virus. Sci Am 256(1):46, 1987

Glatt AE, Chirgwin K, Landesman SH: Treatment of infections associated with human immunodeficiency virus. N Engl J Med 318:1439, 1988

Grady C: HIV: Epidemiology, immunopathogenesis, and clinical consequences. Nurs Clin North Am 23:683, 1988

Haseltine WA, Wong-Staal F: The molecular biology of the AIDS virus. Sci Am 259(10):52, 1988

Henderson DJ: HIV infection: Risks to health care workers and infection control. Nurs Clin North Am 23:767, 1988

Heyward WL, Curran JW: The epidemiology of AIDS in the U.S. Sci Am 259(10): 72, 1988

Kaminski MA, Hartman PM: HIV testing: Issues for the family physician. Am Fam Phys 38(1):117, 1988

Laboratory diagnostic tests for detection of HIV infection, Wisconsin Division of Health, AIDS Update (July):13, 1988

Lovejoy NC: The pathophysiology of AIDS. Oncol Nurs Forum 15:563, 1988

Miles SA: Diagnosis and staging of HIV infection. Am Fam Pract 38:248, 1988

Mitsuya H, Broder S: Strategies of antiviral therapy in AIDS. Nature 325:773, 1987

Weber JN, Weiss RA: HIV infection: The cellular picture. Sci Am 2599(10):100, 1988

Yarchoan R, Mitsuya H, Broder S: AIDS therapies. Sci Am 259(10):110, 1988

Yarchoan R, Broder S: Development of antiretroviral therapy for the acquired immunodeficiency syndrome and related disorders: A progress report. N Engl J Med 316:557, 1987

CHAPTER 14

Disorders of White Blood Cells and Lymphoid Tissues

Objectives

After you have studied this chapter, you should be able to meet the following objectives:

_____ List the cells and tissues of the lymphoreticular system.

_____ Describe the production and life span of the granulocytes.

_____ Define *leukopenia*.

_____ Cite two general causes of granulocytosis.

_____ Describe three mechanisms of drug-induced granulocytosis.

_____ Describe the mechanism of symptom production in agranulocytosis.

_____ Describe the pathogenesis of infectious mononucleosis.

_____ Compare the manifestations of acute infectious mononucleosis and chronic mononucleosis or chronic Epstein-Barr virus infection.

_____ Use the predominant cell type and classification as acute or chronic to describe the four general types of leukemia.

_____ Explain the manifestations of leukemia in terms of altered cell differentiation.

_____ State the warning signs of acute leukemia.

_____ State the major treatment modalities used in leukemia.

_____ Discuss the prognosis associated with different types of leukemia.

_____ Describe the signs and symptoms of Hodgkin's disease.

_____ Discuss the prognosis of Hodgkin's disease in relation to the stage of the disease.

_____ Cite the major treatment modalities used in Hodgkin's disease.

_____ Describe the lymphoproliferative disorder that occurs with multiple myeloma.

_____ Explain the origin of the Bence Jones protein that appears in the urine in multiple myeloma.

The white blood cells and lymphoid system serve to protect the body against invasion by foreign agents. The functions of the granular leukocytes is discussed in Chapter 10, and the functions of lymphocytes is discussed in Chapter 11. In this chapter neutropenia and lymphoproliferative disorders are discussed.

Hemopoietic and lymphoid tissue

The lymphoreticular system includes the white blood cells, their precursors, and their derivatives. It includes the *myeloid,* or bone marrow, tissue in which the white blood cells are formed and the *lymphoid tissues* of the lymph nodes, thymus, spleen, tonsils, and adenoids. Aggregates of lymphoid tissue are also found in the lungs and gastrointestinal tract.

—— White blood cells

White blood cells have their origin in the bone marrow as multipotential hemopoietic stem cells (Figure 14-1). These stem cells are capable of providing progenitor cells for both lymphopoiesis and hemopoiesis (processes by which mature lymph and blood cells are made). Several levels of differentiation

lead to the development of committed unipotential cells, which are the progenitor or parent cells for each of the blood cell types. These committed cells develop into the precursors of blood cells such as the myeloblast from which the granulocytes develop. The myeloblasts differentiate into promyelocytes and then myelocytes (Figure 14-2). At this point it should be emphasized that immature, or blast, forms of blood cells do not normally appear in the peripheral circulation. Generally, a cell is not called a myelocyte until it has at least 12 granules.[1] The myelocytes mature to become metamyelocytes (Greek *meta,* "beyond"), at which point they lose their capacity for mitosis. Subsequent development of the neutrophil involves reduction in size, with transformation from an indented to an oval to a horseshoe-shaped nucleus (band cell), and then to a mature cell with a segmented nucleus. At this point the neutrophil enters the bloodstream. Neutrophil development (from stem cell to mature neutrophil) takes about 2 weeks.

After release from the marrow, the neutrophils spend only a short time (1–2 days) in the circulation before moving into the tissues. Their survival in the tissues is short (about 5 days). They die either in discharging their function or of senescence. The pool of circulating neutrophils (those that appear in the blood count) are in rapid equilibrium with a similar-sized pool of cells marginating along the walls of small blood vessels.[2] Epinephrine, exercise, and corti-

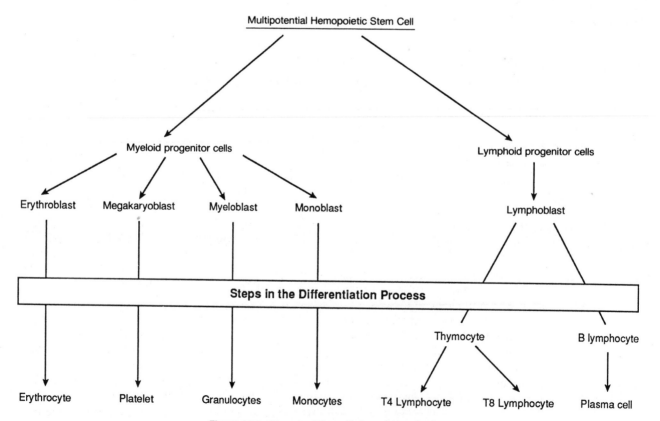

Figure 14-1 Steps in differentiation of blood cells.

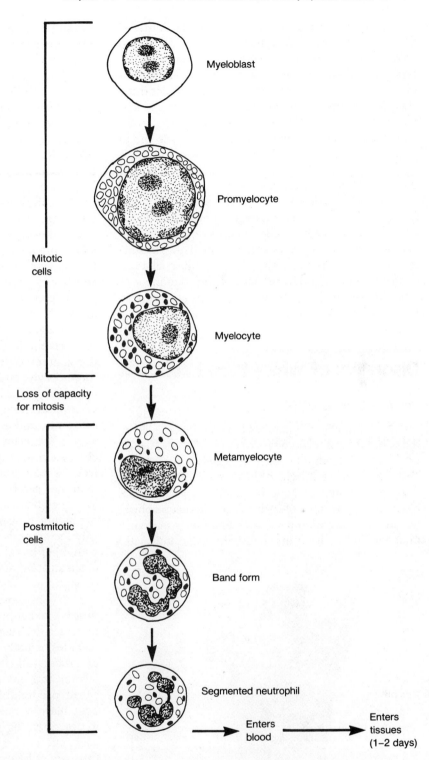

Myeloblast

Promyelocyte

Mitotic cells

Myelocyte

Loss of capacity for mitosis

Metamyelocyte

Postmitotic cells

Band form

Segmented neutrophil

Enters blood

Enters tissues (1–2 days)

Figure 14-2 Schematic diagram of maturation in the neutrophil series. Azurophilic granules appear at the promyelocyte stage, and specific granules (shown in color) appear at the myelocyte stage. (*Cormack DH: Ham's Histology, 9th ed, p 227. Philadelphia, JB Lippincott, 1987. Based on Bainton, et al*)

costeroid drug therapy can cause rapid increases in the circulating neutrophil count by shifting cells from the marginating to the circulating pool. Endotoxins have the opposite effect, producing a transient decrease in neutrophils.

The T-lymphocytes and B-lymphocytes develop in the lymphatic tissue (thymus gland and bursa equivalent) from committed stem cells that originated in the bone marrow.

Lymphoid tissues

Lymphoid tissues make up the body's lymphatic system, which consists of the lymphatic vessels, the lymph nodes, the spleen, and the thymus. Lymph is body fluid that originates as excess fluid from the capillaries (see Chapter 28). It is returned to the vascular compartment and right heart through lymphatic vessels.

Lymph nodes are situated along the course of the lymphatic channels and serve to filter the lymph before it is returned to the circulation (Figure 14-3). Lymph enters a lymph node through afferent lymphatic channels, percolates through a labyrinthine system of minute channels lined with endothelial and phagocytic cells, and then emerges through efferent lymphatic vessels. A number of efferent vessels join to form collecting trunks. Each collecting trunk drains a definite area of the body. By filtering bacteria and other particulate matter, the lymph nodes serve as a secondary line of defense even when clinical disease is not present. In the event of malignant neoplasm development, cancer cells are filtered and retained by the lymph nodes for a period of time before being disseminated to other parts of the body. Because of their contribution to the development of the immune system, the lymph nodes are relatively large at birth and undergo progressive atrophy throughout life.

Disorders of white blood cells

Leukopenia

Normally, the number of white blood cells in the peripheral circulation ranges from 5,000 to 10,000 per mm³ of blood. The term *leukopenia* describes an absolute decrease in white blood cell numbers. The disorder may affect any of the specific types of white blood cells, but most often it affects the neutrophils, which are the predominant type of granulocyte. Lymphopenia, when it occurs, is usually associated with

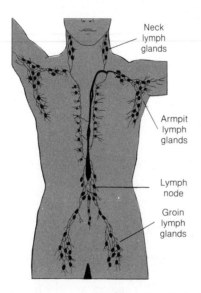

Figure 14-3 Location of some of the lymph nodes in the human body. (*What You Need to Know About Hodgkin's Disease. Washington, DC, Department of Health and Human Services, July 1981*)

Neck lymph glands

Armpit lymph glands

Lymph node

Groin lymph glands

specific clinical conditions such as Hodgkin's disease or corticosteroid therapy.

Agranulocytosis

Agranulocytosis refers specifically to a decrease in the granulocytes, mainly the neutrophils. It is usually defined as a circulating neutrophil count of below 1000 cells per mm³. It can occur because (1) neutrophil production fails to keep pace with granulocyte turnover or (2) accelerated destruction removes neutrophils from the circulating blood. Impairment of granulopoiesis occurs in conditions such as cancer chemotherapy, irradiation, and aplastic anemia, which interfere with the formation of all blood cells. Overgrowth of neoplastic cells in nonmyelocytic leukemia and lymphoma may crowd out the granulopoietic precursors. Because of the very short life span of the neutrophil (less than a day in the peripheral blood), agranulocytosis occurs rapidly when there is impairment of granulopoiesis. Under these conditions, granulocytopenia is usually accompanied by thrombocytopenia (platelet deficiency). *Aplastic anemia* refers to the condition in which there is failure of all myeloid stem cells resulting in anemia, thrombocytopenia, and agranulocytosis.

Accelerated removal of neutrophils from the circulation may occur in a number of conditions. Infections may drain neutrophils from the blood faster than they can be replaced. Autoimmune disorders or idiosyncratic drug reactions may cause increased and premature destruction of neutrophils. In splenomegaly, neutrophils may be trapped in the spleen along with other blood cells. In Felty's syndrome (a variant of rheumatoid arthritis) there is increased destruction of neutrophils in the spleen.

The most common cause of agranulocytosis is drug-related suppression of bone marrow function or increased destruction of neutrophils. Implicated drugs include chemotherapeutic drugs used in the treatment of cancer (alkalating agents, antimetabolites, and others) and chloramphenicol (an antibiotic), which cause predictable dose-dependent depression of bone-marrow function. The term *idiosyncratic* is used to describe drug reactions that are different from the usual effects obtained in the majority of persons and that cannot be explained in terms of allergy. A number of drugs such as phenothiazine tranquilizers, propylthiouracil (used in treatment of hyperthyroidism), phenylbutazone (used in the treatment of arthritis), and many other drugs may cause idiosyncratic depression of bone-marrow function. Some drugs, such as hydantoins and primidone (used in the treatment of epilepsy) can cause intramedullary destruction of granulocytes and thereby impair production. In addition, many idiosyncratic cases of drug-induced neutropenia are thought to be caused by immunologic mechanisms, with the drug or its metabolites acting as an antigen (or hapten) to incite production of antibodies reactive against the neutrophils. It is known that neutrophils possess not only HLA antigens but other antigens specific to a given leukocyte line. Antibodies to these specific antigens have been identified in some cases of drug-induced neutropenia.[3] The causes of agranulocytosis are summarized in Table 14-1.

Because the neutrophil is essential to the cellular phase of inflammation, infections are common in persons with agranulocytosis, and extreme caution is needed to protect them from exposure to infectious organisms. Infections that might go unnoticed in a person with a normal neutrophil count may prove fatal in a person with agranulocytosis.

The symptoms of agranulocytosis usually stem from severe infections that are characteristic of the disorder. These infections commonly occur with organisms that colonize the skin and gastrointestinal tract. Initially there are malaise, chills, and fever, followed by extreme weakness and fatigability. The white blood cell count is often reduced to 1000 cells per mm[3] and may in certain cases fall to 200 to 300 cells per mm[3].[3] Ulcerative necrotizing lesions of the mouth are common in agranulocytosis. Ulcerations of the skin, vagina, and gastrointestinal tract may also occur.

Treatment with antibiotics provides a means of controlling infections in those situations in which the destruction of neutrophils can be controlled or recovery of granulopoietic function of the bone marrow is possible. The prognosis is variable and depends on the cause.

In summary, one of the major disorders of the white blood cells is agranulocytosis, with marked reduction of the circulating neutrophils. Agranulocytosis can occur as the result of defective production or accelerated removal of neutrophils from the circulation. Severe agranulocytosis can occur in lymphoproliferative diseases, in which neoplastic cells crowd out granulocyte precursor cells, and during radiation therapy or treatment with cytotoxic drugs, which destroy granulocyte precursor cells. Because the neutrophil is essential to the cellular stage of inflammation, severe and often life-threatening infections are common in persons with agranulocytosis.

Lymphoproliferative disorders

The term *lymphoproliferative* is used to describe a number of localized and systemic disorders of white blood cells and lymphoid tissues. The discussion in this section focuses on infectious mononucleosis, the leukemias, lymphomas, and plasma cell dyscrasias. Leukocytosis, a common reaction to a variety of inflammatory diseases, is discussed in Chapter 10.

Table 14–1. Causes of agranulocytopenia/granulocytosis

Cause	Mechanism
Accelerated removal (*e.g.*, inflammation and infection)	Removal of neutrophils from the circulation exceeds production
Drug-induced granulocytopenia	
Defective production	
Cytotoxic drugs used in cancer therapy and chloramphenicol	Predictable damage to precursor cells, usually dose dependent
Phenothiazine, thiouracil, phenylbutazone, and others	Idiosyncratic depression of bone-marrow function
Hydantoinates, primidone, others	Intramedullary destruction of granulocytes
Immune destruction	
Aminopyrine, others	Immunologic mechanisms with cytoloysis or leukoagglutination
Periodic or cyclic neutropenia (occurs during infancy and later)	Unknown
Neoplasms involving bone marrow (*e.g.*, leukemias and lymphomas)	Overgrowth of neoplastic cells, which crowd out granulopoietic precursors
Idiopathic neutropenia that occurs in the absence of other disease or provoking influence	Autoimmune reaction
Felty's syndrome	Intrasplenic destruction of neutrophils

Infectious mononucleosis

Infectious mononucleosis is for the most part a benign lymphoproliferative syndrome caused by the Epstein-Barr virus (EBV), one of the herpesviruses. The highest incidence is in adolescents and young adults. The disease tends to be seen more frequently in the upper socioeconomic classes of developed countries. This is probably because the disease, which is relatively asymptomatic when it occurs during childhood, confers complete immunity to the virus. In upper socioeconomic families, exposure to the virus may be delayed until late adolescence or early adulthood. In such individuals, the mode of infection, size of the viral pool, and physiologic and immunologic condition of the host may determine whether the infection occurs or not. Recently, a chronic form of mononucleosis has been recognized.[4]

The mode of transmission of the virus is unclear. Infectious mononucleosis has been called the "kissing disease," and evidence suggests that virally contaminated saliva is one of the main modes of transfer. The virus exhibits selective tropism for the pharyngeal and salivary gland cells, and the saliva is the only body fluid reproducibly shown to contain viral particles.[4]

Acute infectious mononucleosis

The acute form of infectious mononucleosis is characterized by fever, generalized lymphadenopathy, sore throat, and the appearance in the blood of atypical lymphocytes. In the course of infection, the EBV invades the B-lymphocytes of oropharyngeal lymphoid tissues.[3] A replication of the virus ensues, with the subsequent death of the B-lymphocytes and release of the virus into the blood, causing the febrile reaction and specific immunologic responses. Concurrent with the febrile response, viral neutralizing antibodies appear and the virus disappears from the blood. However, some EBV-transformed B-lymphocytes remain in the circulation with the genome of the virus integrated into their genetic structure. The presence of virus-determined antigens on the surface of these B-lymphocytes is recognized by killer T cells and stimulates their multiplication. These killer T cells are the atypical lymphocytes seen in the blood of persons with infectious mononucleosis. The stimulation of the T-lymphocytes throughout the body is responsible for the lymphadenopathy and hepatosplenomegaly.

The signs and symptoms of infectious mononucleosis are usually insidious in onset, with a prodromal period of 1 to 2 weeks during which there is fever, fatigue, general malaise, and anorexia. Occasionally, the onset is abrupt with a high fever. Lymph-adenopathy is present in 90% of cases, with symmetrically enlarged and often tender lymph nodes.[5] Splenomegaly or hepatomegaly occurs in about 50% of cases. Splenomegaly occasionally leads to the rupture of the spleen. This is associated with severe abdominal pain. Fewer than 1% of cases, usually in the adult age group, develop symptoms referable to the central nervous system. These symptoms can include cranial nerve palsies, encephalitis, meningitis, transverse myelitis, and the Guillain-Barré syndrome. Occasionally, severe toxic pharyngotonsillitis may cause airway obstruction. Most cases of infectious mononucleosis recover without incident. Usually the acute phase of the illness lasts for 2 to 3 weeks, after which recovery occurs rapidly. However, some degree of debility and lethargy may persist for 2 to 3 months.

The peripheral blood usually shows an increase in leukocytes, with a white blood cell count between 12,000 and 18,000, 95% of which are lymphocytes. The rise in white blood cells begins during the first week, rises even higher during the second week of the infection, and then returns to normal around the fourth week. Although leukocytosis is common, leukopenia may be seen in some persons during the first 3 days of the illness. Atypical lymphocytes are frequent, constituting over 20% of the total lymphocyte count. A number of circulating immunoglobulins, including heteroantibodies (sheep red cell agglutinins), are found in persons with infectious mononucleosis. These antibodies are typically not absorbed by guinea pig kidneys but are absorbed by beef erythrocytes, a means used to differentiate the antibodies due to the EBV from other disorders that produce antibodies that react with sheep red blood cells.[6]

The treatment of infectious mononucleosis is usually symptomatic and supportive. It includes bedrest and analgesic agents such as aspirin to control fever, headache, and sore throat. In cases of severe pharyngotonsillitis, corticosteroid drugs are given to reduce inflammation.

Chronic mononucleosis

Recently, considerable attention has focused on a disorder variously called *chronic Epstein-Barr virus infection* or *chronic mononucleosis*.[4,7,8] Thousands of affected persons have formed support groups throughout the United States, and *Newsweek* has termed it "the malaise of the 80s."[7]

The illness involves chronic recurring flulike symptoms with chronic fatigue lasting months or years. It typically affects young adults, with women being affected more frequently than men. The manifestations of chronic mononucleosis include recurrent symptoms of upper respiratory infection, myalgias, and low-grade fever. In addition to the overwhelming fatigue, there is often neurologic manifestations including lack of ability to concentrate, disorders of fine motor control, depression, and sleep disorders. Because many of the symptoms resemble psychoneurotic disease, the disease tends to be unrecognized or be misdiagnosed.

It has been proposed that chronic mononucleosis may arise as the result of a reactivation of the Epstein-Barr virus in persons who are made susceptible by a combination of genetic and environmental conditions or as the result of infection with a particular strain of Epstein-Barr or another B-lymphocyte virus that produces chronic infection.

At present there are no definitive diagnostic tests for chronic mononucleosis. Usually there are elevated levels of anti-Epstein-Barr antibody that are higher than those seen in the asymptomatic persons. The management of the disorder is largely symptomatic.

Leukemias

The leukemias are malignant neoplasms of white blood cells and their precursors. The term *leukemia (white blood)* was first used by Virchow to describe a reversal of the usual ratio of red to white blood cells. Because they involve blood cells, the leukemias are disseminated throughout the body from their earliest recognizable stages. They are characterized by: (1) diffuse replacement of bone marrow with leukemic cells, (2) appearance of abnormal immature white blood cells in the peripheral circulation, and (3) widespread infiltration of the liver, spleen, lymph nodes, and other tissues throughout the body.[3] During the past 20 years, advances in molecular biology have contributed greatly to an understanding of leukemic cell types, including the early stages of cell differentiation and gene function. This information has greatly influenced the diagnosis, treatment, and prognosis of persons with leukemia.

Leukemia strikes about 27,000 persons in the United States each year. In 1987, there were an estimated 26,400 new cases and 17,800 deaths from leukemia.[9] The disease strikes more children than any other form of cancer and is the leading cause of death in children ages 3 to 14. Although leukemia is commonly thought of as childhood disease, it strikes more adults than children (24,600 adults per year as compared with 2,000 children).

Classification

There are several types of leukemias. The leukemias are usually classified according to the predominant cell type (lymphocytic or myelocytic) and whether the condition is acute or chronic. Thus, a rudimentary classification system divides leukemia into four types: acute lymphocytic (lymphoblastic) leukemia (ALL), chronic lymphocytic leukemia (CLL), acute myelocytic (myeloblastic) leukemia (AML), and chronic myelocytic leukemia (CML). The myelocytic leukemias, which involve the bone marrow, interfere with the maturation of all blood cells including the granulocytes, erythrocytes, and thrombocytes. ALL is the most frequent leukemia in childhood with a peak incidence between ages 2 and 4 years. AML is seen most often between ages 13 and 39 years and CML between ages 30 and 50 years. CLL is a disorder of older persons and fewer than 10% of persons who develop the disease are less than 50 years of age.

Causes

The causes of leukemia are unknown. There is an unusually high incidence of leukemia among persons exposed to high levels of radiation. The number of cases of leukemia in the most heavily exposed survivors of the atomic blasts at Hiroshima and Nagasaki during the 20-year period from 1950 to 1970 was nearly 30 times the expected rate.[10] There is also an increased incidence of leukemia associated with exposure to benzene and use of antitumor drugs and chloramphenicol.[11,12] There are hints of genetic predisposition. It is known that persons with Down's syndrome have a higher incidence of leukemia, and leukemia has been seen in a significant number of twins. There are chromosomal changes in many forms of leukemia. For example, the Philadelphia chromosome (translocation from chromosome 22 to 9) is evident in approximately 90% of persons with chronic myelogenous leukemia.[3] Interest in the role of viruses as etiologic agents in leukemia is also increasing. Leukemia viruses have been identified in a number of animal species.

Clinical manifestations

Leukemic cells are an immature and mobile type of white blood cell. In Chapter 5 it was explained that differentiation of a cell line determines its structure, function, and life span. Because leukemic cells are immature and poorly differentiated, they are capable of an increased rate of proliferation and a prolonged life span. They are also unable to perform the functions of mature leukocytes, that is, they are ineffective as phagocytes or immune cells. Because they are rapidly proliferating, leukemic cells tend to interfere with the maturation of the normal bone-marrow cells, including the erythroblasts (red blood cells) and the megakaryoblasts (platelets). Being mobile, they are able to travel throughout the circulatory system, cross the blood–brain barrier, and infiltrate many body organs.

Acute leukemias

Acute leukemia is a malignancy of the hemopoietic progenitor cells and usually presents with a sudden and stormy onset of signs and symptoms related to depression of bone-marrow function (Table 14-2). Laboratory findings in acute leukemia reveal the presence of immature (blast) white blood cells in the circulation and bone marrow, where they often constitute 60% to 100% of the cells.[3] They replace the normal marrow elements with proliferating blast cells that do not undergo normal maturation. Consequently, there is a loss of mature myeloid cells such as erythrocytes, granulocytes, and platelets. The platelet count is often decreased to less than 20,000 per mm[3]. Generalized lymphadenopathy, splenomegaly, and hepatomegaly due to infiltration by leukemic cells are characteristic of ALL but are not usually predominant in AML.[3]

The warning signs of acute leukemia, published by the American Cancer Society, are fatigue, paleness, weight loss, repeated infections, easy bruising, nose bleeds and other hemorrhages.[9] Both ALL and AML are characterized by fatigue due to anemia, bleeding secondary to decreased platelets, bone-marrow involvement including subperiosteal infiltration, marrow expansion, and bone resorption causing bone tenderness and pain. Signs of central nervous system involvement occur in both ALL and AML and include headache, nausea and vomiting, cranial nerve palsies, and sometimes seizures and coma. Hyperuricemia occurs as the result of increased proliferation and metabolic alterations of the leukemic cells. Hyperuricemia may increase prior to and during treatment and may require treatment with allopurinol to prevent renal complications secondary to uric acid crystallization in the urine.

The diagnosis of leukemia is based on blood and bone-marrow studies. More than 30% blasts is required to make a diagnosis of acute leukemia.

Acute lymphoblastic leukemia is treated with combination chemotherapy. It includes induction therapy designed to effect a remission, intensification therapy to reduce further the leukemic cell population, and maintenance therapy to maintain remissions. Systemic chemotherapeutic agents are not able to cross the blood–brain barrier and eradicate leukemic cells that have entered the central nervous system (CNS). Cranial irradiation combined with intrathecal chemo-

---

Table 14–2. Clinical manifestations of leukemia and their pathologic basis*

Clinical manifestations	Pathologic basis
Bone-marrow depression	
Malaise, easy fatigability	Anemia
Fever	Infection or increased metabolism by neoplastic cells
Bleeding	Decreased thrombocytes
Petechiae	
Ecchymosis	
Gingival bleeding	
Epistaxis	
Bone pain and tenderness on palpation	Subperiosteal bone infiltration, bone-marrow expansion, and bone resorption
Headache, nausea, vomiting, papilledema, cranial nerve palsies, seizures, coma	Leukemic infiltration of central nervous system
Abdominal discomfort	Generalized lymphadenopathy, hepatomegaly, splenomegaly due to leukemic cell infiltration
Increased vulnerability to infections	Immaturity of the white cells and ineffective phagocytic and immune function
Hematologic abnormalities	
Anemia	Physical and metabolic encroachment of leukemic cells on red blood cell and thrombocyte precursors
Thrombocytopenia	
Hyperuricemia and other metabolic disorders	Abnormal proliferation and metabolism of leukemic cells

* The manifestations will vary with the type of leukemia.

therapy is often used as a prophylactic measure to prevent CNS recurrence.

Acute myeloid leukemia is treated with intensive chemotherapy to effect aplasia of the bone marrow. During this period supportive transfusion and antibiotic therapy are often needed. If remission is achieved, some type of continuing chemotherapy is used. In some cases, a bone-marrow transplant may be used.

Acute leukemia is one of the outstanding examples of a once fatal disease that is now treatable and potentially curable with combination chemotherapy. More than 90% of children with ALL have complete remission, and more than 50% to 60% are alive 5 years later.[13] The treatment response in adults is more variable. It has been reported that chemotherapy induces complete remission in 70% of all persons with AML, about one fourth of whom achieve long-term disease-free survival or cure.[13]

Chronic leukemias

Chronic leukemias have a more insidious onset than acute leukemias and may be discovered during a routine medical exam with blood count. Although CML is usually a disorder of adults, it can affect children as well. CLL is a disorder of older adults.

CML is a myeloproliferative disorder and involves expansion of all bone-marrow elements. The bone-marrow cells of the CML line have the Philadelphia chromosome, suggesting a mutation in the multipotential stem cell as the initiating event. Persons with CML are often asymptomatic when diagnosed. Leukocytosis with immature cell types in the peripheral blood and splenomegaly are early manifestations of the disorder. Anemia and, eventually, thrombocytopenia develop. Anemia causes weakness, easy fatigability, and exertional dyspnea. Low-grade fever, night sweats, and weight loss are usually related to hypermetabolism of the leukemic cells. Hepatomegaly, splenomegaly, and lymphadenopathy often cause a feeling of abdominal fullness and discomfort. Eventually, the white cell maturation ceases, so that increasing numbers of immature myeloblasts appear in the peripheral blood. This is called the *blast phase* and indicates a downward trajectory and poor prognosis.

CLL is a disorder of immunologically incompetent lymphocytes. Abnormal small lymphocytes of the CLL lineage are detected in the peripheral blood. Abnormal findings in peripheral blood and bone marrow are prerequisites for the diagnosis of CLL, except when complete remission has occurred. There is a predisposition to infection and development of autoimmune phenomenon due to the immunologic incompetence of the expanding lymphocyte population. Generalized lymphadenopathy with palpable lymph nodes in the cervical, axillary, inguinal, and femoral regions is common. There may be enlargement of the spleen and liver. Anemia, thrombocytopenia, and neutropenia may result from bone-marrow infiltration.

The treatment of chronic leukemia varies with the type of leukemic cell that is present, the extent of the disease, other health problems, and the person's age. Often the treatment is palliative. Curative treatment for CML involves high-dose chemotherapy and possible bone-marrow transplantation. Bone-marrow transplantation is usually reserved for persons under age 50 who have a HLA-compatible sibling. CLL is mainly a disease of older persons and often follows a slow chronic course; for these persons reassurance that they can live a normal life for many years is important. Complications such as autoimmune thrombocytopenia or hemolytic anemia may be managed with corticosteroid treatment, or a splenectomy may be necessary.

Lymphomas

There are two types of lymphomas: Hodgkin's disease and non-Hodgkin's lymphomas. The most common of these two types is Hodgkin's disease.

Hodgkin's disease

Hodgkin's disease is a malignant neoplasm of the lymphatic structures, named after an English physician, Thomas Hodgkin, who first described the disease in 1832. This disease constitutes 40% of malignant lymphomas. There were an estimated 7300 new cases of Hodgkin's disease in 1987, resulting in 1500 deaths.[9] About 50% of the cases occur in persons between the ages of 20 and 40 years.[14] Recent reports suggest that, in contrast with patients with many types of cancer, the majority of cases of Hodgkin's disease can be cured with appropriate therapy if diagnosed early. In 60% to 90% of persons with localized Hodgkin's disease there is the possibility of a definitive "cure" (normal life expectancy for age, 10 or more years after treatment).[14]

Hodgkin's disease is characterized by painless and progressive enlargement of lymphoid tissue, usually a single node or group of nodes. It is believed to originate within one area of the lymphatic system and, if unchecked, it will spread throughout the lymphatic network. Splenic enlargement usually occurs early in the course of the disease. The malignant proliferating cells may invade almost any area of the body and may produce a wide variety of symptoms. Low-grade fever, night sweats, unexplained weight loss, fatigue, pruritus, and anemia are indicative of disease spread. In its advanced stages, the liver, lungs, digestive tract, and occasionally the central nervous system may be affected.

As the disease progresses, the rapid proliferation of abnormal lymphocytes leads to an immunologic defect, particularly in cell-mediated responses, rendering the person more susceptible to bacterial, viral, fungal, and protozoal infections. Neutrophilic leukocytosis and mild normocytic normochromic anemia are common. Eosinophilia may also occur. Leukopenia is usually a late manifestation. Hypergammaglobulinemia is common during the early stages of the disease, whereas hypogammaglobulinemia may develop in advanced disease.

Lymph node biopsy is used to diagnose the disease. Characteristic of Hodgkin's disease is the presence of a distinctive giant tumor cell known as the Reed-Sternberg (RS) cell, which can be detected on microscopic examination. Computerized tomography (CT) scans of the abdomen are commonly used in screening for involvement of abdominal and pelvic lymph nodes. Radiologic visualization of the abdominal and pelvic lymph structures can be achieved through the use of lymphangiography. A staging laparotomy, in which the abdominal and pelvic lymph nodes are biopsied, is usually done when involvement of these nodes is suspected. Because the spleen is a frequent site of extralymphatic spread, it is often removed during a staging laparotomy.

The staging of Hodgkin's disease is of great clinical importance because the choice of treatment and prognosis are ultimately related to the distribution of the disease. Both radiation and chemotherapy are used in treating the disease. Persons with localized disease are usually treated with radiation therapy. Disseminated Hodgkin's disease is usually treated with combination therapy.

The cause of Hodgkin's disease is unknown. There is a longstanding suspicion that the disease may begin as an inflammatory reaction to an infectious agent. This belief is supported by epidemiologic data that include the clustering of the disease among family members and among students who have attended the same school. There also seems to be an association between the presence of the disease and a deficient immune state. As with other forms of cancer, it is likely that no single agent is responsible for the development of Hodgkin's disease.

Non-Hodgkin's lymphomas

The non-Hodgkin's lymphomas are a group of neoplastic disorders of the lymphoid tissue. There are about 15,000 new cases of non-Hodgkin's lymphoma each year in the United States and about 13,200 related deaths.[14]

The non-Hodgkin's lymphomas are divided into three main groups according to the type of cell involved: lymphocytic lymphoma (or lymphosarcoma), histiocytic lymphoma (or reticulum cell sarcoma), and mixed cell lymphoma.

A viral etiology is suspected in at least some of the lymphomas. Cell cultures and immunologic studies of one type of lymphoma, Burkitt's lymphoma, found in some parts of Africa, have implicated the Epstein-Barr herpes-like virus without proving a causal relationship.[15] There is also a reported increase in lymphomas in persons treated with chronic immunosuppressive therapy and in other immune deficiency states.

The signs and symptoms of non-Hodgkin's lymphoma are similar to those of Hodgkin's disease except for the early involvement of the oropharyngeal lymphoid tissue, skin, gastrointestinal tract, and bone marrow. Leukemic transformation with high peripheral lymphocyte counts occurs in about 13% of persons with non-Hodgkin's lymphoma. There is increased susceptibility to bacterial, viral, and fungal infections associated with hypogammaglobulinemia and poor humoral antibody response, rather than impaired cellular immunity as seen in Hodgkin's disease.

As with Hodgkin's disease, a lymph node biopsy is used to confirm the diagnosis. Treatment depends on the stage of the disease. It may include surgical resection of the diseased tissue, combination chemotherapy, and irradiation.

Multiple myeloma

Multiple myeloma is a plasma cell cancer of the osseous tissue, which in the course of its dissemination may involve other nonosseous sites. It is characterized by the uncontrolled proliferation of an abnormal clone of plasma cells, usually of the IgG or IgA type. In 1985 there were an estimated 9900 new cases of the disease in the United States.[3] Over 90% of cases occur in persons over age 40.[14] The disease carries a mean survival rate of 2 to 3 years with standard therapy.

In multiple myeloma, plasma cells that are seldom found in healthy bone marrow proliferate and erode into the hard bone, predisposing to pathologic fractures and hypercalcemia due to bone dissolution. Paraproteins secreted by the plasma cells may cause a hyperviscosity of body fluids, and they may break down into amyloid, a proteinaceous substance deposited between cells, causing heart failure and neuropathy. In some forms of multiple myeloma, the plasma cells produce only the light chains of the immunoglobulin molecule, which, because of their low molecular weight, are excreted in the urine, where they are termed *Bence Jones proteins*. Many of the Bence Jones proteins are directly toxic to renal tubular structures leading to tubular destruction and eventual renal failure. The malignant plasma cells can also form tumors (plasmacytomas) that have a tendency to cause spinal cord compression.

Bone pain, concentrated in the back, is often one of the first symptoms present in this form of cancer. Bone destruction also impairs the production of erythrocytes and leukocytes and predisposes to anemia and recurrent infections. There is often weight loss and a feeling of weakness. There may be neurologic manifestations due to neuropathy or spinal cord compression and signs of renal failure may be present. The most effective treatment for multiple myeloma is chemotherapy.

In summary, lymphoproliferative disorders affect the cells of the lymphoreticular system, including the lymphocytes and plasma cells. Infectious mononucleosis is a benign lymphoproliferative disorder caused by the Epstein-Barr virus. Malignant lymphoproliferative disorders include the leukemias, Hodgkin's disease, non-Hodgkin's lymphomas, and multiple myeloma. Leukemias are classified according to the cell type (lymphocytic, myelocytic [myelogenous], or monocytic) and whether the disease is acute or chronic. Acute lymphocytic leukemia occurs most often in children. In adults, acute granulocytic and chronic lymphocytic leukemias are most common. Because leukemic cells are immature and poorly differentiated, they proliferate rapidly and crowd out precursors of other blood cells (thrombocytes, granulocytes, and erythrocytes) and they are unable to perform the functions of mature leukocytes. Hodgkin's disease is a malignant neoplasm of the lymphatic structures. It usually begins in a single lymph node or group of lymph nodes and, if unchecked, it invades the spleen and other lymphatic structures. Multiple myeloma results in the uncontrolled proliferation of plasma cells, usually a single clone of IgG- or IgA-producing cells.

References

1. Cormack DH: Ham's Histology 9th ed, p 314. Philadelphia, JB Lippincott, 1987
2. Smith LH, Their SO: Pathophysiology, pp 421. Philadelphia, WB Saunders, 1981
3. Robbins SL, Cotran RS, Kumar V: Pathologic Basis of Disease, 3rd ed, pp 654, 288, 674, 684. Philadelphia, WB Saunders, 1984
4. Jones JF: Chronic Epstein-Barr virus infection. Annu Rev Med 38:195, 1987
5. Henle GE, Horwitz CA: Epstein-Barr virus specific diagnostic test in infectious mononucleosis. Human Pathol 5:551, 1974
6. Lai PK: Infectious mononucleosis: Recognition and management. Hosp Pract 12(8):47, 1977
7. Komaroff AL: The 'chronic mononucleosis' syndromes. Hosp Pract 22(5A):71, 1987
8. Straus SE, Tosato G, Armstrong G, et al: Persisting illness and fatigue in adults with evidence of Epstein-Barr virus infection. Ann Intern Med 102:7, 1985
9. Cancer Facts and Figures 1987. Atlanta, American Cancer Society, 1987
10. Jablon S, Kato H: Studies of the mortality of A-bomb survivors. Radiat Res 50:658, 1972
11. Pederson-Bjergaard J, Larsen SO: Incidence of acute nonlymphocytic leukemia, preleukemia and acute myeloproliferative syndrome up to 10 years after treatment for Hodgkin's disease. N Engl J Med 307:964, 1982
12. Boise JD, Greene MH, Killen JY et al: Leukemia and preleukemia after adjuvant treatment of gastrointestinal cancer with Semustine. N Engl J Med 309:107, 1983
13. Linker C: Blood. In Schroeder SA, Krupp MA, Tierney LM: Current Medical Diagnosis and Treatment, p 319. Norwalk, Connecticut, Appleton & Lange, 1988
14. Rubin P (ed): Clinical Oncology, 6th ed, pp 346, 354, 355, 361. New York, American Cancer Society, 1983
15. Ziegler JL: Burkitt's lymphoma. N Engl J Med, 305(13):735, 1981

Bibliography

Arlin ZA, Clarkson BD: The treatment of acute nonlymphoblastic leukemia in adults. Adv Intern Med 28:303, 1983

Bacigalupo A, Fassoni F, Van Lint MT et al: Bone marrow transplantation in chronic granulocytic leukemia. Cancer 58:2307, 1986

Cassileth PA: Adult acute leukemia. Med Clin North Am 68(3):675, 1984

Coglian-Shutta NA, Broda EJ, Gress JS: Bone marrow transplantation. Nurs Clin North Am 20(1):49, 1984

Desforges JF: Blast crisis—Reversing the direction. N Engl J Med 315:1478, 1986

DeVita V, Hubbard SM, Moxley JH: The cure of Hodgkin's disease with drugs. Adv Intern Med 28:277, 1983

Ersek MT: The adult leukemia patient in the intensive care unit. Heart & Lung 13:183, 1984

Freireich EJ: Hematologic malignances: Adult acute leukemia. Hosp Pract 21(6):91, 1986

Gaynor ER, Ultmann JE: Non-Hodgkin's lymphoma: Management strategies. N Engl J Med 311:1506, 1984

Haller DG: Non-Hodgkins lymphoma. Med Clin North Am 68(3):741, 1984

Jacobs AD, Gale RP: Recent advances in biology and treatment of acute lymphoblastic leukemia in adults. N Engl J Med 311:1219, 1984

Kamani N, August CS: Bone marrow transplantations: Problems and prospects. Med Clin North Am 68:657, 1984

Kyle RA: Diagnosis and management of multiple myeloma and related disorders. Prog Hematol 14:257, 1986

Lehrer RI (Moderator): UCLA Conference: Neutrophils and host defense. Ann Intern Med 109(2):127, 1988

Mauer AM: New directions in the treatment of acute lymphoblastic leukemia in children. N Engl J Med 315:316, 1986

Murray BJ: Medical complication of infectious mononucleosis. Am Fam Pract 30(5):195, 1984

Niederman JC: Infectious mononucleosis: Observations on transmission. Yale J Biol Med 55:259, 1982

Oken MM: Multiple myeloma. Med Clin North Am 68:789, 1984

Portlock CS: Hodgkin's disease. Med Clin North Am 68(3):729, 1984

Rai KR, Sawitsky A, Kandasamy J et al: Chronic lymphocytic leukemia. Med Clin North Am 68(3):697, 1984

Rappeport JM: Sowing hematopoietic seeds. N Engl J Med 309:1385, 1983

Snugden B: Epstein-Barr virus: A human pathogen inducing lymphoproliferation in vivo and in vitro. Rev Infect Dis 4:1048, 1982

Spiers ASD: Chronic granulocytic leukemia. Med Clin North Am 68(3):713, 1984

Thomas ED, Clift RA, Fefer A et al: Marrow transplantation for the treatment of chronic myelogenous leukemia. Ann Intern Med 104:155, 1986

Kathryn J. Gaspard

CHAPTER 15

Alterations in Blood Coagulation and Hemostasis

Mechanisms of hemostasis
Vessel spasm
Formation of the platelet plug
Blood coagulation
Clot retraction
Clot dissolution (fibrinolysis)

Disorders of hemostasis and blood coagulation
Hypercoagulability states
Hyperreactivity of platelet function
Increased clotting activity

Bleeding disorders
Platelet defects
Coagulation defects
Vascular disorders
Effects of drugs on hemostasis
Warfarin
Heparin
Thrombolytic agents

Objectives

After you have studied this chapter, you should be able to meet the following objectives:

_____ State the five stages of hemostasis.

_____ Describe the formation of the platelet plug.

_____ State the purpose of coagulation.

_____ State the function of clot retraction.

_____ Trace the process of fibrinolysis.

_____ Compare normal and abnormal clotting.

_____ State the causes of platelet hyperreactivity.

_____ State two conditions that contribute to increased clotting activity.

_____ State two causes of impaired platelet function.

_____ Describe the role of vitamin K in coagulation.

_____ State three common defects of coagulation factors and the distribution of each.

_____ Describe the physiologic basis of acute disseminated intravascular clotting.

_____ Describe the effect of vascular disorders on hemostasis.

_____ State the mechanism by which warfarin, heparin, and thrombolytic agents inhibit blood clotting.

The term *hemostasis* refers to the stoppage of blood flow. Hemostasis is designed to maintain the integrity of the vascular system and to prevent blood from leaving its channels. Disorders of hemostasis fall into two main categories: (1) the inappropriate formation of clots within the vascular system and (2) the failure of blood to clot in response to an appropriate stimulus.

Mechanisms of hemostasis

Hemostasis is generally divided into five stages: (1) vessel spasm, (2) formation of the platelet plug, (3) blood coagulation or development of an insoluble fibrin clot, (4) clot retraction, and (5) clot dissolution. These steps are summarized in Chart 15-1.

Vessel spasm

Vessel spasm is the first of the stages involved in the formation of a blood clot; it is caused by local and humoral mechanisms. Vessel spasm constricts the vessel and reduces blood flow. It is a transient event that usually lasts less than a minute. Thromboxane A_2, released from the platelets, contributes to vasoconstriction.[1]

Formation of the platelet plug

The platelet plug is the second line of defense, which is initiated as platelets come in contact with the vessel wall. Platelets, or thrombocytes, are large fragments from the cytoplasm of bone stem cells called the megakaryocytes. They are enclosed in a membrane, but they have no nucleus. They have a life span of only 5 to 9 days. Platelet production is controlled by a substance called thrombopoietin. The source of thrombopoietin is unknown, but it appears that its production and release are regulated by the number of platelets in the circulation. The newly formed platelets that are released from the bone marrow spend 24 to 36 hours in the spleen before they are released into the blood.

Platelets are attracted to a damaged vessel wall and in the process change from smooth disks to spiny spheres. Formation of a platelet plug involves both adhesion and aggregation of platelets. Adhesion to the subendothelium requires von Willebrand's factor and platelet receptor sites. Platelet aggregation occurs as bridges of fibrinogen attach platelets to each other, forming a meshwork. Aggregating agents, including adenosine diphosphate (ADP), thrombin, and thromboxane A_2 (a prostaglandin), induce the aggregation process. Defective platelet plug formation causes bleeding in persons who are deficient in receptor sites or von Willebrand's factor.[2]

The unstable platelet plug is cemented together with fibrin converted from fibrinogen through the action of thrombin released from the platelets. This is the final product of coagulation and consolidates the plug.

When vessel injury is slight, the platelet plug may be all that is needed to close the defect; when this happens, the formation of the fibrin clot is not needed. In addition to sealing vascular breaks, platelets play an almost continuous role in maintaining normal vascular integrity. Persons with platelet deficiency have decreased capillary resistance and develop small skin hemorrhages, which result from the slightest trauma or change in blood pressure.

Blood coagulation

Blood coagulation is the third stage of hemostasis. This is the process by which fibrin strands form and create a meshwork that cements blood components together (Figure 15-1). Blood coagulation occurs as a result of activation of either the intrinsic or extrinsic coagulation pathways (Figure 15-2). The intrinsic pathway, which is a relatively slow process, occurs in the vascular system; the extrinsic pathway, which is a much faster process, occurs in the tissues. The terminal steps in both pathways are the same, consisting of the interaction between thrombin and the plasma protein fibrinogen. A final interaction for both pathways converts fibrinogen to fibrin, the material that forms the structural matrix of the clot. Both pathways are needed for normal hemostasis. Bleeding, however, when it occurs because of defects in the extrinsic system, is usually not as severe as that which results from defects in the intrinsic pathway. Both systems are activated when blood passes out of the vascular system. The intrinsic system is activated as blood comes in contact with the injured vessel wall and the extrinsic system when blood is exposed to tissue extracts.

The purpose of the coagulation process is to form an insoluble fibrin clot. This process may involve

---

Chart 15–1: Steps in hemostasis

Vessel spasm
Formation of the platelet plug
  Platelet adherence to the vessel wall
  Platelet aggregation to form the platelet plug
Blood coagulation
  Activation of the intrinsic or extrinsic coagulation pathway
  Conversion of prothrombin to thrombin
  Conversion of fibrinogen to fibrin
Clot retraction
Clot dissolution (fibrinolysis)

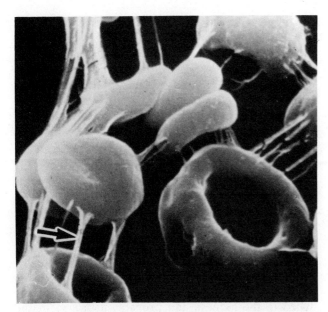

Figure 15-1 Scanning electron micrograph of a blood clot (×5000). The fibrous bridges (indicated by the *arrow*) that form a meshwork between red blood cells are fibrin fibers. (*Chaffee EE, Lytle IM: Basic Physiology and Anatomy, 4th ed. Philadelphia, JB Lippincott, 1980*)

as many as 30 different substances that either promote clotting (procoagulation factors) or inhibit it (anticoagulation factors). The procoagulation factors are identified by Roman numerals (Table 15-1).

Each of the procoagulation factors performs a specific step in the coagulation process. The action of one coagulation factor is usually designed to activate the next factor in the sequence (cascade effect). Some sources identify the activated form of the factor by inserting the subscript *a* after the factor number (factor V_a). Because most of the inactive procoagulation factors are present in the blood at all times, the multistep coagulation process ensures that a massive episode of intravascular clotting does not occur by chance. It also means that abnormalities of the clotting process will occur when one or more of the factors are deficient or when conditions lead to inappropriate activation of any of the steps.

Calcium (factor IV) is required in all but the first two steps of the clotting process. Fortunately, the living body almost always has sufficient calcium to interact in the clotting process. The inactivation of the calcium ion is used to prevent blood that has been removed from the body from clotting. The addition of a citrate-phosphate-dextrose solution to blood stored for transfusion purposes prevents clotting by combining with the calcium ions. Both oxalate and citrate are often added to blood samples used for analysis in the clinical laboratory.

Clot retraction

Clot retraction occurs immediately after the clot has formed. Clot retraction, which requires large

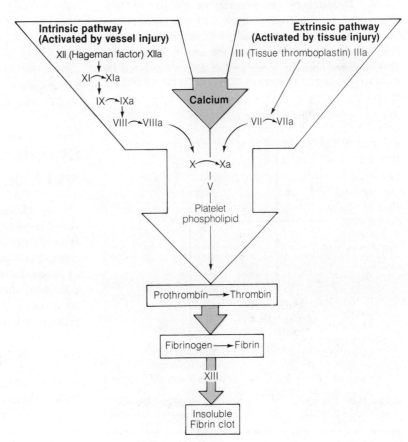

Figure 15-2 The intrinsic and extrinsic coagulation pathways. The terminal steps in both pathways are the same. Calcium, factors X and V, and platelet phospholipids combine to form prothrombin activator; which then converts prothrombin to thrombin. This interaction, in turn, causes conversion of fibrinogen into the fibrin strands that create the insoluble blood clot.

Table 15–1. Procoagulation factors

Factor I	Fibrinogen
Factor II	Prothrombin
Factor III	Tissue thromboplastin
Factor IV	Calcium
Factor V	Proaccelerin, labile factor, A-C globulin
Factor VII	Proconvertin, serum prothrombin conversion accelerator (SPCA)
Factor VIII	Antihemophilic factor (AHF)
Factor IX	Plasma thromboplastin component (PTC), antihemophilic factor B (AH-B), Christmas factor
Factor X	Stuart factor, Stuart–Power factor
Factor XI	Plasma thromboplastin antecedent (PTA)
Factor XII	Hageman factor
Factor XIII	Fibrin stabilizing factor

numbers of platelets, contributes to hemostasis by pulling the edges of the broken vessel together.

Clot dissolution (fibrinolysis)

The dissolution of a blood clot begins shortly after its formation; this allows blood flow to be reestablished and allows tissue repair to take place. The process by which a blood clot dissolves is called fibrinolysis. As with clot formation, clot dissolution requires a sequence of steps (Figure 15-3).

Plasminogen, the proenzyme for the fibrinolytic process, is normally present in the blood in its inactive form. It is converted to its active form, *plasmin,* by plasminogen activators formed in the vascular endothelium and the liver, and is also modulated by

inhibitors. The plasmin formed from plasminogen digests the fibrin strands of the clot as well as other proteins. It also digests certain clotting factors such as fibrinogen, factor V, and factor VIII. Circulating plasmin is rapidly inactivated by alpha$_2$ plasmin inhibitor, which is normally present in high concentrations. This high level of inhibitor protects the clotting factors.

There are two main types of plasminogen activators: tissue-type plasminogen activator (t-PA) and urokinase-type (u-PA).[3] The liver, plasma, and vascular endothelium are the major sources of physiologic activators. They are released in response to a number of stimuli, including vasoactive drugs, elevated body temperature, and exercise. The activators are unstable and rapidly inactivated by inhibitors in the blood and by the liver. For this reason, chronic liver disease may cause altered fibrinolytic activity. Urokinase is produced in the kidneys and probably assists in maintaining the patency of the renal tract by dissolving fibrin deposits in urine.

In summary, hemostasis is designed to maintain the integrity of the vascular compartment. The process is divided into five phases: (1) vessel spasm, which constricts the size of the vessel and reduces blood flow; (2) platelet adherence and formation of the platelet plug; (3) formation of the fibrin clot, which cements the platelet plug together; (4) clot retraction, which pulls the edges of the injured vessel together; and (5) clot dissolution, which involves the action of fibrinolysins that dissolve the clot and allow blood flow to be reestablished and healing of tissues to take place. The process of blood coagulation requires the stepwise activation of coagulation factors, which ensures that the process is not activated by chance.

Disorders of hemostasis and blood coagulation

Hemostasis is normal when it seals a blood vessel thereby preventing blood loss and hemorrhage. It is abnormal when it causes inappropriate blood clotting or when clotting is insufficient to stop the flow of blood from the vascular compartment. Clotting disorders, discussed in the following sections, have been divided into two groups: (1) the hypercoagulability states and (2) bleeding diatheses (disorders).

Hypercoagulability states

All of the components or factors necessary to trigger the intrinsic coagulation pathway are present in the blood at all times. There are two general forms

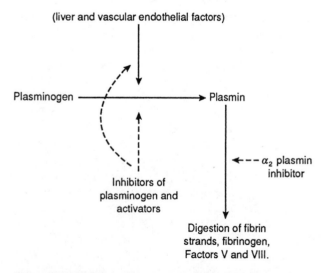

Plasminogen activators

(liver and vascular endothelial factors)

Figure 15-3 The fibrinolytic system and its modifiers. The *solid lines* indicate activation, and the *broken lines* indicate inactivation.

of hypercoagulability states: (1) conditions that create hyperreactivity of the platelet system and (2) conditions that cause accelerated activity of the coagulation system. Current evidence suggests that hyperreactivity of the platelet system results in arterial thrombosis and that increased activity of the clotting system causes venous thrombosis and its sequelae.[4] Chart 15-2 summarizes conditions commonly associated with hypercoagulability states.

Hyperreactivity of platelet function

The causes of increased platelet function tend to be twofold: (1) disturbances in flow and changes in the vessel wall and (2) increased sensitivity of platelets to factors that cause adhesiveness and aggregation. Atherosclerotic plaques disturb flow and render the inner lining of the arterial wall more susceptible to platelet adherence.

Platelets adhering to the vessel wall release growth factors that cause proliferation of smooth muscle and thereby contribute to the development of atherosclerosis. Smoking, elevated levels of blood lipids and cholesterol, hemodynamic stress, and immune mechanisms may cause vessel damage, platelet adherence, and eventually thrombosis. Diabetes mellitus increases the incidence of atherosclerosis by these vessel and platelet mechanisms.

Increased clotting activity

Factors that increase the activation of the coagulation system are (1) stasis of flow and (2) alterations in the coagulation components of the blood (either an increase in procoagulation factors or a decrease in anticoagulation factors). Stasis reduces the clearance of activated clotting factors by the liver and prevents their interactions with inhibitors. Venous thrombosis usually begins in regions of slow and disturbed flow. Venous thrombosis is a common event in the immobilized and postsurgical patient. Heart failure also contributes to venous congestion and thrombosis. Blood coagulation factors have been found to be increased in women using oral contraceptive agents. The incidence of stroke, thromboemboli, and myocardial infarction is greater among women who use oral contraceptives than among those who do not. Clotting factors are also increased during normal pregnancy; these changes, along with limited activity during the puerperium, predispose to venous thrombosis. Another condition that predisposes to hypercoagulability is malignant disease. Many tumor cells are thought to release procoagulation factors, which, along with the increased immobility and sepsis seen in patients with malignant disease, contribute to the increased incidence of thrombosis in these patients.

A reduction in anticoagulants such as antithrombin III, protein C and protein S predisposes to venous thrombosis.[5] Deficiencies of these inhibitor proteins may be inherited, but they are also found in liver disease and protein-losing disorders.

Bleeding disorders

As with hypercoagulability states, bleeding disorders or impairment of blood coagulation can result from defects in any of the factors that contribute to hemostasis. Defects are associated with platelets, coagulation factors, and vascular integrity.

Platelet defects

Bleeding can occur as a result of a decrease in the number of circulating platelets (thrombocytopenia) or impaired platelet function (thrombocytopathia).

Platelets are produced by cells in the bone marrow and are then stored in the spleen before being released into the circulation. Consequently, a decrease in the number of circulating platelets can result from a decrease in platelet production by the bone marrow, an increased pooling of platelets in the spleen, or decreased platelet survival. Replacement of bone marrow by malignant cells, such as occurs in leukemia, impairs the bone marrow's ability to produce platelets. Radiation and drugs such as those used in the treatment of cancer often depress bone-marrow function and cause reduced platelet production (thrombocytopenia). On the other hand, there may be normal production of platelets but excessive pooling of platelets in the spleen. Normally the spleen sequesters about 30% to 40% of the platelets. When the spleen is enlarged (splenomegaly), however, as many as 80% of the platelets can be sequestered in the spleen.

Another cause of thrombocytopenia is the ab-

Chart 15–2: Conditions associated with hypercoagulability states

Hyperreactivity of platelets
  Atherosclerosis
  Diabetes mellitus
  Smoking
  Elevated blood lipids and cholesterol
  Increased platelet levels

Accelerated activity of the clotting system
  Pregnancy and the puerperium
  Use of oral contraceptives
  Postsurgical state
  Immobility
  Congestive heart failure
  Malignant diseases

normal destruction of platelets that is thought to result from an autoimmune response in which the body produces antibodies against its own platelets. Immune thrombocytopenia may follow a viral infection, ingestion of certain drugs, or may be idiopathic, that is, unrelated to any known cause. In acute disseminated intravascular clotting, discussed later, excessive platelet consumption leads to a deficiency.

Thrombocytopathia is a failure of platelet adherence and aggregation and is seen in a number of conditions. Aspirin, which inhibits the production of thromboxane A_2 required for platelet aggregation, is one of the most common causes of this impairment. The effect of aspirin on platelet aggregation lasts for the life of the platelet—usually about 7 to 8 days. In a study in which maternal ingestion of aspirin occurred within 5 days of delivery, six of ten mothers and nine of ten infants had bleeding tendencies.[6] The recent interest in aspirin's effect on hemostasis has been not so much in its ability to cause bleeding as its ability to prevent blood clotting. Chart 15-3 describes other drugs that impair platelet function.

The depletion of platelets must be relatively severe (10,000–20,000 per mm^3 compared with the normal values of 150,000–200,000 per mm^3) before hemorrhagic tendencies become evident. Bleeding that results from platelet deficiencies is usually spontaneous and affects the small vessels of the skin and mucous membranes. Bleeding of the intracranial vessels is also a danger with severe platelet depletion.

—— Coagulation defects

Impairment of blood coagulation can result from deficiencies in one or more of the known clotting factors. Deficiencies can arise because of defective synthesis, production of inactive factors, or increased consumption of the clotting factors.

Impaired synthesis. Coagulation factors V, VII, IX, X, and XIII, prothrombin, fibrinogen, and probably factors XI and XII are synthesized in the liver. Factor VIII is synthesized in the endothelial cells.

Of the coagulation factors synthesized in the liver, factors VII, IX, and X, and prothrombin require the presence of vitamin K for normal activity. In liver disease synthesis of these clotting factors is reduced. In vitamin K deficiency, the liver produces the clotting factor but in an inactive form. Vitamin K is a fat-soluble vitamin that is being continuously synthesized by intestinal bacteria. This means that a deficiency in vitamin K is not likely to occur unless intestinal synthesis is interrupted or absorption of the vitamin is impaired. Vitamin K deficiency can occur in the newborn infant prior to establishment of the intestinal flora and can also occur as a result of treatment with broad-spectrum antibiotics that cause destruction of

---

Chart 15–3: Drugs that may predispose to bleeding

Interference with platelet production or function

Acetazolamide
Alcohol
Antihistamines
Antimetabolite and anticancer drugs
Aspirin and salicylates
Chloramphenicol
Clofibrate
Colchicine
Dextran
Dipyridamole
Diuretics (furosemide, ethacrynic acid, and the thiazide diuretics)
Gold therapy
Heparin
Lidocaine
Nonsteroidal anti-inflammatory drugs
Penicillins
Phenylbutazone
Propranolol
Quinine derivatives (quinidine and hydroxychloroquine)
Sulfonamides
Theophylline
Tricyclic antidepressants
Vitamin E

Interference with coagulation factors

Amiodarone
Anabolic steroids
Coumadin
Heparin
Thyroid preparations

Decrease in Vitamin K levels

Antibiotics
Clofibrate

(Data from Hansten P [ed]: Drug Interactions, 6th ed. Philadelphia, Lea & Febiger, 1989; Koda-Kimble MA [ed]: Applied Therapeutics for Clinical Pharmacists, 4th ed, p 260. San Francisco, Applied Therapeutics, 1988; and Packman MA, Mustard JF: Clinical pharmacology of platelets. Blood 50 [4], 1977)

---

intestinal flora. Because vitamin K is a fat-soluble vitamin, its absorption requires bile salts. A vitamin K deficiency, therefore, may result from impaired fat absorption due to liver or gallbladder disease.

Hereditary defects. Hereditary defects have been reported for each of the clotting factors; most, however, are rare diseases. The two most common defects are hemophilia A (factor VIII deficiency) and hemophilia B (factor IX deficiency). Factor VIII defects account for 80% to 85% of the total cases of hemophilia, while factor IX defects make up the remainder of cases. The clinical manifestations and genetics are similar for both diseases.

Hemophilia is a sex-linked recessive disorder that primarily affects males. Although it is a hereditary disorder, there is no family history of the disorder in about one-third of newly diagnosed cases, suggesting that it has arisen as a new mutation.[7] Factor VIII is probably produced by the endothelial cells and the liver. About 90% of persons with hemophilia produce insufficient quantities of the factor, and 10% produce a defective form. An individual with normal coagulation function possesses 50% to 200% of factor VIII or factor IX levels.[8] In hemophilia, the amount is only 1% to 20%, with 5% to 20% in mild hemophilia, 1% to 5% in moderate hemophilia, and 1% or less in severe forms of hemophilia.[8] In mild or moderate forms of the disease, bleeding usually does not occur unless there is a local lesion or trauma. The disorder may not be detected in childhood. On the other hand, in severe hemophilia, bleeding is usually present in childhood (it may be noted at the time of circumcision) and tends to be both spontaneous and severe. Spontaneous hemorrhage into joints is damaging and is a frequent cause of disability. Prevention of bleeding is the primary concern with hemophilia. In childhood, attempts should be made to avoid or minimize injury by providing safe clothing and toys and encouraging participation in noncontact sports. When bleeding occurs, factor VIII replacement therapy is initiated.

Cryoprecipitate, which is prepared from fresh-frozen plasma, contains factor VIII in concentrated form. Prior to infectious disease testing of blood products, cryoprecipitate prepared from multiple donor samples carried the risk of exposure to viruses for hepatitis B; non-A, non-B hepatitis; and AIDS. Cryoprecipitate is now safer, but should be used only for newly diagnosed children and preferably should be prepared from a small number of tested donors.[7] Safer, highly purified factor VIII and factor IX concentrates are now available for persons with severe deficiencies. Pasteurized or antibody-purified concentrates have reduced the transmission of hepatitis viruses and human immunodeficiency virus (HIV). In addition, the lyophilized concentrates make self-administration at home very convenient. In the future, synthetic factor VIII will likely be produced by recombinant DNA techniques and will eliminate the risk of disease transmission.

Von Willebrand's disease is a common hereditary bleeding disorder most often diagnosed in adulthood. It is transmitted as an autosomal trait and is due to a deficiency of von Willebrand (vW) factor. This factor acts as a carrier protein for factor VIII and causes platelets to adhere to the subendothelial tissue. Deficiency of vW factor is often accompanied by reduced levels of factor VIII and results in defective clot formation. Symptoms include bruising and bleeding from the nose, mouth and gastrointestinal tract, and excessive menstrual flow. Persons with the disorder are often diagnosed when surgery or dental extraction results in prolonged bleeding.[7] In severe cases, cryoprecipitate is infused to replace vW factor and factor VIII. Many persons can now be treated with desmopressin acetate (DDAVP), a synthetic analogue of the hormone vasopressin, which stimulates the endothelial cells to release the deficient vW factor and factor VIII.[9] DDAVP can also be used to treat mild hemophilia A.

Abnormal consumption. Acute disseminated intravascular clotting (DIC) is a paradox in the hemostatic sequence in which blood coagulation, clot dissolution, and bleeding all take place at the same time. The condition begins with activation of the coagulation system with formation of microemboli and is accompanied by consumption of specific clotting factors, aggregation, and loss of platelets and activation of the fibrinolytic mechanisms responsible for clot dissolution.

Disseminated intravascular clotting is not a primary disorder; it occurs as a complication in a variety of disease conditions. The coagulation process can be initiated by activation of either the extrinsic coagulation pathway, through liberation of tissue factors, or the intrinsic pathway, through extensive endothelial damage or stasis of blood. Among the clinical conditions known to incite DIC are massive trauma, burns, sepsis, shock, meningococcemia, and malignant disease. About 50% of individuals with DIC are patients with obstetrical complications. Chart 15-4 summarizes the conditions that have been associated with DIC.

Chart 15–4: Conditions that have been associated with disseminated intravascular clotting (DIC)

Obstetric conditions
Abruptio placenta
Dead fetus syndrome
Preeclampsia and eclampsia
Amniotic fluid embolism

Malignancies
Metastatic cancer
Leukemia

Infections
Acute bacterial infection (*e.g.,* meningococcal meningitis)
Acute viral infections
Rickettsial infections (*e.g.,* Rocky Mountain spotted fever)
Parasitic infections (*e.g.,* malaria)

Shock
Septic shock
Severe hypovolemic shock

Trauma or surgery
Burns
Massive trauma
Surgery involving extracorporeal circulation
Snake bite
Heat stroke

Hematologic conditions
Blood transfusion reactions

Secondary activation of the fibrinolytic system is localized at the sites of intravascular clotting. Breakdown of the fibrin, however, leads to release of products that prevent conversion of fibrinogen to fibrin and thus to further bleeding problems.

Although the coagulation and formation of microemboli initiate the events that occur in DIC, its acute manifestations are usually more directly related to the bleeding problems that occur. The bleeding may be present as petechiae, purpura, or severe hemorrhage. Uncontrolled postpartum bleeding may indicate DIC. Microemboli may cause tissue hypoxia and damage to organ structures. The kidney is usually the most severely damaged organ, but there may also be damage to the heart, lungs, and brain. A form of hemolytic anemia may develop as red cells become damaged when they pass through vessels partially blocked by thrombus.

The treatment for DIC is directed toward the primary disease, correcting the bleeding, and preventing further activation of clotting mechanisms. Heparin may be given to decrease blood coagulation, thereby interrupting the process that leads to consumption of coagulation factors and secondary activation of the fibrinolytic system. It is usually given as a continuous intravenous infusion that can be interrupted promptly if bleeding is accentuated. Fresh coagulation factors in the form of platelets, cryoprecipitate, or fresh-frozen plasma may be used in case of uncontrolled hemorrhage. E-aminocaproic acid, which is a powerful antifibrinolytic agent, may be used when hemorrhage is severe.[10]

Vascular disorders

Vascular disorders cause easy bruising and spontaneous bleeding from small blood vessels. These disorders occur because of structurally weak vessels or vessels that have been damaged by inflammation or immune responses. Among the vascular disorders that cause bleeding are hemorrhagic telangiectasia (an uncommon autosomal dominant trait in which there are dilatations of capillaries and arterioles), vitamin C deficiency (scurvy), Cushing's disease, and senile purpura (bruising in the elderly). Vascular defects also occur in the course of DIC as a result of the presence of the microthrombi and corticosteroid therapy. Vascular disorders are characterized by easy bruising and spontaneous appearance of petechiae and purpura of the skin and mucous membranes. In persons with bleeding disorders due to vascular defects, the platelet count and other tests for coagulation defects are normal.

Effects of drugs on hemostasis

A number of drugs serve to either enhance or impair hemostasis. Oral contraceptives and the corticosteroid drugs are associated with an increase in coagulation factors. Drugs that impair platelet production or function and those that interfere with coagulation are summarized in Chart 15-3. Two drugs are commonly used as anticoagulant agents—heparin and Coumadin, and several newer drugs are used to treat or prevent thrombosis.

Warfarin

The oral anticoagulant drug warfarin acts by decreasing prothrombin and other procoagulation factors that require vitamin K for biologic activity. Warfarin acts at the level of the liver and competes with vitamin K during the synthesis of the vitamin K-dependent coagulation factors. Because the relationship between vitamin K and warfarin is competitive, vitamin K is used as the antidote for warfarin overdose.

Heparin

Heparin is an anticoagulant found in many body cells. It is formed in large quantities in mast cells located in the pericapillary connective tissues and in the basophilic cells of the blood. Pharmacologic preparations of heparin are extracted from animal tissues. Heparin must be injected because it is not absorbed in the gastrointestinal tract. Heparin requires the presence of antithrombin III for its ability to inhibit blood clotting. The heparin–antithrombin III complex accelerates the inactivation of the clotting factors of the intrinsic pathway and inhibits the action of thrombin on fibrinogen.

Thrombolytic agents

A number of thrombolytic enzymes have been purified to treat thrombi and emboli. Two of the plasminogen activators used are streptokinase and urokinase. Streptokinase, a protein elaborated by certain β-hemolytic streptococci, is used in the treatment of coronary artery occlusion (see Chapter 21). The enzyme combines with plasminogen to form plasmin and activate the fibrinolytic pathway. Normal urine contains urokinase, which is elaborated and excreted by the kidneys. A new generation of potent, fibrin-specific agents include t-PA as well as other forms of streptokinase and urokinase. Genetically engineered t-PA can be used in low doses to treat pulmonary embolism and venous thrombosis, and to limit acute myocardial infarction.[11]

In summary, there are two types of disorders of hemostasis and blood clotting: (1) hypercoagulability states and (2) bleeding disorders. Hypercoagulability causes excessive clotting and contributes to thrombus formation. It results from conditions that cause hyperreactivity of platelets or accelerated activity of the clotting system. Bleeding disorders result from impaired formation of the platelet plug that seals the vessels or from defects in the coagulation process. The formation of the platelet plug is impaired when the number of platelets is deficient (because of inadequate production, excessive pooling in the spleen, or excessive destruction) or adherence or aggregation is defective (because of aspirin and other drug effects). Deficiencies of clotting factors can arise because of inadequate synthesis (resulting from liver disease or vitamin K deficiency), production of inactive factors (from hemophilia), or increased consumption (from DIC).

References

1. Hirsh J, Brain EA: Hemostasis and Thrombosis: A Conceptual Approach, 2nd ed, pp 105, 146. New York, Churchill Livingstone, 1983
2. Hawiger J: Adhesive interactions of blood cells and the vessel wall. In Colman RW, Hirsh J, Marder VJ et al (eds): Hemostasis and Thrombosis, 2nd ed, p 182. Philadelphia, JB Lippincott, 1987
3. Robbins KC: The plasminogen-plasmin enzyme system. In Colman RW, Hirsh J, Marder VJ et al (eds): Hemostasis and Thrombosis, 2nd ed, p 343. Philadelphia, JB Lippincott, 1987
4. Arkin CF, Hartman AS: The hypercoagulability states. CRC Crit Rev Clin Lab Sci 10:397, 1979
5. Comp PC, Clouse L: Plasma proteins C and S: The function and assay of two natural anticoagulants. Lab Man 23:29, 1985
6. Stuart MJ, Gross MJ, Elrad H et al: Effects of acetylsalicylic-acid ingestion on maternal or neonatal hemostasis. N Engl J Med 307:909, 1982
7. Rapaport SI: Introduction to Hematology, 2nd ed, pp 510, 528. Philadelphia, JB Lippincott, 1987
8. Levine PH: Clinical manifestations and therapy of hemophilias A and B. In Colman RW, Hirsh J, Marder VJ et al: Hemostasis and Thrombosis, 2nd ed, p 97. Philadelphia, JB Lippincott, 1987
9. Lusher JM: Desmopressin acetate (DDAVP): Its use in disorders of hemostasis. Thromb Haemost 6:385, 1984
10. Merskey C: DIC: Identification and management. Hosp Pract 17:83, 1982
11. Collen D, Stump DC, Gold HK: Thrombolytic therapy. Annu Rev Med 39:405, 1988

Bibliography

Beller FK, Ebert C: Effects of oral contraceptives on blood coagulation. A review. Obstet Gynecol Surv 40:425, 1985

Bennett JS: Blood coagulation and coagulation tests. Med Clin North Am 68:557, 1984

Blanchard RA, Furie BC, Jorgensen M et al: Acquired vitamin K-dependent carboxylation deficiency in liver disease. N Engl J Med 305:242, 1981

Carr ME: Disseminated intravascular coagulation: Pathogenesis, diagnosis, and therapy. J Emerg Med 5:311, 1987

Chang JC: White clot syndrome associated with heparin-induced thrombocytopenia: A review of 23 cases. Heart Lung 16:403, 1987

Clouse LH, Comp PC: The regulation of hemostasis: The protein C system. N Engl J Med 314:1298, 1986

Gerrard JM: Platelet aggregation: Cellular regulation and physiologic role. Hosp Pract 23:89, 1988

Gill FM: Congenital bleeding disorders: Hemophilia and von Willebrand's disease. Med Clin North Am 68:601, 1984

Harrington WJ, Ahn YN, Byrnes JJ et al: Treatment of idiopathic thrombocytopenic purpura. Hosp Pract 18(9):205, 1983

Hoyer LW: Factor VIII: New perspectives. Transfusion Med Rev 1:113, 1987

Jaffe EA: Physiologic functions of normal endothelial cells. Ann NY Acad Sci 454:279, 1985

Larner AJ: The molecular pathology of haemophilia. Q J Med 63:473, 1987

Levine PH: Acquired immunodeficiency syndrome in persons with hemophilia. Ann Intern Med 103:723, 1985

Marcus AJ: Aspirin as an antithrombotic medication. N Engl J Med 309:1515, 1983

Mielke CH: Influence of aspirin on platelets and the bleeding time. Am J Med 72:72, 1983

Moroose R, Hoyer LW: Von Willebrand factor and platelet function. Annu Rev Med 37:157, 1986

Oberle I, Camerino G, Heilig R et al: Genetic screening for hemophilia A (classic hemophilia) with a polymorphic DNA probe. N Engl J Med 312:682, 1985

Ragni NI, Tegtmeier GE, Levy JA et al: AIDS retrovirus antibodies in hemophiliacs treated with factor VIII or factor IX concentrates, cryoprecipitate or fresh frozen plasma: Prevalence, seroconversion rate and clinical correlations. Blood 67:592, 1986

Schafer AI: Bleeding disorders: Finding the cause. Hosp Pract 19(11):88K, 1984

Sharma GV, Cella G, Parisi AF et al: Thrombolytic therapy. N Engl J Med 306:1268, 1982

Van de Werf F, Vanhaecke J, DeGeest H et al: Coronary thrombolysis with recombinant single-chain urokinase-type plasminogen activator in patients with acute myocardial infarction. Circulation 74:1066, 1986

Weintrub PS: Hemophilia A: Virus transmission and immunity in factor VIII therapy. Lab Man 25:53, 1987

Wessler S, Gitel SN: Warfarin: From bedside to bench. N Engl J Med 311:645, 1984

Alterations in Oxygenation of Tissues

The Red Blood Cell and Alterations in Oxygen Transport

Objectives

After you have studied this chapter, you should be able to meet the following objectives:

_____ Trace the development of a red blood cell from erythroblast to erythrocyte.

_____ Describe the formation, transport, and elimination of bilirubin.

_____ Explain the function of the enzyme G6PD in the red blood cell.

_____ Describe the manifestations of anemia and their mechanisms.

_____ Explain the difference between intravascular and extravascular hemolysis.

_____ Cite the factors that predispose to hyperbilirubinemia in the infant.

_____ Explain the action of phototherapy in the treatment of hyperbilirubinemia in the newborn.

_____ Describe the pathogenesis of hemolytic disease of the newborn.

_____ Compare conjugated and unconjugated bilirubin in terms of production of encephalopathy in the neonate.

_____ Compare the hemoglobinopathies associated with sickle cell anemia and thalassemia.

_____ Explain the cause of sickling in sickle cell anemia.

_____ Cite the criteria for nutritional anemia.

_____ Cite common causes of iron-deficiency anemia in infancy and adolescence.

_____ Describe the relationship between vitamin B_{12} deficiency and megaloblastic anemia.

_____ List three causes of bone-marrow depression.

_____ Compare characteristics of the red blood cells in acute blood loss, hereditary spherocytosis, sickle cell anemia, iron-deficiency anemia, and aplastic anemia.

_____ Compare polycythemia vera and secondary polycythemia.

_____ Differentiate between red cell antigens and antibodies in persons with type A, B, AB, and O blood.

_____ Explain the determination of the Rh factor.

_____ List signs and symptoms of a blood transfusion reaction.

Although the lungs provide the means for gas exchange between the external and internal environment, it is the hemoglobin in the red blood cells that transports oxygen to the tissues. The red blood cells also function as carriers of carbon dioxide and participate in acid–base balance. The function of the red blood cells, in terms of oxygen transport, is discussed in Chapter 24, and acid–base balance is covered in Chapter 29. This chapter presents a discussion of the red blood cell, anemia, and polycythemia.

The red blood cell

The red blood cell (erythrocyte) is a concave, spherical disk (Figure 16-1). This shape serves to increase the surface area available for diffusion of oxygen and allows the cell to change in volume and shape without rupturing its membrane. The biconcave form presents the plasma with a surface 20 to 30 times greater than if the red blood cell were an absolute sphere. The erythrocytes, 500 to 1000 times more numerous than other blood cells, are the most common type of blood cell.

The function of the red blood cell, facilitated by the hemoglobin molecule, is to transport oxygen to the tissues. In addition, hemoglobin binds some carbon dioxide and carries it from the tissues to the lungs. The hemoglobin molecule is composed of two pairs of structurally different polypeptide chains. Each of the four polypeptide chains is attached to a heme unit,

which, in turn, surrounds an atom of iron that binds oxygen. The rate at which hemoglobin is synthesized depends on the availability of iron for heme synthesis. Lack of iron results in relatively small amounts of hemoglobin in the red blood cells.

There are two types of normal hemoglobin: adult hemoglobin (HbA) and fetal hemoglobin (HbF). *Adult hemoglobin* consists of a pair of α chains and a pair of β chains. *Fetal hemoglobin* is the predominant hemoglobin in the fetus from the third through the ninth month of gestation. It has a pair of γ chains substituted for the β chains. Because of this chain substitution, fetal hemoglobin has a high affinity for oxygen. This facilitates the transfer of oxygen across the placenta. Fetal hemoglobin is replaced soon after birth with adult hemoglobin.

Red cell production and regulation

Erythropoiesis is the production of red blood cells. After birth, the red cells are produced in the red bone marrow. Until the age of 5 years, almost all bones produce red cells to meet growth needs. Following this period, bone-marrow activity gradually declines; after age 20, red cell production takes place mainly in the membranous bones of the vertebrae, sternum, ribs, and pelvis. With this lessened activity, the red bone marrow is replaced with fatty yellow bone marrow.

The red cells derive from the erythroblasts, which are continuously being formed from the primordial stem cells in the bone marrow. In developing into a mature red cell, the primordial stem cell moves through a series of stages—*erythroblast* to *normoblast* to *reticulocyte* and finally to *erythrocyte* (Figure 16-2). Hemoglobin synthesis begins at the erythroblast stage and continues until the cell becomes an erythrocyte. During its transformation from normoblast to reticulocyte, the red blood cell loses its nucleus. Normally, the period from stem cell to emergence of the reticulocyte in the circulation takes about a week. Maturation of reticulocyte to erythrocyte takes about 24 to 48 hours, and during this process the red cell loses its mitochondria and ribosomes along with its ability to produce hemoglobin and engage in oxidative metabolism. Most maturing red cells enter the blood as reticulocytes. Normally about 1% of the red blood cells are generated from bone marrow each day, and therefore the reticulocyte count serves as an index of the erythropoietic activity of the bone marrow.

The red cell relies on glucose and the glycolytic pathway for its metabolic needs. It relies on the enzyme-mediated anaerobic metabolism of glucose for the generation of the adenosine triphosphate (ATP) needed for normal membrane function and ion trans-

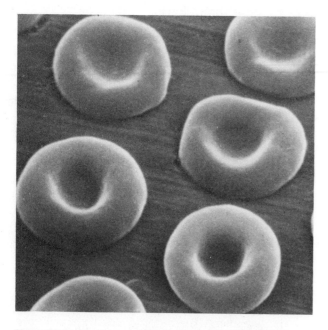

Figure 16-1 Scanning micrograph of normal red blood cells (×5000). The normal concave disk appearance of these cells is apparent. (*Courtesy of STEM Laboratories and Fischer Scientific Company*)

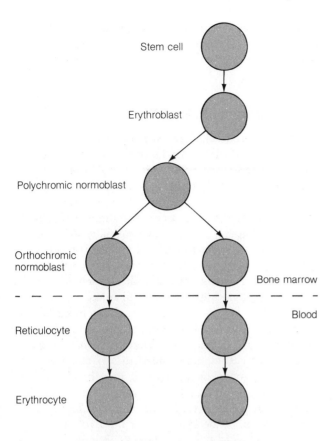

Stem cell

Erythroblast

Polychromic normoblast

Orthochromic normoblast

Bone marrow

Blood

Reticulocyte

Erythrocyte

Figure 16-2 Red blood cell development.

port. Depletion of glucose or the functional deficiency of one of the glycolytic enzymes leads to the premature death of the red blood cell. Another essential enzyme pathway in the red cell is needed to maintain hemoglobin in the reduced state and prevent the formation of methemoglobin, which is nonfunctional and reduces oxygen transport. The enzyme glucose 6-phosphate dehydrogenase (G6PD) is essential to the function of this pathway. A deficiency of this enzyme can lead to denaturing of hemoglobin with hemolysis of the red blood cell. A third pathway provides a large amount of 2,3-diphosphoglycerate (2,3-DPG), which plays an important role in reducing the affinity of hemoglobin for oxygen, thereby facilitating its release at the tissue level.[1]

Erythropoiesis is governed, for the most part, by tissue oxygen needs. *Hypoxia is the main stimulus for red cell production.* Hypoxia does not, however, act directly on the bone marrow. Instead, red cell production by the bone marrow is regulated by the hormone *erythropoietin.* Erythropoietin, a glycoprotein with a molecular weight of about 40,000, is released in response to hypoxia, although the precise mechanism of its formation is unclear. It is known that erythropoietin levels are lower in persons with impaired kidney function and in those who have had a kidney removed. The kidneys, responding to hypoxia, produce

the majority of the hormone. About 5% to 10% is probably released by the liver.[2]

Erythropoietin takes several days to effect release of red blood cells from the bone marrow, and only after 5 or more days does red blood cell production reach maximum. Because red blood cells are released into the blood as reticulocytes, the percentage of these cells in relation to the total red blood cell count is higher when there is a marked increase in red blood cell production. In some severe anemias, for example, the reticulocytes may account for as much as 30% to 50% of the total.[3] In some situations, red cell production is so accelerated that numerous normoblasts appear in the blood. Human erythropoietin, produced by DNA-recombinant technology, is now available for use in treating anemia in persons with end-stage renal disease and may have potential use in persons with sickle cell anemia and those anticipating blood loss during surgery.[4]

Red cell destruction

Mature red blood cells have a life span of about 4 months or 120 days. As the red blood cell ages, a number of changes occur. The metabolic activities within the cell decrease; enzyme activity falls off; and ATP, potassium, and membrane lipids decrease. Normally the rate of red cell destruction (1% per day) is equal to red cell production, but in some conditions, such as hemolytic anemia, the cell's life span may be shorter.

Destruction of red blood cells is accomplished by a group of large phagocytic cells found in the spleen, liver, bone marrow, and lymph nodes. These phagocytic cells ingest and destroy the erythrocytes in a series of enzymatic reactions during which the amino acids from the globulin chains and iron from the heme units are salvaged and reutilized. The bulk of the heme unit is converted to bilirubin (the pigment of bile), which is insoluble in plasma and attaches to the plasma proteins for transport. Bilirubin is removed from the blood by the liver and conjugated with glucuronide to render it water-soluble so that it can be excreted in the bile. The plasma-insoluble form of bilirubin is referred to as unconjugated bilirubin, and the water-soluble form is referred to as conjugated bilirubin. Serum levels of conjugated and unconjugated bilirubin can be measured in the laboratory using the Van der Bergh test, which is described in Chapter 41.[5]

If the rate of bilirubin production is excessive and the ability to conjugate and excrete bilirubin is deficient, excess unconjugated bilirubin will accumulate in the blood. This not only results in a yellow discoloration of the skin (jaundice), but because unconjugated bilirubin is lipid-soluble it can cross neuronal cell membranes. In infants this can cause bilirubin encephalopathy. Such damage may be subtle and may not be apparent for several years, or it may cause a severe neurologic condition called *kernicterus,* which can cause visual–motor defects, deafness, cerebral palsy, mental retardation, and even death. Hyperbilirubinemia is most apt to occur in sick and immature infants, but it can occur in normal newborns as well. The condition affects 50% of newborns, but only 10% require treatment.[5] Unconjugated bilirubin cannot cross the cell membrane as long as it remains bound to albumin or other plasma proteins. Many factors combine to raise serum bilirubin levels in the newborn, including hypoalbuminemia (common in the newborn), acidosis, sepsis, hypoxia, hemolytic disease of the newborn (to be discussed), dehydration, and certain drugs that compete for bilirubin-binding sites on albumin.

Two types of treatment are used for hyperbilirubinemia in the newborn: exchange transfusions and phototherapy. Bilirubin is photolabile. Under visible light in the absorption range of 450 nm to 500 nm, bilirubin is broken down to a less lipid-soluble form, which is readily excreted by the liver. Whole body radiation can be used. Phototherapy units, consisting of banks of eight to ten fluorescent lamps placed about 2 feet above the skin surface of the infant, are generally used.

When red blood cell destruction takes place in the vascular circulation, as in hemolytic anemia, the hemoglobin remains in the plasma. The plasma contains a hemoglobin-binding protein called haptoglobin. Other plasma proteins, such as albumin, may also bind hemoglobin. With extensive intravascular destruction of red blood cells, hemoglobin levels may exceed the hemoglobin-binding capacity of haptoglobin. When this happens, free hemoglobin appears in the blood (hemoglobinemia) and is excreted in the urine (hemoglobinuria). Because this can occur in hemolytic transfusion reactions, urine samples are tested for free hemoglobin following a transfusion reaction.

Laboratory tests

The red cells can be studied by means of a sample of blood (Table 16-1). In the laboratory, modern automated blood cell counters provide rapid and accurate measurements of red cell content and cell indices. The *red blood cell count (RBC)* measures the *total number* of RBCs in a cubic millimeter of blood. The *percentage of reticulocytes* (normally about 1%) provides an index of the rate of red cell production. The *hemoglobin* (grams per 100 ml of blood) measures the *hemoglobin content* of the blood. The major components of the blood are the red cell mass and plasma volume. The *hematocrit* measures the volume of red cell mass in 100 ml of plasma volume. To determine the hematocrit, a sample of blood is placed in a glass tube, which is then centrifuged to separate the cells and the plasma. The hematocrit may be deceptive, because it varies with the quantity of extracellular fluid present, rising with dehydration and falling with overexpansion of the extracellular fluid volume.

The word *corpuscle* means "little body." The *mean corpuscular volume (MCV)* reflects the *volume* or *size* of the red cells. The MCV falls in microcytic anemia and rises in macrocytic anemia. The *mean corpuscular hemoglobin concentration (MCHC)* is the *concentration of hemoglobin* in each cell, and it decreases in hypochromic anemia. Mean cell hemoglobin (MCH) refers to the mass of the red cell and is less useful in classifying anemias. A stained red cell study gives information about the size, color, and shape of the red blood cells. They may be normocytic (of nor-

Table 16–1. Standard laboratory values for red blood cells

Test	Normal values	Significance
Red blood cell count (RBC)		
Men	4.2–5.4 million/mm³	Number of red cells in the blood
Women	3.6–5 million/mm³	
Reticulocytes	1.0%–1.5% of total RBC	Rate of red cell production
Hemoglobin (Hb)		
Men	14–16.5 g/100 ml	Hemoglobin content of the blood
Women	12–15 g/100 ml	
Hematocrit (HCT)		
Men	40%–50%	Volume of cells in 100 ml of blood
Women	37%–47%	
Mean corpuscular volume (MCV)	85–100 fL/red cell	Size of the red cell
Mean corpuscular hemoglobin concentration (MCHC)	31–35 g/100 ml	Concentration of hemoglobin in the red cell
Mean cell hemoglobin (MCH)	27–34 pg/cell	Red cell mass

mal size), microcytic (of small size), or macrocytic (of large size); normochromic (of normal color) or hypochromic (of decreased color).

Bone-marrow function in blood cell production is studied by means of the *bone-marrow smear,* in which the marrow is aspirated with a short, rigid sharp-pointed needle equipped with a stylet.

In summary, the red blood cell provides the means for transport of oxygen from the lungs to the tissues. The red cells develop from stem cells in the bone marrow and are released into the blood as reticulocytes, where they become mature erythrocytes. The life span of a red cell is about 120 days. Red cell destruction normally occurs in the spleen, liver, bone marrow, and lymph nodes. In the process of destruction the heme portion of the hemoglobin molecule is converted to bilirubin. Bilirubin, which is insoluble in plasma, attaches to plasma proteins for transport in the blood. It is removed from the blood by the liver and conjugated to a water-soluble form so that it can be excreted in the bile.

Anemia

Anemia is a condition in which an abnormally low number of circulating red blood cells, abnormally low hemoglobin, or both occur. There may be (1) excessive loss (bleeding) or destruction (hemolysis) of red blood cells or (2) deficient red cell production because of a lack of iron or other nutritional elements or bone-marrow failure (aplastic anemia).

Manifestations

Anemia is not a disease but rather an indication of some disease process or alteration in body function. The manifestations of anemia can be grouped into three categories: (1) impaired oxygen transport, (2) alterations in red cell structure, and (3) signs and symptoms associated with the pathologic process causing the anemia. The manifestations of anemia also depend on its severity and the rapidity of its development. With rapid blood loss, circulatory shock and circulatory collapse may occur. On the other hand, the body tends to adapt to slowly developing anemia, and the loss of red cell mass may be considerable without any signs and symptoms.

Anemia reduces oxygen-carrying capacity and causes tissue hypoxia. The production of 2,3-DPG is a compensatory mechanism that reduces the hemoglobin affinity for oxygen as evidenced by a shift in the oxygen–hemoglobin saturation curve; this causes more oxygen to be released to the tissues rather than remaining bound to hemoglobin.[6] Tissue hypoxia can give rise to angina and night cramps. Fatigue and weakness are common complaints. A redistribution of the blood from the cutaneous tissues causes pallor of the skin, mucous membranes, conjuctiva, and nail beds. Tachycardia and palpitations may occur as the body tries to compensate with a highly metabolic increase in cardiac output. A flow-type systolic murmur, resulting from changes in blood viscosity, may occur. Ventricular hypertrophy and high-output heart failure may develop in severe anemia. Erythropoietin activity is accelerated and may be recognized by diffuse bone pain and sternal tenderness. In addition to the common anemic manifestations, hemolytic anemia is accompanied by jaundice due to increased bilirubin in the blood. In aplastic anemia, petechiae and purpura (red spots due to small vessel bleeding) are the result of reduced platelet function.

Blood loss anemia

With anemia due to bleeding, iron and other components of the erythrocyte are lost from the body. Blood loss may be acute or chronic. In the acute form, there is a risk of hypovolemia and shock rather than anemia (see Chapter 23). The red cells are normal in size and color. A fall in the red blood cell count, hematocrit, and hemoglobin results from hemodilution caused by movement of fluid into the vascular compartment. The hypoxia resulting from blood loss stimulates red cell production by the bone marrow. If the bleeding is controlled and sufficient iron stores are available, the red cell concentration returns to normal within 3 to 4 weeks. Chronic blood loss does not affect the blood volume but instead leads to iron-deficiency anemia (discussed later). Red blood cells are produced with too little hemoglobin, giving rise to microcytic hypochromic anemia.

Hemolytic anemias

Hemolytic anemia is characterized by the premature destruction of red cells with retention in the body of iron and the other products of red cell destruction. Virtually all types of hemolytic anemia are characterized by normocytic and normochromic red cells. Because of the shortened life span of the red cell, the bone marrow is usually hyperactive, resulting in increased numbers of reticulocytes in the circulating blood. As with other types of anemias there is easy fatigability, dyspnea, and other signs of impaired oxygen transport. In addition, mild jaundice is often present. In hemolytic anemia, red cell breakdown can occur within the vascular compartment or it can result from phagocytosis by the reticuloendothelial system. Intravascular hemolysis is manifest by hemoglobinemia and hemoglobinuria.

Hemolytic anemias result from a wide variety of causes. These disorders can be either intrinsic or extrinsic to the red cell. The intrinsic disorders include defects of the red cell membrane, the various hemoglobinopathies, and inherited enzyme defects that cause hemolytic anemia. There are also acquired forms of hemolytic anemia caused by agents extrinsic to the red cell, such as drugs, bacterial and other toxins, antibodies, and trauma.[7] Although all of these disorders cause premature and accelerated destruction of red cells, they cannot all be treated in the same way. Some respond to splenectomy and others to the adrenocorticosteroid hormones, whereas still others do not resolve until the primary disorder is corrected.

Inherited disorders of the red cell membrane

Hereditary spherocytosis, which is inherited as an autosomal dominant trait, is the most common inherited disorder of the red cell membrane. The disorder leads to gradual loss of the membrane surface during the life span of the red blood cell, resulting in a tight sphere instead of a concave disk. While the spherical cell retains its ability to transport oxygen, its shape renders it susceptible to destruction as it passes through the venous sinuses of the splenic circulation.

An aplastic crisis may occur. In the face of a shortened life span, a sudden disruption of red cell production (in most cases caused by a viral infection) causes a rapid drop in hematocrit and hemoglobin levels and a worsening of the anemia, which may be life threatening.

The disorder is usually treated with splenectomy to reduce the red cell destruction. In children, this is usually not done until after age 4 to 5 years to avoid the risk of infectious complications, including septicemia.[7]

Hemoglobinopathies

Abnormalities in hemoglobin structure can lead to accelerated red cell destruction. Two main types of hemoglobinopathies can cause red cell hemolysis: (1) the abnormal substitution of an amino acid in the hemoglobin molecule as in sickle cell anemia and (2) defective synthesis of one of the polypeptide chains that form the globin portion of hemoglobin, as in the thalassemias.

Sickle cell anemia. Sickle cell anemia, affecting approximately 50,000 Americans, is largely a disease of blacks. About one out of every ten black Americans is estimated to carry the trait.[8] In sickle cell anemia, there is a defect of the β chain of the hemoglobin molecule, with an abnormal substitution of a single amino acid. Sickle hemoglobin (HbS) is transmitted by recessive inheritance and can present as either sickle cell trait (heterozygote) or sickle cell disease (homozygote). In the heterozygote only about 40% of the hemoglobin is HgS, whereas in the homozygote almost all of the hemoglobin is HbS. Sickle cell trait is not a mild form of sickle cell anemia, although in severe hypoxia, persons with sickle cell trait may experience some sickling.

In the homozygote, the HbS becomes sickled when deoxygenated. These deformed red blood cells obstruct blood flow in the microcirculation. In order for sickling to occur, one HbS molecule must interact with another. Thus, the person with sickle cell trait who has 60% HbA has little tendency to sickle except in hypoxia. Fetal hemoglobin does not interact with HbS, and therefore the child with sickle cell anemia does not usually begin to experience the effects of the sickling until sometime after 4 to 6 months of age when the fetal hemoglobin has been replaced by HbS.

Factors that precipitate sickling are exertion, infection, other illnesses, hypoxia, acidosis, dehydration, or even such trivial incidents as reduced oxygen tension induced by sleep. Hardly an organ is spared in sickle cell anemia. Affected persons develop severe anemia, painful crises, organ damage, and chronic hyperbilirubinemia. A painful crisis results from vessel occlusion and can appear suddenly in almost any part of the body. The common sites are the abdomen, the chest, and the joints. Infarctions due to sluggish blood flow may cause chronic damage to the liver, spleen, heart, kidney, and other organs. The hyperbilirubinemia resulting from the breakdown products of hemoglobin often leads to production of pigment stones in the gallbladder.

At present, there is no known cure or therapeutic regimen that prevents the problems associated with sickle cell anemia, and treatment is largely supportive. There is an emphasis on avoiding situations that precipitate sickling episodes, such as infections, cold exposure, severe physical exertion, acidosis, and dehydration. Genetic counseling may be of value in family planning.

Thalassemias. In contrast to sickle cell anemia, which involves a single amino acid on the β chain of the hemoglobin molecule, the thalassemias are the result of absent or defective synthesis of either the α or β chains of Hb.[9] The β-thalassemias represent a defect in β-chain synthesis, and the α-thalassemias represent a defect in α-chain synthesis. The defect is inherited as a mendelian trait, and a person may be heterozygous for the trait and have a mild form of the disease or be homozygous and have the full-blown disease. Like sickle cell anemia, the thalassemias occur with high frequency in certain populations. They are most prevalent in Mediterranean populations (e.g., southern Italy and Greece) and in Asian populations (*e.g.,* Thailand, China, and the Philippines). The β-thalassemias, sometimes called *Cooley's anemia* or *Mediterranean anemia,* are most common in Mediterranean populations, and the α-thalassemias are most common among Asians. Both α- and β-thalassemias are common in Africans and American blacks.

Two factors contribute to the anemia that occurs in thalassemia: reduced hemoglobin synthesis and an imbalance in globin chain production. In both α- and β-thalassemia, defective globin chain production leads to deficient hemoglobin production and the development of a hypochromic microcytic anemia. Because only one type of globin chain (either the α chain or the β chain) is affected in the thalassemias, the unaffected type of chain is unable to find a complementary chain for binding. The unpaired chains accumulate in the red cell, contributing to red cell destruction and anemia.

The clinical manifestations of β-thalassemias are based on the severity of the anemia. The presence of one normal gene in heterozygous persons usually results in sufficient normal hemoglobin synthesis to prevent severe anemia. Persons who are homozygous for the trait have very severe transfusion-dependent anemia. The unpaired synthesis of α chains leads to the precipitation of insoluble aggregates or inclusion bodies (Heinz bodies) within the bone-marrow red cell precursors.[10] These inclusion bodies impair DNA synthesis and cause damage to the red cell membrane. Severely affected red cell precursors are destroyed in the bone marrow, and those that escape intramedullary death are at increased risk of destruction in the spleen. Severe growth retardation is present in children with the disorder. With transfusions, survival to the second or third decade is possible.[10] An increased stimulus for hematopoiesis causes bone-marrow expansion and increased iron absorption, and splenomegaly and hepatomegaly result from increased red cell destruction. Bone-marrow expansion leads to thinning of the cortical bone, with new bone formation on the external aspect. Changes are evident on the maxilla and frontal bones of the face. The long bones, ribs, and vertebrae may become vulnerable to fracture. Excess iron stores, which accumulate secondary to increased dietary absorption and intake from repeated transfusions, become deposited in the myocardium, liver, and pancreas to induce organ injury.

Synthesis of the α-globin chains of hemoglobin is controlled by two pairs of (four) genes; hence, the severity of α-thalassemia shows great variations. Silent carriers have deletion of a single α-globin gene. As with β-thalassemia, anemia results from defective hemoglobin production and the accumulation of unpaired globin chains, in this case the β chains. The most severe form of α-thalassemia occurs in infants in whom all four α-globin genes are deleted. Such a defect results in a hemoglobin molecule (Hb Bart's) that is formed exclusively from the α chains of fetal hemoglobin. Hb Bart's, which has an extremely high oxygen affinity, is unable to release oxygen in the tissues. Affected infants suffer from severe hypoxia and are either stillborn or die shortly after birth. Deletion of three of the four α-chain genes leads to unstable aggregates of β chains called *hemoglobin H* (HbH). The β chains are more soluble than the α chains; therefore, their accumulation tends to be less toxic to the red cells, so that senescent rather than precursor red cells are affected. Persons with HbH usually have only mild to moderate hemolytic anemia, and manifestations of ineffective erythropoiesis (bone-marrow expansion and iron overload) are absent.

Inherited enzyme defects

The most common inherited enzyme defect resulting in hemolytic anemia is a deficiency of G6PD. The disorder causes direct oxidation of hemoglobin to methemoglobin and denaturing of the hemoglobin molecule to form *Heinz* bodies. Hemolysis usually occurs as the damaged red blood cells move through the narrow vessels of the spleen causing hemoglobinemia, hemoglobinuria, and jaundice. The gene determining this enzyme is located on the X chromosome, and the defect is expressed only in males and homozygous females. There are a number of genetic variants of this disorder. The African variant has been found in 10% of American blacks.[10] A deficiency of G6PD is thought to protect against malaria, and this may be one of the reasons that the genetic trait has persisted. In blacks, the defect is mildly expressed and is not associated with chronic hemolytic anemia unless exposed to oxidant drugs or chemicals. Numerous oxidant drugs may trigger a hemolytic crisis, principally the antimalarial drugs (primaquine phosphate and Atabrine), the sulfonamides, nitrofurantoin, aspirin, and phenacetin, among others. A more severe deficiency of G6PD is found in peoples of Mediterranean descent (Sardinians, Sephardic Jews, Arabs, and others). In some of these persons chronic hemolysis occurs in the absence of exposure to oxidants. The disorder can be diagnosed through the use of a G6PD assay or screening test.

Acquired hemolytic anemias

A number of acquired factors, exogenous to the red blood cell, produce hemolysis. These include various drugs, chemicals, toxins, venoms, and infections such as malaria. Antibodies that cause premature destruction of red cells may develop. Hemolytic anemia may also be caused by mechanical factors such as prosthetic heart valves, vasculitis, severe burns, and other conditions that directly injure the red cell. In all types of drug-related hemolytic anemia, discontinuance of the drug results in the eventual disappearance of the antibody.

The antibodies that cause red cell destruction fall into two categories: warm-reacting antibodies of the IgG type, which are maximally active at 37°C, and cold-reacting antibodies of the IgM type, which are optimally active at or near 4°C.

The warm antibodies cause no morphologic or metabolic alteration in the red cell. Instead, they react with antigens on the red cell membrane, causing destructive changes that lead to spherocytosis, with subsequent phagocytic destruction in the spleen or reticuloendothelial system. They lack specificity for the ABO antigens but may react with the Rh antigens. The hemolytic reactions associated with the warm-reacting antibodies have varied etiologies; about 60% are idiopathic, 25% to 30% are drug-induced, and the remainder are often related to malignancies of the lymphoproliferative system (chronic lymphocytic leukemia and lymphoma) or collagen diseases (systemic lupus erythematosus).[11] Treatment with the antihypertensive drug alpha-methyldopa produces an antibody that closely resembles the warm-reacting antibodies found in nondrug hemolytic anemias. The diagnosis of warm-reacting antibody hemolytic anemia is made through use of the Coombs' test, or antiglobulin test.

The *Coombs' test* detects the presence of antibody or complement on the surface of the red cell. A *direct Coombs' test* detects the antibody on red blood cells. In this test red cells, which have been washed free of serum, are mixed with Coombs' antiserum. The red cells will agglutinate if the Coombs' reagent binds to and bridges the antibody or complement on adjacent red cells. The direct Coombs' test is positive in autoimmune hemolytic anemia, erythroblastosis fetalis (Rh disease of the newborn), transfusion reactions, and following exposure to certain drugs such as large doses of penicillin, cephalothin, and the antihypertensive drug alpha-methyldopa. The *indirect Coombs' test* detects the presence of antibody in the serum and is positive in the presence of specific antibodies resulting from previous transfusions or pregnancy.

The cold-reacting antibodies activate complement. Chronic hemolytic anemia due to cold-reacting antibodies occurs with lymphoproliferative disorders and as an idiopathic disorder of unknown etiology. The hemolytic process occurs in distal body parts where the temperature may fall below 30°C. Vascular obstruction by red cells results in pallor, cyanosis of the body parts exposed to cold temperatures, and Raynaud's phenomenon (see Chapter 18). Hemolytic anemia develops in only a few persons. In contrast to hemolytic anemia caused by warm-reacting antibodies, the direct Coombs' test is only weakly positive with hemolytic conditions caused by cold-reacting antibodies.

Hemolytic disease of the newborn

Erythroblastosis fetalis, or hemolytic disease of the newborn, occurs in Rh-positive infants of Rh-negative mothers who have been sensitized by previous pregnancies in which the infants are Rh-positive or by blood transfusions of Rh-positive blood. The Rh-negative mother usually becomes sensitized during the first few days following delivery. During this time the antigens from the placental site are released into the maternal circulation. Because the development of the antibodies requires several weeks, the first Rh-positive infant of an Rh-negative mother is usually not affected. Infants with Rh-negative blood have no antigens on their red cells to react with the maternal antibodies and are also not affected.

Once an Rh-negative mother has been sensitized, the Rh antibodies from her blood are transferred to subsequent babies through the placental circulation. These antibodies react with the red cell antigens of the Rh-positive infant, causing agglutination and hemolysis. This leads to severe anemia with compensatory hyperplasia and enlargement of the blood-forming organs, including the spleen and liver, in the fetus. Liver function may be impaired, with decreased production of albumin, and cardiac failure develops with massive edema called *hydrops fetalis.* Blood levels of unconjugated *bilirubin* are abnormally high due to red cell hemolysis, and with these elevated levels there is danger that the bilirubin will precipitate in neuronal tissue and cause the destructive changes of kernicterus.

Not all babies born to Rh-negative mothers are Rh-positive, and those that are Rh-negative are not likely to develop erythroblastosis. If, for example, the father carries a complex of both Rh-positive and Rh-negative genes, there is a chance that the baby will be Rh-negative.

Three recent advances have served to decrease the threat to babies born to Rh-negative mothers: (1) prevention of sensitization, (2) intrauterine transfusion to the affected fetus, and (3) exchange transfusion. Injection of *Rh immune globulin* (gamma globulin containing Rh antibody) prevents sensitization in Rh-negative mothers who have given birth to Rh-positive infants if administered within 72 hours of delivery. The Rh immune globulin must be given after each delivery, abortion, genetic amniocentesis, or fetal–maternal bleed to prevent sensitization. Once sensitization has developed, the immune globulin is of no value.

In the past, about 20% of erythroblastotic fetuses died *in utero*. It is now possible to increase their chances of survival by studying the amniotic fluid to determine the bilirubin concentration, which reflects the severity of the disease. If the fetus is erythroblastotic, intrauterine transfusions of red cells are given into the peritoneal cavity of the fetus.[12] Exchange transfusions are given after birth. In this technique, 10 ml to 20 ml of the infant's blood is removed and replaced with an equal amount of type O, unsensitized Rh-negative blood. This procedure is repeated until twice the blood volume of the infant has been exchanged. The purpose of the exchange transfusion is to prevent hyperbilirubinemia with consequent damage to the brain.

Since 1968, the year Rh immune globulin was introduced, sensitization of Rh-negative women has dropped by more than 80%.[13] Early prenatal care and screening of maternal blood will continue to be important in reducing immunization. Efforts to improve therapy are aimed at production of monoclonal anti-D, the Rh antibody.

Nutritional anemias

A true nutritional anemia must meet two criteria: (1) deficiency or lack of a nutrient alone must produce the anemia and (2) providing the nutrient must correct the anemia.[14] The common types of nutritional anemias are iron-deficiency anemia and megaloblastic anemia due to vitamin B_{12} or folic acid deficiencies.

Iron-deficiency anemia

Iron is an integral constituent of the heme in the hemoglobin molecule, and its deficiency leads to a decrease in hemoglobin synthesis. In iron-deficiency anemia there is a decrease in serum iron. The red cells are decreased in number and are microcytic, hypochromic, and often malformed (poikilocytosis). The lab values will include reduced MCHC and MCV. Membrane changes may predispose to hemolysis causing further loss of red cells.

Body iron is repeatedly reused. When red cells become senescent and are broken down, their iron is released and reused in the production of new red cells. The normal diet contains about 12 mg to 15 mg iron of which normally only 5% to 10% is absorbed. In iron deficiency, the absorption increases. Normally, less than 1 mg iron is lost from the body daily. About 30% of body iron is stored in the bone marrow, the spleen, muscle, and other organs; the remainder is present in the form of hemoglobin.

In the adult, a blood loss of 2 ml to 4 ml per day is the usual reason for an iron deficiency.[15] This blood loss may be due to gastrointestinal bleeding, such as occurs with peptic ulcer, intestinal polyps, hemorrhoids, or malignancy. Excessive aspirin intake may cause undetected gastrointestinal bleeding. In women, blood is lost during menstruation. Although cessation of menstruation spares iron loss in the pregnant woman, iron requirements increase at this time; the expansion of the mother's blood volume requires about 480 mg of additional iron, and the growing fetus requires about 390 mg.

A child's growth places extra demands on the body: blood volume increases, with a greater need for iron. Iron requirements are proportionally higher in infancy (3–24 months) than at any other age, although childhood and adolescence also bring increased requirements.

In infancy the two main causes of iron-deficiency anemia are low iron levels at birth (due to maternal deficiency) and a diet consisting mainly of cow's milk, which is low in absorbable iron. It has been reported that 30% of infants in low-income populations were anemic.[16]

The peak increase in iron deficiency during adolescence stems from increased body requirements resulting from growth spurts and menstrual blood loss at the same time dietary intake may be inadequate.

The signs and symptoms of iron-deficiency anemia are related to the cause and impairment of oxygen transport and lack of hemoglobin. Depending on its severity, fatigability, palpitations, dyspnea, angina, and tachycardia may occur. Late signs are waxy pallor, brittle hair and nails, smooth tongue, and sores in the corners of the mouth. A poorly understood symptom sometimes seen is pica, the bizarre compulsive eating of ice or dirt. Also there may be extreme dysphagia.

The treatment of iron-deficiency anemia is directed toward controlling chronic blood loss, increasing dietary intake of iron, and administering supplemental iron. Parenteral iron may be given if oral forms are not tolerated. Special care is required when administering an iron preparation (Imferon) intramuscularly; it must be injected deeply by pulling the skin to one side before inserting the needle (Z track) to prevent leakage with skin discoloration.

Megaloblastic anemias

Megaloblastic anemias are characterized by a mean corpuscular volume above 100 with increase in red cell size due to abnormalities of maturation in the bone marrow. There may be a vitamin B_{12} deficiency (pernicious anemia) or a folic acid deficiency. (One form of megaloblastic anemia, unresponsive to either vitamin B_{12} or folic acid therapy, is not discussed here.) Because megaloblastic anemias develop slowly, there are often few symptoms until the anemia is far advanced.

Vitamin B_{12} deficiency anemia. Vitamin B_{12} (*cyanocobalamin*) is an essential nutrient required for synthesis of DNA; when it is deficient, failure of nuclear maturation and cell division occurs, especially of the rapidly proliferating red cells. Moreover, when B_{12} is deficient, the red cells that are produced are abnormally large, have flimsy membranes, and are oval rather than the normal biconcave disk shape. These odd-shaped cells have a short life span, which can be measured in weeks rather than months. The MCV is elevated and MCHC is normal. The resulting condition is called pernicious anemia. It is the most common form of anemia due to vitamin B_{12} deficiency. Pernicious anemia is also accompanied by neurologic changes in which degeneration of the dorsal and lateral columns of the spinal cord causes symmetrical paresthesias of the feet and fingers, which eventually progress to spastic ataxia. Vitamin B_{12} is found in foods of animal origin, and dietary deficiency is relatively rare except in vegetarians.

Absorption of vitamin B_{12} in the intestine requires the presence of *intrinsic factor,* which is produced by the gastric mucosa. A decrease in intrinsic factor leads to pernicious anemia. Intrinsic factor binds to vitamin B_{12} in food and protects it from the enzymatic actions of the gut and facilitates its absorption. As discussed in Chapter 40, production of intrinsic factor is impaired in chronic gastritis (in which atrophic changes occur in the gastric mucosa) and following total removal of the stomach. Treatment consists of intramuscular injections of vitamin B_{12}.

Folic acid deficiency anemia. *Folic acid* is also required for red cell maturation, and its deficiency produces the same type of red cell changes that occur in vitamin B_{12} deficiency anemia (*i.e.,* increased MCV and normal MCHC). Symptoms are also similar, but the neurologic manifestations are not present.

Folic acid is readily absorbed from the intestine. It is found in vegetables (particularly the green leafy types), fruits, cereals, and meats. However, much of the vitamin is lost in cooking. The most common cause of a folic acid deficiency is malnutrition, especially in association with alcoholism; it is also seen with malabsorption syndromes such as sprue. Pregnancy increases the need for folic acid five- to tenfold, so a deficiency can occur at this time. Poor dietary habits, anorexia, and nausea are other reasons for a folic acid deficiency during pregnancy. Several groups

of drugs may also contribute to a deficiency. Primidone, phenytoin, and phenobarbital (drugs used to treat seizure disorders) and triamterene (a diuretic) predispose to a deficiency by interfering with its absorption. Methotrexate (a folic acid analogue used in treatment of cancer) impairs the action of folic acid by blocking its conversion to the active form.

Bone-marrow depression (aplastic anemia)

Bone-marrow depression or failure usually is an outcome of stem cell dysfunction with failure to produce blood cells. True red cell aplasia (failure to develop) can occur, but is rare. More commonly there is a reduction in circulating leukocytes, thrombocytes, and erythrocytes, and the bone marrow is replaced with fatty tissue.

Anemia results from the failure of the marrow to replace senescent red cells that are destroyed and leave the circulation, although the cells that remain are of normal size and color. At the same time, because the leukocytes, particularly the neutrophils, and the thrombocytes have a short life span, a deficiency of these cells usually is apparent before the anemia becomes severe.

Aplastic anemia can occur at any age. It may be insidious in onset, or it may strike with suddenness and great severity. Weakness, fatigability, and pallor are present. Thrombocytopenia (decrease in the number of platelets) develops and leads to purpura; and the decrease in neutrophils increases susceptibility to infection.

Among the causes of bone-marrow depression are exposure to radiation, infections, and chemical agents that are toxic to bone marrow. The best-documented of the identified toxic agents are benzene, the antibiotic chloramphenicol, and the alkylating agents and antimetabolites used in the treatment of cancer (see Chapter 5). Bone-marrow depression due to exposure to a chemical agent may sometimes be an idiosyncratic reaction, that is, it affects only certain susceptible persons. Such reactions are often severe and sometimes irreversible and fatal. Although aplastic anemia can develop in the course of many infections, it has been reported most often following non-A, non-B hepatitis, mononucleosis, and other viral illnesses. In two-thirds of the cases there is no known cause, and these are termed *idiopathic aplastic anemia.*[12] Current therapy for aplastic anemia in the young and severely affected includes bone-marrow transplantation.[12] Histocompatible donors supply stem cells to replace the patient's destroyed marrow cells. Graft-versus-host disease and infections are major risks of the procedure, yet up to 70% survival is reported. Immunosuppression with anti-lymphocyte globulin is also a promising therapy that eliminates T cells and prevents suppression of proliferating stem cells. Patients with aplastic anemia should avoid the offending agents, should be treated with antibiotics for infection, and may require blood cell transfusions to correct the anemia.

In summary, anemia describes a condition in which a decrease in red cell mass occurs. It is not a disease but a manifestation of some disease process or alteration in body function. It is generally caused by excess loss of red cells (blood loss or hemolytic anemias) or by impaired production (nutritional and aplastic anemias). The manifestations of anemia include those associated with (1) impaired oxygen transport, (2) alterations in red blood cell structure, and (3) signs and symptoms of the underlying process causing the anemia.

Polycythemia

Polycythemia is an abnormally high total red blood cell mass. It is categorized as relative, primary, or secondary. In *relative polycythemia* the hematocrit rises because of a loss of plasma volume without a corresponding decrease in red cells. *Polycythemia vera (primary polycythemia)* is a proliferative disease of the bone marrow characterized by an absolute increase in total red blood cell mass and volume. It is seen most commonly in men aged 40 to 60 years. *Secondary polycythemia* results from an increase in the level of erythropoietin. This elevation is related to living at high altitudes and to chronic heart and lung disease, both of which cause hypoxia. Smoking more than one and a half packs of cigarettes daily may also cause secondary polycythemia.

In polycythemia vera, signs and symptoms are those related to increased blood viscosity, hypermetabolism, and increase in red cell count, hemoglobin, and hematocrit. The increased blood volume gives rise to hypertension. There may be complaints of headache, inability to concentrate, and some difficulty in hearing due to decreased cerebral blood flow. There is a plethoric appearance, or dusky redness—even cyanosis—particularly of the lips, fingernails, and mucous membranes. Because of the concentration of blood cells, the person may experience itching and pain in the fingers or toes, and the hypermetabolism may induce night sweats and weight loss. With the elevated blood viscosity and stagnation of blood flow, thrombosis and hemorrhage are possible.

Relative polycythemia is corrected by increasing the vascular fluid volume. Treatment of secondary polycythemia focuses on relieving the hypoxia.

For example, the use of continuous low-flow oxygen therapy is a means of correcting the severe hypoxia that occurs in some persons with chronic obstructive lung disease. This form of treatment is thought to relieve the pulmonary hypertension and polycythemia and delay the onset of cor pulmonale. The goal in primary polycythemia is a reduction in blood viscosity. This can be done by phlebotomy (withdrawal of blood) or chemotherapy or radiation to suppress bone-marrow function.

In summary, polycythemia describes a condition in which there is an increase in red blood cell mass. It may be relative in type, with red cell mass increased due to a loss of vascular fluid; primary, with proliferative changes in the bone marrow; or secondary, with elevation of erythropoietin levels due to hypoxia.

Transfusion therapy

Transfusion therapy provides the patient with the deficient blood component. Component therapy, which was introduced in the 1960s, allows a variety of blood constituents to be derived from a single unit of whole blood.[17] Components such as red cells, platelets, antihemophilic factors, and fresh-frozen plasma are now available to correct a specific deficiency. This provides a more efficient use of blood for a greater number of recipients and reduces the transfusion of unneeded components. This discussion focuses on the administration of whole blood and the red cell component. Plasma or its components (platelets, granulocytes, albumin, clotting factors) may be administered separately. Table 16-2 describes the red cell components used for transfusion.

Prior to transfusion, compatibility testing, a series of procedures to ensure the best results of blood transfusion, is required. Donor and recipient samples are typed (ABO group and Rh type) and screened for unexpected antibodies. Appropriate donor samples are then cross-matched with the recipient sample. In cross-matching, cells and serum from the donor and recipient are selectively combined and observed for agglutination following direct mixing, addition of a high-protein solution to promote agglutination, and addition of Coombs' reagent following thorough washing of red cells (direct Coombs').

ABO types

There are four major ABO blood groups as determined by the presence or absence of two red cell antigens (A and B). Persons who have neither A nor B antigens are classified as having type O blood, those with A antigens as having type A blood, those with B antigens as having type B blood, and those with both A and B antigens as having type AB blood (Table 16-3). The ABO blood types are genetically determined. The type O gene is apparently functionless in production of a red cell antigen. Each of the other genes is expressed by the presence of a strong antigen on the surface of the red cell. Six genotypes, or gene combinations, result in four phenotypes or blood type expressions.

Normally, the body does not develop antibodies to its own tissues or blood cells. When an ABO antigen is not present on the red cell, antibodies develop in the plasma. Thus, persons with type A antigens on their red cells develop type B antibodies in their serum; persons with type B antigens develop type A antibodies in their serum; persons with type O blood develop both type A and type B antibodies; and persons with type AB blood develop neither A nor B antibodies. The ABO antibodies are usually not present at birth but begin to develop at age 3 months to 6 months and reach maximum levels at 5 years to 10 years of age.[18]

─── Rh types

The D antigen of the Rh system is also important in transfusion compatibility. The Rh type is coded by three closely linked genes: C, c, D, d, and E, e. Each gene, with the exception of d, codes for a specific antigen. The D antigen is the most immunogenic. Persons expressing the D antigen are termed Rh-positive, while those who do not express the D antigen are Rh-negative. Unlike serum antibodies for the ABO blood types that develop spontaneously after birth, development of Rh antibodies requires exposure to one or more of the Rh antigens. About 70% of Rh-negative persons will develop the antibody to D antigen if exposed to Rh-positive blood.[19] Because it takes several weeks to produce antibodies, a reaction may be delayed and is usually mild. If, however, subsequent transfusions of Rh-positive blood are given to

Table 16–2. Red blood cell components used in transfusion therapy

Component	Preparation	Use	Limitations
Whole blood	Drawn from donor Anti-coagulant-preservative solutions added, usually acid-citrate-dextrose (ACD), citrate-phosphate-dextrose (CPD), or CPD-adenine. Stored at 1–6°C until expiration up to 35 days.	Replacement of blood volume and oxygen-carrying capacity lost in massive bleeding.	Contains few viable platelets or granulocytes and is deficient in coagulation factors V and VIII. May cause hypervolemia, febrile and allergic reactions and infectious disease (i.e., hepatitis and AIDS).
Red blood cells	Removal of two-thirds of plasma by centrifugation. Additive solution contains adenine to extend shelf life up to 42 days and maintain ATP levels.	Standard transfusion to increase oxygen-carrying capacity in chronic anemia and slow hemorrhage. Reduces danger of hypervolemia.	Contains no viable platelets or granulocytes. Risk of reactions and infectious disease.
Leukocyte-poor red blood cells	Removal of 70%–90% of leukocytes, platelets, and debris by centrifugation or filtration.	Reduces risk of nonhemolytic febrile reactions in susceptible individuals.	Preparation may reduce red cell mass to 70%. 24-hr shelf life; infectious disease risk.
Washed red blood cells	Red cells are washed in normal saline and centrifuged several times to remove plasma and constituents.	Reduces risk of febrile and allergic reactions.	Loss of red cell mass, 24-hr shelf life, costly preparation, and infectious disease risk.
Frozen red blood cells	Red cells are mixed with glycerol to prevent ice crystals from forming and rupturing the cell membrane. Cells must be thawed, deglycerolized, and washed before transfusing.	Reduces risk of severe febrile reactions. Preserves rare and autologous (self-donated) units for transfusion up to 7 years.	Costly and lengthy preparation. Loss of red cell mass, short shelf life and infectious disease risk.

(Data from Reynolds A, Steckler D: Practical Aspects of Blood Administration, pp 43–93. Arlington, VA, American Association of Blood Banks, 1986; and Widmann FK [ed]: Technical Manual, 9th ed, pp 35–58. Arlington, VA, American Association of Blood Banks, 1985)

Table 16–3. ABO system for blood typing

Genotype	Red cell antigens	Blood type	Serum antibodies
OO	None	O	AB
AO	A	A	B
AA	A	A	B
BO	B	B	A
BB	B	B	A
AB	AB	AB	None

a person who has now become sensitized, there may be a severe immediate reaction.

Blood transfusion reactions

The seriousness of blood transfusion reactions prompts the need for extreme caution when blood is administered. Care should be taken to ensure proper identification of the recipient and transfusion source, because most transfusion reactions are due to clerical errors or misidentification.[18] Once the transfusion has been started, monitoring of vital signs and careful observation for signs of transfusion reaction are imperative.

The most feared and lethal transfusion reaction is the destruction of donor red cells by the reaction with antibody in the recipient's serum. This immediate hemolytic reaction is usually due to ABO incompatibility. The signs and symptoms of such a reaction include sensation of heat along the vein where the blood is being infused, flushing of the face, urticaria, headache, pain in the lumbar area, chills and fever, constricting pain in the chest, cramping pain in the abdomen, nausea and vomiting, tachycardia, hypotension, and dyspnea. The transfusion should be stopped immediately should any of these signs occur. Access to a vein should be maintained, because it may be necessary to administer intravenous medications and take blood samples. The blood must be saved for studies to determine the cause of the reaction. Hemoglobin that is released from the hemolyzed donor cells is filtered in glomeruli of the kidneys. One of the possible complications of a blood transfusion reaction is oliguria and renal shutdown due to the adverse effects of the filtered hemoglobin on renal tubular flow. Therefore, the urine should be examined for hemoglobin, urobilinogen, and red blood cells.

A febrile reaction is the most common transfusion reaction occurring in about 2% of transfusions.[19] Patient antibodies directed against the donor's white cells cause chills and fever. Antihistamines treat the reaction, and use of leukocyte-poor blood will avoid future reactions.

Allergic reactions are due to patient antibodies against donor proteins, particularly IgA. Hives and itching occur and can be treated with antihistamines. Susceptible persons may be transfused with washed red cells to prevent reactions.

Delayed hemolytic reactions may occur more than 10 days after transfusion and are due to undetected antibodies in the recipient's serum. Usually no symptoms are evident, but the reaction is accompanied by a fall in the hematocrit.

In summary, transfusion therapy provides the means for replacement of red blood cells and other blood components. Red blood cells contain surface antigens, and reciprocal antibodies are found in the serum. Four major ABO blood types are determined by the presence or absence of two red cell antigens: A and B. The presence of the D antigen determines the Rh-positive type; absence of the D antigen determines the Rh-negative type. ABO and Rh types must be determined in recipient and donor blood prior to transfusion and must be cross-matched to prevent transfusion reactions.

References

1. Bunn HF: Hemoglobin I. Structure and function. In Beck WS: Hematology, 4th ed, p 140. Cambridge, MIT Press, 1985
2. Erslev AJ: Production of erythrocytes. In Williams WJ, Beutler E, Erslev AJ et al (eds): Hematology, 3rd ed, p 371. New York, McGraw-Hill, 1983
3. Guyton A: Textbook of Medical Physiology, 7th ed, pp 44, 45. Philadelphia, WB Saunders, 1986
4. Eschbach JW, Egrie JC, Downing MR et al: Correction of the anemia of end-stage renal disease with recombinant human erythropoietin. N Engl J Med 316:73, 1987
5. Sisson RC: Molecular basis of hyperbilirubinemia and phototherapy. J Invest Dermatol 77:158, 1981
6. Erslev AJ: Clinical manifestations of erythrocyte disorders. In Williams WJ, Beutler E, Erslev AJ et al (eds): Hematology, 3rd ed, p 58. New York, McGraw-Hill, 1983
7. Forget BG: Hemolytic anemias: Congenital and acquired. Hosp Pract 15(4):67, 1980
8. Proceedings of the First National Sickle Cell Education Symposium, p 6. Department of Health, Education and Welfare DHEW publication No. NIH76-1007, 1976
9. Azen EA: Sicklemia and thalassemia. In MacKinney AA (ed): Pathophysiology of Blood, p 121. New York, John Wiley and Sons, 1984
10. Robbins SL, Cotran R, Kumar V: Pathologic Basis of Disease, 3rd ed, pp 625, 639. Philadelphia, WB Saunders, 1984
11. Jandl JH: Hemolytic anemia II. Immunohemolytic anemia. In Beck WS: Hematology, 4th ed, p 191. Cambridge, MIT Press, 1985

12. Rapaport SI: Introduction to Hematology, 2nd ed, p 152, 167. Philadelphia, JB Lippincott, 1987

13. Bowman JM: The prevention of Rh immunization. Transfusion Med Rev 2:129, 1988

14. Herbert V: The nutritional anemias. Hosp Pract 15(3):65, 1980

15. Beck WS: Hypochromic anemia I. Iron deficiency and excess. In Beck WS: Hematology, 4th ed, p 118. Cambridge, MIT Press, 1985

16. Lane M, Johnson CL: Prevalence of iron deficiency. In Oski FA, Pearson HA (eds): Iron Nutrition Revisited—Infancy, Childhood, Adolescence: Report of the Eighty-Second Ross Conference on Pediatric Research, p 31. Columbus, OH, Ross Laboratories, 1981

17. Swisher SN, Petz LD: An overview of blood transfusion. In Petz LD, Swisher SN (eds): Clinical Practice of Blood Transfusion, p 3. New York, Churchill Livingstone, 1981

18. Pittiglio DH (ed): Modern Blood Banking and Transfusion Practices, p 91. Philadelphia, FA Davis, 1983

19. Kelton JG, Heddle NM, Blajchman MA: Blood Transfusion, A Conceptual Approach, pp 50, 117. New York, Churchill Livingstone, 1984

Bibliography

Adamson JW: Hemoglobin—from F to A, and back. N Engl J Med 310:917, 1984

Alavi JB: Sickle cell anemia: Pathophysiology and treatment. Med Clin North Am 68:545, 1984

Camitta BM, Storb R, Thomas ED: Aplastic anemia: Parts 1 and 2. N Engl J Med 306:645, 712, 1982

Dallman PR: Manifestations of iron deficiency. Semin Hematol 19:19, 1982

Embury SH: The clinical pathophysiology of sickle cell disease. Annu Rev Med 37:361, 1986

Erslev A: Erythropoietin coming of age. N Engl J Med 316:101, 1987

Gaston MH, Verter JI, Woods G, et al: Prophylaxis with oral penicillin in children with sickle cell anemia. N Engl J Med 314:1593, 1986

Green R, Kuhl W, Jacobson R et al: Masking of macrocytes by thalassemia in blacks with pernicious anemia. N Engl J Med 307:1322, 1982

Halberg L: Iron nutrition and food iron fortification. Semin Hematol 19:31, 1982

Herbert V: Biology of disease: Megaloblastic anemias. Lab Invest 52:3, 1985

Kellermeyer RW: General principles of evaluation and therapy of anemias. Med Clin North Am 68:533, 1984

Mohandas N, Phillips WM, Bessis M: Red blood cell deformability and hemolytic anemias. Semin Hematol 16:95, 1979

Petz LD: Drug-induced immune hemolysis. N Engl J Med 313:510, 1985

Pineda AA, Taswell HF, Brzica SM: Delayed hemolytic transfusion reaction. An immunologic hazard of blood transfusion. Transfusion 18:1, 1978

Platt OS, Rosenstock W, Espeland MA: Influence of sickle hemoglobinopathies on growth and development. N Engl J Med 311:7, 1984

Recny MA, Scobe HA, Kim Y: Structural characterization of natural human urinary and recombinant DNA-derived erythropoietin. J Biol Chem 262:17156, 1987

Scrimshaw NS: Iron deficiency and its functional consequences. Compr Ther 11:40, 1985

Slichter SJ: Transfusion and bone marrow transplantation. Transfusion Med Rev 2:1, 1988

Spaet TH: Anemia is a symptom. Hosp Pract 17(2):17, 1980

Steinberg MH, Hebbel RP: Clinical diversity of sickle cell anemia: Genetic and cellular modulation of disease severity. Am J Hematol 14:405, 1983

Valentine WN: Hemolytic anemias and erythrocyte enzymopathies. Ann Intern Med 103:245, 1985

CHAPTER 17

The Circulatory System and Control of Blood Flow

Organization of the circulatory system
  Systemic and pulmonary circulations
  Pressure and volume distribution
  Blood vessel structure and function
    Vascular smooth muscle
    Arteries and arterioles
    Veins and venules
    Capillaries

Principles of blood flow
  Pressure, resistance, and flow
    Peripheral vascular resistance
  Velocity and cross-sectional area
  Wall tension, radius, and pressure
  Laminar and turbulent flow

Control of blood flow
  Arterial pressure pulses
  Flow in the venous system
  The microcirculation
    Local control of blood flow
    Neural control of blood flow
    Collateral circulation

Objectives

After you have studied this chapter, you should be able to meet the following objectives:

_____ Describe the organization of the circulatory system.

_____ Compare the distribution of blood flow and blood pressure in the systemic and pulmonary circulations.

_____ State how beta-blocking agents and calcium-channel blocking drugs produce relaxation of vascular smooth muscle.

_____ Compare the structure of arteries, arterioles, veins, and capillaries.

_____ Relate the function of capillaries in various organ systems to the size of the capillary pores.

_____ State the formula for total peripheral resistance.

_____ Explain how vessel radius, vessel length, blood viscosity, and blood pressure affect blood flow.

_____ Relate the cross-sectional area to pressure and the velocity of flow in a blood vessel.

_____ Relate kinetic energy and potential energy to lateral wall pressure and the velocity of blood flow in a vessel.

_____ Use Laplace's law to explain the effect of radius size on the pressure and wall tension in a vessel.

_____ Compare laminar and streamlined flow in terms of the development of turbulent flow in the vascular system.

_____ Describe the origin of the pressure pulse.

_____ Define _mean arterial blood pressure_ and state the rationale for its use.

_____ Relate the effects of gravity to mechanisms of venous flow.

_____ State the relationship between intrathoracic pressure and venous return to the right heart.

_____ Define _microcirculation._

_____ State the difference between nutrient and non-nutrient blood flow.

_____ Explain how the endothelium is thought to interact with various blood-borne substances in producing blood vessel dilatation or constriction.

_____ Describe the regulation of blood flow in terms of local, neural, and humoral components.

_____ Define _hyperemia._

The circulatory system, which consists of the heart and blood vessels, has one main function—transport. It delivers oxygen and nutrients needed for metabolic processes to the tissues, carries waste products from cellular metabolism to the kidneys and other excretory organs for elimination, and circulates electrolytes and hormones needed to regulate body function. Temperature regulation relies on the circulatory system for transport of core heat to the periphery, where it can be dissipated into the external environment. In addition, the circulatory system plays a vital role in the transport of various immune substances that contribute to the body's defense mechanisms. The purpose of this chapter is to discuss the functional components of the circulatory system and the control of blood flow. Control of blood pressure is discussed in Chapter 19, and control of cardiac function is discussed in Chapter 20.

Organization of the circulatory system

Systemic and pulmonary circulations

The circulatory system can be divided into two parts: the systemic and the pulmonary circulations. The systemic circulation supplies all of the body's tissues except the lungs, which are supplied by the pulmonary circulation. The systemic circulation is often referred to as the *peripheral circulation*. Because it must transport blood to distant parts of the body, often against gravity, the systemic circulation functions as a high-pressure system (mean arterial blood pressure approximately 90–100 mmHg). The pulmonary circulation along with the blood that is in the heart is often called the *central circulation*. The pulmonary circulation links the gas exchange function of the lungs with the transport function of the circulatory system; its location is the chest in close proximity to the heart, which propels blood through it. In contrast to the systemic circulation, the pulmonary circulation functions as a low-pressure system (mean arterial blood pressure is approximately 12 mmHg).

Each division of the circulation has a pump, an arterial system, capillaries, and a venous system. The heart is the pump that propels blood through both divisions. It is divided into a right heart, which pumps blood to the pulmonary circulation, and a left heart, which pumps blood to the systemic circulation (Figure 17-1). Each side of the heart is further divided into two chambers, an atrium and a ventricle. The ventricles are the main pumping chambers of the heart. The atria act as collection chambers for blood

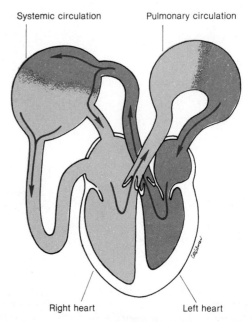

Systemic circulation   Pulmonary circulation

Right heart   Left heart

Figure 17-1 Systemic and pulmonary circulations. The right side of the heart pumps blood to the lungs and the left side of the heart pumps blood to the systemic circulation.

returning to the heart and as axillary pumps for the ventricles. In both the pulmonary and systemic circulations, the arteries and arterioles function as a distribution system to move blood to the tissues, the capillaries as an exchange system where the transfer of gases, nutrients, and waste products takes place, and the venules and veins as a collection system for blood as it returns to the heart.

The circulation of blood through the heart and blood vessels will function effectively only as long as that flow is unidirectional and if the outputs of the right and left hearts are equal. Unidirectional flow through the heart is ensured by the heart valves. The distribution of pressure and volumes throughout the circulatory system requires that both sides of the heart pump equal amounts of blood. If the output of the left heart were to fall below that of the right heart, blood would accumulate in the pulmonary circulation. If the right side of the heart pumped less than the left, blood would accumulate in the systemic circulation.

Pressure and volume distribution

The systemic circulation contains about 84% of the total blood volume, the pulmonary circulation contains 8%, and the heart contains 8%. Of the blood in the heart and systemic circulation, 4% of the total blood volume is in the left heart, 16% is in the arteries and arterioles, 4% is in the capillaries, 64% is in the veins and venules, and 4% is in the right heart (Figure 17-2).[1]

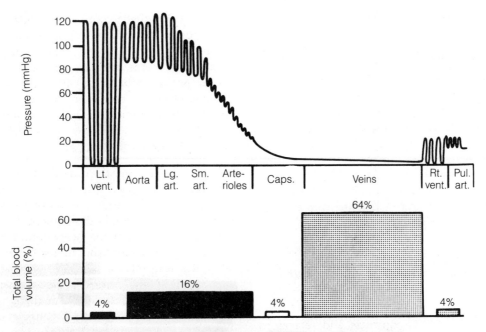

Figure 17-2 Pressure and volume distribution in the systemic circulation. The graphs illustrate the inverse relationship between internal pressure and volume in different portions of the circulatory system. (*Smith JJ, Kampine JP: Circulatory Physiology: The Essentials, 2nd ed. Baltimore, Williams & Wilkins, 1984*)

In the systemic circulation, as pictured in Figure 17-2, the pressure distribution is opposite of its volume distribution. The mean arterial pressure in the arterial side of the circulation, which contains only about one-sixth of the blood volume, is much greater than the pressure on the venous side of the circulation, which contains about two-thirds of the blood.

Blood moves from the arterial to the venous side of the circulation along a pressure gradient, moving from an area of higher to an area of lower pressure. Because arterial flow is pulsatile with pressures that range from a lower diastolic value to a higher systolic value, the average or *mean arterial pressure* is often used to describe arterial pressure. Mean arterial pressure can be estimated by adding one-third of the pulse pressure (difference between systolic and diastolic blood pressures) to the diastolic blood pressure. Both capillary and venous flow are nonpulsatile, and, hence, there is no need to convert these pressures to a mean pressure. The mean arterial blood pressure (in a young adult) is about 90 mmHg, and vena caval pressure is about 6 mmHg. It is this difference in pressure between the arterial and venous sides of the circulation (about 84 mmHg) that provides the driving force for flow of blood in the systemic circulation. The pulmonary circulation has similar arterial–venous pressure differences, albeit of a lesser magnitude, that facilitate blood flow.

Because the pulmonary and systemic circulations are connected and function as a closed system, blood can be shifted from one circulation to the other.

In the pulmonary circulation, the blood volume (about 450 ml in the adult) can vary from as low as 50% of normal to as high as 200% of normal.[2] Increases in intrathoracic pressure, which interfere with venous return to the right heart, can cause a shift from the pulmonary to the systemic circulation of as much as 250 ml of blood. Hemorrhage or loss of blood volume also produces a shift in blood from the pulmonary to the systemic circulation. With narrowing of the mitral valve due to stenosis there is obstruction to outflow of blood from the pulmonary circulation, which produces an increase in pulmonary blood volume. Left-sided heart failure has a similar effect on pulmonary blood volume; in this situation, the pumping action of the left ventricle is inadequate to move blood from the pulmonary to the systemic circulation. Because the volume of the systemic circulation is about seven times that of the pulmonary circulation, a shift of blood from one system to the other has a much greater effect in the pulmonary than in the systemic circulation.

Blood vessel structure and function

All of the blood vessels, except the capillaries, have walls composed of three layers (Figure 17-3). The *tunica externa,* or *tunica adventitia,* is the outermost covering of the vessel. This layer is composed of fibrous and connective tissue that serves to support the vessel. The *tunica media,* or *middle layer,* is largely a

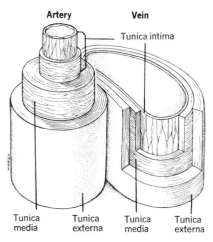

Figure 17-3 Medium-sized artery and vein showing the relative thickness of the three layers. (*Chaffee EE, Lytle IM: Basic Physiology and Anatomy, 4th ed. Philadelphia, JB Lippincott, 1980*)

smooth muscle layer that constricts and relaxes in order to control the diameter of the vessel. The *tunica intima, or inner layer,* has an elastic layer that joins the media and a thin layer of endothelial cells that lie adjacent to the blood. The endothelial layer provides a smooth and slippery inner surface for the vessel. This smooth inner lining, as long as it remains intact, prevents blood clotting.

Vascular smooth muscle

Smooth muscle contracts slowly and generates high forces for long periods of time with low energy requirements; it uses only $^1/_{40}$ to $^1/_{400}$ the energy of skeletal muscle. These characteristics are important in structures, such as blood vessels, that must maintain their tone day in and day out.

Although smooth muscle contains both actin and myosin filaments, these filaments do not form striations as in skeletal and cardiac muscle. Smooth muscle also lacks the fast sodium channels that function in the depolarization of skeletal and cardiac muscle (see Chapter 1). Instead, the calcium ion is responsible for initiating contraction in smooth muscle. Calcium is either released from intracellular stores or enters through calcium channels in the cell membrane. Contraction can be initiated by either a change in the membrane potential or activation of membrane receptors. When smooth muscle is directly depolarized (electrically stimulated), a change in voltage across the cell membrane causes calcium channels to open, allowing extracellular calcium to enter and initiate contraction. With receptor activation the calcium comes from intracellular stores. Receptor-mediated contraction involves the use of a second messenger such as cyclic adenine monophosphate (cAMP) and can be either excitatory or inhibitory.

Sympathetic control of vascular smooth muscle occurs via receptors. Alpha-adrenergic receptors produce vasoconstriction via release of calcium from intracellular stores, and beta receptors produce vasodilatation via inhibition of calcium release. Calcium-channel blocking drugs exert their action by blocking calcium entry through the calcium channels.

Arteries and arterioles

The layers of the different types of blood vessels vary with vessel function. Arteries are thick-walled vessels with large amounts of elastic fibers. The elasticity of these vessels allows them to stretch during cardiac systole when the heart contracts and blood enters the circulation and to recoil during diastole when the heart relaxes. The arterioles, which are predominantly smooth muscle, serve as resistance vessels for the circulatory system. Sympathetic vasoconstrictor tone enables these vessels to constrict or to relax as needed to maintain blood pressure. The mean arterial pressure in the large arteries of the systemic circulation is normally about 90 mmHg to 100 mmHg; in the small arteries it is 60 mmHg to 90 mmHg; and in the arterioles it is 40 mmHg to 60 mmHg.

Veins and venules

The veins and venules are thin-walled, distensible, and collapsible vessels. The structure of the veins allows these vessels to act as a reservoir or blood storage system. The venous system is a low-pressure system that relies on changes in intra-abdominal pressure and the action of muscle pumps to assist in the movement of blood back to the heart. Their pressure ranges from about 10 mmHg at the end of the venules to about 0 mmHg at the entrance of the vena cavae into the heart. The peripheral veins have valves that prevent the retrograde, or backward, flow of blood and aid in the return of blood to the heart (Figure 17-4).

Capillaries

The interchange of gases, nutrients, and cellular wastes between the tissues and the circulatory system occurs in the capillary bed (Figure 17-5). The capillaries are microscopic, single-cell-thick vessels that connect the arterial and venous segments of the circulation. There are about 10 billion capillaries with a surface area of 500 to 700 m^2.[2]

The capillary wall is composed of a single layer of endothelial cells surrounded by a basement membrane. Intracellular junctions join the capillary endothelial cells—these are called the *capillary pores.* Lipid-soluble materials diffuse directly through the capillary cell membrane. Water and water-soluble

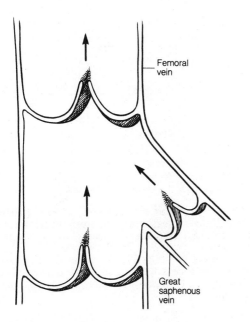

Figure 17-4 Venous valves located at the junction of the great saphenous and the common femoral veins. *Arrows* indicate direction of blood flow.

lary. In organs that process blood contents, such as the liver, capillaries have large pores so substances can pass easily through the capillary wall. In the kidney, the glomerular capillaries have small openings called *fenestrations*, which pass directly through the middle of the endothelial cells. Fenestrated capillary walls are consistent with the filtration function of the glomerulus.

The movement of fluids through the capillary pores occurs along a pressure gradient. At the arterial end, the intracapillary pressure (in the systemic circulation) is about 25 mmHg, and it drops to about 10 mmHg at the venous end. Because of this pressure gradient, fluids are pushed out of the capillary at the arterial end and pulled back in at the venous end. Plasma proteins and other nondiffusible particles that remain in the capillary exert an osmotic force that contributes to pulling of fluid back into the venous end of the capillary. The mechanisms that control the distribution of fluids between the capillaries and the tissues are discussed in Chapter 28.

materials leave and enter the capillary through the capillary pores. The size of the capillary pores varies with capillary function. In the brain, the endothelial cells are joined by tight junctions that form the blood–brain barrier. This prevents substances that would alter neural excitability from leaving the capil-

In summary, the circulatory system is designed to deliver nutrients and remove waste products for body tissues. The heart pumps blood throughout the system. The blood vessels serve as tubes through which blood flows; the arterial system carries fluids from the heart to the tissues, and the veins carry them back to the heart. The circulatory system can be di-

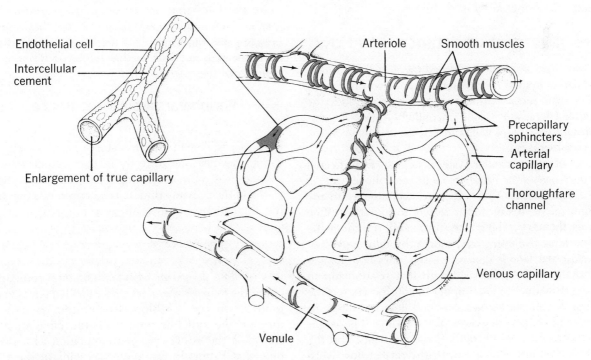

Figure 17-5 A capillary bed. Precapillary sphincters are relaxed, thus permitting the flow of blood through the capillary network. A greatly magnified portion of capillary wall is shown in the inset (*upper left*). (*Chaffee EE, Lytle IM: Basic Physiology and Anatomy, 4th ed. Philadelphia, JB Lippincott, 1980*)

vided into two parts: the systemic and the pulmonary circulations. The systemic circulation, which is served by the left heart, supplies all of the tissues except the lungs, which are served by the right heart and the pulmonary circulation. Blood moves throughout the circulation along a pressure gradient, moving from the high-pressure arterial system to the low-pressure venous system.

The walls of all blood vessels, except the capillaries, are composed of three layers: the tunica externa, tunica media, and tunica intima. The layers of the vessel vary with its function. Arteries are thick-walled vessels with large amounts of elastic fibers. The walls of the arterioles, which control blood pressure, have large amounts of smooth muscle. Veins are thin-walled, distensible, and collapsible vessels. Capillaries are single-cell-thick vessels designed for the exchange of gases, nutrients, and waste materials.

Principles of blood flow

The circulation of the blood in the cardiovascular system is determined by blood vessel diameter, velocity of flow, and resistance to flow. Blood flow is brought about by a pressure difference, or gradient, between the various parts of the circulatory system. This pressure difference provides the force that overcomes the resistance to blood flow. Blood pressure is measured in millimeters of mercury (mmHg), and blood flow is measured in milliliters.

Pressure, resistance, and flow

Resistance is the impediment to flow. In the circulatory system it is the force that blood must overcome as it moves through a vessel. It includes the frictional forces the blood encounters during its contact with the vessel wall and interaction between the various blood cells.

In the vascular system, resistance is affected by the *length of the vessel*, its *radius*, and the *viscosity of the blood* (Figure 17-6). It is related directly to the length of the vessel and inversely to its radius. The longer the vessel, the greater the overall resistance the blood must overcome as it moves through the vessel. Because the length of most vessels does not change, we shall not be concerned with that relationship in this discussion. A more important consideration is the radius of the vessel. Resistance to flow is related inversely to the fourth power of the radius. The larger the radius of a vessel, the less the resistance and the greater the flow. For example, the rate of flow is 16 times greater in a vessel with a radius of 2 cm than in one with a radius of 1 cm. Thus, even small changes in a vessel's diameter can produce marked changes in

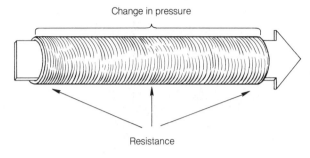

$$\text{Flow } Q = \frac{\text{Change in pressure} \times \pi \text{ radius}^4}{8 \times \text{length} \times \text{viscosity}}$$

Figure 17-6 The factors that affect blood flow (Poiseuille's law). Increasing the pressure difference between the two ends of the vessel or enlarging the radius of the vessel causes flow to increase. Increasing the length of the vessel or the viscosity of the blood causes flow to decrease. Flow diminishes as resistance increases. Resistance is directly proportional to blood viscosity and the length of the vessel and inversely proportional to the fourth power of the radius.

blood flow. The reader is asked to consider the consequences of a 25%, 50%, and 75% narrowing of a coronary artery in terms of blood flow to the myocardium.

The term *viscosity* refers to the ease with which molecules of fluid slide over each other when the fluid is moving. Water flows more rapidly through a tube than syrup does because the water molecules slide over each other more easily. As a general rule, the viscosity of a fluid is related to its thickness. The more particles that are present in a solution, the greater the interaction and friction forces that develop between the molecules. It is the blood cells (particularly, the red blood cells) that largely determine the viscosity of the blood.

Peripheral vascular resistance

Blood pressure (BP) is needed to overcome resistance to flow in the circulatory system. Resistance cannot be measured directly in the vascular system. Instead, it is estimated, using measurements of blood flow and the pressure difference between two points of the circulation.

$$\text{Resistance} = \frac{\text{Pressure Difference}}{\text{Flow}}$$

The *peripheral vascular resistance*, sometimes called the *total peripheral resistance* (TPR), refers to the total resistance the blood encounters as it flows through the systemic, or peripheral, circulation. It considers the entire systemic circulation as a single tube that begins in the aorta and ends in the right atrium. The pressure difference between these two points (about 100 mmHg) is the mean arterial blood pressure (about 100 mmHg) minus the right atrial pressure (about 0 mmHg). The cardiac output (CO), which is about 100 ml/sec at rest, is the flow through the system. Thus the TPR is $^{100}/_{100}$ or 1 peripheral resistance unit (PRU). The total resistance in the pulmonary circulation is only about 0.12 PRU. In this case, the blood flow is the same as in the systemic circulation, but the pressure difference between the pulmonary artery and the left atrium (16 mmHg minus 4 mmHg) is much less.

Because pressure is needed to overcome the resistance to blood flow, blood pressure is influenced greatly by the vascular resistance. Accordingly, arterial blood pressure is equal to the cardiac output multiplied by the total peripheral resistance (BP = CO × TPR).

Velocity and cross-sectional area

The characteristics of blood movement in the circulatory system are determined by both flow and velocity. Velocity is a distance measurement; it refers to linear movement with time or the speed (centimeters per second) with which blood flows through a vessel. Flow is a volume measurement (milliliters per second); it is determined by both the cross-sectional area of a vessel and the velocity of flow (Figure 17-7). When the flow through a given segment of the circulatory system is constant as it must be for continuous flow, the velocity will be inversely proportional to the cross-sectional area (*e.g.*, the smaller the vessel, the greater the velocity). It is like pursing your lips to whistle. In this case the small diameter of the mouth opening increases the velocity of airflow to the point where turbulent flow produces a whistling sound.

The total energy in a system is equal to the sum of the system's potential and kinetic energies. Both types of energy contribute to flow and pressure in the circulatory system; one produces forward flow and the other produces lateral pressure on vessel walls (Figure 17-8). Kinetic energy (Mass × Velocity^2

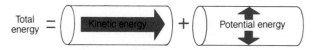

Figure 17-8 Total energy in the vascular system is spent either in moving blood forward (*kinetic energy*) or in stretching the vessel wall (*potential energy*).

[MV^2]) involves motion. Potential energy is energy that can be stored and that has potential for later use. In areas of the circulation where the cross-sectional area is reduced, as in a narrowed blood vessel or stenotic heart valve, both the kinetic energy expenditure and the velocity of flow are increased and the amount of total energy that can be stored as potential energy is reduced. Potential energy involves lateral pressure exerted against the sides of a blood vessel; it produces stretching of the elastic components of the vessel wall. Potential energy is converted to active energy when the vessel wall recoils after being stretched. The exertion of lateral pressure against a vessel wall can be damaging to blood vessels that have been weakened as in an aneurysm.

Wall tension, radius, and pressure

In a blood vessel, wall tension is the force per unit length tangential to the vessel wall that opposes the distending pressure.[3] The relationship among wall tension, pressure, and the radius of a vessel or sphere was described more than 200 years ago by the French astronomer and mathematician *Pierre de Laplace*.[3] This relationship, which is expressed by the following formula, pressure (P) = tension (T)/radius (R), has come to be known as LaPlace's law (Figure 17-9). Laplace's law states that the tension in the wall of a sphere is equal to the product of its radius and its intraluminal pressure. As discussed in Chapter 18, the principles related to wall thickness, wall tension, radius, and intraluminal pressure contribute to the progress and often the eventual rupture of arterial aneurysms. Wall tension is related inversely to wall thickness—the thicker the wall, the less the tension, and the thinner the wall, the greater the tension. Therefore, Laplace's law applies mainly to a sphere (or tube) with an infinitely thin wall.[3] In hypertension, arterial vessel walls hypertrophy and become thicker; thereby minimizing wall stress.

Laplace's law can also be applied to the pressure required to maintain the patency of small blood vessels. Providing that the thickness of a vessel wall and its tension remain constant, it takes more pressure to keep a vessel open as its radius decreases in size. This is analogous to blowing up a balloon. When the balloon is small it takes more effort to inflate the bal-

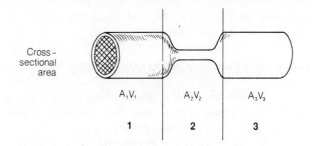

Figure 17-7 Effect of cross-sectional area on velocity of flow. In section 1, velocity is low because of an increase in cross-sectional area. In section 2, velocity is increased because of a decrease in cross-sectional area. In section 3, velocity is again reduced because of an increase in cross-sectional area.

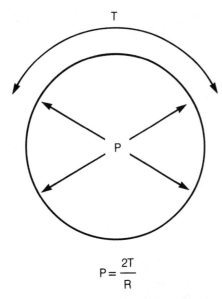

$$P = \frac{2T}{R}$$

Figure 17-9 Law of Laplace (for a sphere $P = 2T\ R$, and for a tube $P = T\ R$), where P = the pressure needed to distend an elastic sphere or tube; T = the tension in the wall of the sphere or tube; and R = the radius of the sphere or tube.

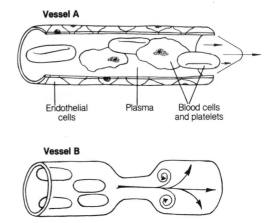

Figure 17-10 Laminar and turbulent flow in blood vessels. Vessel *A* illustrates streamlined or laminar flow in which the plasma layer is adjacent to the vessel endothelial layer and blood cells are in the center of the bloodstream. Vessel *B* depicts the presence of turbulent flow. The axial location of the platelets and other blood cells is disturbed.

loon than it does when the balloon is larger. The critical closing pressure refers to the pressure at which blood vessels close to the point where blood can no longer flow through them. In circulatory shock, for example, many of the small vessels collapse as blood pressure drops to the point where it can no longer overcome the tension in the vessels' walls.

Laminar and turbulent flow

Laminar is layered or *streamlined flow* in which friction is overcome by layering the blood components so that the plasma is adjacent to the smooth, slippery surface of the blood vessel and the cellular components, including the platelets, are in the center or axis of the bloodstream (Figure 17-10). This arrangement reduces friction by allowing the blood layers to slide smoothly over each other with the axial layer having the most rapid rate of flow.

Structural changes in the vessel wall often disrupt flow and produce turbulence (Figure 17-10). Turbulence means that blood flows crosswise as well as lengthwise along a vessel in a manner similar to the eddy currents seen in a rapidly flowing river at a point of obstruction. The tendency for turbulence to occur increases in direct proportion to the velocity of flow. Atherosclerotic narrowing of a vessel increases the velocity of flow leading to turbulent flow, which can often be heard through a stethoscope. An audible murmur in a blood vessel is referred to as a bruit. Turbulent flow also predisposes to clot formation as platelets and other coagulation factors come in contact with the endothelial lining of the vessel.

In summary, blood flow is controlled by many of the same mechanisms that control fluid flow in other systems. It is influenced by vessel length, vessel radius, the viscosity of the blood, the pressure difference between the two ends, cross-sectional area, and wall tension. The rate of flow is directly related to the pressure difference between the two ends of the vessel and the vessel radius and inversely related to vessel length and blood viscosity. The cross-sectional area of a vessel influences the velocity of flow; as the cross-sectional area decreases, the velocity is increased, and vice versa. The relationship among wall tension, pressure, and radius is described by Laplace's law, which states that wall tension becomes greater as the radius increases.

Control of blood flow

Although the physics of blood flow has many similarities to flow in nonbiologic systems, it differs in many respects including the intermittent pumping action of the heart, the elastic characteristics of blood vessels, and the mechanisms of control.

Arterial pressure pulses

Blood enters the arterial circulation during ventricular systole. The intermittent pumping action of the ventricles produces a pressure pulse that serves as the driving force for the circulation. In the systemic circulation, the pressure pulse has its origin in the rapid ejection of blood from the left ventricle into the aorta at the onset of systole. This creates an impulse that is transmitted from molecule to molecule along the length of the vessel. In the aorta, this impulse, or pressure wave, is transmitted at a velocity of 4 m to 6 m per second, which is about 20 times faster than the actual flow of blood. These pressure waves are similar to those created by splashing water in a basin or tub. When taking a pulse it is the pressure pulses that are felt, and it is the pressure pulses that produce the Korotkoff sounds heard during blood pressure measurement. The tip or maximum deflection of the pressure pulse coincides with the systolic blood pressure, and the minimum point of deflection coincides with the diastolic pressure.

As the pressure wave moves out through the aorta into the arteries, it is reflected backward and thus collides with the next advancing pressure wave (Figure 17-11). Just as the waves created by splashing water in a tub increase in amplitude as they hit the edge of the tub and reverse their direction of flow, the pressure pulse increases as it moves to the peripheral arteries; therefore, the pulse pressure in the femoral artery, for example, is usually greater than that in the aorta. With peripheral arterial disease, resistance to transmission of the pressure wave increases and a delay occurs in the transmission of the reflected wave, so that the pulse decreases in amplitude.

Following its initial amplification, the pressure pulse becomes smaller and smaller as it moves through the smaller arteries and arterioles, until it disappears entirely in the capillaries. This damping of the pressure pulse is caused by the resistance and distensibility characteristics of these vessels. The increased resistance of these small vessels impedes the flow that carries the pressure waves. Their distensibility is great enough, however, that any small change in flow does not cause a pressure change. Although the pressure pulses are not usually transmitted to the capillaries, there are situations in which this does occur. For example, injury to a finger or other area of the body often results in a throbbing sensation. In this case, extreme dilatation of the small vessels in the injured area produce a reduction in the damping of the pressure pulse. Capillary pulsations also occur in conditions that cause exaggeration of aortic pressure pulses, such as aortic regurgitation or patent ductus arteriosus (see Chapter 21).

Flow in the venous system

Venous flow is designed to return the blood to the heart. The veins are capable of enlarging and storing large quantities of blood, which can be made available to the circulation as needed. Veins are innervated by the sympathetic nervous system. When blood is lost from the circulation, sympathetic stimulation causes veins to constrict as a means of maintaining intravascular volume. The venous system is a low pressure system and when a person is in the upright position, blood flow in the venous system must oppose the effects of gravity. Valves in the veins of extremities prevent the retrograde flow, and with the help of skeletal muscles that surround and intermittently compress the veins in a milking fashion, blood is moved forward to the heart. There are no valves in the abdominal or thoracic veins, and blood flow in these veins is influenced heavily by the pressure in the surrounding cavities.

As explained earlier in the chapter, flow in the circulatory system occurs along a pressure gradient, moving from the high pressure arterial system to the low pressure venous system. As blood enters the right atrium from the central veins the pressure in the circulation normally drops to about 0 mmHg; it is this low atrial pressure that maintains the movement of blood into the right heart. Right atrial pressure is regulated by a balance between the ability of the heart to pump blood out of the right atrium and through the left heart into the systemic circulation and the tendency of blood to flow from the peripheral veins into the right heart (called venous return). The difference between venous and right atrial pressure is called the *atrial filling pressure*. When the heart pumps strongly, the right atrial pressure decreases and atrial filling is enhanced. When atrial pressure rises, venous flow backs up.

Breathing and respiratory maneuvers also affect blood flow in the central veins and right atrium.

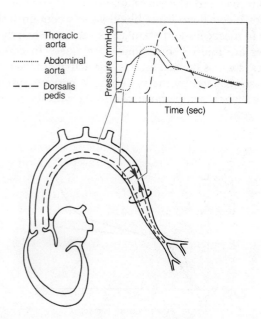

Figure 17-11 Amplification of the arterial pressure wave as it moves forward in the peripheral arteries. This amplification occurs as a forward-moving pressure wave merges with a backward-moving reflected pressure wave. The inset at upper right illustrates the increasing amplitude of the pressure pulse in the thoracic aorta, abdominal aorta, and dorsalis pedis.

— Thoracic aorta

········· Abdominal aorta

--- Dorsalis pedis

Pressure (mmHg)

Time (sec)

The negative pressure generated during inspiration is transmitted to the right atrium; this decreases right atrial pressure and increases atrial filling pressure, and blood flow into the thoracic veins and right heart is increased. During expiration when intrathoracic pressures are increased, blood flow is decreased.

The microcirculation

The capillaries, venules, and metarterioles of the circulatory system are collectively referred to as the *microcirculation*. It is here that the exchange of gases, nutrients, metabolites, and heat occurs. Blood enters the capillary through an arteriole and leaves by way of a small venule. The metarterioles serve as thoroughfare channels that link arterioles and capillaries. Precapillary sphincters control the flow of blood in the microcirculation. When the precapillary sphincters are open, blood flows through the capillary channels. Blood flow through capillary channels designed for exchange of nutrients and metabolites is called *nutritional flow*. In some parts of the microcirculation, blood flow bypasses the nutrient capillary bed moving through a connection called an *arteriovenous (AV) shunt*, which directly connects an arteriole and a venule. This type of blood flow is called *nonnutrient flow* because it does not allow for nutrient exchange. Nonnutrient channels are important in terms of heat exchange. The AV shunts found in the microcirculation of the skin are important in terms of temperature regulation.

The control of blood flow through the microcirculation performs two functions: (1) it provides for the tissue exchange of gases, nutrients, and metabolites and (2) it controls the total peripheral resistance of the circulatory system. The total cardiac output travels through the microcirculation; therefore, the tone of these vessels, particularly the arterioles, determines the total peripheral resistance and, as will be discussed later, the arterial blood pressure. If, for example, all of the arterioles were to open fully, the total peripheral resistance, and thus the blood pressure, would fall catastrophically. These two somewhat conflicting functions require a degree of independent control over arteriole resistance and flow in the capillaries of the microcirculation. The nervous system controls the peripheral resistance by regulating the smooth muscle tone of the arterioles, and local factors control the precapillary sphincters, which regulate flow through the nutrient channels of the capillary bed.

Local control of blood flow

Local control is governed largely by the nutritional needs of the tissue. For example, blood flow to organs such as the heart, brain, and kidney remains relatively constant, although blood pressure may vary over a range of 60 mmHg to 180 mmHg (Figure 17-12). The ability of the tissues to regulate their own blood flow is called *autoregulation*. Autoregulation of blood flow is controlled by local tissue factors, such as oxygen lack or accumulation of tissue metabolites. It involves the selective opening and closing of capillary channels. Local control is particularly important in tissues such as skeletal muscle, which has varying blood flow requirements according to the level of activity.

An increase in local blood flow is called *hyperemia*. When the blood supply to an area has been occluded and then restored, local blood flow through the tissues increases within seconds to restore the metabolic equilibrium of the tissues. This increased flow is called *reactive hyperemia*. The transient redness seen after leaning an arm on a hard surface is an example of reactive hyperemia. The ability of tissues to increase blood flow in situations of increased activity, such as exercising, is called *functional hyperemia*. Local control mechanisms rely on a continuous flow from the main arteries and, therefore, hyperemia cannot occur when the arteries supplying the capillary beds are narrowed. For example, if a major coronary artery becomes occluded, the opening of channels supplied by that vessel cannot restore blood flow.

Vasodilator substances, formed in tissues in response to a need for increased blood flow, aid in the local control of blood flow. The most important of these are histamine, serotonin (5-hydroxytryptamine), the kinins, and the prostaglandins. *Histamine* increases blood flow. Most blood vessels contain histamine in mast cells and nonmast cell stores; when these tissues are injured, histamine is released. In certain tissues, such as skeletal muscle, the activity of the mast cells is mediated by the sympathetic nervous system; that is, when sympathetic control is withdrawn, the

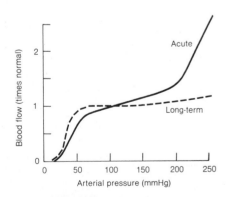

Figure 17-12 Effect on blood flow through a muscle of increasing arterial pressure. *The solid curve* shows the effect if pressure is raised over a period of a few minutes. *The dashed curve* shows the effect if the arterial pressure is raised slowly over a period of many weeks. *(Guyton A: Medical Physiology, 7th ed. Philadelphia, WB Saunders, 1986)*

mast cells release histamine. This mechanism is augmented with withdrawal of vasoconstrictor activity. *Serotonin* is liberated from aggregating platelets during the clotting process; it causes vasoconstriction and plays a major role in control of bleeding. Serotonin is found in brain and lung tissues, and there is some speculation that it may be involved in the vascular spasm associated with some allergic pulmonary reactions and migraine headaches. The *kinins* (*kallidins* and *bradykinin*) are liberated from the globulin kininogen, which is present in body fluids. The kinins cause relaxation of arteriole smooth muscle, increase capillary permeability, and constrict the venules. In exocrine glands, the formation of kinins contributes to the vasodilatation needed for glandular secretion. *Prostaglandins* are synthesized from constituents (the long-chain fatty acid, arachidonic acid) of the cell membrane. Tissue injury incites the release of arachidonic acid from the cell membrane, which initiates prostaglandin synthesis. There are several prostaglandins (E_2, F_2, and D_2), which are subgrouped according to their solubility; some produce vasoconstriction and some produce vasodilatation. As a general rule of thumb, those in the E group are vasodilators and those in the F group are vasoconstrictors. The adrenal glucocorticoid hormones can produce an anti-inflammatory response by blocking the release of arachidonic acid, and thus preventing prostaglandin synthesis.

Endothelial factors. The endothelium, which lies between the blood and vascular smooth muscle, serves as a physical barrier for vasoactive substances that circulate in the blood. Once thought to be nothing more than a single layer of cells that line blood vessels, it is now known that endothelium plays an active role in controlling vascular function.

In capillaries, which are composed of a single layer of endothelial cells, the endothelium is active in transport of cell nutrients and wastes. In addition to its function in capillary transport, the endothelium removes vasoactive agents such as norepinephrine from the blood; it converts precursors such as angiotensin I to angiotensin II, which is a potent vasoconstrictor; and it secretes vasoactive substances such as prostacyline, which inhibits platelet aggregation and produces vasodilatation.

Of particular importance was the discovery, first reported in 1980, that the intact endothelium was able to produce a factor that caused relaxation of vascular smooth muscle. This factor was named *endothelial-derived relaxing factor (EDRF)*.[4,5] The discovery was an outcome of laboratory observations in which strips of vascular smooth muscle were exposed to agents known to produce relaxation. It was found that relaxation only occurred in vessel strips with an intact endothelium. Although the original discovery was made using acetylcholine, a number of other agents have since been shown to produce vascular relaxation in the same way. Thrombin was one of the first blood constituents shown to trigger EDRF. Aggregating platelets and the products they release also evoke endothelium-dependent vessel relaxation. This probably contributes to the protective role the endothelium plays in controlling platelet aggregation and thrombus formation. It also raises the question as to what happens in atherosclerotic vessels in which the endothelium has been injured or lost. In these vessels, the absence or dysfunction of the endothelium may favor the occurrence of abnormal vasoconstriction.

Recent evidence suggests the presence of an endothelial-derived contracting factor (EDCF). A reported stimulus for EDCF is hypoxia. In the pulmonary circulation, the production of EDCF could help to explain the vasoconstriction and pulmonary hypertension that occurs with hypoxia.

Neural control of blood flow

The neural control centers for regulation of cardiovascular function are located in the reticular formation of the lower pons and medulla of the brain. The area of the reticular formation in the brain that controls vasomotor function is called the *vasomotor center*. The sympathetic nervous system serves as the final common pathway for controlling the smooth muscle tone of the blood vessels. Most of the sympathetic preganglionic fibers that control vessel function travel in the intermediolateral column of the spinal cord and exit with the ventral nerves; they then synapse with postganglionic fibers in the paravertebral ganglia. The sympathetic neurons that supply the blood vessels maintain them in a state of tonic activity, so that even under resting conditions the blood vessels are partially constricted. Vessel constriction and relaxation are accomplished by altering this basal input. Increasing sympathetic activity causes constriction of some vessels, such as those of the skin, the gastrointestinal tract, and the kidney. Some blood vessels are supplied by both vasoconstrictor and vasodilator fibers. Skeletal muscle, for example, is innervated by both types of fibers; activation of sympathetic vasodilator fibers provides the muscles with increased blood flow during exercise. Although the parasympathetic nervous system contributes to the regulation of heart function, it has little, if any, control over blood vessels.

Collateral circulation

Collateral circulation is a mechanism for the long-term regulation of local blood flow. In the heart and other vital structures, anastomotic channels exist between some of the smaller arteries. These channels permit perfusion of an area by more than one artery. When one artery becomes occluded, these anastomotic channels increase in size, allowing blood from a patent artery to perfuse the area supplied by the occluded vessel. For example, persons with extensive obstruction of a coronary blood vessel may rely on collateral circulation to meet the oxygen needs of the myocardial tissue normally supplied by that vessel. As with other long-term compensatory mechanisms, the recruitment of collateral circulation is most efficient when obstruction to flow is gradual rather than sudden.

In summary, arterial flow is pulsatile in nature; it reflects the intermittent contraction and relaxation of the heart. The pressure pulses that result from the pumping action of the heart are transmitted throughout the arterial system and reflect the energy that is imparted to the blood during systole. Venous flow is designed to return blood to the heart. It is a low pressure system and relies on venous valves and the action of muscle pumps to offset the effects of gravity.

The mechanisms that control blood flow are designed to ensure delivery of blood to the capillaries in the microcirculation where the exchange of cellular nutrients and wastes occurs. Local control is governed largely by the needs of the tissues and is regulated by local tissue factors such as lack of oxygen or the accumulation of metabolites. Hyperemia is a local increase in blood flow that occurs following a temporary occlusion of blood flow. It is a compensatory mechanism that serves to decrease the oxygen debt of the deprived tissues. The vasomotor center of the reticular formation of the lower pons and medulla provides for neural control of blood flow by the sympathetic nervous system. Collateral circulation is a mechanism for long-term regulation of local blood flow involving the development of collateral vessels.

References

1. Smith JJ, Kampine JP: Circulatory Physiology, 2nd ed, p 10. Baltimore, Williams & Wilkins, 1984
2. Guyton A: Medical Physiology, 7th ed, pp 289, 348. Philadelphia, WB Saunders, 1986
3. Johansen K: Aneurysms. Sci Am 247(1):110, 1982
4. Furchgott RF, Zawadzki JV: The obligatory role of endothelial cells in relaxation of arterial smooth muscle by acetylcholine. Nature 288:373, 1980
5. Vanhoutte PM: Endothelium and the control of vascular tissue. NIPS 2(2):21, 1987

CHAPTER 18

Alterations in Blood Flow

Objectives

After you have studied this chapter, you should be able to meet the following objectives:

_____ List five mechanisms of blood vessel obstruction.

_____ Describe vessel changes that occur in atherosclerosis.

_____ Use the principles of blood flow from Chapter 17 to explain why atherosclerosis is usually a silent disease until extensive vessel occlusion has occurred.

_____ Cite two current theories used to explain the pathogenesis of atherosclerosis.

_____ List three established risk factors in atherosclerosis.

_____ List the five types of lipoproteins and state their function in terms of lipid transport.

_____ State the proposed function of the apoproteins in terms of lipoprotein function.

_____ Describe the effects of a hereditary absence or defect in LDL receptors.

_____ State two possible mechanisms for the beneficial effects of controlling the fat and cholesterol content of the diet.

_____ State three general ways in which lipid-lowering drugs exert their actions.

_____ Distinguish among berry aneurysms, aortic aneurysms, and dissecting aneurysms.

_____ Relate the Laplace's law to wall tension in an aneurysm.

_____ List the signs and symptoms associated with thoracic and abdominal aneurysms.

_____ State the signs and symptoms of acute arterial occlusion.

(continued)

_____ State a method for describing gradations in pulse volume.

_____ Differentiate between the mechanisms of ischemia in Raynaud's syndrome and thromboangiitis obliterans (Buerger's disease).

_____ State the signs and symptoms of chronic peripheral vascular disease.

_____ Describe the effect of gravity on the venous system.

_____ State the signs and symptoms of venous insufficiency.

_____ Describe the pathology involved in venous thrombosis.

_____ Cite two causes of pressure sores.

_____ Explain how shearing forces contribute to ischemic skin damage.

_____ Explain why pressure sores are more apt to develop over bony prominences.

_____ List four measures that contribute to the prevention of pressure sores.

Interruption of blood flow in either the arterial or the venous system interferes with delivery of oxygen and nutrients to the tissues. Alterations in arterial flow produce ischemia or the temporary holding back of blood from the tissues. Venous obstruction, on the other hand, causes congestion and edema. This chapter is organized into four sections: (1) mechanisms of vessel obstruction, (2) disorders of the arterial circulation, (3) alterations of the venous circulation, and (4) pressure sores caused by localized interruption of blood flow.

Mechanisms of vessel obstruction

Occlusion of flow within a vessel can result from (1) thrombus formation, (2) emboli, (3) compression, (4) vasospasm, or (5) structural defects in the vessel (Figure 18-1). Each of these mechanisms is discussed briefly in preparation for the discussion on specific alterations in arterial and venous flow.

—— Thrombi

A thrombus is a blood clot. Blood clotting is a homeostatic mechanism intended to seal off blood vessels, to prevent bleeding, and to maintain the continuity of the vascular system. Thrombi can develop in either the arterial or the venous system and obstruct flow. Alterations in hemostasis are discussed in Chapter 15.

—— Emboli

An embolus is a foreign mass transported in the bloodstream. Although an embolus moves freely in the larger blood vessels, it becomes lodged and obstructs flow once it reaches a smaller vessel. An embolus can be a dislodged thrombus or can consist of air, fat, tumor cells, or other materials. Approximately 95% of venous thrombi that become emboli have their origin in the veins of the legs. These emboli move

through the venous system, into the right heart, and then into the pulmonary circulation where they can become lodged and obstruct blood flow. Arterial emboli commonly have their origin in the heart itself and can travel to the brain, spleen, kidney, or vessels of the lower extremity before they become lodged and obstruct flow.

—— Compression

The lumen of a blood vessel can be occluded by external forces. The external pressure of a tourniquet, for example, is intended to compress blood vessels and interrupt blood flow. Likewise, casts and circular dressings predispose to vessel compression,

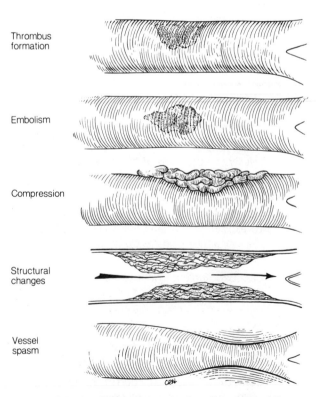

Thrombus formation

Embolism

Compression

Structural changes

Vessel spasm

Figure 18-1 Conditions that cause disruption of blood flow.

particularly when swelling occurs after these devices have been applied. Tumors may encroach on blood vessels as they grow. Blood vessels may be compressed between bony structures such as the sacrum and the supporting surfaces of a chair or bed.

Vasospasm

Vasospasm may result from locally or neurally mediated reflexes. Exposure to cold causes severe vasoconstriction in many of the superficial blood vessels. Fortunately, local control mechanisms produce brief periods of vasodilatation designed to maintain tissue oxygen needs. Those who have spent time on the ski slopes, or elsewhere in the cold, may have noticed the intermittent redness of their companions' noses during these periods of vasodilatation. In certain disease states, vasospasm from exposure to cold or other stimuli is excessive and may lead to ischemia and tissue injury.

Structural defects

Structural changes in blood vessels can take many forms. Defects in venous valves may impair blood flow in the venous system, causing varicose veins. Arteriosclerosis causes rigidity and narrowing of the arterioles. Aneurysms are dilatations in arteries that appear at points where the vessel wall has been weakened.

In summary, interruption of flow in either the arterial or the venous system interferes with the flow of oxygen and nutrients to the tissues. Occlusion of flow can result from (1) the presence of a thrombus, (2) emboli, (3) vessel compression, (4) vasospasm, or (5) structural changes within the vessel.

Alterations in arterial flow

The arterial system distributes blood to all of the various tissues of the body. Pathology of the arterial system affects body function through impaired blood flow. The discussion in this section focuses on arteriosclerosis, aneurysms, acute arterial occlusion, peripheral vascular diseases—Raynaud's syndrome and Buerger's disease—and assessment of arterial flow.

Vascular disease is a relatively silent disorder. To be more explicit, the diseased vessel itself seldom gives rise to symptoms that warn of its presence. Rather, signs and symptoms arise because of ischemia in the body part served by the vessel. The pain associated with coronary heart disease (angina pectoris) and intermittent claudication (pain and weakness in

the leg occurring with exercise and relieved by rest) provide evidence of impaired blood flow. Unfortunately, arterial disease is usually far advanced by the time these symptoms occur.

Atherosclerosis

Arteriosclerosis is a general term that literally means *hardening of the arteries*. The term describes several conditions. One form of arteriosclerosis, Mönckeberg's medial sclerosis, affects the media of medium-sized arteries and is characterized by a hyaline thickening of the arterioles and small blood vessels. This form of arteriosclerosis increases vessel rigidity but does not encroach on the lumen of the vessel and obstruct blood flow. Atherosclerosis, a form of arteriosclerosis, is characterized by the formation of intimal fibrofatty lesions, called atherosclerotic plaques, which narrow the vessel lumen.

Atherosclerosis affects the large and medium-sized arteries—the aorta and its branches, the coronaries, and the large vessels that supply the brain. In 1985, atherosclerosis was a leading contributor to as many as 693,500 heart attack and stroke deaths.[1] In 1988, the estimated cost of coronary heart disease and stroke was $48.7 billion in health-care expenditures and lost productivity. The bright side of this grim picture is the recent decline in death rates from coronary heart disease. In 1978 alone, there were 114,000 fewer deaths among people ages 35 to 74 years than would have been expected had the rate not declined from its high level in the 1960s.[2] This decline probably reflects new and improved methods of medical treatment as well as improved health-care practices resulting from an increased public awareness of the factors that predispose to development of the disorder.

Atherosclerosis begins as an insidious process, and clinical manifestations of the disease often do not become evident for 20 to 40 years or longer. Fibrous plaques often begin to appear in the arteries of Americans in their twenties. Among 300 American soldiers (average age 22 years) killed during the Korean war, 77% were found to have gross evidence of atherosclerosis.[3]

Atherosclerotic lesions are characterized by (1) the accumulation of intracellular and extracellular lipids, (2) proliferation of vascular smooth muscle cells, and (3) formation of large amounts of scar tissue and connective tissue proteins.[4] The lesion begins as a gray to pearly white elevated thickening of the vessel intima with a core of extracellular lipid (mainly cholesterol, which is usually complexed to proteins) covered by a fibrous cap of connective tissue and smooth muscle. Later lesions contain hemorrhage, ulceration, and scar tissue deposits. As the lesions increase in size, they encroach on the lumen of the artery and

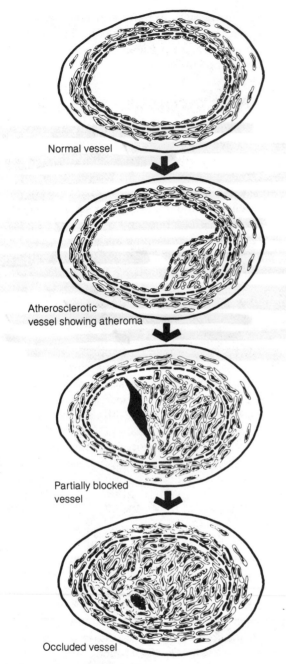

Figure 18-2 Evolution of occlusion in an atherosclerotic vessel. (*Report of the 1981 Working Group to Review the Report by the National Heart and Lung Institute Task Force on Arteriosclerosis: Arteriosclerosis. DHEW Publication No. NIH 1526*)

eventually may either occlude the vessel or predispose to thrombus formation, causing reduction of blood flow (Figure 18-2). Because blood flow is related to the fourth power of the radius (see Chapter 17), reduction in blood flow becomes more severe as the disease progresses.

Risk factors

To date, the cause or causes of atherosclerosis have not been determined with certainty. However, epidemiologic studies have identified predisposing risk factors, which are listed in Table 18-1. Some of these risk factors can be changed and others cannot.

Risk factors such as heredity, male sex, and increasing age cannot be changed. It appears that the tendency to develop atherosclerosis runs in families. A number of genetically determined alterations in lipoprotein and cholesterol metabolism have been identified, and it seems likely that others will continue to be identified in the future. Race is also an inherited risk factor. Black Americans have hypertension more often than whites and consequently their risk of atherosclerosis and coronary heart disease is increased.[1] The incidence of atherosclerosis increases with age. Men are at greater risk for developing coronary heart disease than women; even though the death rate of women increases after menopause, it never reaches that of men.

The major risk factors that can be changed include cigarette smoking, high blood pressure (see Chapter 19), and high blood cholesterol levels (to be discussed in this chapter). Cigarette smoking is linked closely with coronary heart disease and sudden death. The risk of death from coronary heart disease is about 60 to 70 times greater for smokers than nonsmokers.[5] The greatest effects of smoking are noted in young men and women, particularly those below the age of 55. The effects are related directly to the number of cigarettes smoked. Risk factors such as high blood pressure and high blood cholesterol levels can often be controlled with the aid of a physician and other health professionals. The responsibility for changing other risk factors such as smoking rests largely with the individual.

Table 18–1.   Risk factors of atherosclerosis

Major risk factors that cannot be changed	Major risk factors that can be changed	Contributing factors
Heredity	Cigarette smoking	Diabetes
Male sex	High blood pressure	Obesity
Increasing age	Blood cholesterol levels	Physical inactivity
		Stress

(From Heart Facts 1988. Dallas, American Heart Association, 1988)

The association between coronary heart disease and contributing risk factors is not as convincing as for the established risk factors. These factors often are linked with the established or other risk factors. For example, obesity and physical inactivity are often observed in the same person. Furthermore, both of these situations are reported to bring about elevations in blood lipid levels. Likewise, smoking patterns, blood pressure levels, and other risk factors are closely associated with stress and personality patterns. Diabetes mellitus (type II) often develops in middle-aged individuals and among persons who are overweight. Diabetes tends to elevate blood lipids and otherwise increase the risk of atherosclerosis (see Chapter 45). Therefore, controlling other risk factors is particularly important in persons with diabetes.

Mechanisms of development

Although the risk factors associated with atherosclerosis have been identified through epidemiologic studies, there are many unanswered questions regarding the mechanisms by which these risk factors contribute to the development of atherosclerosis. In the past several decades two broad theories of atherogenesis have emerged: (1) the vessel injury hypothesis, and (2) the lipid infiltration hypothesis (vessel response to lipoproteins and cholesterol).

Vessel injury.   The vascular endothelial layer acts as a selective barrier that protects the subendothelial layers from interacting with blood cells and blood components. The endothelial cells determine the nature of lipoproteins and other plasma constituents that reach the subendothelial space and vascular smooth muscle. They bind low-density lipoproteins (LDLs) and modify them so that the LDLs can be ingested by macrophages; they produce vasoactive agents, growth factors, and growth inhibitors. The vascular endothelial cells are arranged in a single layer with cell-to-cell attachments. It has been suggested that with repeated injury, there may be impaired ability of the endothelium to regenerate. A number of factors are regarded as possible injurious agents, including products associated with smoking, immune mechanisms, and mechanical stress such as that associated with hypertension. If the injury is a single event, the lesion is usually reversible. However, if the original mechanism that led to vessel injury persists, there is less time for healing to occur and the lesion may become chronic.

Normally there are interactions between the arterial endothelium and the white blood cells, particularly the monocytes (macrophages), that occur throughout life; however, this interaction is increased when blood cholesterol levels are elevated (hypercholesterolemia). It has been reported that one of the earliest responses to hypercholesterolemia is the attachment of clusters of monocytes throughout the arterial tree.[6] The monocytes have been observed to move through the intercellular attachments of the endothelial cells into the subendothelial spaces where they contribute to the formation of fatty streaks. With continued enlargement of the fatty streaks, the endothelial cells are pulled apart, exposing the underlying connective tissue; this may provide the opportunity for platelet adherence, aggregation, and thrombosis.

Proliferation of smooth muscle is a feature in atherosclerotic plaque formation. A current hypothesis of atheroma formation is that injury to the arterial endothelium is the initiating factor that permits platelets, cholesterol, and other blood components to come in contact with and stimulate abnormal proliferation of muscle cells and connective tissue in the vessel wall (Figure 18-3). Platelets contain a potent smooth-muscle mitogenic factor (a substance that induces cell mi-

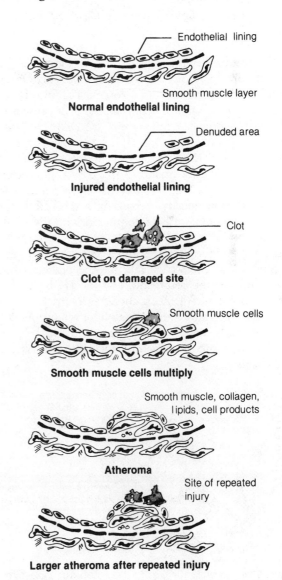

Figure 18-3 A theory for evolution of atheroma. (*Report of the 1977 Working Group to Review the Report by the National Heart and Lung Institute Task Force on Arteriosclerosis: Arteriosclerosis. DHEW Publication No. NIH 81-2034*)

tosis and cell transformation). According to current theory, this factor is released from platelets when they aggregate over a denuded area on the vessel wall. Recent evidence suggests that the LDLs act as the cofactors necessary for growth and proliferation of vascular smooth muscle cells, but are not able to stimulate the process by themselves.[7]

Cholesterol and the lipoproteins. There is considerable evidence linking hypercholesterolemia to atherogenesis and its sequelae—coronary heart disease, stroke, peripheral vascular disease, and sudden death. According to the guidelines developed by the National Cholesterol Education Program's Expert Panel on Detection, Evaluation, and Treatment of High Blood Cholesterol in Adults, a cholesterol level of 200 mg/dl to 239 mg/dl represents borderline high risk of coronary heart disease.[8]

Because lipids are insoluble in plasma, they are encapsulated by certain fat-carrying proteins—the lipoproteins—for transportation in the blood. The cholesterol esters and triglycerides are located in the hydrophobic core of the macromolecule, surrounded by phospholipids and apoproteins (Figure 18-4). There are five classes of lipoproteins: (1) chylomicron, (2) very low-density lipoprotein (VLDL), (3) intermediate-density lipoprotein (IDL), (4) low-density lipoprotein, and (5) high-density lipoprotein (HDL). The naming of these lipoproteins is based on ultracentrifugation, by which the proteins are separated according to their density. Accordingly, the VLDL carries large amounts of lipid compared with the HDL. The lipoproteins can also be separated by electrophoresis, a technique that uses an electrical field to separate proteins. The VLDL fall into the prebeta band, the LDL into the beta band, and the HDL into the alpha band. Beta-VLDL, a cholesterol-enriched form of VLDL, migrates with the beta-lipoproteins on electrophoresis. It is elevated in persons with an inherited form of hyperlipoproteinemia called *familial dysbetaproteinemia.*

Each type of lipoprotein consists of a large molecular complex of lipids and proteins called *apoproteins.*[9,10] The major lipid constituents are cholesterol, cholesterol esters, triglycerides, and phospholipids. There are five major classes of apoproteins, designated A through E, the major types being A, B-48, B-100, C, and E.[11] The apoproteins control the interactions and ultimate metabolic fate of the lipoproteins. Some of the apoproteins activate lipolytic enzymes that facilitate the removal of lipids from the lipoproteins; others serve as a reactive site that cellular receptors can recognize and use in the process of endocytosis and metabolism of the lipoproteins. The major apoprotein in LDL is B-100. The lipoproteins are synthesized in the small intestine and in the liver. The chylomicrons, which are the largest lipoprotein molecules, are synthesized in the wall of the small intestine. They are involved in the transport of exogenous triglycerides and cholesterol that has been absorbed from the gastrointestinal tract. Chylomicrons travel to the capillaries of adipose tissue and skeletal muscle; there they transfer their triglycerides to fat and muscle cells. The remaining cholesterol-containing chylomicron remnant particles are taken up by the liver. In this way, the chylomicrons transport dietary triglycerides to the tissues and cholesterol to the liver.

The liver synthesizes and secretes VLDL and HDL. The VLDL particles contain triglycerides, cholesterol, and numerous apoproteins; they are the primary endogenous pathway for transport of triglycerides that are already in the body. Like chylomicrons, VLDLs carry triglycerides to tissue capillaries for entry into fat and muscle cells. The IDL constitute the lipoprotein remnants that remain when the triglycerides are removed from the VLDL; these are either taken up and broken down by the liver or they are converted to LDLs by an intravascular process that removes most of the triglycerides, leaving the cholesterol esters in the core. Both the IDL and the LDL are atherogenic.[9]

The LDLs are the major carriers of cholesterol. About two-thirds of plasma cholesterol is carried by LDLs so that its measurement provides a good estimate of blood cholesterol in most people. Cholesterol is an important constituent of cell membranes and also is used by some cells in the synthesis of steroid hormones. Although most cells can synthesize their own cholesterol, they prefer to remove it from the plasma. The LDL can be catabolized by a number of cell types by both receptor-dependent and nonreceptor-dependent mechanisms. The liver contains cells with highly specific LDL surface receptors. About two-thirds of the circulating LDL is removed by the liver by means of the LDL receptors. The remainder is taken up and broken down in the peripheral tissues by a degradative process, which includes macro-

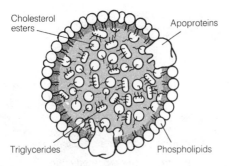

Figure 18-4 General structure of a lipoprotein. The cholesterol esters and triglycerides are located in the hydrophobic core of the macromolecule, surrounded by phospholipids and aproproteins.

Cholesterol esters

Apoproteins

Triglycerides

Phospholipids

phages of the reticuloendothelial system. Macrophage uptake of LDL within the arterial wall can result in the accummulation of cholesterol ester, the formation of foam cells, and the development of atherosclerosis. When there is a decrease in LDL receptors in the liver or when LDL levels exceed receptor availability, the amount of LDL that must be removed by the peripheral tissues is increased.

Cholesterol is not metabolized in the peripheral tissues, and amounts not used in the synthesis of cell membranes would accumulate if there were no mechanism for its removal. It is now believed that HDLs serve as carriers that remove cholesterol from the peripheral tissues and transport it back to the liver for catabolism and excretion.[12] The HDLs are also believed to inhibit cellular uptake of LDLs. These two mechanisms could help to explain the protective effect that the HDL have been observed to provide relative to the risk of coronary heart disease.

Recent epidemiologic studies suggest the potentially serious effects of hyperlipidemia depend not so much on the level of serum lipids but on the type of lipoproteins present. High levels of LDLs contribute to the development of atherosclerosis; whereas, high levels of HDLs appear to provide some protection against the disorder. It has been observed that HDL levels are increased in trained individuals who exercise regularly, in women who take estrogens, and in persons who consume a moderate amount of alcohol. Smoking and diabetes, which are in themselves risk factors for atherosclerosis, are associated with high levels of LDLs and low levels of HDLs.

Plasma cholesterol can become elevated as a result of an increase in any of the lipoproteins: the chylomicrons, VLDL, IDL, LDL, or HDL. The commonly used classification system for hyperlipid-emias is based on the type of lipoprotein involved (Table 18-2). Three factors—nutrition, genetics, and metabolic diseases—can raise blood lipid levels. Most cases of elevated levels of LDL cholesterol are probably multifactorial. Some persons may have increased sensitivity to dietary cholesterol; others may have altered synthesis of the apoproteins including oversynthesis of apoprotein B-100, the major apoprotein in the LDL. Causes of secondary hyperlipoproteinemia include obesity with high-caloric intake and diabetes. High-calorie diets increase the production of VLDL with triglyceride elevation and high conversion of VLDLs to LDLs. Excess ingestion of cholesterol may reduce formation of LDL receptors. It has been suggested that large amounts of dietary cholesterol may suppress the synthesis of LDL receptors in the liver, because the liver will require less cholesterol from circulating LDL.[13]

Many types of hypercholesterolemia have a genetic basis. There may be a defective synthesis of the apoproteins, a lack of receptors, defective receptors, or defects in the handling of cholesterol within the cell that are genetically determined. For example, the normal LDL receptor is deficient or defective in the genetic disorder known as familial hypercholesterolemia (type IIA). This autosomal dominant type of hyperlipoproteinemias results from a mutation in the gene specifying the receptor for LDL. Because most of the circulating cholesterol is removed by receptor-dependent mechanisms, blood cholesterol is markedly elevated in persons with this disorder. The disorder is probably one of the most frequent of all mendelian disorders; the frequency of heterozygotes is 1 in 500 in the general population.[11] Heterozygotes have a two- to threefold elevation of plasma cholesterol levels, and in homozygotes the elevation may be fivefold or greater.

Table 18-2. Classification of hyperlipoproteinemias

Type	Familiar name	Lipoprotein abnormality	Cause
Type I	Exogenous dietary hypertriglyceridemia	Elevated chylomicrons; triglycerides. Normal cholesterol	Dietary fat not cleared from the plasma
Type IIA	Hypercholesterolemia (familial)	Elevated LDL, cholesterol. Normal triglycerides	Hereditary metabolic defect
Type IIB	Combined hyperlipidemia	Elevated LDL, VLDL, cholesterol, triglycerides	Possible long-term dietary excess; hereditary component
Type III	Remnant hyperlipidemia	Increased beta-VLDL, cholesterol, triglycerides	Hereditary metabolic defect (familial dysbetalipoproteinemia)
Type IV	Endogenous hypertriglyceridemia	Elevated VLDL, triglycerides. Cholesterol normal or elevated	Excessive carbohydrate intake
Type V	Mixed hypertriglyceridemia	Elevated chylomicrons, VLDL, cholesterol. Triglycerides greatly increased	Possible metabolic defect

(Data from Robbins SL, Kumar V: Basic Pathology, 4th ed, p 289. Philadelphia, WB Saunders, 1987; and Gotto AM: Lipoprotein metabolism and etiology of hyperlipidemia. Hosp Pract 23(Suppl 1):4, 1988)

Although the heterozygotes commonly have an elevated cholesterol from birth, they do not develop symptoms until adult life when they develop xanthomas (cholesterol deposits) along the tendons and atherosclerosis. Myocardial infarction before age 40 is common. The homozygote is much more severely affected, developing cutaneous xanthomas in childhood and frequently dying of myocardial infarction by the age of 20.[11]

Diagnosis and treatment of hyperlipidemia

The National Institutes of Health Consensus Development Conference on Lowering Blood Cholesterol to Prevent Heart Disease recommended: (1) that all Americans attempt to reduce their cholesterol intake, (2) that individuals at moderate risk for coronary heart disease (cholesterol levels above the 75th percentile for Americans) and those at high risk (levels above the 90th percentile) be treated aggressively with diet, and (3) that drugs be added to the regimen, particularly for high-risk persons, if diet alone fails to lower cholesterol.[14]

Capillary-blood cholesterol testing methods have provided a means for mass screening for hypercholesterolemia. In most adults, a fasting serum using a venous blood sample is indicated. In those at high risk, such as relatives of persons with a strong family history of coronary heart disease, children as well as adult family members should be tested. In persons with cholesterol levels above 200 mg/dl, repeat measurements of serum cholesterol along with direct HDL-cholesterol and serum triglyceride levels are usually indicated. LDL-cholesterol can be estimated using this approach.

The treatment of hypercholesterolemia focuses on dietary and life-style modifications, and when these are unsuccessful, pharmacologic treatment is necessary. Three dietary elements affecting dietary cholesterol and its lipoprotein fractions are excess calorie intake leading to obesity, saturated fats, and cholesterol.[15] Excess calories consistently lower HDLs and less consistently elevate LDLs. Saturated fats in the diet can strongly influence cholesterol levels. Each 1% of saturated fat, relative to calorie intake, has been estimated to increase the cholesterol level on an average of 2.8 mg/dl. Depending on individual differences, it tends to raise both the VLDLs and the LDLs. Dietary cholesterol has a tendency to increase the LDL cholesterol. On an average, each 100 mg/day of ingested cholesterol raises the serum cholesterol 8 to 10 mg/dl.[15]

Soluble fiber in the diet (pectin, bran, and guar) is another dietary intervention that has been shown to have moderate LDL-lowering effects. How-

Table 18–3. Lipid-lowering drugs: actions and common side-effects

Drug	Mechanism of action	Common side-effects
Nicotinic acid	Reduces VLDL synthesis (with subsequent decrease in LDL) and decreases HDL removal by inhibiting lipolysis in adipocytes and hepatic triglyceride production	Flushing, pruritis, nausea, and gastrointestinal tract distress. Carbohydrate tolerance, hyperuricemia, and liver dysfunction may occur.
Fibric acid derivatives (clofibrate, gemfibrozil)	Enhanced intravascular catabolism and removal of VLDL and increased HDL synthesis through increased lipoprotein lipase activity	Nausea and abdominal discomfort, myalgia (muscle cramps and tenderness), and skin rashes. Displaces acidic drugs from albumin-binding sites and can enhance the action of drugs such as the oral anticoagulant, warfarin. Enhances gallstone formation.
Bile acid sequestrants (cholestyramine, colestipol)	These drugs are insoluble hydrophilic resins that are not absorbed from the gastrointestinal tract. They bind and increase the fecal elimination of bile acids. This results in increased removal of cholesterol from the circulation.	Gastrointestinal side-effects, including nausea, vomiting, abdominal discomfort, constipation, and indigestion, may result from sequestering of bile acids. A high fluid intake, increased dietary bulk, and stool softeners are used to alleviate these side-effects.
Probucol	Removes LDL from the circulation independent of LDL receptor activity	Diarrhea, flatulence, nausea, abdominal discomfort. Increases HDL levels. The drug is lipid soluble and becomes sequestered and remains in body fat stores for months after discontinuation. Its safety for use with children and pregnant women has not been established.

ever, most studies that have reported beneficial effects have used large amounts of fiber, which tend to produce gastrointestinal side-effects, although tolerance tends to improve with prolonged usage.

Recently, fish oils (omega-3 fatty acids) have received attention as a preventive measure for atherosclerosis. The research finding on the value of fish oils on lipoprotein levels is inconclusive. In fact, the anti-atherogenic effects of fish oils may be more related to their effects on platelet aggregation and impaired prostaglandin synthesis than on lowering blood lipids. There is concern over side-effects from the use of fish oils such as glucose intolerance, action on immune function, and bleeding. Also, although purified oils are now available, capsules of unpurified oil containing the cholesterol that is present in fish oil extract are still available. Ingestion of large amounts of the unpurified oil may actually raise, rather than lower cholesterol levels.[16]

Three types of medications are available for treatment of hypercholesterolemia: niacin and its congeners, fibric acid agents, and bile acid-binding resins. Lipid-lowering drugs ultimately work by affecting lipoprotein production, intravascular breakdown, or removal from the bloodstream. Nicotinic acid (a niacin congener) blocks the synthesis and release of VLDL by the liver, thereby lowering not only VLDL levels, but IDL and LDL levels as well. The fibric acid derivatives enhance intravascular lipolysis of VLDL and IDL. The bile acid-binding resins enhance LDL removal. Many of these drugs have significant side-effects, so they are usually only used in persons with significant hyperlipidemia that cannot be controlled by other means, such as diet. Table 18-3 lists some of the common lipid-lowering drugs, their effect on lipoprotein metabolism, and side-effects.

Arterial aneurysms

An aneurysm is an abnormal localized vessel dilatation caused by weakness of the arterial wall. Aneurysms can assume several forms and may be classified according to their etiology, location, and anatomical features (Figure 18-5). A *berry aneurysm* consists of

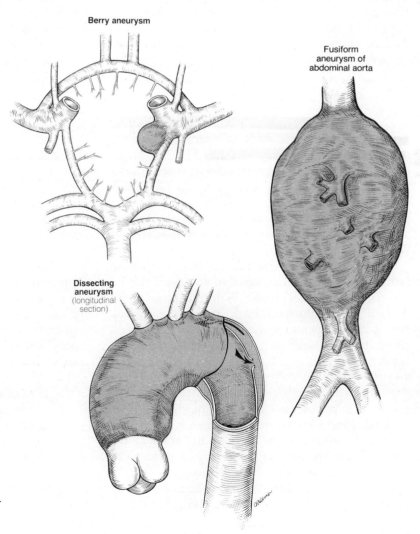

Berry aneurysm

Fusiform aneurysm of abdominal aorta

Dissecting aneurysm (longitudinal section)

Figure 18-5 Three forms of aneurysms—berry aneurysm in the circle of Willis, fusiform-type aneurysm of the abdominal aorta, and a dissecting aortic aneurysm.

a small, spherical dilatation of the vessel, rarely exceeding 1 cm to 1.5 cm in diameter.[17] They are usually found in the circle of Willis in the cerebral circulation. A *fusiform aneurysm* involves the entire circumference of the vessel and is characterized by a gradual and progressive dilatation of the vessel. These aneurysms, which vary in diameter (up to 20 cm) and length, may involve the entire ascending and transverse portions of the thoracic aorta or may extend over large segments of the abdominal aorta. A *saccular aneurysm* extends over part of the circumference of the vessel and appears saclike. They can vary in size up to 15 cm to 20 cm but are frequently about 5 cm to 10 cm in diameter.[17] In a *dissecting aneurysm*, vessel dilatation occurs because of the accumulated blood within the layers of the vessel wall. This occurs when blood enters the wall of the artery, dissecting its layers to create a blood-filled cavity.

The weakness that leads to aneurysm formation may be due to several factors, including congenital defects, trauma, infections, and arteriosclerosis. Once initiated, the size of the aneurysm tends to progress as the tension on the vessel wall increases. Untreated, the aneurysm may burst because of internal pressure. Even an unruptured aneurysm can cause damage by exerting pressure on adjacent structures and interrupting blood flow.

Aortic aneurysms

Aortic aneurysms may involve any part of the aorta: the ascending aorta, aortic arch, descending aorta, or thoracic-abdominal aorta. Multiple aneurysms may be present. Aortic aneurysms were, until recently, caused largely by tertiary syphilis. Now, with better control of syphilis, atherosclerosis has become the leading cause of aneurysmal development. Atherosclerotic aneurysms are most common in men over 50 years of age.

Aortic aneurysms may or may not cause symptoms. The first evidence of an aneurysm may be associated with vessel rupture. With aneurysms of the thoracic aorta, substernal, back, and neck pain may occur. There may also be dyspnea, stridor, or a brassy cough due to pressure on the trachea. Hoarseness may result from pressure on the recurrent laryngeal nerve, and there may be difficulty swallowing because of pressure on the esophagus. The aneurysm can compress the superior vena cava causing distention of neck veins and edema of the face and neck. It may also cause enlargement of the aorta in the areas of the aortic valve to the point of preventing complete valve closure and causing aortic regurgitation.

Aneurysms of the abdominal aorta are usually below the level of the renal artery and generally involve the bifurcation of the aorta and proximal end of the common iliac arteries. Because an aneurysm is of arterial origin, a pulsating mass may provide the first evidence of the disorder. This mass may be discovered during a routine physical examination, or the affected person may complain of its presence. Calcification, which frequently exists on the wall of the aneurysm, may be detected during abdominal x-ray examination. Pain may be present and varies from mild midabdominal or lumbar discomfort to severe abdominal and back pain. The aneurysm may extend to and impinge on the renal, iliac, or mesenteric arteries. Stasis of blood favors thrombus formation along the wall of the vessel, and peripheral emboli may develop causing symptomatic arterial insufficiency. With both thoracic and abdominal aneurysms the most dreaded complication is rupture—the danger of which correlates with aneurysm size.

Arteriography, using a radiopaque dye to render the aneurysm visible on x-ray, may be used in diagnosis. Recently, several noninvasive diagnostic techniques have come into use: ultrasound, magnetic resonance imaging (MRI), and computerized axial tomography (CT scan). Surgical repair, in which the involved section of the aorta is replaced with a synthetic graft of woven Dacron, is frequently the treatment of choice. Hypertension, if present, should be controlled.

Dissecting aneurysms

A dissecting aneurysm is an acute life-threatening condition. It involves hemorrhage into the vessel wall with longitudinal tearing (dissection) of the vessel wall to form a blood-filled channel. Unlike syphilitic or atherosclerotic aneurysms, dissecting aneurysms often occur without evidence of previous vessel dilatation.

Dissecting aneurysms are caused by conditions that weaken or cause degenerative changes in the elastic and smooth muscle of the medial layer of the aorta. They are seen most often in the 40- to 60-year-old age group and are more common in men than women.[17] There is a history of hypertension in 94% of cases.[17] Dissecting aneurysms are also associated with connective tissue diseases such as Marfan's syndrome and during pregnancy due to histochemical changes in the aorta that occur during this time.

Dissecting aortic aneurysms can occur anywhere along the length of the aorta. Approximately 75% of dissections have their origin in the ascending aorta. The most common site in the ascending aorta is within a few centimeters of the aortic valve. The second most common site is the thoracic aorta just distal to the origin of the subclavian artery.[18] Dissection is usually bidirectional, moving proximally toward the heart and distally into the descending aorta. When the ascending aorta is involved, expansion of the vessel wall may impair closure of the aortic valve. Although the length of dissection varies, it is possible for the abdominal aorta to be involved, with, finally, progression into the renal, iliac, or femoral arteries.

A major symptom of a dissecting aneurysm is the abrupt appearance of excruciating pain described as tearing or ripping. The location of the pain may point to the site of dissection. Pain associated with dissection of the ascending aorta is frequently located in the anterior chest; whereas pain associated with dissection of the descending aorta is often located in the back. In the early stages, blood pressure is often moderately or markedly elevated. Later, both the blood pressure and the pulse become unobtainable in one or both arms as the dissection disrupts arterial flow to the arms.

Mortality due to dissecting aneurysm is high. Within the first 48 hours, 50% of all untreated patients die, and 90% die within 6 weeks.[19] Aortic angiography, echocardiography, and CT scans aid in the diagnosis of aortic aneurysm. Treatment may be medical or surgical. Surgical treatment consists of resection of the involved segment of the aorta and replacement with a prosthetic graft. Medical treatment involves control of hypertension and drugs to lessen the force of systolic blood ejection from the heart.

Acute arterial occlusion

Acute arterial occlusion usually results from a thrombus or from emboli originating in the heart. It is usually a complication of heart disease—ischemic heart disease with or without infarction, atrial fibrillation, or rheumatic heart disease. Trauma or arterial spasm due to arterial cannulation is another cause.

The signs and symptoms of acute arterial occlusion depend on the artery involved and the adequacy of the collateral circulation. Emboli tend to lodge in bifurcations of the major arteries, including the aorta and iliac and the femoral and popliteal arteries. Occlusion in an extremity causes sudden onset of acute pain with numbness, tingling, weakness, pallor, and coldness. These changes are followed rapidly by cyanosis, mottling, and loss of sensory, reflex, and motor function. Pulses are absent below the level of the occlusion.

Treatment of acute arterial occlusion is aimed at restoring blood flow. Thrombolytic therapy (streptokinase or tissue plasminogen activator) may be used in an attempt to dissolve the clot. Anticoagulant therapy (heparin) is usually given to prevent extension of the embolus. An embolectomy—surgical removal of the embolus—may be indicated. It is important that application of heat and cold be avoided and that the extremity be protected from hard surfaces and overlying bedclothes.

Peripheral arterial disease

The peripheral arterial circulation is usually described as arterial circulation outside the heart. For our purposes, we will consider the peripheral circulation as that outside the pulmonary and cerebral circulation. Arteriosclerosis, discussed earlier, is a major cause of peripheral vascular disorders. Two other conditions, Raynaud's phenomenon and thromboangiitis obliterans (Buerger's disease) will serve as prototypes of peripheral arterial disease.

Raynaud's syndrome

Raynaud's syndrome is a functional disorder caused by intense vasospasm of the arteries and arterioles in the fingers and, less often, in the toes. Raynaud's syndrome is divided into two types: Raynaud's disease, which occurs without demonstrable cause, and Raynaud's phenomenon, which occurs secondary to some other disease condition. Raynaud's disease is seen most frequently in otherwise healthy young women, and it is often precipitated by exposure to cold or by strong emotions. Raynaud's phenomenon is associated with previous vessel injury such as frostbite, occupational trauma associated with the use of heavy vibrating tools, neurologic disorders, and chronic arterial occlusive disorders. Another occupational-related cause is the exposure to alternating hot and cold temperatures such as that experienced by butchers and food preparers.[20] Raynaud's phenomenon is often the first symptom of collagen diseases. In 70% of persons with scleroderma, it is the first symptom; and in lupus erythematosus, it is the presenting problem in 8% to 16% of cases.[21]

In Raynaud's disease or phenomenon, ischemia due to vasospasm causes changes in skin color that progress from pallor to cyanosis, a sensation of cold, and changes in sensory perception such as numbness or tingling. The color changes are usually first noted in the tips of the fingers, later moving into one or more of the distal phalanges. Following the ischemic episode, there is a period of hyperemia with intense rubor, throbbing, and paresthesias. The period of hyperemia is followed by a return to normal color. If Raynaud's disease begins asymmetrically (does not affect both hands in the same manner) it usually becomes symmetrical within 4 to 6 months.[21] During the attack there may be slight swelling. With repeated episodes of ischemia, the nails may become brittle, and the skin over the tips of the affected fingers may become thickened. Nutritional impairment of these structures may give rise to arthritis. Ulceration and superficial gangrene of the fingers, although infrequent, may occur.

In primary Raynaud's disease, the anatomy of the blood vessels appears normal and the cause of the vasospasm is unknown. It appears that local circulatory control mechanisms such as disorder of prostaglandin release may be involved. Raynaud's phenomenon is usually characterized by anatomical abnormalities of the vessels.

Treatment measures are directed toward eliminating factors that cause vasospasm and protecting the digits from trauma during an ischemic episode. Abstinence from smoking and protection from cold are first priorities. Avoidance of emotional stress is another important factor in controlling the disorder because anxiety and stress may precipitate a vascular spasm in predisposed individuals. Vasoconstrictor medications such as the decongestants contained in allergy and cold preparations should be avoided. Treatment with vasodilator drugs may be indicated, particularly if episodes are frequent, because frequency tends to encourage the potential for development of thrombosis and gangrene. The calcium-channel blocking drugs that exert a vasodilator effect on vascular smooth muscle are currently being tested. Intravenous infusion of prostaglandin E seems to be beneficial during an acute attack of vasospasm, and its effects may last for several weeks. The McIntyre maneuver, which is used by skiers to warm their hands, has been shown to be helpful in the early stages of the vasospastic attack.[22] To do this maneuver, the person assumes standing position and briskly swings the hands downward and behind the body and then upward and in front of the body at a rate of about 180 times per minute. The centrifugal force of this maneuver moves blood into the fingers. Biofeedback training may be helpful in persons with Raynaud's disease but does not seem to be as effective in those with Raynaud's phenomenon.[23] In the past, surgical interruption of sympathetic nerve pathways (sympathectomy) was an accepted form of therapy for persons with severe symptomatology. However, the results were poor, and the procedure is seldom done today.

Thromboangiitis obliterans (Buerger's disease)

Thromboangiitis obliterans is, as the name implies, an inflammatory arterial disorder that causes thrombus formation. The disorder affects the medium-sized arteries, usually the plantar and digital vessels in the foot and in the lower leg. Arteries in the arm and hand may also be affected. Although primarily an arterial disorder, the inflammatory process often extends to involve adjacent veins and nerves. The cause of Buerger's disease is unknown. It is a disease of men between 25 and 40 years of age who are heavy cigarette smokers.

Pain is the predominant symptom. During the early stages of the disease, there is intermittent claudication of the calf muscles and the arch of the foot. In severe cases, pain is present even when the person is at rest. The impaired circulation increases sensitivity to cold. The peripheral pulses are diminished or absent, and there are changes in the color of the extremity. In moderately advanced cases, the extremity becomes cyanotic when the person assumes a dependent position, and the digits may turn reddish blue in color even when in a nondependent position. With lack of blood flow, the skin assumes a thin, shiny look, and hair growth and skin nutrition suffer. Chronic ischemia causes thick malformed nails. If the disease continues to progress, tissues will eventually ulcerate, and gangrenous changes will arise that may necessitate amputation.

In the treatment program for thromboangiitis obliterans, it is mandatory that the person stop smoking cigarettes. Other treatment measures are of secondary importance and focus on methods for producing vasodilatation and for preventing tissue injury. Sympathectomy may be done to alleviate the vasospastic manifestations of the disease. Buerger's exercises take advantage of the gravitational effects of position change to improve blood flow to the affected part. The exercises consist of a cycle of approximately 2-minute positional changes: horizontal, legs elevated 45 degrees, legs in a dependent position, and then horizontal again. The exercises are usually repeated five times and are done three times a day. Patients are usually instructed to wiggle their toes while performing the exercises.

Atherosclerotic occlusive disease

Atherosclerosis is an important cause of peripheral-vessel vascular disease. The superficial femoral and popliteal arteries are the most frequent sites for development of atherosclerotic occlusive disease. When it occurs in the lower leg and foot, the tibial, common peroneal, or pedal vessels are the most commonly affected arteries. As with atherosclerosis in other locations, the signs of vessel occlusion are gradual. The signs include intermittent claudication, atrophic changes and thinning of the skin and subcutaneous tissues of the lower leg, and diminution in the size of the leg muscles. The foot is often cool, and the popliteal and pedal pulses are weak or absent. Limb color blanches with elevation and becomes a deep red color when in the dependent position. Walking (slowly) to the point of claudication is usually encouraged because it increases the collateral circulation. Surgery (femoropopliteal bypass grafting using a section of saphenous vein) may be indicated in severe cases. Thromboendarterectomy with removal of the occluding core of atherosclerotic tissue may be done if the section of diseased vessel is short. Percutaneous transluminal angioplasty, in which a balloon catheter is inserted into the area of stenosis and the balloon inflated to increase vessel diameter, is another form of treatment.

Assessment of arterial flow

There are a number of methods for assessing arterial flow and detecting arterial disease. These include monitoring of arterial pulses, angiography, Doppler ultrasound flow studies, magnetic resonance imaging (MRI), impedance plethysmography, and thermography.

The volume of the peripheral pulses and capillary refill time are useful indirect methods for assessing peripheral perfusion.

Peripheral arterial pulses are palpated over vessels in the head, neck, and extremities. In situations associated with potential vessel spasm or thrombus formation, it may be necessary only to check for the presence of pulses. In many situations, however, the pulse volume provides useful information about vascular volume and the condition of the arterial circulation. Pulse volume can be graded on a scale of 0 to +4.

0—Pulse is not palpable.

+1—Pulse is thready, weak, and difficult to palpate; it may fade in and out and is easily obliterated with pressure.

+2—Pulse is difficult to palpate and may be obliterated with pressure, so light palpation is required. Once located, however, it is stronger than +1.

+3—Pulse is easily palpable, does not fade in and out, and is not easily obliterated by pressure. This pulse is considered to have normal volume.

+4—Pulse is strong, bounding, hyperactive, easily palpated, and not obliterated with pressure. In some cases, such as aortic regurgitation, it may be considered pathologic.[24]

Arterial auscultation is used to listen to the flow of blood with a stethoscope. A *bruit* is an audible murmur that can be heard over a peripheral artery. It is caused by turbulent blood flow and is suggestive of obstructive arterial disease.

Capillary refill time is an indicator of the efficiency of the microcirculation. It is measured by depressing the nailbed of a finger or toe until the underlying skin blanches. The refill time is normal if the capillary vessels refill within 3 seconds following release of the pressure.[24]

Angiography involves the injection of a radiopaque dye into the vascular system to allow visualization of the blood vessels on x-ray.

Ultrasonic Doppler flow studies use reflected ultrasound waves, which are transmitted back to the skin surface where they are sensed by an appropriate transducer. With moving objects such as blood cells, the frequency of the reflected sound is shifted in relation to the transmitted signal. This frequency shift is used in determining both the velocity and direction of blood flow.

Magnetic resonance imaging is a new noninvasive technique that can be used to study blood flow. The method uses a magnetic field to align the charges on blood components as they move through blood vessels. The aligned charges emit measurable radio frequency signals, which can be detected electronically and recorded.

Impedance plethysmography estimates blood flow in a limb or digit using measurements of resistance (impedance) changes that occur as the fluid volume of the limb changes due to the pulsatile nature of arterial blood flow. With this method four electrodes are placed in a row along the limb. A high-frequency AC voltage of very low amplitude is transmitted across the skin by the two outer electrodes, while the two inner electrodes monitor the changes in electrical resistance that occur because of changes in blood flow.

The temperature of the skin is determined by many factors, including arterial blood flow. One of the observations in atherosclerotic and acute arterial occlusion is that the affected area is colder than normal. Skin temperature may be measured with a skin thermometer. Infrared *thermography* uses an infrared camera to map the skin temperature of an area.

In summary, there are two types of arterial disorders: (1) diseases such as atherosclerosis and peripheral arterial diseases that obstruct blood flow and (2) disorders such as aneurysms that weaken the vessel wall. Atherosclerosis, a leading cause of death in the United States, affects large and medium-sized arteries such as the coronary and cerebral arteries. It has an insidious onset, and its lesions are usually far advanced before symptoms appear. Although the mechanisms of atherosclerosis are uncertain, risk factors associated with its development have been identified. These include (1) factors such as heredity, sex, and age, which cannot be controlled; (2) factors such as smoking, high blood pressure, high serum cholesterol levels, and diabetes, which can be controlled; and (3) other contributing factors such as obesity, lack of exercise, and stress. Aneurysms are abnormal vessel dilatations of an artery. The weakness that leads to aneurysm formation can be caused by several factors including congenital defects in vessel structure, trauma, infections, and atherosclerosis. Peripheral arterial diseases affect blood vessels outside the heart and thorax. They include Raynaud's phenomenon, caused by vessel spasm, and thromboangiitis obliterans (Buerger's disease), characterized by an inflammatory process that involves medium-sized arteries and adjacent veins and nerves of the lower extremities.

Alterations in venous flow

Veins are low-pressure, thin-walled vessels that rely on the ancillary action of skeletal muscle pumps and changes in abdominal and intrathoracic pressure to return blood to the heart. Unlike the arterial system, the venous system is equipped with valves that prevent retrograde flow of blood. Although its structure enables the venous system to serve as a storage area for blood, it also renders the system susceptible to problems related to stasis and venous insufficiency. This section focuses on two common problems of the venous system: varicose veins and venous thrombosis. Pulmonary embolism, a complication of deep vein thrombosis, is discussed in Chapter 25.

——— Varicose veins

Varicose, or dilated, tortuous veins of the lower extremities, are common and often lead to secondary problems of venous insufficiency. Estimates suggest that 10% of the adult population is affected by varicose veins and another 40% or 50% have slight asymptomatic varicosities.[25] Customarily, varicose veins are described as being primary or secondary. Primary varicosities originate in the superficial saphenous veins, and secondary varicose veins result from impaired flow in the deep venous channels.

A brief review of the anatomy of the venous system of the legs explains why varicosities may develop. The venous system in the legs might well be described as being composed of two venous channels: the superficial (saphenous and its tributaries) veins and the deep venous channels (Figure 18-6). Perforating or communicating veins connect these two systems. Blood from the skin and subcutaneous tissues in the leg collects in the superficial veins and is then transported across the communicating veins into the deeper venous channels for return to the heart. When a person walks, the action of the muscle pumps produces an increase in flow in the deep channels and facilitates movement of blood from the superficial to the deep veins.

Valves present in the veins prevent the retrograde flow of blood and play an important role in the function of the venous system. Although these valves are irregularly located along the length of the veins, they are almost always found at junctions where the communicating veins merge with the larger deep veins and where two veins meet. The number of venous valves differs somewhat from one individual to another as does the structural competence, factors that may help to explain the familial predisposition to development of varicose veins.

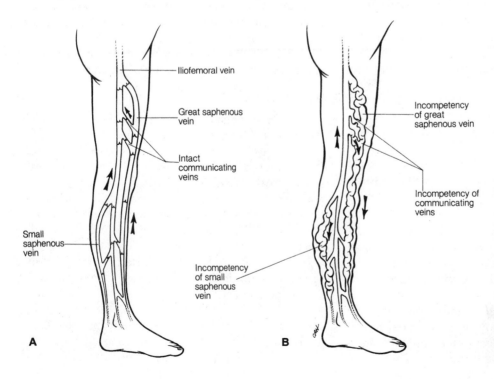

Figure 18-6 The superficial and deep venous channels of the leg. View **A** represents normal venous structures and flow patterns. View **B** illustrates varicosities in the superficial venous system that are the result of incompetent valves in the communicating veins. The *arrows* in both views indicate the direction of blood flow. (*Modified from Abramson DI: Vascular Disorders of the Extremities, 2nd ed. New York, Harper & Row, 1974*)

Causes

Varicose veins result from prolonged dilatation and stretching of the vascular wall as a result of increased venous pressure. One of the most important factors in the elevation of venous pressure is the hydrostatic effect associated with the standing position. When a person is in the erect position, the full weight of the venous columns of blood is transmitted to the leg veins. The effects of gravity are compounded in persons who stand for long periods of time without using their leg muscles to assist in pumping blood back to the heart. Because there are no valves in the inferior vena cava or common iliac veins, blood in the abdominal veins must be supported by the valves located in the external iliac or femoral veins. When intra-abdominal pressure increases, as it does during pregnancy, or when the valves in these two veins are absent or defective, the stress on the saphenofemoral junction is increased. The high incidence of varicose veins in women who have been pregnant also suggests a hormonal effect on venous smooth muscle leading to venous dilatation and valvular incompetence.

Prolonged exposure to increases in pressure causes the venous valves to become incompetent so they no longer close properly. When this happens, blood regurgitates into the superficial veins. Furthermore, once varicose veins have developed, the venous structures become deformed, promoting further dilatation.

Another consideration is that the superficial veins have only subcutaneous fat and superficial fascia for support, whereas the deep venous channels are supported by muscle, bone, and connective tissue. Therefore, obesity tends to increase the risk for varicose veins.

Normally, about 80% to 90% of venous blood from the lower extremities is transported through the deep channels. The development of secondary varicose veins becomes inevitable when flow in these channels is impaired or blocked. Among the causes of secondary varicose veins are thrombophlebitis, congenital or acquired arteriovenous fistulas, congenital venous malformations, and pressure on the abdominal veins due to pregnancy or a tumor.

Venous insufficiency

Signs and symptoms associated with varicose veins vary. Most women complain of their unsightly appearance. In addition to their cosmetic effects, varicose veins tend to impair venous emptying giving rise to a condition known as venous insufficiency. This often causes a sensation of progressive heaviness and, with prolonged standing, aching legs. In contrast to the ischemia due to arterial insufficiency, venous insufficiency tends to lead to tissue congestion, edema, and eventual impairment of tissue nutrition. The edema is exacerbated by long periods of standing. In its advanced form, impairment of tissue nutrition causes stasis dermatitis and the development of stasis or varicose ulcers. Stasis dermatitis is characterized by the presence of thin, shiny bluish brown, irregularly pigmented desquamative skin that lacks the support of the underlying subcutaneous tissues. Minor injury leads to relatively painless ulcerations that are difficult to heal. The lower part of the leg is particularly prone to develop stasis dermatitis and varicose ulcers.

Diagnosis and treatment

Several procedures are used to assess the extent of venous involvement associated with varicose veins. One of these, Trendelenburg's test, involves the use of a tourniquet in the following manner. A tourniquet is applied to the affected leg while it is elevated and the veins are empty. The person then assumes the standing position, and the tourniquet is removed. If the superficial veins are involved, the veins distend quickly. To assess the deep channels, the tourniquet is applied while the person is standing and the veins are filled. The person then lies down and the affected leg is elevated. Emptying of the superficial veins indicates that the deep channels are patent. The Doppler ultrasonic flow probe may also be used to assess the flow in the large vessels. Angiographic studies employing a radiopaque contrast medium are also used to assess venous function.

Ideally, measures should be taken to prevent the development and progression of varicose veins. Once the venous channels have been repeatedly stretched and the valves rendered incompetent, little can be done to restore normal venous tone and function. These measures center on avoiding any activities that involve prolonged elevation of venous pressure.

Treatment measures for varicose veins focus on improving venous flow and preventing tissue injury, such as avoiding prolonged standing and providing for frequent leg elevation. When properly fitted, elastic support stockings compress the superficial veins and thus prevent distention. These stockings should be applied before the standing position is assumed at a time when the leg veins are empty. Surgical treatment consists of removing the varicosities and the incompetent perforating veins, but it is limited to persons with patent, deep venous channels. Sclerotherapy, which is usually done on small residual varicosities, is another treatment measure; it involves injection of a sclerosing agent into the collapsed superficial veins in order to produce fibrosis of the vessel lumen.

Venous thrombosis

In thrombophlebitis there is inflammation of a vein with subsequent thrombus formation; while in phlebothrombosis, thrombus formation is followed by inflammation. In phlebothrombosis, the clot is less firmly attached to the vessel wall than is the case in thrombophlebitis, so that embolization is a greater risk. From a clinical standpoint, it is often difficult to determine which came first—the inflammation or the clot. Therefore, this discussion treats thrombophlebitis and phlebothrombosis as one and the same.

In 1846, Virchow described the triad that has come to be associated with thrombosis: (1) stasis of blood, (2) increased blood coagulability, and (3) vessel-wall injury.[26] It is thought that two of the three factors must be present for thrombi to form. Thrombi can develop in either the superficial or the deep veins (DVT). Thrombus formation in deep veins is a precursor to venous insufficiency and embolus formation.

A number of factors may be present that promote venous thrombosis (Chart 18-1). Immobilization, trauma, and surgery are definite risk factors, as are aging, heart failure, hypercoagulability states, and a previous history of venous disorders. The patient immobilized by a hip fracture or joint replacement is particularly vulnerable to DVT. Persons in the older age groups (over 40 years) are more susceptible than younger people. Although there is no single explanation for it, factors known to promote venous stasis, such as heart failure, venous pathology, and cancer occur more frequently in older individuals. Hypercoagulability is in itself a homeostatic mechanism invoked in conditions of stress or injury. It may be that thrombi form as a result of changes in clotting factors or in the fibrinolytic system (see Chapter 15). When body fluid is lost because of injury or disease, the resulting hemoconcentration will cause the clotting factors to become more concentrated. Certain malignancies are associated with increased clotting tendencies, and although the reason for this is largely unknown, substances that promote blood coagulation may be released from the tissues due to the cancerous growth. In congestive heart failure and shock, there is impaired circulation with stasis of coagulation factors.

What part oral contraceptive agents play in promoting blood coagulation and, as a consequence, a predisposition to venous thrombosis and pulmonary embolism is controversial. Certainly, if other risk factors are present, both the risk and benefits of oral contraceptives need to be carefully weighed.

Signs and symptoms

The most common signs of thrombophlebitis are those related to the inflammatory process: pain, swelling, deep muscle tenderness, and fever. Generally, the pain is described as localized, deep, aching, and throbbing and is exacerbated by walking. A positive Homans' sign—pain in the popliteal area when the foot is forcefully dorsiflexed—suggests thrombophlebitis. Swelling of the leg usually occurs soon after the onset of pain. How much swelling there is depends on the extent to which venous flow is impaired. Fever, general malaise, and an elevated white blood cell count and sedimentation rate are accompanying signs of inflammation.

Phlebothrombosis differs from thrombophlebitis in that the early signs of inflammation are often absent. Frequently, a positive Homans' sign or manifestations of pulmonary embolism are the only evidence that thrombosis has occurred.

Diagnosis and treatment

The risk of pulmonary embolism emphasizes the need for early detection and treatment of thrombophlebitis. Several tests are useful for this purpose: ascending venography, contrast DVT scans, Doppler ultrasonic flowmeter studies, and impedance plethysmography. The DVT scan involves the intravenous injection of radioactive fibrinogen (^{125}I), which becomes incorporated into any developing thrombus. The thrombus is then detected by a scintillation counter, which records the radioactivity at selected points in the extremity.

These methods provide means for assessment of venous flow or fibrinogen accumulation and are useful in monitoring persons at risk for developing venous thrombosis.

Chart 18–1: Risk factors associated with venous thrombosis

Aging
Anesthesia and surgery
Circulatory failure
  Congestive heart failure
  Shock
Dehydration
Hematologic disorders
  Polycythemia
  Disorders of blood clotting
  Disorders of fibrinolytic activity
Malignancy
Massive trauma or infection
Obesity
Reproductive processes
  Pregnancy
  Parturition
  Oral contraceptive therapy
Venous disorders
  Venous insufficiency
  Vascular trauma
  Venous obstruction

Whenever possible, venous thrombosis should be prevented, in preference to being treated. Early ambulation following childbirth and surgery is one measure that decreases the risk of thrombus formation. Exercising the legs and wearing support stockings also improve venous flow. A further precautionary measure is to avoid assuming body positions that favor venous pooling. For example, in the hospitalized patient, if both the head and knees of the hospital bed are raised, blood will tend to pool in the pelvic veins. Long unbroken auto and plane trips also promote venous pooling and thrombus formation.

In both thrombophlebitis and phlebothrombosis, bedrest with elevation of the affected extremity is prescribed. In one study, contrast medium remained in the soleus veins, on the average, for 10 minutes in supine patients whose legs were in horizontal position.[27] This may explain why postoperative thrombi frequently originate in the soleus vein. A 20-degree elevation of the legs will prevent stasis.[28] It is important that the entire lower extremity or extremities be carefully extended to avoid acute flexion of the knee or hip. Heat is often applied to the leg to relieve venospasm and to aid in the resolution of the inflammatory process. Measures are also taken to prevent the bed coverings from resting on the leg because this increases discomfort.

Two anticoagulants, warfarin and heparin, are used both to treat and to prevent thrombophlebitis. *Treatment* is usually initiated with either continuous or periodic intravenous heparin infusions. This is followed by *prophylactic* therapy with either subcutaneous minidose heparin injections or oral warfarin sodium to prevent further thrombus formation. Minidose heparin is usually injected into the subcutaneous tissue of the lower abdomen or laterally above the iliac crest.[29,30] Prophylactic therapy is usually continued for 6 to 10 weeks following uncomplicated DVT and for up to 6 months following pulmonary embolism. The mechanisms of action of the anticoagulant drugs are discussed in Chapter 15. Thrombolytic therapy (streptokinase or tissue plasminogen activator) may be used in an attempt to dissolve the clot.

In summary, the storage function of the venous system renders it susceptible to venous insufficiency, stasis, and thrombus formation. Varicose veins occur with prolonged distention and stretching of the superficial veins due to venous insufficiency. Varicosities can arise because of defects in the superficial veins (primary varicose veins) or because of impaired blood flow in the deep venous channels (secondary varicose veins). Venous thrombosis, thrombophlebitis, and pulmonary embolism are associated with three factors: vessel injury, stasis of venous flow, and hypercoagulability states.

Impairment of local blood flow: pressure sores

Pressure sores are ischemic lesions of the skin and underlying structures caused by external pressure, which impairs the flow of blood and lymph. *Decubitus* comes from the Latin term meaning "lying down"; pressure sores are often referred to as decubitus ulcers or bedsores. However, a pressure sore may result from pressure exerted in either the seated or supine positions. It is most likely to develop over a bony prominence, but it may occur on any part of the body that is subjected to external pressure, friction, or shearing forces.

Sources of tissue injury

Shearing forces

Shearing forces are caused by the sliding of one tissue layer over another with stretching and angulation of blood vessels causing injury and thrombosis. Clinically, injury due to shearing forces commonly occurs when the head of the bed is elevated, causing the torso to slide down thus transmitting pressure to the sacrum and deep fascia; at the same time, friction and perspiration cause the sacral skin to remain fixed to the bed. Another source of shearing forces is pulling rather than lifting a patient up in bed. In this case the skin remains fixed to the sheet while the fascia and muscles are pulled upward.

Pressure

External pressure that exceeds capillary pressure interrupts the blood flow in the capillary beds. When this pressure is greater than the pressure in the arterioles, it also interrupts the flow in these vessels. The average blood pressure of the normal skin capillaries is about 25 mmHg. A pressure exceeding 50 mmHg applied to the skin over a bony prominence is sufficient to interrupt the blood flow and cause ischemia.[31] Approximately 7 lb of pressure per square inch of tissue surface is sufficient to shut off blood flow.[32] Great pressure distributed over a small area will cause more rapid breakdown of tissue than a small amount distributed over a larger area. If this pressure is applied constantly for 2 hours, oxygen deprivation coupled with an accumulation of metabolic end products leads to irreversible tissue damage. Altering the distribution of pressure from one skin area to another prevents tissue damage. If a person weighing 70 kg with a total surface area of 1.8 m^2 were in the supine position, with pressure evenly distributed, the pressure at any given point would be 5.7 mmHg.[32] Normally, pressure on the skin and underlying tissues is continually shifted to prevent ischemia. During the night, for example, frequent turning prevents ischemic injury of tissues overlying the bony prominences that support the weight of the body; the same is true for sitting for any length of time. The movements needed to shift the body weight are made unconsciously, and only when movement is restricted do we become aware of discomfort. Pressure ulcers occur most commonly with conditions, such as spinal cord injury, in which normal sensation and movement to effect redistribution of body weight are impaired.

Whether a person is sitting or lying down, the weight of the body is borne by tissues covering the bony prominences. Ninety-six percent of pressure sores are located on the lower part of the body, most often over the sacrum, the coccygeal areas, the ischial tuberosities, and the greater trochanter.[33] Pressure over a bony area is transmitted from the surface to the underlying dense bone; all the underlying tissue is compressed with the greatest pressure at the surface of the bone and dissipating in conelike fashion toward the surface of the skin (Figure 18-7). The skin lesion is often just the tip of the iceberg; extensive underlying tissue damage is often present when a small superficial skin lesion is first noted.

Grading of pressure sores

Pressure sores can be graded according to four categories developed by Shea.[34] Grade 1 lesions are characterized by a hardened, warm, reddish brown swelling. These lesions are essentially reversible and will resolve in 5 to 10 days if treated by relieving pressure and taking measures to prevent bacterial contamination. Grade 2 lesions involve all of the soft tissue, with development of a shallow, full-thickness skin ulcer with pigmented edges that blend into a broad area that is warm, swollen and hardened, and reddish brown in color. Grade 2 ulcers are also reversible; they take longer to heal than grade 1 ulcers, however, and require treatment directed toward pre-

venting further breakdown. Grade 3 pressure sores extend through the skin into the subcutaneous fat with extensive undermining; they are frequently infected and foul smelling. There may be profound loss of fluid and protein from these open draining wounds. Although grade 3 pressure sores will heal by second intention, the resulting scar tissue is thin and subject to easy breakdown. A grade 4 ulcer includes penetration of the deep fascia with involvement of muscle and bone. Dislocation, resulting from septic joints and osteomyelitis, may occur. Septicemia is a frequent cause of death in persons with grade 4 pressure ulcers.[35]

Prevention and treatment

Prevention of pressure ulcers is preferable to treatment. In 1978 it was estimated that the cost of treating a pressure ulcer ranged from $6,000 for less severe ulcers to $17,500 for severe ulcers requiring extensive care and convalescent time, not to mention the discomfort and other problems arising from their occurrence.[31] Risk factors identified as contributing to the development of pressure sores are unconsciousness, dehydration, paralysis, restricted mobility, circulatory impairment, and emaciation. The elderly are particularly prone to develop pressure sores; in one institution, 76% of the pressure ulcers that occurred during two 6-month periods of time were in persons over 70 years of age.[36] Identifying patients who are at risk for development of decubitus ulcers allows health-care facilities to focus prevention measures on this group, and this has been shown to reduce the incidence of pressure sores.[32,37]

Prevention includes frequent position change, meticulous skin care, and careful and frequent observation to detect early signs of skin breakdown. Bed linens should be kept clean, dry, and wrinkle free. A natural or synthetic sheepskin that is soft and resilient, does not wrinkle, and distributes weight evenly may be used. Usually a synthetic sheepskin that is easily laundered is used. Special pads and mattresses that

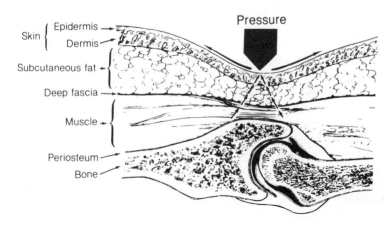

Figure 18-7 Pressure over a bony prominence compresses all intervening soft tissue, with a resulting wide, three-dimensional pressure gradient that causes varying degrees of ischemia and damage. *(Shea JD: Pressure sores: Classification and management. Clin Orthop 112:90, 1975)*

distribute weight more evenly may be used. Such items as silicone-filled pads, egg-crate cushions, turning frames, flotation pads, and other devices minimize contact pressure. Adequate exposure of the skin to air is necessary to avoid the buildup of heat and perspiration. A bed cradle may be used to keep bedclothes away from the skin. Care should be taken to maintain the individual at a position of 30 degrees to 40 degrees to minimize slipping and shearing forces from sliding against the sheets. It is also important that the person be lifted and not dragged across the sheet. A lifting sheet works well for this purpose. Elevation of the ankles and heels off the sheets with foam pads can reduce skin breakdown in these areas of the body.

Casts, braces, and splints can exert extreme pressure on underlying tissues, and persons with these devices require special attention to avoid skin breakdown.

Prevention of dehydration improves the circulation; reduces the concentration of urine, minimizing skin irritation in incontinent patients; and reduces urinary problems contributing to incontinence. Maintenance of adequate nutrition is important. Anemia and malnutrition contribute to tissue breakdown and delay healing once tissue injury has occurred.

Once skin breakdown has occurred, special treatment measures are needed to prevent further ischemic damage, reduce bacterial contamination and infection, and promote healing. Frequent cleansing and irrigation with sterile water, normal saline, or other cleansing agents are done to remove drainage and any other contamination that has occurred.

Numerous topical agents have been used as adjuvants in the treatment of pressure sores. Some of the more widely used are enzyme preparations, such as fibrinolysin and desoxyribonuclease (Elase) and sutilains ointment (Travase), which are used to assist in debridement of the ulcer. A preparation of trypsin, balsam of Peru, and castor oil (Granulex) may also be used for this purpose. Dextranomer (Debrisan) is a long-chain polysaccharide that is used to absorb the products of collagen and tissue breakdown and contaminating bacteria and allows the wound to heal without crusting.

Op-site is a self-adhesive transparent dressing that seals in the body's own defenses against invasion —leukocytes, plasma, and fibrin.[38] It promotes natural healing without the usual formation of a dry crust over the wound. Although Op-site is nonporous and prevents the escape of fluid, it is permeable to air and water vapor and prevents the growth of anaerobic bacteria.

In summary, pressure sores are caused by ischemia of the skin and underlying tissues. They are caused by external pressure, which disrupts blood flow, or by shearing forces, which cause stretching and injury to blood vessels. Pressure sores are divided into four grades: grade 1 lesions, which are reversible and are characterized by hardened, warm, reddish brown swelling; grade 2 lesions, which involve all the soft tissue with development of a shallow, full-thickness skin ulcer; grade 3 lesions, which extend through the skin into the subcutaneous fat with extensive undermining and are frequently infected; grade 4 lesions, which penetrate the deep fascia and involve bone and muscle. Pressure sores can be prevented by frequent change of position, careful skin care, adequate nutrition and hydration, and use of special pads and mattresses that aid in the distribution of weight.

References

1. 1988 Heart Facts. Dallas, Texas. American Heart Association, 1988
2. Report of the 1981 Working Group to Review the Report by the National Heart and Lung Institute Task Force on Arteriosclerosis. DHEW Publication No. NIH 81-2034, p 37, 1981
3. Enos WF, Beyer JC, Holmes RF: Pathogenesis of coronary artery disease in American soldiers killed in Korea. JAMA 158:912, 1955
4. Campbell GR, Chambley-Campbell JH: Invited review: The cellular pathobiology of atherosclerosis. Pathology 13:424, 1981
5. Report of the 1977 Working Group to Review the Report of the National Heart and Lung Institute on Arteriosclerosis. DHEW Publication No. NIH 78-1526, p 20, 1977
6. Ross R: The pathogenesis of atherosclerosis—An update. N Engl J Med 314(8):488, 1986
7. Smith LH, Thier SO: Pathophysiology, p 1163. Philadelphia, WB Saunders, 1981
8. Report of the National Cholesterol Education Program's Expert Panel on Detection, Evaluation, and Treatment of High Blood Cholesterol in Adults. Arch Intern Med 148:36, 1988
9. Gotto AM: Lipoprotein metabolism and the etiology of hyperlipidemia. Hosp Pract 23(Suppl 1):4, 1988
10. Gwynne JT: Lipoprotein structure and metabolism. Consultant 28(6):6, 1988
11. Robbins SL, Kumar V: Basic Pathology, 4th ed, pp 105, 288. Philadelphia, WB Saunders, 1987
12. Steinberg D: Research related to underlying mechanisms in atherosclerosis. Circulation 60:1562, 1979
13. Grundy SM: Pathogenesis of hyperlipidproteinemia. J Lipid Res 25:1611, 1984
14. Consensus Conference: Treatment of hypertriglyceridemia. JAMA 251:1196, 1984
15. Goldberg RB: Dietary modification of cholesterol levels. Consultant 28(6;Suppl):35, 1988
16. Knopp RH: New approaches to cholesterol lowering: Efficacy and safety. Hosp Pract 23(Suppl 1):22, 1988
17. Robbins SL, Cotran RS, Kumar V: Pathologic Basis of Disease, 3rd ed, pp 529, 532. Philadelphia, WB Saunders, 1984

18. DeSanchis RW, Doroghazi RM, Austen WG et al: Aortic dissection. N Engl J Med 317:1060, 1987
19. Webb RW, Bunswick RA: Management of acute dissection of the aorta. Heart Lung 9:284, 1980
20. Lennihan R, Porter JM, Summer DS et al: Raynaud's phenomenon: A wrap-up. Patient Care 22(3):94, 1988
21. Lipsmeyer EA: Raynaud's syndrome. J Arkansas Med Soc 79:63, 1982
22. McIntyre DR: A maneuver to reverse Raynaud's vasospasm. JAMA 240:2760, 1978
23. Gordon RS: From National Institutes of Health. Biofeedback for patients with Raynaud's vasospasm. JAMA 242:509, 1979
24. Miller KM: Assessing peripheral perfusion. Am J Nurs 78:1673, 1978
25. Lofgren KA: Varicose veins: Their symptoms, complications and management. Postgrad Med 65(6):131, 1979
26. Virchow R: Weinere untersuchungen uber dic verstropfung der lungenrarterie und ihre folgen. Beitr Exp Pathol Physiol 2:21, 1846
27. Nicolaides AN, Kakkar VV, Renney JTG: Soleal sinuses and stasis. Br J Surg 58:307, 1971
28. Nicolaides AN, Gordon-Smith I: The prevention of deep venous thrombosis. In Hobbs JT (ed): The Treatment of Venous Disorders, A Comprehensive Review of Current Practice in the Management of Varicose Veins and Postthrombotic Syndrome. Philadelphia, JB Lippincott, 1977
29. Caprini JA, Zoellner JL, Weisman M: Heparin therapy—Part II. Cardiovasc Nurs 13(4):17, 1977
30. Chamberlain SL: Low-dose heparin therapy. Am J Nurs 80:1115, 1980
31. Terry C, Silverstein P (eds): Management of Dermal Ulcers. Deerfield, IL, Travenol Laboratories, Inc., 1981
32. Beland I, Passos JY: Clinical Nursing, 4th ed, p 1112. New York, Macmillan, 1981
33. Reuler JB, Cooney TG: The pressure sore: Pathophysiology and principles of management. Ann Intern Med 94:661, 1981
34. Shea JD: Pressure sores. Clin Orthop 12:89,1975
35. Galpin JE, Chow AW, Bayer AS et al: Sepsis associated with decubitus ulcers. Am J Med 61:346, 1976
36. Anderson KE, Korning SA: Medical aspects of decubitus ulcer. Int J Dermatol 5:265, 1982
37. Ameis A, Chiarcossi A, Jimenez J: Management of pressure sores. Postgrad Med 67(2):177, 1980
38. Ahmed MC: Op-site for decubitus care. AJN 82:61, 1982

Bibliography

Atherosclerosis and arterial pathology

Barter PH, Hopkins GJ, Ying CH: The role of lipid transfer problems in plasma lipoprotein metabolism. Am Heart J 113:538, 1987

Bernstein EF, Fronek A: Current status of noninvasive tests in the diagnosis of peripheral arterial disease. Surg Clin North Am 62(3):473, 1982

Brown WV: Focus on fenofibrate. Hosp Pract 23(Suppl 1):31, 1988

Farrell PA, Barboriak J: The time course of alterations of plasma lipid and lipoprotein concentrations during eight weeks of endurance training. Atherosclerosis 37:231, 1980

Goldstein JL, Brown MS: The LDL receptor defect in familial hypercholesteremia. Med Clin North Am 66:335, 1982

Goldstein JL, Kita T, Brown MS: Defective lipoprotein receptors and atherosclerosis. N Engl J Med 309:288, 1983

Hazard WR: Dyslipidemia and accelerated atherosclerosis. Hosp Pract 23(May 30):41, 1988

Hoffman GS: Raynaud's disease and phenomenon. Am Fam Physician 21(1):91, 1980

Johansen K: Aneurysms. Sci Am 247(1):101, 1982

Less RS, Myers GS: Noninvasive diagnosis of arterial disease. Adv Intern Med 27:475, 1982

Lennihan R, Porter JM, Sumner DS et al: Raynaud's phenomonen: A wrap-up. Patient Care 22(3):94, 1988

Levy RI: Current status of the cholesterol controversy. Am J Med 72:1, 1983

Levy RI: Currently available lipid-lowering agents. Hosp Pract 23(Suppl 1):14, 1988

Olin JW, Graor RA: Thrombolytic therapy in treatment of peripheral arterial occlusions. Ann Emerg Med 17:1210, 1988

Roenigk HH Jr: Leg ulcers in the elderly. Geriatrics 34:21, 1979

Samuel P, McNamara DJ, Shapiro J: The role of diet in the etiology and treatment of atherosclerosis. Annu Rev Med 34:179, 1983

Schaefer EJ, Levy RI: Pathogenesis and management of lipoprotein disorders. N Engl J Med 312:1300, 1985

Stump DC, Mann DC: Mechanisms of thrombus formation and lysis. Ann Emerg Med 17:1138, 1988

Shionoya S, Hirai M, Kawai S, et al: Pattern of arterial occlusion in Buerger's disease. Angiology 31:375, 1982

Spittell JA Jr: Diagnosis and treatment of occlusive peripheral arterial disease. Geriatrics 37(1): 57, 1982

Spittel JA Jr: Occlusive peripheral arterial disease: Guidelines for office management. Postgrad Med 719(2):137, 1982

Stadel BV: Oral contraceptives and cardiovascular disease. N Engl J Med 3059(11):612, 1981

Weingarten J, Teirney LM Jr: Aortic dissection. West J Med 144:728, 1987

Pressure sores

Resch CS, Kerner E, Robson MC et al: Pressure sore volume measurement. J Am Geriatr Soc 36:444, 1988

Seiler WO, Stahelin HB: Recent findings on decubitus ulcer pathology: Implications for care. Geriatrics 41(1):47, 1986

Seiler WO, Stahelin HB: Decubitus ulcers: Treatment through five therapeutic principles. Geriatrics 40(9):30, 1985

Sugarman B: Infection and pressure sores. Arch Phys Med Rehab 66:177, 1985

Xakellis GC, Garzone P: Pressure ulcers. Am Fam Pract 35:159, 1987

Venous pathology

Barnes RW: Current status of noninvasive tests in the diagnosis of venous disease. Surg Clin North Am 62(3):489, 1982

Bennison J: The support of the venous circulation. Angiology 32:442, 1982

CHAPTER 19

Alterations in Blood Pressure: Hypertension and Orthostatic Hypotension

Objectives

After you have studied this chapter, you should be able to meet the following objectives:

_____ State the physiologic origin of the arterial pressure pulse.

_____ Use the hemodynamic changes in arterial flow that occur during indirect blood pressure measurements using an inflatable cuff to explain the origin of the Korotkoff sounds.

_____ State the correct methods for obtaining indirect blood pressure measurements in children, adults, and elderly persons.

_____ Explain how cardiac output and peripheral vascular resistance interact in determining blood pressure levels.

_____ Relate the determinants of blood pressure (cardiac output and peripheral vascular resistance) to systolic blood pressure, diastolic blood pressure, pulse pressure, and mean arterial blood pressure.

_____ Construct a diagram illustrating the neural pathways involved in the baroreflex control of heart rate and peripheral vascular resistance.

_____ Trace the physiology of the renin–angiotensin–aldosterone system and state its effects on blood vessel and renal function.

_____ State the effect of vasopressin on blood pressure regulation.

_____ Describe the effects of salt and water intake and mechanisms of renal elimination on the long-term regulation of blood pressure.

_____ Cite the current definition of _hypertension_ put forth by the Joint National Committee (JNC) on Detection, Evaluation, and Treatment of Hypertension.

(continued)

_____ Define *systolic hypertension*.

_____ Differentiate among essential, secondary, and malignant forms of hypertension.

_____ Describe the possible influence of age, race, obesity, salt and other cation (potassium, calcium, and magnesium) intake, alcohol consumption, stress, and oral contraceptive medications on development of essential hypertension.

_____ Explain the circulatory changes that occur during pregnancy.

_____ Describe the four types of hypertension that can occur during pregnancy.

_____ Cite the criteria for the diagnosis of high blood pressure in children.

_____ Relate the circulatory changes that occur with aging to the development of systolic hypertension.

_____ Describe modifications for blood pressure measurement in elderly persons as related to the auscultatory gap, pseudohypertension, and detection of orthostatic hypotension.

_____ Describe the physiologic causes of blood pressure elevation in renal disease, adrenocortical endocrine disorders, pheochromocytoma, brain ischemia, and coarctation of the aorta.

_____ Cite the benefits of the stepped-care approach to treatment of hypertension.

_____ List the nonpharmacologic treatments for hypertension and explain their benefits in reducing blood pressure.

_____ State the actions of diuretics, adrenergic-inhibiting drugs, vasodilating drugs, angiotensin-converting enzyme inhibitors, and calcium-channel blocking drugs in terms of blood pressure control.

_____ List major side effects of commonly used antihypertensive drugs.

_____ Describe the effects of malignant hypertension on the vascular system.

_____ List the three categories of drugs used to treat hypertension and the chief characteristics of each.

_____ Define *orthostatic hypotension*.

_____ Describe the pathologic changes that culminate in orthostatic hypotension.

_____ State why older persons are more likely than younger ones to experience orthostatic hypotension.

_____ State the relationship between orthostatic hypotension and fluid deficit.

_____ Describe the mechanisms of drug action that may induce orthostatic hypotension.

_____ Describe treatment measures in orthostatic hypotension.

The importance of measuring blood pressure and treating high blood pressure has been recognized for over 50 years. A speaker at the 1938 meeting of the Chicago Society of Internal Medicine stated:

> ... while it [measurement of blood pressure] does not carry an immediate purport in cases of acute illness as do the temperature and pulse; yet for long-term evaluation of health of the average person it is far more significant. No other commonly used test gives such quick and reasonably exact information regarding life expectancy.[1]

The discussion in this chapter focuses on control of blood pressure, and conditions of altered arterial pressure—hypertension and orthostatic hypotension.

Control of blood pressure

The arterial blood pressure is the driving force for blood in the circulatory system. Although blood pressure varies from moment to moment, it is perhaps the most controlled variable in the circulatory system.

The pressure pulse

The arterial pressure reflects the intermittent ejection of blood from the left ventricle into the aorta. It rises as the left ventricle contracts, and falls as it relaxes, giving rise to what is called a pressure wave. This pressure wave is responsible for the Korotkoff sounds heard when blood pressure is measured using a blood pressure cuff. The ejection of blood from the right ventricle into the pulmonary artery also produces pressure pulses, albeit of lesser magnitude than those of the systemic arterial pressure.

The contour of the arterial pressure tracing shown in Figure 19-1 is typical of the pressure changes that occur in the large arteries of the systemic circulation. There is a rapid rise in the pulse contour during left ventricular contraction (systole), followed by a slower rise to peak pressure. About 70% of the blood that leaves the left ventricle is ejected during the first one-third of systole (called the *rapid ejection period*); this accounts for the rapid rise in the pulse contour. The end of systole is marked by a brief downward deflection and formation of the dicrotic notch, which occurs when ventricular pressure falls below that in the aorta. The sudden closure of the aortic valve and the rebound energy it produces cause a brief rise in pressure immediately following the

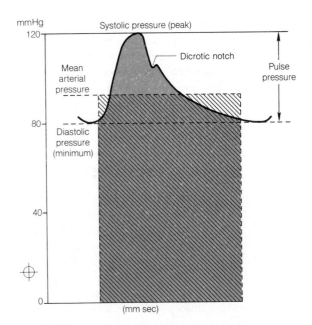

Figure 19-1 Intra-arterial pressure tracing made from the brachial artery. Pulse pressure is the difference between systolic and diastolic pressures. The *cross-hatched area* under the pressure tracing represents the mean arterial pressure, which can be calculated by using the formula:

$$\text{mean arterial pressure} = \text{diastolic pressure} + \frac{\text{pulse pressure}}{3}$$

notch. As the ventricles relax and blood flows into the peripheral vessels during diastole, the pressure falls rapidly at first and then declines slowly as the driving force decreases.

In healthy young adults, the pressure at the height of the pressure pulse (systolic pressure) is about 120 mmHg and 80 mmHg at the lowest pressure (diastolic pressure).[2] The pulse pressure (about 40 mmHg) is the difference between the systolic and diastolic pressures. It reflects the magnitude or height of the pressure pulse. The mean arterial pressure represents the average pressure in the arterial system during both ventricular contraction and relaxation (about 90–100 mmHg) and is depicted by the cross-hatched areas under the pressure tracing in Figure 19-1.

Determinants of blood pressure

Arterial blood pressure is determined by the cardiac output (stroke volume × heart rate) and the total peripheral resistance and can be expressed as the product of the two.

blood pressure =
cardiac output × total peripheral resistance

The total peripheral vascular resistance reflects the tone of the resistance vessels and the viscosity of the blood: it is increased when resistance vessels constrict and when blood viscosity is increased. The term *total peripheral resistance* (also called *peripheral vascular resistance*) is used to describe the sum of all the resistive forces that impede flow in the circulatory system. The body maintains its blood pressure by adjusting the cardiac output to compensate for changes in total peripheral resistance, and it changes the total peripheral resistance to compensate for changes in cardiac output.

In hypertension and disease conditions that affect blood pressure, changes in blood pressure are often described in terms of systolic, diastolic, pulse pressure, and mean arterial blood pressures. Each of these pressures contributes individually and collectively to blood flow in the various tissue beds of the body. The level to which each of these pressures rises and falls is influenced by the stroke volume, elastic properties of the aorta, and the total peripheral resistance.

Systolic blood pressure

The systolic pressure reflects the intermittent ejection of blood into the aorta (Figure 19-2). As blood is ejected into the aorta, it stretches the vessel wall and produces a rise in aortic pressure. The extent to which the systolic pressure rises or falls is determined by the amount of blood ejected into the aorta (stroke volume), the velocity of ejection, and the elastic properties of the aorta. Systolic pressure increases when there is a rapid ejection of a large stroke volume or when the stroke volume is ejected into a rigid aorta. Only about one-third of the ejected blood leaves the aorta during ventricular systole. Normally, the elastic walls of the aorta stretch to accommodate the blood that remains in the aorta; this prevents the pressure from rising excessively during systole and serves to maintain pressure during diastole. In some elderly people, the elastic fibers of the aorta lose some of their resiliency and the aorta becomes more rigid as a result of the aging process. When this occurs, the aorta is less able to stretch and buffer the pressure that is generated as blood is ejected into the aorta. This results in an elevated systolic pressure.

Diastolic blood pressure

The diastolic pressure is maintained by the pressure that has been stored in the elastic walls of the aorta during systole (Figure 19-2). The level at which the diastolic pressure is maintained depends on: (1) the condition of the arteries and their ability to stretch and store energy, (2) competency of the aortic valve, and (3) the resistance of the arterioles. The arteries are located between the outlet of the left heart (aortic valve) and the arterioles, which control the total pe-

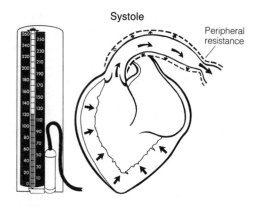

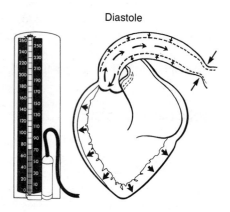

Figure 19-2 Diagram of the left side of the heart. Systolic blood pressure (*top*) represents the ejection of blood into the aorta during ventricular systole; it reflects the stroke volume, the distensibility of the aorta, and the velocity with which blood is ejected from the heart. Diastolic blood pressure (*bottom*) represents the pressure in the arterial system during diastole; it is largely determined by the peripheral vascular resistance.

ripheral resistance and runoff of blood from the arterial circulation. When there is an increase in total peripheral resistance, as with sympathetic stimulation, diastolic blood pressure rises. With atherosclerosis, the smaller arteries may become rigid and unable to accept the runoff of blood from the aorta without producing an increase in diastolic pressure.

Closure of the aortic valve at the onset of diastole is essential to the maintenance of the diastolic pressure. When there is incomplete closure of the aortic valve, as in aortic regurgitation (see Chapter 21), the diastolic pressure drops as blood flows backward into the left ventricle.

Pulse pressure

The pulse pressure (systolic minus diastolic pressure) reflects the pulsatile nature of the arterial blood flow and is an important component of blood pressure. During the rapid ejection period of ventricular systole, the volume of blood that is introduced into the arterial system exceeds the volume that exits. The

pulse pressure reflects this difference. The pulse pressure rises when additional amounts of blood are ejected into the arterial circulation, and it falls when the resistance to outflow is decreased. In hypovolemic shock, the pulse pressure declines due to a decrease in stroke volume and systolic pressure. This occurs despite an increase in peripheral resistance, which serves to maintain the diastolic pressure.

Mean arterial blood pressure

The mean arterial blood pressure represents the average blood pressure in the systemic circulation. The mean arterial pressure determines tissue blood flow. Mean arterial pressure can be estimated by adding one-third of the pulse pressure to the diastolic pressure (diastolic blood pressure + pulse pressure/3). Hemodynamic monitoring equipment in intensive and coronary care units usually compute mean arterial pressure automatically. Because it is a good indicator of tissue perfusion, the mean arterial pressure is often monitored, along with systolic and diastolic blood pressures, in critically ill patients.

Blood pressure measurement

Clinically, arterial blood pressure measurements are usually obtained by the indirect method using a sphygmomanometer and the auscultatory method. In the measurement of blood pressure, a cuff, which contains a rubber bladder, is placed around the upper arm. The bladder of the cuff is then inflated to a point at which its pressure exceeds that of the artery, thus occluding the blood flow. The cuff is then slowly deflated until the pressure in the vessel once again exceeds the pressure in the cuff. At this time, a small amount of blood is forced through the partially obstructed artery; by placing a stethoscope over the brachial artery distal to the cuff, one can audibly monitor the tapping sounds that are produced.

Blood pressure is recorded in terms of both systolic and diastolic pressures, for example, 120/70 mmHg. The initial tapping sound heard as blood is forced through the artery is the systolic pressure. Diastolic pressure reflects the point at which the sounds become muffled or are no longer heard; it represents the point at which arterial pressure is sufficient to prevent vessel compression by the cuff. The auscultatory sounds, or tapping sounds, heard during blood pressure measurement are often referred to as Korotkoff sounds after the Russian physician who first described them (Table 19-1). It is recommended that the disappearance of sound (phase V) should be used for the diastolic reading.[3]

Accuracy of blood pressure measurement requires that the equipment be properly calibrated, the

Table 19–1. Korotkoff sounds

Phase I: That period marked by the first tapping sounds, which gradually increase in intensity.

Phase II: The period during which a murmur or swishing sound is heard.

Phase III: The period during which sounds are crisper and greater in intensity.

Phase IV: The period marked by distinct, abrupt muffling or by a soft blowing sound.

Phase V: The point at which sounds disappear.

correct cuff size be used, the arm be properly positioned, and the cuff be inflated and deflated correctly. The room should be free of distracting noises, and the blood pressure gauge should be at eye level. The appropriate size cuff is essential for accurate blood pressure measurement—too large a cuff is apt to give low readings whereas an inappropriately small cuff may give too high a reading. In adults, the bladder of the cuff should encircle at least two-thirds of the arm.[3] The arm to be used should be placed so that the cuff is at the level of heart. Deflation should be slow enough so that accurate measurements can be obtained (2 mmHg/heart beat).

Blood pressure can also be measured in the legs using a thigh cuff or in the forearm. When blood pressure is measured in the forearm, an appropriate sized cuff is placed below the elbow and the Korotkoff sounds are monitored over the radial artery.[4] Forearm blood pressures are particularly useful in obese individuals, particularly when an appropriate sized cuff is not available for the upper arm. Automated or semiautomated methods of blood pressure measurement use a microphone, pulse sensor, or Doppler methods for detecting the equivalent of the Korotkoff sounds.

Intra-arterial methods provide for direct measurement of blood pressure. Intra-arterial measurement requires the insertion of a catheter into a peripheral artery. The arterial catheter is connected to a pressure transducer, which converts pressure into a digital signal that can be measured, displayed, and recorded.

Blood pressure measurement in infants and children

In children, as in adults, accuracy of blood pressure measurements depends on having the child relaxed and in a comfortable position with proper positioning of the arm and appropriate cuff size. It has been recommended that the cuff bladder should cover at least two-thirds of the arm circumference.[5] Devices using Doppler or oscillometric principles are available for measuring blood pressure in infants and small

children. In the Doppler method, blood movement through the artery is interpreted audibly by a special transducer contained in the cuff. The oscillometric technique relies on sensing, or feeling, the arterial pulse. Although these methods provide accurate measurement of systolic pressure, their reliability for diastolic pressures has not been established. It is recommended that phase IV Korotkoff sounds be used as an indicator of diastolic pressure when the auscultatory method is used for children ages 3 to 12 years; this is because Korotkoff sounds are often audible throughout deflation of the cuff.

Mechanisms of blood pressure control

Under ordinary conditions there are moment-by-moment variations in blood pressure related to activities of daily living such as moving from the supine to standing position, exercise, and emotional stress. Normally, blood pressure is regulated at levels sufficient to ensure adequate tissue perfusion. Blood pressure regulation requires the use of both short-term and long-term mechanisms.

Short-term regulation of blood pressure

The short-term adjustments (those occurring over seconds, minutes, or hours) are intended to correct temporary imbalances in blood pressure that occur with situations such as postural change, exercise, or hemorrhage. They involve neural and hormonal mechanisms.

The neural mechanisms of blood pressure control, which are largely vested in the autonomic nervous system (ANS), include intrinsic circulatory reflexes, extrinsic reflexes, and higher center influences. The intrinsic reflexes, including the baroreflex and chemoreceptor-mediated reflex, are located within the circulatory system and are essential for rapid and short-term regulation of blood pressure. The extrinsic reflexes are found outside the circulation. They include blood pressure responses associated with such things as pain, cold, and isometric handgrip exercise. The neural pathways for these reactions are largely unknown, and their responses are less consistent than those of the intrinsic reflexes. Among higher center responses are the central nervous system (CNS) ischemic response and those due to changes in mood and emotion. There are also a number of hormones and humoral mechanisms that contribute to blood pressure regulation, including the renin–angiotensin–aldosterone mechanism and vasopressin. Of recent interest are the renal prostaglandins and the atrial natriuretic factor.

Baroreceptors. The baroreceptors are pressure-sensitive receptors located in the walls of blood vessels and the heart. The carotid and aortic baroreceptors are located in strategic positions between the heart and the brain (Figure 19-3). The baroreceptors respond to a change in the stretch of the vessel wall by sending impulses to cardiovascular centers in the brain to effect appropriate changes in heart action and vascular smooth muscle tone. For example, a fall in blood pressure on moving from the lying to the standing position produces a decrease in the stretch of the aortic and carotid baroreceptors with a resultant increase in heart rate and vasoconstriction. The rapidity with which the baroreflex response occurs is such that a change in heart rate can often be observed within one or two heartbeats. The vasoconstrictor response may take several seconds to occur.

The carotid and aortic baroreceptors are often referred to as the high-pressure baroreceptors because they are located in the arterial side of the circulation. There are also low-pressure baroreceptors, which are located in the right atria and pulmonary artery (the low-pressure side of the circulation). As with other neural receptors, the baroreceptors adapt to prolonged changes in blood pressure and are probably of little importance in the long-term regulation of blood pressure.

Chemoreceptors. The chemoreceptors are sensitive to changes in the oxygen, the carbon dioxide, and the hydrogen ion content of the blood. The arterial chemoreceptors are located in the carotid bodies, which lie in the bifurcation of the two common carotids, and in the aortic bodies of the aorta (Figure 19-3). Because of their location, these chemoreceptors are always in close contact with the arterial blood. Although the main function of the chemoreceptors is to regulate ventilation, they also communicate with the vasomotor center and can induce widespread vasoconstriction. Whenever the arterial pressure drops below a critical level, the chemoreceptors are stimulated because of a diminished oxygen supply and a buildup of carbon dioxide and hydrogen ions. As we shall see in Chapter 25, persons with hypoxemia due to chronic lung disease may develop both systemic and pulmonary hypertension.

The autonomic nervous system. The efferent mechanisms for the neural control of blood pressure are vested in the parasympathetic and sympathetic divisions of the autonomic nervous system (ANS). The efferent output from the ANS is linked to visceral sensory (e.g., visceral pain, nausea, and bladder fullness), somatic sensory (somatic pain and thermal sensations), and special sensory (vision and hearing) afferent input. The neural control centers for the regulation of blood pressure are located in the reticular formation of the lower pons and medulla of the brain stem where the integration and modulation of autonomic nervous system responses occur. The area of the reticular formation that controls blood vessel tone is called the *vasomotor center*. These brain stem centers receive information from many areas of the nervous system including the hypothalamus.

The ANS contributes to blood pressure control through both cardiac (heart rate and cardiac contractility) and vascular (peripheral vascular resistance) mechanisms. The heart is innervated by both the parasympathetic and sympathetic nervous systems. Parasympathetic innervation of the heart is by means of the vagus nerve. The effect of vagal stimulation on heart function is largely limited to heart rate, with increased vagal activity producing a slowing of the pulse. Stimulation of the sympathetic nervous system produces an increase in both heart rate and cardiac contractility. The sympathetic nervous system controls blood vessel tone. Even under resting or basal conditions the resistance vessels of the arterial system are partially constricted. The peripheral vascular resistance, a determinant of blood pressure, is controlled by altering this basal tone. The parasympathetic ner-

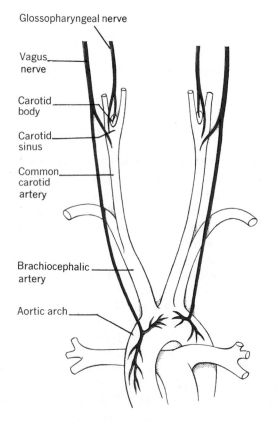

Glossopharyngeal nerve

Vagus nerve

Carotid body

Carotid sinus

Common carotid artery

Brachiocephalic artery

Aortic arch

Figure 19-3 Location and innervation of the aortic arch and carotid sinus baroreceptors and the carotid body chemoreceptors. (Chaffee EE, Lytle IM: Basic Physiology and Anatomy, 4th ed. Philadelphia, JB Lippincott, 1980)

vous system exerts little, if any, control over blood vessel function.

The actions of the autonomic nervous system are mediated by chemical neurotransmitters. Acetylcholine is the postganglionic neurotransmitter for parasympathetic neurons, and norepinephrine is the main neurotransmitter for postganglionic sympathetic neurons. Sympathetic neurons also respond to epinephrine, which is released into the bloodstream by the adrenal medulla. The neurotransmitter dopamine can also act as a neuromediator for some sympathetic neurons.

The neuromediators exert their effect through membrane proteins called *receptors*. The neuromediators and receptors interact in a lock and key fashion, which ensures specificity of action. Receptors that interact with acetylcholine are called *cholinergic* receptors, and those that interact with the sympathetic neuromediators, *adrenergic* receptors. There are two types of adrenergic receptors: alpha and beta receptors. In vascular smooth muscle, stimulation of alpha receptors produces vasoconstriction; stimulation of beta receptors, vasodilatation. Alpha receptors have been further subdivided into alpha$_1$ and alpha$_2$ receptors. Alpha$_1$ receptors are found primarily at postsynaptic effector sites such as vascular smooth muscle. Alpha$_2$ receptors are abundant in the central nervous system and act at presynaptic sites to produce feedback inhibition of sympathetic outflow. Beta$_1$ receptors are found primarily in the heart, and beta$_2$ receptors, in the bronchioles and in other sites that have beta-mediated functions. In many tissues, the response that occurs is determined by the presence of a particular receptor type, which can vary from tissue to tissue. For example, in vascular smooth muscle that has alpha$_1$ receptors, sympathetic stimulation produces vasoconstriction; similar stimulation produces vasodilatation in other vessels that have beta$_2$ receptors. The actions of the autonomic nervous system are further discussed in Chapter 48.

The role of the autonomic nervous system in control of blood pressure is only now beginning to be understood. For example, central alpha^2-adrenergic receptors are now known to inhibit sympathetic outflow from the brain. Several antihypertensive medications exert their effect at this level. Alpha- and beta-adrenergic receptors respond to endogenous or exogenous catecholamines (*e.g.*, drugs). Drugs that can selectively activate or block specific types of adrenergic receptors have been developed to treat high blood pressure.

The central nervous system responses. It is not surprising that the central nervous system, which plays an essential role in regulating vasomotor tone and blood pressure, would have a mechanism for con-

trolling the blood flow to the cardiovascular centers that control circulatory function. When the blood flow to the brain has been sufficiently interrupted to cause ischemia of the vasomotor center, these vasomotor neurons become strongly excited, causing massive vasoconstriction as a means of raising the blood pressure to levels as high as the heart can pump against. This response is called the CNS ischemic response, and it can raise the blood pressure to levels as high as 270 mmHg for as long as 10 minutes.[6] The CNS ischemic response is a last-ditch stand to preserve the blood flow to vital brain centers; it does not become activated until blood pressure has fallen to at least 50 mmHg and it is most effective in the range of 15 mmHg to 20 mmHg. If the cerebral circulation is not reestablished within 3 to 10 minutes, the neurons of the vasomotor center cease to function, so that the tonic impulses to the blood vessels stop and the blood pressure falls precipitously.

The Cushing reflex is a special type of CNS reflex resulting from an increase in intracranial pressure. When the intracranial pressure rises to levels that equal intra-arterial pressure, blood vessels to the vasomotor center become compressed, initiating the CNS ischemic response. The purpose of this reflex is to produce a rise in arterial pressure to levels above intracranial pressure so that the blood flow to the vasomotor center can be reestablished.

Renin–angiotensin–aldosterone mechanism. Along with the autonomic nervous system, renal function, and hormones that are salt-losing or salt-retaining, the renin–angiotensin–aldosterone system plays a central role in blood pressure regulation. Renin is an enzyme that is synthesized and released from the kidneys. Factors that control renin release include renal blood flow and renal artery pressure. Renin levels increase as renal blood flow and renal artery pressure fall. Renin is also released in response to sympathetic stimulation.

Renin combines with a plasma protein (*angiotensinogen*) that is present in the bloodstream to form angiotensin I (Figure 19-4). Angiotensin I enters the circulation and travels to the lung, where it is converted to angiotensin II by the angiotensin-converting enzyme. There are several potential pathways whereby angiotensin II, the active component of the renin–angiotensin–aldosterone mechanism, could influence short-term and long-term regulation of blood pressure: through vasoconstriction of blood vessels; through activation of the sympathetic nervous system or by potentiation of its effects; or through influence of fluid volume by thirst, direct renal mechanisms, or aldosterone.[7] Although angiotensin II has a short half-life of minutes, it is one of the most potent vasoconstrictors known. Angiotensin II exerts a direct ef-

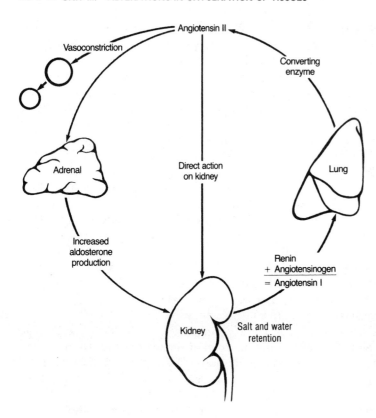

Figure 19-4 Control of blood pressure by the renin–angiotensin–aldosterone system. Renin combines with the plasma protein angiotensinogen to form angiotensin I; angiotensin-converting enzyme in the lung changes angiotensin I to angiotensin II; angiotensin II produces vasoconstriction and increases salt and water retention through direct action on the kidney and through increased aldosterone secretion by the adrenal cortex.

fect on the kidneys to decrease the elimination of salt and water. It acts in a feedback manner to decrease renin release, and it stimulates the production and release of aldosterone from the adrenal cortex. Aldosterone provides more long-term regulation of blood pressure through salt and water retention.

Among persons with hypertension, there is a subgroup that has high renin levels and another subgroup that has low renin levels with normal angiotensin and aldosterone levels. It has been proposed that the elevation of blood pressure in persons in the high renin group is due to vasoconstriction, and in the low renin group it is due to volume expansion. Angiotensin-converting enzyme (ACE) inhibitors are used in the treatment of some persons with hypertension, particularly those with high renin levels.[8] The ACE inhibitors not only reduce blood pressure, but they increase renal blood flow and the glomerular filtration, which is advantageous in certain types of hypertension.

Renal prostaglandins. Renal prostaglandins attenuate the renal response to various vasoconstrictor stimuli including angiotensin, norepinephrine, and renal nerve stimulation. It is thought that these hormones play a role in preserving renal circulation whenever it is threatened and in modulating rises in systemic blood pressure from various mechanisms. Inhibitors of prostaglandin synthesis such as the nonsteroidal anti-inflammatory drugs (NSAID) have the potential for decreasing renal blood flow in persons with impaired renal function. Whether a renal prostaglandin deficiency can contribute to hypertension is unknown.

Vasopressin. Vasopressin, or antidiuretic hormone (ADH), is released from the posterior pituitary gland in response to decreases in blood volume and blood pressure. Its release is mediated by the osmolality of body fluids and other stimuli. The antidiuretic actions of vasopressin are discussed in Chapter 27. Vasopressin has a direct vasoconstrictor effect on blood vessels, particularly those of the splanchnic circulation. However, long-term increases in vasopressin cannot maintain volume expansion or hypertension, and it does not enhance hypertension produced by sodium-retaining hormones or other vasoconstricting substances. Rather, it has been suggested that vasopressin plays a permissive role in hypertension by its fluid-retaining properties or that it acts as a neurotransmitter that serves to modify autonomic nervous system function.[9]

Atrial natriuretic factor. Of recent interest is a hormone called the *atrial natriuretic factor,* which may affect blood pressure control. The hormone is thought to inhibit sodium transport out of cells in exchange for potassium. In the kidney, inhibition of sodium–potassium transport causes increased sodium excretion. In vascular smooth muscle, it results in a net uptake of calcium and, in turn, increased vascular tone. In sympathetic neurons, the inhibition of sodium transport enhances norepinephrine release and inhibits its uptake. It is thought that some individuals who are prone to develop hypertension have a congenital or acquired defect in sodium excretion by the kidney and that excess sodium ingestion in these individuals stimulates increased secretion of the natriuretic factor as a compensatory mechanism. In these individuals hypertension develops as a side effect of the natriuretic factor and its action on vascular smooth muscle and the sympathetic nervous system.[10,11]

Long-term regulation of blood pressure

Both neural and hormonal regulation of blood pressure are short-term mechanisms that act rapidly to restore blood pressure. Short-term mechanisms are capable of completely correcting changes in blood pressure that occur during the performance of normal, everyday activities such as physical exercise and changes in posture. These mechanisms are also responsible for the maintenance of blood pressure at survival levels during acute life-threatening situations. They are, however, ineffective in the long-term regulation of blood pressure; the day-by-day, week-by-week, and month-by-month regulation of blood pressure is vested in what Guyton terms the "renal-body fluid pressure control system."[6]

In the renal-body fluid system for the long-term regulation of blood pressure, the kidneys respond to a change in arterial pressure by either increasing or decreasing salt and water excretion. For example, an increase in arterial pressure greatly increases the rate at which both water (pressure diuresis) and sodium (pressure natriuresis) are excreted by the kidney. Figure 19-5 illustrates the control of blood pressure by renal output mechanisms. The only point on the graph at which the intake and output are balanced is at point A. At point B, where intake has increased almost fourfold, the blood pressure has increased to only 106 mmHg, demonstrating that the kidney adjusts the output of urine to balance the input. The function of the kidney in regulating body fluids is discussed in Chapter 30.

The only way to change the long-term regulation of blood pressure using the concept of the renal-body fluid control system is to change either the pressure range of the renal output curve or the net rate of intake. For example, kidney disease, which impairs salt and water excretion, results in a shift of the curve to the right so that points A and B occur at a higher arterial pressure. It is important to consider that the renal mechanisms will control the blood volume at a level required to attain the blood pressure needed to balance the intake and output. In some situations such

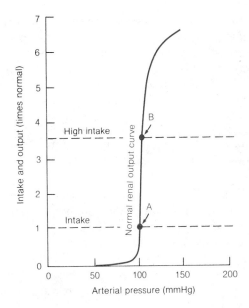

Figure 19-5 Graphic representation of long-term regulation of blood pressure based on the renal–body fluid mechanism for pressure control. The steep part of the curve is the normal urinary output curve and indicates that a 3.5 times normal intake will only increase arterial pressure from a level of 100 mmHg to 106 mmHg. *(Guyton A: Medical Physiology, 6th ed. Philadelphia, WB Saunders, 1981)*

as hot weather, which produces vasodilatation, more volume is required to attain this balance.

It is often difficult to imagine how small a change in body fluid is needed to cause a marked change in blood pressure. For example, a 3% to 5% (about 500 ml) chronic increase in body fluid is sufficient to increase the blood pressure by as much as 20 to 40 mmHg.[6] This example demonstrates how treatment measures that decrease body fluid levels can effect a reduction in blood pressure in some persons with hypertension. On the other hand, it is difficult to understand how a large volume of fluid can be acutely infused into a patient without causing a marked elevation in blood pressure unless one remembers that neural reflexes such as vasodilatation and other short-term mechanisms prevent significant changes in blood pressure for short periods of time.

In summary, the alternating contraction and relaxation of the heart produce a pressure pulse that moves the blood through the circulatory system. The elastic walls of the aorta stretch during systole and relax during diastole to maintain the diastolic pressure. The pressure pulse is responsible for the Korotkoff sounds heard when blood pressure is measured using a blood pressure cuff, and it is this impulse that is felt when the pulse is taken. Systolic pressure denotes the highest point of the pulse pressure, and diastolic, the lowest point. The pulse pressure is the difference between these two pressures. The mean arterial pressure reflects the average pressure throughout the cardiac cycle. It can be estimated by adding one-third of the pulse pressure to the diastolic pressure. Systolic pressure is determined primarily by the characteristics of the stroke volume, whereas diastolic pressure is determined largely by the conditions of the arteries and arterioles and their abilities to accept the runoff of blood from the aorta. Blood pressure is determined by the cardiac output and total peripheral resistance.

Blood pressure can be measured either directly or indirectly. Direct measurement requires the insertion of a catheter into an artery. Clinical measurement of blood pressure is usually done by the indirect method using a blood pressure cuff and either the auscultatory or Doppler method. Special methods are required for measurement of blood pressure in infants and small children.

Short-term and long-term mechanisms for blood pressure control normally maintain the mean arterial blood pressure within a range that is adequate for tissue perfusion. Short-term mechanisms occur over minutes or hours and are intended to correct temporary imbalances in blood pressure, such as those caused by postural changes, exercise, or hemorrhage. These involve neural and hormonal mechanisms. Long-term mechanisms control the day-by-day, week-by-week, and month-by-month regulation of blood pressure and involve the excretion of salt and water by the kidneys (the renal-body fluid pressure control system).

Hypertension

Hypertension, or high blood pressure, is probably the most common of all cardiovascular disorders. Almost 60 million persons in the United States have an elevated blood pressure (140/90 mmHg or greater) or have reported being told by a physician that they have high blood pressure. The prevalence of hypertension increases with age, and the rate among black Americans is higher than among white Americans.[12] It occurs in all geographic areas of the country and affects individuals from low-, middle-, and upper-income groups. Hypertension is credited with causing 30,700 deaths annually; it takes its toll mainly through vascular complications that lead to stroke, coronary heart disease, and chronic renal failure.[13]

Hypertension is commonly divided into the categories of primary and secondary hypertension. In primary hypertension, often called essential hypertension, the chronic elevation in blood pressure occurs without evidence of other disease. In secondary hy-

pertension, the elevation of blood pressure accompanies some other disorder, such as kidney disease. Malignant hypertension, as the name implies, is an accelerated form of hypertension. The discussion that follows focuses on these forms of hypertension, hypertension in children and the elderly, and the complications and treatment of hypertension.

Essential hypertension

The 1988 report of the Joint National Committee (JNC) on Detection, Evaluation, and Treatment of High Blood Pressure of the National Institutes of Health has recommended criteria for the diagnosis of high blood pressure in those individuals aged 18 years and older.[3] The diagnosis of hypertension is made if the diastolic blood pressure measurement is 90 mmHg or higher or the systolic blood pressure measurement is 140 mmHg or higher when at least two blood pressure measurements are averaged on two or more successive visits. High blood pressure may be further categorized into high normal blood pressure, mild hypertension, moderate hypertension, severe hypertension, borderline isolated systolic hypertension, and isolated systolic hypertension (Table 19-2). The report emphasizes that obtaining one elevated blood pressure reading should not constitute the diagnosis of hypertension. Blood pressure measure-

Table 19–2. Classification of blood pressure (BP) in adults aged 18 years or older*

BP range (mmHg)	Category†
Diastolic	
<85	Normal blood pressure
85–89	High normal blood pressure
90–104	Mild hypertension
105–114	Moderate hypertension
≥115	Severe hypertension
Systolic (diastolic BP <90)	
<140	Normal BP
140–159	Borderline isolated systolic hypertension
≥160	Isolated systolic hypertension

* Classification based on the average of two or more readings on two or more occasions.

† A classification of borderline isolated systolic hypertension (systolic BP = 140–159 mmHg) or isolated systolic hypertension (systolic BP ≥160 mmHg) takes precedence over a classification of high normal BP (diastolic BP = 85–89 mmHg) when both occur in the same person. A classification of high normal BP (diastolic BP = 85–89 mmHg) takes precedence over a classification of normal BP (systolic BP < 140 mmHg) when both occur in the same person.

(The 1988 Report of the Joint National Committee on Detection, Evaluation, and Treatment of High Blood Pressure. NIH Pub No 88-1088. Washington, DC, US Department of Health and Human Services, 1988)

ments should be taken when the individual is relaxed and has rested for at least 5 minutes and has not smoked or ingested caffeine within 30 minutes. A mercury manometer with the appropriately sized cuff or an aneroid manometer that is accurately calibrated should be used for blood pressure measurements. At least two measurements should be made at each visit in the same arm while the individual is seated. The diastolic pressure is recorded at the disappearance of sound, or phase V of the Korotkoff sounds.[3]

Causes of hypertension

The causes of the condition called *essential hypertension* are complex and largely unknown. It is known, however, that a number of factors interact in producing long-term elevations in blood pressure; these factors include hemodynamic, neural, humoral, and renal mechanisms. As with other disease conditions, it is improbable that there is a single cause responsible for the development of essential hypertension or, for that matter, that the condition is a single disease.

Because arterial blood pressure is the product of cardiac output and total peripheral resistance, all forms of hypertension involve hemodynamic mechanisms—either an increase in cardiac output or total peripheral resistance or a combination of the two. Many other factors such as the autonomic nervous system, the kidneys, the electrolyte composition of the intracellular and extracellular fluids, cell membrane transport mechanisms, and humoral substances play either an active or permissive role in regulating the hemodynamic mechanisms that control blood pressure.

Risk factors

Although the cause or causes of essential hypertension are largely unknown, several risk factors have been implicated as contributing to its development. These risk factors include family history, advancing age, race, and high salt intake. Other life-style factors can contribute to the development of hypertension by interacting with the risk factors. These life-style factors include obesity; excess alcohol consumption; intake of potassium, calcium, magnesium; stress; and use of oral contraceptive drugs.

Family history. The inclusion of heredity as a contributing factor in the development of hypertension is supported by the fact that hypertension is seen most frequently among persons with a family history of hypertension. Current studies suggest that in persons with a positive family history the risk for developing essential hypertension is approximately twice that of persons with a negative family history. The inher-

ited predisposition does not seem to rely on other risk factors, but when they are present the risk is apparently additive. This is particularly true of obesity. When obesity and a genetic predisposition are both present, the risk of developing hypertension becomes three to four times higher.[14] The pattern of heredity is unclear (*i.e.*, it is not known whether a single gene or multiple genes are involved). Whatever the explanation, the high incidence of hypertension among close family members seems significant enough to be presented as a case for recommending that persons from so-called high-risk families be encouraged to participate in hypertensive screening programs.

Advancing age. Maturation and growth are known to cause predictable increases in blood pressure. For example, in the newborn, arterial blood pressure is normally only about 50 mmHg systolic and 40 mmHg diastolic. Sequentially, blood pressure increases with physical growth from a value of 78 mmHg systolic at 10 days of age to 120 mmHg at the end of adolescence. Blood pressure usually continues to undergo a slow rate of increase during the adult years. The relationship between the aging process and hypertension is commonly accepted. The author can recall many older persons describing the normal range of blood pressure as being "100 plus your age." While this definition is not entirely correct, it is quite possible that the cardiovascular and autonomic nervous system changes that are part of the normal aging process do, in fact, contribute to the increased blood pressures observed in older persons. It must be remembered that individuals tend to age differently; this factor undoubtedly accounts for some of the great variations in blood pressure among elderly persons. However, the finding of isolated systolic hypertension is common in the elderly population and will be discussed later in this chapter.

Race. Hypertension is not only more prevalent in blacks than whites, but it is also more severe. The National Health and Nutrition Examination Survey II, 1976–1980 reported that diastolic blood pressures were significantly greater for black than white men and women in age groups 35 years and above and that systolic pressures of black women at every age were greater than those of white women.[15] Furthermore, it has been reported that hypertension in blacks tends to appear earlier than in whites, and it is often not treated early enough or aggressively enough.[16] The result is a higher incidence of more severe hypertension in blacks.

The reasons for the increased incidence of hypertension in blacks is unknown. Studies have shown that black persons with hypertension have lower renin levels than white persons with hypertension.[16] It has been suggested that environmental stresses associated with poverty, low education, low occupational status, socioeconomic stress, and eating habits that include foods high in salt and fat and other nutritionally contraindicated foods may contribute to the risk of hypertension in blacks.[17] Because of their low-renin profile, blacks are reported to respond better to drugs, such as diuretics and calcium-channel blocking drugs, that don't exert their primary actions through renin mechanisms.[18]

High salt intake. Increased salt intake has long been suspected as an etiologic factor in the development of hypertension. The relationship between body levels of sodium and hypertension is based, at least partially, on the finding of a decreased incidence of hypertension among primitive, unacculturated people from widely differing parts of the world.[19,20] For example, among the Yanomamo Indians of northern Brazil, who excrete only about 1 mEq of sodium per day, the average blood pressure in men 40 to 49 years of age is 107/67 mmHg and 98/62 mmHg in women of the same age.[21] From childhood through adult life, acculturated societies consume 10 g to 20 g of salt daily. Drinking water may be another source of increased sodium intake; in some cities there is considerable sodium in the water supply. Of recent interest is the relationship between the feeding practices of infants who are exposed to high salt intake at a very early age and the development of hypertension. Findings from one study indicate that on a weight basis, infants consumed more sodium (through prepared formula and baby foods) than older children.[22]

Just how increased salt intake contributes to the development of hypertension is still unclear. Evidence to support individual and group susceptibility to the hypertensive effects of sodium comes from observations made from the development of a strain of spontaneously hypertensive rats. These rats develop hypertension earlier than other strains, and their hypertension is more severe when extra salt is added to their diet. It may be that salt causes an elevation in blood volume, increases the sensitivity of cardiovascular or renal mechanisms to adrenergic influences, or exerts its effects through some other mechanism such as the renin–angiotensin–aldosterone mechanism. Interestingly, it has been observed that excessive salt intake does not cause hypertension in all persons, nor does the reduction in salt intake reduce blood pressure in all hypertensives. This probably means that some people are more susceptible than others to the effects of increased sodium intake. The impact of long-term nationwide restriction of sodium consumption is not known; it could, for example, create problems in persons who respond poorly to volume-depleting stresses in the absence of readily available salt in their diet.[23] Identification of persons at risk who would specifically

benefit from salt reduction would facilitate hypertension management.

Obesity. Excessive weight is commonly observed in association with hypertension. In a large nationwide screening program of more than a million persons, it was found that the frequency of hypertension in overweight persons 20 to 39 years of age was double that of persons of normal weight and triple that of underweight persons.[24] It has been suggested that fat distribution might be a more critical indicator of hypertension risk than actual overweight. The waist-to-hip ratio is commonly used to distinguish between waist (fat cell deposits in the abdomen) and hip or gluteal gynecoid obesity (fat cell deposits in the buttocks and legs). Studies have shown that there is a relationship between hypertension and increased waist-to-hip ratio even when body-mass index and skinfold thickness are taken into account.[25,26] The exact mechanism by which obesity contributes to the development of hypertension is largely unknown, although it may be that mechanisms responsible for elevating blood pressure in the overweight person are related to the metabolic needs of the excess adipose tissue, along with the increased demands on the cardiovascular system to provide adequate blood flow through the enlarged tissue mass. It is also quite possible that the dietary habits of the overweight person include the ingestion of excessive amounts of salt along with increased caloric intake. Hyperinsulinemia (excess insulin in the blood), which reduces sodium excretion and causes neuroendocrine disturbances such as abnormalities of the sympathetic nervous system, may also contribute to the development of hypertension in obese individuals.[27] Whatever the cause, it is known that weight loss is effective in reducing blood pressure in a significant number of obese hypertensive individuals. In one study, it was shown that weight loss or sodium restriction in hypertensives controlled for 5 years more than doubled the success of withdrawal of drug therapy.[28]

Excess alcohol consumption. Studies have shown a significant relationship between alcohol consumption and hypertension;[29] it has been suggested that as much as 10% of hypertension cases can be related to alcohol consumption.[30] One of the first reports of a link between alcohol consumption and hypertension came from the Oakland-San Francisco Kaiser-Permanente Medical Care Program study of 84,000 persons that correlated known drinking patterns and blood pressure levels.[31] This study revealed that the regular consumption of three or more drinks per day increased the risk of hypertension. Systolic pressures were more markedly affected than diastolic pressures. Alcohol has been shown to inhibit acutely vasopressin release, to increase heart rate and cardiac output, and to decrease peripheral vascular resistance. It has been suggested that these acute hemodynamic responses may reflect a rapid rise in plasma epinephrine and cortisol levels and a slower rise in norepinephrine.[8] It can be assumed the repeated occurrence of these acute responses results in a continued elevation in blood pressure. Blood pressure control may improve or return to normal when alcohol consumption is decreased or eliminated.

Intake of potassium, calcium, and magnesium.

Recently, it has been proposed that it is the ratio of sodium to potassium in the diet, rather than increased sodium intake alone, that influences blood pressure.[32-34] In terms of food intake, a diet high in sodium is generally low in potassium; and conversely, a diet high in potassium is generally low in sodium. One of the major benefits of increased potassium intake is increased elimination of sodium. Other effects include a dampening of vasoconstrictor responses that are induced by norepinephrine and other vasoactive agents. A high-potassium diet does not appear to alter blood pressure in normotensive persons, nor is there evidence to suggest a significant effect from giving potassium to hypertensives with normal potassium levels. The use of potassium supplements is expensive and possibly even hazardous for some persons. Instead, it is recommended that high-potassium,low-sodium foods be substituted for high-sodium, low-potassium foods in the diet.[8]

The interrelationship of high blood pressure, calcium, and magnesium levels has been investigated.[35] Although there have been reports of high blood pressure in persons with low calcium intake or lowering of blood pressure with increased calcium intake, at present the link between low calcium intake and hypertension is inconclusive.[36] Magnesium, which has been described as "nature's physiologic calcium blocker," is credited with blocking calcium entry into vascular smooth muscle cells, thereby decreasing vascular reactivity.[37] As with calcium, however, the benefits of supplementing magnesium intake in persons with hypertension are controversial.

Stress.

Physical and emotional stress undoubtedly contribute to transient alterations in blood pressure. Studies in which arterial blood pressure was continually monitored on a 24-hour basis as individuals performed their normal activities showed marked fluctuations in pressure associated with normal life stresses—increasing during periods of physical discomfort and family crisis and declining during rest and sleep.[38,39] As with other risk factors, the role of stress-related episodes of transient hypertension in producing the chronically elevated pressures seen in essential hypertension is still speculative. It may be that vascular smooth muscle hypertrophies with increased activity in a manner similar to that of skeletal muscle or that the central integrative pathways in the brain become adapted to the frequent stress-related input.

Psychologic techniques involving biofeedback, relaxation, and transcendental meditation have emerged as methods to control alterations in blood pressure. It is still too early to tell whether these techniques will offer information about the role of stress in the production of hypertension or will prove useful in its treatment.

Use of oral contraceptive drugs.

Oral contraceptives cause a mild increase in blood pressure in many women and overt hypertension in about 5%.[40] Why this occurs is largely unknown, although it has been suggested that estrogen and progesterone are responsible for the effect. The fact that various contraceptive drugs contain different amounts and combinations of estrogen and progestational agents may contribute to the incidence of hypertension among different women. Fortunately, the hypertension associated with oral contraceptives usually disappears once the drug has been discontinued, although it may take as long as 6 months for this to happen. However, in some women the blood pressure may not return to normal; they may be among populations at risk for developing hypertension. The risk of hypertension-associated cardiovascular complications are found primarily in women over 35 years of age and in those who smoke.[40]

Signs and symptoms

Essential hypertension is frequently asymptomatic, and diagnosis is often made by chance during screening procedures or when an individual seeks medical care for other purposes. Although headache is often considered to be an early symptom of hypertension, it is present only in a small number of hypertensives at the time of diagnosis. When present, the headache associated with hypertension is believed to be due to intense vasodilatation. It occurs most frequently on awakening and is usually felt in the back of the head or neck. A common early symptom of long-term hypertension is nocturia, which indicates that the kidney is losing its ability to concentrate urine. Epistaxis (nosebleeds), tinnitus (ringing in the ears), and vertigo (dizziness), although often claimed to be characteristic of hypertension, have been found to be no more frequent among persons with recognized hypertension than among those with normal blood pressures.

Other commonly associated signs and symptoms are probably related to the complications of hypertension—the long-term effects of blood pressure elevation on other organ systems in the body, such as the kidneys, eyes, heart, and blood vessels.

Aside from elevated blood pressure measurements, few diagnostic tests are useful in detecting and diagnosing essential hypertension. In this respect, the increased availability of hypertensive screening clinics provides a means for early detection. Blood pressure varies in response to stress, time of day, and other factors; therefore, a diagnosis of essential hypertension is never based on a single blood pressure reading. Contributing factors such as a family history of hypertension or the presence of obesity often assist in confirming the diagnosis. Laboratory tests, x-ray films, and other diagnostic tests are usually done to rule out secondary hypertension or associated complications.

Effects

The complications and mortality associated with primary and secondary hypertension can be explained as the increased wear and tear on the heart and blood vessels.

The increase in the workload of the left ventricle as it pumps against the elevated pressures in the systemic circulation is directly related to the degree and duration of the hypertension. This increased work is the stimulus for ventricular muscle hypertrophy, and it increases the heart's need for oxygen. If the increased work demands exceed the heart's compensatory efforts, heart failure occurs because the heart can no longer pump effectively. (Heart failure is discussed in Chapter 22.) The individual who develops coronary artery disease along with hypertension is at especially high risk, because the heart's oxygen transport facilities are impaired in the presence of increased oxygen needs. Surprisingly, many people seem to tolerate elevated levels of blood pressure for many years before its detrimental effects on cardiac function are detected. The hypertrophied left ventricle is usually visible on an x-ray film and shows a characteristic left axis deviation on the electrocardiogram.

Arteries and arterioles throughout the body experience the effects of the mechanical stress associated with hypertension. Again, the severity and duration of the increase largely determine the extent of vascular changes. In general, hypertension has been implicated in accelerating the development of atherosclerosis, which causes a narrowing of the vessel lumen, and in weakening the vessels. Also, there is greater risk of aortic aneurysm, coronary heart disease, renal complications, retinopathy, and cerebral vascular disease.

High blood pressure in pregnancy

About 10% of all pregnancies are accompanied by hypertension.[41] The American College of Obstetricians and Gynecologists has established four criteria for the diagnosis of hypertension in pregnancy: (1) systolic pressure greater than 140 mmHg, (2) increase of 30 mmHg in systolic pressure, (3) diastolic pressure greater than 90 mmHg, (4) increase of 15 mmHg in diastolic pressure.[42] Any of these criteria must be present on at least two occasions not less than 6 hours apart. Hypertension in pregnancy is classified into four groups: preeclampsia-eclampsia, chronic hypertension, chronic hypertension with superimposed preeclampsia-eclampsia, and late or transient hypertension.[43]

Preeclampsia, sometimes called *pregnancy-induced hypertension,* is characterized by the triad of hypertension of pregnancy as previously defined, proteinuria (300 mg/liter in 24 hours), and edema (weight gain in excess of 2 lb/week) developing after the 20th week of pregnancy. Eclampsia is an exaggerated form of preeclampsia that has progressed to include convulsions and finally coma. Preeclampsia usually presents after the 20th week of gestation but may occur earlier in pregnancy. The condition occurs primarily during first pregnancies and during subsequent pregnancies in women with chronic hypertension, multiple fetuses, diabetes mellitus, or coexisting renal disease. It is associated with a condition called a *hydatidiform mole* (abnormal pregnancy caused by a pathologic ovum, resulting in a mass of cysts). Of interest is the reversal of the diurnal pattern of blood pressure in preeclamptic hypertension—it is often highest during the night.

Chronic hypertension is considered as hypertension that is unrelated to the pregnancy. It is defined as (1) history of high blood pressure prior to pregnancy, (2) identification of hypertension before 20 weeks of pregnancy, (3) hypertension that persists after pregnancy. In women with chronic hypertension, blood pressure often decreases in early pregnancy and then increases during the last trimester (3 months) of pregnancy, resembling preeclampsia. Consequently, women with undiagnosed chronic hypertension who do not present for medical care until the later months of pregnancy may be incorrectly diagnosed as having preeclampsia. Furthermore, women with chronic hypertension are at increased risk for developing preeclampsia-eclampsia. Late or transient hypertension is a condition of high blood pressure that occurs during the last trimester or early post-delivery period, but resolves to normotensive levels within 10 days after delivery.

Defining the causes of hypertension in pregnancy is difficult because of the normal circulatory changes that occur.[43] Blood pressure normally decreases during the first trimester, reaches its lowest point during the second trimester, and gradually rises during the third trimester. The fact that there is a 40% to 60% increase in cardiac output during early pregnancy means the fall in blood pressure that occurs during the first part of pregnancy must be due to a decrease in peripheral vascular resistance. Because the cardiac output remains high throughout pregnancy, the gradual rise in blood pressure that begins during the second trimester probably represents a return of the peripheral vascular resistance to normal. Also, pregnancy is normally accompanied by increased levels of renin, angiotensin I and II, estrogen, progesterone, prolactin, and aldosterone, all of which may alter vascular reactivity. Although there are differences of opinion, it has also been reported that volume contraction usually precedes development of overt clinical preeclampsia. There is a concern as to whether volume contraction is a primary or secondary event in preeclampsia, and this has led to contrasting methods of treatment: volume expansion versus use of diuretics and salt restriction.[44]

High blood pressure in children

The incidence of high blood pressure in children is not known. Only recently have population studies of blood pressure in children been undertaken. The results of these studies are just now being analyzed and interpreted.

Blood pressure is known to rise from infancy to late adolescence. During childhood, blood pressure is influenced by growth and maturation; therefore, blood pressure norms have been established using age (and height), race, and sex-specific percentiles to identify children for further follow-up and treatment.

The National Heart, Lung, and Blood Institute (NHLBI) convened its second task force in 1985 to (1) identify proper techniques for measuring blood pressure in infants (birth to 2 years), children (2 to 12 years), and adolescents (13 to 18 years); (2) to characterize the existing base on blood pressure distribution throughout childhood and prepare distribution curves of blood pressure by height and weight information; (3) recommend blood pressure ranges for children denoting normal, high normal, and hypertensive; (4) present guidelines for detecting children with hypertension and, at the same time, guard against inappropriate labeling of children as hypertensive who are not hypertensive; (5) identify the appropriate diagnostic steps to be taken in the evaluation of children with hypertension; and (6) to delineate nonpharmacologic and pharmacologic treatment strategies for management of children with hypertension.[45]

The task force classified blood pressure into three ranges: normal (systolic and diastolic pressures less than the 90th percentile for age and sex); high normal (systolic and/or diastolic blood pressures between the 90th and 95th percentile for age and sex); and high blood pressures or hypertension (average systolic and diastolic blood pressures equal to or greater than the 95th percentile for age and sex on at least three

Table 19–3. Classification of hypertension in the young, by age group

Age group	95th percentile (mmHg)	99th percentile (mmHg)
Newborns— 7 days	SBP ≥ 96	SBP ≥ 106
Newborns (8–30 days)	SBP ≥ 104	SBP ≥ 110
Infants (<2 years)	SBP ≥ 112 DBP ≥ 74	SBP ≥ 118 DBP ≥ 82
Children (3–5 years)	SBP ≥ 116 DBP ≥ 76	SBP ≥ 124 DBP ≥ 84
Children (6–9 years)	SBP ≥ 122 DBP ≥ 78	SBP ≥ 130 DBP ≥ 86
Children (10–12 years)	SBP ≥ 126 DBP ≥ 82	SBP ≥ 134 DBP ≥ 90
Adolescents (13–15 years)	SBP ≥ 136 DBP ≥ 86	SBP ≥ 144 DBP ≥ 92
Adolescents (16–18 years)	SBP ≥ 142 DBP ≥ 92	SBP ≥ 150 DBP ≥ 98

(Report of the Second Task Force on Blood Pressure Control in Children—1987. Pediatrics 79:1, 1987)

occasions). High blood pressure was further defined as significant hypertension (blood pressure between the 95th and 99th percentile for age and sex) and severe hypertension (blood pressure above the 99th percentile for age and sex). Table 19-3 presents classification of significant and severe blood pressure by age; the source of age-specific percentiles for blood pressure measurements in children appears in the references.

The Task Force recommended further that children 3 years of age through adolescence should have their blood pressure taken once a year. It is recommended that phase IV Korotkoff sounds are used for diastolic pressure in infants and children 3 to 12 years of age. The phase V Korotkoff sound is used with adolescents 13 to 18 years. As with adults, blood pressure should be obtained using the proper sized cuff and a well-functioning manometer. Repeated measurements over time, rather than a single isolated determination, are required to establish consistent and significant observations. Accurate blood pressure measurements are often difficult to obtain in infants and children who are restless; errors are easily generated in Korotkoff sounds if heavy pressure is exerted on the stethoscope. Doppler and oscillometric techniques can be used in infants and children to provide accurate systolic measurements; however, diastolic measurements are more difficult to obtain.

Children with high blood pressure, significant high blood pressure, or severe high blood pressure should be referred for medical evaluation and treatment as indicated. Treatment includes nonpharmacologic methods and, if necessary, pharmacologic therapy. The Task Force suggested use of the stepped-care approach for drug treatment of children who require antihypertensive medications.

High blood pressure in the elderly

Isolated systolic hypertension (systolic pressure > 160 mmHg and/or diastolic pressure < 95 mmHg) is considered an abnormal clinical finding in old age.[46,47] The prevalence of hypertension (both systolic and diastolic) in the elderly population of the United States ranges from 44% to 63% for whites and 60% to 76% for blacks, depending on the criteria used (*e.g.*, 160 mmHg or 140 mmHg systolic and 95 mmHg or 90 mmHg diastolic pressure).[48] For years, systolic hypertension was considered innocuous and was not treated. The results of the Framingham study have shown, however, that there is approximately a twofold to fivefold increase in death from cardiovascular disease associated with isolated systolic hypertension.[49]

Data from the Framingham study also indicate that hypertension, whether systolic or diastolic, is a risk factor for cardiovascular morbidity and mortality in older as well as younger persons.[50] Stroke is two to three times more common in elderly hypertensives than in age-matched normotensive subjects.[51,52]

The aging processes that tend to increase blood pressure are stiffening of the arteries, decreased baroreceptor sensitivity, increased peripheral vascular resistance, and decreased renal blood flow. Normally, other aging processes such as an increased volume capacity of the aorta, decrease in blood volume, and a decrease in cardiac output tend to counteract the rise in pressure.[53] The disproportionate rise in systolic pressure observed in some elderly persons is explained in terms of the increased rigidity of the aorta and peripheral arteries that accompanies the aging process; this is caused by a loss of elastic fibers in the media, an increase in the amount of collagen, calcium deposition in the media, and atheroma formation in the intima.[54] Normally the elastic properties of the aorta allow it to stretch during systole as a means of buffering the rise in pressure that occurs as blood is ejected from the heart. Then, during diastole the recoil of the elastin fibers serves to transmit the stored pressure to the peripheral arterioles as a means of maintaining the diastolic blood pressure. As the aorta loses its elasticity and becomes more rigid as a result of the aging process, the pressure generated during ventricular systole is transmitted to the peripheral arteries practically unchanged.

The Working Group on Hypertension in the Elderly, which met in 1985, recommended that blood pressure measurements in the elderly should be similar to those for the rest of the population.[45] For elderly persons with elevations in both systolic and diastolic pressures, recommendations for detection and confirmation are the same as for younger persons as stated in the 1988 Report of the Joint National Committee (JNC) on Detection, Evaluation, and Treatment of High Blood Pressure.[3] For persons with a systolic blood pressure greater than 160 mmHg and normal diastolic pressure on two separate visits, referral to a physician for further evaluation is recommended.

Blood pressure measurement methods require special considerations in the elderly. The indirect measurement of blood pressure (using a blood pressure cuff and the Korotkoff sounds), when compared to the direct intra-arterial method, has been reported to give falsely elevated readings, especially of diastolic pressure, by as high as 15 to 30 mmHg.[54] This is because excessive cuff-pressure is needed to compress the sclerotic arteries of some older persons. A simple procedure called *Osler's maneuver* has been reported to differentiate persons with true hypertension from those whose blood pressure is spuriously elevated because of excessive sclerosis of the large arteries.[55] This procedure involves inflating the blood-pressure cuff above systolic pressure and carefully palpating the radial or brachial artery. Whenever either of these arteries remains clearly palpable (despite being pulseless), the person is said to be Osler-positive; when the artery is collapsed and not palpable, the person is said to be Osler-negative. On the other hand, in elderly persons with hypertension, a silent interval, called the auscultatory gap, may occur between the end of the first and beginning of the third phases of the Korotkoff sounds, providing the potential for underestimating the systolic pressure, sometimes by as high as 50 mmHg.[56] Because the gap occurs only with auscultation, it is recommended that a preliminary determination of systolic blood pressure be made by palpation and the cuff then be inflated above this value for auscultatory measurement of blood pressure. It is also recommended that the cuff be deflated slowly to avoid missing the first Korotkoff sounds.

There is often a transient fall in blood pressure during the first 2 to 3 minutes of standing, after which reflex-mediated increases in heart rate and total peripheral resistance (vascular constriction) usually return blood pressure to normal values. Because these reflexes are often less responsive in the elderly and may be impaired by hypertensive medications, it has been recommended that blood pressure be recorded 2 to 5 minutes after assumption of the standing position, as well as in the seated position.[3] This should be done not only during pretreatment examinations but during follow-up examinations once treatment has been instituted. This is done to detect the complication of postural hypotension, which can occur with some medications. If standing blood pressures are consistently lower than sitting pressures, the standing blood pressure should be used to titrate drug doses during treatment.[3]

Secondary hypertension

Only 5% to 10% of hypertensive cases are currently classified as secondary hypertension—that is, hypertension due to another disease condition. In secondary hypertension, as with other alterations in physiologic function, the presence of an elevation in blood pressure may be a homeostatic response that is recruited in an effort to maintain body function at least partially; or the elevated pressure may be due to an actual alteration in body structures that control or affect blood pressure. The disease states that most frequently give rise to secondary hypertension are (1) renal disease, (2) vascular disorders, (3) alterations in endocrine function and hormone levels, and (4) acute brain lesions. To avoid duplication in descriptions, the mechanisms associated with elevations of blood pressure in these disorders are discussed briefly, and a more detailed discussion of specific disease disorders is reserved for other sections of the book.

Renal disease

With the dominant role that the kidney assumes in blood pressure regulation, it is not surprising that the largest single cause of secondary hypertension is renal disease. By controlling salt and water levels, the kidney is probably involved in virtually all types of hypertension. In renal disease, salt and water retention undoubtedly plays a major role in elevated blood pressure. Also implicated in the development of renal hypertension is an imbalance between the vasoconstrictor and vasodepressor substances produced by the kidney.

Renovascular hypertension is a common cause of secondary hypertension; its prevalence has been estimated as 1% to 6% of all hypertensives.[57] This condition involves renal artery stenosis due to fibrous, fibromuscular, or atherosclerotic disease. In contrast to atherosclerosis, which most commonly occurs in older persons, fibrous or fibromuscular renal artery disease is more common in women and tends to occur in younger age groups (30- and 40-year-olds).

Diagnosis of renovascular disease often involves the use of angiographic studies. Angioplasty repair has been shown to be an effective long-term treatment for the disorder. Medical treatment includes the use of angiotensin II antagonists (captopril and saralasin).

Vascular disorders

Arteriosclerosis. As mentioned earlier in this chapter, hypertension itself predisposes to vascular disorders and vascular pathology tends to produce or perpetuate hypertension. The effects of arteriosclerosis on blood pressure are generally interpreted as changes in total peripheral resistance. In arteriosclerosis of the aorta and large arteries, the rigid vessel walls resist the runoff of blood ejected from the heart during systole, so the blood pressure rises and remains elevated during diastole. When renal blood vessels are affected, additional renal mechanisms contribute to the blood pressure elevation. The exaggerated vascular changes seen in malignant hypertension are discussed later in this chapter.

Coarctation of the aorta. An unusual form of hypertension occurs in coarctation of the aorta (adult form) in which there is a narrowing of that vessel as it exits from the heart, most commonly beyond the subclavian arteries (see Chapter 21). In the infantile form, the narrowing occurs proximal to the ductus arteriosus, in which case heart failure and other problems are present. As a result, many affected babies die within their first year of life. In the adult form of coarctation, there is often an increase in cardiac output that results from renal compensatory mechanisms. The ejection of a large stroke volume into a narrowed aorta with limited ability to accept the runoff results in an increase in systolic blood pressure and blood flow to the upper part of the body. Blood pressure in the lower extremities may be normal, although it is frequently low. For this reason, blood pressures in the legs may be assessed as a screening method for this disorder. The pulse pressure in the legs is almost always narrowed, and the femoral pulses are weak. Because the aortic capacity is diminished, there is usually a marked increase in systolic pressure (measured in the arms) during exercise when both stroke volume and heart rate are exaggerated.

Alterations in endocrine function

Secondary hypertension due to endocrine disorders is rare; when it does occur it is usually of adrenal origin and involves either the adrenal medullary or cortical tissue.

Pheochromocytoma. A *pheochromocytoma* is a tumor of chromaffin tissue usually found in the adrenal medulla; but it may also arise in other sites where there is chromaffin tissue, such as the sympathetic ganglia. Like adrenal medullary cells, the tumor cells of a pheochromocytoma produce and secrete the catecholamines epinephrine and norepinephrine. Thus, the hypertension results from the massive release of these catecholamines. Often their release is paroxysmal rather than continuous, causing periodic episodes of hypertension, tachycardia, sweating, anxiety, and other signs of excessive sympathetic activity. Several tests are available to differentiate this type of hypertension from other types.

Currently the most commonly used diagnostic measure is the determination of urinary catecholamines and their metabolites, including vanillylmandelic acid (VMA).

Elevated levels of adrenocortical hormones. Increased levels of *adrenal cortical hormones* can also give rise to hypertension. Both primary hyperaldosteronism (excess production of aldosterone by the adrenal cortex) and excess levels of glucocorticoids (Cushing's disease or syndrome) tend to raise the blood pressure (see Chapter 44). These hormones facilitate salt and water retention by the kidney; the hypertension that accompanies excessive levels of either hormone is probably related to this factor. It has been observed that in primary hyperaldosteronism a salt-restricted diet often brings the blood pressure down. Because aldosterone acts on the distal renal tubule to promote sodium exchange for the potassium lost in the urine, persons with hyperaldosteronism usually have decreased potassium levels. The drug spironolactone is an aldosterone antagonist and is therefore used in the medical management of patients with an excess of this hormone. The drug increases sodium excretion and potassium retention.

Brain lesions

The hypertension associated with brain lesions is usually of short duration and should be considered a protective homeostatic mechanism. It is mentioned here because it tells us quite a bit about intracranial pressure and cerebral blood flow. The brain and other cerebral structures are located within the rigid confines of the skull with no room for expansion, and any increase in intracranial pressure tends to compress the blood vessels that supply the brain. Because adequate blood flow is essential to life, it is not surprising that brain lesions that increase intracranial pressure and impede cerebral blood flow trigger a vasoconstrictor response (Cushing's phenomenon) designed to elevate blood pressure as a way to restore blood flow to the brain. This flow is reestablished when the arterial pressure increases to a level higher than the increase in the intracranial pressure that caused the compression of the vessels. Should the intracranial pressure rise to the point that the blood supply to the vasomotor center becomes inadequate, vasoconstrictor tone is lost, and the blood pressure begins to fall.

Malignant hypertension

A small number of persons with secondary hypertension develop an accelerated and potentially fatal form of the disease—malignant hypertension. This is usually a disease of younger persons, particularly young black men, women with toxemia of pregnancy, and persons with renal and collagen diseases.

Malignant hypertension is characterized by marked elevations in blood pressure with diastolic values above 120 mmHg, renal disorders, vascular changes, and retinopathy. There may be intense arterial spasm of the cerebral arteries with hypertensive encephalopathy. Cerebral vasoconstriction is probably an exaggerated homeostatic response designed to protect the brain from excesses of blood pressure and flow. The regulatory mechanisms are often insufficient to protect the capillaries, and cerebral edema frequently develops. As it advances, papilledema (swelling of the optic nerve at its point of entrance into the eye) ensues, giving evidence of the effects of pressure on the optic nerve and retinal vessels. There may be headache, restlessness, confusion, stupor, motor and sensory deficits, and visual disturbances. In severe cases, convulsions and coma follow.

Prolonged and severe exposure to exaggerated levels of blood pressure in malignant hypertension injures the walls of the arterioles, and intravascular coagulation and fragmentation of red blood cells may occur. The renal blood vessels are particularly vulnerable to hypertensive damage. In fact, renal damage due to vascular changes is probably the most important prognostic determinant in malignant hypertension. Elevated levels of blood urea nitrogen and serum creatinine, metabolic acidosis, hypocalcemia, and proteinuria provide evidence of renal impairment.

The complications associated with a hypertensive crisis demand immediate and rigorous medical treatment. With proper therapy, the death rate from this cause can be markedly reduced, as can further episodes. Two drugs to treat hypertensive emergencies are mentioned here, although others also may be required to bring the blood pressure down to a safe level. These two drugs—diazoxide, which causes arteriolar dilatation, and sodium nitroprusside, a vasodilator that also affects the venous system—are administered intravenously.

Treatment of hypertension

In secondary hypertension, efforts are made to correct or control the disease condition that is causing the hypertension. Antihypertensive medications and other measures supplement the treatment for the underlying disease.

Figure 19-6 Individualized step-care therapy for hypertension. For some patients, nonpharmacologic therapy should be tried first. If blood pressure goal is not achieved, add pharmacologic therapy. Other patients may require pharmacologic therapy initially. In these instances, nonpharmacologic therapy may be helpful adjunct. *ACE* indicates angiotensin-converting enzyme. (*After The 1988 Report of the Joint National Committee on Detection, Evaluation, and Treatment of High Blood Pressure. US Department of Health and Human Services, NIH Publication No. 88-1088, 1988)*

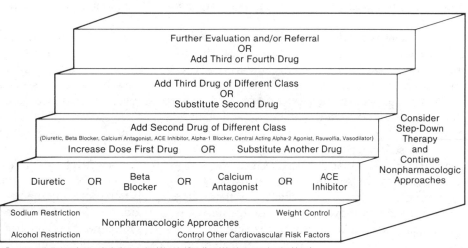

Nonpharmacologic treatment

The recommendation for the first step or stage of hypertension treatment is the use of nonpharmacologic methods either singly or as an adjunct to pharmacologic treatment. In recognizing that nonpharmacologic methods, particularly weight reduction, salt restriction, and moderation of alcohol consumption, may lower blood pressure and improve the efficacy of pharmacologic agents, the 1988 JNC recommended the use of nonpharmacologic methods as the first step in treatment of high blood pressure. Increased potassium intake, biofeedback and relaxation procedures, as well as controlling cardiovascular risk factors such as smoking, dietary fats, and sedentary life-style, were considered nonpharmacologic methods.

Recognizing obesity as a major risk factor in essential hypertension, the committee recommended that all obese hypertensive adults be encouraged to participate in weight reduction programs with the goal of achieving a body weight within 15% of their desirable weight.

Because of its association with high blood pressure, The JNC recommended restriction of eth-

The main objective for treatment of essential hypertension is to achieve and maintain arterial blood pressure below 140/90 mmHg, with the goal of preventing morbidity and mortality.[3] The Joint National Committee (JNC) on Detection, Evaluation, and Treatment of High Blood Pressure has recommended the stepwise approach to treatment of hypertension (Figure 19-6). The stepped-care recommendations of the 1988 JNC include both nonpharmacologic and pharmacologic methods.

anol consumption to no more than 1 oz per day (equal to 2 oz of 100-proof whiskey, approximately 8 oz of wine, or 24 oz of beer).

A high-salt diet may play a critical role in maintaining blood pressure elevation, and it may limit the effectiveness of some antihypertensive drugs. It was recommended that persons with hypertension limit their salt intake to 70 to 100 mEq per day (*i.e.*, 1.5 to 2.5 grams sodium or 4 to 6 grams of salt). Because many prepared foods are high in sodium, merely refraining from use of the saltshaker is usually not sufficient. Instead, it was recommended that people consult package labels for the sodium content of canned foods, frozen foods, soft drinks, and other foods and beverages to reduce sodium intake adequately. Studies have suggested that in addition to excess salt intake, a reduction in potassium intake may contribute to elevated blood pressure levels. Therefore, an increased potassium intake is recommended for persons with normal renal function. Although inadequate intake of calcium and magnesium has been reported to influence blood pressure, there is insufficient evidence in terms of the benefits and risks associated with increased intake of these two cations to suggest their supplementation.

Although nicotine has not been associated with long-term elevations in blood pressure as in essential hypertension, it has been shown to increase the risk of heart disease. The fact that both smoking and hypertension are major cardiovascular risk factors should be reason enough to encourage the hypertensive smoker to quit. In addition, studies have also reported an interaction between smoking and the antihypertensive drug propranolol, in which smokers required larger doses of the drug to achieve similar reductions in blood pressure as compared to non-smokers.

There is conflicting evidence as to the direct effects of dietary fats on blood pressure. As with smoking, however, the interactive effects of saturated fats and high blood pressure as cardiovascular risk factors would seem to warrant dietary modification to reduce the intake of foods high in cholesterol and saturated fats.

A sedentary life-style has been cited as a risk factor in cardiovascular disease. Accordingly, a regular program of physical exercise (walking, biking, swimming) is protective, especially for those at increased risk for cardiovascular disease because of hypertension. Exercise may have further indirect benefits, such as weight loss or motivation for changing other risk factors. Persons with hypertension should be evaluated before beginning an exercise program of appropriate types of exercise. Weight lifting and other forms of isometric exercise can raise blood pressure acutely and should be done with caution.

Although biofeedback and relaxation methods have shown benefits for selective groups of persons with hypertension, these methods have not been subjected to rigorous clinical investigation. Therefore, they may be suggested as adjunctive therapy rather than the sole treatment for hypertension.

Pharmacologic treatment

The use of drugs in the treatment of hypertension is indicated when nonpharmacologic methods are not adequate. Among the drugs used in the stepped-care approach to treatment of hypertension are: diuretics, adrenergic inhibitors, vasodilators, angiotensin-converting enzyme inhibitors, and calcium-channel blocking drugs.

When a pharmacologic agent is needed, step 2 drugs (a diuretic, beta-blocker, calcium antagonist, or ACE inhibitor) are prescribed. Direct-acting vasodilating drugs produce reflex sympathetic stimulation and fluid retention and are not well suited as initial step 2 drugs. If after a 1- to 3-month interval, the response to the initial drug is not adequate, one of three approaches is used: (1) the dose can be increased if the initial dose was below the maximum recommended, (2) an agent from another class can be added, or (3) the initial drug can be discontinued and another drug substituted. The purpose of the stepped-care approach is to achieve blood pressure control with the least amount of medication and the fewest side effects at the lowest cost. Combining antihypertensive drugs with different modes of action will often allow smaller doses of drugs to be used to achieve blood pressure control, thereby minimizing the possibility of dose-dependent side effects from any one drug.

Diuretics, such as the thiazides, loop-diuretics, and the aldosterone antagonist (potassium-sparing) diuretics, produce a reduction in vascular volume and subsequent decrease in cardiac output and peripheral vascular resistance. The thiazide diuretics appear to have a direct blood pressure-lowering effect separate from their diuretic action.

The *adrenergic inhibitors* exert their effects at various levels of the sympathetic nervous system. Some of the main actions of the beta-blockers are on beta receptors in the heart and on renin release by the kidneys. The centrally acting adrenergic agents block sympathetic outflow from the central nervous system. Peripherally acting inhibitors depress the function of postganglionic neurons. Alpha$_1$-adrenergic blockers reduce the effect of the sympathetic nervous system on vascular smooth muscle cells by blocking alpha receptors. Inhibition of sympathetic activity often affects functions other than those related to blood pressure. The two divisions of the autonomic nervous system have opposing and antagonistic actions. When the sympathetic nervous system is inhibited, the restraining effects on the parasympathetic nervous system are removed and manifestations of enhanced parasympathetic function such as increased gastrointestinal motility may occur. Accordingly, many of the side effects of adrenergic-inhibiting drugs are related to the altered autonomic responses—either decreased sympathetic function or increased parasympathetic function —they induce. The side effects of the various drugs are listed in Table 19-4.

Vasodilator drugs promote a decrease in total peripheral resistance by directly producing relaxation of vascular smooth muscle, particularly of the arterioles. These drugs often produce initial stimulation of the sympathetic nervous system and tachycardia and salt and water retention as a result of the decreased filling of the vascular compartment.

The angiotensin-converting enzyme inhibitors act by decreasing angiotensin II levels and reducing its effect on vasoconstriction, aldosterone levels, intrarenal blood flow, and the glomerular filtration rate.

The calcium-channel blockers inhibit the movement of calcium into cardiac and vascular smooth muscle. Each of the different agents in this group acts in a slightly different way. They probably reduce blood pressure by several mechanisms, including a reduction of smooth muscle tone in the venous and arterial systems.[58] Some calcium blockers have a direct myocardial effect that reduces the cardiac output through a decrease in cardiac contractility and a fall in heart rate. Other drugs influence venous tone and reduce the cardiac output through a decrease in venous return. Still others influence arterial vascular smooth muscle by either inhibiting calcium transport across the cell membrane channels or inhibiting the vascular response to norepinephrine or angiotensin.

Drugs are added in stepwise approach until the blood pressure is reduced to goal level, and then maintenance doses of drugs are established. Drugs are selected using the guideline of the stepped-care approach. Among the factors considered when hypertensive drugs are prescribed are the person's (1) lifestyle (persons with a busy schedule may have problems with medications that must be taken three times a day), (2) demographics (some drugs are more effective in elderly or black persons), (3) motivation for adhering to the drug regimen (some drugs can produce undesirable and even life-threatening consequences if discontinued abruptly), (4) other disease conditions and therapies, (5) potential for side effects (*e.g.*, some drugs may impair sexual functioning or mental acuity; others have not been proven safe for women of childbearing age), and (6) cost of the drug in relation to financial resources. There is a wide variation in the price of the different antihypertensive medications that should be considered when medications are prescribed. This is particularly important for low-income persons with moderate to severe hypertension, because keeping costs at an affordable level may be the key to compliance. Recent studies by a nationwide Gallup survey revealed that 25% of persons reported that paying for medication to treat their high blood pressure is "very much" or "somewhat" of a problem.[59]

For persons with mild hypertension who have satisfactorily controlled their blood pressure through treatment for at least 1 year, reduction of medication using a reverse stepwise approach may be used, particularly if there has been successful adherence to nonpharmacologic methods of treatment. Table 19-4 lists the drugs in the stepped-care approach, their mechanism of action, and common side effects. (See an up-to-date pharmacology text for further information on each of these drugs.)

In summary, hypertension is probably one of the most common cardiovascular disorders. It may occur as a primary disorder (essential hypertension) or as a symptom of some other disease (secondary hypertension). Hypertension can affect persons of all age groups including children, pregnant women, and elderly persons. The incidence of hypertension increases with age, is seen more frequently among blacks, and is linked to a family history of high blood pressure, obesity, and increased salt intake. Uncon-

trolled hypertension increases the risk of heart disease, renal complications, retinopathy, and stroke. Because hypertension occurs as a silent disorder, screening programs provide an effective means of early detection. The importance of screening lies in the fact that hypertension can usually be controlled and its complications prevented or minimized with appropriate treatment measures. The Joint National Committee on Detection, Evaluation, and Treatment of High Blood Pressure recommends a stepped-care approach to treatment of hypertension that includes both non-pharmacologic and pharmacologic methods.

Orthostatic hypotension

The term *orthostatic hypotension* refers to a fall in both systolic and diastolic blood pressure on standing. In the absence of normal baroreflex function, blood pools in the lower part of the body when the standing position is assumed, cardiac output falls, and blood flow to the brain is inadequate. Dizziness, fainting, or both may then occur.

When the upright position is assumed, there is usually a momentary shift in blood to the lower part of the body with an accompanying fall in central blood volume and arterial pressure. Normally, this fall in blood pressure is transient, lasting through several cardiac cycles. This is because the baroreceptors located in the thorax and carotid sinus area sense the fall in blood pressure and initiate reflex constriction of the veins and arterioles as well as an increase in heart rate, which brings blood pressure back to normal. Within a few minutes of standing, blood levels of ADH and sympathetic neuromediators increase as a secondary means of ensuring maintenance of normal blood pressure in the standing position. Muscle movement in the lower extremities also aids venous return to the heart by pumping blood out of the legs.

In persons with healthy blood vessels and normal autonomic function, cerebral blood flow is usually not reduced in the upright position unless arterial pressure falls below 70 mmHg. The strategic location of the arterial baroreceptors between the heart and brain is designed to ensure that the arterial pressure is maintained within a range sufficient to prevent a reduction in cerebral blood flow.

Causes

In orthostatic hypotension, the mean arterial and pulse pressure are decreased by at least 30 mmHg to 35 mmHg after 10 minutes of standing.[60] It has been reported to occur with (1) increased age, (2)

Table 19–4. Adverse drug effects

Drugs	Selected side effects*	Precautions and special considerations

Adrenergic inhibitors
  β-adrenergic blockers†
    Acebutolol
    Atenolol
    Metoprolol
    Nadolol
    Penbutolol sulfate
    Pindolol
    Propranolol hydrochloride
    Timolol
	Bronchospasm, peripheral arterial insufficiency, fatigue, insomnia, sexual dysfunction, exacerbation of congestive heart failure, masking of symptoms of hypoglycemia, hypertriglyceridemia, decreased HDL cholesterol (except for pindolol and acebutolol)	Should not be used in patients with asthma, COPD, congestive heart failure, heart block (>first-degree), and sick sinus syndrome; use with caution in insulin-treated diabetic patients and patients with peripheral vascular disease; should not be discontinued abruptly in patients with ischemic heart disease

Centrally acting adrenergic inhibitors Clonidine	Drowsiness, sedation, dry mouth, fatigue, sexual dysfunction	Rebound hypertension may occur with abrupt discontinuance, particularly with prior administration of high doses or with continuation of concomitant β-blocker therapy
Guanabenz	As above	As above
Guanfacine hydrochloride	As above	As above
Methyldopa	As above	May cause liver damage and Coombs'-positive hemolytic anemia; use cautiously in elderly patients because of orthostatic hypotension; interferes with measurements of urinary catecholamine levels.
Peripherally acting adrenergic inhibitors Guanadrel sulfate	Diarrhea, sexual dysfunction, orthostatic hypotension	Use cautiously because of orthostatic hypotension
Guanethidine monosulfate	Same as for guanadrel	Same as for guanadrel
Rauwolfia alkaloids	Lethargy, nasal congestion, depression	Contraindicated in patients with history of mental depression; use with caution in patients with history of peptic ulcer
Reserpine	Same as for rauwolfia alkaloids	Same as for rauwolfia alkaloids
α₁-adrenergic blockers Prazosin hydrochloride	"First-dose" syncope, orthostatic hypotension, weakness, palpitations	Use cautiously in elderly patients because of orthostatic hypotension
Terazosin hydrochloride	As above	As above
Combined α-β-adrenergic blocker Labetalol†	Bronchospasm, peripheral vascular insufficiency, orthostatic hypotension	Should not be used in patients with asthma, COPD, congestive heart failure, heart block (>first-degree), and sick sinus syndrome; use with caution in insulin-treated diabetic patients and patients with peripheral vascular disease
Vasodilators	Headache, tachycardia, fluid retention	May precipitate angina pectoris in patients with coronary artery disease
Hydralazine	Positive antinuclear antibody test	Lupus syndrome may occur (rare at recommended doses)
Minoxidil	Hypertrichosis	May cause or aggravate pleural and pericardial effusions; may precipitate angina pectoris in patients with coronary artery disease

Angiotensin-converting enzyme inhibitors
  Captopril
  Enalapril
  Lisinopril
	Rash, cough, angioneurotic edema, hyperkalemia, dysgeusia	Can cause reversible, acute renal failure in patients with bilateral renal arterial stenosis or unilateral stenosis in a solitary kidney; proteinuria may occur (rare at recommended doses); hyperkalemia can develop, particularly in patients with renal insufficiency; rarely can induce neutropenia; hypotension has been observed with initiation of ACE inhibitors, especially in patients with high plasma renin activity or in those receiving diuretic therapy

Table 19–4. Adverse drug effects (continued)

Drugs	Selected side effects*	Precautions and special considerations
Calcium antagonists	Edema, headache	Use with caution in patients with congestive heart failure; contraindicated in patients with second- or third-degree heart block
Verapamil	Constipation	May cause liver dysfunction
Diltiazem hydrochloride	Constipation	May cause liver dysfunction
Nifedipine	Tachycardia	
Nitrendipine	Tachycardia	
Nicardipine	Tachycardia	

* The listing of side effects is not all-inclusive, and health practitioners are urged to refer to the package insert for a more detailed listing.
† Sudden withdrawal of these drugs may be hazardous in patients with heart disease.
(The 1988 Report of the Joint National Committee on Detection, Evaluation, and Treatment of High Blood Pressure. NIH Pub No 88-1088. Washington, DC, US Department of Health and Human Services, 1988)

decreased blood volume, (3) defective autonomic function, (4) severe varicose veins, and (5) immobility or impaired function of the skeletal muscle pumps.

Aging

Weakness and dizziness on standing are common complaints of the elderly. It has been reported that about 10% of persons over the age of 65 have a fall in systolic pressure of 20 mmHg or more on assumption of the upright position.[61] Because cerebral blood flow is primarily dependent on systolic pressure, patients with impaired cerebral circulation may experience symptoms of weakness, ataxia, dizziness, and syncope when their arterial pressure falls even slightly. This may happen in older persons who are immobilized for brief periods of time or whose blood volume is decreased due to inadequate fluid intake or overzealous use of diuretics.

Fluid deficit

Orthostatic hypotension is often an early sign of fluid deficit. When blood volume is decreased, the vascular compartment is only partially filled; although cardiac output may be adequate when a person is in the recumbent position, it often decreases to the point of causing weakness and fainting when the person assumes the standing position. Common causes of orthostatic hypotension related to hypovolemia are (1) excessive use of diuretics, (2) excessive diaphoresis, (3) loss of gastrointestinal fluids through vomiting and diarrhea, and (4) loss of fluid volume associated with prolonged bedrest.

Autonomic dysfunction

The sympathetic nervous system plays an essential role in adjustment to the upright position. Sympathetic stimulation increases heart rate and cardiac contractility and causes constriction of peripheral veins and arterioles. Orthostatic hypotension caused by altered autonomic function is common in peripheral neuropathies associated with diabetes mellitus, following injury or disease of the spinal cord, or as the result of a cerebral vascular accident in which sympathetic outflow from the brain stem is disrupted. Another cause of autonomically mediated orthostatic hypotension is the use of drugs that interfere with sympathetic activity (Table 19-5).

Bedrest

With prolonged bedrest there is a reduction in plasma volume, a decrease in venous tone, failure of peripheral vasoconstriction, and weakness of the skeletal muscles that support the veins and assist in returning blood to the heart. Orthostatic intolerance is a recognized problem of space flight—a potential risk upon reentry into the earth's gravitational field. Physical deconditioning follows even short periods of bedrest. After 3 to 4 days, the blood volume is decreased. Loss of vascular and skeletal muscle tone is less predictable but probably becomes maximal after about 2 weeks of bedrest.

Idiopathic orthostatic hypotension

Idiopathic orthostatic hypotension is unrelated to drug therapy or pathologic conditions. It may be of two types: (1) idiopathic orthostatic hypotension not accompanied by other signs of neurologic deficits and (2) idiopathic hypotension accompanied by multiple neurologic deficits (Shy-Drager syndrome). The Shy-Drager syndrome is characterized by upper motor neuron damage with uncoordinated movements, urinary incontinence, constipation, and other signs of neurologic pathology.

Table 19–5. Drugs known to cause orthostatic hypotension*

Drug groups	Specific drugs	Mechanism of action
Antihypertensive drugs	Pentolinium (Ansolysen)	Blocks transmission of sympathetic impulses at the autonomic ganglia
	Trimetaphan (Arfonad)	
	Guanethidine (Ismelin)	Blocks sympathetic impulses at the postganglionic sites
	Methyldopa (Aldomet)	Decreases sympathetic outflow from the central nervous system
	Clonidin (Catapres)	
	Hydralazine (Apresoline)	Direct vasodilator action
	Prazosin (Minipres)	
	Minoxidil (Loniten)	
Antiparkinsonian drugs	Levodopa preparation	Vasodilatation due to beta-adrenergic stimulation or alpha blockade of the peripheral vascular system
	Amantadine (Symmetrel)	
Antipsychotic drugs	Chlorpromazine (Thorazine)	Loss of reflex vasoconstriction due to blocking of alpha receptors; these drugs also impair sympathetic outflow from the brain
	Thiethylperazine (Torecan)	
	Thioridazine (Mellaril)	
Calcium-channel blockers	Diltiazem (Cardizem)	Direct vasodilator action
	Nifedipine (Procardia)	
	Verapamil (Calan, Isoptin)	
Tricyclic and related antidepressant drugs	Amitriptyline (Elavil, Endep, Amitid, Amtril, others)	Blocks norepinephrine uptake in central adrenergic neurons, with a resultant increase in stimulation of central alpha-adrenergic receptors, causing a decrease in peripheral sympathetic nervous system activity
	Amoxapine (Asendin)	
	Desipramine (Norepramine, Pertofrane)	
	Doxepin (Adapin, Sinequan)	
	Imipramine (Tofranil, Imavate, others)	
	Nortriptyline (Aventyl, Pamelor)	
	Maprotiline (Ludiomil)	
	Traxodone (Desyrel)	
Vasodilator drugs	Nitrates (nitroglycerin and long-acting nitrates)	Direct vasodilator action

* This list is not intended to be inclusive; it encompasses some of the widely prescribed drugs.

—— Diagnosis and treatment

Orthostatic hypotension can be assessed with the blood pressure cuff. A reading should be made when the patient is supine, immediately upon assumption of the seated or upright position, and at 2-minute to 3-minute intervals for a period of 10 minutes to 15 minutes. It is strongly recommended that a second person be available when blood pressure is measured in the standing position, to prevent injury should the patient become faint. A tilt table can also be used for this purpose. With a tilt table, the recumbent patient can be moved to a head-up position without voluntary movement when the table is tilted.

Treatment of orthostatic hypotension is usually directed toward alleviating the cause or, if this is not possible, toward helping the patient cope. Correcting the fluid deficit and trying a different antihypertensive medication are examples of measures designed to correct the cause. Measures designed to help the patients cope are (1) gradual ambulation, that is, sitting on the edge of the bed for several minutes before standing to allow the circulatory system to adjust, (2) avoidance of situations that encourage excessive vasodilatation (such as drinking alcohol or exercising vigorously in a warm environment), and (3) avoidance of excess diuresis (use of diuretics), diaphoresis, or loss of body fluids. Tight-fitting elastic support hose or an abdominal support garment may help prevent pooling of blood in the lower extremities and abdomen.

In summary, orthostatic hypotension refers to an abnormal fall in both systolic and diastolic blood pressures that occurs on assumption of the upright position. Among the factors that contribute to its occurrence are (1) advanced age, (2) decreased blood volume, (3) defective function of the autonomic nervous system, (4) severe varicose veins, and (5) the effects of immobility.

References

1. Robinson SC, Brucer M: Range of normal blood pressure: A statistical study of 11,383 persons. Arch Intern Med 64(3):409, 1939
2. US Department of Health and Human Services: Blood pressure levels in persons 18–74 years of age in

1976–80, and trends in blood pressure from 1960–80 in the United States. Vital Health Stat [11], No 234, Publication No (PHS) 86–1684, 1986

3. The 1988 Report of the Joint National Committee on Detection, Evaluation, and Treatment of High Blood Pressure. Arch Intern Med 148(5):1023, 1988. Also as NIH Publication No 88–1088, May 1988

4. Trout KW, Bertrand CA, Williams MH: Measurement of blood pressure in obese persons. JAMA 162(10):970, 1956

5. Committee Members, Second International Symposium on Hypertension in Children: Recommendations for management of hypertension in children. Hypertension: Clin and Exper Theory and Practice, A8(4&5):901, 1986

6. Guyton A: Textbook of Medical Physiology, 7th ed, pp 251, 257, 259. Philadelphia, WB Saunders, 1986

7. Hall JH, Mizette L, Woods LL: The renin–angiotensin system and long-term regulation of arterial hypertension. J Hypertension 4:387, 1986

8. Weinberger MH: Angiotensin-converting enzyme inhibitors. Med Clin North Am 71(5):979, 1987

9. Cowley AW, Liard JF: Vasopressin and arterial pressure regulation. Hypertension 11(Suppl I):I-25, 1988

10. New natriuretic hormone, Key to essential hypertension? Hosp Pract 19(9):39, 1983

11. Blaustein MP, Hamlyn JM: Role of natriuretic factor in essential hypertension: An hypothesis. Ann Intern Med 98(Part 2):785, 1983

12. Rowlands M, Roberts J: Blood pressure levels in persons 6–74 years: United States 1967–1980, Advancedata. National Center for Health Statistics No 84. Washington, DC, US Dept of Health and Human Services, Public Health Service, Oct 8, 1982

13. Heart Facts 1988. Dallas, American Heart Association, 1988

14. Stamler J, Stamler R, Riedinger WF et al: Hypertension screening in 1 million Americans. JAMA 235(21):2299, 1976

15. US Department of Health and Human Services: Blood pressure levels in persons 18–74 years of age in 1976–80, and trends in blood pressure from 1960–80 in the United States. Vital Health Stat [11], No 234:6–7, 1986

16. Saunders E: Hypertension in blacks. Med Clin North Am 71(5):1013, 1987

17. Saunders E: Special techniques in management of blacks. In Hall WD, Saunders E, Shulman NB (eds): Hypertension in Blacks, Pathophysiology and Treatment. Chicago, Year Book Medical Publishers, 1985

18. Saunders E: Stepped care and profiled care in the treatment of hypertension: Considerations for black Americans. Am J Med 81(Suppl 6C):39, 1986

19. Berglund G: The role of salt in hypertension. Acta Med Scand Suppl 672:117, 1983

20. Hunt JC: Sodium intake and hypertension: A cause for concern. Ann Intern Med 98(Part 2):724, 1983

21. Oliver WJ, Cohen EL, Neel JV: Blood pressure, sodium intake, and sodium related hormones in the Yanomamo indians, a "no-salt" culture. Circulation 52(1):146, 1975

22. Berensen GS, Voors AW, Frank GC et al: Studies of blood pressure and dietary sodium intake in children in semi-rural southern United States: The Bogalusa Heart Study. Ann Intern Med 98(part 2):735, 1983

23. Laragh JH, Pecker MS: Dietary sodium and essential hypertension: Some myths, hopes, and truths. Ann Intern Med 98(part 2):735, 1983

24. Stamler R, Stamler J, Riedlinger WR: Weight and blood pressure. JAMA 240:1607, 1978

25. Lapidus L, Bengtsson C, Larsson B et al: Distribution of adipose tissue and risk of cardiovascular disease and death: A 12 year follow-up study in the population of Gothenburg, Sweden. Br Med J 289:1257, 1984

26. Larrson B, Svardsudd K, Welin L et al: Abdominal adipose tissue distribution, obesity, and risk of cardiovascular disease: 13-year follow-up of participants in the study of men born in 1913. Br Med J 288:1401, 1984

27. Dustan HP: Mechanisms of hypertension associated with obesity. Ann Intern Med 98(Part 2):860, 1983

28. Langford HG, Blaufox D, Oberman A et al: Dietary therapy slows the return of hypertension after stopping prolonged medication. JAMA 253(5):657, 1985

29. Gruchow HW, Sobocinski KA, Barboriak JJ: Alcohol, nutrient intake, and hypertension in US adults. JAMA 253(11):1567, 1985

30. Kaplan NM: Clinical Hypertension, 4th ed, pp 294, 156, 112, 113. Baltimore, Williams & Wilkins, 1986

31. Klatsky AL, Freidman GD, Siegelaub AB: Alcohol consumption and blood pressure. N Engl J Med 296(21):1194, 1977

32. Meneely GR, Battarbee HD: High sodium–low potassium environment and hypertension. Am J Cardiol 38:768, 1976

33. Lanford GH: Dietary potassium and hypertension: Epidemiologic data. Ann Intern Med 98(Part 2):770, 1983

34. Fregly MJ: Estimates of sodium and potassium intake. Ann Intern Med 98(Part 2):792, 1983

35. McCarron DA: Calcium and magnesium in human hypertension. Ann Intern Med 98(Part 2):800, 1983

36. Kaplan NM, Meese RS: The calcium deficiency hypothesis of hypertension: A critique. Ann Intern Med 105:947, 1986

37. Iseri LT, French JH: Magnesium: Nature's physiologic calcium blocker. Am Heart J 108(1):188, 1984

38. Bevan AT, Hanour AJ, Stott FH: Direct arterial pressure recording in unrestricted man. Clin Sci Molec Med 36:329, 1969

39. Pickering T, Harshfield GA, Kleinert HD et al: Blood pressure during normal daily activities, sleep, and exercise. JAMA 247(7):992, 1982

40. Woods JW: Oral contraceptives and hypertension. Hypertension 11(Suppl II):II-11, 1988

41. Kaunitz AM, Hughes JM, Grimes DA et al: Causes of maternal mortality in the United States. Obstet Gynecol 65:605, 1985

42. Maikranz P, Lindheimer MD: Hypertension in pregnancy. Med Clin North Am 71(5):1031, 1987

43. Lindheimer MD, Katz AI: Hypertension in pregnancy. N Engl J Med 313(11):675, 1985

44. Gallery EDM, Hynyor SN, Gyory AZ: Plasma volume contraction: A significant factor in both pregnancy associated pre-eclampsia and chronic hypertension in pregnancy. Q J Med 192:593, 1979

45. National Heart, Lung and Blood Institute: Report of the Second Task Force on Blood Pressure Control in Children. Pediatrics 79(1):1, 1987

46. Working Group on Hypertension in the Elderly: State-

ment on hypertension in the elderly. JAMA 256(1):70, 1986

47. Emerau JP, DeCamps A, Manciet A et al: Hypertension in the elderly. Am J Med 84(Suppl 1B):92, 1988
48. Kannel WB, Dawber TR, McGee DL: Perspectives in systolic hypertension: The Framingham Study. Circulation 61:1179, 1980
49. Kannel WB, Gordon T: Evaluation of cardiovascular risk in the elderly: The Framingham Study. Bull NY Acad Med 54:573, 1978
50. Ostfeld AM, Shekelle RB, Kawans H et al: Epidemiology of stroke in an elderly welfare population. Am J Public Health 64:450, 1974
51. Shekelle RB, Ostfeld AM, Klawans HI, Jr: Hypertension and risk of stroke in an elderly population. Stroke 5:71, 1974
52. Kohn RR: Heart and cardiovascular system. In Finch CE, Hayflick L (eds): Handbook of the Biology of Aging, pp 300–301. New York, Van Nostrand Rheinhold, 1977
53. Niarchos AP, Laragh JH: Hypertension in the elderly: Pathophysiology. Mod Concepts Cardiovasc Dis 49(8): 43, 1980
54. Spence JD, Sibbald WJ, Cape RD: Pseudohypertension in the elderly. Clin Sci Molec Med 55:399s, 1978
55. Messerli FH, Ventura HO, Amodeo C: Osler's maneuver and pseudohypertension. N Engl J Med 312(24): 1548, 1985
56. Niarchos AP, Laragh JH: Hypertension in the elderly: Diagnosis and treatment. Mod Concepts Cardiovasc Dis 69:49, 1980
57. Re RN: The renin–angiotensin system. Med Clin North Am 71(5):880, 1987
58. Cohn JN: Calcium, vascular smooth muscle, and calcium entry blockers in hypertension. Ann Intern Med 98(Part 2):806, 1983
59. Pauley MV, Stason WB: Contemporary considerations in the treatment of hypertension. Am J Med 81(Suppl 6C):1, 1986
60. Ziegler MG, Lake CR, Kopin IJ: The sympathetic nervous-system deficit in primary orthostatic hypotension. N Engl J Med 296(6):293, 1977
61. Johnson RH, Smith AC, Spalding JMK, et al: Effect of posture on blood pressure in elderly patients. Lancet 1:731, 1965

Bibliography

Agras S: Relaxation therapy and hypertension. Hosp Pract 17:129, 1983

Beauchamp GK, Bertino M, Engelman K: Modification of salt taste. Ann Intern Med 98:763, 1983

Bravo EL, Gifford RW: Pheochromocytoma: Diagnosis, localization, and management. N Engl J Med 311(20): 1298, 1984

Cottier C, Shapiro K, Julius S: Treatment of mild hypertension with progressive muscle relaxation. Arch Intern Med 144:1954, 1984

Cruickshank JM, Thorp JM, Zacharias FJ: Benefits and potential harm of lowering high blood pressure. Lancet 1:581, 1987

Davidman M, Opsahl J: Mechanisms of elevated blood pres-

sure in human essential hypertension. Med Clin North Am 68(2):301, 1984

Ferris TF: The kidney and hypertension. Arch Intern Med 142:1889, 1982

Frohlich ED: Cardiac hypertrophy in hypertension. N Engl J Med 317:831, 1987

Frohlich ED: The heart in hypertension: Unresolved conceptual challenges. Hypertension 10:(Suppl I):I-19, 1988

Friedman GD, Klatsky AL, Siegelaub AB: Alcohol intake and hypertension. Ann Intern Med 98:846, 1983

Gifford RW: Myths about hypertension in the elderly. Med Clin North Am 71:1003, 1987

Hall WD: Isolated systolic hypertension in the elderly. Mod Conc Cardiovasc Dis 56:29, 1987

Health and Public Policy Committee, American College of Physicians: Biofeedback for hypertension. Ann Intern Med 102:709, 1985

Hunt JC, Frohlich ED, Moser M et al: Devices used for self-measurement of blood pressure: Revised statement of the National High Blood Pressure Education Program. Arch Intern Med 147:820, 1987

James WPT, Ralph A, Sanchez-Castillo CP: The dominance of salt in manufactured food in the sodium of affluent societies. Lancet 1:426, 1987

Kaplan NM: Renal dysfunction in essential hypertension. N Engl J Med 309(17):1052, 1983

Kaplan NM: Nonpharmacologic therapy of hypertension. Med Clin North Am 71:921, 1987

Kaplan NM, Meese RS: The calcium deficiency hypothesis of hypertension: A critique. Ann Intern Med 105:947, 1986

Langford HG, Blaufox D, Oberman A: Diet therapy slows the return of hypertension after stopping prolonged medication. JAMA 253:657, 1985

Leumann EP, Haller V, Spiess B et al: Cuff-associated errors of blood pressure recording in infants and toddlers. Clin Exper Theory Pract A8(4&5):605, 1986

Levine DM, Green LW, Deeds SG et al: Health education for hypertensive patients. JAMA 241:1700, 1986

Linas S: Potassium: Weighing the evidence for supplementation. Hosp Pract 23(12):73, 1988

MacMahon SW, Norton RN: Alcohol and hypertension: Implications for prevention and treatment. Ann Intern Med 105:124, 1986

Messerli FH: Essential hypertension in the elderly: Haemodynamics, intravascular volume, plasma renin activity, and circulating catecholamine levels. Lancet 2(8357):983, 1983

Messerli FH, Schneider RE, Nunez BD: Heterogeneous pathophysiology of hypertension: Implications for therapy. Am Heart J 112:886, 1986

Perloff D, Sokolow M, Cowan R: The prognostic value of ambulatory blood pressures. JAMA 249(20):2792, 1983

Pickering TG: Blood pressure monitoring outside the office for the evaluation of patients with resistant hypertension. Hypertension II(Suppl II):II-96, 1988

Rakel RE: Antihypertensive therapy and quality of life. Am Family Pract 35:221, 1987

Robertson D, Hollister AS, Kincaid D et al: Caffeine and hypertension. Am J Med 77:54, 1984

Roccella EJ, Bowler AE, Horan M: Epidemiologic considerations in defining hypertension. Med Clin North Am 71:785, 1987

Schneider RE, Messerli FH: Obesity hypertension. Med Clin North Am 71:991, 1987

Schulman NB, Martinez B, Brogan D et al: Financial cost as an obstacle to hypertensive therapy. Am J Public Health 76:1105, 1986

Stason WB, Pauly MV (guest eds): Contemporary considerations in treatment of hypertension: Cost efficacy, and preference. (Symposium) Am J Med 81:(entire issue), 1986

Tarazi RC: Pathophysiology of essential hypertension: Role of the autonomic nervous system. Am J Med 72:2, 1983

Tunbridge RDG, Donnai P: Pregnancy-associated hypertension, a comparison of its prediction by 'roll-over test' and plasma noradrenaline measurement in 100 primigravidae. Br J Obstet Gynecol 90:1027, 1983

Weisman DN: Systolic or diastolic blood pressure significance. Pediatrics 82:112, 1988

Worley RJ: Pathophysiology of pregnancy-induced hypertension. Clin Obstet Gynecol 27:821, 1984

Orthostatic hypotension

Cunha UV: Management of orthostatic hypotension in the elderly. Geriatrics 42(9):61, 1987

Hoeldtke RD, Carabello B: Hemodynamic changes during food ingestion in a patient with postprandial hypotension. J Am Geriatr Soc 35:354, 1987

Khurana RK: Orthostatic hypotension. NY State J Med 88:570, 1988

Memmer MK: Acute orthostatic hypotension. Heart Lung 17:134, 1988

Robbins AS, Rubenstein LZ: Postural hypotension in the elderly. J Am Geriatr Soc 32:769, 1984

Rousseau PC: Postural hypotension in the elderly. Hosp Pract 23(Oct 30):74, 1988

Schatz IJ: Orthostatic hypotension II: Clinical diagnosis, testing, treatment. Arch Intern Med 144:1037, 1984

Susman J: Orthostatic hypotension. Am Family Pract 37(6):115, 1988

Ziegler MG: Choosing therapy for postural hypotension. Drug Ther 11(10):49, 1981

CHAPTER 20

Control of Cardiac Function

Objectives

After you have studied this chapter, you should be able to meet the following objectives:

_____ Describe how the ventricular wall thickness and the pressure generated by the right and left ventricles are related.

_____ Describe the sequential development of the embryonic heart.

_____ State the function of the pericardium.

_____ Cite the function of the valvular structures of the heart.

_____ State the function of the intercalated disks in cardiac muscle.

_____ Trace an impulse that is generated in the SA node through the conduction system of the heart.

_____ Relate systolic and diastolic changes in the left ventricular pressure and volume to changes in the ECG and phonocardiogram.

_____ Define the terms _preload_ and _afterload_.

_____ Explain the effects that increased and decreased venous return to the heart have on cardiac output using Starling's law of the heart.

_____ Describe the permeability characteristics of cells in the ventricular conduction system to sodium, potassium, and calcium ions during the five phases of an action potential.

_____ Explain the importance of the plateau and length of the refractory period in cardiac muscle.

_____ State the formula for calculating the cardiac output.

_____ Define _cardiac reserve_.

(continued)

_____ Explain the effect of postural stress and the increased intrathoracic pressure associated with the Valsalva's maneuver on venous return, heart rate, and blood pressure.

_____ Explain the function of the vessel endothelium in controlling blood vessel relaxation and contraction.

_____ Cite the distribution of sympathetic and parasympathetic nervous system innervation and the effects on heart rate and cardiac contractility.

_____ Describe the determinants of oxygen consumption by the myocardium.

The heart is a four-chambered muscular pump about the size of a man's fist that beats an average of 70 times a minute, 24 hours a day, 365 days a year for a lifetime. In one day this pump moves over 1,800 gallons of blood throughout the body, and the work performed by the heart over a lifetime would lift 30 tons to a height of 30,000 ft. In this chapter, the embryonic development of the heart, its overall structure and function, and diagnostic methods for assessing cardiac function are discussed.

Functional anatomy of the heart

The heart is located between the lungs, in the mediastinal space of the intrathoracic cavity, within a loose-fitting sac called the pericardium. It is suspended by the great vessels, with its broader side (base) facing upward and its tip (apex) pointing downward, forward, and to the left. The heart is positioned obliquely, so that the right heart is almost fully in front of the left heart with only a small portion of the lateral left ventricle on the frontal plane of the heart (Figure 20-1). The impact of the heart's contraction is felt against the chest wall at a point between the fifth and sixth ribs, a little below the nipple and about 3 inches to the left of the midline. This is called the point of maximum impulse (PMI).

The heart is divided longitudinally into a right and a left pump, each composed of two muscular chambers: a thin-walled atrium, which serves as a reservoir for blood coming into the heart, and a thick-walled ventricle, which pumps blood out of the heart. The two halves of the heart are separated by the interatrial and interventricular septa.

The right heart delivers blood to the lungs where the blood is oxygenated and carbon dioxide is removed. Because of the close proximity of the lungs to the heart and the low resistance to flow in the pulmonary circulation, the right heart operates as a low-pressure pump (pulmonary artery pressure is about 22/8 mmHg).

In contrast to the right heart, the left heart must pump blood throughout the entire systemic circulation. Because of the distance the blood must travel and the resistance to blood flow, this side must operate as a high-pressure pump (systemic arterial blood pressure is approximately 120/70 mmHg). The increased thickness of the left ventricular wall results from the additional work that this ventricle is required to perform.

Although the right heart and the left heart function under different pressure requirements, both must pump the same amount of blood over a period of time. This concept has a particular meaning in relation to both right-sided and left-sided heart failure (see Chapter 22).

— Embryonic development of the heart

The heart is the first functioning organ in the embryo; its first pulsative movements begin during the third week following conception. This early development of the heart is essential for the rapidly growing embryo, because the embryo soon outgrows its ability to meet its nutritional and elimination needs through diffusion alone.

The developing heart begins to function as a single tubular structure and then rapidly undergoes a series of synchronized folding and positional changes as both it and the embryo continue to grow and develop (Figure 20-2). As it changes externally, the tubular embryonic heart also changes internally, partitioning into two parts, a right and a left heart.

The atrial and ventricular septa divide the tubular heart into separate right and left hearts. The development of a closed ventricular septum is usually completed by the end of the seventh week. The formation of a closed atrial septum is more complex, and closure does not occur until after birth. During the formation of the atrial septum, an opening called the foramen ovale develops to establish a communicating channel between the two upper chambers of the heart. This opening allows blood from the umbilical vein to pass directly into the left heart, bypassing the lungs (Figure 20-3). As the lungs expand following birth, the pulmonary and systemic circulations separate into two systems and the foramen ovale closes.

Separation of the heart occurs as the tissue bundles, called the *endocardial cushions,* begin to form in the mid-portion of the dorsal and ventral walls and

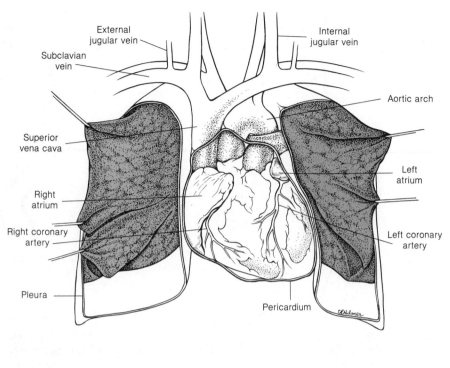

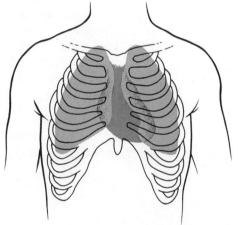

Figure 20-1 (*Top*) Anterior view of the heart and great vessels; (*bottom*) position of the heart in relation to the skeletal structures of the chest cage.

grow inward. As the endocardial cushions enlarge, they meet and fuse to form a right and left atrioventricular channel (Figure 20-4). The mitral and tricuspid valves develop in these channels.

To complete the transformation into a four-chambered heart, provision must be made for separating the blood pumped from the right heart, which is to be diverted into the pulmonary circulation, from the blood pumped from the left heart, which is to be pumped to the systemic circulation. This separation of blood flow is accomplished by developmental changes in the outlet channels of the tubular heart, the bulbus cordis and the truncus arteriosus, which undergo spiral twisting and vertical partitioning (Figure 20-5). In the process of forming a separate pulmonary trunk and aorta, the ductus arteriosus arises to allow the blood entering the pulmonary trunk to be shunted

into the aorta as a way of bypassing the lungs. Like the foramen ovale, the ductus arteriosus usually closes shortly after birth.

Structures of the heart

The wall of the heart is composed of an outer epicardium, which lines the pericardial cavity; a fibrous skeleton; the myocardium or muscle layer; and the smooth endocardium, which lines the chambers of the heart.

Pericardium

The pericardium forms a fibrous covering around the heart, holding it in a fixed position in the thorax. It provides both physical protection and a

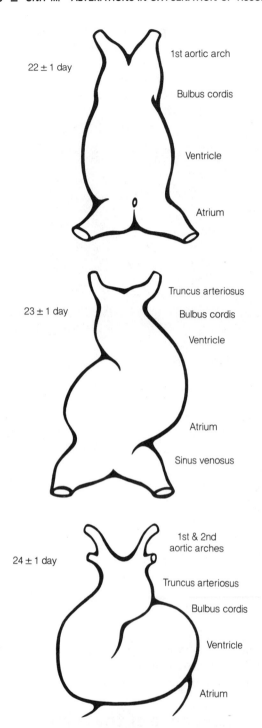

Figure 20-2 Ventral views of the developing heart (20–25 days). *(Adapted from Moore KL: The Developing Human, 4th ed. Philadelphia, WB Saunders, 1988)*

barrier to infection. The pericardium consists of a tough outer fibrous layer and an inner serous layer. The outer layer is attached to the great vessels that enter and leave the heart, the sternum, and the diaphragm. The fibrous pericardium is highly resistive to distention; it prevents acute dilatation of the heart chambers and exerts a restraining effect on the left ventricle. The serous layer consists of a visceral layer

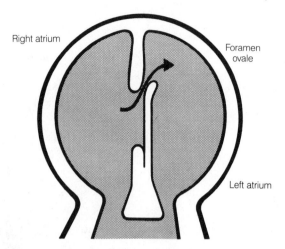

Figure 20-3 The foramen ovale. *(Adapted from Moore KL: The Developing Human, 4th ed. Philadelphia, WB Saunders, 1988)*

and a parietal layer. The visceral layer, also known as the epicardium, covers the entire heart and great vessels and then folds over to form the parietal layer that lines the fibrous pericardium (Figure 20-6). Between the visceral and parietal layers is the pericardial cavity, a potential space containing 30 ml to 50 ml of serous fluid that acts as a lubricant to minimize friction as the heart contracts and relaxes.

Fibrous skeleton

An important structural feature of the heart is its fibrous skeleton, which consists of four interconnecting valve rings and surrounding connective tissue.

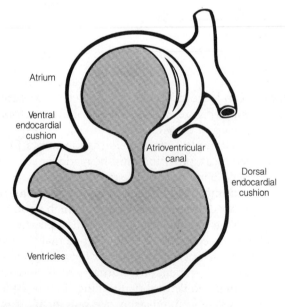

Figure 20-4 Development of the endocardial cushions. *(Adapted from Moore KL: The Developing Human, 4th ed. Philadelphia, WB Saunders, 1988)*

lated disks, which are low-resistance pathways for the passage of ions and electrical currents from one cardiac cell to another. The myocardium, therefore, behaves as a single unit, or syncytium, rather than as a group of isolated units, as does skeletal muscle. When one myocardial cell becomes excited, the impulse travels rapidly to all of the other cells.

Endocardium

The endocardium is a thin, three-layered membrane that lines the heart. The innermost layer consists of smooth endothelial cells supported by a thin layer of connective tissue. The endothelial lining of the endocardium is continuous with the lining of the blood vessels that enter and leave the heart. The middle layer consists of dense connective tissue with elastic fibers. The outer layer, composed of irregularly arranged connective tissue cells, contains blood vessels and branches of the conduction system and is continuous with the myocardium.

Heart valves

In order for the heart to function effectively, blood must move forward through its chambers. This directional control is provided by the heart's two atrioventricular (tricuspid and mitral) and two semilunar (aortic and pulmonic) valves (Figure 20-9).

The atrioventricular (AV) valves control the flow of blood between the atria and the ventricles. The thin edges of the AV valves form cusps, two on the left (bicuspid) side of the heart and three on the right (tricuspid) side. The bicuspid valve is also known as the mitral valve. The atrioventricular valves are supported by the papillary muscles, which project from the wall of the ventricles, and the chordae tendineae, which attach to the valve. Contraction of the papillary

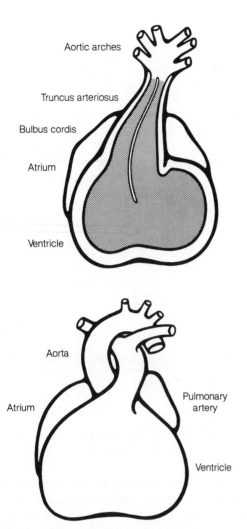

Figure 20-5 Separation and twisting of the truncus arteriosus to form the pulmonary artery and aorta. *(Adapted from Moore KL: The Developing Human, 4th ed. Philadelphia, WB Saunders, 1988)*

It separates the atria and ventricles and forms a rigid support for attachment of the valves and insertion of the cardiac muscle (Figure 20-7). The tops of the valve rings are attached to the muscle masses of the atria, pulmonary trunks, and aorta. The bottoms are attached to the ventricular walls.

Myocardium

The myocardium, the muscular portion of the heart, includes the atrial and ventricular muscle fibers (which contract in a manner similar to skeletal muscle) and the specialized muscle fibers of the conduction system (which contract only slightly). Cardiac muscle cells have properties somewhere between those of skeletal and smooth muscle. They are small striated and branched cells with interconnecting fibers (Figure 20-8). The cell membranes of the interconnecting fibers fuse to form tight junctions, or interca-

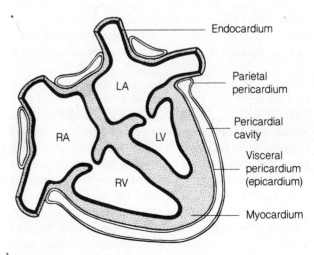

Figure 20-6 The layers of the heart showing the visceral pericardium, the pericardial cavity, and the parietal pericardium.

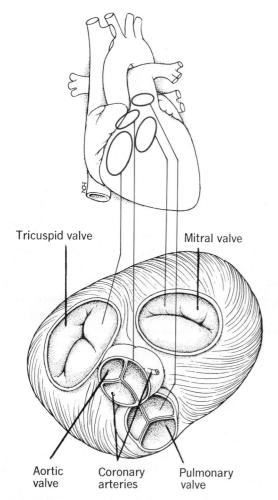

Figure 20-7 Fibrous skeleton of the heart, which forms the four interconnecting valve rings and support for attachment of the valves and insertion of cardiac muscle. *(Chaffee EE, Lytle IM: Basic Physiology and Anatomy, 4th ed. Philadelphia, JB Lippincott, 1980)*

muscles at the onset of systole ensures closure by producing tension on the leaflets of the AV valves before the full force of ventricular contraction pushes against them. The chordae tendineae are cordlike structures that support the AV valves and prevent them from turning inside out and everting into the atria during systole.

The aortic valve controls the flow of blood into the aorta; the pulmonic valve controls blood flow into the pulmonary artery. The aortic and pulmonic valves are often referred to as the semilunar valves because their flaps are shaped like half-moons. Both the pulmonic and aortic valves have three leaflets shaped like little teacups. These cuplike structures collect the retrograde, or backward, flow of blood that occurs toward the end of systole, enhancing closure. For the development of a perfect seal along the free edges of the semilunar valves, each valve cusp must have a triangular shape when it is closed, which is caused by a nodular thickening at the apex of each

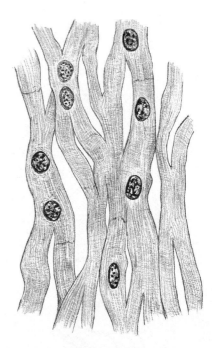

Figure 20-8 Cardiac muscle. Branching fibers, centrally placed nuclei, and intercalated disks can be seen. *(Chaffee EE, Lytle IM: Basic Physiology and Anatomy, 4th ed. Philadelphia, JB Lippincott, 1980)*

leaflet (Figure 20-10). The openings for the coronary arteries are located in the aorta just above the aortic valve.

There are no valves at the atrial sites (venae cavae and pulmonary veins) where blood enters the

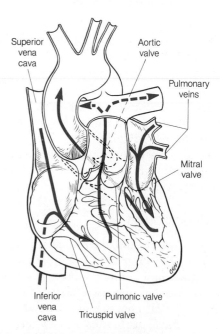

Figure 20-9 The valvular structures of the heart. The atrioventricular valves are in an open position, and the semilunar valves are closed. There are no valves to control the flow of blood at the inflow channels (vena cava and pulmonary veins) to the heart.

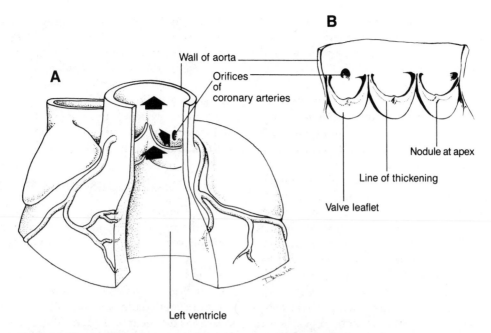

Figure 20-10 Diagrammatic representation of the aortic valve. Its position at the base of the ascending aorta is indicated in **A**, and the appearance of its three leaflets when the aorta is cut open and spread out flat is depicted in **B**.(Cormack DH: Ham's Histology, 9th ed p 432, Philadelphia, JB Lippincott, 1987)

heart. This means that excess blood will be pushed back into the veins when the atria become distended. For example, the jugular veins often become prominent in severe right-sided heart failure when they normally should be flat or collapsed. Likewise, the pulmonary venous system becomes congested when outflow from the left atrium is impeded.

In summary, the heart is a four-chambered muscular pump that lies in the pericardial sac within the mediastinal space of the intrathoracic cavity. The embryonic development of the heart occurs during the third to eighth weeks following conception. During this time, development of the atrial and ventricular septa divides the embryonic tubular heart into a right heart and a left heart. The endocardial cushions develop to form the AV valves, which separate the atria and ventricles. The wall of the heart is composed of an outer epicardium, which lines the pericardial cavity; a fibrous skeleton; the myocardium, or muscle layer; and the smooth endocardium, which lines the chambers of the heart. The right heart pumps blood to the pulmonary circulation and the left heart pumps blood to the systemic circulation. The four heart valves control the direction of blood flow as it moves through the heart. The AV valves control the flow of blood between the atria and ventricles; the pulmonic valve controls the flow of blood from the right ventricle into the pulmonary artery; and the aortic valve controls the flow of blood from the left ventricle into the aorta. There are no valves at the atrial sites (venae cavae and pulmonary veins) where blood enters the heart; blood flows into the heart along a pressure gradient.

Conduction system and electrical activity of the heart

Heart muscle differs from skeletal muscle in its ability to generate and rapidly conduct its own action potentials (electrical impulses). This unique rhythmic property allows the heart to continue beating independently of the nervous system.

In certain areas of the heart, the myocardium has been modified to form the specialized cells of the conduction system. Although most myocardial cells are capable of initiating and conducting impulses, it is the heart's conduction system that maintains its pumping efficiency. Specialized pacemaker cells *generate* impulses at a faster rate than other types of heart tissue, and the conduction tissue *transmits* impulses at a faster rate than other types of heart tissue. It is because of these properties that the conduction system is able to control the rhythm of the heart.

Each cardiac contraction is initiated by an impulse that originates in the sinoatrial (SA) node, which is located in the posterior wall of the right atrium near the entrance to the superior vena cava. The SA node is called the *pacemaker* of the heart because it has the fastest inherent firing rate in the conduction system. Impulses from the SA node travel through the atria to the atrioventricular (AV) node (Figure 20-11). There are at least four intra-atrial pathways, including Bachmann's bundle, that connect the SA and AV nodes.[1]

The heart has essentially two separate conduction systems—one controls atrial activity and the other controls ventricular activity. These two systems are connected by the AV node. Within the AV node, atrial fibers connect with the very small junctional fibers of the node itself. The velocity of conduction through these fibers is very slow (about 1/25th that of normal cardiac muscle), which greatly delays transmission of the impulse into the AV node.[2] A further delay occurs as the impulse travels through the AV node into the transitional fibers and finally into the bundle of His (also called the AV bundle). The delay in transmission of impulses through the AV node is important in that it allows the atria to empty before the ventricle contracts. Because the AV node provides the only connection between the two conduction systems, the atria and the ventricles will beat independently of each other if the transmission of impulses through the AV node is blocked.

The Purkinje system, which supplies the ventricles, has large fibers that allow for rapid conduction and almost simultaneous excitation of the entire right and left ventricles. This rapid rate of conduction throughout the Purkinje system is necessary for the rapid and efficient ejection of blood from the heart. The Purkinje fibers originate in the AV node and then form the bundle of His, which extends through the fibrous tissue between the valves of the heart and into the ventricular system. The bundle of His divides almost immediately into right and left bundle branches as it reaches the interventricular septum. The bundle branches move through the subendocardial tissues toward the papillary muscles and then subdivide into the Purkinje fibers, which branch out and supply the outer walls of the ventricle. The left bundle branch fans out as it enters the septal area and divides further into two segments: the left posterior and left anterior fascicles.

Cardiac muscle contraction

Cardiac muscle, like skeletal muscle, is composed of sarcomeres containing myosin and actin filaments (see discussion of muscle tissue in Chapter 1).

Calcium ions are of particular importance in the regulation of cardiac muscle contraction. During an action potential, calcium is released from the sarcoplasmic reticulum and the transverse (T) tubules; these ions diffuse into the area of the actin and myosin filaments where they provide the signal for the contraction process to begin. Muscular relaxation results from cessation of the calcium influx, its removal from the actin-myosin sites, and its energy-dependent reuptake from the cytoplasm into the sarcoplasmic reticulum and other storage sites. Compared with skeletal muscle cells, cardiac muscle cells are smaller, have less-well-defined sarcoplasmic reticulum, and have a shorter distance from the cell membrane to the myofibrils. Because of this, cardiac muscle relies more heavily than skeletal muscle on extracellular calcium ions for participation in the contractile process. The entry of extracellular calcium into myocardial cells is facilitated by two important mechanisms that have been identified. Calcium enters the cell through the cell membrane, particularly during the plateau of the action potential. Calcium for cardiac muscle contraction also enters by means of the nonenergy-dependent sodium–calcium exchange, in which two internal calcium ions are exchanged for one external sodium ion. Because of the normally low concentration of sodium within the cell, this mechanism is usually not an important source of calcium for cardiac contraction, but it may become important in conditions such as heart failure. Drugs such as digitalis, which block the sodium pump, increase the contractile properties of cardiac muscle by making more calcium available through this exchange system.

Action potentials

The action potential of a cardiac muscle is divided into five phases: phase 0 is depolarization, which is characterized by the rapid upstroke of the action potential; phase 1 is the brief period of repolarization; phase 2 is the plateau, which lasts for 0.1

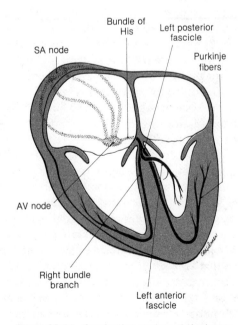

Figure 20-11 Conduction system of the heart.

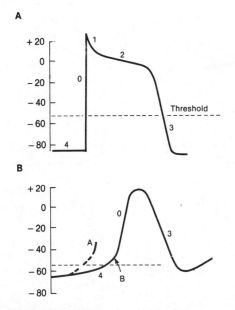

A

B

Figure 20-12 Action of cardiac muscle and pacemaker cells. **(A)** Fast action potential that occurs in myocardial cells of atrial and ventricular muscle. The phases are identified by numbers: phase 4, resting membrane potential; phase 0, depolarization; phase 1, brief period of repolarization; phase 2, plateau; and phase 3, repolarization. **(B)** Slow response, SA and AV nodes. The slow response is characterized by a slow, spontaneous rise in the phase 4 membrane potential to threshold levels; it has a lesser amplitude and shorter duration than the fast response. Increased automaticity (A) occurs when rate of phase 4 depolarization is increased.

second to 0.2 second; phase 3 is the period of repolarization; and phase 4 is the resting membrane potential (Figure 20-12). The plateau, or phase 2, of the action potential contributes to the unique electrical properties of cardiac muscle. It causes the action potential of cardiac muscle to last 20 to 50 times longer than that of skeletal muscle and causes a corresponding increased period of contraction.[1]

The electrical activity of the myocardial cell depends on changes in the permeability of the cell membrane to cations, primarily sodium, potassium, and calcium. There are two types of membrane channels through which ions flow during the depolarization phase of the action potential: the fast and slow channels. During phase 0, the membrane permeability to sodium increases rapidly, resulting in the fast inward movement of current through the fast channels. With phase 1, immediately following this rapid increase in sodium permeability, an abrupt decrease in sodium permeability occurs. If the sodium permeability remained low and potassium permeability increased to its resting level, the cell would rapidly repolarize. This is not the case. Instead, when the membrane has become partially depolarized, a second slow inward current develops and continues throughout the plateau of phase 2. The slow channels, which are much more permeable to calcium than sodium,

are sometimes called the calcium channels. During the phase 3 repolarization period, there is a sharp rise in the membrane permeability to potassium as the slow inward movement of sodium and calcium is inactivated. The rapid outward movement of the potassium ions during this phase facilitates the reestablishment of the resting membrane potential. Phase 4 corresponds to diastole; it is the period during which the membrane is impermeable to sodium.

Action potentials from the contracting cells of the atria and ventricles, the specialized intracardiac conduction system, and the distal portion of the AV node depend on both the fast and slow channels. There are, however, two main types of action potentials in the heart (Figure 20-12). One type, the so-called fast response, occurs in the normal myocardial cells of the atria and ventricles and in the conducting fibers (internodal conduction fibers and Purkinje fibers) of these chambers. The amplitude and the rate rise of phase 1 is important to the conduction velocity of the fast response. The other type, the so-called slow response, is found in the SA node, which is the natural pacemaker of the heart, and conduction fibers of the AV node. The hallmark of these pacemaker cells is a spontaneous phase 4 depolarization. The membrane permeability of these cells allows a slow inward leak of current to occur through the slow channels during phase 4; this leak continues until the threshold for firing is reached, at which point the cell spontaneously depolarizes. The rate of pacemaker cell discharge varies with the resting membrane potential and the slope of phase 4 depolarization. The catecholamines (epinephrine and norepinephrine) increase heart rate by increasing the slope or rate of phase 4. Acetylcholine, which is released during vagal stimulation of the heart, decreases the slope of phase 4.

The fast response of atrial and ventricular muscle can be converted to a slow pacemaker response under certain conditions. For example, such conversions may occur spontaneously in persons with severe coronary artery disease, in areas of the heart in which blood supply has been severely curtailed. Impulses generated by these cells can lead to ectopic beats and serious arrhythmias.

── Refractory period of the heart

The pumping action of the heart requires alternating contraction and relaxation. Following an action potential, there is a refractory period during which the membrane is resistant to a second stimulus. During the absolute refractory period, the membrane is completely insensitive to stimulation. This period is followed by the relative refractory period during which a more intense stimulus is needed to initiate an action potential. In skeletal muscle, the refractory period is very short compared with the duration of the contraction, so that a second contraction can be initiated before the first is over. This results in a summated tetanized contraction. In cardiac muscle, the absolute refractory period is almost as long as the contraction, and a second contraction cannot be stimulated until the first is over. The longer length of the absolute refractory period of cardiac muscle is important in maintaining the alternating contraction and relaxation that is essential to the pumping action of the heart and for the prevention of fatal arrhythmias.

In summary, the rhythmic contraction and relaxation of the heart relies on the specialized cells of the heart's conduction system. Specialized cells in the SA node have the fastest inherent rate of impulse generation and act as the pacemaker of the heart. Impulses from the SA node travel through the atria to the AV node, and then to the AV bundle and the ventricular Purkinje system. The AV node provides the only connection between the atrial and ventricular conduction systems. The atria and ventricles are independent of each other when AV node conduction is blocked.

The action potential of cardiac muscle is divided into five phases: phase 0 represents depolarization and is characterized by the rapid upstroke of the action potential; phase 1 is characterized by a brief period of repolarization; phase 2 consists of a plateau, which prolongs the duration of the action potential; phase 3 represents repolarization; and phase 4 is the resting membrane potential. The calcium ions contribute to the unique electrical properties of the heart and help in cardiac muscle contraction. Calcium ions enter the cardiac cells through special channels called the slow channels, or calcium channels. Drugs that selectively block the calcium channels are used in the treatment of heart disease.

The cardiac cycle

The cardiac cycle can be divided into two parts: systole, the period during which the ventricles are contracting and blood is being ejected from the heart, and diastole, the period during which the ventricles are relaxed and the heart is filling with blood.

During diastole, the ventricles normally increase their volume to about 120 ml (called the end-diastolic volume), and at the end of systole about 50 ml of blood remains in the ventricles (end-systolic volume). The difference between the end-diastolic volume and the end-systolic volume is the stroke volume. The portion of blood ejected during systole (stroke volume) divided by the end-diastolic volume is

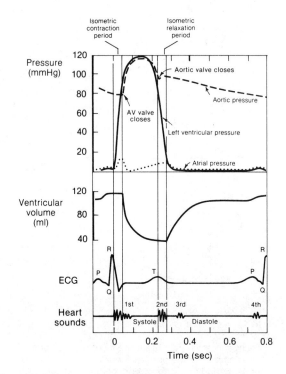

Figure 20-13 Events in the cardiac cycle, showing changes in aortic pressure, left ventricular pressure, atrial pressure, left ventricular volume, the electrocardiogram, and heart sounds.

called the ejection fraction. There are simultaneous changes in left atrial pressure, left ventricular pressure, aortic pressure, ventricular volume, the electrocardiogram (ECG), and phonocardiogram during the cardiac cycle (Figure 20-13).

Ventricular systole and diastole

During ventricular systole, the ventricles are contracting and blood is leaving the heart. The electrical activity, recorded on the ECG, precedes the mechanical events of the cardiac cycle. As the wave of depolarization (the QRS complex on the ECG) passes through the ventricles, it triggers a contraction. As the ventricles begin to contract, the AV valves close giving rise to the first heart sound. Following the closure of the AV valves, there is an additional 0.02 second to 0.03 second during which contraction is occurring in the ventricles, but the volume remains the same because both sets of valves are closed and no blood is leaving the heart. This period of the cardiac cycle, during which the heart muscle is undergoing isometric contraction, is called the isovolumetric period. The ventricular pressures rise abruptly during isometric contraction until left ventricular pressure is slightly above aortic pressure (and right ventricular pressure is above pulmonary artery pressure). At this point, the semilunar valves open and blood is ejected from the heart. About 60% of the stroke volume is ejected during the first quarter of systole, and the remaining 40% is ejected during the next two quarters of systole. Little blood is ejected from the heart during the last quarter of systole although the ventricle remains contracted. At the end of systole, there is a precipitous fall in intraventricular pressures due to the relaxation of the ventricles. As this occurs, blood from the large arteries flows back toward the ventricles causing the aortic and pulmonic valves to snap shut; an event that is marked by the second heart sound. The T wave on the ECG occurs during the last half of systole and represents repolarization of the ventricles.

The movement of blood into the aorta at the onset of systole causes the elastic fibers in the walls of the vessel to stretch and the pressure to rise. During the last quarter of systole, the aortic pressure begins to fall as blood flows out of the aorta into the peripheral vessels. At the end of ejection, the left ventricle begins to relax and its pressure falls below that in the aorta, at which point the aortic valve closes. The incisura, or notch, in the aortic pressure tracing represents closure of the aortic valve. Recoil of the elastic fibers in the aorta that were stretched during systole serve to maintain arterial blood pressure during the diastolic phase of the cardiac cycle.

Following the closure of the semilunar valves, the ventricles continue to relax for another 0.03 second to 0.06 second (the isometric relaxation or isovolumetric period); during this time the volume remains the same but the ventricular pressure drops until it becomes less than atrial pressure. At this time, the AV valves open and the blood that has been accumulating in the atria during systole flows into the ventricles. Most of ventricular filling occurs during the first third of diastole, or the rapid filling period. During the middle third of diastole, inflow into the ventricles is almost at a standstill. The last third of diastole is marked by the atrial contraction, which gives an additional thrust to ventricular filling. When audible, the third heart sound is heard during the rapid filling period of diastole as blood flows into a distended or noncompliant ventricle. The fourth heart sound occurs during the last third of diastole.

—— Atrial systole and diastole

Atrial contraction occurs during the last third of diastole. It is preceded by the P wave on the ECG, which represents depolarization of the atria. There are three main atrial pressure waves that occur during the cardiac cycle. The *a* wave is caused by atrial contraction. The *c* wave occurs as the ventricles begin to contract, and their increased pressure causes the AV valves to bulge into the atria. The *v* wave results from a slow buildup of blood in the atria toward the end of systole when the AV valves are still closed. The atrial pressure waves are transmitted to the internal jugular veins as pulsations. These pulsations can be observed visually and may be used to assess cardiac function. For example, exaggerated *a* waves occur when the right atrium has difficulty emptying into the right ventricle.

Although the main function of the atria is to store blood as it enters the heart, these chambers also act as primer pumps that aid in ventricular filling. This function becomes more important during periods of increased activity when the diastolic filling time is decreased or when heart disease impairs ventricular filling. In these two situations, the cardiac output would fall drastically were it not for the action of the atria. It has been estimated that atrial contraction can contribute as much as 30% to cardiac reserve during periods of stress, while having little or no effect on cardiac output during rest.

In summary, the cardiac cycle is divided into two parts: systole, during which the ventricles contract and blood is ejected from the heart, and diastole, during which the ventricles are relaxed and blood is filling the heart. The stroke volume (about 70 ml) represents the difference between the end-diastolic volume (about 120 ml) and the end-systolic volume (about 50 ml). The electrical activity of the heart, as represented on the electrocardiogram, precedes the mechanical events of the cardiac cycle. The heart sounds signal the closing of the heart valves during the cardiac cycle. Atrial contraction occurs during the last third of diastole. Although the main function of the atria is to store blood as it enters the heart, atrial contractions act to increase cardiac output during periods of increased activity when the filling time is reduced or in disease conditions in which ventricular filling is impaired.

Regulation of cardiac performance

The efficiency of the heart as a pump is often measured in terms of cardiac output. Cardiac output is the product of the stroke volume and the heart rate:

$$\text{cardiac output} = \text{stroke volume} \times \text{heart rate}$$

The cardiac output varies with body size and the metabolic needs of the tissues. It increases with physical activity and decreases during rest and sleep. The normal average cardiac output in an adult ranges from 3.5 liters to 8.0 liters/minute. In the trained athlete, this value can increase to levels as high as 35 liters/minute during exercise. The *cardiac reserve* refers to the maximum percentage of increase in cardiac output that can be achieved above the normal resting level.

The normal young adult has a cardiac reserve of about 300% to 400%.[2]

Factors affecting cardiac output

The heart's ability to increase its output according to body needs is mainly dependent on four factors: (1) the preload, or ventricular filling; (2) the afterload, or resistance to ejection of blood from the heart; (3) cardiac contractility; and (4) the heart rate.

Preload

The volume achieved during diastolic filling of the ventricles is referred to as the preload because it is work imposed on the heart before the contraction begins. The preload varies with venous return to the heart, which, in turn, is determined by the right atrial pressure and mean systemic pressure. It contributes to the force of ventricular contraction by means of the Frank-Starling mechanism.

Right atrial and systemic filling pressures. During diastole, the ventricles fill with venous blood that has been returned to the atria. Venous return to the right atrium is determined by the right atrial and mean systemic filling pressures. The mean systemic filling pressure refers to the degree of filling of the systemic circulation. It is the force that moves blood back to the heart. Venous return is greatest when the right atrial pressure is low and the mean systemic filling pressure is high. Because the heart is in the thoracic cavity, the right atrial pressure reflects the intrathoracic pressure. Therefore, venous return is increased during inspiration when the intrathoracic and right atrial pressures are decreased, and it is decreased during expiration when the intrathoracic and right atrial pressures are increased.

Starling's law of the heart. The anatomical arrangement of the actin and myosin filaments in the myocardial muscle fibers is such that the tension or force of contraction is greatest when the muscle fibers are stretched just before the heart begins to contract. The maximum force of contraction is achieved when venous return produces an increase in ventricular filling (preload) such that the muscle fibers are stretched about two and one-half times their normal resting length. When the muscle fibers are stretched to this degree, the actin and myosin filaments are in an optimal position for maximum contraction. The increased force of contraction that accompanies an increase in ventricular end-diastolic volume is referred to as the *Frank-Starling mechanism* or *Starling's law of the heart.* The Frank-Starling mechanism allows the heart to adjust its pumping ability to accommodate various

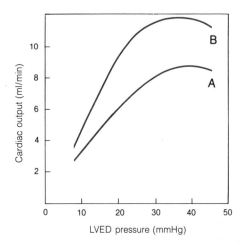

Figure 20-14 The Starling ventricular function curve. An increase in left end-diastolic pressure (volume) produces an increase in cardiac output (*curve A*) by means of the Frank-Starling mechanism. The maximum force of contraction and increased stroke volume are achieved when diastolic filling causes the muscle fibers to be stretched about two and one-half times their resting length. In *curve B,* an increase in cardiac contractility produces an increase in cardiac output without a change in LVED volume and pressure.

levels of venous return. The Frank-Starling mechanism can be graphically represented on the Starling curve (Figure 20-14).

Afterload

The afterload is the force, or resistance, against which the heart must pump to eject blood. It is the work that is presented to the heart after the contraction has commenced. The arterial blood pressure is the main source of afterload strain on the heart. The afterload of the left ventricle is increased with narrowing (stenosis) of the aortic valve, and the afterload of the right ventricle is increased when stenosis of the pulmonic valve is present. In the late stages of aortic stenosis, the left ventricle may need to generate systolic pressures up to 300 mmHg in order to move blood through the diseased valve.[3]

Cardiac contractility

Cardiac contractility refers to the ability of the heart to change its force of contraction without changing its resting (diastolic) length. The contractile state of the myocardial muscle is determined by biochemical and biophysical properties that govern the actin and myosin interactions within the myocardial cells. An *inotropic* influence is one that modifies the contractile state of the myocardium. For instance, hypoxia exerts a negative inotropic effect by decreasing cardiac contractility, whereas sympathetic stimulation produces a positive inotropic effect by increasing it.

Heart rate

The heart rate increases the cardiac output by increasing the frequency with which blood is ejected from the heart. As the heart rate increases, however, the time spent in diastole is reduced, and there is less time for the filling of the ventricles before the onset of systole. At a heart rate of 75 beats/minute, one cardiac cycle lasts 0.8 second, of which about 0.3 second is spent in systole and about 0.5 second in diastole. As the heart rate increases, the time spent in systole remains about the same while that spent in diastole decreases. This leads to a decrease in stroke volume; and at high heart rates, it may actually cause a decrease in cardiac output. In fact, one of the dangers of ventricular tachycardia is a reduction in cardiac output because the heart does not have time to fill adequately.

Autonomic control of cardiac function

The autonomic nervous system modifies the activity of the conduction system and the contractile properties of the heart. The autonomic control of cardiac function is mediated by a number of sensors located throughout the circulatory system. For example, the baroreceptors, located in the aortic arch and carotid sinus, monitor blood pressure and effect changes in heart rate through the autonomic nervous system (see Chapter 19). There are also atrial and ventricular receptors that respond to distention and other stimuli.

Parasympathetic control of cardiac function

The parasympathetic outflow to the heart originates from the vagal nucleus in the medulla. The axons of these neurons pass to the heart in the cardiac branches of the vagus nerve. The parasympathetic nervous system has two effects on heart action: it slows the rate of impulse generation in the SA node, and it slows transmission of impulses through the AV node. As a consequence, there is a slowing of heart rate. Normally, the parasympathetic nervous system is tonically active and has a restraining effect on heart rate. Strong vagal stimulation can actually stop impulse formation in the SA node or block transmission in the AV node. When this happens, there is a delay of about 10 to 15 seconds after which a ventricular pacemaker takes over, causing the ventricles to begin beating at a rate of 15 to 40 beats/minute. The neuromediator for the parasympathetic control of the heart is acetylcholine (cholinergic). The drug atropine, which has an anticholinergic action, blocks vagal stimulation to the heart and causes heart rate to increase.

Sympathetic control of cardiac function

Sympathetic outflow to the heart and blood vessels arises from neurons located in the reticular formation of the brain stem. The axons of these neurons descend in the intermediolateral columns of the spinal cord; they exit from the upper thoracic segments of the spinal cord and synapse in the paravertebral ganglia with the postganglionic neurons that innervate the heart (see Chapter 48). Cardiac sympathetic fibers are widely distributed to the SA and AV nodes as well as the myocardium. Increased sympathetic activity produces an increase in both the heart rate and the velocity and force of cardiac contraction. The sympathetic control of cardiac function is mediated by the catecholamines. The actions of the sympathetic nervous system are mediated via beta$_1$-adrenergic receptors. These receptors respond to norepinephrine released from the sympathetic neurons that innervate the heart and to catecholamines (epinephrine and norepinephrine) from the adrenal gland that circulate in the bloodstream. Beta-adrenergic blocking drugs are used to inhibit the effects of sympathetic stimulation on the heart.

Autonomic response to circulatory stresses

The response of the cardiovascular system to the stresses of everyday living is mediated largely through the autonomic nervous system. These stresses include postural stress, Valsalva's maneuver, and face immersion.

Postural stress. During movement from the supine to the standing position, about 20% of the blood in the heart and lungs is displaced into the legs.[3] The venous filling of the heart is decreased, the stroke volume falls, and blood pressure decreases. As the blood pressure drops, the baroreceptors are stimulated and produce a reflex-mediated increase in heart rate and peripheral vascular resistance. These responses prevent the blood pressure from falling excessively when the standing position is assumed. With prolonged standing, an increase in plasma volume and the action of the skeletal muscle pumps aid in the return of blood to the heart. Decreased tolerance of the upright position causes orthostatic hypotension, which is discussed in Chapter 19.

Valsalva's maneuver. Valsalva's maneuver, which involves forced expiration against a closed glottis, incites a sequence of rapid changes in preload and afterload stresses along with autonomically mediated changes in the heart rate and total peripheral resistance.[4] Valsalva's maneuver is a normal accompaniment of many everyday activities. It is used in coughing, lifting, pushing, vomiting, and straining at stool. The pushing that occurs during the final stages of childbirth makes extensive use of the maneuver. The rise in intrathoracic pressure (often to levels of 40 mmHg or greater) during the strain of Valsalva's maneuver causes a decrease in venous return to the heart, with a resultant decrease in stroke volume output from the heart, a decrease in systolic and pulse pressures, and a baroreflex-mediated increase in the heart rate and the total peripheral resistance. Following the release of the strain, venous return is suddenly reestablished; both stroke volume and arterial blood pressure undergo marked, but transient, elevations. The sudden rise in arterial pressure that occurs at a time when reflex vasoconstriction is still present gives rise to a vagal slowing of the heart rate that normally lasts for several beats. Valsalva's maneuver may be used as a method of testing circulatory reflexes, because the increase in heart rate and total peripheral resistance that occurs during Valsalva's strain, as well as the bradycardia that follows its release, are mediated through the baroreceptors and the autonomic nervous system.

Face immersion (diving reflex).

The diving reflex is a potent protective mechanism against asphyxia in birds and submerged vertebrates; it allows for gross redistribution of the circulation in order to ensure the oxygenation of the brain and the heart. The diving response has three main features: (1) apnea, (2) an intense vagal slowing of heart rate, and (3) a powerful peripheral vasoconstriction. Except for the coronary and cerebral blood vessels, there is massive vasoconstriction to the extent that the circulation becomes, in effect, a heart–brain circuit.[5] Because of the severe vasoconstriction, arterial pressure remains relatively unchanged. The reflex enables the duck to remain submerged for 15 minutes, the sea lion for 30 minutes, and the whale for 2 hours.[5]

In humans, application of cold water to the face produces a similar reduction in the heart rate and the skin and muscle blood flow. The slowing of the heart rate is greater with ice water than cool water and greater with cool water than cool air. Because of the powerful vagal effects, pathologic arrhythmias such as premature ventricular contractions can occur after only 30 seconds of diving.[5] Immersion of the face in ice water may be used clinically to terminate supraventricular paroxysmal tachycardia. Because the reflex is potent in the newborn, it may protect against asphyxia during the birth process. It has also been credited with increasing the survival of children who have accidentally fallen into cold water and remained submerged for longer periods of time than are normally associated with survival.

In summary, the efficiency of the heart as a pump is often measured in terms of cardiac output (the product of stroke volume and heart rate). The heart's ability to increase its output according to body needs is dependent on: (1) the preload, or filling of the ventricles (end-diastolic volume); (2) the afterload, or resistance to ejection of blood from the heart; (3) cardiac contractility, which is determined by the interaction of the actin and the myosin filaments of cardiac muscle fibers; and (4) the heart rate, which determines the frequency with which blood is ejected from the heart. The maximum force of cardiac contraction occurs when an increase in preload stretches muscle fibers of the heart to approximately two and one-half times their resting length (Frank-Starling mechanism). The autonomic nervous system contributes to the regulation of cardiac output by altering the heart rate, cardiac contractility, the preload, and the afterload. Activation of the parasympathetic nervous system slows the heart rate. The sympathetic nervous system innervates the conduction system of the heart, the arterioles, and the veins; its stimulation produces an increase in heart rate and cardiac contractility, in preload (venous constriction), and in afterload (arterial vasoconstriction). The autonomic nervous system plays a major role in regulatory circulatory responses to everyday activities such as postural stress, Valsalva's maneuver, and exposure to cold.

Coronary circulation

The blood supply for the heart is provided by the coronary arteries, which arise in the aorta just distal to the aortic valve. There are two coronary arteries: the right coronary artery, which mainly supplies the right ventricle and atrium, and the left coronary artery, which divides near its origin to form the left circumflex artery and the anterior descending artery. The left coronary artery mainly supplies the left ventricle and atrium. After passage through the arteries and capillary beds, most of the venous blood from the myocardium returns to the right atrium through the coronary sinus; some blood returns to the right atrium by way of the anterior coronary veins. There are also vascular channels that communicate directly between the vessels of the myocardium and the chambers of the heart; these are the arteriosinusoidal, the arterioluminal, and the thebesian vessels.

Regulation of coronary blood flow

Blood flow in the coronary arteries is regulated by the metabolic and oxygen needs of the heart muscle. The mechanisms for controlling coronary blood flow have not as yet been fully determined. Numerous agents, generally referred to as metabolites, have been suggested as mediators of coronary artery vasodilatation observed during increased cardiac work.[1] Among the substances implicated are carbon dioxide, reduced oxygen tension, lactic acid, hydrogen ions, histamine, potassium ions, increased osmolality, and adenine nucleotides. These substances are released from myocardial cells when there is an increased need for oxygen delivery.

The autonomic nervous system exerts both direct and indirect effects on coronary blood flow. The direct effects result from the actions of the neuromediators of the autonomic nervous system. The indirect effects arise because of increased metabolic activity that occurs with autonomically mediated changes in heart rate and contractility. Both alpha-adrenergic receptors, which cause vessel constriction, and beta-adrenergic receptors, which produce vessel dilatation, are known to exist in the coronary vessels.

Recently, it has been shown that the intact endothelium of blood vessels produces vasodilator and vasoconstrictor substances, called *endothelium-derived relaxing factor (EDRF)* and *endothelium-derived contracting factors (EDCF)*.[6] These substances, which are discussed in Chapter 17, interact with substances in the blood to produce local relaxation or constriction of blood vessels.

Contraction of myocardial muscle fibers affects the flow of blood through the coronary arteries. During systole, the contraction of myocardial muscle compresses the coronary arteries and causes a reduction in blood flow. Because of the high pressure that the left ventricle must generate, the decrease in flow is greatest in the arteries that supply this chamber. It has been estimated that about 70% of blood flow through the coronaries occurs during diastole. This is particularly significant in tachycardia when the increase in heart rate causes an increase in oxygen consumption, while the time spent in diastole is markedly reduced. An increase in heart rate probably has little effect on oxygen delivery in the normal heart because the process of autoregulation causes the coronary arteries to dilate. On the other hand, rigid atherosclerotic vessels probably have a limited capacity for dilatation, in which case an increase in heart rate may impair oxygen delivery to the myocardium.

Metabolic needs of the myocardium

The energy expended for myocardial contraction requires constant utilization of oxygen and other nutrients (fatty acids, glucose, and ketones). Although muscles can store limited supplies of nutrients, they are unable to store oxygen. Oxygen must, instead, be supplied continuously for metabolic processes to continue. The oxygen supply for the heart is derived from the blood that flows through the coronary arteries. Under normal conditions, the heart extracts and uses about 60% to 80% of the oxygen from the blood flowing through the coronary arteries, compared with the 25% to 30% that is extracted by skeletal muscles. Because there is little oxygen reserve in the blood, the coronary arteries must increase their flow to meet the metabolic needs of the myocardium during periods of increased activity. The normal resting blood flow through the coronary arteries averages about 225 ml/min.[1] During strenuous exercise, coronary blood flow must increase four- to fivefold to meet the energy requirements of the heart.

Normally, the heart uses fats as a fuel source; about 70% of the heart's energy supply is derived from fatty acids, which must be metabolized by aerobic mechanisms.[1] Under conditions of oxygen deprivation, the heart must convert to the anaerobic metabolism of glucose, with subsequent production of lactic acid, to meet its energy needs. Lactic acid is thought to be the source of pain stimulation during myocardial ischemia.

Determinants of oxygen consumption

The oxygen needs of the heart are determined by the tension that the heart must generate to pump blood, the stroke volume that is ejected, the contractile state of the heart, and the heart rate.

Oxygen consumption and the need for oxygen delivery by the coronary arteries are determined largely by the tension that the heart muscle must generate during contraction to eject blood into the aorta (left ventricle) and pulmonary artery (right ventricle) and the length of time that this tension must be maintained (tension × time). When the heart is dilated at the onset of systole, it must use additional energy just to overcome the wall tension and decrease its size before it can generate the pressure needed to eject blood. When some cardiac muscle fibers are damaged, others must take up the load. They do this by increasing their length so that the heart dilates and the wall tension is increased (see Chapter 17, Laplace's law). The oxygen consumption is therefore greater for the same workload.

The stroke work is the effort the heart expends to pump blood. Work is generally defined as force multiplied by distance. For example, the work required to carry a heavy box up a flight of stairs is equal to the weight of the box times the height of the stairs. The main (external) work of the heart is determined by the amount of blood (like the weight of the box) that is pumped with each beat and the pressure (like the height of the stairs) that the ventricle must develop to move the blood into the aorta or pulmonary artery.

$$\text{stroke work} =$$
$$\text{stroke volume} \times \text{mean arterial blood pressure}$$

The stroke work of the left ventricle pumping against a mean systemic pressure of 85 mmHg is going to be greater than the stroke work of the right ventricle pumping against a mean pulmonary artery pressure of 15 mmHg. Stroke work is increased in the presence of hypertension and in valvular disorders that reduce the size of the valve opening through which blood must be pumped.

The contractile state of the heart refers to its ability to change its force of contraction without a change in end-diastolic volume, the heart rate, or arterial pressure. Oxygen consumed during the contractile state is used to produce and maintain the interactions between the actin and myosin filaments of the myocardial fibers. The cardiac glycosides (digitalis drugs) increase the myocardial contractility, allowing the heart to increase its stroke volume without an increase in metabolic demands. The catecholamines increase cardiac contractility, but they also increase the metabolic requirements of the myocardium.

The heart rate increases the myocardial oxygen requirements by increasing the frequency with which the heart goes through the processes that require oxygen consumption.

In summary, the blood supply for the heart is provided by the coronary arteries, which arise in the aorta just distal to the aortic valve. Coronary blood flow is regulated by the metabolic and oxygen needs of the heart muscle. Contraction of myocardial muscle fibers compresses the coronary arteries so that blood flow is greatest during diastole. Under normal conditions, the heart extracts 60% to 80% of the oxygen from the blood flowing through the coronary arteries, compared with the 25% to 30% that is extracted by skeletal muscle. Because the blood that flows through the coronary arteries contains little reserve oxygen, the coronary arteries must increase their flow during periods of increased activity. The oxygen needs of the heart are determined by the tension that the heart must generate to pump blood, the stroke volume that is ejected, and the heart rate.

References

1. Berne RM, Levy MN: Physiology, pp 457, 443, 601, 602. St Louis, CV Mosby, 1983
2. Guyton A: Textbook of Medical Physiology, 7th ed, p 322, 312. Philadelphia, WB Saunders, 1986
3. Shepard JT, VanHoutte PM: The Human Cardiovascular System, p 158. New York, Raven Press, 1979
4. Porth CJM, Bamrah VS, Tristani FE et al: The Valsalva: Mechanisms and clinical implications. Heart Lung 13(5):507, 1984
5. Smith JJ, Kampine JP: Circulatory Physiology, 2nd ed, pp 255–56. Baltimore, Williams & Wilkins, 1984
6. Vanhoutte P: The endothelium and control of vascular tissue. NIPS 2(1):18, 1987

Alterations in Cardiac Function

Objectives

After you have studied this chapter, you should be able to meet the following objectives:

_____ List at least five causes of pericarditis.

_____ Compare the manifestations of acute pericarditis with those of chronic pericarditis with effusion.

_____ State the characteristics of constrictive pericarditis.

_____ Relate the cardiac compression that occurs with cardiac tamponade to the clinical manifestations of the disorder including pulsus paradoxus.

_____ Describe the anatomy of the coronary blood vessels and the control of coronary blood flow.

(continued)

_____ Explain the significance of atherosclerosis in the pathogenesis of coronary heart disease.

_____ State the physiologic cause of myocardial ischemia.

_____ Distinguish among classic angina, variant angina, unstable angina, silent myocardial ischemia, and myocardial infarction in terms of pathophysiology and symptomatology.

_____ State the purpose of treadmill stress testing as it relates to the diagnosis of myocardial ischemia.

_____ Compare the treatment goals for angina and silent myocardial ischemia with those for myocardial infarction.

_____ Describe the actions of nitroglycerin, the beta-adrenergic blocking agents, and the calcium-channel blocking drugs as they relate to the treatment of myocardial ischemia.

_____ Compare infarct nuclear imaging, myocardial perfusion imaging, and radionuclide ventriculography.

_____ Briefly explain the procedure used in cardiac catheterization and diagnostic information that can be obtained from the procedure.

_____ Compare the procedures used in percutaneous transluminal coronary angioplasty and coronary bypass surgery.

_____ Explain the mechanism(s), criteria for use, and benefits of thrombolytic therapy in persons with myocardial infarction.

_____ Cite the benefits of an exercise program in persons with coronary heart disease.

_____ Describe the origin of the ECG signal, and explain the rationale for use of the 12-lead ECG.

_____ Diagram the normal origin and conduction sequence of electrical activity in the heart and relate to a lead II ECG tracing.

_____ Relate the activity of the cardiac conduction system to the mechanical functioning of the heart.

_____ Cite the types of cardiac conditions that can be diagnosed using the ECG.

_____ Compare sinus dysrhythmia with atrial dysrhythmia.

_____ Describe the characteristics of first-, second-, and third-degree heart block.

_____ State the potential complications associated with premature ventricular contractions.

_____ List the four classes of antidysrhythmic drugs.

_____ State the major manifestations of acute rheumatic fever.

_____ State the probable sequence of events in rheumatic fever.

_____ State the predisposing factors in bacterial endocarditis and the significance of each.

_____ Distinguish between the role of infectious organisms in the production of rheumatic fever and of bacterial endocarditis.

_____ Relate the pathologic changes that occur with bacterial endocarditis to production of signs and symptoms of the disease.

_____ Relate the presence of valvular disease to cardiac function.

_____ State the differences in blood flow and cardiac function that occur with a stenotic and regurgitant heart valve.

_____ Compare the hemodynamic derangements that occur with aortic stenosis and aortic regurgitation.

_____ Describe the clinical findings in mitral valve defects.

_____ Discuss the epidemiology of mitral valve prolapse.

_____ Compare the methods of and diagnostic information obtained from cardiac auscultation, phonocardiography, and echocardiography as they relate to valvular heart disease.

_____ State the causes and symptoms of myocarditis.

_____ Compare the heart changes that occur with dilated, hypertrophic, and constrictive cardiomyopathies.

_____ Relate the occurrence of Down's syndrome to congenital heart defects.

_____ State the effect of altered pulmonary blood flow on congenital heart disease.

_____ Compare the features of atrial septal defects with those of ventricular septal defects.

_____ Explain why the phrase ''blue baby'' is used to describe a baby with tetralogy of Fallot.

_____ State the effect of congenital pulmonary stenosis on pulmonary blood flow.

_____ Explain the significance of endocardial cushion defects.

_____ Describe the anatomical situation in transposition of the great vessels.

_____ Explain the function of the ductus arteriosus in fetal life.

_____ Describe the effect on blood flow of preductal and postductal coarctation of the aorta.

The latest estimates indicate that more than 42 million persons in the United States have some form of cardiovascular disease. About 50% of all deaths, 991,332 in 1988, result from cardiovascular disease.[1] Heart attack is the nation's number one killer; it is responsible for more than one-third of all deaths and is the predominant cause of early disability in the American labor force. Each year, about 25,000 children are born with congenital heart defects and 100,000 children and 2,050,000 adults are affected with rheumatic fever. In 1988, it was estimated that heart and blood vessel disease cost the nation an average of 83.7 billion dollars. In an attempt to focus on common heart problems that affect persons in all age groups, this chapter has been organized into seven sections: (1) disorders of the pericardium, (2) coronary heart disease, (3) disorders of cardiac rhythm and conduction, (4) diseases of the myocardium, (5) disorders of the endocardium, (6) valvular heart disease, and (7) congenital heart disease.

Disorders of the pericardium

The pericardium isolates the heart from the other thoracic structures, maintains its position in the thorax, and prevents it from overfilling. The two layers of the pericardium are separated by a thin layer of serous fluid, which serves to prevent frictional forces from developing as the inner visceral layer, or epicardium, comes in contact with the outer parietal layer of the fibrous pericardium. The mechanisms that control the movement of fluid between the capillaries and the pericardial space are the same as those that control fluid movement between the capillaries and the interstitial spaces of other body tissues (see Chapter 28). Normally, the pericardial sac contains 30 ml to 50 ml of clear straw-colored fluid.[2] Conditions, such as kidney disease and heart failure, that produce edema in other structures of the body may also produce an accumulation of fluid in the pericardial sac. This is called *pericardial effusion*. In hydropericardium, the excess pericardial fluid is a serous transudate with a low specific gravity. Although a liter or more of transudate may accumulate, volumes of over 500 ml are uncommon.

The pericardium is subject to many of the pathologic processes such as inflammation, neoplastic disease, and congenital disorders that affect other structures of the body (Chart 21-1). Pericardial disease is usually associated with or occurs secondary to another disease, either within the heart or in the surrounding structures.[2] The discussion in this chapter focuses on the pathologic processes associated with acute inflammation of the pericardium (pericarditis), pericardial effusion, cardiac tamponade, and constrictive pericarditis.

Types of pericardial disorders

Acute pericarditis

Acute pericarditis is an inflammation of the pericardium characterized by chest pain, a pericardial friction rub, and serial electrocardiogram abnormalities.[3] It can result from a number of diverse causes. In many cases, the condition is self-limited, resolving in a period of 2 to 6 weeks; in other cases, the same cause

---

Chart 21–1: Classification of disorders of the pericardium

Inflammation

Acute inflammatory pericarditis
1. Infectious
   Viral (echo, coxsackie and others)
   Bacterial (tuberculosis, staphylococcus, streptococcus, and so forth)
   Fungal
2. Immune and collagen disorders
   Rheumatic fever
   Rheumatoid arthritis
   Systemic lupus erythematosus
3. Metabolic disorders
   Uremia and dialysis
   Myxedema
4. Ischemia and tissue injury
   Myocardial infarction
   Cardiac surgery
   Chest trauma
5. Physical and chemical agents
   Radiation therapy
   Untoward reactions to drugs, such as hydralazine, procainamide, and anticoagulants

Chronic inflammatory pericarditis
   Can be associated with most of the agents causing an acute inflammatory response

Neoplastic Disease
1. Primary
2. Secondary (carcinoma of the lung or breast, lymphoma, and so forth)

Congenital Disorders
1. Complete or partial absence of the pericardium
2. Congenital pericardial cysts

---

may persist over time and produce a recurrent subacute or chronic disease. Although not common, cardiac tamponade may develop, causing serious, lifethreatening hemodynamic derangements.

Acute pericarditis can be classified according to etiology (infections, trauma, or rheumatic fever) or the nature of the exudate (fibrinous, purulent, hemorrhagic). Like other inflammatory conditions, acute pericarditis is often associated with increased capillary permeability. The capillaries that supply the serous pericardium become permeable, allowing plasma proteins, including fibrinogen, to leave the capillaries and enter the pericardial space. This results in an exudate that varies in type and amount depending on the causative agent. The most common type of exudate in acute pericarditis is fibrinous or serofibrinous (serous fluid mixed with fibrinous exudate). If the exudate contains red cells it is hemorrhagic, and if it contains pus cells it is purulent. Acute pericarditis is frequently associated with a fibrous exudate, which has been described as having a shaggy bread-and-butter appearance because it resembles the surfaces of a bread-and-butter sandwich that has been pulled apart. Acute fibrinous pericarditis may heal by resolution or progress to organization of the fibrin strands with deposition of scar tissue and formation of adhesions between the layers of the serous pericardium.

The most common causes of acute pericarditis include idiopathic or viral etiology, uremia, bacterial infection, and acute myocardial infarction.[3] The disorder is seen more frequently in men than women and is often preceded by a prodromal phase during which fever, malaise, and other flulike symptoms are present. The condition usually lasts for several weeks, during which precordial pain, friction rub, and electrocardiographic (ECG) changes are present. Although the acute symptoms may subside shortly, easy fatigability often continues for several months.

Other causes of acute pericarditis are rheumatic fever, the postpericardiotomy syndrome, posttraumatic pericarditis, metabolic disorders, physical and chemical agents, and pericarditis associated with connective tissue diseases. With the increased use of open-heart surgery in the treatment of various heart disorders, the postpericardiotomy syndrome has become a commonly recognized form of pericarditis. Although this type of pericarditis is thought to be due to an inflammatory response resulting from the presence of blood in the pericardium, it has been suggested that a viral agent, possibly arising from the multiple transfusions required during this type of surgery, may also play a role. Among the connective tissue diseases that cause acute pericarditis are rheumatic fever and systemic lupus erythematosus. In childhood, the most common cause is rheumatic fever. Among the metabolic disorders that cause pericarditis are myxedema and uremia. Pericarditis with effusion is a common complication in persons being maintained on hemodialysis for the treatment of renal failure.

Manifestations of acute pericarditis. The manifestations of acute pericarditis include a triad of chest pain, friction rub, and ECG changes. The clinical findings and other manifestations may vary according to the etiologic agent. Leukocytosis and elevation in sedimentation rate are common.

Nearly all persons with acute pericarditis have chest pain. The pain is usually abrupt in onset, occurs in the precordial area, and is described as sharp. It may radiate to the neck, back, abdomen, or side. It is usually worse with deep breathing, coughing, swallowing, and positional changes. Often the patient will seek relief by sitting up and leaning forward. Only a small portion of the pericardium, the outer layer of the lower parietal pericardium below the fifth and sixth intercostal spaces, is sensitive to pain. This means that pericardial pain probably results from inflammation of the surrounding structures, particularly the pleura. Pain is more common when considerable effusion of fluid is present in the pericardial sac, probably because of the increased stretching of the lower parietal pericardium. Acute pericarditis may also cause dyspnea.

A pericardial friction rub, which is heard when a stethoscope is placed on the chest, results from rubbing and friction between the inflamed pericardial surfaces. The sound associated with a friction rub has been described as leathery or close to the ear. It is usually heard best when the patient is leaning forward in the seated position and the diaphragm of the stethoscope is placed firmly along the left sternal border over the xiphoid process or near the lower border of the sternum. There are usually three components to the pericardial friction rub: the first occurs during atrial contraction, the second during the rapid filling phase of diastole, and the third during ventricular systole.[4] The two diastolic components of the friction rub may become merged to produce what has been termed a to-and-fro rub. In some patients, only a systolic rub is present. The friction rub associated with acute pericarditis usually lasts from 7 to 10 days.

Four stages of ECG changes occur during acute pericarditis: (1) stage 1 in which there is an acute elevation of the ST segment, (2) stage 2 in which the ST segment becomes isoelectric; (3) stage 3 in which the T wave becomes inverted; and (4) stage 4 in which the ECG returns to normal.[5] The ST segment changes begin within hours to days following the onset of acute pericarditis. Serial ECGs are useful in differentiating between myocardial infarction in which the ST segment does not return to the isoelectric line before the T-wave inversion occurs, and acute pericarditis, in which T-wave inversion occurs after the ST segment has returned to normal. (See a specialty text for a more complete description of these ECG changes.)

—— Pericardial effusion

Pericardial effusion refers to the presence of exudate in the pericardial cavity. The amount of exudate, the rapidity with which it accumulates, and the elasticity of the pericardium will determine the effect the effusion has on cardiac function. Small pericardial effusions may produce no symptoms or abnormal clinical findings. Even a large effusion that develops slowly may cause few, if any, symptoms, providing the pericardium is able to stretch and avoid compressing the heart. On the other hand, a sudden accumulation of 200 ml may raise intracardiac pressure to levels that seriously limit the venous return to the heart. Signs of cardiac compression may also occur with relatively small accumulations of fluid when the pericardium has become thickened by scar tissue or neoplastic infiltrations.

Cardiac tamponade. Cardiac tamponade is defined as cardiac compression due to excess fluid or blood in the pericardial sac. It can occur as the result of trauma, effusion, cardiac rupture, or dissecting aneurysm. The seriousness of the condition results from restriction in ventricular filling with a subsequent critical reduction in stroke volume and depends on the amount of fluid present and the rate at which it accumulates. A rapid accumulation of fluid results in an increase in central venous pressure, a decrease in venous return to the heart, distention of the jugular veins, a decrease in cardiac output despite an increase in heart rate, a decrease in systolic blood pressure, and signs of circulatory shock.

Pulsus paradoxus refers to an exaggeration of the normal inspiratory decrease in systolic blood pressure and is a clinical indicator of cardiac tamponade. Pulsus paradoxus is easiest to detect when the blood pressure cuff is inflated to a value above the systolic pressure and then deflated slowly at a rate of 2 mmHg/sec until the first Korotkoff sound is detected with expiration. Following the notation of this pressure, the cuff is deflated until the Korotkoff sounds can be heard throughout the respiratory cycle. A difference greater than 10 mmHg between the two readings is indicative of pulsus paradoxus. In cardiac tamponade, this implies a large reduction in ventricular volume. The decreased intrathoracic pressure that occurs during inspiration normally accelerates venous flow, increasing right atrial and ventricular filling; this causes the interventricular septum to bulge to the left, producing internal compression of the left ventricle. In cardiac tamponade, the left ventricle is compressed from within by movement of the interventricular septum and from without by fluid in the pericardium (Figure 21-1). With pulsus paradoxus, left ventricular output can decrease within a beat of the beginning of inspiration.

Chronic pericarditis with effusion. Chronic pericarditis with effusion is characterized by an increase in inflammatory exudate that continues beyond the anticipated period of time. In some cases, the exudate will persist for several years. In most cases of chronic pericarditis, no specific pathogen can be identified. The process is commonly associated with other forms of heart disease, such as rheumatic fever, congenital heart lesions, or hypertensive heart disease. Systemic diseases such as lupus erythematosus, rheumatoid arthritis, scleroderma, and myxedema are also causes of chronic pericarditis, as are metabolic disturbances associated with acute and chronic renal failure. Unlike those of acute pericarditis, the signs and

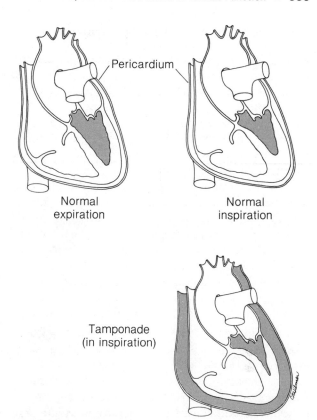

Figure 21-1 Effect of respiration and cardiac tamponade on ventricular filling and cardiac output. During inspiration venous flow into the right heart increases, causing the interventricular septum to bulge into the left ventricle. This produces a decrease in left ventricular volume, with a subsequent decrease in stroke volume output. In cardiac tamponade, the fluid in the pericardial sac produces further compression of the left ventricle, causing an exaggeration of the normal inspiratory decrease in stroke volume and systolic blood pressure.

symptoms of chronic pericarditis are often minimal; many times the disease is detected for the first time on routine chest film. As the condition progresses, the fluid may accumulate and compress the adjacent cardiac structures and impair cardiac filling.

Constrictive pericarditis

In constrictive pericarditis, scar tissue develops between the visceral and parietal layers of the serous pericardium. In time, the scar tissue contracts and interferes with cardiac filling, at which point cardiac output and cardiac reserve become fixed. Ascites is a prominent early finding, often occurring without signs of accompanying peripheral edema. The jugular veins are also distended. Kussmaul's sign is an inspiratory distention of the jugular veins due to the inability of the right atrium, encased in its rigid pericardium, to accommodate the increase in venous return that occurs with inspiration.

—— Diagnosis and treatment

Various diagnostic tests are used to confirm the presence of pericardial disease. These measures include auscultation, chest x-ray, electrocardiogram, echocardiography, radiation-scanning procedures, and computerized tomography. The echocardiogram is the most definitive of these studies. Aspiration and laboratory analysis of the pericardial fluid may be used to identify the causative agent.

Treatment is dependent on the etiology. When infection is present, antibiotics specific for the causative agent are usually prescribed. Anti-inflammatory drugs may be given to minimize the inflammatory response and the accompanying undesirable effects. Pericardiocentesis, the removal of fluid from the pericardial sac, may be a life-saving measure in severe cardiac tamponade. Surgical treatment may be required in traumatic lesions of the heart or in constrictive pericarditis in which cardiac filling is severely impaired.

In summary, disorders of the pericardium include acute pericarditis, pericardial effusion, cardiac tamponade, and constrictive pericarditis. Acute pericarditis is characterized by chest pain, ECG changes, and a friction rub. Among the causes of acute pericarditis are infections, uremia, rheumatic fever, connective tissue diseases, and myocardial infarction. Pericardial effusion refers to the presence of an exudate in the pericardial cavity and can be either acute or chronic. Pericardial effusion can increase intracardiac pressure, compress the heart, and interfere with venous return to the heart. The amount of exudate, the rapidity with which it accumulates, and the elasticity of the pericardium determine the effect that the effusion has on cardiac function. Cardiac tamponade is a life-threatening cardiac compression resulting from excess fluid in the pericardial sac. In constrictive pericarditis, scar tissue develops between the visceral and parietal layers of the serous pericardium. In time, the scar tissue contracts and interferes with cardiac filling.

Coronary heart disease

Heart disorders caused by impaired coronary blood flow are called coronary heart disease; they include ischemic heart disease and myocardial infarction. Disease of the coronary vessels can cause angina, myocardial infarction, cardiac dysrhythmias, conduction defects, heart failure, and sudden death. Almost half of all cardiovascular deaths are due to coronary heart disease. In 1985, coronary heart disease caused 540,800 deaths; 4,870,000 persons have a history of angina, heart attack, or both.[1]

In most cases, coronary heart disease is caused by atherosclerosis. Epidemiologic studies have identified three treatable risk factors: hypertension, elevated blood lipids, and cigarette smoking. A number of additional contributing factors in the development of coronary heart disease, such as family history of heart disease, obesity, physical inactivity, male gender, and certain personality types, have been implicated. Coronary heart disease is often a silent disorder; most men and women over 50 years of age have moderately far advanced coronary atherosclerosis although most of them have no symptoms of heart disease.[6]

Coronary heart disease can affect one or all of the coronary arteries (one-, two-, or three-vessel disease) and can be diffuse or localized to one area of a single vessel. Usually 75% or more of the vessel lumen must be occluded before there is a significant reduction in blood flow.

—— Coronary arteries and distribution of blood flow

There are two main coronary arteries, the left and right, which arise from the coronary sinus just above the aortic valve (Figure 21-2). The left coronary artery extends for approximately 3.5 cm as the *left main coronary artery* and then divides into the anterior descending and circumflex branches. The *left anterior descending artery* passes down through the groove between the two ventricles, giving off diagonal branches, which supply the left ventricle, and perforating branches, which supply the anterior portion of the interventricular septum and the anterior papillary muscle of the left ventricle. The *circumflex* branch of the left coronary artery passes to the left and moves posteriorly in the groove that separates the left atrium and ventricle, giving off branches that supply the left lateral wall of the left ventricle. The *right coronary artery* lies in the right atrioventricular groove, and its branches supply the right ventricle. The right coronary artery usually moves to the back of the heart where it forms the *posterior descending artery,* which supplies the posterior portion of the heart (the interventricular septum, atrioventricular node, and posterior papillary muscle). The sinoatrial node is also usually supplied by the right coronary artery. In about 10% of persons, the left circumflex rather than the right coronary artery moves posteriorly to form the posterior descending artery. The term *dominant* designates the main coronary artery that extends to form the posterior descending artery. Dominant left circulation tells us that the posterior descending artery is a branch of the left circumflex, and dominant right tells us that the posterior descending artery is a branch of the right coronary artery.

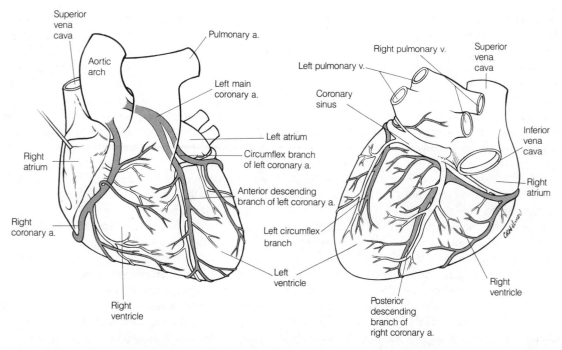

Figure 21-2 Coronary arteries and some of the coronary sinus veins.

Many factors interact in the control of coronary blood flow including vessel diameter, aortic pressure, extravascular compression, presence of collateral channels, and vasodilator responses.

As explained in Chapter 17, the flow of fluids through a tube is directly related to the fourth power of its radius. Translated, this means that if the radius of a vessel is changed by a factor of two, there will be a 16-fold change in flow ($2 \times 2 \times 2 \times 2 = 16$). Consequently, either a reduction in vessel radius due to atherosclerosis or an increase in vessel radius due to medical interventions such as vasodilator drugs or angioplasty can have significant effects on blood flow.

The coronary arteries originate in the aorta just outside the aortic valve. The primary factor responsible for perfusion of the coronary arteries is the aortic pressure, which is generated by the heart itself. Changes in aortic pressure generally produce parallel changes in coronary blood flow.

In addition to providing the aortic pressure that drives blood through the coronary vessels, the heart also influences blood supply by the squeezing effect that the contracting myocardium has on its intramuscular blood vessels. The large epicardial coronary arteries lie on the surface of the heart, with smaller intramyocardial branches coming off and penetrating the myocardium and traveling to a network or plexus of subendocardial vessels. The intramyocardial vessels, which lie between cardiac muscle fibers, are compressed as the heart contracts during systole, and, as a result, subendocardial blood flow becomes proportionally less than blood flow in the epicardial vessels (Figure 21-3). The subendocardial vessels are more extensive, however, than the vessels that supply the outer layers of the heart, and they fill during diastole to compensate for the decreased flow that occurs during systole. Because subendocardial blood flow occurs during diastole, there is risk of myocardial ischemia and infarction when diastolic pressure is low and there is an elevation in diastolic intraventricular pressure sufficient to compress the vessels in the subendocardial plexus.[7] Intramyocardial

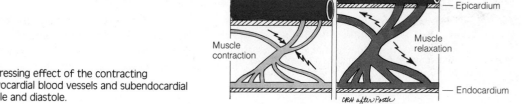

Figure 21-3 The compressing effect of the contracting myocardium on intramyocardial blood vessels and subendocardial blood flow during systole and diastole.

blood flow is also affected by heart rate because at rapid heart rates the time spent in diastole is greatly reduced.

Although there are no connections between the large coronary arteries, there are anastomotic channels that join the small arteries (Figure 21-4). With gradual occlusion of the larger vessels, the smaller collateral vessels increase in size and provide alternative channels for blood flow.[8] One of the reasons coronary artery disease does not produce symptoms until it is far advanced is that the collateral channels develop at the same time that the atherosclerotic changes are occurring.

One of the characteristics of the coronary circulation is the ability of its vessels to dilate in the presence of increased metabolic activity. This mechanism has been observed in the denervated as well as innervated heart, suggesting that the mechanism is controlled by local factors, such as metabolites released during increased metabolism. Although the mechanism remains unsettled, numerous agents such as oxygen (hypoxia), carbon dioxide, lactic acid, potassium, and prostaglandins have been suggested.

Recent research has shown that the endothelial cells lining the arterial walls normally synthesize and release chemical mediators that produce vasodilatation (endothelium-derived relaxing factor [EDRF]) and vasoconstriction (endothelium-derived constricting factor [EDCF]).[9] This suggests that the

intact endothelium may have a protective role in regulating blood flow. Endothelium-derived relaxing factor maintains circulation of the blood by relaxing smooth muscle and promoting antiaggregation of platelets in arteries with intact endothelial cells. Some of the reported stimuli for release of EDRF in coronary blood vessels are acetylcholine, thrombin, norepinephrine, and vessel distention. For example, it has been shown that the endothelial cells of coronary arteries possess alpha$_2$-adrenergic receptors, which, when activated, cause release of EDRF. In laboratory experiments in which the endothelium has been removed, aggregating platelets produce massive vasoconstriction. This vasoconstriction does not occur when an intact endothelium is present, suggesting that aggregating platelets release substances that can trigger potent EDRF responses. One of the main stimuli for EDCF is hypoxia. From these research observations it has been proposed that the intact endothelium contributes to the regulation of blood flow by both (1) releasing factors that produce relaxation or constriction of vascular smooth muscle and (2) preventing aggregation and release of platelet factors that promote thrombus formation.

Myocardial ischemia

The term *ischemia* means to suppress or withhold blood flow. Myocardial ischemia occurs when the ability of the coronary arteries to supply blood is inadequate to meet the metabolic demands of the heart. Myocardial ischemia due to an inadequate blood supply may be caused by atherosclerotic lesions of the coronary vessels, vasospasm of the coronary vessels, or a combination of the two conditions. Metabolic demands of the heart are increased with everyday activities such as mental stress, exercise, and exposure to cold. In certain disease states, such as thyrotoxicosis, the metabolic demands may be so excessive that blood supply is inadequate despite normal coronary arteries. In other situations such as aortic stenosis, the coronary arteries may not be diseased, but the perfusion pressure may be insufficient to provide adequate blood flow. Both symptomatic myocardial ischemia (angina pectoris) and silent (painless) myocardial ischemia are important functional indicators of active coronary heart disease and increased risk of myocardial infarction or sudden death.

Angina pectoris

The term *angina* (Latin) means to choke. Angina pectoris is a symptomatic paroxysmal pain or pressure sensation associated with transient myocardial ischemia. Typically, the pain is described as constricting, squeezing, or suffocating. It is usually steady,

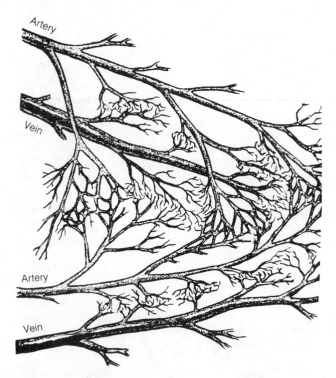

Figure 21-4 Anastomoses of the smaller coronary arterial vessels. *(Guyton AC: Textbook of Medical Physiology, 6th ed. Philadelphia, WB Saunders, 1981)*

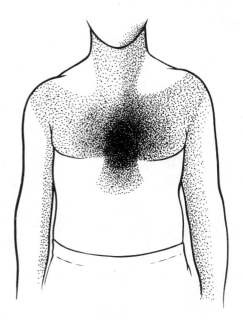

Figure 21-5 Areas of pain due to angina. *(Adapted from Heart Facts 1984. American Heart Association, 1984)*

increasing in intensity only at the onset and end of the attack. The pain of angina is usually located in the precordial or substernal area; it is similar to myocardial infarction in that it may radiate to the left shoulder, jaw, arm, or other areas of the chest (Figure 21-5). In some persons, the arm or shoulder pain may be confused with arthritis; in others, epigastric pain is confused with indigestion. The duration of angina is brief—seldom does it last more than 5 minutes. There are three types of angina: classic angina, variant angina, and unstable angina.

Classic angina. Classic angina, sometimes called exertional angina, is associated with atherosclerotic disease of the coronary arteries and occurs when the metabolic needs of the myocardium exceed the ability of the occluded coronary arteries to deliver adequate blood flow. Despite the fact that the overwhelming majority of persons with angina have atherosclerotic heart disease, angina does not develop in a considerable number of persons with advanced coronary atherosclerosis. This is probably due to their sedentary life-style, the development of adequate collateral circulation, or the inability of these persons to perceive pain. In many instances, myocardial infarction occurs without a prior history of angina. Pain is usually precipitated by situations that increase the work demands of the heart, such as physical exertion, exposure to cold, and emotional stress.

Variant angina. The syndrome of variant angina was first described by Prinzmetal and associates in 1959 and is sometimes referred to as Prinzmetal's angina.[10] Subsequent evidence suggests that

variant angina is caused by spasms of the coronary arteries; thus, the condition is also called vasospastic angina. In most instances, the spasms occur in the presence of coronary artery stenosis; however, variant angina has been shown to occur in the absence of visible disease. Unlike the classic form of angina, which occurs with exertion or stress, variant angina usually occurs during rest or with minimal exercise and is frequently nocturnal. It may be associated with rapid eye movement (REM) sleep. It commonly follows a cyclic or regular pattern of occurrence (*e.g.,* it happens at the same time each day). Dysrhythmias are often present when the pain is severe, and the individual suffering the attack is often aware of their presence. Electrocardiographic changes are significant if recorded during an attack. Typically the ST segment is elevated on the same lead during each attack, suggesting the involvement of a single vessel. The mechanism of coronary vasospasm is uncertain. It has been suggested that it may result from hyperactive sympathetic nervous system responses, from a defect in the handling of calcium in vascular smooth muscle, or from a reduced production of prostaglandin I_2. The calcium-channel blocking drugs have proved extraordinarily effective in treating variant angina.

Unstable angina. Unstable angina is an accelerated form of angina in which the pain is characterized by a changing pattern. It begins to appear more frequently, is more severe, lasts longer, and may appear at rest. Unstable angina is sometimes called preinfarction angina because of its propensity for accelerating to myocardial infarction.

Unstable angina is usually triggered by a subtle or minor injury to a coronary atherosclerotic plaque. Although plaque disruption may occur with or without thrombosis, it increases the degree of coronary artery obstruction. When the original injury is mild, intermittent thrombotic occlusions may occur and cause episodes of anginal pain at rest. Additionally, there is release of vasoconstricting factors (thromboxane, serotonin, and platelet-derived growth factor) from platelets that aggregate at the site of injury. These platelet factors contribute, even at rest, to episodes of reduced coronary blood flow and either silent or symptomatic myocardial ischemia. Thrombus formation can progress until the coronary artery becomes occluded, leading to myocardial infarction. Ischemic episodes may also be precipitated by factors that increase blood flow needs of the myocardium.[11]

Silent ischemia

Silent myocardial ischemia occurs in the absence of anginal pain. The factors that cause silent myocardial ischemia appear to be the same as those responsible for angina—impaired blood flow due to the effects of coronary atherosclerosis and/or vasospasm. Silent myocardial ischemia affects three populations: (1) persons who are asymptomatic without other evidence of coronary heart disease, (2) persons who have had a myocardial infarct and continue to have episodes of silent ischemia, and (3) persons with angina who also have episodes of silent ischemia.

Diagnostic methods

The diagnosis of myocardial ischemia is based on history, electrocardiogram, response to administration of nitroglycerin, and the results of exercise stress testing. Nuclear imaging and/or cardiac catheterization may be used to describe the location and extent of the disease.

Exercise stress testing. Exercise stress testing is a means of observing cardiac function under stress. Three types of tests are used: the step test, the bicycle ergometer, and the treadmill. The treadmill is used most frequently in the United States. Many people are not accustomed to riding bicycles, and the usefulness of the step test is limited because it requires considerable motivation on the part of the patient and it also produces greater distortion of the ECG than the other tests. During treadmill testing, the person walks or runs on a moving belt. The level of physical activity, or workload, that the person performs can be gradually increased by changing the speed and the incline of the belt; this is usually done in stages. The ECG is monitored continuously during the test, and the blood pressure is taken at predetermined intervals. It is also possible to monitor oxygen consumption. A person is assumed to have reached the limit for oxygen uptake at the point of exhaustion. Usually the person being tested continues to exercise, completing successive stages of the test, until exhaustion or a predetermined heart rate is reached. The maximal heart rate is estimated by age. Tables of maximal heart rate by age are available, but, as a general rule, the predicted maximal heart rate can be estimated by subtracting age from 220 (e.g., the target heart rate for a 30-year-old would be 190 beats/minute). The person may be asked to continue until the predicted maximum heart rate is achieved or until a percentage (i.e., 85%–90%) of the predicted maximal rate is reached.

The presence of chest pain, severe shortness of breath, dysrhythmias, ST-segment changes on the ECG, or a decrease in blood pressure is suggestive of coronary heart disease, and if one or more of these signs are present, the test is usually terminated.

Metabolic equivalents (METs), which are multiples of the basal metabolic rate, are commonly used to express the workload at various stages of the exercise protocols. A MET is equivalent to the energy expended in resting in a supine position, sitting, standing, eating, or having an ordinary conversation. Walking at 4 miles per hour (mph), cycling at 11 mph, playing tennis (singles), digging a garden, or doing heavy carpentry requires 5 to 6 METs. Running 6 mph requires 10 METs, and running 10 mph requires 17 METs. Physically trained individuals can achieve workloads beyond 16 METs. Healthy sedentary individuals, however, seldom exercise beyond 10 or 11 METs; and in persons with coronary heart disease workloads of 8 METs are usually sufficient to produce angina.

Nuclear imaging. Nuclear cardiology techniques involve the use of radionuclides (radioactive substances) and are essentially noninvasive. Three types of nuclear cardiology tests are commonly used: infarct imaging, myocardial perfusion imaging, and ventriculography. With all three types of tests, a scintillation camera is used to record the radiation emitted from the radionuclide.

Acute infarct imaging uses a radionuclide (e.g., technetium pyrophosphate) that is taken up by the cells in the infarcted zone. With this method, the radionuclide becomes concentrated in the damaged myocardium, allowing its visualization as a hot spot, or positive area, of increased uptake of the radionuclide.

Myocardial perfusion imaging uses radionuclides that are extracted from the blood and taken up by functioning myocardial cells. Thallium-201, an analogue of potassium, is usually used for this purpose. The physical half-life of thallium-201 is 72 hours. Thallium-201 is distributed to the myocardium in proportion to the magnitude of blood flow. Following injection, an external detection device describes the distribution of the radioactive material. An ischemic area appears as a "cold spot" that lacks radioactive uptake. Thallium-201 can be used to assess myocardial blood flow during both rest and exercise.

Radionuclide ventriculography provides actual visualization of ventricular structures during systole and diastole and provides a means for evaluating ventricular function during rest and exercise. A radioisotope such as technetium-labeled albumin, which does not leave the capillaries but remains in the blood and is not bound to the myocardium, is used for this type of imaging. This type of nuclear imaging can be used to determine right and left ventricular volumes, ejection fractions, regional wall motion, and cardiac contractility. This method is also useful in the diagnosis of intracardiac shunts.

Radionuclide ventriculography can be performed using first-pass techniques in which the initial transit of the radioactive material is used in evaluating cardiovascular function. With this technique, the radionuclide bolus can be localized as it passes through the cardiac chambers, making it possible to visualize one side of the heart at a time. A second technique, called multigated acquisition (MUGA), produces computerized composite images of the heart that have been accumulated over hundreds of cardiac cycles. The distribution of these images is regulated by a gating signal from the ECG that controls the scintillation camera so that repeated images are taken during a designated portion of the cardiac cycle. This allows for calculation of left ventricular end-diastolic volumes, left ventricular end-systolic volumes, and left ventricular ejection fractions.

Cardiac catheterization.

Cardiac catheterization involves the passage of flexible catheters into the great vessels and chambers of the heart. In right heart catheterization, the catheters are inserted into a peripheral vein (usually the basilic or femoral) and then advanced into the right heart. The left heart catheter is inserted retrograde through a peripheral artery (usually the brachial or femoral) into the aorta and left heart. The cardiac catheterization laboratory, where the procedure is done, is equipped for viewing and recording fluoroscopic images of the heart and vessels in the chest and for measuring pressures within the heart and great vessels. There is also equipment for cardiac output studies and for obtaining samples of blood for blood gas analysis. Angiographic studies are made by injecting a contrast medium into the heart, so that an outline of the moving structures can be visualized and filmed. Coronary arteriography involves the injection of a contrast medium into the coronary arteries; this permits visualization of lesions within these vessels.

Treatment measures

Measures for the treatment of myocardial ischemia are usually directed toward reducing the work demands of the heart and/or vessel constriction when coronary spasm is present. Treatment measures include nonpharmacologic and pharmacologic methods directed at reducing the preload and afterload work of the heart and measures such as percutaneous transluminal coronary angioplasty and coronary artery bypass surgery, which are used to improve blood flow to the myocardium.

Nonpharmacologic methods.

Nonpharmacologic treatment methods include the selective pacing of physical activities, stress reduction, avoidance of cold or other stresses that produce vasoconstriction, and weight reduction if obesity is present. Immediate cessation of activity is often sufficient to abort an anginal attack. Sitting down or standing quietly is often preferable to lying down, because these positions tend to decrease preload by producing pooling of blood in the lower extremities. Sudden exposure to cold tends to increase vasoconstriction and afterload stress; thus, persons with myocardial ischemia are cautioned against rapidly drinking large amounts of cold liquids (greater than 240 ml) and breathing extremely cold air. Anxiety often precipitates angina and silent myocardial ischemia because it causes an increase in both heart rate and blood pressure.

Pharmacologic methods.

Pharmacologic methods include the selective use of antiplatelet aggregating drugs, nitroglycerin and long-acting nitrates, beta-adrenergic blocking drugs, and calcium-channel blocking drugs. Nitrates are the initial treatment of choice for relief or prevention of the acute episode of anginal pain. The calcium-channel blocking drugs have proved extraordinarily effective in treating variant angina, particularly in persons in whom spasms occur spontaneously and those in whom it can be stimulated by effort or cold. Beta-adrenergic blocking drugs can be helpful for those who present with accompanying effort angina, suggesting a hemodynamically compromising atherosclerotic obstruction along with spasm.

Nitroglycerin (glycerol trinitrate) provides prompt relief of anginal pain and silent myocardial ischemia. It is a vasodilating drug that causes relaxation of both venous and arterial vessels. Venous dilatation reduces venous return to the heart (preload), thereby reducing ventricular volume and compression of the subendocardial vessels, and returns the end-diastolic length of the ventricular muscle fibers to a more favorable position on the Starling curve. It also decreases the tension in the wall of the ventricle so that less pressure is needed to pump blood, and it reduces the amount of blood that needs to be pumped. Relaxation of the arteries reduces the pressure against which the heart must pump (afterload). Nitroglycerin is destroyed by the liver when it is taken orally; therefore, it is administered sublingually either as a pill or spray. Sublingual absorption is rapid, and relief of pain usually begins in 30 seconds. Nitroglycerin is also available in ointment and adhesive patch forms for topical application. Ointment has a duration of 4 to 6 hours. The adhesive patches have a longer duration of action (24 hours). Although they are more costly than the ointment, they tend to increase compliance in many individuals. Topical forms of nitroglycerin are used prophylactically because of their prolonged action.

The *beta-adrenergic blocking drugs* act as antagonists that block beta receptor-mediated functions of the sympathetic nervous system. There are two types of beta receptors: $beta_1$ and $beta_2$ receptors. $Beta_1$ receptors are found in the heart, and $beta_2$ receptors are found in other parts of the body. At present, there are seven beta-blocking drugs approved by the Food and Drug Administration (FDA): propranolol, nadolol, timolol, pindolol, acebutolol, atenolol, and metoprolol. Of these drugs, atenolol and metoprolol are cardioselective in low doses (preferentially block beta$_1$ receptors), whereas the other five drugs block both beta$_1$ and beta$_2$ receptors and are nonselective in their actions. Blockade of beta receptors in the heart reduces the heart rate, cardiac contractility, and myocardial oxygen consumption.

The *calcium-channel blocking drugs* are sometimes called calcium antagonists. Diltiazem, nifedipine, and verapamil are currently approved for treatment of angina pectoris and cardiac dysrhythmias; they are being investigated for treating cardiomyopathy and hypertension. Although these three drugs have different chemical structures, they are effective in blocking a number of calcium-dependent functions; that is, they block the function of the calcium channels or enter the cell and substitute for calcium at intracellular receptor sites.[12]

Free intracellular calcium serves to link many membrane-initiated events with cellular responses, such as action potential generation and muscle contraction. Vascular smooth muscle lacks the sarcoplasmic reticulum and other structures necessary for intracellular storage of calcium; instead, it relies on the influx of calcium from the extracellular fluid into the cell to initiate and sustain contraction. In cardiac muscle, the slow inward calcium current contributes to the plateau of the action potential and to cardiac contractility. The slow calcium current is particularly important in the pacemaker activity of the SA node and the conduction properties of the AV node. The therapeutic effect of the calcium antagonists results from coronary and peripheral artery dilatation and decreased myocardial metabolism associated with the decrease in myocardial contractility. The calcium-channel blockers are particularly effective in reducing vasospasm; in patients with variant angina, nifedipine has proven to have a efficacy of 82% to 94%, and verapamil, 61% to 86%.[12] In clinical doses, verapamil and diltiazem depress the SA and AV nodes. The extent of slowing depends on the dose, the route of administration, and concomitant use of other drugs. Verapamil may be administered intravenously for the termination of paroxysmal supraventricular tachycardia. Nifedipine, in the usual clinical doses, has no direct effect on AV node conduction.

Percutaneous transluminal coronary artery angioplasty (PTCA) and bypass surgery. PTCA or bypass surgery may be done to relieve coronary artery obstruction. Surgery for coronary spasm is usually only indicated when angiographic tests demonstrate that spasm occurs around an area of fixed obstruction, but not in other coronary vessels or distal to the site of obstruction. It is not indicated for primary vasospastic angina because spontaneous remission of variant angina has been noted to occur 6 months to 12 months after the acute phase, primarily in persons with normal coronaries or with less than 70% diameter obstruction.[13–15]

Percutaneous transluminal coronary angioplasty involves the dilatation of a stenotic coronary vessel. The procedure is similar to cardiac catheterization for coronary angiography. With PTCA, a double lumen balloon dilatation catheter is introduced percutaneously into the femoral or brachial artery and then advanced under fluoroscopic view to the coronary ostium. It is then directed into the affected coronary artery and advanced until the balloon segment is within the stenotic area of the vessel. Once in place, the balloon is inflated for 3 seconds to 5 seconds using a pressure-controlled pump. The inflation may be repeated several times if needed. The mechanism for reduction of stenosis is not completely understood. It has been suggested that compression of the lipids and loose connective tissue with the atheromatous lesion may occur or that splitting and separation of the smooth muscle fibers may produce a controlled injury to the vessel that serves to increase the outer diameter of the vessel.[16] If dilatation is successful, the patient is monitored for 6 to 8 hours and then discharged in 1 to 2 days.

Current criteria for PTCA treatment include demonstrated evidence of myocardial ischemia or infarction, single or multiple vessel disease with some or all stenoses amenable to dilatation, acute coronary arterial occlusion during a myocardial infarction, less than 3 months' duration of a chronic coronary arterial occlusion, stenosis of vein grafts from previous coronary bypass surgery, and suitable candidacy for coronary bypass surgery.[17] Use of PTCA has been reported to be successful in 90% of patients who meet these criteria.[17] Restenosis rates during the first 6 months are high (30%–40%).[18–20] Placement of a stent (hollow tube) within the vessel is being tested as a method of improving artery patency after PTCA. Initial studies show that the self-expanding stainless steel endoprosthesis has a dilating as well as stenting role.[21] The use of PTCA combined with laser and thermal ablation devices is also currently under investigation. Although laser thermal techniques have been useful additions to balloon dilatation in peripheral vessels, additional research is needed to determine their effectiveness on coronary artery obstruction.[22]

The surgical treatment of angina—*coronary artery bypass surgery*—remains popular for patients who have significant coronary artery disease. In this surgical procedure, revascularization of the myocardium is effected by placing a saphenous vein graft between the aorta and the affected coronary artery distal to the site of occlusion or by using the internal mammary artery as a means of revascularizing the left anterior descending artery or its branches. Figure 21-6 illustrates the placement of a saphenous vein graft and a mammary artery graft. Although it cannot be documented that this surgery significantly alters the progress of the disease, it does relieve pain, so that patients may have a more productive life. In three studies that examined the effect of bypass surgery on morbidity and mortality in persons with mild to moderate angina, it was found that there was a significant reduction in angina, an improvement in exercise tolerance, and improved quality of life. However, there was no significant decrease in myocardial infarction incidence.[23-26] Another study reported a 6-year chance of survival in 89% of bypass surgery patients who had a diagnosis of severe angina, two-vessel disease with at least one significant proximal lesion, and poor left ventricular function; this compared to a 76% chance of a 6-year survival in persons with similar pathology who underwent medical treatment.[27]

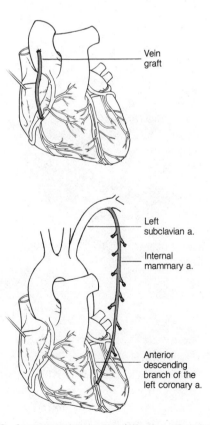

Figure 21-6 Coronary artery revascularization. *(Top)* Saphenous vein bypass graft. The vein segment is sutured to the ascending aorta and the right coronary artery at a point distal to the occluding lesion. *(Bottom)* Mammary artery bypass. The mammary artery is anastomosed to the anterior descending left coronary artery, bypassing the obstructing lesion.

Myocardial infarction

Myocardial infarction refers to the ischemic death of myocardial tissue associated with impaired blood flow sufficient to produce lethal cell injury. Obstructed blood flow can be caused by thrombosis, ulceration and hemorrhage in an atherosclerotic plaque, or prolonged vasospasm. It is also possible that a sudden increase in oxygen demand by the myocardium may contribute to the ischemic event. Research has shown that 80% to 90% of transmural infarctions are caused by thrombosis of a coronary artery.[28] As discussed under unstable angina, it is possible that the event responsible for the infarct—vessel spasm or excessive myocardial oxygen demand—may also predispose to thrombus formation. Even though thrombosis may not be the initiating event in myocardial infarction, almost all patients dying of myocardial infarction have been found to have severe coronary atherosclerosis.[2]

An infarct may involve the endocardium, myocardium, epicardium, or a combination of these. An intramural infarct is one that is contained within the myocardium, whereas a transmural infarct involves all three layers of the heart. Most infarcts are transmural, involving the free wall of the left ventricle and the interventricular septum. The increased vulnerability of the the left ventricle is probably related to its increased work demands. According to Robbins and Kumar,[2] about 30% to 40% of infarcts affect the right coronary artery, 40% to 50% affect the left anterior descending artery, and the remaining 15% to 20% affect the left circumflex artery. This distribution is depicted in Figure 21-7.

Although gross tissue changes are not apparent for hours following myocardial infarction (Table 21-1), it has been reported that the ischemic area ceases to function within a matter of minutes and that irreversible damage to cells occurs in about 40 minutes. There is also evidence that an area of injury and ischemic zone borders the necrotic area (Figure 21-8).

Manifestations

The manifestations of myocardial infarction can be categorized into four groups: (1) pain and autonomic responses associated with the ischemic event, (2) weakness and signs related to impaired myocardial function, (3) dysrhythmias and electrocardiographic changes associated with ischemia and death of myocardial cells, and (4) signs of inflammation and elevated serum enzyme levels indicative of tissue death.

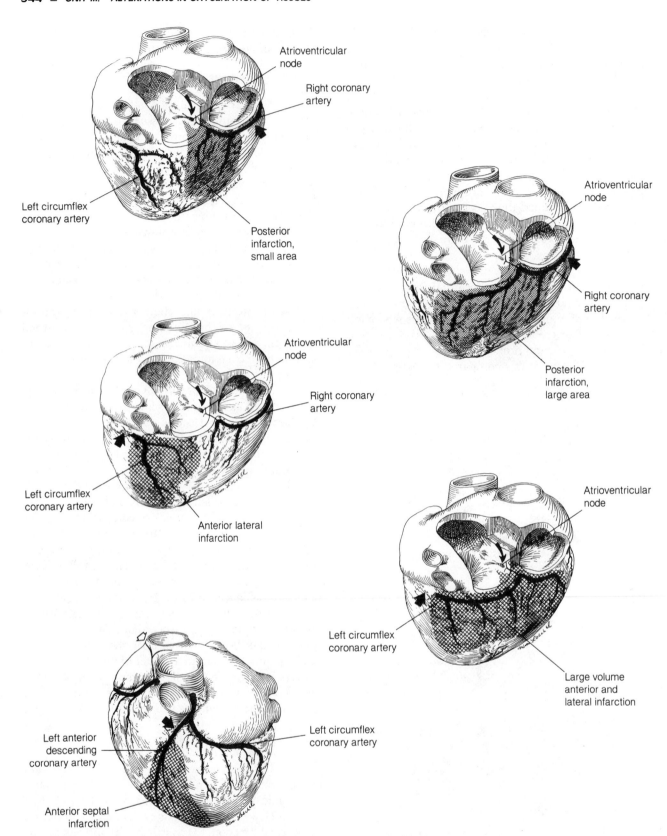

Figure 21-7 Anatomy and distribution of the coronary arteries and the topography of infarction. *Shaded areas* represent extent of infarction. *Arrows* point to affected arteries. Percentages relate to persons with described involvement of right, left circumflex, or left anterior descending coronary artery. *(James TN: Arrhythmias and conduction disturbances in acute myocardial infarction. Am Heart J 64[3]:416, 1962)*

The onset of myocardial infarction is usually abrupt, with pain as the significant symptom. Typically, the pain is severe and crushing, often described as being constricting, suffocating, or like "someone sitting on my chest." The pain is usually substernal, radiating to the left arm, neck, or jaw, although it may be experienced in other areas of the chest. Unlike that of angina, the pain associated with myocardial infarction is more prolonged and is not relieved by rest or nitroglycerin, and narcotics are frequently required.

Gastrointestinal complaints are common. There may be a sensation of epigastric distress; nausea and vomiting may occur. These symptoms are thought to be related to the severity of the pain and vagal stimulation. The epigastric distress may be mistaken for indigestion, and the patient may seek relief with antacids or other home remedies, which only delays getting medical attention. Frequently there are complaints of fatigue and weakness, especially of the arms and legs. Pain and sympathetic stimulation combine to give rise to tachycardia, anxiety, restlessness, and feelings of impending doom. The skin is often pale, cool, and moist. The impaired myocardial function may lead to hypotension and shock.

Electrocardiographic (ECG) changes may not be present immediately following the onset of symptoms, except as dysrhythmias. Premature ventricular contractions are common dysrhythmias following myocardial infarction. The occurrence of other dysrhythmias and conduction defects depends on the areas of the heart and conduction pathways that are included in the necrotic myocardium.

Following a myocardial infarction, there are usually three zones of tissue damage: (1) a zone of myocardial tissue that becomes necrotic because of an absolute lack of blood flow, (2) a surrounding zone of injured cells, some of which will recover, and (3) an outer zone in which cells are ischemic and can be salvaged if blood flow can be reestablished (Figure 21-8). The boundaries of these zones may change with time post-infarct and with success of treatment measures to reestablish flow.

During the period of impaired blood flow, injured and ischemic cells revert to anaerobic metabolism with a resultant increase in lactic acid production, much of which is released into the local extracellular fluid. In addition, the necrotic cells become electrically inactive and their membranes become disrupted so that their intracellular contents, including potassium, are released into the surrounding extracellular fluid. This causes local areas of hyperkalemia, which can affect the membrane potentials of functioning myocardial cells. As a result of membrane injury and local changes in extracellular potassium and pH, some parts of the infarcted heart are unable to conduct or generate impulses, some areas are more difficult to excite, and still others are overly excitable. These different levels of membrane excitability in the necrotic, injured, and ischemic zones of the infarcted area set the stage for the development of dysrhythmias and conduction defects following myocardial infarction. Furthermore, each of these zones in the infarcted area conducts impulses differently. These changes in impulse conduction can be detected on the ECG and are the basis for determining whether an infarct has occurred and the area of the heart in which it is located. Typical ECG changes associated with death of myocardial tissue include prolongation of the Q wave, elevation of the ST segment, and inversion of the T wave. (The ECG changes are variable and complex, and interested readers and those intending to work in the coronary care unit are referred to specialty texts.)

Table 21-1. Tissue changes following myocardial infarction

Time following onset	Gross tissue changes
6–12 hours	No gross changes
18–24 hours	Pale to gray-brown Slight pallor of area
2–4 days	Necrosis of area is apparent. Area is yellow-brown in center and hyperemic around the edges
4–10 days	Area becomes soft; fatty changes in the center are well developed Hemorrhagic areas are present in the infarcted area. Rupture of the heart, when it occurs, happens during this period
10 days or more	Fibrotic (scar) tissue replacement and revascularization commences
6 weeks	Scar tissue replacement of necrotic tissue is usually complete, depends on size of infarct

(Developed from data in Robbins SL, Cotran R, Kumar V: Pathologic Basis of Disease, 3rd ed, pp 559–560. Philadelphia, WB Saunders, 1984)

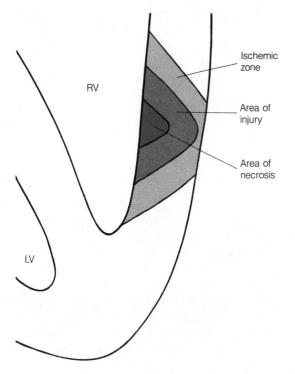

Figure 21-8 Areas of tissue damage after myocardial infarction.

In the infarcted area, cell death causes inflammation and the release of intracellular enzymes into the extracellular fluid. Fever and leukocytosis usually develop within about 24 hours and continue for 3 days to 7 days. The sedimentation rate rises on the second and third days and remains elevated for 1 week to 3 weeks. Enzymes released include creatine phosphokinase (CPK), lactic dehydrogenase (LDH), and glutamine oxaloacetic transaminase (GOT). As indicated in Table 21-2, these enzymes become elevated at different times after infarction and provide useful diagnostic information. The enzyme CPK (MB band), which is one of three isoenzymes of CPK, has been found to be a more reliable indicator of myocardial infarction than other enzymes (singly or in combination) or the electrocardiogram.[29]

Complications

The stages of recovery are closely related to the size of the infarct and the changes that have taken place within the infarcted area. Fibrous scar tissue lacks the contractile, elastic, and conductive properties of normal myocardial cells; hence, the residual effects as well as the complications are determined essentially by the extent and location of the injury. Among the complications of myocardial infarction are sudden death, heart failure and cardiogenic shock, pericarditis and Dressler's syndrome, thromboemboli, rupture of the heart, and ventricular aneurysms.

Sudden death due to coronary heart disease is death occurring within an hour of the onset of symptoms, and it is usually attributed to fatal dysrhythmias, which may occur without evidence of infarction. Approximately 30% to 50% of persons with acute myocardial infarction die of ventricular fibrillation within the first few hours after symptoms begin. Early hospitalization after onset of symptoms greatly improves chances of survival from sudden death. This is because the appropriate resuscitation facilities are immediately available at the time that the fatal ventricular dysrhythmia occurs.[30]

Depending on its severity, myocardial infarction has the potential for compromising the pumping action of the heart. Both heart failure (see Chapter 22) and cardiogenic shock (see Chapter 23) are dreaded complications of myocardial infarction.

Pericarditis may complicate the course of acute myocardial infarction. It usually appears on the second or third day postinfarction. At this time, the patient experiences a new type of pain, which is sharp and stabbing in nature and aggravated with deep inspiration and positional changes. A pericardial rub may or may not be heard in all patients who have postinfarction pericarditis, and often it is transitory, usually resolving uneventfully. Dressler's syndrome describes signs and symptoms associated with pericarditis, pleurisy, and pneumonitis: fever, chest pain, dyspnea, and abnormal laboratory (elevated white blood cell count and sedimentation rate) and ECG

Enzyme	Time postinfarction		
	Exceeds normal value	Reaches peak value	Returns to normal
CPK (Creatine phosphokinase)*	4–8 hours	24 hours	3–4 days
GOT (Glutamine oxaloacetic transaminase)	8–12 hours	24–48 hours	4–7 days
LDH (Lactic dehydrogenase)†	12–24 hours	3–6 days	8–14 days

Table 21–2. Elevation of serum enzymes postmyocardial infarction

  * There are three isoenzymes of CPK; myocardial cells possess the isoenzyme MB.
  † There are five isoenzymes of LDH; myocardial cells have both LDH_1 and LDH_2. Normally the ratio of LDH_1 go LDH_2 is less than 1; following myocardial infarction, this ratio is reversed.

findings. The symptoms may arise between 1 day and several weeks following infarction and are thought to represent a hypersensitivity response to tissue necrosis. Anti-inflammatory agents or corticosteroid drugs may be used to reduce the inflammatory response.

Thromboemboli are a potential complication, arising either as venous thrombi or, occasionally, as a clot from the wall of the ventricle. Immobility and impaired cardiac function contribute to the stasis of blood in the venous system. Elastic stockings, along with active and passive leg exercises, are usually included in the postinfarction treatment plan as a means of preventing thrombus formation. If a clot is detected on the wall of the ventricle (usually by echocardiography), treatment with anticoagulants is used.

The acute postmyocardial infarction period can be complicated by rupture of the myocardium, the interventricular septum, or a papillary muscle. Myocardial rupture is usually fatal, occurring at the time when the injured ventricular tissue is soft and weak, about the seventh to the tenth day. Necrosis of the septal wall or papillary muscle may also lead to the rupture of either of these structures with a worsening of ventricular performance. Surgical repair is usually indicated, but, whenever possible, it is delayed until the heart has had time to recover from the initial infarction. Vasodilator therapy and the aortic balloon counterpulsation pump may provide supportive assistance during this period.

Scar tissue does not have the characteristics of normal myocardial tissue. When a large section of ventricular muscle is replaced by scar tissue, that section does not contract with the rest of the ventricle; instead there is outpouching—*aneurysm*—of the ventricle during systole, which diminishes myocardial pumping efficiency (Figure 21-9). This increases the work of the left ventricle and predisposes to heart failure. The ischemia in the surrounding area predisposes to the development of dysrhythmias; and within the aneurysm, stasis of blood can lead to thrombus formation. Surgical resection is often corrective.

Diagnosis and treatment

The diagnosis of myocardial infarction is based on the presence of prolonged chest pain and other signs of distress, changes in heart rate and blood pressure, ECG changes, and elevation in serum enzymes. Nuclear imaging, specifically acute infarction imaging using technetium pyrophosphate, may be used to confirm the diagnosis.

If a person presents for medical treatment within 6 hours of symptom onset, a cardiac catheterization may be done to determine the location of the occlusion, the extent of injury, and the advisability of

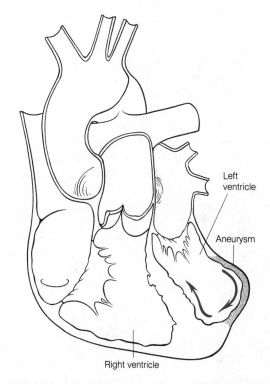

Figure 21-9 Paradoxical movement of a ventricular aneurysm during systole.

treatment using intracoronary infusion of a thrombolytic agent, PTCA, or coronary artery bypass surgery.

The treatment of myocardial infarction has changed drastically within the past several decades. Patients are ambulated earlier, leave the hospitals sooner, and are encouraged to return to an active and productive life; this contrasts with the requirements for prolonged activity restriction and limited return to work that were imposed in the past. The current treatment methods for myocardial infarction are directed toward: (1) symptom relief and management of life-threatening events, (2) limiting heart damage by increasing the circulation to the heart and decreasing the workload of the heart, and (3) rehabilitation to maximize physical and psychologic well-being during and following recovery. All patients with myocardial infarction require ECG monitoring, oxygen therapy, and pain relief. Treatment measures such as thrombolytic therapy, PTCA, and coronary bypass surgery may be appropriate if the patient presents within 6 hours of symptom onset because myocardial cells may still be viable and salvageable. Beta-adrenergic blocking drugs are effective in limiting morbidity and mortality after myocardial infarction because of their ability to decrease the sympathetic stimulation of the heart and the development of dysrhythmias. Rehabilitation in the form of rest, exercise, and cardiac risk factor modification is essential for regaining physical and psychologic well-being.

Administration of oxygen augments the oxygen content of inspired air and increases the oxygen saturation of hemoglobin. Arterial oxygen levels may fall precipitously following myocardial infarction, and oxygen administration helps to maintain the oxygen content of the blood perfusing the coronary circulation.

The severe pain of myocardial infarction gives rise to anxiety and recruitment of autonomic nervous system responses, both of which increase the work demands of the heart. Morphine and meperidine (Demerol) are often given intravenously for pain relief because they have a rapid onset of action and the intravenous route does not elevate enzyme levels. Also, the intravenous route bypasses the variable rate of absorption of subcutaneous or intramuscular sites, which are often underperfused because of a decrease in cardiac output that occurs following infarction. Vasodilating drugs are often given because they decrease venous return (reduce preload) and arterial blood pressure (afterload) and, thereby, reduce oxygen consumption. Morphine has vasodilator properties and is often used as the narcotic of choice in treatment of acute myocardial infarction. Intravenous nitroglycerin, another vasodilator, is also given to limit infarction size and is most effective if given with 4 hours of symptom onset.

Thrombolytic drugs are used to dissolve blood clots; they react with plasminogen to create plasmin, which lyses fibrin clots and digests clotting factors V, VIII, prothrombin, and fibrinogen.[28,31] Intravenous or intracoronary artery infusion of thrombolytic agents is used as a treatment for persons in whom myocardial infarctions are caused by intracoronary thrombi. Several thrombolytic agents are approved by the Federal Drug Administration including streptokinase, acylated plasminogen-streptokinase activator complex (APSAC), recombinant tissue plasminogen activator (r-tPA), and urokinase. This therapy acts directly to improve myocardial blood supply. The treatment usually requires 20 minutes to 40 minutes to reestablish blood flow; to be effective, the treatment must be done within 3 hours to 6 hours following the onset of the acute myocardial infarction period at a time when the heart tissue that is supplied by the affected vessel can still be salvaged. The patient must be a low-risk candidate for complications due to bleeding.[32] When the drug is administered by intracoronary infusion, the procedure is carried out during cardiac catheterization using coronary arteriographic studies. The optimal dose and the combination of thrombolytic agents with each other and with mechanical therapies are still under investigation.

It is now possible to open or dilate total and partial occlusions of coronary arteries with an inflatable balloon-tipped catheter (PTCA). This has the effect of directly improving circulation to the myocardium. Depending on the skills of the physician and patient selection criteria, success rates for reperfusion after acute myocardial infarction range from 80% to 90%.[17] Restenosis is the most common problem, occurring in 33.6% of all patients who have been dilated.[33] Recent studies have suggested that patients who present within the first 6 hours of symptom onset may benefit from elective rather than emergency PTCA following successful thrombolysis.[34,35] Further studies on the progress of PTCA and thrombolytic therapy are in progress.

Coronary bypass surgery is used to improve directly circulation to the myocardium as described earlier in the chapter. Lower postoperative and long-term mortality rates have been reported for persons with acute myocardial infarction who had coronary bypass surgery performed within 6 hours of symptom onset.[36]

Because sympathetic activity increases the metabolic activity of the myocardium and, consequently, myocardial oxygen consumption, beta-adrenergic blocking drugs may be used to reduce sympathetic stimulation of the heart following myocardial infarction. These drugs decrease myocardial contractility (and cardiac workload), alter resting myocardial membrane potentials (and decrease dysrhythmia frequency), and may also redistribute coronary artery blood flow and improve myocardial blood supply.

Rehabilitation programs for persons with myocardial infarction incorporate rest, exercise, and risk factor modification. Protecting the oxygen supply of the heart and decreasing the myocardial oxygen consumption as much as possible are concerns during the early treatment of myocardial infarction. Persons with myocardial infarction are usually maintained on bedrest for a period of at least 48 hours, although the use of a bedside commode for elimination purposes may be allowed. This 48-hour period of time is followed by a gradual increase in activity depending on the severity of the infarction and the presence of complications. Modifying the diet to include foods that are low in salt and cholesterol and are easy to digest is another treatment measure used to decrease cardiac work. Stool softeners are often prescribed to prevent constipation and straining with defecation.

An exercise program is an integral part of a cardiac rehabilitation program. It includes such activities as walking, swimming, and bicycling. These exercises involve changes in muscle length and rhythmic contractions of muscle groups. Exercise programs are usually individually designed to meet each person's physical and psychologic needs. The goal of the exercise program is to increase the maximal oxygen consumption by the muscle tissues, so that these persons are able to perform more work at a lower heart rate and blood pressure. In addition to exercise, cardiac risk factor modification incorporates strategies for smoking cessation, weight loss, stress reduction, and control of hypertension and diabetes.

In summary, coronary heart disease is usually due to atherosclerosis. It is frequently a silent disorder, and symptoms do not occur until the disease is far advanced. Myocardial ischemia occurs when there is a disparity between the metabolic needs of the myocardium and the amount of blood that the coronary arteries can deliver and may manifest itself as angina. There are three types of angina. Classic angina is associated with atherosclerosis of the coronary arteries, in which pain is precipitated by increased work demands on the heart and is relieved by rest; variant angina is due to spasms of the coronary arteries; and unstable angina is an accelerated form of angina in which the pain occurs more frequently, is more severe, and lasts longer. Silent myocardial ischemia occurs without symptoms. Myocardial infarction refers to the ischemic death of myocardial tissue associated with obstructed blood flow in the coronary arteries. The infarct can involve the endocardium, myocardium, epicardium, or a combination of all three layers as well as the pericardium. The complications of myocardial infarction include potentially fatal dysrhythmias, heart failure, cardiogenic shock, pericarditis, thromboemboli, rupture of cardiac structures, and ventricular aneurysms.

Disorders of cardiac rhythm and conduction

The specialized cells in the conduction system manifest four inherent properties: (1) automaticity, (2) excitability, (3) conductivity, and (4) refractoriness (see Chapter 20). The term *dysrhythmia* refers to an alteration in cardiac rhythm. An alteration in any of these properties may produce dysrhythmias or conduction defects. There are many causes of altered cardiac rhythms, including congenital defects of the conduction system, degenerative changes, ischemia and myocardial infarction, fluid and electrolyte imbalances, and the effects of drug ingestion. Dysrhythmias are not necessarily pathologic; they can occur in the healthy as well as the diseased heart. Disturbances in cardiac rhythms exert their harmful effects by interfering with the heart's pumping ability. Rapid heart rates reduce the diastolic filling time, causing a subsequent decrease in the stroke volume output and in coronary perfusion while increasing the myocardial oxygen needs. Abnormally slow heart rates may impair the blood flow to vital organs such as the brain.

The electrocardiogram

The electrocardiogram (ECG) provides a practical, relatively inexpensive, and noninvasive method of viewing the electrical activity of the heart. No other area of cardiac function is so readily and easily monitored on a moment-by-moment basis. A description of the ECG is presented in this section of the chapter to help the reader understand disorders of cardiac rhythm and conduction.

The ECG is a recording of the electrical activity of the heart. The electrical currents generated by the heart spread through the body to the skin, where they can be sensed by appropriately placed electrodes, amplified, and then recorded on an oscilloscope or chart recorder. The horizontal axis of the ECG measures time (seconds), and the vertical axis measures the amplitude of the impulse (millivolts). Each heavy vertical black line represents 0.2 second and each thin black line, 0.04 second (Figure 21-10). On the horizontal axis, each heavy horizontal line represents 0.05 mV. The connections of the ECG are such that an upright deflection indicates a positive potential, and a downward deflection indicates a negative potential.

The deflection points of an ECG are designated by the letters P, Q, R, S, and T. The P wave represents SA node and atrial depolarization; the QRS complex (beginning of the Q wave to the end of the S wave) represents ventricular depolarization; and the T wave represents ventricular repolarization. Atrial repolarization occurs during ventricular depolarization and is hidden in the QRS complex.

The process of impulse generation in the heart and other excitable tissue involves the movement or flow of electrically charged ions at the level of the cell membrane. The ECG represents the sum of all these impulses as they are conducted through the body fluids to the skin surface. The ECG records three types of electrical events: the resting membrane potential, depolarization, and repolarization. During the resting state, the membrane is impermeable to the flow of charge and charges of opposite polarity (positive on the outside and negative on the inside) become aligned along the membrane (Figure 21-11). Depolarization occurs when the cell membrane becomes selectively permeable to a current-carrying ion such as sodium. During the process of repolarization, electrical charges move inward across the cell membrane and the membrane potential becomes reversed so that the inside becomes positive in relation to the outside. Repolarization involves the reestablishment of the resting membrane potential. During repolarization, membrane conductance or permeability for potassium becomes greatly increased, allowing the positively charged potassium ions to move outward across the membrane; this removes positive charges from inside

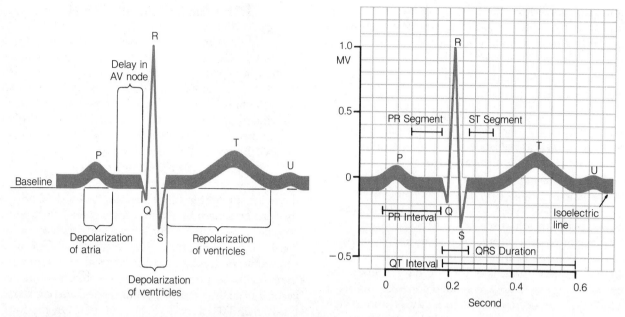

Figure 21-10 Diagram of the electrocardiogram (lead II) and representative depolarization and repolarization of the atria and ventricle. The P wave represents atrial depolarization, the QRS complex ventricular depolarization, and the T wave ventricular repolarization. Atrial repolarization occurs during ventricular depolarization and is hidden under the QRS complex.

the membrane, and the cell membrane again becomes negative on the inside and positive on the outside. The sodium–potassium membrane pump also assists in repolarization by pumping positively charged sodium ions out across the cell membrane.

The ECG records the potential difference in charge (in millivolts [mV]) that occurs between two electrodes as the depolarization and repolarization waves move through the heart and are conducted to the skin surface. The shape of the recorder tracing is determined by the direction in which the impulse spreads through the heart muscle in relation to electrode placement. A depolarization wave that moves toward the recording electrode will register as a positive, or upward, deflection. Conversely, if the impulse moves away from the recording electrode, the deflec-

tion will be downward, or negative. When there is no flow of charge between electrodes, the potential is zero and a straight line is recorded at the baseline of the chart. If the direction of current flow is perpendicular to the recording electrode, the recorder will also register zero because the electrode cannot detect the direction of current flow. The electrocardiograph recorder is much like a camera in that it can record different views of the electrical activity of the heart depending on where the recording electrode is placed.

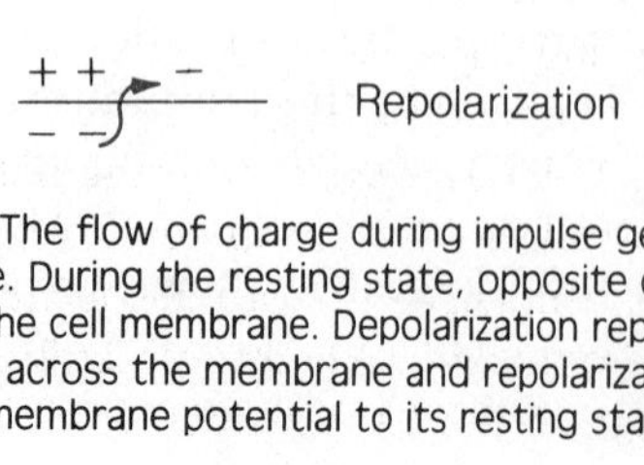

Unlike laboratory experiments, which record from a single nerve or muscle fiber, the ECG records the sum of all the electrical activity of the heart. A force that has both magnitude and direction is referred to as a vector. The electrical vector of the heart, which can be measured using the ECG, designates all of the electromotive forces of the heart: it has magnitude, direction, and polarity. A vector can be represented by an arrow in which the length of the shaft represents the magnitude of the force and the tip of the arrow represents the direction of the force. The mean QRS vector can be estimated from the standard leads of the ECG and is used in describing the size and position of the heart.

Conventionally, 12 leads are recorded for a diagnostic ECG, each viewing the electrical forces of the heart from a different position on the body's surface. The electrodes are attached to the four extremities or representative areas on the body (near the shoulders and lower chest or abdomen). The electrical

+ + + + +
— — — — —   Resting state

+ +
— —⌐— +   Depolarization

+ + —
— —⌐— ⌐   Repolarization

Figure 21-11 The flow of charge during impulse generation in excitable tissue. During the resting state, opposite charges are separated by the cell membrane. Depolarization represents the flow of charge across the membrane and repolarization of the return of the membrane potential to its resting state.

potential recorded from any one extremity should be the same no matter where the electrode is placed on the extremity.[7] Chest electrodes are moved to different positions on the chest. The right limb lead is used as a ground electrode. Additional electrodes may be applied to other areas of the body, such as the back, when indicated.

Bipolar limb leads. The three standard, or bipolar, limb leads record the potential difference between two electrodes (the indifferent [−] electrode and the recording [+] electrode). Lead I records the difference in potential between the left and right arms, with the right arm negative in relation to the left arm (Figure 21-12). Lead II records the potential difference between the right arm, which is negative, and the left leg, which is positive. Lead III records the potential difference between the left arm (negative) and the left leg (positive). The relationship among the three leads is expressed algebraically by Einthoven's equation: lead II = lead I + lead III. This equation is based on Kirchoff's law, which states that the algebraic sum of all the potential differences in a closed circuit is equal to zero. The equation is used to obtain the mean electrical vector for the heart.

Augmented unipolar limb leads. The augmented unipolar limb leads measure impulses from the heart without being influenced by an indifferent electrode as in the bipolar limb leads. The augmented leads actually record a potential difference, but from infinity. Lead aVr records the potential from the right arm, aVl records the potential from the left arm, and aVf records the potential from the left leg (foot). Recordings from these sites are of very small magnitude, thus they are amplified or augmented. Instead of lead II = lead I + lead III, lead aVf equals the total electri-

cal vector from the heart as recorded from the foot. Likewise, aVl equals the total electrical vector from the heart, as recorded from the left arm, and aVR equals the total vector, as recorded from the right arm.

Unipolar chest leads. Usually six unipolar chest leads are recorded with an electrode that can be moved to specific areas of the chest. As with the unipolar limb leads, the chest leads record the potential from the heart without being influenced by an indifferent electrode.

Vectorcardiography. A vectorcardiogram is a three-dimensional ECG. It displays a vector loop of impulses on the frontal (right to left and head to toe), sagittal (front to back and head to toe), or horizontal (front to back and left to right) planes of the body. Whereas an electrocardiographic lead records in one single axis, a vectorcardiograph records the same electrical event simultaneously in two perpendicular axes.

Mechanisms of dysrhythmias and conduction disorders

Automaticity is the ability of certain cells of the conduction system to initiate spontaneously an impulse or action potential. The SA node has an inherent discharge rate of 60 times to 100 times a minute; normally it acts as the pacemaker of the heart because it reaches the threshold for excitation before other parts of the conduction system have recovered sufficiently to be depolarized. If the sinus node fires more slowly, or if the SA node conduction is blocked, another site that is capable of automaticity will take over as pacemaker. Other regions that are capable of automaticity include the atrial fibers that have plateau-type action potentials, the AV node, the bundle of His, and the bundle-branch Purkinje fibers. These pacemakers generally have a slower rate of discharge. The AV node has an inherent firing rate of 40 to 60 times per minute, and the Purkinje system, 30 to 40 times per minute. Even though the SA node is functioning properly, other cardiac cells can assume accelerated properties of automaticity and begin to initiate impulses when they are injured, oxygen-deprived, or exposed to certain chemicals or drugs.

An *ectopic pacemaker* is an excitable focus outside the normally functioning SA node. These pacemakers can reside in other parts of the conduction system or in muscle cells of the atria or ventricles. A premature contraction occurs when an ectopic pacemaker initiates a beat. In general, premature contractions do not follow the normal conduction pathways, they are not coupled with normal mechanical events, and they often render the heart refractory or incapable of responding to the next normal impulse arising in

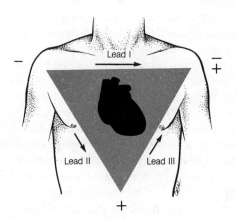

Figure 21-12 Einthoven's triangle, illustrating the connections of the bipolar limb leads. The heart is the center of the triangle. Lead I records the potential difference between the left arm and the right arm. Lead II records the potential difference between the right arm and the left leg. Lead III registers the difference between the left arm and left leg.

the SA node. Premature contractions occur without incident in persons with healthy hearts in response to sympathetic stimulation or to stimulants such as caffeine. In the diseased heart, the premature contraction may lead to more serious dysrhythmias.

Excitability describes the ability of a cell to respond to an impulse and generate an action potential. Myocardial cells that have been injured or replaced by scar tissue do not possess normal excitability. For example, cells within the ischemic zone become depolarized during the acute phase of myocardial ischemia. These ischemic cells remain electrically coupled to the adjacent nonischemic area, and, thus, current from the ischemic zone can induce reexcitation of cells in the nonischemic zone.

Conductivity is the ability to conduct impulses, and *refractoriness* is the inability to respond to an incoming stimulus. The refractory period of cardiac muscle is the interval in the repolarization period during which an excitable cell has not recovered sufficiently to be reexcited. Disturbances in either conductivity or refractoriness predispose to dysrhythmias.

An important condition in the development of dysrhythmias is the phenomenon of reentry. Reentry occurs when an impulse reexcites an area through which it previously traveled, disrupting the normal conduction sequence. For reentry to occur, there must be a unidirectional, or one-way, block in one limb of a conduction pathway (Figure 21-13). When this occurs, the impulse is conducted through the unaf-

fected limb of the pathway and then reenters the affected limb from the reverse direction; if sufficient time has elapsed for the refractory period in the reentered area to have ended, a self-perpetuating "circuitous-type" movement can be initiated. The functional components of a reentry circuit can be large and include an entire specialized conduction system or it can be microscopic; it can include myocardial tissue, AV nodal cells, or junctional cells.

Types of dysrhythmias

Sinus node dysrhythmias

The normal rhythm of the heart with the sinus node in command is regular and ranges from 60 beats/minute to 100 beats/minute. On the electrocardiogram, a P wave may be observed to precede every QRS complex.

Alterations in the function of the SA node lead to a change in the rate and regularity of the heartbeat. *Sinus bradycardia* describes a slow heart rate (less than 60 beats/minute). In sinus bradycardia, a P wave precedes each QRS; this confirms that the impulse is originating in the SA node rather than in a part of the conduction system that has a slower heart rate. Vagal stimulation decreases the firing rate of the SA node and conduction through the AV node to cause a decrease in the heart rate. A slow resting rate of 50 beats/minute to 60 beats/minute may be normal in a well-trained athlete who maintains a large stroke volume. *Sinus tachycardia* refers to a rapid heart rate (100–160 beats/minute) that has its origin in the SA node (a P wave precedes every QRS complex). Sympathetic stimulation or withdrawal of vagal tone incites an increase in heart rate. Sinus tachycardia is normal during fever, exercise, and in situations that incite sympathetic stimulation. *Sinus dysrhythmia* is a condition in which the heart rate speeds up and then slows down in an irregular, but cyclic, pattern; it is often associated with respiration and alterations in autonomic control. It is common and normal in young people. *Sinus arrest* refers to failure of the SA node to discharge and results in an irregular pulse. An escape rhythm develops as another pacemaker takes over. Sinus arrest may result in prolonged periods of asystole and often predisposes to other dysrhythmias. Causes of sinus arrest include disease of the SA node, digitalis toxicity, and excess vagal tone. The *sick sinus syndrome* is a term that describes a condition of periods of bradycardia alternating with tachycardia. The bradycardia is caused by disease of the sinus node (or other intra-atrial conduction pathways) and the tachycardia, by paroxysmal atrial or junctional dysrhythmias.

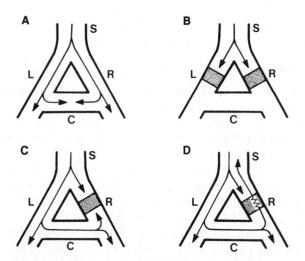

Figure 21-13 The role of unidirectional block in reentry. (**A**) An excitation wave traveling down a single bundle (*S*) of fibers continues down the left (*L*) and right (*R*) branches. The depolarization wave enters the connecting branch (*C*) from both ends and is extinguished at the zone of collision. (**B**) The wave is blocked in the *L* and *R* branches. (**C**) Bidirectional block exists in Branch *R*. (**D**) Unidirectional block exists in branch *R*. The antegrade impulse is blocked, but the retrograde impulse is conducted through and reenters bundle *S*. (Berne RM, Levy MN: *Physiology,* 2nd ed. St Louis, CV Mosby, 1988)

Dysrhythmias originating in the atria

The impulse from the SA node passes through the conductive pathways in the atria to the AV node. An *atrial premature contraction* can originate in the atrial conduction pathways or in atrial muscle cells. This contraction is transmitted to the ventricle as well as back to the SA node. The retrograde transmission to the SA node often interrupts the timing of the next sinus beat so that a pause occurs between the two normally conducted beats. *Atrial flutter* describes an atrial rate of 160 beats/minute to 350 beats/minute. There is a delay in conduction through the AV node, and the ventricles respond to every second, third, or fourth beat (*e.g.*, when conduction from the atria to the ventricles is 3:1, an atrial flutter rate of 225 will result in a ventricular rate of only 75). *Atrial fibrillation* describes an atrial rate in excess of 350, usually 450 beats/minute to 600 beats/minute. Here, conduction through the AV node is totally disorganized, the peripheral pulse is grossly irregular, and a pulse deficit can be observed. The pulse deficit is the difference between the apical and peripheral pulses. In atrial fibrillation, the rate may be such that there is not sufficient stroke output with some beats to be felt at the wrist, causing a difference between the apical heartbeat and peripheral pulses. Atrial fibrillation can occur as the result of left atrial distention due to mitral stenosis. It is the most common atrial dysrhythmia in the elderly. Atrial fibrillation predisposes to thrombus formation in the atria, with subsequent risk of formation of systemic emboli. Figure 21-14 illustrates the electrocardiographic changes that occur with atrial dysrhythmias.

During rest and moderate activity, ventricular filling is not dependent on atrial contraction. Atrial contraction contributes only about 25% to 30% of cardiac reserve; therefore, atrial dysrhythmias may go unnoticed unless they are transmitted to the ventricle. In persons with marginal cardiac output, however, the loss of atrial function may result in a sufficient decrease in cardiac output to produce symptoms.

Disorders of atrioventricular conduction

The AV node provides the only connection for transmission of impulses between the atrial and the ventricular conduction systems. Junctional fibers in the AV node have high resistance characteristics, which cause a delay in the transmission of impulses from the atria to the ventricles; this allows for filling of the ventricles and protects them from abnormally rapid rates that arise in the atria. Conduction defects are most commonly due to fibrosis or scar tissue in the

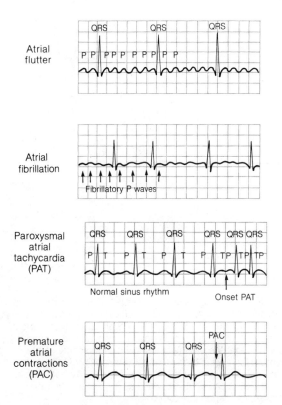

Figure 21-14 Electrocardiographic (ECG) tracings of atrial dysrhythmias. On the top is a tracing of atrial flutter, characterized by the presence of atrial flutter (P) waves occurring at a rate of 160 to 350 beats per minute. The ventricular rate remains regular because of the conduction of every sixth atrial contraction. In atrial fibrillation (*second tracing*) there is an atrial rate of in excess of 350 beats per minute; the P waves are no longer distinct and the ventricular rate becomes irregular. The *third tracing* illustrates paroxysmal atrial tachycardia (PAT), preceded by a normal sinus rhythm. The *fourth tracing* illustrates a premature atrial contraction (PAC).

fibers of the conduction system. Conduction defects of the AV node can also occur as the result of digitalis toxicity.

Heart block occurs when conduction through the AV node is delayed or interrupted. It may occur in the AV nodal fibers or in the AV bundle (bundle of His), which is continuous with the Purkinje conduction system that supplies the ventricles. The PR interval on the ECG corresponds with the time that it takes for the cardiac impulse to travel from the SA node to the ventricular pathways; the normal range is 0.12 second to 0.20 second.

A *first-degree heart block* occurs when conduction through the AV pathway is delayed and the PR interval is longer than 0.20 second (Figure 21-15). In *second-degree block*, one or more of the atrial impulses are blocked. There are two types of second-degree block: the *Mobitz type I*, or *Wenckebach phenomenon*, describes a progressive increase in the PR interval until the point at which one P wave is totally blocked;

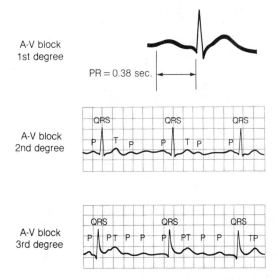

A-V block
1st degree

PR = 0.38 sec.

A-V block
2nd degree

A-V block
3rd degree

Figure 21-15 Electrocardiographic (ECG) changes that occur with alterations in AV node conduction. The *top tracing* shows the prolongation of the PR interval, which is characteristic of first-degree AV block. The second tracing illustrates Mobitz type II second-degree AV block, in which the conduction of one or more P waves is blocked. In third-degree AV block, complete block in conduction of impulses through the AV node occurs, and the atria and ventricles each develop their own rate of impulse generation (*bottom tracing*).

the *Mobitz type II block* (Figure 21-15) describes the situation in which there is a sudden block in one or more atrial impulses without an antecedent prolongation of the PR interval. In a Mobitz type II block, the ventricular rate is regular and reflects the degree of block; this type of block is significant because it often precedes complete heart block.

Third-degree, or *complete,* heart block occurs when the conduction link between the atria and ventricles is completely lost (Figure 21-15); the atria continue to beat at a normal rate and the ventricles develop their own rate, which is normally slow (30–40 beats/minute). Complete heart block causes a decrease in cardiac output with possible periods of syncope (called a Stokes-Adams attack). Patients with complete heart block usually require a pacemaker.

—— Junctional dysrhythmias

The AV node can act as a pacemaker in the event that the SA node fails to initiate an impulse. Junctional fibers in the AV node or bundle can also serve as ectopic pacemakers, producing *premature junctional contractions (PJC).*

—— Disorders of ventricular rhythm and conduction

The junctional fibers in the AV node join with the bundle of His, which divides to form the right and left bundle branches; they then branch to form

the Purkinje fibers, which supply the walls of the ventricles (see Figure 20-11). On leaving the junctional fibers, the cardiac impulse travels through the AV bundle, moves down the right and left bundle branches that lie beneath the endocardium on either side of the septum, and then spreads out through the walls of the ventricles. Interruption of impulse conduction through the bundle branches, called a *bundle branch block,* does not usually cause alterations in the rhythm of the heartbeat; this is because the impulse is usually conducted along an alternate or detour pathway. It does, however, take longer for the impulse to be transmitted through the Purkinje system when there is a conduction defect; this produces changes in the QRS complex of the ECG and causes the QRS complex to be wider than the normal 0.08 second to 0.12 second. The left bundle branch is divided into two parts called fascicles. A *hemiblock* refers to interruption of impulse conduction of one of the fascicles of the left bundle branch.

Dysrhythmias arising in the ventricles are usually considered more serious than those arising in the atria because they afford the potential for interfering with the pumping action of the heart. A *premature ventricular contraction* (PVC) is caused by a ventricular ectopic pacemaker. Following a PVC, the ventricle is usually not able to repolarize sufficiently to respond to the next impulse that arises in the SA node; this causes the "compensatory pause," which occurs while the ventricle waits to reestablish its previous rhythm (Figure 21-16). With a PVC, the diastolic volume is usually insufficient for ejection of blood into the arterial system; this causes a skipped beat. In the absence of heart disease, PVCs are usually not of great clinical significance. They can also occur in digitalis toxicity and in myocardial ischemia and infarction. A special pattern of PVC called *ventricular bigeminy,* occurs in such a way that each normal beat is followed by or paired with a PVC. It is often an indication of digitalis toxicity or heart disease. The occurrence of frequent PVCs in the diseased heart predisposes to other more serious dysrhythmias, including ventricular tachycardia and fibrillation. *Ventricular tachycardia* describes a ventricular rate of 160 beats/minute to 250 beats/minute; it is dangerous because it causes a reduction in the diastolic filling time to the point at which the cardiac output is severely diminished or nonexistent (Figure 21-16). In *ventricular fibrillation,* the ventricle quivers but does not contract; with the cessation of cardiac output, no pulse is palpable or audible (Figure 21-16).

—— Diagnosis and treatment

Diagnosis of disorders of cardiac rhythm and conduction is usually made on the basis of the ECG. Further clarification of conduction defects and cardiac

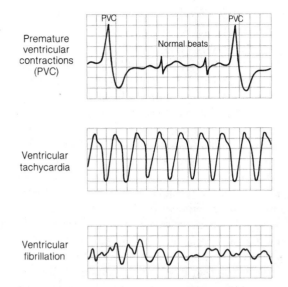

Figure 21-16 Electrocardiographic (ECG) tracings of ventricular dysrhythmias. Premature ventricular contractions (PVCs) originate from an ectopic focus in the ventricles, causing a distortion of the QRS complex (*top tracing*). Because the ventricle usually cannot repolarize sufficiently to respond to the next impulse that arises in the SA node, a PVC is followed by a compensatory pause. Ventricular tachycardia is characterized by a rapid ventricular rate of 160 to 250 beats per minute and the absence of P waves (*middle tracing*). In ventricular fibrillation, which is illustrated in the *bottom tracing,* there are no regular or effective ventricular contractions, and the ECG tracing is totally disorganized.

dysrhythmias can be done using electrophysiologic studies.

A resting ECG records the impulses of the heart as they occur during a limited period of time and during periods of inactivity. The resting ECG is the first approach to the clinical diagnosis of disorders of cardiac rhythm and conduction; it is limited, however, to events that occur during the time period that the ECG is being monitored.

Holter monitoring is one form of long-term monitoring, during which a person wears a 12-lead ECG recording device for 24 hours. During this time, the person also keeps a diary of his/her activities, which are later correlated with the ECG recording. Holter monitoring is useful for documenting rhythm and conduction abnormalities in persons who have predictable symptoms.

Intermittent ECG recorders are also used in the diagnosis of dysrhythmias and conduction defects. With intermittent ECG recording, a monitoring lead ECG recording device, which either records or transmits by telephone the ECG to a recording machine, is worn. Some of these recorders have a patient-activated memory component to record the electrical events that precede the onset of symptoms. These types of ECG recordings are useful in persons who have very transient and unpredictable symptoms.

The exercise stress test is useful in determining exercise-induced disorders of cardiac rhythm, particularly premature ventricular contractions (PVCs), because these dysrhythmias indicate a poorer prognosis in persons with known coronary disease and recent myocardial infarction. Bicycle and treadmill exercise are equally effective in detecting exercise-induced PVCs.

An electrophysiology study involves the passage of flexible catheters into the great vessels and chambers of the heart. Two or more multipolar catheters are inserted into the femoral, subclavian, or antecubital veins and positioned with fluoroscopy into the right atrium and right ventricle. Multipolar catheters can also be inserted into the left heart chambers by way of a peripheral artery. The catheter tips are positioned at several different sites, and the endocardium is stimulated. Multiple atrial, AV junctional, and ventricular electrocardiograms are recorded during the electrical stimulation. The catheters may also be used to pace the heart as part of the test. Overdrive pacing, cardioversion, or defibrillation may be necessary during the test to terminate tachycardia induced during the stimulation procedures. Electrophysiology tests may be done to identify the location of additional electrical pathways between the ventricles and atrial or ventricular tissue sites in which tachycardias originate. These tests may also be done repeatedly to test patient responses to drugs, devices such as implantable defibrillators, and surgical interventions used in treatment of dysrhythmias.

The treatment of cardiac rhythm or conduction disorders is directed toward controlling the dysrhythmia, correcting the cause, and preventing more serious or fatal dysrhythmias. Correction may involve simply adjusting an electrolyte disturbance or withholding a medication such as digitalis. Preventing more serious dysrhythmias often involves drug therapy, electrical stimulation, or surgical intervention.

Antidysrhythmic drugs act by modifying disordered formation and conduction of impulses that induce cardiac muscle contraction. These drugs are currently classified into four groups. Table 21-3 lists the drugs in each of these four classes and summarizes their actions on cardiac action potentials and the ECG. The cardiac glycosides (*e.g.,* digitalis drugs) are also used in the management of dysrhythmias such as atrial tachycardia, flutter and fibrillation.

Correction of conduction defects, bradycardias, and tachycardias can involve the use of an electronic pacemaker, cardioversion, or defibrillation. Electrical interventions can be used in both emergency and elective situations. A pacemaker is an electronic device that delivers an electrical stimulus to the heart. It is used to initiate heart beats in situations when the normal pacemaker of the heart is defective or in complete heart block in which the rate of cardiac contraction and consequent cardiac output is inadequate to perfuse vital tissues. A pacemaker may be used as a temporary or a permanent measure. Internal temporary pacing involves the passage, under fluoroscopic or electrocardiographic direction, of a venous catheter with electrodes on its tip into the right atrium or ventricle, where it is wedged against the endocardium. External temporary pacing involves the placement of large patch electrodes on the chest wall. Permanent pacing requires the direct insertion of pacemaker electrodes into the epicardium, or the transvenous insertion into the apex of the right ventricle, where the electrode comes in contact with the endocardium.

Defibrillation or DC cardioversion is the only reliable method for treating ventricular fibrillation and is one of the effective methods of treating ventricular tachycardias as well. Defibrillation or DC cardioversion can be delivered externally through large patch electrodes on the chest or internally through small patch electrodes sewn into the epicardium and/or transvenous wires placed in the right ventricle. The electric current from the defibrillator or cardioverter interrupts the disorganized impulses, allowing the SA node to regain control of the heart.

Surgical interventions such as coronary bypass surgery, ventriculotomy, endocardial resection, and cryoablation may be used to improve myocardial oxygenation, remove dysrhythmogenic foci, or alter electrical conduction pathways. Coronary bypass surgery improves myocardial oxygenation. Ventriculotomy involves removal of aneurysm tissue and resuturing of the myocardial walls to eliminate the paradoxical ventricular movement and to eliminate foci of dysrhythmias. In endocardial resection, endocardial tissue that has been identified as dysrhythmogenic through use of diagnostic tests is peeled away. Cryoablation causes freezing and necrosis of defective or aberrant electrical conduction pathways. The tech-

Table 21–3. Antidysrythmic drugs and their electrophysiologic properties

Class name	Class	Drug	Action on cardiac action potential*	Action on ECG
Fast sodium-channel blocking agents	IA	Quinidine Procainamide (Pronestyl) Disopyramide (Norpace) Propafenone (Rythmonorm)	Depress phase 4 (decrease automaticity) Moderately depress phase 0 (decrease conductivity) Moderately prolong phase 3 (prolong repolarization)	Little effect on QRS interval; prolongation of QT interval
	IB	Lidocaine (Xylocaine) Phenytoin (Dilantin) Tocainide (Tonocard) Mexiletine (Mexitil) Aprindine (Fibocil) Cibenzoline Moricizine (Ethmozine)	Depress phase 4 (depress automaticity) Little effect on conductivity Decrease phase 2 (decrease refractoriness) Decrease phase 3 (shorten repolarization)	No effect on QRS or QT intervals
	IC	Flecainide (Tambocar) Encainide (Enkaid) Lorcainide	Markedly depress phase 0 (decrease conductivity) Little effect on refractoriness Little effect on repolarization	Prolong QRS interval; no effect on QT interval
Beta-blocking drugs	II	Propranolol (Inderal) Nadolol (Corgard) Atenolol (Tenormin) Timolol (Blocadren, Timoptic) Acebutolol (Sectral) Metoprolol (Lopressor) Pindolol (Visken)	Depress phase 4 (decrease automaticity) Decrease heart rate and myocardial contractility Blunt catecholamine effect	No effect on QRS or QT interval
Action potential extending drugs	III	Amiodarone (Cordarone) Bretylium (Bretylol) Sotalol	Prolong phase 3 (prolong repolarization)	Mild prolongation of QRS interval; marked prolongation of QT interval
Slow calcium-channel blocking agents	IV	Verapamil (Calan, Isoptin) Diltiazem (Cardizem) Nifedipine (Procardia) Bepridil	Depress phase 4 Lengthen phases 1 and 2	No effect on QRS or QT intervals

* The phases of the cardiac action potential are illustrated in Figure 20-12.
(Reprinted from Burke LJ, Norris SO: Nursing Care of the Patient with Recurrent Dysrhythmias. In Kern LS (ed): Cardiac Critical Care Nursing, p. 165, with permission of Aspen Publishers, Inc., © 1988)

nique is used to treat recurrent life-threatening supraventricular or ventricular tachycardias. Other surgical techniques including transvenous electrocoagulation and laser ablation are under investigation as potential treatment interventions for recurrent tachycardias.

In summary, disorders of cardiac rhythm arise as the result of disturbances in impulse generation or conduction of impulses in the heart. Cardiac dysrhythmias are not necessarily pathologic—they occur in healthy as well as diseased hearts. Sinus dysrhythmias have their origin in the SA node. They include sinus bradycardia (heart rate less than 60 beats/minute); sinus tachycardia (heart rate 100–160 beats/minute); sinus dysrhythmia, in which the heart rate speeds up and slows down; sinus arrest, in which there are prolonged periods of asystole; and the sick sinus syndrome, a condition characterized by periods of bradycardia alternating with tachycardia. Atrial dysrhythmias arise from alterations in impulse generation that occur within the conduction pathways or muscle of the atria. They include atrial premature contractions, atrial flutter (atrial depolarization rate of 160–350 beats/minute), and atrial fibrillation (atrial depolarization rate in excess of 350 beats/minute). Atrial dysrhythmias often go unnoticed unless they are transmitted to the ventricles. Alterations in the conduction of impulses through the AV node lead to disturbances in the transmission of impulses from the atria to the ventricles. There can be a delay in transmission (first-degree heart block), failure to conduct one or more impulses (second-degree heart block), or complete failure to conduct impulses between the atria and ventricles (third-degree heart block). Conduction disorders of the bundle of His, called bundle branch blocks, cause a widening of and changes in the configuration of the QRS complex of the ECG. Because of their potential for interfering with the pumping action of the heart, dysrhythmias arising in the ventricles are usually considered more serious than those arising in the atria. Premature ventricular contraction (PVC) is caused by a ventricular ectopic pacemaker. Ventricular tachycardia is characterized by a ventricular rate of 160 beats/minute to 250 beats/minute. Ventricular fibrillation (ventricular rate in excess of 350 beats/minute) is a fatal dysrhythmia unless it is successfully treated with defibrillation.

Diseases of the myocardium

The myocardium, which is made up of thick muscular columns, lies between the endocardium and the epicardium. It is responsible for the pumping action of the heart. This section discusses two diseases of the myocardium—myocarditis and cardiomypathies.

Myocarditis

Myocarditis is an acute inflammation of the myocardium. It can occur as a primary disease or as a secondary disorder as in rheumatic fever. Viral myocarditis accounts for approximately 80% of cases and is the one that most often presents as a primary infection.[37] Bacterial myocarditis is relatively rare in relation to viral forms of the disease, the most common forms being associated with rheumatic fever and diphtheria toxins. Other causes of myocarditis are radiation therapy, hypersensitivity reactions, and any chemical or physical agent that induces acute myocardial necrosis and secondary inflammatory changes.

Etiology and manifestations

Viral myocarditis is most often caused by the coxsackie group of viruses, principally coxsackie B.[2] Viral infections, particularly of coxsackie group B origin, are also associated with dilated cardiomyopathies. The question has arisen as to whether such infections may initiate immunologic damage to the myocardium, possibly involving antimyocardial antibodies, that leads to changes later identified as cardiomyopathy.

Clinical manifestations of myocarditis vary from an absence of symptoms to profound heart failure or sudden death. When coxsackie myocarditis occurs in children or young adults, it is often symptomatic. It affects twice as many males as females.[2] Acute symptomatic myocarditis often presents as malaise, dyspnea, low-grade fever, and a tachycardia that is more pronounced than would be expected with the level of fever that is present. Often there is a history of an upper respiratory tract infection, followed by a latent period of several days. In young adults, sudden death may occasionally be caused by viral myocarditis. Among adults, the disorder is more likely to be self-limited and benign. The ECG changes of acute myocarditis include ECG conduction disturbances such as ventricular dysrhythmias, AV junctional block, ST-segment elevation, T-wave inversion, and transient Q waves. Clinical symptoms include a flulike syndrome, fever, leukocytosis, and elevations in serum enzymes (SGOT, SGPT, and LDH). Cardiac auscultation may reveal an S_3 ventricular gallop rhythm and a transient pericardial or pleurocardial rub. In most cases, myocarditis is transient and symptoms subside in 1 to 2 months. With advanced disease, there is congestive heart failure involving both ventricles.

Diagnosis and treatment

Diagnosis of myocarditis involves viral antigen detection, serologic testing, and myocardial biopsy. Detection of the virus antigen or IgM antibody response has been quite successful. Serologic testing allows determination of the stage of viral infection. IgG antibody titers peak after the first month of the disease. Myofibril degeneration and increased interstitial lymphocytes confirm active inflammatory disease on myocardial biopsy.

Current treatment focuses on symptom management and immunosuppressive therapy. Immunosuppressive therapy has been reported to be successful in resolving inflammation as shown by repeated biopsies. Persons with chronic myocarditis show much greater improvement than those who have an acute form of the disease.

Cardiomyopathies

The cardiomyopathies are a group of disorders that affect the heart muscle. They can develop as either primary or secondary disorders. The primary cardiomyopathies, which are discussed in this chapter, are heart muscle diseases of unknown cause. Secondary cardiomyopathies are conditions in which the cardiac abnormality is due to another cardiovascular disease, such as myocardial infarction. In the United States, an estimated 1% of cardiac deaths can be attributed to primary cardiomyopathies. The onset of the primary cardiomyopathies is often silent, and the symptoms do not occur until the disease is well advanced. The diagnosis is suspected when a young, previously healthy normotensive individual develops cardiomegaly and heart failure.

The International Society and Federation of Cardiology/World Health Organization has categorized the primary cardiomyopathies into three groups: (1) dilated, (2) hypertrophic, and (3) restrictive cardiomyopathies (Figure 21-17).[38]

Dilated cardiomyopathies

The dilated, or congestive, cardiomyopathies are recognized by the dilatation of the heart chambers (often all four) and the impaired pumping function of the ventricles, with increases in both end-systolic and end-diastolic volumes of the heart. There is a profound reduction in the left ventricular ejection fraction (the ratio of stroke volume to end-diastolic volume) to 40% or less, compared with a normal value of about 67%. Microscopically, there is evidence of scarring and atrophy of myocardial cells. The ventricular wall is usually thickened, and mural thrombi are common, most often in the left ventricle but also in the right ventricle or in either atrium.

The cause of dilated cardiomyopathy is unknown. The disease itself is probably the result of several factors acting in concert, in a susceptible person, with alcohol, viral infections, the puerperium,

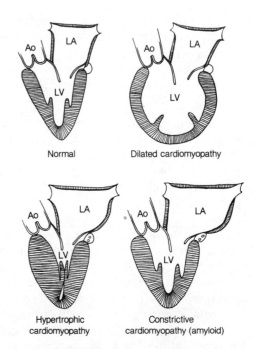

Figure 21-17 The various types of cardiomyopathies compared to the normal heart. *(Roberts WC, Ferrans VJ: Pathologic anatomy of the cardiomyopathies. Hum Pathol 6:289, 1975)*

and other causes acting as risk factors. In one study, 20% of persons with the disorder had a history of excessive alcohol consumption, 20% had had a severe influenza-like syndrome within 60 days of the appearance of the cardiac manifestations, and another 8% had a previous history of rheumatic fever without valvular involvement.[39]

There is considerable evidence that acute alcohol consumption reduces cardiac contractility and can produce dysrhythmias and conduction disorders. In the heart, the presence of alcohol or its metabolite, acetaldehyde, interferes with a number of cellular functions that involve the transport and binding of calcium. With chronic alcohol consumption, the toxic effects of alcohol on the myocardium can persist after the alcohol has been metabolized.

Although it is rare, congestive cardiomyopathy can also develop during the peripartum period. Most cases of peripartal cardiomyopathy have their onset 1 to 6 weeks after delivery, but a few women begin to develop symptoms during the last month of pregnancy.[40] The incidence of peripartal cardiomyopathy is significantly higher in women over 30 years of age, in a third or subsequent pregnancy, and in the presence of twins or toxemia.[41] The cause of the condition is unknown.

There are two possible outcomes of peripartal cardiomyopathy. In approximately half of the cases, the heart returns to normal within 6 months and the chances for long-term survival are good. In these women, heart failure returns only during subsequent pregnancies. In the other half of the cases, the cardiomegaly persists, and the prognosis is poor and death is very probable if another pregnancy occurs.[40]

In dilated cardiomyopathy, heart failure occurs because impairment of left ventricular ejection requires that the left ventricle dilate (Starling mechanism) to compensate for the fall in stroke volume that would otherwise occur. Dilation of the heart and pump failure may be present for years before symptoms are noted. However, once symptoms have developed, the course of the disorder is distinguished by a propensity for development of heart failure, embolism, and poor prognosis. Three-fourths of persons will die in 4 years to 5 years from the time of diagnosis. One-fourth, however, will do well for some unexplained reason.[38] The most striking symptoms are both right- and left-sided heart failure, dyspnea on exertion, paroxysmal nocturnal dyspnea, orthopnea, weakness, fatigue, ascites, and peripheral edema. On physical examination, an enlarged apical beat with the presence of a third and fourth heart sound, and a murmur associated with regurgitation of one or both atrioventricular valves are frequently found. The systolic pressure is either normal or low, and the peripheral pulses are often of low amplitude. Pulsus alternans, in which the pulse regularly alternates between weaker and stronger, may be present. Basilar rales are frequently present. Sinus tachycardia, atrial fibrillation, and complex ventricular dysrhythmias are common.

The treatment of dilated cardiomyopathy is directed toward relieving the symptoms of heart failure; relieving the workload of the heart; or, in select cases, heart transplantation (see Chapter 23). Digoxin, diuretics, and afterload-reducing drugs are used to improve myocardial contractility and decrease left-ventricular filling pressures. Avoidance of myocardial depressants, including alcohol, and pacing rest with asymptomatic levels of exercise or activity are imperative.

Hypertrophic cardiomyopathies

Hypertrophic cardiomyopathy is characterized by a small left-ventricular volume with hypertrophy of ventricular muscle mass. Although the hypertrophy may be symmetric, the involvement of the ventricular septum is often disproportionate in some patients, producing obstruction of the left-ventricular outflow channel. Synonyms for this disorder include idiopathic hypertrophic subaortic stenosis (IHSS) and asymmetric septal hypertrophy (ASH).

A distinctive finding in hypertrophic cardiomyopathy is the microscopic presence of myofibril disarray. Instead of the normal parallel arrangement of myofibrils, the myofibrils branch off at random angles, sometimes at right angles to an adjacent fiber with which they may connect. Small bundles of fibers may course haphazardly through normally arranged muscle fibers.[2] It is thought that the presence of these disordered fibers may produce abnormal movements of the ventricles with uncoordinated contraction and impaired relaxation.[42]

The cause of hypertrophic cardiomyopathy is unknown. Often it is of familial origin, the disorder being inherited as an autosomal dominant trait.

The manifestations of hypertrophic cardiomyopathy are variable; for reasons that are unclear, some persons with the disorder remain asymptomatic, whereas others become incapacitated. Symptomatic hypertrophic cardiomyopathy is commonly a disease of young adulthood. The most common symptom is dyspnea associated with an elevation in left-ventricular diastolic pressure resulting from impaired ventricular filling and increased wall stiffness secondary to ventricular hypertrophy.[43] Because of the obstruction to outflow from the left ventricle, the systolic pressure difference between the left ventricle and the aorta increases. Chest pain, fatigue, and syncope are also common and become worse during exertion. Dysrhythmias, both atrial and ventricular, may occur. Sudden death can occur and is especially common in certain families.

The treatment of hypertrophic cardiomyopathy includes medical and surgical management. The goal of medical management is to relieve the symptoms by lessening the pressure difference between the left ventricle and the aorta, thereby improving cardiac output. Beta-adrenergic receptor blocking drugs may be used in persons with chest pain, dysrhythmias, or dyspnea. These drugs reduce the heart rate and myocardial contractility, allowing more time for ventricular filling and reduction of ventricular stiffness. Recent use of the calcium-channel blocking drug verapamil has proved useful in relieving the symptoms of dyspnea, chest pain, and syncope.[44] Increased calcium uptake and increased intracellular calcium content are associated with an increased contractile state, a characteristic finding in persons with hypertrophic cardiomyopathy. Disopyramide and amiodarone are effective in controlling the supraventricular and complex ventricular tachydysrhythmias associated with hypertrophic cardiomyopathies. Both drugs may also reduce the subaortic gradient due to their negative inotropic effects.[44] Surgical treatment may be used if severe symptoms persist despite medical treatment. It involves incision of the septum (myotomy) with or without the removal of part of the tissue (myectomy) and it is accompanied by all of the risks of open-heart surgery.

Restrictive cardiomyopathies

Of the three categories of cardiomyopathies, the restrictive type is the least common in the Western countries. With this form of cardiomyopathy, ventricular filling is restricted due to excessive rigidity of the ventricular walls, while the contractile properties of the heart remain relatively normal. The most common causes of restrictive cardiomyopathy are endocardial fibroelastosis and infiltrations, such as amyloidosis. Although the cause of fibroelastosis is unknown, about one-third of the cases are associated with congenital heart defects. The extent of the manifestations is dependent on the extent of the involvement. When there are only focal lesions, there may be few effects and normal longevity. On the other hand, when the lesions are diffuse, cardiac decompensation and death may result. The manifestations of restrictive cardiomyopathy resemble those of constrictive pericarditis.

In summary, the myocardium contains the muscle fibers of the heart. Myocarditis is an acute inflammation of the myocardium, most often of viral origin. The manifestations of viral myocarditis range from absence of symptoms to sudden death. Most often the disease is benign and self limiting. The cardiomyopathies represent disorders of the heart muscle. Cardiomyopathies may present as primary or secondary disorders. Secondary cardiomyopathies are conditions in which damage to the cardiac muscle occurs as the result of another disease process, such as myocardial infarction. There are three main types of primary cardiomyopathies: (1) dilated or congestive cardiomyopathy, in which fibrosis and atrophy of myocardial cells with dilatation of all four heart chambers occur; (2) hypertrophic cardiomyopathy, which is characterized by a disproportionate involvement of the ventricular septum, causing obstruction of the left-ventricular outflow channel, and a disarray in the organization of myocardial fibers and ventricular hypertrophy; and (3) restrictive cardiomyopathy, in which there is excessive rigidity of the ventricular wall. The cause of the primary cardiomyopathies is largely unknown. The disease is suspected when a young, previously healthy individual develops cardiomegaly and heart failure.

Disorders of the endocardium

The endocardium has a smooth surface that interfaces with blood moving through the heart. The endocardium covers the septum, the papillary muscles, the latticework of muscular columns called the trabeculae carneae, and the valvular structures. The smoothness of this layer is an essential characteristic in preventing platelet aggregation and clot formation. This section discusses two diseases of the endocardium, rheumatic fever and endocarditis.

Rheumatic fever

Rheumatic fever is an important disease because of its potential for causing chronic heart problems. It currently affects 2,150,000 adults and children in the United States. Although it is generally a preventable disease, the death rate from rheumatic fever in 1985 was 6,200.[1] Although, rheumatic fever is more prevalent in groups subjected to poor nutrition, crowded living conditions, and inadequate health care, there has been a recent resurgence of rheumatic fever in both underprivileged and middle class families. The recent outbreaks are due to throat infections caused by a new strain of group A beta-hemolytic streptococcus.

Age plays an important role in the epidemiology of rheumatic fever. It is most prevalent in school-age children. The incidence of acute rheumatic fever peaks between ages 5 and 15 years.[2]

Etiology and manifestations

Rheumatic fever is associated with infection due to group A beta-hemolytic streptococcus and usually follows an inciting pharyngeal infection by 1 to 4 weeks. It is of particular significance that rheumatic fever and its cardiac complications can be prevented by antibiotic treatment of the initial streptococcal infection.

The pathogenesis of the disease is unclear, and why only 3% of persons with uncomplicated streptococcal infections develop rheumatic fever remains to be answered. The timeframe for development of symptoms in relation to the sore throat, as well as the presence of antibodies to the streptococcus organism, strongly suggests an immunologic origin. Like other immunologic phenomena, rheumatic fever requires an initial sensitizing exposure to the offending (streptococcus) agent, and the risk of recurrence is high following each subsequent exposure. Rheumatic fever can present as an acute, recurrent, or chronic disorder.

The acute stage includes a history of an initiating streptococcal infection and subsequent involvement of the mesenchymal connective tissue of the heart, blood vessels, joints, and subcutaneous tissues. Common to all is the presence of a lesion called the *Aschoff body*. The Aschoff body is a localized area of tissue necrosis containing fibrinoid material. The recurrent phase usually involves extension of the cardiac effects of the disease. The chronic problems are associated with valvular defects due to the disease.

The child with rheumatic fever usually has

had a history of sore throat, headache, fever, abdominal pain, nausea and vomiting, swollen glands (usually at the angle of the jaw), and other signs of a streptococcal infection. Throat cultures taken at the time of the acute infection are positive for streptococcus. The sedimentation rate, C-reactive protein, and white blood cell count are usually elevated at the time that heart or joint manifestations begin to appear. A high or rising antistreptolysin O titer is also suggestive of rheumatic fever. Streptolysin O is a hemolytic factor produced by most strains of group A beta-hemolytic streptococci; antistreptolysin O (ASO) is an antibody against the hemolytic factor produced by the streptococci. Other signs and symptoms associated with an acute episode of rheumatic fever are related to the structures involved in the disease process.

Rheumatic fever can affect any of the three layers of the heart: pericardium, myocardium, and endocardium. Usually all three layers are involved. Rheumatic pericarditis causes the production of a fibrinous or serofibrinous exudate. For the most part, myocardial changes are reversible and produce minimal changes in cardiac function. It is the involvement of the endocardium and valvular structures that produces the permanent and disabling effects of the disease. Although any of the four valves can be involved, the mitral and aortic valves are affected most often. During the acute inflammatory stage of the disease, the valvular structures become reddened and swollen; small vegetative lesions develop on the valve leaflets. Gradually, the acute inflammatory changes proceed to fibrous scar tissue development, which tends to contract and cause deformity of the valve leaflets and shortening of the chordae tendineae. In some cases, the edges or commissures of the leaflets fuse together as healing occurs.

The manifestations of rheumatic carditis include a heart murmur in a child without a previous history of rheumatic fever, change in the character of a murmur in a person with a previous history of the disease, cardiomegaly or enlargement of the heart, friction rub or other signs of pericarditis, and congestive heart failure in a child without discernible cause.[45]

Polyarthritis, although not a cause of permanent disability, is the most common finding in rheumatic fever. The inflammatory process affects the synovial membrane of the joint, causing swelling, heat, redness, pain, tenderness, and limitation of motion. The arthritis is almost always migratory, affecting one joint and then moving to another. The joints most frequently affected are the larger ones, particularly the knees, ankles, elbows, and wrists.

The *skin lesions* seen in rheumatic fever are of two types, subcutaneous nodules and erythema marginatum. The *subcutaneous nodules* range in size from 1 cm to 4 cm; they are hard, painless, and freely movable, and usually overlie the extensor muscles of the wrist, elbow, ankle, and knee joints. *Erythema marginatum* lesions are maplike macular areas, seen most commonly on the trunk or inner aspects of the upper arm and thigh. Skin lesions are present only in about 10% of patients who have rheumatic fever; they are transitory and disappear during the course of the disease.

Chorea (Sydenham's chorea), sometimes called St. Vitus' dance, is the major central nervous system manifestation. It is seen most frequently in girls. Typically, there is an insidious onset of irritability and other behavior problems. The child is often fidgety, cries easily, begins to walk clumsily, and tends to drop things. The choreic movements are spontaneous, rapid, purposeless jerking movements, which tend to interfere with voluntary activities. Facial grimaces are common, and even speech may be affected. Fortunately, the chorea is self-limiting, usually running its course within a matter of weeks or months.

Recurrent nosebleeds (epistaxis) are thought to be a subclinical manifestation of rheumatic fever.

Diagnosis and treatment

The diagnosis of rheumatic fever is based on clinical and laboratory findings. The Jones Criteria for guidance in diagnosis of rheumatic fever were initially proposed in 1955 and revised in 1965 by a committee of the American Heart Association. The criteria were developed because no single laboratory test, sign, or symptom is pathognomonic of the disease, although several combinations of them are diagnostic. The criteria group the signs and symptoms into major and minor categories. The presence of two major signs or one major and two minor signs indicates a high probability of the presence of rheumatic fever, if supported by a history of a preceding group A streptococcal infection. The revised criteria are summarized in Chart 21-2.

Treatment is designed to control the acute inflammatory process and to prevent cardiac complications and recurrence of the disease. During the acute phase, prevention of residual cardiac effects is of primary concern. Administration of antibiotics and anti-inflammatory drugs and selective restriction of physical activities are usually carried out during the acute stage of illness. Secondary prevention involves the prophylactic use of penicillin (or another antibiotic in penicillin-sensitive patients) for a period of at least 5 years to prevent recurrence. Penicillin is also the antibiotic of choice for treating the acute illness. Salicylates and corticosteroids are also widely used.

Secondary prevention and compliance with a plan for prophylactic administration of penicillin require that the patient and the family understand the rationale for such measures as well as the measures

Chart 21–2: Jones criteria (revised) for guidance in diagnosis of rheumatic fever*

Major manifestations	Minor manifestations
Carditis	History of previous rheumatic
Polyarthritis	fever or rheumatic heart
Chorea	disease
Erythema marginatum	Arthralgia
Subcutaneous nodules	Fever
	Laboratory findings
	Acute phase reactants
	Erythrocyte sedimentation
	rate, C-reactive protein,
	leukocytosis
	Prolonged PR interval on ECG

Supporting evidence of streptococcal infection

Increased titer of antistreptolysin antibodies, ASO (antistreptolysin O), others
Positive throat culture for group A streptococcus
Recent scarlet fever

* The presence of two major criteria, or of one major and two minor criteria, indicates a high probability of acute rheumatic fever, if supported by evidence of preceding group A streptococcal infection.
(Reprinted with permission. American Heart Association, 1982)[45]

themselves. Patients also need to be instructed to report possible streptococcal infections to their physician. They should be instructed to inform their dentist about the disease so that they can be adequately protected during dental procedures that might traumatize the oral mucosa.

Bacterial endocarditis

Etiology and manifestations

The significance of bacterial endocarditis lies in its tendency to develop in persons with a damaged heart. It can be caused by almost any pathogen, the most common being *Streptococcus viridans*. Staphylococci, gram-negative bacteria, and fungi have also been isolated as causes of endocarditis.

Two predisposing factors contribute to the development of endocarditis—a *damaged endocardial surface* and a *portal of entry* by which the organism gains access to the bloodstream. The presence of valvular disease, rheumatic heart disease, or congenital heart defects provides an environment conducive to bacterial growth. The second factor, bacteremia, may emerge in the course of seemingly minor health problems, such as an upper respiratory tract infection, a skin lesion, or a dental procedure. Simple gum massage or an innocuous oral lesion may afford the patho-

genic bacteria access to the bloodstream. Bacterial endocarditis is reported to be a significant potential disease in narcotic addicts who "mainline," and it is a potential complication in patients with intravascular catheters that remain in place for long periods of time.

The vegetative lesion characteristic of bacterial endocarditis consists of a collection of pathogens and cellular debris enmeshed in the fibrin strands of clotted blood. These lesions may be singular or multiple, may reach a size of several centimeters, and are usually found loosely attached to the free edges of the valve surface. The loose organization of the lesion permits the organisms to disseminate, and fragments are carried by the blood to give rise to small hemorrhages, abscesses, and infarcted areas in other parts of the body—kidneys, spleen, brain, and joints.

Bacterial endocarditis may occur in an acute or subacute form. *Acute bacterial endocarditis* is thought to affect primarily persons with normal hearts, whereas *subacute bacterial endocarditis* (SBE) is seen most frequently in patients with damaged hearts. The signs and symptoms include fever, change in the character of an existing heart murmur, and evidence of embolic distribution of the vegetative lesions. In the acute form, the fever is usually spiking and accompanied by chills. In the subacute form, the fever is usually low grade and of gradual onset and is frequently accompanied by other systemic signs of inflammation such as anorexia, malaise, and lethargy. Small petechial hemorrhages frequently result when emboli lodge in the small vessels of the skin, nailbeds, and mucous membranes.

Diagnosis and treatment

The blood culture is the most significant diagnostic aid in bacterial endocarditis. Usually a series of three to six cultures are obtained during a 36- to 48-hour period to ensure adequate sampling.

The focus of treatment is toward identifying and destroying the causative organism, minimizing the residual cardiac effects, and treating the pathology induced by the emboli. The blood cultures usually identify the organism so its sensitivity to antibiotics can be assessed. An appropriate antibiotic is prescribed to eradicate the pathogen. Surgery is indicated in the presence of moderate to severe heart failure, progressive renal failure, significant emboli, dysrhythmias, or left-sided endocarditis. This active treatment stands in contrast to preantibiotic days when bacterial endocarditis often was fatal. Of even greater importance is prevention in persons known to be at risk. Prevention can be largely accomplished through prophylactic administration of an antibiotic prior to dental and other procedures that may cause bacteremia.

In summary, the endocardium lines the heart and covers the valvular structure; it provides a smooth surface that interfaces with the blood. Rheumatic fever, which is associated with an antecedent group A streptococcal infection, is an important cause of heart disease. Its most serious and disabling effects result from involvement of the heart valves. Because there is no single laboratory test, sign, or symptom that is pathognomonic of acute rheumatic fever, the Jones Criteria are used to establish the diagnosis during the acute stage of the disease. Bacterial endocarditis involves the invasion of the endocardium by pathogens that produce vegetative lesions of the endocardial surface. The loose organization of these lesions permits the organisms and fragments of the lesions to be disseminated throughout the systemic circulation. It can be caused by a number of organisms. Two predisposing factors contribute to the development of endocarditis: (1) a damaged endocardium and (2) a portal of entry through which the organisms gain access to the bloodstream.

Valvular heart disease

Dysfunction of the heart valves can result from a number of disorders, including congenital defects, trauma, ischemic damage, degenerative changes, and inflammation. Rheumatic endocarditis is the most common cause. Its inflammatory changes cause scar tissue to form on the valve leaflets and the chordae tendineae with a subsequent shortening of the chordae and deformation of the valve structure. Two types of mechanical disruptions may occur in valvular disease: (1) narrowing or stenosis of the valve opening or (2) failure of a valve to close completely (Figure 21-18). Although any of the four heart valves can become diseased, the most commonly affected are the mitral and aortic valves.

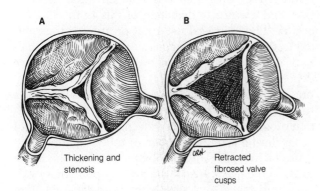

Figure 21-18 Disease of the aortic valve as viewed from the aorta; (**A**) Stenosis of the valve opening and (**B**) an incompetent or regurgitant valve that is unable to close completely.

Hemodynamic derangements

Valvular disease can be either stenotic (failure to open completely) or regurgitant (failure to close completely), but often there is a combination of stenotic and regurgitant effects. The influence of valvular disease on cardiac function is related to alterations in blood flow and increased work demands on the heart.

Stenosis causes a decrease in flow through the valve, with an increased work demand on the heart chamber in front of the diseased valve. In mitral stenosis, for example, the left atrium becomes distended and the work output required of this chamber is increased. As the condition advances, blood return from the lungs is impeded, and the pulmonary circulation becomes congested. Blood flow through a normal valve can increase to five to seven times the resting value; consequently, valvular stenosis must be severe before it causes life-threatening problems.[45] The first evidence of symptoms usually is noted during situations of increased flow such as exercise.

An incompetent (regurgitant) valve permits blood flow to continue while the valve is closed, flowing into the left ventricle during diastole when the aortic valve is affected, and into the left atrium during systole when the mitral valve is diseased. With an incompetent valve, the work demands of both the heart chamber in front and that in back of the affected valve are increased. In mitral regurgitation, the left atrium is presented with an increased volume and the left ventricle with a bidirectional flow pattern such that blood is propelled into both the left atrium and the aorta during systole.

Types of valvular disorders

Aortic valve defects

The orifices of the coronary arteries are strategically located in the aorta, just distal to the aortic valve leaflets (Figure 21-19). In aortic stenosis, the velocity of flow through the narrowed valve orifice is increased at the expense of the lateral pressure needed to perfuse the coronary arteries. In aortic regurgitation, failure of aortic valve closure during diastole causes diastolic pressure to fall; this decreases the pressure needed to perfuse the coronary arteries.

Aortic valve stenosis. *Aortic stenosis* causes resistance to ejection of blood into the aorta, so the work demands on the left ventricle are increased and the volume of blood ejected into the systemic circulation is decreased. The most common causes of aortic stenosis are rheumatic fever and congenital heart defects. In the elderly, it may be related to degenerative atherosclerotic changes of the valve leaflets.

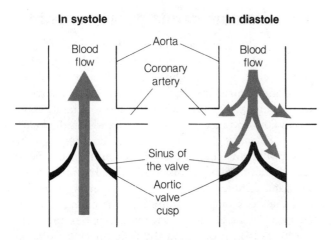

Figure 21-19 Location of the orifices for the coronary arteries and the direction of blood flow during systole and diastole.

Obstruction to aortic outflow causes a decrease in stroke volume, in which systolic blood pressure and pulse pressure are reduced. It takes a longer time for the heart to eject blood; the heart rate is often slow and the pulse is of low amplitude. Resistance to flow through the aortic valve gives rise to an auscultatory murmur in systole.

The onset of signs and symptoms depends, to a large extent, on the person's activity level; in one who leads a sedentary life, the disease may be far advanced before symptoms are noted. Exertional dyspnea is a common presenting symptom. It is characterized by vertigo and syncope when the stroke volume falls to levels insufficient for cerebral needs. Also, the combination of increased work demands on the hypertrophied left ventricle and decreased perfusion of the coronary vessels may cause angina.

Aortic valve regurgitation. An *incompetent aortic valve* allows blood to return to the left ventricle during diastole. This defect may result from conditions that cause scarring of the valve leaflets or from enlargement of the valve orifice to the extent that the valve leaflets no longer meet. Rheumatic fever ranks first on the list of causes of aortic regurgitation.

A widening of the pulse pressure, the result of an increased systolic pressure and decreased diastolic pressure, is characteristic of aortic regurgitation. Widening of the pulse pressure has two underlying mechanisms: first, there is an increase in the stroke volume (and systolic blood pressure) as the left ventricle ejects blood entering from the lungs, as well as the blood that has leaked back across the aortic valve into the ventricle during diastole; second, because the aortic valve fails to close completely, diastolic pressure cannot be maintained. The left ventricle hypertrophies because of the increased volume load on this chamber.

Turbulence of flow across the aortic valve during diastole produces a high-pitched or blowing type of murmur.

The large stroke volume, wide pulse pressure, and rapid runoff of blood from the aorta produce characteristic changes in the peripheral pulses: prominent carotid pulsations in the neck, throbbing peripheral pulses, and a left-ventricular impulse that causes the chest to move with each beat. The term *water-hammer* pulse is often used to describe the hyperkinetic peripheral pulse found in persons with aortic regurgitation.

Symptoms of aortic regurgitation are those associated with heart failure: exertional dyspnea, dizziness, pulmonary edema, and orthopnea. Angina follows the impaired coronary perfusion due to a low diastolic pressure and the increased work demands on the left ventricle. Patients with significant aortic regurgitation complain of throbbing of the chest due to the hyperdynamic left ventricle.

Mitral valve defects

The mitral valve controls the directional flow of blood between the left atrium and the left ventricle. The cusps of the atrioventricular valves are thinner than those of the semilunar valves; they are anchored to the papillary muscles by the chordae tendineae. During much of systole, the mitral valve is subjected to the high pressure generated by the left ventricle as it pumps blood into the systemic circulation, and the chordae tendineae prevent the eversion of the valve leaflets into the left atrium.

Mitral valve stenosis. Mitral valve stenosis is characterized by fibrous replacement of valvular tissue, along with stiffness and fusion of valve commissures. Involvement of the chordae tendineae causes shortening, which pulls the valvular structures more deeply into the ventricles. As the impediment to flow through the valve increases, the left atrial pressure rises and eventually dilatation of this heart chamber occurs. The increased left atrial pressure is transmitted to the pulmonary venous system, causing pulmonary congestion. The rate of flow across the valve depends on the size of the valve orifice, the driving pressure (atrial minus ventricular pressure), and the time available for flow during diastole. As the condition progresses, symptoms of decreased cardiac output occur during extreme exertion or other situations that cause tachycardia and thereby reduce diastolic filling time. In the late stages of the disease, pulmonary vascular resistance increases with the development of pulmonary hypertension; this increases the arterial pressure against which the right heart must pump and eventually leads to failure of this side of the heart.

The signs and symptoms of mitral valve stenosis depend on the severity of the obstruction and are generally related to (1) elevation in left atrial pressure and pulmonary congestion, (2) decreased cardiac output due to impaired left-ventricular filling, and (3) left atrial enlargement with development of atrial arrhythmias and mural thrombi. The symptoms are those of pulmonary congestion, including nocturnal paroxysmal dyspnea and orthopnea. Premature atrial beats, paroxysmal atrial tachycardia, and atrial fibrillation may occur as a result of distention of the left atria. Together, the fibrillation and distention predispose to mural thrombus formation, from which systemic emboli may form. Palpitations, chest pain, weakness, and fatigue are common complaints. The murmur of mitral valve stenosis is found during diastole when blood is flowing through the constricted valve orifice; it is characteristically a low-pitched rumbling murmur, best heard at the apex of the heart. The first heart sound is often accentuated and somewhat delayed because of the increased left atrial pressure; an opening snap often precedes the diastolic murmur as a result of the elevation in left atrial pressure.

Mitral valve regurgitation. In addition to rheumatic fever, the causes of mitral regurgitation are rupture of the chordae tendineae, which is commonly caused by bacterial endocarditis, papillary muscle dysfunction, or rupture due to coronary heart disease, and secondary stretching of the valve structures due to dilatation of the left ventricle. With mitral valve insufficiency, blood from the left ventricle is forced back into the left atrium during systole; this blood is then returned to the left ventricle during diastole. With chronic regurgitation, dilatation of the left ventricle occurs as a result of the increased volume and muscle mass needed to eject a much larger stroke volume (the forward stroke volume that is ejected into the aorta and the regurgitant stroke volume that is ejected into the left atrium). As the disorder progresses, left-ventricular function becomes impaired and the left atrial pressure increases with the subsequent development of pulmonary hypertension. The increased volume work associated with mitral regurgitation is relatively well tolerated and persons with the disorder often remain asymptomatic for 10 years to 20 years despite severe regurgitation. A characteristic feature of mitral valve regurgitation is an enlarged left ventricle and a pansystolic or holosystolic (throughout systole) murmur.

Mitral valve prolapse. Mitral valve prolapse, sometimes referred to as the floppy mitral valve syndrome, has been reported to be present in 2.5% of males and 7.6% of females in the general population.[46,47] The disorder is seen three times more frequently in women than men and may have a familial basis. Although the cause of the disorder is unknown, it has been associated with Marfan's syndrome, osteogenesis imperfecta, and other connective tissue disorders, as well as cardiac, hematologic, neuroendocrine, metabolic, and psychologic disorders.

Pathologic findings in mitral valve prolapse include a myxedematous (mucinous) degeneration of the spongiosum, which lies between the collagen and elastic tissue covering the atrial aspect of the valve and the thick layer of connective tissue that provides the main support for the valve, causing a redundancy of valve tissue and ballooning of the valve leaflets into the left atrium during systole when the ventricular pressure is high. It has also been suggested that certain forms of the disorder may arise from disorders of the myocardium that result in abnormal movement of the ventricular wall or papillary muscle; this places undue stress on the mitral valve. In epidemiologic survey studies, the majority of persons with the disorder were unaware that they had it. The most commonly encountered symptoms in the clinical setting are chest pain, weakness, dyspnea, fatigue, anxiety, palpitations, and lightheadedness. The chest pain differs from angina in that it is often prolonged, ill-defined, and not associated with exercise or exertion. The pain has been attributed to ischemia resulting from traction of the prolapsing valve leaflets. It has recently been suggested that the anxiety, palpitations, and dysrhythmias that accompany the disorder may be due to an abnormal function of the autonomic nervous system that accompanies the disorder. Rare cases of sudden death have been reported in persons with mitral valve prolapse, mainly in persons with a family history of similar occurrences.

The disorder is characterized by a spectrum of auscultatory findings, ranging from a silent form to one or more midsystolic clicks followed by a late systolic murmur.[47] A variety of abnormal electrocardiographic changes can occur. Dysrhythmias may be brought out by exercise stress testing or 24-hour ECG monitoring. Echocardiographic studies have become a method for the diagnosis of mitral valve prolapse, and the availability of this technique has undoubtedly contributed to increased recognition of the problem, particularly in its asymptomatic form.

The treatment of mitral valve prolapse focuses on the relief of symptoms and the prevention of complications. The beta-adrenergic blocking drugs have proved useful in treating the autonomic manifestations, chest discomfort, and dysrhythmias that occur in the symptomatic form of the disease. Infective endocarditis is an uncommon complication in patients with a murmur; antibiotic prophylaxis is usually recommended before dental treatments or surgery.

Diagnostic methods

Valvular defects are usually detected through cardiac auscultation. Diagnosis is aided by the use of cardiac auscultation (heart sounds), phonocardiography, echocardiography, and cardiac catheterization.

Heart sounds

Closure of the heart valves produces vibrations of the surrounding heart tissues and blood that can be detected as the audible "lub dup" sounds heard with a stethoscope during cardiac auscultation. There are four heart sounds. The first and second are heard normally in all healthy individuals. The third and fourth heart sounds are not usually heard and may or may not indicate pathology.

The first and second heart sounds represent closure of the AV and the semilunar valves, respectively. The first heart sound (lub), which has a lower pitch and lasts longer (about 0.14 second) than the second sound, marks the onset of systole and the closure of the AV valves. The second heart sound (dup) occurs with the closure of the semilunar valves; it is shorter (0.10 second) and has a higher pitch than the first heart sound. The second heart sound is a composite sound resulting from the closure of both the aortic and the pulmonic valves. Normally, the aortic valve closes slightly before the pulmonic valve, causing a separation of the two components of the second heart sound. During expiration, aortic valve closure precedes pulmonic valve closure by 0.02 second to 0.04 second; during inspiration this difference is increased to 0.04 second to 0.06 second. This is because during inspiration there is an increase in venous return to the right heart, and as a result it takes longer for the right ventricle to empty and for the pulmonic valve to close. At the same time, less blood is returning to the left ventricle, causing the aortic valve to close slightly earlier. An audible widening of the second heart sound that occurs with inspiration is a normal finding. It is often referred to as a physiologic splitting and can be heard only in the left second intercostal space.

The third heart sound is low pitched and occurs during rapid filling of the ventricles early in diastole, about 0.12 second after the second heart sound. It is usually only heard in young individuals or in persons with heart failure. The fourth heart sound is produced by atrial contraction during the last third of diastole; it is audible only in conditions in which resistance to ventricular filling occurs during late diastole. The heart sounds and their relationship to the cardiac cycle are illustrated in Figure 20-13.

The loudness of the first and second heart sounds depends on the rate of change in pressure across the valve. At high heart rates, intraventricular pressures rise rapidly, whereas atrial pressures remain relatively low. As a result, the first heart sound is intensified. The same principle occurs during exercise when the force of ventricular contraction is increased. Conversely, the intensity of the first heart sound is decreased when ventricular contractions are sluggish as a result of a weakened heart muscle. The loudness of the second heart sound is related to the rate of decrease in ventricular pressure at the end of systole. In persons with hypertension, the second heart sound is accentuated because ventricular pressure is high at the time the aortic valve closes, and, therefore, the rate at which ventricular pressure falls is accelerated.

Heart murmurs are caused by abnormal vibrations produced by turbulent blood flow. In the heart, turbulence occurs when the velocity of blood flow is increased, the valve diameter is decreased, or the viscosity of the blood is decreased. For example, very high velocities of flow may be reached when blood is ejected through a narrowed, or stenotic, heart valve. Severe anemia may reduce blood viscosity to the point at which turbulence occurs.

Auscultation to detect murmurs or abnormalities of the heart sounds is a valuable diagnostic procedure. Although auscultation of the heart does not involve the use of expensive equipment, it does require a trained ear and a thorough understanding of the physiologic events associated with valvular function and the cardiac cycle.

Phonocardiography

A permanent recording of the heart sounds can be obtained through use of a recording called a *phonocardiogram*. This is obtained by placing a high fidelity microphone on the chest wall over the heart while a recording is being made. Usually, an electrocardiographic tracing is recorded simultaneously for timing purposes.

Echocardiography

Echocardiography uses ultrasound to record an image of heart structures. An ultrasound signal has a frequency greater than 20,000 Hz (cycles per second) and is inaudible to the human ear. Echocardiography uses ultrasound signals in the range of 2 million Hz to 5 million Hz. The ultrasound signal is reflected (echoes) whenever tissue resistance to the transmission of the sound beam changes. It is possible to image the internal structures of the heart, because the chest wall, the blood, and the different heart structures all reflect ultrasound differently.

The echocardiograph transducer, which is placed on the chest, serves as both transmitter for the ultrasound waves and receiver for the echoes reflected back from the heart structures. The transducer emits pulses of microwaves, each lasting 1 μsec (1 millionth of a second) at a rate of 1000 times/second; the remaining 99.9% of the time is used in receiving the echo. When the echo reaches the transducer, it is converted to an electronic signal and recorded. The ultrasound signal travels through different tissues at variable speeds depending on the density. The time that has elapsed between the emission of the signal and the return of the echo is converted automatically into a measurement of distance from the chest wall. In this manner, an echocardiograph can record a dynamic, or moving, image of the heart, with the depth of the structures on the vertical axis and time on the horizontal axis (M-mode echo). An ECG is recorded simultaneously for timing purposes. A second and more recent method (two-dimensional, or 2D, echo) permits examination of larger areas of the heart in multiple planes (Figure 21-20).

The echocardiogram is useful for determining ventricular dimensions and valve movements, obtaining data on the movement of the left-ventricular wall and septum, estimating diastolic and systolic volumes, and viewing the motion of individual segments of the left-ventricular wall during systole and diastole. It can also be used for studying valvular disease and detecting pericardial effusion.

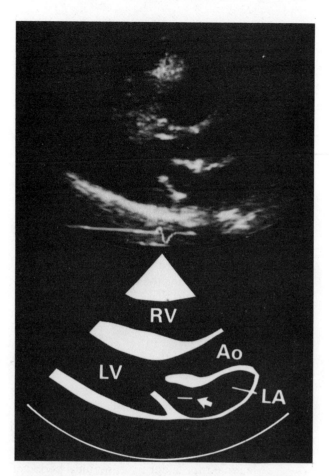

Figure 21-20 A two-dimensional echocardiogram. Parasternal long-axis view of a patient with a Hancock porcine mitral valve prosthesis. (*RV* = right ventricle; *LV* = left ventricle; *Ao* = aorta; *LA* = left atrium; *arrow* points to the valve leaflets.) *(Courtesy of LS Wann, M.D., Zablocki Veterans Administration Medical Center, Wood, Wisconsin)*

Treatment

The treatment of valvular defects consists of (1) medical management of heart failure and associated problems and (2) surgical intervention to either repair or replace the defective valve. Mitral commissurotomy is the surgical enlargement of a stenotic valve. It may be performed as either an open or a closed procedure. The open procedure requires extracorporeal circulation (cardiopulmonary bypass) but has the advantage of affording the surgeon direct visualization of the operative site. Valvular replacement, either with a prosthetic device or a homograft, is usually reserved for severe disease, because the ideal substitute valve has not yet been invented. Percutaneous balloon valvuloplasty involves the opening of a stenotic valve by guiding an inflated balloon through the valve orifice. The procedure is done in the cardiac catheterization laboratory and involves the insertion of a balloon catheter into the heart by way of a peripheral blood vessel. Pulmonary valvuloplasty has been approved by the Federal Drug Administration; valvuloplasty for other valves is still investigational.

In summary, dysfunction of the heart valves can result from a number of disorders, including congenital defects, trauma, ischemic heart disease, de-

generative changes, and inflammation. Rheumatic endocarditis is a common cause. Valvular heart disease produces its effects through disturbances in the blood flow. A stenotic valvular defect is one that causes a decrease in blood flow through a valve, resulting in impaired emptying and increased work demands on the heart chamber in front of the diseased valve. A regurgitant valvular defect permits the blood flow to continue when the valve is closed; it increases the work demands of the chamber in front and in back of the affected valve. Valvular heart disorders produce blood flow turbulence and are often detected through cardiac auscultation.

Congenital heart disease

Normal development of the heart requires a precise and orderly sequence of differentiation and growth. Congenital heart defects can arise at any stage of development, with structural abnormalities reflecting growth that was occurring at the time the disturbance arose. Table 21-4 is designed to assist the reader in understanding the embryonic origin of specific defects.

Approximately 8 out of every 1000 babies are born with a congenital heart defect. About one-third of these have a severe defect that would cause death within the first year if it were not corrected. This section of the chapter is designed to provide an overview of congenital heart defects, including the hemodynamic changes that accompany congenital heart disorders and the more common defects. Depending on the type of defect present, children with congenital heart disease will experience varying signs and symptoms associated with altered heart action, heart failure, and difficulty in supplying the peripheral tissues with oxygen and other nutrients.

Causes

Development of the heart and major blood vessels is usually completed by the end of the eighth week of gestation. Included in this brief span of time is the critical period between the third and eighth weeks with its complex changes in cardiac development. Congenital heart defects have been attributed to environmental, genetic, and chromosomal causes.

Maternal rubella during this critical period of fetal development is associated with an increased incidence of heart defects; in one study, congenital heart disease was identified in 52% of babies who were born with congenital rubella during the 1964–65 New York City epidemic.[49] Also, it appears that other vi-

ruses, some drugs, and radiation can cause congenital heart defects.

Chromosomal and genetic factors are thought to account for about 5% of congenital heart defects. Characteristic of these influences is the number of cardiac lesions observed in children born with Down's syndrome (trisomy of chromosome 21). The familial clustering of a number of congenital heart defects suggests that these defects are polygenic in origin. The 3% risk of polygenic recurrence that occurs with the presence of one affected child increases substantially as a second and third child are found to have similar defects.

Although both environmental and genetic influences have been cited as causes of congenital heart disease, the cause is often unknown, and it has been postulated that perhaps genetic and environmental factors interact and contribute to the defect.

Hemodynamic derangements

Congenital heart defects produce their major effects through (1) the shunting or mixing of arterial and venous blood and (2) the alterations in pulmonary blood flow and production of pulmonary hypertension.

Shunting of blood

Shunting of blood refers to the diverting of blood flow from one system to the other—from the arterial to the venous or the venous to the arterial system. The shunting of blood in congenital heart defects usually originates with the presence of an ab-

Table 21–4. Classification of congenital heart defects according to site of embryonic origin

Stage of embryonic development	Defect
Development of the atrial septum	Atrial septal defect of septum secondum
	Atrial septal defect of septum primum
Development of the ventricular septum	Ventricular septal defect of muscular septum
	Ventricular septal defect of membranous septum
Development of the endocardial cushions	Ebstein's anomaly of the tricuspid valve
	Abnormalities of the tricuspid and mitral valve
	Defect in ostium primum
	Defect in membranous portion of the ventricular septum
Spiraling and partitioning of the truncus arteriosus and bulbus cordis	Transposition of the great vessels
	Persistent truncus
	Tetralogy of Fallot
	Pulmonary stenosis
	Pulmonary outflow obstruction
Development of the aortic arches	Coarctation of the aorta
	Patent ductus arteriosus

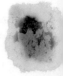

normal opening between the right and left circulations and the presence of a *pressure difference* that facilitates flow.

In atrial defects, blood usually moves from the left atrium into the right atrium because of the higher pressure in the left heart. In a more complicated pressure-flow situation, such as a ventricular septal defect accompanied by obstruction of the pulmonary outflow channel, pressure builds up in the right ventricle to the extent that it may exceed left-ventricular pressure; in this case, blood is pushed from the right side of the heart to the left side. The presence of a right-to-left shunt results in unoxygenated blood being ejected into the systemic circulation, causing cyanosis. In the left-to-right shunt, blood intended for ejection into the systemic circulation is recirculated through the right heart and back through the lungs; the increased volume distends the right heart and pulmonary circulation and increases the workload placed on the right ventricle. Children with a septal defect that causes left-to-right shunting usually have an enlarged right heart and pulmonary blood vessels.

Changes in blood flow and pressure

Many of the complications of congenital heart disorders result from their effect on the pulmonary circulation, which may be exposed to either an increase or a decrease in blood flow.

In contrast to the arterioles in the systemic circulation, the mature pulmonary arterioles are thin-walled vessels, so they can accommodate various levels of stroke volume from the right heart. The maturation process that produces thinning of the smooth muscle layer in these vessels is delayed until after birth. In many forms of congenital heart disease, increased pulmonary blood flow during the early neonatal period results in delay or impairment of maturation. If vascular disease is allowed to progress, pulmonary vascular resistance increases and pulmonary hypertension develops. How damaging this blood flow will be to the maturing pulmonary vessels depends on the time of onset and the extent of the increased flow. In many instances, the volume overload occurs after the pulmonary vessels have already developed their low-resistance properties.

In situations in which the shunting of systemic blood flow into the pulmonary circulation threatens permanent injury to the pulmonary vessels, a surgical procedure may be done in an attempt to reduce the flow by increasing resistance to outflow from the right ventricle. This procedure, called pulmonary banding, consists of placing a constrictive band around the main pulmonary artery. The banding technique is often used as a temporary measure to alleviate the symptoms and protect the pulmonary vessels in anticipation of later surgical repair of the defect.

There are also defects that decrease pulmonary blood flow, producing inadequate oxygenation of blood. The affected child often experiences fatigue, exertional dyspnea, impaired growth, and even syncope.

Types of defects

Atrial septal defects

Atrial septal defects are more common in girls than in boys. Embryologically, division of the atria is facilitated by the development of two separate septa, which lie side by side; the septum primum is formed first and the septum secondum develops later. Neither septum completely separates the atria, and an oblique opening, the foramen ovale, allows blood to flow from the right atria into the left heart as a means of bypassing the uninflated lungs. The septum primum acts as a one-way valve to prevent the backward flow of blood. At birth, the lungs expand, umbilical blood flow is interrupted, and left atrial pressure rises, pushing the septum primum against the septum secondum. The continued contact of septum primum with septum secondum induces permanent closure of the foramen ovale, which is usually completely closed by the second or third month of extrauterine life.

Atrial septal defect occurs with the aberrant development of the septum primum or septum secondum or, more frequently, because the foramen ovale fails to close. The affected child often is asymptomatic because the defect is so small. In the case of an isolated septal defect that is large enough to allow shunting, the flow of blood will usually be from the left to the right side of the heart (remember that the pressure in the left heart is greater than that in the right); when this happens, there is an increase in the volume of the right heart and pulmonary artery (Figure 21-21, **A**). This increased blood volume that must be ejected from the right heart prolongs closure of the pulmonic valve and produces a separation, or fixed splitting, of the aortic and pulmonic components of the second heart sound.

Ventricular septal defects

Ventricular septal defects are the most common form of congenital heart defect; in 20% of all persons with congenital heart disease a ventricular defect is the only abnormality, and males are affected more frequently than females. These defects vary in size and can be located in almost any part of the structure, the site being determined by the embryologic event that was occurring at the time that growth

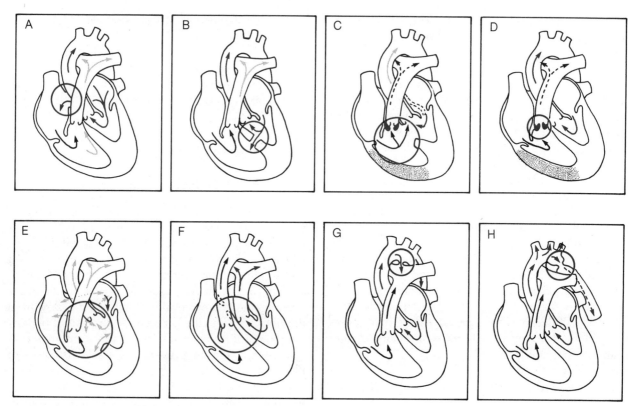

Figure 21-21 Congenital heart defects. (**A**) Atrial septal defect. Blood is shunted from left to right. (**B**) Ventricular septal defect. Blood is usually shunted from left to right. (**C**) Tetralogy of Fallot. This involves a ventricular septal defect, dextroposition of the aorta, right ventricular outflow obstruction, and right ventricular hypertrophy. Blood is shunted from right to left. (**D**) Pulmonary stenosis, with decreased pulmonary blood flow and right ventricular hypertrophy. (**E**) Endocardial cushion defects. Blood flows between the chambers of the heart. (**F**) Transposition of the great vessels. The pulmonary artery is attached to the left side of the heart and the aorta to the right side. (**G**) Patent ductus arteriosus. The high pressure blood of the aorta is shunted back to the pulmonary artery. (**H**) Postductal coarctation of the aorta.

was interrupted. The ventricular septum originates from two sources: the interventricular groove of the folded tubular heart gives rise to the muscular part of the septum, and the endocardial cushions fuse to separate the atria and extend to form the membranous portion of the septum. The upper membranous portion of the septum is the last area to close and it is here that most defects occur.

A ventricular septal defect may be the only cardiac defect or may be one of multiple cardiac anomalies. Many defects of medium or small size in the muscular septum close spontaneously.

As with atrial septal defects, the alterations in cardiac function related to openings in the ventricular septum depend on the presence of other heart defects and their size and location. The shunting of blood across the defect is determined largely by the pressures within the two ventricles. Flow is usually left to right because of the higher pressure in the left ventricle (Figure 21-21, **B**). In situations in which an obstruction to pulmonary outflow accompanies a ventricular defect, right ventricular pressure may exceed

left-ventricular pressure, and then the flow will be from right to left. Depending on the size of the opening, the signs and symptoms may range from the presence of an asymptomatic systolic murmur to frank congestive heart failure. Often, ventricular septal defects are a component of a defect of greater complexity, such as tetralogy of Fallot.

Tetralogy of Fallot

As the name implies, tetralogy of Fallot consists of four associated congenital heart defects: (1) ventricular septal defects involving the membranous septum and the anterior portion of the muscular septum; (2) dextroposition or shifting to the right of the aorta, so that it overrides the right ventricle and is in communication with the septal defect; (3) obstruction or narrowing of the pulmonary outflow channel, including a pulmonic valve stenosis, a decrease in the size of the pulmonary trunk, or both; and (4) hypertrophy of the right ventricle due to the increased work required to pump blood through the obstructed pulmonary channels (Figure 21-21, **C**).

Most children with tetralogy of Fallot display varying degrees of cyanosis—hence the term *blue babies.* The cyanosis develops as the result of decreased pulmonary blood flow and because the right-to-left shunt causes mixing of unoxygenated blood with the oxygenated blood being ejected into the peripheral circulation. Because of the decreased availability of oxygen, these children have limited exercise tolerance. As a means of coping with this exercise intolerance, the child often is observed to assume spontaneously the squatting position, though just how the squatting effects an increase in blood oxygen levels is still conjectural. Some authorities suggest that the position increases blood flow to the brain and other vital organs by temporarily reducing blood flow to the lower extremities, while others suggest that the compression of vessels in the lower extremities may incite a vasoconstrictor response that serves to elevate blood pressure.

Because of the hypoxemia that occurs in these children, palliative surgery designed to increase pulmonary blood flow is often needed during early infancy, with corrective surgery being done at a later age.[3]

Pulmonary stenosis

Pulmonary stenosis may occur as an isolated valvular lesion or in conjunction with more complex defects, such as tetralogy of Fallot. In isolated valvular defects, the pulmonary cusps may be absent or malformed or may remain fused at their commissural edges; often, all three abnormalities are present. Pulmonic valvular defects usually cause some impairment of pulmonary blood flow and increase the workload imposed on the right heart (Figure 21-21, **D**). In infants with severe defects causing marked impairment of pulmonary blood flow, the ductus arteriosus may provide the vital accessory route for perfusing the lungs during early postnatal life. Medical treatment efforts designed to maintain the patency of the ductus arteriosus may be used to maintain or increase pulmonary blood flow. If pulmonary stenosis is extreme, increased pressures in the right heart may delay closure of the foramen ovale. Pulmonary valvotomy is often the treatment of choice. Transcatheter balloon valvuloplasty may be used in some infants with moderate degrees of obstruction. The procedure provides palliative improvement, although it is not known if the improvement is permanent.[3]

Endocardial cushion defects

Children with Down's syndrome have a high incidence of endocardial cushion defects, with estimates indicating that as many as 50% of such children have some form of endocardial cushion defect. The endocardial cushions form the atrioventricular canals, the upper part of the ventricular septum, and the lower part of the atrial septum. Considering the embryologic contributions of the endocardial cushions to heart development, it is easy to see why the defect can cause so many different types of problems. In its most severe form, the defect involves both the atrial and ventricular septa and the tricuspid and mitral valves. When growth is halted at a later stage of development, there may be a septum primum defect and a cleft in the mitral valve. Any single defect or combination of endocardial defects is possible (Figure 21-21, **E**).

Ebstein's anomaly is a defect in endocardial cushion development characterized by displacement of tricuspid valvular tissue into the ventricle. The displaced tricuspid leaflets are attached either directly to the right ventricular endocardial surface or to shortened or malformed chordae tendineae.

Transposition of the great vessels

In complete transposition of the great vessels, the aorta originates in the right ventricle and the pulmonary trunk in the left. The structural defect present in this anomaly suggests that during embryonic partitioning of the aorta and pulmonary trunk there was failure in the spiral movement of the bulbus cordis and truncus arteriosus (Figure 21-21, **F**). In infants born with this defect, survival depends on communication between the right and left heart, either in the form of a septal defect or as a patent ductus arteriosus. A procedure called a balloon atrial septostomy may be done to increase the blood flow between the two sides of the heart. This is done by inserting a balloon-tipped catheter into the heart through the vena cava, then passing the catheter through the foramen ovale into the left atrium. The balloon is then inflated, and as it is brought back through the foramen ovale, the opening is enlarged.

A surgical procedure, the Mustard operation, in which the atrial septum is removed and a new wall is created so that blood is directed into the proper outflow channels, corrects the defect.

Patent ductus arteriosus

In fetal life, the ductus arteriosus is the vital link by which blood from the right heart bypasses the lungs and enters the systemic circulation (Figure 21-21, **G**). Following birth, this passage is no longer needed, and it usually closes during the first 24 to 72 hours. The physiologic stimulus and mechanisms associated with permanent closure of the ductus are not entirely known, but the fact that infant hypoxia predisposes to a delayed closure suggests that arterial oxygen levels play a role. Many preterm infants lack the normal mechanisms for closure because of prematurity. As is true of other heart and circulatory defects, patency of the ductus arteriosus may be present in various forms; the opening may be small, medium-sized, or large.

The function of the ductus arteriosus in providing a right-to-left shunt in prenatal life has prompted the surgical creation of an aortic-pulmonary shunt as a means of improving pulmonary blood flow in children with severe pulmonary outflow disorders. Research has focused on the role of type E prostaglandins in maintaining the patency of the ductus; it has been found that, by injecting prostaglandin E into the umbilical vein of infants who require a ductal shunt, closure has been delayed or prevented.[50] Administration of indomethacin, an inhibitor of prostaglandin synthesis, is used as a treatment to induce closure of a patent ductus arteriosus. When this method of treatment fails, surgical ligation may be needed.[3]

Coarctation of the aorta

Coarctation of the aorta can be described as a localized narrowing of the aorta, either proximal to (preductal) or distal to the ductus (postductal). (See Figure 21-21, **H**.)

In *preductal* coarctation, the ductus remains open and shunts blood from the pulmonary artery, through the ductus arteriosus, into the aorta. It is frequently seen with other cardiac anomalies and carries a high mortality. Because of the position of the defect, blood flow throughout the systemic circulation is reduced, and the affected infant develops heart failure at an early age due to the increased workload imposed on the left ventricle.

In *postductal* coarctation, symptoms often do not arise until late adolescence or adult life. In these persons, the narrowing of the aorta distal to the subclavian artery and proximal to the descending aorta creates disparity between the pulses and blood pressure of the upper and lower extremities (see Chapter 19).

Manifestations and treatment

Congenital heart defects present with numerous signs and symptoms. Some defects, such as patent ductus arteriosus and small ventricular septal defects, often close spontaneously, and in other less severe defects, there are no signs and symptoms. Often, the disorder is discovered during a routine health examination. Pulmonary congestion, cardiac failure, and decreased peripheral perfusion are the chief concerns in children with more severe defects. Such defects often cause problems shortly after birth or in early infancy. The child often exhibits cyanosis, respiratory

difficulty, and fatigability, and is likely to have difficulty with feeding and failure to thrive. A generalized cyanosis that persists more than 3 hours following birth is suggestive of congenital heart disease.

One technique for evaluating the infant consists of administering 100% oxygen for 10 minutes. If the infant "pinks up," the cyanosis is probably due to respiratory problems. Because infant cyanosis may appear as a duskiness, it is important to assess the color of the mucous membranes, fingernails, toenails, tongue, and lips. Pulmonary congestion in the infant causes an increase in respiratory rate, orthopnea, grunting, wheezing, coughing, and rales. The baby whose peripheral perfusion is markedly decreased may appear to be in a shocklike state. The manifestations and treatment of heart failure in the infant and small child are similar in many ways to those in the adult (see Chapter 22), but the infant's small size and limited physical reserve make them more serious and treatment more difficult. The treatment plan usually includes supportive therapy designed to help the infant compensate for the limitations in cardiac reserve and to prevent complications. Surgical intervention is often required in severe defects, and it may be done in the early weeks of life or, conditions permitting, may be delayed until the child is older. (See a pediatric textbook for a complete description of treatment.)

In summary, congenital heart defects affect about 8 out of every 1000 neonates. The fetal heart develops during the third to eighth weeks following conception, and it is during this period that defects in its development arise. The defect reflects the stage of development at the time when the causative event occurred. A number of factors are thought to contribute to the development of congenital heart defects, including genetic and chromosomal influences, viruses, and environmental agents such as drugs and radiation. Often the cause of the defect is unknown. The defect may produce no effects or it may markedly affect cardiac function. Infants with severe congenital heart defects often suffer from pulmonary congestion, heart failure, and decreased peripheral perfusion.

References

1. Facts 1989. Dallas, Texas, American Heart Association, 1988
2. Robbins SL, Kumar V: Pathologic Basis of Disease, 4th ed, pp 316, 322, 328, 342, 343. Philadelphia, WB Saunders, 1987
3. Braunwald E: Heart Disease, 3rd ed, pp 924, 944, 948, 1487–91. Philadelphia, WB Saunders, 1988
4. Spodick D: Acoustic phenomena in pericardial disease. Am Heart J 81:114, 1971

5. Spodick D: The normal and diseased pericardium: Current concepts of pericardial physiology, diagnosis, and treatment. J Am Coll Cardiol 1:240, 1983

6. Arteriosclerosis. Report of the 1977 Working Group to Review the Report of the National Heart and Lung Institute Task Force on Arteriosclerosis, p 14. U.S. Department of Health, Education and Welfare, 1977.

7. Guyton A: Medical Physiology, 7th ed, p 300. Philadelphia, WB Saunders, 1986

8. Gregg DE, Patterson RE: Functional importance of coronary collaterals. N Engl J Med 303(24):1404, 1980

9. Vanhoutte PM: The endothelium and control of coronary artery tone. Hosp Pract 23(5):77, 1988

10. Prinzmetal M, Kennamer R, Merliss R et al: A variant form of angina pectoris. Am J Med 27:375, 1959

11. Adams PC, Fuster V, Badimon L et al: Platelet/vessel wall interactions, rheologic factors and thrombogenic substrate in acute coronary syndromes: Preventive strategies. Am J Cardiol 60:9G, 1987

12. Breland BD, Boland MF: Use of calcium channel blocking drugs in angina pectoris. J Miss State Med Assoc 25:57, 1984

13. Conti CR: Large vessel coronary vasospasm: Diagnosis, natural history and treatment. Am J Cardiol 55:41B, 1985

14. Freedman SB, Richmond DR, Alwyn M et al: Late follow-up (41 to 102 months) of medically treated patients with coronary artery spasm and minor atherosclerotic coronary obstructions. Am J Cardiol 57:1261, 1987

15. Previtali M, Panciroli C, Ardissino D et al: Spontaneous remission of variant angina documented with Holter monitoring and ergonovine testing in patients treated with calcium antagonists. Am J Cardiol 59:235, 1987

16. Block PC, Baughman KL, Pasternak RC et al: Transluminal angioplasty: Correlation of morphologic and angiographic findings in an experimental model. Circulation 61:778, 1980

17. Holmes DR, Vlietsta RE: Percutaneous transluminal coronary angioplasty: Current status and future trends. Mayo Clin Proc 61:865–76, 1986

18. Bertrand ME, Marco J, Cherrier F et al: French percutaneous transluminal coronary angioplasty (PTCA) registry: Four years experience (Abstr) JACC 7:21, 1986

19. Holmes DR, Vlietstra RE, Smith HC et al: Restenosis after percutaneous transluminal coronary angioplasty (PTCA): A report from the PTCA registry of the NHLBI. Am J Cardiol 53:77c–81c, 1984

20. Leimgruber PP, Reubin GS, Hollman J et al: Restenosis after successful coronary angioplasty in patients with single vessel disease. Circulation 73:710–17, 1986

21. Serruys PW, Julliere Y, Bertrand ME et al: Additional improvement of stenosis geometry in human coronary arteries by stenting after balloon dilatation. Am J Cardiol 61:716, 1988

22. Litvack F, Gunfest WS, Papaicannou T et al: Role of laser and thermal ablation devices in the treatment of vascular diseases. Am J Cardiol 61:816–66, 1988

23. CASS Principal Investigators and Associates: Myocardial infarction and mortality in the Coronary Artery Surgery Study (CASS) randomized trial. N Engl J Med 310:750, 1984

24. Varnaushas E: The European Coronary Surgery Study Group: Survival, myocardial infarction, and employment status in a prospective randomized study of coronary artery bypass surgery. Circulation (Suppl) 72:90–101, 1985

25. Detre KM, Taharo T, Hultgren H et al: Long-term mortality and morbidity results of the Veterans Administration randomized trial of coronary artery bypass surgery. Circulation (Suppl) 72:84–89, 1985

26. CASS Principal Investigators and Associates: Coronary Artery Surgery Study (CASS): A randomized trial of coronary artery bypass surgery. Quality of life in patients randomly assigned to treatment groups. Circulation 68:951–60, 1983

27. Mock MB, Fisher LD, Holmes DR et al: Comparison of effects of medical and surgical survival in severe angina pectoris and two-vessel coronary artery disease with and without left ventricular dysfunction: A coronary artery surgery study. Am J Cardiol 61:1198, 1988

28. DeWood MA, Spores J, Notske C et al: Prevalence of total coronary occlusion during the early hours of transmural myocardial infarction. N Engl J Med 303:897, 1980

29. Grande P, Christiansen C, Peterson A et al: Optimal diagnosis in acute myocardial infarction. Circulation 61:723, 1980

30. Panidis IP, Morganrath J: Initiating events in sudden death. Cardiovascular Clin 15:81, 1985

31. Sharma CV: Thrombolytic therapy. N Engl J Med 306:1268, 1982

32. Gorlin R: Balancing the benefits, risks and unknowns of thrombolytic therapy in acute myocardial infarction. JACC 11:1349, 1988

33. Holmes DR, Van Raden MJ, Smith HC et al: Restenosis after percutaneous transluminal coronary angioplasty (PTCA): A report from the PTCA registry of the National Heart, Lung, and Blood Institute. Am J Cardiol 53:77C, 1984

34. Topol EJ, Califf RM, George BS et al: A randomized trial of immediate versus delayed elective angioplasty after intravenous tissue plasminogen activator in acute myocardial infarction. N Engl J Med 317:581, 1987

35. Guerci AD, Gerstenblith G, Brinker JA et al: A randomized trial of intravenous tissue plaminogen activator for acute myocardial infarction with subsequent randomization to elective coronary angioplasty. N Engl J Med 317:1614, 1987

36. DeWood M, Berg R: The role of surgical reperfusion in myocardial infarction. Cardiol Clin 2:113, 1987

37. Kawai C, Matsumori A, Fujiwara H et al: Myocarditis and cardiomyopathy. Ann Rev Med 38:227, 1987

38. Brandenburg RO, Nishimura RA: Clinical differentiation of the cardiomyopathies. Practical Cardiol 11:149, 1985

39. Fuster V, Gersh BJ, Giulianti ER et al: The natural history of dilated cardiomyopathy. Am J Cardiol 47:525, 1981

40. Johnson AR, Palacios I: Dilated cardiomyopathies of the adult. N Engl J Med 307:1051, 1982

41. Demakis JG, Shahbudin H, Rahimtoola MB et al: Natural course of peripartum cardiomyopathy. Circulation 44:1053, 1971

42. Bohachick P, Rongaus AM: Hypertrophic cardiomyopathy. Am J Nurs 84:320, 1984

43. Braunwald, E (ed): Heart Disease: A Textbook of Cardiovascular Medicine, vol 2, p 1451. Philadelphia, WB Saunders, 1980

44. Maron BJ, Bonow RD, Cannon RD et al: Hypertrophic cardiomyopathy: Interrelations of clinical manifestations, pathophysiology, and therapy. N Engl J Med 316:844, 1987

45. Schluman S (Chair), Committee on Rheumatic Fever and Bacterial Endocarditis: Jones Criteria (Revised) for Guidance in the Diagnosis of Rheumatic Fever. Dallas, American Heart Association, 1982

46. Sololow M, McIlroy MB: Clinical Cardiology, p 351. Los Altos, Lange Medical Publications, 1977

47. Savage DD, Garrison RJ, Devereaux RD et al: Mitral valve prolapse in the general population. I. Epidemiologic features: The Framingham Study. Am Heart J 106:571, 1983

48. Levy D, Savage D: Prevalence and clinical features of mitral valve prolapse. Am Heart J 113:1281, 1987

49. Engle MA, Adams F, Betson C et al: Primary prevention of congenital heart disease. Circulation 41:A26, June, 1970

50. Rudolph AM, Heymann MA: Medical treatment of ductus arteriosus. Hosp Pract 12(2):57, 1977

Bibliography

Congenital heart disease

Baker EJ: Valvulopasty, angioplasty and embolotherapy in congenital heart disease. Int J Cardiol 12:139, 1986

Fisk R: Management of pediatric cardiovascular patients after surgery. Crit Care Q 9:75, 1986

Girando RM: Coarctation of the aorta. Crit Care Nurse 8(1):38, 1988

Givens L, Ricks J: Assessment of clinical manifestations of cyanotic and acyanotic heart disease in infants and children. Heart Lung 14:200, 1985

Lawrence P, Wieczorek B: Congenital valvular disease. J Cardiovasc Nurs 1:18, 1987

Page GG: Tetralogy of Fallot. Heart Lung 15(4):390, 1986

Phillips JM, Raviele AA: Diagnostic and therapeutic techniques in pediatric cardiology: Past, present, and future. Crit Care Q 8:1, 1985

Vincent RN, Collins GF: Cardiac embryology and fetal cardiovascular physiology. Crit Care Q 9:1, 1986

Coronary heart disease

Cohn PF: Silent myocardial ischemia: Present status. Mod Concepts Cardiovasc Dis 56(1): 1987

Cohn PF: Silent myocardial ischemia: Dimensions of the problem with and without angina. Am J Med 80(Suppl 4C):3, 1986

Eliot RS, Buell JC: Role of emotions and stress in the genesis of sudden death. JACC 5(6):95B, 1985

Eliot RS, Buell JC, Dembroski TM: Bio-behavioral perspectives on coronary heart disease and sudden cardiac death. Acta Med Scand (Suppl) 660:203, 1982

Fuster V, Badimon L, Cohen M et al: Insights in the pathogenesis of acute ischemic syndromes. Circulation 77:1213, 1988

Fuster V, Steele PM, Chesebro JH: Role of platelets and thrombosis in coronary atherosclerotic disease and sudden death. JACC 5(6):175B, 1985

Hillis D, Frishman W, Leon M et al: Current perspectives in

angina: Therapeutic approaches. Cardiovasc Rev Rep 6(6):709, 1985

Jenkins CD; Psychosocial risk factors in coronary heart disease. Acta Med Scand (Suppl) 660:123, 1982

Kennedy JW: Thrombolytic therapy for acute myocardial infarction. Heart Lung 16(6 [part 2]):740, 1987

Maseri A: Pathogenetic classification of unstable angina as a guideline to individual patient management and prognosis. Am J Med 80(Suppl 4C):48, 1986

McBride W, Lange RA, Hillis LD: Restenosis after successful coronary angioplasty: Pathophysiology and prevention. N Engl J Med 318:1734, 1988

Muller JE, Stone PH, Turi ZG et al: Circadian variation in the frequency of onset of acute myocardial infarction. N Engl J Med 313(21):1315, 1985

Perchalski DL, Pepine CJ: Patient with coronary artery spasm and role of the critical care nurse. Heart Lung 16:392, 1987

Robison JS: Acute right ventricular infarction: Recognition, evaluation, and treatment. Crit Care Nurs 7:42, 1987

Rozanski A, Berman DS: Silent myocardial ischemia, I and II. Am Heart J 114:615, 627, 1987

Sakallaris BR: Laser therapy for cardiovascular disease. Heart Lung 16(5):465, 1987

Schiro AG, Curtis DG: Asymptomatic coronary artery disease. Heart Lung 17(2):144, 1988

Sigwart U, Puel J, Mirkovitch V et al: Intravascular stents to prevent occlusion and restenosis after transluminal angioplasty. N Engl J Med 316:701, 1987

Stein B, Israel DH, Cohen M et al: Pathogenesis of coronary occlusion. Hosp Pract 23:87, 1988

Topol EJ: Clinical use of streptokinase and urokinase therapy for acute myocardial infarction. Heart Lung 16(6 [part 2]):760, 1987

Willerson JT, Hillis LD, Winniford M et al: Speculation regarding mechanisms responsible for acute ischemic heart disease syndromes. JACC 8(1):245, 1986

Conduction system disorders

Burke LJ, Norris SO: Nursing care of the patient with recurrent ventricular dysrhythmias. In Kern LS (ed): Cardiac Critical Care Nursing, p 143. Rockville, Maryland, Aspen Publishers, 1988

Click LA: Cardiac arrhythmias in infants and children. Crit Care Q 8:9, 1985

Dance D, Yates M: Nursing assessment and care of children with complications of congenital heart disease. Heart Lung 14:209, 1985

Featherston RG: Care of sudden death survivors: The aberrant cardiac patients. Heart Lung 17:242, 1988

Karnes N: Differentiation of aberrant ventricular conduction from ventricular ectopic beats. Crit Care Nurs 7:56, 1987

Mancini CBJ: Cardioversion of atrial fibrillation: Consideration of embolization, anticoagulation, prophylactic pacemaker, and long-term success. Am Heart J 104(3):617, 1982

McGovern BA, Ruskin JN: Ventricular tachycardia: Initial assessment and approach to treatment. Mod Concepts Cardiovasc Dis 56:13, 1987

Olshansky B, Waldo AL: Atrial fibrillation: Update on mechanism, diagnosis, and management. Mod Concepts Cardiovasc Dis 56(5):23, 1987

Parsonnet V, Bernstein AD: Pacing in perspective: Concepts and controversies. Circulation 73(6):1087, 1986

Porterfield LM, Porterfield JG, DuVall C: Insertion of a permanent pacemaker. Crit Care Nurse 7(4):30, 1987

Rahimtoola SH, Zipes DP, Akhtar M et al: Consensus statement of the conference on the state of the art of electrophysiologic testing in the diagnosis and treatment of patients with cardiac arrhythmias (Part 1 and Part 2). Mod Concepts Cardiovasc Dis 56(10, 11):55, 60, 1987

Ruskin JN: Primary ventricular fibrillation. N Engl J Med 317(5):307, 1987

Zimmaro DM: Catheter ablation of ventricular tachycardia and related nursing interventions. Crit Care Nurse 7(4):20, 1987

Drugs: cardiovascular

Catalano JT: Antiarrhythmic medications classified by their autonomic properties. Crit Care Nurse 6:44, 1986

Curran CC, Mathewson M: Use of cardiac glycosides in the critically ill. Crit Care Nurse 7:31, 1987

Frishman WH: Clinical differences between beta-adrenergic blocking agents: Implications for therapeutic substitution. Am Heart J 113:1190, 1987

Goldman L, Sia ST, Cook EF et al: Costs and effectiveness of routine therapy with long-term beta-adrenergic antagonists after acute myocardial infarction. N Engl J Med 319:152, 1988

Gorlin R: Balancing the benefits, risks and unknowns of thrombolytic therapy in acute myocardial infarction. JACC 11:1349, 1988

Marder VJ, Sherry S: Thrombolytic therapy (parts 1 and 2). N Engl J Med 318(24):1512 and (25):1585, 1988

Mason JW: Amiodarone. N Engl J Med 316(8):455, 1987

Parker JO: Drug therapy: Nitrate therapy in stable angina pectoris. N Engl J Med 316(26):1635, 1987

Rodriguez SW, Reed RL: Thrombolytic therapy in MI. Am J Nurs 87:631, 1987

Schwartz, Bourassa MG, Lesperence J et al: Aspirin and dipyridamole in the prevention of restenosis after percutaneous transluminal angioplasty. N Engl J Med 318:1714, 1988

Sobel BE: Fibrinolysis and activators of plasminogen. Heart Lung 16(6 [part 2]):775, 1987

Thiebar S: Antiarrhythmic drug therapy: An overview. Crit Care Q 7:21, 1984–5

Touloukian JE: Calcium channel blocking agents: Physiologic basis of nursing interventions. Heart Lung 14:342, 1985

Endocardial disorders: endocarditis and rheumatic fever

Chadwich EG, Shulman ST: Prevention of infective endocarditis. Mod Concepts Cardiovasc Dis 55:11, 1986

Gillum RF: Trends in acute rheumatic fever and chronic rheumatic heart disease: A national perspective. Am Heart J 111:430, 1986

Karp RB: Role of surgery in infective endocarditis. Cardiovasc Clin 17:141, 1987

Kaye D: Prophylaxis for infective endocarditis: An update. Ann Intern Med 104:419, 1986

Kaye D: Infective carditis: An overview. Am J Med 78(Suppl 6B):107, 1985

Markowitz M: Rheumatic fever in the Eighties. Pediatr Rheumatol 33:1141, 1986

Marrie TJ: Infective endocarditis: A serious and changing disease. Crit Care Nurse 7:31, 1987

Massel BF, Chute CG, Walker Am et al: Penicillin and the marked decrease in morbidity and mortality from rheumatic fever in the United States. N Engl J Med 318:280, 1988

Robbins MJ, Eisenberg ES, Frishman WH: Infective endocarditis: A pathophysiolgic approach to therapy. Cardiol Clin 5:545, 1987

Scrima DA: Infective endocarditis: Nursing considerations. Crit Care Nurse 7(2):47, 1987

Sullman PM, Drake TA, Sande MA: Pathogenesis of endocarditis. Am J Med 78(Suppl 6B):110, 1985

Williams RC: Rheumatic fever and the streptococcus: Another look at molecular mimicry. Am J Med 75(5):727, 1983

Zabriskie JB: Rheumatic fever: The interplay between host, genetics, and microbe. Circulation 71(6):1077, 1986

Exercise, exercise testing, and cardiac rehabilitation

Fletcher GF: Exercise and exercise testing—A symposium. Heart Lung 13:5, 1984

Huston TP, Puffer JC, Rodney WM: The athletic heart syndrome. N Engl J Med 313(1):24, 1985

Johnston BL: Exercise testing for patients with myocardial infarction and coronary bypass surgery: Emphasis on predischarge phase. Heart Lung 13:18, 1984

Marshall JA: Rehabilitation of the coronary bypass patient. Cardiovasc Nurs 21:19, 1985

Price MS: Cardiac rehabilitation prescription for an inpatient program. Focus Crit Care 14:58, 1987

Wingate S: Rehabilitation of the patient with valvular heart disease. J Cardiovasc Nurs 1:52, 1987

Myocardial disorders: myocarditis and cardiomyopathies

Bohanchick P, Rongaus AM: Hypertrophic cardiomyopathy. Am J Nurs 84:4, 1984

Brandenberg RO, Nishimura RA: Clinical differentiation of the cardiomyopathies. Pract Cardiol 11:149, 1985

Bulkley NH: The cardiomyopathies. Hosp Pract 19(6):59, 1984

Cunningham JL: Assessment and care of the patient with myocardial contusion. Crit Care Nurse 7:68, 1987

Fowles RE, Mason JW: Role of cardiac biopsy in the diagnosis and management of cardiac disease. Prog Cardiovasc Dis 27(3):153, 1984

Gillum RF: Idiopathic cardiomyopathy in the United States, 1970–1982. Am Heart J 111:752, 1986

Homans DC: Peripartum cardiomyopathy. N Engl J Med 312(22):1432, 1985

Maron BJ, Bonow RO, Cannon RO et al: Hypertrophic cardiomyopathy: Interrelationships of clinical manifestations, pathophysiology and therapy (second of two parts). N Engl J Med 316(13, 14):844, 1987

Mersch J: End-stage cardiac disease: Cardiomyopathy. In Douglas MK, Shinn JA (eds): Advances in Cardiovascular Nursing, pp 117–39. Rockville, Maryland, Aspen Systems, 1985

Miracle VA: Idiopathic hypertrophic subaortic stenosis. Crit Care Nurse 8(3):102, 1988

Nicod R, Polikar R, Peterson KL: Hypertrophic cardiomyopathy and sudden death. N Engl J Med 318(19):1255, 1988

Olson EG: The pathophysiology of cardiomyopathies: A critical analysis. Am Heart J 98:385, 1979

—— Pericardial disorders

Kralstein J, Frishman WH: Malignant pericardial diseases: Diagnosis and treatment. Cardiol Clin 5:583, 1987

Spodick DH: Acute pericardial disease. Heart Lung 14(6):599, 1985

—— Valvular heart disease

Baddour LM, Bisno AL: Mitral valve prolapse: Multifactorial etiologies and variable prognosis. Am Heart J 112:1359, 1986

Block PC: Aortic valvuloplasty—A valid alternative. N Engl J Med 319(3):169, 1988

Chelton SZ, Williams WH: Heart valve replacement in infants and children. Crit Care Q 8:29, 1985

Cullen L, Laxon C: Ballooning open a stenotic valve. Am J Nurs 88(7):987, 1988

DeUbago JL, DePrada JA, Bardaji JL et al: Percutaneous balloon valvulotomy for calcific rheumatic mitral stenosis. Am J Cardiol 59:1007, 1987

Georges J, Stotts N: Reducing cardiac cachexia before cardiac valve replacement. Dimensions Crit Care Nurse 4:349, 1985

Grass S, Utz S: Mitral valve prolapse: A review of the scientific and medical literature. Heart Lung 15:507, 1986

Lamb L, DiGiacomo B: What to expect when your patient's scheduled for mitral valve replacement. Am J Nurs 85:58, 1985

Morgan R, Davis J, Fraker T: Current status of valve prosthesis. Surg Clin North Am 65:699, 1985

Safian RD, Berman AD, Diver DJ et al: Balloon aortic valvuloplasty in 170 consecutive patients. N Engl J Med 319:125, 1988

Seifert P: Surgery for acquired valvular heart disease. J Cardiovasc Nurs 1:26, 1987

Selzer A: Changing aspects of the natural history of valvular aortic stenosis. N Engl J Med 317(2):91, 1987

Utz S, Grass S: Mitral valve prolapse: Self-care needs, nursing diagnosis, and interventions. Heart Lung 16:77, 1985

CHAPTER 22

Heart Failure

Compensatory mechanisms
   The Frank-Starling mechanism
   Sympathetic stimulation
   Myocardial hypertrophy
Congestive heart failure

Manifestations of heart failure
   Right-sided failure
   Left-sided failure
   Nocturia
   Increased sympathetic activity
   Cardiac cachexia
   Cheyne-Stokes respirations
Acute pulmonary edema

Diagnosis and treatment
   Diagnostic methods
   Treatment methods
     Pharmacologic treatment
     Treatment of acute pulmonary
      edema
     Heart transplant

Objectives

After you have studied this chapter, you should be able to meet the following objectives:

_____ Explain the effect of cardiac reserve on symptom development in heart failure.

_____ Explain how the compensatory mechanisms of increased sympathetic stimulation, fluid retention, and myocardial hypertrophy maintain cardiac reserve.

_____ Describe the effects of backward and forward failure on the circulation.

_____ Compare the hemodynamic and clinical manifestations of right-sided heart failure and left-sided heart failure.

_____ State why the presence of cyanosis is not a good indicator of hypoxia in persons with severe anemia.

_____ Use the Starling curve to explain the development of dyspnea in heart failure.

_____ Explain the mechanisms involved in paroxysmal nocturnal dyspnea.

_____ Explain the cause of nocturia, cardiac cachexia, and Cheyne-Stokes breathing in persons with congestive heart failure.

_____ Relate the effect of left ventricular failure to the development of pulmonary edema.

_____ Describe the clinical picture of pulmonary edema.

_____ Describe the actions of digitalis and their effects on cardiac function.

_____ Explain the action of furosemide (Lasix) in relieving the signs and symptoms of acute pulmonary edema.

_____ Describe the action of vasodilating drugs in relieving the symptoms of heart failure and acute pulmonary edema.

_____ Relate the action of angiotensin II enzyme inhibitors to the improvement of cardiac function in persons with heart failure.

_____ Explain the rationale for placing a person with pulmonary edema in the seated position.

_____ List donor and recipient criteria for heart transplantation.

Heart failure is a major health problem. It has been estimated that 2.3 million persons in the United States are afflicted with heart failure.[1] Whereas the incidence of other cardiovascular disorders has decreased over the past 10 to 20 years, heart failure has increased at a dramatic rate because more persons who normally would die of acute myocardial infarction are surviving, but with compromised ventricular function.[2] Although heart failure affects all age groups, 75% of persons with heart failure are over 60 years of age.[3]

Heart failure is not a specific disease, but rather it is the inability of the heart to pump blood commensurate with the metabolic needs of body tissues. It may result either from a diseased heart that is unable to pump blood or from excessive demands placed on a normal heart, as in the case of thyrotoxicosis. Heart failure may present as an acute or chronic disorder. In persons with asymptomatic heart disease, heart failure may be precipitated by an unrelated illness or stress. The discussion in this chapter focuses on congestive heart failure and acute pulmonary edema.

Primary disorders of the heart, such as coronary heart disease, valvular heart disease, and cardiomyopathies, clearly account for most cases of heart failure. Of the various types of primary heart disease, most involve abnormalities of the contractile properties of the left ventricle. A normal ventricle ejects about two-thirds of the blood that is present in the ventricle at the end of diastole (ejection fraction). In heart failure, the ejection fraction declines progressively with increasing degrees of myocardial dysfunction. In very severe forms of heart failure, the ejection fraction may be as low as 20% to 25%.[4] The resultant increased residual volume leads to cardiac dilatation and a rise in diastolic filling pressure. This leads to a passive congestion of organs proximal to the failing ventricle (the lungs when it is the left ventricle, and the liver and extremities when it is the right). Cardiac dilatation also increases the tension in the wall of the ventricle, and, as a result, more work is needed to eject blood from the heart (see Laplace's law, Chapter 17).

Compensatory mechanisms

The heart has the amazing capacity to adjust its activity to meet the varying needs of the body—during sleep its output declines, and during exercise it increases markedly. This ability to increase output during increased activity is called the *cardiac reserve*. For example, competitive swimmers and long-distance runners have large cardiac reserves. During exercise, the cardiac output of these athletes rapidly increases to as much as five to six times the normal level.

In sharp contrast with the healthy athlete, persons with heart failure often use their cardiac reserve even at rest. For them, even such simple activities as climbing a flight of stairs may cause shortness of breath because they have exceeded their cardiac reserve.

Cardiac reserve is maintained mainly through three processes: (1) the Frank-Starling mechanism, (2) increased sympathetic nervous system activity, and (3) myocardial hypertrophy. The diseased as well as the healthy heart employs these mechanisms. In many forms of heart disease, early decreases in cardiac function go unnoticed because these compensatory mechanisms maintain the cardiac output. Unfortunately, the mechanisms were not intended for long-term use, and in severe and prolonged heart failure, the compensatory mechanisms themselves begin to cause problems (Figure 22-1).

The Frank-Starling mechanism

As we discussed in Chapter 20, the Frank-Starling mechanism produces an increase in stroke volume by means of an increase in ventricular end-diastolic volume. The increased volume leads to increased filling and stretching of the myocardial fibers during diastole and a resultant increase in the force of the next contraction (Figure 22-2). In heart failure, the increase in ventricular end-diastolic volume results from an increase in vascular volume, which yields a subsequent increase in venous return to the heart.

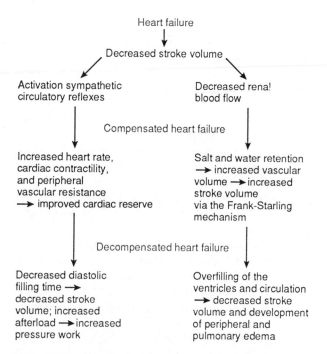

Figure 22-1 Sequence of events in compensated and decompensated heart failure.

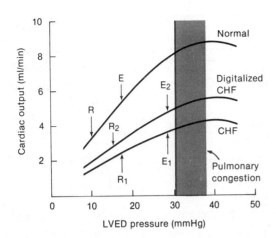

Figure 22-2 Frank-Starling curves (*R* = resting; *E* = exercise; *LVED* = left ventricular end-diastolic; *CHF* = congestive heart failure.) *(Iseri LT, Benvenuti DJ: Pathogenesis and management of congestive heart failure—revisited. Am Heart J 105(2):346, 1983)*

Several mechanisms contribute to fluid retention in heart failure. Normally, the kidneys receive about 25% of the cardiac output. With heart failure and the sympathetic-mediated vasoconstriction of the renal blood vessels that accompanies a decrease in cardiac output, this amount may be decreased to as low as 8% to 10%; the result is an increase in sodium and water retention by means of the renin–angiotensin–aldosterone mechanism.[4] A second mechanism involves the metabolism in the liver of aldosterone, which stimulates the retention of sodium and water by the kidneys. In heart failure, passive congestion of the liver leads to decreased destruction of aldosterone, and thus to sodium and water retention. Also, there is evidence of abnormal secretion of antidiuretic hormone in heart failure, which may contribute to water retention.

A newly identified hormone called the atrial natriuretic factor, or atriopeptin, has been shown to affect fluid balance in heart failure.[5,6] Atrial natriuretic factor (ANF) is a peptide hormone released from atrial cells in the heart in response to increased atrial pressure. The hormone produces rapid and transient natriuresis, diuresis, and moderate loss of potassium in the urine. Increased ANF has been found in adults with congestive heart failure, but the role of ANF in compensating for alterations in cardiac function that occur with heart failure is still unclear.

Cardiac output may be normal at rest in persons with heart failure due to increased ventricular end-diastolic volume and the Frank-Starling mechanism. This mechanism becomes ineffective, however, when the heart becomes overfilled and the muscle fibers overstretched. With the deterioration of myocardial contractility, the ventricular function curve depicted in Figure 22-2 flattens out, so that with any given increase in cardiac output, such as occurs with increased physical activity, there is a greater rise in left ventricular end-diastolic volume and pressure, with an elevation of pulmonary capillary pressure and development of dyspnea.[7] Overfilling of the ventricle also results in an increase in wall tension; as a result, more contractile force is needed to overcome the tension and generate the same pressure as a smaller ventricle (see Laplace's law, Chapter 17). Because the increased wall tension increases myocardial oxygen requirements, it contributes to the impairment of cardiac function.

Sympathetic stimulation

The importance of the sympathetic nervous system in the control of cardiac function is well established. Beta-adrenergic (β_1) mechanisms increase cardiac output by raising heart rate and increasing myocardial contractile force. Although sympathetic activity does not appear to contribute to the intrinsic contractile state of the heart, it augments contractility during periods of stress. Persons with heart failure have been shown to have increased concentration of plasma norepinephrine at rest and during exercise, compared with persons without heart failure.[8] In addition, 24-hour urine norepinephrine levels were markedly increased in persons with heart failure, which indicates increased activity of the sympathetic nervous system, including the adrenal medulla.[9] There is evidence that in cardiac failure the sympathetic receptors in the heart remain functional and able to respond to norepinephrine. The failing heart, however, is unable to synthesize the neuromediator and must depend on increased catecholamines in the blood. Studies have suggested that the density of beta receptors may decrease in persons with advanced heart failure and may contribute to a further decrease in cardiac contractility.[10]

Increased sympathetic activity also causes vasoconstriction and a compensatory redistribution of cardiac output. Blood from the skin, kidneys, and gastrointestinal tract is diverted to the more critical cerebral and coronary circulations. This general increase in sympathetic tone produces an increase in vascular resistance and the afterload against which the heart must pump.

Myocardial hypertrophy

Myocardial hypertrophy is a long-term compensatory mechanism. Cardiac muscle, like skeletal muscle, responds to an increase in work demands by undergoing hypertrophy. Heart diseases that increase resistance to the ejection of blood from the ventricles are the greatest stimulus for hypertrophy; for example, the left ventricle may increase in size to six times normal in severe aortic stenosis. If portions of the heart muscle are damaged and replaced with scar tissue, the undamaged part of the myocardium often hypertrophies as a means of improving the pumping capacity of the ventricle. However, myocardial hypertrophy is no longer beneficial when the oxygen requirements of the increased muscle mass exceed the ability of the coronary vessels to bring blood to the area. Myocardial hypertrophy can cause stiffness of the ventricle and contribute to ventricular dysfunction.

In summary, heart failure is characterized by the impaired pumping ability of the heart and represents the outcome of many forms of heart disease or other conditions that place excessive demands on the heart. The cardiac reserve represents the heart's ability to increase its output according to the needs of the body. Three compensatory mechanisms contribute to the cardiac reserve: the Frank-Starling mechanism, the activity of the sympathetic nervous system, and myocardial hypertrophy. In many forms of heart disease, early decreases in cardiac function go unnoticed because of these compensatory mechanisms. As heart failure progresses, however, the compensatory mechanisms may contribute to the production of signs and symptoms and a worsening of cardiac function.

Congestive heart failure

Heart failure occurs when the heart fails to pump sufficient blood to meet the metabolic needs of body tissues. The hemodynamic hallmarks of heart failure are a decrease in cardiac output and an increase in right and left ventricular pressures. In congestive heart failure, there is a decrease in cardiac output along with fluid accumulation in body tissues. Table 22-1 lists the causes of heart failure.

When the heart fails as a pump, there may be two direct effects on the circulation: backward or forward failure. *Backward failure* refers to signs and symptoms that arise from inadequate emptying, which allows blood to accumulate in vessels or heart chambers located behind the failing ventricles (in the lungs when there is failure of the left ventricle and in the systemic circulation when there is failure of the right ventricle), resulting in congestion of the pulmonary and venous systemic circulations. *Forward failure* results in impaired output of blood into the vessels emerging from the heart. Heart failure may also be classified according to the side of the heart (right or left) that is affected. Although the initial event that leads to heart failure may be primarily right-sided or left-sided in origin, long-term heart failure usually involves both sides. It is easier, however, to understand the physiologic mechanisms associated with heart failure when right- and left-sided failure are discussed separately.

Table 22–1. Causes of heart failure

Impaired cardiac function	Excess work demands
Myocardial disease	**Increased pressure work**
Cardiomyopathies	Systemic hypertension
Myocarditis	Pulmonary hypertension
Coronary insufficiency	Coarctation of the aorta
Myocardial infarction	
Valvular heart disease	**Increased volume work**
Stenotic valvular disease	Arteriovenous shunt
Regurgitant valvular disease	Excessive administration of intravenous fluids
Congenital heart defects	**Increased perfusion work**
	Thyrotoxicosis
	Anemia
Constrictive pericarditis	

Manifestations of heart failure

Right-sided failure

The right side of the heart moves deoxygenated blood from the systemic circulation into the pulmonary circulation. Right-sided heart failure is characterized by an accumulation or damming back of blood in the systemic venous system. This causes an increase in right atrial and peripheral venous pressures, with subsequent development of edema in the peripheral tissues and congestion of the abdominal organs. Fluid accumulation also produces a gain in weight. One pint of accumulated fluid results in a weight gain of 1 pound. Thus, daily measurement of weight can be used as a means of assessing fluid accumulation in heart failure.

The peripheral edema is most pronounced in the lower extremities and in the area over the sacrum. As venous distention progresses, blood backs up in the hepatic veins that drain into the inferior vena cava, and the liver becomes engorged. In severe and prolonged right-sided failure, liver function is frequently impaired, and liver cells may die. Congestion of the portal circulation may also lead to enlargement of the spleen with transudation of fluid into the peritoneal cavity (ascites). Congestion of the gut may cause gastrointestinal disturbances, including anorexia, abdominal pain, and loss of weight. In longstanding heart failure, severe weight loss may progress to a condition called *cardiac cachexia,* in which there is wasting of body tissues.

Left-sided failure

The left side of the heart moves blood from the low-pressure pulmonary circulation into the high-pressure arterial side of the systemic circulation. With impairment of the left heart function, the blood tends to accumulate in the pulmonary circulation. An increase in pulmonary capillary pressure reflects the increased left atrial pressure and leads to pulmonary edema. In severe pulmonary edema, capillary fluid moves into the alveoli. The accumulated fluid in the alveoli and respiratory passages impairs the gas exchange function of the lung. With the decreased ability of the lungs to oxygenate the blood, the hemoglobin leaves the pulmonary circulation without being fully oxygenated. Cyanosis and shortness of breath result.

Shortness of breath due to congestion and increased pressure in the capillaries of the lung is one of the major manifestations of left-sided heart failure. A perceived shortness of breath (breathlessness) is called *dyspnea*. Dyspnea related to an increase in activity is called *exertional dyspnea*. *Orthopnea* is shortness of breath that occurs when a person is supine, or lying down. The gravitational forces that cause fluid to become sequestered in the lower legs and feet when the person is standing or sitting are not operational when the person is supine; the fluid is then mobilized from the legs and dependent parts of the body and redistributed to an already distended pulmonary circulation. *Paroxysmal nocturnal dyspnea* is a sudden attack of dyspnea during sleep. It disrupts sleep, and the person awakens with a feeling of extreme suffocation. Bronchospasm due to congestion of the bronchial mucosa may be present, causing wheezing and difficulty in breathing. This condition is sometimes referred to as *cardiac asthma*.

Fatigue and limb weakness often accompany diminished output from the left ventricle. Cardiac fatigue is different from emotional fatigue in that it is not present in the morning but appears and progresses as activity increases during the day. In acute or severe left-sided failure, cardiac output may fall to levels that are insufficient for providing the brain with adequate oxygen, and there are indications of mental confusion and disturbed behavior. Confusion, impairment of memory, anxiety, restlessness, and insomnia are common in elderly persons with advanced heart failure, particularly in those with cerebral atherosclerosis.

Nocturia

Nocturia occurs relatively early in the course of congestive heart failure. During the day, when the person is in an upright position, the blood flow is redistributed away from the kidneys. At night, resting in the recumbent position produces an increase in

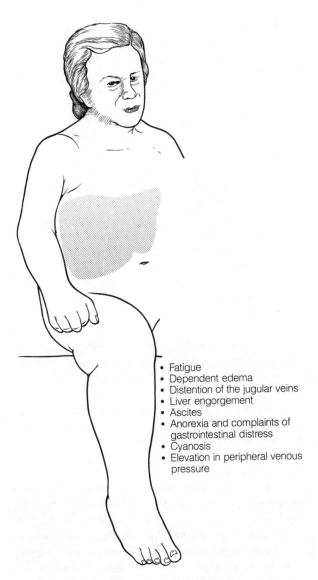

- Fatigue
- Dependent edema
- Distention of the jugular veins
- Liver engorgement
- Ascites
- Anorexia and complaints of gastrointestinal distress
- Cyanosis
- Elevation in peripheral venous pressure

Figure 22-3 Manifestations of right-sided heart failure.

Cyanosis may occur in either right- or left-sided heart failure. In right-sided failure, the blood flow is sluggish and extraction of oxygen from the blood as it passes through the capillaries is increased; the quantity of deoxygenated hemoglobin in the blood then increases.*

The jugular veins are above the level of the heart and are normally collapsed in the standing position. In severe right-sided failure, the external jugular veins become distended and can be visualized when the person is standing. The manifestations of right-sided heart failure are depicted in Figure 22-3.

* The blue discoloration associated with cyanosis requires the presence of 5 g of deoxygenated hemoglobin. A severely anemic person may not have sufficient hemoglobin to permit 5 g to become deoxygenated. Some of the success credited to the bloodletting practices of the 18th and 19th centuries probably resulted from treating cyanosis by causing anemia.

cardiac output and blood flow to the kidneys as edema fluids from the dependent parts of the body are mobilized. Renal vasoconstriction diminishes, and urine formation increases. When oliguria occurs, it is a late sign related to a severely reduced cardiac output.

Increased sympathetic activity

Increased sympathetic activity, although a principal compensatory mechanism in heart failure, is also responsible for a number of physical signs. Peripheral vasoconstriction is manifested by pallor and coldness of the extremities and cyanosis of the digits. There may also be diaphoresis and tachycardia. Vasoconstriction may impede the loss of body heat and result in low-grade fever.

Cardiac cachexia

Cardiac cachexia is a condition of malnutrition and tissue wasting that occurs in persons with end-stage heart failure. A number of factors probably contribute to its development, including fatigue and depression that interfere with food intake, congestion of the liver and gastrointestinal structures that impair digestion and absorption and produce feelings of fullness, and circulating toxins and mediators released from poorly perfused tissues that impair appetite and contribute to tissue wasting.

Cheyne-Stokes respirations

Cheyne-Stokes respirations are a form of periodic breathing (see Chapter 24) with a waxing and waning of respirations interspersed with periods of apnea. This type of breathing may occur in persons with heart failure and is thought to result from a discrepancy between arterial and alveolar oxygen and carbon dioxide levels—the consequence of a prolonged circulation time between the heart and the respiratory center in the brain.

Acute pulmonary edema

Pulmonary edema refers to the condition in which fluid accumulates in the interstitial spaces and alveoli of the lung. Pulmonary edema causes stiffness of the lungs, making lung expansion more difficult, and it can produce hypoxemia by interfering with the gas exchange function of the lung. Acute pulmonary edema is a life-threatening condition. Although pulmonary edema is often associated with left heart failure, it can also result from increased permeability of the pulmonary capillary membrane, which in turn may be due to an infectious process, exposure to toxic gases, drug reactions, or other conditions. Hypervolemia due to rapid infusion of intravenous fluids or a blood transfusion in an elderly person or in a person

with limited cardiac reserve may precipitate an episode of pulmonary edema. The following discussion centers on pulmonary edema due to heart failure.

With pulmonary edema due to heart failure, the contractile properties of the left ventricle are inadequate to eject all of the blood that enters from the lungs; this causes a sharp rise in left end-diastolic volume and pressure and a resultant increase in pulmonary venous and capillary pressures. Normally fluid does not leave the pulmonary capillaries and enter the lung spaces. This is because the pulmonary capillary pressure that serves to push fluid into the lung tissue is much lower than the capillary osmotic pressure, which pulls fluid back into the capillary (see Chapter 28). In situations where the pumping ability of the left ventricle is impaired to the extent that the pulmonary capillary pressure exceeds the capillary osmotic pressure, fluids move from the capillary into the interstitial tissues and alveoli.

An episode of pulmonary edema usually occurs at night when the person has been reclining for a period of time; gravitational forces are removed from the circulatory system, so edema fluid that had been sequestered in the lower extremities when they were in the dependent position is returned to the vascular compartment and redistributed to the pulmonary circulation. An acute episode may also occur as a complication of impaired cardiac pumping ability in myocardial infarction.

A person with pulmonary edema is usually seen sitting and gasping for air (Figure 22-4). The apprehension is obvious. The pulse is rapid; the skin is moist and cool, and the lips and nailbeds are cyanotic. As the lung edema worsens and oxygen supply to the brain falls off, confusion and stupor appear. Dyspnea and air hunger are accompanied by a cough productive of frothy and often blood-tinged sputum —the effect of air mixing with the plasma and blood cells that have exuded into the alveoli. The movement of air through the alveolar fluid produces a fine crepitant sound, called *rales,* which can be heard through a stethoscope placed on the chest. As fluid moves into the larger airways, the breathing is louder. In the terminal stage, it is called the *death rattle.* In severe pulmonary edema, persons literally drown in their own secretions.

In summary, congestive heart failure implies an accumulation of body fluids due to decreased cardiac function. In right-sided failure, congestion of the systemic venous system occurs, and in left-sided failure, pulmonary congestion occurs. Because the circulation forms a closed system, heart failure eventually affects both sides of the heart. Acute pulmonary edema represents a life-threatening accumulation of fluid in the lungs resulting from failure of the left ventricle.

shape of the heart and pulmonary vasculature. The cardiac silhouette can be used to detect cardiac hypertrophy and dilatation. Evidence of pulmonary venous hypertension and pulmonary congestion can also be detected on x-ray. Echocardiographic studies are used to reveal the size and function of cardiac valvular structures and the size and motion of both ventricles. It will also indicate pericardial effusion. Radionuclide angiography and cardiac catheterization are other diagnostic tests used in describing the underlying causes of heart failure.

Invasive hemodynamic monitoring is often used in the management of acute life-threatening episodes of heart failure. These methods include the use of central venous pressure measurements, pulmonary capillary wedge pressures, thermodilution cardiac output measurements, and intra-arterial measurements of blood pressure.

Central venous pressure reflects the amount of blood returning to the heart and the ability of the heart to pump the blood forward into the arterial system. Measurements of central venous pressure can be obtained by means of a catheter inserted into the superior vena cava through a peripheral vein. This pressure is decreased in hypovolemia and increased in heart failure. The changes that occur in central venous pressure over time are usually more significant than

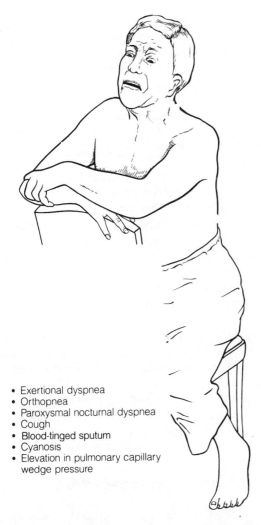

- Exertional dyspnea
- Orthopnea
- Paroxysmal nocturnal dyspnea
- Cough
- Blood-tinged sputum
- Cyanosis
- Elevation in pulmonary capillary wedge pressure

Figure 22-4 Manifestations of acute left-sided heart failure.

Diagnosis and treatment

—— Diagnostic methods

As stated earlier, heart failure represents the failure of the heart as a pump and can occur in the course of a number of heart diseases or other systemic pathologies. It can present as a chronic disorder with insidious onset, as an acute phenomenon with sudden onset, or as an end-stage disease. The diagnosis of heart failure is based on signs and symptoms related to the failing heart itself, such as shortness of breath and fatigue, or to the compensatory mechanisms, which represent excessive compensatory efforts, such as edema. The Functional Classification of the New York Heart Association is one guide to classifying the extent of dysfunction (Table 22-2).

Electrocardiography findings may indicate underlying disorders of cardiac rhythm or conduction. Chest x-rays provide information about the size and

Table 22-2. New York Heart Association functional classification of patients with heart disease

Classification	Characteristics
Class I	Patients with cardiac disease but without the resulting limitations in physical activity. Ordinary activity does not cause undue fatigue, palpitation, dyspnea, or anginal pain.
Class II	Patients with heart disease resulting in slight limitations of physical activity. They are comfortable at rest. Ordinary physical activity results in fatigue, palpitation, dyspnea, or anginal pain.
Class III	Patients with cardiac disease resulting in marked limitation of physical activity. They are comfortable at rest. Less than ordinary physical activity causes fatigue, palpitation, dyspnea, or anginal pain.
Class IV	Patients with cardiac disease resulting in inability to carry on any physical activity without discomfort. The symptoms of cardiac insufficiency or of the anginal syndrome may be present even at rest. If any physical activity is undertaken, discomfort increases.

(Criteria Committee of the New York Heart Association. Diseases of the Heart and Blood Vessels: Nomenclature and Criteria for Diagnosis, 6th ed, pp 112–113. Boston, Little, Brown, 1964)

the absolute numerical values obtained during a single reading.

Pulmonary capillary wedge pressure (PCWP) is obtained by means of a flow-directed, balloon-tipped Swan-Ganz catheter. This catheter is introduced through a peripheral vein and is then advanced into the superior vena cava. The balloon is inflated with air once the catheter is in the thorax; it then floats through the right heart and pulmonary artery until it becomes wedged in one of the small pulmonary arteries (Figure 22-5). Once the catheter is in place, the balloon is inflated *only* when the PCWP is being measured, to prevent necrosis of pulmonary tissue. With the balloon inflated, the catheter monitors pulmonary capillary pressures in direct communication with pressures from the left heart. The pulmonary capillary pressures provide a means of assessing the pumping ability of the left heart.

One type of Swan-Ganz catheter is equipped with a thermistor probe to obtain *thermodilution measurements of cardiac output.* In this method, a known amount of solution of a known temperature (iced or room temperature) is injected into the right atrium through an opening in the catheter, and the temperature of the blood is measured downstream in the pulmonary artery by means of a thermistor probe located at the end of that catheter. A microcomputer calculates blood flow (and cardiac output) using the difference between the temperatures recorded from the two sites.

Intra-arterial blood pressure measurements are obtained through the use of a small catheter inserted into a peripheral artery, usually the radial artery. The catheter is connected to a pressure transducer and beat-by-beat measurements of blood pressure are recorded. Depending on the system used, both the contour of the pressure pulse and a digital reading of the systolic, diastolic, and mean arterial pressures are displayed on the bedside monitor along with the electrocardiograph.

Treatment methods

The treatment of heart failure is directed toward the secondary consequences of circulatory failure as well as the primary source of the failure. The goals of treatment focus on: (1) limiting the progress of the primary disease or workload imposed on the heart, (2) supporting the function of the failing heart, (3) limiting excessive compensatory mechanisms, and (4) arriving at an activity pattern consistent with the limitations of the declining cardiac reserve.[11,12] It includes: (1) the pharmacologic and nonpharmacologic control of afterload stresses such as hypertension, (2) the surgical repair of a ventricular defect or improperly functioning stenotic valve, (3) the use of medications to improve cardiac function and limit excessive compensatory mechanisms, and (4) the instruction and counseling in terms of the selective modification of activities and life-style to a level consistent with the functional limitations of a reduced cardiac reserve.

Pharmacologic treatment

Medications such as digitalis preparations, diuretics, arterial and venous vasodilators, and angiotensin II-converting enzyme inhibitors are prescribed. Digitalis is often prescribed to increase the heart's pumping efficiency. Restriction of salt intake and diuretic therapy facilitate the excretion of edema fluid. Counseling, health teaching, and other assistive measures help persons with heart failure to manage their activity patterns appropriately.

Digitalis. *Digitalis* has been a recognized treatment for congestive heart failure for the past 200 years. The various forms of digitalis are called *cardiac glycosides.* They improve cardiac function by increasing the force and strength of ventricular contraction. In addition, they slow the heart rate by decreasing SA node activity and decreasing conduction through the AV node, thus slowing heart rate and increasing diastolic filling time. These drugs cause a partial inhibition of the enzyme that activates the adenosine triphosphate (ATP) that supplies the energy for the operation of the sodium–potassium membrane pump. This causes decreased extrusion of calcium from cardiac cells following muscle contraction and results in increased availability of intracellular calcium for con-

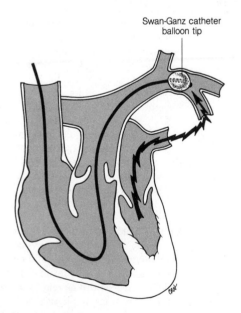

Figure 22-5 Swan-Ganz balloon-tip catheter positioned in a pulmonary capillary. The pulmonary capillary wedge pressure, which reflects the left ventricular diastolic pressure, is measured with the balloon inflated.

Swan-Ganz catheter balloon tip

tractile processes and the development of muscle tension. Although not a diuretic, digitalis promotes urine output by improving renal blood flow.

The margin between therapeutic and toxic doses of digitalis is very narrow. Low potassium, high calcium, and low magnesium blood levels predispose patients to digitalis toxicity, an important consideration in patients who are on digitalis because many of them are also taking diuretics, which promote potassium and magnesium losses. A number of drugs have been shown to affect digitalis levels. Cholestyramine, some broad-spectrum antibiotics, antacids, and kaolin–pectin mixtures (*e.g.,* Kaopectate) may decrease absorption of the drug. Quinidine, verapamil, and amiodarone increase plasma levels of the drug by reducing both the volume of distribution and the excretion of the drug by the kidneys.

Digitalis toxicity can be described by its effect on three body systems—the cardiovascular, gastrointestinal tract, and central nervous system. The most serious effect is digitalis-induced cardiac dysrhythmias. These cardiac dysrhythmias can take many forms and can mimic most disturbances of cardiac rhythm. Anorexia, nausea, and vomiting are common gastrointestinal indications of toxicity. They may occur in patients receiving parenteral digitalis, which suggests that they are a result of disturbances in the central nervous system rather than direct irritation of the gastrointestinal tract. Psychic and visual problems are signs of toxicity to the central nervous system. Some patients have described the visual disturbance as "looking through yellow-green glasses." Confusion is a common sign of digitalis toxicity in the elderly. A recent advance in laboratory methods allows the monitoring of serum digitalis levels.

Newer positive-inotropic drugs that increase cardiac contractility are available for use in situations of acute heart failure. These include beta-adrenergic agonists, dopaminergic agents, and a group of nondigitalis noncatecholamine agents that increase cardiac contractility by inhibiting myocardial phosphodiesterase. However, none of these agents are available in oral form. One of the phosphodiesterase agents, amrinone, has been approved for intravenous use.

Diuretics. Diuretics promote the excretion of edema fluid, and in emergencies they are often administered intravenously. The diuretic furosemide (Lasix) appears to have a biphasic effect on pulmonary congestion. When given intravenously, it appears to produce venous dilatation almost immediately, with increased venous pooling of blood and a decrease in venous return to the right heart. The decrease in venous tone that occurs when furosemide is administered intravenously precedes its diuretic action by about 30 to 60 minutes.[13]

Vasodilator drugs. Vasodilator drugs cause relaxation of vascular smooth muscle. These drugs induce venous pooling of blood, relax the pulmonary arterial and venous vessels, and reduce the peripheral vascular resistance. With pooling of blood in the peripheral veins, there is less blood available to the right heart for delivery to the pulmonary circulation. Relaxation of the pulmonary vessels diminishes the pressure in the pulmonary capillaries and allows fluid to be reabsorbed from the interstitium of the lung and from the alveoli. (See Chapter 28 for a discussion of edema formation.) With a decrease in peripheral vascular resistance, there is less pressure against which the left heart must pump, and thus the work of the left ventricle is decreased.

Among the vasodilators currently in use are the nitrates, hydralazine, prazosin, and the angiotensin-converting enzyme inhibitors. The nitrates produce relaxation of both arteriolar and venous smooth muscle. Sodium nitroprusside is a form of nitroglycerin given by continuous intravenous infusion in situations of acute heart failure. Oral and topical forms of nitroglycerin are used in the long-term management of heart disease and heart failure (see Chapter 21). Hydralazine is a potent arteriolar dilator; it markedly reduces afterload and increases cardiac output. The combination of nitrates and oral hydralazine has proved effective in the management of persons with mild to moderate heart failure symptoms. However, the side effects of hydralazine (gastrointestinal upset, headaches, tachycardia, hypotension, and drug-induced lupus syndrome) limit its use in some persons. Prazosin, an oral alpha-adrenergic blocking drug that relaxes arterial smooth muscle, is being used selectively in the treatment of heart failure. However, its long-term benefits are not known.

In heart failure, renin activity is frequently elevated because of decreased renal blood flow. The net result is an increase in angiotensin II, which causes vasoconstriction and increased aldosterone production (see Chapter 19). Both of these mechanisms increase the workload of the heart. Converting enzyme inhibitors (captopril or enalapril), which prevent the conversion of angiotensin I to angiotensin II, may be used in the treatment of heart failure.

Treatment of acute pulmonary edema

Treatment is directed toward reducing the fluid volume in the pulmonary circulation. This can be accomplished by reducing the amount of blood that the right heart delivers to the lungs or by improving the work performance of the left heart.

A number of measures are available that decrease the blood volume in the pulmonary circulation;

the seriousness of the pulmonary edema will determine which are to be used. One of the simplest measures to relieve orthopnea is to assume the seated position. For many persons, sitting up or standing is almost instinctive and may be sufficient to relieve the symptoms associated with mild accumulation of fluid.

Measures to improve left heart performance focus on (1) decreasing the preload by reducing the filling pressure of the left ventricle and (2) reducing the afterload against which the left heart must pump. This can be accomplished through the use of vasodilator drugs, treatment of arrhythmias that impair cardiac function, and improvement of the contractile properties of the left ventricle with digitalis. Rapid digitalization may be accomplished with intravenous administration of the drug.

Oxygen therapy increases the oxygen content of the blood and helps relieve anxiety. Positive-pressure breathing increases the intra-alveolar pressure and opposes the capillary filtration pressure in the pulmonary capillaries and is sometimes used as a temporary measure to decrease the amount of fluid moving into the alveoli.

Although its mechanisms of action are unclear, morphine sulfate is usually a drug of choice in acute pulmonary edema. Morphine relieves anxiety and depresses the pulmonary reflexes that cause spasm of the pulmonary vessels. It also increases venous pooling. Aminophylline is another drug, administered intravenously, that may be useful. It reduces bronchospasm, increases the glomerular filtration rate, and promotes urinary excretion of sodium and water. This drug relieves Cheyne-Stokes respirations, which sometimes occur in severe heart failure. Relief is due not to the theophylline itself, but to the ethylenediamine in which the theophylline is solubilized.

Another means of reducing pulmonary blood volume in severe life-threatening situations is venesection or alternating tourniquets. Fortunately, with modern pharmacologic treatments, there is less need for these treatment methods. Venesection consists of removing 300 ml to 500 ml of blood from the body. (It seems likely that the success of the barbershop surgeon with his bloodletting practices was due at least partly to the temporary relief of symptoms of pulmonary congestion.) Alternating tourniquets afford a means of trapping venous blood in the extremities. The aortic balloon pump (see Chapter 23) or ventricular assist devices may be used as temporary support measures for severe heart failure.[14]

Heart transplant

Heart transplant, once a scientific curiosity, has now become an established method of treatment for some persons with end-stage heart disease. Many of the successes of heart transplantation can be credited to improved methods of immunosuppressive therapy, which optimize survival and rehabilitation. In 1987, more than 1,400 heart transplants were performed in the United States. The survival rate for heart transplantations performed in high-volume transplant centers approaches 80%.[15] Despite the overall success of heart transplantation, donor availability and complications from infection, rejection, and immunosuppression drug therapy remain as problems.

Persons are considered for heart transplantation when they are less than 60 years of age and have (1) end-stage ischemic, valvular, or congenital heart disease with maximal medical treatment, not amenable to conventional or high-risk surgery; (2) New York Heart Association class III to IV congestive heart failure; (3) intractable, recurrent, malignant ventricular arrhythmias; (4) an expected survival of less than 6 months; (5) no systemic infections, cancer, serious impairment of liver, kidney, or respiratory function, recent pulmonary embolism, recent cerebrovascular accident or neurologic deficits, or other disease that would limit transplant survival; and (6) no history of drug or alcohol abuse. Emotional, financial, and other costs must also be carefully considered.[15,16] Donor hearts are obtained from persons who are less than 40 years of age and have (1) been declared brain dead, (2) a compatible ABO blood type, (3) comparable size to the recipient (so the heart is of an appropriate size), (4) experienced no cardiac arrest, heart contusion, or abnormal heart wall motion, (5) minimal prolonged hypotension or inotropic support, and (6) no evidence of systemic infection.

Surgery is performed by placing the recipient on cardiopulmonary bypass and excising the diseased heart. An orthotopic cardiac approach is usually used to attach the donor heart (Figure 22-6). Pacing wires are implanted into the right ventricle to assist with temporary pacing of the heartbeat.

Immediate postoperative care is directed toward maintaining hemodynamic stability, observing for bradyrhythmias and postoperative hemorrhage, and monitoring for transient renal failure. Subsequent postoperative management focuses on recognition and prevention of infection or rejection of the donor heart, and monitoring of immunosuppressive therapy.

In summary, heart failure is the end result of a number of different types of heart disorders. Therefore, identification of the cause of heart failure is an important part of the treatment plan. Treatment is directed toward (1) correcting the cause whenever possible, (2) improving cardiac function, (3) maintaining the fluid volume within a compensatory level, and (4) developing an activity pattern consistent with

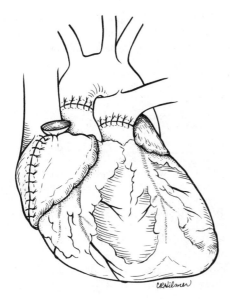

Figure 22-6 Heart transplantation and sites of donor heart attachment.

individual limitations in cardiac reserve. Among the medications used in the treatment of heart failure are digitalis, diuretics, vasodilator drugs, and angiotensin II-converting enzyme inhibitors. Treatment of acute pulmonary edema is directed toward reducing the fluid volume in the pulmonary circulation. Emergency measures often focus on translocating the excess fluid from the pulmonary to the systemic circulations. Heart transplantation may be indicated in selected cases.

References

1. American Heart Association: 1988 Heart Facts, p 22. Dallas, 1988
2. Packer M: Prolonging life in patients with congestive heart failure: The new frontier. Circulation 75(Suppl IV):IV–1, 1987
3. Sidd JJ: Congestive heart failure. Orthop Clin North Am 9(3):744, 1978
4. Iseri LT, Benvenuti DJ: Pathogenesis and management of congestive heart failure—Revisited. Am Heart J 105:346, 1983
5. Needleman P, Greenwald JE: Atriopeptin: A cardiac hormone intimately involved in fluid, electrolyte, and blood-pressure homeostasis. N Engl J Med 314(13):828, 1986
6. Raine AEG, Pil D, Erne P et al: Atrial natriuretic peptide and atrial pressure in patients with congestive heart failure. N Engl J Med 315(9):533, 1986
7. Chidsey CA, Harrison DC, Braunwald E: Augmentation of plasma norepinephrine response to exercise in patients with congestive heart failure. N Engl J Med 267:650, 1962
8. Chidsey CA, Braunwald E, Morrow AG: Catecholamine excretion and cardiac stores of norepinephrine in congestive heart failure. Am J Med 39:442, 1965
9. Braunwald E: The sympathetic nervous system in heart failure. Hosp Pract 12:31, 1970
10. Bristow MR, Ginsburg R, Minobe W et al: Decreased catecholamine sensitivity and β-adrenergic-receptor density in failing hearts. N Engl J Med 307(4):205, 1982
11. Pramaley WW: Medical treatment of congestive heart failure. Circulation 7S(Suppl IV):IV–4, 1987
12. Gorlin R: Treatment of congestive heart failure: Where are we going? Circulation 75(Suppl IV):IV–108, 1987
13. Ditshit K, Vyden JK, Forrester JS et al: Renal and extrarenal effects of furosemide in congestive heart failure. N Engl J Med 288:1087, 1973
14. Silvay G: Mechanical support of the failing heart. Mt Sinai J Med 52(7):548, 1985
15. Futterman LG: Cardiac transplantation: A comprehensive nursing perspective. Part 1. Heart Lung 17:499, 1988
16. Painvin GA, Frazier OH, Chandler LB et al: Cardiac transplantation: Indications, procurement, operation, and management. Heart Lung 14:484, 1985

Bibliography

Alpert MA: Cardiac failure in the elderly. Am Family Pract Sept:123, 1984

Artman M, Graham TP: Congestive heart failure in infancy: Recognition and management. Am Heart J 103:1040, 1982

Atlas SA: Atrial natriuretic factor: Renal and systemic effects. Hosp Pract 21(7):67, 1986

Bing RJ: The biochemical basis of myocardial failure. Hosp Pract 9:93, 1983

Blasco VV: Features of hepatic involvement in congestive heart failure. Cardiol Rev Rep 4:963, 1983

Braunwald E: Mechanism of action of calcium-channel blocking agents. N Engl J Med 307(26):1618, 1982

Braunwald E, Colucci WS: Vasodilator therapy of heart failure. N Engl J Med 310(7):459, 1984

Cannon PJ: The kidney in heart failure. N Engl J Med 296:26, 1977

Chatterjee K: Vasodilators and angiotensin-converting enzyme inhibitors in the treatment of heart failure. Cardio Rev Rep 4:779, 1983

Cohn JR: Treatment by modification of circulatory dynamics. Hosp Pract 19(8):37, 1984

Colucci WS, Wright RF, Braunwald E: New positive inotropic agents in treatment of congestive heart failure, Parts I and II. N Engl J Med 314(5, 6):290, 349, 1986

Franciosa JA: Why patients with heart failure die: Hemodynamic and functional determinants of survival. Circulation 75(Suppl IV):IV–20, 1987

Francis GS, Cohn J: The autonomic nervous system in congestive heart failure. Annu Rev Med 37:235, 1986

Hedges JR: Preload and afterload revisited. Emerg Nurs 9(5):262, 1983

Katz AM: The physiologic approach to the treatment of heart failure. Hosp Pract 22(2):117, 1987

Lurie K, Billingham ME, Harrison DC et al: Decreased catecholamine sensitivity and adrenergic-receptor density in failing human hearts. N Engl J Med 307:205, 1982

Maskin CS, Jemtel TH, Kugler J et al: Inotropic therapy in the management of congestive heart failure. Cardio Rev Rep 3:837, 1982

Massie BM, Conway M: Survival of patients with congestive heart failure: Past, present, and future prospects. Circulation 75(Suppl IV):IV-11, 1987

Murray JF: The lungs and heart failure. Hosp Pract 20(4):55, 1985

Packer M: Prolonging life in patients with congestive heart failure: The next frontier. Circulation 75(Suppl IV):IV-1, 1987

Recent developments in pulmonary edema. UCLA Conference, reprinted in Ann Intern Med 99:808, 1983

Ross J: The failing heart and the circulation. Hosp Pract 18:151, 1983

Scholz H: Inotropic drugs in the treatment of heart failure. Hosp Pract 19(5):57, 1984

Silvay G, Koffsky RM: Mechanical support of the failing heart. Mt Sinai J Med 52(7):548, 1985

Smith TW: Digitalis in the management of heart failure. Hosp Pract 19(3):67, 1984

Smith TW: Digitalis: Mechanisms of action and clinical use. N Engl J Med 318(6):358, 1988

Sonnenblick EH, Factor S, Le Jemtel TH: The rationale for inotropic therapy in heart failure. Cardio Rev Rep 4:910, 1983

Sparkes RS: The adrenergic nervous system in heart failure. N Engl J Med 311:850, 1984

Sullivan JM: Drug suppression of the angiotensin system in congestive heart failure. Annu Rev Med 34:169, 1983

Warren JV: Early diagnosis of congestive heart failure. Hosp Pract 22(5):43, 1987

Willerson JT: What is wrong with the failing heart? N Engl J Med 307:243, 1982

Zak R: Cardiac hypertrophy: Biochemical and cellular relationships. Hosp Pract 18(3):85, 1983

Circulatory Shock

Objectives

After you have studied this chapter, you should be able to meet the following objectives:

_____ State a clinical definition of *shock*.

_____ List the chief characteristics of hypovolemic shock, cardiogenic shock, obstructive shock, distributive shock, and septic shock.

_____ List and describe the four stages of hypovolemic shock.

_____ Trace the compensatory mechanisms that are activated in hypovolemic shock.

_____ State the basis of cardiogenic shock.

_____ State the rationale for the use of the vasodilator drugs and the intra-aortic balloon pump in cardiogenic shock.

_____ State the common features of normovolemic shock, neurogenic shock, and anaphylactic shock.

_____ State a proposed mechanism for the development of toxic shock.

_____ List immediate treatment measures that healthcare professionals should take in anaphylactic shock.

_____ Differentiate nutrient flow from nonnutrient flow.

_____ Trace the conversion of oxygen and fuel substrates to ATP.

_____ State the physiologic basis of thirst in shock.

_____ State the manifestations of shock revealed in the skin and the body temperature.

_____ Describe the central problem involved in measuring blood pressure in shock.

_____ Describe changes in pulse rate, urinary output, and sensorium that are indicative of shock.

_____ Describe the pathology seen in shock lung.

_____ Describe the damage to the renal system and the gastrointestinal system associated with shock.

_____ State the rationale for treatment measures to correct and reverse shock.

Circulatory shock is not a specific disease; it can occur in the course of many life-threatening, traumatic or disease states. Nor is shock a simple state of hypotension. Rather, circulatory shock implies a failure of the circulatory system. It has been defined as a clinical condition characterized by "an inadequate blood flow to vital organs or the inability of the body cell mass to metabolize nutrients normally."[1]

Although blood flow relies on blood pressure, the two are not synonymous. Blood flow relies not only on pressure, but on a vessel diameter that is large enough to facilitate flow and on sufficient blood volume to fill the vascular compartment. In shock, compensatory mechanisms that cause vasoconstriction often serve to maintain blood pressure while compromising blood flow.

In 1895 a Harvard surgeon published what has come to be recognized as the classic manifestations of irreversible shock.

> A patient is brought into the hospital with a compound comminuted fracture ..., where the bleeding has been slight. As the litter is gently deposited on the floor he makes no effort to move or look about him. He lies staring at the surgeon with an expression of complete indifference as to his condition. There is no movement of the muscles of the face; the eyes, which are deeply sunken in their sockets, have a weird, uncanny look. The features are pinched and the face shrunken. A cold, clammy sweat exudes from the pores of the skin, which has an appearance of profound anaemia. The lips are bloodless and the fingers and nails are blue. The pulse is almost imperceptible; a weak, threadlike stream may, however, be detected in the radial artery. The thermometer, placed in the rectum, registers 96° or 97°F. The muscles are not paralyzed anywhere, but the patient seems disinclined to make any muscular effort. Even respiratory movements seem for the time to be reduced to a minimum. Occasionally the patient may feebly throw about one of his limbs and give vent to a hoarse, weak groan. There is no insensibility ..., but he is strangely apathetic, and seems to realize but imperfectly the full meaning of the questions put to him. There is no use to attempt an operation until appropriate remedies have brought about a reaction. The pulse, however, does not respond; it grows feebler and finally disappears, and "this momentary pause in the act of death" is soon followed by the grim reality. A postmortem examination reveals no visible changes in the internal organs.[1]

Types of shock

Adequate perfusion of body tissues depends on the pumping ability of the heart, a vascular circuit that transports blood to the cell and back to the heart, a sufficient amount of blood to fill the circulatory system, and tissues that are able to use and extract oxygen and nutrients from the blood delivered to the capillaries of the microcirculation. There are several ways to classify shock. For our purposes the following classification is useful: (1) hypovolemic, (2) cardiogenic, (3) obstructive, and (4) distributive. The four types of shock are summarized in Chart 23-1.

Hypovolemic shock

Hypovolemic shock occurs when there is an acute loss of 15% to 20% of the circulating blood volume. The decrease may be due to a loss of whole blood (hemorrhage), plasma (severe burns), or extracellular fluid (gastrointestinal fluids lost in vomiting or diarrhea). Hypovolemic shock can also occur with third-space losses, when extracellular fluid is trapped outside the vascular compartment. Often blood and fluid losses are concealed. One source cites the case of an elderly man who suffered severe crushing injuries of both legs. The patient had no external evidence of bleeding yet required 8 liters of blood over a period of 7 hours for stabilization of vital signs.[1]

Of the four types of shock, hypovolemic shock has been the most widely studied and usually serves as a prototype in discussions of the manifestations of shock. The severity and clinical findings associated with hypovolemic shock are summarized in Table 23-1.

The progression of hypovolemic shock can be divided into four stages. There is an *initial stage* during which the circulatory blood volume is decreased but not enough to cause serious effects. The second

---

Chart 23-1: Classification of shock

1. Hypovolemic
   Loss of whole blood
   Loss of plasma
   Loss of extracellular fluid
2. Cardiogenic
   Failure of the heart as a pump (myocardial damage or deterioration)
   Severe alterations in rhythm (heart block or severe bradycardia)
   Mechanical defect (papillary muscle dysfunction/rupture, ventricular aneurysm, or ventricular septal defect)
3. Obstructive
   Inability to fill properly (cardiac tamponade)
   Obstruction to outflow (pulmonary embolus, cardiac myxoma, pneumothorax, or dissecting aneurysm)
4. Distributive
   Loss of sympathetic vasomotor tone
   Presence of vasodilating substances in the blood (anaphylactic, septic, or toxic shock syndrome)
   Arteriovenous shunting
   Failure of body cells to utilize oxygen

stage is the *compensatory stage;* although the circulating blood volume is reduced, compensatory mechanisms are able to maintain blood pressure and tissue perfusion at a level sufficient to prevent cell damage. The third stage is the *progressive stage* or *stage of decompensated shock.* At this point unfavorable signs begin to appear: the blood pressure begins to fall, blood flow to the heart and brain is impaired, capillary permeability is increased, fluid begins to leave the capillary, blood flow becomes sluggish, and the body cells and their enzyme systems are damaged. The fourth and final stage of shock is the *irreversible stage.* In irreversible shock, even though the blood volume may have been temporarily restored and vital signs stabilized, death ensues eventually. Although the factors that determine recovery from severe shock have not been clearly identified, it appears that they are related to blood flow at the level of the microcirculation.

Compensatory mechanisms

Three major compensatory mechanisms are activated in hypovolemic shock: (1) vasoconstrictor response, (2) shift of fluid from the interstitial to the intravascular compartment, and (3) increased pumping efficiency of the heart. The compensatory mechanisms in hypovolemic shock are summarized in Figure 23-1.

Within seconds after the onset of hemorrhage or the loss of blood volume, signs of sympathetic and adrenal medullary activity appear. During the early stages, vasoconstriction causes a reduction in the size of the vascular compartment and an increase in peripheral vascular resistance. This response is usually all that is needed when the injury is slight, and blood loss is arrested at this point. Ten percent of a person's total volume of blood can be removed without significantly affecting blood pressure—the reader is reminded that the average blood donor loses a pint of blood without suffering adverse effects. Figure 23-2 shows how blood loss influences cardiac output and blood pressure. It can be seen that the changes in blood pressure lag behind the drop in cardiac output. This is due to the vasoconstriction and increase in heart rate that occur as blood leaves the circulatory system. It is also apparent that cardiac output and tissue blood flow will decrease before signs of hypotension occur.

As shock progresses, the heart rate and cardiac contractility increase and vasoconstriction becomes more intense. The blood flow to the skin, skeletal muscles, kidneys, and abdominal organs decreases. The sympathetic vasoconstrictor response affects both the arterioles and the veins. Arteriolar constriction helps to maintain blood pressure by increasing the

Table 23-1. Correlation of clinical findings and the magnitude of volume deficit in hemorrhagic shock

Severity of shock	Clinical findings	Percent reduction in blood volume* (ml in parentheses)
None	None; normal blood donation	Up to 10 (500 ml)†
Mild	Minimal tachycardia	15–25 (750–1250)
	Slight decrease in blood pressure	
	Mild evidence of peripheral vasoconstriction with cool hands and feet	
Moderate	Tachycardia, 100–120 bpm	25–35 (1250–1750)
	Decrease in pulse pressure	
	Systolic pressure, 90–100 mmHg	
	Restlessness	
	Increased sweating	
	Pallor	
	Oliguria	
Severe	Tachycardia over 120 bpm	Up to 50 (2500)
	Blood pressure below 60 mmHg systolic and frequently unobtainable by cuff	
	Mental stupor	
	Extreme pallor, cold extremities	
	Anuria	

* Blood volume changes based on the clinical observations of Beecher et al.
† Based on blood volume of 7% in a 70-kg male of medium build.
(Weil M, Shubin H: Diagnosis and Treatment of Shock, p 118. Baltimore, Williams & Wilkins, 1967)

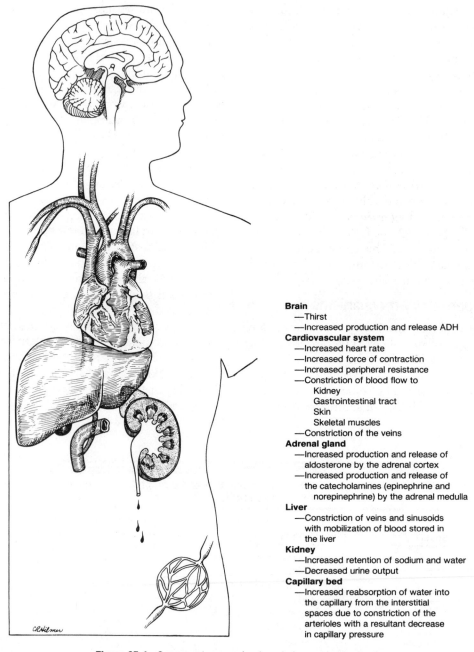

Brain
—Thirst
—Increased production and release ADH
Cardiovascular system
—Increased heart rate
—Increased force of contraction
—Increased peripheral resistance
—Constriction of blood flow to
  Kidney
  Gastrointestinal tract
  Skin
  Skeletal muscles
—Constriction of the veins
Adrenal gland
—Increased production and release of
  aldosterone by the adrenal cortex
—Increased production and release of
  the catecholamines (epinephrine and
    norepinephrine) by the adrenal medulla
Liver
—Constriction of veins and sinusoids
  with mobilization of blood stored in
  the liver
Kidney
—Increased retention of sodium and water
—Decreased urine output
Capillary bed
—Increased reabsorption of water into
  the capillary from the interstitial
  spaces due to constriction of the
  arterioles with a resultant decrease
  in capillary pressure

Figure 23-1 Conpensatory mechanisms in hypovolemic shock.

systemic vascular resistance, whereas venous constriction mobilizes blood that has been stored in the capacitance side of the circulation and increases venous return to the heart. There is considerable capacity for blood storage in the large veins of the abdomen and the liver. About 350 ml of blood that can be mobilized in shock is stored in the liver.

The compensatory changes in heart rate, cardiac contractility, and vascular tone developing in shock are mediated through the sympathetic nervous system. In the absence of sympathetic reflexes, only about 15% to 20% of the blood can be removed over a period of 30 minutes before death occurs, compared with the 30% to 40% that can be removed over a similar time period with intact sympathetic innervation.[2] Sympathetic stimulation does not cause constriction of the cerebral and coronary vessels, and blood flow through the heart and brain is maintained at essentially normal levels as long as the mean arterial pressure remains above 70 mmHg.[2]

Vasoconstriction causes a reduction in the size of the vascular compartment, so that it can be adequately filled by a smaller blood volume. Compensatory mechanisms designed to replace fluid lost from the vascular compartment also exist. During shock, a decline in capillary pressure causes water to be drawn

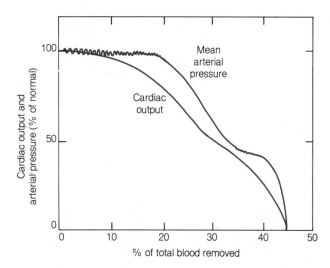

Figure 23-2 Effect of hemorrhage on cardiac output and arterial pressure. *(Guyton AC: Textbook of Medical Physiology, 7th ed. Philadelphia, WB Saunders, 1986)*

into the vascular compartment from the interstitial spaces. The maintenance of vascular volume is further enhanced by renal mechanisms that conserve fluid. The previously described decrease in renal blood flow resulting from sympathetic vasoconstriction causes both a decrease in the glomerular filtration rate and an increase in the reabsorption of sodium and water, due to activation of the renin–angiotensin–aldosterone mechanism. The decrease in blood volume also stimulates the centers in the hypothalamus that regulate the antidiuretic hormone (ADH) and thirst; a decrease in blood volume of 10% is sufficient to activate both of these mechanisms.[3]

—— Cardiogenic shock

Cardiogenic shock implies failure of the heart to pump blood adequately. It differs from hemorrhagic shock in that cardiac output falls despite a normal or elevated blood volume and cardiac pressures. Cardiogenic shock can occur because of the damage to the heart that occurs during myocardial infarction, ineffective pumping due to cardiac dysrhythmias, mechanical defects that may occur as a complication of myocardial infarction such as ventricular septal defect, ventricular aneurysm, acute disruption of valvular function, or problems associated with open-heart surgery. Cardiomyopathy, whether due to hypertension, alcohol, bacterial or viral infection, ischemia, or unknown etiology, is another major cause of cardiogenic shock. In all cases there is failure to eject blood from the heart, hypotension, and inadequate cardiac output. Often increased peripheral vascular resistance is present and contributes to the deterioration of cardiac function by increasing afterload or the resistance to ventricular systole. The filling pressure, or preload of the heart, is also increased. De-

creased cardiac output results in increased end-systolic ventricular volume. Added to the usual venous return, the presystolic load of the heart is increased and further complicates the cardiac status.

The most common cause of cardiogenic shock is myocardial infarction. It develops in 15% to 20% of persons admitted to hospitals with a diagnosis of myocardial infarction, and its severity and progression appear to be related to the amount of myocardium involved.[3,4] Patients dying of cardiogenic shock generally have lost at least 40% of the contracting muscle of the left ventricle because of either a recent infarct or a combination of recent and old infarcts.

Cardiogenic shock can also follow other types of shock associated with inadequate coronary blood flow, or it can develop because substances released from ischemic tissues impair cardiac function. One such substance, myocardial toxic factor (MTF), is released into the circulation during severe shock. The MTF has a severe depressant effect on myocardial contractility, frequently reducing the cardiac contractile efficiency by as much as 50%. The MTF is thought to originate in the pancreas as the result of cellular ischemia in that organ.[2]

Treatment of cardiogenic shock requires a precarious balance between improving cardiac output, reducing the workload (and oxygen needs) of the myocardium, and preserving coronary perfusion. There is a need to regulate fluid volume within a level that maintains the filling pressure (venous return) of the heart and maximum utilization of the Frank-Starling mechanism without causing pulmonary congestion. Use of the Swan-Ganz balloon-tipped catheter has provided a means for monitoring the circulatory filling pressure by measuring pulmonary capillary wedge pressure (see Chapter 22). When the catheter is properly positioned and the balloon is inflated, the catheter will obstruct forward blood flow, allowing left heart pressures to be reflected through the catheter tip. The catecholamines increase cardiac contractility but must be used with caution, because they also produce vasoconstriction and increase the afterload. The openings for the coronary arteries are located in the aorta just distal to the aortic valve. The major portion of coronary blood flow occurs during diastole and depends largely on aortic diastolic pressure. Unfortunately, an increase in aortic pressure needed to improve coronary perfusion produces an increase in the afterload and myocardial oxygen consumption that may cause further myocardial ischemia and necrosis. The aortic balloon pump (to be discussed later) provides a means of increasing aortic diastolic pressure so as to maintain coronary and peripheral blood flow without increasing systolic pressure and the afterload, against which the left ventricle must pump.

Obstructive shock

Any condition that causes mechanical obstruction to the flow of blood through the central circulation (great veins, heart, or lungs) may result in shock. Although obstructive shock can be caused by a number of conditions including dissecting aortic aneurysm, cardiac tamponade, pneumothorax, atrial myxoma, or evisceration of abdominal contents into the thoracic cavity due to a ruptured hemidiaphragm, its most frequent cause is a pulmonary embolus. The primary physiologic result of obstructive shock is elevated right heart pressure and/or impaired venous return to the heart. Treatment modalities focus on correcting the cause of the disorder, frequently with surgical interventions or invasive procedures such as pericardicentesis (removal of fluid from the pericardial sac) for tamponade or the insertion of a chest tube for correction of a tension pneumothorax.

Distributive shock

With loss of blood vessel tone, the capacity of the vascular compartment expands to the extent that a normal volume of blood does not fill the circulatory system. Loss of vessel tone has two main causes: (1) a decrease in the sympathetic control of vasomotor tone and (2) the presence of vasodilator substances in the blood. There is a decrease in venous return in distributive shock, which leads to a diminished cardiac output, but no decrease in the total blood volume; hence this type of shock is often referred to as *normovolemic shock.*

Neurogenic shock

The term *neurogenic shock* describes shock due to decreased sympathetic control of blood vessel tone; there may be a defect in vasomotor center function in the brain stem or in the sympathetic outflow to the blood vessels. Output from the vasomotor center can be interrupted by brain injury, the depressant action of drugs, hypoxia, or lack of glucose (*e.g.,* insulin reaction). Fainting due to emotional causes is a transient form of neurogenic shock. General anesthetic agents can depress the vasomotor center, and spinal anesthesia or spinal cord injury can interrupt the transmission of outflow from the vasomotor center. In contrast to hypovolemic shock, in neurogenic shock the heart rate is often slower than normal and the skin is dry and warm.

Anaphylactic shock

Vasodilator substances in the blood can produce massive vasodilatation with peripheral blood pooling. This, in fact, is what happens in *anaphylactic shock.* This type of shock is due to a hypersensitivity reaction in which histamine and histamine-like substances are released into the blood (see Chapter 12). These substances cause dilatation of both arterioles and venules along with a marked increase in capillary permeability. The vascular response in anaphylactic shock is accompanied by the contraction of other nonvascular smooth muscle such as the bronchioles. Penicillin, shellfish, insect stings, animal sera, and nuts are antigens that are common causes of anaphylactic shock.

Anaphylactic shock is usually of sudden origin; death can occur within a matter of minutes unless appropriate medical intervention is promptly instituted. Signs and symptoms associated with impending anaphylactic shock include abdominal cramps, apprehension, burning and warm sensation of the skin, itching, urticaria (hives), coughing, choking, wheezing, tightness of the chest, and difficulty in breathing. Once blood begins to pool peripherally, there is a precipitous drop in blood pressure and the pulse becomes so weak that it is difficult to detect. Airway obstruction may ensue as a result of laryngeal edema.

Prevention of anaphylactic shock is always preferable to treatment. Once a person has been sensitized to an antigen, the risk of a fatal outcome always exists. All persons with known hypersensitivities should carry some form of warning to alert medical personnel should they become unconscious or unable to relate this information. Information about Medic-Alert bracelets and tags is available through most pharmacies. Patients should be carefully questioned about any earlier drug reactions and should be told what medications they are to receive before the medications are administered. It is also recommended that persons being treated as outpatients remain in the facility for 30 minutes following any injection of medication known to produce anaphylaxis, because most serious reactions occur within this period of time.

Unfortunately, it is not always possible to prevent anaphylactic shock. Therefore, all health-care personnel should be aware of the characteristic signs and symptoms so that appropriate care can be instituted promptly. Epinephrine constricts the blood vessels and relaxes the smooth muscle in the bronchioles; it is usually the first drug to be given to a patient believed to be experiencing an anaphylactic reaction. Other treatment measures include the administration of oxygen, antihistamine drugs, and hydrocortisone. Resuscitation measures may be required. It is often helpful to institute measures to decrease absorption when the antigenic agent has been injected into the tissues. This can be accomplished by application of ice, which constricts the blood vessels. Measures to reduce absorption should not replace other treatment measures, but they may be particularly helpful in situations in which medical treatment is not immediately available; for example, application of ice may delay the absorption of the antigen from a bee sting so that there is time to secure medical attention.

—— Septic shock

Septic shock has only come to be recognized as a clinical entity in the past 40 years. Its incidence has increased in recent years. At present, it has a mortality rate of about 50%. Septic shock is most frequently associated with gram-negative bacteremia, although it can be caused by gram-positive bacilli and other microorganisms.[5]

Unlike other types of shock, septic shock is often associated with pathologic complications such as pulmonary insufficiency (shock lung), disseminated intravascular clotting (DIC), and multiple organ failure. Septic shock often presents with fever, vasodilatation, and warm, flushed skin. Mild hyperventilation, respiratory alkalosis, and abrupt alterations in personality and inappropriate behavior (due to reduction in cerebral blood flow) may be the earliest signs of septic shock. These signs, which are thought to be a primary response to the bacteremia, often precede the usual signs and symptoms of sepsis by several hours or days.

Two major predisposing factors are involved in the development of septic shock: access to the vascular compartment by an infectious agent and a susceptible host. The elderly and those with extensive trauma and burns, neoplastic disease, and diabetes are particularly susceptible to infection and the development of septic shock. Another cause is the presence of an indwelling urinary or intravenous catheter. It has been proposed that the rising incidence of septic shock is related to (1) the widespread use of antibiotics, with development of a reservoir of virulent and resistant organisms; (2) concentration in hospitals of larger numbers of infections; (3) more extensive operations on elderly and high-risk patients; (4) an increase in the number of patients suffering from severe trauma; and (5) use of steroids and immunosuppressant and anticancer drugs.[6]

There appear to be two basic hemodynamic patterns associated with septic shock, dependent on the patient's vascular volume at the onset of shock.[1] The first pattern is a hyperdynamic circulatory response in patients with a normal blood volume at the onset of sepsis. These patients have a high cardiac output, normal or increased central venous pressure, increased pulse pressure, and warm and flushed skin. This response is seen most frequently in young healthy persons, for example, young women who have had a septic abortion. The second response pattern is seen in patients who have a decreased blood volume at the onset of sepsis. They present with a low cardiac

output, low central venous pressure, and cold, cyanotic extremities.

The causes of septic shock are unclear. There is evidence suggesting that sepsis causes a cellular defect that inhibits oxygen utilization and occurs before hemodynamic changes such as hypotension occur.[1] In this situation, a hyperdynamic circulatory response is probably a compensatory mechanism to increase the blood flow and oxygen supply to the deficient cells. Another possibility is that toxins from the sepsis-producing organisms incite an immune reaction, which leads to changes in the vascular tone and permeability. The resulting vasodilatation and third spacing of extracellular fluids combine to magnify the hypotensive effects of septic shock and increase the mortality. In experimental animals, shock may be induced by the injection of purified endotoxin, which has a protein lipopolysaccharide composition.[7] The polysaccharide component of the endotoxin produces a complement-consuming anaphylaxis-like reaction during which vasoactive substances such as histamine and serotonin are liberated. Whether or not the reactions to endotoxins seen in animals hold true for humans is at present a subject of controversy.

It seems probable that various organisms may produce septic shock through different mechanisms; this would account for the different hemodynamic responses seen in hyperdynamic, or warm, septic shock and those seen in hypodynamic, or cold, septic shock.

In recent years, a condition called *toxic shock syndrome* has become recognized as a life-threatening event. It is characterized by extreme hypotension, high fever, headache, dizziness, myalgia, confusion, skin rash, conjunctivitis, sore throat, vomiting, and watery diarrhea. Desquamation (peeling) of the skin on the hands and feet frequently occurs during convalescence.

Although some cases of toxic shock syndrome have been reported in men and children, by far the greatest number of cases occur in menstruating women. In one study of 37 cases reported during a 5-year period in Wisconsin, 35 occurred in menstruating women, and at least 10 of these women had one recurrent episode during subsequent menstrual periods.[8] The majority of these women were tampon users. *Staphylococcus aureus* was the organism most frequently cultured from the cervix and vagina.[9] Onset of menstrual toxic shock syndrome occurs 1 to 11 days after vaginal bleeding begins, the median interval being 2 days.[10] Nonmenstrual toxic shock syndrome has been associated with surgical infections; nonsurgical infections of the skin, subcutaneous, or osseous tissues; and childbirth or abortion.

Although the pathogenesis of toxic shock syndrome is not fully understood, several contributing factors have been postulated.[9] The acute febrile illness, which is similar to endotoxic shock, suggests a toxin-mediated process. Toxins produced by *Staphylococcus aureus* are known to produce fever, hypotension, and death in laboratory animals. It seems possible that toxin-producing staphylococci previously colonized in nasal passages or on the skin could be introduced into the vagina by way of the fingers or tampon applicator. Because the menstrual flow is a good medium for bacterial growth, multiplication of the bacteria occurs, with production of large quantities of the toxin. The toxin then diffuses from the hyperemic vaginal mucosa into the circulation, triggering complement, coagulation, kallikrein, and prostaglandin mechanisms that act in concert to produce the hypotension and other manifestations of toxic shock syndrome. The skin rash characteristic of the disorder may represent a hypersensitivity reaction to the toxin.

In summary, shock is an acute emergency situation in which body tissues are either deprived of oxygen or cellular nutrients or are unable to use these materials in their metabolic processes. Shock may develop because there is not enough blood in the circulatory system (hypovolemic shock), because the heart fails as a pump (cardiogenic shock), because blood flow or venous return is obstructed (obstructive shock), or because the tissues are unable to utilize oxygen and nutrients (distributive).

Manifestations

Pathophysiologic changes

The compensatory mechanisms that the body recruits in shock are not intended for long-term use. When injury is severe or its effects are prolonged, the compensatory mechanisms begin to have detrimental effects. The intense vasoconstriction causes a decrease in tissue perfusion, impaired cellular metabolism, liberation of lactic acid, and cell death. Once circulatory function has been reestablished at the onset of shock, whether the shock will be irreversible or the patient will survive is determined largely at the cellular level.

Flow in the microcirculation

Delivery of oxygen and nutrients to body cells and removal of metabolic waste products depend on adequate blood flow throughout the capillaries of the microcirculation. There are two types of capillary flow—*nutrient flow* and *nonnutrient flow* (see Figure 17-11). Nutrient flow describes flow in the true capillary pathways that supply cells with oxygen and nutrients. In nonnutrient flow, blood is shunted directly from the arterial to the venous side of the circulation without passing through the true capillary pathways. Nonnutrient flow provides warmth, but not oxygen and nutrients, to the tissues. In septic shock, nonnutrient flow is increased and the skin is warm and flushed. On the other hand, both nutrient and nonnutrient flow are decreased in hypovolemic shock and the skin is cool and clammy.

In severe and prolonged shock, the vascular system fails. When this occurs, there is relaxation of the arterioles and venules, a fall in arterial pressure, and venous pooling of blood. At the capillary level, hypoxia and products of cell deterioration cause increased capillary permeability, stagnation of blood flow, the formation of small blood clots, and trapping of intravascular volume in the interstitium due to third spacing of extracellular fluids.

Cellular changes

At the cellular level, oxygen and nutrients supply the energy needed to maintain cellular function. Within the cell, oxygen and fuel substrates are converted to adenosine triphosphate (ATP), the cell's energy source. The cell uses ATP for a number of purposes including protein synthesis and operation of the sodium and potassium membrane pump that extrudes sodium from the cell while returning potassium to its interior.

The cell uses two pathways to convert nutrients to energy (see Chapter 1). The first is the *anaerobic* (nonoxygen) *glycolytic* pathway, which is located in the cytoplasm. Glycolysis converts glucose to ATP and pyruvate. The second pathway is the *aerobic citric acid cycle* (Krebs' cycle), which is located in the mitochondria. When oxygen is available, pyruvate from the glycolytic pathway moves into the mitochondria and enters the citric acid cycle where it is transformed into ATP and metabolic by-products (carbon dioxide and water). Breakdown products of fatty acids and proteins can also be metabolized in the mitochondrial pathway. When oxygen is lacking, pyruvate does not enter the citric acid cycle; instead, it is converted to ATP and lactic acid. In severe shock, cellular metabolic processes are essentially anaerobic, which means that excess amounts of lactic acid accumulate in both the cellular and extracellular compartments. Measurements of lactate levels greater than 4.4 nmol/liter have been associated with significantly higher mortality.[11]

The anaerobic pathway, while allowing energy production to continue in the absence of oxygen, is relatively inefficient—it produces only 2 ATP units, whereas the citric acid cycle produces 36 ATP units.

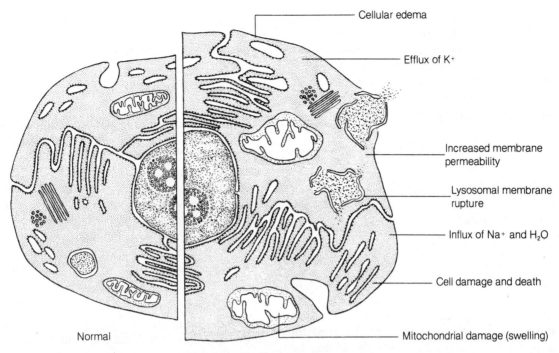

Figure 23-3 Cellular effects of shock.

Without sufficient energy production, normal cell function cannot be maintained (Figure 23-3). The activity of the sodium–potassium membrane pump is impaired—potassium leaves the cell and there is an influx of sodium and water. The cell swells and the membrane becomes more permeable. The mitochondria swell and the lysosomal membranes rupture. This is followed by cell death and the release of intracellular contents into the extracellular spaces. Last, there is reason to believe that the release of lysosomal enzymes and their products (*e.g.,* MTF from pancreatic enzymes) and vasoactive peptides leads to changes in the microcirculation that adversely affect recovery from shock.

Signs and symptoms

The signs and symptoms of shock are closely related to low peripheral blood flow and excessive sympathetic stimulation. For purposes of discussion, the manifestations of shock have been divided into the following categories: (1) thirst, (2) skin and body temperature changes, (3) arterial and venous pressure, (4) pulse, (5) urine output, and (6) changes in sensorium.

Thirst

Thirst is an early symptom in hypovolemic shock, easily overlooked in situations in which concealed bleeding occurs. Explanations regarding the causes of thirst are many, although the underlying cause is probably related to decreased blood volume and increased serum osmolarity (see Chapter 27). Pa-

tients with trauma frequently have a decreased renal blood flow, due to an intense adrenal medullary response, along with an increase in ADH levels, which causes water retention. Water should, therefore, be given cautiously because water intoxication can occur in a patient who continues to drink water in the face of altered renal function.

Skin and body temperature

The skin reflects the existence of two different peripheral responses to shock. In one, sympathetic stimulation leads to intense vasoconstriction of the skin vessels with activation of the sweat glands—the skin is cool and moist. In the other, there is vasodilatation—the skin is warm and flushed. The former can be observed in hypovolemic and cardiogenic shock, the latter in hyperdynamic septic shock. In cardiogenic shock, the lips, nailbeds, and skin are cyanotic because of stagnation of blood flow and increased extraction of oxygen from the hemoglobin as it passes through the capillary bed. In hemorrhagic shock, the loss of red blood cells leaves the skin and mucous membranes pale.

The decrease in body temperature, often observed in shock, reflects a decrease in the body's metabolic rate. There is a reported correlation between the temperature in the great toe (great toe temperature minus environmental temperature) and the survival rate in shock, in that patients who had increases in toe temperature during dopamine treatment for shock had the highest survival rate. These differences were not accounted for by a simultaneous increase in rectal temperature and were therefore thought to reflect differences in peripheral blood flow to the distal extremities.[12] In septic shock, body temperature may be elevated because of infection and the skin may be warm because of nonnutrient shunting of blood flow in the capillary beds of the skin and peripheral tissues.

Pressures and pulses

There has been considerable controversy over the value of blood pressure measurements in the diagnosis and management of shock. This is because compensatory mechanisms tend to preserve blood pressure until shock is relatively far advanced. Furthermore, an adequate arterial pressure does not ensure the adequate perfusion of vital structures such as the liver and kidneys. This is not to imply that blood pressure should not be measured in patients at risk for developing shock, but it does indicate the need for other assessment measures by which shock may be detected at an earlier stage.

In shock, blood pressure is often measured intra-arterially, as the sphygmomanometer may not always provide an accurate means; systolic pressures measured by the cuff method are often lower than those measured intra-arterially. This is because, in shock, the increased vascular resistance in the upper extremities prevents the hemodynamic events that normally produce Korotkoff sounds. Thus, the first tapping sounds detectable with the stethoscope will be heard at a pressure considerably lower than that measured from the artery. The *Doppler method,* in which blood pressure is measured noninvasively by ultrasound, often provides a more accurate estimate of Korotkoff sounds when they are no longer audible through the stethoscope. In some instances, this method may be used as an alternative to continuous intra-arterial monitoring.

An increase in heart rate is often an early sign of shock. Like vasoconstriction, the tachycardia of early shock is a sign of sympathetic nervous system response to injury. Tachycardia may also reflect emotional aspects surrounding the injury or the pain associated with the trauma. Blood volume and vessel tone are reflected in the quality of the pulse. A weak and thready pulse indicates vasoconstriction and a reduction in filling of the vascular compartment.

Urine output

Urine output decreases in the initial stages of shock, as was discussed earlier. Compensatory mechanisms decrease renal blood flow as a means of diverting blood flow to the heart and brain. Oliguria of 20 ml/hour or less is indicative of severe shock and inadequate renal perfusion. Continuous measurement of urine output is essential for assessing the circulatory status of the patient in shock.

Sensorium

Restlessness and apprehension are common behaviors in early hypovolemic shock. As the shock progresses and blood flow to the brain decreases, the restlessness of an earlier stage is replaced by apathy and stupor. During this latter stage, there is no longer an expression of concern about the outcome of the injury, and complaints of pain and discomfort cease. If shock is unchecked, the apathy will progress to coma. Coma due to blood loss alone and not related to head injury or other factors is usually an unfavorable sign; it usually means that the patient has sustained a lethal blood loss.[5]

In summary, the manifestations of shock are related to a low peripheral blood flow and excessive sympathetic stimulation. The low peripheral blood flow produces (1) thirst, (2) changes in skin temperature, (3) a fall in blood pressure and an increase in heart rate, (4) changes in venous pressure, (5) decreased urine output, and (6) changes in the sensorium. Signs and symptoms such as changes in skin temperature (increased in septic shock and decreased in hypovolemic and other forms of shock) may differ with the type of shock. The intense vasoconstriction that serves to maintain blood flow to the heart and brain causes a decrease in tissue perfusion, impaired cellular metabolism, liberation of lactic acid, and eventual cell death. Once circulatory function has been reestablished at the onset of shock, whether the shock will be irreversible or the patient will survive is determined largely by changes that occur at the cellular level.

Complications of shock

Wiggers, a noted circulatory physiologist, has aptly stated, "Shock not only stops the machine, but it wrecks the machinery."[13] Indeed, many body systems are wrecked by severe shock. Five major complications of severe shock are (1) shock lung, (2) acute renal failure, (3) gastrointestinal ulceration, (4) disseminated intravascular clotting, and (5) multiorgan failure. Thus, the complications of shock are serious and often fatal.

Shock lung

Shock lung or adult respiratory distress syndrome (ARDS) is a potentially lethal form of respiratory failure that can follow severe shock (see Chapter

26). The term *shock lung* was introduced during the Vietnam War to describe the progressive pulmonary failure seen in soldiers who suffered major trauma. The symptoms do not usually develop until 24 to 48 hours after the initial trauma, in some instances later. ARDS is thought to result from increased permeability of the pulmonary capillaries to water and plasma proteins. Protein-rich fluids leak into the alveolar and interstitial spaces, impairing gas exchange and making the lung stiffer and more difficult to inflate. Some patients develop a hyaline membrane syndrome similar to that seen in respiratory distress syndrome in the newborn. The respiratory rate and effort of breathing increase. Arterial blood gases establish the presence of profound hypoxemia with hypercarbia, resulting from impaired matching of ventilation and perfusion and from the greatly reduced diffusion of blood gases across the thickened alveolar membranes.

The exact cause of ARDS is unknown. It has been suggested that the problem results from (1) a decrease in lung perfusion and ischemia of the type II alveolar cells, which produce surfactant, (2) oxygen toxicity, (3) neurogenic factors that cause pulmonary venoconstriction and pulmonary edema due to sympathetic nervous factors, (4) fluid overload with stretching and disruption of the pulmonary capillaries, (5) damage to the lung by endotoxins and substances released as the result of sepsis, or (6) prolonged hypotension. One widely accepted cause of ARDS is disseminated intravascular clotting—the presence of thromboemboli in the pulmonary microcirculation. It is possible that multiple mechanisms operate to cause a similar pattern of injury or to trigger a common response (*e.g.*, intravascular clotting), which, in turn, produces the pulmonary damage.

Acute renal failure

The renal tubules are particularly vulnerable to ischemia, and *renal failure* is one important late cause of death in severe shock. In fact, sepsis and trauma account for the majority of cases of acute renal failure. The endotoxins implicated in septic shock are powerful vasoconstrictors, capable of activating the sympathetic nervous system and causing intravascular clotting. They have been shown to trigger all of the separate physiologic mechanisms that contribute to the onset of acute renal failure. The degree of renal damage is related to the severity and duration of shock; the normal kidney is able to tolerate severe ischemia for a period of 15 to 20 minutes. The renal lesion most frequently seen after severe shock is *acute tubular necrosis*. Acute tubular necrosis is usually reversible, although return to normal renal function may require weeks or months (see Chapter 32 for further discussion). Continuous monitoring of urine output during shock provides a means of assessing renal blood flow.

Gastrointestinal ulceration

The gastrointestinal tract is particularly vulnerable to ischemia because of the circulatory pattern of its mucosal surface. In shock there is widespread constriction of blood vessels supplying the gastrointestinal tract; this causes a redistribution of blood flow such that mucosal perfusion is severely diminished. In fact, there is growing evidence that the splanchnic and mesenteric vascular beds experience disproportionately greater vasoconstriction in response to circulating catecholamines and angiotensin II than other vascular beds.[14] As a result, superficial mucosal lesions of the stomach and duodenum can develop within hours of severe trauma, sepsis, or burn. (Stress ulcers associated with burns are called Curling's ulcers.) Bleeding is a common sign of gastrointestinal ulceration due to shock. Hemorrhage has its onset usually within 2 to 10 days following the original insult, and often it gives no warning.

Disseminated intravascular clotting (DIC)

Disseminated intravascular clotting, a complication of septic shock, is characterized by the formation of small clots in the microcirculation. Consumption and depletion of platelets, fibrinogen, and other clotting factors occur, leading to the disruption of the normal clotting process with abnormal bleeding or hemorrhage (see Chapter 15).

Multiple organ failure

Multiple organ failure is a particularly life-threatening complication of shock, especially septic shock. Mortality rates vary from 30% to 100% depending on the number of organs involved.[15] If required for long periods of time, many of the compensatory mechanisms stimulated by shock become the cause of multiple organ failure. Selectively severe vasospasm such as occurs in the hepatic and mesenteric circulations and the release of endorphins that potentiate the hypotensive effects of vasodilatation are just two of many mechanisms that contribute to failure of multiple organ systems.[14,16] Interventions for multiple organ failure are focused on support of the affected systems.

In summary, the complications of shock result from the deprivation of circulation to vital organs or systems such as the lungs, kidneys, gastrointestinal tract, and blood coagulation system. Shock lung or adult respiratory distress syndrome produces lung changes that occur with shock. It is characterized by changes in permeability of the alveolar-capillary membrane with the development of interstitial edema and severe hypoxia that does not respond to oxygen therapy. The renal tubules are particularly vulnerable to ischemia, and acute renal failure is an important complication of shock. Gastrointestinal bleeding occurs as a complication of gastrointestinal ischemia. Disseminated intravascular clotting is characterized by the formation of small clots in the circulation. It is thought to be caused by sluggish blood flow in the microcirculation or inappropriate activation of the coagulation cascade because of toxins or other products released as a result of the shock state. Multiple organ failure, perhaps the most ominous complication of shock, rapidly depletes the ability of the body to compensate and recover from a shock state.

Treatment measures

The treatment of shock is directed toward correcting or controlling the underlying cause and improving tissue perfusion. This discussion presents an overview of commonly employed treatments.

In hypovolemic shock, the goal of treatment is to restore vascular volume. This can be accomplished through intravenous administration of fluids and blood. The plasma expanders (*dextrans and colloidal albumin solutions*) have a high molecular weight, do not necessitate blood typing, and remain in the circulation for longer periods of time than the crystalloids such as glucose and saline. The dextrans must be used with caution, however, because they may induce serious or fatal reactions, including anaphylaxis.

── Circulatory assistance

In hypovolemic shock, a pneumatic compression suit called *military antishock trousers (MAST)* may be used.[17] The MAST suit, which encases the legs and abdomen and can be inflated separately or wholly, compresses the blood vessels of the legs and/or abdomen and increases venous return to the heart. This *autotransfusion* effect is particularly life-saving when used in the field to manage hemorrhagic shock or traumatic shock. The MAST suit is absolutely contraindicated in cardiogenic shock, however, because the increased venous return further overloads the failing heart.

In cardiogenic shock, treatment measures are directed toward reducing the work of the heart while improving its pumping efficiency. An intra-aortic bal-

Table 23–2. Vasoactive drugs used in treatment of shock

Drug	Mechanism	Action*
Epinephrine (Adrenalin)	Alpha Beta$_1$ and $_2$	Vasoconstriction (specific for anaphylactic shock) Increase in heart rate and cardiac contractility Causes a decrease in renal and splanchnic blood flow while increasing skeletal muscle flow
Norepinephrine (Levophed)	Alpha Beta$_1$	Vasoconstriction Increase in heart rate and cardiac contractility
Phenylephrine (Neo-Synephrine)	Alpha	Vasoconstriction
Isoproterenol (Isuprel)	Beta$_1$ Beta$_2$	Increase in heart rate and cardiac contractility Vasodilatation and perfusion of cerebral and renal tissue
Metaraminol (Aramine)	Alpha Beta$_1$	Vasoconstriction Increase in heart rate and cardiac contractility
Dopamine (Intropin)	Alpha Beta$_1$ Dopaminergic	Vasoconstriction with large doses Increased heart rate and cardiac contractility Vasodilatation of splanchnic and renal vessels
Dobutamine	Beta$_1$	Increases cardiac contractility with minimal increase in heart rate (specific in cardiogenic shock)
Nitroprusside (Nipride)	Dilator of venous and arterial smooth muscle	Decreases venous return to the heart causing a decrease in end-diastolic volume and pressure Decreases systemic vascular resistance with a resultant decrease in left ventricular stroke work (specific for cardiogenic shock)
Nitroglycerin (Tridil)	Dilator of venous smooth muscle at any dose Dilator of arterial smooth muscle at high doses	Same as nitroprusside

* This list is not intended to be inclusive; it encompasses the drug actions related only to treatment of shock.

loon pump may be used to supplement cardiac pumping in situations of severe cardiogenic shock. The balloon pump is inserted retrograde into the thoracic aorta through a peripheral artery. The balloon, filled with helium, is synchronized to inflate during diastole and deflate during systole. Diastolic inflation creates a diastolic pressure wave that results in increased perfusion to all the organs, including the myocardium. The sudden release of pressure at the onset of systole lowers resistance to ejection of blood from the left ventricle, thereby increasing the heart's pumping efficiency without increasing the afterload and myocardial oxygen consumption.

—— Vasoactive drugs

Vasoactive drugs are agents capable of either constricting or dilating blood vessels. Currently, there is considerable controversy about the advantages or disadvantages related to use of these drugs. The major vasoactive drugs used to treat shock are summarized in Table 23-2.

There are two types of receptors for the sympathetic nervous system—alpha and beta. Beta receptors are further subdivided into beta$_1$ and beta$_2$. In the cardiorespiratory system, stimulation of the alpha receptors causes vasoconstriction; stimulation of beta$_1$ receptors causes an increase in heart rate and the force of myocardial contraction; and stimulation of beta$_2$ receptors produces vasodilatation of the skeletal muscle beds and relaxation of the bronchioles. Currently, dopamine is prescribed to treat shock because it induces a more favorable array of alpha and beta receptor actions than many of the adrenergic drugs. Dopamine is thought to increase blood flow to the kidneys, liver, and other abdominal organs while maintaining vasoconstriction of less vital structures such as the skin and skeletal muscles. *Nitroprusside* (Nipride) and nitroglycerin, vasodilator drugs, are used to treat cardiogenic shock. Nipride causes both arterial and venous dilatation, thus producing a decrease in venous return to the heart with a reduction in arterial resistance against which the left heart must pump. Nitroglycerin focuses its effects on the venous vascular beds until, at high doses, it begins to dilate the arterial beds as well. The arterial pressure is maintained by an increased ventricular stroke volume ejected against a lowered peripheral vascular resistance; this allows blood to be redistributed from the pulmonary vascular bed to the systemic circulation.

In summary, the treatment of shock depends on the cause and type of shock that is present. It focuses on correcting or controlling the cause and improving tissue perfusion. In hypovolemic shock, the goal of treatment is to restore vascular volume. In cardiogenic shock, treatment is directed toward reducing the workload of the heart while improving its pumping efficiency. Vasoactive drugs, capable of either constricting or dilating blood vessels, may be used.

References

1. MacLean FL: Shock: Causes and management of circulatory shock. In Sabiston DC (ed): Davis-Christopher's Textbook of Surgery, 12th ed, pp 58, 59. Philadelphia, WB Saunders, 1981
2. Guyton AC: Textbook of Medical Physiology, 6th ed, p 333, 336, 441. Philadelphia, WB Saunders, 1981
3. Makabali C, Weil M, Henning RJ: An update on the therapy for shock: Current concepts in mechanisms and management of circulatory shock. Cardiovasc Rev Rep 3:899, 1982
4. Whitman G: Tissue perfusion. In McKinney M, Packa D, Dunbar S (eds): AACN Clinical Reference for Critical-Care Nursing, 2nd ed, p 129. New York, McGraw-Hill, 1988
5. Parker MM, Parillo JE: Septic shock: Hemodynamics and pathogenesis. JAMA 250:3324, 1983
6. Septic shock: A threat to the threatened. Emerg Med 19(18):24, 1987
7. Weil M: Current understanding of mechanisms and treatment of circulatory shock caused by bacterial infection. Ann Clin Res 9:181, 1977
8. Davis JP, Chesney MD, Wand PJ et al: Toxic-shock syndrome. N Engl J Med 303:1429, 1980
9. Tofte RW, Williams DN: Toxic shock syndrome. Postgrad Med 73(1):175, 1983
10. Shands KN, Schmid GP, Bruce BD: Association of tampon use and *Staphylococcus aureus* and clinical features in 52 cases. N Engl J Med 303:1436, 1980
11. Vincent JL, DuFaye P: Serial lactate determination during circulatory shock. Crit Care Med 11:449, 1983
12. Ruiz CE, Weil MH, Carlson RW: Treatment of circulatory shock with dopamine. JAMA 242(2):167, 1979
13. As cited in Smith JJ, Kampine JP: Circulatory Physiology, p 298. Baltimore, Williams & Wilkins, 1980
14. Buckley GB, Oshima A, Bailey RW: Pathophysiology of hepatic ischemia in cardiogenic shock. Am J Surg 151:87, 1986
15. Carrico CJ, Meakins JL, Marshall JC et al: Multiple organ failure syndrome. Arch Surg 121:196, 1986
16. Napolitano L, Chernou B: Endorphins in circulatory shock. Crit Care Med 16:566, 1988
17. Alfaro R: Pneumatic antishock suits: When and how to use them. Dimen Crit Care Nurs 1(1):9, 1982

Bibliography

Ayers SM: The prevention and treatment of shock in acute myocardial infarction. Chest 93:175–215, 1988

Beall GN, Cesaburi R, Singer A: Anaphyaxis—Everyone's problem. West J Med 144:329, 1986

Beckwith N: Fundamentals of fluid resuscitation. Nursing Life 7(3):49–56, 1987

Bennett BR: Positive and negative feedback mechanisms as a result of shock. Emerg Care Q 1(2):11–17, 1985

Bond RF, Johnson G: Vascular adrenergic interactions during hemorrhagic shock. Fed Proc 44:281, 1985

Brossack MA, Raffin TA: Importance of venous return, venous resistance and mean circulatory pressure in the physiology and management of shock. Chest 5:906–12, 1987

Chaudry IH: Cellular mechanisms in shock and ischemia and their correction. Am J Physiol 245:R117, 1983

Filkines JP: Monokines and the metabolic pathophysiology of septic shock. Fed Proc 44:300, 1985

Ganem D: Toxic shock syndrome. Medical Staff Conference, University of California, San Francisco. West J Med 135:383, 1981

Greenberg MD: Shock: Its pathophysiology and treatment. Emergency 18(6):52–53, 1986

Gysler M: Toxic shock syndrome—A synopsis. Pediatr Clin North Am 28:422, 1981

Jacobson MA, Young CS: New developments in the treatment of gram-negative bacteremia. West J Med 144:185, 1986

Loegering DJ: Intravascular hemolysis and RES phagocytic and host defense functions. Circ Shock 10:383, 1983

MacLean LD: Shock: A century of progress. Ann Surg 201:407, 1985

McSwain NE: Pneumatic anti-shock garment: State of the art 1988. Ann Emerg Med 17:506, 1988

Mizock B: Septic shock: A metabolic perspective. Arch Intern Med 144:579, 1984

Pinsky MR: Cause-specific management of shock. Postgrad Med 73:127, 1983

Rackow EC, Falk JL, Fein IA et al: Fluid resuscitation in circulatory shock: A comparison of the cardiorespiratory effects of albumin, hetastarch, and saline solutions, in patients with hypovolemic and septic shock. Crit Care Med 11:839, 1983

Rice V: Shock management. Part II. Pharmacologic intervention. Crit Care Nurse 5(1):42, 1985

Rice V: The clinical continuum of septic shock. Crit Care Nurse 4(4):86, 1984

Rice V: Shock management. Part I. Fluid replacement. Crit Care Nurse 4(6):69, 1984

CHAPTER 24

Control of Respiratory Function

Structural organization of the respiratory system
  Conducting airways
    Nasal passages
    Mouth and pharynx
    Larynx
    Tracheobronchial tree
  Respiratory tissues
  Pleura
Exchange of gases between the atmosphere and the alveoli
  Respiratory environment
    Atmospheric and respiratory pressures
    Pressure–volume relationships
    Law of partial pressures
    Water vapor pressure

Ventilation
  Mechanics of breathing
  Lung compliance
  Surface tension
  Airway resistance
  Efficiency and work of breathing
  Dead air space
Exchange and transport of gases in the body
Pulmonary blood flow
Ventilation–perfusion relationships
  Distribution of blood flow
  Distribution of ventilation
  Ventilation–perfusion ratio
Alveolar gas exchange

Gas transport
  Oxygen transport
  Carbon dioxide transport
  Blood gases
Hypoxia
  Acute hypoxia
  Chronic hypoxia
Control of respiration
  Neural control mechanisms
    Chemoreceptors
    Lung receptors
  Alterations in breathing patterns
    Periodic breathing
  Dyspnea
  Cough reflex
    Sputum
    Cough suppressants (antitussive drugs)
    Expectorants

Objectives

After you have studied this chapter, you should be able to meet the following objectives:

_____ State the three major components of respiration.

_____ List the structures of the conducting airways and respiratory tissues.

_____ Describe the function of the mucociliary blanket.

_____ Define *water vapor pressure*.

_____ Cite the source of water for humidification of air as it moves through the airways.

_____ Explain the mechanisms whereby fever causes an increase in the viscosity of respiratory secretions.

_____ Relate the differences in anatomical structure of the right and left primary bronchi to the effect of foreign body aspiration and displacement of an endotracheal tube.

_____ Compare the supporting structures of the large and small airways in terms of cartilaginous and smooth muscle support.

_____ Describe the autonomic nervous system innervation of the airways.

_____ Relate the elastic properties of the lungs and chest wall to the creation of a negative intrapleural pressure.

_____ State the function of the three types of alveolar cells.

_____ Relate Boyle's law to inspiration and expiration.

(continued)

_____ Explain how the law of partial pressures can be used to determine the pressure of a gas when its percentage of the total is known.

_____ Explain the effect that water vapor pressure has on the partial pressure of other alveolar gases.

_____ Compare atmospheric, airway, alveolar, and intrapleural pressures during the inspiratory and expiratory phases of ventilation.

_____ Define inspiratory reserve, expiratory reserve, vital capacity, and residual volume.

_____ Describe the method for measuring FEV_1.

_____ State the formula for determining lung compliance.

_____ Use Laplace's law to explain the need for surfactant in maintaining the inflation of small alveoli.

_____ State the major determinant of airway resistance.

_____ Explain why increasing lung volume (taking deep breaths) reduces airway resistance.

_____ Explain the effect of forced and normal expiratory effort on the volume of air that can be exhaled in a given period of time.

_____ Cite the difference between physiologic and anatomical dead air space.

_____ Trace the exchange of gases in the alveoli.

_____ Compare the distribution of blood flow and ventilation in the top and the bottom of the lungs in the standing and lying positions.

_____ Explain why ventilation and perfusion must be matched.

_____ List four factors that affect alveolar–capillary gas exchange.

_____ Explain the difference between Po_2 and hemoglobin-bound oxygen.

_____ Describe the transport of oxygen by hemoglobin.

_____ Explain the significance of shift to the right versus shift to the left in the oxygen-dissociation curve.

_____ State the significance of blood hemoglobin levels and the development of cyanosis.

_____ Explain why venous blood samples are not usually used for the measurement of blood gases.

_____ Define hypoxia.

_____ List the four types of hypoxia.

_____ State the manifestations of acute hypoxia.

_____ Explain how the body adapts to chronic hypoxia.

_____ Describe the difference between automatic and voluntary control of ventilation.

_____ Compare the role of the central and peripheral chemoreceptors in monitoring the Po_2 and Pco_2 levels of the blood.

_____ Cite the function of the lung receptors.

_____ Define four terms used to denote alterations in normal breathing.

_____ Describe the type of periodic breathing known as Cheyne-Stokes breathing.

_____ Define dyspnea.

_____ List three types of conditions in which dyspnea occurs.

_____ State the purpose of the cough reflex.

_____ Trace the physiologic mechanisms involved in coughing from the inhalation of an irritating substance to the actual expulsion effort of the cough.

_____ List four conditions that interfere with coughing.

_____ Compare the physiologic basis for the use of cough suppressants with that for the use of expectorants.

Respiration provides the body with a means for gas exchange. Respiration includes gas exchange at the cellular level (internal respiration), as well as the exchange of gases between the internal and external environments (external respiration). Respiration can be divided into three parts: (1) ventilation; (2) perfusion, or flow of blood in the pulmonary circulation; and (3) diffusion of gases between the alveoli and the blood in the pulmonary circulation. The discussion in this chapter focuses on the structure and function of the respiratory system as it relates to these three aspects of respiration. Included in the chapter is a discussion of breathing, breathing assessment, and coughing, which is needed for an understanding of the content in subsequent chapters.

Structural organization of the respiratory system

The respiratory system consists of the airways (nasal passages, mouth, nasopharynx, larynx, and trachea), the lungs, and the chest cage. The chest cage is a closed compartment, bounded at the top by the neck muscles and at the bottom by the diaphragm. The outer walls of the chest cage are formed by the 12 pairs of ribs, the sternum, the thoracic vertebrae, and the intercostal muscles that lie between the ribs. The inside of the chest cage is called the thoracic, or chest, cavity. The lungs are cone-shaped organs located side by side in the thoracic cavity (Figure 24-1). They are separated from each other by the mediastinum (the space between the lungs) and its contents (the heart, great vessels, esophagus, thymus, lymph nodes, and the vagus, cardiac, and phrenic nerves). The lungs lie free, invested in a transparent serous membrane called the pleura, except for attachments to the heart and trachea. The upper part of the lung, which lies against the top of the thoracic cavity, is called the apex, and the lower part, which lies against the diaphragm, is called the base. The right lung is divided into three lobes, and the left lung, into two lobes.

The respiratory system can be divided into two parts: the conducting airways and the respiratory tissues, where gas exchange takes place. The conducting portion of the respiratory tract consists of the

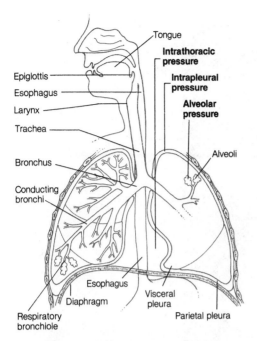

Figure 24-1 Structures of the respiratory system and respiratory pressures.

nose, nasopharynx, larynx, trachea, bronchi, and bronchioles (see Figure 24-1). The true respiratory portion of the lung consists of the alveolar structures and the pulmonary capillaries.

Conducting airways

The conducting airways are lined with a pseudostratified columnar epithelium, which contains serous glands, mucus-secreting goblet cells, and hair-like projections called cilia (Figure 24-2). The mucus produced by these cells forms a blanket-like layer, the *mucociliary blanket,* which protects the respiratory system and entraps dust and other foreign particles as they move through the conducting airways. The cilia, which are in constant motion, move the mucous blanket with its entrapped particles escalator fashion toward the pharynx from where it is either expectorated or swallowed.

The function of the mucous escalator in clearing the lower airways and alveoli is optimal at normal oxygen levels and is impaired by hypoxia and hyperoxia. Clearance is stimulated by coughing and adrenergic bronchodilators such as epinephrine. It is impaired by drying, for example, by heated but unhumidified indoor air during winter. Cigarette smoking also slows down or paralyzes the mucociliary escalator.[1] This slowing allows the residue from tobacco smoke, dust, and other particles to accumulate in the lungs, decreasing the efficiency of this pulmonary defense mechanism. There is also evidence that smoking causes hyperplasia of the goblet cells, which results in an increase in respiratory tract secretions, and increases the susceptibility and incidence of respiratory infections in smokers, as opposed to nonsmokers. As is discussed in Chapter 25, these changes are thought to contribute to the development of chronic bronchitis and emphysema.

Nasal passages

The nose is the preferred airway for the entrance of air into the respiratory tract during normal breathing. As air passes through the nasal passages, it is filtered, warmed, and humidified. The outer part of the nasal passages is lined with coarse hair, which aids in filtering dust and large particles from the air. The upper portion of the nasal cavity is lined with mucous membrane supplied with a rich network of small blood vessels; this portion of the nasal cavity supplies warmth and moisture to the air breathed.

The capacity of the air to contain water vapor without condensation occurring increases as the temperature rises. The *relative humidity* is the percentage of water vapor in the air at a specific temperature in relation to the maximum capacity of the air at that same temperature. The air in the alveoli, which is maintained at body temperature, is completely saturated with water vapor (relative humidity 100%) and usually contains considerably more water than is present in the air breathed. The difference between the water vapor contained in the air breathed and that found in the alveoli is drawn from the moist surface of the mucous membranes that line the respiratory passages and is a source of insensible water loss (see Chapter 27). Under normal conditions, about a pint of water per day is lost in the process of humidifying the air breathed.[2] The amount of moisture required to humidify the air is increased when a person breathes dry air. It is also increased during fever due to the temperature-associated increase in water vapor pressure within the lungs. In addition, an increase in the respiratory rate usually accompanies fever, so that more air passes through the airways, withdrawing moisture from its mucosal surface. As water is removed from these secretions to humidify the air, the respiratory secretions often become thick, preventing free movement of the cilia. Thus, the protective function of the mucociliary blanket may become impaired. This is particularly true of persons in whom the water intake is inadequate. With mouth breathing or breathing through a tracheotomy (opening in the throat), air entering the lungs is not warmed, filtered, or humidified as it would be when breathing through the nose. On the other hand, continuous airway ventilation (using humidified air) can lead to fluid overload by decreasing or eliminating the normal insensible water losses that occur with respiration.

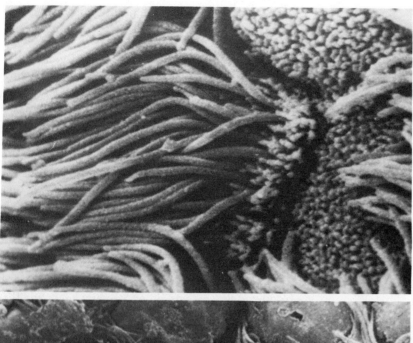

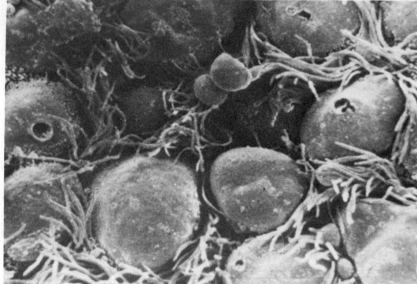

Figure 24-2 (Top) Scanning electron micrograph showing cilia (longer projections) that are in constant motion, moving the mucociliary blanket upward in a conveyor-belt fashion toward the pharynx. The small, flat clusters are the microvilli, which transport fluid across the bronchial lining. **(Bottom)** Scanning electron micrograph of the small, round goblet cells that secrete mucus. *(Courtesy of Janice Nowell of the University of California, Santa Cruz, California)*

Mouth and pharynx

The mouth serves as an alternative airway when the nasal passages are plugged or when there is need for the exchange of large amounts of air, such as occurs during exercise. The pharynx is the only opening between the nasal and mouth openings and the lungs. Consequently, obstruction of the pharynx leads to immediate cessation of ventilation. Neural control of the tongue and pharyngeal muscles is impaired in coma and in certain types of neurologic disease. In these conditions, the tongue tends to fall back into the pharynx and obstruct the airway, particularly if the person is lying on the back. Swelling of the pharyngeal structures due to injury or infection also predisposes a person to airway obstruction, as does the presence of a foreign body.

Larynx

The larynx connects the pharynx with the trachea. The epiglottis is a thin leaf-shaped structure that aids in covering the larynx during the act of swallowing to prevent food and fluids from entering the larynx and trachea. The walls of the larynx are supported by cartilaginous structures that prevent collapse during inspiration. The functions of the larynx can be divided into two categories: (1) those associated with speech and (2) those associated with protecting the lungs by preventing the entrance of substances other than air.

The larynx is located in a strategic position between the upper airways and the lungs, and is sometimes referred to as the watchdog of the lungs. When confronted with a substance other than air, the laryngeal muscles contract and close off the airway. At the same time, the cough reflex is initiated as a means of removing the foreign substance from the airway. Paralysis of the laryngeal muscles predisposes to aspiration of foreign materials into the lungs.

Tracheobronchial tree

The trachea, or windpipe, is a continuous tube that connects the larynx and the major bronchi of the lungs (Figure 24-3). It is about 2.0 cm to 2.5 cm in diameter and about 10 cm to 12 cm in length. The walls of the trachea are supported by horseshoe-shaped cartilages, which prevent it from collapsing during inspiration when the pressure in the thorax is negative.

The trachea divides to form the right and left *primary* bronchi. Each bronchus enters the lung through a slit called the *hilus*. The point at which the trachea divides is called the *carina*. The carina is heavily innervated with sensory neurons, and coughing and bronchospasm may result when this area is stimulated, as in tracheal suctioning. The right primary bronchus is shorter and wider and continues at a more vertical angle with the trachea than the left primary bronchus, which is longer and narrower, and continues from the trachea at a more acute angle. This makes it easier for foreign bodies to enter the right main bronchus rather than the left. For this reason, when an endotracheal tube is inserted to maintain a patent airway and facilitate ventilation, it is essential to secure the tube properly. If the tube should slip into the right main bronchus, it would prevent air from entering the left lung, causing it to collapse (atelectasis).

Each primary bronchus divides into *secondary*, or *lobar*, *bronchi*, which supply each of the lobes of the lungs—three in the right lung and two in the left. The right middle lobe bronchus is of relatively small caliber and length and sometimes bends sharply near its bifurcation. It is surrounded by a collar of lymph nodes that drain both the middle and lower lobes and is particularly subject to obstruction, recurrent infection, and atelectasis. The secondary bronchi divide to form the *segmental bronchi*, which supply the bronchopulmonary segments of the lung. There are ten segments in the right lung and nine segments in the left lung. These segments are identified according to their location in the lung (*e.g.*, the apical segment of the right upper lobe) and are the smallest named units in the lung. Lung lesions such as atelectasis and pneumonia are often localized to a particular bronchopulmonary segment.

The bronchi continue to branch, forming smaller bronchi, until they become the *terminal bronchioles*, the smallest of the conducting airways. The structure of the primary bronchi is similar to that of the trachea in that both of these airways are supported by cartilaginous rings. As the bronchi become smaller, however, the cartilaginous support thins out until it disappears at the level of the bronchioles. Instead, the bronchioles are encircled with a spiraling layer of smooth muscle fibers (Figure 24-4). Bronchospasm,

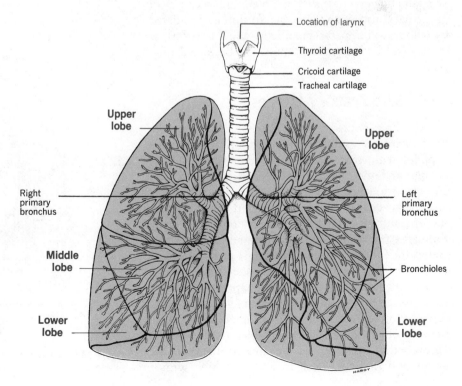

Figure 24-3   The larynx, trachea, and bronchial tree (anterior view). *(Chaffee EE, Lytle IM: Basic Physiology and Anatomy, 4th ed. Philadelphia, JB Lippincott, 1980)*

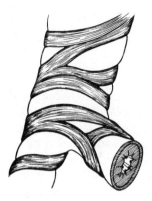

Figure 24-4 Arrangement of smooth muscle fibers that surround the bronchioles.

or contraction, of these muscles causes narrowing of the bronchioles and impairs air flow.

Bronchial smooth muscle tone is controlled by the autonomic nervous system. Afferent fibers from receptors in the smooth muscle are carried in the vagus nerve to respiratory control centers in the brain stem. Activation of parasympathetic outflow to bronchial smooth muscle through vagal efferent fibers produces bronchoconstriction. Sympathetic stimulation produces relaxation of bronchial smooth muscle and is mediated by means of beta-adrenergic receptors (beta$_2$). Studies have shown that few, if any, sympathetic nerve fibers directly innervate the airways and release neuromediators.[3] The beta receptors are stimulated by exogenous catecholamines or by endogenous epinephrine and norepinephrine that have been produced in the adrenal gland. Normally the parasympathetic nervous system maintains a low degree of bronchial constriction. Bronchial dilatation is initiated by withdrawal of parasympathetic tone that is further augmented by sympathetic-mediated bronchial dilatation.

Respiratory tissues

The lobules are the functional units of the lung where gas exchange takes place. Each lobule is supplied with structures that provide for both gas exchange and the circulation of blood (Figure 24-5). The gas exchange structures consist of a bronchiole and the alveolar ducts and sacs. Blood enters the lobule through a pulmonary artery and then exits through a pulmonary vein. Lymphatic structures surround the lobule and aid in removal of plasma proteins and other particles from the interstitial spaces.

The alveolar sacs are cup-shaped, thin-walled structures separated from each other by thin alveolar septa. Most of the septa are occupied by a single network of capillaries, so that the blood is exposed to air on both sides. It has been estimated that there are about 300 million alveoli in an adult lung with a

surface area of about 50 m^2 to 100 m^2.[4] Unlike the bronchioles, which are tubes with their own separate walls, the alveoli are interconnecting spaces that have no separate walls (Figure 24-6). As a result of this arrangement, the air between the alveolar structures mixes continually. Small discontinuities in the alveolar wall, the pores of Kohn, probably contribute to the mixing of air under certain conditions.

The alveolar structures are composed of three types of cells—the alveolar macrophages, the type I alveolar cells, and the type II alveolar cells. The alveolar macrophages are responsible for the removal of offending matter from the alveolar epithelium. Available evidence suggests that smoking impairs the function of the macrophages. The type I alveolar cells are flat squamous epithelial cells, across which gas exchange takes place. The type II alveolar cells produce surfactant, a lipoprotein substance that decreases the surface tension within the alveoli. This action allows for greater ease of lung inflation and helps to prevent the collapse of the smaller airways (to be discussed later).

Pleura

A thin, transparent, double-layered serous membrane, called the pleura, lines the thoracic cavity and encases the lungs. The outer, parietal layer lies adjacent to the chest wall, and the inner, visceral layer adheres to the surface of the lung. A thin film of serous fluid separates the two pleural layers, and this allows

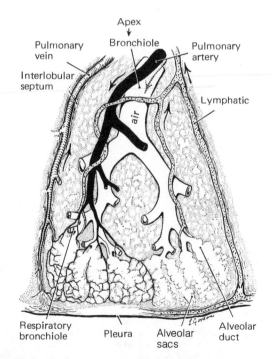

Figure 24-5 A lobule of the lung. *(Chaffee EE, Lytle IM: Basic Physiology and Anatomy, 4th ed. Philadelphia, JB Lippincott, 1980)*

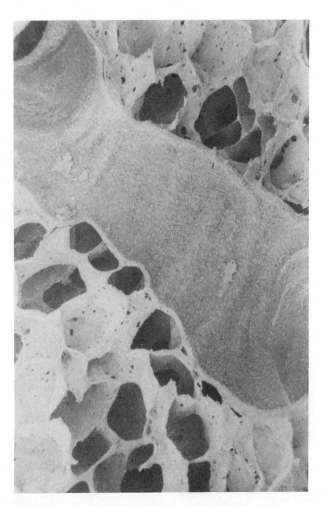

Figure 24-6 A close-up of a cross-section of a small bronchus and surrounding alveoli. *(Courtesy of Janice A. Nowell of the University of California, Santa Cruz, California)*

the two layers to glide over each other and yet hold together, so that there is no separation between the lungs and the chest wall. This adherence is similar to what occurs when a glass of water is placed on a thin film of water that has been spilled on a table top. The pleural cavity is a potential space in which serous fluid or inflammatory exudate can accumulate. *Pleural effusion* is an abnormal collection of excess fluid or exudate in the pleural cavity.

The pressure within the pleural cavity is always negative in relation to alveolar pressure (about -4 mmHg when the alveolar spaces are open to the atmosphere; *i.e.,* between breaths when the glottis is open). Both the lungs and the chest wall have elastic properties, each pulling in the opposite direction. If removed from the chest, the lungs would contract to a smaller size; and the chest wall, if freed from the lungs, would expand. The opposing forces of the chest wall and lungs create a pull against the visceral and parietal layers of the pleura, causing the pressure within the pleural cavity to become negative. During

inspiration, the elastic recoil of the lung increases, causing intrapleural pressure to become more negative than during expiration. Without the negative intrapleural pressure holding the lungs against the chest wall, their elastic recoil properties would cause them to collapse. Collapse of the lungs due to air in the pleural cavity is called *pneumothorax.*

In summary, the function of the respiratory system is to oxygenate and remove carbon dioxide from the blood. The respiratory system can be divided into two parts: the conducting airways and the respiratory tissues where gas exchange takes place. The conducting airways include the nasal passages, mouth, nasopharynx, larynx, and tracheobronchial tree. The conducting airways are lined with pseudostratified columnar epithelium, which contains serous glands, goblet cells, and hairlike projections called cilia. The mucus produced by these cells forms the mucociliary blanket, which aids in removing dust and other foreign particles from the respiratory tract. The exchange of gases between the external environment and the blood takes place in the lobules of the lungs, which are supplied with gas exchange structures (bronchiole, alveolar duct, and alveolar sac) and capillary blood flow, which enters through a pulmonary artery and exits through a pulmonary vein. The pleura, which is a transparent double-layered membrane, invests the lungs. A thin layer of fluid separates the two layers of the pleura and allows them to adhere and slide effortlessly over each other. The opposing elastic forces of the lungs and chest wall pull on the pleura, creating a negative pressure within the pleural cavity. Without this negative pressure, which holds the lungs against the chest wall, the elastic properties of the lungs would cause them to collapse.

Exchange of gases between the atmosphere and the alveoli

Respiratory environment

There is nothing mystical about ventilation; it is a purely mechanical event that obeys the laws of physics as they relate to the behavior of gases. Some of these principles are summarized for the reader's review.

Atmospheric and respiratory pressures

At sea level, the atmospheric pressure is 760 mmHg, or 14.7 pounds per square inch (PSI). In measuring respiratory pressure, atmospheric pressure is assigned a value of zero. A pressure of +15 mmHg means that the pressure is 15 mmHg above atmospheric pressure, and a pressure of −15 mmHg is 15 mmHg less than atmospheric. Respiratory pressures are often expressed in cmH$_2$O, which can be converted to mmHg by multiplying by 1.35. (The specific gravity of mercury is 13.546.)

Pressure–volume relationship

Boyle's law states that the pressure of a gas will vary inversely with the volume of the container, provided the temperature is kept constant. This means that if equal amounts of a gas are placed into two containers, one with a smaller volume than the other, the pressure of the gas in the container with the smaller volume will be greater than the pressure of the gas in that with the larger volume. The movement of gases is always from an area of greater pressure to one of lesser pressure. In the example just given, if a connection were placed between the two containers, air would move from the smaller volume to the larger volume.

Law of partial pressures

The pressure resulting from any particular gas is called the *partial pressure,* or *tension.* The capital letter P followed by the subscript for the chemical name of the gas (PO_2) is used to denote its partial pressure. The law of partial pressures states that the total pressure of a mixture of gases is equal to the sum of the partial pressures of the separate gases in the mixture. If the concentration of oxygen at 760 mmHg is 20%, then its partial pressure is 152 mmHg (760 × 0.20).

Water vapor pressure

The amount of water vapor contained in a gas mixture is determined by the temperature of the gas and is unrelated to atmospheric pressure. Air in the lungs is completely saturated (100% humidity) with water vapor. At a normal body temperature of 98.6°F, the pressure of water vapor in the lungs is 47 mmHg. The water vapor pressure must be included in the sum of the total pressure of the gases in the alveoli (*i.e.,* the total pressure of other gases in the alveoli is 760 − 47 = 713 mmHg).

Ventilation

Ventilation is concerned with the movement of gases into and out of the lung. It depends on a system of open airways and movement of the thoracic cage by the respiratory muscles—diaphragm, intercostals, and accessory muscles. The diaphragm is the principal muscle of inspiration. It is innervated by the phrenic nerve roots that arise from the cervical level of the spinal cord—mainly from C4, but also from C3 and C5. The intercostal muscles receive their innervation from the thoracic level of the spinal cord. When speaking of ventilation, the combined function of neuromuscular components and skeletal structures of the thoracic cage is often referred to as the *respiratory pump.*

Mechanics of breathing

During inspiration, an increase in thoracic volume causes a decrease in thoracic pressure, which, in turn, leads to air movement into the chest. This increase in volume is brought about mainly by contraction of the diaphragm. When the diaphragm contracts, the abdominal contents are forced downward and the chest expands from top to bottom (Figure 24-7). During normal levels of inspiration, the diaphragm moves about 1 cm, but this can be increased up to 10 cm on forced inspiration and expiration. Paralysis of the diaphragm causes it to move up rather than down during inspiration because of the negative pressure in the chest. This is called *paradoxical movement* and can be demonstrated on fluoroscopy when the patient sniffs.

The external intercostal muscles connect to the adjacent ribs and slope downward and forward.

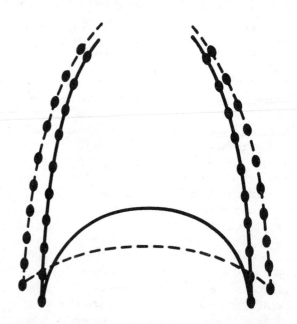

Figure 24-7 Action of the diaphragm. The diaphragm is shown as a curved line across the bottom of the rib cage. At end-expiration, indicated by *solid lines,* the rib cage diameter is small and the dome of the diaphragm is sharply curved. As the diaphragm contracts, the dome descends and becomes flatter, while the lower border of the rib cage is simultaneously pushed upward and outward. *(Guenter CA, Welch MH: Pulmonary Medicine, 2nd ed. Philadelphia, JB Lippincott, 1982)*

When they contract, they raise the ribs and rotate them slightly so that the sternum is pushed forward; this enlarges the chest from side to side and from front to back. Paralysis of the intercostal nerves does not seriously affect respiration because of the effectiveness of the diaphragm.

The accessory muscles of inspiration include the scaline muscles, which elevate the first two ribs, and the sternocleidomastoid muscles, which raise the sternum. These muscles contribute little to quiet breathing but contract vigorously during exercise. Other muscles that play a minor role in inspiration are the alae nasi, which produce flaring of the nostrils during obstructed breathing.

During expiration, the elastic components of the chest wall and the lung structures that were stretched during inspiration recoil passively, causing lung volume to decrease so that the pressure within the lungs is greater than the atmospheric pressure; therefore, air moves out of the lungs. Normally, expiration is a passive event that contributes little to the work of breathing. Instead, energy is expended in the work of enlarging the chest during inspiration. When needed, the abdominal and internal intercostal muscles can be used to increase expiratory effort. The increase in intra-abdominal pressure that accompanies the forceful contraction of the abdominal muscles pushes the diaphragm upward and results in an increase in intrathoracic pressure. The internal intercostals move inward, pulling the chest downward, and are also used to increase expiratory effort.

Respiratory pressures. The pressure inside the airways and the alveoli of the lung is called the *intrapulmonary pressure*. The pressure within the alveoli can also be called the *alveolar pressure*. The gases within this area of the lung are in communication with atmospheric pressure. When the glottis is open and no air is moving into or out of the lungs (prior to inspiration or expiration) the intrapulmonary pressure is equal to atmospheric pressure. The pressure in the pleural cavity is called the *intrapleural pressure*. It is always less than, or negative in relation to, the intrapulmonary and atmospheric pressures. It is this negative pressure that overcomes the elastic recoil properties of the lungs and prevents the lungs from collapsing. The *intrathoracic* pressure is the pressure within the thoracic cavity. It is equal to intrapleural pressure and is the pressure to which the heart and great vessels are exposed. The locations of the different respiratory pressures are illustrated in Figure 24-1.

The intrapulmonary and intrapleural pressures change with ventilation (Figure 24-8). They become more negative as the chest enlarges during inspiration and less negative as the chest becomes smaller during expiration. During inspiration, there is a

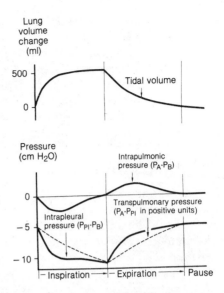

Figure 24-8 Changes and interrelationships of lung volume, intrapulmonary pressure, intrapleural pressure, and transpulmonary pressure during a breathing cycle. (P_B = barometric pressure; P_A = alveolar pressure; P_{Pl} = pleural pressure.) *(Slonin NB, Hamilton LH: Respiratory Physiology, 5th ed. St Louis, CV Mosby, 1985)*

greater decrease in intrapleural pressure than in intrapulmonary pressure. The resultant increase in transpulmonary pressure (difference between airway and intrapleural pressure) pulls the airways open, facilitating the air flow. During expiration the reverse is true: there is a proportionately greater decrease in the airway pressure than in the intrapleural pressure; the transpulmonary pressure is less and the airways become smaller.

Lung compliance

Lung compliance describes the ease with which the lungs can be inflated and is related to their elasticity.

Specifically, it refers to a change in lung volume that occurs with a given change in respiratory pressures.

$$\text{compliance} = \frac{\text{change in volume}}{\text{change in pressure}}$$

For example, it takes less negative pressure, and thus less inspiratory effort, to inflate a compliant lung than it does to inflate a stiff and noncompliant lung. It is similar to blowing up a new and noncompliant balloon and one that is compliant from having been blown up before. Lung compliance is decreased in lung diseases such as interstitial lung disease and pulmonary fibrosis, which cause the lungs to become stiff and lose their elasticity. Pulmonary congestion and edema produce a reversible decrease in pulmonary compliance. Pulmonary compliance is increased in the elderly and in persons with emphysema, probably because of changes in elastic tissues.

Lung compliance can be evaluated by using lung volumes and esophageal pressures, which are used as a measurement for intrapleural pressure. Lung volumes are measured using the spirometer, and esophageal pressures are measured by passing a tube with a small balloon attached into the esophagus.

Surface tension

An important factor in lung inflation is the surface tension of the liquid film that lines the alveoli. It arises because the forces that hold the molecules of the liquid film together are much stronger than those between the liquid–gas interface; the result is that the surface area of the liquid film tends to become as small as possible. The same behavior is seen in soap bubbles. The surface of the bubble contracts to form a sphere as the bubble is being blown. The pressure in the alveoli (which are modeled as spheres with open airways leading from them) can be predicted using Laplace's law (pressure = 2 × surface tension/radius). Thus, if the surface tension was equal throughout the lung, the alveoli with the smallest radii would have the greatest pressure, and this would cause them to empty into the larger alveoli. This does not occur, however, because of the surface-tension-reducing properties of the surfactant molecules that line the inner surface of the alveoli.

The pulmonary surfactants are a group of phospholipids that are synthesized within the type II alveolar cells and secreted into the alveoli where they become part of the lining layer. The surfactant molecule has two ends: a hydrophobic (water-insoluble) end and a hydrophilic (water-soluble) end. The hydrophilic end attaches to fluid molecules, and the hydrophobic end, to the gas molecules, interrupting the forces between the fluid molecules that are responsible for creating the surface tension. Surfactant exerts three important effects on lung inflation: (1) it increases lung compliance, or ease of inflation; (2) it provides stability and more even inflation of the alveoli; and (3) it assists in keeping the alveoli dry. Without surfactant, lung inflation would be extremely difficult, requiring intrapleural pressures of −20 mmHg to −30 mmHg, compared with the −3 mmHg to −5 mmHg normally needed to maintain inflation of the alveoli.[5] Surfactant not only reduces the surface tension in the alveoli, but it does so more effectively in the small alveoli, which have the greatest tendency to empty into the larger alveoli and collapse. It is thought that the surface-active molecules of surfactant are more densely packed at the surface of the small alveoli, and hence the surface-tension-reducing ability is greater than in larger alveoli where the density of the molecules is less. Surfactant also helps to keep the alveoli dry. The surface tension forces tend to pull fluid into the alveoli from the capillaries; by reducing these forces, surfactant prevents the transudation of this fluid across the alveolar–capillary membrane.

The type II alveolar cells that produce surfactant do not begin to mature until the 26th to 28th weeks of gestation, and consequently, many premature babies are born with poorly functioning type II alveolar cells and have difficulty producing sufficient amounts of surfactant. In these babies, the collapse of the lungs because of a lack of surfactant is called respiratory distress syndrome (RDS), or hyaline membrane disease. The production of surfactant also requires adequate amounts of oxygen and blood flow for delivery of substrates such as fatty acids. Among infants predisposed to develop RDS are premature infants, infants of diabetic mothers, infants born by cesarean section (when performed prior to the 38th week of gestation), and those suffering from hypoxia, acidosis, and hypothermia.

When it is necessary to consider the early delivery of an infant, an estimate of the maturity of the type II alveolar cells can be obtained by measuring the *lecithin* to *sphingomyelin* (L/S) ratio in the amniotic fluid through amniocentesis. In this way, it is often possible to delay the delivery of an infant until the type II alveolar cells are sufficiently mature to permit its survival. The incidence of RDS among premature babies born through vaginal delivery appears to be less than among those born by cesarean section, and it has been hypothesized that the stress of vaginal delivery may increase the babies' cortisol levels. A number of studies have shown that cortisol can accelerate the maturation of type II cells.[6] These observations have led to the clinical use of corticosteroid drugs before delivery in mothers with babies at high risk for developing RDS. Human surfactant is now available and studies are being conducted to determine the effects of its administration on pulmonary function in premature infants.[7]

Surfactant production is also impaired in adult respiratory distress syndrome (ARDS), or shock lung, discussed in Chapter 23.

Airway resistance

Airway resistance refers to the impediment that air encounters as it moves through the airways. The volume of air that moves into and out of the alveoli is directly related to the pressure gradient between the alveoli and the atmosphere and inversely related to the resistance of the airways. The resistance of the airways, in turn, is inversely proportional to the fourth power of the airway radius. Normally, resistance to airflow is so small that only minute changes in pressure are needed to move large volumes of air into the lungs. For example, the average pressure change, from pharynx to alveoli, during a normal breath of 500 ml of air is less than 1 mmHg. Because a change in the size of the airway radius produces a 16-fold change in airflow, small changes in airway caliber, such as those caused by pulmonary secretions or bronchospasm, can produce a marked increase in airway resistance. For persons with these conditions to maintain the same rate of airflow as before the onset of increased airway resistance, an increase in driving pressure (respiratory effort) is needed.

The airway resistance is greatly affected by lung volumes, being less during inspiration than during expiration. This is because the airways are pulled open by traction from the surrounding lung tissue; as the lungs expand the airways are pulled open, and as the lungs deflate the elastic fibers of the airways recoil and their diameters decrease in size. This is one of the reasons persons with conditions such as bronchial asthma, which cause abnormal airway resistance, often have less difficulty in inhaling than exhaling.

Laminar and turbulent airflow. There are two types of airflow: laminar and turbulent. Laminar, or streamlined, airflow occurs in straight circular tubes with the gas in the center of the tube moving twice as fast as the average velocity because the gas at the periphery must overcome the resistance to flow. In contrast to laminar flow, turbulent flow is disorganized flow in which the molecules of the gas move laterally, collide with each other, and change their velocities. Whether or not turbulence develops depends on the radius of the airways, the interaction of the gas molecules, and the velocity of airflow. It is most apt to occur when the radius of the airways is large and the velocity of flow is high. Turbulent flow occurs regularly in the trachea. Turbulence of airflow accounts for the breath sounds that are heard during

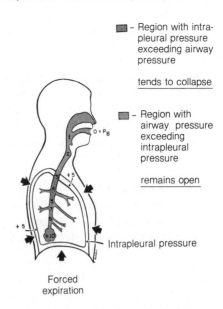

Figure 24-10 Mechanism that limits maximal expiratory flow rate. Forced expiration increases intrapleural pressure, reversing the transpulmonary pressure relationship. This reversal collapses nonrigid airways to produce an expiratory "check-valve." *(Slonin NB, Hamilton LH: Respiratory Physiology, 5th ed. St Louis, CV Mosby, 1985)*

chest auscultation (listening to the chest with a stethoscope).

In the bronchial tree with its many branches, laminar airflow probably occurs only in the very small airways where velocity of flow is low. Because the small airways contribute so little resistance, they constitute a silent zone. In small airway disease, it is probable that considerable abnormalities are present before the condition can be detected using the usual measurements of airway resistance.

Dynamic airway compression. Whether one starts to exhale forcefully or begins to exhale slowly and then accelerates, the volume of air that is exhaled over a given period of time remains the same (Figure 24-9). This occurs because the forced expiratory effort reduces the transpulmonary pressure (intrapleural pressure − airway pressure) needed to hold the airways open. Before inspiration has begun, the transpulmonary pressure is about −4 mmH$_2$O. The traction forces associated with increased lung expansion produce further increases in transpulmonary pressure during inspiration. During forced expiration, transpulmonary pressure is decreased because of a disproportionate increase in intrapleural pressure compared with airway pressure. As air moves out of the lung the drop in airway pressure causes a further decrease in the transpulmonary pressure (Figure 24-10). If this drop in pressure is sufficiently great, the surrounding intrapleural pressure will compress the nonrigid airways, interrupting the airflow and trapping air in the alveoli. Although this type of expiratory flow limitation is seen only during forced expiration in normal

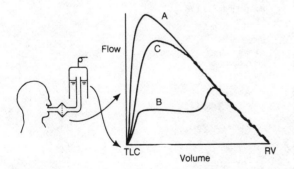

Figure 24-9 Flow-volume curves. In *A*, a maximal inspiration was followed by a forced expiration. In *B*, expiration was initially slow and then forced. In *C*, expiratory effort was submaximal. The descending portions of all three curves are almost superimposed. *(West JB: Respiratory Physiology, 2nd ed. Baltimore, Williams & Wilkins, 1979)*

persons, it may occur during normal breathing in persons with lung diseases such as emphysema, which magnify the pressure drop along the smaller airways and increase the intrabronchial pressure needed to maintain airway patency. Measures such as pursed lip breathing increase the airway pressure and improve the expiratory flow rates. Another factor that increases airway closure is low lung volumes, which reduce the transpulmonary driving pressure.

Lung volumes and capacities. The amount of air that is inhaled or exhaled from various lung volumes can be measured with a spirometer (Figure 24-11). With the type of spirometer depicted, the bell,

which is inverted over a water bath, moves down during inspiration and up during expiration, causing the pen to move up and down and mark the chart paper.

Lung volumes can be subdivided into four components: tidal volume, inspiratory reserve volume, expiratory reserve volume, and residual volume. The *tidal volume* (TV), usually about 500 ml, is the amount of air that moves into and out of the lungs during normal breathing. The maximum amount of air that can be inspired in excess of the normal tidal volume is called the *inspiratory reserve volume* (IRV), and the maximum amount that can be exhaled in excess of the normal tidal volume is the *expiratory reserve volume*

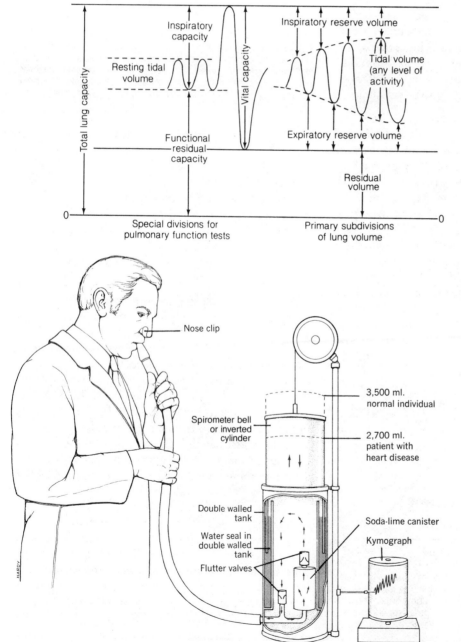

Figure 24-11 Measurement of vital capacity using a spirometer. *(Chaffee EE, Lytle IM: Basic Physiology and Anatomy, 4th ed. Philadelphia, JB Lippincott, 1980)*

(ERV). Some air always remains in the lungs following forced expiration—approximately 1200 ml; this air is the *residual volume* (RV). The residual volume tends to increase with age because more air is trapped in the lungs at the end of expiration.

The *total lung capacity* (TLC) is the sum of all the volumes in the lung. The residual volume cannot be measured with the spirometer because this air cannot be expressed from the lungs. The RV is measured by indirect methods such as the helium dilution method, the nitrogen washout method, or body plethysmography (see a respiratory physiology text for a description of these tests). Lung volumes and capacities are summarized in Table 24-1.

Lung capacities include two or more components of the total lung capacity. The *vital capacity* (VC) equals the IRV plus the TV plus the ERV and is the amount of air that can be exhaled from the point of maximal inspiration. The *inspiratory capacity* (IC) equals the TV plus the IRV. It is the amount of air that a person can breathe beginning at the normal expiratory level and distending the lungs to the maximal amount. The *functional residual capacity* (FRC) is the sum of the RV and ERV; it is the volume of air remaining in the lungs at the end of normal expiration.

Pulmonary function studies. The previously mentioned lung volumes and capacities are anatomical or static lung volumes, measured without relation to time. The spirometer is also used to measure dynamic lung function (ventilation with respect to time);

these tests are often used in assessing pulmonary function. Pulmonary function is measured for a variety of clinical purposes, including diagnosis of respiratory disease, preoperative surgical and anesthetic risk evaluation, and symptom and disability evaluation for legal or insurance purposes. The tests are often used in the evaluation of dyspnea, cough, wheezing, and abnormal x-ray or laboratory findings.

The *maximum voluntary ventilation (MVV)* measures the volume of air that a person can move into and out of the lungs during maximum effort lasting for 12 to 15 seconds. This measurement is usually converted to liters per minute. The *forced expiratory vital capacity (FVC)* involves full inspiration to total lung capacity followed by forceful maximal expiration. Obstruction of airways will produce an FVC that is lower than that observed with more slowly performed vital capacity measurements. The expired volume is plotted against time. The $FEV_{1.0}$ is the *forced expiratory volume* that can be exhaled in 1 second. Frequently, the $FEV_{1.0}$ is expressed as a percentage of the FVC. The $FEV_{1.0}$ and the FVC are used in the diagnosis of obstructive lung disorders. The *forced inspiratory vital flow (FIF)* measures the respiratory response during rapid maximal inspiration. Calculation of the airflow during the middle half of inspiration (FIF 25%–75%) relative to the forced midexpiratory flow rate (FEF 25%–75%) is used as a measure of respiratory muscle dysfunction, because the inspiratory flow is more dependent on effort than expiration. The pulmonary function tests are summarized in Table 24-2.

Table 24–1. Lung volumes and capacities

Volume	Symbol	Measurement
Tidal volume (about 500 ml at rest)	TV	Amount of air that moves into and out of the lungs with each breath
Inspiratory reserve volume (approximately 3000 ml)	IRV	Maximum amount of air that can be inhaled from the point of maximum expiration
Expiratory reserve volume (approximately 1100 ml)	ERV	Maximum volume of air that can be exhaled from the resting end-expiratory level
Residual volume (approximately 1200 ml)	RV	Volume of air remaining in the lungs after maximum expiration. This volume cannot be measured with the spirometer; it is measured indirectly using methods such as the helium dilution method, the nitrogen washout technique, or body plethysmography
Functional residual capacity (approximately 2300 ml)	FRC	Volume of air remaining in the lungs at end-expiration (sum of RV and ERV)
Inspiratory capacity (approximately 3500 ml)	IC	Sum of IRV and TV
Vital capacity (approximately 4600 ml)	VC	Maximum amount of air that can be exhaled from the point of maximum inspiration
Total lung capacity (approximately 5800 ml)	TLC	Total amount of air that the lungs can hold; it is the sum of all the volume components after maximal inspiration. This value is about 20% to 25% less in females than in males.

Efficiency and work of breathing

The *minute volume* is the amount of air that is exchanged in 1 minute; it is determined by the metabolic needs of the body. The minute volume is equal to the tidal volume multiplied by the respiratory rate, which is about 6000 ml (500 ml tidal volume × respiratory rate of 12 breaths per minute) during normal activity. The pattern of breathing—the tidal volume and the rate of breathing—is usually determined by the ease of lung expansion (compliance) and the effort needed to move air through the conducting airways. For example, in persons with stiff and noncompliant lungs, expansion of the lungs is difficult, and these persons usually find it easier to breathe if they keep their tidal volume low and breathe at a more rapid rate (*i.e.,* 300 × 20 = 6000 ml) to achieve their minute volume and meet their oxygen needs.

minute volume = tidal volume × respiratory rate

On the other hand, persons with airway disease usually find it less difficult to inflate the lungs but expend more energy in moving air through the airways. As a result, these persons tend to take deeper breaths and to breathe at a slower rate (*i.e.,* 600 × 10 = 6000 ml) to achieve their oxygen needs.

Dead air space

Dead air space refers to the air that must be moved with each breath but *does not participate in gas exchange.* Movement of air through dead air space contributes to the work of breathing but not to gas exchange. There are two types of dead air space: that contained in the *conducting airways (anatomic),* and that contained in the *respiratory portion of the lung (alveolar).* The physiologic dead space includes the anatomical dead space plus the alveolar dead space. The volume of anatomic airway dead space is fixed and is approximately 150 ml to 200 ml, depending on body size. It constitutes air contained in the nose, pharynx, trachea, and bronchi. The alveolar dead space is normally about 5 ml to 10 ml. If alveoli are ventilated but deprived of blood flow, they do not contribute to gas exchange and thus constitute alveolar dead space. The alveolar ventilation is equal to the minute ventilation minus the physiologic dead space ventilation. Creation of a tracheotomy decreases the dead space ventilation and can have the effect of decreasing the work of breathing.

In summary, ventilation provides the means for the exchange of gases (renewal of oxygen and removal of carbon dioxide) between the lungs and the atmosphere. It is dependent on a system of open airways and movement of the thoracic cage by the respiratory muscles—the diaphragm and intercostals. The energy that is used for respiration is expended in enlarging the chest during inspiration. Expiration involves the recoil of the elastic components of the chest wall that were stretched during inspiration and is largely passive, thus contributing very little to the work of breathing. Lung compliance describes the ease with which the lungs can be inflated. A spirometer is used to measure lung volumes and capacities. Pulmonary function tests measure ventilation with respect to time.

Table 24–2. Pulmonary function tests*

Test	Symbol	Measurement
Maximal voluntary ventilation	MVV	Maximum amount of air that can be breathed in a given time
Forced vital capacity	FVC	Maximum amount of air that can be rapidly and forcefully exhaled from the lungs following full inspiration. The expired volume is plotted against time.
Forced expiratory volume achieved in 1 sec	$FEV_{1.0}$	Volume of air expired in the first second of FVC
Percentage of forced vital capacity	$FEV_{1.0}/FVC\%$	Volume of air expired in the first second, expressed as a percentage of FVC
Forced midexpiratory flow rate	FEF25–75%	The forced midexpiratory flow rate determined by locating the points on the volume–time curve recording obtained during FVC corresponding to 25% and 75% of FVC and drawing a straight line through these points. The slope of this line represents the average midexpiratory flow rate.
Forced inspiratory flow rate	FIF25–75%	FIF is volume inspired from RV at the point of measurement. FIF25–75% is the slope of a line between the points on the volume pressure tracing corresponding to 25% and 75% of the inspired volume.

* By convention, all the lung volumes and rates of flow are expressed in terms of body temperature and pressure and saturated with water vapor (BTPS), which allows for a comparison of the pulmonary function data from laboratories with different ambient temperatures and altitudes.

Exchange and transport of gases in the body

—— Pulmonary blood flow

The lungs have a dual blood supply, the bronchial and the pulmonary circulations. The *pulmonary circulation* provides for the gas exchange function of the lungs, whereas the *bronchial circulation* provides cells of the lungs with blood to meet their nutritional needs.

The *bronchial arteries* arise from the thoracic aorta and enter the lungs with the major bronchi, dividing and subdividing along with the bronchial tubes supplying them and the other lung structures with oxygen. The capillaries of the bronchial circulation drain into the *bronchial veins,* the larger of which empties into the vena cava and returns blood to the right heart. The smaller of the bronchial veins empties into the pulmonary veins. This blood is unoxygenated, because the bronchial circulation does not participate in gas exchange. As a result, this blood dilutes the oxygenated blood returning to the left heart from the lungs.

The primary function of the pulmonary circulation is to facilitate gas exchange. The pulmonary circulation serves several important functions in addition to gas exchange: it filters all the blood that moves from the right to the left side of the circulation; it removes most of the thromboemboli; and it serves as a reservoir of blood for the left side of the heart. In order to accomplish this, there must be a continuous flow of blood through the respiratory portion of the lungs. Unoxygenated blood enters the lung through the pulmonary artery, which has its origin in the right heart and enters the lung at the hilus, along with the primary bronchus. The pulmonary arteries branch in a manner similar to that of the airways. The small pulmonary arteries accompany the bronchi as they move down the lobules and branch to supply the capillary network that surrounds the alveoli (see Figure 24-5).

The meshwork of capillaries in the respiratory portion of the lung is so dense that the flow in these vessels is often described as being similar to a sheet of flowing blood. The oxygenated capillary blood is collected in the small pulmonary veins of the lobules, and from there it moves to the larger veins to be collected finally in the four large pulmonary veins that empty into the left atrium. The term *perfusion* is used to describe the flow of blood through the pulmonary capillary bed.

The pulmonary vessels are thinner and more compliant than those in the systemic circulation, and the pressures in the pulmonary system are much lower (22/8 mmHg versus 120/70 mmHg). The low-pressure, low-resistance characteristics of this system serve to accommodate the delivery of varying amounts of blood from the systemic circulation without producing signs and symptoms of congestion. The volume in the pulmonary circulation is about 500 ml, with about 100 ml of this volume being located in the pulmonary capillary bed. When the output of the right ventricle and the input of the left ventricle are equal, the pulmonary blood flow remains constant. However, small differences between the input and output can result in large changes in the pulmonary volume if the differences continue for many heartbeats. The movement of blood through the pulmonary capillary bed requires that the mean pulmonary arterial pressure be greater than the mean pulmonary venous pressure. Pulmonary venous pressure increases in left-sided heart failure, and this causes the blood to accumulate in the pulmonary capillary bed, resulting in transudation of capillary fluid into the alveoli. Acute pulmonary edema is discussed in Chapter 22.

—— Ventilation–perfusion relationships

The distribution of pulmonary blood flow and ventilation differs along the distance of the lung from top to bottom. This distribution is normally altered by changes in position and exercise. It is also altered by bedrest and diseases of the heart and lungs.

—— Distribution of blood flow

The distribution of pulmonary blood flow is greatly affected by body position. In the upright position, the distance of the upper apices of the lung above the level of the heart often exceeds the perfusion capabilities of the mean pulmonary arterial pressure (about 12 mmHg), and therefore blood flow in the upper part of the lung is less than in the base or bottom part of the lung. In the supine position, the lungs and heart are at the same level and blood flow to the apices and base of the lung become more uniform. In this position, however, blood flow to the posterior or dependent portions (*e.g.,* bottom of the lung when lying on the side) exceeds the flow in the anterior or nondependent portions of the lung. In persons with pulmonary vascular congestion, rales develop in the dependent portions of the lungs exposed to increased blood flow.

Pulmonary blood flow can be markedly altered by disease conditions of the lung. Persons with chronic lung disease often have marked alterations in the pulmonary blood flow that contribute to problems with oxygenating blood (see Chapter 25). Alveolar hypoxia is a potent constrictor of pulmonary vasculature. Bronchial asthma often causes marked reduction in the blood flow to regions of the lung because of the hypoxic vasoconstriction of the poorly ventilated areas. Clinically, the effect of hypoxia on pulmonary blood vessels may result in the marked elevation of pulmonary arterial blood pressure.

Distribution of ventilation

Changes in posture affect ventilation as well as blood flow. During inspiration, the movement of the ribs increases the lung volume proportionately more at the base of the lung than at the apex and the downward movement of the diaphragm expands the lower lobes of the lung more than the upper lobes. As a result, more air moves into the lower portions of the lung. As with blood flow, the difference in ventilation is abolished in the supine position, and the posterior (bottom) portion of the lung is better ventilated than the anterior (upper) portion. The same holds true for the lateral position.

At low lung volumes, however, the pattern of ventilation that occurs at normal and high lung volumes is reversed. With a small inspiration air goes to the apex rather than the base of the lung. As with blood flow, this uneven distribution of ventilation is thought to result from gravity and from distortion of the lungs and chest wall by their weight, which causes changes in lung expansion and the intrapleural pressure. At the end of maximal expiration at low lung volumes, the intrapleural pressure at the base of the lung exceeds the airway pressure, causing airway collapse, so that air moves into the top part of the lungs. At larger lung volumes, there is greater chest expansion with greater decreases in the intrapleural pressure at the base of the lung, so that the airways remain open and air moves preferentially into that portion of the lung.

It is important to recognize that even at low lung volumes some air remains in the alveoli of the lower portion of the lungs, preventing their collapse. According to Laplace's law (discussed previously), the pressure needed to overcome the tension in the wall of a sphere or an elastic tube is inversely related to its radius (pressure = 2 × tension/radius); therefore, the small airways close first, trapping some gas in the alveoli. Trapping of air in the alveoli of the lower part of the lungs may be increased in older individuals and in persons with lung disease (e.g., emphysema). This is thought to be due to a loss in the elastic recoil properties of the lungs, so that the intrapleural pressure (created by the elastic recoil of the lung and chest wall) becomes less negative. In these persons, airway closure occurs at the end of normal lung volumes, trapping larger amounts of air. Eventually, the air trapping causes an increase in the anterior-posterior chest dimensions.

Ventilation–perfusion ratio

The gas exchange properties of the lung depend on the matching of ventilation and perfusion, so that there are equal amounts of air and blood entering the respiratory portion of the lungs. Two factors may interfere with the matching of ventilation and perfusion—dead air space and shunt. Dead air space, as discussed previously, refers to an area of the lung that is perfused but not ventilated. Shunt refers to blood that moves from the venous to the arterial system without being oxygenated. There are two types of shunts: physiologic and anatomic. In a physiologic shunt, there is mismatching of ventilation and perfusion and, as a result, there is not enough ventilation to provide the oxygen needed to oxygenate the blood flowing through the alveolar capillaries. In an anatomic shunt, the blood moves from the venous to the arterial side of the circulation without moving through the lung. Anatomic intracardiac shunting of blood because of congenital heart defects is discussed in Chapter 21. Physiologic shunting of blood usually results from destructive lung disease, which impairs ventilation, or from heart failure in which there is interference with the movement of blood through sections of the lungs.

There are many causes of mismatched ventilation and perfusion, of which the most obvious are illustrated in Figure 24-12. Part **A** illustrates the desired ventilation and perfusion pattern in which normal ventilation of the alveoli and normal blood flow through the pulmonary capillary that surrounds it occur. Part **B** illustrates a situation (shunt) of hypoventilation in which perfusion is normal while ventilation is lacking because of airway obstruction. This is the type of situation that occurs in atelectasis (see Chapter 25). In part **C** ventilation (dead air space) is normal, but the pulmonary artery supplying the lobule is obstructed. An example of this situation is pulmonary embolism. Most of the situations in which ventilation and perfusion are mismatched are less obvious. In lung disease, for example, there may be altered ventilation in one area of the lung and altered perfusion in another area.

Alveolar gas exchange

Gas exchange takes place in the alveoli. Here gases diffuse across the alveolar–capillary membrane moving from an area of higher partial pressure to one of lower partial pressure. Oxygen moves from the alveoli into the capillary, and carbon dioxide moves from the capillary network into the alveoli. There is rapid equilibration between the gases in the alveoli and those in the blood, so that the partial pressure of the blood gas at the venous end of the pulmonary

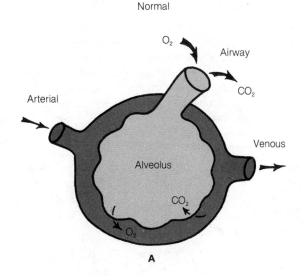

Normal

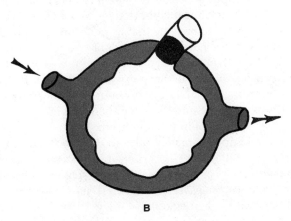

Perfusion without ventilation

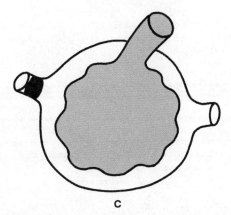

Ventilation without perfusion

Figure 24-12 Matching of ventilation and perfusion. **A,** normal matching of ventilation and perfusion; **B,** perfusion without ventilation (shunt); **C,** ventilation without perfusion (dead air space).

capillary is approximately the same as that in the alveoli.

The diffusion of gases in the lung is influenced by four factors: (1) the surface area available for diffusion, (2) the thickness of the alveolar–capillary membrane through which the gases diffuse, (3) the differences in the partial pressure of the gas on either side of the membrane, and (4) the characteristics of the gas. Diseases that destroy lung tissue or increase the thickness of the alveolar–capillary membrane influence the diffusing capacity of the lung. Removal of one lung, for example, reduces the diffusing surface by one-half. The thickness of the alveolar–capillary membrane and the distance for diffusion are increased in pulmonary edema and pneumonia. Administration of high concentrations of oxygen increases the difference in pressure on the two sides of the alveolar–capillary membrane and increases the diffusion of the gas. The characteristics of the gas and its molecular weight and solubility determine how rapidly it diffuses through the respiratory membranes. Carbon dioxide diffuses 20 times more rapidly than oxygen, because of its greater solubility in the respiratory membranes and plasma. The factors that affect alveolar–capillary gas exchange are summarized in Table 24-3.

The *diffusing capacity of the lung* (D_L) is a measure of the rate of transfer of gases through the alveolar–capillary membrane (measured in milliliters per minute). It is measured using a gas that readily diffuses across the membrane, is easily analyzed, and is affected by the same factors that influence oxygen diffusion. Carbon monoxide, which meets these criteria, is usually used for this purpose. The test is done by having a person breathe a known concentration of carbon monoxide (usually for a 10-second breathhold or short measured interval of time). The volume of carbon monoxide that diffuses across the alveolar–capillary membrane is calculated from measurements of lung volume and changes in carbon monoxide level of inspired and expired air. Because blood levels of carbon monoxide are usually zero, there is no back diffusion of the gas and the difference between the inspired and expired carbon monoxide reflects the diffusion of the gas. The diffusing capacity for oxygen can be calculated using the diffusing capacity for carbon monoxide and known information about the solubility of the two gases. Persons who smoke or are exposed to carbon monoxide may have appreciable amounts of the gas in their lungs, invalidating the test results. The diffusing capacity of the lung is affected by conditions that alter the permeability of the alveolar–capillary membrane and the ability of the red blood cells to bind and transport the gas.

—— Gas transport

The lungs enable inhaled air to come in close proximity to blood flowing through the pulmonary capillaries so that exchange of gases between the internal environment of the body and the external environment can take place. They thus restore the oxygen content of the arterial blood and remove the carbon dioxide from the venous blood. The red blood cells, in turn, facilitate transport of gases as they move between the lungs and the tissues.

—— Oxygen transport

Oxygen is transported in two forms—in chemical combination with hemoglobin and physically dissolved in blood plasma. The *partial pressure* (PO_2), or *oxygen tension*, is the level of the *dissolved gas*, much like the dissolved carbon dioxide in a capped bottle of a carbonated soft drink. It is the dissolved form of oxygen that crosses the cell membrane and participates in cell metabolism. Hemoglobin in the red blood cell is the transport vehicle, binding oxygen in the pulmonary capillaries and releasing it into the tissue capillaries. The released oxygen becomes dissolved in the plasma as it moves between the red blood cell and the tissue cells.

Dissolved oxygen. Only about 1% of the oxygen carried in the blood is in the dissolved state; the remainder is carried with the hemoglobin. The amount of oxygen that will dissolve in plasma is determined by two factors: (1) the solubility of oxygen in plasma and (2) the partial pressure of the gas in the alveoli. The solubility of oxygen in plasma is fixed and is very small. For every *1 mmHg* PO_2 present in the alveoli, *0.003 ml of oxygen becomes dissolved in 100 ml of plasma.* This means that at a normal alveolar PO_2 of 100 mmHg the blood carries only 0.3 ml of dissolved oxygen in every 100 ml of plasma. As will be discussed, this amount is very small compared with the amount that can be carried in an equal amount of blood when oxygen is attached to hemoglobin.

Although the oxygen carried in plasma is insignificant, as just described, it may be a lifesaving mode of transport in carbon monoxide poisoning when most of the hemoglobin sites are occupied by carbon monoxide and are unavailable for transport of oxygen. The hyperbaric chamber, in which 100% oxygen at high atmospheric pressures is administered to treat certain disorders, increases the amount of oxygen that can be carried in the dissolved state, so that sufficient oxygen may be made available to prevent the death of vital structures such as brain cells. The reader may want to calculate the amount of oxygen that can be carried in the plasma when a person breathes 100% oxygen at 3 atmospheres, the pressure frequently employed in hyperbaric chambers.*

Hemoglobin transport. In the lung, oxygen moves across the alveolar–capillary membrane, through the plasma, and into the red blood cell where it forms a loose and reversible bond with the hemoglobin molecule (Figure 24-13). In the normal lung, this process is rapid, so that even with a fast heart rate, the hemoglobin is almost completely saturated with oxygen during the short time that it spends in the pulmonary capillary bed. A small amount of unoxygenated blood from the bronchial circulation is mixed with the oxygenated blood in the pulmonary veins and as a result, the hemoglobin is only about 95% to 97% saturated as it moves into the arterial circulation.

Hemoglobin is a highly efficient carrier of oxygen, and approximately 98% to 99% of the oxygen used by body tissues is carried in this manner. *Each gram of hemoglobin is capable of carrying about 1.34 ml of oxygen when completely saturated.* This means that a person with a hemoglobin of 14 g/100 ml of blood carries 18.8 ml of oxygen in each 100 ml of blood in the form of oxyhemoglobin.

---

* 2280 (760 mmHg × 3 atmospheres) × 0.003 (solubility of O_2 in plasma) = 6.8 ml/100 ml of plasma. The actual value would be slightly less than this, because the calculation does not take into account the partial pressure of carbon dioxide or water vapor pressure in the alveoli.

Table 24–3. Factors affecting alveolar–capillary gas exchange

Factors affecting gas exchange	Examples
Surface area available for diffusion	Removal of a lung or diseases such as emphysema and chronic bronchitis, which destroy lung tissue or cause mismatching of ventilation and perfusion
Thickness of the alveolar–capillary membrane	Conditions such as pneumonia, interstitial lung disease, and pulmonary edema, which increase membrane thickness
Partial pressure of alveolar gases	Ascent to high altitudes where the partial pressure of oxygen is reduced. In the opposite direction, increasing the partial pressure of a gas in the inspired air (*e.g.,* oxygen therapy) will increase the gradient for diffusion
Solubility and molecular weight of the gas	Carbon dioxide, which is more soluble in the cell membranes, diffuses across the alveolar–capillary membrane more rapidly than oxygen

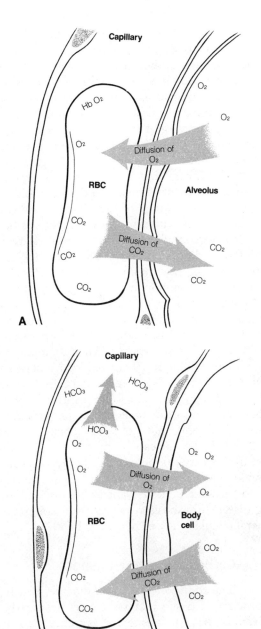

Figure 24-13 Transport of oxygen by the red blood cell. (**A**) In the lung, oxygen moves from the alveoli to the hemoglobin, and carbon dioxide moves from the red cell to the alveoli. (**B**) In the tissues, oxygen moves from the red blood cell to the capillary fluid and then into the interstitial fluid, where it becomes available to the cell, while carbon dioxide moves in the opposite direction.

The oxygenated hemoglobin is transported in the arterial blood to the peripheral capillaries where the oxygen is released and made available to the tissues for use in cell metabolism. As the oxygen moves out of the capillaries in response to the needs of the tissues, the hemoglobin saturation, which was about 95% to 97% as the blood left the left heart, drops to about 75% as the mixed venous blood returns to the right heart.

Oxygen–hemoglobin dissociation. Oxygen that remains bound to hemoglobin cannot participate in tissue metabolism. The efficiency of the oxygen transport system depends on the ability of the hemoglobin molecule to bind oxygen in the lung and release it on demand. The affinity of hemoglobin refers to its capacity to bind oxygen, thus, the hemoglobin binds oxygen readily when affinity is increased and releases oxygen when affinity is decreased.

Hemoglobin's affinity for oxygen is influenced by pH, in that it binds oxygen more strongly under alkaline conditions and releases it more easily under acid conditions. Carbon dioxide moves out of the blood in the lungs, raising the pH and thereby increasing the oxygen affinity. In the tissues, a decrease in pH because of cellular release of carbon dioxide and metabolic acids lowers hemoglobin affinity for oxygen and thereby enhances its release.

The relationship between the oxygen carried in combination with hemoglobin and the P_{O_2} of the blood is described by the *oxygen–hemoglobin dissociation curve*, which is pictured in Figure 24-14. The curve is S-shaped, with the top *flat portion* representing the binding of oxygen to the *hemoglobin in the lung* and the *steep portion* representing its *release into the tissue capillaries*. At about 100 mmHg P_{O_2}, a plateau occurs at which point the hemoglobin is about 98% saturated. Increasing the alveolar P_{O_2} above this level

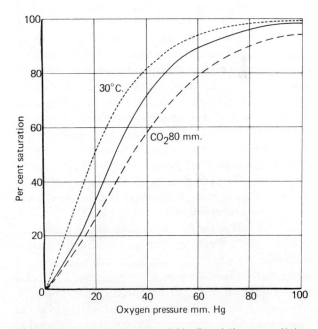

Figure 24-14 The oxygen–hemoglobin dissociation curve. Note that when the carbon dioxide is increased or when the blood pH is decreased, the curve is shifted to the right, and therefore the hemoglobin binds less oxygen for any partial pressure of oxygen. When the curve is shifted to the left, as occurs when the carbon dioxide is decreased or the pH is increased, the opposite occurs. *(Chaffee EE, Lytle IM: Basic Physiology and Anatomy, 4th ed. Philadelphia, JB Lippincott, 1980)*

will have no further effect in increasing hemoglobin saturation. Even at high altitudes, when the partial pressure of oxygen is considerably decreased, the hemoglobin remains relatively well saturated. At 60 mmHg PO_2 the hemoglobin is still 89% saturated.

The steep portion of the dissociation curve—between 60 mmHg and 40 mmHg—represents the removal of oxygen from the hemoglobin as it moves through the tissue capillaries. This portion of the curve is of great importance because it permits considerable transfer of oxygen from hemoglobin to the tissues with only a small drop in oxygen tension. Normally the tissues remove about 5 ml of oxygen per 100 ml of blood, and the hemoglobin of mixed venous blood as it returns to the right heart is about 75% saturated (PO_2 40 mmHg). In this portion of the dissociation curve, the rate at which oxygen is released from the hemoglobin is determined largely by tissue utilization. During strenuous exercise, for example, the muscle cells may remove as much as 15 ml of oxygen per 100 ml of blood from the hemoglobin.

Hemoglobin can be regarded as an oxygen buffer system that regulates oxygen pressure in the tissues. Thus, hemoglobin affinity for oxygen must change with the metabolic needs of the tissues. This change is represented by a shift in the dissociation curve to the right or the left as pictured in Figure 24-13.

As the curve shifts to the right, the tissue PO_2 is greater for any given level of hemoglobin saturation. A shift to the right is usually caused by conditions such as fever, acidosis, or an increase in PCO_2, which reflects increased tissue metabolism. Chronic hypoxia also causes the dissociation curve to shift to the right. The red blood cells, unlike other tissues, contain high levels of the glycolytic intermediate 2,3-diphosphoglycerate (2,3-DPG), the levels of which increase during hypoxia; this reduces hemoglobin affinity for oxygen and favors its release to the tissues. A shift to the right because of an increase in 2,3-DPG occurs in various conditions of hypoxia, including those resulting from high altitude, pulmonary insufficiency, heart failure, and severe anemia.

A shift to the left of the dissociation curve represents an enhanced affinity of hemoglobin for oxygen and occurs in situations associated with a decrease in tissue metabolism, such as alkalosis, decreased body temperature, and decreased carbon dioxide levels. The degree of change in affinity is indicated by the P_{50}, or the partial pressure of oxygen that is needed to achieve a 50% saturation of hemoglobin. Returning to Figure 24-13, the reader will note that the dissociation curve on the left has a P_{50} of about 20 mmHg; the normal curve, a P_{50} of 26; and the curve on the right, a P_{50} of 35 mmHg.

Cyanosis. Reduced hemoglobin—hemoglobin from which the oxygen has been removed—is purple. Cyanosis is the purplish discoloration of the skin, nailbeds, and mucous membranes because of the presence of excessive reduced hemoglobin in the superficial capillaries. Cyanosis does not occur until there are at least 5 g of reduced hemoglobin per 100 ml of blood in these capillaries. The appearance of cyanosis depends on the thickness and pigment of the skin, the peripheral blood flow, and the amount of hemoglobin present. Consequently, cyanosis is not always a sensitive index of hypoxia. It is difficult to detect in persons with dark skin. Cyanosis is deceiving; it can occur when there is a local decrease in blood flow and does not necessarily reflect the oxygen content of blood flow in other parts of the body. For example, it is common for the fingers to turn blue during exposure to cold. This is because of the sluggish blood flow with increased extraction of oxygen from the blood as it flows through the superficial vessels. Because cyanosis appears when there are 5 g of reduced hemoglobin in 100 ml of blood, a person with polycythemia (an excess of red blood cells) may easily carry 5 g of reduced hemoglobin per 100 ml of blood without evidence of hypoxia. A person with anemia, on the other hand, may not have sufficient hemoglobin that 5 g/100 ml can be present in the reduced state; in this case the person will be hypoxic but not cyanotic. The undersurface of the tongue is a reliable area to check for central cyanosis because of heart or lung disease[8] (cyanosis resulting from abnormal peripheral circulation does not occur here).

Carbon dioxide transport

The transport of carbon dioxide, which is a by-product of tissue metabolism, is not nearly the problem of oxygen transport. It is transported in the blood in three forms—attached to hemoglobin, as dissolved carbon dioxide, and as bicarbonate. The amount of carbon dioxide in the blood does influence the acid–base balance of the extracellular fluids (see Chapter 29).

As carbon dioxide is formed during metabolic processes, it diffuses out of cells into the tissue spaces and capillaries. Upon entering a capillary, carbon dioxide undergoes chemical and physical reactions that are essential for its transport. A small portion of the carbon dioxide is carried in the dissolved state (PCO_2) to the lungs. The PCO_2 of the arterial blood is about 40 mmHg, and the PCO_2 of the venous blood is about 45 mmHg; the difference between the two values represents the amount of dissolved carbon dioxide carried in the plasma. The amount of dissolved carbon dioxide that can be carried in the plasma is determined by the partial pressure of the gas and the solubility coefficient for the gas (0.03 ml/100 ml/mmHg). Dissolved carbon dioxide combines with water to form carbonic acid (H^+ HCO_3^-). This would be a slow reaction were it not for the enzyme *carbonic anhydrase*. Carbonic anhydrase, which increases the reaction between carbon dioxide and water about 5000-fold, is present in large quantities in red blood cells. Therefore, most of the carbon dioxide reacts with carbonic anhydrase in the red cell before it leaves the capillaries. In the red cell, the hydrogen ion that is generated from the carbonic anhydrase-mediated reaction combines with the hemoglobin, which is a powerful acid–base buffer. The bicarbonate ion that is formed from the reaction diffuses into the plasma, replaced by the chloride ion in a bicarbonate-chloride shift. This is made possible by a special bicarbonate-chloride carrier protein in the red cell membrane. As a result of the bicarbonate-chloride shift, the chloride content of the red cell is greater in venous blood than in arterial blood. The reversible combination of carbon dioxide with water in the red cell accounts for about 70% of all carbon dioxide transport.[5]

In addition to the carbonic anhydrase-mediated reaction with water, carbon dioxide also reacts directly with hemoglobin to form *carbaminohemoglobin*. The combination of carbon dioxide with hemoglobin is a reversible reaction, involving a loose bond, that allows for transport of carbon dioxide from the tissues to the lung where it is released into the alveoli for exchange with the external environment. The release of oxygen from hemoglobin enhances the binding of carbon dioxide in the peripheral tissues; in the lungs, the combination of oxygen with hemoglobin displaces carbon dioxide. This is because the combination of oxygen with hemoglobin causes the hemoglobin to become a stronger acid. In the lungs, the highly acidic hemoglobin has a lesser tendency to form carbaminohemoglobin, and carbon dioxide is released from the blood into the alveoli. In the tissues, the release of oxygen from hemoglobin decreases its acidity and increases its ability to form carbaminohemoglobin.

Blood gases

To accurately measure blood gases, arterial blood is required. Venous blood is not used because venous levels of oxygen and carbon dioxide reflect the metabolic requirements of the tissues rather than the gas exchange properties of the lungs. The P_{O_2} of arterial blood is normally above 80 mmHg, and the P_{CO_2} is in the range of 35 mmHg to 45 mmHg.

Hypoxia

Hypoxia refers to a reduction in tissue oxygenation. It can result from an inadequate amount of oxygen in the air, disease of the respiratory system, alterations in circulatory function, anemia, or the inability of the cells to utilize oxygen. The causes of hypoxia can be divided into four categories: (1) hypoxemic hypoxia in which the oxygen content of the blood is reduced; (2) stagnant, or ischemic hypoxia, in which circulation of oxygen in the blood is impaired; (3) anemic hypoxia, in which the ability to transport oxygen in the blood decreases; and (4) histotoxic hyp-

Table 24–4. Types, mechanisms of production, and causes of hypoxia

Type	Mechanisms of production	Causes
Hypoxemic hypoxia	Insufficient oxygen reaching the blood	Decreased oxygen in the atmosphere Pulmonary disease Airway obstruction Neuromuscular disease
Stagnant hypoxia	Failure to transport oxygen because of impaired blood flow	Heart failure Circulatory shock Local disruption of blood flow
Anemic hypoxia	Reduction in the oxygen-carrying capacity of the blood	Decrease in red blood cells Abnormal hemoglobin Carbon monoxide poisoning
Histotoxic hypoxia	Impaired utilization of oxygen by the cell	Cellular poisons such as cyanide Tissue edema Abnormal tissue needs

oxia, in which the cells are unable to utilize oxygen (*e.g.*, cyanide poisoning). The categories, mechanisms of production, and causes of hypoxia are summarized in Table 24-4.

Acute hypoxia

The partial pressure of oxygen decreases as one ascends above sea level and much of what is known about acute hypoxia has been learned from high altitude and aviation studies. The partial pressure of oxygen, which constitutes 21% of the total gases in the air, falls from 159 mmHg at sea level (760 mmHg barometric pressure) to 110 mmHg at 10,000 feet to 73 mmHg at 20,000 feet.[5] Denver, Colorado, with an altitude of 5,250 feet, has partial pressure of oxygen of 121 mmHg. Atmospheric oxygen is diluted with water vapor and carbon dioxide in the lung. As a result, alveolar oxygen pressure is less than that in the environment; it falls from about 104 mmHg at sea level to 67 mmHg at 10,000 feet to 40 mmHg at 20,000 feet. The ceiling for breathing air is approximately 23,000 feet; this can be doubled to about 47,000 feet when breathing pure oxygen. The use of pressurized cabins in aircraft allows for safe travel at high altitudes. In the clinical setting, acute hypoxia can occur at sea level in persons with sudden blood loss, carbon monoxide poisoning, acute circulatory disorders, respiratory disease, or other disorders that interfere with the exchange or transport of oxygen.

Severe hypoxia causes cyanosis, cardiovascular signs such as tachycardia, and central nervous system signs such as mental clouding. The signs of hypoxia are usually mild until the PO_2 falls below 60 mmHg, and the symptoms do not become severe until the PO_2 falls to 40 mmHg to 50 mmHg. One of the earliest signs of acute hypoxia is a chemoreceptor-mediated increase in ventilation. The chemoreceptors (to be discussed later in this chapter) are particularly sensitive to changes in PO_2 (blood oxygen levels) in the range of 60 mmHg to 30 mmHg. Important early effects of acute hypoxia are decreases in judgment and motor proficiency. These manifestations become more acute with prolonged exposure to hypoxic conditions. For example, mental proficiency is decreased to half of normal after 1 hour of sudden exposure to the barometric pressures at 15,000 feet and decreased to one-fifth after 18 hours.[5] Other signs of acute hypoxia include dyspnea, fatigue, headache, nausea and vomiting, and decreased visual acuity. Cyanosis of the lips and nailbeds is usually present in persons with adequate hemoglobin levels. Cheyne-Stokes breathing and insomnia are common problems in unacclimated persons during the first several days of exposure to high altitudes. Disorientation, hallucinations, convulsions, and coma occur with extreme levels of hypoxia.

It has been speculated that some of the symptoms, such as insomnia and Cheyne-Stokes breathing, associated with ascent to high altitudes are related to the decreased carbon dioxide levels resulting from hyperventilation.

Chronic hypoxia

Chronic hypoxia induces changes similar, albeit of a lesser degree, to those observed in acute hypoxia. Dyspnea, fatigue, and cyanosis are common problems associated with a long-term impairment in the oxygenation of tissues. In addition, there is evidence of adaptive mechanisms, such as pulmonary hypertension and polycythemia.

The body adapts to hypoxia by increased ventilation, pulmonary vasoconstriction, and increased production of red blood cells. Hyperventilation results from the hypoxic stimulation of the chemoreceptors. The stimulus for the increased production of red blood cells results from the release of erythropoietin from the kidneys in response to hypoxia (see Chapter 16). Polycythemia increases the red blood cell concentration and the oxygen-carrying capacity of the blood. Pulmonary vasoconstriction occurs as a local response to alveolar hypoxia; it increases pulmonary arterial pressure and serves to improve the matching of ventilation and blood flow. Other adaptive mechanisms include a shift to the right in the oxygen dissociation curve due to increased 2,3-DPG, as a means of increasing oxygen release to the tissues. An increase in oxidative enzymes in the cell serves as a means of increasing the efficiency of oxygen utilization.

In summary, the lungs enable inhaled air to come in close proximity with the blood flowing through the pulmonary capillaries, so that the exchange of gases between the internal environment of the body and the external environment can take place. The blood provides the means for the transport of gases in the body. Oxygen is transported in two forms: (1) in chemical combination with hemoglobin and (2) physically dissolved in plasma (PO_2). Hemoglobin is an efficient carrier of oxygen, and about 98% to 99% of oxygen is transported in this manner. Carbon dioxide is carried in three forms—as carbaminohemoglobin, dissolved carbon dioxide, and bicarbonate. Hypoxia refers to an acute or chronic reduction in tissue oxygenation. It can result from decreased oxygen content of the blood (hypoxemic hypoxia), impaired blood flow (stagnant hypoxia), reduced oxygen-carrying capacity of the blood (anemic hypoxia), or impaired cellular utilization of oxygen (histotoxic hypoxia).

Control of respiration

Neural control mechanisms

Unlike the heart, which has inherent rhythmic properties and can beat independently of the nervous system, muscles controlling respiration require continuous input from the nervous system. The movement of the diaphragm, intercostal muscles, sternocleidomastoid, and other accessory muscles controlling ventilation is integrated by neurons located in the pons and medulla. These neurons are collectively referred to as the *respiratory center*. Previous beliefs regarding separate inspiratory and expiratory centers are probably no longer applicable. Instead, it is now believed that the respiratory center consists of two dense bilateral aggregates of respiratory neurons involved in both initiating inspiration and expiration and incorporating afferent impulses into motor responses of the respiratory muscles. The first, or dorsal, group of neurons in the respiratory center is concerned primarily with inspiration. These neurons control the activity of the phrenic nerves and drive the second, or ventral, group of respiratory neurons. In addition, they probably integrate impulses from the lungs and airways into the ventilatory response. The second group of neurons, which contains both inspiratory and expiratory neurons, controls the spinal motor neurons of the intercostal and abdominal muscles. The pacemaker properties of the respiratory center result from the cycling of the two groups of respiratory neurons. The nature and mechanism of this cycling is still under investigation.

Axons from the neurons in the respiratory center cross in the midline and descend in the ventrolateral columns of the spinal cord. The tracts that control expiration and inspiration are spatially separated in the cord, as are the tracts that transmit specialized reflexes (*e.g.*, coughing and hiccuping) and voluntary control of ventilation. Only at the level of the spinal cord are the respiratory impulses integrated to produce a reflex response. The neural control of ventilation is depicted in Figure 24-15.

The control of breathing has both automatic and voluntary components. The automatic regulation of ventilation is controlled by input from two types of sensors or receptors: chemoreceptors, which monitor the blood levels of oxygen, carbon dioxide, and *p*H and adjust ventilation to meet the changing metabolic needs of the body; and lung receptors, which monitor breathing patterns and lung function. Voluntary regulation of ventilation integrates breathing with voluntary acts such as speaking, blowing, and singing. These acts, initiated by the motor and premotor cor-

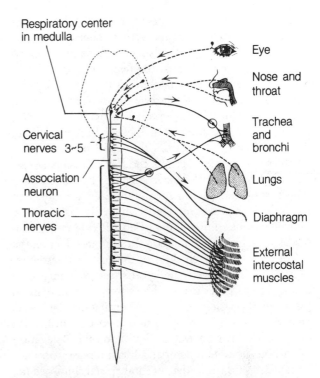

Figure 24-15 Activity in the respiratory center. Impulses traveling over afferent neurons activate central neurons, which in turn activate the efferent neurons that supply the muscles of respiration. Thus, respiratory movements may be altered by a variety of stimuli. *(Chaffee EE, Greisheimer EM: Basic Physiology and Anatomy, 3rd ed. Philadelphia, JB Lippincott, 1974)*

tex, cause the temporary suspension of automatic breathing. It has been suggested that alterations in the control of automatic and voluntary regulation of breathing may contribute to various forms of sleep apnea. This is discussed in Chapter 26.

The automatic and voluntary components of respiration are regulated by afferent impulses coming to the respiratory center from a number of sources. Afferent input from higher brain centers is evidenced by the ability to consciously alter the depth and rate of respiration. Fever, pain, and emotion exert their influence through lower brain centers. Vagal afferents from sensory receptors in the lungs and airways are integrated in the dorsal area of the respiratory center.

Chemoreceptors

Tissue needs for oxygen and the removal of carbon dioxide are regulated by chemoreceptors that monitor blood levels of these gases. Input from these sensors is transmitted to the respiratory center, and ventilation is adjusted to maintain the arterial blood gases within a normal range.

There are two types of chemoreceptors: central and peripheral chemoreceptors. The most important chemoreceptors for sensing changes in blood carbon dioxide content are the central chemoreceptors. These receptors are actually chemosensitive regions located in the medulla near the respiratory center and are bathed in cerebrospinal fluid. Although the central chemoreceptors monitor carbon dioxide levels, the actual stimulus for these receptors is provided by hydrogen ions that are present in the cerebrospinal fluid. This fluid is separated from the blood by the blood–brain barrier, which permits the free diffusion of carbon dioxide but not of bicarbonate or hydrogen ions. The carbon dioxide, in turn, combines rapidly with water to form carbonic acid, which dissociates into hydrogen ions. Thus, the carbon dioxide content in the blood regulates ventilation through its effect on the pH of the extracellular fluid of the brain. These chemoreceptors are extremely sensitive to short-term changes in carbon dioxide. The effect of an increase in plasma carbon dioxide levels on ventilation reaches its peak within a minute or so and then declines if the CO_2 level remains elevated. With long-term elevation in carbon dioxide, a compensatory increase in bicarbonate secretion into the cerebral spinal fluid occurs, which acts as a buffer for the hydrogen ions. Thus, persons with chronically elevated levels of carbon dioxide no longer respond to this stimulus for increased ventilation but rely on the stimulus provided by a decrease in the blood oxygen levels.

The arterial oxygen levels are monitored by peripheral chemoreceptors located in the carotid and aortic bodies. Although these chemoreceptors also monitor carbon dioxide, they play a much more important role in monitoring arterial blood oxygen levels. These receptors exert little control over ventilation until the PO_2 has dropped to below 60 mmHg. Hypoxia is the main stimulus for ventilation in persons with chronic hypercarbia. If these persons are given oxygen therapy at a level sufficient to increase the PO_2 above that needed to stimulate the peripheral chemoreceptors, their ventilation may be seriously depressed.

Lung receptors

There are three types of lung receptors: stretch, irritant, and juxtacapillary (J) receptors. Stretch receptors are located in the smooth muscle layers of the conducting airways. They respond to changes in pressure within the walls of the airways. When the lung is inflated, these receptors inhibit inspiration and promote expiration (Hering-Breuer reflex). They are important in establishing breathing patterns and in minimizing the work of breathing by adjusting the respiratory rate and tidal volume to accommodate changes in lung compliance and airway resistance. Irritant receptors have a distribution similar to that of the stretch receptors. They can be mechanically stimulated by increases in airway pressure, changes in lung inflation, and changes in bronchial smooth muscle tone. Stimulation of the irritant receptors leads to airway constriction and a pattern of rapid, shallow breathing. This pattern of breathing probably protects respiratory tissues from the damaging effects of toxic inhalants. It is also thought that the mechanical stimulation of receptors may serve to ensure more uniform lung expansion by initiating periodic sighing and yawning. The function of the J receptors is uncertain; at present, it is thought that they sense lung congestion. These receptors may be responsible for the rapid, shallow breathing that occurs with pulmonary edema, pulmonary embolism, and pneumonia.

Alterations in breathing patterns

The act of breathing is normally effortless and does not require conscious thought. In an adult, the normal rate of respiration is about 16 to 18 per minute, with about one breath for every four heartbeats. This rate increases with exercise and other activities that increase body metabolism. In normal breathing, expiration is largely passive and is accomplished within 4 to 6 seconds.

Respiratory movements are normally smooth, with equal expansion of both sides of the chest. In men, respiratory movements tend to be primarily diaphragmatic, whereas in women, there tends to be greater movement of the intercostal muscles. When breathing becomes labored, the accessory muscles of the neck come into play, and there may be flaring of the nares.

The suffix -pnea denotes a relationship to breathing. *Tachypnea* is rapid breathing, and *hyperpnea* is an increase in both the rate and depth of respiration. Hyperpnea is normal during exercise. *Bradypnea* is an abnormally slow respiratory rate. *Hyperventilation* is ventilation in excess of that needed to maintain a normal level of arterial P_{CO_2}. Hyperventilation causes a decrease in P_{CO_2} and tends to lead to respiratory alkalosis (see Chapter 29).

Periodic breathing

Periodic breathing describes a breathing pattern in which there are episodes of apnea, or absence of breathing. *Cheyne-Stokes breathing* is a type of periodic breathing characterized by periods of slowly waxing and waning respirations, separated by a period of apnea that lasts up to 30 seconds. Cheyne-Stokes breathing is thought to be caused by impaired function of the central feedback mechanisms that buffer the respiratory center's response to carbon dioxide. In order for Cheyne-Stokes respirations to occur, the hyperpneic and apneic phases of the breathing pattern must be long enough for sufficient changes in the carbon dioxide content of the blood to occur. During the hyperpneic phase of Cheyne-Stokes breathing, carbon dioxide levels fall, leading to a decreased stimulus for ventilation and finally to apnea. The period of apnea, in turn, causes the carbon dioxide content of the blood to accumulate, and this leads to the hyperpneic phase of the respiratory pattern. Two types of disease conditions cause predisposition to Cheyne-Stokes breathing. One is congestive heart failure, in which there is a great delay in moving blood with its altered carbon dioxide content from the lungs to the chemoreceptors in the brain that control ventilation. The other is impaired function of the brain centers regulating the feedback mechanisms that control respiration. An area of the brain stem controls the feedback gain of the respiratory center in response to changes in carbon dioxide level. Cheyne-Stokes respirations may be seen in persons who have brain lesions that affect this area. Cheyne-Stokes breathing is also seen in healthy individuals as an adaptive response to high altitudes, especially during sleep.

—— Dyspnea

Dyspnea is a subjective sensation of difficulty in breathing that includes both the perception of labored breathing and the reaction to that sensation.[9] The terms *dyspnea, breathlessness,* and *shortness of breath* are often used interchangeably. Dyspnea is observed in at least three different major cardiopulmonary disease states: primary lung diseases such as pneumonia, asthma, and emphysema; heart disease that is characterized by pulmonary congestion; and neuromuscular disorders such as myasthenia gravis and muscular dystrophy that affect the respiratory muscles. Although dyspnea is often associated with respiratory disease, its presence does not necessarily imply pathology; dyspnea occurs during exercise, particularly in untrained individuals.

The cause of dyspnea is unknown. Four types of mechanisms have been proposed to explain the sensation: (1) stimulation of lung receptors, (2) increased sensitivity to changes in ventilation perceived through central nervous system mechanisms, (3) reduced ventilatory capacity or breathing reserve, and (4) stimulation of neural receptors in the muscle fibers of the intercostals and diaphragm and of receptors in the skeletal joints.[10] The first of the suggested mechanisms is stimulation of the previously described lung receptors. These receptors are stimulated by the contraction of bronchial smooth muscle, the stretch of the bronchial wall, pulmonary congestion, and conditions that decrease lung compliance. The second category

of proposed mechanisms focuses on central nervous system mechanisms that transmit information to the cortex regarding respiratory muscle weakness or a discrepancy between the increased effort of breathing and inadequate respiratory muscle contraction. The third type of mechanism focuses on a reduction in ventilatory capacity or breathing reserve. As a general rule, a reduction in breathing reserve (maximum voluntary ventilation not being used during a given activity) to less than 65% to 75% correlates well with dyspnea. The fourth possible mechanism is stimulation of muscle and joint receptors in the respiratory musculature because of a discrepancy in the tension generated by these muscles and the tidal volume that results. These receptors, once stimulated, transmit signals that bring about an awareness of the breathing discrepancy.

Like other subjective symptoms, such as fatigue and pain, dyspnea is difficult to quantify because it relies on a person's perception of the problem. The most common method for measuring dyspnea is a retrospective determination of the level of daily activity at which a person experiences dyspnea. A number of scales are available for this use. One of these uses four grades of dyspnea to evaluate disability (Table 24-5).[10] The visual analog scale is used to assess breathing difficulty that occurs with a given activity such as walking a certain distance. It can also be used to assess dyspnea over time. The treatment of dyspnea depends on the cause. The techniques used clinically to reduce dyspnea include those to reduce anxiety, breathing retraining, and energy conservation measures.

—— Cough reflex

The cough reflex protects the lung from accumulation of secretions and from entry of irritating and destructive substances; it is one of the primary defense mechanisms of the respiratory tract.

The cough reflex is initiated by receptors located in the tracheobronchial wall; they are extremely sensitive to irritating substances and to the presence of excess secretions. Afferent impulses from these receptors are transmitted through the vagus to the medullary center, which integrates the cough response.

Coughing itself requires the rapid inspiration of a large volume of air (usually about 2.5 liters), followed by rapid closure of the glottis. This is followed by forceful contraction of the abdominal and expiratory muscles. As these muscles contract, there is a marked elevation of intrathoracic pressures to levels of 100 mmHg or more. The rapid opening of the glottis, at this point, leads to an explosive expulsion of air.

Many conditions may interfere with the cough reflex and its protective function. The reflex is impaired in persons with weakness of the abdominal or respiratory muscles. This can be caused by disease conditions that lead to muscle weakness or paralysis, by prolonged inactivity, or as an outcome of surgery involving these muscles. Bedrest interferes with expansion of the chest and limits the amount of air that can be taken into the lungs in preparation for coughing, so the cough is weak and ineffective. Disease conditions that prevent effective closure of the glottis and laryngeal muscles interfere with accomplishment of the marked increase in intrathoracic pressure that is needed for effective coughing. The presence of a nasogastric tube, for example, may prevent closure of the upper airway structures. The presence of such a tube may also fatigue the receptors for the cough reflex that are located in the area. Last, the cough reflex is impaired when there is depressed function of the medullary centers in the brain that integrate the cough reflex. Interruption of the central integration aspect of the cough reflex can arise as the result of disease of this part of the brain or the action of drugs that depress the cough center.

Although the cough reflex is basically a protective mechanism, frequent and prolonged coughing can be exhausting and painful and can exert undesirable effects on the cardiovascular and respiratory systems and on the elastic tissues of the lungs. This is particularly true in young children and the elderly.

—— Sputum

Sputum consists of respiratory secretions that are ejected from the mouth during coughing and expectoration. A cough is said to be productive or non-productive depending on the amount of sputum produced.

Sputum contains mucus produced by the epithelial cells that line the respiratory tract as well as any debris that has been inhaled. The normal adult produces about 100 ml of sputum per day, most of which is swallowed as it is propelled into the pharynx by the action of the mucociliary blanket. With infection of the respiratory tract, the sputum often contains infecting organisms and inflammatory debris and becomes purulent. The color of the sputum is an important sign. Yellow sputum, for example, may indicate infection. The presence of verdoperoxidase, liberated from the polymorphonuclear cells in the sputum, causes stagnant pus to turn green. Patients with lower respiratory tract infections may report having a green sputum upon arising in the morning that turns yellow as the day progresses. Pulmonary edema often causes exudation of red blood cells into the alveoli, thus producing frothy blood-tinged sputum. The coughing up of blood-tinged sputum is called hemoptysis.

Methods of cough relief fall into three categories. The first is *correction of the underlying cause.* When this fails or cannot be accomplished immediately, a second method, *administration of a drug with a cough suppressant action,* may be initiated, as long as the agent does not disrupt elimination of tracheobronchial secretions. The third method relies on the *use of expectorant drugs (or procedures),* to increase the quantity of bronchial secretions or to liquefy them; this facilitates removal of secretions from the respiratory system and hence diminishes the need to cough. Table 24-6 lists various cough preparations and summarizes their mechanism of action.

Table 24–5. Instrument to measure dyspnea*

A. Degree of shortness of breath graded from 0 to 3

Grade	Description
0	No unusual shortness of breath compared to other persons of same age, height, and sex
1	More shortness of breath than a person of same age when walking up hills or hurrying on level ground
2	Shortness of breath when walking on level ground
3	Shortness of breath at rest or while dressing

B. Visual analog scale

0 _____ 10
                        10 cm
No difficulty   Unable to
breathing   breathe

* For use in illness trajectory.
(Carrieri VK, Jansen-Bjerklie S, Jacobs S: The sensation of dyspnea: A review. Heart Lung 13(4):441, 1984)

Cough suppressants (antitussive drugs)

Narcotics such as morphine, hydromorphone, and levorphanol cause potent suppression of the cough reflex at the level of the medullary cough center. These drugs also inhibit the ciliary action of the respiratory mucous membrane and depress respiration. Therefore, persons receiving these drugs for control of pain need to be observed for development of respiratory complications, which can arise from depression of respiration and impairment of the cough reflex and other respiratory defense mechanisms.

The narcotics codeine and hydrocodone also act as cough suppressants but have fewer side effects and are therefore sometimes used as antitussive drugs. Some of the non-narcotic agents such as dextromethorphan are effective in suppressing the cough without creating drug dependence or other undesirable effects. It is these centrally acting non-narcotic antitussive drugs that are usually contained in over-the-counter preparations.

Another group of drugs act peripherally to reduce stimulation of the afferent receptors of the cough reflex. One of these, benzonatate (Tessalon), is believed to have a local anesthetic effect. Another group of locally acting agents are the demulcents, such as glycerin and honey, which act by coating the irritated pharyngeal structures. Many cough syrups and lozenges contain a demulcent.

Expectorants

Expectorants are drugs or substances that increase the secretion of mucus in the bronchi and reduce its viscosity, making it easier to move the secretions toward the mouth so that they can be disposed of.

Water is probably one of the most effective and is certainly one of the best expectorants. In addition to its use to increase hydration, water is also effective in the form of inhaled steam or moisture.

A number of expectorants are believed to act reflexly by causing gastric irritation, which, in turn, stimulates respiratory tract secretions. The reader is undoubtedly familiar with the increase in salivation and respiratory tract secretions that accompanies nausea and vomiting. Among the expectorants that act by causing gastric irritation are potassium iodide, ammonium chloride, syrup of ipecac, and guaifenesin (Table 24-6). Potassium iodide preparations leave a brassy taste in the mouth and lead to unpleasant hypersecretion from the eyes, nose, and mouth. They can also cause painful swelling of the parotid gland

Table 24-6. Medications used in the treatment of cough

Classification of preparations	Mechanism of action
Antitussive drugs	

Narcotics
  Codeine
  Hydrocodone
	Act centrally on the medullary cough center to suppress the cough

Non-narcotic Dextromethorphan	Acts centrally on the medullary cough center to suppress the cough
Antihistamine Diphenhydramine	Acts centrally on the cough center
Peripherally and centrally acting antitussive Benzonatate	Local anesthetic that acts peripherally on the stretch receptors in the lung and centrally to suppress the cough reflex

Peripherally acting demulcents
  Honey
  Glycerin
	Coat the irritated mucosal surface of the pharynx

Expectorants	

Gastric reflex stimulants
  Potassium iodide
  Syrup of ipecac
  Guaifenesin
  Ammonium chloride
	Increase the production of respiratory tract secretions by causing gastric irritation, which stimulates the gastric reflex and production of respiratory secretions

Bronchial secretory cell stimulant Elixir of terpin hydrate	Acts on bronchial secretory glands to stimulate increased production of respiratory tract secretions
Mucolytic agent Acetylcysteine (Mucomyst)	Reduces the viscosity of mucus by depolymerizing (breaking down) mucopolysaccharides in mucus

and an acneiform skin rash. Iodine preparations influence thyroid function and persons who use these medications over long periods may have changes in thyroid function. Syrup of ipecac is nauseating and is a useful emetic in small children. It is included, in dilute forms, in some cough preparations. Guaifenesin is incorporated into many over-the-counter cough medications, although its effectiveness as an expectorant is controversial. Elixir of terpin hydrate is thought to have a direct stimulatory effect on the bronchial secreting cells and is often combined with codeine in cough syrups. The mucolytic agent acetylcysteine is administered to liquefy the viscid mucus seen in cystic fibrosis.

In summary, the respiratory system requires continuous input from the nervous system. The movement of the diaphragm, intercostal muscles, and other respiratory muscles is controlled by neurons of the respiratory center located in the pons and medulla. The control of breathing has both automatic and voluntary components. The automatic regulation of ventilation is controlled by two types of receptors: lung receptors, which protect respiratory structures, and the chemoreceptors, which monitor the gas exchange function of the lung by sensing changes in blood levels of carbon dioxide, oxygen, and *pH*. There are three types of lung receptors: stretch receptors, which monitor lung inflation; irritant receptors, which protect against the damaging effects of toxic inhalants; and J receptors, which are thought to sense lung congestion. There are two groups of chemoreceptors: central chemoreceptors and peripheral chemoreceptors. The central chemoreceptors are the most important in sensing changes in carbon dioxide levels; and the peripheral chemoreceptors, in sensing arterial blood oxygen levels. Voluntary respiratory control is needed for integrating breathing and actions such as speaking, blowing, and singing. These acts, which are initiated by the motor and premotor cortex, cause temporary suspension of automatic breathing.

Alterations in breathing patterns include tachypnea (rapid breathing), hyperpnea (increase in both the rate and depth of respiration), bradypnea (abnormally slow respiratory rate), and hyperventilation (respiration in excess of that needed to maintain a normal level of P_{CO_2}). Periodic breathing is manifested by periods of apnea. Dyspnea is a subjective sensation of difficulty in breathing. The cough reflex protects the lungs from accumulation of secretions and injury from irritating substances. It is initiated by

airway receptors and transmitted to the medullary cough center, which integrates the cough response. The protective functions of the cough reflex are impaired by weakness of the expiratory muscles, by conditions that prevent closure of the glottis, and by depressed function of the medullary cough center. The cough reflex can be suppressed by medications that (1) depress the medullary cough center, (2) soothe the irritated mucosal surface of the pharynx, or (3) act peripherally on the stretch receptors in the lung. Expectorants are drugs that decrease the viscosity of the respiratory tract secretions and thereby facilitate their expulsion from the respiratory tract.

References

1. Ayres SM: Cigarette smoking and lung diseases. Basics of RD 5(5), (entire issue), 1975
2. Ham AW: Histology, 7th ed, p 719. Philadelphia, JB Lippincott, 1979
3. Berne RM, Levy MN: Physiology, 2nd ed, p 587. St Louis, CV Mosby, 1988
4. West JB: Respiratory Physiology, p 10. Baltimore, Williams & Wilkins, 1974
5. Guyton A: Textbook of Medical Physiology, 7th ed, pp 467, 501, 528, 530. Philadelphia, WB Saunders, 1986
6. Robbins SL, Cotran RS, Kumar V: Pathologic Basis of Disease, 5th ed, p 484. Philadelphia, WB Saunders, 1984
7. Davis JM, Venes-Meehan K, Notter RH et al: Changes in pulmonary mechanics after the administration of surfactant to infants with respiratory distress syndrome. N Engl J Med 319:476, 1988
8. Branin PK: Physical assessment in acute respiratory failure. Crit Care Q 1:27, 1979
9. Howell JBL (ed): Breathlessness. Philadelphia, FA Davis, 1966
10. Carrieri VK, Jansen-Berjklie S: The sensation of dyspnea: A critical review. Heart Lung 13:437, 1984

Bibliography

Carrieri VK, Jansen-Bjerklie S: Strategies patients use to manage the sensation of dyspnea. West J Nurs Res 8:284, 1986

Reischman RR: Review of ventilation and perfusion physiology. Crit Care Nurse 8(7):24, 1988

Thomas HM, Lefrak SS, Irwin RS et al: The oxyhemoglobin dissociation curve in health and disease. Am J Med 57:331, 1974

Wasserman K, Casaburi R: Dyspnea: Physiological and pathophysiological mechanisms. Annu Rev Med 39:503, 1988

CHAPTER 25

Alterations in Respiratory Function

Objectives

After you have studied this chapter, you should be able to meet the following objectives:

_____ Describe the transmission of the common cold from one person to another.

_____ Explain why respiratory infections are common in young children.

_____ Compare croup, epiglottitis, and bronchiolitis in terms of incidence by age, site of infection, and signs and symptoms.

_____ Define the terms *wheezing* and *stridor*.

_____ Explain the mechanisms of sternal and chest wall retraction in small children with upper airway obstruction due to infection.

_____ Give the reason that children with epiglottitis require immediate medical care.

_____ List the signs of impending respiratory failure in small children.

(continued)

_____ Differentiate between areas of the lung that are involved in lobar, bronchial, and viral pneumonias.

_____ Explain why bronchopneumonia is often seen at the extremes of age.

_____ Describe the four stages of lung involvement in lobar pneumonia.

_____ Explain why the formulation of the influenza vaccine must be changed from year to year.

_____ Cite the characteristics of three groups of persons for whom influenza vaccine is recommended.

_____ State why revaccination with pneumococcal vaccine is not recommended.

_____ Describe the transmission of tuberculosis.

_____ Differentiate between primary tuberculosis and secondary tuberculosis on the basis of their pathophysiology.

_____ State the significance of a positive reaction to the skin test for tuberculosis.

_____ Explain why multiple drug regimens are used in treatment of tuberculosis.

_____ State the mechanism for the transmission of fungal infections of the lung.

_____ State the characteristics of pleural pain.

_____ Explain why tension pneumothorax is a life-threatening emergency

_____ Describe five mechanisms that cause pleural effusion.

_____ Relate the pathologic changes that occur with pleural effusion to the production of signs and symptoms.

_____ Define the terms *hydrothorax, chylothorax,* and *hemothorax.*

_____ Explain why surgery increases the risk of atelectasis.

_____ State the feature common to chronic obstructive pulmonary diseases.

_____ State the effect that stimulation of the sympathetic and parasympathetic nervous systems have on bronchial smooth muscle.

_____ State the difference between extrinsic and intrinsic asthma.

_____ Relate the pathology that occurs in bronchial asthma to the production of signs and symptoms.

_____ Explain the distinction between chronic bronchitis and emphysema.

_____ State the function of alpha$_1$-antitrypsin in the prevention of chronic obstructive lung disease.

_____ State the difference between chronic obstructive pulmonary diseases and interstitial lung diseases.

_____ Explain the rationale for inspiratory muscle training in persons with chronic obstructive pulmonary disease.

_____ Describe the rationale for the use of low-flow oxygen in patients with severe hypoxemia due to chronic obstructive pulmonary disease.

_____ State the changes in ventilation that cause nocturnal hypoxemia in some persons with chronic obstructive pulmonary disease.

_____ Describe the abnormalities characteristic of cystic fibrosis.

_____ State the chief manifestations of bronchiectasis.

_____ Cite the characteristics of occupational dusts that determine their pathogenicity in terms of the production of pneumoconioses.

_____ Compare the hypersensitivity reactions that occur with bronchial asthma with those that occur in the hypersensitivity form of occupational lung diseases.

_____ State the immediate effects of pulmonary embolism.

_____ State three causes of pulmonary hypertension.

_____ Describe the alterations in cardiovascular function that are characteristic of cor pulmonale.

_____ State two environmental factors that may cause bronchogenic cancer.

_____ List two symptoms of lung cancer that are related to the invasion of the mediastinum.

_____ Cite three paraneoplastic manifestations of lung cancer.

Respiratory illnesses represent one of the more common reasons for visits to the physician, admission to the hospital, and forced inactivity among all age groups. Forty-seven million Americans—children and adults—suffer from one or more chronic respiratory diseases. For purposes of discussion, the respiratory disorders included in this chapter have been divided into six groups: (1) infections, (2) disorders of the pleura, (3) obstructive lung disorders, (4) interstitial lung disease, (5) pulmonary vascular disease, and (6) lung cancer. Alterations in ventilation and respiratory failure are discussed in Chapter 26.

Respiratory infections

The respiratory tract is susceptible to infectious processes caused by many types of microorganisms. For the most part, the signs and symptoms of respiratory tract infections depend on the function of the structure involved, the severity of the infectious process, and the person's age and general health. The discussion in this section of the chapter focuses on the common cold, acute respiratory tract infections in children, pneumonia, tuberculosis, and fungal infections of the lung.

—— The common cold

The common cold occurs more frequently than any other respiratory tract infection. Most adults have 2 to 4 colds per year; children may have up to 10 per year.[1] The 1985 over-the-counter market for common cold preparations was estimated as $556 million.[2] The condition usually begins with a feeling of dryness and stuffiness affecting mainly the nasopharynx; it is accompanied by excessive production of nasal secretions and lacrimation, or tearing of the eyes. Usually the secretions remain clear and watery. The mucous membranes of the upper respiratory tract become reddened, swollen, and bathed in mucous secretions. Involvement of the pharynx and larynx causes sore throat and hoarseness. Headache and generalized malaise may be present. In severe cases there may be chills, fever, and marked prostration. The disease process is usually self-limiting, lasting about 7 days.

Although the condition can be caused by a number of viruses, the rhinovirus has been shown to cause the greatest percentage of diagnosed colds.[3] The first step in the spreading of a cold is the shedding of viruses, the area of greatest potential being the nasal mucosa. In infected individuals, the number of rhinoviruses was found to be 10 to 100 times greater in the nasal mucus than in pharyngeal secretions.[4] Studies have shown that colds are spread most frequently in the home or school.[5,6] The fingers are the most incriminated source of spread and the nasal mucosa and conjunctival surface of the eyes the most important portals of entry of the virus. Cold viruses have been found to survive for 3.5 hours on the skin and hard surfaces, such as wood and plastic; survival is poor on facial tissue and porous cloth. The most highly contagious period is during the first 3 days following the onset of symptoms, and the incubation period is about 5 days. Studies suggest that the aerosol spread of colds through coughing and sneezing is much less important than the spread by fingers picking up the virus from contaminated surfaces and carrying it to the nasal membranes and eyes.[6,7] This suggests that careful attention to hand washing is one of the most important preventive measures for avoiding the common cold.

A large number of over-the-counter remedies are available for treating the common cold. Because the common cold is an acute and self-limiting illness in persons who are otherwise healthy, treatment with antibiotics and other medications that are potentially harmful is contraindicated. Symptomatic treatment with rest and antipyretic drugs is all that is usually needed. There is some controversy about the use of vitamin C to reduce the incidence and severity of colds and influenza. Several studies have found an association between vitamin C intake and a reduced incidence,[8,9] whereas others have found that vitamin C had no effect on the number or severity of colds.[10] Antihistamines are popular over-the-counter drugs because of their action in drying nasal secretions. However, they may dry up bronchial secretions and worsen the cough, and in addition they may cause dizziness, drowsiness, and impaired judgment. As with vitamin C, there is no evidence that they shorten the duration of the cold. Decongestant drugs (sympathomimetic agents) are available in over-the-counter nasal sprays, drops, and oral cold medications. These drugs constrict the blood vessels in the swollen nasal mucosa and reduce nasal swelling. Rebound nasal swelling can occur with indiscriminate use of nasal drops and sprays. Oral preparations containing decongestants may cause systemic vasoconstriction and elevation of blood pressure when given in doses large enough to relieve nasal congestion; therefore, they should be avoided by persons with hypertension, heart disease, hyperthyroidism, diabetes mellitus, and other health problems.

—— Acute respiratory infections in children

In children, respiratory tract infections are common; although they are troublesome, they are usually not serious. Frequent infections occur because the immune system of infants and small children has not been exposed to many common pathogens; consequently, they tend to develop infections with each new exposure. Although most such infections are not serious, the small size of an infant or child's airways tends to promote impaired airflow and obstruction. For example, an infection that causes only sore throat and hoarseness in an adult may result in serious airway obstruction in a small child.

—— Upper airway infections

Obstruction of the upper airways secondary to infection tends to exert its greatest effect during the inspiratory phase of respiration. Movement of air through an obstructed upper airway, particularly the vocal cords in the larynx, tends to produce a crowing sound called *stridor*. Impairment of the expiratory phase of respiration can also occur; this causes a *wheezing* (whistling) sound as air moves through the obstructed area. With mild to moderate obstruction, inspiratory stridor is more prominent than expiratory wheezing because the airways tend to dilate with expiration. When the swelling and obstruction become severe, the airways can no longer dilate during expiration and both stridor and wheezing occur.

Cartilaginous support of the trachea and the larynx is poorly developed in infants and small children. As a result, these structures are soft and tend to collapse when the airway is obstructed and the child cries, causing the inspiratory pressures to become more negative. When this happens, both the stridor and inspiratory effort are increased. The phenomenon of airway collapse in the small child is analogous to what happens when a thick beverage, such as a milkshake, is drunk through a soft paper straw. The straw will collapse when the negative pressure produced by the sucking effort exceeds the flow of liquid through the straw.

The marked decrease in intrathoracic pressure resulting from increased inspiratory effort in the presence of airway obstruction also tends to cause retraction (sucking in) of the softer chest structures, such as the supraclavicular spaces, the sternum, the epigastrium, and the intercostal spaces. The increased inspiratory effort also causes flaring of the nares.

There are two upper respiratory tract infections of early childhood that are serious—croup and epiglottitis. Croup is the more common one, and it is usually benign and self-limiting. Epiglottitis, on the other hand, is rapidly progressive and life-threatening. The characteristics of both infections are described in Table 25-1.

Croup. Croup is a viral infection that affects the larynx, trachea, and bronchi. It is generally seen in children aged 3 months to 3 years. Because the sub-glottic area is normally the narrowest part of the respiratory tree in this age group, the obstruction is usually greatest in this area.[11]

Croup is characterized by inspiratory stridor, hoarseness, and a barking cough. The British use the term *croup* to describe the cry of the crow or raven, and this is undoubtedly how the term originated. One form of croup, spasmodic croup, characteristically occurs at night. The episode usually lasts several hours and may recur several nights in a row. Spasmodic croup tends to recur with subsequent respiratory infections.

Although the respiratory manifestations of croup often appear suddenly, they are usually preceded by upper respiratory infections that cause rhinorrhea (runny nose), coryza (common cold), hoarseness, and a low-grade fever. The symptoms usually subside when the child is exposed to moist air. For example, letting the bathroom shower run and then taking the child into the bathroom often brings prompt and dramatic relief of symptoms. A mist tent or vaporizer is used for more continuous treatment. Exposure to cold air also seems to relieve the airway spasm; often, the severe symptoms will be relieved simply because the child is exposed to cold air on the way to the hospital emergency room.

Other treatments may be required when a mist tent is ineffective. One method is to administer a racemic mixture of epinephrine (L-epinephrine and D-epinephrine) by positive pressure breathing through a face mask. A second method involves administration of the anti-inflammatory adrenal corticosteroid hormones. Establishment of an artificial air-

Table 25–1. Characteristics of epiglottitis, croup, and bronchiolitis in small children

Characteristics	Epiglottitis	Croup	Bronchiolitis
Common causative agent	*Hemophilus influenzae*, type B, bacterium	Parainfluenza virus	Respiratory syncytial virus most common
Most commonly affected age group	1–5 years	3 months to 3 years	Less than 18 months (most severe in infants under 6 months)
Onset and preceding history	Sudden onset	Usually follows symptoms of a cold	Preceded by stuffy nose and other signs
Prominent features	Child appears very sick and toxic Sits with mouth open and chin thrust forward Low-pitch stridor, difficulty swallowing, fever, drooling, anxiety *Danger of airway obstruction and asphyxia*	Stridor and a wet, barking cough Usually occurs at night Relieved by exposure to cold or moist air	Breathlessness, rapid shallow breathing, wheezing, cough, and retractions of lower ribs and sternum during inspiration
Usual treatment	Intubation or tracheotomy Treatment with appropriate antibiotic	Mist tent or vaporizor Administration of oxygen	Suportive treatment, administration of oxygen and hydration

way may become necessary in severe airway obstruction.

Epiglottitis. Acute epiglottitis is caused by *Hemophilus influenzae,* type B, bacterium. It is characterized by inflammatory edema of the supraglottic area, which includes the epiglottis and pharyngeal structures. It comes on suddenly, bringing danger of airway obstruction and asphyxia; the child with epiglottitis often requires immediate hospitalization.

The child appears pale, toxic, and lethargic and assumes a distinctive position—sitting up with the mouth open and the chin thrust forward. Difficulty in swallowing, a muffled voice, drooling, fever, and extreme anxiety are present.

Immediate establishment of an airway by either endotracheal tube or tracheotomy is usually needed. If epiglottitis is suspected, the child should never be forced to lie down because this causes the epiglottis to fall backward and may lead to complete airway obstruction. Examination of the throat with a tongue blade or other instrument may cause fatal airway obstruction and should be done only by medical personnel experienced in intubation of small children. It is also unwise to attempt any procedure, such as drawing blood, that would heighten the child's anxiety because this, too, could precipitate airway spasm and cause death.

Recovery from epiglottitis is usually rapid and uneventful once an adequate airway has been established and appropriate antibiotic therapy has been initiated.

It should be pointed out that epiglottitis can occur in adults as well as children. At present, the incidence is small (an estimated 9.7 cases per million) but appears to be increasing. In adults, epiglottitis may present with acute respiratory compromise or as a milder form of disease. Although the causative agent or agents have not been identified, *H. influenzae* does not appear to be a primary causative agent in adults. Also, airway closure is less of a threat in adults; it does occur, however, and provision for emergency tracheotomy should be available.[12]

——— Lower airway infections

Lower airway infections produce air trapping with prolonged expiration. Wheezing results from bronchospasm, mucosal inflammation, and edema. The child presents with increased expiratory effort, increased respiratory rate, and wheezing. If the infection is severe, there will also be marked intercostal retractions and signs of impending respiratory failure.

Bronchiolitis. Bronchiolitis is a viral infection of the lower airways, most commonly caused by the respiratory syncytial virus. Other viruses, such as adenovirus, parainfluenza, and rhinovirus, have also been implicated as causative agents. The infection produces inflammatory obstruction of the small airways and necrosis of the cells lining the lower airways. The child is usually able to take in sufficient air but has trouble exhaling it. Air becomes trapped in the lung distal to the site of obstruction and interferes with gas exchange. Hypoxemia and, in severe cases, hypercapnia may develop. Airway obstruction may produce air trapping and hyperinflation of the lungs or collapse of the alveoli. Bronchiolitis is usually seen in children under 18 months of age, the most serious cases occurring in babies under 6 months of age.

Babies with acute bronchiolitis have a typical appearance, marked by breathlessness with rapid respirations, a distressing cough, and retraction (drawing in) of the lower ribs and sternum. Crying, feeding, and activity exaggerate these signs. Wheezing and rales may or may not be present depending on the degree of airway obstruction. In infants with severe airway obstruction, wheezing decreases as the airflow diminishes. Generally the most critical phase of the disease is the first 24 to 72 hours.[13] Cyanosis, pallor, listlessness, and sudden diminution or absence of breath sounds indicate impending respiratory failure. The characteristics of bronchiolitis are described in Table 25-1.

Treatment is supportive and includes administration of humidified oxygen to relieve hypoxia. A position that facilitates respiratory movements (elevation of the head) and avoids airway compression is used. Unnecessary handling is kept at a minimum to avoid tiring. Because the infection is viral, antibiotics are not effective and are given only for a secondary bacterial infection. Dehydration may occur as the result of increased insensible water losses because of the rapid respiratory rate and feeding difficulties, and measures to ensure adequate hydration are needed. Recovery begins after the first 48 to 72 hours and is usually rapid and complete.[14]

——— Signs of impending respiratory failure

Respiratory problems of infants and small children are often of sudden origin, and recovery is usually rapid and complete. However, children are at risk for development of airway obstruction and respiratory failure resulting from obstructive disorders or lung infection. The child with epiglottitis is at risk for development of airway obstruction; the child with bronchiolitis, for development of respiratory failure resulting from impaired gas exchange. The signs and symptoms of impending respiratory failure are listed in Chart 25-1.

Pneumonias

The term *pneumonia* describes inflammation of parenchymal structures of the lung, such as the alveoli and the bronchioles. Etiologic agents include both infectious and noninfectious agents. For example, inhalation of irritating fumes or aspiration of gastric contents can result in severe pneumonia. Recently subtle changes have occurred in the spectrum of microorganisms causing infectious pneumonias, namely, a decrease in pneumonias caused by *Streptococcus pneumoniae* and an increase in pneumonias caused by other microorganisms such as *Pseudomonas, Candida* and other fungi, and nonspecific viruses. Many of these pneumonias occur in persons with impaired immune defenses. *Pneumocystis carinii*, a virulent type of pneumonia, has recently surfaced as a disease associated with acquired immunodeficiency syndrome (AIDS).

Pneumonias are usually classified according to their etiologic agent and their anatomic distribution. The anatomic distribution can be considered under three general headings: (1) lobar, (2) bronchial, and (3) interstitial. In *lobar pneumonia*, there is involvement of a large portion or an entire lobe of a lung (Figure 25-1). With *bronchopneumonia*, there is a patchy consolidation with involvement of several lobules. These lesions vary in size from 3 cm to 4 cm and, because of gravity, are more common in the lower and posterior portions of the lung. In *interstitial pneumonia*, the inflammatory process is more or less confined within the wall that surrounds the alveoli and bronchioles. This type of pneumonia is generally caused by viral or mycoplasmal infections.

Although antibiotics have significantly reduced mortality due to pneumonias, these diseases remain an important immediate cause of death in the elderly and in persons with debilitating diseases. In 1981 pneumonia was the sixth leading cause of death in the United States.[15]

The normal lung is sterile. Most of the agents that cause pneumonia are inhaled into the lung in the air breathed. Depending on the population being examined, pneumococci have been shown to be present in the nasopharynx in 5% to 59% of healthy persons.[16] Normally, respiratory tract defense mechanisms would prevent these organisms from entering the lung. Loss of the cough reflex, damage to the ciliated endothelium that lines the respiratory tract, and lowered resistance to infection all increase susceptibility to pneumonia. Persons with immunologic deficiencies, congestive heart failure, or hypostatic pulmonary edema are particularly prone to develop pneumonia. Table 25-2 summarizes respiratory tract defense mechanisms along with factors that impair their effectiveness and thereby predispose to pneumonia.

Lobar pneumonia

Approximately 90% to 95% of cases of lobar pneumonia are caused by *Streptococcus pneumoniae*.[17] Classically, lobar pneumonia occurs in otherwise healthy adults and is relatively uncommon in infants and the elderly.

The tissue changes in lobar pneumonia are consistent with signs of acute inflammation. This acute inflammatory response can be divided into four stages: (1) congestion, (2) red hepatization, (3) gray hepatization, and (4) resolution. Often its progress is modified by antibiotic therapy. The *congestive stage* represents the initial inflammatory response and is characterized by vascular engorgement of the alveolar vessels and transudation of serous fluid into the alveoli. The period of congestion lasts for about 24 hours and is followed by the stage of *red hepatization*.

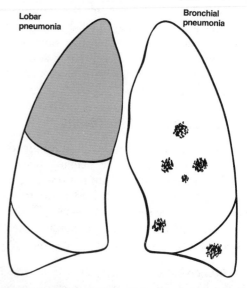

Figure 25-1 Distribution of lung involvement in lobar and bronchial pneumonia.

During this stage, there is extravasation of red blood cells and fibrin into the alveoli, and the lungs become firm and red with a liver-like appearance—hence the term red hepatization. The stage of *gray hepatization* is characterized by an accumulation of fibrin and the beginning disintegration of the inflammatory white and red cells. Sometimes the infection extends into the pleural cavity causing *empyema*—pus in the pleural cavity. In untreated pneumonia, the stage of *resolution* occurs in about 8 to 10 days and represents the enzymatic digestion and removal of the inflammatory exudate from the infected lung area. The exudate is either coughed up or removed from the lung by macrophages.

The signs and symptoms of lobar pneumonia coincide with the stage of the disease. The onset is usually sudden and is characterized by malaise, a severe shaking chill, and fever. The temperature may go as high as 106°F. During the congestive stage, coughing brings up a watery sputum and breath sounds are limited, with fine crepitant rales. As the disease progresses, the character of the sputum changes; it may be blood-tinged (or rust-colored) to purulent. Pleuritic pain, a sharp pain that is more severe with respiratory movements, is common. With antibiotic therapy, fever usually subsides in about 48 to 72 hours and recovery is uneventful.

Bronchopneumonia

Bronchopneumonia is considered to be a disease of the very young, the very old, and the debilitated—the very young because their immunologic reserve and respiratory defense mechanisms have not as yet developed and the very old because of a decline in immunity and because many have other diseases that predispose them to pneumonia.

Virtually any pathogenic organism can cause bronchopneumonia. Hospitalized patients are susceptible to bacteria present in the environment. These nosocomial (hospital-acquired) infections are usually due to gram-negative microorganisms and are resistant to microbial therapy. Proper hand washing and decontamination of inhalation equipment is important in preventing these infections.

In contrast to lobar pneumonia, which has a rapid onset, the early manifestations of bronchopneumonia are often insidious and in most cases include a low-grade fever along with a cough and inspiratory rales. Complications include formation of a lung abscess, empyema, and bacteremia.

Legionnaires' disease

Legionnaires' disease is a form of bronchopneumonia caused by the hard-to-isolate gram-negative bacillus *Legionella pneumophila,* a member of the *Legionella* species. The organism is almost ubiquitous in water, particularly warm standing water.[18] The disease was first recognized and received its name after an epidemic of severe and frequently fatal pneumonia among delegates to an American Legion convention in a Philadelphia hotel. The spread of infection was traced to a water-cooled air-conditioning system. Although healthy people can develop the infection, the risk is greatest among persons with chronic diseases or impaired cell-mediated immunity.

Symptoms of the disease typically begin about 2 to 10 days after infection with malaise, weakness, lethargy, fever, and dry cough. Depending on the severity of the disease, the initial manifestations are followed by recurring chills, dyspnea, weakness, confusion, pleuritic pain, and blood-stained sputum. Other manifestations include disturbances of central nervous system function, gastrointestinal tract involvement, arthralgias, and elevation in body temperature, sometimes to over 104°F. The disease causes consolidation of lung tissues and impairs gas exchange. The

Table 25–2. Respiratory defense mechanisms and conditions that impair their effectiveness

Defense mechanism	Function	Factors that impair effectiveness
Nasopharyngeal defenses	Remove particles from the air; contact with surface lysosomes and immunoglobulins (IgA) protects against infection	IgA deficiency state, hay fever, common cold, trauma to the nose, others
Glottic and cough reflexes	Protect against aspiration into tracheobronchial tree	Loss of cough reflex due to stroke or neural lesion, neuromuscular disease, abdominal or chest surgery, depression of the cough reflex due to sedation or anesthesia, presence of a nasogastric tube (tends to cause adaptation of afferent receptors)
Mucociliary blanket	Removes particles from the respiratory tract	Smoking, viral diseases, chilling, inhalation of irritating gases
Pulmonary macrophages	Remove microorganisms and foreign particles from the lung	Chilling, alcohol intoxication, smoking, anoxia

mortality rate can be as high as 20% to 30% in previously healthy persons and 80% in immunocompromised persons.[19]

Pneumocystis pneumonia

Pneumocystis carinii pneumonia is an opportunistic, often fatal, form of infection seen in debilitated persons and those with impaired immune function, particularly those with impaired cell-mediated immunity. The immunosuppression associated with corticosteroid drugs seems to be more important than cytotoxic therapy in predisposing to infection.[19] Currently, pneumocystis is a major pulmonary infection in persons with AIDS. The infection, which is airborne, usually produces an initial random and patchy involvement of the lungs. In vulnerable hosts, the disease spreads rapidly throughout the lungs, producing involvement similar to that of adult respiratory syndrome (see Chapter 26). Microscopically, the walls of the involved alveoli become thickened and edematous and alveoli become filled with a foamy, protein-rich fluid.[18] As the disease progresses the gas-exchange function of the lungs becomes severely impaired.

Viral and mycoplasmal pneumonias

Viral pneumonias can occur as a primary infection or as a complication of other diseases, such as chickenpox and measles. The influenza virus is the most common cause of viral pneumonia. In the adult, chickenpox is associated with pneumonia in 10% to 15% of cases, with a mortality rate of about 20%.[20] The mycoplasmas are the smallest free-living agents of disease, having characteristics of both viruses and bacteria. Pneumonias due to the mycoplasmas are sometimes called *primary atypical pneumonias.*

Viral or atypical pneumonias involve the interstitium of the lung and may masquerade as chest colds, with manifestations often confined to fever, headache, and muscle aches and pains. Viruses impair the respiratory tract defenses and predispose to secondary bacterial infections.

Immunization

Vaccines are available to protect against the influenzal infections and pneumococcal pneumonia. These vaccines are recommended for high-risk groups who, because of their age or underlying health problems, are unable to cope well with these infections and often require medical attention, including hospitalization. For example, influenza outbreaks in nursing homes resulted in infection rates as high as 60%, with mortality rates of 30% or more.[21]

Influenza immunization. Several strains of the influenza virus are responsible for epidemics of the disease. These strains undergo small changes over time that affect their antigenicity and the host protection afforded by previous immunization. Influenza's impact is normally greatest when new strains appear against which the population lacks immunity. Therefore, the formulation of the influenza vaccine must be changed yearly in response to changes in the influenza virus. Each year the Public Health Advisory Committee on Immunization Practices updates its recommendations for the composition of the vaccine.

Currently, the Immunization Practices Advisory Committee recommends annual vaccination using inactivated influenza vaccine to prevent or minimize the effect of influenza infections in high-risk groups.[21,22] The high-risk group has been classified into three categories according to priority of need. The highest-priority groups are adults and children with chronic cardiovascular or pulmonary system disorders severe enough to have required regular medical follow-ups or hospitalization during the preceding year and residents of nursing homes and other chronic-care facilities. Of second priority are medical personnel working with high-risk patients. Although not proven, it is believed that these personnel may transfer influenza infections to their patients. The third-priority group includes otherwise healthy individuals who are over 65 years of age and adults and children with chronic metabolic diseases, such as diabetes mellitus, kidney dysfunction, anemia, or asthma severe enough to have required regular medical checkups or hospitalization during the previous year.

Pneumococcal immunization. Like influenza, pneumococcal pneumonia causes significant morbidity and mortality in high-risk groups. A 23-valent pneumococcal vaccine, composed of antigens from 23 types of *Streptococcus Pneumoniae* (pneumococcus), was licensed in the United States in 1983, replacing the 14-valent type licensed in 1977. At present, pneumococcal vaccine is given only once; revaccination is not recommended. This is because local and systemic reactions are common among persons who receive second doses. It is also recommended at present that persons who have received the 14-valent type of vaccine should not be revaccinated with the 23-valent vaccine.[23]

Vaccination with the pneumococcal vaccine is recommended for adults with chronic illnesses, particularly cardiovascular and pulmonary diseases, who sustain increased morbidity with respiratory infections. Vaccination is also recommended for adults with other chronic illnesses associated with increased risk of pneumococcal infections and for otherwise healthy older adults, especially those aged 65 and over. Children aged 2 years and older with chronic illnesses such as sickle cell disease, splenectomy, nephrotic syndrome, cerebrospinal fluid leaks, or conditions associated with immunosuppression should also be immunized.[23]

Tuberculosis

Tuberculosis is an infectious disease caused by *Mycobacterium tuberculosis*. The mycobacteria are slender, rod-shaped, acid-fast, aerobic organisms. There are two forms of tuberculosis that pose a particular threat in humans—*Mycobacterium tuberculosis* and *Mycobacterium bovis*. Bovine tuberculosis is acquired by drinking milk from infected cows and initially affects the gastrointestinal tract. This form of tuberculosis has been virtually eradicated in North America and other developed countries as a result of rigorous controls on dairy herds and the pasteurization of milk. There has been a recent increase in the United States of atypical mycobacterial infections, including those caused by *Mycobacterium kansasii* and *Mycobacterium intracellularis*.

The incidence of tuberculosis in the United States has decreased markedly during the past several decades, with active cases falling from 76.7 per 100,000 in 1932 to 11.0 per 100,000 in 1982.[24] Nevertheless, there were nearly 25,000 new cases reported in the United States in 1983.[25] Regrettably, 6% of new cases die of the disease. Furthermore, the number of new cases of extrapulmonary tuberculosis remains unchanged. Tuberculosis is more common in the homeless, among refugees from Asia and Central America, and among persons infected with the AIDS virus. The elderly are also more vulnerable to the infection. It was originally thought that the case rates among the elderly were higher because the majority of such persons were infected years ago, when tuberculosis was more common. However, a recent study of 223 Arkansas nursing homes revealed that the prevalence of the disease among newly admitted elderly residents as determined by tuberculin skin testing was less than expected for their age. However, the rate of infection increased with each year spent in the home, with the highest rates occurring in homes with recent infectious cases.[26] These findings suggest that many previously infected persons have outlived their initial infecting organism, as indicated by the negative results on skin testing, and that they are vulnerable to reinfection.

Transmission

Tuberculosis is an airborne infection spread by *droplet nuclei*—minute, invisible particles harbored in the respiratory secretions of persons with active tuberculosis. Although the secretions often contain many larger particles, these larger particles tend to be filtered out of the air by gravity. If the larger particles are inhaled, they are usually trapped in the nasopharyngeal area and are removed by the action of the mucociliary blanket. Consequently, it is only the droplet nuclei that contribute to the transmission of the disease. These nuclei remain suspended in air and are circulated by air currents. They are so small that when inhaled they travel directly to the alveoli.

Pathogenesis

The destructiveness of tuberculosis is due not to the inherently destructive tubercle bacillus, but to the hypersensitivity response it evokes. For purposes of discussion, tuberculosis can be divided into primary and secondary infections; the initial infection is classified as primary tuberculosis and subsequent infections as secondary tuberculosis.

Primary tuberculosis is usually initiated in the alveolar wall as a result of inhaling tubercle bacilli. Primary tuberculosis has sometimes been called *childhood tuberculosis,* probably because contact with the disease occurred during childhood. The process begins as an acute inflammatory response and progresses to a chronic granulomatous inflammation (see Chapter 10). Cell-mediated immunity and hypersensitivity reactions contribute to the evolution of the disease.

The initial response of the involved alveolar tissue is a local nonspecific pneumonitis. With initiation of the inflammatory response, polymorphonuclear leukocytes enter the area and phagocytize the bacilli but do not kill them. Within about 24 to 48 hours the polymorphonuclear cells are replaced by macrophages (histiocytes). Many of the bacilli engulfed by the macrophages remain viable and proliferate. At some time, approximately days 10 to 20, the infiltrating macrophages begin to elongate and fuse together to form an epithelioid cell tubercle, which becomes surrounded by lymphocytes. One or more tubercles may form. Following this period of time, the central portion of the lesion undergoes necrosis and forms a yellow cheesy mass called *caseous necrosis.* The tuberculin skin test becomes positive at about the time that the caseous necrosis occurs, suggesting that the necrosis results from the hypersensitivity response. Healing of the tubercular lesion occurs as collagenous scar tissue forms and encapsulates the lesion. In time most of these lesions become calcified and are visible on a chest x-ray film. The primary lesion is known as a *Ghon focus,* and the combination of the tubercle lesion and the involved lymph nodes is the *Ghon complex.* The Ghon complex may contain viable organisms.

Occasionally, primary tuberculosis may progress, eroding into a bronchus and there discharging the contents of its necrotic center. An air-filled cavity forms, permitting bronchogenic spread of the disease. In rare instances, tuberculosis may erode into a blood vessel, giving rise to hematogenous dissemination. *Miliary tuberculosis* describes minute lesions resulting from this type of dissemination and may involve almost any organ, particularly the brain, meninges, liver, kidney, and bone marrow.

Secondary tuberculosis usually results from reactivation of a previously healed primary lesion. It often occurs in situations of impaired body defense mechanisms. The partial immunity that follows initial exposure affords protection against reinfection and to some extent aids in localizing the disease should secondary infection occur. The hypersensitivity reaction, on the other hand, is an aggravating factor in secondary tuberculosis, as evidenced by the frequency of cavitation and bronchial dissemination. The cavities may coalesce to a size of up to 10 cm to 15 cm in diameter. Pleural effusion and tuberculous empyema are common as the disease progresses.

Manifestations

Primary tuberculosis is usually asymptomatic, the only evidence of the disease being a positive tuberculin skin test and the presence of calcified lesions on the chest x-ray film. Secondary tuberculosis may also be asymptomatic, particularly when the lesion is confined to the apexes or upper portions of the lung. Often, however, there is an insidious onset of afternoon elevation of temperature, night sweats, slight cough with mucoid sputum, weakness, fatigability, and loss of appetite and weight. As the disease advances, there may be dyspnea and orthopnea.

Diagnosis and treatment

Diagnostic methods.   The most frequently used screening methods for tuberculosis are the tuberculin skin tests and chest x-ray studies. Cultures (bacteriologic studies) of the sputum or gastric contents determine the presence of the organism. Gastric contents are aspirated after a fast of 8 to 10 hours, usually as the patient arises in the morning. These secretions contain tubercle bacilli swallowed during the night.

The tuberculin skin test was introduced by Robert Koch in the late 19th century. The test measures delayed hypersensitivity (cell-mediated, type IV) that follows exposure to the tubercle bacillus. It is important to recognize that a positive reaction to the skin test does not mean that a person has tuberculosis, only that there has been exposure to the bacillus and that cell-mediated immunity to the organism has developed.

There are two skin tests, the multiple puncture technique and the intercutaneous technique. In the multiple puncture technique, use of purified protein derivative (PPD)—for example, the Aplitest, Slavo Test PPD, Heaf test, or old tuberculin (Tine, Mono Vacc) test—is the preferred method. A positive response is manifested by vesicle formation at the test site. The quantity of tuberculin introduced under the skin using the multiple puncture technique cannot be precisely controlled. For this reason the multiple puncture methods are not intended as diagnostic tests but are used as initial screening procedures in asymptomatic persons who have not been exposed to someone with tuberculosis. Verification of the reaction to a multiple puncture test is recommended by the standard Mantoux test unless vesicle formation is present.[27] The intercutaneous or Mantoux test (Aplisol or Tubersol) is the standard test for suspected tuberculosis. A positive reaction is evidenced by a discrete area of skin elevation of 10 mm or more. In tuberculosis, the areas of induration usually are between 15 mm and 20 mm or more.

Treatment methods.   Tuberculosis is an unusual disease in that chemotherapy is required for a long time. The tubercle bacillus is an aerobic organism that multiplies slowly and remains relatively dormant in oxygen-poor caseous material. It undergoes a high rate of mutation and tends to develop a resistance to any one drug. For this reason, multiple drug regimens are used, except for prophylaxis. The primary drugs used in the treatment of tuberculosis are isoniazid (INH), rifampin, ethambutol, and streptomycin. Secondary drugs include aminosalicylic acid (PAS), ethionamide, capreomycin, kanamycin, pyrazinamide, and viomycin. The secondary drugs are usually considered only when resistance to the primary choice drugs develops. All of these drugs act by inhibiting the growth of the tubercle bacillus.

Isoniazid is remarkably potent against the tubercle bacillus and is probably the most widely used drug in tuberculosis. Although its exact mechanism of action is unknown, it apparently combines with an enzyme that is needed by the INH-susceptible strains of the tuberculous bacillus. Resistance to the drug develops rapidly, and combination with other effective drugs delays the development of resistance. Rifampin inhibits RNA synthesis in bacteria. Although ethambutol is known to inhibit the growth of the tubercle bacillus, its mechanism of action is unknown. Streptomycin, the first drug found to be effective against tuberculosis, must be given parenterally, which limits its usefulness particularly in long-term therapy. It remains an important drug in tuberculosis therapy and is used primarily in individuals with severe, possibly life-threatening forms of tuberculosis.

Based on several recent trials, a marked change in chemotherapy for uncomplicated tuberculosis has developed. Short-course programs of therapy (usually 9 months) have replaced the traditional 18-to-24-month traditional multidrug regimens.

Two groups of persons meet the criteria established for the use of antimycobacterial therapy for tuberculosis: the first consists of those who have contact with cases of active tuberculosis and who are at risk for developing an active form of the disease (classification 1 or 2); the second group includes persons with active tuberculosis (classification 3).

INH is commonly used prophylactically in the first group. This group includes persons with a positive skin test who (1) have had close contact with active cases of tuberculosis, (2) have converted from a negative to positive skin test within two years, (3) have a history of untreated tuberculosis or x-ray evidence of asymptomatic tuberculosis, (4) have special risk factors such as end-stage renal disease, immunosuppression, or silicosis, and (5) are 35 years of age or under with a positive reaction of unknown duration. Because INH can cause hepatitis, persons being treated with the drug should be followed closely and warned of symptoms of the disease.[28,29]

Fungal infections

Although the spores of fungi are constantly present in the air we breathe, only a few reach the lung and cause disease. The most common of these are histoplasmosis, coccidioidomycosis, and blastomycosis. These infections are usually mild and self-limiting and are seldom noticed unless they produce local complications or progressive dissemination occurs. The signs and symptoms of these infections commonly resemble those of tuberculosis.

Histoplasmosis

Histoplasmosis, caused by the dimorphic fungus (see Chapter 9) *Histoplasma capsulatum,* is the most common fungal infection in the United States. Skin testing surveys suggest that 18% to 20% of persons in the United States have been infected with the disease.[30] Most cases occur along the major river valleys of the Midwest—the Ohio, the Mississippi, and the Missouri. The organism grows in soil and other areas that have been enriched with bird excreta: old chicken houses, pigeon lofts, barns, and trees where birds roost. The infection is acquired by inhaling the fungal spores that are released when the dirt or dust from the infected areas is disturbed. The spores convert to the parasitic yeast phase when exposed to body temperature in the alveoli. The organisms are then carried to the regional lymphatics and from there are

disseminated throughout the body in the bloodstream. They are removed from the circulation by fixed macrophages of the reticuloendothelial system. When delayed hypersensitivity develops (see Chapter 12), the macrophages are usually able to destroy the fungi.

The manifestations of histoplasmosis are strikingly similar to those of tuberculosis. Depending on the host's resistance and immunocompetence, the disease usually takes one of four forms: (1) latent asymptomatic disease, (2) self-limiting primary disease, (3) chronic pulmonary disease, or (4) disseminated infection. The average incubation period for the infection is about 14 days. Only 40% of infected persons have symptoms and only about 10% of these are ill enough to see a physician.[31] *Asymptomatic latent histoplasmosis* is characterized by evidence of healed lesions in the lungs or hilar lymph nodes accompanied by a positive histoplasmin skin test (analogous to the tuberculin test). *Primary pulmonary histoplasmosis* occurs in otherwise healthy people as a mild, self-limiting, febrile, respiratory infection. Its symptoms include muscle and joint pains and a nonproductive cough. Erythema nodosum (subcutaneous nodules) or erythema multiforme (hivelike lesions) sometimes appear. During this stage of the disease, chest x-rays usually show single or multiple infiltrates.

Chronic histoplasmosis resembles secondary tuberculosis. Infiltration of the upper lobes of one or both lungs with cavitation occurs. This form of the disease is more common in middle-aged men who smoke and in persons with chronic lung disease. The most common manifestations are productive cough, fever, night sweats, and weight loss. In many persons, the disease is self-limiting. In others, there is progressive destruction of lung tissue and dissemination of the disease.

Disseminated histoplasmosis can follow either primary or chronic histoplasmosis but most often develops as an acute and fulminating infection in the very old or the very young, or in persons with compromised immune function. Although the macrophages of the reticuloendothelial system can remove the fungi from the bloodstream, they are unable to destroy them.[31] Characteristically this form of the disease produces a high fever, generalized lymph node enlargement, hepatosplenomegaly, muscle wasting, anemia, leukopenia, and thrombocytopenia. There may be hoarseness, ulcerations of the mouth and tongue, nausea, vomiting, diarrhea, and abdominal pain. Often, meningitis becomes a dominant feature of the disease.

Absolute diagnosis of histoplasmosis requires identification of the organism on culture. The infection incites a delayed hypersensitivity immune response and the histoplasmin skin test is used to test for exposure to the organism. This test remains positive after the initial infection has occurred and does not indicate whether the disease is of recent or past origin. In addition to the delayed response, the humoral immune system responds to the acute infection by producing antibodies. Though these antibodies are not protective, they serve as markers of infection. These antibodies can be measured by means of the complement fixation (CF) test. An immunodiffusion (ID) test can also be used as a test for the antibodies. Both the CF and ID tests become positive 2 weeks after the onset of symptoms. The antifungal drugs amphotericin B and ketoconazole are used for persons with disease severe enough to require treatment or those with compromised immune function who are at risk for developing disseminated disease. Amphotericin B is given intravenously and is usually the drug of choice in severe disease. The drug can impair kidney and liver function and produce anemia. Ketoconazole is given orally and takes up to 3 weeks to produce its effect.

Coccidioidomycosis

Coccidioidomycosis is a common fungal infection caused by inhaling the spores of *Coccidioides immitis*. An estimated 100,000 new cases occur annually.[31] It is most prevalent in the southwestern United States. About 80% of persons in the San Joaquin Valley are coccidioidin-positive.[17] Because of its prevalence in this area, the disease is sometimes referred to as "San Joaquin fever" or "valley fever." The disease resembles tuberculosis, and its mechanisms of infection are similar to those of histoplasmosis.

The disease most commonly occurs as an acute, primary self-limiting pulmonary infection with or without systemic involvement, but in some cases it progresses to a disseminated disease. About 60% of exposed persons only manifest a positive skin test (either coccidioidin skin test or spherulin skin test) and are unaware of the infection.[31] In the other 40% the illness usually resembles influenza. There may be fever, a cough, and pleuritic pain, accompanied by erythema multiforme or erythema nodosum. The skin lesions are usually accompanied by arthralgias or arthritis without effusion, particularly of the ankles and knees. The terms "desert bumps" and "desert arthritis" are used to describe these manifestations. The presence of skin and joint manifestations indicates strong host defenses, because persons who have had such manifestations seldom develop disseminated disease. Disseminated disease occurs in 1 out of 6000 infected persons and in fewer than 0.5% of persons with symptomatic disease. The commonly affected structures in disseminated disease are the lymph nodes, meninges, spleen, liver, kidney, skin, and adrenals. Meningitis is the most common cause of death.

Positive diagnosis of coccidioidomycosis can be made by direct visualization of spherules (multinucleated parasitic *Coccidioides immitis* cells) in the expectorated sputum after application of 10% potassium hydroxide. Although cultures can be used to identify the fungus, the results are positive in only about half of the cases. Furthermore, extreme caution is needed when handling this fungus because laboratory personnel can be easily infected. Two serologic tests, the tube-precipitin (TP) test and the complement-fixation (CF) test, are considered to be extremely useful in establishing a diagnosis of coccidioidomycosis. The CF test may be used in following the progress of the disease; an elevated CF titer is considered to indicate risk of disease dissemination. The skin tests with coccidioidin and spherulin do not indicate whether the disease is recent or has occurred in the past. Their main value is in epidemiologic studies and in confirming the diagnosis in persons who convert from a negative to a positive test during an illness. As with histoplasmosis, the antifungal drugs amphotericin B and ketoconazole are used in the treatment of progressive or disseminated diseases.

Blastomycosis

Blastomycosis is caused by the organism *Blastomyces dermatitidis*. It is characterized by local suppurative and granulomatous lesions of the lungs and skin. The disease is most commonly found in North America and is particularly prevalent in the southeastern and south central states.

The symptoms of acute infection are similar to those of acute histoplasmosis, including fever, cough, aching of the joints and muscles, and, uncommonly, pleuritic pain. In contrast to histoplasmosis, the cough in blastomycosis is often productive and the sputum is purulent. Acute pulmonary infections are usually self-limiting or progressive. Extrapulmonary spread most commonly involves the skin, bones, or prostate gland. These lesions may provide the first evidence of the disease.

The diagnosis of blastomycosis is more difficult than that of histoplasmosis. Visualization of the yeast in the sputum after application of 10% potassium hydroxide provides a presumptive diagnosis. When this fails, cultural isolation of the fungus is often attempted. The blastomycin skin test lacks specificity and is no longer available. The treatment of the progressive or disseminated form of the disease includes the use of amphotericin B or ketoconazole.

In summary, respiratory infections are the most common cause of respiratory illness. They include the common cold, respiratory infections common to children, pneumonias, and tuberculosis. The common cold occurs more frequently than any other respiratory infection. The fingers are the most incriminated source of transmission, and the most common portals of entry are the nasal mucosa and the conjunctiva of the eye. Because of the smallness of the airway of infants and children, respiratory tract infections in these groups are often more serious. Infections that may cause only a sore throat and hoarseness in the adult may produce serious obstruction in the child. Among the respiratory tract infections that affect small children are croup, epiglottitis, and bronchiolitis. Epiglottitis is a life-threatening supraglottic infection carrying the danger of airway obstruction and asphyxia.

Pneumonia describes an infection of the parenchymal tissues of the lung. Lobar pneumonia involves a large portion or lobe of the lung and is usually caused by the *Streptococcus pneumoniae*. Bronchopneumonia is caused by a number of agents. It is characterized by patchy consolidation of several lobes of the lung and often affects persons with other debilitating diseases. Legionnaires' disease is a form of bronchopneumonia caused by the gram-negative bacillus *Legionella pneumophila*. *Pneumocystis carinii* pneumonia is an opportunistic infection that occurs in debilitated and persons with impaired immune function, including persons with AIDS. Viral or atypical pneumonia can occur as a primary infection, such as that caused by influenza virus, or as a complication of other viral infections, such as measles. Viral and atypical pneumonias involve the interstitium of the lung and often masquerade as chest colds. Vaccines are available for the immunization of persons in groups at high risk for the development of influenzal or pneumococcal pneumonias.

Tuberculosis is a chronic respiratory infection caused by *Mycobacterium tuberculosis*. The incidence of tuberculosis, which is now being treated effectively with chemotherapeutic drugs, has decreased sharply in the past four to five decades. Infections caused by the fungi *Histoplasma capsulatum* (histoplasmosis), *Coccidioides immitis* (coccidioidomycosis), and *Blastomyces dermatitidis* (blastomycosis) resemble tuberculosis. These infections are common but seldom serious unless they produce progressive destruction of lung tissue or the infection disseminates outside the lungs.

Disorders of the pleura

The pleura is a thin double-layered membrane that encases the lungs. The inner visceral pleura lies adjacent to the lung; the outer parietal layer covers the inner aspect of the chest wall, the superior aspect of the diaphragm, and the mediastinum. The visceral and parietal pleurae are separated by a thin layer of serous fluid, and the potential space between the two layers is called the *pleural cavity*. The right and left pleural cavities are separated by the mediastinum, which contains the heart and other thoracic structures. Because of the inward elastic recoil forces of the lung and the outward elastic recoil of the chest wall, the pressure within the pleural space is negative. It becomes more negative as the chest expands during inspiration and less negative as the chest contracts during expiration. It is the negative pressure within the pleural cavity that keeps the lungs from collapsing. Disorders of the pleura include pain, pneumothorax, and pleural effusion.

Pleural pain

Pain is one of the most common symptoms of conditions that cause inflammation of the pleura. Most commonly the pain is abrupt in onset: the person experiencing it can cite almost to the minute when the pain started. It is usually unilateral, and tends to be localized to the lower and lateral part of the chest. Although the pain may radiate to the shoulder or abdomen, it does not usually originate from the substernal, paravertebral, or any other central part of the chest. The pain is usually made worse by chest movements, such as coughing and deep breathing, that exaggerate pressure changes within the pleural cavity and increase movement of the inflamed or injured pleural surfaces. Because deep breathing is painful, tidal volumes are usually kept small and breathing becomes rapid. Reflex muscle splinting usually occurs on the affected side, causing a lesser excursion of the affected side during respiration and development of atelectasis.

It is usually important to differentiate pleural pain from pain produced by other conditions, such as musculoskeletal strain of chest muscles, bronchial irritation, and myocardial disease. Musculoskeletal pain may occur as the result of frequent forceful coughing. This type of pain is usually bilateral and located in the inferior portions of the rib cage where the abdominal muscles insert into the anterior rib cage. It is usually made worse by movements associated with contraction of the abdominal muscles. The pain associated with irritation of the bronchi is usually substernal and dull in character, rather than sharp; it is usually worse with coughing but is not affected by deep breathing. Myocardial pain, which is discussed in Chapter 21, is usually located in the substernal area and is not associated with respiratory movements.

Although analgesic and narcotic drugs reduce awareness of pleural pain, they usually do not entirely relieve the discomfort associated with coughing and deep breathing. The nonsteroidal antiinflammatory drug indomethacin has been used successfully to relieve pain and facilitate effective coughing.[30]

Pneumothorax

Pneumothorax refers to an accumulation of air within the pleural cavity with a resultant partial or complete collapse of the affected lung. *Spontaneous pneumothorax* occurs when an air-filled bleb, or blister, on the lung surface ruptures and air leaks into the pleural cavity. In *secondary pneumothorax*, air enters the pleural space as the result of injury to the chest wall, respiratory structures, or esophagus. *Tension pneumothorax* describes the condition in which the pressure within the pleural space is greater than the atmospheric pressure during the entire respiratory cycle.

What causes the air-filled blebs responsible for spontaneous pneumothorax and why they rupture are unknown. Spontaneous pneumothorax most often occurs in young men. It may also occur in conjunction with lung diseases, such as chronic obstructive lung disease, that cause trapping of gases and destruction of lung tissue. Because the pressure in the pleural space is normally negative in relation to the pressure within the alveoli, rupture of the lung surface allows air to enter the pleural space; the lung collapses as a result of its own recoil. The air leak will usually continue until the decline in lung size causes it to seal.

Secondary pneumothorax may be caused by penetrating or nonpenetrating injuries. Fractured or dislocated ribs that penetrate the pleura are the most common cause of pneumothorax due to nonpenetrating chest injuries. Hemothorax often accompanies these injuries. Pneumothorax may also accompany fracture of the trachea or major bronchus or rupture of the esophagus. Persons with pneumothorax due to chest trauma frequently have other complications and may require chest surgery.

A tension pneumothorax is a life-threatening condition. It occurs when injury to the chest or respiratory structures permits air to enter but not leave the pleural space, so that the lesion acts as a one-way valve (Figure 25-2). This results in a rapid increase in pressure within the chest, a compression atelectasis of the unaffected lung, a shift in the mediastinum to the opposite side of the chest, and compression of the vena cava with impairment of venous return to the heart. Emergency treatment of tension pneumothorax involves the prompt insertion of a large-bore needle or chest tube into the affected side of the chest along with water-seal drainage or continuous chest suction to aid in lung reexpansion. The sucking of air into the thoracic cavity through an open chest wound can often be prevented by promptly covering the area with an airtight covering (*e.g.*, Vaseline gauze or a firm piece of

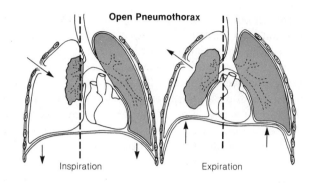

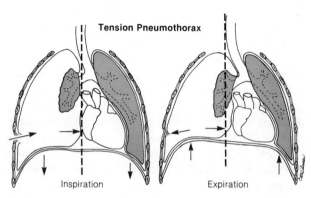

Figure 25-2 Open or communicating pneumothorax (*top*) and tension pneumothorax (*bottom*). In an open pneumothorax, air enters the chest during inspiration and exits during expiration. There may be slight inflation of the affected lung due to a decrease in pressure as air moves out of the chest. In tension pneumothorax, air can enter but not leave the chest. As the pressure in the chest increases, the heart and great vessels are compressed and the mediastinal structures are shifted toward the unaffected side of the chest. The trachea is pushed from its normal midline position toward the unaffected side of the chest and the unaffected lung is compressed.

plastic). It is essential, however, that the covering be secured in a manner that seals the wound during inspiration and allows any air that has entered the thorax to exit during expiration.

Manifestations

The manifestations of pneumothorax depend on its size and the integrity of the underlying lung. In spontaneous pneumothorax, manifestations of the disorder include development of pleuritic pain in an otherwise healthy individual. There is an almost immediate increase in respiratory rate as a result of the activation of receptors that monitor lung volume; this may be accompanied by dyspnea. An asymmetry of the chest may be present because of the air trapped in the pleural cavity on the affected side. This asymmetry may be evidenced during inspiration as a lag in the movement of the affected side (the affected side of the chest does not begin to move until the unaffected lung reaches the same degree of inspiration as the lung with the air trapped in the pleural space). Percussion of the chest produces a more hyperresonant sound because of an increased air-to-fluid ratio, and breath sounds are decreased over the area of the pneumothorax. If the pneumothorax is large, the structures in the mediastinal space will shift toward the unaffected side of the chest (Figure 25-2). When this occurs, the position of the trachea, normally located in the midline of the neck, deviates with the mediastinum. The position of the trachea can be used as a means of assessing this portion of the chest. There may be distention of the neck veins and subcutaneous emphysema (movement of air into the subcutaneous tissues of the chest and neck) and clinical signs of shock.

Hypoxemia usually develops immediately after a large pneumothorax, followed by vasoconstriction of the blood vessels in the affected lung, causing the blood flow to shift to the unaffected lung. In persons with spontaneous pneumothorax, this mechanism usually returns oxygen saturation to normal within about 24 hours.

Diagnosis and treatment

Diagnosis of pneumothorax can be confirmed by chest x-ray. The treatment varies with the extent of the disorder. Even without treatment, air within the pleural space usually reabsorbs once the pleural leak seals. In small spontaneous pneumothoraces, the air usually reabsorbs spontaneously and only observation and follow-up chest x-rays are required. In larger pneumothoraces, the air is removed by needle aspiration or underwater seal drainage with or without an aspiration pump. This type of drainage system allows the air to exit the pleural space through a tube that is immersed in water, with the water acting as a one-way valve to prevent the air from reentering the chest. In secondary pneumothorax, surgical closure of the chest wall defect, ruptured airway, or perforated esophagus may be required.

Pleural effusion

Normally only a thin layer (usually less than 10–20 ml) of serous fluid separates the visceral and parietal layers of the pleural cavity. *Pleural effusion* refers to a collection of fluid in the pleural cavity. The fluid may be a transudate, exudate, chyle, or blood.

Like edema developing elsewhere in the body, pleural effusion occurs when the rate of fluid formation exceeds the rate of its removal (see Chapter 28). Five mechanisms have been linked to the abnormal collection of fluid in the pleural cavity: (1) increased capillary pressure, as in congestive heart failure; (2) increased capillary permeability, which occurs with inflammatory conditions; (3) decreased colloidal osmotic pressure, such as the hypoalbuminemia occurring with liver disease and nephrosis; (4) increased intrapleural negative pressure, which develops with atelectasis; and (5) impaired lymphatic drainage of the pleural space, which is usually due to obstructive processes such as mediastinal carcinoma.[32]

Pleural effusion may involve the presence of a transudate or exudate, depending on the protein content of the fluid. A transudate has a protein content of less than 3.0 g/ml and an exudate a protein content greater than 3.0 g/ml. Additional criteria that may be used to define a pleural exudate are (1) a pleural fluid-to-serum-protein ratio greater than 0.5, (2) a pleural fluid LDH level greater than the upper two-thirds limit of normal or (3) a pleural fluid-to-serum-LDH ratio exceeding 0.6.[33] LDH (lactate dehydrogenase) is a protein marker and is easily measured. Conditions that produce exudative pleural effusions are infections, pulmonary infarction, malignancies, rheumatoid arthritis, and lupus erythematosus. *Empyema* refers to pus in the pleural cavity; it can be caused by direct spread from adjacent bacterial pneumonia, rupture of a lung abscess into the pleural space, invasion from a subphrenic infection, or infection associated with trauma.

Noninflammatory collections of serous fluid are called *hydrothorax*. The condition may be either unilateral or bilateral. The most common cause of hydrothorax is congestive heart failure. Other causes are renal failure, nephrosis, liver failure, malignancy, and myxedema.

Chylothorax refers to the presence of chyle in the thoracic cavity. Chyle, a milky fluid containing chylomicrons, is found in the lymph fluid originating in the gastrointestinal tract. The thoracic duct transports chyle to the central circulation. Chylothorax results from trauma, inflammation, or malignant infiltration obstructing chyle transport from the thoracic duct into the central circulation.

Hemothorax is the presence of blood in the thoracic cavity. Bleeding may arise from chest injury, a complication of chest surgery, malignancies, or rupture of a great vessel such as an aortic aneurysm. Hemothorax may be classified as minimal, moderate, or large.[30] A minimal hemothorax involves the presence of 300 ml to 500 ml of blood in the pleural space. Small amounts of blood are generally absorbed from the pleural space and a minimal hemothorax generally clears in 10 to 14 days without complication. A moderate hemothorax (500–1000 ml blood) fills about one-third of the pleural space and may produce signs of lung compression and loss of intravascular volume. It requires immediate drainage and replacement of intravascular fluids. A large hemothorax fills half or more of one side of the chest; it indicates the presence of 1000 ml or more of blood in the thorax and is usually caused by bleeding from a high-pressure vessel such as an intercostal or mammary artery. It requires immediate drainage and, if the bleeding continues, surgery to control the bleeding. One of the complications of untreated moderate or large hemothorax is fibrothorax—or the fusion of the pleural surfaces by fibrin, hyalin, and connective tissue—and in some cases calcification of the fibrous tissue, which causes restriction in lung expansion.

Manifestations

The manifestations of pleural effusion vary with the cause. Hemothorax may be accompanied by signs of blood loss, and empyema by fever and other signs of inflammation. Fluid in the pleural cavity acts as a space-occupying mass; it causes a decrease in lung volume on the affected side that is proportional to the amount of fluid collected. The effusion causes a mediastinal shift toward the contralateral side with a decrease in lung volume on that side as well. Characteristic signs of pleural effusion are dullness or flatness to percussion and diminished breath sounds. Pleuritic pain usually occurs only when inflammation is present, although a constant type of discomfort may be felt with large effusions. Usually 2000 ml or more of fluid must be present before dyspnea occurs. A minimum of 250 ml of unilateral fluid accumulation must be present before the condition can be detected on chest x-ray.

Treatment

Thoracentesis, the aspiration of fluid from the pleural space, is used for both diagnostic and therapeutic purposes. It is often used to obtain a sample of pleural fluid for diagnostic studies. The treatment of pleural effusion is directed at the cause of the disorder. With large effusions, thoracentesis may be used to allow reexpansion of the lung. A palliative method of treatment used when pleural effusion is due to a malignancy is the injection of a sclerosing agent into the pleural cavity; this causes obliteration of the pleural space and prevents the reaccumulation of fluid.

In summary, disorders of the pleura include pain, pneumothorax, and pleural effusion. Pain is commonly associated with conditions that produce inflammation of the pleura. Characteristically, it is unilateral, abrupt in onset, and exaggerated by respiratory movements. *Pneumothorax* refers to an accumulation of air in the pleural cavity with the partial or complete collapse of the lung. It can result from rupture of an air-filled bleb on the lung surface or from penetrating or nonpenetrating injuries. A tension pneumothorax is a life-threatening event in which air progressively accumulates within the thorax, causing not only the collapse of the lung on the injured side but also a progressive shift of the mediastinum to the opposite side of the thorax, producing severe cardiorespiratory impairment. *Pleural effusion* refers to the collection of fluid in the pleural cavity. The fluid may be a transudate (hydrothorax), exudate (empyema), blood (hemothorax), or chyle (chylothorax).

Obstructive lung disorders

The function of the airways is to facilitate the movement of gases into and out of the lungs. As the airways branch out from the major bronchi they decrease in size and lose their cartilaginous support. At the point where the cartilaginous support disappears and the diameter is reduced to about 1 mm, the bronchi become bronchioles. Rings of smooth muscle joined by diagonal muscle fibers surround the epithelial lining of the bronchioles. Contraction and relaxation of the smooth muscle layer, which extends into the wall of the alveolar ducts, controls the resistance to airflow through the bronchioles. The bronchioles are lined with simple columnar and cuboidal epithelium, which contains ciliated and secretory cells. The smooth muscle layer of the bronchioles is richly innervated and sensitive to catecholamines and other chemical mediators. Airway obstruction can result in thickened secretions (mucous plugs), spasm of the bronchial smooth muscle (bronchospasm), or disease conditions that disrupt the structure of the bronchioles and alveoli. This section of the chapter includes a discussion of atelectasis, bronchial asthma, and chronic lung disease.

Atelectasis

Atelectasis refers to the incomplete expansion of a lung or portion of a lung. It can be caused by airway obstruction, lung compression such as occurs in pneumothorax or pleural effusion, or the increased recoil of the lung because of loss of pulmonary surfactant (discussed in Chapter 24). The disorder may be present at birth (primary atelectasis), or it may develop in the neonatal period or in later life (secondary atelectasis). Primary atelectasis of the newborn implies that the lung has never been inflated. It is seen most frequently in premature and high-risk infants. A secondary form of atelectasis can occur in infants who established respiration and subsequently developed impairment of lung expansion. Among the causes of secondary atelectasis in the newborn are the respiratory distress syndrome associated with lack of surfactant and airway obstruction due to aspiration of amniotic fluid or blood.

In the older child or adult, atelectasis is commonly caused by airway obstruction. Complete obstruction of the airway is followed by the absorption of oxygen from the dependent alveoli and collapse of that portion of the lung. A bronchus can be obstructed by a mucous plug within the airway or by external compression due to fluid, tumor mass, exudate, or other matter in the area surrounding the airway. A small segment of lung or an entire lung lobe may be involved in atelectasis. Both chest expansion and breath sounds are decreased on the affected side. If the collapsed area is large, the trachea will deviate to the affected side. Signs of respiratory distress will be proportional to the extent of lung collapse.

The danger of atelectasis increases following surgery. Anesthesia, pain, administration of narcotics, and immobility tend to promote retention of viscid bronchial secretions and hence airway obstruction. Encouraging a patient to cough and to take deep breaths, frequent changes of position, adequate hydration, and early ambulation decrease the likelihood of atelectasis developing.

Bronchial asthma

Conservative estimates indicate that between 8 million and 10 million Americans suffer from asthma. The disease affects people of all ages and is the most common cause of chronic illness in children under age 17. Furthermore, there is a reported increase in deaths from asthma.[34]

The disease is characterized by bronchial hyperreactivity to various stimuli, causing reversible bronchospasm, edema of the mucosal surface of the bronchioles, and increased production of mucus. Airway obstruction leads to wheezing and dyspnea. In severe cases there is hyperinflation of the lungs and an imbalance between ventilation and perfusion, with impairment of gas exchange. The attacks differ from person to person, and between attacks many persons are symptom-free. Both immune mechanisms (extrinsic asthma) and autonomic nervous system imbalances (intrinsic asthma) play a role in the associated bronchospasm; these are described in the section entitled Types of Asthma.

Etiologic mechanisms

Persons with asthma react to low concentrations of agents that do not normally cause bronchoconstriction. Bronchoconstriction may result from allergen exposure, from direct irritation by industrial chemicals or airborne pollutants, from respiratory tract infections, from drugs, from exercise, and from emotions. The list of agents that can cause bronchial asthma is long and growing. A recent addition to the list is the metabisulfites used in food processing and as an additive to beer, wine, and fresh vegetables.[35]

Immune response. Allergic asthma results primarily from a type I, IgE immune response (see Chapter 12). The mast cells of the bronchial tissues contain granules of chemical mediators—histamine, slow-reacting substance of anaphylaxis (SRS-A), eosinophil chemotactic factor, platelet-activating factor, and prostaglandins—that can provoke bronchospasm, enhance vascular permeability, and increase mucus secretion and in other ways trigger an asthmatic attack. The granules from the sensitized mast cells are released on exposure to the offending allergen. Common allergens include house dust; pollen from trees, grass, and weeds; animal danders; and mold spores.

Autonomic nervous system imbalance. The autonomic nervous system (ANS) influences both bronchial smooth muscle and mediator release from the mast cells. The ANS parasympathetic component produces bronchoconstriction and promotes mediator release, whereas the sympathetic component produces bronchial relaxation and inhibits mediator release. Normally no chronically active bronchial relaxant (sympathetic) forces are in operation; rather, a slight, vagally mediated bronchoconstrictor tone predominates. Hence a modest increase in sympathetic activity during periods of stress and increased oxygen need can bring about a marked decrease in airway resistance; this makes breathing easier and allows for increased ventilation.

The effect of the sympathetic nervous system on bronchial smooth muscle tone and mast cell function is mediated by beta$_2$-adrenergic nervous system receptors. Smooth muscle tone and the release of inflammatory mediators from the mast cells are modulated by intracellular levels of the cyclic nucleotides, particularly cyclic adenosine monophosphate (cAMP). When the level of this second messenger (cAMP) falls, bronchial smooth muscle contracts. Beta-adrenergic agonists such as epinephrine augment the cAMP levels in the mast cells so there is less mediator release from the mast cell granules. The interaction between autonomic nervous system influences, cAMP levels, and drugs used for asthma is depicted in Figure 25-3.

Types of asthma

There are two types of asthma, extrinsic and intrinsic. *Extrinsic asthma* (allergic asthma) is caused by release of inflammatory mediators from sensitized mast cells. Generally, this form of asthma is seen in persons with a family history of allergy and its onset occurs during childhood or adolescence. Persons with allergic asthma may also have other allergies, such as hay fever. Attacks are related to exposure to specific

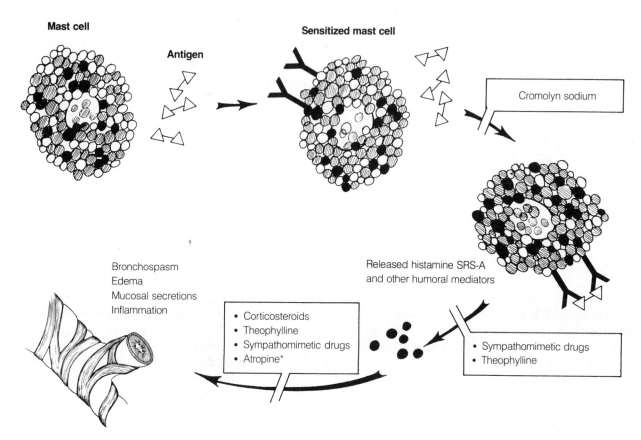

Figure 25-3 The site of action of drugs used in the treatment of bronchial asthma. Cromolyn sodium prevents mast cell degranulation and mediator release. The sympathomimetic drugs (beta-adrenergic agonists) and theophylline inhibit mediator production by the mast cells. The adrenal corticosteroid hormones, theophylline, sympathomimetic drugs, and atropine reduce or prevent bronchospasm, edema, excess mucosal secretions, and inflammation.

allergens. Skin tests for the offending allergens are positive. *Intrinsic asthma* is characterized by an absence of clearly defined precipitating factors. Onset is usually after age 35. The attacks are frequently precipitated by factors such as infection, weather changes, exercise, emotion, exposure to bronchial irritants, and various drugs, including aspirin.

There is a small group of asthmatics in whom aspirin sensitivity is associated with severe asthmatic attacks, presence of nasal polyps, and recurrent episodes of rhinitis.[36] In addition, the yellow food dye tartrazine and nonsteroidal anti-inflammatory drugs, such as aminopyrine, phenylbutazone, ibuprofen, and indomethacin, may provoke attacks.

Exercise-induced asthma occurs in 70% to 80% of persons with bronchial asthma.[37] It occurs in both intrinsic and extrinsic asthma. The cause of exercise-induced asthma is unclear. The condition may be only an intermittent response, depending on various environmental conditions. It has been suggested that during exercise, bronchospasm is due to increased airway cooling caused by an increased minute ventilation or, alternatively, by water loss from the airway mucosa.[37,38] The response is often exaggerated when the person exercises in a cold environment; wearing a mask over the nose and mouth often minimizes the attack or prevents it. It appears that the proper selection of a mask could be important for persons subject to exercise-induced asthma, because it has been shown that increasing the humidity of the inhaled air is more important than simply heating the air.[39] A proper warm-up period is also important.

Manifestations

Persons with asthma exhibit a wide range of signs and symptoms, from chest tightness to an acute immobilizing attack. Many sufferers are asymptomatic between attacks.

With progressive airway obstruction occurring during an attack, expiration becomes prolonged. The amount of air that can be forcibly expired in 1 second (forced expiratory volume$_{1.0}$, or $FEV_{1.0}$) is decreased. Air becomes trapped in the lungs, increasing the residual volume (see Chapter 24). The asthmatic must now breathe at a higher residual lung volume, and more energy is needed to overcome the tension already present in the lungs. Fatigue follows. Both inspiratory reserve capacity and vital capacity diminish. Because air is trapped in the alveoli and inspiration is occurring at higher lung volumes, the cough becomes less effective. As the condition progresses, the effectiveness of alveolar ventilation declines, and mismatching between ventilation and perfusion causes hypoxemia and hypercapnia.

During an *acute attack,* the asthmatic generally prefers to sit up. There is visible use of the accessory muscles. The skin is often moist, and anxiety and apprehension are obvious. The person wheezes during both inspiration and expiration, often audibly. The breath sounds may be coarse and loud. Vesicular breath sounds become more distant because of trapping of air. Dyspnea may be severe, and often the person is able to speak only one or two words before taking a breath. A cough may accompany the wheezing. At the point where airflow is markedly decreased, the cough becomes ineffective despite being repetitive and hacking; this point often marks the onset of respiratory failure.

—— Treatment

Two modalities are used in the management of bronchial asthma. One method focuses on prevention, the other on treatment during an attack. Figure 25-3 diagrams the action of various therapeutic drugs in relieving asthmatic bronchospasm.

Preventive measures include avoidance of bronchial irritants, such as allergens or breathing of cold air, that are known to precipitate an attack. A careful history is often needed to identify all the contributory factors. When the offending agent cannot be avoided (*e.g.,* house dust), a program of desensitization may be undertaken (see Chapter 12). The drug cromolyn sodium is sometimes effective in preventing allergic reactions. The drug is administered by inhalation. It stabilizes the mast cells, thereby preventing release of the inflammatory mediators that cause the attack. This drug must be given prophylactically and is of no benefit when taken during an attack.

During the attack itself, bronchodilators are used. These include the beta-adrenergic agonists (*e.g.,* epinephrine) and theophylline preparations. The adrenergic agents relax bronchial smooth muscle and relieve congestion of the bronchial mucosa. Certain forms of these drugs may be given by inhalation for rapid onset of action.

However, the efficacy of the aerosol preparations depends on the manner of inhalation. It is important that the medication be broken into small droplets so it can penetrate deeply into the respiratory tract to reach the small airways; this is difficult to achieve when the nebulizer is held at the level of the mouth.

When the medication is administered in this position, large droplets tend to be delivered to the oropharynx and throat, rather than moving down into the small airways. The use of a flexible extender or spacer placed between the nebulizer and the mouthpiece helps to insure delivery of smaller droplets, thereby enhancing delivery of the medication to the smaller obstructed airways. With the extender in place, the medication is delivered during slow inhalation from functional residual capacity (FRC); the mouthpiece is removed; the breath is held for about 10 seconds and then exhaled through pursed lips.[35]

Ipratropium is a synthetic atropine analog that is administered by inhalation. It produces bronchodilatation by direct action on the large airways and does not change the composition or viscosity of the bronchial mucus. Theophylline also acts by relaxing smooth muscle. Theophylline preparations can be administered by oral, rectal, or intravenous route. The adrenergic drugs and theophylline preparations have different mechanisms of action and are therefore complementary. The adrenergic drugs directly increase the levels of cAMP in the bronchial smooth muscle, whereas theophylline decreases the metabolism of cAMP and increases diaphragmatic contractility.[40] The adrenocorticosteroid drugs are also used to treat acute asthmatic attacks. It is thought that these drugs stabilize the lysosomes of the inflammatory cells, prevent the accumulation of histamine in mast cells, sensitize the beta-adrenergic receptors, and exert other antiinflammatory actions. The actions of these drugs are described in greater detail in Table 25-3.

Relaxation techniques and controlled breathing help to allay the panic and anxiety that aggravate breathing difficulties. In a child, measures to encourage independence as it relates to symptom control, along with those directed at helping to develop a positive self-concept, are essential.

—— Chronic obstructive pulmonary diseases

Thirty million Americans have some degree of airway obstruction and chronic obstructive pulmonary disease.[41] Chronic lung disease ranks second to coronary heart disease as a cause of disability subject to social security payment and serves as the fifth leading cause of death. The term *chronic obstructive pulmonary disease* (COPD) denotes a group of respiratory disorders characterized by small airway obstruction and reduction in expiratory flow rate. The most prevalent of these disorders are emphysema and chronic bronchitis. In addition to these two types of COPD, this section presents two other forms of chronic obstructive lung disease—bronchiectasis and cystic fibrosis.

Since the most common cause of COPD is smoking, the disease is largely preventable. Unfortunately, clinical findings are completely absent during the early stages of the COPD and by the time symptoms appear, the disease is usually well advanced. For smokers with early signs of airway disease, there is hope that early recognition combined with appropriate treatment and smoking cessation may prevent the usually relentless progression of the disease.

The mechanisms of airway obstruction in COPD are usually multiple. They include a reduction in the elasticity of lung structures, bronchoconstriction, and chronic inflammation. Normally, the elastic recoil of the lung provides the driving pressure for expiration. Thus, a loss of elasticity decreases the expiratory flow rate. The elastic recoil also exerts a radial traction effect on the airways during expiration to prevent their compression. Bronchoconstriction usually results from hyperreactivity of bronchial smooth muscle, as in bronchial asthma. Chronic inflammation causes narrowing of the airways and production of excessive, thick secretions that produce further obstruction.

Airway obstruction prolongs the expiratory phase of respiration and affords the potential for impaired gas exchange due to mismatching of ventilation and perfusion. The forced vital capacity (FVC) is the amount of air that can be forcibly exhaled following maximal inspiration. In an adult with normal respiratory function, this should be achieved in 4 to 6 seconds.[42] As mentioned earlier, the forced expiratory volume (FEV) that can be achieved in 1 second is termed the $FEV_{1.0}$. In chronic lung disease the time required for FVC is increased, the $FEV_{1.0}$ is de-

Table 25–3. Bronchodilator drugs used in the treatment of asthma and chronic obstructive pulmonary diseases

Drug	Action	Route of administration
Adrenergic Drugs	Drugs with a beta$_2$ action produce relaxation of the bronchial smooth muscle by acting at the level of adenyl cyclase to increase cAMP; beta$_1$ agonists stimulate the heart, causing tachycardia and danger of arrhythmias; drugs with an alpha action cause vasoconstriction and raise blood pressure	
Epinephrine	Stimulates both alpha and beta receptors, producing tachycardia and blood pressure changes as well as bronchial dilatation	Usually given by inhalation or subcutaneous injection Intramuscular suspension preparations are available
Ephedrine (and related preparations such as pseudo-ephedrine)	Not a catecholamine; acts by inducing catecholamine release; has disadvantage of causing central nervous system stimulation and cardiovascular side effects	Usually given orally, often in combination with theophylline and a sedative
Isoproterenol	Both beta$_1$ and beta$_2$ actions	Usually given by inhalation Can be given sublingually
Bitolterol	Mainly beta$_2$	Inhalation
Metaproterenol	Mainly beta$_2$; can cause troublesome muscle tremors; may produce tachycardia and blood pressure changes	Oral and inhalation
Pirbuterol	Mainly beta$_2$	Inhalation
Terbutaline	Beta$_2$ actions; may produce troublesome muscle tremors. May also produce tachycardia and blood pressure changes	Oral, subcutaneous, inhalation
Isoetharine	Mainly beta$_2$	Inhalation
Albuterol	Mainly beta$_2$	Inhalation
Theophylline preparations		
Theophylline Aminophylline (86% theophylline) Oxtriphylline (65% theophylline)	Produce bronchodilation by inhibiting metabolism of cAMP; can cause nausea and vomiting, which is mediated through the central nervous system; may produce seizures at high levels, particularly in children	Usually given orally as a single agent, or occasionally as a combination preparation with an adrenergic drug and a sedative May be given intravenously or rectally
Anticholinergic Drugs		
Ipratroprium (Atrovent)	Produces bronchodilation by inhibiting parasympathetic (anticholinergic) control of bronchial smooth muscle contraction	Inhalation
Atropine sulfate	Anticholinergic action; side effects common; contraindicated in narrow-angle glaucoma and prostatic hypertrophy	Inhalation

creased, and the ratio of $FEV_{1.0}$ to FVC is decreased. These and other measurements of expiratory flow are determined by spirometry and are used in the diagnosis of COPD (see Chapter 24).

A simple test to assess the severity of obstructive airway disease is the *match test*. In this test, a lit match is held 6 inches from the mouth, and the patient is asked to blow it out. Ability to extinguish the match indicates a maximum voluntary ventilation of 60 liter/minute and a $FEV_{1.0}$ of 1.6 liters.[30]

—— Emphysema

Emphysema is characterized by a loss of lung elasticity and abnormal dilatation of the air spaces distal to the terminal bronchioles with destruction of the alveolar walls and capillary beds (Figure 25-4). There is hyperinflation of the lungs, and breath sounds are decreased. There are two principal types of emphysema: centrilobular and panlobular (Figure 25-5). The centrilobular type affects the respiratory bronchioles, with initial preservation of the alveolar ducts and sacs. In the panlobular form the peripheral alveoli are involved.

Persons with emphysema have marked dyspnea and struggle to maintain normal blood gas levels

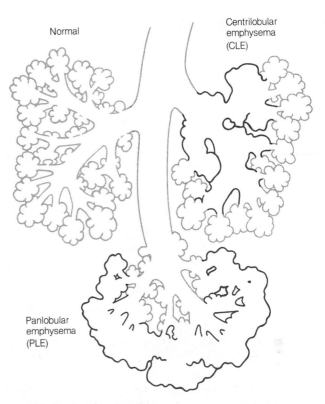

Figure 25-5 The changes in alveolar structure associated with centrilobular and panlobular emphysema.

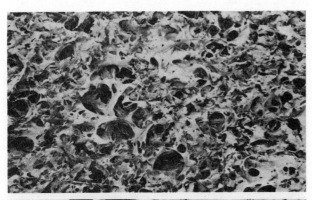
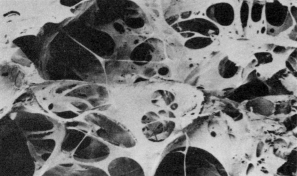

Figure 25-4 Scanning electron micrographs of lung tissue. **(Top)** Normal tissue; **(bottom)** emphysematous tissue (both at same magnification). Note the enlargement of air spaces in the emphysematous lung. *(Courtesy of Kenneth Siegesmund, PhD. Anatomy Department, The Medical College of Wisconsin)*

with increased ventilatory effort, including prominent use of the accessory muscles. The work of breathing is greatly increased and eating is often difficult. As a result, there is often considerable weight loss. An increase in the anterior-posterior dimensions of the chest due to hyperinflation of the lungs produces the so-called barrel chest that is typical of persons with emphysema. Usually the seated position, which stabilizes chest structures and allows for maximum chest expansion, is preferred. Expiration is often accomplished through pursed lips. With loss of lung elasticity and hyperinflation of the lungs, the airways often collapse during expiration because the pressure in the surrounding lung tissues exceeds airway pressure. Pursed-lip breathing increases the resistance to outflow of air, producing a back pressure in the airways sufficient to prevent their collapse. Cough is not a prominent feature in emphysema.

There are several known or suspected causes of emphysema, the most important of which is cigarette smoking. The risk of emphysema increases with the number of cigarettes smoked.[43] A second cause of emphysema is a deficiency of alpha$_1$-antitrypsin. Alpha$_1$-antitrypsin is a proteinase inhibitor; it blocks the action of the proteolytic enzymes that are destructive to elastin and other tissue components in the alveolar wall. The deficiency is an inherited autosomal recessive disorder. Approximately 70% to 80% of persons with a homozygous pattern of inheritance for alpha$_1$-antitrypsin deficiency have COPD.[44] The severity of the condition and age at onset may vary from individual to individual. There is now evidence that cigarette smoking reduces the body stores of alpha$_1$-antitrypsin over time. Therefore, smoking and repeated respiratory tract infections (which also impede normal production) tend to contribute to the development of emphysema in persons with an alpha$_1$-antitrypsin deficiency.

Chronic bronchitis

In chronic bronchitis, airway obstruction is caused by inflammation of both major and small airways. There is edema and hyperplasia of bronchial structures and excessive production of mucus. A history of a chronic productive cough that has persisted for at least 2 successive years in the absence of other disease is necessary for diagnosis of chronic bronchitis. Typically, the cough has been present for many years, with a gradual increase in acute exacerbations that produce a frankly purulent sputum.

The disease is seen most commonly in middle-aged men and is associated with chronic irritation from smoking and recurrent infections. In the United States, smoking is the most important cause of chronic bronchitis. Viral and bacterial infections are common and are thought to be a result rather than a cause of the problem. In contrast to persons with emphysema, those with chronic bronchitis tend to maintain their weight. There is shortness of breath with a progressive decrease in exercise tolerance. Hypoxemia, hypercapnia, and cyanosis develop, reflecting an imbalance between ventilation and perfusion. The marked hypoxemia acts as a stimulus for increased pulmonary vascular resistance and red cell production. Polycythemia and pulmonary hypertension ensue, associated with right heart failure and peripheral edema.

As the disease progresses, breathing becomes more labored, even at rest. The expiratory phase of respiration is prolonged, and expiratory rhonchi and rales can be heard on auscultation. A common finding is clubbing of the fingers, a condition in which the tips of the fingers become bulbous, resembling drumsticks (Figure 25-6).

Manifestations

The mnemonics "pink puffer" and "blue bloater" have been used to differentiate the clinical manifestations of emphysema and chronic bronchitis. The manifestations of the two conditions are also designated type A (pink puffers) and type B (blue bloaters). The important features of these two forms of COPD are described in Table 25-4. In actual practice

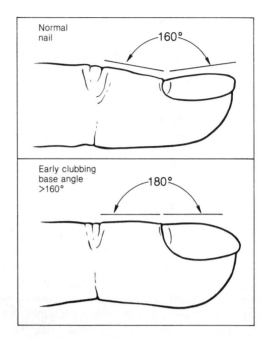

Figure 25-6 Clubbing of the finger. Normally there is an obtuse angle of about 160° between the base of the nail and the adjacent dorsal surface of the finger; with clubbing, this angle exceeds 180°.

the differentiation between the two types is not as vivid as presented here.

A major difference between the pink puffers and the blue bloaters is the responsiveness to the hypoxic stimuli. With pulmonary emphysema there is a proportionate loss of both ventilation and perfusion area in the lung. For whatever reason, these persons are "pink puffers" or "fighters"—able to struggle and overventilate, and thus maintain relatively normal blood gas levels until late in the disease. On the other hand, the excessive bronchial secretions and airway obstruction that is characteristic of chronic bronchitis causes mismatching of ventilation and perfusion. For some unknown reason, these persons do not compensate by increasing their ventilation; consequently, they develop hypoxemia, cyanosis, and eventually cor pulmonale with peripheral edema. These are the "blue bloaters" or "nonfighters."

Although emphysema and chronic bronchitis are diagnosed and treated as specific diseases, most persons with COPD have features of both conditions. Persons with combined forms of COPD characteristically seek medical attention in the fifth or sixth decade of life complaining of cough, sputum production, and shortness of breath. Often the symptoms have been present to some extent for 10 years or more. The productive cough usually occurs in the morning. Dyspnea becomes more severe as the disease progresses. Frequent exacerbations of infection and respiratory insufficiency are common, with absence from work and eventual disability. The late stages of COPD are characterized by pulmonary hypertension, cor pulmonale, recurrent respiratory infections, and chronic respiratory failure. Death usually occurs during an exacerbation of illness associated with infection and respiratory failure.

Treatment. Maintaining or improving physical and psychosocial functioning is an essential part of the treatment plan for persons with COPD. The treatment methods include measures to prevent and control environmental irritants and infection, maintenance of nutrition and fluid balance, use of bronchodilator drugs, and mobilization of secretions. A long-term pulmonary rehabilitation program can significantly reduce episodes of hospitalization and add measurably to a person's ability to manage and cope with his or her impairment in a positive way. Breathing exercises and retraining focus on restoring the function of the diaphragm, reducing the work of breathing, and improving gas exchange. Physical conditioning, with a gradual increase in activity, improves exercise tolerance. Psychosocial rehabilitation must be individualized to meet the specific needs of persons with COPD and their families. These needs will vary with age, occupation, financial resources, social and recreational interest, and interpersonal and family relationships. Work simplification strategies may be needed when impairment is severe.

Oxygen therapy is prescribed in selected persons with significant hypoxemia. Obviously, not all persons with COPD have the same treatment needs.

Because COPD is a chronic disease, the results of treatment depend largely on self-care measures that involve both the afflicted person and the family members. These persons need to have a complete understanding of the disease process and the manner in which it affects respiratory function, as well as the purpose of the prescribed treatment measures.

Environmental irritants and infection. Avoidance of cigarette smoke and other environmental airway irritants is a must. Vocational counseling may be needed if there is occupational exposure. Monitoring of air pollution levels and adjusting activities accordingly will aid in controlling shortness of breath. Wearing a cold weather mask often prevents dyspnea and bronchospasm due to cold air and wind exposure. Respiratory tract infections can prove fatal to persons with severe COPD. A person with COPD should avoid exposure to others with known respiratory tract infections and should avoid attending large gatherings during periods of the year when influenza or respiratory tract infections are prevalent. Immunization for influenza and pneumococcal infections will decrease the likelihood of their occurrence. Persons with COPD should be taught to monitor their sputum for signs of infection, so that treatment can be instituted at the earliest sign of infection.

Table 25–4. Characteristics of chronic bronchitis and emphysematous types of chronic lung disease

Characteristic	Type A pulmonary emphysema ("pink puffers")	Type B chronic bronchitis ("blue bloaters")
Smoking history	Usual	Usual
Age of onset	Relatively later in life	Relatively earlier in life
Clinical features		
Barrel chest (hyperinflation of the lungs)	Often dramatic	May be present
Weight loss	May be severe in advanced disease	Infrequent
Shortness of breath	May be absent early in disease	Predominant early symptom, insidious in onset, exertional
Decreased breath sounds	Characteristic	Variable
Wheezing	Usually absent	Variable
Rhonchi	Usually absent or minimal	Often prominent
Sputum	May be absent or may develop late in the course	Frequent early manifestation, frequent infections, abundant purulent sputum
Cyanosis	Often absent, even late in the disease when there is low PO_2	Often dramatic
Blood gases	Relatively normal until late in the disease process	Hypercapnia may be present Hypoxemia may be present
Cor pulmonale	Only in advanced cases	Frequent Peripheral edema
Polycythemia	Only in advanced cases	Frequent
Prognosis	Slowly debilitating disease	Numerous life-threatening episodes due to acute exacerbations

Maintenance of nutrition and fluid balance. Because persons with COPD expend so much effort on breathing, many find it difficult to chew their food and manage the effort of a large meal. This situation, combined with impaired diaphragm descent, air-swallowing, and medications that cause anorexia and nausea, impairs nutrition and promotes weight loss. Small, frequent, nutritious, and easily swallowed feedings aid in maintaining good nutrition and preventing weight loss. Vitamin supplements may be called for. Water is the most readily available expectorant for liquefying secretions, so fluid intake should be encouraged, particularly in persons who have thick, tenacious sputum. Fluid that is either too hot or too cold may aggravate breathing problems.

Bronchodilator drugs. Bronchodilators, including adrenergic drugs, theophylline preparations, and anticholinergic drugs, are probably the most widely prescribed medications for use in treatment of COPD. As previously discussed, both adrenergic drugs and theophylline produce relaxation of bronchial smooth muscle by increasing cAMP levels. Beta$_2$-specific agents have a more specific action than earlier adrenergic drugs and produce fewer cardiac effects. Theophylline preparations can be administered orally, rectally, or intravenously. Long-acting oral preparations are available. There is a wide variability from case to case in the absorption and metabolism of these preparations; therefore, theophylline blood levels are used as a guide in arriving at an effective dose schedule. The newly available anticholinergic aerosol ipratropium produces bronchodilation by blocking parasympathetic cholinergic receptors that produce contraction of bronchial smooth muscle. In combination with other bronchodilators, the drug enhances and prolongs bronchodilation. Table 25-3 lists and describes the action of commonly prescribed bronchodilator drugs.

Many adrenergic drugs are available in aerosol form for inhalation, and in this form they are particularly useful in controlling bronchospasm. Because they are convenient and effective, they can be abused by improper administration and overuse.

Although the adrenal corticosteroids are not routinely prescribed for long-term treatment of COPD, some persons do require them. The adrenal corticosteroids are available for local use in aerosol form minimizing the undesirable effects that often accompany systemic use.

Mobilization of secretions. Postural drainage provides a means for removing excess secretions from the lungs. It is done by positioning the patient's body according to the distribution and configuration of the tracheobronchial tree so that gravity causes secretions to drain into the larger airways, from which they can be removed with relative ease. The effectiveness of postural drainage may be enhanced by percussion or vibration of the chest wall, done with vibrating or tapping motions of the hands or electronic vibrators or ultrasound generators. The reader is referred to other reference sources, some of which are listed at the end of the chapter, for a more complete description of these exercises and treatments.

Exercise and breathing retraining. Graded exercise programs help to prevent deterioration of physical condition and to improve the person's ability to carry out the activities of daily living. Most exercise programs use free or treadmill walking or stationary bicycling. The activities should be performed at least three to four times a week and should be limited by the person's dyspnea and not by a target heart rate. Pursed-lip breathing to prevent airway collapse and abdominal breathing exercises improve ventilation, relieve fatigue of accessory muscles, and sometimes help prevent dyspnea. The purpose of abdominal breathing is to relax the abdominal muscles during inspiration; this produces a decrease in intraabdominal pressure and allows for fuller descent of the diaphragm.

Breathing exercises and retraining are designed to increase respiratory muscle strength and endurance, thereby improving exercise performance. The diaphragm and other inspiratory muscles form a muscle pump that is as vital to the respiratory functions of the body as the heart is to the circulatory functions. During inspiration the diaphragm contracts and descends; during expiration it passively ascends, causing air to leave the lungs. In normal respiration, the diaphragm does 65% of the work of breathing, while the accessory muscles do about 35%.[45] In emphysema, the contribution of the diaphragm to the work of breathing is diminished because of loss of lung elasticity, with consequent air trapping and lung distention. In order to compensate for this deficiency, persons with emphysema use their accessory muscles for breathing. Breathing is laborious, and the work of breathing increases. This labored breathing pattern may progress to the point that the diaphragm contributes only about 30% to the effort of breathing, and the accessory muscles carry 70% of the load.[42] Recent studies have shown that although respiratory muscles may be weakened in COPD, it is possible to strengthen them through inspiratory muscle training using either resistive loading during inspiration or isocapnic hyperpnea.[46,47] Resistive loading is accomplished by having the person breathe through an inspiratory breathing device that increases the resistance to airflow during inspiration. Hand-held devices that can be used at home are available for this purpose. Isocapnic hyperpneic exercise uses exercises that increase ventilation, trains expiratory as well as inspiratory muscles, and is best suited for developing respiratory muscle endurance. Isocapnic hyperpneic exercise requires the use of a special rebreathing circuit to maintain normal carbon dioxide levels. At present, the rebreathing equipment needed for this type of exercise is not available for home use, which limits the usefulness of this type of exercise.

Oxygen therapy. In advanced cases of COPD, the imbalance between ventilation and perfusion causes hypoxemia. Hypoxemia in which arterial PO_2 levels fall below 55 mm Hg causes polycythemia and reflex vasoconstriction of the pulmonary vessels, with resultant pulmonary hypertension and further impairment of gas exchange in the lung. Those affected are at risk for developing cor pulmonale.

In such severe cases, administration of continuous low-flow (1–2 liter/min) oxygen often increases the arterial oxygen levels, decreases dyspnea and pulmonary hypertension, and improves neuropsychological function and exercise tolerance. Portable oxygen administration units, which allow for mobility and the performance of activities of daily living, are usually used. The Nocturnal Oxygen Therapy Trial Group study of persons with advanced disease—particularly those with heart failure associated with COPD—performed at six centers in the United States and Canada has clearly shown that oxygen is more effective when given almost continuously than when it is given roughly 50% of the time. The survival rate of persons receiving continuous oxygen therapy was almost two times that of those receiving 12-hour nocturnal therapy.[48]

It has been found that persons with COPD may have episodes of hypoxemia both at night and during daytime naps. These persons do not, however, experience the daytime hypersomnolence and loud snoring that is usually associated with sleep apnea (see Chapter 26). The hypoxemia that occurs during sleep in persons with COPD is usually associated with slow and shallow breathing rather than with periods of apnea. Cardiac arrhythmias and other electrocardiographic evidence of myocardial ischemia may accompany the episodes of hypoxemia.[49] Sleep studies, in which arterial oxygen saturation is measured using an ear oximeter, may be done when nocturnal hypoxemia is suspected in a person with COPD. Although these persons do not usually experience severe hypoxemia during waking hours and do not meet the criteria for continuous low-flow oxygen therapy, they may benefit from nocturnal oxygen therapy.[50]

Oxygen administration in persons with COPD must be undertaken with a certain amount of caution. The saying, "A little bit is good, a whole lot is better," does not hold true for oxygen administration

in COPD. The flow rate (in liters per minute) is usually titrated to provide an arterial PO_2 of about 60 mm Hg. Because the ventilatory drive associated with hypoxic stimulation of the peripheral chemoreceptors does not occur until the arterial PO_2 has been reduced to about 60 mm Hg or less, increasing the arterial oxygen above that level tends to depress stimulation for ventilation and often leads to hypoventilation and carbon dioxide retention.

Cystic fibrosis

Cystic fibrosis is a hereditary disease transmitted as an autosomal recessive trait. It affects approximately 1 in 2000 children. Homozygotes (persons with two defective genes) have all, or substantially all, of the clinical symptoms of the disease, whereas heterozygotes are carriers of the disease but have no recognizable symptoms. It is an exocrine gland disorder involving both the mucus-secreting and the eccrine sweat glands. Because cystic fibrosis involves production of a thick tenacious mucus, it is sometimes referred to as *mucoviscidosis*.

Clinically, cystic fibrosis is characterized by elevation of sodium chloride levels in the sweat, pancreatic insufficiency, and chronic lung disease. Abnormalities in pancreatic function are present in about 80% of affected children. The pancreatic insufficiency gives rise to malabsorption and steatorrhea. In the newborn, meconium ileus may cause intestinal obstruction. Respiratory manifestations are due to an accumulation of viscid mucus in the bronchi, which produces bronchial obstruction and dilatation. Mucus plugs can result in the total obstruction of an airway, causing atelectasis.

Diagnosis and treatment

Early diagnosis and treatment of cystic fibrosis are important in that they may delay the onset of chronic illness. The diagnosis is generally based on an abnormal pilocarpine iontophoresis sweat chloride test. The test is usually done on sweat obtained from a child's forearm or from an infant's thigh. A small electric current is used to carry the drug pilocarpine, which increases sweat production, into the skin. Sweat is collected using an absorbent paper or gauze sponge and then analyzed in the laboratory. The test is often inaccurate in newborns because the quantity of sweat produced is insufficient for testing. Babies with the disorder often taste salty when kissed. A new device that simplifies the sweat test and reduces its cost has recently been introduced. The battery-operated device, which looks like an oversized wristwatch, uses pilocarpine iontophoresis to induce sweating. Disposable patches change color when chloride levels in the sweat are elevated.

The treatment of cystic fibrosis usually consists of replacement of pancreatic enzymes, physical measures to improve the clearance of tracheobronchial secretions (postural drainage and chest percussion), and prompt treatment of respiratory tract infections. Progress of the disease is variable. Improved medical management has led to longer survival—currently, to about age 20.

—— Bronchiectasis

Bronchiectasis is an abnormal dilatation of the bronchioles associated with chronic necrotizing infection of the bronchi. To be diagnosed as bronchiectasis the dilatation must be permanent, because reversible bronchial dilatation may accompany viral and bronchial pneumonias. There are a number of causes of bronchiectasis, including bronchial obstruction due to conditions such as tumors and foreign bodies; congenital abnormalities associated with abnormal development of the bronchi; cystic fibrosis, in which airway obstruction is caused by impairment of normal mucociliary function; immunologic deficiencies, which predispose to respiratory tract infections; and exposure to toxic gases, which cause airway obstruction. Two conditions, obstruction and infection, are present in all of these disorders, and both contribute to the development and progression of the disease. Bronchial obstruction causes atelectasis, which results in smooth muscle relaxation and dilatation of the walls of the airways that remain patent. Infection produces inflammation, weakening, and further dilatation of the walls of the bronchioles.

—— Diagnosis and treatment

Bronchiectasis is associated with an assortment of abnormalities that profoundly affect respiratory function, including atelectasis, obstruction of the smaller airways, and diffuse bronchitis. There is coughing, fever, recurrent bronchopulmonary infection, and expectoration of foul-smelling, purulent sputum. The daily quantity of sputum can amount to cupsful. The physiological abnormalities that occur in bronchiectasis are similar to those seen in chronic bronchitis and emphysema. As in both of these conditions, chronic bronchial obstruction leads to marked dyspnea and cyanosis. Clubbing of the fingers sometimes develops.

The basic therapy consists of early recognition and treatment of infection along with regular postural drainage and chest physical therapy. Persons with this disorder benefit from many of the rehabilitation and treatment measures used in the treatment of chronic bronchitis and emphysema.

In summary, airway obstruction occurs in a number of reversible and chronic conditions. Atelectasis refers to an incomplete expansion of the lung. Although it is often caused by airway obstruction, it can also result from the compression of lung structures, such as occurs in pneumothorax, or from recoil of the lung due to loss of surfactant. Bronchial asthma is characterized by hypersensitivity of the bronchial smooth muscle to various stimuli. It causes reversible bronchospasm, edema of the mucosal surface of the bronchioles, and increased production of mucus. Chronic obstructive pulmonary disease describes a group of conditions characterized by obstruction to airflow in the lungs. Among the conditions associated with COPD are chronic bronchitis, emphysema, cystic fibrosis, and bronchiectasis. The condition is manifested by hyperinflation of the lungs, increased time required for the expiratory phase of respiration, and mismatching of ventilation and perfusion. As the condition advances, signs of respiratory distress and impaired gas exchange become evident, with development of hypercapnia and hypoxemia.

Interstitial lung diseases

The interstitial lung diseases are a diverse group of lung disorders with similar clinical and pathophysiologic features. They include the occupational lung diseases, lung diseases caused by toxic drugs and radiation, and lung diseases of unknown etiology. These lung diseases are currently thought to affect more than 10 million people in the United States.[51]

The interstitial lung diseases produce varying degrees of inflammation, fibrosis, and disability. The disorders may be acute or insidious in onset; they may be rapidly progressive, slowly progressive, or static in their course. Because they result in a stiff and noncompliant lung, they are commonly classified as fibrotic or restrictive lung disorders. The most common of the interstitial lung diseases are those caused by exposure to occupational and environmental inhalants and sarcoidosis, the cause of which is unknown. Examples of interstitial lung diseases and their etiologies are listed in Table 25-5.

In contrast to the obstructive lung diseases, which primarily involve the airways of the lung, the restrictive lung disorders exert their effect on the collagen and elastic connective tissue found between the airways and the blood vessels of the lung. In addition, many of these diseases also involve the airways, arteries, and veins. In general, these lung diseases share a pattern of lung dysfunction that includes diminished lung volumes, reduced diffusing capacity of the lung, and varying degrees of hypoxemia.

Current theory suggests that most interstitial lung diseases, regardless of the cause, have a common pathogenesis. It is thought that these disorders are initiated by some type of injury to the alveolar epithelium, followed by an inflammatory process that involves the alveoli and interstitium of the lung. An accumulation of inflammatory and immune cells causes continued damage of lung tissue and the replacement of normal, functioning lung tissue with fibrous scar tissue.[52]

Manifestations

Interstitial lung disease is characterized by an insidious onset of breathlessness; it initially occurs during exercise and may progress to the point that the person is totally incapacitated. Typically, a person with a restrictive lung disease breathes with a pattern of rapid, shallow respirations. This tachypneic pattern of breathing, in which the respiratory rate is increased and the tidal volume is decreased, leads to a reduction in the work of breathing, because it takes less work to move air through the airways at an increased rate than it does to stretch a stiff lung to accommodate a larger tidal volume. A nonproductive cough is also present

in many individuals, particularly if there is continued exposure to the inhaled irritant. Basilar rales may be present in the lungs, and clubbing of the fingers and toes may occur.

Lung volumes, including vital capacity and total lung capacity, are reduced in interstitial lung disease. In contrast to chronic obstructive lung disease, in which expiratory flow rates are reduced, the $FEV_{1.0}$ is usually preserved, though the ratio between the $FEV_{1.0}$ and the vital capacity may increase. Although resting arterial blood gases are usually normal early in the course of the disease, arterial oxygen levels may fall during exercise, and in cases of advanced disease, hypoxemia is often present even at rest. In the late stages of the disease, hypercapnia and respiratory acidosis develop. The impaired diffusion of gases that occurs in persons with interstitial lung disease is thought to be due primarily to an increase in physiologic dead space resulting from unventilated regions of the lung.

Diagnosis and treatment

The diagnosis of interstitial lung disease requires a careful personal and family history, with particular emphasis on exposure to environmental, occupational, and other injurious agents. Chest x-rays may

Table 25–5. Causes of interstitial lung diseases

Etiology	Examples
Known	
Occupational and environmental inhalants	
Inorganic dusts	Silicosis
	Asbestosis
	Talcosis
	Coal miner's pneumoconiosis
	Berylliosis
Organic dusts	Farmer's lung (moldy hay)
	Pigeon breeder's lung (bird serum, excreta, and feathers)
	Air-conditioner lung (bacteria found in humidifiers and air conditioners)
	Bagassosis (contaminated sugarcane)
Gases, fumes, aerosols	Silo filler's lung (nitrogen dioxide, chlorine, ammonia, phosgene, sulfur dioxide)
Drugs	Cancer chemotherapeutic drugs (*e.g.*, bleomycin), nitrofurantoin
Radiation	External radiation, inhaled radioactive materials
Infections	Widespread tuberculosis
Poisons	Paraquat
Diseases of other organ systems	Chronic pulmonary edema
	Chronic uremia
Unknown	
	Sarcoidosis
	Idiopathic pulmonary fibrosis
	Connective tissue diseases, such as lupus erythematosus, scleroderma, and rheumatoid arthritis

be used as an initial diagnostic method, and serial chest films are often used in following the progress of the disease. A biopsy specimen for histologic study and culture may be obtained by means of surgical incision or by bronchoscopy using a fiberoptic bronchoscope. In bronchoalveolar lavage, fluid is instilled into the alveoli through a bronchoscope and then removed by suction in order to obtain inflammatory and immune cells for laboratory study. Gallium lung scans are often used to detect and quantify the chronic alveolitis that occurs in interstitial lung disease. Gallium does not localize in normal lung tissue, but uptake of the radionuclide is increased in interstitial lung disease and other diffuse lung diseases.

The treatment goals for interstitial lung diseases focus on identifying and removing the injurious agent, suppressing the inflammatory response, preventing progression of the disease, and providing supportive therapy for persons with advanced disease. Generally, the treatment measures vary with the type of lung disease that is present. Corticosteroid drugs are frequently used to suppress the inflammatory response. Many of the supportive treatment measures used in the late stages of the disease, such as oxygen therapy and measures to prevent infection, are similar to those discussed for persons with chronic obstructive lung disease.

Occupational lung diseases

The occupational lung diseases can be divided into two major groups: the pneumoconioses and the hypersensitivity diseases. The pneumoconioses are caused by the inhalation of inorganic dusts and particulate matter. The hypersensitivity diseases result from the inhalation of organic dusts and related occupational antigens. A third type of occupational lung disease, byssinosis, a disease that affects cotton workers, has characteristics of both the pneumoconioses and hypersensitivity lung disease.

Among the pneumoconioses are silicosis (found in hard-rock miners, foundry workers, sandblasters, pottery makers, and workers in the slate industry), coal miner's pneumoconiosis (found in coal miners), asbestosis (in asbestos miners, manufacturers of asbestos products, and installers and removers of asbestos insulation), talcosis (in talc miners or millers and in infants and small children who accidentally inhale powder containing talc), and berylliosis (in ore extraction workers and alloy production workers). The danger of exposure to asbestos dust is not confined to the workplace. The dust pervades the general environment because it was used in the construction of buildings and in other applications before its health hazards were realized. It has been mixed into paints and plaster, wrapped around water and heating pipes,

used to insulate hair dryers, and woven into theater curtains, hot pads, and ironing-board covers.

Important etiologic determinants in the development of the pneumoconioses are (1) the size of the dust particle, its chemical nature, and its ability to incite lung destruction and (2) the concentration of dust and the length of exposure to it. The most dangerous particles are those in the range of 1 to 5 μm. These small particles are carried through the inspired air into the alveolar structures, whereas larger particles are trapped in the nose or mucous linings of the airways and removed by the mucociliary blanket. Exceptions are asbestos and talc particles, which range in size from 30 to 60 μm but find their way into the alveoli because of their density. All particles within the alveoli must be cleared by the lung macrophages. Macrophages are thought to transport engulfed particles from the small bronchioles and the alveoli, which have neither cilia nor mucus-secreting cells, to the mucociliary escalator or to the lymphatic channels for removal from the lung. This clearing function is hampered when the function of the macrophage is impaired by factors such as cigarette smoking, consumption of alcohol, and hypersensitivity reactions. This helps to explain the increased incidence of lung disease among smokers exposed to asbestos. In silicosis the ingestion of silica particles leads to the destruction of the lung macrophages and the release of substances that produce fibrosis. Tuberculosis and other diseases caused by the mycobacteria are common in persons with silicosis. Because the macrophages are responsible for protecting the lungs from tuberculosis, the destruction of macrophages accounts for the increased susceptibility of persons with silicosis to tuberculosis.

With some dusts the concentration of dust in the environment strongly influences the effect on the lung. For example, acute silicosis is seen only in persons whose occupations entail intense exposure to silica dust over a short period. It is seen in sandblasters, who use a high-speed jet of sand to clean and polish bricks and the insides of corroded tanks, in tunnelers, and in rock drillers, particularly if they drill through sandstone.[53] Acute silicosis is a rapidly progressive disease, usually leading to severe disability and death within 5 years of diagnosis. In contrast to acute silicosis, which is caused by exposure to extremely high concentrations of silica dust, the symptoms related to chronic low-level exposure to silica dust often do not begin to develop until after many years of exposure, and then the symptoms are often insidious in onset and slow to progress.

The hypersensitivity occupational lung disorders (hypersensitivity pneumonitis) are caused by intense and often prolonged exposure to inhaled organic dusts and related occupational antigens. Affected persons have a heightened sensitivity to the antigen. Unlike bronchial asthma, this type of hypersensitivity reaction involves primarily the alveoli. These disorders cause progressive fibrotic lung disease, which can be prevented by the removal of the environmental agent. The most common forms of hypersensitivity pneumonitis are farmers' lung, which results from exposure to moldy hay; pigeon breeders' lung, provoked by exposure to the serum, excreta, or feathers of birds; bagassosis, from contaminated sugarcane; and humidifier or air-conditioner lung, caused by bacteria in the water reservoirs of these appliances.

── Sarcoidosis

Sarcoidosis, sometimes called *Boeck's sarcoid,* is a multisystem granulomatous disorder of unknown etiology. An alteration in T-lymphocyte function is thought to contribute to the disorder.[54]

The disease predominantly affects young adults, aged 20 to 40 years, although it may occur in older groups. The annual incidence of sarcoidosis in the United States is about 22,500 cases; it is 10 to 20 times more common in blacks and is more prevalent in both blacks and whites living in the southeastern part of the country.[55]

Sarcoidosis has variable manifestations and an unpredictable course of progression in which any organ system can be affected. The three systems that most commonly present symptoms are the lungs, the skin, and the eyes. Table 25-6 lists the sites of extrathoracic involvement in sarcoidosis. More than 40% of persons with sarcoidosis report nonspecific symptoms such as fever, sweating, anorexia, weight loss, fatigue, and myalgia. Although only about 60% of persons with sarcoidosis have respiratory symptoms, almost all have abnormal chest x-rays. In about 25% of cases, the disease is first detected on a routine chest x-ray. The roentgenographic manifestations of the disorder can be classified into four stages.[56]

Stage 0: no roentgenographic abnormalities.
Stage 1: bilateral hilar adenopathy.
Stage 2: bilateral hilar adenopathy with parenchymal infiltrates.
Stage 3: parenchymal infiltrates without hilar adenopathy.

In persons with stage 0 disease—that is, with other symptomatology but no abnormal findings on radiography—the rate of spontaneous recovery approaches 100%. The x-ray abnormalities will clear in about 65% of persons with stage 1, 50% of persons with stage 2, and 20% of persons with stage 3 disease.

The diagnosis of sarcoidosis is usually made using the transbronchial lung biopsy, bronchial lavage, the Kveim skin test, and serum angiotensin-converting enzyme (SACE) test. The Kveim test is a skin test that uses antigen from human sarcoid tissue injected intradermally into the flexor surface of the forearm. The injection site is observed for the development of a nodule during the 6 weeks following injection of the antigen. If a nodule develops, it is examined through biopsy for sarcoid tissue. In active sarcoidosis the SACE level is elevated. The SACE test is used to evaluate the progress of the disease and the effectiveness of treatment. When treatment is indicated, the corticosteroid drugs are used. These agents produce clearing of the chest x-ray and improve pulmonary function, but it is not known whether they affect the long-term outcome of the disease.

In summary, the interstitial lung diseases are characterized by fibrosis and decreased compliance of the lung. They include the occupational lung diseases, lung diseases caused by toxic drugs and radiation, and lung diseases of unknown etiology, such as sarcoidosis. These disorders are thought to result from an inflammatory process that begins in the alveoli and extends to involve the interstitial tissues of the lung. In

Table 25–6. Sites of extrathoracic involvement in sarcoidosis

Site	Approximate incidence (%)	Manifestations
Liver	90 (biopsy)	Hepatomegaly, abnormal liver function tests
Eye	15–20	Lacrimal gland involvement, iridocyclitis, keratoconjunctivitis, cataract formation, glaucoma
Skin	20	Erythema nodosum, cosmetically unattractive and disfiguring skin lesions
Spleen	10	Splenomegaly, abdominal pain, anemia, leukopenia, thrombocytopenia
Central nervous system	5	Chronic meningitis, involvement of cranial nerves, *e.g.,* Bell's palsy; endocrine disorders due to involvement of hypothalamus or pituitary gland, *e.g.,* diabetes insipidus
Bone	4	Arthritis of large weight-bearing joints, bone cysts
Abnormal calcium metabolism	15	Hypercalcemia, hypercalciuria

contrast with chronic obstructive pulmonary diseases, which affect the airways, interstitial lung diseases affect the supporting collagen and elastic tissues that lie between the airways and blood vessels. These lung diseases produce a decrease in lung volumes, a reduction in the diffusing capacity of the lung, and varying degrees of hypoxia. Because lung compliance is reduced, persons with this form of lung disease have a rapid, shallow breathing pattern.

Pulmonary vascular disorders

As blood moves through the lung, blood oxygen levels are raised and carbon dioxide is removed. These processes depend on the matching of ventilation (gas exchange) and perfusion (blood flow). This section discusses two major problems of the pulmonary circulation, pulmonary embolism and pulmonary hypertension. Pulmonary edema, another major problem of the pulmonary circulation, is discussed in Chapter 22.

Pulmonary embolism

Pulmonary embolism develops when a blood-borne substance lodges in a branch of the pulmonary artery and obstructs the flow. The embolism may consist of a thrombus, air that has accidentally been injected during intravenous infusion, fat that has been mobilized from the bone marrow following a fracture or from a traumatized fat depot,[54] or amniotic fluid that has entered the maternal circulation following rupture of the membranes at the time of delivery. This discussion is limited to the most common form of pulmonary embolism, thromboembolism.

In the United States, approximately 630,000 cases of thromboembolism occur annually.[57] About 67,000 of these persons die within the first hour, before a diagnosis can be made and treatment instituted. Another 120,000 die before the condition is recognized. Pulmonary embolism is uncommon before adulthood and increases in incidence with age, so that at age 80, about 70% of autopsied patients have emboli.[30]

Almost all pulmonary emboli are due to deep vein thrombosis. Therefore, persons at risk for developing venous thrombosis are the same persons who are at risk for developing thromboemboli.

The effect of an embolism on cardiopulmonary function depends on the size and location of the obstruction. Small emboli that become lodged in the peripheral branches of the pulmonary artery may exert little effect, whereas sudden death occurs when a large embolus causes total occlusion of the pulmonary artery. Depending on size, pulmonary embolism causes (1) obstruction of pulmonary blood flow, with pulmonary arterial hypertension and right heart failure, (2) breathlessness, (3) hypoxemia, and (4) lung infarction.

Manifestations

Dyspnea, abrupt in onset, is the most common symptom of pulmonary embolism, and the breathing pattern is often rapid and shallow. With obstruction of pulmonary blood flow, there is severe apprehension and crushing substernal chest pain resembling that of myocardial infarction; the neck veins are distended, and cyanosis, diaphoresis, syncope, mental confusion, and other signs of shock follow. Pulmonary infarction often causes pleuritic pain that changes with respiration, being more severe on inspiration and less severe on expiration. With lung infarction there may be hemoptysis.

Diagnosis and treatment

Diagnosis of pulmonary embolism is based on blood gases, lung scan, laboratory studies, chest x-ray films, electrocardiogram (ECG), and, in selected cases, angiography. The arterial oxygen tension (PO_2) is almost always decreased when emboli of significant size are present in the lung. This is because of the mismatching of ventilation and perfusion. The lung scan is a widely used diagnostic test. In this test, radioactive iodinated serum albumin is injected intravenously and collects in the pulmonary circulation. A scintillation counter is passed over the chest to provide a picture of blood flow in the various lung segments. The laboratory studies and chest x-ray films are useful in ruling out other conditions that might give rise to similar symptoms. The ECG may show signs of right heart strain, since emboli can cause an increase in pulmonary vascular resistance. Angiography involves the passage of a venous catheter through the heart and into the pulmonary artery under fluoroscopy. An embolectomy is sometimes performed during this procedure.

The treatment goals for pulmonary emboli focus on (1) preventing deep vein thrombosis and the development of thromboemboli, (2) protecting the lungs from exposure to thromboemboli when they occur, and (3) in the case of large and life-threatening pulmonary emboli, sustaining life and restoring pulmonary blood flow.

Prevention focuses on (1) identification of persons at risk, (2) avoidance of venous stasis and hypercoagulability states, and (3) early detection of venous thrombosis. In patients at risk, low-dose subcutaneous heparin may be administered to decrease the likelihood of deep vein thrombosis, thromboembolism, and fatal pulmonary embolism following major surgical procedures.

There are two surgical procedures for protecting the lung from thromboemboli: venous ligation to prevent the embolus from traveling to the lung and vena caval plication. The plication, done with a suture, or by insertion of a clip, filter, or sieve, permits blood to flow while trapping the embolus.

Restoration of blood flow in persons with life-threatening pulmonary emboli can be accomplished through the surgical removal of the embolus or emboli. In the case of multiple pulmonary emboli, the thrombolytic drug streptokinase may be used. The drug is administered intravenously or directly into the pulmonary artery. Thrombolytic therapy is followed by administration of heparin and then warfarin.

Pulmonary hypertension

Pulmonary hypertension describes the elevation of pressure in the pulmonary arterial system. The pulmonary circulation is a low pressure system designed to accommodate varying amounts of blood delivered from the right heart and to facilitate gas exchange. The normal mean pulmonary artery pressure is about 15 mmHg (28 systolic/8 diastolic). Pulmonary artery hypertension can be caused by an elevation in left atrial pressure, increased pulmonary blood flow, or increased pulmonary vascular resistance. Although pulmonary hypertension can develop as a primary disorder, most cases develop secondary to some other condition.

Etiologic mechanisms

Increased left atrial pressure. In conditions such as mitral valve stenosis and left ventricular heart failure, the elevation in left atrial pressure is transmitted to the pulmonary circulation and results in a passive elevation of pulmonary aterial pressures. Continued increases in left atrial pressure can lead to medial hypertrophy and intimal thickening of the small pulmonary arteries, causing sustained hypertension.

Increased pulmonary blood flow. Increased pulmonary blood flow results from increased flow through left-to-right shunts in congenital heart diseases such as atrial or ventricular septal defects and patent ductus arteriosus. If the high flow state is allowed to continue, morphologic changes will occur in the pulmonary vessels, leading to sustained pulmonary hypertension. The pulmonary vascular changes that occur with congenital heart disorders are discussed in Chapter 21.

Increased pulmonary vascular resistance. Unlike the vessels in the systemic circulation, which generally dilate in response to hypoxemia and hypercapnia, the pulmonary vessels constrict. The stimulus for constriction seems to originate in the air spaces in the vicinity of the small branches of the pulmonary arteries. In situations in which certain regions of the lung are hypoventilated, the response is adaptive in that it diverts blood flow away from the poorly ventilated areas to more adequately ventilated portions of the lung. This effect, however, becomes less beneficial as more and more areas of the lung become poorly ventilated.

Pulmonary hypertension may develop at high altitudes in persons with normal lungs. It is also a common problem in persons with advanced chronic bronchitis and emphysema. In interstitial lung diseases, the fibrotic process may actually cause obliteration of pulmonary vessels, leading to pulmonary hypertension. Persons who experience marked hypoxemia during sleep—that is, those with sleep apnea—may experience marked elevations in pulmonary arterial pressure.

Primary pulmonary hypertension. Primary pulmonary hypertension is a rare, often lethal, form of pulmonary hypertension, the etiology of which is unknown. It is characterized by marked intimal fibrosis of the pulmonary arteries and arterioles. The disease can occur at any age, and familial occurrences have been reported. Persons with the disorder usually have a steadily progressive downhill course, with death occurring in 3 to 4 years. The recent use of the vasodilators hydralazine and diazoxide for the treatment of this form of pulmonary hypertension has met with some degree of success.

Cor pulmonale

The term *cor pulmonale* refers to heart failure resulting from primary lung disease and long-standing pulmonary hypertension. It involves hypertrophy and the eventual failure of the right ventricle. The manifestations of cor pulmonale include the signs and symptoms of the primary lung disease and the signs of right-sided heart failure. There is shortness of breath and a productive cough, which becomes worse during periods of heart failure. Failure of the right ventricle and elevation of intrathoracic pressure resulting from airway obstruction cause venous distention and peripheral edema. Plethora (redness) and cyanosis and warm, moist skin may be present because of the compensatory polycythemia and desaturation of arterial blood that accompany chronic lung disease. Drowsiness and altered consciousness may occur as the result of carbon dioxide retention. Management of cor pulmonale focuses on the treatment of both the lung disease and the heart failure (see Chapter 22). Low-flow oxygen therapy may be used to reduce the pulmonary hypertension and polycythemia associated with severe hypoxemia due to chronic lung disease.

In summary, pulmonary vascular disorders include pulmonary embolism and pulmonary hypertension. Pulmonary embolism develops when a blood-borne substance lodges in a branch of the pulmonary artery and obstructs blood flow. The embolus can consist of a thrombus, air, fat, or amniotic fluid. The most common form is a thromboembolus arising from the deep venous channels of the lower extremities. Pulmonary hypertension is the elevation of pulmonary arterial pressure. It can be caused by an elevated left atrial pressure, increased pulmonary blood flow, or increased pulmonary vascular resistance secondary to lung disease. The term cor pulmonale describes right heart failure caused by primary pulmonary disease and long-standing pulmonary hypertension.

Cancer of the lung

In the United States, lung cancer strikes an estimated 150,000 persons every year,[57] most commonly those between 40 and 70 years of age. Lung cancer is a leading cause of death among men and a steadily increasing cause among women. These consistent increases over the past 50 years have coincided closely with the increase in cigarette smoking over the same span. It has been estimated that 85% of lung cancer cases are due to cigarette smoking.[58] Many studies have shown that the risk of developing lung cancer increases with the number of cigarettes smoked and that the average male smoker is ten times more likely to develop lung cancer than the nonsmoker.[59] Industrial hazards also contribute to the incidence of lung cancer. A commonly recognized hazard is exposure to asbestos, with the mean risk of lung cancer being significantly greater in asbestos workers than in the general population. Tobacco smoke contributes heavily to the development of lung cancer in persons exposed to asbestos; the risk in this population group is estimated to be 92 times greater than that for non-smokers.[60]

Bronchogenic carcinoma is the cancer type seen in 90% to 95% of cases. These tumors can be further subdivided into epidermoid or squamous cell carcinoma (35%–50%); adenocarcinoma (15%–35%); small cell anaplastic (oat cell) carcinoma (20%–25%); and large cell carcinoma (10%–15%).[17]

The tracheobronchial tree is lined with at least five types of epithelial cells, which form the pseudostratified cell layer of these airways (see Chapter 1). There are three types of columnar cells— the mucus-secreting goblet cells, the ciliated cells, and the brush cells. The basal cells are small, multipotential stem cells parallel to the basement membrane on which the pseudostratified cell layer rests. One group of basal cells probably acts as reserve cells for the columnar cells; the other group, termed *Kulchitsky's* (or K-type) *cells,* appears to be neuroendocrine in origin and is believed to have the capacity to secrete hormones. These cell characteristics would account for the paraneoplastic syndromes that occur in some forms of bronchogenic carcinoma. Squamous cell carcinoma probably arises from the basal reserve cells, adenocarcinoma from the mucus-secreting cells, and small cell and bronchial carcinoid cancers from the K-type cells.[60]

—— Manifestations

Cancer of the lung develops insidiously, often giving little or no warning of its presence. Because its symptoms are similar to those associated with smoking and chronic bronchitis, they are often disregarded.

The manifestations of lung cancer can be divided into four categories: (1) local respiratory disturbances, (2) the effects of local spread and metastasis, (3) nonspecific effects such as weight loss, and (4) the nonmetastatic endocrine, neurologic, and connective tissue disorders.[30]

Lung cancers produce their local effects by irritation and obstruction of the airways and invasion of the mediastinum and pleural space. The earliest symptoms are chronic cough, shortness of breath, and wheezing due to airway irritation and obstruction. Hemoptysis (blood in the sputum) occurs when the lesion erodes blood vessels. Pain receptors in the chest are limited to the parietal pleura, mediastinum, larger blood vessels, and peribronchial afferent vagal fibers.[30] Dull, intermittent, poorly localized retrosternal pain is common in tumors that involve the mediastinum. Pain becomes persistent, localized, and more severe when the disease invades the pleura.

Tumors that invade the mediastinum may cause hoarseness (because of the involvement of the recurrent laryngeal nerve) and difficulty in swallowing (due to compression of the esophagus). An uncommon complication called the *superior vena cava syndrome* can occur in some persons with mediastinal involvement. Interruption of flow in this vessel usually results from compression by the tumor or involved lymph nodes. The disorder can interfere with venous drainage from the head, neck, and chest wall. The outcome is determined by the speed with which the disorder develops and the adequacy of the collateral circulation.

Tumors adjacent to the visceral pleura often insidiously produce pleural effusion. This effusion can compress the lung and cause atelectasis and dyspnea. It is less apt to cause fever, pleural friction rub, or pain than pleural effusion resulting from other causes.

Metastases already exist in 50% of patients presenting with evidence of lung cancer and develop inexorably in the majority (90%) of patients.[61] The most common sites of these metastases are the brain, bone, and liver.

Paraneoplastic disorders are those that are unrelated to metastasis. No other type of cancer produces such disorders as frequently as lung cancer. Neurologic or muscular symptoms often develop 6 months to 4 years before the lung tumor is detected. One of the more common of these problems is weakness and wasting of the proximal muscles of the pelvic and shoulder girdles with decreased deep tendon reflexes, but without sensory changes.[30]

Certain bronchogenic carcinomas produce hormones. It has been estimated that approximately 10% of persons with bronchogenic cancer have evidence of ectopic hormone production.[30] The most frequently produced hormones are parathormone (causing hypercalcemia, see Chapter 27), antidiuretic hormone (syndrome of inappropriate secretion of ADH, see Chapter 27), and ACTH (clinical Cushing's syndrome, see Chapter 44).

Because cancer of the lung is usually far advanced before it is discovered, the prognosis is generally poor, with a 5-year survival rate of only 5% to 10%. The hope for the future rests with methods of earlier detection and with prevention.

Diagnosis and treatment

The diagnosis of lung cancer is based on a careful history and physical examination and other tests such as chest radiography, bronchoscopy, cytologic studies (Papanicolaou's test) of the sputum or bronchial washings, percutaneous needle biopsy of lung tissue, scalene lymph node biopsy, radioisotope studies, and carcinoembryonic antigen enzyme titers. Radioisotope studies include technetium-99, which is used to detect superior vena caval obstruction and study pulmonary blood flow. Gallium and bleomycin scans become fixed to the tumor and can be used to detect its presence. The carcinoembryonic antigen (CEA) is produced by undifferentiated lung tumor cells; high CEA titers usually correlate with extensive disease. This test is often used to follow the progress of the disease and its response to treatment.

Like other types of cancer, lung cancers are classified according to cell type (squamous cell carcinoma, adenocarcinoma, small cell anaplastic carcinoma, and large cell carcinoma) and staged according to the TNM system (see Chapter 5). These classifications are used for treatment planning.

Treatment methods for lung cancer include surgery, radiotherapy, and chemotherapy.[62] These treatments may be used singly or in combination. Surgery is usually used for the removal of small localized tumors. It can involve a lobectomy, pneumonectomy, or segmental resection of the lung. Radiation can be used as a definitive or main treatment modality, as part of a combined treatment plan, or for palliation of symptoms. Because of the frequency of metastases, chemotherapy is often used in treating lung cancer. Combination chemotherapy, which uses a regimen of several drugs, is usually employed. Immunotherapy, using the bacille Calmette-Guérin (BCG) of the *Mycobacterium bovis*, has been used as an adjuvant treatment. Several other immunotherapy regimens are under investigation. The mechanisms of these treatment methods are discussed in Chapter 5.

In summary, cancer of the lung is a leading cause of death among men ages 40 to 70, and the death rate is increasing among women. In the United States this increase in death rate has coincided with the increase in cigarette smoking. Industrial hazards, such as exposure to asbestos, increase the risk of developing lung cancer. Of all forms of lung cancer, bronchogenic carcinoma is the most common, accounting for 90% to 95% of cases. Because lung cancer develops insidiously, it is often far advanced before it is diagnosed, a fact that is used to explain the poor 5-year survival rate—only 5% to 10% of affected persons are alive and well 5 years after treatment.

References

1. Lowenstein SR, Parrino TA: Management of the common cold. Adv Intern Med 32:207, 1987
2. Douglas RG: The common cold—Relief at last. N Engl J Med 314:114, 1986
3. Hendley JA, Gwaltney JM Jr, Jordon WS: Rhinovirus infections in an industrial population. IV. Infections within the families of employees during two fall peaks of respiratory illness. Am J Epidemiol 89:184, 1969
4. Beem, MO: Acute respiratory illness in nursery school children: A longitudinal study of occurrence of illness and respiratory viruses. Am J Epidemiol 90:30, 1969
5. Klumpp TG: The common cold. Med Times 98:1s, 1980

_464_ ■ _UNIT III: ALTERATIONS IN OXYGENATION OF TISSUES_

6. Hendley JO, Wenzel RP, Gwaltney JM Jr: Transmission of rhinovirus colds by self-inoculation. N Engl J Med 288:1361, 1973

7. Gwaltney JM Jr, Moskalski PB, Hendley JO: Hand-to-hand transmission of rhinovirus colds. Ann Intern Med 88:464, 1978

8. Anderson TW, Reid BW, Beaton GH: Vitamin C and the common cold: A double blind study. Can Med Assoc J 107:503, 1974

9. Miller JZ, Nance WE, Norton JA, et al: Therapeutic effect of vitamin C: A co-twin study. JAMA 237:248, 1977

10. Carr B, Einstein R, Lai LY, Martin NG, Starmer GA: Vitamin C and the common cold. Med J Aust 2:411, 1981

11. Simkins R: Croup and epiglottitis: Am J Nurs 81:519, 1981

12. Baker AS, Eavey RD: Adult supraglottitis (epiglottitis). N Engl J Med 314:1185, 1986

13. Sims DG: Acute bronchiolitis in infancy. Nurs Times 75:1842, 1979

14. Simkins R: The crisis of bronchiolitis. Am J Nurs 81:514, 1981

15. Vital Statistics Report: Annual Summary of the United States, 1979, Vol 28, No 13. Washington DC, US Department of Health and Human Services, 1980

16. Dowling JN, Sheehe PR, Feldman H: Pharyngeal pneumococcal acquisitions in "normal" families: A longitudinal study. J Infect Dis 124(1):9, 1971

17. Robbins SL, Cotran R, Kumar V: Pathologic Basis of Disease, 3rd ed, pp 734, 357, 751. Philadelphia, WB Saunders, 1984

18. Robbins SL, Kumar V: Basic Pathology, 4th ed, pp 433–434. Philadelphia, WB Saunders, 1987

19. Andreoli TE, Carpenter CCJ, Plum F, Smith LH: Cecil Essentials of Medicine, pp 164–165. Philadelphia, WB Saunders, 1986

20. Jones DA: Viral infection of the respiratory system. Chest Heart Stroke J 3(5):48, 1979

21. Centers for Disease Control: Prevention and control of influenza. MMWR 33(9), 1984

22. Prevention and control of influenza. Ann Intern Med 101:218, 1984

23. Centers for Disease Control: Update: Pneumococcus polysaccharide vaccine usage—United States. MMWR 33(2), 1984

24. Tuberculosis Statistics, DHHS Publication No (CDC) 81-8241. Bethesda, MD, US Department of Health and Human Services, 1980

25. Davidson P: Tuberculosis: New views of an old disease, N Engl J Med 312:1514, 1985

26. Stead WW, Lofgren JP, Warren E, et al: Tuberculosis as endemic and nosocomial infection among elderly in nursing homes. N Engl J Med 312:1483, 1985

27. American Thoracic Society, Ad Hoc Committee of the Scientific Assembly on Tuberculosis, Comstock GW Chr: The tuberculin skin test. Am Rev Respir Dis 124:356, 1982

28. Ad·Hoc Committee of the American Thoracic Society: Statement on preventive therapy of tuberculosis infection. Am Rev Respir Dis 110:371, 1974

29. Johnson JR: Chemoprophylaxis of pulmonary tuberculosis. Postgrad Med 74(3):64, 1983

30. Guenther CA, Welch MH: Pulmonary Medicine, 2nd ed, pp 109, 433, 476, 526, 556, 810, 812, 821. Philadelphia, JB Lippincott, 1982

31. Davies SF, Sarosi GA: Fungal infections of the lung. Postgrad Med 73(6):242, 1983

32. Sahn SA: Pleural manifestations of pulmonary disease. Hosp Pract 16(3):73, 1981

33. Stauffer JL: Pulmonary diseases. In Schroeder SA, Krupp MA, Tierney LM (eds): Current Medical Diagnosis and Treatment, p 184. Norwalk CO, Appleton Lange, 1988

34. Sly RM: Increases in deaths from asthma. Ann Allergy 53:20, 1984

35. Cherniack RM: Continuity of care in asthma management. Hosp Pract 22(18):119, 1987

36. Samter M, Beers RR: Intolerance to aspirin: Clinical studies and considerations of pathogenesis. Ann Intern Med 68:975, 1968

37. Roberts JA: Exercise-induced asthma in athletes. Sports Med 6:193, 1988

38. Haltom JR, Strunk RC: Pathogenesis of exercise-induced asthma: Implications for treatment. Annu Rev Med 37:143, 1986

39. McFadden ER, Ingram RH Jr: Exercise-induced asthma. N Engl J Med 301:763, 1979

40. Auber M, DeTroyer A, Sampson M: Aminophylline improves diaphragmatic contractility. N Engl J Med 305:249, 1981

41. Petty TL: COPD in the setting of "multidimensional" illness. Hosp Pract 23(2):39, 1988

42. Chronic Obstructive Pulmonary Disease, 5th ed, inside front cover. American Lung Association and Medical Section, American Thoracic Society, 1977

43. The Health Consequences of Smoking. Washington DC, US Department of Health, Education and Welfare, 1971

44. Kueppers F, Black LP: Alpha-antitrypsin and its deficiency. Am Rev Respir Dis 110:176, 1974

45. Hodgkin JE, et al: Chronic obstructive airway diseases: Current concepts in diagnosis and comprehensive care. JAMA 232:1253, 1975

46. Kim MJ: Respiratory muscle training: Implications for patient care. Heart Lung 13:333, 1984

47. Pardy RL, Rivington R, Daspas PJ, et al: Inspiratory muscle training compared with physiotherapy in patients with chronic airflow limitations. Am Rev Respir Dis 123:421, 1981

48. Nocturnal Oxygen Therapy Group Trial: Continuous or nocturnal oxygen therapy in hypoxemic chronic obstructive lung disease. Ann Intern Med 93:391, 1980

49. Tirlapur DTM, Mir MA: Nocturnal hypoxemia associated with electrocardiographic changes in patients with chronic obstructive airways disease. N Engl J Med 306:125, 1982

50. Fletcher EC, Levin DC: Cardiopulmonary hemodynamics during sleep in subjects with chronic obstructive pulmonary disease. Chest 85:6, 1984

51. Luce JM: Interstitial lung disease. Hosp Pract 18(7):173, 1983

52. Crystal RG, Gadek JE, Ferrans VJ, et al: Interstitial lung disease. Am J Med 70:542, 1981

53. Occupational Lung Disease: An Introduction. New York, American Lung Association, 1983
54. Crystal RG, Roberts WC, Hunninghake GW, et al (moderators): Pulmonary sarcoidosis: A disease characterized and perpetuated by activated lung T-lymphocytes (report of the NIH conference). Ann Intern Med 94:73, 1981
55. Daniele RP: Sarcoidosis: Diagnosis and management. Hosp Pract 18(6):113, 1983
56. Whitcomb ME: The Lung: Normal and Diseased, p 150. St. Louis, CV Mosby, 1982
57. Dalen JE, Alpert JS: Natural history of pulmonary embolism. Prog Cardiovasc Dis 17:259, 1975
58. Cancer Facts 1987. New York, American Cancer Society, 1987
59. Smoking and cancer. MMWR 31, No 11:77 1982
60. Carr DT: Bronchiogenic carcinoma. Basics of RD 5(5):55, 1977
61. Van Houte P, Salazar OM, Phillips CE, et al: Lung Cancer. In Rubin P (ed): Clinical Oncology, 6th ed, p 142. New York, American Cancer Society, 1983

Bibliography

Chronic lung disease

Barnes PJ, Chung KF, Page CP: Inflammatory mediators and asthma. Pharm Rev 40:49, 1988
Bascom R, Johns CJ: The natural history and management of sarcoidosis. Adv Intern Med 31:213, 1986
Benatar SR: Fatal asthma. N Engl J Med 314:423, 1986
Canny GJ, Levison H: Exercise response and rehabilitation in cystic fibrosis. Sports Med 4:143, 1987
Crystal RG, Bitterman PB, Rennard SI: Interstitial lung diseases of unknown cause (parts 1 and 2). N Engl J Med 310:154,435, 1984
Geha RS: Regulation of IgE synthesis in atopic disease. Hosp Pract 23(3):91, 1988
Gross NJ, Skorodin MS: Role of parasympathetic system in airway obstruction due to emphysema. N Engl J Med 311:421, 1984
Hale KA: Chronic airflow obstruction. Postgrad Med 73:259, 1983
Hiller FC, Wilson FJ: Evaluation and management of acute asthma. Med Clin North Am 63:669, 1983
Hopp LJ: Ineffective breathing pattern related to decreased lung expansion. Nurs Clin North Am 22:193, 1987
Krohmer JR: Asthma out of control. Emerg Med 20 (May 15):97, 1988
Lareau S, Larson JL: Ineffective breathing pattern related to airflow limitation. Nurs Clin North Am 22:179, 1987
Lee M, Gentry AF, Schwartz R, et al: Tartarazine-containing drugs. Drug Intell Clin Pharm 15:782, 1981
Lieberman P: Rhinitis: Allergic and nonallergic. Hosp Pract 23(9):117, 1988
Mathews LW, Drotar D: Cystic fibrosis—A long-term chronic disease. Med Clin North Am 31:133, 1984

McFadden ER: Exercise and asthma. N Engl J Med 317:502, 1987
Nadel JA: Bronchial reactivity. Adv Intern Med 28:207, 1983
Newhouse MT, Dolovich MB: Control of asthma by aerosols. N Engl J Med. 315:870, 1986
Paloucek FP, Rodvold KA: Evaluation of theophylline overdoses and toxicities. Ann Emerg Med 17:135, 1988
Rubio TT: Infection in patients with cystic fibrosis. Am J Med 81(1A):73, 1986
Tepper RS, Zander JE, Eigen H: Chronic respiratory problems in infancy. Curr Probl Pediatr 16:305, 1986
Thomas PD, Hunninghake GW: Current concepts of the pathogenesis of sarcoidosis. Am Rev Respir Dis 135:747, 1987
Weis JE: Atopy and airways responsiveness in chronic obstructive lung disease. N Engl J Med 317:1345, 1987
Wilson DO, Rogers RM, Hoffman RM: Nutrition and chronic lung disease. Am Rev Respir Dis 132:1347, 1985

Respiratory infections

Australian R: Pneumococcal pneumonia: Diagnosis, epidemiologic, therapeutic, and prophylactic considerations. Chest 90:738, 1986
American Thoracic Society: Treatment of tuberculosis in adults and children. Am Rev Respir Dis 134:355, 1986
Centers for Disease Control: Diagnosis and management of mycobacterial infection and disease in persons with human immunodeficiency virus disease. Ann Intern Med 106:254, 1987
Dismukes WE: Blastomycosis: Leave it to beaver. N Engl J Med 314:575, 1986
Edelstein PH, Meyer RD. Legionnaires disease: A review. Chest 85:114, 1984
Hamrick RM, Yeager H: Tuberculosis update. Am Fam Pract 38:205, 1988
Hughes W: Pneumocystis carinii pneumonitis. N Engl J Med 317:1021, 1987
LaForce FM, Eickhoff TC: Pneumococcal vaccine: An emerging consensus. Ann Intern Med 108:757, 1988
Lowenstein SR: Management of the common cold. Adv Intern Med 32:207, 1987
Mendelsohn J: Pediatric respiratory emergencies. Topics Emerg Med 2:25, 1980
Milner AD: Acute airway obstruction in children under 5. Thorax 37:641, 1982
Page HS: Croup and epiglottitis: Sudden trouble for young children. Am Lung Assoc Bull 67(2):9, 1981

Pulmonary vascular disorders

Hirsch J (ed): Venous thromboembolism: Prevention, diagnosis and treatment. Chest 89(Suppl):369 (entire issue), 1986
Hurewitz AN, Bergofsky EH: Pathogenic mechanisms in chronic pulmonary hypertension. Heart Lung 15:327, 1986
Peter RH, Rubin L: The pharamacologic control of the pulmonary circulation in pulmonary hypertension. Adv Intern Med 29:495, 1984

Reid LM: Structure and function in pulmonary hypertension. Chest 89:279, 1986

Valenzuela T: Pulmonary embolism. Ann Emerg Med 17:209, 1988

Voelkel NF: Mechanisms of hypoxic pulmonary vasoconstriction: New perspectives. Chest 89:279, 1986

Wollschlager CM, Khan F: Secondary pulmonary hypertension. Heart Lung 15:336, 1986

—— Lung cancer

Carr DT: Lung cancer: Pitfalls and controversies in diagnosis and management. Consultant 28:33, 1988

MacMahon H, et al: Diagnostic methods in lung cancer. Semin Oncol 10:20, 1983

Whimster WF: Lung tumors: Differentiation and Classification. Pathol Annu 18(1):121, 1983

CHAPTER 26

Alterations in Control of Ventilation and Respiratory Failure

---

Objectives

After you have studied this chapter, you should be able to meet the following objectives:

_____ List at least three categories of drugs that can depress respiratory function.

_____ Cite a common characteristic of ventilatory impairment that occurs in disorders of the respiratory muscles.

_____ Define *sleep apnea*.

_____ Compare the respiratory activities in each of the four stages of sleep.

_____ List the behaviors that are characteristic of REM sleep.

_____ State the signs and symptoms of sleep apnea.

_____ Differentiate between the alterations in respiratory function that account for the cessation of breathing in central and obstructive sleep apnea.

_____ Compare the characteristics of persons at risk for developing obstructive sleep apnea with those of persons at risk for developing central sleep apnea.

_____ Describe methods that might be used in the diagnosis of sleep apnea.

_____ Compare the control of breathing and response to hypoxia in infants and adults.

_____ Cite four general causes of hyperventilation syndrome.

_____ State the signs and symptoms of hyperventilation syndrome.

_____ Relate the alterations in arterial carbon dioxide levels to the production of altered body function in hyperventilation syndrome.

_____ Describe the measures used in the treatment of hyperventilation syndrome.

_____ State a general definition for *acute respiratory failure*.

_____ Explain the pathology of respiratory failure by citing clinical examples.

_____ Describe the clinical manifestations of hypoxemia and hypercapnia.

_____ Explain why cyanosis may not be an accurate diagnostic criterion for hypoxemia.

_____ Describe the pathologic lung changes that occur in ARDS.

_____ List the conditions that are associated with ARDS.

_____ Relate the clinical manifestations of ARDS to the pathologic changes associated with it.

The major function of the lungs is to oxygenate and remove carbon dioxide from the blood as a means of supporting the metabolic functions of body cells. Hypoventilation and respiratory failure result in hypoxia and hypercapnia, whereas hyperventilation causes hypocapnia. The discussion in this chapter focuses on alterations in ventilatory control and on respiratory failure.

Alterations in control of ventilation

Normally breathing involves a smooth and regular sequence of inspiration and expiration at a rate and depth regulated to maintain the arterial partial pressures of O_2 and CO_2 at relatively constant levels. Unlike the action of the heart, which beats independently of the nervous system, the inflation and deflation of the lungs require continuous input from the nervous system (see Chapter 24). A number of different types of disorders may alter neural control of ventilation. The ventilatory drive can be depressed by drugs, rendered ineffective in neuromuscular disorders affecting the respiratory muscles, and increased in hyperventilation syndrome. In sleep apnea, abnormalities in the coordination of ventilation occur during sleep. Sudden infant death syndrome (SIDS) has been attributed to abnormalities in ventilatory drive.

Drug-induced respiratory depression

The function of the respiratory muscles can be impaired by drugs that depress the central nervous system and the respiratory center; by neuromuscular blocking drugs such as *d*-tubocurarine and succinylcholine (used to effect muscle relaxation during surgery) that block the transmission of impulses at the level of the myoneural junction; or by drugs that act peripherally at a site beyond the myoneural junction, possibly by interfering with calcium release from the sarcoplasmic reticulum (Table 26-1).

Almost all the drugs known to cause depression of the central nervous system have been associated with decreased alveolar ventilation. Stupor and coma caused by depressant drug poisoning present as a picture of coma, progressing from class 0 to IV (see Chapter 50). Overdoses of barbiturates, hypnotics, narcotics, and antidepressant drugs are common causes of admission to respiratory intensive care units. Airway obstruction due to involvement of the muscles of the oropharynx and loss of the cough reflex precedes or accompanies loss of ventilatory drive and complicates the condition. Insertion of an endotra-

Table 26–1. Drugs with respiratory depressant actions*

Functional drug groups†	Mechanisms of action
Anesthetic agents	
General anesthesia	Depression of CNS function including medullary respiratory center
Spinal anesthesia	Production of ascending muscle paralysis to level of respiratory muscles
Drugs affecting brain stem respiratory mechanisms	
Opiates and narcotic analgesics Barbiturates and sedatives Tricyclic antidepressants Alcohol	Depression of brain stem respiratory mechanisms, causing a decrease in ventilatory drive
Drugs affecting myoneural junction	
Muscle relaxants Aminoglycoside antibiotics‡ Polymyxin antibiotics‡ Quinine‡ Quinidine‡	Production of impulse blockade at level of myoneural junction in skeletal muscle, including respiratory muscles
Drugs affecting muscle contraction	
Dantrolene	Reduction of excitation–contraction coupling within skeletal muscle fiber, causing muscle weakness

* The respiratory effects of these drugs are usually dose dependent.
† This list of drugs is not inclusive.
‡ The respiratory effects of these drugs usually occur at toxic doses.

cheal tube with mechanical ventilatory support may be needed when hypoventilation causes hypercapnia. It is important to recognize that small doses of drugs that depress the respiratory center may cause further impairment of ventilation and lead to hypercapnia in persons with preexisting respiratory disease. Therefore, these drugs should be used with great caution in persons with chronic lung disease and respiratory muscle weakness.

Weakness of the respiratory muscles

Weakness of the respiratory muscles can result from conditions that denervate the muscles (*e.g.,* spinal cord injury or poliomyelitis), affect the myoneural junction (*e.g.,* myasthenia gravis), or cause direct involvement of the muscles themselves (*e.g.,* muscular dystrophy). Disorders of the respiratory muscles are characterized by decreases in vital capacity and maximum voluntary ventilation, while measures of expiratory flow are well maintained. Many persons with these disorders may be able to maintain adequate ventilation for brief periods, but sustaining normal minute ventilation (respiration rate × tidal volume) may impose an excessive load on the weakened and fatigued muscles, and hypoventilation may result. Persons with impaired respiratory muscle function show extreme sensitivity to respiratory depressant drugs.

Sleep apnea

Apnea is defined as the cessation of airflow through the nose and mouth for a period of 10 seconds or longer. The diagnosis of sleep apnea depends on the occurrence of 30 or more apneic periods during 7 hours of sleep.[1] Typically, the apneic periods last for 15 to 120 seconds and some persons may have as many as 500 apneic periods per night.

Sleep stages and respiration

Sleep is not a constant, uniform state, but rather a pattern of sequential stages with a periodicity of about 90 minutes. These stages are associated with electroencephalographic (EEG), behavioral, and physiological changes that affect the control of breathing. Two sleep states have been defined: rapid eye movement (REM) sleep, also referred to as active sleep, and non-REM sleep, or quiet sleep.

Non-REM sleep is encountered when one first becomes drowsy; it has four stages reflecting an increasing depth of sleep. Stage 1 consists primarily of low-voltage, mixed-frequency EEG activity; it reflects the drowsy state. Stage 2 is a deeper sleep during which EEG activity is characterized by bursts of high-frequency (12–14 cycles/second) and high-am-

plitude waves called K complexes. Stages 3 and 4 are often referred to as slow-wave sleep because the EEG is dominated by high-voltage, low-frequency (1–2 cycles/second) waves. Stages 1 and 2 of non-REM sleep are often characterized by a pattern of breathing in which there is cyclic waning and waxing of tidal volume and respiratory rate, which may include brief periods (5–15 seconds) of apnea. This breathing pattern is known as *periodic breathing*. Although the amount of periodic breathing that occurs during the first two stages of non-REM sleep differs among healthy persons, it is more common in persons over age 40.[2] Periodic breathing during sleep is very common at high altitudes because of a change in the set point of the PO_2 chemoreceptors. Once sleep becomes stabilized during stages 3 and 4 of non-REM sleep, breathing becomes more regular. During slow-wave sleep, ventilation is usually 1 liter to 2 liters/minute less than during quiet wakefulness; the PCO_2 levels are 4 mmHg to 8 mmHg greater; the PO_2 levels are 3 mmHg to 10 mmHg less; and the *p*H is 0.03 to 0.05 units less.[2] Control of breathing during non-REM sleep is dominated by automatic (involuntary reflex) control mechanisms—responses to hypercapnia, hypoxia, and lung inflation are intact and critically important to maintaining ventilation.

REM sleep resembles wakefulness in many ways: the EEG displays unsynchronized, low-voltage, mixed-frequency waves, and there are frequent muscular and rapid eye movements. Autonomic nervous system activity changes during REM sleep: the heart rate and blood pressure may fluctuate rapidly and the cerebral blood flow and metabolic rate decrease. Respiration becomes irregular (but not periodic) and may include periods of apnea lasting as long as 15 to 20 seconds in healthy adults and 10 seconds in infants. Breathing during REM sleep has many of the features of the voluntary type of control that integrates breathing with voluntary acts such as talking, walking, and swallowing. Automatic control of breathing remains during REM sleep, but its influence is diminished.

In all stages of sleep most skeletal muscles, with the exception of the diaphragm, undergo a decrease in tone.[3] This loss of muscle tone is most pronounced during REM sleep. In the awake state, intercostal muscle activity tends to stiffen the rib cage. With the absence of this tone during sleep, the negative intrapleural pressure caused by contraction of the diaphragm can cause paradoxical motion of the rib cage (the rib cage moves inward during inspiration rather than outward) and a decrease in functional residual capacity. The loss of tone in the upper airways can cause airway obstruction. Negative airway pressure produced by contraction of the diaphragm tends to bring the vocal cords together, collapse the pharyngeal wall, and suck the tongue back into the throat. Airway collapse is accentuated in persons with conditions that cause narrowing of the upper airway or weakness of the throat muscles.

Types of sleep apnea

Sleep apnea can be classified as obstructive, central, or mixed. Obstructive apnea is caused by the obstruction of the upper airway. With central apnea the respiratory drive ceases and there is no movement of the chest or abdominal muscle. Mixed apnea constitutes a mixture of central and obstructive apnea. Because breathing seems to be controlled by different mechanisms during REM and non-REM sleep, different causes are associated with the different types of sleep apnea.

Obstructive sleep apnea. Obstructive sleep apnea is commonly associated with obesity and disorders that compromise the patency of the airway. It occurs most commonly in middle-aged men. Although androgens are suspected of contributing to the disorder, their mechanism of action is at present unknown. The pickwickian syndrome, named after the fat boy in Charles Dickens' *The Posthumous Papers of the Pickwick Club,* published in 1837, is characterized by obesity, hypersomnolence, periodic breathing, hypoxemia, and right heart failure. Alcohol and other drugs that depress the central nervous system seem to increase the severity of obstructive apneic episodes.

Obstructive sleep apnea is characterized by loud snoring interrupted by periods of silence. Abnormal gross motor movements during sleep are common. In many cases, the snoring precedes by many years the onset of other signs of sleep apnea. There are often complaints of morning headache and nausea and persistent daytime sleepiness. The hypersomnolence can lead to occupational and driving accidents. Psychological problems associated with impotence, intellectual deterioration, and depression are also part of the symptom complex. The signs and symptoms of sleep apnea are summarized in Chart 26-1. In children, a decline in school performance may be the only indication of the problem.

Chart 26–1: Signs and symptoms of sleep apnea

Noisy snoring
Insomnia
Abnormal movements during sleep
Morning headaches
Excessive daytime sleepiness
Intellectual and personality changes
Sexual impotence
Systemic hypertension
Pulmonary hypertension, cor pulmonale
Polycythemia

In addition to the sleep disturbances, a number of cardiovascular problems are associated with sleep apnea syndromes. A number of cardiac arrhythmias have been observed in individuals with sleep apnea. Frequent apneic periods may result in increased pulmonary and systemic blood pressures. More than two-thirds of the sleep apneic patients in one study had daytime hypertension.[4] In severe cases, pulmonary hypertension, polycythemia, and cor pulmonale may develop.

Sleep apnea and sleep-related periodic leg movements appear to be more widespread among the elderly. One study reported a 24% prevalence of sleep apnea among subjects aged 60 to 95 years.[5] However, sleep apnea tends to be mild in the elderly, with few sleep-wake complaints and only small changes in heart rate (mean 10 beats or less) and oxygen desaturation (mean less than 5%). At present, it is not known if this type of sleep apnea in the elderly contributes to conditions such as hypertension.

Central sleep apnea. Central sleep apnea is associated with disorders that affect the central nervous system and respiratory neurons, such as encephalitis, brain stem infarction, and bulbar poliomyelitis. With central sleep apnea, sleep is difficult to maintain and several awakenings occur during the night. There may be some daytime fatigue, depression, and impaired sexual functioning. In contrast to persons with obstructive sleep apnea, persons with central sleep apnea tend to be of normal weight.

Diagnosis and treatment

Sleep apnea is usually suspected from a history of snoring, disturbed sleep, and daytime sleepiness. A definitive diagnosis is accomplished with sleep studies done in a sleep laboratory using polysomnography.[6] This procedure consists of (1) an EEG and electro-oculogram to determine the sleep stages, (2) monitoring of the airflow, (3) an ECG to detect arrhythmias, (4) impedance pneumography, intercostal electromyography, or esophageal manometry to monitor respiratory effort, and (5) ear oximetry or transcutaneous oxygen monitoring to detect changes in oxygen saturation.

The treatment of sleep apnea is determined by the type of apnea that is present. Weight loss is often beneficial in persons with obstructive apnea. Severe cases may require a tracheostomy. Applying pressure on the nasal airways at night has been reported to help in obstructive sleep apnea.[7] Protriptyline, a nonsedative tricyclic antidepressant that reduces REM sleep, has also been used successfully to reduce apneic episodes in some persons.[8] In cases of central apnea, a variety of medications have been used to increase the central respiratory drive, including theophylline, acetazolamide, clomipramine, and medroxyprogesterone. In severe cases, the most effective treatment is electrical stimulation of the phrenic nerves with implanted electrodes.

Sudden infant death syndrome

Sudden infant death syndrome (SIDS), or crib death, is the most common cause of death in infants 1 to 12 months of age and is most common between the ages of 3 and 18 weeks.[9] The incidence is about 2 per 1000 infants; it is less common in whites, greater in blacks, and greatest in Native Americans.[10] Male infants are at greater risk than female infants, and infants born prematurely are at greater risk than full-term infants. There is an increased incidence of SIDS among infants born to young unmarried mothers who had little prenatal care, as well as among infants of mothers addicted to narcotics. Although there is no evidence of genetic transmission, SIDS has occurred three and even four times in the same family, and twins and triplets have a greater incidence of SIDS.[10] Since SIDS is essentially a diagnosis of exclusion, it is also possible that infant deaths attributed to SIDS resulted from other causes.[11]

The usual history of an infant with SIDS is one of a previously healthy infant who is found dead after going to sleep for a nap or for the night. In the past, these deaths have often been attributed to infanticide, allergic responses, infections, or suffocation. Current theory, however, suggests that an abnormal control of ventilation places the infant at particular risk for this disorder. The ventilatory response of an infant varies from that of the adult in several ways.[12] Unlike the adult, the newborn infant responds to hypoxemia with a temporary increase in ventilation, followed by a sustained decrease in ventilation. The hypoxemia may induce periodic breathing with periods of apnea lasting from 10 to 20 seconds. Even before birth, hypoxemia such as that produced by cigarette smoking in the mother has been observed to cause a decrease in the breathing movements of the fetus. Episodes of periodic breathing are most severe in premature and high-risk infants. Periodic breathing in infants occurs primarily during sleep and may be partly related to the compliant chest wall of the infant. During REM sleep, which constitutes about 50% to 80% of sleep in infants, there is a loss of intercostal muscle tone; this leads to an exaggeration of the paradoxical chest motion and airway collapse as the diaphragm contracts and pulls the chest cage inward. It has been suggested that partial obstruction of the airways or inadequacy of the ventilatory pump of infants at risk for SIDS causes alveolar hypoxia, which leads to hyperplasia of pulmonary vascular smooth muscle and hypoxemia, which leads to changes in brain stem cells.[10] Both pulmonary vascular hyperplasia and changes in the brain stem cells have been observed on autopsy in infants who died of SIDS. As the pulmonary vascular muscularity increases, pulmonary vasoconstriction becomes more intense, increasing the afterload burden of the right heart enough to promote cardiac failure and even more severe hypoxia. The brain stem changes promote hypoventilation and hypoxemia, causing further brain stem injury.

Diagnosis and treatment

Measures for the management and treatment of SIDS have focused on methods of identifying those infants at risk. High-risk infants (*e.g.*, those with near-miss SIDS and infants who have been successfully resuscitated) are placed on home monitoring programs, and the parents are trained in both monitoring and cardiorespiratory resuscitation methods.

Hyperventilation syndrome

The hyperventilation syndrome involves overbreathing, reduction in PCO_2, and respiratory alkalosis. In 1871, De Costa provided the first account of the syndrome in the medical literature when he reported on the cases of 300 Civil War soldiers affected with the disorder. The disorder has subsequently been labeled soldier's heart, irritable heart, De Costa's syndrome, and neurocirculatory asthenia. De Costa noted that the affected soldier "got out of breath, could not keep up with his comrades, was annoyed with dizziness and palpitation, and with pain in the chest; his accouterments oppressed him, and all through this he appeared well and healthy." The nervous manifestations of the syndrome were "headache, dizziness, and disturbed sleep."[12] Removal from the stress of active duty along with enforced rest reduced the symptoms, but even with removal from active duty, the "irritability of the heart remained."[12]

Causes

The causes of hyperventilation syndrome have been categorized into four groups: (1) organic, (2) physiological, (3) emotional, and (4) habitual.[13] Organic causes include such things as drug effects and central nervous system lesions, such as meningitis. Responses to high altitude, heat, and exercise constitute physiological causes of hyperventilation.[14] Emotional states that predispose to hyperventilation are hysteria, anxiety, depression, and anger. Although stress may trigger the initial event, anxiety and fear over the symptoms may perpetuate the syndrome.[15] Because the symptoms of hyperventilation syndrome commonly involve the heart and head, the person experiences intense anxiety, often accompanied by a fear of death or of losing control. The condition occurs in children as well as adults.[16]

Manifestations

The hyperventilation syndrome commonly causes symptoms such as headache, dyspnea, numbness and tingling sensations, lightheadedness, chest pain, palpitations, and sometimes syncope. There are often complaints of dyspnea and being unable to take a full deep breath. Persons with a full constellation of the syndrome breathe with rapid, shallow breaths marked by irregularity in the depth and rate of respiration. Sighing is common. Hyperventilators are primarily thoracic rather than abdominal breathers. There is a tendency to breathe using the upper chest wall intercostal muscles, which may cause dull aching soreness in the left precordial area, mimicking angina. It has been suggested that the alkalosis associated with hyperventilation syndrome can induce coronary artery spasm in persons with Prinzmetal's angina[17,18] and in some individuals with atherosclerotic coronary artery disease.[18,19] It has also been observed that S–T wave changes can occur with hyperventilation.[16]

Many persons afflicted with the hyperventilation syndrome have not a continuously symptomatic state but rather recurrences of symptoms with or without recognizable provocative stresses. Others have a more chronic form of the disorder in which the respiratory center is reset to enable high levels of PCO_2 to persist in spite of a normal pH.[20] This may explain the chronicity of the disorder and the ease with which symptoms associated with hyperventilation can be provoked in individuals who are chronically hypocapnic. Sympathetic nervous system stimulation provokes a hyperventilatory response and may increase the occurrence of symptoms in persons with chronic hyperventilation problems.

It has recently been observed that panic disorder and hyperventilation syndrome have similar manifestations. Hyperventilation has been demonstrated in persons with panic episodes, and panic is a frequent manifestation of hyperventilation. It has been suggested that some persons with either diagnosis have the same disorder and share a biologically and often genetically determined hypersensitivity of a central nervous system alarm system.[21]

Diagnosis and treatment

A provocative test, in which a person deliberately hyperventilates, can be done to demonstrate occurrence of the symptoms.[13] Arterial blood gases may be obtained to study the pH and carbon dioxide levels. Electrocardiograph monitoring is done during the test on persons who have complained of chest pain, and caution should be used when performing the test on persons with known or suspected coronary heart disease. The treatment focuses on educating the person and his family about the disorder, relaxation therapy, and training to overcome faulty breathing patterns. Rebreathing into a paper bag can be used to control the symptoms. For many individuals, the realization that they can control their symptoms and nothing is seriously wrong reduces their anxiety and helps them to control the disorder.

In summary, alterations in the control of ventilation include drug-induced disorders, respiratory muscle weakness, sleep apnea, SIDS, and the hyperventilation syndrome. Almost all the drugs known to cause depression of the respiratory system have been associated with impairment of ventilation. Drugs can act centrally to depress the respiratory center, or they may act peripherally at the level of the myoneural junction. Weakness of the respiratory muscles can result from conditions that denervate the muscles, affect the myoneural junction, or directly involve muscle tissue. Sleep apnea involves 30 or more apneic spells characterized by the cessation of airflow through the nose and mouth for a period of 10 seconds or longer. It can result from disorders that compromise the patency of the airways during sleep (obstructive sleep apnea) or disorders that affect the central nervous system and respiratory neurons (central sleep apnea). SIDS is the most common cause of death in infants 1 to 12 months of age. Although its cause is unknown, current theory suggests that these infants have immature or impaired ventilatory control mechanisms. The hyperventilation syndrome consists of overbreathing, reduction in PCO_2, and respiratory alkalosis. It can result from organic causes such as drug effects and central nervous system lesions, physiological changes due to heat exposure and exercise, emotional states, or habit. It can cause headache, dyspnea, numbness and tingling sensations, lightheadedness, palpitations, and sometimes syncope.

Acute respiratory failure

Respiratory failure occurs when the lungs are unable to adequately oxygenate the blood or prevent undue retention of carbon dioxide even at rest. Respiratory failure can develop acutely in persons whose lungs previously had been normal or may be superimposed on chronic disease of the lung or chest wall. It has been reported that obstructive lung disease accounts for about one-third of the cases of acute respiratory failure in intensive care units.[22]

There is no absolute definition of the levels of

arterial PO_2 and PCO_2 that indicate respiratory failure. As a general rule, *respiratory failure* refers to a PO_2 level of 50 mmHg or less and *hypercapnia* (hypercarbia) to a PCO_2 level greater than 50 mmHg. These values are not altogether reliable when dealing with persons who have chronic lung disease, because many of these persons are alert and functioning with blood gas levels outside this range. Table 26-2 compares the normal values for blood gases with those of respiratory failure.

Causes

Respiratory failure is not a specific disease. It is associated with a number of disorders in which the lungs fail to deliver sufficient oxygen to the arterial blood or to remove sufficient carbon dioxide. Three types of conditions contribute to the hypoxemia in respiratory failure: hypoventilation, impaired diffusion across the alveolar capillary membrane, and mismatching of ventilation and perfusion. These conditions include impaired ventilation due to upper airway obstruction, weakness or paralysis of the respiratory muscles, chest wall injury, and disease of the pulmonary airways and lungs. The causes of respiratory failure are summarized in Table 26-3; many are discussed in other parts of the text.

Manifestations

Respiratory failure may be seen in previously healthy persons as the result of acute disease or trauma involving the respiratory system, or it may develop in the course of a chronic respiratory disease. The presenting signs and symptoms are different in each of these situations. The common manifestations of respiratory failure are hypoxemia and hypercapnia. Various types of respiratory failure are associated with different degrees of hypoxemia and carbon dioxide retention. In the respiratory syndrome that causes impaired diffusion across the alveolar capillary membrane, hypoxemia becomes severe, whereas arterial PCO_2 decreases or remains normal because carbon dioxide is more soluble in the alveolar capillary membrane than oxygen. In conditions, such as chronic obstructive pulmonary disease, in which respiratory failure is superimposed on lung disease, severe mis-

Table 26-2. Blood gases in respiratory failure compared with normal values

Arterial blood gas value	Normal value	Respiratory failure
PO_2	Above 80 mmHg	50 mmHg or less
PCO_2	35–45 mmHg	50 mmHg or above

Table 26-3. Causes of respiratory failure

Category of impairment	Examples
Impaired ventilation	
Upper airway obstruction	Laryngospasm
	Foreign body aspiration
	Tumor of the upper airways
	Infection of the upper airways (*e.g.*, epiglottitis)
Weakness or paralysis of the respiratory muscles	Drug overdose
	Injury to the spinal cord
	Poliomyelitis
	Guillain-Barré syndrome
	Muscular dystrophy
	Disease of the brain stem
Chest wall injury	Rib fracture
	Burn eschar
Impaired matching of ventilation and perfusion	
	Chronic obstructive lung disease
	Restrictive lung disease
	Severe pneumonia
	Atelectasis
Impaired diffusion	
Pulmonary edema	Left heart failure
	Inhalation of toxic materials
Respiratory distress syndrome	Respiratory distress syndrome in the newborn
	Adult respiratory distress syndrome (shock lung)

matching of ventilation and perfusion often results in both hypoxemia and hypercapnia.

Hypoxemia

In hypoxemia, the blood oxygen levels are insufficient to meet the oxidative requirements of body tissues. These tissues vary considerably in their vulnerability to hypoxia; those with the greatest need are the nervous system and heart.

The signs and symptoms of hypoxemia can be grouped into two categories: those resulting from impaired function of vital centers and those resulting from the activation of compensatory mechanisms. Central nervous system hypoxia produces symptoms similar to acute intoxication. There may be personality changes, restlessness, agitated or combative behavior, muscle incoordination, euphoria, impaired judgment, delirium, and eventual coma. The neurologic manifestations are frequently the presenting clinical features in acute respiratory failure. Tachycardia, cool skin (peripheral vasoconstriction), diaphoresis, and a mild increase in blood pressure result from the recruitment of sympathetic compensatory mechanisms. Although cyanosis may be evident, its presence cannot be relied on. Its detection requires a concentration of approximately 5 g/dL of hemoglobin in the circulating blood (see Chapter 24). When the hemoglobin concentration is normal, this means that the arterial saturation must be reduced to below 70% and the arterial PO_2 reduced to less than 35 mmHg before cyanosis develops, hence it is a late sign of hypoxemia.[22] This is especially critical in persons with anemia, since they may be severely hypoxic but lack the hemoglobin necessary for development of cyanosis. Hypotension and bradycardia are often preterminal events in hypoxemia, indicating the failure of compensatory mechanisms. The signs and symptoms of hypoxemia are listed in Chart 26-2.

Hypoxemia may be insidious in onset, and its symptoms may be attributed to other causes, particularly in chronic lung disease. Decreased sensory function, such as impaired vision or fewer complaints of pain, may be an early sign of hypoxia. This is probably because the involved sensory neurons have the same need for high levels of oxygen as do other parts of the nervous system.

Hypercapnia

Carbon dioxide has a direct vasodilatory effect on many blood vessels and a sedative effect on the nervous system. When the cerebral vessels are dilated, headache will develop. The conjunctiva are hyperemic and the skin flushed. Hypercapnia has nervous system effects similar to those of an anesthetic—hence the term *carbon dioxide narcosis*. There is progressive somnolence, disorientation, and, if untreated, coma. Mild to moderate increases in blood pressure are common. The signs and symptoms of hypercapnia are summarized in Chart 26-3. The body adapts to chronic increases in blood levels of carbon dioxide, hence persons with chronic hypercapnia may not develop symptoms until the PCO_2 is markedly elevated. Elevated levels of PCO_2 are characterized by respiratory acidosis, discussed in Chapter 29.

Chart 26-2: Signs and symptoms of hypoxemia

Arterial PO_2 below 50 mmHg	Loss of judgment
Tachycardia	Euphoria
Mild increase in blood pressure	Unruly or combative behavior
Cool and moist skin	Sensory impairment
Confusion	Mental fatigue
Delirium	Drowsiness
Difficulty in problem solving	Stupor and coma (late)
	Hypotension (late)
	Bradycardia (late)

Chart 26-3: Signs and symptoms of hypercapnia

Increased PCO_2
Headache
Conjunctival hyperemia
Flushed skin
Increased sedation
  Drowsiness
  Disorientation
  Coma
Tachycardia
Diaphoresis
Mild to moderate increase in blood pressure

Treatment

Treatment of respiratory failure is directed toward correcting the cause and relieving the hypoxemia and hypercapnia; and for this purpose a number of treatment modalities are available, including establishment of an airway, use of bronchodilators, antibiotics for respiratory infections, and others. Controlled oxygen therapy and mechanical ventilation are used in treating blood gas abnormalities associated with respiratory failure.

Oxygen therapy

Oxygen may be given by nasal cannula, catheter, Venturi mask, or mask–bag combination. Oxygen may also be administered directly into an endotracheal or tracheostomy tube. A high-flow administration system is one in which the flow rate and reserve capacity are sufficient to provide all of the inspired air. A low-flow oxygen system delivers less than the total inspired air. The oxygen must be humidified as it is being administered. The flow rate (liters per minute) is based on the arterial PO_2. The rate must be carefully monitored in persons with chronic lung disease because marked increases in PO_2 (above 60 mmHg) are apt to depress the ventilatory drive. There is also the danger of oxygen toxicity with high concentrations of oxygen. Continuous breathing of oxygen at high concentrations can lead to diffuse parenchymal lung injury. Persons with normal lungs begin to experience respiratory symptoms ranging from substernal distress to paresthesias, nausea and vomiting, general malaise, and fatigue after breathing 100% oxygen (at 1 atmosphere) for 6 to 30 hours.[23]

Mechanical ventilation

When alveolar ventilation is inadequate to maintain PO_2 or PCO_2 levels because of either respiratory or neurologic failure, mechanical ventilation may be life-saving. There are two types of positive pressure mechanical ventilators—pressure-controlled units and volume-controlled units. The pressure-controlled ventilator delivers a tidal volume determined by the airway pressure while the flow rate is being controlled. The volume-controlled ventilator delivers a preselected tidal volume while the pressure is monitored. The tidal volume and respiratory rate are adjusted to maintain ventilation at a given minute volume. A nasotracheal, orotracheal, or tracheotomy tube is inserted into the trachea to provide the patient with the airway needed for mechanical ventilation.

A third type of ventilator (iron lung, Cuirass, Poncho, and Body wrap) use negative pressure to expand the chest. They do not require an artificial airway. One of the disadvantages of the negative pressure ventilators is the fact that the application of negative pressure to the abdominal cavity causes blood returning to the right atrium to pool in the large abdominal veins, causing a transient decrease in venous return and cardiac output.[24]

—— Adult respiratory distress syndrome

The adult respiratory distress syndrome (ARDS) is an extreme form of noncardiac pulmonary edema and is the final common pathway through which many serious localized and systemic disorders exert their effect on the respiratory system. At least 50% of persons with ARDS die despite the most sophisticated intensive medical care.[25]

The exact cause of ARDS is unknown. It is thought to result from injury to the microcirculation (small blood vessels and capillaries) of the lung. Numerous insults are associated with its development. The term *shock lung* (see Chapter 23) has been used to describe the respiratory distress syndrome associated with trauma and hypovolemic or septic shock. It may also result from aspiration, infectious processes, hematologic disorders, metabolic events, and reactions to drugs and toxins (Chart 26-4). It is not known whether the condition results from several distinct pathogenic mechanisms that operate to cause a similar pattern of injury or whether a similar pattern of injury is triggered by different mechanisms.[25]

Although a number of conditions may lead to ARDS, they all produce similar pathologic lung changes. The permeability of the alveolar capillary membrane increases, which permits large protein molecules to move out of the vascular compartment into the interstitium and alveoli of the lung. The increased protein concentration in the interstitial spaces contributes to the entry of water. The surface tension in the alveoli may increase markedly because of the inactivation of surfactant by the plasma proteins and

---

Chart 26–4: Conditions in which the respiratory distress syndrome can develop*

Aspiration
Gastric acid
Near-drowning

Reaction to drugs and toxins
Chlordiazepoxide
Heroin
Methadone
Propoxyphene
Chloroform
Colchicine
Barbiturates
Inhaled gases
  Ammonia
  Phosgene
  Ozone
  Oxygen (high concentrations)
  Smoke

Hematologic disorders
Multiple blood transfusions
Disseminated intravascular clotting (DIC)
Exposure to cardiopulmonary bypass

Infectious causes
Bacterial pneumonia
Fungal and *Pneumocystis carinii* pneumonias
Gram-negative sepsis
Tuberculosis
Viral pneumonia

Immune reactions
Anaphylactic shock
Allergic reactions to inhaled substances

Metabolic disorders
Diabetic ketoacidosis
Uremia

Trauma
Burns
Fat embolus
Head trauma
Chest trauma and lung injury
Shock

* This list not intended to be inclusive.

---

injury to the surfactant-producing alveolar cells. This and the increased pressure caused by excess fluid in the interstitial spaces cause alveolar collapse and make the lung stiff and difficult to inflate. The compliance of the lung decreases, and the work of breathing increases. Hyaline membranes develop and line the alveolar ducts and alveoli, compromising the diffusion of respiratory gases.

Clinically, the syndrome consists of progressive respiratory distress, an increase in respiratory rate, and signs of respiratory failure. X-ray findings usually show extensive bilateral consolidation of the lung tissue. Severe hypoxemia persists in spite of increased inspired oxygen levels.

The treatment goals in ARDS are to supply oxygen to vital organs and provide supportive care until the condition causing the pathologic process has been reversed and the lungs have had a chance to heal. Assisted ventilation using high concentrations of oxygen may be required to overcome the hypoxemia. Positive end-expiratory pressure (PEEP) breathing, which increases the pressure in the airways during expiration, may be used to assist in reinflating the collapsed areas of the lung and improve the matching of ventilation and perfusion.

In summary, respiratory failure is a condition in which the lungs fail to adequately oxygenate the blood or prevent undue retention of carbon dioxide. The causes of respiratory failure are many: it may arise acutely in persons with previously healthy lungs or may be superimposed in chronic lung disease. It is generally defined as a PO_2 of 50 mmHg or less and a PCO_2 of 50 mmHg or more. Hypoxemia incites sympathetic nervous system responses such as tachycardia and produces symptoms similar to those of alcohol intoxication. Hypercapnia causes vasodilation of blood vessels, including those in the brain, and has an anesthetic effect (carbon dioxide narcosis). Adult respiratory distress syndrome (ARDS) is an extreme form of noncardiogenic pulmonary edema that results in respiratory failure. The condition can be caused by a number of serious localized and systemic disorders that cause damage to the alveolar capillary membrane of the lung. It results in interstitial edema of lung tissue, an increase in surface tension due to inactivation of surfactant, collapse of the alveolar structures, a stiff and noncompliant lung that is difficult to inflate, and impaired diffusion of the respiratory gases with severe hypoxemia that is resistant to oxygen therapy.

References

1. Kales A, Vela-Bueno A, Kales J: Sleep disorders: Sleep apnea and narcolepsy. Ann Intern Med 106:434, 1987
2. Phillipson EA: Breathing disorders during sleep. Basics of RD 7(3):102, 1979
3. Cherniack NA: Respiratory dysrhythmias during sleep. N Engl J Med 305:325, 1981
4. Gulleminault C, Cummeninsky J, Dement WC: Sleep Apnea: Recent Advances. Adv Int Med 25:347, 1980
5. Mosko SS, Dickel MJ, Paul T, et al: Sleep apnea and sleep-related periodic leg movements in community resident seniors. J Am Geriatr Soc 36:502, 1988
6. Burroughs BJ, Knudson RJ, Quan SF: Respiratory Disorders, 2nd ed, p 132, St. Louis: CV Mosby, 1983
7. Rapoport DM, Sorkin B, Garay SM, et al: Reversal of the "Pickwickian syndrome" by long-term use of nocturnal nasal-airway pressure. N Engl J Med 307:931, 1982
8. Brownell LG, West P, Sweatman P, et al: Protriptyline in obstructive sleep apnea. N Engl J Med 307:1038, 1982
9. Valdes-Dapena MA: Sudden infant death syndrome: A review of the medical literature 1974-1979. Pediatrics 66: 597, 1980
10. Shannon DC, Kelly DH: SIDS and Near-SIDS. N Engl J Med 307:1022, 1982
11. Thach BT: Sudden infant death. N Engl J Med 315:126, 1986
12. Kryger MH (ed): Pathophysiology of Respiration, p 265. New York, John Wiley, 1981
13. Magarian GJ: Hyperventilation syndromes: Infrequently recognized common expression of anxiety and stress. Medicine 61:219, 1982
14. Pfeffer JM: The aetiology of the hyperventilation syndrome. Psychosomatics 30:47, 1978
15. Lum LC: Hyperventilation: The tip of the iceberg. J Psychosom Res 19:375, 1975
16. Herman SP, Stickler GB, Lucas AR: Hyperventilation syndromes in children and adolescents: Long-term follow-up. Pediatrics 67:183, 1981
17. Mortenson SA, Vihelmson R, Sande E: Prinzmetal's variant angina (PVA), circadian variation in response to hyperventilation. Acta Med Scand (suppl) 644:38, 1981
18. Yasue H, Nagao M, Omote S, et al: Coronary artery spasm and Prinzmetal's variant form of angina induced by hyperventilation and tris-buffer infusion. Circulation 58:56, 1978
19. Yasue H, Omote S, Takizawa A, et al: Alkalosis-induced coronary vasoconstriction: Effects of calcium, diltiazem, nitroglycerin and propranolol. Am Heart J 102:206, 1981
20. Gennari FJ, Goldstein MB, Schwartz WB: The nature of renal adaptation to chronic hypocapnia. J Clin Invest 51:1722, 1972
21. Cowley DS, Roy-Byrne PP: Hyperventilation and panic disorder. Am J Med 83:929, 1987
22. Rogers RM, Weiler C, Ruppenthal B: The impact of intensive care unit on survival of patients with acute respiratory failure. Heart Lung 1:475, 1973
23. Pierce AK: Oxygen toxicity. Basics of RD 1(2)1972
24. Vasbinder-Dillon D: Understanding mechanical ventilation. Crit Care Nurs 8(7):42, 1988
25. Brandstetter RD: The adult respiratory distress syndrome—1986. Heart Lung 15:155, 1986

Bibliography

Balk R, Bone RC: The adult respiratory distress syndrome. Med Clin North Am 67:685, 1983

Balk R, Bone RC: Classification of acute respiratory failure. Med Clin North Am 67 (3):551, 1983

Block AJ: Dangerous sleep: Oxygen therapy for nocturnal hypoxemia. N Engl J Med 306:166, 1982

Block AJ: Respiratory disorder during sleep. Heart Lung 9:1011, 1980

Bonds DR, Crosby LO: Sudden death syndrome: Old causes rediscovered. N Engl J Med 315:126, 1986

Cane RD, Shapiro BA: Mechanical ventilatory support. JAMA 254:87, 1987

Compernolle T, Hoogduin K, Loele L: Diagnosis and treatment of the hyperventilation syndrome. Psychosomatics 20:612, 1979

Cowley DS, Roy-Byrne PP: Hyperventilation and panic disorder. Med Clin North Am 83:929, 1987

Demling DH, Nerlich M: Acute respiratory failure. Surg Clin North Am 63:337, 1983

Fanburg BL: Oxygen toxicity: Why can't a human be more like a turtle? J Intensive Care Med 3:134, 1988

Fletcher EC, Levin DC: Cardiopulmonary hemodynamics during sleep in subjects with chronic obstructive pulmonary disease. Chest 85:6, 1984

Guilleminault C, Quera-Salva MA, Nino-Murcia G, et al: Central sleep apnea and partial obstruction of the upper airway. Ann Neurol 21:465, 1987

Harman E, Wynne JW, Block AJ, et al: Sleep-disordered breathing and oxygen desaturation in obese patients. Chest 79:256, 1981

Jenkinson SG: Oxygen toxicity. J Intensive Care Med 3:137, 1988

Kryger MH (ed): Sleep disorders. (Symposium) Clin Chest Med 6:553 (entire issue), 1985

Luce JM: Respiratory complications of obesity. Chest 78:626, 1980

Marshall JR: Hyperventilation syndrome or panic disorder— What's in a name. Hosp Pract, Oct 15, p 105, 1987

Massaro D. Oxygen toxicity and tolerance. Hosp Pract, July 15, p 95, 1986

Mechanical ventilation (A series of 4 articles). Am J Nurs 84:1372, 1984

Noll ML: SVO$_2$ monitoring. Crit Care Nurs 8(7):11, 1988

Vasbinder-Dillon D: Understanding mechanical ventilators. Crit Care Nurs 8(7):42, 1988

Remolina C, Khan AU, Santiago TV et al: Positional hypoxemia in unilateral lung disease. N Engl J Med 304:523, 1981

Reischman RR: Impaired gas exchange related to intrapulmonary shunting. Crit Care Nurs 8(8):35, 1988

Rinaldo JE, Rogers RM: Adult respiratory distress syndrome. N Engl J Med 315:578, 1986

Rochester DF, Arora NS: Respiratory muscle failure. Med Clin North Am 67 no 3, 1983

Schroeder CH: Pulse oximetry: A nursing care plan. Crit Care Nurs 8(8): 50, 1988

Sprung CL, Pons G, Elser B, et al: The adult respiratory distress syndrome. Postgrad Med 74(1):253, 1983

Valdes-Depena MA: Sudden death syndrome: A review of the literature 1974–1979. Pediatrics 66:597, 1979

Hoffman LA: Ineffective airway clearance related to neuromuscular dysfunction. Nurs Clin North Am 22:151, 1987

Hurewitz AN, Bergofsky EH: Pathogenetic mechanisms in chronic pulmonary hypertension. Heart Lung 14:327, 1986

Kelson SG: The effects of undernutrition on the respiratory muscles. Clin Chest Med 7:101, 1986

Kim MJ, Larson JL: Ineffective airway clearance and ineffective breathing patterns. Nurs Clin North Am 22:125, 1987

Massaro D: Oxygen: Toxicity and tolerance. Hosp Pract 21, July 15, p 95, 1986

Openbrier DR, Covey M: Ineffective breathing pattern related to malnutrition. Nurs Clin North Am 22:225, 1987

Rochester DF: Malnutrition and the respiratory muscles. Clin Chest Med 7:91, 1986

Rochester DF, Enson Y: Current concepts in the pathogenesis of the obesity-hypoventilation 57:402, 1974

Skelton ME, Nield M: Ineffective airway clearance related to artificial airway. Nurs Clin North Am 22:167, 1987

Wissing DR, Romero MD, George RB: Comparing the newer modes of mechanical ventilation. J Crit Illness 2:41, 1987

Alterations in Body Fluids

Alterations in Body Fluids and Electrolytes

Objectives

After you have studied this chapter, you should be able to meet the following objectives:

_____ Differentiate between the intracellular and extracellular compartments in terms of distribution of body fluids and electrolytes.

_____ Define the term _electrolyte_.

_____ State the advantage of using milliequivalents or millimols to describe electrolyte concentrations in body fluids or pharmacological solutions.

_____ Relate the concept of a concentration gradient to the processes of diffusion and osmosis.

_____ List the determinants of body water and electrolytes levels.

_____ Cite the sources of all body secretions.

_____ Explain why water is essential to life by summarizing its functions in the body.

_____ List major sources of body water gain and loss.

_____ State the function and stimuli of thirst.

_____ List the major stimuli for release of ADH by the posterior pituitary.

_____ Explain how ADH regulates the urine concentrating ability of the kidneys.

_____ Compare the pathology and manifestations of diabetes insipidus and the syndrome of inappropriate antidiuretic hormone (SIADH).

_____ Describe the causes of fluid volume deficit with reference to the skin, gastrointestinal tract, third spaces, and the kidneys.

_____ Describe the effects of fluid volume deficit on the skin, circulatory system, brain and nervous system, urinary system, and gastrointestinal system.

(continued)

_____ Differentiate between fluid volume excess and water intoxication in terms of their causes and manifestations.

_____ Describe the effect of body water levels on the sodium concentration in the extracellular fluids.

_____ State the functions of sodium.

_____ Describe the effect of aldosterone on renal regulation of body sodium levels.

_____ Cite the causes of hyponatremia and hypernatremia in terms of altered intake, output, and regulation mechanisms.

_____ Relate the functions of sodium to the clinical manifestations of hyponatremia and hypernatremia.

_____ Explain the functions of potassium.

_____ Explain the role of the kidneys in regulating potassium levels.

_____ Describe the relationship of pH to potassium balance.

_____ State the causes of hypokalemia and hyperkalemia in terms of altered intake, output, and intracellular vs extracellular distribution mechanisms.

_____ Relate the functions of potassium to the clinical manifestations of hypokalemia and hyperkalemia.

_____ Explain the interaction of serum calcium and phosphate.

_____ Describe the role of vitamin D in regulating serum calcium and phosphate levels.

_____ Describe the role of parathyroid hormone and calcitonin in regulating serum calcium levels.

_____ Explain the difference between protein-bound, citrate and other calcium salts, and ionized calcium.

_____ List the functions of calcium.

_____ Describe the causes of hypocalcemia in terms of altered gastrointestinal tract absorption, mobilization of bone stores, renal losses, and protein or citrate binding.

_____ Relate the manifestions of hypocalcemia and hypercalcemia to the functions of ionized calcium.

_____ List the functions of phosphate.

_____ Describe the causes of hypophosphatemia and hyperphosphatemia in terms of altered intake and elimination.

_____ Relate the manifestations of hypophosphatemia and hyperphosphatemia to the functions of phosphate.

_____ List the major functions of magnesium.

_____ Explain the interactions between magnesium, calcium, and potassium.

_____ State the rationale for the neurologic and cardiovascular manifestations of magnesium deficits.

Body fluids contain water, electrolytes, proteins, and other substances. The precise regulation of these fluids within a very narrow physiologic range is essential to life. Normally, the volume and composition of these fluids remain relatively constant in the presence of a wide range of changes in intake and output. Environmental stresses and disease conditions often increase losses, impair intake, and otherwise interfere with mechanisms that regulate body fluid volume, composition, and distribution. The discussion in this chapter, which is limited to the water and electrolyte composition of body fluids, is divided into three parts: (1) regulation of body fluids, (2) alterations in body water, and (3) alterations in the electrolyte composition of body fluids.

Properties of body water

—— Distribution

Body fluids are distributed between two body compartments. The *intracellular compartment* consists of the fluid contained within all of the body's billions of cells (Figure 27-1). The *extracellular compartment* contains all of the fluid located outside of the cells. Included in the extracellular compartment are the interstitial fluids (fluids that surround the cells), intravascular fluids, cerebral spinal fluid, and fluid contained within the various body spaces such as the pleural cavity and the joint spaces. Even the water contained in the anterior chamber of the eye is considered to be extracellular fluid.

—— Electrical properties

Body fluids contain both water and chemical compounds. In solution, these chemical compounds can either remain intact or separate in a process known as *dissociation*. Electrolytes are substances that dissociate in solution to form *charged particles,* or *ions.* For example, a sodium chloride molecule dissociates to form a positively charged sodium (Na^+) and a negatively charged chloride (Cl^-) ion. Particles such as glucose and urea do not dissociate into ions and are called *nonelectrolytes.*

Positively charged ions are called *cations* because they are attracted to the cathode of a wet electric cell. Similarly, negatively charged ions are called *anions* because they are attracted to the anode. The ions found in body fluids carry either one charge (*a monovalent ion*) or two charges (*a divalent ion*). Polyvalent ions are present in some body fluids. These are not discussed in this chapter.

The location of electrolytes is influenced by their electrical charges. You will recall that ions with like charges repel and ions with opposite charges attract. This attraction or repulsion can cause electro-

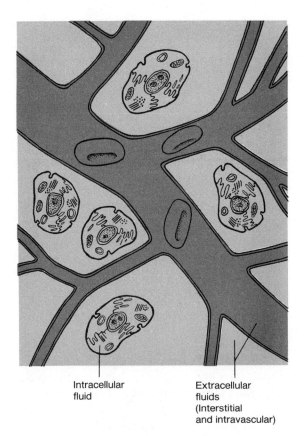

Figure 27-1 Distribution of body water—the extracellular space includes the vascular compartment and the interstitial spaces.

Intracellular fluid

Extracellular fluids (Interstitial and intravascular)

lytes to move from one body compartment to another. In other words, an excess of positively charged ions in a body compartment attracts negatively charged ions in an attempt to balance the electrical charge.

As a general rule, the total number of cations in the body equals the total number of anions. The unit that expresses the charge equivalency of a given weight of an electrolyte is milliequivalents per liter (mEq/liter). One milliequivalent of sodium will have the same number of charges as 1 mEq of chloride regardless of molecular weight (though sodium will be positive and chloride will be negative). The number of milliequivalents in a substance can be derived from the following formula:

$$\text{mEq/liter} = \frac{\text{mg/100 ml} \times 10 \times \text{valence}}{\text{atomic weight}}$$

The International System of Units expresses electrolytes as millimoles per liter (mmol/liter).

$$\text{mmol/liter} = \frac{\text{mEq/liter}}{\text{valence}}$$

This means that 1 mEq will equal 1 mmol of a monovalent electrolyte. Laboratory reports of serum electrolytes and electrolyte composition of intravenous solutions and other medications are expressed as either mEq/liter or mmol/liter. Some electrolytes such as calcium, phosphate, and magnesium are expressed in mg/dl.

Chemical properties

In a biologic system, the concentration of dissolved particles in a solution influences water movement and controls cell size. Diffusion is the movement of charged or uncharged particles along a concentration gradient. The behavior of sugar added to a container of water is an example of diffusion. Initially, the concentration of sugar will be greatest at the point where it comes in contact with the water. Moments later, however, the sugar will have diffused so that its concentration has been equalized throughout the container. Many small molecules diffuse through fluid-filled channels from one body compartment to another along a concentration gradient.

Most of the membranes in the body are semipermeable. This means that they allow water and small uncharged particles to diffuse freely through their pores while partially or completely preventing the passage of charged ions and large molecules. In diffusing through a semipermeable membrane, water moves from the side with the lesser number of nondiffusible particles to the side that has the greater number (Figure 27-2). The pressure due to water movement is called the *osmotic pressure*.

The osmotic activity, or work potential, that the nondiffusible particles exert in drawing water

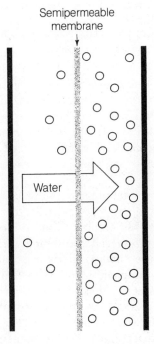

Figure 27-2 Movement of water across a semipermeable membrane. Water movement is from the side that has the lesser number of nondiffusible particles to the side that has the greater number.

Semipermeable membrane

Water

from one side of the semipermeable membrane to the other is measured through the use of a unit called an *osmol.* The osmol is the standard unit of osmotic pressure and is derived from the gram molecular weight —one gram mol of a nondiffusible and nonionizable substance is equal to 1 osmol. In the clinical setting, osmotic activity is usually expressed in milliosmols (one-thousandths of an osmol) per liter. Each nondiffusible particle, large or small, is equally effective in its ability to pull water through a semipermeable membrane. Thus, the osmotic activity of a solution is determined by the number, rather than the size, of the nondiffusible particles.

The osmotic activity of a solution may be expressed as either osmolarity or osmolality. Osmolarity refers to the osmolar concentration in 1 liter of solution (mOsm/liter), whereas osmolality refers to the osmols dissolved in 1 kg of water (mOsm/kg H_2O). Although the terms *osmolarity* and *osmolality* are often used interchangeably, most clinical laboratories report osmotic activity as osmolality. The normal serum osmolality of body serum is approximately 275 mOsm/kg H_2O to 295 mOsm/kg H_2O.

The predominant osmotically active particles within the cell are potassium and its attendant anions. In the extracellular fluid, sodium and its attendant anions account for 90% to 95% of the osmotic pressure. Urea and glucose normally account for less than 5% of the total osmotic pressure in the extracellular compartment. This can change, however, as when blood glucose is elevated in persons with diabetes mellitus or when blood urea nitrogen rises in persons with renal failure.[1]

The cell is enclosed in a flexible membrane; therefore, any change in its volume produces a change in cell size. The term *tonicity* refers to the tension or effect that the osmotic pressure of a solution exerts on cell size because of water movement across the cell membrane. By definition, a *hypertonic* solution is one that causes a cell to shrink or become *crenated* (Figure 27-3). A *hypotonic* solution causes a cell to swell. An *isotonic* solution is one that does not cause a change in cell size.

The osmotic pressure in the extracellular and intracellular compartments is usually the same, except for momentary differences. This is because water moves freely across cell membranes in response to osmotic pressure changes. Body cells may shrink or swell, but the osmolality of the intracellular fluid will remain the same as that of the extracellular fluid. When water is lost from the extracellular compartment, water diffuses out of the intracellular compartment into the extracellular compartment until an equilibrium is reached.

As a general rule, the volume and composition of body fluids at any given time are directly re-

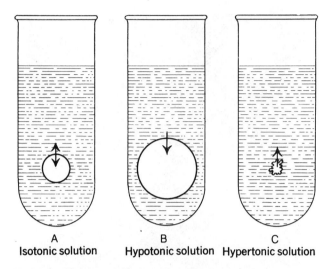

| A | B | C |
| Isotonic solution | Hypotonic solution | Hypertonic solution |

Figure 27-3 Osmosis: (**A**) red cells undergo no change in size in isotonic solutions, (**B**) they increase in size in hypotonic solutions, and (**C**) they decrease in size in hypertonic solutions. *(Chaffee EE, Greisheimer EM: Basic Physiology and Anatomy, 3rd ed. Philadelphia, JB Lippincott, 1974)*

lated to the amount of water or electrolyte that is taken into or added to body fluids minus the amount that is lost from the body. For example, the total amount of sodium chloride that is present in the body at any given time will reflect the oral or parenteral intake, or both, minus what has been lost from the body through the skin, kidneys, and bowel.

As a method for approaching the study of fluids and electrolytes, it is recommended that the reader consider the following categories of information: (1) the purpose or function that water or a given electrolyte serves in relation to overall body function; (2) body requirements, including those related to age differences; (3) sources of gain and loss; and (4) body mechanisms for regulating water and electrolyte levels. When this framework is used to place the causes and manifestations of fluid and electrolyte disorders in context, understanding of the subject is facilitated.

In summary, body fluids are distributed between the intracellular and extracellular compartments of the body. The extracellular fluid compartment contains the intravascular fluid, the interstitial fluid, and the fluid contained in the extracellular spaces, such as the pleural cavity. Body fluids contain water, charged particles called *electrolytes,* and noncharged particles called *nonelectrolytes.* Electrolytes are measured in *mEq* per liter or mmol per liter, measurement units, that express the charge equivalency of a given weight of an electrolyte. Diffusion is the movement of charged and noncharged particles along a concentration gradient. Both electrolytes and nonelectrolytes move between body compartments by diffusion. The movement of water across the semipermeable membranes of the body is controlled by the nondiffusible particles on either side of the membrane in a process called *osmosis*. Osmosis is regulated by the number rather than the size of the nondiffusible particles. The tension or effect that the osmotic pressure of a solution exerts on body cells is called tonicity. When cells are exposed to a hypotonic solution, they swell; when they are exposed to a hypertonic solution, they shrink.

Alterations in fluid volume

Body water is distributed between the intracellular and extracellular compartments. The intracellular compartment contains about two-thirds of the body's water and the extracellular compartment about one-third. In the adult, intracellular water constitutes about 45% of body weight and extracellular fluid about 15% (Figure 27-4). The distribution of body water is determined by the osmotic properties of body fluids and the concentration of electrolytes. Water provides about 90% to 93% of the volume in the extracellular fluid compartment.

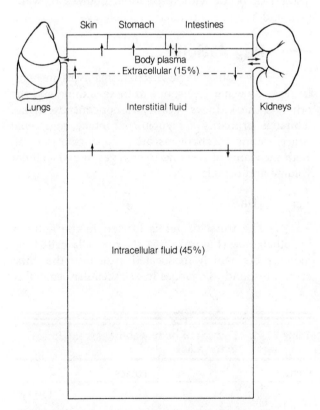

Figure 27-4 Fluid compartments in the adult. Fluid in the intracellular compartment constitutes about 45% of body weight, whereas fluid in the extracellular compartment constitutes about 15% of body weight. Fluid from the extracellular compartment moves into the gastrointestinal tract, skin, lungs, and kidneys.

Chart 27–1: Functions of water
Provides form for body structures
Acts as a transport vehicle for
nutrients
electrolytes
blood gases
metabolic wastes
heat
electrical currents
Provides insulation
Aids in the hydrolysis of food
Acts as a medium and reactant for chemical reactions
Acts as a lubricant
Cushions and acts as a shock absorber

Functions

The functions of water in the human body are many (Chart 27-1). Water adds to the structure of the body, acts as a transport vehicle, lubricates and cushions, acts to hydrolyze food in the digestive system, and is necessary for chemical reactions that occur within the cell.

It is water that gives the body its structure. One has only to compare the dry and wrinkled skin of an elderly person with that of a child to become aware of the extent to which water contributes to the overall form and appearance of the body. Water adds a resiliency to the skin and underlying tissues that is often referred to as *skin* or *tissue turgor*. Tissue turgor is assessed by pinching a fold of skin between the thumb and forefinger. Normally, the skin immediately returns to its normal configuration when the fingers are released. A loss of 3% to 5% of body water causes the resiliency of the skin to be lost, and the tissue will remain raised for several seconds.

The transport of body nutrients, wastes, electrical currents, and heat depends on fluid movement both in the interstitial spaces and in the vascular compartment. In relation to body temperature, water not only transports heat from the inner core of the body to the periphery where it can be released into the external environment, but it also insulates the body against changes in the external temperature. Were it not for the insulation afforded the body by its water content, the body would be much like a rock, gaining heat during the day and losing it at night.

Water also lubricates and cushions. Synovial fluid lubricates the joints, and pericardial fluid prevents the heart from rubbing against the pericardial sac. The act of swallowing would be difficult, if not impossible, were it not for the lubricating properties of the mucus that lines the gastrointestinal tract. The cerebral spinal fluid acts to cushion the brain. During pregnancy, amniotic fluid acts as a shock absorber and protects the delicate fetus.

Water hydrolyzes the food eaten, breaking it down into particles that can be digested and then absorbed across the gastrointestinal tract wall. In addition, many of the chemical reactions that occur within the body require water as a medium or reactant.

Requirements

The body is largely water, and therefore body water is usually expressed as a percentage of body weight. Total body water varies with age, decreasing from infancy to old age. In the full-term infant, body water constitutes as much as 75% to 80% of body weight, whereas body water accounts for only 60% to 70% of body weight in the adult. The premature infant has even greater amounts of body water than the full term infant; the elderly person has much less water in relation to body weight than the younger adult. Because fat is essentially water free, obesity tends to decrease the percentage of water that the body contains, sometimes reducing these levels to values as low as 45% of body weight.

Despite its greater body water content, the infant is more likely to develop fluid imbalances than the adult. This is because the infant has both a higher metabolic rate and a larger surface area in relation to its body mass than an older child or adult. Also, the infant has more difficulty in concentrating its urine because its kidney structures are immature. This means that the infant has greater skin and urine losses and that more water is needed to transport metabolic wastes. The infant, therefore, both ingests and excretes greater volumes of water in relation to its size than the adult. For example, an infant may exchange one-half of its extracellular fluid volume in a single day, whereas an adult exchanges only about one-sixth of this volume during the same period. By the third year of life, the percentages and distribution of body water in the young child approach those of the adult.

Regardless of age, all normal individuals require approximately 100 ml of water per 100 calories metabolized. This means that a person expending 1800 calories for energy requires approximately 1800 ml of water for metabolic purposes. The metabolic rate increases with fever: there is a 12% increase in metabolic rate for every 1°C (7%/1°F) increase in body temperature.

Gains and losses

The main source of water gain is absorption from the gastrointestinal tract; the water gained in this manner includes that obtained from fluids, ingested foods, tube feedings, parenterally administered fluids, and sometimes the water used in rectal irrigation.

Water is also derived from cellular oxidation of foodstuffs. The quantity gained in this manner varies from 150 ml to 250 ml depending on the rate of metabolism.

Water losses occur through the kidneys, skin, lungs, and gastrointestinal tract. Even when oral and parenteral intake has been withheld, the kidneys continue to produce urine as a means of ridding the body of metabolic wastes. The urine output that is required to eliminate these wastes is called the *obligatory urine output*. The obligatory urine loss is about 300 ml to 500 ml/day.

Water losses that occur from the skin and respiratory tract are termed *insensible water losses* because the individual is not aware of them. Under normal conditions, water vapor lost from the skin and lungs approximates 500 ml/m^2 of surface area per day. Skin losses include the water that continually diffuses through the pores in the skin as well as the water lost in the process of sweating. Respiratory losses consist of water vapor that is withdrawn from the mucous membranes to humidify the inspired air and then is lost to the environment during expiration. For readers who have lived in a cold climate, the frosty breath that they see on a cold day is evidence of water losses that occur with respiration. Sources of water gain and loss are illustrated in Table 27-1.

Regulation

Two physiologic mechanisms assist in regulating body water levels; one of these is thirst and the other is the kidneys' ability to concentrate urine. Thirst is primarily a regulator of intake, and renal concentrating mechanisms are regulators of output. Both mechanisms respond to changes in extracellular volume and osmolality.

Thirst

The thirst center is located in the anterior hypothalamus (Figure 27-5). Nerve cells called osmoreceptors, which are located in or near the thirst center, respond to changes in extracellular osmolality

Table 27-1. Sources of body water gains and losses in the adult

Gains		Losses	
		Urine	1500 ml
Oral intake		Insensible losses	
As water	1000 ml	Lungs	300 ml
In food	1300 ml	Skin	500 ml
Water of oxidation	200 ml	Feces	200 ml
Total	2500 ml	Total	2500 ml

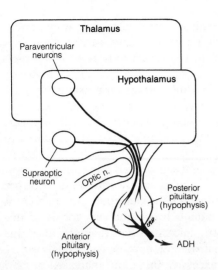

Figure 27-5 The centers of the hypothalamus and pituitary gland, which are involved in water balance. ADH is synthesized by cells in supraoptic and paraventricular nuclei of the hypothalamus; it travels along a neural pathway to the posterior pituitary where it is stored for future release. The thirst center also is located in the anterior hypothalamus.

by either swelling or shrinking. Thirst occurs when an increase in extracellular osmolality causes these cells to shrink. Thirst is one of the earliest symptoms of water loss, occurring when water loss is equal to 2% of body weight.

The most common cause of thirst is an increase in the osmolality of the extracellular fluids. A second cause of thirst is severe hypokalemia, which significantly lessens the kidneys' ability to concentrate urine. This results in polyuria followed by *polydipsia,* excessive thirst. Hypokalemia is known to stimulate the synthesis of prostaglandin E. Inasmuch as prostaglandin E is known to stimulate thirst, it is also possible that polydipsia secondary to hypokalemia is mediated by prostaglandins. A third cause of thirst is a decrease in blood volume, which may or may not be associated with a decrease in serum osmolality. Thirst is one of the earliest symptoms of hemorrhage, often being present long before other signs of blood loss begin to appear. Last, dryness of the mouth produces a sensation of thirst that is not necessarily associated with the body's state of hydration; for example, the thirst that a lecturer experiences as the mouth dries during speaking. It is interesting to note that in animal experiments in which salivary secretion was blocked, excessive drinking did not occur unless the animals were eating food.[2] This same effect has been reported in humans with salivary glands that did not secrete saliva, suggesting that the lubricating properties of water are needed for swallowing food.

Polydipsia is normal when it accompanies conditions of water deficit. Although infrequent, a water excess can occur as the result of excess intake that is unrelated to need. An example of excessive water intake occurs in psychogenic polydipsia. Persons afflicted with this disorder drink water in excess of what the kidneys can excrete. A 1977 news story related the fatal outcome of a 29-year-old woman with a diagnosis of chronic schizophrenia who was drinking 4 gallons of water a day to "cleanse her body of cancer."[3] The thirst mechanism may also be depressed. This sometimes occurs in elderly individuals, particularly following a stroke.

Renal concentrating mechanisms

The kidneys control the concentration of most of the constituents in body fluids, including water and electrolytes. Each kidney has about 1 million functional units called nephrons (see Chapter 30). Water and electrolytes are filtered from the blood in the glomerulus and are then selectively reabsorbed in the tubules. The rate at which water and electrolytes can be removed from the body is determined by renal blood flow and the glomerular filtration rate; urine output declines during shock as renal blood flow falls. As the urine filtrate moves through the tubule, water and electrolytes that are needed for maintaining the volume and composition of body fluids are reabsorbed into the extracellular fluid and those that are not needed are excreted in the urine.

Antidiuretic hormone (ADH)

The reabsorption of water by the kidneys is regulated by the antidiuretic hormone (ADH), also known as *vasopressin.* ADH is synthesized by cells in the supraoptic and paraventricular nuclei of the hypothalamus (Figure 27-5). The hormone is transported along a neural pathway (the hypophyseal tract) to the neurohypophysis (posterior pituitary) and is then stored for future release. A rise in ADH levels produces an increase in water reabsorption from the distal tubules and collecting ducts of the kidneys. As with thirst, ADH levels are controlled by volume and osmolar changes in the extracellular fluids. Osmoreceptors in the hypothalamus sense changes in extracellular osmolality and stimulate the production and release of ADH. A small increase in serum osmolality of 1% to 2% is sufficient to cause ADH release. Likewise, stretch receptors in the great veins, atria, and carotid sinus area sense changes in blood volume or blood pressure, and input from these receptors aids in regulation of ADH release.

A blood volume decrease of 10% to 15% produces a maximal increase in ADH levels, and blood pressure reductions of 5% to 10% are needed to increase ADH levels.[1] As with many other homeostatic mechanisms, acute conditions tend to produce greater changes in ADH levels than chronic conditions; long-term changes in blood volume or blood pressure may exist without affecting ADH levels.

Many stress situations increase the synthesis and release of ADH. Severe pain, nausea, trauma, surgery, certain anesthetic agents, and some analgesic drugs increase ADH levels. Nausea can increase ADH levels 10 times to 1000 times those required for maximal diuresis.[1] Interestingly, vomiting that occurs in the absence of nausea does not affect ADH levels. Among the drugs that affect ADH are nicotine, which stimulates its release, and alcohol, which inhibits it. Table 27-2 lists drugs that are known to affect ADH levels.

Two important conditions serve to alter ADH levels: diabetes insipidus and inappropriate secretion of ADH. Because of their effects on water balance, both of these conditions are discussed in this chapter.

Diabetes insipidus. Diabetes insipidus means "tasteless diabetes" as opposed to diabetes mellitus, or "sweet diabetes." Diabetes insipidus occurs because of a defect in the synthesis or release of ADH *(central diabetes insipidus)* or because the kidneys do not respond to ADH *(nephrogenic diabetes insipidus)*. About 60% of diabetes insipidus seen clinically results from tumors or lesions in the hypophyseal tract.[4] Temporary diabetes insipidus can follow head injury or surgery near the hypophyseal tract. Nephrogenic diabetes insipidus may occur as an X-linked recessive trait or, more commonly, as a result of kidney disease, potassium depletion, or chronic hypercalcemia.

Persons with diabetes insipidus are unable to concentrate their urine during periods of water restriction; they excrete large volumes of urine, usually 3 to 5 liters per day. This large urine output is accompanied by excessive thirst; as long as the thirst mechanism is normal and fluid is readily available, there is little or

no alteration in the fluid levels in persons with diabetes insipidus. The danger arises when the condition develops in an unconscious person, because an inadequate fluid intake rapidly leads to hypertonic dehydration and increased serum osmolality.

Diagnosis of diabetes insipidus is based on measurements of urine and serum osmolality. These tests may be used to evaluate the response to an infusion of a hypertonic saline solution or to pharmacologic preparations of ADH. Persons with nephrogenic diabetes insipidus do not respond to pharmacologic preparations of the hormone; this method is used to differentiate between the two forms of the disease. Diagnostic measures for diabetes insipidus include those that rule out psychogenic polydipsia as a reason for the excessive thirst and increased urine output. A recently developed radioimmunoassay test for ADH can be used for this purpose. When central diabetes insipidus is suspected, diagnostic methods such as skull x-rays and computed tomographic (CT) scans of the pituitary hypothalamic area are used to determine the cause of the disorder.

The treatment of central diabetes insipidus consists of treating any underlying disorder and supplying the body with pharmacologic preparations that contain the missing hormone. These preparations must be administered parenterally or nasally; they are not given by mouth because they are destroyed in the gastrointestinal tract. New nonhormonal forms of therapy have recently been introduced for cases in which ADH release is still present. The oral hypoglycemic agent chlorpropamide (Diabinese) may be used to stimulate ADH release in central diabetes insipidus. Other drugs that are used to treat this form of diabetes insipidus are carbamazepine (Tegretol) and clofibrate. In nephrogenic diabetes insipidus, the thiazide diuretics are now the specific form of therapy. These drugs probably act predominantly by causing an increase in sodium excretion by the kidneys, which lowers the glomerular filtration rate and increases reabsorption of fluid in the proximal tubule.[5]

Syndrome of inappropriate ADH. The syndrome of inappropriate ADH (SIADH) results from a failure of the negative feedback system that regulates the release and inhibition of ADH. When this syndrome is present, the secretion of ADH continues even when serum osmolality is decreased; this leads to a marked retention of water in excess of sodium, causing a dilutional hyponatremia. An increase in the glomerular filtration rate resulting from an increased plasma volume causes further increases in sodium loss. Urine osmolality is high and serum osmolality low. Urine output decreases despite adequate or increased fluid intake and the resultant water retention produces a rapid gain in body weight. Serum sodium, hematocrit, and blood urea nitrogen levels are all de-

Table 27-2. Drugs that affect ADH levels

Drugs that decrease ADH levels/action	Drugs that increase ADH levels/action
Demeclocycline	Acetaminophen
Ethanol	Analgesics (morphine and meperidine)
Glucocorticoids	Anesthetics (most)
Lithium carbonate	Antipsychotic tranquilizers
Morphine antagonists	Cancer drugs (vincristine and cyclophosphamide)
Norepinephrine	Carbamazepine
Phenytoin	Chlorpropamide
Reserpine, chlorpromazine	Clofibrate
	Isoproterenol
	Nicotine
	Phenobarbital
	Thiazide diuretics (chorothiazide)
	Tricyclic antidepressants

creased because of the expansion of the extracellular fluid volume.

The SIADH can be caused by a number of conditions, including lung tumors and chest lesions, central nervous system (CNS) disorders, and various pharmacologic agents. The first report of SIADH was made in the late 1950s in association with lung cancer. Tumors, particularly bronchogenic carcinoma, are known to produce and release ADH independent of hypothalamic control mechanisms. Other intrathoracic conditions, such as tuberculosis, pneumonia, and positive pressure breathing, are also known to cause SIADH. The suggested mechanism for SIADH in these cases is activation of the atrial volume receptors in response to decreased atrial filling with activation of atrial receptors that incite ADH release. Disease and injury to the CNS can cause direct pressure on or direct involvement of the hypothalamic-posterior pituitary structures. Examples include brain tumors, hydrocephalus, head injury, meningitis, and encephalitis. Other stimuli, such as pain, stress, and temperature changes, are capable of stimulating ADH release through the limbic system. Drugs induce SIADH in different ways; some drugs are thought to increase hypothalamic production and release, whereas others are believed to act directly on the renal tubules to potentiate the action of ADH.

SIADH may occur as a transient condition, as in a stress situation, or as a chronic condition resulting from conditions such as a lung tumor. The severity of symptoms is usually proportional to the extent of sodium depletion and water intoxication. Symptoms of mild SIADH (serum sodium levels around 130 mEq/liter) include headache, anorexia, muscle cramps, general fatigue, and dulling of the sensorium. In severe SIADH (serum sodium levels below 126 mEq/liter) neurologic symptoms of acute water intoxication begin to appear; they include nausea, vomiting, muscular twitching, seizure, and coma.

The treatment of SIADH depends on its severity. In mild cases the treatment consists of fluid restriction. If fluid restriction is not sufficient, diuretics such as mannitol or furosemide (Lasix) may be given to promote diuresis and free water clearance. Lithium and the antibiotic demeclocycline inhibit the action of ADH on the renal collecting ducts and are sometimes used in treating the disorder. In cases of severe sodium depletion, a hypertonic (3% or 5%) sodium chloride solution may be administered intravenously.

Fluid volume deficit

The extracellular fluid compartment is the source of all body secretions, including sweat, urine, and gastrointestinal tract secretions. Fluid volume deficit occurs when loss of body fluids exceeds fluid intake. Water moves rapidly between body compartments; because of this, an extracellular fluid volume deficit is usually accompanied by a deficit of intracellular fluids. Fluid deficit is a serious threat, especially those with limited ability to conserve water. Dehydration caused by diarrhea continues to be one of the leading causes of death among small children in certain parts of the world.

Causes

There are two main causes of fluid volume deficit: inadequate intake and increased losses (Table 27-3).

Impaired intake. Fluid intake may be reduced because of a lack of access to water, impaired thirst, unconsciousness, or neuromuscular problems that prevent water access or impair swallowing. Access to water is commonly taken for granted. However, for someone with impaired movement, water availability becomes a problem. With hypodipsia, or impaired thirst, the need for water intake does not activate the thirst stimulus. The inability to swallow impairs water intake.

Excessive losses
Gastrointestinal losses. There is a continuous exchange of fluid between the extracellular compartment and the lumen of the gastrointestinal tract. In a single day, 8 to 10 liters of extracellular fluid is secreted into the gastrointestinal tract; most of this fluid is reabsorbed as the bowel contents move toward the anus. Vomiting and diarrhea interrupt the reabsorption process and in some situations lead to increased secretion of fluid (in excess of 8–10 liters) into the gastrointestinal tract; the presence of irritating or hypertonic contents increases the movement of fluid into the bowel, exaggerating fluid losses. In many forms of diarrhea, the rate of fluid secretion into the gastrointestinal tract is increased because of the osmotic or irritating effects of the causative agent. In Asiatic cholera, death can occur within a matter of hours as irritating substances formed by the cholera organism cause excessive amounts of fluid to be secreted into the bowel; these fluids are then lost as vomitus or diarrheal fluid.

Urine losses. The kidneys normally regulate the volume and solute concentration of the extracellular fluid—promoting diuresis in conditions of fluid excess and conserving water when extracellular fluid volume is decreased. Extracellular fluid deficit can result from osmotic diuresis or the injudicious use of diuretic therapy. In hyperglycemia, serum sodium is diluted as the osmotic effects of the elevated glucose cause water to be pulled out of body cells. The presence of glucose in the urine filtrate prevents reabsorption of water by the renal tubules; this causes increased losses of both sodium and water. The degree of hyponatremia, or serum sodium decrease, resulting from hyperglycemia can be estimated by assuming a 1.6 mEq/liter decrease in serum sodium for every 100 mg/ml rise in blood sugar above normal values.[6]

Surface area losses.   The skin acts as an exchange surface for body heat and as a vapor barrier to prevent water from leaving the body. Body surface losses of sodium and water increase when there is excessive sweating or when large areas of the skin have been damaged. Fever and hot weather increase sweating. In very hot weather, water losses through sweating may be increased as much as 1.5 liters/hour to 2.0 liters/hour.[2] Both respiratory rate and sweating are usually increased as body temperature rises. As much as 3 liters of water may be lost in a single day as a result of fever. Burns are another cause of excess fluid loss. Evaporative losses range from 0.8 ml to 2.6 ml/kg for every percentage point burn area. This loss can approach a level of 6 to 8 liters per day.[6]

Third space losses.   Third space losses refer to the sequestering of extracellular fluids in an area that is physiologically unavailable to the body—in the serous cavities, extracellular spaces in injured tissues, or the lumen of the gut. For example, fluid deficits can develop in intestinal obstruction as water and electrolytes pool in the distended bowel. Third spacing results from increased capillary permeability; there is a concomitant movement of plasma proteins into the sequestered area. The osmotic gradient associated with the presence of these colloids causes additional water to move into the third space area.

Manifestations

The signs and symptoms of fluid volume deficit are closely associated with the functions of water that were discussed earlier in the chapter. A discussion of the signs and symptoms associated with extracellular fluid deficit is complicated by the fact that fluid deficit may present as an isotonic depletion of fluid volume in which both water and sodium are lost or as a condition in which water losses exceed sodium

Table 27–3.   Fluid deficit

Causes	Signs and symptoms
Inadequate fluid intake	**Acute weight loss (% body weight)**
Unconsciousness or inability to express thirst	Mild extracellular deficit: 2% loss
Oral trauma or inability to swallow	Moderate extracellular deficit: 2–5% loss
Impaired thirst mechanism	Severe extracellular deficit: 6% or more loss
Withholding of fluids for therapeutic reasons	**Thirst**
Excessive fluid losses	**Decreased urine output**
Gastrointestinal losses	Increased urine osmolality
Vomiting	Increased specific gravity
Diarrhea	**Increased serum osmolality**
Gastrointestinal suction	Increased hematocrit
Fistula drainage	Increased BUN
Urine losses	**Decreased vascular volume**
Diuretic therapy	Tachycardia
Osmotic diuresis (hyperglycemia)	Weak and thready pulse
Adrenal insufficiency	Postural hypotension
Salt-wasting renal disease	Decreased vein filling and increased vein refill time
Skin losses (salt and water)	Hypotension and shock
Fever	**Decreased volume in extracellular spaces**
Exposure to hot environment	Depressed fontanel in an infant
Burns and wounds that remove skin	Sunken eyes and soft eyeballs
Third space losses (sodium and water)	**Loss of intracellular fluid**
Intestinal obstruction	Dry skin and mucous membrane
Edema	Cracked and fissured tongue
Ascites	Decreased salivation and lacrimation
Burns (first several days)	Neuromuscular weakness
	Fatigue
	Increased body temperature

loss. The signs and symptoms presented in this section of the chapter apply in both circumstances. The signs and symptoms of fluid volume deficit are summarized in Table 27-3.

Body weight.   A decrease in body weight is one of the best indicators of fluid loss. One liter of water weighs 1 kg (2.2 lb). A mild extracellular fluid deficit exists when weight loss equals 2% of body weight; in a person weighing 68 kg (150 lb) this percentage weight loss equals 1.4 liters of water. Severe fluid deficit exists when weight loss is in excess of 6% of body weight. To be accurate, weight must be measured at the same time each day, with an equal amount of clothing being worn. Because extracellular fluid is trapped within the body in persons with third space losses, body weight may not decrease when extracellular fluid loss occurs for this reason.

Intake and output.   Intake and output measurements afford a second method for assessing fluid balance. Although these measurements provide insight into the causes of fluid imbalance, they are often inadequate in measuring actual losses and gains. This is because accurate measurements of intake and output are often difficult to obtain and insensible losses are difficult to estimate. Pflaum reported a mean error in intake and output calculations of 800 ml per day compared with daily weight measurements.[8]

Thirst.   Thirst is an early symptom of water deficit, occurring when water losses are equal to 1% to 2% of body weight. Unfortunately, infants and persons who are unconscious or who cannot communicate are unable to express this need. Also, thirst is not always present in isotonic fluid deficit that is caused by sodium depletion.

Urine output.   Urine output usually decreases and urine osmolality and specific gravity increase during periods of water deficit. An exception to this rule occurs when the fluid deficit follows either an impairment in the kidneys' ability to concentrate urine or diuresis occurring for other reasons. Normally, the ratio of urine osmolality to serum osmolality in a 24-hour urine sample exceeds 1 to 1 and after an overnight fast should be greater than 3 to 1. A dehydrated patient (one who has a loss of water) may have a urine-to-serum ratio that approaches 4 to 1. In these patients, urine osmolality may exceed 1000 mOsm/kg H_2O. In persons who have difficulty concentrating their urine—for example, those with diabetes insipidus or chronic renal failure—the urine-to-serum ratio is often less or equal to 1 to 1. Urine specific gravity compares the weight of urine with that of water, providing an index for solute concentration. A change in specific gravity of 1.010 to 1.020 (water is considered to be 1.000) is an increase of 400 mOsm/

kg H_2O. In the sodium-depleted state, the kidney will usually try to conserve sodium; urine specific gravity will be normal and urine sodium and chloride concentrations will be low.

Serum osmolality.   The normal serum osmolality is 275 mOsm/kg H_2O to 295 mOsm/kg H_2O. Because the serum in the extracellular compartment is roughly 90% to 93% water, the concentration of blood cells and other solutes will increase as extracellular water decreases. This is true of hematocrit and blood urea nitrogen (BUN). Serum sodium concentration will also increase when fluid deficit is due primarily to a water loss.

Extracellular volume.   Arterial and venous volumes decline during periods of fluid deficit. Both the pulse and the blood pressure change as the volume in the arterial system declines: The heart rate increases and the pulse becomes weak and thready. Postural hypotension is an early sign of fluid deficit, characterized by a blood pressure that is at least 10 mm Hg lower when one is sitting and standing than lying down. When volume depletion becomes severe, signs of shock and vascular collapse appear. On the venous side of the circulation, the veins become less prominent and venous refill time increases. A simple test to determine venous refill time consists of compressing the distal end of a vein on the dorsal aspect of the hand (when the hand is not in the dependent position). The vein is then emptied by "milking" the blood toward the heart. Normally, the vein will refill almost immediately when the occluding finger is removed. When venous volume is decreased, as occurs in fluid deficit, the venous refill time will increase.

The amount of fluid in all of the body spaces decreases in fluid volume deficit. Although most body spaces are not visible, a decrease in cerebral spinal fluid in the infant causes depression of the anterior fontanel. Likewise, the eyes assume a sunken appearance and feel softer than normal when the fluid content in the anterior chamber of the eye is decreased.

Intracellular volume.   As fluid is lost from the extracellular compartment in excess of solute, the extracellular fluid becomes hypertonic in relation to the fluid in the intracellular compartment. When this happens, the water is pulled out of body cells. The skin and mucous membranes become dry, and there is a decrease in the activity of the cells in the salivary and lacrimal glands. The tongue becomes dry and fissured. Swallowing is difficult. A reliable method for testing for dryness of the mouth is to place your finger on the mucous membranes where the gums and the cheek meet. When a fluid deficit is present, you will find that your finger does not glide easily because of the dryness. This method works well in infants and in persons who are unconscious.

One of the most serious aspects of a fluid deficit is the dehydration of brain and nerve cells. Generalized muscle weakness, muscle rigidity, and muscle tremors often occur in severe fluid deficit as water is removed from the cells in the nervous system. Delirium, hallucinations, and maniacal behavior may also develop when the fluid deficit is severe.

Body temperature. Dehydration is known to produce a rise in body temperature. Part of this elevation in temperature probably results from a lack of available fluid for sweating. Loss of vascular volume impairs the transport of core body heat to the periphery for exchange with the external environment. It also appears that dehydration has a direct effect on the hypothalamus, because dehydration can cause fever even in a cold environment. Body temperature may reach 105° when dehydration is severe.[9]

Treatment

The treatment of fluid deficit consists of replacement therapy, which includes replacing both the water and the electrolytes that have been lost. Replacement fluids can be given orally or intravenously. The oral route is usually preferable.

Oral glucose-electrolyte replacement solutions are available for the treatment of infants with diarrhea.[10] Until recently, these solutions were prescribed either early in the diarrhea illness to prevent dehydration or as a first step in reestablishing oral intake after parenteral replacement therapy. These solutions are now being widely used as replacements for intravenous fluids in the treatment of dehydration due to diarrhea in small children, especially in developing countries where the availability of intravenous fluids is limited and diarrhea is the leading cause of

death.[11] Although cola drinks are often recommended as folk remedies for dehydration caused by acute diarrhea, their electrolyte content is often inadequate for replacement purposes and their high sugar content may complicate the situation by inducing an osmotic diarrhea.[12] Intravenous replacement solutions continue to be the treatment of choice in severe fluid deficit.

Fluid volume excess

Fluid volume excess can result from retention of both sodium and water that produces an isotonic expansion of the extracellular fluid compartment or from water retention in excess of sodium (water intoxication). For purposes of clarification, an isotonic expansion of extracellular fluid volume will be referred as *fluid volume excess* and water retention in excess of sodium as *water volume excess*. Fluid volume excess involves an increase in both interstitial and vascular volumes. Water volume excess is accompanied by solute dilution and hypotonicity of the extracellular fluids.

Causes

An increase in body fluids usually results from decreased excretion, particularly if it is coupled with increased intake. With fluid volume excess, both sodium and water are usually retained. Among the causes of decreased sodium and water elimination are heart failure, cirrhosis of the liver, and decreased kidney function (Table 27-4). A condition called *circulatory overload* results from an increase in intravascular blood volume; it can occur during infusion of intravenous fluids or transfusion of blood if the amount or rate of administration is excessive. The elderly and persons with heart disease require careful observation

---

Table 27-4. Fluid excess

Causes	Signs and symptoms
Excessive sodium and water intake	**Acute weight gain (% body weight) in excess of 5%**
Excessive dietary intake	
Excessive ingestion of medications or home remedies containing sodium	**Increased extracellular fluid**
Excessive administration of parenteral solutions containing sodium	Pitting edema of the extremities
	Puffy eyelids
Inadequate renal losses	Pulmonary edema
Renal disease	Shortness of breath
Increased corticosteroid levels	Rales
Aldosterone	Dyspnea
Glucocorticoids	Cough
Congestive heart failure	Full and bounding pulse
Cirrhosis of the liver	Venous distention

because even small amounts of blood may overload the circulatory system. Although an increase in fluid volume often accompanies disease, this is not always true. For example, a compensatory isotonic expansion of body fluids occurs during hot weather as a mechanism for increasing body heat loss. As discussed previously, water retention that occurs with SIADH can produce hyponatremia and a hypotonic expansion of body fluids.

Manifestations

The manifestations of fluid or water excess depend on the effect of the excess fluid on serum osmolality. *Edema*, or excess fluid in the interstitial spaces, is characteristic of isotonic fluid excess (see Chapter 28). Just as weight loss is a good indicator of fluid volume deficit, so also is weight gain an indicator of fluid excess. In circumstances where the fluid excess accumulates gradually, edema fluid may mask weight loss that is due to actual loss of tissue mass; this often happens in debilitating disease conditions and in starvation. The edema associated with extracellular fluid excess may be generalized or it may be confined to dependent areas of the body such as the legs and feet. Often the eyelids are puffy when the person awakens. When excess fluid accumulates in the lungs, there is shortness of breath, complaints of difficult breathing, respiratory rales, and a productive cough (see Chapter 22). An increase in vascular volume causes the pulse to have a full and bounding quality.

The manifestations of water volume excess are largely related to solute dilution, decreased serum osmolality, and cellular swelling. The signs and symptoms may be acute (severe water intoxication) or more insidious in onset and less severe. Severe water intoxication is manifested by headache, nausea, vomiting, abdominal cramps, weakness, and stupor. Convulsions and coma may develop as a result of changes in the water content of brain cells. The manifestations of water volume excess are similar to those for hyponatremia that are summarized in Table 27-6.

Treatment

The treatment of fluid volume excess focuses on providing a more favorable balance between sodium and water intake and output. Diuretics are often used to increase sodium elimination. When there is need for intravenous fluid administration or transfusion of blood components, these should be carefully monitored to prevent fluid overload.

The treatment of water excess depends on its cause and severity. Water restriction may be sufficient (see treatment for SIADH). Hypertonic saline solutions may be used to reduce cellular swelling in cases of severe water intoxication.

In summary, body water is distributed between the intracellular and extracellular fluid compartments. Body water levels are regulated by thirst (intake) and by renal mechanisms that control urine concentration (output). Renal mechanisms for concentrating urine are mediated by ADH. Diabetes insipidus is a condition of inadequate ADH levels or function, and SIADH one of inappropriate secretion of the hormone. A fluid volume deficit is characterized by a reduction in intracellular and extracellular fluids. Fluid volume deficit causes thirst, a decrease in vascular volume and circulatory function, decreased urine output and increased urine specific gravity, and signs related to loss of fluid from the cellular compartment. The causes and manifestations of fluid volume deficit are summarized in Table 27-3. Fluid volume excess can exist as an isotonic expansion of body fluids or as a disproportionate increase in water volume (Table 27-4). Fluid volume excess is characterized by increases in both interstitial and intravascular fluids. Water volume excess, which is characterized by decreased serum osmolality and cellular swelling, occurs when water is retained in excess of sodium salts (as in SIADH).

Electrolyte disorders

Although water provides volume for the body fluids, it is the electrolytes that contribute to the function of these fluids. Electrolytes serve many functions. They (1) assist in regulating water balance, (2) participate in acid–base regulation, (3) contribute to enzyme reactions, and (4) play an essential role in neuromuscular activity. This section focuses on the alterations in body function that are associated with disturbances in sodium, potassium, calcium, phosphate, and magnesium balance. Alterations in bicarbonate and chloride concentrations are discussed in Chapter 29.

There are marked differences in the composition of intracellular and extracellular electrolytes (Table 27-5). The reader will note that the sodium concentration is greatest in the extracellular compartment, whereas potassium is concentrated within the cells. Blood (serum) tests measure the concentration of electrolytes in the extracellular compartment rather than the intracellular compartment. The suffix *-emia* refers to blood. Hyponatremia, for example, denotes a decreased sodium concentration in the blood. Although blood levels are usually representative of the total body levels of an electrolyte, this is not always the case, particularly with potassium, which is approximately 28 times more concentrated inside the cell than outside.

Table 27–5. Concentration of intracellular and extracellular electrolytes

Electrolytes	Intracellular concentration (mEq/l)	Intracellular concentration (mmol/l)	Extracellular concentration (mEq/l)	Extracellular concentration (mmol/l)
Sodium	10	10	137–147	137–147
Potassium	141	141	3.5–5.0	3.5–5.0
Chloride	4	4	100–106	100–106
Bicarbonate	10	10	24–31	24–31
Phosphate	75	38	2.0–3.0	1.0–1.5
Calcium	1	0.5	4.5–5.3	2.25–2.65
Magnesium	58	29	1.5–2.5	0.75–1.25

Alterations in sodium balance

Sodium affects many body functions. Regulation of serum sodium is essential for maintaining (1) the osmolality of the extracellular fluids, (2) normal neuromuscular function, (3) acid–base balance, and (4) numerous vital chemical reactions. As the major cation in the extracellular compartment, sodium and its attendant anions (chloride and bicarbonate) account for about 90% to 95% of the osmotic activity that is present in the extracellular fluids. Sodium is a component of sodium bicarbonate and, as such, is very important in regulating acid–base balance.

Causes. Sodium intake is normally derived from dietary sources. Body needs can usually be met by as little as 500 mg/day.* In the United States, the average salt intake is about 6 g to 15 g/day, or 12 to 30 times the daily requirement. Other sources of sodium are intravenous saline infusions and medications that contain sodium. An often-forgotten source of sodium is the sodium bicarbonate or other sodium-containing home remedies that are used to treat upset stomach or other ailments. Sodium ingestion in excess of what the kidneys can excrete is an unlikely occurrence in healthy individuals, probably because taste prohibits this from occurring and because of the kidney's remarkable ability to regulate sodium. Sodium excess has occurred, however, in persons receiving intravenous saline infusions and in persons unable to monitor their oral intake. The accidental substitution of salt for sugar in infant formulas has been known to produce severe hypernatremia, causing brain damage and death.

The body loses sodium through the kidneys, skin, and gastrointestinal tract. The kidneys are extremely efficient in regulating sodium output, and when sodium intake is limited or conservation of sodium is needed, the kidneys are able to reabsorb almost all of the sodium that has been filtered by the glomerulus. This results in an essentially sodium-free urine. Conversely, urinary losses of sodium will increase as intake is increased. For practical purposes, the 24-hour urinary excretion of sodium is assumed to be equal to sodium intake.

Alterations in kidney function can cause either an increase or a decrease in sodium losses. Sodium deficit with an accompanying loss of extracellular fluid occurs in salt-wasting kidney disease. On the other hand, many forms of kidney disease cause sodium retention. A decrease in renal blood flow causes increased sodium retention by means of the renin–angiotensin–aldosterone mechanism (discussed later in this chapter). For this reason, sodium retention is increased in nonrenal diseases that cause a decrease in renal blood flow. In congestive heart failure, renal blood flow is decreased because the heart does not pump properly.

Although skin losses of sodium are usually negligible, sweat losses can be extensive during exercise and periods of exposure to a hot environment. A person who sweats profusely can lose as much as 15 g to 30 g of sodium per day; this amount decreases to as little as 3 g to 5 g with acclimatization.[2] Loss of skin surface, such as occurs in extensive burns, also leads to excessive skin losses of sodium.

Sodium moves freely between the extracellular fluid and the contents of the gastrointestinal tract. In the upper part of the gastrointestinal tract, the concentration of sodium is very similar to that of serum. Sodium is reabsorbed as the contents of the gut move through the lower part of the bowel, so that the concentration of sodium in the stool is normally only about 32 mEq/liter. Sodium losses increase with vomiting, diarrhea, fistula drainage, and gastrointestinal suction. Irrigation of gastrointestinal tubes with distilled water removes sodium from the gastrointestinal tract, as do repeated tap water enemas.

Regulation

The normal serum concentration of sodium ranges from 135 mEq/liter to 147 mEq/liter (135 mmol/liter to 147 mmol/liter). It is important for the reader to recognize that serum sodium values reflect the concentration of sodium in the extracellular fluids, expressed as milliequivalents per liter, rather than an absolute amount. This means that dehydration will cause the concentration of sodium to increase even though the total body sodium remains unchanged. Likewise, fluid excess will cause sodium levels to decrease even though sodium has not been lost from the body.

Aldosterone regulation. The reabsorption of sodium by the kidneys is largely regulated by aldosterone. Aldosterone is a mineralocorticoid hormone

* In the absence of sweating.

(remember that sodium and potassium are minerals) that is produced by the adrenal cortex. In the distal tubules of the kidney, aldosterone promotes the reabsorption of sodium into the blood, and in exchange, potassium is secreted into the distal tubular fluid so that it can be eliminated in the urine. The aldosterone mechanism allows for fine tuning of serum sodium and potassium levels. When serum sodium levels are low or potassium levels are high, aldosterone levels become increased.

Several mechanisms are known to control aldosterone levels: (1) extracellular sodium levels, (2) extracellular potassium levels, (3) angiotensin II, and (4) the adrenocorticotropic hormone (ACTH). A reduction in renal blood flow increases aldosterone levels by means of the renin–angiotensin–aldosterone mechanism. When renal blood flow decreases, renin is released. Renin promotes the conversion of a circulating polypeptide, angiotensinogen, to angiotensin I. Angiotensin I is converted to angiotensin II in the lung. It is angiotensin II that increases aldosterone levels.

Although aldosterone increases sodium reabsorption by the kidney and thereby contributes to what might be called short-term regulation of sodium balance, it is thought to play only a minor role in long-term regulation of sodium levels. This is because an increase in sodium reabsorption through the aldosterone mechanism ultimately leads to an increase in renal blood flow and glomerular filtration rate, with a subsequent decrease in renin release.

In Addison's disease, a condition of chronic adrenal cortical insufficiency, there is unregulated loss of sodium in the urine accompanied by increased potassium retention due to impaired mineralocorticoid function. The glucocorticoid hormones produced in the adrenal cortex also have mineralocorticoid activity. Cushing's syndrome is a condition in which levels of glucocorticoid hormones are increased. The fact that these hormones increase salt and water retention helps to explain why persons who are being treated with drugs that contain exogenous forms of these hormones often develop hypertension and edema. Alterations in adrenocortical hormones are discussed in Chapter 44.

Sodium deficit

Sodium deficit in the extracellular fluids (hyponatremia) occurs when the sodium concentration in the blood falls below 137 mEq/liter (137 mmol/liter). Sodium deficit may result from an actual loss of sodium from the body, or from a dilution caused by a gain in extracellular water. Usually, sodium is lost from the body.

Causes. Excessive sodium losses occur with excessive sweating, gastrointestinal losses, and diuresis. Excessive sweating in hot weather leads to loss of sodium and water. Hyponatremia develops when tap water is used to replace fluids lost in sweating. (Salt tablets [0.5 g/500 ml water] or commercially available electrolyte solutions can be used to replace water and electrolytes lost through excessive perspiration.) Repeated tap water enemas or frequent gastrointestinal irrigations with distilled water remove sodium chloride from the gastrointestinal tract. Salt depletion also occurs with adrenal insufficiency and with diuresis due to vigorous use of diuretics (Table 27-6). Hyperglycemia, too, depresses serum sodium concentration. Because sodium is largely an extracellular cation, it becomes diluted as water moves out of cells in response to the osmotic effects of the elevated blood sugar level. It has been estimated that there is a 1.6 mEq/liter decrease in serum sodium for every 100 mg/dl rise in serum glucose above the normal level (100 mg/dl).

Normally, homeostatic mechanisms make it almost impossible to produce an increase in body water when renal function is adequate and ADH and aldosterone levels are normal. Excess water is retained, however, when a person has elevated ADH levels. Although uncommon, water excess can occur as the result of excessive water intake. As was mentioned earlier in the chapter, patients with psychogenic polydipsia drink water in excess of what the kidneys can excrete. Water intoxication in the psychiatric patient may be aggravated by treatment with antipsychotic drugs that increase ADH levels.

Manifestations. In hyponatremia, the osmotic pressure of the extracellular fluids becomes less than that in the cells and water moves from the extracellular compartment into the cells. The signs and symptoms of hyponatremia depend on the rapidity of onset and the severity of the sodium dilution. If the condition develops slowly, the signs and symptoms are usually not apparent until serum sodium levels approach 125 mEq/liter (125 mmol/liter). The brain and nervous system are the most seriously affected by increases in intracellular water, and neurologic signs and symptoms progress rapidly once serum sodium levels fall below 120 mEq/liter (120 mmol/liter). Gastrointestinal symptoms include anorexia, nausea and vomiting, abdominal cramps, and diarrhea. Swelling of brain tissue can cause headache, lethargy and weakness, mental depression, apprehension, confusion, personality changes, gross motor weakness, and even hemiplegia. Convulsions and coma occur when serum sodium levels reach extremely low levels. An acute increase in intracellular water is often of sudden onset and should be suspected in any postoperative or post-trauma patient who suddenly behaves in a bizarre fashion.

An increase in intracellular water produces another significant observation. The increased intracellular water content causes tissues to have a plastic consistency resembling that of modeling clay. This permits fingerprinting of the skin. If you roll your finger over the sternum, your fingerprint will become visible on the patient's skin. This is different from the tissue indentation that occurs with pitting edema.

—— Sodium excess

Sodium excess (hypernatremia) occurs when serum levels rise above 147 mEq/liter (147 mmol/liter).

Causes. Serum sodium excess almost always follows a loss of body fluids that have a lower than normal concentration of sodium so that water is lost in excess of sodium. This can occur (1) in diabetes insipidus, in which urinary losses of water are increased; (2) when respiratory losses are increased, as in tracheobronchitis; (3) during episodes of watery diarrhea; and (4) when osmotically active tube feedings are given with inadequate amounts of water. The therapeutic administration of sodium-containing solutions may also cause hypernatremia. Cardiopulmonary resuscitation may require the administration of large doses of sodium bicarbonate (50 mEq/50 ml vial). Hypernatremia will develop unless an additional 850

ml of water accompanies each set of three ampules that is administered.[6] Hypertonic saline intended for intraamniotic instillation for therapeutic abortion may inadvertently be injected intravenously, causing hypernatremia.

Generally hypernatremia, with an accompanying water deficit, will stimulate thirst and increase water intake. Hypernatremia is therefore more apt to occur in infants and persons who are unable to express their thirst or obtain water to drink. The unconscious person is particularly at risk for developing hypernatremia (Table 27-7).

Manifestations. The clinical manifestations of hypernatremia are largely related to an increase in serum osmolality; this causes water to be pulled out of body cells. Urine output is decreased because of renal conserving mechanisms. Thirst is excessive. Body temperature is frequently elevated, and the skin becomes warm and flushed. The mucous membranes are dry and sticky, and the tongue is rough and dry. The subcutaneous tissues assume a firm and rubbery texture. The vascular volume decreases; the pulse becomes rapid; and the blood pressure drops. Most significantly, water is pulled out of the cells in the central nervous system; this causes decreased reflexes, agitation, and restlessness. Coma and convulsions may develop as hypernatremia progresses. Permanent brain damage has occurred in infants recovering from severe hypernatremia.

Table 27–6. Sodium deficit (hyponatremia)

Causes	Signs and symptoms
Excessive sodium losses	**Laboratory values**
Sweating	Serum sodium below 137 mEq/liter (137
Gastrointestinal losses	mmol/liter)
Diuresis	Decreased serum osmolality
Sodium dilution	Dilution of other blood components, including
Excess administration of sodium-free	chloride, hematocrit, and BUN
parenteral solutions	**Increased water content of brain and nerve cells**
Psychogenic polydipsia	Headache
Ingestion of tap water during periods	Mental depression
of sodium deficit	Personality changes
Repeated administration of tap water	Confusion
enemas	Apprehension and feeling of impending doom
Kidney disease that impairs water	Lethargy, weakness
elimination	Stupor
Increased ADH levels	Coma
Trauma, stress, pain	Convulsions
SIADH	**Gastrointestinal disturbances**
Use of medications that increase	Anorexia, nausea and vomiting
ADH	Abdominal cramps
	Diarrhea
	Increased intracellular fluid
	Fingerprinting over sternum

Alterations in potassium balance

Potassium is the major cation in the intracellular compartment. Potassium affects many body functions and (1) contributes to maintenance of intracellular osmolality, (2) is necessary for neuromuscular control and the precise regulation of skeletal, cardiac, and smooth muscle activity, (3) influences acid–base balance, and (4) participates in many intracellular enzyme reactions. For example, potassium contributes to the intricate chemical reactions that transform carbohydrates into energy, change glucose into glycogen, and convert amino acids to proteins.

Causes. Potassium intake is normally derived from dietary sources. In healthy individuals, potassium balance can usually be maintained by a daily dietary intake of 50 mEq to 100 mEq. Additional amounts of potassium are needed during periods of trauma and stress. The kidneys are the main source of potassium loss. Renal losses of potassium are influenced by the urine flow rate, serum sodium concentration, potassium intake, acid–base balance, and aldosterone levels. Potassium is filtered in the glomerulus, reabsorbed with sodium and water in the proximal tubule and with sodium and chloride in the descending limb of Henle, and secreted into the distal tubule and collecting duct for elimination in the urine. Normally about 80% to 90% of potassium losses occur in the urine and the rest occur in the stool or sweat.

Regulation

Potassium is essentially an intracellular cation; all but about 2% of body potassium is contained within body cells.[14] This means that serum levels of potassium, which normally range from 3.5 mEq/liter to 5.0 mEq/liter (3.5 mmol/liter to 5.0 mmol/liter), do not always accurately reflect intracellular levels. Serum levels of potassium are mainly regulated by renal mechanisms and redistribution between the intracellular and extracellular compartments. When body cells are injured or when cellular activity becomes catabolic, potassium is released into the extracellular compartment and is then lost in the urine. Subsequently, with chronic potassium deficiency, the kidneys' ability to conserve potassium improves and the urine loss is reduced to as little as 5 mEq/liter (5 mmol/liter). When this happens, serum levels of potassium are likely to remain within normal levels even though total body potassium has decreased. However, serum potassium levels tend to fall when tissue breakdown ceases and cellular activity becomes anabolic,

Table 27–7. Sodium excess (hypernatremia)

Causes	Signs and symptoms
Excessive sodium intake	**Laboratory findings**
Rapid or excessive administration of parenteral sodium chloride or sodium bicarbonate solutions	Serum sodium above 147 mEq/liter (147 mmol/liter)
Excessive oral intake	Increased serum osmolality
Decreased extracellular water	**Thirst**
Increased water losses	**Urine output**
Diuretic therapy	Oliguria or anuria
Adrenal cortical hormone excess	High specific gravity
Diabetes insipidus	**Intracellular dehydration**
Tracheobronchitis	Skin and mucous membranes
Watery diarrhea	Skin dry and flushed
Hypertonic tube feedings	Mucous membranes dry and sticky
Decreased water intake	Tongue rough and dry
Unconsciousness or inability to express thirst	Subcutaneous tissue
Oral trauma or inability to swallow	Firm and rubbery
Impaired thirst mechanism	Central nervous system
Withholding of water for therapeutic reasons	Agitation and restlessness
	Decreased reflexes
	Maniacal behavior
	Convulsions and coma
	Increased body temperature
	Decreased vascular volume
	Tachycardia
	Decreased blood pressure
	Weak and thready pulse

causing potassium to move back into the cellular compartment. This is because potassium is needed for glycogen storage and protein synthesis. It has recently been shown that magnesium deficiency causes intracellular potassium depletion, whether or not there is adequate potassium intake. This is discussed in the section on alterations in magnesium.

Aldosterone regulation.   Aldosterone plays an essential role in regulating the extracellular potassium concentration. Urinary losses of potassium increase under the influence of aldosterone, whereas sodium retention is increased. The feedback regulation of aldosterone levels, in turn, is strongly regulated by serum potassium levels; for example, an increase in potassium ion concentration of less than 1 mEq/liter will cause aldosterone levels to triple. Furthermore, this increased secretion will continue for as long as the elevated potassium levels are present.

Potassium balance can be seriously affected by disorders of aldosterone secretion. *Primary aldosteronism* is caused by a tumor in the cells of the adrenal cortex (in the zona glomerulosa) that secrete aldosterone. Excess secretion of aldosterone by the tumor cells causes severe potassium losses and a decrease in serum potassium levels. Patients with this disorder may develop muscle paralysis as a result of the low serum levels of potassium. Adrenal insufficiency (Addison's disease) causes the opposite effect; persons with this disorder have elevated serum potassium levels due to an aldosterone deficiency.

Potassium-hydrogen ion exchange.   The hydrogen ion concentration (*p*H) of the extracellular fluid contributes to compartmental shifts of potassium. In acidosis, the movement of hydrogen ions into body cells is used as a means of buffering *p*H changes in the extracellular fluids. Generally, the serum potassium concentration rises 0.6 mEq/liter for each 0.1 unit fall in blood *p*H. When a hydrogen ion moves into the cell, another positively charged ion (potassium) must move out into the extracellular fluid. This means that potassium tends to move out of the intracellular compartment in acidosis and into the intracellular compartment in alkalosis.

A potassium and hydrogen exchange also occurs in the distal tubule of the kidney. When the extracellular concentration of potassium is high, tubular secretion of potassium into the urine is increased and hydrogen excretion is decreased, causing a decrease in serum *p*H (metabolic acidosis). Conversely, when extracellular concentrations of potassium are low, tubular secretion of potassium into the urine is decreased and hydrogen ion secretion is increased; this tends to lead to metabolic alkalosis. Metabolic alkalosis tends to exaggerate urine losses of potassium. This is because the excess negatively charged bicarbonate ions that are present in the urine must be accompanied by positively charged ions as they are eliminated. Some sodium ions are excreted with the bicarbonate, but some are also reabsorbed in exchange for potassium ions, which are then lost in the urine.

Potassium deficit

Hypokalemia refers to a decrease in serum potassium levels below 3.5 mEq/liter (3.5 mmol/liter). Because potassium moves freely between the intracellular and extracellular compartments, hypokalemia can occur as the result of a loss of total body potassium or because extracellular potassium has moved into the intracellular compartment. Usually both intracellular and extracellular potassium concentrations are decreased simultaneously.

Causes.   The causes of potassium deficit can be grouped into three categories: (1) inadequate intake, (2) excessive losses, and (3) redistribution between the intracellular and extracellular fluid compartments (Table 27-8).

The kidneys are unable to conserve potassium during periods of acute potassium loss, and continue to excrete it even in time of great need. This means that a potassium deficit can develop rather quickly if intake is inadequate. Unfortunately, intake is frequently impaired at the time that potassium losses are increased, as following surgery or during prolonged diarrhea. The elderly are particularly likely to develop a potassium deficit. This is because they often have poor eating habits as a consequence of living alone; they may have limited income, which makes buying foods high in potassium difficult; they may have difficulty in chewing many of the foods that have a high potassium content because of poorly fitting dentures; or they may have problems with swallowing. Furthermore, medical problems in the elderly often require treatment with drugs, such as diuretics, that tend to increase potassium losses.

The kidneys are the main source of potassium loss. Normally about 80% to 90% of potassium losses occur in the urine, with the remaining losses in the stool and sweat. Unfortunately, the kidneys do not have the homeostatic mechanisms needed to conserve potassium during brief periods of insufficient intake. An adult on a potassium-free diet will continue to lose approximately 5 mEq to 15 mEq of potassium daily. Following trauma, and in stress situations, urinary losses of potassium are greatly increased, sometimes approaching levels of 150 mEq/day to 200 mEq/day (150 mmol/liter to 200 mmol/liter). Diuretic therapy (with the exception of potassium-sparing diuretics such as spironolactone) results in additional urinary losses of potassium. Some antibiotics, particularly amphotericin B and gentamicin, are impermeable anions that require the presence of positively charged cations for elimination in the urine; this causes potassium wasting.

Although potassium losses from the skin and gastrointestinal tract are usually minimal, these losses can become excessive under certain conditions. For instance, burns increase surface losses of potassium, and sweat losses can become markedly increased in persons who are acclimated to a hot climate. This is partly because increased secretion of aldosterone during heat acclimatization increases the loss of potassium in both urine and sweat.[2] Gastrointestinal losses can also become excessive; this occurs with vomiting and diarrhea and when gastrointestinal suction is being used. The potassium content of liquid stools, for example, is about 40 mEq/liter to 60 mEq/liter (40 mmol/liter to 60 mmol/liter).[14]

Because of the high ratio of intracellular to extracellular potassium, a redistribution of potassium from the extracellular to intracellular compartment can produce a marked fall in serum levels. One cause of a potassium redistribution is insulin. Following insulin administration, there is increased movement of both glucose and potassium into cells. Potent beta-adrenergic drugs such as epinephrine and albuterol have a similar effect on potassium distribution. In a condition known as *familial periodic paralysis,* acute episodes of hypokalemia, sufficient to cause paralysis, are caused by redistribution of potassium.

Manifestations. Potassium deficit causes altered renal function and produces changes in skeletal, cardiac, and smooth muscle function. Often the signs and symptoms of potassium deficit are gradual in onset and for that reason go undetected for a long time.

Hypokalemia leads to an impairment in the kidneys' ability to concentrate urine and an increase in ammonia production. Urine output is increased, urine specific gravity is decreased, and serum osmolality is increased. There are complaints of polyuria, nocturia, and thirst. Increased ammonia production appears to

Table 27–8. Potassium deficit (hypokalemia)

Causes	Signs and symptoms
Inadequate intake	**Laboratory values**
Inability to eat	Serum potassium below 3.5 mEq/liter
Diet deficient in potassium	(3.5 mmol/liter)
Administration of potassium-free parenteral solutions	**Skeletal muscles**
Excessive gastrointestinal losses	Muscle tenderness, paresthesias, or cramps
Vomiting	Weakness
Diarrhea	Muscle flabbiness
Suction	Paralysis
Fistula drainage	**Cardiovascular system**
Excessive renal losses	Postural hypotension
Diuretic phase of renal failure	Increased sensitivity to digitalis
Diuretic therapy (except aldosterone antagonists)	Arrhythmias
Increased mineralocorticoid levels	**Gastrointestinal tract**
Cushing's syndrome	Anorexia
Primary aldosteronism	Vomiting
Treatment with glucocorticoid hormones	Abdominal distension
Intracellular shift	Paralytic ileus
Treatment for diabetic acidosis	**Respiratory muscles**
Alkalosis, either metabolic or respiratory	Shortness of breath
	Shallow breathing
	Kidneys
	Polyuria
	Low osmolality and specific gravity of urine
	Nocturia
	Thirst
	Central nervous system function
	Confusion
	Depression
	Acid–base balance
	Metabolic alkalosis

be a compensatory mechanism that occurs in response to a decrease in intracellular pH resulting from a potassium-hydrogen exchange that occurs with hypokalemia. As the intracellular pH falls, renal synthesis of ammonia is increased. Since ammonia is obtained through the deamination of amino acids, nitrogen balance becomes negative and protein synthesis is impaired. For this reason, children who need proteins for growth and persons who need amino acids for tissue repair are particularly vulnerable to prolonged periods of hypokalemia. Ammonia is eliminated through the liver. For persons with advanced liver disease, hypokalemia can lead to disturbing elevations in blood ammonia. At the level of the kidney, increased ammonia levels are thought to interfere with inflammatory and immune responses and to predispose to kidney infections.

Hypokalemia causes numerous signs and symptoms associated with gastrointestinal function. These include anorexia, nausea, vomiting, abdominal distention, absence of bowel sounds, and paralytic ileus. When gastrointestinal symptoms occur gradually and are not severe, they often serve to impair potassium intake and exaggerate the condition.

At least three defects in skeletal muscle function occur with potassium deficiency: (1) alterations in the resting membrane potential (see Chapter 1), (2) alterations in glycogen synthesis and storage, and (3) impaired ability to increase blood flow during strenuous exercise.[15] With hypokalemia there is hyperpolarization of neuromuscular tissue with decreased responsiveness to stimulation. Neuromuscular signs and symptoms appear when serum potassium levels fall to approximately 2.5 mEq/liter (2.5 mmol/liter). The clinical manifestations include muscle weakness, fatigue, and cramps, particularly during exercise. Paralysis can occur with severe hypokalemia. Leg muscles, particularly the quadriceps, are most prominently affected. Some patients complain of muscle tenderness and paresthesias rather than weakness. In chronic potassium deficiency, actual muscle atrophy may occur and contribute to muscle weakness. In familial periodic paralysis, episodes of hypokalemia cause attacks of flaccid paralysis that last from a few minutes to several hours. The paralysis may be precipitated by situations that cause severe hypokalemia by producing an intracellular shift in potassium, such as a high-carbohydrate meal or administration of insulin, epinephrine, or glucocorticoid drugs. The paralysis is often reversed by potassium therapy. Severe hypokalemia may affect the respiratory muscles. When this happens, the diaphragm is usually affected earlier than the intercostal muscles.

Normal concentrations of intracellular potassium are necessary for glycogen synthesis in muscle cells. This means that potassium deficiency can interfere not only with the electrical activity of skeletal muscle but also with muscle metabolism, especially under exercise conditions that rely heavily on anaerobic pathways. Release of potassium from muscle is thought to contribute to the autoregulation of blood flow during exercise, and potassium deficiency can interfere with the release of potassium ions from exercising muscle. Thus, potassium deficiency can lead to impaired blood flow and consequent ischemic injury to muscle cells during intense physical exercise.[15]

Potassium deficiency also affects cardiovascular function. Postural hypotension is common. Serious cardiac arrhythmias can result from hypokalemia. *Of particular importance is the fact that hypokalemia increases the risk of digitalis toxicity.* The dangers associated with digitalis toxicity are compounded in patients who are receiving both digitalis and diuretics.

Treatment. Potassium deficits are treated by increasing the intake of foods high in potassium content—meats, dried fruits, fruit juices (particularly orange juice), and bananas. The reader is referred to a nutrition text for a description of foods that are high in potassium. Oral potassium supplements are prescribed for persons whose intake of potassium is insufficient in relation to losses. This is particularly true of persons who are on diuretic therapy and who are taking digitalis. Many of these supplements are caustic and bitter-tasting. Granules, liquids, and powders need to be adequately diluted before administering. A wax-matrix, slow-release tablet form of the drug is available; it does not have a bitter taste and is often less offensive to take.

Potassium is given intravenously when the oral route is not tolerated or when rapid replacement is needed. The rapid infusion of a concentrated potassium solution has been known to cause death due to cardiac arrest. Health personnel who assume responsibility for administering intravenous solutions containing potassium should be fully aware of all the precautions pertaining to its dilution and flow rate. Pharmacology texts, drug company package inserts, fluid and electrolyte texts, and pharmacists serve as useful resources for this information.

Potassium excess

Hyperkalemia refers to an increase in blood levels of potassium in excess of 5.5 mEq/liter (5.5 mmol/liter). In general it can be said that serum potassium excess occurs whenever potassium gains exceed losses.

Causes. The major causes of potassium excess are (1) renal failure, (2) adrenal insufficiency, and (3) excess potassium gains due to tissue trauma or administration of potassium (oral or intravenous) at a rate that exceeds the kidneys' ability to control serum potassium levels (Table 27-9). It is difficult to increase dietary potassium intake to the point of causing hyperkalemia when sufficient aldosterone is present and renal function is adequate. An exception to this rule is when potassium solutions are being infused intravenously—*severe and fatal incidents of hyperkalemia have resulted from the intravenous infusion of potassium. Intravenous solutions containing potassium should never be started until urine output has been assessed and renal function has been deemed to be adequate;* this is because the kidneys control potassium losses. Movement of potassium out of body cells into the extracellular fluids also can lead to elevated blood potassium levels. For example, burns and crushing injuries cause potassium to be liberated into the extracellular fluid. Often these same injuries cause a decrease in renal function, which contributes to the development of hyperkalemia.

Manifestations. The signs and symptoms of potassium excess are closely related to the alterations in neuromuscular function that accompany potassium deficit. Although the mechanisms responsible for the altered neuromuscular function observed in hypo- and hyperkalemia are different, the end results are similar. The first symptom associated with hyperkalemia is often a paresthesia; this may appear when potassium levels reach 6 mEq/liter (6 mmol/liter). The most serious effect of hyperkalemia is cardiac arrest. The electrocardiographic changes that occur with alterations in serum potassium levels are described in Figure 27-6.

Treatment. The treatment of potassium excess focuses on (1) decreasing or curtailing intake, (2) increasing renal excretion, and (3) increasing cellular uptake. Decreased intake can be achieved by restricting dietary sources of potassium. It should be mentioned here that the major ingredient in most salt substitutes is potassium chloride, and they should not be given to patients with renal problems. Increasing potassium output is often more difficult. Persons with renal failure may require hemodialysis or peritoneal dialysis to reduce the serum potassium levels. A sodium polystyrene sulfonate resin may also be used to remove potassium ions from the colon. The sodium ions in the resin are replaced by potassium ions and then the potassium-containing resin is excreted in the stool.

Emergency methods usually focus on measures that cause serum potassium to move into the cell. The intravenous infusion of insulin and glucose is sometimes used for this purpose.

Alterations in calcium and phosphate balance

There is a close link between the regulation of the divalent calcium and phosphate ions in the body. A change in the concentration of one ion leads to a change in the concentration of the other. Therefore, calcium and phosphate are discussed together in this chapter.

Calcium and phosphate salts are deposited in the organic matrix of bone—bone is essentially 30% matrix and 70% salts. In the extracellular fluid the concentration of calcium and phosphate is reciprocally regulated—when calcium levels are high, phosphate levels are low and *vice versa*. Normal serum levels of calcium (9.0–10.6 mg/dl) and phosphate (3.0–4.5 mg/dl) are regulated so that their product (calcium × phosphate) is maintained at a value of approximately 35. Maintenance of this reciprocal re-

---

Table 27-9. Potassium excess (hyperkalemia)

Causes	Signs and symptoms
Excessive intake or gain	**Laboratory values**
Excessive oral intake	Serum potassium above 5.5 mEq/liter
Excessive or rapid parenteral infusion	(5.5 mmol/liter)
Tissue trauma, burns, and massive crushing injuries	**Neural and skeletal muscle activity**
	Paresthesias
Inadequate renal losses	Weakness and dizziness
Renal failure	Muscle cramps
Adrenal insufficiency	**Smooth muscle activity of the gastrointestinal tract**
Addison's disease	Nausea, diarrhea
Potassium-sparing diuretics	Intestinal colic and gastrointestinal distress
	Cardiac electrophysiology
	Peaked T waves, depressed S–T segment
	Depressed P wave and widening of QRS segment
	Cardiac arrest

Hyperkalemia   **Normal**   **Hypokalemia**

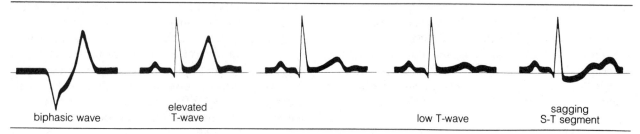

biphasic wave   elevated T-wave   low T-wave   sagging S-T segment

Figure 27-6 ECG changes with hyper- and hypokalemia.

lationship is important in preventing tissue precipitation. Precipitation of calcium and phosphate salts is also prevented by inhibitors that are present in most tissues.

Gains and losses

Calcium and phosphate enter the body through the gastrointestinal tract, are stored in bone, and are excreted through the kidney. The major sources of calcium are milk and milk products. Phosphate is derived from many sources, including milk and meats. Only about 30% to 50% of dietary calcium is absorbed into the body from the duodenum and upper jejunum; the remainder is excreted in the stool. Phosphate, on the other hand, is absorbed exceedingly well.

Normally, the kidneys control calcium and phosphate losses. The two ions are filtered in the glomerulus and are selectively reabsorbed in the renal tubules. Renal elimination of phosphate is regulated by an overflow mechanism in which the amount of phosphate that is lost in the urine is directly related to phosphate concentrations in the blood. When serum phosphate levels rise above a critical level, the rate of phosphate loss in the urine reflects the excess blood phosphate levels. Calcium excretion is reciprocally related to phosphate excretion. In renal failure, phosphate excretion is impaired and as a result serum calcium levels decline as blood phosphate levels rise.

Regulation

Serum calcium and phosphate are regulated by vitamin D, parathyroid hormone, and calcitonin. The body contains a supply of exchangeable calcium that is in equilibrium with calcium in the extracellular fluids. Most of this exchangeable calcium is found in bone. It is this exchangeable pool that serves as a storage site for calcium. Movement of calcium between the extracellular fluids and the exchangeable pool is rapid—it usually occurs within minutes to 1 hour. The regulation of phosphate levels is closely linked to calcium metabolism. The phosphate ion is freely absorbed from the intestine, and changing the serum phosphate levels to as high as three to four times the normal value does not seem to have an immediate effect on body function. Bone metabolism and the actions of vitamin D, parathyroid hormone, and calcitonin are discussed in Chapter 57.

Extracellular calcium levels

Calcium can be found in several forms in the body. About 99% of body calcium is found in bone, where it provides the strength and stability for the collagen and ground substance that form the structural matrix of the skeletal system. The other 1% is located in the tissues and extracellular fluids. The calcium salts in bone serve as a reservoir of tissue and serum calcium.

Extracellular calcium exists in three forms. About 40% of serum calcium is bound to plasma proteins and cannot pass through the capillary wall to leave the vascular compartment. About 10% of serum calcium is combined with substances such as citrate, phosphate, and sulfate. This form is not ionized. The remaining 50% of serum calcium is ionized. It is the ionized calcium that is able to leave the capillary and enter the intercellular spaces, and it is this form of calcium that is physiologically important.

Most of the nondiffusible calcium is bound to albumin; only about 10% to 15% of the protein-bound fraction is associated with globulin. Thus, the total serum calcium will change with changes in serum albumin. As a general rule, the total serum calcium level is decreased 0.8 mg/dl for every 1 g/dl change from normal in the serum albumin level. Hypocalcemia associated with decreased serum albumin levels results in a decrease in protein-bound rather than ionized calcium and is usually asymptomatic. An alkaline *p*H will increase binding of calcium to protein, lowering the ionized calcium while the total serum calcium remains unchanged. Hyperventilation can produce an effective hypocalcemia with tetany by increasing the protein-binding of calcium without altering the total calcium concentrations.[16]

Ionized calcium serves a number of functions: it participates in many enzyme reactions; it exerts an important effect on cell membrane potentials and permeability; it is necessary for contraction in skeletal, cardiac, and smooth muscle; it controls the synaptic release of acetylcholine; it influences cardiac contractility and automaticity via slow calcium channels; and it is essential for blood clotting. The use of calcium channel blocking drugs in circulatory disorders demonstrates the importance of the calcium ion in the normal function of the heart and blood vessels. Calcium is required for all but the first two steps of the intrinsic pathway for blood coagulation. Removal of ionized calcium is often used as a method to prevent clotting of blood that has been removed from the body: Citrate is often used to combine with calcium and prevent clotting in blood that is to be used for transfusions.

Calcium deficit

Serum calcium levels are protected by bone stores and do not usually require a continual daily intake.

Causes. The causes of hypocalcemia, or deficit in ionized calcium, are (1) impaired ability to mobilize calcium from bone stores, (2) abnormal binding of calcium so that greater proportions of calcium are in the unionized form, (3) abnormal losses of calcium from the kidneys, and (4) decreased absorption of calcium from the intestine (Table 27-10).

The ability to mobilize calcium from bone stores is impaired in hypoparathyroidism. A parathyroid hormone (PTH) deficiency occurs with primary hypoparathyroidism; it can occur secondary to neck surgery, particularly if the surgery involves removal of a parathyroid adenoma, thyroidectomy, or bilateral neck resection for cancer. Parathyroid suppression may result from gland suppression (after parathyroid surgery) or from interference with blood supply. The hypocalcemia may occur immediately or from 1 to 2 days after surgery and is usually transient.

The electrolyte or ionized form of calcium is decreased as serum calcium binds to plasma proteins or other substances. For example, serum pH affects the ionization of calcium; ionization is increased in acidosis and decreased in alkalosis. Free fatty acids (FFA) increase binding of calcium to albumin.[17] Elevations in FFA sufficient to alter calcium binding may occur during stressful situations that cause elevations of epinephrine, glucagon, growth hormone, or ACTH. Heparin, beta-adrenergic drugs (epinephrine, isoproterenol, norepinephrine), and alcohol can also produce elevations in FFA sufficient to increase calcium binding. As mentioned previously, citrate combines with calcium and is often used as an anticoagulant for blood transfusions. Theoretically, excess citrate in donor blood could combine with the calcium in a recipient's blood, causing hypocalcemia and tetany. Normally, however, this does not occur because the liver removes the citrate within a matter of minutes. Therefore, when blood transfusions are administered at a slow rate (less than 1 liter/hour in the adult) there is little danger of hypocalcemia due to citrate binding.[2] Hypocalcemia is a common finding in acute pancreatitis. It is not known whether the

---

Table 27–10. Calcium (Ca^{++}) deficit (hypocalcemia)

Causes	Signs and symptoms
Impaired ability to mobilize calcium from bone	**Laboratory values**
Hypoparathyroidism	Serum calcium below 8.5 mg/dl
Abnormal calcium binding	**Increased nerve excitability**
Decreased serum albumin	Paresthesias, especially numbness or tingling
Decreased pH	Skeletal muscle cramps
Increased free fatty acids	Abdominal spasms and cramps
Rapid transfusion of citrated blood	Hyperactive reflexes
Acute pancreatitis	Carpopedal spasm
Abnormal losses	Tetany
Renal failure	Laryngeal spasm
Inadequate vitamin D	Positive Chvostek's test
Impaired absorption	Positive Trousseau's test
Renal failure	**Cardiovascular manifestations**
Liver disease	Hypotension
	Cardiac insufficiency
	Failure to respond to drug that acts via calcium-mediated mechanisms

calcium is precipitated in the pancreas as a result of fat necrosis or is sequestered elsewhere.

There is an inverse relationship between calcium and phosphate excretion by the kidneys. Phosphate is retained in renal failure, causing serum calcium levels to decrease and PTH levels to increase. Hypocalcemia and hyperphosphatemia occur when the glomerular filtration rate falls below 25 ml to 30 ml/minute, the normal being 100 ml to 120 ml/minute.

Intestinal absorption of calcium decreases with a deficiency of vitamin D. Vitamin D deficiency stemming from low intake is seldom seen today because many foods are fortified with vitamin D. Vitamin D deficiency is more apt to occur in malabsorption states, such as biliary obstruction, pancreatic insufficiency, and celiac disease, in which the ability to absorb fat and fat-soluble vitamins is impaired. Vitamin D (inactivated form) is stored in the liver. In subsequent steps the liver and the kidneys convert inactive vitamin D to the activated form (1,25-dihydroxycholecalciferol). Vitamin D remains in the body only a short time once it has been activated. This means that patients with renal failure will have problems with the absorption of calcium because of impaired activation of vitamin D. Fortunately, the activated form of the hormone (calcitriol) has been synthesized and is now available for use in the treatment of calcium deficit in patients with renal failure.

Manifestations. The manifestations of acute hypocalcemia relate to increased neural excitability and cardiovascular effects. Ionized calcium stabilizes neuromuscular excitability. In severe hypocalcemia, increased neuromuscular excitability can cause tetany, laryngeal spasm, convulsions, and death. Both Chvostek's and Trousseau's signs are used in checking for an increase in neuromuscular excitability and tetany. Chvostek's sign is elicited by tapping the face just below the temple at the point where the facial nerve emerges. Tapping the face over the facial nerve causes spasm of the lip, nose, or face when the test is positive. An inflated blood pressure cuff is used to test for Trousseau's sign. The cuff is inflated to a point where it temporarily occludes the circulation of the hand, usually for a period of 1 to 5 minutes. Contraction of the fingers and hands (carpopedal spasm) indicates the presence of tetany. Cardiovascular effects of acute hypocalcemia include hypotension, cardiac insufficiency, cardiac dysrhythmias, and failure to respond to drugs such as digitalis, norepinephrine, and dopamine that act through calcium-mediated mechanisms.

Treatment. The treatment of calcium deficit is directed toward increasing the intake or absorption from the intestine. One glass of milk contains about 300 mg of calcium. An intravenous infusion containing calcium gluconate is used when tetany or acute symptoms are present or anticipated because of a decrease in serum calcium. The active form of vitamin D is administered when the liver or kidney mechanisms needed for hormone activation are impaired.

Calcium excess

A serum calcium excess (hypercalcemia) results from excessive bone resorption and from intestinal absorption that exceeds the ability of the kidney to excrete the excess calcium ions (Table 27-11).

Causes. The most common causes of increased bone resorption (or destruction) are neoplasms, hyperparathyroidism, and prolonged immobility. There are a number of malignant tumors, including carcinoma of the lungs, that have been associated with hypercalcemia. Some tumors actually destroy the bone, whereas others produce an osteoclast-activating factor, and some are sites of ectopic parathyroid hormone production. Hyperparathyroidism may be mild or severe. It is more common in postmenopausal women because estrogen tends to increase the effect of parathyroid hormone on bone. Lithium is associated with increased parathyroid hormone levels.

Intestinal absorption of calcium increases with excessive doses of vitamin D. Fortunately, the liver can store vitamin D; and it is reported that 1000 times the normal quantities can be ingested with only a threefold increase in serum levels of the active hormone.[1] Granulomatous conditions such as sarcoidosis, tuberculosis, silicosis, and histoplasmosis produce an increase in vitamin D. In such conditions, vitamin D is produced by the monocytes that compose the granuloma. Another cause of excessive calcium absorption is the milk–alkali syndrome. The milk–alkali syndrome occurs in patients with peptic ulcers who are being treated with excessive amounts of milk and alkaline antacids, particularly calcium carbonate preparations.

Alkalosis causes the kidneys to decrease calcium elimination. Excess calcium carbonate taken without milk has also been known to produce an increase in calcium levels. The thiazide diuretics can produce an increase in total serum calcium of 0.5 mg/dl to 1.0 mg/dl in otherwise healthy persons.[16] This reflects the indirect effects of hemoconcentration and the direct effects of bone resorption. In most persons, the calcium levels return to normal after several weeks of therapy. However, the thiazide diuretics may cause hypercalcemia in persons with underlying bone disorders and increased bone resorption.

Manifestations. The signs and symptoms associated with calcium excess originate from three sources: (1) a decrease in neuromuscular activity, (2) reabsorption of calcium from bone, and (3) exposure of the kidney to high concentrations of calcium. Neural excitability is decreased in hypercalcemia. There may be a dulling of consciousness, stupor, weakness, and muscle flaccidity. Acute psychoses are common when calcium levels rise above 16 mg/dl. The heart responds to elevated levels of calcium with increased contractility and ventricular arrhythmias. Digitalis causes these responses to be accentuated. High calcium concentrations in the urine impair the ability of the kidney to concentrate urine by interfering with the action of ADH. This causes salt and water diuresis and an increased sensation of thirst. Hypercalciuria also predisposes to the development of renal calculi.

Hypercalcemic crisis describes an acute increase in serum calcium levels above 8 mEq/liter to 9 mEq/liter or (4–4.5 mmol/liter). Malignant disease and hyperparathyroidism are major causes of hypercalcemic crisis. In hypercalcemic crisis, polyuria, excessive thirst, volume depletion, fever, altered levels of consciousness, azotemia (nitrogenous wastes in the blood), and a disturbed mental state accompany other signs of calcium excess. Symptomatic hypercalcemia is associated with a high mortality rate; death is often due to cardiac arrest.

Treatment. The treatment of calcium excess is usually directed toward correcting or controlling the condition that is causing the disorder. Excretion of sodium is accompanied by calcium excretion. Diuretics and sodium chloride can be administered in emergency treatment of hypercalcemia. Corticosteroids and mithramycin are used to treat hypercalcemia due to malignancy. Diphosphonates have been recently introduced as a treatment method.[18]

Extracellular phosphate levels

Phosphate is an integral part of all body tissues. About 85% of phosphorus is located in bone; most of the remaining 15% is located intracellularly. In the adult, the normal serum phosphate level is 3.0 mg/dl to 4.5 mg/dl of serum. These values are slightly higher in children (4.0–7.0 mg/dl).

Table 27–11. Calcium (Ca^{++}) excess (hypercalcemia)

Causes	Signs and symptoms
Excessive gains	Serum calcium above 10.5 mg/dl altered neural and muscular acting
Increased intestinal absorption	
Excessive vitamin D	Muscle weakness and atrophy
Excessive calcium in diet	Ataxia, loss of muscle tone
Milk–alkali syndrome	Lethargy
Increased bone resorption	Stupor and coma
Immobility	Personality or behavioral changes
Increased levels of parathyroid	**Associated with increased bone resorption**
hormone	
Malignant neoplasms	Deep bone pain
Thiazide diuretics	Pathologic fractures
Inadequate losses	**Renal**
Hyperparathyroidism	Signs of renal insufficiency
	(acute reversible)
	Polyuria
	Flank pain
	Signs of kidney stones
	Increased losses of sodium
	and potassium
	Cardiovascular
	Hypertension
	Shortening of the QT interval,
	AV block on electrocardiogram
	Gastrointestinal
	Anorexia
	Nausea
	Vomiting
	Constipation

The functions of phosphate can be grouped into four categories: (1) phosphate plays a major role in bone formation; (2) it is essential to metabolic processes—that is, it is incorporated into adenosine triphosphate (ATP) as well as into enzymes needed for metabolism of glucose, fat, and protein; (3) it is an essential component of several vital parts of the cell, being incorporated into the nucleic acids and into the cell membrane; and (4) it acts as an acid–base buffer in the extracellular fluid and in renal excretion of hydrogen ions. Delivery of oxygen by the red cell depends on organic phosphates in ATP and 2,3-diphosphoglycerate (2,3-DPG). Phosphate is also needed for normal function of other blood cells, including the white cells and platelets.

Phosphate deficit

Only recently has the importance of phosphate depletion been recognized.

Causes.   Phosphate depletion is associated with antacid use, malnutrition, alcoholism, ketoacidosis, and hyperthyroidism. Antacids that contain aluminum hydroxide, aluminum carbonate, and calcium carbonate bind with phosphate, causing increased phosphate losses in the stool. Aluminum hydroxide is sometimes used therapeutically to decrease phosphate levels in chronic renal failure. Alcoholism is commonly recognized as a cause of hypophosphatemia. The mechanisms underlying hypophosphatemia in the alcoholic are not clearly understood; they may be related to malnutrition or to hypomagnesemia. Hypophosphatemia can occur during prolonged courses of intravenous fluids or nutritional repletion.[19] Malnutrition and diabetic ketoacidosis increase phosphate excretion and phosphate loss from the body. Refeeding of malnourished patients increases the incorporation of phosphate into nucleic acids and phosphorylated compounds in the cell. The same thing happens when diabetic ketoacidosis is reversed with insulin therapy. The intracellular shift of phosphate causes the serum phosphate levels to drop. Parathyroid hormone decreases the serum phosphate levels through a different mechanism: it increases the renal excretion of phosphate. Alkalosis has an indirect effect on serum phosphate levels. The increase in *p*H causes increased binding of calcium, which in turn leads to a decrease in ionized calcium and an increase in the release of PTH.

Manifestations.   Hypophosphatemia causes signs and symptoms related to altered neural function, disturbed musculoskeletal function, and hematologic disorders. Neural manifestations include intentional tremors, paresthesias, hyporeflexia, stupor, coma, and seizures (Table 27-12). Anorexia and dysphagia can occur. There may be muscle weakness, stiffness of the joints, bone pain, and osteomalacia. Red cell metabolism is impaired in phosphate deficiency; the cells become rigid and have increased hemolysis and diminished ATP and 2,3-DPG levels. Chemotaxis and phagocytosis by white blood cells is impaired. Platelet function is also disturbed. Respiratory insufficiency due to impaired function of the respiratory muscles can develop in severe hypophosphatemia.[20]

Treatment.   The treatment of hypophosphatemia includes replacement therapy. This may be accomplished with dietary sources high in phosphate (one glassful of milk contains about 250 mg phosphate) or with oral or intravenous replacement solutions. Phosphate supplements are usually contraindicated in hypercalcemia and renal failure. Treatment with phosphate supplements can lead to disseminated calcification.

Phosphate excess

Hyperphosphatemia usually results from renal failure or a decrease in PTH. Hyperphosphatemia has been reported in children following use of a single sodium phosphate/biphosphate enema.[21]

Hyperphosphatemia is associated with a decrease in serum calcium; thus, many of the signs and symptoms of a phosphate excess may be related to a calcium deficit (see Table 27-10).

Alterations in magnesium

Magnesium is the second most abundant intracellular cation. Of the total, 50% is stored in bone, 49% is contained in the body cells, and the remaining 1% is dispersed in the extracellular fluids. The normal serum concentration of magnesium is 1.8 mg/dl to 3.0 mg/dl.

Only recently has the importance of magnesium to the overall function of the body been recognized. Magnesium acts as a cofactor in many enzyme reactions. It is essential in all enzyme systems known to be catalyzed by ATP, so that profound disruption of cell function occurs in magnesium-deficient tissues. Magnesium is necessary for protein and DNA synthesis, DNA and RNA transcription, and translation of RNA. Maintenance of normal intracellular levels of potassium depends on magnesium: Magnesium deficiency causes intracellular potassium depletion. Magnesium can bind to calcium receptors; it has been suggested that alterations in magnesium levels may exert their effects through calcium-mediated mechanisms. Magnesium may bind competitively to calcium binding sites, producing the appropriate response; it may compete with calcium for a binding site, but not exert an effect; or it may alter the distribution of calcium by interfering with its movement across the cell membrane.[22]

Regulation.   The average American diet contains about 180 mg to 300 mg of magnesium. All green vegetables contain abundant amounts of magnesium. Although some controversy remains, it is generally agreed that the minimum daily requirement for magnesium in the adult is 250 mg (150 mg in the infant and 400 mg in pregnant or lactating women).[23]

Magnesium is absorbed from the intestine and excreted by the kidneys. Intestinal absorption is not closely regulated, and it has been estimated that 25% to 65% of dietary magnesium is absorbed. Calcium and magnesium compete for reabsorption in both the intestines and the renal tubules; factors that tend to increase calcium absorption will cause a decrease in magnesium absorption. Parathyroid hormone is thought to enhance renal reabsorption of magnesium, although this action is often outweighed by the effects of hypercalcemia, which act to inhibit reabsorption.

Magnesium deficit (hypomagnesemia)

Hypomagnesemia can be expected in 6.9% to 11% of hospitalized patients in whom serum electrolyte determinations are routinely performed,[24] and 38% to 42% of patients with hypokalemia have concurrent hypomagnesemia.[25,26] Magnesium deficiency usually results from impaired absorption in the intestine or from increased urinary losses. Although the kidneys are able to defend against hypermagnesemia, they are less able to conserve magnesium and prevent hypomagnesemia. Urine losses of magnesium are increased with diuresis, and diuretics are the most common cause of increased renal losses.

One of the most common causes of magnesium deficiency is chronic alcoholism.[16] Many factors contribute to hypomagnesemia in alcoholism, including low intake and gastrointestinal losses from diarrhea. The effects of hypomagnesemia are exaggerated by other electrolyte disorders, such as hypokalemia, hypocalcemia, and metabolic acidosis, often seen in chronic alcoholism.

Magnesium levels are also decreased in conditions that cause malabsorption, in malnutrition, and in patients receiving parenteral hyperalimentation in which the magnesium content is inadequate. Prolonged diarrhea or laxative abuse may also lead to severe magnesium deficiency. Excessive calcium intake will impair magnesium absorption by competing for the same transport site. Magnesium losses are increased in diabetic ketoacidosis, diuretic therapy, and hyperaldosteronism (Table 27-13).

Table 27–12.   Phosphate deficit (hypophosphatemia)

Causes	Signs and symptoms
Increased loss from the gastrointestinal tract	Serum levels below 3.0 mg/dl in adults and 4.0 mg/dl in children
Antacids (aluminum and calcium)	**Altered neural function**
Severe diarrhea	Intention tremor
Lack of vitamin D	Ataxia
Increased renal excretion	Paresthesias
Alkalosis	Hyporeflexia
Hyperparathyroidism	Confusion
Diabetic ketoacidosis	Stupor
Renal tubular defects	Coma
Decreased intake	Seizures
Malnutrition	**Altered musculoskeletal function**
Alcoholism	Muscle weakness
Increased movement into the cell	Joint stiffness
Intravenous hyperalimentation	Bone pain
Recovery from malnutrition	Osteomalacia
Administration of insulin for ketoacidosis	**Gastrointestinal symptoms**
	Anorexia
	Dysphagia
	Hematologic disorders
	Hemolytic anemia
	Platelet dysfunction with bleeding disorders
	Impaired function of white blood cells

Manifestations. The signs and symptoms of magnesium deficit are characterized by personality change; neuromuscular irritability; tremors; athetoid or choreiform movements; positive Babinski's, Chvostek's, or Trousseau's signs; tachycardia; hypertension; and ventricular dysrhythmias. There is an accelerated loss of potassium from cardiac and skeletal muscle fibers. Hypokalemia has long been associated with diuretic therapy and digitalis toxicity. More recently, magnesium deficiency has been implicated in aggravating potassium deficiency and interfering with potassium repletion. Electrocardiographic changes are associated with both hypomagnesemia and hypokalemia.[23]

Magnesium excess

Magnesium excess is rare. When it does occur it is usually related to renal insufficiency or to injudicious use of magnesium sulfate as a laxative. The signs and symptoms occur only when serum magnesium levels exceed 4 mEq/liter (2 mmol/liter).[15] Hypermagnesemia causes sedation of the nervous system with muscle weakness, confusion, and respiratory paralysis. Blood pressure is decreased and the electrocardiogram shows an increase in the PR interval, a broadening of the QRS complex, and elevation of the T wave. The treatment of hypermagnesemia includes cessation of magnesium administration. Calcium is a direct antagonist of magnesium, and intravenous administration of calcium may be used. Peritoneal dialysis or hemodialysis may be required.

In summary, electrolytes serve many functions. They (1) assist in regulating body water balance, (2) participate in acid–base balance, (3) contribute to enzyme reactions, and (4) play an essential role in neuromuscular activity. Serum levels of an electrolyte represent its concentration (mEq/liter) in the extracellular compartment.

Sodium is the major cation in the extracellular fluid. Serum sodium levels are strongly affected by extracellular water levels: sodium concentration is increased in water deficit and decreased in water excess. Normal levels of sodium are essential to maintenance of the osmolality of the extracellular fluids; many of the manifestations of altered sodium balance are caused by swelling (hyponatremia) or shrinking (hypernatremia) of body cells, including those of the central nervous system. Sodium also contributes to neuromuscular excitability, acid–base balance, and numerous chemical reactions that occur in the body.

Potassium is the major intracellular cation. It contributes to the maintenance of intracellular osmolality, is necessary for normal neuromuscular function, and influences acid–base balance. Because potassium is poorly conserved by the body, adequate daily intake is needed. Most of the body's potassium loss occurs through the kidneys; hence, potassium imbalances can occur rapidly in diuresis (hypokalemia) or renal failure (hyperkalemia). Alterations in potassium balance affect skeletal, cardiac, and smooth muscle function.

There is a close link between the regulation of calcium and the regulation of phosphate in the body (*e.g.*, an elevation of serum phosphate produces a decrease in serum calcium). Of the three forms of extracellular calcium (protein bound, citrate bound, and ionized), only the ionized form can cross the cell membrane and contribute to cellular function. Ionized calcium has a number of functions: it contributes to neuromuscular function, serves a vital function in the

---

Table 27–13. Magnesium deficit (hypomagnesemia)

Causes	Signs and symptoms
Impaired intake or absorption	**Laboratory findings**
Alcoholism	Serum magnesium less than
Malabsorption	1.8 mg/dl
Small-bowel bypass surgery	**Neuromuscular hyperirritability**
Malnutrition or starvation	Personality change
Parenteral hyperalimentation of	Athetoid or choreiform movements
inadequate Mg^{++}	Positive Babinski's sign
High dietary intake of calcium without	Nystagmus
concomitant increase in Mg^{++}	Tetany
Increased losses	Positive Chvostek's or Trousseau's
Diabetic ketoacidosis	signs
Diuretic therapy	**Cardiovascular manifestations**
Hyperparathyroidism	Tachycardia
Hyperaldosteronism	Hypertension
Magnesium-wasting renal disease	Ventricular arrhythmias

blood clotting process, and participates in a number of enzyme reactions. Alterations in ionized calcium levels produce neural effects: neural excitability is increased in hypocalcemia and decreased in hypercalcemia. Phosphate is largely an intracellular anion. It is incorporated into the nucleic acids and into ATP. A phosphate deficit causes signs and symptoms of altered neural function, disturbed musculoskeletal function, and hematologic disorders. Phosphate excess occurs with renal failure and PTH deficit; it is associated with decreased serum calcium levels. Magnesium is the second most abundant intracellular cation. It acts as a cofactor in many enzyme reactions and affects neuromuscular function in the same manner as the calcium ion.

References

1. Robertson GL: Thirst and vasopressin function in normal and disordered states of water balance. J Lab Clin Med 101(3):351, 1983
2. Guyton A: Textbook of Medical Physiology, 7th ed, pp 846, 431, 383, 853, 85, 1018. Philadelphia, WB Saunders, 1986
3. Lawrence SV: Woman's death by water intoxication ruled suicide. Clin Psych News 5:3, 1977
4. Baker AB, Baker LH: Clinical Neurology, vol 2. In Haymaker W, Anderson E (eds): Disorders of the Hypothalamus and Pituitary Gland, pp 18, 24, 25. Hagerstown, MD, Harper & Row, 1976
5. Moses M, Miller M, Streeten DHP: Pathology and pharmacologic alterations in release and actions of ADH. Metabolism 25:705, 1976
6. Narins RG, Jones ER, Stom MC: Diagnostic strategies in disorders of fluid, electrolyte, and acid–base disorders. Am J Med 72:496, 1982
7. Pruit BA: Other complications of burn injury. In Artz CP, et al: Burns, p 518. Philadelphia, WB Saunders, 1979
8. Pflaum SS. Investigation of intake-output as a means of assessing body fluid balance. Heart & Lung 8:498, 1979
9. Goldberger E: A Primer on Water, Electrolytes, and Acid–Base Syndromes, 6th ed, p 34. Philadelphia, Lea & Febiger, 1980
10. Snyder JD: From pedialyte to popsicles: A look at oral rehydration therapy in the United States. Am J Clin Nutr 35:157, 1982
11. The Medical Letter vol 25, no 629:19, 1983
12. Weisman Z. Cola drinks and rehydration in acute diarrhea (letter). N Engl J Med 315:768, 1986
13. Katz MA: Hyperglycemic-induced hypernatremia—calculations of expected serum sodium depression. N Engl J Med 293:843, 1975
14. Knockel JF: Etiology and management of potassium deficiency. Hosp Pract 22(1):153, 1987
15. Knockel JP: Neuromuscular manifestations of electrolyte disorders. Am J Med 72:521, 1982
16. Agus LS, Wasserstein A, Goldfarb S: Disorders of calcium and magnesium homeostasis. Am J Med 72:473, 1982
17. Zaloga GP, Chennow B: Hypocalcemia in critical illness. JAMA 256:1924, 1986
18. Harinck H, Plantingh AST, Elte JW, et al: Role of bone and kidney in tumor-induced hypercalcemia and its treatment with bisphosphate and sodium chloride. Am J Med 82(6):1133, 1987
19. Knockel JP: The clinical status of hypophosphatemia. N Engl J Med 313:447, 1985
20. Aubier M, Murciano D, Lecocquic Y, et al: Effect of hypophosphatemia on diaphragmatic contractility in patients with acute respiratory failure. N Engl J Med 313:420, 1985
21. Davis RF, Eichner J, Archie W, et al: Hypocalcemia, hyperphosphatemia and dehydration following a single hypertonic phosphate enema. J Pediatr 90:484, 1977
22. Levine BS, Coburn JW: Magnesium, the mimic/agonist of calcium. N Engl J Med 310:1253, 1984
23. Metheny NM, Snively WD: Nurses' Handbook of Fluid Balance, p 79. Philadelphia, JB Lippincott, 1979
24. Whang R: Magnesium deficiency: Pathogenesis, prevalence, and clinical complications. Am J Med 82(suppl 3A):24, 1987
25. Whang R, Oei TO, Aikawa J, et al: Predictors of clinical hypomagnesemia—hypokalemia, hypophosphatemia, hyponatremia, hypocalcemia. Arch Intern Med 144:1794, 1984
26. Boyd JC, Bruns DE, Wills MR: Frequency of hypomagnesemia in hypokalemic states. Clin Chem 29:178, 1983

Bibliography

Arieff AI: Osmotic failure: Physiology and strategies for treatment. Hosp Pract 23(6):173, 1988
Chenevey B: Overview of fluids and electrolytes. Nurs Clin North Am 22:749, 1987
Cronin RE: Psychogenic polydipsia with hyponatremia: Report of eleven cases. Am J Kidney Dis 9:410, 1987
Gennari FJ: Serum osmolality: Uses and limitations. N Engl J Med 310:102, 1984
Hammond DN, Moll GW, Robertson GL, et al: Hypodipsia with normal osmoregulation of vasopressin. N Engl J Med 315:433, 1986
Jacobson HR: Diuretics: Mechanisms of action and uses. Hosp Pract 22 (Dec 15):129, 1987
Knochel JP: Neuromuscular manifestations of electrolyte disorders. Am J Med 72:521, 1982
Miller PR, Krebs RA, Neal BJ, et al: Hypodipsia in geriatric patients. Am J Med 73:354, 1982
Robertson GL: Thirst and vasopressin function in normal and disordered states of water balance. J Lab Clin Med 101:351, 1983
Skorecki KL, Brenner BM: Body fluid homeostasis in man: A contemporary overview. Am J Med 70:77, 1981
Valle GA, Lemberg L: Electrolyte imbalances in cardiovascular disease: The forgotten factor. Heart Lung 17:324, 1988

—— Calcium and phosphorus

Flier JS, Moore MJ: The hypercalcemia of cancer. N Engl J Med 310:1718, 1984
Knockel JP: The clinical status of hypophosphatemia: An update. N Engl J Med 313:447, 1985

Levine MM, Kleeman CR: Hypercalcemia: pathophysiology and treatment. Hosp Pract 22(7):93, 1987

Mundry GR, Ibbotson KJ, D'Souza SM, et al: The hypercalcemia of cancer. N Engl J Med 310:1718, 1984

Spencer H, Kramer L: The calcium requirement and factors causing calcium loss. Fed Proc 45:2758, 1986

Strewler GL, Nissenson RA: Nonparathyroid hypercalcemia. Adv Intern Med 32:235, 1987

—— Magnesium

Dyckner T, Wester P: Clinical significance of diuretic-induced magnesium loss. Pract Cardiology 10(6):12, 1984

Gumz JG: Clinical significance of magnesium: A review. Drug Intell Clin Pharm 21:240, 1987

Hollenberg NK, Hollifield JW (eds): Potassium/magnesium depletion: Is your patient at risk of sudden death? Am J Med 82(3A) (entire issue), 1987

Swales JD: Magnesium deficiency and diuretics. Br Med J 2:1377, 1982

Whang R, Tjien O, Watanabe A: Frequency of hypomagnesemia in hospitalized patients receiving digitalis. Arch Intern Med 145:655, 1985

—— Potassium

Adrogue HJ, Madias NE: Changes in potassium concentrations during acute acidosis. Am J Med 71:456, 1981

Cannon-Babb ML, Schwartz AB: Drug-induced hyperkalemia. Hosp Pract 21(9):99, 1986

Clive DM, Stoff JS: Hyperkalemia: The potential for harm. J Intensive Care Med 3(1):1, 1988

Harrington JT, Isner JM, Kassirer JP: Our national obsession with potassium. Am J Med 73:155, 1982

Hollenberg NK (ed): Potassium, magnesium, and cardiovascular mortality. Am J Med 80(suppl 4A) (entire issue), 1986

Kassirer JP, Harrington JT: Fending off the potassium pushers. N Engl J Med 312:785,1985

Layzer RB: Periodic paralysis and the sodium-potassium pump. Ann Neurol 11:547, 1982

Morgan DB, Davidson C: Hypokalemia and diuretics: An analysis of publications. Br Med J 1:905, 1980

Rao TL, Mathru KM, Salem MR, et al: Serum potassium levels following transfusion of frozen erythrocytes. Anesthesiology 52:170, 1982

Thier SO: Potassium physiology. Am J Med 80(suppl 4A):3, 1986

Sopko JA, Freeman RM: Salt substitutes as a source of potassium. JAMA 238:608, 1977

Stein JH: Hypokalemia: Common and uncommon causes. Hosp Pract 23(3):55, 1988

Sterns RH, Cox M, Feig PU, et al: Internal potassium balance and the control of the plasma potassium concentration. Medicine 60:339, 1981

Tannen RL: Effects of potassium on blood pressure control. Ann Intern Med 98(part 2):773, 1983

Vee Rice: The role of potassium in health and disease. Crit Care Nurs 2(3):54, 1982

Williams ME, Rosa RM, Epstein FH: Hyperkalemia. Adv Intern Med 31:265, 1986

Williams ME, Rosa RM: Hyperkalemia: disorders of internal and external potassium balance. J Intensive Care Med 3(1):52, 1988

—— Sodium

Anderson RJ, Chung H, Kluge R, et al: Hyponatremia: A prospective analysis of its epidemiology and the pathogenetic role of vasopressin. Ann Intern Med 102:164, 1985

Arief AI: Hyponatremia associated with permanent brain damage. Adv Intern Med 32:325, 1987

Buckalew VM Jr: Hyponatremia: Pathogenesis and management. Hosp Pract 21 (Nov 30):49, 1986

Moran SM, Jamison RL: The variable hyponatremic response to hyperglycemia. West J Med 142:49, 1985

Schrier RW: Treatment of hyponatremia. N Engl J Med 312:1121, 1985

Sterns RH: Severe symptomatic hyponatremia: treatment and outcomes. Ann Intern Med 107:656, 1987

CHAPTER 28

Alterations in Distribution of Body Fluids: Edema

**Regulation of interstitial fluid
  volume**
  Capillary filtration pressure
  Colloidal osmotic pressure
  Lymph flow

Edema
  Causes
    Increased capillary pressure
    Decreased colloidal osmotic
      pressure
    Increased capillary permeability
    Obstruction of lymphatic flow

Effects
  Pitting edema
  Nonpitting edema
Assessment
Treatment
**Accumulation of fluid in the
  serous cavities**

Objectives

After you have studied this chapter, you should
be able to meet the following objectives:

_____ Describe the role of the capillaries in regulating
interstitial fluid volume.

_____ Describe the factors that control fluid exchange
at the capillary level.

_____ Define the term _hydrostatic pressure._

_____ Differentiate between colloidal osmotic pressure
and osmotic pressure due to crystalloids.

_____ Explain the function of lymph flow in capillary fluid
dynamics.

_____ Describe the causes of increased capillary pressure.

_____ Explain the relationship between plasma protein
levels and edema formation.

_____ List the causes of increased capillary permeability.

_____ State the causes of lymphedema.

_____ Describe the physiological effects of edema.

_____ Compare pitting edema and nonpitting edema.

_____ State the three goals that apply to the treatment
of edema.

_____ Relate the principles of edema to the accumulation of fluids in serous cavities.

Normally, about 25% of the total body water is contained in the interstitial, or tissue, spaces. This water acts as a transport vehicle for gases, nutrients, wastes, and other materials that need to be transported between body cells and the vascular compartment. Interstitial fluid also provides a reservoir from which vascular volume can be maintained during periods of hemorrhage or loss of vascular volume. A tissue gel, or spongelike material composed of large quantities of mucopolysaccharides, fills the tissue spaces and aids in the even distribution of interstitial fluid. The decrease in tissue gel that occurs with age is thought to account in part for the wrinkles that accompany aging.

Several factors contribute to alterations in the distribution of extracellular water. Because of the nonspecific nature of these alterations and the frequency with which they occur, this chapter focuses on increases in interstitial fluid, or edema.

Regulation of interstitial fluid volume

The interchange of cellular and vascular fluid occurs at the capillary level, with fluid leaving the capillary bed, traversing the interstitial spaces, and entering the cell and vice versa. Normally, the movement of fluid between the capillary bed and the interstitial spaces is continuous. A state of equilibrium exists as long as equal amounts of fluid enter and leave the interstitial spaces. White blood cells, plasma proteins, and other molecules that are too large to reenter the capillary rely on the loosely structured wall of the lymphatic vessels for return to the vascular compartment. About 10% of the filtered fluid is returned to the circulation through the lymphatics.

fluid leaving the capillary =
fluid reentering the capillary + lymphatic flow

Capillaries are microscopic vessels one layer thick that connect the arterioles of the arterial system with venules of the venous system (Figure 28-1). Small cuffs of smooth muscle, the precapillary sphincters, are positioned at the arterial end of the capillary. The smooth muscle tone of the arterioles, venules, and precapillary sphincters serves to control blood flow through the capillary bed.

Two types of mechanisms control the movement of capillary fluid—outward and inward forces. The outward forces, those that cause fluid to move out of the capillary into the tissue spaces, include (1) the capillary filtration (or capillary) pressure, (2) the tissue fluid pressure, and (3) the colloid osmotic pressure exerted by plasma proteins that are in the tissue spaces. The inward movement of fluid is controlled largely by the colloid osmotic pressure within the capillary.

Capillary filtration pressure

The capillary filtration pressure is the force that pushes water through the capillary pores into the interstitial spaces. Capillary filtration pressure reflects the arterial pressure, the venous pressure, and the hydrostatic effects of gravity (Figure 28-2).

The arterial pressure decreases as blood moves away from the heart. Nevertheless, the pressure

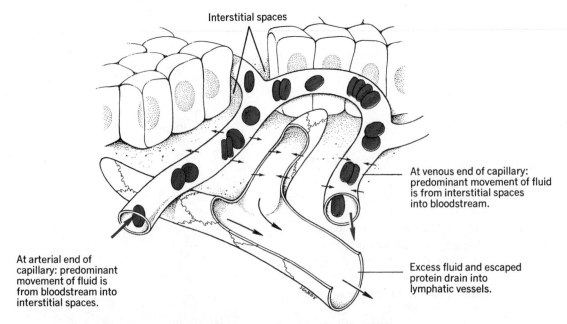

Interstitial spaces

At venous end of capillary: predominant movement of fluid is from interstitial spaces into bloodstream.

At arterial end of capillary: predominant movement of fluid is from bloodstream into interstitial spaces.

Excess fluid and escaped protein drain into lymphatic vessels.

Figure 28-1 Exchanges through capillary membranes in the formation and removal of interstitial fluid. (Chaffee EE, Lytle IM: Basic Physiology and Anatomy, 4th ed. Philadelphia, JB Lippincott, 1980)

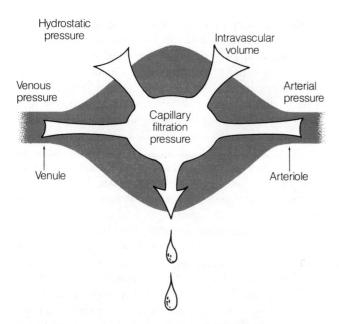

Figure 28-2 The forces that influence capillary filtration pressure.

at the arterial end of the capillary is normally higher than the pressure at its venous end. This pressure difference, or gradient, contributes to the exchange of fluid at the capillary level. Venous pressure can also be transmitted back to the capillary because there are no sphincters at this end of the capillary. This means that increases in venous pressure, such as those that occur with heart failure, will eventually lead to an increase in intracapillary pressure. Capillary pressure also reflects changes in capillary volume. Capillary volume is controlled by the precapillary flow (tone of the precapillary sphincters and the arterioles that supply the capillary) and the postcapillary (venule and small vein) resistances. Selective constriction of the venules will cause capillary pressures to rise, whereas constriction of the arterioles and precapillary sphincters leads to a decrease in pressure.

The pressure due to gravity is called the *hydrostatic pressure*. In a person in the standing position, the weight of the blood in the vascular column causes an increase of 1 mmHg in pressure for every 13.6 mm of distance below the level of the heart.* Gravity has no effect on blood pressure in a person in the recumbent position because the blood vessels are then at the level of the heart. Often the terms *capillary pressure* and *hydrostatic pressure* are used interchangeably; this is because of the passive nature of pressure in the capillary bed. In this chapter, for purposes of discussion, hydrostatic pressure is considered to be the result of gravity and is presented separately from other factors that affect capillary pressure.

Colloidal osmotic pressure

A colloid solution is one in which there are evenly dispersed particles, much as cream particles become dispersed when milk is homogenized. The term *colloidal osmotic pressure* is used to distinguish the osmotic effects of the particles in a colloidal solution from those of the dissolved crystalloids such as sodium. The plasma proteins are large molecules that disperse in the blood and occasionally escape into the tissue spaces. Because the capillary membrane is almost impermeable to the plasma proteins, these particles exert a force that draws fluid into the capillary and offsets the pushing force of the capillary filtration pressure. The plasma contains a mixture of plasma proteins, including albumin, the globulins, and fibrinogen. Albumin, which is the smallest and most abundant of the plasma proteins, accounts for about 70% of the total osmotic pressure. The reader is reminded that it is the number, and not the size of the particles in solution, that controls the osmotic pressure. One gram of albumin (molecular weight 69,000) contains almost six times as many molecules as 1 g of fibrinogen (molecular weight 400,000).**

Lymph flow

Normally, slightly more fluid leaves the capillary than can be reabsorbed at the venous end. This excess fluid is returned to the circulation by way of the lymph channels; almost all body tissues have lymph channels. The structure of the lymph capillary is unique in that the junctions between the endothelial cells of the vessels are loosely connected to form valves and are attached by anchoring filaments to the surrounding tissue (Figure 28-3). These valves allow fluid to enter the lymph channel. The anchoring filaments serve to pull the valves open when tissue fluid increases. Once the fluid has entered the lymph channel, however, it cannot leave because the valve prevents backward flow. Contraction of smooth muscles in the lymph channels (lymph pump) causes the lymph fluid to empty into the veins in the chest. Compression of tissues and muscle movements contributes to the movement of fluid in the lymph channels.

In summary, exchange of fluids between the vascular compartment and the interstitial spaces occurs at the capillary level. The capillary filtration pressure pushes fluids out of the capillaries, and the colloidal osmotic pressure exerted by the plasma proteins pulls fluids back into the capillaries. Albumin,

---

* The hydrostatic pressure in the veins of an adult male can reach a level of 90 mmHg. This pressure is then transmitted to the capillary bed.

** The normal values for the plasma proteins are (1) albumin 4.5 g per 100 ml, (2) globulins 2.5 g per dL, and (3) fibrinogen 0.3 g per dL.

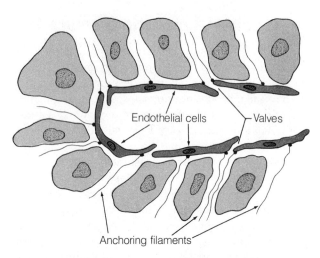

Figure 28-3 Special structure of the lymphatic capillaries that permits passage of substances of high molecular weight back into the circulation. *(Guyton AC: Textbook of Medical Physiology, 6th ed. Philadelphia, WB Saunders, 1981)*

which is the smallest and most abundant of the plasma proteins, provides the major osmotic force for return of fluid to the vascular compartment. Normally, slightly more fluid leaves the capillary bed than can be reabsorbed. This excess fluid is returned to the circulation by way of the lymphatic channels.

Edema

Edema refers to excess interstitial fluid in the tissues. Edema is not a disease but rather the manifestation of altered physiological function.

Causes

The alterations in physiological function that lead to edema are (1) increases in capillary filtration pressure, (2) decreases in capillary colloidal osmotic pressure, (3) increases in capillary permeability, and (4) obstruction to lymph flow. Edema can occur in healthy as well as sick individuals: for example, the swelling of the hands and feet that occurs in hot weather. The causes of edema are summarized in Chart 28-1.

Increased capillary pressure

Edema develops when an increase in capillary pressure causes excess movement of fluid from the capillary bed into the interstitial spaces. Among the factors that cause an increase in capillary pressures are (1) decreased resistance to flow through the arterioles and capillary sphincters that supply the capillary bed, (2) increased resistance to outflow at the venous end

of the capillary bed, (3) increased extracellular fluid volume associated with an increase in intravascular volume, and (4) increased gravitational forces. In hives and other allergic or inflammatory conditions, localized edema develops because of a histamine-induced dilatation of the precapillary sphincters and arterioles that supply the swollen area. Impaired venous outflow from the capillary causes a retrograde increase in capillary pressure. Thrombophlebitis, or the presence of venous blood clots, leads to edema of the affected part. In right-sided heart failure, blood dams up throughout the entire systemic venous system, causing organ congestion and edema of the dependent extremities. Increased reabsorption of sodium and water by the kidney leads to an increase in extracellular volume with an increase in capillary pressure and subsequent movement of fluid into the tissue spaces. In hot weather the superficial blood vessels dilate and sodium and water retention increases, which causes swelling of the hands and feet. Edema of the ankles and feet becomes more pronounced during prolonged periods of standing, when the forces of gravity are superimposed on the heat-induced vasodilatation and the increase in extracellular fluid volume.

Chart 28–1:   Causes of edema

Increased capillary pressure
  Arteriolar dilatation
    Allergic responses (hives and angioneurotic edema)
    Inflammation
  Venous obstruction
    Hepatic obstruction
    Heart failure
    Thrombophlebitis
  Increased vascular volume
    Heart failure
    Increased levels of adrenal cortical hormones
    Increased premenstrual sodium retention
    Pregnancy
    Environmental heat stress
  Effects of gravity
    Prolonged standing
Decreased colloid osmotic pressure
  Decreased production of plasma proteins
    Liver disease
    Starvation or severe protein deficiency
  Increased loss of plasma proteins
    Protein-losing kidney diseases
    Extensive burns
Increased capillary permeability
  Inflammation
  Immune responses
  Neoplastic disease
  Tissue injury and burns
Obstruction of lymphatic flow
  Infection or disease of the lymphatic structures
  Surgical removal of lymph nodes

Decreased colloidal osmotic pressure

The plasma proteins exert the osmotic force that is needed to move fluid back into the capillary from the tissue spaces. Edema develops when plasma protein levels become inadequate because of abnormal losses or inadequate production. The glomerulus of the kidney nephron is a network of capillaries. In certain conditions, these capillaries may become permeable to the plasma proteins. When this happens, large amounts of plasma proteins are filtered out of the blood and then lost in the urine. An excess loss of plasma proteins also occurs when large areas of skin are injured or destroyed. Edema is a common problem during the early stages of a burn, resulting from both capillary injury and loss of plasma proteins.

Plasma proteins are synthesized from amino acids. In starvation and malnutrition, edema develops because of a lack of amino acids for use in plasma protein production. In starvation, edema may actually mask the loss of tissue mass. Finally, because plasma proteins are synthesized in the liver, severe liver dysfunction causes decreased plasma protein synthesis with the development of edema and ascites. Liver disease also contributes to edema formation by causing obstruction to venous flow through the portal circulation and through impaired metabolism of hormones, such as aldosterone, which increase sodium retention.

It is now possible to measure the colloid osmotic pressure of the plasma (25.4 mmHg is normal).[1] Infusion of albumin can be used to raise colloidal osmotic pressure as a means of restoring intravascular volume or reversing interstitial fluid losses.

Increased capillary permeability

When the capillary pores become enlarged or the integrity of the capillary wall is destroyed, capillary permeability is increased. Injury due to burns, mechanical distention, inflammation, and immune responses are known to increase capillary permeability. Once an increase in capillary permeability has been established, plasma proteins and other osmotically active particles leak out into the interstitial spaces and perpetuate the accumulation of tissue fluid.

Obstruction of lymphatic flow

The osmotically active plasma proteins and other large particles rely on the lymphatics for movement back into the circulatory system from the interstitial spaces. When lymph flow is obstructed, lymphedema occurs. Malignant involvement of lymph structures and removal of lymph nodes at the time of cancer surgery are common causes of lymphedema. Another cause of lymphedema is infection. Elephantiasis (filariasis) is a tropical infection in which nematodes of the superfamily Filarioidea invade the lymph nodes, causing massive swelling of a body part. This infection has been reported to cause a single leg to swell to such proportions that it weighs almost as much as the rest of the body.

Effects

The effects of edema are determined largely by its location. Edema of the brain, larynx, or lung is an acute, life-threatening condition. On the other hand, swelling of the ankles and feet is often insidious in onset and may or may not be associated with disease. Edema may interfere with movement, limiting motion or making opening of the eyes difficult. Edema can also be disfiguring. In terms of psychological effects and self-concept, edema often causes a distortion of body features, creating problems in obtaining proper-fitting clothing and shoes.

At the tissue level, edema increases the distance for diffusion of oxygen, nutrients, and wastes. Edematous tissues are usually more susceptible to injury and to development of ischemic tissue damage, including pressure sores. The skin of a severely swollen finger can act as a tourniquet, shutting off the blood flow to the finger.

In chronic edema, the intercellular fibers in the tissue spaces become stretched out like an old balloon so that less filtration pressure is needed to push fluids into the interstitial spaces. The stretching of the tissue spaces makes correction or permanent reversal of edema difficult.

Pitting edema

Pitting edema occurs when the accumulation of interstitial fluid exceeds the absorptive capacity of the tissue gel. In pitting edema, the tissue water is mobile and can be translocated with pressure exerted by a finger. Imagine, if you will, a sponge that is supersaturated with water. To test for pitting edema, the observer applies firm finger pressure to the edematous areas. Pitting edema is present if an indentation remains after the finger has been removed.

Nonpitting edema

Nonpitting edema usually reflects a condition in which serum proteins have accumulated in the tissue spaces and coagulated. Often the area is firm and discolored. Brawny edema is a type of nonpitting edema in which the skin thickens and hardens. Nonpitting edema is seen most frequently following local infection or trauma.

Assessment

Methods for assessing edema include visual inspection, including the use of finger pressure to determine the degree of pitting that is present. Pitting edema is evaluated on a scale of +1 to +4. Daily weight is also a useful index of interstitial fluid gain. A third assessment measure involves measuring the circumference of an extremity (or the abdomen).

Treatment

The treatment of edema is usually directed toward (1) maintaining life when the swelling involves vital structures, (2) correcting or controlling the cause, and (3) preventing tissue injury. Diuretic therapy is often used to treat edema. The reader is again reminded that edema is not always associated with disease and that normal compensatory increases in tissue fluid may respond to such simple measures as elevating the feet.

Elastic support stockings and sleeves increase tissue pressure and resistance of the capillary walls to outward movement of fluid, and thus decrease the movement of fluid from the capillary into the tissue spaces. These support devices are often prescribed in conditions such as lymphatic or venous obstruction and are most efficient if applied before the tissue spaces have filled with fluid—in the morning, for example, before the effects of gravity have caused fluid to move into the ankles.

Accumulation of fluid in the serous cavities

The serous cavities are potential spaces located in strategic body areas where there is continual movement of body structures—the joints, the pericardial sac, and the pleural cavity. The exchange of extracellular fluid between the capillaries, the interstitial spaces, and the potential space of the serous cavity resembles capillary exchange elsewhere in the body. The potential spaces are closely linked with lymphatic drainage systems. The milking action of the moving structures continually forces fluid and plasma proteins back into the circulation, keeping these cavities empty. Any obstruction to lymph flow will tend to cause fluid accumulation in the serous cavities.

The prefix *hydro-* may be used to indicate the presence of excessive fluid, as in *hydrothorax,* which means excessive fluid in the pleural cavity. Or the term *effusion* may be used, as in *pleural effusion,* referring to an accumulation of fluid in the pleural cavity.

The fluid accumulated in a serous cavity may be either serous or exudative. A common cause of fluid accumulation in serous cavities is infection. In infection, white cells and cellular debris collect and obstruct lymph flow, causing osmotically active proteins to accumulate. A second cause of fluid accumulation is a malignant tumor; malignant tumors may invade the lymph channels that drain the serous cavity, and thus contribute to fluid accumulation.

Ascites is an accumulation of fluid in the peritoneal cavity. Because of its proximity to the portal circulation, the peritoneal cavity is more susceptible to excess fluid accumulation than are other body cavities. This is because anytime there is a significant increase in pressure in the liver sinusoids, serum exudes through the capillaries on the surface of the liver and passes into the peritoneal cavity. Congestive heart failure, cirrhosis, and carcinoma of the liver are examples of conditions that obstruct hepatic blood flow and cause fluid to move into the peritoneal cavity. Because the portal vein receives blood from the peritoneal surface, portal hypertension creates an increase in the filtration pressure of the capillaries that line the peritoneal cavity.

Excess fluid may be aspirated or removed from a serous cavity. The term *paracentesis* refers to puncture of a cavity for removal of fluid. Usually a needle or similar instrument is inserted into the cavity and the fluid is withdrawn. Analysis of the fluid for the presence of infectious organisms and malignant cells often aids in diagnosis of the disease responsible for the fluid accumulation.

In summary, edema occurs in healthy as well as sick individuals. The physiologic mechanisms that predispose to edema formation are (1) increased capillary pressure, (2) decreased capillary colloidal osmotic pressure, (3) increased capillary permeability, and (4) obstruction of lymphatic flow. The effect that edema exerts on body function is determined by its location—cerebral edema can be a life-threatening situation, whereas swollen feet can be a normal discomfort that accompanies hot weather.

Reference

1. Morissette MP: Colloid osmotic pressure: Its measurement and clinical value. Can Med Assoc J 116:897, 1977

CHAPTER 29

Alterations in Acid–Base Balance

Objectives

After you have studied this chapter, you should be able to meet the following objectives:

_____ Define the terms *acid* and *base*.

_____ Cite the source of the body's volatile and metabolic acids.

_____ Describe the three forms of carbon dioxide transport and their contribution to acid–base balance.

_____ Compare the role of the kidneys and respiratory system in regulation of acid–base balance.

_____ State the Henderson-Hasselbalch equation and explain its use.

_____ Describe the blood buffer systems.

_____ Describe the renal phosphate buffer system and the ammonia buffer system.

_____ State the difference between acidemia and acidosis.

_____ Compare corrective and compensatory mechanisms for regulating body pH.

_____ Explain how potassium ions and hydrogen ions interact in pH regulation.

_____ Use the example of the postprandial alkaline tide to explain the bicarbonate ion/chloride ion interaction in pH regulation.

_____ State the definitions of *metabolic acidosis, metabolic alkalosis, respiratory acidosis,* and *respiratory alkalosis.*

_____ List the common causes of metabolic acidosis, metabolic alkalosis, respiratory acidosis, and respiratory alkalosis.

_____ Compare the neurologic manifestations of acidosis and alkalosis.

_____ Describe a clinical situation involving an acid–base disorder in which both primary and compensatory mechanisms might be active.

_____ Contrast and compare the clinical manifestations of acidosis and alkalosis.

Normal body function depends on acid–base balance being regulated within a narrow physiologic range. The metabolic activities that take place in the body require the precise regulation of pH so that membrane excitability, enzyme systems, and chemical reactions can function in an optimal way. Two types of acids are produced during the metabolic processes that transform carbohydrates, fats, and proteins into cellular energy: volatile respiratory acids and nonvolatile metabolic acids. Carbonic acid, which is volatile, results from dissolved carbon dioxide, which is eliminated through the lungs. All the other acids that are formed in the body or that enter the body through the gastrointestinal tract or parenteral route are referred to as *metabolic acids*. The use of the term metabolic acids may seem confusing, since carbonic acid is also derived from metabolic processes. By convention, however, the nonvolatile acids are referred to as metabolic acids to differentiate them from carbonic acid, which is called a *respiratory acid*. The hydrogen ions from the fixed metabolic acids are eliminated through the kidneys.

When one speaks of regulation of pH, it implies the regulation of the hydrogen ion (H⁺). Many conditions, pathologic or otherwise, can alter body pH. This chapter focuses on metabolic and respiratory-induced changes in acid–base balance.

Determination of pH

An *acid* is a molecule that can contribute a H⁺ ion and a *base* is a molecule that can accept or remove a H⁺ ion. An *alkali* is a combination of one or more alkali metals such as sodium or potassium with a highly basic ion such as a hydroxyl ion (OH⁻). Sodium bicarbonate is the main alkali in the extracellular fluid. Although the definitions differ somewhat, the terms *alkali* and *base* are often used interchangeably. Hence the term alkalosis has come to mean the opposite of acidosis.

The degree to which an acid dissociates and acts as a hydrogen donor determines whether it is a strong or weak acid. The same is true of a base and its ability to dissociate and accept a hydrogen ion. Most of the body's acids and bases are weak acids and bases; the most important of these are carbonic acid and bicarbonate.

The symbol pH refers to the concentration of hydrogen ions, or more specifically to the negative logarithm (*p*) of the hydrogen ion (H⁺) in equivalents per liter (pH of 7.0 implies a hydrogen concentration of 10^{-7} equivalents per liter). The hydrogen ion and carbon dioxide content of the body are normally regulated so that the pH of the extracellular fluids is maintained within the narrow range of 7.35 to 7.45.

Both hydrogen and bicarbonate are by-products of metabolic processes. Hydrogen ions are continuously formed as body fuels are oxidized. Persons in western society, with their large protein and fat intake, produce considerable amounts of nonvolatile acids. The catabolism of proteins yields two strong inorganic acids–sulfuric and phosphoric. Incomplete oxidation of glucose results in the formation of lactic acid, and oxidation of fats, in ketoacids. In all, the average diet yields about 40 mmol to 80 mmol of hydrogen ions that must be eliminated each day.

Despite the substantial amount of fixed metabolic acids that result from protein and fat metabolism, by far the largest source of metabolic acids is the oxidation of glucose and other carbohydrates that yield carbon dioxide. One molecule of glucose, for example, yields six molecules of carbon dioxide.

Carbon dioxide combines with water to form bicarbonate ($CO_2 + H_2O = H^+ + HCO_3^-$). This reaction is catalyzed by an enzyme called *carbonic anhydrase*, which is present in large quantities in red blood cells, renal tubular cells, and other tissues in the body. The rate of the reaction between carbon dioxide and water is increased about 5000 times by the presence of carbonic anhydrase. Were it not for this enzyme, the reaction would occur too slowly to be of any significance.

The carbon dioxide in the blood is transported in three forms: (1) attached to hemoglobin, (2) as dissolved carbon dioxide, and (3) as bicarbonate (Figure 29-1). Normally, about 23% of the carbon dioxide is transported in the red blood cell, where it is attached to the hemoglobin molecule. A small percentage of carbon dioxide dissolves in the plasma; it is the source of carbonic acid (H_2CO_3). The remaining carbon dioxide is carried as the bicarbonate ion (HCO_3^-). Collectively, dissolved carbon dioxide and HCO_3^- constitute about 77% of the carbon dioxide that is transported in the extracellular fluid.

The dissolved carbon dioxide content of the blood can be calculated using the partial pressure of carbon dioxide (P_{CO_2}) and its solubility coefficient.

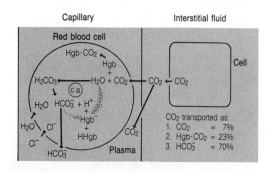

Figure 29-1 Mechanisms of carbon dioxide transport. (*After Guyton AC: Textbook of Medical Physiology, 7th ed. Philadelphia, WB Saunders, 1986*)

Under normal physiologic conditions, the solubility coefficient for carbon dioxide is 0.03. This means that the dissolved carbon dioxide concentration in the venous blood, which normally has a P_{CO_2} value of about 45 mm Hg, will be 1.35 mEq/liter or 1.35 mmol/liter ($45 \times 0.03 = 1.35$). The dissolved carbon dioxide and carbonic acid in a solution are in a reversible equilibrium state, with the amount of carbonic acid that is present being proportional to the amount of dissolved carbon dioxide. Because it is almost impossible to measure undissociated carbonic acid, dissolved carbon dioxide (CO_2) is usually used instead of carbonic acid in calculating pH.

The pH of the extracellular fluid is determined by the ratio of bicarbonate to carbonic acid and the degree to which carbonic acid dissociates to form a hydrogen ion and a bicarbonate ion. The dissociation constant (K) is used to describe the degree to which an acid or base dissociates. The symbol pK refers to the negative logarithm of the dissociation constant. At normal body temperature the pK for the bicarbonate buffer system is 6.1. The use of a negative logarithm for the dissociation constant allows pH to be expressed as a positive value.

The Henderson-Hasselbalch equation calculates the serum pH by using the logarithm of the dissociation constant and the logarithm of the bicarbonate to dissolved CO_2 ratio. In its simplest form this equation states that

$$pH = pK + \log \frac{HCO_3^-}{CO_2}$$

As a point of emphasis, it is the ratio rather than the absolute values for bicarbonate and dissolved CO_2 (carbonic acid) that determines pH. Let us consider two examples to emphasize this point. The first situation uses normal serum values and the second uses increased concentrations of both bicarbonate and dissolved CO_2

Situation 1

$$pH\ 7.4 = 6.1 + \log \frac{27\ \text{mEq/liter}\ HCO_3}{1.35\ \text{mEq/liter}\ CO_2}$$

ratio 27:1.35 = 20:1*

Situation 2

$$pH\ 7.4 = 6.1 + \log \frac{48\ \text{mEq/liter}\ HCO_3}{2.40\ \text{mEq/liter}\ CO_2}$$

ratio 48:2.4 = 20:1*

These examples demonstrate that pH will remain relatively stable over a wide range of changes in bicarbonate and dissolved CO_2 concentrations as long as

* The log of 20 is 1.3.

the two concentrations approach a ratio value of 20 to 1. Plasma pH will decrease when the ratio is less than 20 to 1 (for example, the log of 10 is 1; when the ratio of bicarbonate to dissolved CO_2 is equal to 10, the pH of the blood will be 7.1), and it will increase when the ratio is greater than 20 to 1.

Regulation of acid–base balance

The pH of body fluids is regulated by buffering mechanisms that prevent large moment-to-moment changes in body pH, by respiratory and renal mechanisms that eliminate excess acids and bases, and by the selective conservation of bicarbonate by the kidneys. The pH is further influenced by the electrolyte composition of the intracellular and extracellular compartments.

Acid–base buffer systems

The second-by-second regulation of body fluid pH is dependent on buffer systems. These buffer systems are immediately available to combine with excess acids or alkalis and thus prevent large changes in pH from occurring while respiratory and renal mechanisms are being recruited.

A buffer system consists of a weak acid and the alkali salt of that acid, or a weak base and its acid salt. In the process of preventing large changes in pH, the system trades a strong acid for a weak acid or a strong base for a weak base. There are three major buffer systems that protect the pH of body fluids: the bicarbonate buffer system, the phosphate buffer system, and protein buffers.

In the *bicarbonate buffer system*, CO_2 is the source of both carbonic acid and bicarbonate. This buffering system substitutes the weak carbonic acid for a strong acid such as hydrochloric acid ($HCl + NaHCO_3 \rightleftharpoons H_2CO_3 + NaCl$) or the weak bicarbonate base for a strong base such as sodium hydroxide ($NaOH + H_2CO_3 \rightleftharpoons NaHCO_3 + H_2O$). The bicarbonate buffering system is unique in that its acid is volatile and can be released into the air through the lungs. The *phosphate buffer system* consists of two elements, $H_2PO_4^-$ and HPO_4^{--}. When a strong acid such as hydrochloric acid is added to a mixture of these two phosphates, a weak acid is formed and the pH changes only slightly ($HCl + Na_2HPO_4 \rightleftharpoons NaH_2PO_4 + NaCl$). Likewise, if a strong base such as sodium hydroxide is added to the solution, a weak base is formed ($NaOH + NaH_2PO_4 \rightleftharpoons Na_2HPO_4 + H_2O$). Because phosphate is eliminated in the urine, this system is particularly important in buffering fluids in the kidney tubules. *Proteins* are composed of amino acids, some of which have free acidic radicals that can dissociate into base and hydrogen ions. The protein buffers are largely located within cells. Both hydrogen and CO_2 can diffuse across cell membranes for buffering by intracellular proteins. The protein buffer system is particularly plentiful and hence it is a very important and powerful system.

Respiratory control mechanisms

The respiratory system provides for the elimination of CO_2 into the air and plays a major role in acid–base regulation. Carbon dioxide crosses the blood-brain barrier with ease and in the process reacts with water to form carbonic acid which dissociates into hydrogen and bicarbonate ions; it is the hydrogen ions that stimulate the respiratory center. Thus, increased levels of CO_2 in the blood induce an almost immediate increase in ventilation, causing an increase in the amount of CO_2 exhaled and thus a rapid correction in CO_2 level.

Renal control mechanisms

The kidneys play an essential role in acid–base regulation. The renal mechanisms for regulating acid–base balance cannot adjust the pH within minutes, as respiratory mechanisms can, but they keep on functioning until the pH has returned to normal or near-normal range.

Hydrogen ion elimination– bicarbonate conservation

The kidneys regulate acid–base balance by eliminating hydrogen ions and reabsorbing bicarbonate ions. Bicarbonate reabsorption can be regarded as a recycling process in which the filtered bicarbonate is reabsorbed and returned to the blood. The process of bicarbonate reabsorption begins when CO_2 moves into a tubular cell and combines with water, in a carbonic anhydrase-mediated reaction, to form a bicarbonate ion and hydrogen ion (Figure 29-2). The hydrogen ion is then secreted into the tubular fluid and a sodium ion is reabsorbed in a coupled transport process. The reabsorbed sodium ion and the newly generated bicarbonate ion move from the tubular cell into the extracellular fluid. In the tubular fluid, the secreted hydrogen ion combines with a filtered bicarbonate ion to yield CO_2 and water. The water eliminated in the urine and the CO_2 diffuses into the tubular cell and combines with water to form another bicarbonate and hydrogen ion.

Normally, only a few of the hydrogen ions remain in the tubular fluid as it moves from the proximal to the distal and collecting tubules to become

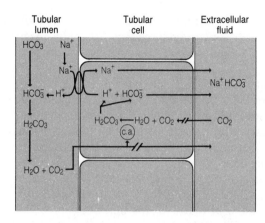

Figure 29-2 Hydrogen ion (H^+) secretion and bicarbonate ion (HCO_3^-) retrieval in a renal tubular cell. Carbon dioxide (CO_2) diffuses into the tubular cell from the blood or urine filtrate where it combines with water in a carbonic anhydrase (c.a.) catalyzed reaction that yields carbonic acid (H_2CO_3). The H_2CO_3 dissociates to form H^+ and HCO_3^-. The H^+ is secreted into the tubular fluid in exchange for Na^+. The Na^+ and HCO_3^- enter the extracellular fluid.

urine. This is because the secretion of hydrogen ions into the tubular fluid is usually roughly equivalent to the number of bicarbonate ions that are filtered in the glomerulus. When excess CO_2 is present, as occurs during respiratory acidosis, hydrogen ion secretion exceeds bicarbonate ion filtration and the urine becomes acidic. On the other hand, filtration of bicarbonate in excess of hydrogen ion secretion results in production of an alkaline urine.

Tubular buffering systems

The pH of the urine can range from as low as about 4.6 to 8.0. An extremely acidic urine would be damaging to structures in the urinary tract; this limits the number of unbuffered hydrogen ions that can be excreted by the kidneys. When the number of hydrogen ions that are secreted into the tubular fluid threaten to cause the pH of the urine to become too acidic, the phosphate and ammonia systems buffer the excess hydrogen ions.

The phosphate buffer system uses monohydrogen phosphate (HPO_4^{--}) and dihydrogen phosphate ($H_2PO_4^-$) that are present in the urine. The combination of H^+ with HPO_4^{--} to form $H_2PO_4^-$ allows the kidneys to increase their excretion of hydrogen ions (Figure 29-3). Because they are poorly absorbed, the phosphates become more concentrated as they move through the tubules. Importantly, this system works best when the renal tubular fluid becomes more acidic.

Renal tubular cells are able to use amino acids to synthesize ammonia and secrete it into the tubular fluid. The ammonia buffer system allows hydrogen ions to combine with ammonia (NH_3) to form an

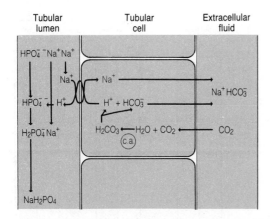

Figure 29-3 The renal phosphate buffer system. The monohydrogen phosphate ion (HPO_4^{--}) enters the renal tubular fluid in the glomerulus. A H^+ combines with the HPO_4^{--} to form $H_2PO_4^-$ and is then excreted into the urine in combination with Na^+. The HCO_3^- moves into the extracellular fluid along with the Na^+ that was exchanged during secretion of the H^+.

ammonium ion (NH_4^+). The tubular fluid contains abundant quantities of chloride ions, and the ammonium ion is excreted in the urine as ammonium chloride (Figure 29-4). Because this process requires large amounts of an enzyme that deaminates the amino acids that are used in ammonia synthesis, it takes 2 or 3 days for the tubular cells to increase enzyme synthesis and for this buffer system to become efficient.

Ion exchange systems and their effect on *p*H

Because of their electrogenic properties, the positively charged hydrogen ion and the negatively charged bicarbonate ion can be exchanged for other ions; this can influence acid–base balance.

Potassium-hydrogen

The potassium ion interacts in important ways with the hydrogen ion. Both ions are positively charged and both ions move freely between the intracellular and extracellular compartments; when excess hydrogen ions are present in the extracellular fluid, they move into the intracellular compartment for buffering. When this happens, another cation—in this case potassium—must leave the cell and move into the extracellular fluid. Hydrogen ions can also be exchanged for potassium ions when the need arises. When extracellular potassium levels fall, potassium moves out of the cell and is replaced by hydrogen ions.

The reciprocity between hydrogen and potassium ion exchange extends to the kidneys. When plasma potassium levels decrease, fewer potassium ions are available for secretion in the urine by the renal tubular cells and consequently hydrogen ion se-

cretion is increased. As hydrogen ion secretion continues, metabolic alkalosis develops. An elevation in plasma potassium has the opposite effect. Acidosis causes a decrease in potassium secretion and alkalosis an increase in potassium secretion.

Chloride-bicarbonate

One of the mechanisms that the kidneys use in regulating the *p*H of the extracellular fluids is to conserve or eliminate bicarbonate ions; in the process, it is often necessary to shuffle anions. Chloride is the most abundant anion in the extracellular fluid and can substitute for bicarbonate when an anion shift is needed. As an example, serum bicarbonate levels normally increase as hydrochloric acid is secreted into the stomach following a heavy meal, causing what is termed the *postprandial alkaline tide*. Later, as the chloride is reabsorbed in the small intestine, the *p*H returns to normal. *Hypochloremic alkalosis* refers to an increase in *p*H that is induced by a decrease in serum chloride levels. *Hyperchloremic acidosis* occurs when excess levels of chloride are present.

Body sodium levels can influence acid–base balance. Sodium reabsorption in the kidneys requires the reabsorption of an accompanying anion. The two major anions in the extracellular fluid are chloride and bicarbonate. If sodium reabsorption is markedly stimulated, as a result of prolonged sodium chloride deprivation or volume contraction, increased bicarbonate reabsorption can produce an alkalosis.

Laboratory tests

The terms *acidemia* and *alkalemia* refer only to the *p*H of the blood as measured on a *p*H meter and give little information about the cause of the acid–base

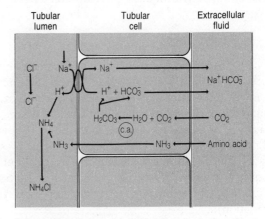

Figure 29-4 The ammonia buffer system in a renal tubular cell. The tubular cell synthesizes ammonia (NH_3) from amino acids. The NH_3 is secreted into the tubular fluid, where it combines with a H^+ to form an ammonium ion (NH_4^+). The ammonium ion combines with chloride for excretion in the urine. The HCO_3^- moves into the extracellular fluid along with the Na^+ that was exchanged during secretion of the H^+.

disorder. It was pointed out earlier that pH can be relatively normal within a wide range of dissolved CO_2 and base bicarbonate levels. A number of laboratory tests can be used to obtain a better description of acid–base disorders.

Carbon dioxide

As mentioned previously, the dissolved CO_2 levels can be determined from blood gas measurements using the PCO_2 and the solubility coefficient for CO_2 (normal arterial PCO_2 is 38–42 mmHg). The total CO_2 content of blood, including that contained in bicarbonate, can be obtained by adding a strong acid to a plasma sample and measuring the amount of CO_2 generated.

Bicarbonate

More than 70% of the CO_2 in the blood is in the form of bicarbonate. The serum bicarbonate concentration can be determined from the total CO_2 content of the blood. The normal range of values for venous bicarbonate is 24 mEq/liter to 33 mEq/liter (24 mmol/liter to 33 mmol/liter).

Base excess or deficit

Base excess or deficit measures the level of all the buffer systems of the blood–hemoglobin, protein, phosphate, and bicarbonate. The normal base excess or deficit describes the amount of a fixed acid or base that must be added to a blood sample to achieve a pH of 7.4 (normal ±3.0 mEq/liter).[1] For practical purposes, base excess/deficit is a measurement of bicarbonate excess or deficit. A positive result (bicarbonate excess) indicates metabolic alkalosis and a negative result (bicarbonate deficit) indicates metabolic acidosis.

Anion gap

The anion gap describes the difference between the sodium ion concentration and the sum of the measured anions (Cl^- and HCO_3^-) in the extracellular fluid. This difference represents the concentration of unmeasured anions, such as phosphates, sulfates, organic acids, and proteins, that is present (Figure 29-5). Normally, the anion gap is about 12 mEq/liter (a value of 16 mEq is normal if both the sodium and potassium concentrations are used in the calculation).

In summary, normal body function depends on the precise regulation of acid–base balance. The pH of the extracellular fluid is normally maintained within the narrow physiologic range of 7.35 to 7.45.

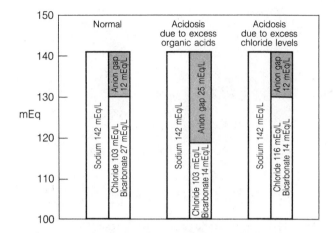

Figure 29-5 The anion gap in acidosis due to excess metabolic acids and excess serum chloride levels. Unmeasured anions such as phosphates, sulfates, and organic acids increase the anion gap because they replace bicarbonate (this assumes there is no change in sodium content).

Metabolic processes produce volatile and fixed metabolic acids that must be buffered and eliminated from the body. The volatile acid, H_2CO_3, is in equilibrium with dissolved CO_2, which is eliminated from the lungs. The fixed metabolic acids, most of which are excreted by the kidneys, are derived mainly from protein and fat metabolism. It is the ratio of the bicarbonate ion concentration to dissolved CO_2 (carbonic acid concentration) that determines body pH. When this ratio is 20:1, the pH is 7.4. The ability of the body to maintain pH within the normal physiologic range depends on respiratory and renal mechanisms as well as blood buffer systems; the most important of these is the bicarbonate buffer system. Potassium and hydrogen ions are interchangeable cations; excess potassium can affect acid–base balance and alterations in acid–base balance can affect potassium levels. Likewise, the bicarbonate and chloride anions can produce changes in acid–base balance as they are interchanged.

Alterations in acid–base balance

The terms *acidosis* and *alkalosis* describe the clinical conditions that arise as a result of changes in dissolved CO_2 and bicarbonate concentration. Any condition that produces a change in pulmonary ventilation sufficient to significantly alter the CO_2 content of the blood is referred to as a *respiratory acid/base disorder*. The term *metabolic acidosis* or *alkalosis* refers to all other types of acid–base disorders that result from a change in bicarbonate levels (Chart 29-1).

Acidosis and alkalosis usually involve both a primary or initiating event and a compensatory state that results from homeostatic mechanisms that attempt to correct or prevent large changes in *p*H. For example, a person may have a primary metabolic acidosis as a result of overproduction of ketoacids and a compensatory respiratory alkalosis because of a compensatory increase in ventilation. Compensatory mechanisms adjust the *p*H toward a more normal level without actually correcting the underlying cause of the the disorder. The respiratory mechanisms, which compensate by either increasing or decreasing ventilation, are rapid but seldom able to return the *p*H to normal. This is because, as the *p*H returns toward normal, the respiratory stimulus is lost. The kidneys compensate by conserving bicarbonate or secreting hydrogen ions. It normally takes longer to recruit renal mechanisms than respiratory mechanisms. Renal mechanisms are more efficient, however, because they continue to operate until the *p*H has returned to normal or a near-normal value.

Compensatory mechanisms usually provide a means to control *p*H in situations where correction is impossible or cannot be immediately achieved. Often, compensatory mechanisms are interim measures that permit survival while the body attempts to correct the primary disorder. It is important to recognize that compensation requires the use of mechanisms that are different from those that caused the primary disorder. In other words, the lungs cannot compensate for respiratory acidosis that is caused by lung disease, nor can the kidneys compensate for metabolic acidosis that occurs because of renal failure. The body can, however, use renal mechanisms to compensate for respiratory-induced changes in *p*H and it can use respiratory mechanisms to compensate for metabolically induced changes in acid–base balance.

As with other conditions, compensatory mechanisms vary in acute and chronic acid–base disorders. Figure 29-6 is a *p*H–bicarbonate diagram that can be used to determine the acute or chronic nature of an acid–base disorder and the compensation that has occurred. From the diagram, it can be seen that a given increase in PCO_2 is associated with a lesser fall in *p*H in chronic compensated respiratory acidosis than in acute uncompensated respiratory acidosis.

Most of the manifestations of acid–base disorders fall into three categories: (1) those associated with the primary disorder that caused the *p*H disturbance, (2) those related to the altered *p*H, and (3) those that occur because of the body's attempt to

compensate for the altered *p*H. Many of the alterations in body function associated with acid–base disturbances are related to the *p*H change and its effect on the excitability of the nervous system. The hydrogen ion tends to stabilize nerve membranes, rendering them less excitable. When the *p*H falls below 7.0, for example, the nervous system becomes so depressed that confusion and coma develop. Alterations in *p*H also affect calcium ionization and thus affect neural excitability, which also contributes to the neurologic manifestations that occur with acid–base disorders. Ionization of calcium and neural excitability are decreased in acidosis and increased in alkalosis.

Metabolic acidosis

Metabolic acidosis refers to a primary deficit in base bicarbonate that results from excess production of fixed metabolic acids. In metabolic acidosis, the blood *p*H falls below 7.35, and the serum bicarbonate decreases to less than 24 mEq/liter.

Causes

There are two major causes of metabolic acidosis: increased gain of metabolic acids or excessive loss of bicarbonate (Table 29-1). The increased gain of unmeasured metabolic acids results in an increased anion gap. Chloride levels increase in situations of bicarbonate loss. Therefore, when metabolic acidosis is due to decreased bicarbonate levels, the anion gap is within normal limits.

Increased metabolic acid gain. Metabolic acids increase when (1) there is an overproduction of ketoacids, (2) lactic acid is formed as body cells are forced to metabolize carbohydrates without a sufficient supply of oxygen, or (3) the kidneys are unable to excrete metabolic acids. The presence of excess metabolic acids leads to a replacement of sodium bicarbonate by the sodium salt of the offending acid (*e.g.*, sodium lactate); this produces an increase in the anion gap.

An overproduction of ketoacids occurs when carbohydrate stores are inadequate or when the body cannot use available carbohydrates as a fuel. Under these conditions, fatty acids are converted to ketones. When ketone production exceeds utilization, ketoacidosis develops.

Chart 29-1: Primary defects in acid–base balance

↓ HCO_3^- Metabolic acidosis represents a decrease in bicarbonate (HCO_3^- deficit)

↑ H_2CO_3 Respiratory acidosis represents an increase in carbonic acid (H_2CO_3 excess)

↑ HCO_3^- Metabolic alkalosis represents an increase in bicarbonate (HCO_3^- excess)

↓ H_2CO_3 Respiratory alkalosis represents a decrease in carbonic acid (H_2CO_3 deficit)

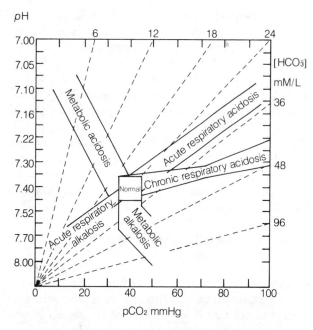

Figure 29-6 Acute and chronic acid–base disorders as determined by Pco_2, bicarbonate, and pH values. *(Adapted from Masoro EJ, Siegel PD: Acid–Base Regulation: Its Physiology, Pathophysiology and Interpretation of Blood Gas Analysis. Philadelphia, WB Saunders, 1977)*

The most common cause of ketoacidosis is uncontrolled diabetes mellitus, in which an insulin deficiency leads to the release of fatty acids from adipose cells with subsequent production of excess ketoacids (see Chapter 45). During periods of fasting or food deprivation, the lack of carbohydrates produces a self-limited state of ketoacidosis. This is because the fall in blood sugar that accompanies fasting promotes the release of insulin, which acts to suppress the release of fatty acids from fat cells. A ketogenic diet is one that is low in carbohydrate and favors ketoacid production. Over the years, various ketogenic diets have been used for weight reduction; part of the success of these diets derives from symptoms such as anorexia that occur with metabolic acidosis.

A condition called *alcoholic ketoacidosis* can develop in alcoholics. It usually follows prolonged alcohol ingestion, particularly if accompanied by decreased food intake and vomiting.[2,3] Ketones are formed during the oxidation of alcohol, a process that occurs in the liver. The ketoacids responsible for alcoholic ketoacidosis are, in part, formed as a result of alcohol metabolism. The condition also develops in response to starvation and extracellular fluid volume depletion caused by vomiting, decreased fluid intake, and the inhibition of antidiuretic hormone by alcohol (see Chapter 27). Ketone formation is enhanced by the hypoglycemia that results from alcohol-induced inhibition of glucose synthesis (gluconeogenesis) by

the liver and impaired ketone elimination by the kidneys due to dehydration. Numerous other factors, such as elevations in cortisol, growth hormone, glucagon, and catecholamines, mediate free fatty acid release and thereby contribute to the development of alcoholic ketoacidosis.

Lactic acid is produced during periods of anaerobic metabolism, which occurs when cells do not receive enough oxygen to convert body fuels to CO_2 and water. Blood flow to the skeletal muscles, liver, and other tissues is decreased during circulatory shock and heart failure. Lactic acid also accumulates during periods of excessive oxygen need, such as strenuous exercise, when blood flow and consequent oxygen delivery cannot keep pace with the increased needs of the exercising muscles.

Aspirin (acetylsalicylic acid) is converted to salicylic acid in the body. Salicylate overdose produces serious toxic effects, including death. Among the effects of salicylate toxicity are two types of acid–base disorders: an initial respiratory alkalosis and a subsequent severe metabolic acidosis. The salicylates cross the blood-brain barrier and directly stimulate the respiratory center, causing a fall in Pco_2 and respiratory alkalosis. The kidneys compensate by excreting increased amounts of bicarbonate, potassium, and sodium. This contributes to the development of metabolic acidosis. Salicylates also interfere with carbohydrate metabolism, which results in increased production of metabolic acids.

One of the treatments for salicylate toxicity is alkalization of the plasma. Salicylic acid, which is a weak acid, exists in equilibrium with the alkaline salicylate anion. It is the salicylic acid that is toxic because of its ability to cross cell membranes and enter brain cells. The salicylate anion crosses membranes poorly and is less toxic. With alkalization of the extracellular fluids, the ratio of salicylic acid to salicylate is greatly reduced. This allows cellular salicylic acid to move out of cells into the extracellular fluid along a concentration gradient. Respiratory alkalosis may be self-protective.[4] The renal elimination of salicylates follows a similar pattern when the urine is alkalinized. Hemodialysis (use of the artificial kidney) may be used to increase the removal of salicylates from the body when salicylate toxicity is life-threatening.

The kidneys both conserve bicarbonate and secrete hydrogen ions for elimination in the urine. In renal failure there is loss of both glomerular and tubular function with retention of nitrogenous wastes and metabolic acids. In a condition called *renal tubular acidosis*, there is normal glomerular function, but the tubular secretion of hydrogen ions or reabsorption of bicarbonate is abnormal. Renal tubular acidosis is discussed in Chapter 31.

Increased bicarbonate losses. Increased bicarbonate losses occur with loss of bicarbonate-rich body fluids or when there is an excess of chloride ions. Intestinal secretions have a high bicarbonate concentration. Consequently, excessive losses of bicarbonate occur with severe diarrhea, small bowel or biliary fistula drainage, iliostomy drainage, and intestinal suction. In diarrhea of microbial origin, bicarbonate is secreted into the bowel to neutralize the metabolic acids that are produced by the microorganisms causing the diarrhea.

When the anion gap is within normal limits, there is a reciprocal relationship between serum chloride concentrations and serum bicarbonate levels; when chloride levels are elevated, the bicarbonate levels decrease. Hyperchloremic acidosis can occur as the result of abnormal absorption of chloride by the kidneys or as a result of treatment with chloride-containing medications (sodium chloride, amino acid-chloride hyperalimentation solutions, and ammonium chloride). Ammonium chloride is broken down into an ammonium (NH_4^+) and a chloride ion. The ammonium ion is converted to urea in the liver, leaving the chloride ion free to react with hydrogen to form hydrochloric acid. The administration of intravenous sodium chloride or parenteral hyperalimentation solutions that contain an amino acid-chloride combination can cause acidosis in a similar manner.

Manifestations

The manifestations of metabolic acidosis fall into three categories: (1) signs and symptoms of the disorder causing the acidosis, (2) alterations in function resulting from the decreased pH, and (3) changes in body function related to recruitment of compensatory mechanisms. The signs and symptoms of metabolic acidosis usually begin to appear when the plasma bicarbonate concentration falls to 20 mEq/liter or less.

Metabolic acidosis is seldom a primary disorder. Rather it usually develops during the course of another disease. Hence the manifestations of metabolic acidosis are frequently superimposed on the symptoms of the contributing health problem. With diabetic ketoacidosis, which is a common cause of

---

Table 29–1. Metabolic acidosis

Causes	Manifestations
Excess metabolic acids (increased anion gap)	pH below 7.35
Excessive production of metabolic acids	Bicarbonate below 24 mEq/liter
Fasting and starvation	(24 mmol/liter)
Ketogenic diet	**Altered gastrointestinal function**
Diabetic ketoacidosis	Anorexia
Lactic acidosis	Nausea
Alcoholic ketoacidosis	Vomiting
Salicylate poisoning	Abdominal pain
Decreased loss of metabolic acids	**Depression of neural function**
Kidney failure or dysfunction	Weakness
Excessive bicarbonate loss (normal anion gap)	Lethargy
	General malaise
Loss of intestinal secretions	Confusion
Diarrhea	Stupor
Intestinal suction	Coma
Intestinal or biliary fistula	Depression of vital functions
Increased renal losses	**Cardiovascular manifestations**
Renal tubular acidosis	Cardiac arrhythmias
Treatment with acetazolamide	Heart unresponsive to catecholamines
Increased chloride levels	Decreased heart rate
Abnormal chloride reabsorption by the kidney	Decreased cardiac output
Sodium chloride infusions	**Skin**
Treatment with ammonium chloride	Warm and flushed
Parenteral hyperalimentation	**Signs of compensation**
	Kussmaul breathing
	Decreased PCO_2
	Acid urine
	Increased ammonia in urine

metabolic acidosis, there is an increase in blood and urine sugars and a characteristic smell of ketones to the breath. In metabolic acidosis that accompanies renal failure, blood urea nitrogen levels are elevated and tests of renal function yield abnormal results.

Changes in pH have a direct effect on body function that can produce signs and symptoms that are common to all types of acidosis, regardless of cause. A person with metabolic acidosis will often complain of weakness, fatigue, general malaise, and a dull headache. There may also be anorexia, nausea, vomiting, and abdominal pain. As mentioned earlier, the anorexia associated with mild metabolic acidosis may be viewed as an advantage to someone on a weight loss ketogenic diet. On the other hand, the gastrointestinal symptoms may be misleading in a person with undiagnosed diabetes mellitus. In this case, the person may be thought to have gastrointestinal flu or other abdominal pathology, such as appendicitis.

Neural activity becomes depressed as body pH declines. The hydrogen ion crosses the blood-brain barrier with ease; as acidosis progresses, the level of consciousness decreases and stupor and coma develop. The skin is often warm and flushed because skin vessels become less responsive to the vasoconstrictor input from the sympathetic nervous system. Tissue turgor is impaired and the skin is dry when fluid deficit accompanies acidosis. When the pH falls to 7.0, cardiac dysrhythmias, including fatal ventricular dysrhythmias, can develop and the heart becomes unresponsive to the catecholamines (norepinephrine and epinephrine). At this point both heart rate and cardiac output decrease.

Metabolic acidosis is accompanied by signs and symptoms related to the recruitment of compensatory mechanisms. When renal mechanisms are operative, the urine pH will decrease and urine ammonia levels will rise. The respiratory system compensates for a decrease in pH by increasing ventilation; this is accomplished through deep and rapid respirations. In diabetic ketoacidosis, this breathing pattern is referred to as *Kussmaul breathing*. For descriptive purposes, it can be said that Kussmaul breathing resembles the hyperpnea of exercise—the person breathes as though he/she had been running. There may be complaints of difficult breathing or dyspnea with exertion; with severe acidosis, dyspnea may be present even at rest.

Treatment

The treatment of metabolic acidosis focuses on correcting the condition that caused the disorder and restoring the fluids and electrolytes that have been lost from the body. The treatment of diabetic ketoacidosis is discussed in Chapter 45.

Metabolic alkalosis

Metabolic alkalosis refers to a primary increase in serum base bicarbonate. In metabolic alkalosis, blood pH is above 7.45, plasma bicarbonate is above 29 mEq/liter (29 mmol/liter), and base excess is above +3.0 mEq/liter (3 mmol/liter).

Causes

Metabolic alkalosis occurs in conditions that either increase the intake of bicarbonate or other bases (carbonate, citrate, acetate), or produce excess retention of bicarbonate by the kidneys (Table 29-2). Most of the body's serum bicarbonate is obtained either from CO_2 that is produced during metabolic processes or from recycling of bicarbonate by the kidneys. Usually bicarbonate production and renal reabsorption are balanced in a manner that prevents alkalosis from occurring. It is only when new bicarbonate is added to the body or excessive amounts of bicarbonate are retained that metabolic alkalosis develops. Calcium increases bicarbonate reabsorption by the kidneys. A condition called the *milk alkali syndrome* may develop in persons who consume excessive amounts of milk along with alkaline antacids.

Hydrogen and chloride losses are associated with increased bicarbonate retention by the kidneys. Chloride is the major anion in the extracellular fluid and when it is lost from the body, bicarbonate is conserved as a replacement anion. Vomiting, removal of gastric secretion through use of nasogastric suction, and diuretics are the most common causes of metabolic alkalosis in hospitalized patients.[5] Bulimia, or self-induced vomiting, is often associated with metabolic alkalosis.[6] In hypokalemia, renal excretion of hydrogen ions is decreased as the kidneys focus on conserving potassium. Sudden decreases in extracellular fluid volume produce an increase in renal reabsorption of sodium and bicarbonate. This is referred to as a *volume contraction* and can occur in the course of diuretic therapy. Diuretics that block chloride reabsorption in the kidney (*e.g.,* chlorothiazide and furosemide) produce a bicarbonate retention through both volume contraction and loss of the chloride ion.

Respiratory acidosis produces a compensatory loss of hydrogen and chloride ions in the urine along with bicarbonate retention. When respiratory acidosis is corrected abruptly, metabolic alkalosis may develop.

Manifestations

Persons with metabolic alkalosis are often asymptomatic or have signs related to volume depletion or hypokalemia. The neurologic signs (hyperexcitability) occur less frequently with metabolic alkalosis than with other acid–base disorders. This is because the bicarbonate ion crosses the blood-brain barrier more slowly than hydrogen or CO_2; therefore, it produces a lesser change in cerebral spinal fluid pH. When neurologic manifestations do occur, as in acute and severe metabolic alkalosis, they include mental confusion, hyperactive reflexes, tetany, and carpopedal spasm. Metabolic alkalosis also leads to a compensatory hypoventilation with development of varying degrees of hypoxemia and respiratory acidosis. Significant morbidity occurs with severe metabolic alkalosis (pH above 7.55), including respiratory failure, dysrhythmias, seizures, and coma.[5]

—— Treatment

The treatment of metabolic alkalosis is usually directed toward correcting the cause of the condition. A chloride deficit requires correction, and potassium chloride is the treatment of choice when there is an accompanying potassium deficit. When potassium chloride is used as a therapy, the chloride anion replaces the bicarbonate anion, and the administration of potassium not only allows for correction of the potassium deficit but also allows the kidneys to conserve hydrogen ions while eliminating the potassium ions. Fluid replacement with normal saline or one-half normal saline is often used in the treatment of persons with volume contraction alkalosis.

—— Respiratory acidosis

Respiratory acidosis is caused by an accumulation of dissolved CO_2. In respiratory acidosis, blood pH is below 7.35 and arterial P_{CO_2} is above 50 mmHg.

—— Causes

Respiratory acidosis can occur as an acute or chronic disorder in acid–base balance. The causes of respiratory acidosis include any respiratory condition that impairs gas exchange. Acute respiratory acidosis can be caused by impaired function of the medullary respiratory center (as in narcotic overdose), chest injury, weakness of the respiratory muscles, or airway obstruction (Table 29-3). Acute respiratory acidosis can also result from breathing air with a high CO_2 content. One of the most common causes of chronic respiratory acidosis is chronic obstructive lung disease (see Chapter 25). Because renal compensatory mechanisms take time to exert their effects, blood pH can drop sharply in persons with acute respiratory acidosis.

Almost all persons with acute respiratory acidosis will be hypoxemic if breathing room air. In many cases, signs of hypoxemia will develop before those of respiratory acidosis. This is because CO_2 diffuses across the alveolar capillary membrane 20 times more rapidly than oxygen. In many lung disorders, there are some areas of the lung that have more

---

Table 29–2. Metabolic alkalosis

Causes	Manifestations
Increase in gain of bicarbonate	pH greater than 7.45
Ingestion of sodium bicarbonate or alkaline salts	Bicarbonate greater than 29 mEq/liter (29 mmol/liter)
Milk-alkali syndrome	Increased excitability of the nervous system (develops late because bicarbonate crosses blood-brain barrier slowly)
Bicarbonate retention	
Loss of chloride (hydrogen) with bicarbonate retention	Confusion
Vomiting	Hyperactive reflexes
Gastric suctioning	Muscle hypertonicity
Diuretic therapy	Tetany
Potassium deficit with hydrogen ion excretion	Convulsions
Excessive levels of adrenal cortical hormones	**Signs of compensation**
Decreased potassium intake	Decreased rate and depth of respiration
Increased potassium losses	Increased urine pH
Contraction alkalosis (loss of body fluids)	Decreased P_{CO_2}
	Manifestations of associated disorders
	Hypokalemia
	Fluid volume deficit

severely compromised gas-exchange function than others. In these circumstances either the respiratory acidosis or hypoxemia stimulates ventilation, so that elimination of CO_2 from the relatively normal areas of the lung is increased, whereas oxygen uptake from the same area is limited by a hemoglobin saturation that approaches 100%.

An acute episode of severe respiratory acidosis can occur in persons with chronic lung disease who have chronically elevated PCO_2 levels. This is sometimes called *CO₂ narcosis*. In these persons, the medullary respiratory center has become adapted to the elevated levels of CO_2 and no longer responds to increases in PCO_2. Instead, the oxygen content of their blood becomes the major stimulus for respiration. If oxygen is administered at a flow rate that is sufficient to suppress this stimulus, the rate and depth of respiration will decrease and the CO_2 content of the blood will increase.

Manifestations

The signs and symptoms of respiratory acidosis depend on the rapidity of onset and on whether the condition is acute or chronic. Because respiratory acidosis is often accompanied by hypoxemia, the manifestations of respiratory acidosis are often intermixed with those of oxygen deficit. Carbon dioxide readily crosses the blood-brain barrier, exerting its effects by changing the pH of brain fluids. It produces an increase in cerebral blood flow. If the condition is severe and prolonged, it can cause an increase in cerebral spinal fluid pressure and papilledema. Headache, blurred vision, irritability, muscle twitching, and psychological disturbances can occur with acute respiratory acidosis. Impairment of consciousness, ranging from lethargy to coma, develops as the PCO_2 rises; hence the term *CO₂ narcosis*. Paralysis of extremities may occur and there may be respiratory depression. Less severe forms of acidosis are often accompanied by warm and flushed skin, weakness, and tachycardia.

Treatment

The treatment of acute and chronic respiratory acidosis is directed toward improving ventilation. In severe cases, mechanical ventilation may be necessary. The treatment of respiratory acidosis due to respiratory failure is discussed in Chapter 26.

Respiratory alkalosis

Respiratory alkalosis is caused by a decrease in dissolved CO_2, or a carbonic acid deficit. In respiratory alkalosis, the pH is above 7.45, arterial PCO_2 is below 35 mmHg, and serum bicarbonate levels are

Table 29–3. Respiratory acidosis

Causes	Manifestations
Impaired ventilation	pH less than 7.35
Depression of the central nervous system	PCO_2 greater than 50 mmHg
Drug overdose	**Depression of neural function**
Head injury	Headache
Diseases of the airways or lungs	Weakness
Bronchial asthma	Confusion and disorientation
Emphysema	Behavioral changes
Chronic bronchitis	Depression
Respiratory distress in the newborn	Paranoia
Pneumonia	Hallucinations
Pulmonary edema	Tremors
Disorders of chest wall or respiratory muscles	Paralysis
Paralysis of respiratory muscles	Stupor and coma
Chest injuries	**Skin**
Kyphoscoliosis	Warm and flushed
Extreme obesity	**Compensatory mechanisms**
Treatment with curare-type drugs	Increased loss of hydrogen in the urine
Upper airway obstruction	
Aspiration of foreign body	
Obstructive sleep apnea	
Laryngospasm	
Increased carbon dioxide inhalation	
Breathing air that is high in carbon dioxide content	

usually below 24 mEq/liter (24 mmol/liter). Because respiratory alkalosis can occur suddenly, bicarbonate level may not change before respiratory correction has been accomplished.

Causes

The causes of respiratory alkalosis center on circumstances that produce hyperventilation. Hyperventilation means that the respiratory rate is in excess of that needed to maintain normal P_{CO_2} levels and should not be confused with the hyperpnea that occurs with exercise. One of the most common causes of hyperventilation is anxiety. The hyperventilation syndrome, which is characterized by recurring episodes of hyperventilation, is described in Chapter 26. Other causes of hyperventilation are fever, oxygen deficiency, early salicylate toxicity, and encephalitis. Hypoxemia exerts its effect through the peripheral chemoreceptors. Salicylate toxicity and encephalitis produce hyperventilation by directly stimulating the medullary respiratory center. Hyperventilation can also occur during anesthesia or with use of mechanical ventilatory devices (Table 29-4).

Manifestations

The signs and symptoms of respiratory alkalosis are associated with hyperexcitability of the nervous system and a decrease in cerebral blood flow. There is often a feeling of lightheadedness, dizziness, tingling, and numbness of the fingers and toes. There may also be sweating, palpitations, panic, air hunger, and dyspnea. Chvostek's and Trousseau's signs may be positive, and tetany and convulsions may occur. Because CO_2 provides the stimulus for short-term regulation of respiration, short periods of apnea may occur in persons with acute episodes of hyperventilation.

Treatment

The treatment of respiratory alkalosis focuses on measures to increase the P_{CO_2}. Attention is directed toward correcting the disorder that caused the overbreathing. Rebreathing of small amounts of expired air (breathing into a paper bag) may prove useful in restoring P_{CO_2} levels in persons with anxiety-produced respiratory alkalosis.

In summary, acidosis describes a decrease in pH, and alkalosis describes an increase in pH. Acid–base disorders may be caused by alterations in the body's volatile acids (respiratory acidosis or respiratory alkalosis) or nonvolatile acids (metabolic acidosis or metabolic alkalosis). Metabolic acidosis is defined as a decrease in bicarbonate, and metabolic alkalosis as an increase in bicarbonate. Metabolic acidosis is caused by either an excessive production and accumulation of metabolic acids or an excessive loss of bicarbonate. Metabolic alkalosis is caused by an increase in bicarbonate or a decrease in hydrogen ion or chloride ion levels. Respiratory acidosis reflects an increase in CO_2 levels and is caused by conditions that produce hypoventilation. Respiratory alkalosis is caused by conditions that cause hyperventilation and a reduction in CO_2 levels. The signs and symptoms of acidosis and alkalosis reflect (1) alterations in body function associated with the disorder causing the acid–base disturbance, (2) the effect of the pH change on body function, and (3) the body's attempt to correct and maintain the pH within a normal physiologic range. In general, neuromuscular excitability is decreased in acidosis and increased in alkalosis.

Table 29–4. Respiratory alkalosis

Causes	Manifestations
Increased ventilation (hyperventilation)	pH above 7.45
Anxiety and psychogenic hyperventilation	Bicarbonate below 24 mEq/l (24 mmol/liter)
Reflex stimulation	Increased excitability of the nervous system
Hypoxemia	
Lung disease that reflexly stimulates ventilation	Numbness and tingling of fingers and toes
Local lung lesions	Dizziness, panic, and lightheadedness
Stimulation of respiratory center	Tetany
Elevated blood ammonia	Positive Chvostek's and Trousseau's signs
Salicylate toxicity	Convulsions
Encephalitis	Cardiovascular manifestations
Anxiety	Cardiac dysrhythmias
Mechanical ventilation	

References

1. Fischbach F: Laboratory Diagnostic Tests, 3rd ed, p 797. Philadelphia, JB Lippincott, 1988
2. Duffens K, Marx JA: Alcoholic ketoacidosis—A review. J Emerg Med 5:399, 1987
3. Williams HE: Alcoholic hypoglycemia and ketoacidosis. Med Clin North Am 68: 33, 1984
4. Rose BD: Clinical Physiology of Acid–Base and Electrolyte Disorders, 2nd ed, p 410. New York, McGraw-Hill, 1984
5. Galla JH, Luke RG: Pathophysiology of metabolic alkalosis. Hosp Pract 22(10): 123, 1987
6. Mennen M: Severe metabolic alkalosis in the emergency department. Ann Emerg Med 17:354, 1988

Bibliography

Atkinson DE, Bourke E: Metabolic aspects of regulation of systemic pH. Am J Physiol 252:F947, 1987

Ackerman GL, Arruda JA: Acid-base and electrolyte imbalance in respiratory failure. Med Clin North Am 67:645, 1983

Adrogue HL, Madias NE: Changes in plasma potassium concentration during acute acid-base disturbances. Am J Med 71:456, 1981

Adrogue HJ, Wilson H, Boyd AE, et al: Plasma acid-base patterns in diabetic ketosis. N Engl J Med 307:1603, 1982

Bishop RL, Weisfeldt ML: Sodium bicarbonate administration during cardiac arrest: Effect on arterial pH, PCO_2, and osmolality. JAMA 235:506, 1976

Cogan MC, Fu-Ying Liu, Berger BE, et al: Metabolic alkalosis. Med Clin North Am 67:903, 1983

Cohen RD, Woods F: Lactic acidosis revisited. Diabetes 32: 181, 1983

Cooper DJ, Worthley LIG: Adverse haemodynamic effects of sodium bicarbonate in metabolic acidosis. Intensive Care Med 13:425, 1987

Dubose TD: Clinical approach to patients with acid-base disorders. Med Clin North Am 67:799, 1983

Duffens K, Marx JA: Alcoholic ketoacidosis. J Emerg Med 5:399, 1987

Emmett M, Narins RG: Clinical use of the anion gap. Medicine 56:38,1977

Felts PW: Ketoacidosis. Med Clin North Am 67:845, 1983

Flier JS, Moore MJ: The metabolic derangement and treatment of diabetic ketoacidosis. N Engl J Med 309:159, 1983

Foster DW, McGarry JD: The metabolic derangements and treatment of diabetic ketoacidosis. N Engl J Med 309:159, 1983

Jenkins JK, Best TR, Nicks SA: Milk-alkali syndrome with a serum calcium level of 22 mg/dl and J waves on the ECG. South Med J 80:1444, 1987

Kaehny WD: Respiratory acid-base disorders. Med Clin North Am 67:915, 1983

Laski ME: Normal regulation of acid-base balance: renal and pulmonary response and other extrarenal buffering mechanisms. Med Clin North Am 67:771, 1983

Narins RG, Jones ER, Stom MC et al: Diagnostic strategies in disorders of fluid, electrolytes and acid-base homeostasis. Am J Med 72:496, 1982

Oh MS, Carroll JH: The anion gap. N Engl J Med 297:814, 1977

Oster JR: The binge-purge syndrome: a common albeit unappreciated cause of acid-base and fluid-electrolyte disturbances. South Med J 80:58, 1987

Stackpoole PW: Lactic acidosis: the case against bicarbonate therapy. Ann Intern Med 105:276, 1986

Tannen RL: Ammonia and acid-base homeostasis. Med Clin North Am 67:781, 1983

Williams HE: Alcoholic hypoglycemia and ketoacidosis. Med Clin N Am 68:33, 1984

CHAPTER 30

Control of Renal Function

Objectives

After you have studied this chapter, you should be able to meet the following objectives:

_____ Describe the anatomy of the normal kidney.

_____ State the reason that injury to the kidney does not usually produce peritonitis.

_____ Describe the structure and function of the glomerular capillary membrane including the endothelial layer, basement membrane, and epithelial layer.

_____ List the parts of the tubule.

_____ Differentiate between glomerular filtration, tubular reabsorption, and tubular secretion.

_____ Trace the elimination of uric acid by the kidney and explain the effect of small doses of aspirin on uric acid elimination.

_____ Describe the determinants of blood flow in the kidney.

_____ Define renal clearance.

_____ Explain how the kidney produces a concentrated urine.

_____ Describe the role of aldosterone in regulating sodium and potassium.

_____ Explain the endocrine function of the kidneys.

_____ Describe the characteristics of normal urine.

_____ Explain the significance of casts in the urine.

_____ Explain the value of the urine specific gravity in evaluating renal function.

_____ Explain the value of serum creatinine levels in evaluating renal function.

_____ Explain the concept of the glomerular filtration rate.

_____ Describe the methods used in cystoscopic examination of the urinary tract, ultrasound studies of the urinary tract, CT scans, IVP studies, and renal artery arteriograms.

(continued)

_____ State the basis for the action of osmotic diuretics.

_____ Describe the actions of acetazolamide.

_____ Explain why mercaptomerin and meralluride alter sodium transport.

_____ Describe the actions of furosemide and ethacrynic acid.

_____ Give another term for aldosterone antagonists and one example of an aldosterone antagonist.

_____ Name and describe three tests of renal function.

It is no exaggeration to say that the composition of the blood is determined not so much by what the mouth takes in as by what the kidneys keep (Homer W. Smith, *From Fish to Philosopher*).[1]

The kidneys are two remarkable organs. Each is smaller than a man's fist, yet in one day they filter about 1700 liters of blood and combine its waste products into about 1 liter of urine. As a part of their function, the kidneys filter physiologically essential substances, such as sodium and potassium ions, from the blood and selectively reabsorb those that are needed to maintain the normal composition of the internal body fluids. Substances not needed for this purpose pass into the urine. In regulating the volume and composition of body fluids, the kidneys perform both excretory and endocrine functions. The renin–angiotensin mechanism participates in the regulation of blood pressure and the maintenance of circulating blood volume, and erythropoietin indirectly stimulates the formation of red blood cells. The discussion in this chapter focuses on the structure and function of the kidneys, tests of renal function, and actions of diuretics.

Kidney structure and function

—— Gross structure

The kidneys are paired, bean-shaped organs that lie outside the peritoneal cavity in the back of the upper abdomen, one on each side of the vertebral column at the level of the twelfth thoracic to third lumbar vertebrae (Figure 30-1). The right kidney is normally lower than the left, presumably because of the position of the liver. In the adult each kidney measures about 10 cm to 12 cm in length, 5 cm to 6 cm in width, and 2.5 cm in depth, and weighs about 4 ounces to 6 ounces. Usually only the lower edge of the right kidney is palpable on abdominal examination. Alterations in kidney size and shape are frequently associated with disease states.

The medial border of the kidney is indented by a deep fissure called the *hilus*. It is here that blood vessels and nerves enter and leave the kidney. The ureters, which connect the kidney with the bladder, also enter the kidney at the hilus.

The kidney is a multilobular structure composed of up to 18 lobes. On longitudinal section it can be divided into an outer cortex and an inner medulla (Figure 30-2). The cortex, which is reddish-brown, contains the glomeruli and convoluted tubules of the nephron and blood vessels (Figure 30-3). The medulla of the kidney consists of light-colored cone-shaped masses, the renal pyramids, that are divided by the columns of the cortex (columns of Bertin) that extend into the medulla. Each pyramid, topped by a region of cortex, forms a lobe of the kidney. The apices of the pyramids form the papillae (8–18 per kidney, corresponding to the number of lobes), which are perforated by the openings of the collecting ducts. The renal pelvis is a wide funnel-shaped structure at the upper end of the ureter. It is made up of the calyces or cuplike structures that drain the upper and lower halves of the kidney.

Each kidney is ensheathed in a fibrous external capsule and is surrounded by a mass of fatty connective tissue, especially at its ends and borders. The adipose tissue protects the kidney from mechanical blows and assists, together with the attached blood

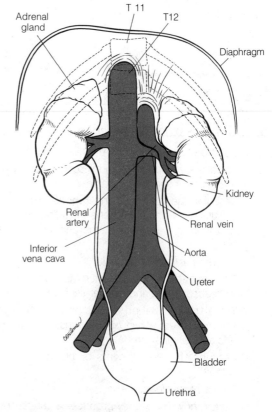

Figure 30-1 The kidneys, ureter, and bladder.

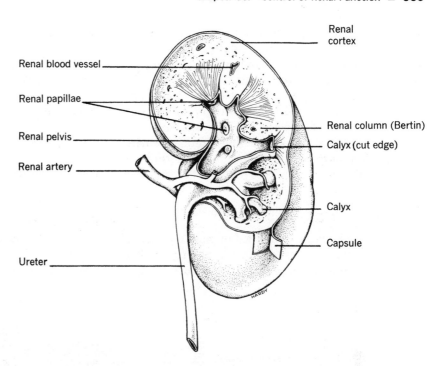

Renal cortex

Renal blood vessel

Renal papillae

Renal pelvis

Renal artery

Renal column (Bertin)

Calyx (cut edge)

Calyx

Capsule

Ureter

Figure 30-2 The internal structure of the kidney. *(Chaffee EE, Lytle IM: Basic Physiology and Anatomy, 4th ed. Philadelphia, JB Lippincott, 1980)*

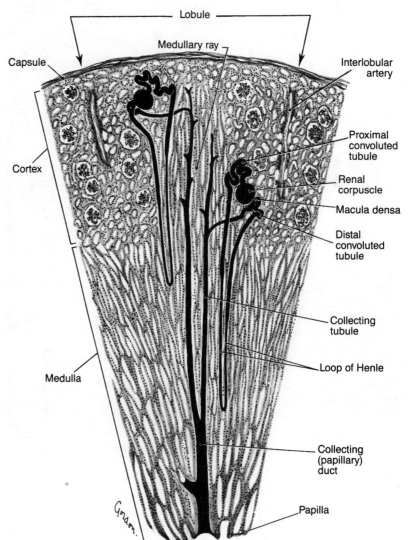

Lobule

Medullary ray

Capsule

Interlobular artery

Cortex

Proximal convoluted tubule

Renal corpuscle

Macula densa

Distal convoluted tubule

Collecting tubule

Loop of Henle

Medulla

Collecting (papillary) duct

Papilla

Figure 30-3 Schematic representation of the basic arrangement of nephrons and collecting tubules in a lobule of the kidney. *(Cormack DH: Ham's Histology, 9th ed. Philadelphia, JB Lippincott, 1987)*

vessels and fascia, in holding the kidney in place. If this fat is absorbed, as can occur during severe weight loss, the kidney may slip out of position, compressing the ureter and obstructing urine flow. Although the kidneys are relatively well protected, they may occasionally be bruised by blows to the loin or by compression between the lower ribs and the ilium. Because the kidneys are outside the peritoneal cavity, injury and rupture do not produce the same threat of peritoneal involvement as does rupture of organs such as the liver or spleen.

── Nephron

Each kidney is composed of more than a million tiny, closely packed functional units called *nephrons*. Each nephron consists of a vascular compo-

nent (a glomerulus) and a tubular component (Figure 30-4). The nephron is supplied by two capillary systems, the glomerulus and the peritubular capillary network. The glomerulus is a unique high-pressure filtration system that is located between two arterioles, the afferent and efferent arterioles, which can selectively dilate or constrict to regulate the glomerular capillary pressure.

The peritubular capillary network is a low-pressure reabsorptive system originating from the efferent arteriole. These capillaries are distributed around all portions of the tubules, an arrangement that permits rapid movement of solutes and water between the tubular lumen and the capillaries. The peritubular capillaries rejoin to form the venous channels by which blood ultimately leaves the kidneys.

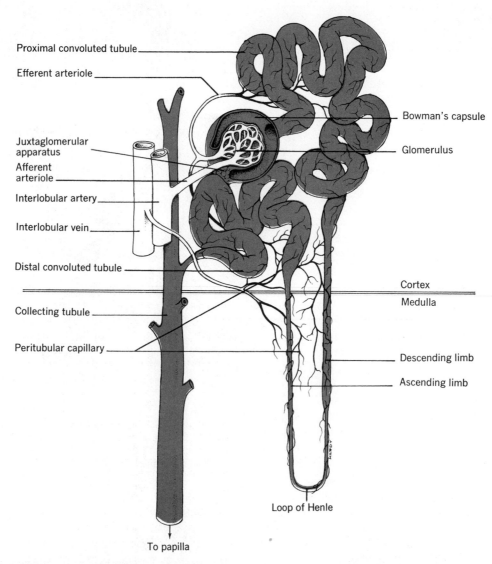

Figure 30-4 The nephron, showing the glomerular and tubular structures along with the blood supply. *(Chaffee EE, Greisheimer EM: Basic Physiology and Anatomy, 3rd ed. Philadelphia, JB Lippincott)*

Glomerular structure and function

The glomerulus consists of a network of capillaries encased in a thin-walled sac, *Bowman's capsule*. Fluid and particles from the blood are filtered through the membrane of the glomerulus into Bowman's capsule, which extends to form the tubules of the nephron. The mass of capillaries and its surrounding epithelial capsule are collectively referred to as the *renal corpuscle* (Figure 30-5 **A**).

The glomerular capillary membrane is composed of three layers: (1) the capillary endothelial layer, (2) the basement membrane, and (3) the single-celled capsular epithelial layer (Figure 30-5 **B**). The endothelial layer lines the glomerulus and interfaces with blood as it moves through the capillary. It is perforated by many small holes called *fenestrations*. The basement membrane consists of a homogeneous acellular meshwork of collagen fibers, glycoproteins, and mu.opolysaccharides (Figure 30-5 **C**). The epithelial layer that covers the glomerulus is continuous with the epithelium that lines Bowman's capsule. The epithelial layer that covers the glomerulus is called the *visceral epithelium* to differentiate it from the *parietal layer* that lines Bowman's capsule. The visceral epithelial cells have unusual octopus-like structures that possess a large number of extensions, or foot processes (podocytes), that are embedded in the basement membrane (Figure 30-6). These foot processes form slit pores through which the glomerular filtrate passes.

Because both the endothelial and epithelial layers of the glomerular capillary have porous structures, it is the basement membrane that determines the permeability of the glomerular capillary membrane.[2] The spaces between the fibers that make up the basement membrane represent the pores of a filter and determine the size-dependent permeability barrier of the glomerulus. The size of the pores in the basement membrane normally prevents red blood cells and plasma proteins from passing through the glomerular membrane into the urine filtrate. There is evidence that the epithelium plays a major role in forming the basement membrane components, and it is probable that the epithelial cells are active in forming new basement membrane material throughout life. Because material is being added to the exterior of the basement membrane, it seems reasonable to assume that equal amounts are being removed from the inner surface to keep it from becoming unduly thick.[3] Alterations in the structure and composition of the glomerular basement membrane are responsible for the leakage of proteins and blood cells that occurs with many forms of glomerular disease.

Another important component of the glomerulus is the mesangium. There are areas where the capillary endothelium and basement membrane do

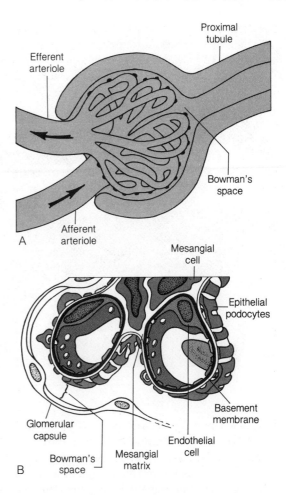

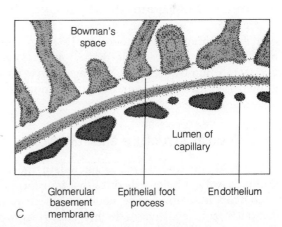

Figure 30-5 Renal corpuscle. (**A**) Structures of the glomerulus. (**B**) Position of the mesangial cells in relation to the capillary loops and Bowman's capsule. (**C**) Cross section of the glomerular membrane illustrating the position of the endothelium, basement membrane, and epithelial foot processes.

not completely surround each capillary. Mesangial cells, which lie between the capillary tufts, provide support for the glomerulus in these areas (see Figure 30-5 **B**). The mesangial cells produce an intercellular substance that is similar to that of the basement membrane, and it is this substance that covers the endothe-

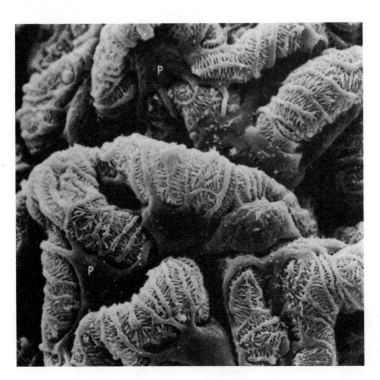

Figure 30-6 Scanning electron micrograph of a glomerulus from the kidney of a normal rat. The visceral epithelial cells, or podocytes (*P*), extend multiple processes outward from the main cell body to wrap around individual capillary loops. Immediately adjacent pedicels, or foot processes, arise from different podocytes (magnification ×4800). *(Brenner BM, Rector FC: The Kidney, Philadelphia, WB Saunders, 1981. Reprinted by permission.)*

lial cells where they are not covered by epithelially derived basement membrane. The mesangial cells possess (or can develop) phagocytic properties and remove macromolecular materials that enter the intercapillary spaces. Mesangial cells also exhibit contractile properties in response to neurohumoral substances and are thought to contribute to the regulation of blood flow through the glomerulus. In normal glomeruli, the mesangial area is narrow and contains only a small number of cells. Mesangial hyperplasia and increased mesangial matrix occur in a number of glomerular diseases.

Tubular structure and function

Although the plasma is filtered in the glomerulus, it is the tubular structures that transform the filtered fluid into urine. The nephron tubule is divided into four segments: a highly coiled segment called the *proximal convoluted tubule*, which originates in Bowman's capsule; a thin, looped structure called the *loop of Henle;* a distal coiled portion called the *distal convoluted tubule;* and the final segment called the *collecting tubule*, which joins with several tubules to collect the urine filtrate. The filtrate passes through each of these segments before reaching the pelvis of the kidney.

Nephrons can be roughly grouped into two categories. About 85% of the nephrons originate in the superficial part of the cortex and are called *cortical nephrons*. They have short and thick loops of Henle that penetrate only a short distance into the medulla. The remaining 15% are called *juxtamedullary nephrons*. They originate deeper in the cortex and have longer and thinner loops of Henle that penetrate the entire length of the medulla. The juxtamedullary nephrons are largely concerned with urine concentration.

Throughout its course, the tubule is composed of a single layer of epithelial cells resting on a basement membrane. The structure of the epithelial cells varies with tubular function. The cells of the proximal tubule have a fine villous structure that increases the surface area for reabsorption; they are also rich in mitochondria, which support active transport processes. The epithelial layer of the thin segment of the loop of Henle is thin, with very few mitochondria, indicating minimal metabolic activity and active reabsorptive function.

About 65% of all reabsorptive and secretory processes that occur in the tubular system take place in the proximal tubule.[4] There is almost complete reabsorption of nutritionally important substances such as glucose, amino acids, and vitamins; electrolytes such as sodium, potassium, chloride, and bicarbonate are 65% to 80% reabsorbed in this tubular segment. As solutes are transported out of the tubular cells, their concentration within the lumen decreases and their concentration outside the tubule increases, providing a concentration gradient for the osmotic reabsorption of water. The proximal tubule is highly permeable to water, and the osmotic movement of water occurs so rapidly that the concentration difference of solutes on either side of the membrane is seldom more than a few milliosmols.

The *thin segment* of the loop of Henle is important in maintaining the concentrating capabilities of the nephron. As its name implies, the epithelial cells of this tubular segment are very thin, which contributes to their permeability characteristics. The descending limb is highly permeable to water and moderately permeable to urea, sodium, and other ions. The ascending limb, in contrast to the descending limb, is only slightly permeable to urea and water but is capable of active sodium transport. As will be explained later, these differences in permeability and sodium transport are responsible for the production of a countercurrent mechanism that concentrates solutes in the interstitial fluids surrounding the collecting ducts, a condition necessary for the antidiuretic hormone (ADH)-mediated reabsorption of water.

The *thick segment* of the loop of Henle begins in the ascending limb of the loop where the epithelial cells become thickened. This segment extends all the way back to the glomerulus from which the tubule originated and then passes between the afferent and efferent arteriole forming the *juxtoglomerular complex* (Figure 30-7). Because of its location, the juxtaglomerular complex is thought to play an essential feedback role in linking the functioning of the afferent and efferent arterioles to the composition of the distal tubular fluid. This hypothesis is supported by the presence in the distal tubule of macula densa cells that

appear to secrete substances toward the arterioles. In addition, juxtaglomerular cells in the afferent and efferent arterioles contain granules of inactive renin, suggesting that the composition of the distal tubular fluid contributes to the control of sodium and water reabsorption through the renin–angiotensin–aldosterone mechanism (discussed later in this chapter and in Chapter 19).

The distal tubule begins at the juxtaglomerular complex, continuing from the thick segment of the ascending loop of Henle. The distal tubule is divided into two segments: the *diluting segment* and the *late distal tubule*. The diluting segment includes the entire thick portion of the loop of Henle and about half of the convoluted portion of the distal tubule. The cells of the thick segment are specifically adapted to reabsorb chloride from the tubular lumen into the extracellular fluid for return to the bloodstream. The reabsorption of the negative chloride ions creates an electrical gradient, which results in the passive reabsorption of sodium. Certain diuretic drugs act by inhibiting this transport system. The diluting segment is almost entirely impermeable to water and urea, and consequently the outward transport of sodium and chloride dilutes the tubular fluid, a condition that is necessary for production of a dilute urine. The later distal tubule is adapted for the active transport of sodium and other positive ions. It is here and in the collecting tubule that potassium ions are secreted into the tubular fluid and aldosterone exerts its effects on sodium and potassium reabsorption.

Like the distal tubule, the collecting duct is divided into two segments: *the cortical collecting tubule* and *the inner medullary collecting duct*. The cortical segment begins in the renal cortex at the termination of the convoluted distal tubule. It fuses with cortical tubules from several other nephrons before it turns down from the cortex toward the renal papillae. As the cortical collecting duct passes through the medullary portion of the kidney, it becomes the inner medullary collecting duct. The epithelium of the collecting duct is well designed to resist extreme changes in the osmotic or *p*H characteristics of tubular fluid, and it is here that the urine becomes highly concentrated, highly diluted, highly alkaline, or highly acidic. The permeability of the epithelium to water in both portions of the collecting duct is determined mainly by the concentration of ADH. When large quantities of the hormone are present, the tubular epithelium becomes very permeable to water, and most of the water that is in the tubular fluid is reabsorbed from the tubule and returned to the blood. Very little water is reabsorbed in the absence of the hormone. Alterations in body fluids due to disorders of ADH levels are discussed in Chapter 27.

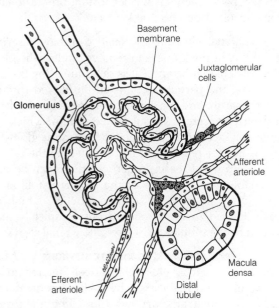

Figure 30-7 The renal capsule, showing the close contact of the distal tubule with the afferent arteriole and the macula densa and juxtaglomerular apparatus.

Urine formation

Urine formation begins with the filtration of essentially protein-free plasma through the glomerular capillaries into Bowman's capsule. The movement of fluid through the glomerular capillary bed is determined by the same factors (capillary pressure and colloidal osmotic pressure) that affect fluid movement through other capillaries in the body (see Chapter 28). About 125 ml of fluid is filtered each minute. This is called the *glomerular filtration rate (GFR)*. This rate can vary from a few ml/min to as high as 200 ml/minute.

The location of the glomerulus, between two arterioles, allows for the maintenance of a high-pressure filtration system. The capillary filtration pressure (about 60 mmHg) in the glomerulus is about two to three times higher than that of other capillary beds in the body. The filtration pressure and the glomerular filtration rate are regulated by the constriction and relaxation of the afferent and efferent arterioles. Constriction of the efferent arteriole increases resistance to outflow from the glomeruli and increases the glomerular pressure and the glomerular filtration rate. On the other hand, constriction of the afferent arteriole causes a reduction in the renal blood flow, glomerular filtration pressure, and glomerular filtration rate. Both the afferent and efferent arterioles are innervated by the sympathetic nervous system. During periods of strong sympathetic stimulation, such as occurs during shock, the filtration pressure can be reduced so far that the glomerular filtration rate falls to almost zero.[4]

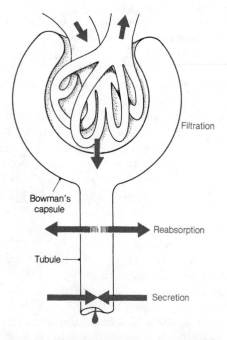

Figure 30-8 Mechanisms of urine formation. The plasma is filtered in the glomerulus, and urine is formed as substances are reabsorbed or secreted into the filtrate.

From Bowman's capsule the glomerular filtrate moves into the tubular segments of the nephron. In its movement through the lumen of the tubular segments, the glomerular filtrate is changed considerably by the transtubular transport of water and solutes. Tubular transport occurs in both inward and outward directions as tubular secretion and tubular reabsorption (Figure 30-8). The basic mechanisms of transport through the tubular membrane are similar to those of other membranes in the body and include both passive and active transport. Water and urea are passively absorbed along concentration gradients. Sodium, potassium, chloride, calcium, phosphate, and urate ions, glucose molecules, and amino acids are actively absorbed through the tubular membrane. Some substances, such as hydrogen, potassium, and urate ions, are actively secreted into the tubular fluids. Under normal conditions only about 1 ml of the 125 ml/minute filtered by the glomerulus is excreted as urine. The other 124 ml are reabsorbed in the tubules. This means that the average output of urine is about 60 ml/hour.

Glomerular tubular balance

One of the most remarkable features of the kidney is its feedback regulation between glomerular filtration and the rate of tubular reabsorption. Although the mechanism is unclear, there is a feedback mechanism that produces a decrease in the glomerular filtration rate when tubular reabsorption is reduced. Likewise, a reduction in tubular reabsorption occurs when the glomerular filtration rate falls. The result of this feedback mechanism is a constant proportionality between filtration and reabsorption.

Renal clearance. *Renal clearance* describes the ability of the kidneys to remove or clear the blood of a particular substance. It is determined by the particle size, the particle's ability to be filtered through the glomeruli, and the capacity of the renal tubules to reabsorb or secrete the substance. Inulin, which is a large polysaccharide, is freely filtered in the glomeruli and is neither reabsorbed nor secreted by the tubular cells. Because of these properties, inulin can be used as a laboratory measure of the glomerular filtration rate. Other substances such as glucose, which are freely filtered in the glomeruli but completely reabsorbed by the tubular cells, have a low renal clearance.

Renal threshold (transport maximum). Many substances such as glucose are freely filtered in the glomerulus and reabsorbed by special energy-dependent tubular transport systems. The maximum amount of substances that these transport systems can reabsorb, called the *transport maximum,* is usually sufficient for all of the filtered substance to be reabsorbed and none to appear in the urine. The point at which the substance appears in the urine is also called the *renal threshold*. There are, however, circumstances in which the amount of substance filtered in the glomerulus exceeds the transport maximum for the substance. For example, when blood sugar is elevated in uncontrolled diabetes mellitus, the amount that is filtered in the glomerulus often exceeds the transport maximum (320 mg/minute) for glucose, and sugar spills into the urine.

Control of urine concentration

The kidneys are able to produce either a concentrated or a dilute urine depending on the composition and volume of the extracellular fluids. The concentration or dilution of the urine occurs in the collecting tubules and depends on (1) the increased solute concentration in the medullary area surrounding the collecting ducts and (2) the selective permeability of the collecting tubules, which is controlled by ADH.

In about one-fifth of the nephrons (juxtamedullary nephrons), the loops of Henle and special peritubular capillaries called the *vasa recta* descend into the renal medulla. Here, a countercurrent mechanism controls water and solute flow. As a result, water is kept out of the peritubular area and sodium and urea are retained. A consequence of these processes is that a high concentration of the osmotically active particles collect in the interstitium of this portion of the kidney (Figure 30-9). It is here, where the kidney interstitium surrounds the collecting tubules, that the presence of these osmotically active particles facilitates the ADH-mediated reabsorption of water.

During periods of dehydration, the kidney plays a major role in maintaining water balance. Osmoreceptors in the hypothalamus sense the increase in osmolality of extracellular fluids and stimulate the release of ADH. The collecting tubules, under the influence of ADH, become permeable to water. Once the permeability of the collecting tubules has been established, water moves out of the tubular lumen and into the interstitium of the medullary area, where it enters the peritubular capillaries for return to the vascular system. This serves to maintain extracellular volume by returning water to the vascular compartment and leads to the production of a concentrated urine by removing water from the tubular filtrate. In the absence of ADH, the renal tubules remain impermeable to water, and a dilute urine is formed.

Sodium elimination

The excretion of sodium by the kidneys is highly variable. The sodium in the blood is freely filtered, so that its concentration in the glomerular

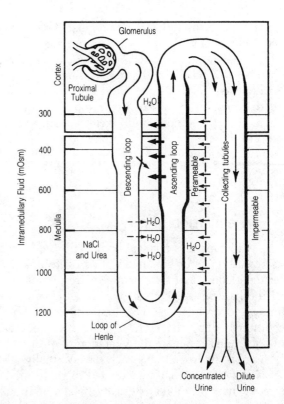

Figure 30-9 The countercurrent mechanism for concentrating urine. Antidiuretic hormone controls the permeability of the collecting tubule.

filtrate approximates that of plasma; it is then actively transported back into the plasma as fluid moves through the tubules. It is important that the tubular reabsorption varies with the glomerular filtration rate. For example, when additional sodium filtration occurs because of an increase in the glomerular filtration rate, reabsorption must increase to maintain serum sodium levels. About 65% of sodium reabsorption takes place in the proximal tubule, 27% in the loop of Henle, and 8% in the distal tubule.

Sodium reabsorption in the distal tubule is highly variable and is dependent on the presence of aldosterone. In the presence of aldosterone, almost all of the sodium from the distal tubular fluid is reabsorbed, and the urine becomes essentially sodium-free. Virtually no sodium is reabsorbed from the distal tubule in the absence of aldosterone. The remarkable ability of the distal tubular cells to alter sodium reabsorption in relation to changes in aldosterone allows the kidney to excrete urine with sodium levels that range from a few tenths of a gram to 40 g.

Potassium elimination

Like sodium, potassium is freely filtered in the glomerulus; but unlike sodium, potassium is both reabsorbed from and secreted into the tubular fluid. The secretion of potassium into the tubular fluid occurs in the distal tubule and is regulated by aldosterone. Only about 70 mEq of potassium are delivered to the distal tubule each day, yet the average person consumes this much and more potassium in the diet. Excess potassium that is not filtered in the glomerulus and delivered to the distal tubule must therefore be secreted into the tubular fluid for elimination from the body. In the absence of aldosterone (as in Addison's disease), potassium secretion becomes minimal. In these circumstances, potassium reabsorption exceeds secretion, and blood levels of potassium increase.

Regulation of pH

The kidneys regulate body pH by conserving base bicarbonate or eliminating hydrogen ions. Neither the blood buffer systems nor the respiratory control mechanisms for carbon dioxide elimination can eliminate hydrogen ions (H^+) from the body. This is accomplished by the kidneys. The average North American diet results in the liberation of 40 mmol to 80 mmol of hydrogen ions each day. Virtually all of the hydrogen ions that are excreted in the urine are secreted into the tubular fluid by means of tubular secretory mechanisms. As described in Chapter 29, the ability of the kidney to excrete hydrogen depends on buffers in the urine that combine with the ion. The three major buffers are bicarbonate (HCO_3^-), phosphate (HPO_4^{--}), and ammonia (NH_3). Bicarbonate is both filtered into the tubular fluid and broken down to form carbon dioxide and water. The carbon dioxide is then absorbed into the tubular cells and bicarbonate is regenerated. The HPO_4^{--} is filtered into the tubular fluid and is not reabsorbed. Ammonia is synthesized in tubular cells by the deamination of certain amino acids. It diffuses into the tubular fluid and combines with the hydrogen ion. An important aspect of this buffer system is that the deamination process increases whenever the body's hydrogen ion concentration remains elevated for 1 to 2 days.

Uric acid elimination

Uric acid is a product of purine metabolism (see Chapter 57). Excessively high blood levels (hyperuricemia) can cause gout, and excessive levels in the urine can cause kidney stones. Uric acid is freely filtered in the glomerulus, completely reabsorbed in the proximal convoluted tubule, secreted into the tubular fluid in the middle section of the proximal tubule, and finally reabsorbed in the loop of Henle. Uric acid uses the same transport systems as other anions such as aspirin, sulfinpyrazone, and probenecid. Small doses of aspirin compete with uric acid for secretion into the tubular fluid and reduce uric acid secretion, whereas large doses compete with uric acid for reabsorption and increase uric acid excretion in the urine. Because of its effect on uric acid secretion, aspirin is not recommended for treatment of gouty arthritis. Thiazide and loop diuretics (furosemide and ethacrynic acid) can also cause hyperuricemia (and gouty arthritis), presumably through a decrease in extracellular fluid volume and enhanced uric acid reabsorption.

Urea elimination

Urea is an end product of protein metabolism. The normal adult produces 25 g to 30 g per day;[1] the quantity rises when a high-protein diet is consumed, when there is excessive tissue breakdown, or in the presence of gastrointestinal bleeding. In the presence of gastrointestinal bleeding, the blood protein is broken down to form ammonia in the intestine; it is then absorbed into the portal circulation and converted to urea by the liver before being released into the blood stream. The kidneys, in their role as regulators of blood urea nitrogen (BUN) levels, filter the urea in the glomeruli and then reabsorb it in the tubules. This allows for maintenance of a normal BUN, which is in the range of 8 mg to 25 mg per dL (2.9 to 8.9 mmol/liter) of blood. Blood urea nitrogen becomes concentrated during periods of dehydration, and its excretion is markedly decreased when the glomerular filtration rate drops. The renal tubules are permeable to urea, which means that the longer the tubular fluid remains in the kidney, the greater the reabsorption of urea into the blood. Hence, only small amounts of urea are reabsorbed into the blood when the glomerular filtration rate is high, whereas relatively large amounts of urea are returned to the blood when the glomerular filtration rate is reduced.

Renal blood flow

Each kidney is supplied by a renal artery that arises on either side of the aorta. Upon entering the kidney, each renal artery divides into the segmental and then the lobar arteries that supply the upper, middle, and lower parts of the kidney. The lobar arteries further subdivide to form the interlobar arteries at the level of the cortical medullary junction (Figure 30-10). These arteries arch across the pyramids to form the arcuate arteries, which give rise to the intralobular arteries. The afferent arterioles that supply the glomeruli arise from the interlobular arteries.

In the adult the kidneys are perfused with about 1300 ml of blood per minute, or about 25% of the cardiac output. This large blood flow is needed not for renal metabolism but to ensure sufficient glomerular filtration for the removal of waste products from the blood. Blood flow to the kidneys remains

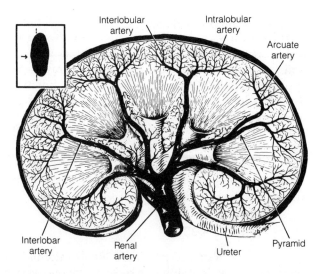

Figure 30-10 Schematic illustration of the arterial supply of the kidney, simplified for clarity. *(Ham AW, Cormack DH: Histology, 9th ed, p 583. Philadelphia, JB Lippincott, 1987)*

relatively constant within a mean arterial blood pressure range of 80 mmHg to 180 mmHg. The constancy of flow is maintained by a process called autoregulation (discussed in Chapter 17). For autoregulation to occur, the resistance of blood flow through the kidney must be varied in direct proportion to the arterial pressure. The exact mechanisms responsible for the intrarenal regulation of blood flow are still unclear. It seems likely that the intrarenal release of substances capable of regulating local vascular resistance may play a role.[5] Although nearly all the blood flow to the kidney passes through the cortex, less than 10% is directed to the medulla, and only about 1% goes to the papillae. Under conditions of decreased renal blood flow or increased sympathetic nervous system stimulation, blood flow is redistributed away from the cortex toward the medulla. This redistribution of blood flow decreases glomerular filtration while maintaining the urine concentrating ability of the kidneys, a factor that is important during conditions such as shock.

Endocrine function

At present it is known that the kidney is concerned with either producing or activating renin, erythropoietin, and vitamin D.

Renin–angiotensin mechanism

Renin is an enzyme released by the juxtaglomerular cells of the afferent and efferent arteriole (see Figure 30-7). Renin is thought to be released in response to a decrease in renal blood flow, a change in the composition of the distal tubular fluid, or as the result of sympathetic nervous system stimulation. It

combines with angiotensinogen, a plasma protein that circulates in the blood, to form angiotensin I. In the lungs, the angiotensin-converting enzyme changes angiotensin I to angiotensin II. Angiotensin II is a potent vasoconstrictor and stimulator of aldosterone release. It is also thought that angiotensin II contributes to the regulation of blood flow within the kidney. The renin–angiotensin–aldosterone mechanism plays an important part in both short-term and long-term regulation of blood pressure (see Chapter 19).

Regulation of red blood cell formation

Erythropoietin, 90% to 95% of which is formed in the kidneys, is a hormone that regulates red blood cell production and is released in response to hypoxia. It is believed that the kidneys respond to hypoxia by producing a substance or enzyme that converts a circulating plasma protein to an active form of erythropoietin. This active form of erythropoietin acts on the bone marrow to stimulate production and release of red blood cells (see Chapter 16). As a result, persons with chronic hypoxia often have increased red blood cell levels (polycythemia). This occurs in conditions such as congestive heart failure and chronic lung disease.

Activation of vitamin D

Vitamin D increases calcium absorption from the gastrointestinal tract and helps control calcium deposition in bone. Vitamin D exists in several forms: natural vitamin D (cholecalciferol), which results from ultraviolet irradiation of the skin, and synthetic vitamin D (ergocalciferol), which is derived from irradiation of ergosterol. Both forms of vitamin D must undergo chemical transformation to become active: first to 25-hydroxycholecalciferol in the liver and then to 1,25-dihydroxycholecalciferol in the kidneys.

In summary, the kidneys perform both excretory and endocrine functions. In the process of excreting wastes, the kidneys filter the blood and then selectively reabsorb those materials that are needed to maintain a stable internal environment. The kidneys (1) rid the body of metabolic wastes, (2) regulate fluid volume, (3) regulate the composition of electrolytes, (4) assist in maintaining acid–base balance, (5) aid in regulation of blood pressure through the renin–angiotensin–aldosterone mechanism and control of extracellular fluid volume, (6) regulate red blood cell production through erythropoietin, and (7) aid in calcium metabolism by activating vitamin D.

Tests of renal function

The function of the kidneys is to filter the blood, selectively reabsorb those substances that are needed to maintain the constancy of body fluid, and excrete metabolic wastes. Therefore, the composition of the urine and blood provides valuable information about the adequacy of renal function. Radiologic tests, endoscopy, and renal biopsy are procedures that afford a means of viewing the gross and microscopic structures of the kidneys and urinary system.

—— Urinalysis

Urine is a clear, amber-colored fluid that is about 95% water and 5% dissolved solids. The kidneys normally produce about 1.5 liters of urine a day. Normal urine contains metabolic wastes and few, if any, plasma proteins, blood cells, or glucose molecules. Urine tests can be performed on a single urine specimen or on a 24-hour urine sample. Table 30-1 describes urinalysis values for normal urine.

Casts are molds of the distal nephron lumen. A gel-like substance called Tamm and Horsfall mucoprotein, which is formed in the tubular epithelium, forms the matrix of casts. Casts composed of this gel but devoid of cells are called *hyaline casts*. These casts tend to develop when the protein concentration of the urine is high (as in nephrotic syndrome), urine osmolality is high, and urine *p*H is low. The inclusion of granules or cells in the matrix of the protein gel leads to formation of various other types of casts.

—— Specific gravity

The *specific gravity* (or osmolality) of urine varies with its concentration of solutes. Urine specific gravity provides a valuable index of the hydration status and functional ability of the kidneys. Although there are more sophisticated methods for measuring specific gravity, it can be easily measured using an inexpensive piece of equipment called a urinometer. Healthy kidneys can produce a concentrated urine with a specific gravity of 1.030 to 1.040. During periods of marked hydration, the specific gravity can approach 1.000. With diminished renal function, there is a loss of renal concentrating ability, and the urine specific gravity may fall to levels of 1.006 to 1.010 (usual range is 1.015 to 1.025 with normal fluid intake). These low levels are particularly significant if they occur during periods that follow a decrease in water intake (*e.g.,* during the first urine specimen on arising in the morning).

—— Blood tests

Blood tests can provide valuable information about the kidney's ability to remove metabolic wastes from the blood and to maintain normal electrolyte and *p*H composition of the blood. Normal blood values are listed in Table 30-2. Serum potassium, phosphate, blood urea nitrogen (BUN), and creatinine tend to increase in renal failure. Serum calcium, *p*H, and bicarbonate tend to decrease in renal failure. The effect of renal failure on the concentration of serum electrolyte and metabolic end products is discussed further in Chapter 32.

—— Creatinine

Creatinine is a product of *creatine* metabolism in muscles; therefore, its formation and release is relatively constant and proportional to the amount of muscle mass present. Because creatinine is filtered in the glomeruli but not reabsorbed in the tubules, its blood values depend closely on the glomerular filtration rate. In addition to its use in calculating the glomerular filtration rate, the creatinine level is useful in estimating the functional capacity of the kidney (Figure 30-11). The normal creatinine value is about 0.7 mg per dL of blood for a woman with a small frame, about 1.0 mg per dL of blood for a normal adult man, and about 1.5 mg per dL of blood (60 to 130 mmol/

Table 30–1. Normal values for routine urinalysis

General characteristics and measurements	Chemical determinations	Microscopic examination of sediment
Color: yellow-amber—indicates a high specific gravity and small output of urine.	Glucose: negative	Casts negative: occasional hyaline casts
Turbidity: clear to slightly hazy	Ketones: negative	Red blood cells negative or rare
Specific gravity: 1.015–1.025 with a normal fluid intake	Blood: negative	Crystals negative
*p*H: 4.6–4.8—average person has a *p*H of about 6 (acid)	Protein: negative	White blood cells negative or rare
	Bilirubin: negative	
	Urobilinogen: 0.1–1	
	Nitrate for bacteria: negative	
	Leukocyte esterase: negative	

(Fishbach F: A Manual of Laboratory Diagnostic Tests, p 124, Philadelphia, JB Lippincott, 1988)

Table 30–2. Normal blood chemistry levels

Substance	Normal value
BUN	8.0–25.0 mg/dl (2.9–8.9 mmol/liter)
Creatinine	0.7–1.5 mg/dl (60–130 μ mol/liter)
Sodium	137–147 mEq/liter (137–147 mmol/liter)
Chloride	100–106 mEq/liter (100–106 mmol/liter)
Potassium	3.5–5 mEq/liter (3.5–5 mmol/liter)
Carbon dioxide (CO_2 content)	24–29 mEq/liter (24–29 mmol/liter)
Calcium	8.5–10.3 mg/dl (2.1–2.6 mmol/liter)
Phosphate	3–4.5 mg/dl (1–1.5 mmol/liter)
Uric acid	3.0–9 mg/dl (0.18–0.54 mmol/liter)
pH	7.35–7.45

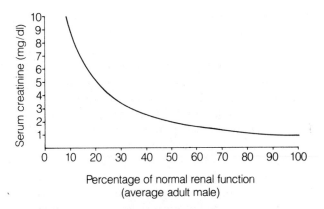

Figure 30-11 Relationship between percentage of renal function and serum creatinine levels. *(Drawn from data in Mitch WE, Walser M: A simple method of estimating progression of chronic renal failure. Lancet 2:1326, 1976)*

liter) for a muscular man. A normal serum creatinine level is usually indicative of normal renal function. If the value doubles, the glomerular filtration rate—and renal function—probably have fallen to half their normal state. A rise in blood creatinine level to three times the normal value suggests that there is a 75% loss of renal function, and with creatinine values of 10 mg per dL or more, it can be assumed that about 90% of renal function has been lost.

Glomerular filtration rate

The glomerular filtration rate (GFR) provides a gauge of renal function. It can be measured clinically by collecting timed samples of blood and urine. Creatinine, a product of creatine metabolism by the muscle, is filtered by the kidneys but not reabsorbed in the renal tubule. Therefore, one of the substances that are measured in calculating the GFR is creatinine. The clearance rate for such a substance is the amount that is completely cleared by the kidneys in 1 minute. The formula is expressed as follows:

$$C = \frac{UV}{P}$$

where C = clearance rate
U = urine concentration
V = urine volume
P = plasma concentration

The normal creatinine clearance is 115 to 125 ml/min and is corrected for body surface area, which reflects the muscle mass where creatinine metabolism takes place. The test may be done on a 24-hour basis, with blood being drawn at the time the urine collection is completed. In another method, two 1-hour urine samples are collected and a blood sample is drawn between.

Cystoscopy

Cystoscopy provides a means for direct visualization of the urethra, bladder, and ureteral orifices. It relies on the use of a cystoscope, an instrument with a lighted lens. The cystoscope is inserted through the urethra into the bladder. Biopsy specimens, lesions, small stones and foreign bodies can be removed from the urethra, bladder, and ureters by this means.

Ultrasound studies

Ultrasound studies use the reflection of ultrasonic (high-frequency) waves to visualize the deep structures of the body. The procedure is painless and noninvasive and it requires no patient preparation. Ultrasound is used to visualize the structures of the kidneys and has been proved useful in the diagnosis of many urinary tract disorders, including congenital anomalies, renal abscesses, hydronephrosis, and kidney stones. It can differentiate between a renal cyst and a renal tumor.[5] The use of ultrasound also enables accurate placement of needles for renal biopsy and catheters for percutaneous nephrostomy.

Radiologic studies

Radiologic studies include a simple flat plate (x-ray) of the kidneys, ureters, and bladder (KUB) that can be used to determine the size, shape, and position of the kidneys and to note any radiopaque stones that may be in the kidney pelvis or ureters. An excretory urogram, or intravenous pyelogram (IVP), is done by injecting a radiopaque dye into a peripheral vein; this dye is then filtered by the glomerulus and excreted into the urine, and x-ray films are taken as it moves through the kidneys and ureters. The IVP is used to detect space-occupying lesions of the kidneys, pyelonephritis, hydronephrosis, vesicoureteral reflux, and kidney stones. Some people are highly allergic to the radiographic dye used for the IVP and may develop an anaphylactic reaction following administration of the dye. Therefore, every person undergoing

IVP studies should be questioned about previous reactions to the dye or to similar dyes. If the test is considered essential in such persons, premedication with antihistamines and corticosteroids may be used. The dye also reduces renal blood flow; acute renal failure can occur, particularly in persons with vascular disease or preexisting renal insufficiency.[5]

Other radiologic tests include computed tomography, radionuclide imaging, and renal arteriograms. Computed tomography (CT) scan refers to x-ray films taken by rotating tubes that sharply delineate tissue at any level they irradiate. CT scans may be used to outline the kidney and detect renal masses and tumors. Radionuclide imaging involves the injection of a radioactive material that is subsequently detected externally by a scintillation camera, which detects the radioactive emissions. Radionuclide imaging is used to evaluate renal function and structures as well as the ureters and bladder. It is particularly useful in evaluating the function of renal transplant kidneys. Renal arteriography provides x-ray pictures of the blood vessels supplying the kidney. It involves the injection of a radiopaque dye directly into the renal artery. Usually a catheter is introduced through the femoral artery and advanced under fluoroscopic view into the abdominal aorta; the catheter tip is then maneuvered into the renal artery and the dye is injected. This test is used in evaluating persons suspected of having renal artery stenosis, abnormalities of renal blood vessels, or vascular damage to the renal arteries following trauma.

In summary, urinalysis and blood tests that measure levels of by-products of metabolism and electrolytes provide information about renal function. Cystoscopic examinations can be used for direct visualization of the urethra, bladder, and ureters. Ultrasound can be used to determine kidney size, and renal radionuclide imaging to evaluate the kidney structures. Radiologic methods such as the excretory urogram or intravenous pyelogram provide a means by which kidney structures such as the renal calyces, pelvis, ureters, and bladder can be outlined.

Action of diuretics

In some disease states, it is desirable to increase the urine output through the use of diuretics. Diuresis is the rapid passage of urine through the kidneys. Water reabsorption in the kidneys is largely passive and is dependent on sodium reabsorption. Therefore, most diuretics exert their action by interfering with sodium reabsorption. Only those substances that have a direct impact on the kidneys are regarded as diuretics. For example, digitalis preparations increase urine output in persons with heart failure by increasing cardiac output, renal blood flow, and the glomerular filtration rate but are not diuretics. Because of diuretics' mechanism of action, it is logical to include a discussion of them in this chapter. There are four types of diuretics: (1) osmotic, (2) inhibitors of urine acidification, (3) inhibitors of sodium trans-

Table 30–3. Diuretic actions*

Diuretic	Mode of action	Untoward actions
Osmotic diuretics	Cause water diuresis by creating an osmotic gradient, which serves to hold water in the tubular fluid; osmotic diuretics are filtered in the glomerulus but not reabsorbed in the tubule	Cause dehydration and electrolyte imbalance
Inhibitors of urine acidification (carbonic anhydrase inhibitors)	Impair hydrogen ion secretion in the tubular exchange system where sodium reabsorption is linked to hydrogen secretion	Increase potassium and bicarbonate losses; cause systemic acidosis
Mercurial diuretics	Prevent sodium reabsorption in the proximal tubule	Cause sodium depletion because of site of action; excess chloride loss can lead to hypochloremic alkalosis
Aldosterone antagonists	Block sodium reabsorption in the potassium-sodium exchange site of the distal tubule	Can increase potassium levels
Thiazide diuretics	Prevent sodium chloride reabsorption at the site between the thick ascending loop of Henle and the distal tubule	Cause increased potassium loss; may increase uric acid levels and impair glucose metabolism
Loop diuretics	Prevent sodium reabsorption in the active transport site of the thick ascending loop of Henle	Increase potassium losses and uric acid retention; ethacrynic acid has been associated with eighth nerve damage and deafness

* The reader is referred to a pharmacology text for specific examples of each of these diuretics.

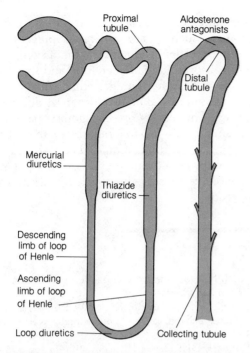

Proximal tubule

Aldosterone antagonists

Distal tubule

Mercurial diuretics

Thiazide diuretics

Descending limb of loop of Henle

Ascending limb of loop of Henle

Loop diuretics

Collecting tubule

Figure 30-12 Sites where diuretics exert their action.

port, and (4) aldosterone antagonists. Table 30-3 and Figure 30-12 describe the sites and mechanisms of action and untoward effects of these classes of diuretics.

Osmotic diuretics

Osmotic diuretics, such as mannitol, are substances that are filtered in the glomerulus but not reabsorbed in the tubules. Because they are not reabsorbed, they serve to increase the osmolality of the tubular filtrate and cause a decrease in water reabsorption. The osmotic diuretics maintain a high urine volume following a hemolytic reaction or the ingestion of toxic substances, such as salicylates or barbiturates, that are excreted in the urine. Osmotic diuretics have a dehydrating effect on body tissues and may be useful in reducing intracranial or intraocular pressure. In diabetes mellitus, the renal tubular cells are unable to reabsorb all of the glucose that is filtered in the glomerulus, and the excess glucose acts as an osmotic diuretic.

Inhibitors of urine acidification

Acetazolamide (Diamox), a carbonic anhydrase inhibitor, impairs the reaction that converts carbon dioxide and water to bicarbonate and hydrogen ions. Bicarbonate is poorly absorbed in the renal tubules; rather, it combines with hydrogen that is secreted into the tubule to form carbon dioxide and water. The carbon dioxide is then reabsorbed into the tubular cells, where it combines with water, in a car-

bonic anhydrase-catalyzed reaction, to form bicarbonate and hydrogen ions. When hydrogen ion secretion is blocked by the action of acetazolamide, both the bicarbonate ion and the sodium ion that accompany it are lost in the urine. The loss of bicarbonate results in a mild systemic acidosis, and as this occurs the kidneys resume secreting hydrogen ions, overcoming the effect of the carbonic anhydrase inhibition. Therefore, the action of acetazolamide is of short duration, and this drug has been replaced by more effective diuretics, such as the thiazides. Acetazolamide also decreases the formation of aqueous humor and cerebral spinal fluid, and it continues to be used for that purpose.

Inhibitors of sodium transport

Sodium reabsorption occurs in the proximal tubule, the thick ascending loop of Henle, and the distal tubule where aldosterone regulates sodium and potassium exchange. Diuretics that alter sodium transport can act at any of these levels.

Mercurial diuretics (e.g., mercaptomerin and meralluride) act to inhibit enzymes needed for sodium transport that are located in the proximal convoluted tubules, where 70% to 80% of the filtered sodium is reabsorbed. The mercurial diuretics also provoke decreased reabsorption of the chloride ion, causing excessive chloride losses in the urine and consequent hypochloremic alkalosis. The mercurial diuretics are poorly absorbed from the gastrointestinal tract and they almost always cause gastrointestinal irritation. Therefore, they are given by injection. These diuretics are seldom used today.

Thiazide diuretics (e.g., chlorothiazide [Diuril], chlorthalidone [Hygroton], and hydrochlorothiazide [Hydrodiuril]) exert their action by preventing the reabsorption of chloride in the section of the tubule that is located between the thick ascending loop of Henle and the distal tubule. A decrease in sodium reabsorption follows the blocking of chloride reabsorption. The thiazides produce increased losses of potassium in the urine, uric acid retention, and some impairment in glucose tolerance. They are given orally and are very suitable for long-term therapy.

Furosemide (Lasix), *ethacrynic acid* (Edecrin), and *bumetanide* (Bumex) are sometimes called *loop diuretics* because they exert their major effect on sodium chloride reabsorption occurring in the thick ascending loop of Henle. About three-fourths of the sodium remaining after passage through the proximal tubule is absorbed in the ascending loop of Henle. This means that diuretics that act at these sites can cause potent diuresis. Impairment of sodium reabsorption in the loop of Henle causes a decrease in the osmolarity of the interstitial fluid surrounding the collecting ducts and further impedes the kidney's ability to concentrate urine. Both of these drugs cause potassium loss, increase uric acid retention, and tend to impair glucose tolerance. Both drugs also can cause hypovolemia. Ethacrynic acid is associated with eighth nerve damage and deafness. Because of its ability to produce arteriolar vasodilatation and diuresis when given intravenously, furosemide is often administered in emergency treatment of pulmonary edema.

—— Aldosterone antagonists

Spironolactone (Aldactone), triamterene (Dyrenium), and amiloride (Moduretic) are *aldosterone antagonists* which block the action of aldosterone on the distal tubular exchange site. In this way they increase the loss of sodium in the urine while enhancing potassium retention. Because of this action, these diuretics are sometimes called *potassium-sparing diuretics.* Spironolactone, in particular, has the potential for causing hyperkalemia.

In summary, diuretics are drugs that increase urine output. Diuretics, with the exception of osmotic diuretics, exert their action by altering sodium transport. Osmotic diuretics are filtered in the glomerulus and reabsorbed in the tubules. They act by increasing the osmolarity of tubular fluid. Inhibitors of urine acidification, such as acetazolamide, prevent bicarbonate reabsorption and with it, the accompanying sodium reabsorption. The mercurial and thiazide diuretics, as well as furosemide, ethacrynic acid, and bumetanide, inhibit sodium transport at different tubular sites. The aldosterone antagonists, spironolactone, triamterene, and amiloride, block the action of aldosterone in the distal tubule. These diuretics decrease sodium reabsorption while causing potassium retention. They are sometimes called potassium-sparing diuretics.

References

1. Smith H: From Fish to Philosopher, p 4. Boston, Little, Brown and Company, 1953
2. Robbins SL, Cotran RS, Kumar V: Pathologic Basis of Disease, 2nd ed, p 993. Philadelphia, WB Saunders, 1987
3. Cormack DH: Ham's Histology, 9th ed, pp 575–576. Philadelphia, JB Lippincott, 1987
4. Guyton A: Textbook of Medical Physiology, 7th ed, p 400. Philadelphia, WB Saunders, 1986
5. McConnell EA, Zimmerman MF: Care of the Patient with Urologic Problems, p 19. Philadelphia, JB Lippincott, 1983

Alterations in Renal Function

Objectives

After you have studied this chapter, you should be able to meet the following objectives:

_____ Cite the effect of urinary obstruction in the fetus.

_____ State the possible effects of kidney position or form on kidney function.

_____ State at least four causes of urinary obstruction.

_____ Describe the effects of urinary tract obstruction on renal structure and function.

_____ Cite three theories that are used to explain the formation of kidney stones.

_____ Explain the mechanisms of pain and infection that occur with kidney stones.

_____ List the four types of kidney stones and describe at least one predisposing factor for each type.

_____ State the difference between the methods of ureterorenoscopy, percutaneous nephrostomy, and extracorporeal lithotripsy for removal of kidney stones.

_____ Cite the organisms most responsible for urinary tract infections.

_____ List three physiological mechanisms that protect against urinary tract infections.

_____ Explain the different degrees of pathogen virulence in terms of urinary tract infections.

_____ Explain the association between increased risk of urinary tract infections in the female and sexual intercourse, pregnancy, old age, urinary stasis and reflux, and differences in bladder and kidney host cells.

_____ Describe measures used to reduce urinary tract infections due to urinary catheters.

(continued)

_____ Use the terms *proliferation, sclerosis, membranous, diffuse, focal, segmental,* and *mesangial* to explain changes in glomerular structure that occur with glomerulonephritis.

_____ Relate the proteinuria, hematuria, pyuria, oliguria, edema, hypertension, and azotemia that occurs with glomerulonephritis to changes in glomerular structure.

_____ Differentiate between the signs and symptoms that occur with the nephrotic syndrome, the nephritic syndromes, rapidly progressive glomerulonephritis, and chronic glomerulonephritis in terms of clinical manifestations and prognosis.

_____ Explain the vulnerability of the kidney to injury due to drugs and toxins.

_____ List the major manifestations of renal cancer.

More than 20 million North Americans suffer from diseases of the kidney and urinary tract; about 80,000 die each year because of these diseases. Kidney and urinary tract diseases are a major cause of work loss among men and women: approximately 10% of America's outpatient visits result from such problems.[1] The number of persons with chronic and disabling renal disease has increased, in part because recent advances in dialysis and renal transplant methods are now keeping persons alive who would formerly have died.

The kidneys are subject to many of the same types of disorders that affect other body structures, including developmental defects, infections, altered immune responses, and neoplasms. The kidneys filter blood from all parts of the body; and although many forms of renal disease, referred to as primary renal disorders, originate in the kidneys, others develop secondary to disorders such as diabetes mellitus and systemic lupus erythematosus. The discussion in this chapter focuses on congenital disorders of the kidney, obstructive disorders, urinary tract infections, disorders of the glomerular function, tubulointerstitial disorders, and neoplasms of the kidney. Acute and chronic renal failure is discussed in Chapter 32 and the effects of other disease conditions, such as hypertension, shock, and diabetes mellitus, are discussed in other sections of the book.

Congenital disorders of the kidney

About 10% of persons are born with potentially significant malformations of the urinary system. Congenital defects of the kidney can take several forms. They can present as a decrease in the amount of kidney tissue (agenesis or hypoplasia) or as alterations in the form and position of the kidneys (kidney displacement or horseshoe kidney). Developmental anomalies of the fetal urinary tract are among the most commonly recognized congenital anomalies. The incidence of lethal anomalies is between 0.3 and 0.7 per 1,000 births.[2]

Agenesis and hypoplasia

The kidneys begin to develop early in the 5th week of gestation and start to function about 3 weeks later. The term *agenesis* refers to the absence of an organ due to a failure to develop. *Dysgenesis* is the failure to develop normally. Unilateral agenesis of the kidneys is relatively common, and persons with this defect are often unaware of its presence as long as the single kidney functions normally. Dysgenesis or agenesis of both kidneys is relatively rare; when it does occur, it is often accompanied by pulmonary hypoplasia. It is incompatible with life, and infants with this defect are stillborn or die shortly after birth of either pulmonary or renal complications. In renal *hypoplasia,* the kidneys do not develop to normal size. Like agenesis, hypoplasia more commonly affects only one kidney. When both kidneys are affected, there is progressive development of renal failure.

The urine produced by the fetal kidneys mixes with the amniotic fluid, and the fetus drinks it and reabsorbs it through the gastrointestinal tract. In pregnancies involving babies with nonfunctional kidneys or outflow obstruction of the kidneys, the amount of amniotic fluid is very small—a condition called *oligohydramnios.* The cause of fetal death in these babies is thought to be cord compression due to the oligohydramnios.[2]

Recent animal experiments have shown that ureteral or bladder outlet obstruction causes renal dysgenesis or agenesis and pulmonary hypoplasia. Obstructions in fetal urinary outflow can now be diagnosed with ultrasound imaging. In the normal fetus, the kidneys can be visualized as early as 12 weeks. The sensitivity with which fetal obstructive uropathy can be diagnosed is low before 20 weeks and high between 35 and 40 weeks. *In utero* surgery has been done to relieve outflow obstructions with the hope of preventing pulmonary hypoplasia and renal dysgenesis. The procedure is experimental, and its success rate is still being determined.[3]

Alterations in kidney position and form

The developmental process can result in kidneys that lie outside their normal position, usually just above the pelvic brim or within the pelvis. Because of the abnormal position, kinking of the ureters and obstruction of urine flow may occur.

One of the most common alterations in kidney form is the horseshoe kidney. This abnormality occurs in about 1 out of every 500 to 1000 persons.[4] In this disorder the upper or lower poles of the two kidneys are fused, producing a horseshoe-shaped structure that is continuous along the midline of the body anterior to the great vessels. Most horseshoe kidneys are fused at the lower pole. Usually, the condition does not cause problems unless there is an associated defect in the renal pelvis or other urinary structures that favors obstruction of urine flow.

In summary, approximately 10% of infants are born with potentially significant malformations of the urinary system. These abnormalities can range from bilateral renal agenesis, which is incompatible with life, to hypogenesis of one kidney, which usually causes no problems unless the function of the single kidney is impaired. The developmental process can result in kidneys that lie outside their normal position. Because of the abnormal position, kinking of the ureters and obstruction of urine flow can occur.

Obstructive disorders

Urinary obstruction can occur in persons of any age and can involve any of the urinary tract structures, from the nephron to the urethral meatus. The conditions that cause urinary tract obstruction include developmental defects, calculi (stones), normal pregnancy, benign prostatic hyperplasia, scar tissue resulting from infection and inflammation, tumors, and neurologic disorders such as spinal cord injury and diabetic neuropathy (Figure 31-1). The causes of urinary tract obstructions are summarized in Table 31-1.

Mechanisms of renal damage in urinary obstruction

The destructive effects of urinary obstruction on kidney structures are determined by the degree (partial vs. complete, unilateral vs. bilateral) and duration of impaired flow. The two most damaging effects of urinary obstruction are (1) the back pressure that

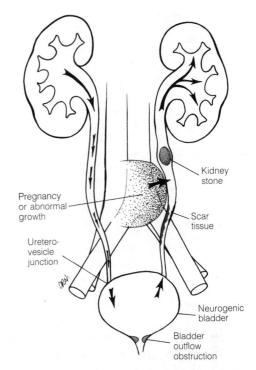

Figure 31-1 Locations and causes of urinary tract obstruction.

develops, which interferes with blood flow and destroys renal tissue, and (2) the stasis of urine, which predisposes to infection. A common complication of urinary tract obstruction is infection. The static urine provides a medium in which bacteria can grow; when present, urinary calculi serve as foreign bodies and contribute to infection. In addition to the direct effects on renal function, urinary tract obstruction can produce a variety of complications, including hypertension, stone formation, and necrosis of the renal papillae. Hypertension is more common in cases of unilateral obstruction in which renin secretion is enhanced, probably secondary to impaired renal blood. In these circumstances, removal of the obstruction often leads to a reduction in blood pressure. When hypertension accompanies bilateral obstruction, renin levels are usually normal and the elevated blood pressure is probably volume-related. Relief of bilateral obstruction leads to loss of volume and a fall in blood pressure.[5] In some cases, relieving the obstruction does not correct the hypertension. Papillary necrosis may occur with acute severe obstruction and is thought to result from ischemia.

Prolonged or severe partial obstruction causes irreversible kidney damage. If obstruction is complete, irreversible damage occurs after 12 weeks.[6] Depending on the degree of obstruction that is present, pressures build up, beginning at the site of obstruction and moving backward into the kidney. Initially, the corti-

Table 31-1. Causes of urinary tract obstruction

Level of obstruction	Cause
Renal pelvis	Renal calculi
	Papillary necrosis
Ureter	Renal calculi
	Pregnancy
	Tumors that compress the ureter
	Ureteral stricture
	Congenital disorders of the ureterovesical junction and ureteropelvic junction strictures
Bladder and urethra	Bladder cancer
	Neurogenic bladder
	Bladder stones
	Prostatic hyperplasia or cancer
	Urethral strictures
	Congenital urethral defects

cal structures of the kidney are subjected to less pressure than medullary and pelvic structures. Usually, the most severe effects occur at the level of the papillae because these structures are subjected to the greatest pressure. Accordingly, impaired concentrating ability due to pressure effects on medullary tubular structures precedes impairment of glomerular filtration, which occurs in the cortex.

The term *hydronephrosis* refers to dilatation of the renal pelvis with progressive renal atrophy caused by obstruction to urine flow through the ureter or lower parts of the urinary tract. The term *hydroureter* is used to describe ureteral dilatation caused by obstructive disorders (Figure 31-2). Bilateral hydronephrosis occurs only when the obstruction is below the level of the ureters. If the obstruction occurs at the level of the ureters or above, hydronephrosis is unilateral.

Signs and symptoms

The signs and symptoms of urinary obstruction depend on the site of obstruction, the cause, and the rapidity with which the condition developed. Signs and symptoms of urinary obstruction include pain, signs of urinary tract infection, hypertension, and signs of renal dysfunction, such as impaired ability to concentrate urine. Changes in urine output may be a misleading sign, since output may be normal or even high in partial obstruction.

Pain, which is often the factor that causes a person to seek medical attention, is the result of distention of the bladder, collecting system, or renal capsule. Its severity is most closely related to the rate, rather than the degree of distention.[5]

Pain occurs most often with acute obstruc-

tion, where the distention of urinary structures is rapid. This is in contrast to chronic obstruction, where distention is gradual and may not cause pain. Instead, gradual obstruction may only produce vague abdominal or back discomfort. When pain occurs, it is related to the site of obstruction. Obstruction of the renal pelvis or upper ureter causes pain and tenderness over the flank area. With lower levels of obstruction, the pain may radiate to the testicles in the male or labia in the female. With partial obstruction, particularly of the ureteropelvic junction, pain may occur during periods of high fluid intake, when a high rate of urine flow causes an acute hydronephrosis. Because of its visceral innervation, ureteral obstruction may produce reflex impairment of gastrointestinal tract peristalsis and motility, with abdominal distention and, in severe cases, paralytic ileus.

Diagnosis and treatment

Early diagnosis of urinary tract obstruction is important because the condition is usually treatable and a delay in therapy may result in permanent dam-

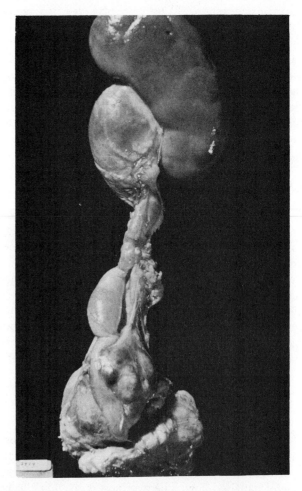

Figure 31-2 Hydroureter caused by ureteral obstruction in a woman with cancer of the uterus.

age to the kidney. Diagnostic methods vary with the symptoms. For example, a distended bladder suggests prostatic hyperplasia in the male. Radiologic methods are often used. The opaque kidney stones are often visible on x-ray films. Intravenous urograms, computed tomographic studies, and renal scans using a radiopharmaceutical agent such as gallium may be used. Ultrasound has proven to be the single most useful noninvasive diagnostic modality for urinary obstruction. Other diagnostic methods, such as urinalysis, are used to determine the extent of renal involvement and the presence of infection.

Treatment of urinary obstruction depends on the cause. Urinary stone removal may be necessary or surgical treatment of structural defects indicated.

—— Renal calculi

The most common cause of urinary tract obstruction is urinary calculi. The term *nephrolithiasis* refers to kidney stones. Although stones can form in any part of the urinary tract, most develop in the kidneys. About 1 million North Americans are hospitalized each year with kidney stones, and an equal number are treated for stones without hospitalization.

Kidney stones are crystalline structures made up of materials that the kidneys normally excrete in the urine. Kidney stones require a nidus, or nucleus, in order to form, and a urinary environment that supports continued precipitation of stone components in order to grow. It is thought that the urine normally contains substances that inhibit precipitation of stone components. Currently three major theories are used to explain stone formation: the saturation theory, the inhibitor deficiency theory, and the matrix theory.[7] It is possible that one or more of these factors contribute to stone formation in the same person. The saturation theory states that the risk of stone formation is increased when the urine is saturated with stone components (calcium salts, uric acid, magnesium ammonium phosphate, or cystine). The inhibitor theory suggests that persons who have a deficiency of endogenous compounds that inhibit stone formation in their urine are at increased risk for stone formation. One such compound has been recently identified and termed *urinocalcin*. The matrix theory proposes that organic materials, such as mucopolysaccharides derived from the epithelial cells that line the tubules, act as a nidus for stone formation. This theory is based on the observation that organic matrix materials can be found in all layers of kidney stones. It is not known whether the matrix material contributes to the initiation of stone formation or the material is merely entrapped as the stone forms.

There are four types of kidney stones: calcium stones (oxalate or phosphate), magnesium ammonium phosphate stones, uric acid stones, and cystine stones. The causes and treatment measures for each of these types of renal stones are described in Table 31-2.

Most kidney stones (80% to 90%) are calcium stones—calcium oxalate, calcium phosphate, or a combination of the two materials. Calcium stones are usually associated with increased concentrations of calcium in the blood and urine. Excessive bone resorption caused by immobility, bone disease, hyperparathyroidism, and renal tubular acidosis are all con-

Table 31-2. Composition, contributing factors, and treatment of kidney stones

Type of stone	Contributing factors	Treatment
Calcium (oxalate and phosphate)	Hypercalcemia and hypercalciuria Immobilization Hyperparathyroidism Vitamin D intoxication Diffuse bone disease Milk-alkali syndrome Renal tubular acidosis Hyperoxaluria Intestinal bypass surgery	Treatment of underlying conditions Thiazide diuretics Increased fluid intake
Magnesium ammonium phosphate (struvite)	Urea-splitting urinary tract infections	Treatment of urinary tract infection Acidification of the urine Increased fluid intake
Uric acid (urate)	Formed in acid urine with *p*H of approximately 5.5 Gout High-purine diet	Increased fluid intake Allopurinal for hyperuricuria Alkalinization of urine
Cystine	Cystinuria (inherited disorder of amino acid metabolism)	Increased fluid intake Alkalinization of urine

tributing conditions. Very high oxalate concentrations in the blood and urine predispose to formation of oxalate stones.

Magnesium ammonium phosphate, or struvite, stones form only in alkaline urine and in the presence of bacteria that possess an enzyme called urease, which splits the urea the kidneys secrete in large amounts to ammonia and carbon dioxide. The ammonia that is formed takes up a hydrogen ion to become an ammonium ion, increasing the pH of the urine so it becomes more alkaline. Phosphate levels are increased in alkaline urine and, since magnesium is always present, struvite stones form. These stones enlarge as the bacterial count grows and can increase in size until they fill an entire kidney pelvis. Because of their shape they are called *staghorn stones*. Staghorn stones are almost always associated with urinary tract infections and a persistently alkaline urine.

Uric acid stones develop in the presence of gout and high concentrations of uric acid in the urine. Unlike radiopaque calcium stones, uric acid stones are not visible on x-ray. Cystine stones are rare. They are seen in cystinuria, which results from a genetic defect in renal transport of cystine.

Renal colic is the term used to describe the colicky pain that accompanies urinary obstruction due to kidney stones. The symptoms of renal colic are due to stones 1 mm to 5 mm in diameter that are able to move into the ureter and obstruct flow. Classic ureteral colic is manifested by acute, intermittent, and excruciating pain in the flank and upper outer quadrant of the abdomen on the affected side. The pain may radiate to the lower abdominal quadrant, the bladder area, the perineum, or the scrotum in the male. The skin may be cool and clammy, and nausea and vomiting are often present.

Treatment of acute renal colic is usually supportive. Pain relief may be needed during acute phases of obstruction and antibiotic therapy may be necessary to treat urinary infections. All urine should be strained during an attack in the hope of retrieving the stone for chemical analysis and determination of stone type. This information, along with a careful history and laboratory tests, affords the basis for long-term preventive measures.

In some cases, stone removal may be necessary. Several methods are available for removal of kidney stones: ureteroscopic removal, percutaneous removal, and extracorporeal lithotripsy. All of these procedures eliminate the need for an open surgical procedure, which is another form of treatment.

Ureteroscopic removal involves the passage of an instrument through the urethra into the bladder and then into the ureter. The development of high-quality optics has improved both the ease with which this procedure is performed and its outcome. The procedure, which is performed under fluoroscopic guidance, involves the use of various instruments for dilating the ureter and for grasping and removing the stone. Usually, preprocedure radiologic studies using a contrast medium (intravenous pyelography) are done to determine the position of the stone and direct the placement of the ureteroscope.[8]

Percutaneous nephrostomy involves the insertion, through the flank, of a small gauge needle into the collecting system of the kidney; the needle tract is then dilated and an instrument called a *nephroscope* is inserted into the kidney pelvis.[8] The procedure is performed under fluoroscopic guidance. Preprocedure radiologic and ultrasound examinations of the kidney and ureter are used in determining the placement of the nephroscope. Stones of up to 1.0 cm can be removed through this method. Larger stones must be broken up with an electrohydraulic or ultrasonic lithotriptor (stone breaker).

A nonsurgical treatment called *extracorporeal shock wave lithotripsy,* introduced in Germany in 1980, received US Food and Drug Administration approval in 1984 for treatment of stones primarily in the renal calyx, pelvis, and upper third of the ureter.[9] The procedure, which is accomplished using a specially constructed water-filled tank, uses shock waves to fragment calculi into sandlike particles. During the procedure, the patient is seated on a chair-type support and immersed in warm water up to the level of the clavicles. The current equipment cannot accommodate persons who weigh over 300 pounds or who are taller than 6 feet 6 inches. Fluoroscopy is used to visualize the stone and determine the point of impact for the shock waves. The shock waves are generated when an electric spark fires across the gap of a special spark plug that is placed in the bottom of a tank of water.[8,9] The spark vaporizes the water in the immediate area of the spark, forming a shock wave that is conveyed through the water toward the patient. The shock wave is propagated through the water and soft tissue of the body, which have similar acoustic impedances, until it reaches the stone, which has a higher acoustic impedance. Because of the stones' high acoustic impedance, the shock wave releases its energy on impact; this fragments and gradually reduces the stone to a sandlike consistency that can be passed in the urine. Bone is not affected because of its high percentage of protein matrix and small crystal size.[8] Typically, a total of 1000 to 2000 shocks are generated to fragment a stone. Electrocardiograph monitoring is done during the procedure, and the spark generations are coordinated with the R wave of the ECG to protect against dysrhythmias during the firing of the spark plug. Each spark lasts one microsecond and the total procedure takes about 60 to 90 seconds. The procedure requires the use of general or epidural anesthesia because of the considerable pain that is produced as the shock waves traverse the body.

In summary, obstruction of urine flow can occur at any level of the urinary tract. Among the causes of urinary tract obstruction are developmental defects, normal pregnancy, infection and inflammation, kidney stones, neurologic defects, and prostatic hypertrophy. Obstructive disorders produce stasis of urine, thereby increasing the risk of infection and calculi formation, and result in back-pressure that is damaging to kidney structures. There are four types of kidney stones: calcium (oxalate and phosphate) stones, which are associated with increased serum calcium levels; magnesium ammonium phosphate stone (struvite) stones, which are associated with urinary tract infection; uric acid stones, which are related to elevated uric acid levels; and cystine stones, which are seen in cystinuria.

Urinary tract infections

Urinary tract infections (UTIs) are the second most common type of bacterial infections seen by the physician (respiratory tract infections are first). The term *urinary tract infection* can refer to several distinct entities, including asymptomatic bacteriuria, catheter-associated urinary tract infection, cystitis, and pyelonephritis.

Urinary tract infections affect persons of all ages. In infants they occur more often in boys than girls. After the first year of life, however, urinary tract infections are more frequent in females because of the short urethra and because the vaginal vestibule can be easily contaminated with fecal flora. About 20% of all adult women will develop at least one urinary tract infection during their lifetime. In men, the length of the urethra and the antibacterial properties of the prostatic fluid provide some protection from ascending urinary tract infections until about age 50 years. After this age, prostatic hypertrophy becomes more common, and with it may come obstruction and urinary tract infection.

There are two routes by which bacteria can enter the kidneys: (1) through the bloodstream, and (2) as an ascending infection from the lower urinary tract. Most infections are of the ascending type. Although the distal portion of the urethra often contains pathogens, the urine formed in the kidneys and found in the bladder is normally sterile or free of bacteria. This is because of the washout phenomenon, in which urine from the bladder normally washes bacteria out of the urethra. When a urinary tract infection occurs, the bacteria that have colonized the urethra, vagina, or perineal area are often responsible. *Escherichia coli* is by far the most common urinary pathogen. Other common pathogens include *Proteus, Klebsiella, Enterobacter,* and *Serratia* species.[10]

Host-agent interaction

Because certain individuals seem to be predisposed to developing urinary tract infections, considerable interest has been focused on studies that relate host-agent interactions and identify factors that increase the risk of urinary tract infection. Studies have shown an increased risk of urinary tract infection in persons with urinary obstruction and reflux; in pregnant and nonpregnant women; and in elderly persons.[11] Furthermore, some conditions, including diabetes mellitus, pregnancy, immunosuppression, and upper urinary tract obstruction, are associated with serious morbidity from urinary tract infections. Instrumentation and urinary catheterization are the most common predisposing factors in nosocomial urinary tract infections.[12]

Host defenses

In the development of a urinary tract infection, host defenses are matched against the virulence of the pathogen. The host defenses of the bladder have several components, including the washout phenomenon (in which bacteria are removed from the bladder and urethra during voiding), the protective mucin layer that lines the bladder and protects against bacterial invasion, and the local immune responses. In the ureters, peristaltic movements normally facilitate the movement of urine from the kidney pelvis through the ureters and into the bladder. Immune mechanisms, particularly secretory IgA immunoglobulins, are considered to provide an important antibacterial defense. Phagocytic blood cells further assist in the removal of bacteria from the urinary tract.

Recently, there has been a growing appreciation of the protective function of the bladder's mucin layer. It is thought that the epithelial cells lining the bladder synthesize protective substances that subsequently become incorporated into the mucin layer that adheres to the bladder wall. One theory proposes that the mucin layer acts by binding water, which then constitutes a protective barrier between the bacteria and the epithelium. Elderly and postmenopausal women have been shown to produce less mucin than younger women, suggesting that estrogen may play a role in its secretion.

Pathogen virulence

Current investigations are focusing on the adherence properties of the bacteria that infect the urinary tract. It has been shown that these bacteria have fine protein filaments that help them adhere to receptors on the lining of urinary tract structures. These filaments are called *fimbriae* or *pili*. Among the factors contributing to bacterial virulence, the type of fimbriae that the bacteria possess may be the most important. Bacteria with certain types of fimbriae are associated primarily with cystitis, and those with other types with a high incidence of pyelonephritis. The bacteria associated with pyelonephritis are thought to have fimbriae that bind to carbohydrates that are specific to the surfaces of epithelial cells in this part of the urinary tract.

Obstruction and reflux

Obstruction and reflux are important contributing factors in the development of urinary tract infections. Normally any microorganisms that enter the bladder are washed out during voiding. When outflow is obstructed, urine remains in the bladder and acts as a medium for microbial growth; the microorganisms in the contaminated urine can then ascend along the ureters to infect the kidney. It has been shown that the presence of residual urine correlates directly with bacteriuria and with its recurrence following treatment.[13] Another aspect of bladder outflow obstruction and bladder distention is increased intravesicular pressure, which tends to compress blood vessels in the wall of the bladder, leading to a decrease in the mucosal defenses of the bladder.

In urinary tract infections associated with stasis of urine flow, the obstruction may be either anatomic or functional in nature. Anatomic obstructions include urinary tract stones; prostatic hyperplasia in elderly men; pregnancy; and obstructions of the posterior urethral valve, ureteropelvic junction, or ureterovesical junction. Anatomic obstructions have been reported in 3% to 21% of children who present with urinary tract infections.[14] Functional obstructions include neurogenic bladder, infrequent voiding, and detrusor (bladder) muscle instability, and constipation.

Reflux occurs when urine from the urethra moves into the bladder (urethrovesical reflux) or from the bladder into the ureters (ureterovesical reflux). In women, a urethrovesical reflux can occur during activities such as coughing or squatting, in which an increase in intraabdominal pressure causes the urine to be squeezed into the urethra and then flow back into the bladder as the pressure decreases. This can also happen when the act of voiding is abruptly interrupted for any reason. Because the urethral orifice is frequently contaminated with bacteria, the reflux mechanism may cause bacteria to be drawn back into the bladder.

A second type of reflux mechanism can occur at the level of the bladder and ureter. This reflux mechanism is called the *vesicoureteral reflux*. Normally, peristaltic movements propel urine from the kidneys to the bladder. In vesicoureteral reflux, urine is propelled from the bladder through the ureters into the kidneys. It is most commonly seen in children with urinary tract infections and is believed to result from congenital defects in length, diameter, muscle structure, or innervation of the submucosal segment of the ureter.[15] It is also seen in adults with obstruction to bladder outflow.

Urinary tract infections in women

In women, the urethra is short and in close proximity to the vagina and rectum, offering little protection against entry of microorganisms into the bladder. There is a peak incidence of these infections in the 15- to 24-year-old age group, suggesting that hormonal and anatomic changes associated with puberty as well as sexual activity contribute to urinary tract infections. Massage of the anterior vagina may be followed by the appearance of bacteria in previously sterile urine, and sexual intercourse often results in an increase of bacterial concentrations in the voided urine.[16]

The role of sexual activity in the development of urethritis and cystitis is controversial. The well-documented "honeymoon cystitis" suggests that sexual activity may contribute to such infections in susceptible women. A nonpharmacologic approach to treatment of frequent urinary tract infections associated with sexual intercourse is increasing fluid intake before intercourse and voiding soon after intercourse. This procedure uses the washout phenomena to remove bacteria from the bladder.

Urinary tract infections during pregnancy. Urinary tract infections occur more commonly during pregnancy. This is particularly true of those women who have bacteriuria during their initial prenatal visit. Normal changes in the functioning of the urinary tract occur during pregnancy that predispose to urinary tract infections. These changes involve the collecting system of the kidneys and include dilatation of the renal calyces, pelves, and ureters that begins during the first trimester and becomes most pronounced during the third trimester. This dilatation of the upper urinary system is accompanied by a reduction in the peristaltic activity of the ureters that is thought to result from the muscle-relaxing effects of progesterone-like hormones and the mechanical obstruction from the enlarging uterus. In addition to the changes in the kidney and ureter, the bladder becomes displaced from its pelvic position to a more abdominal position, producing further alterations in ureteral position.[17]

The complications of urinary tract infection during pregnancy include acute pyelonephritis, toxemia, persistent bacteriuria, and chronic pyelonephritis. Because bacteriuria may occur as an asymptomatic condition in pregnant women, it is recommended that women be screened by quantitative urine culture on the first prenatal visit. Women who are uninfected on their initial prenatal visit have a low incidence of bacteriuria during pregnancy. Women with bacteriuria should be followed closely, and infections should be properly treated to prevent complications.[18]

Urinary tract infections in the elderly

Urinary tract infections are relatively common in the elderly. One study of 100 consecutive episodes of community-acquired bacteremia in the elderly found that the urinary tract was the source of infection in 34% of these persons.[19] Several factors predispose the elderly to urinary tract infections: (1) immobility resulting in poor bladder emptying, (2) bladder outflow obstruction due to prostatic hyperplasia or kidney stones, (3) bladder ischemia due to urinary retention, (4) senile vaginitis, (5) constipation, and (6) diminished bactericidal activity of urine and prostatic secretions.[19] Added to these risks are other health problems that necessitate instrumentation of the urinary tract. Furthermore, elderly persons may not present with the usual symptoms of urinary tract infection. Instead, they may experience incontinence, confusion, vague abdominal pain, and anorexia or nausea. Sometimes there may be no symptoms until the infection is far advanced.

Types of urinary tract infection

Urinary tract infections include presence of bacteria in the urine, cystitis, and catheter-induced infections. Pyelonephritis and upper urinary tract infection are discussed with tubulointerstitial disorders.

Bacteriuria

Bacteriuria, or the presence of bacteria in the urine, is often used in diagnosing urinary tract infections. The source of bacteria in the urine can be contamination of the urine specimen, simple colonization of the urinary tract, or bacterial invasion of urinary structures. Colonization is usually defined as multiplication of microorganisms in or on a host without apparent evidence of invasiveness or tissue injury. A commonly accepted criterion for diagnosis of a urinary tract infection is the presence of more than 100,000 (10^5) organisms per ml of urine. The accuracy of the diagnosis is strengthened if such numbers are found in two consecutive urine samples and if the bacteria are of a single type. Contaminated urine specimens often contain several types of microorganisms.

Cystitis

An acute episode of cystitis or bladder infection is characterized by frequency of urination (sometimes as often as every 20 minutes), lower abdominal discomfort, and burning and pain on urination (dysuria). There also may be systemic signs of infection, with fever and generalized malaise. If there are no complications, the symptoms disappear within 48 hours. This type of cystitis is mainly a disorder of young women. Symptoms of cystitis may also represent urethritis or vaginitis attributable to *Trichomonas*, bacterial vaginosis, chlamydia, or gonorrhea.

Catheter-associated infections

Urinary catheters are tubes made of latex or plastic. They are inserted through the urethra into the bladder for the purpose of urinary drainage. They are a source of urethral irritation and provide a means for entry of microorganisms into the urinary tract. Indwelling catheters are used in about 10% of patients admitted to general hospitals.[18] A closed drainage system (closed to air and other sources of contamination) and careful attention to perineal hygiene (cleansing of the area around the urethral meatus) will help to prevent infections in persons who require an indwelling catheter. Careful handwashing and early detection and treatment of urinary tract infections are also essential. When an indwelling catheter is employed, the risk of infection is increased with use of broad-spectrum antibiotics and catheter irrigations—in fact, hospital patients themselves are cited as the most common reservoir of infection.[20] The Centers for Disease Control recommend that patients with urinary catheters not share a room unless special requirements for intensive care make this necessary.[20] This recommendation follows the observation that an increased incidence of urinary tract infections has been reported in catheterized patients sharing a room.

Diagnosis and treatment

Early diagnosis and treatment of urinary tract infection is essential for preventing permanent kidney damage. Screening of high-risk groups and attention to care of persons with indwelling catheters are important measures. Pregnant women and persons with diabetes or renal problems who are at risk for developing urinary tract infections can usually be managed in the physician's office.

The diagnosis of urinary tract infection is usually based on symptoms and on examination of the urine for the presence of microorganisms. Care is needed in collecting urine specimens representative of bladder urine. Specimens kept for longer than 1 hour must be refrigerated to prevent the contaminating organisms from multiplying. Catheterized specimens, once common, have been largely replaced with clean voided specimens. To obtain a clean voided specimen, the area around the urethra is carefully cleansed and a midstream specimen is obtained by having the person void directly into a sterile container. This method is usually adequate and eliminates the risk of introducing microorganisms into the bladder during insertion of a catheter. In infants, and sometimes in other age groups, a suprapubic aspiration may be done to obtain a sample of bladder urine.

As well as the bacterial count, the urine leukocyte count is also used: the presence of pyuria (more than 10 leukocytes/mm^3 uncentrifuged urine) indicates host injury as opposed to asymptomatic bacterial colonization. When necessary, x-rays, ultrasound, and CT and renal scans are used to identify contributing factors, such as obstruction.

Immunofluorescence studies may be done to determine whether the infection involves the upper urinary tract.[21] This test is expensive, however, and is usually not done on a routine basis. Detailed identification and antibiotic sensitivity tests are often done in cases of chronic infection. The treatment of urinary tract infection is based on the type of infection that is present (lower or upper urinary tract infection) and the presence of contributing host-agent factors.

Antibiotics are usually used to treat acute infection. The forcing of fluids may relieve signs and symptoms and is used as an adjunct to antibiotic treatment.

Lower urinary tract infection is usually treated successfully with a single-dose antimicrobial therapy and increased fluid intake.[22] A follow-up urine culture is essential when single-dose therapy is used. Because failure of single-dose therapy is suggestive of renal infection, this method of treatment can be used as a means of localizing urinary tract infection. With pyelonephritis, there is risk of permanent kidney damage, so these infections are treated more aggressively. Treatment with an appropriate antimicrobial agent is usually continued for 10 to 14 days. Hospitalization may be recommended during the early stages of infection until a response to treatment is observed. Chronic infection is more difficult to treat.

Because it is often associated with obstructive uropathy or reflux flow of urine, diagnostic tests are usually performed to detect such abnormalities. When possible the condition causing the reflux flow or obstruction is corrected. Persons with recurrent urinary tract infection are usually treated with antibiotics for 10 to 14 days in doses sufficient to maintain high urine levels and investigated for obstruction or other causes of infection. Men, in particular, should be investigated for obstructive disorders or a prostatic focus of infection.

In summary, urinary tract infection is the second most common type of bacterial infection seen by the practicing physician. Infections can range from simple bacteriuria to severe kidney infections that cause irreversible kidney damage. Most upper urinary tract infections ascend from the urethra and bladder. A number of factors interact in determining the predisposition to development of urinary tract infections, including urinary tract obstruction, urine stasis and reflux; pregnancy-induced changes in urinary tract function; age-related changes in the urinary tract; changes in the protective mechanisms of the bladder and ureters; impaired immune function; and the virulence of the pathogen. Urinary tract catheters and urinary instrumentation contribute to the incidence of urinary tract infections. Early diagnosis and treatment of urinary tract infection are essential to preventing permanent kidney damage.

Disorders of glomerular function

The glomeruli are tufts of capillaries that lie between two arterioles: the afferent and efferent arterioles. The capillaries of the glomeruli are arranged in lobules and supported by a stalk consisting of mesangial cells and a basement membrane–like extracellular matrix. The glomerulus contains four types of cells: epithelial, endothelial, mesangial, and the recently identified resident nephrophages (macrophages). The glomerular membrane is composed of three layers: (1) an endothelial layer lining the capillary, (2) a basement membrane, and (3) a layer of epithelial cells forming the outer surface of the capillary and also lining the Bowman's capsule. The epithelial cells are attached to the basement membrane by discrete cytoplasmic extensions, the foot processes (podocytes). Within the glomeruli, blood is filtered and the urine filtrate formed. The capillary membrane is selectively permeable: it allows water, electrolytes, and dissolved particles, such as glucose and amino acids, to leave the capillary and enter Bowman's space and prevents larger particles, such as plasma proteins and blood cells, from leaving the blood.

Glomerulonephritis, an inflammatory process involving glomerular structures, is the leading cause of chronic renal failure in the United States, accounting for one-half of persons who need dialysis. The disorder causes 12,000 deaths a year and is responsible for $20 million in work loss.[1] There is no one cause of glomerular disease. The disease may occur as a primary condition in which the glomerular pathology is the only disease present or it may occur as a secondary condition in which the glomerular pathology occurs secondary to another disease, such as vasculitis or systemic lupus erythematosus. An understanding of the various forms of glomerular pathology has emerged only recently. Much of this understanding can be attributed to advances in immunobiology and electron microscopy, development of animal models, and increased use of renal biopsy during the early stages of glomerular disease.

Although little is known about the etiologic agents or triggering events that produce glomerular disease, it is clear that most cases of primary glomerular disease and many cases of secondary disease have an immune origin.[23,24] Two types of immune mechanisms have been implicated from research studies: (1) injury resulting from deposition of soluble circulating antigen-antibody complexes in the glomeruli and (2) injury resulting from antibodies reacting with insoluble fixed glomerular antigens. With circulating immune complexes, the kidney is the "innocent bystander" because the antigen is not of glomerular origin and the kidney did not initiate the event.[5] The antigen of the immune complexes may be of endogenous origin, as in systemic lupus erythematosus (DNA), or it may be of exogenous origin, as in poststreptococcal glomerulonephritis (streptococcal membrane antigens). Frequently, the antigen is unknown. Whatever the inciting antigen, the antigen-antibody complex is formed in the circulation and becomes trapped in the glomerular membrane as blood is being filtered. The antigen-antibody complexes probably produce injury through complement-mediated mechanisms such as cell lysis or chemotaxis, which draws leukocytes to the area.[25] Once deposited, the immune complexes are eventually degraded by infiltrating monocytes and phagocytic mesangial cells. If the inciting antigen is short-lived, as in poststreptococcal glomerulonephritis, the inflammatory changes subside. If however, the antigen is being continuously produced, repeated inflammatory reactions may occur, leading to chronic glomerulonephritis.

The fixed antigens that cause glomerular disease may have their origin in the glomerulus or may be planted there from another source. The best-known model is the so-called antiglomerular membrane antibodies implicated in Goodpasture's syndrome. With this type of injury, antibodies are directed against glomerular basement membrane antigens. Damage to the glomeruli is probably complement- and leukocyte-mediated, although other mechanisms may be involved. Activation of complement initiates the generation of chemotactic agents (anaphylatoxins) and recruitment of neutrophils. The neutrophils release proteases that cause breakdown of the glomerular basement membrane and release of free radicals that cause cell damage. Injury may also occur without complement involvement. In these cases, other factors, such as platelet interactions, arachidonic acid metabolites, and free radicals, have been suggested as injurious agents. There is also evidence that intraglomerular hemodynamic changes such as increased intracapillary pressures or filtration rates may contribute to glomerular injury and progression of glomerulonephritis.

The cellular changes that occur with glomerular disease include proliferative, sclerotic, membranous changes. The term *proliferation* refers to an increase in cells in the glomerulus, regardless of origin; *sclerosis*, to an increase in the noncellular components of the glomerulus (primarily collagen); and *membranous*, to an increase in the thickness of the glomerular capillary wall, often due to immune complex deposition. Glomerular changes can be *diffuse*, involving all glomeruli and all parts of the glomeruli; *focal*, where only some glomeruli are affected and others are essentially normal; *segmental*, involving only a certain segment of each glomeruli; or *mesangial*, affecting only the mesangial cell.[5] Figure 31-3 illustrates changes associated with glomerular disease.

Diseases of the glomeruli disrupt glomerular filtration and alter the capillary membrane so that it becomes permeable to plasma proteins and blood cells. Increased glomerular capillary permeability leads to proteinuria, hematuria, pyuria, oliguria, edema, hypertension, and azotemia. In many cases, early glomerular disease is asymptomatic and the condition is often discovered incidentally through abnormal findings on urinalysis (primarily proteinuria, azotemia, or elevated blood pressure).

Proteinuria, predominantly albuminuria, provides the most important evidence of glomerular injury. With progression from mild to severe glomerular injury, progressively increased amounts of larger plasma proteins, such as gamma globulins, are found in the urine. Hematuria can result from bleeding anywhere in the urinary tract. With glomerular disease, hematuria develops because of active inflammatory disease and damage to the capillary membrane. The hematuria may be minimal and only detected on microscopic examination or it may be sufficient to discolor the urine. The red blood cells are either entrapped in casts or else degraded by tubular enzymes so that the urine is smoke- or cola-colored. Red blood

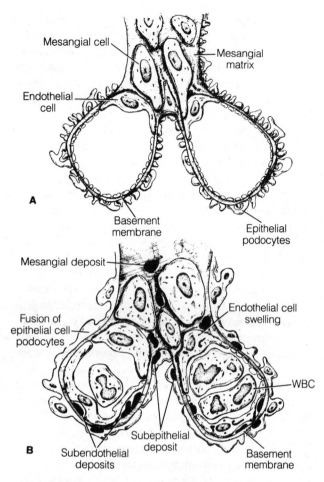

Figure 31-3 Schematic representation of glomerulus: (**A**) normal; (**B**) localization of immune deposits (mesangial, subendothelial, subepithelial) and changes in glomerular architecture associated with injury. (*Whitley K, Keane WF, Vernier RL: Acute glomerulonephritis: A clinical overview. Med Clin North Am 68(2):263, 1984*)

cells in the urine sediment are pathognomonic of glomerular inflammation (glomerulonephritis). Passage of polymorphonuclear leukocytes through the glomerular membrane causes pyuria.

Oliguria, edema, and hypertension often accompany glomerular injury. Oliguria occurs when glomerular injury is severe enough to produce a marked decrease in glomerular filtration. The hypoalbuminemia of glomerular disease has two causes: loss of albumin in the urine and dilution due to retention of sodium and water. The effect is to lower plasma colloidal osmotic pressure, causing edema (see Chapter 28). The hypertension is due to the increase in vascular volume caused by sodium and water retention and possibly to increased synthesis of vasoconstrictor compounds by the kidney. Azotemia, or increased levels of nitrogenous wastes in the blood, results from both a reduction in the filtration of urea and other nitrogenous wastes in the glomeruli and an increase in tubular reabsorption of these substances due to renal hypoperfusion.

Glomerular pathologies have been grouped into four categories: (1) nephrotic syndrome, which affects the integrity of the glomerular capillary membrane; (2) nephritic syndrome, which is caused by diseases that evoke an inflammatory response within the glomeruli; (3) rapidly progressive glomerulonephritis, which is a distinctive form of nephritic syndrome that is rapidly progressive; and (4) chronic glomerulonephritis, in which there is an insidious onset of uremia or renal failure.

The nephrotic syndrome

The nephrotic syndrome is not a specific glomerular disease, but a constellation of clinical findings that result from increased glomerular permeability to protein. It is characterized by massive proteinuria (a daily loss of 3.5 g or more) and lipiduria. There is an associated hypoalbuminemia (less than 3 g per dL), generalized edema, and hyperlipidemia.

The generalized edema, which is usually the first manifestation and can be so severe as to be incapacitating, results from the decrease in colloidal osmotic pressure that accompanies the loss of plasma proteins. Other factors, such as increased salt and water retention, may also play a role in edema formation. The hyperlipidemia is characterized by elevated levels of both triglycerides and cholesterol. It is believed that hyperlipidemia results when a compensatory increase in albumin synthesis by the liver serves as a stimulus for increased synthesis of low-density lipoproteins. Because of the elevated levels of low-density lipoproteins, persons with nephrotic syndrome are at increased risk of developing atherosclerosis. The loss of immunoglobulins in the urine is believed to increase susceptibility to infection, especially those due to staphylococcus and pneumococcus. Another problem that arises in persons with nephrosis is thrombosis (arterial and venous), presumably from an imbalance in coagulation factors that accompanies loss of plasma proteins in the urine. In general, low-molecular-weight plasma proteins, such as factors IX, X, XI, XII, prothrombin, plasminogen, antiplasmin, antithrombin III, and alpha-antitrypsin, are lost in the urine. In contrast, those of high molecular weight—such as factor VIII, von Willebrand factor, factor V, factor VII, and macroglobulin—remain in the circulation.[26] It is thought that an imbalance between procoagulation and anticoagulation factors may be responsible for the high incidence of thrombosis.

Nephrosis can occur as a primary disease or secondary to glomerular changes caused by systemic diseases such as diabetes mellitus or systemic lupus erythematosus. The relative frequency of these causes varies with age. In children under age 15, nephrotic syndrome is almost always caused by primary glomerular disease, whereas in adults it often occurs as a secondary disorder.

Among the primary glomerular lesions leading to nephrosis are (1) minimal change disease, which is characterized by diffuse loss (fusion) of foot processes from the epithelial layer of the glomerular membrane; (2) focal sclerosis, in which there is sclerosis (increased collagen deposition) of some of the tufts within a glomerulus; (3) membranous glomerulopathy, in which there is diffuse thickening of the glomerular basement membrane due to deposition of immune complexes; and (4) membranoproliferative glomerulonephritis, in which there is both basement membrane thickening and cellular proliferation.

The nephritic syndromes

The nephritic syndromes are characterized by hematuria with red cell casts in the urine, a diminished glomerular filtration rate, usually some degree of oliguria, azotemia, and hypertension. Although there may also be proteinuria and edema, these are not sufficient to cause the nephrotic syndrome. It is caused by diseases that provoke a proliferative inflammatory response of the endothelial, mesangial, or epithelial cells of the glomeruli. The inflammatory process damages the capillary wall, permitting escape of red blood cells into the urine (hematuria) and producing hemodynamic changes that cause a decrease in the glomerular filtration rate.

The nephritic syndrome may occur as a primary disorder of the glomerulus or as a secondary effect of another disease condition such as vasculitis or systemic lupus erythematosus. It can be initiated by immune complexes, antiglomerular basement antibodies, cellular mechanisms alone, or blood-borne leukocytes (neutrophils, monocytes, and lymphocytes). Among the most common glomerular causes of nephritic syndrome is diffuse proliferative glomerulonephritis, especially poststreptococcal glomerulonephritis.

Acute proliferative glomerulonephritis

The most commonly recognized form of acute glomerulonephritis is diffuse proliferative glomerulonephritis, which follows infections by strains of group A, beta-hemolytic streptococci. Diffuse proliferative glomerulonephritis may also occur following infections by other organisms, including staphylococci and a number of viral agents, such as those responsible for mumps, measles, and chicken pox. With this type of nephritis, the inflammatory response is caused by an immune reaction that occurs when circulating immune complexes become entrapped in the glomerular membrane. Proliferation of the endothelial cells lining the glomerular capillary (endocapillary form of the disease) and the mesangial cells lying between the endothelium and epithelium follows (see Figure 31-3). The capillary membrane swells and becomes permeable to plasma proteins and blood cells. Although the disease is seen primarily in children, adults of any age can also be affected.

The classic case of poststreptococcal glomerulonephritis follows a streptococcal infection by about 10 days to 2 weeks—the time needed for development of antibodies. Oliguria, which develops as glomerular filtration rate decreases, is one of the first symptoms. Proteinuria and hematuria follow due to increased glomerular capillary wall permeability. The blood is degraded by materials in the urine, and a cola-colored urine may be the first sign of the disorder. Salt and water retention gives rise to edema (particularly of the face and hands) and hypertension. Important laboratory findings include an elevated streptococcal exoenzyme (antistreptolysin-O) titer, a decline in C3 complement (see Chapter 11), and the presence of cryoglobulins (large immune complexes) in the serum.

Treatment for acute poststreptococcal glomerulonephritis is largely symptomatic. The acute symptoms usually begin to subside in about 10 days to 2 weeks, although in some children the proteinuria may persist for several months. The immediate prognosis is favorable, and approximately 95% of children recover spontaneously. The outlook for adults is less favorable. About 60% recover completely. In the remainder of cases, the lesions resolve eventually but there may be permanent kidney damage.

Rapidly progressive glomerulonephritis

Like the nephrotic and nephritic syndromes, rapidly progressive glomerulonephritis does not have a single, specific etiology. As its name implies, this type of glomerulonephritis is rapidly progressive: it involves a 50% decrease in the glomerular filtration rate (GFR) within 3 months. About 90% of those affected develop renal failure and require dialysis or transplantation.[5] The disorder is characterized by focal and segmental proliferation of endogenous glomerular cells as well as activation and recruitment of monocytes (macrophages) with formation of crescent-shaped structures that obliterate the Bowman's space. Persons with this disorder often have evidence of antibodies directed against the basement membrane. Among the systemic diseases associated with this form of glomerulonephritis are vasculitis, systemic lupus erythematosus, acute poststreptococcal glomerulonephritis (usually in adults), and primary glomerular diseases such as Goodpasture's syndrome.

Chronic glomerulonephritis

Chronic glomerulonephritis represents the end-stage of the many different types of glomerulonephritis. Histologically, it is characterized by small kidneys with sclerosed glomeruli. It rarely develops in children with acute poststreptococcal glomerulonephritis and is frequently seen in persons who survive the acute phase of rapidly progressive glomerulonephritis. However, in about one-fourth of the persons who present with chronic glomerulonephritis, there is no history of glomerular disease.[4] In most cases, chronic glomerulonephritis develops insidiously and is characterized by signs of chronic renal failure (see Chapter 32). The disease is progressive, but at widely varying rates.

Diabetic glomerulosclerosis

Diabetic nephropathy, or kidney disease, is a major complication of diabetes mellitus. It has been estimated that 55% of persons with type I, insulin-dependent diabetes and 30% of persons with type II, noninsulin-dependent diabetes develop end-stage renal disease.[4] The glomerulus is the most commonly affected structure in diabetic nephropathy; thickening of the glomerular basement membrane and development of diffuse or nodular glomerulosclerosis being the most prominent types of pathology. Widespread thickening of the glomerular capillary basement membrane occurs in almost all persons with diabetes and can occur without evidence of proteinuria.[4] Diffuse glomerulosclerosis involves an increase in mesangial matrix and thickening of the glomerular basement membrane. In nodular glomerulosclerosis, also known as *Kimmelstiel-Wilson syndrome*, there is nodular deposition of hyaline in the mesangial portion of the glomerulus. As the sclerotic process progesses in both the diffuse and nodular forms of glomerulosclerosis, there is complete obliteration of the glomerulus with impairment of renal function. Although the mechanisms of glomerular changes in diabetes are uncertain, they are thought to represent enhanced and/or defective synthesis of the basement membrane and mesangial matrix with an inappropriate incorporation of glucose into the noncellular components (collagen) of these glomerular structures.

The manifestations of diabetic glomerulosclerosis include recurrent proteinuria with slow but steady progression to renal failure. The condition occurs more frequently in persons with poorly controlled diabetes, which emphasizes the need for adherence to treatment methods that improve metabolic control.

Hypertensive glomerular disease

Renal failure and azotemia occur in 1% to 5% of persons with longstanding hypertension.[4] Hypertension is associated with a number of changes in glomerular structures, including sclerotic changes. As the glomerular vascular structures thicken and perfusion diminishes, the blood supply to the nephron decreases, causing the kidney to lose some of its ability to concentrate the urine. This may be evidenced by nocturia. Blood urea nitrogen (BUN) levels may also become elevated, particularly during periods of water deprivation. Proteinuria may occur as a result of changes in glomerular structure.

In summary, diseases of the glomerulus disrupt glomerular filtration and alter the permeability of glomerular capillary membrane to plasma proteins and blood cells. *Glomerulonephritis* is a term used to describe a group of diseases that cause inflammation and injury of the glomerulus. These diseases disrupt the capillary membrane and cause proteinuria, hematuria, pyuria, oliguria, edema, hypertension, and azotemia. Almost all, if not all, types of glomerulonephritis are due to immune mechanisms. Chronic glomerulonephritis represents the end-stage of the many types of glomerulonephritis and is characterized by an insidious onset of renal failure. Glomerulosclerosis is a major complication of diabetes mellitus and hypertension.

Tubulointerstitial disorders

A number of disorders affect renal tubular structures, including the proximal and distal tubules. Most also affect the interstitial tissue surrounding the tubules, and thus the disorders are often called *tubulointerstitial diseases*. These disorders include acute tubular necrosis (see Chapter 32), renal tubular acidosis, pyelonephritis, renal cystic disease, and the effects of drugs and toxins.

Tubulointerstitial renal diseases may be divided into acute and chronic disorders. The acute disorders are characterized by their sudden onset and by signs of interstitial edema; they include acute pyelonephritis and acute hypersensitivity reaction to drugs. The chronic disorders produce interstitial fibrosis, atrophy, and mononuclear infiltrates; persons are often asymptomatic until late in the course of the disease. In the early stages, tubulointerstitial diseases are commonly manifested by fluid and electrolyte disorders that reflect subtle changes in tubular function. These manifestations can include inability to concentrate the urine, as evidenced by polyuria and nocturia; interference with acidification of the urine resulting in metabolic acidosis; and diminished tubular reabsorption of sodium and other substances. [27]

Renal tubular acidosis

Renal tubular acidosis refers to a group of tubular disorders that result in acidosis and its subsequent complications, including metabolic bone disease, kidney stones, and growth failure in children. There are two main types of renal tubular acidosis: proximal tubular disorders that affect bicarbonate reabsorption and distal tubular defects that affect the secretion of fixed metabolic acids. [28,29]

The proximal tubule is the site where 90% to 95% of the filtered bicarbonate is reabsorbed. With the onset of impaired tubular bicarbonate absorption, there is a loss of bicarbonate in the urine that reduces plasma bicarbonate levels. There is a concomitant loss of sodium in the urine that accompanies the bicarbonate loss; this leads to contraction of the extracellular fluid volume with increased aldosterone secretion and a resultant decrease in serum potassium levels (see Chapter 27). With proximal tubular defects in acid–base regulation, the distal tubular sites for secretion of the fixed acids into the urine continue to function and eventually the reabsorption of bicarbonate by the proximal cells resumes, albeit at a lower level of serum bicarbonate. Whenever serum levels rise above this decreased level, bicarbonate is lost in the urine. The proximal tubular defect in bicarbonate reabsorption can extend to other substances, such as glucose, amino acids, and phosphate. Defects in calcium and phosphate reabsorption may accentuate bicarbonate losses.

Distal tubular acidosis involves a defect in the secretion of fixed acids that leads to failure to acidify the urine. The secretion of hydrogen ions in the distal tubules is linked to sodium reabsorption; failure to secrete hydrogen ions results in a loss of sodium bicarbonate in the urine. The extracellular fluid volume compartment contracts, aldosterone production increases, and hypokalemia develops. The persistent acidosis causes calcium to be released from bone to buffer the excess hydrogen ions. Increased losses of calcium in the urine lead to increased levels of parathyroid hormone, resorption of bone, bone pain, and development of kidney stones.

The treatment of renal tubular acidosis depends on the defect and may require administration of bicarbonate and potassium. The selective use of diuretics may also be indicated.

Renal cystic disease

A renal cyst is a fluid-filled sac or segment of a dilated nephron. Renal cystic disease may be inherited or acquired and the cysts may be single or multiple and can vary in size from microscopic to several centimeters in diameter. Renal cystic disease is thought to result from tubular obstructions that increase intratubular pressure or from changes in the basement membrane of the renal tubules that predispose to cystic dilatation. Once the cyst begins to form, continued fluid accumulation contributes to its persistent growth. Renal cystic diseases probably exert their effects by compressing renal blood vessels, producing degeneration of functional renal tissue and obstructing tubular flow.

There are essentially four types of renal cystic disease: Polycystic kidney disease, medullary sponge kidney, acquired cystic disease, and single or multiple kidney cysts. [30] Polycystic disease develops as an inherited trait. Medullary sponge kidney is a congenital lesion affecting the distal and collecting ducts. Medullary sponge kidney does not cause progressive renal failure; it does, however, produce stasis of urine and predisposes to kidney infections and nephrolithiasis. Acquired renal cystic disease occurs in persons with advanced renal failure and is caused by degenerative changes in the kidney. Simple cysts are the most common cystic disease of the kidney. These can be single or multiple, unilateral or bilateral, and are usually less than 1 cm in diameter although they may grow larger. Most simple cysts do not produce symptoms, and they do not compromise renal function. When they are symptomatic they may cause flank pain, hematuria, urinary tract infection, and hypertension related to ischemia-produced stimulation of the renin-angiotensin system. They are most commonly seen in older people.

Polycystic kidney disease. The most common form of renal cystic disease is polycystic kidney disease that develops as a hereditary trait. There are two types of polycystic disease: autosomal recessive and autosomal dominant. Autosomal recessive polycystic disease is relatively rare; often the condition is present at birth, hence it was formerly called infantile polycystic disease. Significant renal dysfunction is usually present, accompanied by variable degrees of liver fibrosis and portal hypertension. The disorder can be diagnosed by ultrasonography. There is no known treatment for the disease and death usually occurs in infancy. Some children may present with less severe kidney problems and more severe liver disease. The disorder is transmitted as a recessive trait, meaning that there is a one in four chance of the parents having another child with the disorder.

Autosomal dominant polycystic kidney disease is relatively common: it is estimated to affect one in every 400 persons[1] and accounts for 10% of persons in the United States with end-stage renal disease. The disorder is transmitted as a dominant trait, which means there is a 50% chance of children of an affected parent developing the disorder. Recently, it has been found that the mutant gene responsible for the defect is located on the short arm of chromosome 16. There is a high degree of penetrance for the defect; persons who inherit the gene are likely to develop the disorder. However, there is considerable variability in gene expression, so that many affected persons do not develop clinical symptoms, or if they do, the symptoms occur very late in life.

The kidneys of persons with polycystic disease eventually become enlarged because of the presence of multiple cysts. Cysts may also be found in the liver and, less commonly, in the pancreas and spleen. Additionally, there may be a weakness in the walls of the cerebral arteries that can lead to aneurysm formation. Subarachnoid hemorrhage occurs in about 10% of persons with polycystic kidney disease.[5]

The manifestations of polycystic kidney disease include flank pain, vague abdominal pain from the enlarged cysts, episodes of gross hematuria from bleeding into a cyst, infected cysts from ascending urinary tract infection, and hypertension resulting from compression of intrarenal blood vessels with activation of the renin-angiotensin mechanism. Persons with polycystic kidney disease are also at risk for development of renal cell carcinoma. The progress of the disease is slow, and end-stage renal failure is uncommon before the age of 40.

The diagnosis of autosomal polycystic kidney disease can be made by radiologic studies such as the intravenous pyelogram or ultrasonography or CT scans. Ultrasound and CT scans have largely replaced intravenous pyelography because they are better able to detect small cysts. Ultrasound is particularly useful as a screening test for the disease. It is currently recommended that first-degree relatives of affected persons be screened for polycystic disease if they are at least 20 years of age. The sensitivity of ultrasonography in this age group is about 95%; before that age, false negatives may occur because the cysts are too small to detect.[30]

The treatment of polycystic kidney disease is largely supportive. Control of hypertension and prevention of ascending urinary tract infection is important. Dialysis and renal transplantation are used for those persons who progress to end-stage renal disease.

Pyelonephritis

Pyelonephritis refers to an infection of the kidneys and renal pelvis. In its earliest stages it is characterized by inflammatory foci that are interspersed throughout the renal interstitium. Small abscesses may form on the surface of the kidney. In time the lesions are replaced by scar tissue. There are two forms of pyelonephritis: acute and chronic. Because pyelonephritis affects the tubules and interstitium of the kidneys, it is classified as a tubulointerstitial kidney disease.

Acute pyelonephritis represents an acute suppurative inflammation of renal tubulointerstitial tissues caused by bacterial infection. Infection may occur through the bloodstream or ascent from the bladder. Factors that contribute to the development of acute pyelonephritis are catheterization and urinary tract instrumentation, vesicoureteral reflux, pregnancy, increased susceptibility to infection, and neurogenic bladder.

The onset of acute pyelonephritis is usually abrupt, with chills and fever, headache, back pain, tenderness over the costovertebral angle, and general malaise. It is usually accompanied by signs of bladder irritation, such as dysuria, frequency, and urgency. Pyuria occurs, but is not diagnostic because it also occurs in lower urinary tract infections. It is now possible to determine whether an infection involves the upper or lower urinary tract through detection of the antibody coating on the bacteria. Antibody coating is an immune response that occurs in the kidney during upper urinary tract infections and is easily detected by the immunofluorescence test. Also, the finding of leukocyte casts in the urine indicates that the infection is in the kidney rather than the lower urinary tract.

Acute pyelonephritis is treated with appropriate antimicrobial drugs. Unless obstruction or other complications are present, the symptoms usually disappear within several days. Hospitalization during initial treatment may be necessary. Depending on the cause, recurrent infections are possible.

Chronic pyelonephritis is both chronic and progressive. There is scarring and deformation of the renal calyces and pelvis. The disorder appears to involve a bacterial infection superimposed on obstructive abnormalities or the vesicoureteral reflux. Although the mechanisms by which the urinary obstruction interacts to produce kidney damage in chronic pyelonephritis are unknown, recent observations suggest some component of the urine may serve as an antigenic determinant to induce an immune response. One of the suspected urine components is the Tamm-Horsfall proteins, which are synthesized in the tubular epithelial cells of the thick ascending loop of Henle and the distal convoluted tubules.[31]

Chronic pyelonephritis may cause many of the same symptoms as acute pyelonephritis, or its onset may be insidious. Loss of tubular function and ability to concentrate urine gives rise to polyuria and nocturia, and mild proteinuria is common. Severe hypertension is often a contributing factor in the progress of the disease. Chronic pyelonephritis is a significant cause of renal failure. It is thought to be responsible for 25% of all cases of renal insufficiency and end-stage renal disease.

Drug-related nephritis

Drug-related nephropathies involve functional or structural changes in the kidney that occur following exposure to a drug. The kidney is exposed to a high rate of delivery of any substance in the blood because of its large blood flow and high filtration pressure. The kidney is also very active in the metabolic transformation of drugs and is therefore exposed to a number of toxic metabolites. Some drugs and toxic substances damage the kidneys by causing a decrease in blood flow, others directly damage tubulointerstitial structures, and still others cause damage by producing hypersensitivity reactions. The tolerance to drugs varies with age and depends on renal function, state of hydration, blood pressure, and the pH of the urine. Because of a decrease in physiologic function, the elderly are particularly susceptible to renal damage due to drugs and toxins. The dangers of nephrotoxicity are increased when two or more drugs capable of producing renal damage are given at the same time.

Acute drug-related hypersensitivity reactions produce tubulointerstitial nephritis, with damage to the tubules and interstitium. It was initially observed in persons who were sensitive to the sulfonamide drugs; currently, it is more often observed to result from use of methicillin and other synthetic antibiotics, as well as furosemide and the thiazide diuretics, by persons who are sensitive to these drugs. The condition begins about 15 days after exposure to the drug (the period may vary from 2 to 40 days).[5] At the onset there is fever, eosinophilia, hematuria, mild proteinuria, and in about one-fourth of the cases a rash. In about 50% of cases oliguria and signs of acute renal failure develop. Withdrawal of the drug is usually followed by complete recovery, but there may be permanent damage in some cases, usually in older persons. Drug nephritis may not be recognized in its very early stage because it is uncommon.

Chronic analgesic nephritis, which is seen in association with analgesic abuse, causes interstitial nephritis with renal papillary necrosis.[5] When first observed, it was attributed to phenacetin, a then-common ingredient of over-the-counter medications containing aspirin, phenacetin, and caffeine. Although phenacetin is no longer contained in these preparations, it has been suggested that other ingredients, such as aspirin and acetaminophen, may also contribute to the disorder. How much analgesic it takes to produce papillary necrosis is not known; ingestion of 2 kg to 30 kg of these analgesic compounds over a period of years has been known to result in papillary necrosis.[5] Headache, anemia, gastrointestinal tract symptoms, and hypertension are associated with the condition.

In summary, tubulointerstitial diseases affect both the tubules and the surrounding interstitium of the kidneys. These disorders include renal tubular acidosis, chronic pyelonephritis, renal cystic disease, and the effects of drugs and toxins. Renal tubular acidosis describes a form of systemic acidosis that results from tubular defects in bicarbonate reabsorption or hydrogen ion secretion. Renal cystic disease is a condition in which there is dilatation of tubular structures to form a cyst. Cysts may be single or multiple. Polycystic kidney disease is an inherited form of renal cystic disease; it can be inherited as a recessive or autosomal trait. Recessive polycystic kidney disease is rare and usually presents as severe renal dysfunction during infancy. Autosomal dominant polycystic disease does not usually become symptomatic until later in life, often after 40 years of age. Pyelonephritis can occur as an acute or chronic condition. Acute pyelonephritis is usually caused by ascending bladder infections or infections that come from the bloodstream; it is usually successfully treated with appropriate antimicrobial drugs. Chronic pyelonephritis is a progressive disease that produces scarring and deformation of the kidney calyces and pelvis. Drug-induced impairment of tubulointerstitial structure and function is usually the result of hypersensitivity reactions.

Neoplasms

There are two major groups of renal neoplasms: embryonic kidney tumors (Wilms' tumor) that occur during childhood and adult kidney cancers.

Adult kidney cancers

Adult kidney cancer accounts for 2% of all cancers. An estimated 18,100 new cases of kidney cancer are diagnosed each year, and approximately 8,300 persons die annually from this type of cancer.[32] The availability of computed tomography (CT) scanning has contributed significantly to earlier diagnosis and more accurate staging of renal cancers.

Renal cell carcinoma (hypernephroma) accounts for approximately 85% of kidney tumors, with transitional or squamous cell cancers of the renal pelvis accounting for most of the remaining cancers. The etiology of hypernephroma remains unclear. It occurs most often in older individuals in the 6th or 7th decade. Males are affected twice as frequently as women. It is thought that some of these tumors may occur as a result of chronic irritation associated with kidney stones. Epidemiologic evidence suggests a correlation between smoking and renal cancer.[32]

The manifestations of kidney cancer include hematuria, costovertebral pain, presence of a palpable mass, polycythemia, and fever. Hematuria, which occurs in 70% to 90% of cases, is the most reliable of these signs. It is, however, intermittent and may be microscopic; as a result, the tumor may reach considerable size before it is detected. In about one-third of the cases, metastases are present at the time of diagnosis.

Renal cancer is suspected when there are findings of hematuria and a renal mass. Renal ultrasonography, CT scanning, intravenous pyelograms, and renal arteriography are used to confirm the diagnosis. Surgery (radical nephrectomy with lymph node dissection) is the treatment of choice for all resectable tumors. Preoperative irradiation may be used. Single-agent and combination chemotherapy have been used with limited success. The 5-year survival rate for hypernephroma ranges from 30% to 50%.

—— Wilms' tumor (nephroblastoma)

Wilms' tumor is one of the most common malignant tumors in children; 75% of cases occur in children under 5 years of age.[32] Epithelial, muscle, and bone tissue are components of the tumor. The common presenting signs are a large abdominal mass and hypertension. Treatment involves surgery, chemotherapy, and radiotherapy (the tumor is radiosensitive). Two-year survival rates for children under 2 years of age have increased to about 73% with this aggressive plan of treatment. The survival rate for older children is less.[32]

In summary, there are two major groups of renal neoplasms: embryonic kidney tumors (Wilms' tumor) that occur during childhood and adult kidney cancers. Adult kidney cancers account for 2% of all cancers. The most common manifestations of kidney cancer is hematuria. Renal ultrasonography has contributed significantly to earlier diagnosis and more accurate staging of renal cancers.

Wilms' tumor is the most common malignant tumor of children. The most common presenting signs are a large abdominal mass and hypertension. The 2-year survival rate for children with Wilms' tumor is about 90% with an aggressive plan of treatment.

References

1. National Kidney Foundation: Facts about transplantation and kidney and urologic diseases. KF News, New York, National Kidney Foundation, 1988
2. Manning FA: Fetal surgery for obstructive uropathy: Rationale considerations. Am J Kidney Dis 10:259, 1987
3. Glassberg KI: Summary of the annual meeting of the section of pediatric urology. Pediatrics 81:588, 1988
4. Robbins SL, Cotran RS, Kumar V: Pathologic Basis of Disease 3rd ed, pp 998, 1020, 1023, 1046, 1036. Philadelphia, WB Saunders, 1984
5. Rose BD: Pathophysiology of Renal Disease, 2nd ed, pp 453, 451, 470, 407. New York, McGraw-Hill, 1987
6. Better OS, Arieff AI, Massry SG, et al: Studies on renal function after relief of complete unilateral obstruction of three months' duration in man. Am J Med 54:234, 1973
7. Abraham PA, Smith CL: Medical evaluation and management of calcium nephrolithiasis. Med Clin North Am 68:281, 1984
8. Rotolo JE, O'Brien WM, Pahira JJ: Urinary Tract Calculi: Three new procedures to replace open surgery. Consultant 28(3):110, 1988
9. Jocham K, Chaussy C, Schmiedt E: Extracorporeal shock wave lithotripsy. Urol Int 41:357, 1987
10. Ludy JP: Urologic sepsis. Urol Clin N Am 9:259, 1982
11. Androle VT: Urinary tract infections: Recent developments. J Infect Dis 156:865, 1987
12. Kunin CM. Genitourinary infections in the patient at risk: Extrinsic risk factors. Am J Med 76:141, 1984
13. Lindberg U, Bjure J, Haugstvedt S, et al: Asymptomatic bacteriuria in schoolgirls: III. Relation between residual urine volume and recurrence. Acta Paediatr Scan 64:437, 1975
14. Spencer JR, Schaeffer AJ: Pediatric urinary tract infections. Urol Clin N Am 13:661, 1986
15. Hodson J, Kincaid-Smith P: Reflux Nephrology, p 3. New York, Masson Publishing, 1979
16. Buckley RM, McGuckin M, MacGreagor RR: Urine bacterial counts after sexual intercourse. N Engl J Med 298:321, 1978
17. Krieger JN. Complications and treatment of urinary tract infections during pregnancy. Urol Clin North Am 13:685, 1986
18. Kunin CM: An overview of urinary tract infections. In Kunin CM: Detection, Prevention, and Management of Urinary Tract Infections, 3rd ed, pp 41, 99, 157. Philadelphia, Lea & Febiger, 1979
19. Zweig S: Urinary tract infections in the elderly. Am Family Pract 35(5):123, 1987
20. Centers for Disease Control: Epidemics of nosocomial urinary tract infections caused by multiply resistant

gram-negative bacilli: Epidemiology and control. J Infect Dis 133:363, 1976

21. Jones SR, Smith JW, Sanford JP: Localization of urinary tract infections caused by detection of antibody-coated bacteria in urine sediment. N Engl J Med 290:591, 1974

22. Stam WE, Turck M: Urinary tract infection. Adv Intern Med 24:141, 1983

23. Glassock RJ: Pathology of acute glomerulonephritis. Hosp Pract 23(2):163, 1988

24. Wilson CB, Dixon FJ: The renal response to immunologic injury. In Brenner BM, Rector FC, Jr(eds): The Kidney, 3rd ed, pp 800-805. Philadelphia, WB Saunders, 1986

25. Micheal AF: Immunologic mechanisms in immune complex disease. Kidney Int 28:569, 1985

26. Cameron JS: The nephrotic syndrome and its complications. Am J Kidney Dis 10:163, 1987

27. Cotran R: Tubulointerstitial nephropathies. Hosp Pract 1:79, 1982

28. Davidman M, Schmitz P: Renal tubular acidosis: A pathophysiologic approach. Hosp Pract 23(1):77, 1988

29. Kurtzman NA: Renal tubular acidosis: A constellation of syndromes. Hosp Pract 22(11):173, 1987

30. Thompson C: The spectrum of renal cystic diseases. Hosp Pract 23(4):165, 1988

31. Andriole VT: The role of Tamm-Horsfall protein in the pathogenesis of reflux nephropathy and chronic pyelonephritis. Yale J Biol Med 58:91, 1985

32. Frank I, Keys M, McCure CS: Urological and male genital cancers. In Rubin P (ed): Clinical Oncology, 6th ed, p 198. New York, American Cancer Society, 1983

Bibliography

Anderson RU: Urinary tract infections in the compromised host. Urol Clin North Am 13:727, 1986

Bahnson RR: Urosepsis. Urol Clin North Am 13:627, 1986

Bauchner H, Phillip B, Dashefsky B, et al: Prevalence of bacteriuria in febrile children. Ped Infect Dis J 6:239, 1987

Benson M, LiPuma JP, Resnick MI: The role of imaging studies in urinary tract infections. Urol Clin North Am 13:605, 1986

Bonventre JV: Mediators of ischemic renal injury. Annu Rev Med 39:531, 1988

Burgener S: Justification of closed intermittent urinary catheter irrigation/instillation: A review of current research and practice. J Adv Nurs 12:229, 1987

Burns MW, Burns JL, Krieger JN: Pediatric urinary tract infection. Pediatr Clin North Am 34:1111, 1987

Clarkson AR, Woodroffe AJ, Aarons I, et al: IgA nephropathy. Annu Rev Med 38:157, 1987

Coe FL, Parks JH: Pathophysiology of kidney stones and strategies for treatment. Hosp Pract 23(3):185, 1988

Couser WG: Rapidly progressive glomerulonephritis: Classification, pathogenesis, mechanisms, and therapy. Am J Kid Dis 11:449, 1988

Couser WG, Abrass CK: Pathogenesis of membranous nephropathy. Annu Rev Med 39:517, 1988

Cullpepper RM, Andreoli TE: The pathophysiology of the glomerulonephropathies. Annu Rev Med 34:161, 1983

Davison JM: Overview: Kidney function in pregnant women. Am J Kidney Dis 14:248, 1987

Fowler JE: Urinary tract infections in women. Urol Clin North Am 13:673, 1986

Gardner KD: Pathogenesis of human cystic renal disease. Annu Rev Med 39:185, 1988

Gibson TP: Renal disease and drug metabolism: An overview. Am J Kid Dis 13:7, 1986

Hanno P: Therapeutic principles of antimicrobial therapy and new antimicrobial agents. Urol Clin North Am 13:577, 1986

Kafetz K: Renal impairment in the elderly: A review. J Royal Soc Med 76:398, 1983

Komaroff AL: Acute dysuria in women. N Engl J Med 310:368, 1984

Larsen EH, Gasser TC, Madsen PO: Antimicrobial prophylaxis in urologic surgery. Urol Clin North Am 13:591, 1986

Leibovivi L, Alpert G, Loar A, et al: Urinary infections and sexual activity in young women. Arch Intern Med 147:345, 1987

Levey AS, Perrone RD, Madias NE: Serum creatinine and renal function. Annu Rev Med 39:465, 1988

Madaio MP, Harrington JT: The diagnosis of acute glomerulonephritis. N Engl J Med 309:1299, 1983

Mannhardt W, Schofer O, Schulte-Wissermann H: Pathogenic factors in recurrent urinary tract infections and renal scar formation in children. Eur J Pediatr 145:330, 1986

Mauer SM, Steffes MW, Brown DM: The kidney in diabetes. Am J Med 70:603, 1981

Mayrer AR, Winter P, Andriole VT: Immunopathogenesis of chronic pyelonephritis. Am J Med 72(7):59, 1983

Mulley AG: Management of nephrolithiasis. Annu Rev Med 39:347, 1988

Pagna KD: The intrigue and challenge of Goodpasture's syndrome. Heart Lung 9:699, 1980

Parsons CL: Pathogenesis of urinary tract infections. Urol Clin N Amer 13:563, 1986

Pirson Y, de Strihou CVY: renal effects of nonsteroidal antiinflammatory drugs: Clinical relevance. Am J Kid Dis 8:338, 1986

Platt R: Quantitative definition of bacteriuria. Am J Med 72(7):44, 1983

Platt R, Polk F, Murdock B: Risk factors for nosocomial urinary tract infections. Am J Epidemiol 124:977, 1987

Reidsenber MM: Kidney function and drug action. N Engl J Med 313:816, 1985

Remis RS, Gurwith MJ, Gurwith D, et al: Risk factors for urinary tract infections. Am J Epidemiol 126:685, 1987

Roberts JA: Pyelonephritic, cortical abscess, and perinephric abscess. Urol Clin North Am 13:637, 1986

Robertson WG: Pathophysiology of stone formation. Urol Int 41:329, 1986

Ruge C: Shock(wave) treatment for kidney stones. Am J Nurs 86:400, 1986

Ronald AR: Current concepts in the management of urinary tract infections in adults. Med Clin North Am 68(2):335, 1984

Schaeffer AJ: Catheter-associated bacteriuria. Urol Clin North Am 13:735, 1986

Schmucki A, Asper R: Clinical significance of stone analysis. Urol Int 41:343, 1986

Shortliffe LMD, Spiegelman SS: Infections stone. Urol Clin North Am 13:717, 1986

Skiar AH, Caruana RJ, Lammers JE: Renal infections in autosomal dominant polycystic disease. Am J Kid Dis 10:81, 1987

Spencer J, Schaeffer AJ: Pediatric Urinary tract infections. Urol Clin North Am 13:661, 1986

Stamm WE: Measurement of pyuria and its relation to bacteriuria. Am J Med 72(7):53, 1983

Stamm WE, Turck M: Urinary tract infections. Adv Intern Med 28:141, 1983

Stillman MT, Napier J, Blackshear JL: Adverse effects of nonsteroidal drugs on the kidney. Med Clin North Am 68:371, 1984

Uehling DT: Future approaches to management of urinary tract infections. Urol Clin North Am 13:749, 1986

Ulshofer B: Clinical aspects of stone formation and conservative treatment. Urol Int 41:348, 1986

White RHR: Management of urinary tract infections. Arch Dis Child 62:421, 1987

Renal Failure

Acute renal failure
  Causes of acute renal failure
    Prerenal conditions
    Intrarenal conditions
    Postrenal conditions
  Clinical manifestations
    Oliguric phase
    Diuretic phase
  Treatment

Chronic renal failure
  Clinical manifestations
    Alterations in fluids and
      electrolytes
    Hematologic abnormalities
    Cardiovascular problems
    Gastrointestinal disturbances
    Neurological disorders
    Osteodystrophy
    Skin disorders
    Altered sexual functioning

Effect of renal failure on
  elimination of drugs
Treatment
  Dialysis and renal
    transplantation
  Dietary management
  Exercise

Objectives

After you have studied this chapter, you should be able to meet the following objectives:

_____ Differentiate between acute and chronic renal failure in terms of onset, etiology, and outcome.

_____ Classify the following conditions as prerenal, intrarenal, or postrenal: acute glomerulonephritis, prostatic hypertrophy, hemorrhage, septicemia, hemolytic reaction.

_____ Describe the clinical manifestations of the oliguric and diuretic phases of acute renal failure.

_____ State the reason for the isosthenuria-polyuria that occur in chronic renal failure.

_____ Compare the renal dysfunction that occurs with renal impairment, renal insufficiency, and end-stage renal disease.

_____ Compare the clinical manifestations of azotemia and uremia.

_____ Describe the alterations in serum sodium, serum phosphate, and potassium regulation that occur in chronic renal failure.

_____ Explain the relationship between end-stage renal disease and the presence of anemia and bleeding disorders.

_____ Describe the alterations in cardiovascular function that occur in end-stage renal disease.

_____ List the gastrointestinal disturbances that occur in end-stage renal disease.

_____ State the possible rationale for neurologic manifestations that occur in end-stage renal disease.

_____ Define the term *osteodystrophy* and relate it to the altered calcium and phosphate balance that occurs in end-stage renal disease.

_____ List the skin disorders that develop in persons with end-stage renal disease.

_____ State the possible alterations in sexual function that occur in end-stage renal disease.

_____ State the basis for adverse drug reactions in persons with end-stage renal disease.

_____ Describe the scientific principles underlying dialysis treatment.

_____ Compare the procedure of hemodialysis with peritoneal dialysis.

_____ Cite the complications of renal transplantation.

_____ State the goals for dietary management of persons with end-stage renal disease as they relate to protein restrictions; carbohydrate, fat, and caloric needs; and potassium, sodium, and fluid intake.

Renal failure is a condition in which the kidneys fail to remove metabolic end-products from the blood and regulate the fluid, electrolyte, and pH balance of the extracellular fluids. The underlying cause may be renal pathology, systemic disease, or urologic defects of nonrenal origin. Renal failure can occur as an acute or chronic disorder. Acute renal failure is abrupt in onset and is often reversible if recognized early and treated appropriately. By contrast, chronic renal failure is the end result of irreparable damage to kidneys. It develops slowly, usually over the course of a number of years.

The term *azotemia* refers to an abnormally high level of nitrogenous wastes (urea nitrogen, uric acid, and creatinine) in the blood. Its presence reflects the inability of the kidneys to filter these waste products from the blood. Azotemia is present in both acute and chronic renal failure. The normal concentrations of urea in the plasma is approximately 26 mg/100 ml. In renal failure this level may rise to as high as 800 mg/100 dl.[1]

Acute renal failure

Acute renal failure refers to an acute suppression of renal function. The true incidence of acute renal failure is unknown, but it is thought to affect at least 10,000 persons annually in the United States.[2] The mortality is, unfortunately, about 60%. This is probably because older persons and those with severe illness and trauma are being kept alive by respirators and other extraordinary means until renal failure supervenes.

Causes of acute renal failure

The conditions responsible for acute renal failure are usually described as prerenal, intrarenal, and postrenal (Chart 32-1). This classification aids in identifying and treating the cause of the disorder.

Prerenal conditions

Prerenal causes of acute renal failure consist of those conditions that impair renal blood flow. This is the most common form of acute renal failure and is considered to be reversible if the basis of renal hypofunction can be identified and corrected within 24 hours.

The kidneys normally filter about 20% to 25% of the cardiac output. With a loss of blood volume or in cardiac failure, this large blood flow to the kidneys may be sharply reduced. When the afferent arterial pressure falls much below 60 mmHg to 70 mmHg, glomerular filtration ceases, and little or no

---

Chart 32-1: Causes of acute renal failure

Prerenal
Hypovolemia
  Dehydration
  Loss of gastrointestinal tract fluid
  Hemorrhage
  Fluid sequestration (*e.g.*, burns)
Septicemia
  Septic shock
Heart failure
Interruption of renal blood flow due to surgery and other causes

Intrarenal
Prolonged renal ischemia
Exposure to nephrotoxic agents
  Aminoglycosides (*e.g.*, gentamicin, kanamycin, colistin)
  Heavy metals (*e.g.*, lead, mercury)
  Organic solvents (*e.g.*, carbon tetrachloride, ethylene glycol)
  Radiopaque contrast media
  Sulfonamides
Acute glomerulonephritis
Intratubular obstruction
  Uric acid crystals
  Hemolytic reactions (*e.g.*, blood transfusion reactions)
  Precipitated proteins resulting from multiple myelomas
  Rhabdomyolysis
Acute inflammatory conditions
  Acute pyelonephritis
  Necrotizing papillitis

Postrenal
Ureteral obstruction (*e.g.*, calculi, tumors)
Bladder outlet obstruction (*e.g.*, prostatic hyperplasia, urethral strictures)

---

urine is formed. Thus, one of the early manifestations of prerenal failure is a sharp decrease in urine output. Normally, the ratio of serum BUN to creatinine is about 20 to 1, but in acute renal failure, there is a disproportionate elevation in BUN compared with serum creatinine. This is because the low glomerular filtration rate allows more time for smaller particles, such as urea, to filter back into the blood. Creatinine, being larger and nondiffusible, remains in the tubular fluid, and the total amount of creatinine that is filtered, although small, is excreted in the urine.

Intrarenal conditions

Intrarenal causes of acute renal failure can be grouped into five categories: ischemia, injury to the glomerular membrane (acute glomerulonephritis), acute tubular necrosis, intratubular obstruction, and acute pyelonephritis and necrotizing papillitis. Acute glomerulonephritis is discussed in Chapter 31, as is pyelonephritis.

Intratubular obstructions are caused by the accumulation of casts and cellular debris that accompanies severe hemolytic reactions or myoglobinuria. Skeletal and cardiac muscles contain myoglobin, which accounts for their rubiginous color. Myoglobin corresponds to hemoglobin in function, serving as an oxygen reservoir within the muscle fibers. Myoglobin is not normally found in the serum or urine. It has a low molecular weight of 17,000; should it escape into the circulation, it is rapidly filtered in the glomerulus. Myoglobinuria is most commonly due to muscle trauma but may result from extreme exertion, hyperthermia, sepsis, prolonged seizures, potassium or phosphate depletion, and alcoholism or drug abuse. Hemoglobin may also escape into the glomerular filtrate when serum levels are markedly increased as a result of a severe hemolytic reaction. Both myoglobin and hemoglobin cause discoloration of the urine, ranging from the color of tea to red, brown, or black.

Acute tubular necrosis is characterized by destructive changes in the tubular epithelium due to ischemia or exposure to nephrotoxic agents. Shock and heart failure, to name two such events, cause prerenal failure, tend to cause renal ischemia, and if allowed to progress, can produce tubular necrosis. As a rule, the blood supply to a normal kidney can be interrupted for about 30 minutes without damage on the kidney,[3] but in acute trauma, sepsis, and heart failure, for example, the interruption in blood flow is often both more severe and longer in duration.

Several drugs and other chemicals, including organic solvents and heavy metals, such as lead and mercury, can injure the renal tubular structures. The aminoglycosides, a group of antibiotics of which gentamicin, kanamycin, and colistin are examples, are all capable of impairing renal function. Several factors contribute to aminoglycoside toxicity, including a decrease in the glomerular filtration rate, which often occurs in the elderly, a preexisting renal disease, hypovolemia, and concurrent administration of other drugs that have a nephrotoxic effect. Contrast media used during cardiac catheterization and intravenous cholangiography, for example, may also be nephrotoxic. The risk of renal damage due to radiopaque contrast media is greatest in elderly persons, in persons with diabetes mellitus, and in persons who for one reason or another are susceptible to kidney disease.

Postrenal conditions

Obstruction of the urinary system at any point from the renal calyces to the urinary meatus is the cause of postrenal failure. Prostatic hyperplasia is the most common underlying problem. Postrenal failure can also be caused by ureteral obstruction in persons who have only one functioning kidney. Obstructive uropathy is responsible for about 10% of cases of acute renal failure.[4]

Clinical manifestations

The manifestations of acute renal failure are frequently superimposed on the signs and symptoms of the condition that caused the kidney failure—heart failure, shock, prostatic hyperplasia, and others. Because acute renal failure is potentially reversible, it is important that early signs be recognized so that appropriate treatment measures can be instituted promptly.

Acute renal failure causes marked impairment in the elimination of nitrogenous wastes, water, and electrolytes. Its course is frequently divided into two phases: the oliguric and the diuretic phase.

Oliguric phase

During the oliguric phase, urine output is greatly reduced. The magnitude of the azotemia that develops depends largely on urine output and on the degree of protein breakdown that is taking place. Although oliguria is usually associated with acute renal failure, there are circumstances in which urine output will be nearly normal, such as when intrarenal dysfunction impairs the ability of the renal tubular structures to concentrate the urine. In severe oliguria, which is accompanied by tissue breakdown, the BUN, creatinine, potassium, and phosphate serum levels increase rapidly, and metabolic acidosis develops. Fluid retention gives rise to edema, water intoxication, and pulmonary congestion. If the period of oliguria is prolonged, hypertension frequently develops and, with it, signs of uremia. When untreated, uremia's neurologic manifestations progress from neuromuscular irritability to convulsions, somnolence, and finally, coma and death. Hyperkalemia is usually asymptomatic until serum levels of potassium rise above 6.0 to 6.5 mEq/liter, at which point characteristic electrocardiographic changes and signs of muscle weakness are seen. Gastrointestinal bleeding and infection are serious complications of acute renal failure.

Diuretic phase

The diuretic phase of acute renal failure usually begins within a few days to 6 weeks after oliguria, indicating that the nephrons have recovered to the point where urine excretion is possible. Diuresis usually occurs before renal function has returned to normal. Consequently, BUN, serum creatinine, potassium, and phosphate may remain elevated or continue to rise even though urine output is increased. In some cases, the diuresis may be due to impaired nephron function and may cause excessive loss of water and electrolytes.

Treatment

A major concern in the treatment of acute renal failure is identifying and correcting the cause by improving renal perfusion or discontinuing nephrotoxic drugs. Fluids are carefully regulated in an effort to maintain normal fluid volume and electrolyte concentrations. Adequate caloric intake is needed to prevent the breakdown of body proteins, which increases nitrogenous wastes. Parenteral hyperalimentation may be used for this purpose. Because secondary infections are a major cause of death in persons with acute renal failure, constant vigilance is needed to detect and prevent such infection. Dialysis may be indicated when nitrogenous wastes and water and electrolyte balance cannot be kept under control by other means.

In summary, acute renal failure is an acute reversible suppression of kidney function. It is generally classified as prerenal, intrarenal, or postrenal in origin. Typically, it progresses through an oliguric phase during which urine output is markedly diminished and fluid and end-products of metabolism accumulate. During the second phase, that of diuresis, urine output increases as renal function begins to return. Usually, correction of the azotemia follows diuresis.

Chronic renal failure

Chronic renal failure represents progressive destruction of kidney structures. Unlike acute renal failure, chronic renal failure is not reversible. As recently as 20 years ago, many persons with chronic renal failure progressed to the final stages of the disease and then died. The high mortality rate was associated not only with the limitations in the treatment of renal disease but with the tremendous cost of on-going treatment. In 1972, federal support for dialysis and transplantation through a Medicare entitlement program began. Continued improvements in dialysis therapy and transplantation have improved the outcomes for persons with renal disease.

Chronic renal failure can result from most of the renal diseases discussed in Chapter 31. Regardless of the cause, chronic renal failure causes progressive deterioration of glomerular filtration, tubular reabsorption, and endocrine functions of the kidneys. All forms of renal failure are characterized by a marked reduction in glomerular filtration rate. The rate of destruction differs from case to case, ranging from several months to many years. The progression of chronic renal failure usually occurs in three stages: renal impairment, renal insufficiency, and end-stage renal failure.[5]

Renal impairment occurs when the glomerular filtration rate falls to 40% to 50% of normal. Signs of renal failure do not begin to appear until over half of the function in both kidneys is lost. This is supported by the fact that many persons survive an entire lifetime with only one kidney. Initially, the kidneys have tremendous adaptive capabilities. As nephrons are destroyed, the remaining nephrons undergo changes to compensate for those that are lost. In the process, each of the remaining nephrons must filter more solute particles from the blood. Because the solute particles are osmotically active, they cause additional water to be lost in the urine. One of the earliest signs of renal failure is *isosthenuria*—polyuria which is almost isotonic with plasma.

Renal insufficiency represents a reduction in the glomerular filtration rate to 20% to 40% of normal. During this stage, azotemia and mild anemia are present. Conservative treatment includes measures to retard deterioration of renal function and assist the body in managing the effects of impaired function. Since in this condition the kidneys have difficulty in eliminating the waste products of protein metabolism, persons on a restricted-protein diet usually have fewer uremic symptoms and a slower progression of renal failure.[6] However, the few remaining nephrons that constitute the functional reserve of the kidneys can be easily disrupted; and at that point, renal failure will progress rapidly.

End-stage renal failure develops when the glomerular filtration rate drops to about 10% to 15% of normal. Histologic findings of an *end-stage* kidney include a reduction in capillaries and scarring in the glomeruli. Atrophy and fibrosis are evident in the tubules. The mass of the kidneys is usually reduced.[6] At this final phase of renal failure, treatment with either dialysis or transplantation is necessary for survival.

Clinical manifestations

Uremia, which literally means "urine in the blood," is the term used to describe the clinical manifestations of end-stage renal disease. Few symptoms of uremia appear until at least two-thirds of the nephrons have been destroyed.[7] Uremia differs from azotemia, which merely indicates the accumulation of nitrogenous wastes in the blood and can occur without symptoms. The uremic condition includes signs of altered fluid and electrolyte balance, alterations in regulatory functions (*e.g.,* hypertension, anemia, osteodystrophy), and accumulation of waste products (*e.g.,* uremic encephalopathy, neuropathy, pruritus). At this stage virtually every organ and structure in the body is affected. Initial symptoms of uremia may be subtle: weakness, fatigue, nausea, and apathy. More severe symptoms include extreme weakness, frequent vomiting, lethargy, and confusion. Without treatment, coma and death will follow.

The signs and symptoms of renal failure can be divided into (1) alterations in electrolyte and fluid balance resulting from impaired nephron function and (2) associated systemic alterations. These changes are summarized in Table 32-1.

Alterations in fluid and electrolytes

Either dehydration or fluid overload can be seen in chronic renal failure, depending on the pathology of the renal disease. In addition to these defects in volume regulation, the kidneys do not correctly filter the blood, reabsorb necessary electrolytes, or concentrate urine. When the glomerular filtration membrane is damaged, larger particles, such as plasma proteins and blood cells, enter the renal tubules and are excreted into the urine.

An early sign of impaired renal function is the inability of the kidneys to regulate the concentration of urine. In renal failure, the specific gravity of the urine becomes fixed (1.008–1.012) and varies little from voiding to voiding. Polyuria and nocturia are common.

The ability to regulate sodium excretion is reduced as renal function declines. Normally, the kidneys tolerate large variations in sodium intake (from 1

Table 32–1. Alterations in body function that occur with chronic renal failure

Body system	Change in function	Manifestation
Body fluids	Compensatory changes in tubular functions	Fixed specific gravity of urine; polyuria and nocturia
	Decreased ability to synthesize ammonia and conserve bicarbonate	Metabolic acidosis
	Inability to excrete potassium	Hyperkalemia
	Inability to regulate sodium excretion	Salt wasting or sodium retention
	Impaired ability to excrete phosphate	Hyperphosphatemia
	Hyperphosphatemia and inability to activate vitamin D	Hypocalcemia and increased levels of parathyroid hormone
Hematologic	Impaired synthesis of erythropoietin and effects of uremia	Anemia
	Impaired platelet function	Bleeding tendencies
Cardiovascular	Activation of renin–angiotensin mechanism, increased vascular volume, and failure to produce vasopressor substances	Hypertension
	Fluid retention and hypoalbuminemia	Edema
	Excess extracellular fluid volume, anemia	Congestive heart failure; pulmonary edema
	Elevated BUN	Uremic pericarditis
Gastrointestinal	Liberation of ammonia	Anorexia, nausea, vomiting
	Decreased platelet function and increased gastric acid secretion due to hyperparathyroidism	Gastrointestinal bleeding
Neurologic	Fluid and electrolyte imbalance	Headache
	Increase in metabolic acids and other small, diffusible particles, such as urea	Signs of uremic encephalopathy: lethargy, decreased alertness, loss of recent memory, delirium, coma, seizures, asterixis, muscle twitching, and tremulousness
		Signs of neuropathy: restless leg syndrome, paresthesias, muscle weakness, and paralysis
Osteodystrophy	Hyperphosphatemia	Osteomalacia
	Hypocalcemia	Osteoporosis
	Hyperparathyroidism	Bone pain and tenderness
		Spontaneous fractures
	Calcium × phosphate product greater than 60	Metastatic calcifications
Skin	Salt wasting	Dry skin and mucous membranes
	Anemia	Pale, sallow complexion
	Hyperparathyroidism	Pruritus
	Decreased platelet function and bleeding tendencies	Ecchymosis and subcutaneous bruises
	High concentration of metabolic end products in body fluids	Uremic frost and odor of urine on skin and breath
Genitourinary	Impaired general health	
	Decreased testosterone	Impotence and loss of libido
	Decreased estrogen	Amenorrhea and loss of libido

mEq to 900 mEq) while maintaining normal serum sodium levels.[8] In chronic kidney failure, the kidneys lose the ability to regulate sodium excretion. There is impaired ability to adjust to a sudden reduction in sodium intake and poor tolerance of an acute sodium overload. Volume depletion with an accompanying decrease in the glomerular filtration rate can occur with a restricted sodium intake or excess sodium loss due to diarrhea and vomiting. Salt wasting is a common problem in advanced renal failure because of impaired tubular reabsorption of sodium. Increasing sodium intake in persons with chronic renal failure often improves the glomerular filtration rate and whatever renal function remains. However, in persons with associated hypertension, the possibility of increasing blood pressure or producing congestive heart failure often rules out supplemental sodium intake.

Abnormalities of calcium, phosphorus, and vitamin D metabolism occur early in the course of chronic renal failure.[9] Regulation of serum phosphate levels requires a daily urinary excretion of an amount equal to that ingested in the diet. With deteriorating renal function, phosphate excretion is impaired and, as a result, serum phosphorus levels rise. Serum calcium levels, which are inversely regulated in relation to serum phosphorus levels, fall (discussed in Chapter 27). The drop in serum calcium, caused by hyperphosphatemia, stimulates parathyroid hormone release with a resultant increase in calcium resorption from bone. Although serum calcium levels are maintained through increased parathyroid function, this adjustment is accomplished at the expense of the skeletal system and other body organs. Persons with chronic renal failure often develop secondary hyperparathyroidism, the result of chronic stimulation of the parathyroid glands.

The hypocalcemia of chronic renal failure is further aggravated by impaired vitamin D function. The kidneys control vitamin D activity by converting the inactive form of vitamin D (25-hydroxycholecalciferol) to its active form (1,25-dihydroxycholecalciferol). Chronic renal failure impairs the ability to convert vitamin D to its active form. With reduced levels of activated vitamin D, calcium absorption from the small intestine is decreased, causing further stimulation of parathyroid function and demineralization of bone.[9]

Early treatment of hypocalcemia and hyperphosphatemia can prevent or slow further long-term complications, such as osteodystrophy. Phosphate-binding antacids are frequently prescribed. They act by increasing fecal losses of phosphate, thereby reducing its absorption from the gastrointestinal tract. Antacids that contain magnesium (i.e., Maalox, Mylanta) are contraindicated because the kidneys regulate the excretion of this mineral. Additionally, milk products and other foods high in phosphorus are restricted in the diet. Calcitriol (1,25-dihydroxycholecaliferol) and calcium supplements are often used to facilitate intestinal absorption of calcium and increase serum calcium levels.

The kidneys are largely responsible for maintaining body pH by eliminating hydrogen ions produced in metabolic processes. This is achieved through hydrogen ion secretion, sodium and bicarbonate reabsorption, and production of ammonia which acts as a buffer for titratable acids. With a decline in renal function, these mechanisms become impaired, and metabolic acidosis results. In chronic renal failure, acidosis seems to stabilize as the disease progresses, probably as a result of the tremendous buffering capacity of bone. This buffering action is thought to increase bone resorption and to contribute to skeletal defects present in chronic renal failure. If hypertension and edema are not problems, the accompanying metabolic acidosis can be treated with appropriate doses of sodium bicarbonate.

About 90% of potassium excretion is through the kidneys. In renal failure, potassium excretion by each nephron increases as the kidneys adapt to a decrease in the glomerular filtration rate. As a result, hyperkalemia usually does not develop until kidney function is severely compromised. Because of this adaptive mechanism, it is not usually necessary to restrict potassium intake in chronic renal failure until urinary output is less than 1000 ml per day and the glomerular filtration rate has dropped below 10 ml per minute.[8]

Azotemia is an early sign of renal failure, usually occurring before other symptoms become evident. Urea is one of the first of the nitrogenous wastes to accumulate in the blood. Blood urea nitrogen (BUN) becomes increasingly elevated as renal failure progresses. Creatinine, a by-product of muscle metabolism, is freely filtered in the glomerulus and is not reabsorbed in the renal tubules. Because creatinine is produced at a relatively constant rate and because any creatinine that is filtered in the glomerulus is lost in the urine rather than being reabsorbed into the blood, serum creatinine can be used as an indirect method for assessing the glomerular filtration rate and extent of renal damage that has occurred in renal failure (see Chapter 30).

Hematologic abnormalities

Chronic anemia is the most profound hematologic alteration that accompanies renal failure. The kidney is the primary site for the production of the hormone erythropoietin which controls red blood cell production. In renal failure, erythropoietin production is usually insufficient to stimulate adequate red blood cell production by the bone marrow. Moreover, the accumulation of uremic toxins further suppresses red cell production in the bone marrow, and the cells that are produced have a shortened life span. Both of these factors contribute to anemia in chronic renal failure.

Persons with renal failure experience a gradual reduction in hematocrit as renal function deteriorates. The hematocrit for a person on hemodialysis may stabilize at about 20%.[10] Persons on peritoneal dialysis have higher serum erythropoietin levels and subsequently have higher hematocrit levels.[11] Folic acid and iron supplements (which are removed during dialysis), androgenic steroids, and blood transfusions may be prescribed to treat anemia. A recombinant erythropoietin has been developed and is now available to decrease the severity of anemia among persons with renal failure.

An estimated 17% to 20% of persons with chronic renal failure have a bleeding tendency.[3] Although platelet production is normal in number, platelet function is impaired, causing bleeding problems. Epistaxis, gastrointestinal bleeding, and bruising of the skin and subcutaneous tissues are seen.

Immunologic abnormalities accompany chronic renal disease, decreasing the efficiency of the immune response to infection. This includes decreases in lymphocyte function, cell-mediated immunity, and granulocyte count.[9] Infection is a common complication and cause of hospitalization and death in chronic renal failure.

Cardiovascular problems

Cardiovascular disorders, including hypertension, congestive heart failure and pericarditis, are commonly seen among persons with chronic renal failure. Hyperkalemia, which often accompanies renal failure, can contribute to cardiovascular problems.

Hypertension is frequently an early manifestation of renal failure. It is caused in part by increased renin production (renin-angiotensin mechanism) by the kidneys coupled with excess extracellular fluid volume. Even in advanced renal failure, enough functioning renal tissue is present to produce renin in quantities sufficient to raise blood pressure.[12] Often, persons with renal insufficiency need to take several antihypertensive medications to control blood pressure. Generally, a diuretic and a beta-adrenergic blocking drug, such as propranolol, are prescribed. In the later stage of renal failure, dialysis is needed to maintain the extracellular fluid volume.

Increased extracellular fluid volume resulting from sodium and water retention, proteinuria, and hypoalbuminemia is clinically identified by the presence of edema. This condition can lead to congestive heart failure and pulmonary edema, especially in the later stages of renal failure.

Pericarditis occurs in as many as 50% of persons with chronic renal failure because of irritation to the pericardial sac by uremic toxins.[13] The danger of pericarditis is death from cardiac tamponade (see Chapter 21). The symptoms depend on the amount of fluid and the rate at which it accumulates in the pericardium.

Hyperkalemia in chronic renal failure often results from failure to follow dietary potassium restrictions, ingestion of medications that contain potassium, blood transfusions, and bleeding. EKG changes indicating hyperkalemia include tall T waves, S-T segment depression, prolonged P-R interval (AV block), and widening of the QRS complex, which can lead to ventricular fibrillation.[10] Hyperkalemia usually results in a medical emergency and requires treatment with intravenous drugs to move potassium from the serum into cells (e.g., sodium bicarbonate, glucose, and insulin) or with Kayexalate to remove potassium from the body.

Gastrointestinal disturbances

Anorexia, nausea, and vomiting are common in uremia, along with a metallic taste in the mouth that further depresses the appetite. Early morning nausea commonly occurs. Ulceration and bleeding of the gastrointestinal mucosa may develop, and hiccoughs are common. A possible cause of nausea and vomiting includes the decomposition of urea by intestinal flora, resulting in a high concentration of ammonia. Parathyroid hormone increases gastric acid secretion and thus contributes to gastrointestinal problems. Nausea and vomiting often improve with restriction of dietary protein and following initiation of dialysis and usually disappear with transplantation.

Neurologic disorders

Neurologic disorders, which are common in uremia, can be categorized as peripheral neuropathies and uremic encephalopathy.

Neuropathy, or involvement of the peripheral nerves, affects the lower limbs more frequently than the upper. It is symmetrical and affects both sensory and motor functions. Neuropathy is caused by atrophy and demyelination of nerve fibers, possibly caused by uremic toxins.[9] The "restless legs syndrome" is a manifestation of peripheral nerve involvement and can be seen in up to two-thirds of persons who are on dialysis.[9] This syndrome is characterized by creeping, prickling, and itching sensations that are usually more intense at rest. Temporary relief is obtained by moving the legs. A burning sensation of the feet, which may be followed by muscle weakness and atrophy, is a manifestation of uremia.

Uremic encephalopathy is poorly understood and may result, at least in part, from an excess of toxic organic acids that alter normal mechanisms preventing their crossing the blood brain-barrier and entering neural tissue. Electrolyte abnormalities, such as sodium shifts, may also contribute.

The central nervous system disturbances in uremia are similar to those caused by other metabolic and toxic disorders, such as portal-systemic encephalopathy, hypoxia, and water intoxication. The manifestations are more closely related to the progress of the uremic disorder than to the level of the metabolic end-products.[14] Generally, profound encephalopathy is common in acute renal failure and less common in chronic renal failure despite the marked blood chemistry abnormalities seen in the latter. Reductions in alertness and awareness are the earliest and most significant indications of uremic encephalopathy. This is often followed by an inability to fix attention, loss of recent memory, and perceptual errors in identifying persons and objects. Delirium and coma occur late in the course, and finally convulsions are the preterminal event.

Disorders of motor function frequently accompany the neurologic manifestations of uremic encephalopathy. During the early stages, there is often difficulty in performing fine movements of the extremities; the gait becomes unsteady and clumsy with *tremulousness* of movement. *Asterixis*, dorsiflexion of the hands and feet, often occurs as the disease progresses. It can be elicited by having the person hyperextend his or her arms at the elbow and wrist with the fingers spread apart. If asterixis is present, this position causes side-to-side flapping movements of the fingers.

Osteodystrophy

Renal osteodystrophy occurs in chronic renal failure because of abnormalities of calcium and phosphorus balance. The condition has sometimes been called *renal rickets*, because its manifestations in children resemble those of a vitamin D deficiency. The primary changes in renal osteodystrophy are osteomalacia and osteoporosis, in which the calcium and phosphate contents of the bone decrease and loss of the supporting structural matrix occurs. Increased parathyroid function causes excessive reabsorption of calcium from long bones, distal ends of the clavicle, and smaller bones, which can be seen on x-ray films. In advanced osteodystrophy, cysts may develop in the bone, a condition called *osteitis fibrosa cystica*. The symptoms of renal osteodystrophy include tenderness, pain, and sometimes spontaneous fractures.

Soft-tissue calcification, or *metastatic calcification* of the cornea, arteries, subcutaneous tissues, and muscle can occur when the phosphate times calcium product rises higher than 60. This is seen after dialysis has been instituted and is usually associated with a rapid rise in the calcium level, which precedes a fall in the phosphate level. Calcium deposits in the eye cause conjunctivitis and are often evidenced by what is called "band" keratopathy. Calcium deposits in the skin cause intense itching.

Skin disorders

The skin is pale in renal failure because of anemia and may have a sallow, yellow-brown hue. The skin and mucous membranes are dry and subcutaneous bruising is common. Skin dryness is caused by a reduction in perspiration due to the decreased size of sweat glands and the diminished activity of oil glands. Pruritus is common; it is secondary to the high serum phosphate levels and the development of phosphate crystals, which occurs with hyperparathyroidism. Severe scratching or repeated needlesticks, especially with hemodialysis, break the skin integrity and increase the risk for infection. Staphylococcus has been identified as the organism most frequently causing sepsis in persons on hemodialysis.[15] In the advanced stages of untreated renal failure, urea crystals may precipitate on the skin—the result of the high urea concentration present in body fluids. The fingernails may become thin and brittle with a dark band just behind the leading edge of the nail, followed by a white band. This appearance is known as *Terry's nails*.

Altered sexual functioning

The etiology of sexual dysfunction in both males and females with chronic renal failure is unclear. The cause most likely is multifactorial and may result from high levels of uremic toxins, neuropathy, altered endocrine function, psychological factors, and medications (*e.g.*, anti-hypertensives). Alterations in physiological sexual responses, reproductive ability, and libido commonly occur.

Impotence occurs in as many as 56% of male dialysis patients.[16] Derangements of the pituitary and gonadal hormones, such as decreases in testosterone levels and increases in prolactin and luteinizing hormone levels, are common, and cause erectile difficulties and decreased spermatocyte counts.[16] Loss of libido may result from chronic anemia as well as decreased testosterone levels. Several drugs, such as exogenous testosterone and bromocriptine, have been used in an attempt to return hormone levels to normal.

Impaired sexual function in females is manifested by abnormal levels of progesterone, luteinizing hormone, and prolactin. Hypofertility, menstrual abnormalities, decreased vaginal lubrication, and various orgasmic problems have been described.[17]

Amenorrhea is common among females who are on dialysis therapy.

Effect of renal failure on elimination of drugs

The incidence of adverse drug reactions is known to increase in persons with renal failure. In considering the effect of various drugs and medications on persons with renal disease, several factors about the drugs need to be taken into account: their absorption, distribution, metabolism, and excretion. The administration of large quantities of phosphate-binding antacids to control hyperphosphatemia and hypocalcemia in persons with advanced renal failure tends to interfere with the absorption of some drugs. Many drugs are bound to plasma proteins, such as albumin, for transport in the body, and the unbound portion of the drug is available to act at the various receptor sites and is free to be metabolized. In many persons there is a decrease in levels of plasma proteins, which are used for the binding and transport of drugs.

In the process of metabolism, some drugs form intermediate metabolites that are toxic if not eliminated. This is true of meperidine, which is metabolized to the toxic intermediate normeperidine, which causes excessive sedation, nausea, and vomiting. Some pathways of drug metabolism, such as hydrolysis, are slowed with uremia. This results in decreased insulin requirements for diabetics as renal function deteriorates.[18]

Decreased elimination by the kidneys allows drugs or their metabolites to accumulate in the body and requires that drug dosages be adjusted accordingly. Some drugs contain unwanted nitrogen, sodium, potassium, and magnesium and must be avoided in persons with renal failure. Penicillin, for example, contains potassium. Nitrofurantoin and ammonium chloride add to the body's nitrogen pool. Many antacids contain magnesium. Patients with renal failure should be cautioned against the use of over-the-counter remedies.

Treatment

The treatment of chronic renal failure can be divided into two stages: conservative management of renal insufficiency and dialysis or renal transplantation. The conservative treatment consists of measures to prevent or retard deterioration in renal function and to assist the body in compensating for the existing impairment. When conservative measures are no longer effective, dialysis or renal transplantation becomes necessary. Dietary management is an important component of treatment for persons with chronic renal failure.

Dialysis and renal transplantation

Trends among the end-stage renal disease population include decreasing mortality rates and an increasing volume of persons requiring dialysis and transplantation. Increasing numbers of persons receiving renal therapy are elderly or have chronic conditions such as diabetes or heart disease. At present, older persons comprise about 40% of persons receiving renal therapy. Approximately 30,000 Americans begin dialysis therapy each year. In 1987, approximately 85,000 people were undergoing dialysis treatments in the United States and approximately 8,300 received a kidney transplant. The average cost of maintenance hemodialysis is $25,000 to $30,000 per year. The cost of transplantation is $35,000 to $40,000, with a cost of $2,000 to $4,000 for maintenance therapy during subsequent years.[19] Thus, successful renal transplantation is proving to be economical as well as superior in offering patients improved quality of life.

The choice between dialysis and transplantation is dictated by age, related health problems, donor availability, and personal preference. Although success rates continue to improve with transplantation, dialysis plays a critical role as a treatment method for end-stage renal disease. It is life-sustaining for persons who are not candidates for transplantation, are awaiting transplantation, or as a backup treatment if transplantation is unsuccessful.

Hemodialysis. The basic principles of hemodialysis have remained unchanged over the years. However, new technology has improved both the efficiency and the speed of dialysis. A hemodialysis system, or artificial kidney, consists of three parts—a blood compartment, a dialysis fluid compartment, and a cellophane membrane that separates the two compartments. There are several types of dialyzers; all incorporate these parts, and all function in a similar fashion. The cellophane membrane is semipermeable, permitting all molecules except blood cells and plasma proteins to move freely in both directions—from the blood into the dialyzing solution and from the dialyzing solution into the blood. The direction of flow is determined by the concentration of the substances contained in the two solutions. Normally, the waste products and the excess electrolytes in the blood diffuse into the dialyzing solution. If there is a need to replace or add substances, such as bicarbonate, to the blood, these can be added to the dialyzing solution (Figure 32-1).

During dialysis, blood moves from an artery through the tubing and blood chamber in the dialysis machine and then back into the body through a vein. Access to the vascular system is through an external AV shunt (tubing implanted into an artery and a vein)

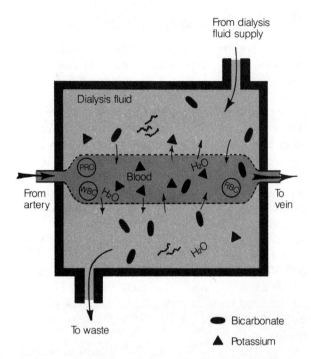

From dialysis
fluid supply

Dialysis fluid

Blood

PRO

WBC H₂O

RBC

H₂O

H₂O

From
artery

To
vein

To waste

⬭ Bicarbonate

▲ Potassium

Figure 32-1 Schematic diagram of a hemodialysis system. The blood compartment and dialysis solution compartment are separated by a cellophane membrane. This membrane is porous enough to allow all of the constituents, except the plasma proteins and blood cells, to diffuse between the two compartments.

or more commonly, through an internal AV fistula (anastomosis of a vein to an artery, usually in the forearm). Heparin is used to prevent clotting during the dialysis treatment; it can be administered continuously, intermittently, or regionally. Problems that may occur during dialysis depending on the blood flow rate and rate of solute removal include hypotension, nausea, vomiting, muscle cramps, headaches, chest pain, and disequilibrium syndrome. Most persons are dialyzed three times a week for 3 to 5 hours. Many dialysis centers provide the option for people to learn to manage hemodialysis at home.

Peritoneal dialysis. The same principles of diffusion, osmosis, and ultrafiltration apply to peritoneal dialysis. However, the thin serous membrane of the peritoneal membrane serves as the dialyzing membrane. A permanent Silastic catheter is surgically placed into the peritoneal cavity below the umbilicus to provide access. The catheter is tunneled through subcutaneous tissue and exits on the side of the abdomen. The dialysis process involves instilling a sterile dialyzing solution (usually 2 liters) through the catheter over 10 minutes. The solution is then allowed to remain, or dwell, in the peritoneal cavity for a prescribed amount of time, during which the metabolic end-products and extracellular fluid diffuse into the dialysis solution. Commercial dialysis solution is available in 1.5%, 2.5%, and 4.25% dextrose concentra-

tions. Solutions with higher dextrose levels will increase osmosis, causing more fluid to be removed. At the end of the dwell time, the dialysis fluid is drained by gravity out of the peritoneal cavity into a sterile bag.

There are a number of ways peritoneal dialysis can be performed—at home versus in-center, automated versus manual system, intermittent versus continuous—all with variations in number of exchanges and dwell time. Individual preference, manual ability, lifestyle, knowledge of the procedure and physiological response to treatment influence the type of dialysis schedule.

Usually, continuous ambulatory peritoneal dialysis (CAPD) is performed. It is a self-care procedure in which the person manages the dialysis procedure and type of solution (dextrose concentration) used at home. The procedure involves instilling dialysate into the peritoneal cavity and rolling up the bag and tubing and securing them under clothing during the dwell. After the dwell time is completed (4 to 6 hours during the day), the bag is unrolled and lowered allowing the waste-containing dialysis solution to drain from the peritoneal cavity into the bag. Each exchange, which involves draining the solution and infusing a new solution, requires about 30 to 45 minutes. Usually four exchanges are performed each day. The continuous rather than intermittent nature of CAPD ensures that the rapid fluctuations in extracellular fluid volume associated with hemodialysis are avoided, and dietary restrictions can be liberalized somewhat.

Potential problems with peritoneal dialysis include infection, catheter malfunction, dehydration due to excessive fluid removal, hyperglycemia, and hernias. The most serious complication is infection, which can occur at the catheter exit site, in the subcutaneous tunnel, or in the peritoneal cavity (peritonitis).

Renal transplantation. Greatly improved success rates have made renal transplantation the treatment of choice for many persons with chronic renal failure. Increasing numbers of kidney transplants are performed nationally each year. Living related family donors account for about 30% of all transplants in the United States; the remainder are cadaver transplants. Donor (cadaver) availability continues to limit the number of transplants performed each year. Transplants from living non-related donors (*e.g.*, spouse) have been performed in cases where suitable ABO and tissue compatibility was present.

The success of transplantation depends primarily on the degree of histocompatibility, adequate organ preservation, and immunologic management. Maintenance immunosuppression therapy includes prednisone, imuran, and cyclosporine. Rejection, which is categorized as acute and chronic, can occur at any time (see Chapter 12). Acute rejection most commonly occurs during the first several months post-transplant and involves a cellular response with the proliferation of T-lymphocytes. Chronic rejection can occur later, months to years after transplant. Because chronic rejection is caused by both cellular and humoral immunity, it does not respond to increased immunosuppression.

Maintenance immunosuppression and increased use of immunosuppression to treat rejection predispose the person to a spectrum of infectious complications. Prophylactic antibiotics are prescribed to decrease the incidence of common infections, such as candidiasis, herpes, and pneumocystis carinii pneumonia. Other infections, such as cytomegalovirus infection and aspergillosis, are seen with chronic immunosuppression.

Dietary management

A major component in the treatment of chronic renal failure is dietary management. The goal of dietary treatment is to provide optimum nutrition while maintaining tolerable levels of metabolic wastes. The specific diet prescription depends on the type and severity of kidney disease and dialysis modality. Because of the severe restrictions placed on food and fluid intake, these diets may be complicated and unappetizing. After renal transplantation a less restrictive diet may be necessary, even when renal function is normal, to control side effects from immunosuppressive medication. Common diet prescriptions are shown in Table 32-2.

Protein. Dietary restriction of protein is necessary with renal insufficiency and dialysis because proteins are broken down to form nitrogenous wastes. At present considerable controversy exists over the degree of restriction needed. Usually, protein need not be restricted until renal insufficiency is relatively far advanced (glomerular filtration rate of 20 ml/min or less).

Generally, a protein restriction with 70% or more of high biological value (containing more essential amino acids) is employed with renal insufficiency. Proteins with a high biologic value are believed to promote the reutilization of endogenous nitrogen, decreasing the amount of nitrogenous wastes that are produced and thus ameliorating the symptoms of uremia. In reutilizing nitrogen, the proteins ingested in the diet are broken down into their constituent amino acids to be utilized in the synthesis of protein required by the body. A 70-kg man synthesizes at least 150 g protein daily while ingesting only 60 g.[20] For this to be accomplished, amino acids must be recycled; and the ingestion of proteins that have a high biologic value makes it possible. Almost all of the amino acids in a whole egg are utilized in the synthesis of essential body proteins; hence, eggs are said to have a high biologic value. In contrast, fewer than half of the amino acids in cereal proteins are reutilized. Amino acids not reutilized to build body proteins are broken down and form the end-product of protein metabolism, such as urea.

Persons on peritoneal dialysis require a greater protein intake because of significant protein losses, ranging from 4 g/day to 13 g/day, through the dialysis.[21] Even higher protein losses can occur with peritonitis. With renal transplantation, high doses of prednisone, especially during the immediate postoperative period or during acute rejection episodes, accelerate protein catabolism.[22] Diets that are high in protein have been shown to reverse steroid-induced negative nitrogen balance.[23]

Carbohydrates, fat, and calories. With renal failure, adequate calories in the form of carbohydrates and fat are required to meet energy needs. This is particularly important when the protein content of the diet is severely restricted. If sufficient calories are not

Table 32-2. Common daily diet recommendations for adults

Nutrient	Renal insufficiency	Maintenance hemodialysis	Maintenance CAPD	Initial post-transplantation
Protein	0.6–0.8 g/kg	0.8–1.0 g/kg	1.2–1.5 g/kg	1.3–2.0 g/kg
Carbohydrate	unrestricted	unrestricted	unrestricted	1.0–1.5 g/kg
Fat	unrestricted	unrestricted	unrestricted	<35% of calories
Calories	40–50 Kcal/kg	40–50 Kcal/kg	restricted by dialysate	30–35 Kcal/kg or to maintain ideal body weight
Potassium	40–70 mEq	40–70 mEq	unrestricted	unrestricted
Sodium	variable	750–1500 mg	750–1500 mg	2000 mg
Phosporus	800–1200 mg	600–1200 mg	600–1200 mg	unrestricted

(Data from Foulks CJ: Nutritional evaluation of patients on maintenance dialysis therapy. Am Nephr Nurs J 15:13, 1988; Gammarino M: Renal transplant diet: Recommendations for the acute phase. Dial Transplant 16:497, 1987; Harum P: Renal nutrition for the renal nurse. Am Nephr Nurs J 8:38, 1984; and Lancaster LE: Renal failure: Pathophysiology, assessment, and intervention. Crit Care Nurs 1:50, 1982)

available, either the limited protein in the diet goes into energy production or body tissue itself will be used for energy purposes.

Caloric intake for persons on CAPD includes food intake as well as calories absorbed from the dialysis solution. A 2-liter bag of 1.5% solution equals 105 calories and a 4.25% solution delivers 289 calories.[24] Therefore, a 70-kg man on CAPD with an ideal caloric intake of 40 Kcal/kg or 2800 calories who uses two 1.5% solutions and two 4.25% solutions per day will only need to ingest about 2000 calories (788 calories from dialysate).

Calories often need to be limited with renal transplantation, since weight gain is common. Lowering the carbohydrate intake reduces the cushingoid side effects caused by corticosteroid drugs that are used to prevent transplant rejection. Reducing the intake of dietary fats and increasing the percentage of polyunsaturated fats can reduce hyperlipidemia after transplantation.[25]

Potassium. When the glomerular filtration rate falls to extremely low levels and when undergoing hemodialysis therapy, dietary restriction of potassium becomes mandatory. Using salt substitutes that contain potassium or ingesting fruits, fruit juice, chocolate, potatoes, or other high-potassium foods can cause hyperkalemia. Persons on continuous peritoneal dialysis usually do not need to limit potassium intake and often may need to increase intake.

Sodium and fluid intake. The sodium and fluid restrictions depend on the kidneys' ability to excrete sodium and water and must be individually determined. Generally, renal disease of glomerular origin is more likely to contribute to sodium retention, whereas tubular dysfunction causes salt wasting.

Fluid intake in excess of what the kidneys can excrete causes circulatory overload, edema, and water intoxication. Inadequate intake, on the other hand, causes volume depletion and hypotension and can cause further decreases in the already compromised glomerular filtration rate. It is common practice to allow a daily fluid intake of 500 ml to 800 ml, which is equal to insensible water loss, plus a quantity equal to the 24-hour urine output.

—— Exercise

The many medical problems that result from renal failure lead to reductions in physical functioning, energy level, and exercise capacity. Variables that strongly affect rehabilitation include age, diabetic status, and treatment mode. With the initiation of dialysis, younger adults usually have higher activity levels than older adults.[26] The physical activity level is much lower among persons with diabetes who are on

dialysis than among persons of the same age who do not have diabetes. Only about one-quarter of persons with diabetes have a level of physical ability beyond that of caring for themselves.[27]

The exercise capacity, as measured by maximal oxygen consumption, for persons treated with hemodialysis or peritoneal dialysis is below that of sedentary healthy individuals and persons who have had successful renal transplants.[28] Factors that have been suggested as causes of this reduction in exercise capacity are anemia, altered peripheral metabolism of lactate, cardiac changes caused by uremia, and general physical deconditioning. Because of this, some dialysis centers have exercise training programs (e.g., cycling) during hemodialysis treatments.

In summary, chronic renal failure results from the destructive effects of many different forms of kidney disease. Regardless of the cause, the consequences of nephron destruction present in end-stage renal disease are alterations in the filtration, reabsorption, and endocrine functions of the kidney. In the advanced stages, renal failure affects almost every system in the body. It causes azotemia and alterations in sodium and water excretion and in body levels of potassium, phosphate, calcium, and magnesium. It also causes anemia, alterations in cardiovascular function, neurologic disturbances, gastrointestinal dysfunction, and discomforting skin changes. Within the past 20 years, dialysis and transplantation have allowed persons with what was once a fatal disease to survive and lead relatively normal and productive lives.

References

1. Guyton A: Textbook of Medical Physiology, 6th ed, p 418, 424. Philadelphia, WB Saunders, 1981
2. Report of the Coordinating Council: Research Needs in Nephrology and Urology, Vol I, p 16. National Institutes of Health, National Institute of Arthritis, Metabolism, and Digestive Diseases, Public Health Service, 1978. DHEW Publication No (NIH) 78–1481
3. Leaf A, Cotran R: Renal Pathophysiology, 2nd ed, pp 174–211. New York, Oxford University Press, 1985
4. Schrier RW: Acute renal failure: Pathogenesis, diagnosis and management. Hosp Pract 16(3):101, 1981
5. Mitchell JC: Axioms on uremia. Hosp Med 14(7):6, 1978
6. Klahr S, Schreiner G, Ichikawa I: The progression of renal failure. N Engl J Med 318:1663, 1657, 1988
7. Bricker NS, Kirschenbaum MA: The Kidney: Diagnosis and Management, p 306. New York, John Wiley & Sons, 1984
8. Orme BM: Chronic renal failure: Guide to management. Hosp Med 14(1):99, 105, 1978
9. Van Stone JC: Dialysis and the Treatment of Renal In-

sufficiency, pp 1, 4, 15, 30, 31. New York, Grune & Stratton, 1983

10. Lancaster LE: Renal failure: Pathophysiology, assessment, and intervention. Crit Care Nurse 1:47, 45, 1982

11. Molzahn AE: Erythropoietin. Dialysis & Transplantation 15:566, 1986

12. Merrill JP, Hampters CL: Uremia. N Engl J Med 282:1014, 1970

13. Zeluff GW, Eknoyan G, Jackson D: Pericarditis in renal failure. Heart Lung 8:1139, 1979

14. Raskin NH, Fisherman RA: Neurological disorders in renal failure. N Engl J Med 294:143, 147, 1976

15. Goldblum SE, Reed WP: Host defenses and immunologic alterations associated with chronic hemodialysis. Annals of Int Med 93:600, 1980

16. Foulks CJ, Cushner HM: Sexual dysfunction in the male dialysis patient: Pathogenesis, evaluation, and therapy. Am J Kidney Dis 8:211, 212, 1986

17. Rickus MA: Sexual dysfunction in the female ESRD patient. Am Nephr Nurses' Assoc J 14(3):185, 186, 1987

18. Bennett WM, McCarron DA: Pharmacotherapy of Renal Disease and Hypertension, p 5. New York, Churchill Livingstone, 1987

19. U.S. Department of Health and Human Services: U.S. Transplant Statistics. Washington D.C., Author, 1987

20. Giordano C: The role of diet in renal disease. Hosp Pract 12(11):115–119, 1977

21. Blumenkrantz MJ, Gahl GM, Kopple JD, Kamdar AV, Jones MR, Kessel M, Coburn JW: Protein loss during peritoneal dialysis. Kidney Int 19:593, 1981

22. Hoy WE, Sargent JA, Hall D, McKenna BA, Pabico RC, Freeman RB, Yarger JM, Byer BM: Protein catabolism during the postoperative course after renal transplantation. Am J Kidney Dis 5:187, 1985

23. Cogan MG, Sargent JA, Yarbrough SG, Vincenti F, Amend WJ: Prevention of prednisone-induced negative nitrogen balance. Ann Int Med 95:160, 1981

24. Harum P: Renal nutrition for the renal nurse. Am Nephr Nurses' J 8:39, 1984

25. Disler PB, Goldberg RB, Kuhn L, Meyers AM, Joffe BI, Seftel HC: The role of diet in the pathogenesis and control of hyperlipidemia after renal transplantation. Clin Nephr 16:31, 1981

26. Carlson DM, Johnson WJ, Kjellstrand CM: Functional status of patients with end-stage renal disease. Mayo Clin Proc 62:340, 1987

27. Gutman RA, Stead WW, Robinson RR: Physical activity and employment status of patients on maintenance dialysis. N Engl J Med 304:310, 1981

28. Painter P, Messer-Rehak D, Hanson P, Zimmerman SW, Glass NR: Exercise capacity in hemodialysis, CAPD, and renal transplant patients. Nephron 42:48, 1986

Bibliography

Badr K, Ichikawa I: Prerenal failure: A deleterious shift from renal compensation to decompensation. N Engl J Med 319:623, 1988

Beck LH: Kidney function and disease in the elderly. Hosp Pract 23:75, 1988

Bonventre JV: Mediators of ischemic renal injury. Ann Rev Med 39:531, 1988

Diamond DR: Nonoliguric acute renal failure. Arch Intern Med 142:1882, 1982

Eggers PW: Effect of transplantation on the Medicare End-Stage Renal Disease Program. N Engl J Med 318:223, 1988

Eknoyan G: Side effects of hemodialysis. N Engl J Med 311:915, 1984

Epstein FH, Brown RS: Acute renal failure: A collection of paradoxes. Hosp Pract 23(1):171, 1988

Erslev A: Erythropoietin coming of age. N Engl J Med 316:101, 1987

Eschbach JW, Adamson JW: Recombinant erythropoietin: Implications for nephrology. Am J Kidney Dis 11:203, 1988

Fine LG: The uremic syndrome: Adaptive mechanisms and therapy. Hosp Pract 22(9):63, 1987

Fraser CL, Arieff AI: Nervous system complications of uremia. Ann Intern Med 109:143, 1988

Goodship THJ, Mitch WE: Nutritional approaches to preserving renal function. Adv Intern Med 33:337, 1988

Hayslett JP: Postpartum renal failure. N Engl J Med 312:1556, 1985

Kanis JA: Osteomalacia and chronic renal failure. J Clin Path 34:1295, 1981

Lee DB, Goodman WG, Coburn JW: Renal osteodystrophy: Some questions on an old disorder. Am J Kidney Dis 11:365, 1988

Levey AS, Perrone RD, Madias NE: Serum creatinine and renal function. Ann Rev Med 39:465, 1988

Maher JF: Uremic pleuritis. Am J Kidney Dis 10(1):19, 1987

Mitch WE, Wilcox CS: Disorders of body fluids, sodium and potassium in chronic renal failure. Am J Med 72:536, 1982

Myers BD, Moran SM: Hemodynamically mediated acute renal failure. N Engl J Med 314:97, 1986

Nolph KD, Lindblad AS, Novak JW: Continuous ambulatory peritoneal dialysis. N Engl J Med 318:1595, 1988

Painter PP: Exercise in end-stage renal disease. Exercise & Sport Sciences Review 16:305, 1988

Reidenberg MM: Kidney function and drug action. N Engl J Med 313:816, 1985

Rosansky SJ, Eggers PW: Trends in US end-stage renal disease population: 1973–1983. Am J Kidney Dis 9(2):91, 1987

Sexauer CL, Matson JR: Anemia in chronic renal failure. Ann Clin Lab Sci 11:484, 1981

Sherwood LM: Vitamin D, parathyroid hormone, and renal disease. N Engl J Med 316:1601, 1987

Strom TB: Summary: Today's biotechnology and tomorrow's antirejection therapy. Am J Kidney Dis 11:163, 1988

Ting A, Morris PJ: The role of HLA matching in renal transplantation. Tissue Antigens 25:225, 1985

Wardle N: Acute renal failure in the 1980's: The importance of septic shock and of endotoxaemia. Nephron 30:193, 1982

Alterations in Genitourinary Function

CHAPTER 33

Alterations in Urine Elimination

Objectives

After you have studied this chapter, you should be able to meet the following objectives:

_____ Cite the two functions of the bladder.

_____ Describe the structure of the bladder.

_____ Trace the innervation of the bladder from the afferent stretch receptors to reflex control of detrusor muscle contraction and voluntary control of the external sphincter.

_____ Explain the influence of the parasympathetic and sympathetic nervous systems on bladder function.

_____ List five classes of autonomic drugs and explain their potential effect on bladder function.

_____ Describe at least three urodynamic studies that can be used to assess bladder function.

_____ State the signs of urinary retention.

_____ State the difference between bladder changes that occur during the spinal shock stage of spinal cord injury and those that occur following recovery of the spinal cord reflexes.

_____ Explain the common cause, symptoms, and dangers of autonomic hyperreflexia in a patient with spinal cord injuries.

_____ Differentiate between lesions that produce detrusor muscle hyperreflexia and those that produce detrusor muscle areflexia in terms of the level of the lesions and their effects on bladder function.

_____ Cite the pathology and causes of nonrelaxing external sphincter.

_____ Describe the symptoms of diabetic bladder neuropathy.

_____ State the rationale for the use of clean self-catheterization in terms of preventing bladder infections.

_____ Describe the difference between bladder training methods used for a neurogenic bladder caused by a lesion of the spinal cord micturition reflex center and one caused by a lesion above the level of the reflex center.

_____ Define the six categories of _incontinence_.

_____ Describe Kegel's exercises and explain their use in the control of stress incontinence.

_____ List at least four special problems of the elderly that contribute to the development of incontinence.

_____ State the most common sign of bladder cancer.

_____ Cite a possible mechanism for the development of bladder cancer.

_____ Describe how the urine Pap smear is used in the detection of bladder cancer.

Although the kidneys control the formation of urine and regulate the composition of body fluids, it is the bladder that stores urine and controls its elimination from the body.[1] Alterations in the storage and expulsion functions of the bladder can result in incontinence, with its accompanying social and hygienic problems, or in obstruction of urinary flow, which has deleterious effects on ureteral and, ultimately, renal function. The discussion in this chapter focuses on normal control of urine elimination, urinary retention, incontinence, and bladder cancer. A discussion of urinary tract infections can be found in Chapter 31.

Control of urine elimination

The bladder (also known as the urinary vesicle) is a freely movable organ located behind the pelvic bone in the male and in front of the vagina in the female. The bladder consists of two parts: the fundus, or body, and the neck, or posterior urethra. In the male, the urethra continues anteriorly through the penis. Urine passes from the kidneys to the bladder through the ureters, which are 4 mm to 5 mm in diameter and about 30 cm in length. The ureters enter the bladder bilaterally at a location toward its base and close to the urethra (Figure 33-1). The triangular area that is bounded by the ureters and the urethra is called the *trigone*. There are no valves at the ureteral openings, but as the pressure of the urine within the bladder rises, the ends of the ureters are compressed against the bladder wall to prevent the backflow of urine.

Bladder structure

The bladder is composed of four layers: (1) an outer serosal layer, which covers the upper surface and is continuous with the peritoneum; (2) a network

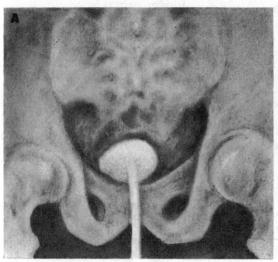
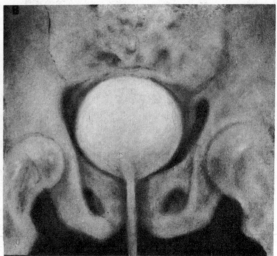

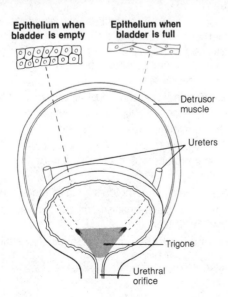

Figure 33-1 **(Top)** Cystogram of male bladder, showing position and filling. **(Bottom)** Diagram of the bladder, showing the detrusor muscle, ureters, trigone area, and urethral orifice. Note the flattening of epithelial cells when the bladder is full and the wall is stretched. (*Chaffee EE, Lytle IM: Basic Physiology and Anatomy, 4th ed. Philadelphia, JB Lippincott, 1980*)

of smooth muscle fibers called the detrusor muscle; (3) a submucosal layer of loose connective tissue; and (4) an inner mucosal lining of transitional epithelium. The tonicity of the urine is often quite different from that of the blood, and the transitional epithelial lining of the bladder acts as an effective barrier to prevent the passage of water between the blood and the bladder contents. The inner elements of the bladder form smooth folds, or rugae. As the bladder expands during filling, these rugae spread out to form a single layer without disrupting the integrity of the epithelial lining.

Muscles in the bladder neck, sometimes referred to as the internal sphincter, are a continuation of the detrusor muscle. They run down obliquely behind the proximal urethra, forming the posterior urethra in males and the entire urethra in females. When the bladder is relaxed, these circular muscle fibers are closed and act as a sphincter. When the detrusor muscle contracts, the sphincter is pulled open simply by the changes that occur in bladder shape. In the female, the urethra (2.5–3.5 cm) is shorter than in the male (16.5–18.5 cm), and the urethral resistance also tends to be less in the female.

Another muscle important to bladder function is the circular skeletal muscle, the external sphincter, that surrounds the urethra distal to the base of the bladder. In general, the external sphincter operates as a reserve mechanism to stop micturition when it is occurring and to maintain continence in the face of unusually high bladder pressure. The skeletal muscle of the pelvic floor also contributes to the support of the bladder and the maintenance of continence. The diaphragm and abdominal muscles play a secondary role in micturition. Their contraction may further increase intravesicular pressure.

── Neural control of bladder function

The innervation of the bladder consists of a peripheral autonomic reflex that is subject to facilitation or inhibition by higher neurologic centers. There are three main levels of neurologic control for bladder function: (1) the spinal cord reflex centers; (2) the micturition center in the brain stem; and (3) the cortical and subcortical centers.

── Spinal cord centers

The centers for reflex control of micturition (passage of urine) are located in the sacral (S2–S4) and thoracolumbar (T11–L1) segments of the spinal cord (Figure 33-2). Motor neurons for the detrusor muscle are located in the sacral cord; their axons travel to the bladder through the pelvic nerve. Lower motor

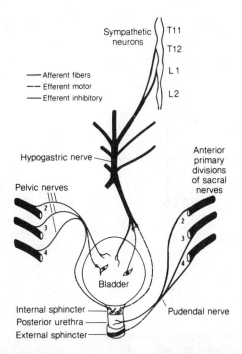

Figure 33-2 Nerve supply to the bladder and the urethra. *(Chaffee EE, Lytle IM: Basic Physiology and anatomy, 4th ed. Philadelphia, JB Lippincott, 1980)*

neurons for the external sphincter are also located in the sacral segments of the spinal cord. These motor neurons communicate with the cerebral cortex via the pyramidal tracts and send impulses to the external sphincter via the pudendal nerve. The sympathetic motor fibers for the trigonal area of the bladder are located in the thoracolumbar segments of the spinal cord. Sensations from the urethra and bladder are returned to the CNS by means of fibers that travel with the parasympathetic (pelvic), somatic (pudendal), and sympathetic (hypogastric) nerves. The pelvic nerve carries sensory fibers from the stretch receptors of the bladder; the pudendal nerve, sensory fibers from the external sphincter and pelvic muscles; and the hypogastric nerve, sensory fibers from the trigonal area.

── Brain stem micturition center

The immediate coordination of the normal micturition reflex occurs in the micturition center of the brain stem, facilitated by ascending and descending pathways from the reflex centers in the spinal cord (Figure 33-3). This center is thought to coordinate the activity of the detrusor muscle and the external sphincter. The detrusor motor neurons of the sacral cord do not respond directly to afferent information generated by bladder filling. Instead, bladder emptying occurs only after afferent generation of a brain-stem–integrated micturition response. Direct reflex detrusor response to afferent pelvic nerve activity de-

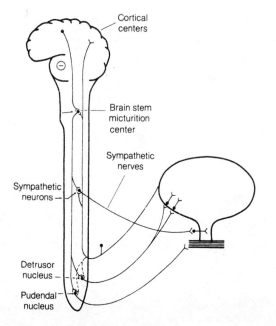

Figure 33-3 Neuronal interactions between lower urinary tract and nervous system. Prior to micturition, the bladder afferents ascend to the micturition center, which is normally inhibited by higher centers. Efferents from the micturition center descend to the thoracolumbar sympathetic center and the detrusor and pudendal nuclei to coordinate vesical contraction with relaxation of the smooth muscle and striated muscle sphincters. (*Krane RJ, Sirosky MB [eds]: Clinical Neuro-Urology, p 145. Boston, Little, Brown, & Co. © 1979. Used with permission.*)

velops after spinal cord injury but does not occur normally.

Cortical and subcortical centers

Cortical brain centers allow for inhibition of the micturition center in the brain stem and conscious control of urination. Neural influences from the subcortical centers in the basal ganglia, which are conveyed by extrapyramidal pathways, modulate the contractile response. They modulate and delay the detrusor contractile response during filling and then modulate the expulsive activity of the bladder to facilitate complete emptying.[2]

Micturition

In infants and small children micturition is an involuntary act that is triggered by a spinal cord reflex; when the bladder fills to a given capacity, the detrusor muscle contracts and the external sphincter relaxes. As the bladder grows and increases in capacity, the tonicity of the external sphincter increases. At age 2 to 3 the child becomes conscious of the need to urinate and can learn to briefly contract the pelvic muscles in order to inhibit contraction of the detrusor muscle and thus delay urination. As the central nervous system continues to mature, inhibition of involuntary detru-

sor muscle activity takes place. Once the child achieves continence, micturition becomes voluntary.

In order to maintain continence, or retention of urine, the bladder must function as a low-pressure storage system; that is, the pressure within the bladder must remain lower than urethral pressure. To ensure that this condition is met, the increase in intravesicular pressure that accompanies bladder filling is almost imperceptible. An increase in bladder volume from 10 ml to 400 ml may be accompanied by only a 5-cm to 10-cm H_2O increase in pressure.[3] Sustained elevations in intravesicular pressures (greater than 40–50 cm H_2O) are associated with ureteral dilatation and development of vesicoureteral reflux. While the pressure within the bladder is maintained at low levels, sphincter pressure remains high (45–65 cm H_2O) as a means of preventing loss of urine as the bladder fills. When the bladder is distended to 150 ml to 300 ml, the sensation of fullness is transmitted to the spinal cord and then to the cerebral cortex, allowing for conscious inhibition of the micturition reflex. During the act of micturition, the detrusor muscle of the bladder fundus and bladder neck contract down on the urine in the fundus; the ureteral orifices are forced shut; the bladder neck is widened and shortened as it is pulled up by the globular muscles in the bladder fundus; and the resistance of the internal sphincter in the bladder neck is decreased as urine moves out of the bladder.

Pharmacology of micturition

Both sympathetic and parasympathetic neuromediators contribute to the micturition reflex. The parasympathetic innervation of the bladder is mediated by the neuromediator acetylcholine. Two types of acetylcholine receptors effect various aspects of micturition—nicotinic and muscarinic. Nicotinic receptors are found in the autonomic ganglia, the neuromuscular end-plates of the external sphincter and pelvic muscles, and the spinal cord. Muscarinic receptors are found in the postganglionic parasympathetic endings of the detrusor muscle.

Although sympathetic innervation is not essential to the act of micturition, it allows the bladder to store a large volume without the involuntary escape of urine—a mechanism that is consistent with the fight-or-flight function subserved by the sympathetic nervous system. The bladder is supplied with both alpha and beta (beta$_2$) sympathetic receptors. The beta receptors are found in the detrusor muscle; they produce relaxation of the detrusor muscle, increasing the bladder volume at which the micturition reflex is triggered.[4] Alpha receptors are found in the trigone area, including the intramural ureteral musculature, bladder neck, and internal sphincter. Activation of alpha receptors produces contraction of these muscles. Sympathetic activity ceases when the micturition reflex is activated. During ejaculation, which is mediated by the sympathetic nervous system, the musculature of the trigone area as well as that of the bladder neck and prostatic urethra contracts and prevents the backflow of seminal fluid into the bladder.

Because of their effect on bladder function, drugs that selectively activate or block autonomic nervous system outflow or receptor activity can impair urine elimination. Table 33-1 describes the action of drugs that can impair bladder function or can be used in the treatment of micturition disorders.

Diagnostic methods of evaluating bladder function

Bladder structure and function can be assessed by a number of methods. Reports or observations of frequency, hesitancy, straining to void, and a weak or interrupted stream are suggestive of outflow obstruction. Palpation and percussion provide information about bladder distention. The presence of bacteriuria or pyuria suggest urinary tract infection and the possibility of urinary tract obstruction.

Bladder structures can be visualized indirectly by use of x-rays of the abdomen and excretory urograms (which involve the use of a radiopaque dye [see Figure 33-1]), computed tomography (CT) scan, magnetic resonance imaging, or ultrasound. Cystoscopy enables direct visualization of the urethra, bladder, and ureteral orifices.

Urodynamic studies

Urodynamic studies are used to study bladder function and voiding problems. Three aspects of bladder function can be assessed by urodynamic studies: (1) bladder, urethral, and intra-abdominal pressure changes; (2) characteristics of urine flow; and (3) the activity of the striated muscles of the external sphincter and pelvic floor. Specific urodynamic tests include uroflometry, cystometrography, urethral pressure profile, sphincter electromyography, and uroflow studies.

Uroflometry. Uroflometry measures the flow rate (milliliters/minute) during urination. It is commonly done using a weight-recording device located at the bottom of a commode receptacle unit. As

Table 33–1. Bladder function and drug actions

Function	Drug groups	Examples
Detrusor muscle		
Increased tone and contraction	Cholinergic drugs (stimulate parasympathetic receptors that cause detrusor muscle contraction)	Bethanechol (Urecholine) Carbachol (Doryl)
	Anticholinesterase drugs (inhibit acetylcholine destruction)	Methacholine (Mechoyl) Furethonium (Furethide) Neostigmine (Prostigmin) Distigmine (Ubretid)
Inhibition of detrusor muscle relaxation during filling	Beta-adrenergic blocking drugs (block beta receptors that cause detrusor muscle relaxation)	Propranolol (Inderal)
Decreased tone	Anticholinergic drugs (block parasympathetic receptors that cause detrusor muscle contraction)	Atropine Methantheline (Banthine) Propantheline (Pro-Banthine) Oxybutynin (Ditropan)
	Adrenergic agonists (activate beta sympathetic receptors that cause detrusor muscle relaxation)	Isoproterenol Baclofen (Lioresal) Hydramitrazine (Lisidonil)
Internal sphincter		
Increased tone	Alpha-adrenergic agonists (activate alpha receptors that cause contraction of muscles of the internal sphincter)	Phenylephrine (Neo-Synephrine) Ephedrine Phenylpropanolamine (Propadrine) Imipramine (Tofranil, Presamine)
Decreased tone	Alpha-adrenergic blocking drugs	Phenoxybenzamine
External sphincter		
Decreased tone	Skeletal muscle relaxants	Baclofen (Lioresal) Dantrolene (Dantrium) Diazepam (Valium)

(Developed from information in Bissada NK, Finkbeiner AE: Pharmacology of continence and micturition. Am Fam Phys 20(5):128, 1979)

the person being tested voids, the weight of the commode receptacle unit increases. This weight change is electronically recorded and then analyzed using both weight (converted to milliliters) and time.

Cystometrography.
The cystometrogram (CMG) is used to measure bladder pressure during both filling and voiding. It provides valuable information about uninhibited bladder contractions, the sensation of bladder fullness and desire to urinate, and the ability to inhibit urination. The test uses either carbon dioxide or sterile water to fill the bladder and some means for continuous recording of pressure during bladder filling and voiding. In a normally functioning bladder, the pressure usually remains constant at 8 cm H_2O to 15 cm H_2O until 350 ml to 450 ml of fluid has been instilled in the bladder. At this point a definite sensation of fullness occurs and the pressure rises sharply to 40 cm H_2O to 100 cm H_2O, and voiding around the catheter occurs. Urinary continence requires that urethral pressure exceed bladder pressure. Usually bladder pressure rises 30 cm H_2O to 40 cm H_2O during voiding. If the urethral resistance is high because of obstruction, greater pressures will be required, a condition that can be detected through use of the CMG.

Urethral pressure profile.
The urethral pressure profile (UPP) is used to evaluate the intraluminal pressure changes along the length of the urethra with the bladder at rest; it provides information about smooth muscle activity along the length of the urethra. This test can be done using the infusion method (the most commonly used), the membrane catheter method, or the microtip transducer. The infusion method involves inserting a small double-lumen urethral catheter, infusing fluid or carbon dioxide into the bladder, and measuring the changes in urethral pressure as the catheter is slowly withdrawn.

Sphincter electromyography.
Sphincter electromyography (EMG) allows the activity of the striated (voluntary) muscles of the perineal area to be studied. Activity is recorded using anal (catheter or plug), urethral (catheter), or perineal (cup or paste) electrodes. Electrode placement is based on the muscle groups that need to be tested. The test is usually done along with urodynamic tests such as the CMG and uroflow studies.

It is often advantageous to evaluate several components of bladder function simultaneously. The most common combinations of studies are CMG, urethral sphincter EMG, and abdominal pressure; UPP and urethral sphincter EMG; and uroflometry, urethral sphincter EMG, and abdominal and bladder pressure (often referred to as a micturition study).[5] Rectal pressure is usually used as a measure of abdominal pressure.

In summary, although the kidneys function in the formation of urine and the regulation of body fluids, it is the bladder that stores and controls the elimination of urine. Micturition is basically a function of the peripheral autonomic nervous system, subject to facilitation or inhibition from higher neurologic centers. The parasympathetic nervous system controls the motor function of the bladder detrusor muscle and the tone of the internal sphincter; its cell bodies are located in the sacral spinal cord and communicate with the bladder through the pelvic nerve. Efferent sympathetic control originates at the level of segments Tll through L1 of the spinal cord and produces relaxation of the detrusor muscle and contraction of the internal sphincter. Skeletal muscle found in the external sphincter and the pelvic muscles that support the bladder are supplied by the pudendal nerve, which exits the spinal cord at the level of segments S2 through S4. The micturition center in the brain stem coordinates the action of the detrusor muscle and the external sphincter, whereas cortical centers permit conscious control of micturition. Bladder function can be evaluated using urodynamic studies that measure bladder, urethral, and abdominal pressures, urine flow characteristics, and skeletal muscle activity of the external sphincter.

Alterations in bladder function

Alterations in bladder function include both urinary obstruction with retention of urine and urinary incontinence with involuntary loss of urine. Although the two conditions have almost opposite effects on urination, they can have similar causes. Both can result either from structural changes in the bladder, urethra, or surrounding organs or from impairment of neurologic control of bladder function.

Urinary retention

In urinary retention, urine is produced normally by the kidneys but is retained in the bladder.[5] The condition has a number of causes, including urethral obstruction, impaired innervation of the bladder (neurogenic bladder), and the effects of drug actions on the control of bladder function. Because it has the potential to produce kidney damage, urinary retention is a serious disorder .

Urethral obstruction

Major structural urinary obstruction is most often due to processes that cause intrinsic narrowing or external compression of the urinary meatus or bladder outlet structures. In males, the most important cause of urinary obstruction is external compression of the urethra due to enlargement of the prostate gland (see Chapter 35). External obstructive processes are less common in females, and when they do occur, they are most often caused by a cystocele of the bladder (see Chapter 37). Bladder tumors and secondary invasion of the bladder by tumors arising in structures that surround the bladder and urethra can compress the bladder neck or urethra and cause obstruction. Narrowing of the urethra due to congenital deformities or scar tissue from injury or infection can also obstruct urine flow. Congenital narrowings of the urinary meatus (meatal stenosis) are more common in boys, and obstructive disorders of the posterior urethra are more common in girls. Gonorrhea and other sexually transmitted diseases contribute to the incidence of infection-produced urethral strictures.

Constipation and fecal impaction can compress the urethra and produce urethral obstruction. This is a particular problem in the elderly.

Compensatory changes. The body normally compensates for the obstruction of urine outflow with mechanisms designed to prevent urine retention. These mechanisms can be divided into three stages: irritability, a compensatory stage, and a decompensatory stage.[6] The degree to which these compensatory changes occur and their effect on bladder structure and urinary function depend on the extent of the obstruction, the rapidity with which it occurs, and the presence of other contributing factors, such as neurologic impairment and infection.

During the early stage of obstruction, the bladder begins to hypertrophy and becomes hypersensitive to afferent stimuli arising from bladder filling. The ability to suppress urination is diminished, and bladder contraction can become so strong it virtually produces bladder spasm. There is urgency, sometimes to the point of incontinence, and frequency both during the day and at night.

With continuation and progression of the obstruction, compensatory changes begin to occur. There is further hypertrophy of the bladder muscle, the thickness of the bladder wall may double, and the pressure generated by detrusor contraction can increase from a normal 20 cm to 40 cm H_2O to 50 cm to 100 cm H_2O in order to overcome the resistance from the obstruction. As the force needed to expel urine from the bladder increases, compensatory mechanisms may become ineffective, causing muscle fatigue before complete emptying can be accomplished. After a few minutes, voiding can again be initiated and completed, accounting for the frequency of urination.[5]

Normally the inner bladder surface forms smooth folds. With continued outflow obstruction, this smooth surface is replaced with coarsely woven structures (hypertrophied smooth muscle fibers) called trabeculae. Small pockets of mucosal tissue, called cellules, commonly develop between the trabecular ridges.[6] These pockets form diverticula when they extend between the actual fibers of the bladder muscle (Figure 33-4). Because the diverticula have no muscle, they are unable to contract and expel their urine into the bladder, and secondary infections due to stasis frequently occur.

Along with hypertrophy of the bladder wall, there is hypertrophy of the trigone area and the interureteric ridge, which is located between the two ureters. This causes back pressure on the kidneys, the development of hydroureters, and eventual kidney damage. In addition, stasis of urine predisposes to urinary tract infections.

When compensatory mechanisms are no longer effective, signs of decompensation begin to occur. The contraction of the detrusor muscle becomes too short to completely expel the urine, and residual urine remains in the bladder. At this point the symptoms of obstruction—frequency of urination, hesitancy, a need to strain to initiate urination, a very weak and small stream, and termination of the stream before the bladder is completely emptied—become pronounced. The amount of residual urine may increase up to 1000 ml to 3000 ml, and overflow incontinence occurs. There may also be acute, or sudden, complete retention of urine. The signs of urinary retention are summarized in Chart 33-1.

Treatment. The immediate treatment of outflow obstruction is relief of bladder distention.

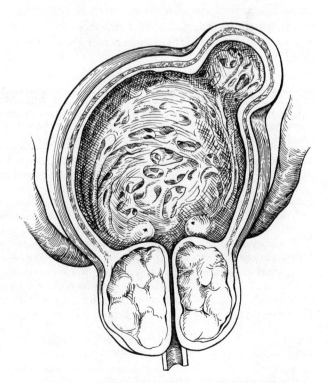

Figure 33-4 Destructive changes of the bladder wall with development of diverticula due to benign prostatic hypertrophy.

Chart 33-1: Signs of urethral obstruction and urine retention

Bladder distention
Hesitancy
Straining when initiating urination
Small and weak stream
Frequency
Feeling of incomplete bladder emptying
Overflow incontinence

This is usually accomplished through urinary catheterization (discussed later in this chapter). If constipation or fecal impaction is present, this should be corrected. Long-term treatment is directed toward correcting the problem causing the obstruction.

Neurogenic bladder

The innervation of the bladder can be interrupted at any level and can selectively involve either sensory or motor innervation or both. Neurogenic disorders of the bladder are usually manifested in one of two ways: by detrusor muscle hyperreflexia or by detrusor muscle areflexia. Detrusor muscle hyperreflexia usually results from neurologic lesions that are located above the level of the micturition reflexes, whereas areflexia results from lesions at the level of the sacral micturition reflex or the peripheral autonomic innervation of the bladder. In addition to detrusor muscle disorders, disruption of micturition occurs when the neurologic control of external sphincter function is impaired. Table 33-2 describes the characteristics of neurogenic bladder according to the level of the lesion.

Detrusor muscle hyperreflexia

The term *reflex neurogenic bladder*, sometimes called *spastic neurogenic bladder, autonomic neurogenic bladder, cord bladder,* or *uninhibited bladder,* is used to describe a neurogenic disorder that causes hyperreflexia of the detrusor muscle. It is caused by any neurologic lesion above the level of the voiding reflex arc. It involves the interruption of the sensory and voluntary control of micturition. Although both pathways are usually affected, the lesion may selectively involve either the sensory or the motor component, and it can occur at different levels of neural control. The most common cause of neurogenic bladder is spinal cord injury (see Chapter 49).

Following the acute stage of spinal cord injury, the micturition response changes from a long-tract reflex to a segmental reflex.[7] Because the sacral reflex arc remains intact, stimuli generated by bladder stretch receptors during filling produce frequent spontaneous contractions of the detrusor muscle. This creates a small hyperactive bladder subject to high-pressure and short-duration uninhibited bladder contractions. Voiding is interrupted, involuntary, or incomplete. Hypertrophy of the trigone develops, often leading to vesicoureteral reflux and renal damage. Dilation of the internal sphincter and spasticity of the perineal muscles innervated by upper motor neurons occur, producing resistance to bladder emptying.

Bladder function during spinal shock. The immediate and early effects of spinal cord injury on bladder function are quite different from those that follow recovery from the impact of the initial injury. During the period immediately following spinal cord injury (see Chapter 49), a state of spinal shock de-

---

Table 33-2. Characteristics and types of neurogenic bladder

Level of lesion	Change in bladder function	Common causes
Cortex or pyramidal tract	Loss of cortical ability to perceive bladder filling results in low volume; physiologically normal micturition occurs suddenly and is difficult to inhibit	Stroke and advanced age
Basal ganglia or extra-pyramidal tract	Detrusor contractions are elicited suddenly without warning and are difficult to control; bladder contraction is shorter than normal and does not produce full bladder emptying	Parkinson's disease
Brain stem micturition center or communicating tracts in the spinal cord	Storage reflexes are provoked during filling, and external sphincter responses are heightened; uninhibited bladder contractions occur at a lower volume than normal and do not continue until the bladder is emptied; antagonistic activity occurs between the detrusor muscle and the external sphincter	Spinal cord injury
Sacral cord or nerve roots	Areflexic bladder fills but does not contract; loss of external sphincter tone occurs when the lesion affects the alpha-adrenergic motor neurons or pudendal nerve	Injury to sacral cord or spinal roots
Pelvic nerve	Increased filling and impaired sphincter control causes increased intravesicular pressure	Radical pelvic surgery
Autonomic peripheral sensory pathways	Bladder overfilling occurs with lack of appreciation of bladder events	Diabetic neuropathies, multiple sclerosis

velops during which all the reflexes, including the micturition reflex, are depressed. During this stage the bladder becomes atonic and cannot contract. Catheterization is necessary to prevent injury to urinary structures associated with overdistention of the bladder. Aseptic intermittent catheterization is the preferred method of catheterization. Depression of reflexes lasts for about 1 to 2 months, after which time the spinal reflexes return and become hyperactive.

Autonomic hyperreflexia. Autonomic hyperreflexia is a life-threatening complication of spinal cord injuries above the level of T6.[7] Normally all viscerovascular reflexes are integrated at supraspinal levels so that a normal blood pressure is maintained. With spinal cord injury, this integration is lost. The condition is characterized by excessive uninhibited autonomic reflexes triggered by stimuli such as overdistention of the viscera and visceral pain. The most common of these stimuli is an overdistended bladder. The manifestations of autonomic hyperreflexia include marked elevations in blood pressure, bradycardia, severe headache, flushing of the skin, diaphoresis below the level of spinal cord injury, blurred vision, nasal congestion, nausea, and spasm of the piloerector muscles (goose bumps). If untreated, the condition can lead to stroke or seizures. The treatment consists of immediate removal of the triggering event—catheterization in cases of bladder distention.

Uninhibited neurogenic bladder. A mild form of reflex neurogenic bladder, sometimes called the uninhibited bladder, can develop following a stroke, during the early stages of multiple sclerosis, or as a result of lesions located in the inhibitory centers of the cortex or the pyramidal tract. With this type of disorder the sacral reflex arc and sensation are retained, the urine stream is normal, and there is no residual urine. However, bladder capacity is diminished.

Detrusor-sphincter dyssynergy. Depending on the level of the lesion, the coordinated activity of the detrusor muscle and the external sphincter may be affected. Lesions that affect the micturition center in the brain stem or impair communication between this center and spinal cord centers interrupt the coordinated activity of the detrusor muscle and the external sphincter. This is called detrusor-sphincter dyssynergy. Instead of relaxing during micturition, the external sphincter becomes more constricted.

—— Detrusor muscle areflexia

Detrusor muscle areflexia, or flaccid neurogenic bladder, occurs when there is injury to the micturition center of the sacral cord, the cauda equina, or the sacral roots that supply the bladder. Atony of the detrusor muscle and loss of the perception of bladder fullness permit the overstretching of the detrusor muscle that contributes to weak and ineffective bladder contractions. External sphincter tone and perineal muscle tone are diminished. Voluntary urination does not occur, but fairly efficient emptying can be achieved by increased intra-abdominal pressure or manual suprapubic pressure. Among the causes of flaccid neurogenic bladder are myelomeningocele and spina bifida.

Bladder neuropathies. In addition to central nervous system (CNS) conditions that disrupt bladder function, disorders of the peripheral (pelvic, pudendal, and hypogastric) neurons that supply the bladder can occur. These neuropathies can selectively interrupt sensory or motor pathways for the bladder or can involve both pathways. The most common causes of bladder neuropathies are diabetes mellitus and multiple sclerosis.

Epidemiologic studies indicate that diabetic bladder neuropathy occurs in 43% to 87% of insulin-dependent diabetics, with no age or sex difference.[8] Initially the disorder affects the sensory axons of the urinary bladder without involvement of the pudendal nerve. There is an insidious onset of bladder dysfunction during which time voidings gradually decrease until urine is passed only once or twice a day.[9] Frequently there is need for straining, accompanied by hesitation, weakness of the stream, dribbling, and a sensation of incomplete bladder emptying. The chief complication is vesicoureteral reflux and ascending urinary tract infection. Because persons with diabetes are already at risk for developing glomerular disease (see Chapter 31), reflux can have serious effects on kidney function. Treatment consists of surgical creation of a temporary urinary diversion, bladder training, and pharmacologic manipulation of bladder function with parasympathetic drugs.[10] To compensate for the decreased contractile properties of the detrusor muscle, the bladder neck may be resected to decrease the resistance to outflow of urine from the bladder. Because the innervation of the external sphincter is not disturbed, continence is maintained.

Nonrelaxing external sphincter. Another condition that affects the peripheral innervation of micturition is called *nonrelaxing external sphincter*.[11] This condition is usually related to a delay in maturation, developmental regression, psychomotor disorders, or locally irritative lesions. Inadequate relaxation of the external sphincter can be the result of anxiety or depression. Any local irritation can produce spasms of the sphincter by means of afferent sensory input from the pudendal nerve; included are vaginitis, perineal inflammation, and inflammation or irritation of the urethra. In men, chronic prostatitis contributes to the impaired relaxation of the external sphincter.

—— Treatment

The goals of treatment for neurogenic bladder disorders center on preventing bladder overdistention, urinary tract infections, and renal damage that can be life-threatening and on reducing the undesirable social and psychological effects of the disorder. The treatment is based on the type of neurologic lesion that is involved, information obtained through use of a health history including fluid intake, report or observation of voiding patterns, urodynamic studies when indicated, presence of other health problems, and the ability of the individual to participate in the treatment. The treatment methods include catheterization, bladder training, pharmacologic manipulation of bladder function, and surgery.

Catheterization. Catheterization involves the insertion of a small-diameter latex or silicon tube into the bladder through the urethra. The catheter may be inserted on a one-time basis to relieve temporary bladder distention, left indwelling (retention catheter), or inserted intermittently. With acute overdistention of the bladder, no more than 1000 ml of urine are removed from the bladder at one time. The theory behind this limitation is that removing more than this amount at one time releases pressure on the pelvic blood vessels and predisposes to shock.[5] Permanent indwelling catheters are sometimes used when there is urinary retention or incontinence in persons who are ill or debilitated or when conservative or surgical methods for the correction of incontinence are not feasible. The use of permanent indwelling bladder catheters in patients with spinal cord injury has been shown to produce a number of complications, including urinary tract infections, urethral irritation and injury, epididymo-orchitis, pyelonephritis, kidney stones, and bladder carcinoma.[12]

Intermittent catheterization is used to treat urinary retention or incomplete emptying secondary to various neurologic or obstructive disorders. Properly used, it prevents bladder overdistention and urethral irritation, allows for more freedom of activity, and provides for periodic distention of the bladder to prevent muscle atony. It is often used with pharmacologic manipulation to achieve continence; and when possible, it is learned and managed as a self-care procedure (intermittent self-catheterization). It may be carried out as either an aseptic (sterile) or a clean procedure. Aseptic intermittent catheterization is used in persons with spinal shock and in persons who need short-term catheterization. The clean procedure is usually for self-catheterization. It is performed at 3-hour to 4-hour intervals to prevent overdistention of the bladder. The best results are obtained if only 300 ml to 400 ml are allowed to collect in the bladder between catheterizations. The use of the clean as opposed to the sterile procedure has been defended on the basis that most urinary tract infections are due to some underlying abnormality of the urinary tract that leads to impaired tissue resistance to bacterial infection, the most common cause of which is decreased blood flow due to overdistention.[13] Overdistention has also been shown to decrease the mucin layer that protects the mucosal surface of the bladder.[14] Studies have shown up to a 48% decrease in bacteriuria after the institution of intermittent self-catheterization.[13] Intermittent self-catheterization has proved particularly effective in children with meningomyelocele.

Bladder training. Bladder training differs with the type of injury that is present. Training includes the use of body positions that facilitate micturition and the monitoring of fluid intake to prevent urinary tract infections and to control urine volume and osmolality.

Among the considerations when monitoring fluid intake is the need to insure adequate fluid intake to prevent an unduly concentrated urine that will stimulate afferent neurons of the micturition reflex. In hyperreflexive bladder or detrusor-sphincter dyssynergy, the stimulation of afferent nerve endings by irritating constituents of the urine results in increased vesicular pressures, vesicoureteral reflux, and overflow incontinence. On the other hand, fluid intake must be balanced to prevent bladder overdistention from occurring during the night. Adequate fluid intake is also needed to prevent urinary tract infections, the irritating effects of which increase bladder irritability and increase the risk of urinary incontinence and renal damage.

The methods used for bladder retraining depend on the type of lesion that is present. In spastic neurogenic bladder, methods designed to trigger the sacral micturition reflex are used; in flaccid neurogenic bladder, manual methods that increase intravesicular pressure are used. *Trigger voiding methods* include manual stimulation of the afferent loop of the micturition reflex through such maneuvers as tapping the suprapubic area, pulling on the pubic hairs, stroking the glans penis, or rubbing the thighs. *Crede's method,* which is done with the person in a sitting position, consists of applying pressure (with four fingers of one hand or both hands) to the suprapubic area as a means of increasing intravesicular pressure. Use of the Valsalva maneuver (bearing down by exhaling against a closed glottis) increases intraabdominal pressure and aids in bladder emptying. This maneuver is repeated until the bladder is empty. For the best results, the patient must cooperate fully with the procedures or, if possible, learn to perform them independently.

Biofeedback methods have been useful for teaching some aspects of bladder control. Biofeedback involves the use of EMG or cystometry as a feedback signal for training a person to control the function of the external sphincter or raise intravesicular pressure enough to overcome outflow resistance.

Pharmacologic manipulation. Pharmacologic manipulation includes the use of drugs to increase the contractile properties of the bladder, decrease the outflow resistance of the internal sphincter, and relax the external sphincter. Often the usefulness of drug therapy is evaluated during cystometric studies. Bethanechol and methacholine may be used to increase detrusor muscle tone in spastic bladder. Methantheline and propantheline are used in spastic bladder to reduce vesical tone and increase bladder capacity. Muscle relaxants such as diazepam (Valium) and baclofen (Lioresal) may be used to decrease the tone of the external sphincter. Table 33-1 describes the drugs that affect bladder function.

Surgical procedures. Among the surgical procedures used in the management of neurogenic bladder are sphincterectomy or transurethral resection of the bladder neck in men with prostatic hypertrophy, reconstruction of the sphincter, nerve resection (the sacral reflex nerves that cause spasticity or the pudendal nerve that controls the external sphincter), and urinary diversion. Extensive work is now being done to find a feasible means of implanting a stimulating electrode in the sacral canal around one or more of the sacral roots to control detrusor activity in persons with flaccid neurogenic bladder.[6]

Urinary diversion can be done by creating an ileal or a colon loop into which the ureters are anastomosed; the distal end of the loop is brought out and attached to the abdominal wall. Other procedures include the attachment of the ureters to the skin of the abdominal wall or the attachment of the ureters to the sigmoid colon with the rectum serving as a receptacle for the urine.

—— Urinary incontinence

The International Continence Society for Standardization of Terminology has defined incontinence as a condition in which involuntary loss of urine is a social or hygienic problem and is objectively demonstrable.[15] Incontinence occurs in all age groups. More than 90% of children are continent by 5 years of age. Many motor skills decline with age, and incontinence, although not a normal accompaniment of the aging process, is seen with increased frequency in the elderly. It has been reported that 10% of men and 17% of women over age 65 have problems with incontinence. The increase in health problems often seen in the elderly, particularly those that interfere with the ability to get to an appropriate place to urinate, probably contributes to the greater frequency of incontinence.

Incontinence can be caused by a number of conditions. It can occur without the person's knowledge, and at other times the person may be aware of the condition but be unable to prevent it. The condition may occur as a transient and correctable phenomenon or it may not be totally correctable and occur with varying degrees of frequency. The International Continence Society for Standardization of Terminology has identified four categories of incontinence based on anatomic or physiological dysfunction: stress incontinence, urge incontinence, overflow incontinence, and reflex incontinence. Other sources use additional or different categories of incontinence, including a category called psychological incontinence and another called environmental or spurious incontinence (Table 33-3).[16]

Stress incontinence. Stress incontinence is the involuntary loss of urine that occurs when intravesicular (bladder) pressure exceeds maximal urethral pressure in the absence of detrusor activity.[15] Stress incontinence commonly occurs with the vesicular pressure changes instituted by coughing, laughing, lifting, or even climbing up and down stairs. It can result from weakness of the urethral sphincter and anatomic changes in the urethrovesical angle. In women, the angle between the bladder and the posterior proximal urethra (urethrovesical junction) is important to continence. Normally this angle is 90 to 100 degrees, with at least one-third of the bladder base contributing to the angle when not voiding (Figure 33-5).[16] During the first stage of voiding this angle is lost as the bladder descends. In women, diminution of

Table 33-3. Types and characteristics of urinary incontinence

Type	Characteristics
Stress	Involuntary loss of urine associated with activities, such as coughing, that increase intra-abdominal pressure
Urge	Involuntary loss of urine associated with the desire to void
Overflow	Involuntary loss of urine when intravesicular pressure exceeds maximal urethral pressure in the absence of detrusor activity
Reflex	Involuntary loss of urine due to abnormal activity of the spinal cord reflex
Psychological	Awareness of need to urinate, but failure to respond appropriately due to conditions such as dementia or confusional state
Environmental or spurious	Impediments to locating, reaching, or receiving assistance to reach an appropriate place to urinate

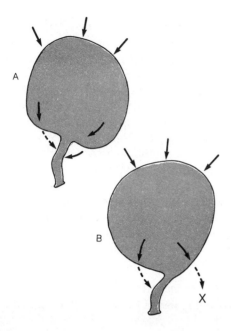

Figure 33-5 Importance of the posterior urethrovesical (PU-V) angle to the continence mechanism. (**A**) In the presence of the normal PU-V angle, sudden changes in intraabdominal pressure are transmitted optimally (indicated by the arrows with dotted lines) to all sides of the proximal urethra. In this way intraurethral pressure is maintained higher than the simultaneously elevated intravesicular pressure. This prevents loss of urine with sudden stress. (**B**) Loss of the PU-V angle results in displacement of the vesicle neck to the most dependent portion of the bladder, preventing the equal transmission of sudden increases in intraabdominal pressure to the lumen of the proximal urethra. Thus, the pressure in the region of the vesical neck rises considerably more than the intraurethral pressure just beyond it, and stress incontinence occurs. (*Green JT, Jr: Obstet Gynecol Surv 23:603, 1968. Reprinted with permission.*)

muscle tone associated with normal aging, childbirth, or surgical procedures can cause weakness of the pelvic floor muscles and result in stress incontinence by obliterating the critical posterior urethrovesical angle. In these women loss of the posterior urethrovesical angle, descent and funneling of the bladder neck, and backward and downward rotation of the bladder occur, so that the bladder and urethra are already in an anatomic position for the first stage of voiding. Therefore, any activity that causes downward pressure on the bladder is sufficient to allow the urine to escape involuntarily.

Local urethral irritation caused by infection or mucous membrane changes can also contribute to incontinence. In men stress incontinence usually occurs only with urinary tract infection, radiation damage, or following surgical procedures such as a prostatectomy.

Urge incontinence. Urge or urgency incontinence is the involuntary loss of urine associated with a strong desire to void. It can be subdivided into motor urge incontinence associated with uninhibited detrusor contractions and sensory urge incontinence that is not caused by uninhibited detrusor contractions or chronic voluntary delay in responding to the urge signal.

Among the causes of urgency incontinence are those conditions in which a partial upper motor neuron lesion makes movement difficult, so that the interval between knowing the bladder needs to be emptied and the ability to stop it from emptying may be less than the time needed to reach the lavatory. Multiple sclerosis is a common cause of this type of incontinence. Musculoskeletal disorders such as arthritis or joint instability may also prevent an otherwise continent person from reaching the toilet in time.

Drugs such as hypnotics, tranquilizers, and sedatives can interfere with the conscious inhibition of voiding, leading to urge incontinence. Diuretics, particularly in the elderly, increase the flow of urine and may contribute to incontinence, particularly in persons with diminished bladder capacity or difficulty reaching the toilet. Urinary infections, increased bladder irritability, urgency, and frequency occur in persons of all ages. In the elderly these conditions often precipitate incontinence.

Overflow incontinence. Overflow incontinence is an involuntary loss of urine that occurs when intravesicular pressure exceeds the maximal urethral pressure because of bladder distention in the absence of detrusor activity. It can occur with retention of urine due to nervous system lesions or obstruction of the bladder neck. With this type of incontinence the bladder is distended, and small amounts of urine are passed, particularly at night. In males, one of the most common causes of obstruction incontinence is enlargement of the prostate gland. Another cause that is often overlooked is fecal impaction (the presence of dry and hard feces in the rectum). When a large amount (bolus) of stool forms in the rectum it can push against the urethra and block the flow of urine.

Reflex incontinence. Reflex incontinence is due to abnormal activity in the spinal cord in the absence of sensation, usually associated with the desire to void. This occurs in persons with severe or complete upper or lower motor neuron lesions. It involves contraction of the bladder wall, with or without connection to the central nervous system, and is the basis for automatic micturition, previously described.

Psychological incontinence. The person with psychological incontinence may be aware of the need to urinate but make no effort to urinate in an appropriate setting. This occurs in dementia and confusional states. Because of the person's decreased mental acuity, it is often difficult to establish whether the need to urinate has not been sensed or the ability to act appropriately is impaired.

Environmental or spurious incontinence. Environmental or spurious incontinence (*i.e.,* that occurring for reasons unrelated to the structure of the urinary tract and its function) results from the inability to locate, reach, or receive assistance in reaching an appropriate place to void.[16] Spurious incontinence is a particular problem in the elderly, who may have problems with mobility and manual dexterity or find themselves in unfamiliar surroundings. It occurs when a person cannot find or reach the bathroom or manipulate clothing quickly enough. Failing vision may contribute to the problem. Embarrassment in front of other people at having to use the bathroom, particularly if the timing seems inappropriate, may cause a person to delay emptying the bladder and may lead to incontinence. Treatment with drugs such as diuretics may cause the bladder to fill more rapidly than usual, making it difficult to reach the bathroom in time if there are problems with mobility or if a bathroom is not readily available. Night sedation may cause a person to sleep through the signal that would normally waken a person so they can get up and empty the bladder and avoid wetting the bed.

—— Diagnosis and treatment

Urinary incontinence is a frequent and major health problem. It increases social isolation, frequently leads to institutionalization in the elderly, and predisposes to infections and skin breakdown.

Urinary incontinence is not a single disease but a symptom with many possible causes. As a symptom it requires full investigation to establish its cause. This is usually accomplished through a careful history and physical examination. Because many drugs affect bladder function, a full drug history is essential. Urodynamic studies may be needed to provide information about urinary pressures and urine flow rates.

The treatment or management depends on the type of incontinence that is present, accompanying health problems, and age. Exercises to strengthen the pelvic muscles and surgical correction of pelvic relaxation disorders are often used in women with stress incontinence. Noncatheter devices to obstruct urine flow or collect urine as it is passed may be used when urine flow cannot be controlled. Urinary incontinence is a major problem in the elderly, who have special treatment needs. Indwelling catheters (discussed earlier in the chapter), though a solution to the problem of urinary incontinence, are usually considered only after all other treatment methods have failed. In some types of incontinence, such as that associated with spinal cord injury or meningomyelocele, self-catheterization provides the means for controlling urine elimination.

Treatment of stress incontinence. Stress incontinence can be treated by physiotherapeutic measures, surgery, or a combination of the two. Surgical correction of cystocele and pelvic relaxation disorders in the female may be needed. Often, however, active muscle-tensing exercises of the pelvic muscles may prove effective. These exercises were first advocated by Kegel, and hence they are often called *Kegel's exercises*.[18] Two groups of muscles are strengthened: (1) those of the back part of the pelvic floor (these are the muscles used to contract the anus and control the passing of stool) and (2) the front muscles of the pelvic floor (these are the muscles used to stop the flow of urine during voiding). In learning the exercises, a woman concentrates on identifying the muscle groups and learning how to control contraction. Once this has been accomplished, she can start an exercise program that consists of slowly contracting the muscles, beginning at the front and working to the back while counting to four and then releasing. The exercises can be done while sitting or standing and should be performed in repetitions of 10, three times a day.[18]

Noncatheter devices. Two types of noncatheter devices are commonly used in the management of urinary incontinence; one obstructs flow, and the other collects urine as it is passed. Obstruction of urine flow is achieved by compressing the urethra or stimulating the contraction of the pelvic floor muscles. Penile clamps are available that occlude the urethra without obstructing blood circulation to the penis. Because these devices obstruct blood flow if they are clamped too tightly, their usefulness is essentially limited to males with dribbling incontinence due to proximal urethral destruction, usually resulting from prostatic surgery. In females, compression of the urethra is usually accomplished by intravaginal devices. Surgically implanted artificial sphincters are available for use in both males and females.[19] These devices consist of an inflatable cuff that surrounds the proximal urethra. The cuff is connected by tubing to an implanted fluid reservoir and an inflation bulb. Pressing the bulb, which is placed in the scrotum in males, inflates the cuff. It is emptied in a similar manner. Another method of occluding the bladder outlet in both males and females is the use of battery-operated electrodes that cause contraction of the pelvic floor muscles. This treatment is most effective in women with stress incontinence due to weakness of the pelvic floor muscles. Implantable electrodes have largely been replaced by those that can be worn in the vagina or in the anus

When urinary incontinence cannot be prevented, various types of urine collection devices or protective pads are used. Men can be fitted with collection devices (condom or sheath urinals) that are worn over the penis and attached to a container at the bedside or body. There are no effective external collection devices for women. Pants and pads are usually used. Dribbling bags (males) and pads (females) in which the urine turns to a non-pourable gel are available for occasional dribbling but are unsuitable for considerable wetting.

Special needs of the elderly. Urinary incontinence is a common problem in the elderly. The incidence is reported to vary from 11% to 42%, depending on whether the survey is taken in the community or in the hospital.[21] Many factors contribute to incontinence in the elderly, and many of these can be altered. Pelvic relaxation disorders occur more frequently in older than in younger females, and prostatic hypertrophy is more common in older than in younger males. Elderly persons often have difficulty in getting to the toilet on time. This can be caused by arthritis that makes walking or removing clothing difficult or by failing vision that makes trips to the bathroom precarious, especially in new and unfamiliar surroundings. Medication prescribed for other health problems may prevent a healthy bladder from functioning normally. Potent, fast-acting diuretics are known for their ability to cause urgency incontinence. Psychoactive drugs such as tranquilizers and sedatives may diminish normal attention to bladder clues. Impaired thirst or limited access to fluids predispose to constipation with urethral obstruction and overflow incontinence and to concentrated and infected urine, which increases bladder excitability.

According to Stanton, "there are two guiding principles in management of incontinence in the elderly. First, growing old does not imply becoming incontinent and, second, incontinence should not be left untreated just because the patient is old."[21] Treatment may involve changes in the physical environment so that the older person can reach the bathroom more easily or remove clothing more quickly. It may require changes in the diet to prevent constipation or a plan for fluid intake that prevents urine from becoming concentrated and irritating to the bladder.

In summary, alterations in bladder function include both urinary obstruction with retention of urine and urinary incontinence with involuntary loss of urine. Urinary retention occurs when the outflow of urine from the bladder is obstructed, because of either urethral obstruction or impaired bladder innervation. Urethral obstruction causes bladder irritability, detrusor muscle hypertrophy, trabeculation and the formation of diverticula, development of hydroureters, and eventual renal failure. Neurogenic bladder is caused by interruption in the innervation of the bladder. It can cause detrusor muscle hyperreflexia or areflexia, depending on the level of the lesion. Urinary incontinence occurs with involuntary loss of urine. It can present as stress incontinence, in which the loss of urine occurs with increases in bladder pressure such as that caused by coughing; urge incontinence, in which there is a strong desire to void; overflow incontinence that results from bladder overdistention; reflex incontinence that is due to uncontrolled reflex activity of the sacral micturition reflex, such as occurs following spinal cord injury; psychological incontinence, in which the person may be aware of the need to void but does not respond appropriately; or spurious or environmental incontinence in which there are impediments to reaching or using an appropriate place to urinate. The treatment of urinary obstruction, neurogenic bladder, and incontinence requires careful diagnosis to determine the cause and contributing factors.

Cancer of the bladder

Bladder cancer is the most frequent form of urinary tract cancer, accounting for 37,000 new cases each year and 2.5% of cancer deaths in 1982.[22] It is seen most frequently in the 50- to 70-year age groups and occurs twice as frequently in men as in women.

Bladder cancers are described as papillary (characterized by polypoid lesions attached by stalks to the bladder mucosa), noninvasive (characterized by thickening of the mucosa but without penetration of the basement membrane), invasive (characterized by penetration into the mucosal basement membrane and possibly into other structures), and flat lesions that lack the well-defined structures of the papillary lesions. Flat lesions may be either in situ or invasive cancers and tend to be more anaplastic than the papillary tumors.[23] Almost 70% of bladder tumors are papillary, noninvasive, low-grade cancers and they have a good prognosis. Hematuria, obstruction, and infection are potential complications that require tumor removal. These tumors frequently recur; with each recurrence 10% to 20% will have a higher cytologic grade, so that the prognosis for any person with papillary lesions may worsen with time.[24] About 25% to 30% of bladder cancers are highly invasive. These tumors may present as in situ lesions or progress rapidly to invasive lesions. The most common sites of metastasis are the pelvic lymph nodes, lungs, bones, and liver.

Although the cause of bladder cancer is unknown, evidence suggests that its origin is related to local influences such as carcinogens that are excreted in the urine and stored in the bladder. This includes the breakdown products of aniline dyes used in the rubber and cable industry. Smoking also deserves attention: it may be responsible for as many as 50% of cases of cancer in men and 33% in women. It has been estimated that 3 mg of 2-naphthylamine, one of the first bladder carcinogens to be identified, is absorbed from the smoke of 20 unfiltered cigarettes.[25] Although earlier studies have suggested an association between bladder cancer and artificial sweeteners such as saccharin and cyclamates, this association has not been proven. Chronic bladder infections and calculus disease also increase the risk of bladder cancer. Bladder cancer occurs among persons harboring the parasite *Schistosoma haematobium* in their bladders. It has been estimated that 85% of Egyptians are infected with the parasites, and bladder tumors represent 10% to 40% of all cancers in Egypt.[23] It is not known whether the parasite excretes a carcinogen or produces its effects through irritation of the bladder.

—— Diagnosis and treatment

The most common sign of bladder cancer is hematuria. Gross hematuria is a presenting sign in 75% of persons with the disease, and microscopic hematuria is present in most others. Occasionally frequency, urgency, and dysuria accompany the hematuria. Because hematuria is often intermittent, the diagnosis is often delayed. Periodic urine cytology is recommended for all persons who are at high risk for the development of bladder cancer because of exposure to urinary tract carcinogens.

The diagnostic methods include cytologic studies, excretory urograms, and cystoscopy and biopsy. High-grade cancers, including in situ lesions, are readily diagnosed in urinary samples using the Papanicolaou's stain (Pap smear). Low-grade tumors are more difficult to detect by this method. Automated systems have been developed and are nearly ready for clinical use. They should be valuable in the detection and follow-up of persons with superficial cancers and may be adapted to the screening of select populations, such as persons with industrial exposure to carcinogenic agents. Ultrasonography and CT scans are used as an aid for staging of the tumor.

The treatment depends on the extent of the lesion and the health of the patient. Endoscopic resection is usually done for diagnostic purposes and may be used as a treatment for superficial lesions. Segmental surgical resection may be used for removing a large single lesion. Intravesicular instillation of chemotherapeutic drugs such as thiotepa, mitomycin C, and doxorubicin (Adriamycin) may be used in persons who present with cancer in situ or multiple superficial lesions.[23,24] When cancer is invasive, cystectomy with resection of the pelvic lymph nodes, prostate, seminal vesicles, and urethra in males is frequently the treatment of choice. Cystectomy requires urinary diversion. Preoperative radiotherapy appears to be beneficial for deeply infiltrating lesions.

In summary, cancer of the bladder is the most common form of urinary tract cancer, accounting for 37,000 new cases each year and 2.5% of all cancer deaths in the United States. Cancer of the bladder can present as low-grade papillary lesions and high-grade flat-type in situ or invasive lesions. The Pap smear is a useful screening test for high-grade carcinomas of the bladder. Although the cause of cancer of the bladder is unknown, evidence suggests that carcinogens excreted in the urine may play a role. Gross hematuria is the most common sign of bladder cancer, occurring in 75% of persons with the disease. Treatment of bladder cancer depends on the cytologic grade of the tumor and the extent of the invasiveness of the lesion.

References

1. McGuire EJ: Physiology of the lower urinary tract. Am J Kidney Dis 2:402, 1983
2. McGuire EJ: Urinary dysfunction in the aged: Neurological considerations. Bull NY Acad Med 56:275, 1980
3. Berne RM, Levy MN: Physiology, 2nd ed, p 814. St Louis, CV Mosby, 1988
4. Mahoney DT, Laferte RL, Blias DJ: Integral storage function and voiding reflexes. Urology 9:95, 1977
5. McConnell EA, Zimmerman MF: Care of Patients with Urologic Problems, p 32. Philadelphia, JB Lippincott, 1983
6. Smith DR: General Urology, 11th ed, p 156. Los Altos, CA, Lange Medical Publishers, 1984
7. Krane RJ, Siroky MB: Clinical Neuro-Urology. Boston, Little, Brown, 1979
8. Frimodt-Miller C: Diabetic cystopathy: Epidemiology and related disorders. Ann Intern Med 92, (P) 2:318, 1980
9. Ellenberg M: Development of urinary bladder dysfunction in diabetes mellitus. Ann Intern Med 92 (2):321, 1980
10. Frimodt-Miller C, Mortenson S: Treatment of diabetic cystopathy. Ann Intern Med 92 (P)2:327, 1980
11. Thon W, Altwein JE: Voiding dysfunction. Urology 23:323, 1984
12. Jacobs SC, Kaufman JM: Complications of permanent bladder catheter drainage in spinal cord injury patients. J Urol 119:740, 1978
13. Lapides J, Diokno AC, Silber SJ: Clean, intermittent self-catheterization in treatment of urinary tract disease. Trans Am Assoc Genitourin Surg 63:92, 1971
14. Perlow DL, Gikas PW, Horwitz EM: Effects of vesicle overdistention on bladder mucin. Urology 18:380, 1981
15. Bates P, Bradley WE, Glen E, et al: The standardization of terminology of lower urinary tract function. J Urol 121:551, 1979

16. Robison J: Incontinence is not a disease. Community Care 399:20, 1982.
17. Green TH: Urinary stress incontinence: Differential diagnosis, pathophysiology, and management. Am J Obstet Gynecol 122:368, 1975
18. Kegel AH: Progressive resistance exercises in the functional restoration of the perineal muscles. Am J Obstet Gynecol 56:238, 1948
19. McCormick K, Scheve AA, Leaby E: Nursing management of urinary incontinence in geriatric inpatients. Nurs Clin North Am 23(1):244, 1988
20. Brocklehurst JC: Noncatheter devices for urinary incontinence in the elderly. Med Instrum 16:167, 1982
21. Stanton SL: Surgical management of female incontinence. In Brocklehurst JC: Urology in the Elderly, p 93. New York, Churchill Livingstone, 1984
22. Frank IN, Keys HM, McCune CS: Urologic and male genital cancers. In Rubin P (ed): Clinical Oncology, 6th ed, p 205. New York, American Cancer Society, 1983
23. Robbins SL, Cotran RS, Kumar V: Pathologic Basis of Disease, 2nd ed, p 1072. Philadelphia, WB Saunders, 1984
24. Murphy WM: Current topics in the pathology of bladder cancer. Pathol Annu 18, P 1:1, 1983
25. Wynder EL, Goldsmith K: The epidemiology of bladder cancer: A second look. Cancer 40:1246, 1977

Bibliography

Abramson AS: Neurogenic bladder: A guide to evaluation and management. Arch Phys Med Rehabil 64:6, 1983

Bissada NK, Finkbeiner AE: Pharmacology of continence and micturition. AFP 20:128, 1979

Burgio KL, Robinson C, Engel BT: The role of biofeedback in Kegel exercise training for stress urinary incontinence. Am J Obstet Gynecol 154:58, 1986

Cella M: The nursing costs of urinary incontinence in a nursing home population. Nurs Clin North Am 23(1):159, 1988

deGroat WC, Booth AM: Physiology of the urinary bladder and urethra. Ann Int Med 92:312, 1980

Fantl JA, Hurt WG, Bump RC, et al: Urethral axis and sphincteric function. Am J Obstet Gynecol 155:554, 1986

Freed SZ: Urinary incontinence in the elderly. Hosp Pract 17:81, 1982

Gershon CR: Rebirth of an old technique—the use of clean, intermittent self-catheterization. J Med Assoc Georgia 71:605, 1982

Hadley EC: Bladder training and related therapies for urinary incontinence in older people. JAMA 256:372, 1986

Helzer MJ, Bartone FF: Intermittent self-catheterization: A revolutionary breakthrough. Nebraska Med J 4:73, 1982

Kaufman JM: Stress urinary incontinence: Current concepts of diagnosis and treatment. J South Carolina Med Assoc 98:671, 1982

Keegan GT, McNichols DW: The evaluation and treatment of urinary incontinence in the elderly. Surg Clin North Am 62:261, 1982

Mastri AR: Neuropathology of diabetic neurogenic bladder. Ann Int Med 92:316, 1980

Mitteness L: The management of urinary incontinence by community-living elderly. Gerontologist 27(2): 185, 1987

Mix LC: Occult neuropathic bladder. Urology 10:1, 1977

Morishita L: Nursing evaluation and treatment of geriatric outpatients with urinary incontinence. Nurs Clin North Am 23(1):189, 1988

Murphy WM, Soloway MS: Developing carcinoma (dysplasia) of the urinary bladder. Pathol Annu 18:197, 1983

Ouslander JG: Diagnostic evaluation of geriatric urinary incontinence. Clin Geriatr Med 2:715, 1986

Ouslander JG: Urinary incontinence. Clin Geriatr Med 2:712, 1986

Ouslander JG, Bruskewitz R: Disorders of micturition in the aging patient. Adv Intern Med 34:165, 1989

Ouslander JG, Sier HC: Drug therapy for geriatric urinary incontinence. Geriatr Clin Med 2:789, 1986

Palmer MH: Incontinence. Nurs Clin North Am 23(1): 139, 1988

Pierson CA: Urinary incontinence: New methods of diagnosis and treatment. JOGN 10:407, 1981

Rawl JC: Clean intermittent catheterization—an update. J South Carolina Med Assoc 78:715, 1982

Resnick NM, Yalla SV: Management of urinary incontinence in the elderly. N Engl J Med 313:800, 1985

Sheperd A, Tribe E, Torrens MJ: Simple practical techniques in the management of urinary incontinence. International Rehab Med 4:15, 1982

Sier H, Ouslander J, Orzeck S: Urinary incontinence among geriatric patients in an acute-care hospital. JAMA 257:1767, 1986

Soloway MS: Bladder cancer: Management of an increasingly common tumor. Bladder Cancer 73:138, 1983

Weiss RM: Clinical correlations of ureteral physiology. Am J Kidney Dis 2:409, 1983

Wells T: Promoting urine control in older adults. Geriatric Nurs 1:236, 1980

Williams ME, Pannill FC: Urinary incontinence in the elderly. Ann Int Med 97:895, 1982

Wyman JF: Nursing assessment of the incontinent geriatric outpatient. Nurs Clin North Am 23(1):169, 1988

Structure and Function of the Male Genitourinary System

Genitourinary structures
  Embryonic development
  Testes and scrotum
    Duct system
    Accessory organs
  Penis

Reproductive function
  Spermatogenesis
  Hormonal control of male reproductive function

Neural control of sexual function
  Aging changes

Objectives

After you have studied this chapter, you should be able to meet the following objectives:

_____ Describe the anatomy of the testes and scrotum.

_____ Describe the anatomy of the duct system and accessory organs.

_____ Cite the rationales that support and oppose circumcision of the male infant.

_____ Describe the process of spermatogenesis.

_____ State the name of the testicular cells that produce testosterone.

_____ State the functions of testosterone.

_____ Draw a diagram illustrating the secretion, site of action, and feedback control of GnRH, LH, and FSH.

_____ Describe the function of FSH in terms of spermatogenesis.

_____ Describe the autonomic nervous system control of erection and ejaculation.

_____ Describe changes in the male reproductive system that occur with aging.

The male genitourinary system consists of a pair of gonads, the testes, a system of excretory ducts, and the accessory organs. The accessory organs include the penis, the bulbourethral glands, the prostate gland, and the seminal vesicles. The system has two basic functions—urine elimination and reproduction. This chapter discusses the embryonic development of the male reproductive structures, the structure of the male genitourinary system, spermatogenesis, sexual performance, hormonal regulation of reproductive function in the male, and changes in genitourinary function that occur at puberty and as a result of the aging process.

Genitourinary structures

—— Embryonic development

The sex of an individual is determined at the time of fertilization by the sex chromosomes. In the early stages of embryonic development the tissues from which the male and female reproductive organs develop are undifferentiated. Until approximately the seventh week of gestation, it is impossible to determine whether the embryo is male or female unless the chromosomes are studied. Until this time, the genital tracts of both the male and the female consist of two wolffian ducts, from which the male genitalia develop, and two müllerian ducts, from which the female genital structures develop. During this period of gestation, the gonads (ovaries and testes) are also undifferentiated.

In the seventh week of embryonic life the gonadal ridge of an embryo with XY chromosomes differentiates to form testes and that of an embryo with XX chromosomes differentiates to form into ovaries. The fetal testes produce two hormones: one stimulates development of the wolffian ducts into structures that form seminal vesicles, vas deferens, and epididymis; the other suppresses the development of female genital structures from the müllerian ducts. Development of

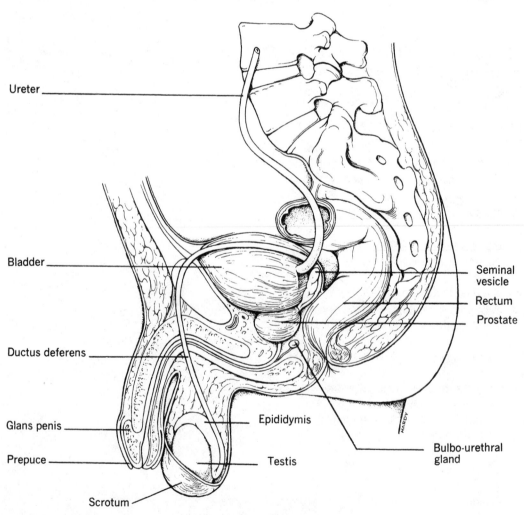

Figure 34-1 The structures of the male reproductive system, including the testes, the scrotum, and the excretory ducts. (*Chaffee EE, Greisheimer EM: Basic Physiology and Anatomy, 3rd ed. Philadelphia, JB Lippincott, 1974*)

the external male genital structures begins during the twelfth week of embryonic life. It is the presence or absence of the androgen testosterone that determines whether an embryo will develop male or female genital structures. In the absence of testosterone, a male embryo with an XY chromosomal pattern will develop female genitalia. It has been hypothesized that the Y chromosome contains a gene that codes for a substance called the H-Y antigen. In the presence of the H-Y antigen, the embryonic gonads develop into testes and in its absence the gonads develop into ovaries.[1]

Testes and scrotum

The testes, or male gonads, are two egg-shaped structures located outside the abdominal cavity in the scrotum, where they are suspended by the spermatic cord (Figure 34-1). The spermatic cord is composed of the arteries, veins, lymphatics, and excretory ducts that supply the testes. The cremaster muscle that suspends the testes and forms the muscle of the scrotum is also contained in the spermatic cord. The testes are responsible for both testosterone and sperm production.

The scrotum, which houses the testes, is made up of an outer skin layer, which forms rugae or folds and is continuous with the perineum and outer skin of the thighs. Under the outer skin lies a thin layer of muscle and fascia, the *tunica dartos.* This layer contains a septum that separates the two testes.

A function of the scrotum is to regulate the temperature of the testes. The optimal temperature for sperm production is about 2°F to 3°F below body temperature. If the testicular temperature is too low, the muscles within the scrotum contract, causing the testes to be brought up tight against the body. On the other hand, when the testicular temperature rises, the muscles relax, which allows the scrotal sac to fall away from the body. Some tight-fitting undergarments hold the testes against the body and are thought to contribute to infertility by interfering with the thermoregulatory function of the scrotum. Cryptorchidism, the failure of the testes to descend into the scrotum, also exposes the testes to the higher temperature of the body.

The testes and epididymis are enclosed in a double-layered membrane, the *tunica vaginalis,* which is derived embryologically from the abdominal peritoneum. An outer covering, the *tunica albuginea,* is a tough white fibrous sheath that resembles the sclera of the eye. The tunica albuginea protects the testes and gives them their ovoid shape.

Embryologically, the testes do not develop within the scrotal sac; they develop in the abdominal cavity and then descend through the inguinal canal into a long pouch of peritoneum (which becomes the tunica vaginalis) in the scrotum during the seventh to the ninth month of fetal life. The descent of the testes is thought to be caused by the male hormone, testosterone, which is very active during this stage of development. Just prior to birth, the inguinal canal closes almost completely. Failure of this canal to close predisposes to the development of an inguinal hernia later in life.

Duct system

Internally, the testes are composed of several hundred compartments or lobules (Figure 34-2). Each lobule contains one or more coiled *seminiferous* tubules. These tubules are the site of sperm production. As the tubules lead into the *efferent ducts,* the seminiferous tubules become the *rete testis.* From the rete testis, 10,000 to 20,000 efferent ducts emerge to join the epididymis, which is the final site for sperm maturation. Interspersed in the connective tissue that fills the spaces between the seminiferous tubules are the epithelial cells—the *cells of Leydig*—which produce *testosterone.*

Accessory organs

Sperm are transported through the reproductive structures by movement of the seminal fluid, which is combined with secretions from the accessory sex glands, epididymis, seminal vesicles, prostate, and Cowper's glands. When sperm is combined with the seminal plasma it is called *semen.*

The sperm enters the epididymis from the efferent ductules in the testes. Because the sperm are

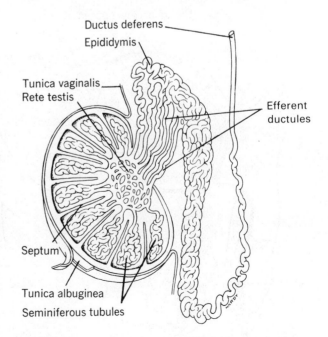

Figure 34-2 The parts of the testes and epididymis. (*Chaffee EE, Lytle IM: Basic Physiology and Anatomy, 4th ed. Philadelphia, JB Lippincott, 1980*)

not motile at this stage of development, peristaltic movements of the ductal walls of the epididymis aid in sperm movement. The sperm continue their migration through the *ductus deferens,* or vas deferens, and enter the *ampulla,* where they are stored until they are released through ejaculation (Figure 34-3). Sperm can be stored in the genital ducts for as long as 42 days and still maintain their fertility.

From the ampulla, the sperm moves to the seminal vesicle, which secretes a fluid containing fructose and other substances required to nourish the sperm. Seminal vesicles are primarily secretory organs. Each of the paired seminal vesicles is lined with secretory epithelium containing an abundance of fructose, prostaglandins, and fibrinogens. The fructose provides nutrients for the ejaculated sperm. The prostaglandins are thought to assist in fertilization by making the cervical mucus more receptive to sperm and by causing reverse peristaltic contractions in the uterus and fallopian tubes to move the sperm toward the ovaries.[2]

The seminal vesicle leads into the ejaculatory duct, which enters the posterior part of the prostate and continues through until it ends in the prostatic portion of the urethra. During emission each vesicle empties fluid into the ejaculatory duct which adds bulk to the semen. The prostate gland, in turn, secretes a thin milky alkaline fluid containing citric acid, calcium, acid phosphate, a clotting enzyme, and a profibrinolysin. During emission the capsule of the prostate contracts, and the added fluid increases the bulk of the semen. The alkaline nature of these secretions is essential for successful fertilization of the ovum, since sperm mobilization occurs at a pH of 6.0 to 6.5. Both vaginal secretions and the fluid from the vas deferens are strongly acidic. The bulbourethral, or Cowper's glands, lie on either side of the membranous urethra. These glands secrete an alkaline mucus which probably aids in neutralizing acids from the urine that remain in the urethra.

A man usually ejaculates about 2 ml to 5 ml of semen. The ejaculate may vary with frequency of intercourse. It is less with frequent ejaculation and may increase two to four times its normal amount during periods of abstinence. The semen that is ejaculated is largely fluid—98% fluid and about 2% sperm.

Penis

The penis is the external genital organ through which the urethra passes. Anatomically, the external penis consists of a shaft that ends in a tip called the *glans* (Figure 34-4). The loose skin of the penis shaft folds to cover the glans, forming the *prepuce,* or *foreskin.* It is this cuff of skin that is removed during circumcision. Recently, there has been mounting opposition to the once routine practice of neonatal circumcision from the medical community and the public alike, based on the argument that the small risks of death and mutilation do not justify circumcision. The American College of Obstetrics and Gynecologists and the American Academy of Pediatrics have concluded that there is no absolute medical indication for routine circumcision. Those supporting the

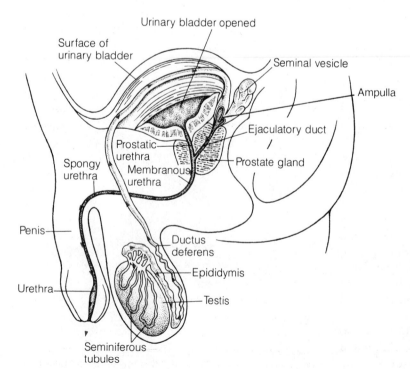

Figure 34-3 The excretory ducts of the male reproductive system and the path that sperm follows as it leaves the testis and travels to the urethra. (*Chaffee EE, Gresheimer EM: Basic Physiology and Anatomy, 3rd ed. Philadelphia, JB Lippincott, 1974*)

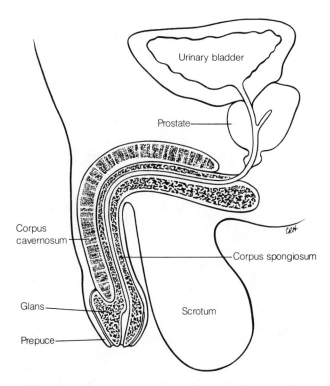

Figure 34-4 Sagittal section of the penis, showing the prepuce, glans, corpus cavernosum, and corpus spongiosum.

practice contend, on the other hand, that the higher rates of infection and penile problems among uncircumcised boys after infancy indicate continued use of the procedure. It is argued that uncircumcized male children have more balanitis and irritation after infancy.[4,5]

The glans of the penis contains many sensory nerves, making this the most sensitive portion of the penile shaft. The cylindrical body or shaft of the penis is composed of three masses of erectile tissue held together by fibrous strands and covered with skin. The two lateral masses of tissue are called the *corpora cavernosa.* The third ventral mass is called the *corpus spongiosum.* The cavernous masses are composed of erectile tissue that distends with blood during penile erection.

In summary, the male genitourinary system functions in both urine elimination and reproduction. The reproductive system consists of a pair of gonads (the testes), a system of excretory ducts (seminiferous tubules and efferent ducts), the accessory organs (epididymis, seminal vesicles, prostate, and Cowper's glands), and the penis. The sex of an individual is determined by the sex chromosomes at the time of fertilization. During the seventh week of gestation, the XY chromosome pattern in the male is responsible for the development of the testes with the subsequent production of testosterone and testosterone-stimulated

development of the internal and external male genital structures. Prior to this period of embryonic development, the tissues from which the reproductive structures of the male and female develop are undifferentiated. In the absence of testosterone production, the male embryo with an XY chromosomal pattern will develop female genitalia.

Reproductive function

At puberty, the male gonads and testes begin to mature and to carry out spermatogenesis and hormone production. Sometime around the age of 10 or 11, the adenohypophysis, or anterior pituitary, begins to secrete the gonadotropins that stimulate testicular function and cause the interstitial cells to begin producing testosterone. About the same time, hormonal stimulation induces mitotic activity of the germ cells that develop in sperm. Once cell maturation has begun, the testes begin to enlarge rapidly as the individual tubules grow. Full maturity and spermatogenesis are usually attained by age 15 or 16.

Spermatogenesis

Spermatogenesis refers to the generation of sperm. It begins at an average age of 13 and continues throughout the reproductive years of a man's life. Spermatogenesis occurs in the seminiferous tubules of the testes. These tubules, if placed end to end, would measure about 750 feet. The outer layer of the seminiferous tubules are made up of connective tissue and smooth muscle; the inner lining is composed of Sertoli cells, within which are embedded the spermatogonia and sperm in various stages of development (Figure 34-5). The Sertoli cells secrete a special fluid that contains nutrients to bathe and nourish the immature germ cells; they provide digestive enzymes that play a role in spermiation (converting the spermatocytes to sperm); and they are thought to play a role in shaping the head and tail of the sperm. In addition the Sertoli cells secrete several hormones, including müllerian inhibitory factor (MIF), which is secreted by the testes during fetal life to inhibit development of fallopian tubes; estradiol, the principal feminizing sex hormone, which seems to be required in the male for spermatogenesis; and inhibin, which serves to control the function of the Sertoli cells through feedback inhibition of follicle-stimulating hormone (FSH) from the anterior pituitary gland.[6]

In the first stage of spermatogenesis, small unspecialized germinal cells located immediately adjacent to the tubular wall, called the *spermatogonia,* undergo rapid mitotic division and provide a continuous source of new germinal cells. As these cells multi-

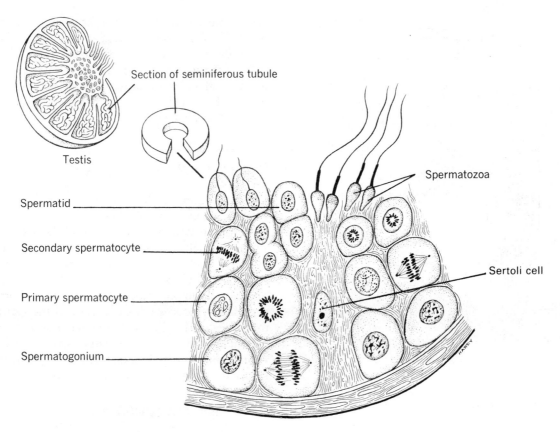

Testis

Section of seminiferous tubule

Spermatozoa

Spermatid

Secondary spermatocyte

Sertoli cell

Primary spermatocyte

Spermatogonium

Figure 34-5 A section of a seminiferous tubule, showing the various stages of spermatogenesis. (*Chaffee EE, Lytle IM: Basic Physiology and Anatomy, 4th ed. Philadelphia, JB Lippincott, 1980*)

ply, the more mature spermatogonia divide into two daughter cells, which grow in size and become the *primary spermatocytes*—the precursors of sperm. Over a period of several weeks, large primary spermatocytes divide by meiosis to form two smaller secondary spermatocytes. Each of the secondary spermatocytes, in turn, divides to form two *spermatids*, or infant sperm.

The spermatid elongates into a *spermatozoon*, or mature sperm cell, with a head and tail (Figure 34-6). The outside of the anterior two-thirds of the head, called the *acrosome*, contains enzymes necessary for penetration and fertilization of the ovum. To-and-fro (flagellar) motion of the tail provides movement for the sperm. The energy for this process is supplied by the mitochondria in the tail. Normal sperm move in a straight line at a velocity of 1 mm to 4 mm per minute. This allows them to move through the female genital tract.

When the sperm grow to full size they move to the epididymis to further mature and gain mobility. A small quantity of sperm can be stored in the epididymis, but most are stored in the vas deferens or the ampulla of the vas deferens. With excessive sexual activity storage may be no longer than a few days. The sperm can live for many weeks in the male genital tract; however, in the female genital tract, their life expectancy is one or two days. Frozen sperm have been preserved for years.

The entire process of spermatogenesis takes about 60 to 70 days. The sperm count in a normal ejaculate is about 100 million to 400 million. Infertility may occur when insufficient numbers of motile, healthy sperm are present.

Hormonal control of male reproductive function

The male sex hormones are called androgens. Testosterone is the main androgen produced in the testes. The adrenal cortex also produces androgens, but in much smaller quantities than the testes. Over 95% of the testosterone is secreted by the testes; the remainder is secreted by the adrenals.

Testosterone is secreted by the interstitial cells of Leydig in the testes. It is metabolized in the liver and then excreted by the kidneys. In the bloodstream testosterone exists in a free or a bound form. The bound form is attached to plasma proteins, including albumin and the sex-hormone binding protein produced by the liver. About 2% is not bound

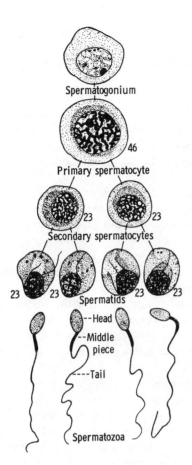

Figure 34-6 The various stages of spermatogenesis. *(Chaffee EE, Lytle IM: Basic Physiology and Anatomy, 4th ed. Philadelphia, JB Lippincott, 1980)*

and is able to enter the cell and exert its metabolic effects. Testosterone exerts a variety of biologic effects in the male (Chart 34-1). In the male embryo, testosterone is essential for the appropriate differentiation of the internal and external genitalia. Testosterone is essential to the development of primary and secondary male sex characteristics during puberty and for the maintenance of these characteristics during adult life. In addition, androgens function as anabolic agents in both males and females to promote metabolism and musculoskeletal growth.

The hypothalamus and the anterior pituitary gland play an essential role in promoting spermatogenic activity in the testes and maintaining endocrine function of the testes by means of the gonadotropic hormones. The release of gonadotropic hormones from the pituitary gland is regulated by the gonadotropin-releasing factor (GnRH), which is synthesized by the hypothalamus and secreted into the hypothalamohypophyseal portal blood (Figure 34-7). Two gonadotropic hormones are secreted by the pituitary gland: follicle-stimulating hormone (FSH) and luteinizing hormone (LH). In the male, LH is also called interstitial cell-stimulating hormone (ICSH).

Chart 34-1. Main actions of testosterone

Induces differentiation of the male genital tract during fetal development
Induces development of primary and secondary sex characteristics:
  Gonadal function
  External genitalia and accessory organs
  Male voice timbre
  Male skin characteristics
  Male hair distribution
Anabolic effects
  Promotes protein metabolism
  Promotes musculoskeletal growth
  Influences subcutaneous fat distribution
Promotes spermatogenesis (in FSH-primed tubules) and maturation of sperm

The production of testosterone by the interstitial cells of Leydig is regulated by LH (Figure 34-7). FSH binds selectively to the Sertoli cells, where it functions in the initiation of spermatogenesis. Although FSH is necessary for the initiation of spermatogenesis, full maturation of the spermatozoa requires testosterone. The Sertoli cells produce an androgen-binding protein that binds testosterone; one of the major actions of FSH may be the regulation of androgen-binding protein production by the Sertoli cells as a means of maintaining high intratubular concentrations of testosterone.

Circulating levels of the gonadotropic hormones are regulated in a negative feedback manner by testosterone. High levels of testosterone produce a

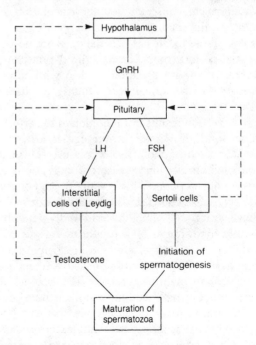

Figure 34-7 Hypothalamic-pituitary feedback control of spermatogenesis and testosterone levels in the male.

negative feedback suppression of LH secretion through a direct action on the pituitary and an inhibitory effect on the hypothalamus. FSH is thought to be inhibited by a substance called *inhibin*, which is produced by the Sertoli cells. Inhibin appears to act mainly at the level of the pituitary gland.[1] Unlike the cyclic hormonal pattern in the female, in the male FSH, LH, and testosterone secretion and spermatogenesis occur at relatively unchanging rates during adulthood.

Neural control of sexual function

In the male, sexual function requires both erection and ejaculation. The physiology of penile erection involves a complex interaction between three systems of the body: the vascular system, the nervous system, and the endocrine system. Although much research has been done on erectile function and dysfunction, many aspects of function remain unclear.

The most important source of impulse stimulation for initiating the male sexual act is the glans penis, which contains a highly organized sensory system. Afferent impulses from sensory receptors in the glans penis pass through the pudendal nerve to ascending fibers in the spinal cord via the sacral plexus. Stimulation of other perineal areas such as the anal epithelium, the scrotum, and the testes can transmit signals to the cord, adding to sexual satisfaction. Ascending fibers from the spinal pathways communicate with undefined areas of the cerebrum. There is a psychic element to sexual stimulation, as thinking sexual thoughts can cause erection and ejaculation. Even though psychic involvement and higher-center functions contribute to the sex act, they are not necessary for sexual performance. Genital stimulation can produce erection and ejaculation in men with complete transection of the spinal cord (this is discussed in Chapter 49).

Erection results from dilation of the arteries in the penis and an increase in intracavernous pressure to levels above the systolic blood pressure. This causes arterial blood under high pressure to build up in erectile tissue of the penis. This erectile tissue consists of large cavernous venous sinusoids, which normally are relatively empty but which fill up rapidly when blood flows into them under high pressure. Various neurotransmitters that control erection are being studied. Several have been identified in penile tissue, including vasoactive intestinal polypeptide (VIP), acetylcholine, and norepinephrine. Erection most likely involves several neurotransmitters. One possibility is that VIP and acetylcholine act synergistically to relax arteriolar and trabecular smooth muscle. Detumescence, or loss of erection, is probably due to the recovery of vascular smooth muscle tone and reactivation of norepinephrine release, which causes contraction of the trabecular muscles and penile arterioles and thereby decreases vascular inflow and increases outflow.[7]

Emission and ejaculation constitute the culmination of the male sexual act. With increasing intensity of the sexual stimulus, the reflex centers of the spinal cord begin to emit sympathetic impulses that leave the cord at the L1 and L2 level and pass through the hypogastric plexus to the genital organs to initiate emission, which is the forerunner of ejaculation. Fluid from the vas deferens, the ampulla, the prostate, and the seminal vesicles is mixed with secretions from the bulbourethral glands and propelled into the internal urethra by contractions of the ischiocavernous and bulbocavernous muscles. The filling of the internal urethra elicits signals that are transmitted through the pudendal nerves from the spinal cord. Increases in pressure in the urethra cause the semen to be propelled to the exterior, resulting in ejaculation. The period of emission and ejaculation is termed *male orgasm*. After ejaculation, erection ceases within one to two minutes.[8]

The role of circulating androgens in regard to sexual function remains unclear. It is apparent that sexual desire and performance is dependent on some threshold level of testosterone; however, this level varies from man to man. Studies of hypogonadal and castrated males show a variety of sexual behavior ranging from complete loss of libido to normal sexual activity. It may be that the role of testosterone in male sexuality is in the area of sexual interest motivation, with individual intrapsychic factors playing a significant role.[9]

Aging changes

Like other body systems, the male reproductive system undergoes degenerative changes as a result of the aging process; it becomes less efficient with age. The declining physiologic efficiency of male reproductive function occurs gradually and involves the endocrine, circulatory, and neuromuscular systems. Compared with the marked physiologic change in aging females, the changes in the aging male are more gradual and less drastic. Gonadal and reproductive failure are not generally related directly to age, because a male remains fertile into advanced age. Eighty- and 90-year-olds have been known to father children.

Contrary to popular belief, many investigators consider that there is no physiological basis for what has been termed the male climacteric. Instead, they attribute its symptomatology to psychologic mechanisms. An aging man may experience midlife crisis with concomitant psychosomatic manifestations that mimic the symptomatology of menopause. Most experts agree that decline in male sexual desire parallels decline in physical vigor and represents the aging of all the body tissues and neural structures.

As the male ages, his reproductive system differs measurably in both structure and function from that of the younger male. Male sex hormone levels, particularly of testosterone, decrease with age, the decline starting later, on the average, than in women. The sex hormones play a part in the structure and function of the reproductive system and other body systems from conception to old age; they affect protein synthesis, salt and water balance, bone growth, and cardiovascular function. Decreasing levels of testosterone affect sexual energy, muscle strength, and the genital tissues. The testes become smaller and lose their firmness. The seminiferous tubules, which produce spermatozoa, thicken and begin a degenerative process which finally inhibits sperm production, resulting in a decrease of viable spermatozoa.[10] The prostate gland enlarges, and its contractions become weaker. The force of ejaculation decreases because of a reduction in the volume and viscosity of the seminal fluid. The seminal vesicle changes little from childhood to puberty. The pubertal increases in the fluid capacity of the gland remain throughout adulthood and then decline after age 60. After 60, the walls of the seminal vesicles thin, the epithelium decreases in height, and the muscle layer is replaced by connective tissue. Age-related changes in the penis consist of fibrotic changes in the trabeculae in the corpus spongiosum, with progressive sclerotic changes in both arteries and veins. Sclerotic changes also follow in the corpora cavernosa, the condition becoming generalized in the 55- to-60-year-old age group.[11]

As a sexual partner, the aging male exhibits some differences in responsiveness and activity from his younger counterpart. Masters and Johnson (1970) studied the significant aging changes in the physiology of the sex act.[12] They noted that frequency of intercourse, intensity of sensation, speed of attaining erection, and force of ejaculation are all reduced.

Many of our social and cultural practices do not support or encourage sexual activity in the elderly. Research, however, indicates that not only does sexual thought and feeling continue into old age but sexual activity also continues for most healthy older individuals.[13] Most gerontologists would agree that continued sexual interest and activity can be therapeutic for the elderly.

Sexual dysfunction in the elderly male is often directly related to the general physical condition of the individual. Diseases that accompany aging can have direct bearing on male reproductive organs. Various cardiovascular, respiratory, hormonal, neurologic, and hematologic disorders can be responsible for secondary impotence. For example, vascular disease affects male potency because it may impair blood flow to the pudendal arteries or their tributaries, resulting in loss of blood volume with subsequent poor distention of the vascular spaces of erectile tissue. Other diseases affecting potency include hypertension, diabetes, cardiac disease, and malignancies of the reproductive organs.[13,14,15]

One of the greatest inhibitors of sexual functioning in older males is loss of self-esteem and development of a negative self-image. The emphasis on youth pervades much of our society both in terms of physical attractiveness and sexuality. The image of success for a man often involves qualities of masculinity and sexual attractiveness. When queried about success, men often mentioned such things as work, managing money well, participating in sports or other activities, discussing politics or world events, advising younger people, and being attractive to women. When a man feels good about himself and expresses self-confidence, sexual attractiveness is communicated regardless of age. Many older men live in environments that are not sensitive to the importance of helping them maintain a positive self-image. Premature cessation of the aforementioned esteem-building activities can contribute to loss of libido and zest for life in the elderly male.[16]

In summary, the function of the male reproductive system is under the negative feedback control of the hypothalamus and the anterior pituitary gonadotropic hormones FSH and LH. Spermatogenesis is initiated by FSH, and the production of testosterone is regulated by LH. Testosterone, the major sex hormone in the male, is produced by the interstitial cells of Leydig in the testes. In addition to the differentiation of the internal and external genitalia in the male embryo, testosterone is essential for the development of secondary male characteristics during puberty, the maintenance of these characteristics during adult life, and spermatozoa maturation.

Like other body systems, the male reproductive system undergoes changes as a result of the aging process. The changes occur gradually and involve parallel changes in endocrine, circulatory, and neuromuscular function. Testosterone levels decrease, the size and firmness of the testes decrease, sperm production declines, and the prostate gland enlarges. There is usually a decrease in frequency of intercourse, intensity of sensation, speed of attaining erection, and force of ejaculation. However, sexual thought, interest, and activity usually continue into old age.

References

1. Greenspan FS, Forshan PH: Basic and Clinical Endocrinology, pp 339–343. Los Altos, CA, Lange Medical Publications, 1983

2. Guyton AC: Textbook of Medical Physiology, 7th ed, pp 954–967. Philadelphia, WB Saunders, 1986

3. Tanagho EA, McAnnick JW: Smith's General Urology, 12th ed, pp 1–15. Norwalk, CT, Appleton and Lange, 1988

4. Fergusson DM, Lawton JM, Shannon JT: Neonatal circumcision and penile problems: An 8-year longitudinal study. Pediatrics 81:537, 1988

5. Herzog LW, Alvarez SR: The frequency of foreskin problems in uncircumcised children. Am J Dis Child 140:254, 1986

6. West JB: Best and Taylor's Physiologic Basis of Medical Practice, 11th ed, pp 907–920. Baltimore, Williams & Wilkins, 1985

7. Lue TF: Male sexual dysfunction. In Smith DR (ed): General Urology, 12th ed, pp 663–677. Norwalk, Appleton and Lange, 1988

8. Aboseif SR: Hemodynamics of penile erection. Urol Clin North Am 15:1, 1988

9. Blackmore C: The impact of orchiectomy upon the sexuality of the man with testicular cancer. Cancer Nurs 11:33, 1988

10. Weg RB: Normal aging changes in the reproductive system. In Burnside IM (ed): Nursing and the Aged, pp 362–374. New York, McGraw-Hill, 1981

11. Croft LH: Physiology of Aging, pp 47–65. Boston, John Wright, 1982

12. Masters WH, Johnson V: Human Sexual Inadequacy, pp 337–338. Boston, Little, Brown, 1970

13. Yeaworth RC, Friedman JS: Sexuality in later life. Nurs Clin North Am 10:565, 1975

14. Steinke EE, Bergen MB: Sexuality and aging: A review of the literature from a nursing perspective. J Gerontol Nurs 12:6, 1986

15. Carnevali DL, Patrick M: Nursing Management of the Elderly, pp 60–61. Philadelphia, JB Lippincott, 1986

16. Breitiung JC: Caring for the Older Adult, pp 100–111. Philadelphia, WB Saunders, 1987

Alterations in Male Genitourinary Function

Disorders of the penis
  Hypospadias and epispadias
  Phimosis and paraphimosis
  Priapism
  Peyronie's disease
  Balanitis xerotica obliterans
  Cancer of the penis
Disorders of the scrotum and
    testes
  Cryptorchidisim
  Hydrocele

Hematocele
Spermatocele
Testicular torsion
Varicocele
Epididymitis
Orchitis
Neoplasms
  Cancer of the scrotum
  Testicular cancer

Disorders of the prostate
  Prostatitis
    Acute bacterial prostatitis
    Chronic bacterial prostatitis
    Nonbacterial prostatitis
    Prostatodynia
  Benign prostatic hyperplasia
  Prostatic cancer

Objectives

After you have studied this chapter, you should be able to meet the following objectives:

_____ State the difference between hypospadias and epispadias.

_____ Cite the significance of phimosis.

_____ Describe the pathology of priapism.

_____ Describe the anatomic changes that occur with Peyronie's disease.

_____ Describe the appearance of balanitis xerotica obliterans.

_____ List the signs of penile cancer.

_____ State the cause of cryptorchidism.

_____ Describe the potential risks associated with cryptorchidism.

_____ Compare the etiology and appearance of hydrocele, hematocele, and spermatocele.

_____ State the difference between extravaginal and intravaginal testicular torsion.

_____ State why testicular torsion of the intravaginal type is a true surgical emergency.

_____ Explain the importance of early treatment of varicocele.

_____ State the major cause of epididymitis in men over 35 years of age.

_____ Describe the symptoms of epididymitis.

_____ State the risk associated with mumps orchitis.

_____ Relate environmental factors to scrotal cancer.

_____ State which age group has the highest incidence of testicular cancer.

_____ Describe testicular self-examination as recommended by the American Cancer Society.

_____ State the cell types involved in seminoma, embryonal carcinoma, teratoma, and choriocarcinoma tumors of the testes.

_____ Relate the recent change in the cure rate for testicular cancers to improvements in detection, diagnosis, clinical staging, and treatment.

_____ Compare the pathology and symptoms of acute bacterial prostatitis, chronic bacterial prostatitis, nonbacterial prostatitis, and prostatodynia.

_____ Describe the physical dysfunction associated with benign prostatic hyperplasia.

_____ List the methods used in the diagnosis and treatment of prostatic cancer.

The male genitourinary system is subject to structural defects, inflammation, and neoplasms, all of which can affect urine elimination, sexual function, and fertility. This chapter discusses disorders of the penis, the scrotum and testes, and the prostate.

Disorders of the penis

The penis houses the urethra and the erectile tissue, which becomes engorged with blood during sexual stimulation. Disorders of the penis include congenital and acquired defects, inflammatory conditions, and neoplasms.

Hypospadias and epispadias

Hypospadias is a congenital defect present in about 1 out of every 400 to 500 male infants. In this disorder, the termination of the urethra is on the ventral surface of the penis. A less common defect is epispadias, in which the opening of the urethra is on the dorsal surface of the penis (Figure 35-1). Both of these abnormalities are often accompanied by other congenital defects, such as undescended testicles and chordee, or ventral bowing, of the penis.

Surgery is required for the correction of both hypospadias and epispadias. Infants born with these disorders are not circumcised because the foreskin is required in the plastic surgery done to correct the defect. When additional deformities such as chordee

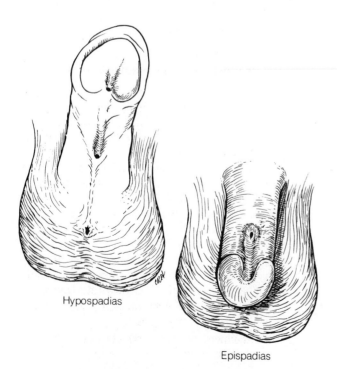

Hypospadias

Epispadias

Figure 35-1 Hypospadias and epispadias.

are present, the surgical repair procedure may be done in stages. Usually, it is suggested that surgical correction be done before the child enters school. The adult male who has not undergone surgery will not have problems with erection or sexual function, but his semen may run out of the vagina during intercourse and thus interfere with impregnation.

Phimosis and paraphimosis

Phimosis refers to a tightening of the penile foreskin that prevents its retraction over the glans. Embryologically the foreskin develops, beginning the 8th week of gestation, as a thickening of the epidermis that eventually grows forward over the base of the glans. By the 16th week of gestation the prepuce and the glans are adherent. Only 4% of newborns have a fully retractable foreskin. With growth, a space develops between the glans and foreskin, and by 6 months, 20% of males have a retractable foreskin; by 1 year, the figure is 50%; and by 3 years, 90%.

Because the foreskin of many males cannot be fully retracted in early childhood, it is important that the area be cleansed thoroughly. There is no need to forcibly retract the foreskin, since this could lead to infection, scarring, or paraphimosis. As the child grows, the foreskin becomes retractable and the glans and foreskin should be cleansed routinely. If symptomatic phimosis occurs after childhood it can cause difficulty with voiding or sexual activity. Circumcision is then the treatment of choice.[1]

In a related condition called paraphimosis, the foreskin is so tight and constricted that it cannot cover the glans. A very tight foreskin can constrict the blood supply to the glans and lead to ischemia and necrosis. Many cases of paraphimosis occur secondary to the foreskin being retracted for an extended period, as in the case of uncircumcised catheterized males.

Priapism

Priapism is a prolonged, painful, nonsexual erection that can persist for hours or days. The condition is caused by impaired hemodynamic conditions in the corpora cavernosa of the penis. Cavernosography of the penis has shown priapism to be divided into two distinct types: *stasis priapism*, in which there is persistent blood stasis, and *high-flow priapism*, in which blood flow is maintained or even increased. In high-flow priapism the penis is less rigid than in stasis priapism; there is also less pain and discomfort.[2]

Priapism has been recorded in all age groups and has many etiologies. Priapism can be classified as primary (idiopathic) or secondary to other disorders, such as neurogenic disorders, trauma, inflammations, infections, hematologic disease (*e.g.*, sickle cell anemia), and congenital defects. Various chemicals and medications such as anticoagulants, methaqualone, adrenal corticosteroids, phenothiazines, guanethidine, hydralazine, exogenous testosterone, and trazodone have been associated with prolonged erection.[3] Any agent affecting impulse transmission at the neuromuscular junction of the corpus cavernosum can induce prolonged erection: thus, drug-induced erection is a frequent cause of priapism. A recent treatment for impotence that includes intracorporeal injection of papaverine has increased the incidence of iatrogenic priapism.[4] Treatment may consist of analgesics, sedation, cold compresses or enemas of cold saline, and aspiration of the corpus cavernosum. If less aggressive treatment does not produce detumescence, a shunt may be established between the corpus cavernosum and the corpus spongiosum, followed by intermittent postoperative compression of the penis.

The prognosis in terms of whether or not fibrosis or erectile failure will occur is determined by the severity and duration of blood stasis. In high-flow priapism lasting for weeks, the damaging stimuli of decreased oxygen tension and intracavernal blood pressure are less pronounced than in stasis priapism. Normal erectile potency can be restored even after a very long duration of high-flow priapism. Persistent stasis priapism, in contrast, is known to result in erectile tissue fibrosis and functional failure unless resolved or surgically treated within 24 hours of onset.[2]

Peyronie's disease

Peyronie's disease involves a localized and progressive fibrosis of unknown etiology that affects the tunica albuginea at the top of the penile shaft (Figure 35-2). It is characterized initially by a perivascular inflammatory cell infiltrate which results in a fibrous plaque containing excessive collagen. This plaque may become calcified and bony.[4] The fibrous tissue prevents lengthening of the involved area during erection, making intercourse difficult and painful. The disease usually occurs in middle-age or elderly men. Recent cytologic evidence indicates random chromosomal changes associated with the plaque tissue, suggesting karyotypic instability. However, it is unclear whether this instability represents multiple pathways for the development of the disease or its secondary consequences.[5]

The treatment may consist of injecting hydrocortisone into the fibrous area, administering vitamin E, using ultrasound wave therapy, or administering fibrolytic agents such as potassium para-aminobenzoate. The fibrous tissue may be removed surgically, although this may impair potency. Many cases of Peyronie's disease are self-limiting. Some practitioners report a 50% or higher spontaneous resolution rate. For this reason, attempts at surgical correction are often delayed.

Balanitis xerotica obliterans (leukoplakia of the penis)

The cause of this disease, which is histologically similar to lichen sclerosus in the female, is unknown. On rare occasions it can cause meatal stenosis that requires surgical intervention. The foreskin shows an expanding area of pigment loss and atrophic sclerotic changes. This is accompanied by atrophy of the skin and poor cohesion of the epidermis to underlying connective tissue, which accounts for the hemorrhagic changes of the glans that accompany even mild trauma. Treatments including local steroids and vitamin E have been relatively unsuccessful. Immediate meatotomy is indicated if meatal stenosis occurs.[6]

Cancer of the penis

Squamous cell cancer of the penis accounts for no more than 1% of male genital tumors in the United States, and it is most common in men between

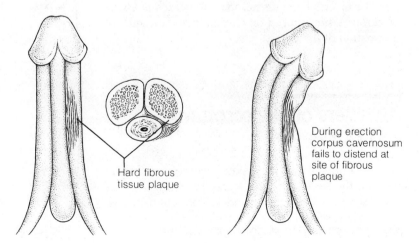

During erection corpus cavernosum fails to distend at site of fibrous plaque

Hard fibrous tissue plaque

Figure 35-2 A hard, fibrous plaque occurs with Peyronie's disease. *(Adapted from Blandy J: Lecture Notes on Urology, 2nd ed. Oxford, Blackwell Scientific Publications, 1977)*

45 and 60 years of age.[1] It is rare in the circumcised male. The protection conferred by circumcision appears to be linked to improvement in genital hygiene, with lessened exposure to potential carcinogens such as smegma or the human papilloma virus. (Human papilloma virus has been associated with cancers of the female reproductive system [see Chapter 38]).[7]

The tumor begins as a small lump or ulcer on the penis. If phimosis is present, there may be painful swelling, purulent drainage, or difficulty in urinating. Palpable lymph nodes in the inguinal region and positive biopsy of the lesion will confirm the diagnosis. Lymphangiography may be done to assess the extent of lymphatic involvement.

Penile cancer tends to follow a slow course. Metastasis to the inguinal nodes is present in only about 25% of men at the time of diagnosis. When diagnosed early, penile cancer is highly curable. Treatment options vary according to stage, size, location, and invasiveness of the tumor. Stage I and II treatment options may include local excision with circumcision, local application of fluorouracil cream, irradiation, laser therapy, and penile amputation.[8] More advanced cancers may necessitate lymph node dissection, irradiation, radiosensitizers or chemotherapy drugs.[9]

In summary, disorders of the penis can be either congenital or acquired. Hypospadias and epispadias are congenital defects in which there is a malposition of the urethral opening: it is located on the ventral surface in hypospadias and on the dorsal surface in epispadias. Phimosis is the condition in which the opening of the foreskin is too tight to permit retraction over the glans. Prolonged, painful, and nonsexual erection that can lead to thrombosis with ischemia and necrosis is called priapism. Peyronie's disease is characterized by the growth of a band of fibrous tissue on top of the penile shaft. Cancer of the penis is relatively rare, accounting for only 1% of male genital cancers. Balanitis xerotica obliterans is a precancerous lesion caused by chronic irritation and inflammation of the penis.

Disorders of the scrotum and testes

The scrotum is a skin-covered pouch that contains the testes and their accessory organs. Defects of the scrotum and testes include cryptorchidism, disorders of the scrotal sac, vascular disorders, inflammation of the scrotum and testes, and neoplasms.

Cryptorchidism

The testes develop intraabdominally in the fetus and usually descend into the scrotum through the inguinal canal during the 8th or 9th month of gestation. Cryptorchidism, or undescended testes, occurs when one or both of the testicles fail to move down into the scrotal sac. The undescended testes may remain within the lower abdomen or at a point of descent within the inguinal canal (Figure 35-3). The cause of cryptorchidism is poorly understood. It may be due to a short spermatic cord, a narrow inguinal ring, or—since a normally functioning hypothalamic-pituitary-testicular axis is considered necessary for testicular development—it may be related to some hormonal imbalance.[7] In a small percentage of cases, it is believed to be hereditary. The incidence of cryptorchidism is directly related to birth weight and gestational age; smaller and shorter-gestational-age infants have a much greater incidence of the disorder. In most children with cryptorchidism, the testes descend into the scrotum within the first 3 to 6 months after birth as a result of a surge in plasma testosterone levels at that time. In 75% of full-term infants and 95% of premature infants born with cryptorchidism, spontaneous testicular descent occurs within the first year of life. Spontaneous descent rarely occurs after this age.

In children with cryptorchidism, histologic abnormalities of the testes occur secondarily to intrinsic defects in the testicle or to adverse effects of the

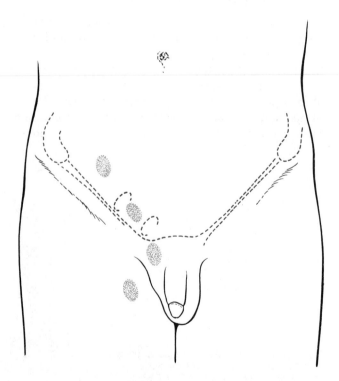

Figure 35-3 Possible locations of undescended testicles.

extrascrotal environment. Temperatures in the inguinal canal are 1°C to 2°C higher than in the scrotum. This increased temperature may damage the undescended testicle; it may even produce morphologic changes in the contralateral testis, possibly reflecting autosensitization through the production of antibodies against spermatozoa, germinal epithelium, or Sertoli's cells. These testicular changes may cause infertility and increase the risk of testicular cancer in later life.

Males with unilateral or bilateral cryptorchidism usually have decreased sperm counts in both the undescended testis and the contralateral testis. At age 3, the number of spermatogonia will have decreased and the seminiferous tubules will be underdeveloped; these changes will be irreversible even with late spontaneous descent or orchiopexy (surgical fixation of an undescended testis in the scrotum). Spermatogonia counts in males with cryptorchidism never reach the normal counts that are found in males whose testes have descended in the usual manner. Studies have shown abnormalities in the sperm density and hormonal levels of men who underwent orchiopexy between the ages of 4 and 12 years. The results of these studies indicate that with cryptorchidism both testes have an inherent defect and that often surgical correction does not bring about fertility correction. The risk of testicular cancer is greatly increased in men with cryptorchidism. This risk is not significantly affected by orchiopexy, hormonal therapy, or late spontaneous descent after the age of 2 years, indicating the importance of treatment before that age.[10]

The testes are not palpable in 15% to 20% of men with cryptorchidism. Improved techniques for testicular localization include ultrasonography (visualization of the testes by recording the pulses of ultrasonic waves directed into the tissues), gonadal venography and arteriography (x-ray of the veins and arteries of the testes after the injection of a contrast medium), and laparoscopy (examination of the interior of the abdomen using a visualization instrument).

The treatment goals for the male with cryptorchidism include measures to (1) enhance fertility, (2) place the gonad in a favorable place for cancer detection, and (3) improve cosmetic appearance. Regardless of the type of treatment that is employed, it should be carried out before the child reaches 2 years of age.[10] Treatment modalities for children with unilateral or bilateral cryptorchidism include initial hormone therapy with human chorionic gonadotropin (HCG). The gonadotropin releasing hormone (GnRH), a hypothalamic hormone that stimulates production of the gonadotropic hormones by the anterior pituitary gland, has been used with considerable success in Europe and has recently been introduced in the United States.[11] For children who do not respond to hormonal treatment, orchiopexy has proved effective.

Hydrocele

The testes and epididymis are almost completely surrounded by the tunica vaginalis, a serous pouch derived from the peritoneum during the fetal descent of the testes from the abdomen into the scrotum. The tunica vaginalis has an outer parietal layer as well as a deeper visceral layer that adheres to the dense fibrous covering of the testes, the tunica albuginea. Normally, the space between these two layers contains only a few milliliters of clear fluid. A scrotal hydrocele is a collection of excess fluid within the layers of the tunica vaginalis.

A hydrocele can develop in the child as a result of a congenital defect or as a process secondary to injury or disorders of the scrotum. A patent processus vaginalis or potential indirect inguinal hernia are often associated with congenital hydroceles. If the hydrocele persists beyond 18 months of age, surgical revision and high ligation of the processus vaginalis at the level of the internal ring is usually recommended.

In the adult, acute hydrocele may be a complication of an infectious process such as gonorrhea, a neoplasm, or trauma to the scrotum that causes the visceral membrane to become more permeable, allowing fluid to accumulate. The tunica vaginalis may also become fluid-filled in persons with conditions, such as heart failure, in which edema is widespread. The fluid is usually serous, but may become a reddish-brown with slight hemorrhage. Transillumination, which is done by shining a light through the scrotum for the purpose of visualizing its internal structures, may be used to reveal the translucent character of the excess fluid and outline the opaque testes within the scrotal sac. Surgical drainage of the fluid may be done to prevent scrotal overheating and consequent sterility.

Hematocele

A hematocele is an accumulation of blood in the tunica vaginalis, which in turn causes the scrotal skin to become dark-red or purple in color. It may develop as a result of an abdominal surgical procedure, scrotal trauma, a bleeding disorder, or a testicular tumor.

Spermatocele

A spermatocele is a painless, sperm-containing cyst that forms at the end of the epididymis. The usual cause is partial obstruction of the ducts that transport sperm from the testes to the urethra. If the cyst is bothersome, it can be evacuated with a hollow needle.

Testicular torsion

Testicular torsion is a twisting of the spermatic cord that suspends the testis. It is the most common acute scrotal disorder in the pediatric and young-adult population. Testicular torsion can be divided into two distinct clinical entities: extravaginal and intravaginal torsion.

In extravaginal torsion, the testicle and the fascial tunicae that surround it rotate around the spermatic cord at a level well above the tunica vaginalis. Extravaginal torsion, the least common form of testicular torsion, occurs almost exclusively in neonates. The torsion probably occurs during fetal or neonatal descent of the testes before the tunica adheres to the scrotal wall. At birth or shortly thereafter a firm, smooth, painless scrotal mass is identified. The scrotal skin appears red and some edema is present. Differential diagnosis is relatively easy since testicular tumors, epididymitis, and orchitis are exceedingly rare in neonates and a hydrocele is softer and can be transilluminated. A physical examination will exclude the presence of hernia. The treatment sometimes includes elective unilateral surgical exploration and orchiectomy (removal of the testis). Contralateral fixation is not usually indicated with extravaginal torsion; however, this is controversial.

Intravaginal torsion (torsion of the testis) is due to the absence of the posterior attachments of the testis within the tunica vaginalis that normally prevent the testis from twisting. It is considerably more common than extravaginal torsion. Although anomalies of suspension vary, in general the tunica vaginalis completely surrounds the testes and epididymis, allowing the testicle to rotate freely within the tunica. At times, the epididymal attachment may be loose enough to permit torsion between the testis and the epididymis. More commonly, however, the testis rotates about the distal spermatic cord. Because this abnormality is developmental, bilateral anomalies are quite common.

Intravaginal torsion occurs most frequently in those aged 8 to 18 years and is rarely seen after age 30. Males usually present in severe distress within hours of onset. Often nausea, vomiting, and tachycardia are present. The affected testis is large and tender with pain radiating to the inguinal area. Extensive cremaster muscle contraction causes a thickening of the spermatic cord.

Testicular torsion must be differentiated from epididymitis orchitis and trauma to the testis. A technetium pertechnetate (^{99m}Tc) scan will demonstrate decreased blood flow with torsion and increased blood flow with epididymitis. Ultrasound studies of the testes may also be helpful.[12] These diagnostic tests are helpful in cases where differential diagnosis is difficult.

Testicular torsion is a true surgical emergency because the viability of testicular tissues diminishes rapidly with time. Surgical intervention involves correcting the abnormal rotation of the testis and "fixing" it in the scrotal sac (orchiopexy). It is important that surgery be performed within 6 hours after the onset of symptoms. The longer the testes remain without blood flow the lower the testicular salvage rate becomes. Subsequent torsion of the contralateral testicle is a well-recognized phenomenon; therefore, bilateral orchiopexy is the treatment of choice. When efforts to restore blood flow fail, orchiectomy is necessary. Studies of males who have had a history of testicular torsion with orchiopexy have demonstrated impaired fertility in the majority of cases. Research has shown that testes prone to torsion are abnormal not only in their suspension system but also in their histologic structure. It is suggested that histologic abnormalities rather than the secondary effects of the torsion may be responsible for the decreased fertility noted in these males.[13]

Varicocele

Varicocele is characterized by varicosities of the pampiniform plexus, a network of veins supplying the testes. A varicocele is found more often on the left side because of the difference in the venous conformation between the right and left testes. The left internal spermatic vein inserts into the left renal vein at a right angle, whereas the right spermatic vein usually enters the inferior vena cava. Varicoceles are rarely found before puberty, and the incidence is highest in men between 15 and 35 years of age.[14]

The possible etiologic mechanisms of varicocele include an insufficiency of the venous valve at the point where the spermatic vein joins the renal vein, causing a reflux of blood back into the veins of the pampiniform plexus. The force of gravity resulting from the upright position and the insertion of the left spermatic vein at a right angle with the renal vein contributes to venous dilatation. If the condition persists, there is a reduction of the elastic fibers and hypertrophy of the vein walls the same as occurs in the formation of leg varices. A hereditary weakness of the connective tissue in the vessel walls may contribute to a predisposition to develop varicocele.

The presence of a varicocele may be associated with male infertility. Although the exact mechanism whereby varicocele produces infertility is not fully understood, several theories of pathogenesis exist. One theory suggests that because a varicocele may be caused by a retrograde flow of blood down the internal spermatic vein, metabolites may be refluxed down the vein, producing adverse effects on both testes. Toxic substances from the renal or adrenal veins may also have an inhibiting effect on sperm production. The data on the role of metabolites in causing infertility are inconclusive. A second theoretical mechanism involves the effect of heat on the testes. This theory proposes that a varicocele can cause an increase in scrotal temperature, a factor that is thought to impair spermatogenesis. A third theory links epididymal factors with infertility. Several factors in the epididymis determine motility and maturation of the spermatozoa, including blood supply, tissue androgens, and electrolyte composition. The retrograde flow of blood in the pampiniform plexus could adversely affect environmental conditions in the epididymis and thereby impair the maturation of the spermatozoa leading to disturbances in motility. There is also the possibility that occult epididymal obstruction accounts for impaired spermatogenesis and infertility. It is possible that several of these factors may interact and impair fertility in the presence of varicocele. The number and combination of these factors may explain why some patients with varicocele are not infertile.[15]

Symptoms of varicocele may also include an abnormal feeling of heaviness in the left scrotum, although many varicoceles are asymptomatic. Usually the presence of varicocele is readily diagnosed on physical examination in both the standing and recumbent positions. Classically, the varicocele will disappear in the lying position due to venous decompression into the renal vein. If the varicocele is secondary to a tumor in the renal vein, it will remain palpable. Scrotal palpation of a varicocele has been compared to feeling a "bag of worms." Small varicoceles may be accentuated by having the patient perform the Valsalva maneuver (forced expiration against a closed glottis) while standing. Diagnostic methods used to confirm varicocele include testicular biopsy, which classically shows germinal cell hypoplasia and premature sloughing of immature sperm forms within the lumen of the seminiferous tubules, venography, scrotal thermography, and Doppler ultrasonography.

Clinical diagnosis of a medium-sized or large varicocele presents little difficulty. However, it is more difficult to diagnose small or subclinical varicoceles. It is important that very small varicoceles be detected early since the extent of testicular damage shows no correlation with the size of the varicocele. The combination of thermography with sonography has proven to be very effective diagnostically.[16]

Surgical repair of varicocele is by far the most common treatment for the disorder. On the average, varicocelectomy is followed by improvement of semen quality in approximately 70% of cases with a concomitant pregnancy rate of 30% to 55%. Percutaneous occlusion of the internal spermatic vein is an alternative to surgery. The spermatic vein can be occluded with sclerosing solutions, steel coils, or balloon-tipped catheter. These techniques avoid general anesthesia and the trauma associated with surgical intervention.[17]

Epididymitis

Epididymitis is an inflammation of the epididymis, the elongated cordlike structure that lies along the posterior border of the testis, whose function is the storage, transport, and maturation of spermatozoa. Epididymitis is the most common cause of intrascrotal pathology in postpubertal males. It is commonly related to infections in the urinary tract that presumably reach the epididymis through either the vas deferens or the lymphatics of the spermatic cord. In rare cases, organisms from other foci of infection reach the epididymis through the blood stream.

A number of organisms are known to cause epididymitis. In men under 35 years of age, *Chlamydia trachomatis* is the major cause of nonspecific epididymitis, and the infection is considered a sexually transmitted disease.[18] In men over 35 years of age, epididymitis is usually related to urinary tract infections caused by gram-negative bacteria or secondary to instrumentation (*e.g.*, catheterization or cystoscopy).

Epididymitis is characterized by unilateral pain and swelling, accompanied by erythema and edema of the overlying scrotal skin that develops over a period of 24 to 48 hours. Initially the swelling and induration are limited to the epididymis. However, the distinction between the testes and epididymis becomes less evident as the inflammation progresses. Fever and complaint of dysuria occur in about half of the cases. Whether urethral discharge is present or not depends on the organism causing the infection. A discharge usually accompanies gonorrheal infections, is common in chlamydial infections, and is less common in infections due to gram-negative organisms. Pyuria may be present depending on the method of urine collection. Because voided specimens contain epididymal secretions, pyuria will be present in voided urine specimens but absent in catheterized specimens.

Treatment consists of bed rest during the acute phase (which usually lasts for 3 to 4 days), scrotal elevation and support, and antibiotics. Gonorrhea is usually treated with intramuscularly administered procaine penicillin and oral probenecid or ceftriaxone (see Chapter 38). Follow-up cultures are needed to ensure successful treatment. Chlamydial infections are treated with tetracycline or doxycycline. Since these infections are sexually transmitted diseases, treatment of the sexual partner is strongly recommended.

In older males with epididymitis, gram-negative bacteria are frequently the etiologic agents. Often benign prostatic hyperplasia, neurogenic bladder, or urethral stricture is present concomitantly and must be considered in the treatment plan. Prostatitis may coexist, so antibiotics that are effective in treating chronic bacterial prostatitis are often used. Antibiotic choice can be adjusted when sensitivity testing is complete.

Most men with epididymitis can be managed successfully as outpatients with oral antibiotics and local measures. Occasionally signs of systemic toxicity occur or outpatient therapy fails. In complicated epididymitis, scrotal ultrasonography can aid in making the decision between continued medical therapy and surgical exploration. Men in whom serial ultrasound studies reveal progressive testicular changes uniformly require orchiectomy.[19]

Orchitis

Orchitis, an infection of the testes, can be precipitated by a primary infection in the genitourinary tract, such as urethritis, cystitis, or seminal vesiculitis. Many infections from other parts of the body spread to the testes through the bloodstream or the lymphatics. Orchitis can develop as a complication of a systemic infection, such as parotitis (mumps), scarlet fever, or pneumonia. Probably the best known of these is orchitis caused by the mumps virus. About 25% to 33% of males 10 years of age or older with mumps develop this form of orchitis.[7] The symptoms usually run their course in 7 to 10 days. Mumps orchitis causes painful enlargement of the testes, with small hemorrhages into the tunica albuginea. Microscopically, an acute inflammatory response is seen in the seminiferous tubules with proliferation of neutrophils, lymphocytes, and histiocytes, causing distention of the tubules. Mumps orchitis causes testicular damage in 30% of males who get the disease after puberty. The residual effects that are seen after the acute phase include hyalinization of the seminiferous tubules, atrophy of the testes, and elevation of follicle-stimulating hormone (FSH) levels due to a lack of testosterone and negative feedback control of FSH. Although there is often some degree of atrophy along with the healing, the patchy nature of the process tends to preserve fertility, even if the process is bilateral. However, if the inflammation and edema has been severe enough to compress the blood supply, sterility may result.[7]

Neoplasms

Tumors can arise from either the scrotum or the testes. Benign scrotal tumors are quite common and often do not require treatment. Carcinoma of the scrotum is rare and is usually associated with exposure to carcinogenic agents. On the other hand, almost all solid tumors of the testes (96%) are malignant.[20]

Although testicular tumors are rare, their vir-ulence and the fact that they develop in relatively young men make them a significant health problem.

Cancer of the scrotum

Cancer of the scrotum is primarily an occupational disease linked to contact with petroleum products, such as tar, pitch, and soot. The malignancy often occurs after 20 to 30 years of exposure. In the early stages, it may appear as a small tumor or wartlike growth that eventually ulcerates. The thin scrotal wall lacks the tissue reactivity needed to block the malignant process; over half of the cases seen involve metastasis to the lymph nodes. The treatment includes wide local excision of the tumor with inguinal and femoral node dissection, because this tumor does not respond well to x-ray treatment.

Testicular cancer

Although relatively rare, accounting for 1% of the cancers in males and for about 3% of the cancers of the male urogenital system, testicular cancer is an important disease because it strikes young men. It is the most common cause of cancer in the 15- to 35-year-old age group and in the past has been a leading cause of death among males entering their most productive years. However, in the past 10 years recent advances in therapy have transformed an almost invariably fatal disease into one in which over 90% of patients can be cured.[21]

The etiology of testicular cancer is unknown. There is a 10- to 40-fold increased risk in males with cryptorchidism.[7] Chronic irritation of the testes, from either infection or other inflammatory processes, is also thought to increase the risk of cancer formation.

Often the first sign of testicular cancer is a slight enlargement of the testicle that may be accompanied by some degree of discomfort. This may be an ache in the abdomen or groin or a sensation of dragging or heaviness in the scrotum. Frank pain may be experienced in the later stages when the tumor is growing rapidly and hemorrhaging occurs. Testicular cancer can spread when the tumor may only be barely palpable.

The American Cancer Society strongly advocates that every young adult male examines his testes at least once a month as a means of early detection of testicular cancer. The examination should be done after a warm bath or shower when the scrotal skin is relaxed. To do this self-examination, each testicle is examined with the fingers of both hands by rolling the testicle between the thumb and fingers to check for the presence of any lumps. If any lump, nodule, or enlargement is noted, it should be brought immediately to the attention of a physician.

The differential diagnosis of testicular cancer

includes consideration of all conditions that produce an intrascrotal mass, such as epididymitis, orchitis, hydrocele, or hematocele. If malignant disease is suspected, surgical exploration via an inguinal incision is performed; and if testicular cancer cannot be excluded, an orchiectomy is done. Scrotal exploration is not performed because the primary lymphatic drainage of the testes is to the retroperitoneal lymph nodes.

Currently, there are several systems for classification of testicular cancer. The Armed Forces Institute of Pathology (AFIP) classification system divides testicular cancer into germinal tumors arising from the spermatozoa and their derivatives and nongerminal cell tumors arising from other cellular components of the testes.[22] Germ cell tumors, which constitute about 95% of all testicular tumors, can be divided into two groups: seminoma and nonseminoma germ cell tumors. Seminomas are thought to arise from the seminiferous epithelium of the testes. They are the most common type of testicular cancer, accounting for approximately 40% of all germ cell tumors. The peak incidence of seminoma occurs in men between 30 and 40 years of age; of nonseminoma, between 20 and 30 years of age.

Nonseminoma germ cell tumors are classified into three histologic types: (1) embryonal carcinoma, (2) teratoma, and (3) choriocarcinoma. Embryonal carcinomas represent about 10% to 20% of all germ cell tumors. They are less differentiated and more aggressive than seminomas. Teratomas are derived from totipotential cells that have the capacity to differentiate into tissues representing any of the three germ layers of the embryo—ectoderm, mesoderm, or endoderm. They constitute less than 10% of germ cell tumors and can occur at any age from infancy to old age. They usually behave as benign tumors in children; in adults they often contain minute foci of cancer cells. Choriocarcinoma, a highly malignant form of cancer that is identical to tumors that arise in the placental tissue, accounts for 1% of testicular cancers. Each of these basic histologic types can occur as a pure form or as a combination of cell types. Forty percent of testicular cancers are of mixed tissue types.[7] The most common mixture is teratocarcinoma, which contains both embryonal carcinoma and teratoma elements.

The clinical staging (TNM classification) for testicular cancer is as follows: stage I, tumor confined to testes; stage II, tumor spread to retroperitoneal lymph nodes; stage III, distant metastases (see Chapter 5). Staging procedures include computed tomography (CT scan) of the chest, abdomen, and pelvis; ultrasonography for detection of bulky inferior nodal metastases; venocavography; and lymphangiography. Tumor markers and radiographic methods are used to detect metastatic spread. Serum markers include alpha-fetoprotein (AFP) and the beta subunit of human chorionic gonadotropin (HCG); they provide information about both the existence of a tumor and the type of tumor present and may detect tumors that are too small to be detected on physical examination or x-ray. Both markers are elevated in 50% to 90% of patients with gross metastases of nonseminomatous germ cell tumors. Except in extremely rare cases AFP is not elevated in seminomas. Moderate elevations of HCG may be detected in 10% of seminomas.

Treatment of testicular cancers includes radical orchiectomy, which is done at the time of diagnostic exploration. Seminomas are very radiosensitive. The treatment of stage I or II seminoma is irradiation of the retroperitoneal and homolateral lymph nodes to the level of the diaphragm. Patients with bulky retroperitoneal or distant metastases are often treated with chemotherapy. Far-advanced seminoma is treated like nonseminoma.

The treatment of nonseminomatous germ cell (stage I) tumor is more controversial and includes the standard retroperitoneal lymphadenectomy, which is followed by either a regimen of adjuvant chemotherapy or observation only. Surgical therapy is advantageous because it enables precise staging, which can improve the outcome for some men with metastatic disease. Surgery is followed by a 2-year period of monthly physical examinations, scheduled tests for tumor markers, and chest x-ray. Observation of stage I tumor avoids the insult of surgery but is more inaccurate in assessment of clinical stage. However, it is an acceptable alternative because systemic therapy is so effective in treating testicular tumors. Even so, the cure rate decreases as the tumor volume increases. It is essential that clients opting for observation are closely followed. This requires physical examination, chest x-ray, and tumor marker assays monthly with abdominal CT scan repeated every 3 months. Any recurrent disease is promptly treated with chemotherapy and/or lymphadenectomy. The overall disease-free survival rate for observation is 98%, which is comparable to the rate following retroperitoneal lymphadenectomy. Patients with small stage II nonseminomatous tumors are treated with retroperitoneal lymphadenectomy. Stage II bulky tumors and stage III tumors are usually treated initially with systemic chemotherapy.[23]

With appropriate treatment, the prognosis of men with testicular cancer is excellent. The 5-year survival rate for patients with stage I and II disease exceeds 90%. Patients with stage III tumors have an overall survival rate of approximately 70%, with prognosis related to the amount of distant metastases present. Even patients with mild or moderate lung metastases have excellent chances for long-term survival. All forms of therapy for testicular cancer can have potentially adverse effects on fertility. For this reason, men with this disorder should be given the opportunity to bank sperm prior to treatment.[23]

In summary, disorders of the scrotum and testes include cryptorchidism, or undescended testicles, hydrocele, testicular torsion, and varicocele. Inflammatory conditions can involve the scrotal sac, epididymis, or testes. Tumors can arise in either the scrotum or the testes. Scrotal cancers are usually associated with exposure to petroleum products such as tar, pitch, and soot. Testicular cancer accounts for 3% of cancers of the male genitourinary system. With present treatment methods a large percentage of men with these tumors can be cured. Testicular self-examination is recommended as a means of early detection of this form of cancer.

Disorders of the prostate

The prostate is a firm glandular structure that surrounds the urethra. It produces a thin, milky alkaline secretion that aids sperm motility by helping to maintain an optimum pH. The contraction of the smooth muscle in the gland promotes semen expulsion during ejaculation.

—— Prostatitis

Prostatitis refers to a variety of inflammatory disorders of the prostate gland, some bacterial in nature and some not. It may occur spontaneously, as a result of catheterization or instrumentation, or secondary to other diseases of the male genitourinary system. There are four types of prostatitis: (1) acute bacterial, (2) chronic bacterial, (3) nonbacterial, and (4) prostatodynia.

—— Acute bacterial prostatitis

Acute bacterial prostatitis is typified by the sudden onset of high fever up to 40°C, chills, marked malaise, and sometimes myalgia to arthralgia. Further symptoms include frequency, urgency, dysuria, and urethral discharge. Dull aching pain is present in the perineum, rectum, or sacrococcygeal region. Rectal examination reveals a swollen, tender, warm prostate with soft scattered areas. Prostatic massage produces a thick discharge with white blood cells that will grow large numbers of pathogens on culture. These pathogens often include gram-negative enteric bacteria such as Pseudomonas, as well as gram-positive staphylococci and streptococci.

Treatment for acute bacterial prostatitis includes bed rest, adequate hydration, antipyretics, and analgesics or spasmolytic drugs to alleviate pain. Usually acute prostatitis will respond to appropriate antimicrobial therapy chosen in accordance with the sensitivity of the causative agents in the urethral discharge. Broad spectrum antibiotic therapy is used until sensitivity tests indicate the drug of choice. Prostatic abscess has been rare since the advent of effective antibacterial therapy but is more common in men with diabetes mellitus.

—— Chronic bacterial prostatitis

In contrast to acute bacterial prostatitis, chronic bacterial prostatitis is a subtle disorder that is difficult to treat. Symptoms include frequency, urgency, and dysuria associated occasionally with perineal discomfort, low-back pain, myalgia, arthralgia and sometimes complicated by epididymitis. Many suffer relapsing lower or upper urinary tract infections because of recurrent invasion of the bladder by the prostatic bacteria. Bacteria may continue to be present in the prostate gland even when the prostatic fluid is sterile. Chronic bacterial prostatitis is accompanied by profound physiochemical alterations in prostatic secretions (alkaline phosphatase) as well as the localization of gram-negative enteric bacteria in the prostate. Long-term therapy (4–6 months) with an appropriate low-dose oral antimicrobial agent such as nitrofurantoin or trimethoprim-sulfamethoxazole is used to treat the infection. Prostatectomy may be done when the infection is not cured or adequately controlled by medical therapy.

—— Nonbacterial prostatitis

A large group of men with prostatitis suffer from pains along the penis, testicles, and scrotum, painful ejaculation, low-back pain, rectal pain, pain along the inner thighs, urinary symptoms, decrease of libido, and impotence but have no bacteria present in the urinary system. Men with nonbacterial prostatitis often have inflammation of the prostate with an elevated white blood cell count and abnormal inflammatory cells in their prostatic secretions. The cause of the disorder is unknown, and efforts to prove unusual pathogens (e.g., mycoplasmas, chlamydiae, trichomonads, and viruses) have been largely unsuccessful. Some researchers believe nonbacterial prostatitis is an autoimmune disorder. Those affected may be treated with tetracycline, with erythromycin, or, if mycosis is present, with an antifungal treatment. Because nonbacterial prostatitis does not usually respond to antibiotic therapy, treatment is often directed toward symptom control. Anti-inflammatory agents such as ibuprofen may be used to provide symptom relief.

—— Prostatodynia

Patients with prostatodynia have symptoms resembling those of nonbacterial prostatitis but display no evidence of inflammation of the prostate.

Some investigators suggest that the symptoms may be due to a tension myalgia of the pelvic floor muscles, whereas others believe that spasm of the external urethral sphincter is causing the symptomatology.[24]

Benign prostatic hyperplasia

Benign prostatic hyperplasia is an age-related nonmalignant enlargement of the prostate gland. Although the condition has traditionally been referred as benign prostatic hypertrophy, or BPH, the basic process is one of hyperplasia rather than hypertrophy. Benign prostatic hyperplasia is a very common process in aging men, occurring in about 8% of men in the 4th decade and rising to an incidence of 75% by the 8th decade. Because of changing demographics and the increasing median age of the United States population, more attention has recently been given to this disorder. Although in most cases this disease is relatively mild, the World Health Association reports a yearly worldwide mortality of 30 deaths per 100,000 population; in the United States the reported yearly mortality is 14.4 deaths per 100,000 population .[25]

Benign prostatic hyperplasia is characterized by the formation of large discrete lesions in the periurethral region of the prostate (Figure 35-4). The exact cause of benign prostatic hyperplasia is unknown. The fact that the condition occurs largely in older men suggests a relationship to changes in hormone balance associated with aging. Both androgens (testosterone) and estrogens appear to contribute to the process. Dihydrotestosterone, which is the biologically active metabolite of testosterone, is thought to be the ultimate mediator of hyperplasia, with estrogen serving to sensitize the prostatic tissue to the growth-producing effects of dihydrotestosterone. Although the exact source is uncertain, small amounts of estrogen are produced in the male. It has been postulated that an increase in levels of estrogen that occurs with aging may facilitate the action of androgens within the prostate despite a decline in testicular output of testosterone.[7]

The clinical significance of benign prostatic hyperplasia resides in its tendency to compress the urethra and cause partial or complete obstruction of urinary outflow. The resulting obstruction to urinary flow can give rise to urinary tract infection, difficulty in voiding, hypertrophy and destructive changes of the bladder wall, hydroureter, and hydronephrosis. Hypertrophy and changes in bladder-wall structure develop in stages. At first, the exaggerated crisscross fibers form trabeculations and then herniations, or sacculations; finally diverticula develop as the herniations extend through the bladder wall (see Chapter 33, Figure 33-4). These diverticula are readily infected, because urine is seldom completely emptied from them. Back pressure on the ureters and collecting system of kidneys promotes hydroureter and hydronephrosis; and as a result, the kidneys develop the physiologic sequelae of atrophy—failure to concentrate urine, to retain sodium, and to remove metabolic acids from the blood. There is danger of eventual renal failure.

The symptoms of benign prostatic hyperplasia are related to the compression of the urethra with accompanying bladder distention and hypertrophy, urinary tract infection, and renal disease. The typical picture includes outflow obstruction with a decreased caliber and force of the urinary stream. As the obstruction increases, acute retention with overdistention of the bladder may occur. The presence of residual urine in the bladder causes frequency of urination and a constant desire to empty the bladder, which becomes worse at night. With marked bladder distention, overflow incontinence may occur with the slightest increase in intraabdominal pressure.

The diagnosis of benign prostatic hyperplasia is based on a history and observation of urinary reten-

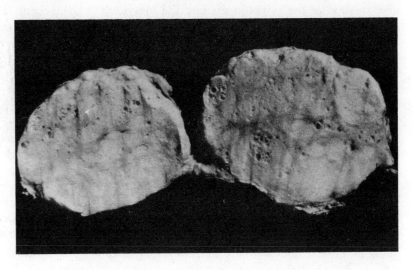

Figure 35-4 Benign nodular hyperplasia of the prostate.

tion. The bladder may be seen and palpated as retention of urine increases. On digital rectal examination, a smooth rubbery enlargement of the prostate is usually detected. Hardened areas of the prostate gland suggest cancer and should be biopsied. Flexible cystoscopy may be beneficial in differential diagnosis since benign prostatic hyperplasia may mimic symptoms of other urinary tract infections. Intravenous urography may be used to reveal the complications of back pressure on the kidney, hydroureteronephrosis, thickening and trabeculation of the bladder, and elevation of the bladder base and trigone by the enlarged prostate. Residual urine can be measured by postvoiding catheterization or estimated by ultrasonography. Urinalysis is used to detect the presence of hematuria, bacteriuria, and pyuria. Serum levels of creatinine and blood urea nitrogen are used to assess renal function.[26]

Acute urinary retention is relieved with catheterization. Urinary tract infections are treated with appropriate antimicrobial agents. Excessive intake of alcohol can result in acute urinary retention and should be avoided. Prolonged periods of urinary retention accompanied by excessive fluid intake may also result in overdistention of the bladder with atony and acute retention.

Benign prostatic hyperplasia that has progressed to the point of producing urinary obstruction and risk of renal complications has traditionally been treated surgically using transurethral resection or an open surgical approach (suprapubic, retropubic, or perineal prostatectomy). Although morbidity and mortality from these procedures are within acceptable limits, acute complications can include priapism, extravasation of urine, urinary retention, epididymitis, and hemorrhage. Reported long-term complications include retrograde ejaculation, impotence, urethral stricture, incontinence, and obstruction.

Recently, excellent short-term results have been demonstrated with retrograde transurethral balloon dilation of the prostatic urethra; the long-term results are under investigation.[27] Medical treatment for benign prostatic hypertrophy, which uses a variety of drugs including hormones and beta-adrenergic blocking agents, has not proven successful for long-term effects but may be useful for patients awaiting surgery.[28]

Prostatic cancer

Next to lung cancer, prostatic cancer is the most common type of cancer in men. It is a potentially lethal disease and is the third most common cause of cancer-related deaths. The incidence of prostatic cancer increases with age, and the disease is rare in men under 50 years of age. One recent study showed an incidence of 10.4% in men 50 to 59 years of age, 18.5 % in those 60 to 69 years, and 28.7% in those 70 to 79 years.[29] The number of men with prostatic cancer, including latent or clinically unrecognized cases, is much larger than would be expected because the disease is relatively slow growing and of low malignant potential.

The precise etiology of prostatic cancer is unknown, but epidemiologic studies suggest that genetics, hormonal factors, diet, chemical carcinogens, and viruses may all play a role in the development of the disease. Prostatic cancer occurs more frequently in some families, and blacks have nearly twice the mortality rate of whites. Hormones appear to influence the induction and promotion of prostate cancer. Studies have noted an association between prostatic cancer and frequency of sexual activity.[30] Further, the response of prostatic cancer to androgen deprivation suggests a direct relationship between the disease and hormones. Diet appears to influence prostatic cancer: intake of green and yellow vegetables appears to have a protective effect, and a diet high in fat appears to contribute to increased incidence. Occupations where there is exposure to certain environmental factors such as cadmium, rubber, and textiles have been linked to higher rates of the disease. Although a direct causal relationship between prostatic cancer and viruses has not been established, a temporal relationship has been identified between the incidence of gonorrhea and the incidence of prostatic cancer. The assumption is that these men may have been exposed to cancer-causing viruses as well. The heterogeneity of this disease suggests that a complex interaction of a variety of substances is responsible for malignancy.[26]

The symptoms of prostatic cancer, when they occur, are similar to those of benign prostatic hyperplasia. The prostate is nodular and fixed on rectal examination. Bone metastasis, when present, is often characterized by low-back pain. Pathologic fractures may occur at the site of metastasis. Outflow obstruction from the bladder may lead to urinary tract infection, urine retention, and renal damage. Anemia may be profound if bone marrow is replaced by tumor.

Laboratory findings that are important in the detection of prostatic cancer include elevations in serum prostatic acid phosphatase, which is associated with poor prognosis in both local and disseminated disease. Prostate-specific antigen (PSA) is an organ-specific marker that because of greater sensitivity and specificity for prostate tissue may prove to be a valuable tumor marker. Detectable levels of PSA after prostatectomy suggest persistent local or metastatic disease. Because PSA is also elevated in benign prostatic hyperplasia and is often elevated after prostate manipulations, it is not suitable for pretreatment screening.[31]

Magnetic resonance imaging (MRI) is a sensitive indicator of the presence of cancer within the prostate. Transrectal ultrasonography can often identify the presence of carcinoma. Radiologic examination of the bones of the skull, ribs, spine, and pelvis can be used to reveal metastases, although radionuclide bone scans are more sensitive. Excretory urograms are used to delineate changes due to urinary tract obstruction and renal involvement. Lymphangiography is often done to determine pelvic node metastases.[32]

Factors affecting survival are the stage of the tumor, the grade, the presence of symptoms, and the physiological age of the man. Cancer of the prostate, like other forms of cancer is both graded and staged (see Chapter 5). Well-differentiated tumors are assigned a grade of 1 and poorly differentiated tumors a grade of 5. Stage A, using the TNM system, describes a latent form of the disease and stage D, metastatic involvement. When the cancer is confined to the prostate gland, the disease is curable, and the great majority of persons will die of something else. When the cancer is locally extensive it is not usually curable, and a substantial fraction will eventually die from the disease. It is important that every effort be made to grade and stage the disease before instituting therapy.

The treatment methods for prostatic cancer remain controversial. Men with stage A low-grade disease have a survival rate close to that of the normal population; nevertheless, some practitioners feel that transurethral resection of the prostate be considered to prevent clinical understaging.[33] Men with stages A_2, B, and C have treatable prostate cancer. Those with a life expectancy of 10 or more years are usually treated aggressively with external radiation therapy (interstitial ^{125}I implantation) or radical prostatectomy. Complications of these treatments can vary. An impotence rate of 20% to 50% and an incontinence rate of 10% is associated with radical prostatectomy. Less impotence is seen with nerve-sparing prostatectomy. External radiation therapy is associated with a 20% to 30% impotence rate and a 10% to 15% rate of major complications. Implantation of ^{125}I is associated with few complications.

Men with late metastatic disease (stage D) are usually treated with antiandrogen therapy. Orchiectomy or estrogen therapy is often effective in reducing symptoms and extending survival. Blocking testosterone production with leutinizing hormone-releasing hormone (LHRH) analogs that inhibit gonadotropin release from the pituitary has proved effective and avoids the side effects of estrogen therapy, including gynecomastia, voice changes, cardiovascular complications, and nausea and vomiting. Systemic chemotherapy has not proven beneficial in this disease.

In summary, the prostate is a firm glandular structure that surrounds the urethra. Inflammation of the prostate occurs as either an acute or a chronic process. Chronic prostatitis is probably the most common cause of relapsing urinary tract infections in the male. Benign prostatic hyperplasia is a common disorder in men over 50 years of age. Because the prostate encircles the urethra, prostatitis tends to cause obstruction of urinary outflow from the bladder. Cancer of the prostate is the most common type of cancer of the male genitourinary system and is the third highest cause of cancer deaths in men 55 to 74 years of age.

References

1. Duckett JW, Snow BW: Disorders of the urethra and penis. In Walsh PC, Gittes RF, Permutter AD (eds): Campbell's Urology, 5th ed, pp 2000-2030. Philadelphia, WB Saunders, 1986
2. Spycher MA, Hauri D: The ultrastructure of the erectile tissue in priapism. J Urol 135:142, 1986
3. Carson CC, Mino RD: Priapism associated with trazodone therapy. J Urology 139:369, 1988
4. Lue TF, Hellstrom JG, McAnnich JW, Tanagho EA: Priapism: A refined approach to diagnosis and treatment. J Urol 136(9):104, 1986
5. Somers KD, Winters BA, Dawson DM, et al: Chromosome abnormalities in Peyronie's disease. J Urol 137:672, 1987
6. Nickel WR, Plumb RT: Cutaneous diseases of the external genitalia. In Walsh PC, et al (eds): Campbell's Urology, 5th ed, pp 956-989. Philadelphia, WB Saunders, 1986
7. Robbins SL, Kumar V: Pathologic Basis of Disease, 4th ed, pp 614–620. Philadelphia, WB Saunders, 1987
8. Mohs FE, Snow SN, Messing EM, et al: Microscopically controlled surgery in the treatment of carcinoma of the penis. J Urol 133:961, 1985
9. McDougal WS, Kirchner FK, Edwards RH, et al: Treatment of carcinoma of the penis: The case for primary lymphadenectomy. J Urol 136:38, 1986
10. Batata MA, Chu FCH, Hilaris BS, et al: Testicular cancer in cryptorchidism. Cancer 49:1023, 1982
11. Raufer J, Handelsman DJ, Swerdloff RS, et al: Hormonal therapy of cryptorchidism. N Engl J Med 314:466, 1986
12. Lee LM, Wright JE, McLoughlin MG: Testicular torsion in the adult. J Urol 130:93, 1983
13. Hadziselimovic F, Snyder H, Duckett J, et al: Testicular histology in children with unilateral testicular torsion. J Urol 136:208, 1986
14. Rodriquez DD, Rodrigues WC, Rivera JJ, et al: Doppler ultrasound versus testicular scanning in evaluation of the acute scrotum. J Urol 125:343, 1981
15. Wirtz J: Epidemiology of idiopathic varicocele. In Jecht

EW, Zietler E (eds): Varicocele and Male Infertility, pp 2-3. New York, Springer-Verlag, 1982

16. Hamm B, Fobbe F, Sorensen R, Felsenberg D: Varicoceles: Combined sonography and thermography in diagnosis and posttherapeutic evaluation. Radiology 160:419,1986

17. Sherins RJ, Howards SS: Male infertility. In Walsh PC, Gittes RF, Permutter AD (eds): Campbell's Urology, 5th ed. Philadelphia, WB Saunders, 1986

18. Berger RE, Alexander ER, Harnich JP, et al: Etiology, manifestations and therapy of acute epididymitis: Prospective study of 50 cases. J Urol 121:750, 1979

19. See WA, Mack LA, Krieger JN: Scrotal ultrasonography: A predictor of complicated epididymitis requiring orchiectomy. J Urol 139:55, 1988

20. Frank IN, Keys HM, McCune CS: Urologic and male genital cancers. In Rubin P (ed): Clinical Oncology, 6th ed, pp 214. New York, American Cancer Society, 1983

21. Einhorn LH: Cancer of the testis: A new paradigm. Hosp Pract 22(4):165, 1986

22. Drasgna RE, Einhorn LH, Williams SD: The chemotherapy of testicular cancer. CA 32:66, 1982

23. Grossmann HB: Malignant tumors of the urogenital tract. In Rakel RE (ed): Conn's Current Therapy. Philadelphia, WB Saunders, 1988

24. Pfau A: Prostatitis, a continuing enigma. Urol Clin N Am 13:695, 1986

25. Smith RH, Wake R, Soloway MS: Benign prostatic hyperplasia: A universal problem among aging men. Postgrad Med 83(6):79, 1988

26. Johnson DE, Swanson DA, VonEschenbach AC: Tumors of the prostate gland. In Tanagho EA, McAninch JW (eds): Smith's General Urology, 12th ed. Norwalk,CT, Appleton & Lang, 1988

27. Casteneda F, Johnson S, Hulbert J, et al: Urethroplasty with balloon catheter in prostatic hypertrophy. Am J Roentgenol 149:313, 1987

28. Casteneda F, Johnson S, Hulbert J, et al: Medical treatment of benign prostatic hypertrophy. Lancet 1:1083, 1988

29. Sheldon CA, Williams RD, Fraley EF: Incidental carcinoma of the prostate: A review of the literature and critical appraisal of classification. J Urol 124:626, 1980

30. Rotkin ID: Epidemiologic studies in prostatic cancer. Cancer Treat Rep 61:173, 1977

31. Hricak H, Dooms GL, Jeffrey RB, et al: Prostatic carcinoma: Staging by clinical assessment, CT, and MR imaging. Radiology 162:331, 1987

32. Seamonds B, Yang N, Anderson K, et al: Evaluation of prostate-specific antigen and prostatic acid phosphatase as prostate cancer markers. Urology 28:479, 1986

33. Epstein JI, Paull G, Eggleston JC, et al: Prognosis of untreated stage A1 prostatic carcinoma: A study of 94 cases with extended follow-up. J Urol 136:837, 1986

Bibliography

Bannister CE: Balloon embolotherapy for varicocele. Nursing 17, No. 2:68, 1987

Blackmore C: The impact of orchidectomy upon the sexuality of the man with testicular cancer. Cancer Nurs 11, No. 1:33, 1988

Campbell ML: Sexual dysfunction in the COPD patient. DCCN 6, No. 2:70, 1987

Casey MP: Testicular cancer: the worst disease at the worst time. RN 50, No. 2:36, 1987

Chodak GW, Eisenberger MA, Scardino PT, Torti FM: Detecting prostate cancer early. Patient Care 21, No. 7:69, 1987

Chodak GW, Eisenberger MA, Scardino PT, Torti FM: Prostate cancer: 1987 options for RX. Patient Care 21, No. 7:74, 1987

Drasga RE, Einhorn LH, Williams SD: The chemotherapy of testicular cancer. CA-A Cancer J Clin 32, No. 2, 1982

Einhorn LH: Cancer of the testes: A new paradigm. Hosp Pract 21 (April 15):165, 1986

Einhorn L: Chemotherapy of testicular cancer. Med Times 110 No. 2:100, 1983

Heinrich-Rynning T: Prostatic cancer treatments and their effects on sexual functioning. Oncol Nurs Forum 14, No. 6:37, 1987

Hesketh PJ: Evaluation and treatment of testicular cancer. Hosp Pract 22, No. 9:87, 1987

Holmes P: Sexuality: New treatments for impotence. Nurs Times 83, No. 34:42, 1987

Hongladarom GC: An overview of current concepts in the management of patients with testicular tumors of germ cell origin—Part 1: Pathophysiology, diagnosis, and staging. Can Nurs 6 No. 1:39, 1983

Hubbard SM, Jenkins J: An overview of current concepts in the management of patients with testicular tumors of germ cell origin—Part II: Treatment strategies by histology and stage. Can Nurs 6 No. 2:125, 1983

Langemo DV: Peyronie's disease. AUAA J 5, No. 3:4, 1985

Lawler PE: Benign prostatic hyperplasia: knowing pathophysiology aids assessment. AORN 40, No. 5:745, 1984

Lee LM, Wright JE, McLoughlin MG: Testicular torsion in the adult. J Urol 130:93, 1983

Melamed AJ: Current concepts in the treatment of prostate cancer. Drug Intell Clin Pharm 21, No. 3:247, 1987

Sharer WC: Acute scrotal pathology. Surg Clin North Am 62 No. 6:1982

Structure and Function of the Female Reproductive System

Objectives

After you have studied this chapter, you should be able to meet the following objectives:

_____ Describe the anatomic relationship of the structures of the external genitalia.

_____ Give the location of the Skene's and Bartholin's glands.

_____ Cite the location of the ovaries in relation to the uterus, fallopian tubes, broad ligaments, and ovarian ligaments.

_____ Explain the function of the fallopian tubes.

_____ Describe the anatomic features of the uterine wall.

_____ State the function of endocervical secretions.

_____ Describe the anatomy of the ovaries.

_____ Describe the feedback control of estrogen and progesterone levels by means of GnRH, LH, FSH, and ovarian follicle function.

_____ List the actions of estrogen and progesterone.

_____ Describe the metabolism and peripheral sources of estrogen.

_____ Cite the function of androgens in the female.

_____ Describe the four functional compartments of the ovary.

_____ Relate FSH and LH levels to the stages of follicle development and to estrogen and progesterone production.

_____ Describe the endometrial changes that occur during the menstrual cycle.

_____ Describe the composition of normal cervical mucus and the changes that occur during the menstrual cycle.

_____ Describe the physiology of normal menopause.

_____ Describe the anatomy of the female breast.

_____ Describe the influence of hormones on breast development.

_____ Explain the effect of estrogen and progesterone on breast changes that occur during pregnancy.

The female genitourinary system consists of the internal paired ovaries, the uterine tubes, the uterus, the vagina and the external mons pubis, the labia majora, the labia minora, the clitoris, the urethra, and the perineal body. Although the female urinary structures are anatomically separate from the genital structures, their anatomic proximity provides a means for cross-contamination and shared symptomatology between the two systems (Figure 36-1). This chapter focuses on the internal and external genitalia. It includes a discussion of hormonal and physical changes that occur throughout the life cycle in response to the gonadotropic hormones. The reader is referred to a specialty text for a discussion of pregnancy.

Reproductive structures

—— External genitalia

The external genitalia are located at the base of the pelvis in the perineal area and include the mons pubis, labia majora, labia minora, clitoris, and perineal body. The urethra and anus, though not genital structures, are usually considered in a discussion of the external genitalia. The external genitalia, also known collectively as the vulva, are diagrammed in Figure 36-2.

—— Mons pubis

The mons pubis is a rounded, skin-covered fat pad located anterior to the symphysis pubis. Puberty stimulates an increase in the amount of fat and the development of darker and coarser hair over the mons. Normal pubic hair distribution in the female follows an inverted triangle with the base centered over the mons. Hair color and texture varies between individuals and racial groups. There is an abundance of sebaceous glands in the skin which can become infected due to normal variations in glandular secretions or poor hygiene. The mons pubis is the most common site of pubic lice infestation in the female.

—— Labia majora

The labia majora (singular: labium majus) are analogous to the male scrotum. These structures are the outermost lips of the vulva, beginning anteriorly at the base of the mons pubis and ending posteriorly at the anus. The labia majora are composed of folds of skin and fat and become covered with hair at the onset of puberty. Prior to puberty, the labia majora have a skin covering similar to that covering the abdomen. With sufficient hormonal stimulation, the labia of a mature woman close over the urethral and vaginal openings; this can change following childbirth or sur-

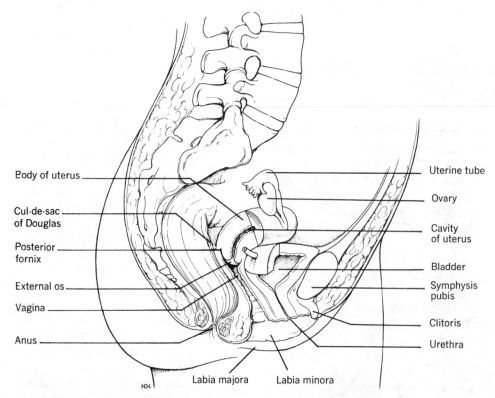

Figure 36-1 Female reproductive system as seen in sagittal section. (*Chaffee EE, Greisheimer EM: Basic Physiology and Anatomy, 3rd ed. Philadelphia, JB Lippincott, 1974*)

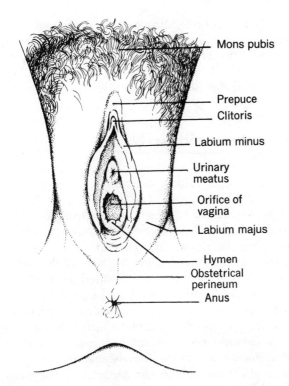

Mons pubis

Prepuce

Clitoris

Labium minus

Urinary meatus

Orifice of vagina

Labium majus

Hymen

Obstetrical perineum

Anus

Figure 36-2 External genitalia of the female. (*Chaffee EE, Lytle IM: Basic Physiology and Anatomy, 4th ed. Philadelphia, JB Lippincott, 1980*)

gery. The labia majora are rich in sebaceous glands. They are subject to the same types of problems as the mons pubis in regard to sebaceous cysts or lice infestations.

Labia minora

The labia minora (singular: labium minus) are located between the labia majora. These delicate cutaneous structures are smaller than the labia majora and are made up of skin, fat, and some erectile tissue. Unlike the skin of the labia majora, that of the labia minora is hairless and usually light pink in color. The edges may be ragged or smooth and may protrude from the labia majora. This is particularly likely after childbearing. The labia minora begin anteriorly at the hood of the clitoris and end posteriorly at the base of the vagina. The area between them is called the vestibule. Within the vestibule are located the urethral and vaginal openings, as well as the Bartholin's lubricating glands. During sexual arousal, the labia minora become distended with blood; with resolution, the labia throb, then return to normal size. The sebaceous glands secrete odoriferous fluid, in both the presence and absence of sexual arousal. The labia majora and labia minora are the most common sites of inflammation and structural changes as the result of certain sexually transmitted diseases.

Clitoris

The clitoris is located below the clitoral hood, or prepuce, which is formed by the joining of the two labia minora. The female clitoris is an erectile organ, rich in blood and nerve supply. Analogous to the male penis, it is a highly sensitive organ that becomes distended during sexual stimulation.

Urethra

The urethra, or urinary meatus, is the external opening of the internal urinary bladder. The urethra is posterior to the clitoris and is usually closer to the vaginal opening than to the clitoris. The urethra, the vaginal opening, and the Bartholin's glands lie within the vestibule.

The urethral opening is the site of the Skene's glands, which have a lubricating function. When infected, these glands or the meatus may become inflamed and painful. The Skene's glands are particularly susceptible to gonococcal infections. Inflammation may occur secondary to trauma, increased sexual activity, or structural defects such as diverticula. Secretions indicating infections may be discharged during urination or gynecologic examination. The close proximity of the urethra to the vagina and rectum predisposes to urethritis and ascending urinary tract infections. Cystitis may develop as a result of contamination with bacteria from the vagina or rectum during intercourse or foreplay.

Introitus and hymen

The vaginal orifice, commonly known as the introitus, is the opening between the external and internal genitalia. The size and shape of the opening is determined by a connective tissue membrane called the hymen that surrounds the introitus. The opening may be oval, circular, or sievelike and may be partially or completely occluded. Occlusion may occur because of the presence of an intact or partially intact hymen. Contrary to popular notion, an intact hymen does not indicate virginity, as this tissue can be stretched without tearing. At puberty, an intact hymen may require surgical intervention to permit discharge of menstrual fluids.

Bartholin's glands

The ducts of the Bartholin's glands are located between the hymenal opening and the posterior labia minora at approximately the 5 o'clock and 7 o'clock positions. These glands lubricate the vestibular area and are particularly active during sexual activity. Bacterial infection of the Bartholin's ducts may cause bilateral or unilateral labial swelling and pain that may become so severe as to inhibit ambulation. Purulent discharge may indicate gonococcal infection, and a culture of the discharge is necessary to rule this out. Infection may progress to abscess formation, which requires excision and drainage. Once incised, the cysts or infections commonly become recurrent. Therefore, perineal hygiene should be emphasized. Bartholin's cysts can develop without evidence of infection and are palpable without tenderness.

Perineal body

The perineal body is that tissue located posterior to the vaginal opening and anterior to the anus. The perineal body is composed of fibrous connective tissue and is the site of insertion of several perineal muscles. To facilitate childbirth, it is sometimes necessary to make an incision, called an episiotomy, in this tissue, as well as in vaginal tissue.

Internal genitalia

Vagina

Connecting the internal and external genitalia is a fibromuscular tube called the *vagina*. The vagina, which is essentially free of nerve-sensation fibers, is located behind the urinary bladder and urethra and anterior to the rectum. The uterine cervix projects into the vagina at its upper end forming recesses called *fornices*. The vagina functions as a route for discharge of menses and other secretions. It also serves as an organ of sexual fulfillment and reproduction.

The membranous vaginal wall forms two longitudinal folds and several transverse folds, or rugae. The vagina is lined with mucus-secreting stratified squamous epithelial cells. Vaginal tissue is usually moist, with a pH maintained within the bacteriostatic range of 3.8 to 4.2. The epithelial cells of the vagina, like other tissues of the reproductive system, respond to changing levels of the ovarian sex hormones. Estrogen stimulates the proliferation and maturation of the vaginal mucosa; this results in a thickening of the vaginal mucosa and an increased glycogen content of the epithelial cells. The glycogen is fermented to lactic acid by the lactobacilli (Döderlein's bacilli) that are part of the normal vaginal flora, accounting for the mildly acid pH of vaginal fluid. The vaginal ecology can be disrupted at many levels, rendering it susceptible to infection. Pregnancy and the use of oral contraceptive agents increase the amount of estrogen within the system. Diabetes or a prediabetic state may increase the glycogen content of the cells. The use of systemic antibiotics may decrease the number of lactobacilli within the vagina. Decreased estrogen stimulation following menopause causes the vaginal mucosa to become thin and dry, often resulting in dyspareunia

(painful intercourse), atrophic vaginitis, and occasionally vaginal bleeding. During a routine pelvic examination, the estrogen level can be estimated by examining the cellular structure and configuration of the vaginal epithelial cells. This test is known as the *maturation index*.

Uterus and cervix

The uterus is a thick-walled muscular organ. This pear-shaped hollow structure is located between the bladder and rectum. The uterus can be divided into three parts: the portion above the insertion of the fallopian tubes, called the *fundus,* the lower constricted part called the *cervix,* and the portion between the fundus and the cervix called the *body* of the uterus (Figure 36-3). The uterus is supported on both sides by four sets of ligaments: the broad ligaments, which run laterally from the body of the uterus to the pelvic sidewalls; the round ligaments, which run from the fundus laterally into each labium majus; the uterosacral ligaments, which run from the uterocervical junction to the sacrum; and the cardinal or transverse cervical ligaments.

The wall of the uterus is composed of three layers: the perimetrium, the myometrium, and the endometrium. The *perimetrium* is the outer serous covering that is derived from the abdominal peritoneum. This outer layer merges with the peritoneum that covers the broad ligaments. Anteriorly, the perimetrium is reflected over the bladder wall, forming the vesicouterine pouch, and posteriorly it extends to form the *cul-de-sac,* or *pouch of Douglas.* Because of the proximity of the perimetrium to the urinary bladder, infection of this organ often causes uterine symptoms, particularly during pregnancy.

The middle muscle layer, the *myometrium,* forms the major portion of the uterine wall. It is continuous with the myometrium of the fallopian tubes and the vagina and extends into all of the supporting ligaments with the exception of the broad ligaments. The inner fibers of the myometrium run in various directions, giving it an interwoven appearance. Contractions of these muscle fibers help to expel menstrual flow and the products of conception during miscarriage or childbirth. When pain accompanies the contractions associated with menses, it is called *dysmenorrhea.* The myometrium has an amazing ability to change length during pregnancy and labor, increasing its capacity more than 4000 times.[1]

The *endometrium,* the inner layer of the uterus, is continuous with the lining of the fallopian tubes and vagina. The endometrium is made up of a basal and a superficial layer. The superficial layer is shed during menstruation and regenerated by cells of the basal layer. Ciliated cells promote the movement

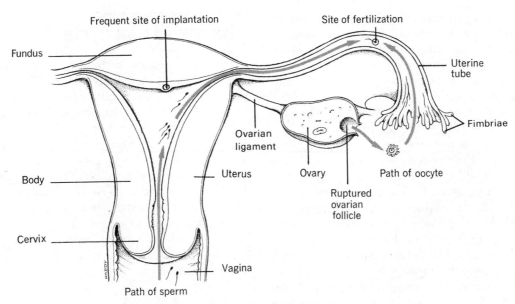

Figure 36-3 Schematic drawing of female reproductive organs, showing the path of the oocyte as it moves from the ovary into the fallopian (uterine) tube; the path of sperm is also shown, as is the usual site of fertilization. (*Chaffee EE, Lytle IM: Basic Physiology and Anatomy, 4th ed. Philadelphia, JB Lippincott, 1980*)

of tubal–uterine secretions out of the uterine cavity into the vagina.

The round cervix is the neck of the uterus that projects into the vagina. The cervix is a firm structure, composed of a connective tissue matrix of glands and muscular tissue elements, that becomes soft and pliable under the influence of hormones produced during pregnancy. Glandular tissue provides a rich supply of protective mucus that changes in character and quantity during the menstrual cycle as well as during pregnancy. The cervix is richly supplied with blood from the uterine artery and can be a site of significant blood loss during delivery.

The opening of the cervix, the *os*, forms a pathway between the uterus and the vagina. The vaginal opening is called the external os and the uterine opening, the internal os. The space between these two openings is the endocervical canal. Secretions from the columnar epithelium of the endocervix protect the uterus from infection, alter receptivity to sperm, and form a mucoid "plug" during pregnancy. The endocervical canal provides a route for menstrual discharge and sperm entrance. Pelvic infection may ascend or descend through the cervix.

Fallopian tubes

The fallopian, or uterine, tubes are slender cylindrical structures attached bilaterally to the uterus and supported by the upper folds of the broad ligament. The end of the fallopian tube nearest the ovary forms a funnel-like opening with fringed fingerlike projections, called *fimbriae*, that actually pick up the

ovum after its release into the peritoneal cavity following ovulation (see Figure 36-3). The fallopian tubes are formed of smooth muscle and lined with a ciliated mucus-producing epithelial layer. The beating of the cilia, along with contractile movements of the smooth muscle, propels the nonmobile ova toward the uterus. If coitus has been recent, fertilization normally occurs in the mid- to outer portion of the fallopian tube. Besides providing a passageway for ova and sperm, the fallopian tubes also provide for drainage of tubal secretions into the uterus. Infection and inflammation may disrupt fallopian tube patency and lead to infertility or, if only partially occluded, to a tubal pregnancy.

Ovaries

By the third month of fetal life, the ovaries of the female have fully developed and have descended to their permanent pelvic position. Remnants of the primitive genital system provide lateral supporting attachments to the uterus, and in the mature female, these supporting structures evolve into the round and suspensory ligaments. Remnants that do not evolve may also form cysts, which may become symptomatic later in life.

Oogenesis is the process of generation of ova by mitotic division that begins at the sixth week of fetal life. These primitive germ cells will ultimately provide the 1 to 2 million or so oocytes that are present in the ovaries at birth. At puberty this number is reduced through cell death to about 300,000.[2]

The newborn's ovaries are smooth, pale, and elongated. They become shorter, thicker, and heavier before the onset of menarche, which is initiated by pituitary influence. The initial hormonal stimulus for this development is believed to come from ovarian rather than systemic estrogen.

In the adult, the ovaries are flat, almond-shaped structures measuring 3 cm to 5 cm in length and weighing approximately 2 g to 3 g. They are located on either side of the uterus below the fimbriated ends of the two oviducts, or fallopian tubes. The ovaries are attached to the posterior surface of the broad ligament and to the uterus by the ovarian ligament. They are covered with a thin layer of surface epithelium, which is continuous with the lining of the peritoneum. The integrity of this covering is periodically broken at the time of ovulation.

The ovaries, like the male testes, have a dual function: they store the female germ cells, or ova, and produce the female sex hormones estrogen and progesterone. Unlike the male gonads, which produce sperm throughout the man's reproductive life, the female gonads contain a fixed number of ova at birth that diminishes throughout the woman's life.

Structurally, the mature ovary is divided into a highly vascular inner medulla, which contains supporting connective tissue, and an outer cortex of stroma and epithelial follicles (vesicles), which contain the primary oocytes, or germ cells. After puberty, the pituitary gonadotropic hormones—follicle stimulating hormone (FSH) and luteinizing hormone (LH)—stimulate primordial follicles to develop into mature graafian follicles. The graafian follicle produces estrogen which begins to stimulate the development of the endometrium in the uterus. Although several follicles begin to develop during each ovulatory cycle, only one or two complete the entire developmental process and rupture to release a mature ovum. After ovulation, the follicle becomes luteinized; and as the corpus luteum, it produces both estrogen and progesterone to support the endometrium until conception occurs or the cycle begins again.

In summary, the female genitourinary system consists of the external and internal genitalia. The genitourinary system as a whole serves both sexual and reproductive functions throughout the life cycle. The gonads, or ovaries, which are internal in the female (unlike the testes in the male) have the dual function of storing the female germ cells, or ova, and producing the female sex hormones. Through the regulation and release of sex hormones the ovaries influence the development of secondary sexual characteristics, the regulation of menstrual cycles, the maintenance of pregnancy, and the advent of menopause.

The menstrual cycle

Between menarche (first menstrual bleeding) and menopause (last menstrual bleeding), the female reproductive system undergoes cyclic changes termed the menstrual cycle. This includes the maturation and release of oocytes from the ovary during ovulation and periodic vaginal bleeding resulting from the shedding of the endometrial lining. However, it is not necessary for a woman to ovulate in order to menstruate; anovulatory cycles do occur. The menstrual cycle produces changes in the breasts, uterus, skin, ovaries, and perhaps other unidentified tissues. The maintenance of the cycle affects biologic and social aspects of a woman's life, including fertility, reproduction, sexuality, and femaleness.

Hormonal control

Normal menstrual function results from interactions among the central nervous system, hypothalamus, anterior pituitary, ovaries, and associated target tissues. Although each part of the system is essential to normal function, the ovaries are primarily responsible for controlling the cyclic changes and the length of the menstrual cycle. In most women in the middle reproductive years, menstrual bleeding occurs every 25 to 35 days, with a median length of 28 days.[3]

The hormonal control of the menstrual cycle is complex. For example, the biosynthesis of estrogens that occurs in adipose tissue may be a significant source of the hormone. There is evidence that a certain minimum body weight (48 kg) and fat content (17%) is necessary for menarche to occur and for the menstrual cycle to be maintained.[2] Although menarche is quite variable, this is supported by the observation of amenorrhea in women with anorexia nervosa, chronic disease, and malnutrition, and women who are long-distance runners. In women with anorexia nervosa, gonadotropin and estriol secretion, including LH release and responsiveness to GnRH, can revert to prepubertal levels.[4] With resumption of weight gain and attainment of sufficient body mass, the normal hormonal pattern is usually reinstated. Obesity or significant weight gain is also associated with oligomenorrhea or amenorrhea and infertility, although the mechanism is not well understood.

Hypothalamic and pituitary hormones

Growth, prepubertal maturation, reproductive cycle, and sex hormone secretion in both males and females are regulated by the follicle-stimulating hormone (FSH) and the luteinizing hormone (LH) from the anterior pituitary gland (Figure 36-4). Because these hormones promote the growth of cells in the ovaries and testes as a means of stimulating the production of sex hormones, they are called the gonadotropic hormones. The secretion of both LH and FSH is stimulated by a single hormone from the hypothalamus called gonadotropin-releasing hormone (GnRH).

In addition to LH and FSH, the anterior pituitary secretes a third hormone—prolactin. Its primary function is the stimulation of lactation in the postpartum period. During pregnancy, prolactin, along with other hormones (estrogen, progesterone, insulin, and cortisol), contributes to breast development in preparation for lactation. Although prolactin does not appear to play a physiologic role in ovarian function, hyperprolactinemia leads to hypogonadism. This may include an initial shortening of the luteal phase with subsequent anovulation, oligomenorrhea or amenorrhea, and infertility. Normally, prolactin production by the pituitary is inhibited by a hypothalamic inhibiting factor. Hyperprolactinemia may occur as a side effect of drug treatment using phenothiazine derivatives (antipsychotic drugs). These drugs are thought to act at the level of the hypothalamus to increase prolactin release by the pituitary.

Ovarian hormones

The ovaries produce estrogens, progesterone, and androgens. Ovarian hormones are secreted in a cyclic pattern as a result of the interaction between the hypothalamic-releasing factors and the pituitary gonadotropic hormones.

The steroid sex hormones enter cells by passive diffusion, bind to specific receptor proteins in the cytoplasm, and then move to the nucleus where they bind to specific sites on the chromosomes (see Chapter 43). These hormones exert their effects through gene–hormone interactions, which stimulate the synthesis of specific messenger RNA (see Chapter 3). The number of hormonal receptor sites on a cell is not fixed; the evidence suggests that they are constantly being removed and replaced. An increase or decrease in the number of receptors can serve as a mechanism for regulating hormone activity. For example, estrogen may induce the development of an increased number of estrogen receptors in some tissues and may also stimulate the synthesis of progesterone receptors. In contrast, progesterone may cause a reduction in the number of estrogen and progesterone receptors.

Estrogens. Estrogens are a family of structurally related female sex hormones synthesized and

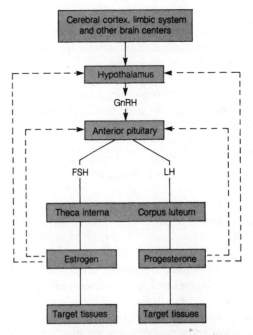

Figure 36-4 Hypothalamic-pituitary feedback control of estrogen and progesterone levels in the female.

secreted by the cells in the ovaries and in small amounts by cells in the adrenal cortex. In addition, androgens can be converted to estrogens peripherally, especially in fat tissue. Three estrogens occur naturally in humans: estrone (E_1), estradiol (E_2), and estriol (E_3). Of these, estradiol is the most biologically potent and the most abundantly secreted product of the ovary. Estrogens are secreted throughout the menstrual cycle; two peaks occur—one before ovulation and one in the middle of the luteal phase. Estrogens are transported in the blood bound to specific plasma globulins (which can also bind testosterone), inactivated and conjugated in the liver, and then excreted in the bile.

Estrogens are necessary for the normal physical maturation of the female. In concert with other hormones, estrogens provide for the reproductive processes of ovulation, implantation, pregnancy, parturition, and lactation by stimulating the development and maintaining the growth of the accessory organs. In the absence of androgens, estrogens stimulate the intrauterine development of the vagina, uterus, and uterine tubes from the embryonic müllerian system. They also stimulate the stromal development and ductal growth of the breasts at puberty, are responsible for the accelerated pubertal skeletal growth phase and for closure of the epiphysis of the long bones, contribute to the growth of axillary and pubic hair, and alter the distribution of body fat to produce the typical female body contours, including the accumulation of body fat around the hips and breasts. Larger quantities also stimulate pigmentation of the skin in the nipple, areolar, and genital regions.

In addition to their effects on the growth of uterine muscle, estrogens also play an important role in the development of the endometrial lining. During anovulatory cycles, continued exposure to estrogens for prolonged periods leads to abnormal hyperplasia of the endometrium and abnormal bleeding patterns. When estrogen production is poorly coordinated during the normal menstrual period, inappropriate bleeding and shedding of the endometrium can also occur.

Estrogens have a number of important extragenital metabolic effects. They are responsible for maintaining the normal structure of skin and blood vessels in women. Estrogens decrease the rate of bone resorption by antagonizing the effects of parathyroid hormone on bone, and for this reason osteoporosis is a common problem in estrogen-deficient postmenopausal women. In the liver, estrogens increase the synthesis of transport proteins for thyroxin, estrogen, testosterone, and other hormones. Estrogens affect the composition of the plasma lipoproteins; they produce an increase in high-density lipoproteins (HDL), a slight reduction in low-density lipoproteins (LDL), and a reduction in cholesterol levels. Plasma triglyceride levels are increased. Estrogens enhance the coagulability of blood by effecting increased circulating levels of plasminogen and factors II, VII, IX, and X.

The estrogens cause moderate retention of sodium and water. Most women retain salt and water and gain weight just before menstruation. This occurs because the estrogens facilitate the loss of intravascular fluids into the extracellular spaces, producing edema and increased sodium and water retention by the kidneys because of the decreased plasma volume. The actions of estrogens are summarized in Table 36-1.

Progesterone. Although the word *progesterone* refers to a substance that maintains pregnancy, progesterone is secreted as a part of the normal menstrual cycle. The corpus luteum of the ovary secretes large amounts of progesterone after ovulation and the adrenal cortex secretes very small amounts. The hormone circulates in the blood attached to a specific plasma protein. It is metabolized in the liver and conjugated for excretion in the bile.

The local effects of progesterone on reproductive organs include the glandular development of the lobular and alveolar tissue of the breasts and the cyclic glandular development of the endometrium. Progesterone can also compete with aldosterone at the level of the renal tubule, causing a decrease in sodium reabsorption with a resultant increase in secretion of aldosterone by the adrenal cortex (such as occurs in pregnancy).[3] Although the mechanism is uncertain, progesterone is known to increase basal body temperature, and is therefore responsible for the increase in body temperature that occurs with ovulation.

Smooth muscle relaxation under the influence of progesterone plays an important role in maintain-

Table 36–1. Actions of estrogens

General function	Specific actions
Growth and development	
Reproductive organs	Stimulate development of vagina, uterus, and fallopian tubes *in utero* and of secondary sex characteristics during puberty
Skeleton	Accelerate growth of long bones and closure of epiphysis at puberty
Reproductive processes	
Ovulation	Promote growth of ovarian follicles
Fertilization	Alter the cervical secretions to favor survival and transport of sperm
	Promote motility of sperm within the fallopian tubes by decreasing mucus viscosity
Implantation	Promote development of endometrial lining in the event of pregnancy
Vagina	Proliferate and cornify vaginal mucosa
Cervix	Increase mucus consistency
Breasts	Stimulate stromal development and ductal growth
General metabolic effects	
Bone resorption	Decrease rate of bone resorption
Plasma proteins	Increase production of thyroid and other binding globulins
Lipoproteins	Increase HDL

ing pregnancy by decreasing uterine contractions and is responsible for many of the common discomforts of pregnancy, such as edema, nausea, constipation, flatulence, and headaches. The increased progesterone present during pregnancy and the luteal phase of the menstrual cycle enhances the ventilatory response to carbon dioxide, leading to a measurable change in arterial and alveolar pCO_2.

Androgens. The normal female produces androgens as well as estrogens and progesterone. About 25% of these androgens are secreted from the ovaries, 25% from the adrenal cortex, and 50% from either ovarian or adrenal precursors. In the female, androgens contribute to normal hair growth at puberty and may have other important metabolic effects.

Ovarian follicle development and ovulation

The tissues of the adult ovary can be conveniently divided into four compartments, or units: (1) the stroma, or supporting tissue; (2) the interstitial cells; (3) the follicles; and (4) the corpus luteum. The stroma is the connective tissue substance of the ovary in which the follicles are distributed. The interstitial cells are estrogen-secreting cells that resemble the Leydig's cells, or interstitial cells, of the testes.

Beginning at puberty, a cyclic rise in the anterior pituitary gonadotropic hormones, follicle-stimulating hormone (FSH) and luteinizing hormone (LH) stimulate the development of several graafian, or mature, follicles. Follicles at all stages of development can be found in both ovaries, except in menopausal women (Figure 36-5).

The vast majority of follicles exist as primary follicles, each of which consists of a round oocyte surrounded by a single layer of flattened epithelial-derived granulosa cells and a basement membrane. The primary follicles constitute an inactive pool of follicles from which all the ovulating follicles develop. Under the influence of endocrine stimulation, 6 to 12 primary follicles develop into secondary follicles once every ovulatory cycle. During the development of the secondary follicle, the primary oocyte increases in size, and the granulosa cells proliferate to form a multilayered wall around it. During this time a membrane called the zona pellucida develops and surrounds the oocyte, and small pockets of fluid begin to appear between the granulosa cells. Blood vessels, however, do not penetrate the basement membrane; the granulosa cell layer remains avascular until after ovulation has occurred.[3]

As the follicles mature, FSH stimulates the development of the cell layers. Cells from the surrounding stromal tissue align themselves to form a

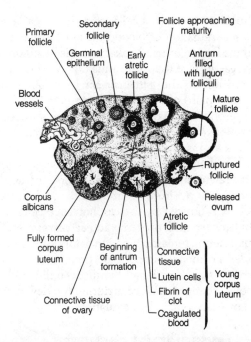

Figure 36-5 Schematic diagram of an ovary, showing the sequence of events in the origin, growth, and rupture of an ovarian follicle, and the formation and retrogression of a corpus luteum. The atretic follicles are those that show signs of degeneration and death. *(Patten BM: Human Embryology. New York, Blakiston, McGraw-Hill)*

cellular wall called the theca. The cells of the theca become differentiated into two layers, an inner theca interna, which lies adjacent to the follicular cells, and an outer theca externa. As the follicle enlarges, a single large cavity, or antrum, is formed and a portion of the granulosa cells and the oocytes are displaced to one side of the follicle by the fluid that accumulates. The secondary oocyte remains surrounded by a crown of granulosa cells, the corona radiata. As the follicle ripens, ovarian estrogen is produced by the granulosa cells. Selection of a dominant follicle occurs with the conversion to an estrogen microenvironment; and the lesser follicles, while continuing to produce some estrogen, will atrophy or become atretic. The dominant follicle accumulates a greater mass of granulosa cells and the theca becomes richly vascular giving the follicle a hyperemic appearance.[2] High levels of estrogen exert a negative feedback on FSH, inhibiting multiple follicular development and causing an increase in LH levels. This represents the follicular stage of the menstrual cycle. As estrogen suppresses FSH, the actions of LH predominate and the mature follicle (measuring approximately 20 mm) bursts; the oocyte, along with the corona radiata, is ejected from the follicle.[5] Normally, the ovum is then picked up and transported through the fallopian tube toward the uterus.

Following ovulation, the follicle collapses and the luteal stage of the menstrual cycle begins. The granulosa cells are invaded by blood vessels and yellow lipochrome-bearing cells from the theca layer. A rapid accumulation of blood and fluid forms a mass called the *corpus luteum*. Leakage of this blood onto the peritoneal surface that surrounds the ovary is thought to contribute to the *mittelschmerz* (middle, or intermenstrual, pain) of ovulation. During the luteal stage, progesterone is secreted from the corpus luteum. If fertilization does not take place, the corpus luteum atrophies and is replaced by white scar tissue (corpus albicans); the hormonal support of the endometrium is withdrawn, and menstruation occurs. In the event of fertilization, human chorionic gonadotropin (HCG) is produced by the trophoblastic cells within the blastocyst and prevents luteal regression. The corpus luteum remains functional for 3 months and provides hormonal support for pregnancy until the placenta is fully functional. Figure 36-6 illustrates the hormonal changes that occur during the development of the ovarian follicle and ovulation.

Endometrial changes

The endometrium consists of two distinct layers, or zones, that are responsive to hormonal stim-

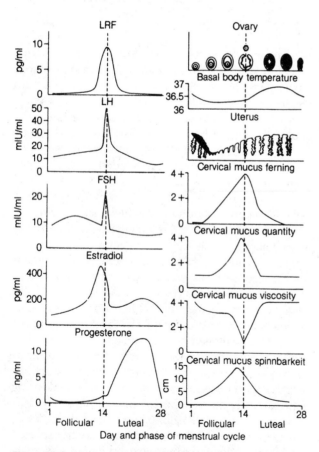

Figure 36-6 Hormonal and morphologic changes during the normal menstrual cycle. (Hershman JM: Endocrine Pathophysiology, 2nd ed. Philadelphia, Lea & Febiger, 1982)

ulation: a basal layer and a functional layer. The basal layer lies adjacent to the myometrium and is not sloughed during menstruation. The functional layer arises from the basal layer and undergoes proliferative changes and menstrual sloughing. It can be subdivided into two components: a thin, superficial, compact layer and a deeper spongiosa layer that makes up most of the secretory and fully developed endometrium. The endometrial cycle can be divided into three phases: (1) the proliferative, or preovulatory phase, during which the glands and stroma of the superficial layer grow rapidly under the influence of estrogen; (2) the secretory, or postovulatory phase, during which progesterone produces glandular dilation and active mucus secretion and the endometrium becomes highly vascular and edematous; and (3) the menstrual phase, during which the superficial layer degenerates and sloughs off.

Cervical mucus

Cervical mucus is a complex heterogeneous secretion produced by the glands of the endocervix. It is composed of 92% to 98% water and 1% inorganic salts, mainly sodium chloride. The mucus also contains simple sugars, polysaccharides, proteins, and glycoproteins. Its *pH* is usually alkaline, ranging from 6.5 to 9.0.[3] Its characteristics are strongly influenced by serum levels of estrogen and progesterone. Estrogen stimulates the production of large amounts of clear, watery mucus through which sperm can penetrate most easily. Progesterone, even in the presence of estrogen, reduces the secretion of mucus. During the luteal phase of the menstrual cycle, mucus is scant, viscous, and cellular (see Figure 36-6).

Two methods are used to examine the properties of cervical mucus and correlate them with hormonal activity. *Spinnbarkeit* is the property that allows cervical mucus to be stretched or drawn into a thread. Spinnbarkeit can be estimated by stretching a sample of cervical mucus between two glass slides and measuring the maximum length of the thread before it breaks. At midcycle, spinnbarkeit usually exceeds 10 cm.[3] A second method of estimating hormonal levels is ferning, or arborization. *Ferning* refers to the characteristic microscopic pattern that results from the crystallization of the inorganic salts in the cervical mucus when it is dried. As the estrogen levels increase, the composition of the cervical mucus changes, so that dried mucus begins to demonstrate ferning in the latter part of the follicular phase. The absence of ferning can indicate inadequate estrogen stimulation of the endocervical glands or inhibition of the endocervical glands by increased secretion of progesterone. Persistent ferning throughout the menstrual cycle suggests anovulatory cycles or insufficient progesterone secretion.

Menopause

Menopause is the cessation of menstrual cycles. It is as much a process as menstruation—not an event. At first the process takes the form of less frequent and lighter menses; it then goes on to culminate in total cessation of menses. This process, also known as the climacteric, may go on for one to several years. The usual age at menopause is 45 to 50 years. However, with improved nutrition, menopause may occur later in life, so that a woman may have a longer reproductive period. A woman who has not menstruated for a full year is said to have completed menopause.

Menopause is due to the gradual cessation of ovarian function and the resultant diminished levels of estrogen. Although estrogens derived from the adrenal cortex continue to circulate in a woman's body, they are insufficient to maintain the secondary sexual characteristics in the same manner as ovarian estrogens. As a result, breast tissue, body hair, skin elasticity, and subcutaneous fat decrease, the ovaries and uterus diminish in size, and the cervix and vagina become pale and friable. The woman may find intercourse painful and traumatic, though some type of vaginal lubrication may be helpful.

Systemically, a woman may experience significant vasomotor instability secondary to the decrease in estrogens and the relative increase in pituitary FSH. This instability may give rise to "hot flashes," palpitations, dizziness, and headaches as the blood vessels dilate. A woman may feel anxious or depressed about these uncontrollable and unpredictable events.

Societal mores influence behaviors. A society that emphasizes youthfulness, fitness, and vigor does not look on aging as a positive process; and menopause is regarded as a hallmark of advancing age. A woman who focuses her energy on beauty and youth may feel frustrated or depressed by the natural aging process. On the other hand, a woman who values her other, nonphysical attributes may welcome advancing age as a time when she may more fully develop as a person.

In summary, between the menarche and menopause, the female reproductive system undergoes cyclic changes termed the menstrual cycle. Normal menstrual function results from complex interactions among the hypothalamus, anterior pituitary gland, ovaries, and associated target tissues such as the endometrium and vaginal mucosa. Although each component of the system is essential for normal function, the ovaries are largely responsible for controlling the cyclic changes and length of the menstrual cycle.

The breast

Although anatomically separate, the breasts are functionally related to the female genitourinary system, in that they respond to the cyclic changes in sex hormones and produce milk for infant nourishment. The breast is also important for its sexual function and for cosmetic appearance. Breast cancer represents one-fifth of all female malignancies. The high rate of breast cancer has drawn even greater attention to the importance of the breast throughout the life span.

Structure

The breast, or mammary tissue, is located between the third and seventh ribs of the anterior chest wall, supported by the pectoral muscles and superficial fascia. Breasts are specialized glandular structures that have an abundant shared nerve, vascular, and lymphatic supply (Figure 36-7). What we commonly call breasts are actually two parts of a single anatomical breast. It is this contiguous nature of breast tissue that is important in both health and illness. Men and women alike are born with rudimentary breast tissue, the ducts lined with epithelium. In women, the pituitary release of FSH, LH, and prolactin at puberty stimulates the ovary to produce and release estrogen. This estrogen stimulates the growth and proliferation of the ductile system. With the onset of ovulatory cycles, progesterone release stimulates the growth and development of ductile and alveolar secretory epithelium. By adolescence the breasts have developed characteristic fat deposition patterns and contours.

Structurally, the breast consists of fat, fibrous connective tissue, and glandular tissue. The superficial fibrous connective tissue is attached to the skin, a fact that is important in the visual observation of skin movement over the breast during breast self-examination. The breast mass is supported by the fascia of the pectoralis major and minor muscles and by the fibrous connective tissue of the breast. Fibrous tissue ligaments, called *Cooper's ligaments,* extend from the outer boundaries of the breast to the nipple area in a radial fashion, like the spokes on a wheel (see Figure 36-7). These ligaments further support the breast and form septa that divide the breast into 15 to 25 lobes. Each lobe consists of grapelike clusters, alveoli or glands, which are interconnected by ducts. The alveoli are

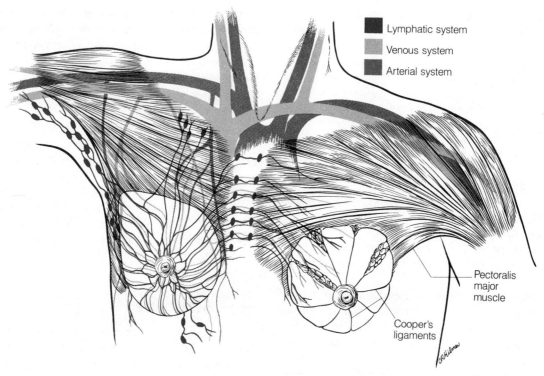

Lymphatic system
Venous system
Arterial system

Pectoralis major muscle

Cooper's ligaments

Figure 36-7 The breasts, showing the shared vascular and lymphatic supply, as well as the pectoral muscles.

lined with secretory cells capable of producing milk or fluid under the proper hormonal conditions (Figure 36-8). The route of descent of milk and other breast secretions is from alveoli to duct, to intralobar duct, to lactiferous duct and reservoir, to nipple. Breast milk is produced secondary to complex hormonal changes associated with pregnancy. Fluid is produced and reabsorbed during the menstrual cycle. The breast responds to the cyclic changes in the menstrual cycle with fullness and discomfort.

The nipple is made up of epithelial, glandular, erectile, and nervous tissue. Areolar tissue sur-

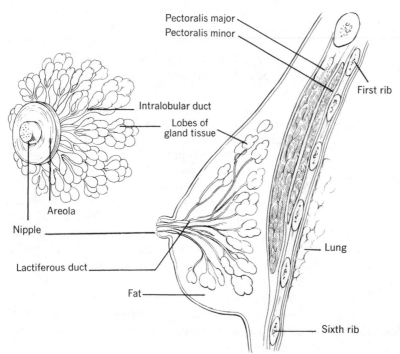

Pectoralis major
Pectoralis minor
First rib

Intralobular duct
Lobes of gland tissue

Areola

Nipple

Lactiferous duct

Fat

Lung

Sixth rib

Figure 36-8 The breast, showing the glandular tissue and ducts of the mammary glands. (*Chaffee EE, Lytle IM: Basic Physiology and Anatomy, 4th ed. Philadelphia, JB Lippincott, 1980*)

rounds the nipple and is recognized as the darker smooth skin between the nipple and the breast. The small bumps or projections on the areolar surface are Montgomery's tubercles, sebaceous glands that keep the nipple area soft and elastic. At puberty and during pregnancy, increased levels of estrogen and progesterone cause the areola and nipple to become darker and more prominent and Montgomery's glands to become more active. The erectile tissue of the nipple is responsive to psychological and tactile stimuli, which contributes to the sexual function of the breast.

There are many individual variations in breast size and shape. The shape and texture vary with hormonal, genetic, nutritional, and endocrine factors, as well as with muscle tone, age, and pregnancy. A well-developed set of pectoralis muscles will support the breast mass higher on the chest wall. Poor posture, significant weight loss, and lack of support may cause the breasts to droop.

Pregnancy

During pregnancy the breast is significantly altered by increased levels of both estrogen and progesterone. Estrogen stimulates increased vascularity of the breast as well as growth and extension of the ductile structures, causing "heaviness" of the breast. Progesterone causes marked budding and growth of the alveolar structures. The alveolar epithelium assumes a secretory state in preparation for lactation. The progesterone-induced changes that occur during pregnancy may confer some protection against cancer. Cellular changes that occur within the alveolar lining are thought to change the susceptibility of these cells to estrogen-mediated changes later in life.

Lactation

During lactation, milk is secreted by alveolar cells, which are under the influence of the anterior pituitary hormone prolactin. Milk ejection from the ductile system occurs in response to the release of oxytocin from the posterior pituitary. The suckling of the infant provides the stimulus for milk ejection.

Suckling produces feedback to the hypothalamus, stimulating the release of oxytocin from the posterior pituitary. Oxytocin in turn causes contraction of the myoepithelial cells lining the alveoli and ejection of milk into the ductal system. A woman may have breast leakage for 3 months to a year after the termination of breast feeding as breast tissue and hormones regress to the nonlactating state. Overzealous breast stimulation with or without pregnancy can likewise cause breast leakage.

Changes with menopause

At the onset of menopause, the levels of estrogen and progesterone are gradually reduced, and the breasts regress secondary to the loss of glandular tissue. The lobular–alveolar structures atrophy, leaving fat, connective tissue, and ducts. The breast generally becomes pendulous with the decrease in tissue mass.

In summary, the breast is a complex structure of variable size, consistency, and composition. Although anatomically distinct, the breasts are functionally related to the female genitourinary system in that they respond to cyclic changes in sex hormones and produce milk for infant nourishment. Breast tissue is not static but changes throughout the life cycle.

References

1. Benson RC: Handbook of Obstetrics and Gynecology, 8th ed, p 20. Los Altos, CA, Lange Medical Publications, 1983
2. Speroff L, Glass RH, Kase NG: Clinical Gynecologic Endocrinology and Infertility, 3rd ed, pp 104, 70. Baltimore, MD, Williams & Wilkins, 1983
3. Greenspan FS, Forsham PH: Basic and Clinical Endocrinology, pp 374, 374, 377, 381, 383. Los Altos, CA, Lange Medical Publications, 1983
4. Hershman JM: Endocrine Pathophysiology, 2nd ed, p 146. Philadelphia, Lea & Febiger, 1982
5. Austin CR, Short RV: Hormonal Control of Reproduction, 2nd ed, p 107. New York, Cambridge Press, 1984

CHAPTER 37

Patricia McCowen Mehring

Alterations in Structure and Function of the Female Reproductive System

Objectives

After you have studied this chapter, you should be able to meet the following objectives:

- _____ Compare the extragenital pathologies associated with vulvulitis, Bartholin's cyst, epidermal cysts, nevi, vulvular dystrophy, and cancer of the vulva.
- _____ State the function of Döderlein's bacilli.
- _____ Describe conditions that predispose to vaginal infections.
- _____ State measures to prevent vaginal infections that a health professional should convey to a client.
- _____ Relate the association between the use of diethylstilbestrol and vaginal carcinoma.
- _____ Define the terms *dysplasia* and *metaplasia*.
- _____ Describe the importance of the cervical transformation zone in the development of cervical cancer.
- _____ Compare the lesions associated with nabothian cysts and cervical polyps.

(continued)

_____ Relate the importance of the Pap smear in early detection and decreased incidence of deaths from cervical cancer.

_____ Define the terms *conization, biopsy, local cautery, cryosurgery,* and *laser therapy* as they relate to the diagnosis and treatment of cervical cancer.

_____ List the complications of untreated cervicitis.

_____ Compare the early signs and symptoms of cancer of the vulva, vagina, cervix, endometrium, fallopian tubes, and ovaries.

_____ Define the term *endometritis.*

_____ Describe the pathology associated with endometriosis.

_____ Briefly describe the treatment methods for endometriosis.

_____ List the symptoms by which the health professional would be able to identify adenomyosis.

_____ Compare the age distribution for cervical and endometrial cancer.

_____ Compare the risk factors for development of cervical and endometrial cancer.

_____ Compare the methods for early detection of cervical and endometrial cancer.

_____ Compare the intramural and subserosal leiomyomas.

_____ List the common causes of pelvic inflammatory disease (PID).

_____ List the common symptoms of PID.

_____ State the etiologic factors associated with tubal pregnancy.

_____ Describe the symptoms of a tubal pregnancy.

_____ State the underlying cause of ovarian cyst.

_____ Differentiate benign ovarian cyst from the Stein-Leventhal syndrome.

_____ List the hormones produced by the three types of functioning ovarian tumors.

_____ State the one reason that ovarian cancer may be difficult to detect in an early stage.

_____ Describe the three types of dysfunction that can result from disorders of pelvic support.

_____ Explain how uterine anteflexion, retroflexion, and retroversion differ from normal uterine position.

_____ Define the terms *amenorrhea, hypomenorrhea, oligomenorrhea, menorrhagia, metrorrhagia,* and *menometrorrhagia.*

_____ State the general cause of most dysfunctional menstrual cycles.

_____ Compare the symptoms of primary dysmenorrhea with those of secondary dysmenorrhea.

_____ Define the condition known as *premenstrual syndrome (PMS).*

_____ List at least ten possible symptoms of PMS.

_____ Describe purposes of the current treatment methods for PMS.

_____ Name and describe four or more benign disorders of the female breast.

Disorders of the female genitourinary system have widespread effects on both physical and psychological function, affecting both sexuality and reproductive function. The reproductive structures are located very close to other pelvic structures, particularly those of the urinary system. Therefore, disorders of the reproductive system may also affect urinary function. This chapter focuses on infection and inflammation, benign conditions, and neoplasms of the female reproductive structures, disorders of pelvic support and uterine position, and alterations in menstruation. A brief overview of infertility is also included.

Disorders of the external genitalia

Vulvitis and folliculitis

Vulvitis, or inflammation of the vulva, is not generally considered a specific disease but tends to develop subsequent to other local and systemic disorders. The cause is often an irritating vaginal discharge. *Candida albicans* (yeast) is the most common cause of chronic vulvar pruritus, particularly in women with diabetes mellitus. Vulvitis may also be a component of sexually transmitted diseases such as herpes genitalis or human papilloma virus infection (condyloma). Local dermatitis reactions to chemical irritants such as laundry products, perfumed soaps or sprays, spermicides, or allergens such as poison ivy can also cause inflammation. Finally, vulvar itching may be due to atrophy that is part of the normal aging process. The management of vulvitis focuses on appropriate treatment of underlying causes and comfort measures to relieve the irritation. These include keeping the area clean and dry, using warm sitz baths with baking soda, wet dressings or Burow's solution soaks (a mild astringent), or applying a mild hydrocortisone cream for the immediate relief of symptoms.

Folliculitis is an infection that involves the hair follicles of the mons or labia majora. The infection, which is characterized by small red papules or pustules surrounding the hair shaft, is relatively common because of the density of bacteria in this area as well as the occlusive nature of clothing covering the genitalia. Treatment includes thorough cleansing of the area with germicidal soap, followed by the appli-

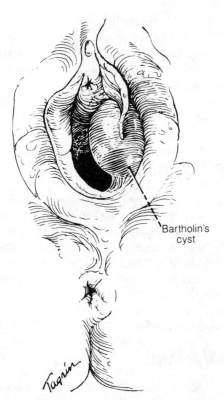

Bartholin's cyst

Figure 37-1 Bartholin's cyst. (*Green TH Jr: Gynecology: Essentials of Clinical Practice, 3rd ed. Boston, Little, Brown & Co, 1977*)

cation of a mild bacterial ointment such as neosporin or polysporin.

Bartholin's cyst/Bartholin abscess

A cyst is a fluid-filled sac. Bartholin's cyst results from the occlusion of the duct system within Bartholin's gland. When the cyst becomes infected, the contents become purulent; if untreated, a Bartholin's abscess can result. The obstruction that causes cyst and abscess formation most commonly follows a bacterial, chlamydial, or gonococcal infection. Cysts can attain the size of an orange, and frequently recur (Figure 37-1). Abscesses can be extremely tender and painful. Asymptomatic cysts require no treatment. The treatment of symptomatic cysts consists of the administration of appropriate antibiotics, local application of moist heat, and incision and drainage. Cysts that are frequently abscessed or are large enough to cause blockage of the introitus may require surgical intervention (marsupialization).

Epidermal cysts

Epidermal cysts (sebaceous or inclusion cysts) are common semisolid tumors of the vulva. These small nodules are lined with keratinizing squamous epithelium and contain cellular debris with a sebaceous appearance and odor. Epidermal cysts may be solitary or multiple and have a yellow appearance when stretched or compressed. They usually resolve spontaneously and treatment is unnecessary unless they become infected or significantly enlarged.[1]

Nevi

Nevi (moles) occur on the vulva as elsewhere on the body. They can be singular or multiple, flat or raised, and may vary in degree of pigmentation from flesh-colored to very dark brown/black. Nevi are asymptomatic, but should be observed for changes that could indicate malignancy. Nevi may resemble melanomas or basal cell carcinomas and excisional biopsy is recommended when doubt exists.

Vulvar dystrophy

Vulvar dystrophy, which is characterized by white lesions of the vulva, is a common condition once considered to be premalignant. These lesions may be categorized as lichen sclerosus, hyperplastic dystrophy, or a mixed classification depending on clinical and histologic characteristics. Clinically, lichen sclerosus patches are thin, parchment-like, and "atrophic," whereas hyperplastic areas are thick, grey-white plaques. Both can be pruritic. Vulvar biopsy is needed for accurate diagnosis. Lichen sclerosus responds best to topical application of testosterone propionate in Vaseline; hyperplastic dystrophy to a combination steroid (betamethasone valerate) and antipruritic (crotamiton [Eurax]) cream. Lichen sclerosus recurs frequently, and lifetime maintenance therapy is suggested. Hyperplastic dystrophy is less common. Mixed dystrophy requires combination therapy over a longer period.[1]

Cancer of the vulva

Carcinoma of the vulva accounts for 3% to 5% of all malignancies of the female genitourinary system. Invasive carcinoma is seen most frequently in women who are 60 years of age or older; almost one-half are over 70 years of age. The mean age for carcinoma in situ is 10 years younger than for invasive carcinoma.[2] Certain sexually transmitted diseases, such as condyloma accuminatum, predispose to vulvar cancer, which may account for the recent rise in incidence of vulvar intraepithelial neoplasia among women in their 20's and 30's.

About 85% to 90% of invasive cancers of the vulva are squamous cell carcinomas. The initial lesion may appear as an inconspicuous thickening of the skin, a small raised area or lump, or an ulceration that fails to heal. These lesions often resemble eczema or dermatitis and may produce few symptoms, other than pruritus, local discomfort, and exudation. A recurrent, persistent, pruritic vulvitis may be the only complaint. Therefore, the symptoms are frequently treated with various home remedies before medical treatment is sought. The lesion often becomes secondarily infected, and this causes pain and discomfort. Gradually the malignant lesion spreads superficially or as a deep furrow involving all of one labial side. Because there are many lymph channels around the vulva, the cancer metastasizes freely to the regional lymph nodes. It seems to make little difference whether the tumor is well differentiated or undifferentiated; lymph node metastases can occur in either case. The most common extension is to the superficial inguinal, deep femoral, and external iliac lymph nodes.

Other types of cancer found on the vulva include intraepithelial cancer (Bowen's disease, erythroplasia of Queyrat, and carcinoma in situ simplex), extramammary Paget's disease (which can be intraepithelial or invasive), carcinoma of Bartholin's gland (5% of vulvar cancer), basal cell carcinoma (2%–3% of vulvar cancer), or malignant melanoma (8%–11% of vulvar cancer).[2]

Early diagnosis is important in the treatment of vulvar carcinoma. Because malignant lesions can vary so much in appearance and are often mistaken for other conditions, biopsy and treatment are often delayed. Treatment is primarily wide surgical excision of the lesion for noninvasive cancer and vulvectomy with node resection for invasive cancer. Local chemotherapeutic agents (fluorouracil [5-FU]) and colposcopically guided laser therapy are used to treat focal areas of malignancy in cases where surgery is contraindicated. The 5-year survival rate for women with lesions of less than 3 cm in diameter and minimal node involvement is 60% to 80% following surgical treatment. Follow-up visits every 3 months for the first 2 years after surgery and then every 6 months thereafter is important to detect recurrent disease or a second primary cancer. The 5-year survival rate for patients who have larger lesions in conjunction with three or more positive nodes is less than 15% following surgical treatment.[2] Once pelvic lymphadenopathy is established, the prognosis is poor.

In summary, the surface of the vulva is affected by disorders that affect skin on other parts of the body. These disorders include inflammation (vulvulitis and folliculitis), epidermal cysts, and nevi. Although these disorders are not serious they can be distressing in that they produce severe discomfort and itching. Bartholin's cysts are the result of occluded ducts within the Bartholin's glands. They are often painful and can become infected. Vulvar dystrophies are characterized by thinning and hyperplastic thickening of vulvar tissues. Cancer of the vulva, which accounts for 3% to 5% of all female genitourinary cancers, is associated with genital herpes infections and human papilloma virus.

Disorders of the vagina

The normal vaginal ecology depends on the delicate balance of hormones and bacterial flora. Normal estrogen levels maintain a thick protective squamous epithelium that contains glycogen. *Döderlein's bacilli,* a part of the normal vaginal flora, metabolize glycogen and in the process produce the lactic acid that normally maintains the vaginal *p*H below 4.5. Disruptions in these normal environmental conditions predispose to infection.

Vaginitis

Vaginitis is an inflammation of the vagina; it is characterized by vaginal discharge and burning, itching, redness, and swelling of vaginal tissues. Pain often occurs with urination and with sexual intercourse. Vaginitis may be caused by chemical irritants, foreign bodies, and infectious agents. The causes of vaginitis differ in various age groups. In premenarchal girls, most vaginal infections are due to nonspecific causes such as poor hygiene, intestinal parasites, or the presence of foreign bodies. *Candida albicans, Trichomonas vaginalis,* and bacterial vaginosis are the most common causes of vaginal discharge in the childbearing years and can be sexually transmitted (see Chapter 38). In postmenopausal women, atrophic vaginitis is the most common form.

Atrophic vaginitis is an inflammation of the vagina that occurs after menopause or removal of the ovaries and their estrogen supply. Estrogen deficiency results in a lack of regenerative growth of the vaginal epithelium, rendering these tissues more susceptible to infection and irritation. Furthermore, *Döderlein's bacilli* disappear, so that the vaginal secretions become less acid. The symptoms of atrophic vaginitis include itching, burning, and painful intercourse. These symptoms can usually be reversed by local application of estrogen creams or vaginal suppositories.

Every woman has a normal vaginal discharge during the menstrual cycle, but it should not cause burning or itching or have an unpleasant odor. These symptoms are suggestive of inflammation or infection. Because these symptoms are common to the different types of vaginitis, precise identification of the organism is essential for proper treatment. A careful history should include information about systemic disease conditions, the use of drugs—such as antibiotics—that foster the growth of yeast, dietary habits, stress, and other factors that alter the resistance of vaginal tissue to infections. A physical examination is usually done to evaluate the nature of the discharge and its effects on the genital structures. Microscopic examination of a saline wet-mount smear (prepared by dipping a cotton-tipped applicator into a test tube of saline solution and transferring a small amount to a slide) is the primary means of identifying the organism responsible for the infection. A small amount of potassium hydroxide (KOH) is added to the solution on the slide to aid in the identification of *C. albicans.* Culture methods may be needed when the organism is not apparent on the wet-mount preparation.

The prevention and treatment of vaginal infections depend on proper health habits and on accurate diagnosis and treatment of ongoing infections. Measures to prevent infection include development of daily hygiene habits that keep the genital area clean and dry, maintenance of normal vaginal flora and healthy vaginal mucosa, and avoidance of contact with organisms known to cause vaginal infections. Perfumed products such as feminine deodorant sprays, douches, bath powders, even soaps and toilet paper can be irritating and may alter the normal vaginal flora. Tight clothing prevents the dissipation of body heat and evaporation of skin moisture and thus promotes favorable conditions for the growth of pathogens, as well as irritation. Nylon and other synthetic undergarments, pantyhose, and swimsuits tend to hold body moisture next to the skin and to harbor infectious organisms, even after they have been washed. Cotton undergarments that withstand hot water and bleach (a fungicide) may be preferable for women to prevent such infections. Swimsuits and other garments that do not withstand hot water or bleaching should be hung in the sunlight to dry. Women should be taught to wipe from front to back to avoid bringing rectal contamination into the vagina. Avoiding sexual contact whenever an infection is known or suspected should limit that route of transmission.

Cancer of the vagina

In general, primary cancers of the vagina are extremely rare. They account for about 1% to 2% of all malignancies of the female reproductive system. Like vulvar carcinoma, carcinoma of the vagina is largely a disease of older women, with a peak incidence between 50 and 70 years of age. The exception to that is clear-cell adenocarcinoma associated with DES exposure *in utero,* which has an age range of 7 to 29 years of age (mean, 19 years).[3] Vaginal cancers

may result from local extension of cervical cancer, from local irritation such as occurs with prolonged use of a pessary, or from exposure to sexually transmitted herpes virus or papillomaviruses.

More than 90% of vaginal cancers are squamous cell carcinomas, with other common types being adenocarcinomas, sarcomas, and melanomas.[2] Maternal ingestion of diethylstilbestrol (DES) in early pregnancy has been clearly associated with the development of clear-cell adenocarcinoma in female offspring who were exposed *in utero.* Between 1940 and 1975, DES, a nonsteroidal synthetic estrogen, was frequently prescribed to prevent miscarriage. Its association with adenocarcinoma of the vagina was not discovered until the late 1960s. A tumor registry of clear-cell adenocarcinoma of the genital tract in young women was established in 1971, and over 400 cases have now been reported. The incidence of clear-cell adenocarcinoma of the vagina is quite low, approximately 0.1% in young women who were exposed *in utero* to synthetic estrogen. This is fortunate, since at the time of the banning of DES, an estimated 4 million American women had taken the drug. Although only a small percentage of girls exposed to estrogen actually develop clear-cell adenocarcinoma, 75% to 90% of them do develop benign adenosis (ectopic extension of cervical columnar epithelium into the vagina, which is normally stratified squamous epithelium), which may predispose to cancer. Any girl exposed to DES should be encouraged to have semiannual gynecologic examinations beginning at age 14 or at menarche with an initial examination that includes careful colposcopic inspection of the cervix and vagina.

The most common symptom of vaginal carcinoma is abnormal bleeding. However, 20% of women are asymptomatic, with the cancer being discovered during a routine pelvic examination. The anatomic proximity of the vagina to other pelvic structures (urethra, bladder and rectum) permits early spread to these areas. Pelvic pain, dysuria, constipation, and vaginal discharge can be associated symptoms. Vaginal squamous cell carcinoma is most often detected in the upper anterior one-third of the vagina, with adenocarcinoma found more often on the lower anterior and lateral vaginal vault.[4] However, malignancy can develop anywhere within the vagina, and visualization during physical examination should always cover the entire vault. Women should continue to have vaginal cytology studies (Pap smears) at least every 2 years following hysterectomy to rule out development of vaginal cancer. Diagnosis requires a biopsy of suspicious lesions or areas. Further studies, such as cystoscopy or proctoscopy, may be necessary.

Treatment of vaginal cancer must take into consideration the size, location, and spread of the lesion, and the woman's age. Radical surgery and radiation are both curative. When there is upper vaginal involvement, radical surgery includes a total hysterectomy, pelvic lymph node dissection, and placement of a graft from the buttock to the area from which the vagina was excised. The ovaries are usually preserved unless they are diseased. Extensive lesions and those located in the middle or lower vaginal area are usually treated by radiation therapy. Newer therapies for isolated lesions include vaporization with the CO_2 laser or intravaginal application of a cream incorporating 5-FU (Efudex).[2,5] The prognosis depends on the stage of the disease, the involvement of lymph nodes, and the degree of mitotic activity of the tumor. With radiotherapy or radical surgery, the 5-year survival rate for cancer not related to DES is 20% to 30%; for DES-related cancers the survival rate is about 80%.[6]

Disorders of the cervix

The cervix is composed of two distinct types of tissue. The exocervix, or visible portion, is covered with stratified squamous epithelium, which also lines the vagina. The endocervical canal is lined with columnar epithelium. The junction of these two tissue types (the squamocolumnar junction) appears at various locations on the cervix at different points in a woman's life (Figure 37-2). During periods of high estrogen production, particularly fetal existence, menarche, and during the first pregnancy, the cervix everts or turns outward, exposing the columnar epithelium to the vaginal environment. The combination of estrogen and low vaginal pH leads to a gradual transformation from columnar to squamous epithelium—a process called *metaplasia*. The dynamic area

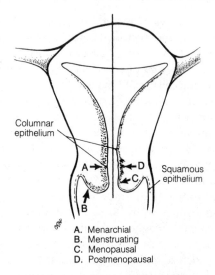

A. Menarchial
B. Menstruating
C. Menopausal
D. Postmenopausal

Figure 37-2 Location of squamocolumnar junction in menarchial, menstruating, menopausal, and postmenopausal women.

of change where metaplasia takes place is called the *transformation zone*.[7]

The transformation zone is a critical area for the development of cervical cancer. During the process of metaplasia the newly developed squamous epithelial cells are vulnerable to genetic change if exposed to carcinogenic agents (cancer-producing substances). *Dysplasia* literally means disordered growth or development. Although initially a reversible cell change, untreated dysplasia can develop into carcinoma.

Metaplasia can result in retention cysts, called *nabothian cysts*, that develop when mucus becomes trapped within the deeper clefts of the columnar epithelial cells. These are benign cysts that require no treatment unless they become so numerous that they cause cervical enlargement. The nabothian cyst farthest away from the external cervical os indicates the outer aspect of the transformation zone. The transformation zone is the area of the cervix that must be sampled to have an adequate Pap smear, and is the area that is most carefully examined during colposcopy.

Cervicitis and cervical polyps

Cervicitis is an acute or chronic inflammation of the cervix. Acute cervicitis may result from the direct infection of the cervix or may be secondary to a vaginal or uterine infection. It may be caused by a variety of infective agents, including *Candida albicans, Trichomonas vaginalis, Neisseria gonorrhoeae, Gardnerella vaginalis, Chlamydia trachomatis, Ureaplasma urealyticum,* or herpes simplex virus. Chlamydia is the organism most commonly associated with mucopurulent cervicitis.[8] Chronic cervicitis represents a low-grade inflammatory process. It is common in parous women and may be a sequela to minute lacerations that occur during childbirth, instrumentation, or other trauma. The organisms are usually of a nonspecific type, often staphylococcus, streptococcus, or coliform bacteria.

With acute cervicitis, the cervix becomes reddened and edematous. Irritation from the infection results in copious mucopurulent drainage and leukorrhea. The symptoms of chronic cervicitis are less well defined: the cervix may be ulcerated or normal in appearance; it may contain nabothian cysts; the cervical os may be distorted by old lacerations or everted to expose areas of columnar epithelium; and a mucopurulent drainage may be present.

Untreated cervicitis may extend to include the development of pelvic cellulitis, low back pain, painful intercourse, cervical stenosis, dysmenorrhea, and further infection of the uterus or fallopian tubes. Depending on the causative agent, acute cervicitis is treated with appropriate antibiotic therapy. Diagnosis of chronic cervicitis is based on vaginal examination, colposcopy, cytologic smears, and occasionally biopsy to rule out malignant changes. The treatment usually involves cryosurgery or cauterization, which causes the tissues to slough and thus leads to eradication of the infection. Colposcopically guided laser vaporization of abnormal epithelium is the newest, but most expensive treatment for cervicitis.

Polyps are the most common lesions of the cervix and can be found in women of all ages, although they are most common during the reproductive years. The polyps are soft, velvety-red lesions; they are usually pedunculated and are often found protruding through the cervical os. They usually develop as a result of inflammatory hyperplasia of the endocervical mucosa. Polyps are often asymptomatic but may have associated postcoital bleeding. Most are benign, but they should be removed and examined by a pathologist to rule out malignant change.

—— Cancer of the cervix

Cervical cancer is the most readily detected and, if detected early, the most easily cured of all the cancers of the female reproductive system. The incidence of invasive cervical cancer has steadily decreased over the years, while that of cancer in situ has risen. Approximately 13,000 cases of cancer of the cervix were diagnosed in 1988 and there were about 7000 deaths from cervical cancer during the same period. The death rate has steadily declined over the past 40 years with the introduction of more sensitive and readily available screening methods (Pap smear, colposcopy, cervicography), consistent use of a standardized grading system that guides treatment, and more effective treatment methods. The 5-year survival rate for all cervical cancer patients is 66%; with early diagnosis the rate is 80% to 90%; for cancer in situ, the rate approaches 100%.[9]

Carcinoma of the cervix is usually considered to be a sexually transmissible disease.[10] It is rare among celibate women. Risk factors include early age at first intercourse, multiple sexual partners, and a promiscuous male partner. An uncircumcised male partner, multiple pregnancies, and use of oral contraceptives—once considered predisposing factors—have all been eliminated from the list of factors that place women at risk for cervical cancer. A relationship between herpes simplex virus 2 (HSV-2) and human papilloma virus with cancer of the cervix has been demonstrated. An HSV-2 antigen (AG-4) has been identified in 90% of cervical carcinoma biopsy samples and HSV-2 DNA sequences have been identified within the DNA molecule of malignant cells. Certain strains of HPV have been identified in invasive carcinoma of the cervix,[11,12] while others are more often associated with dysplasia or cancer in situ.[13,14] Because these viruses are spread by sexual contact, their association with cervical cancer provides a tempting hypotheses to explain the relationship between sexual practices and cervical cancer.

One of the most important advances in the early diagnosis and treatment of cancer of the cervix was made possible by the observation that this cancer arises from precursor lesions, which begin with the development of atypical cervical cells. These gradually progress to cancer in situ and finally to invasive cancer of the cervix. Atypical cells differ from normal cervical squamous epithelium. There are changes in the nuclear and cytoplasmic parts of the cell and more variation in cell size and shape (dysplasia). Cancer in situ is localized to the epithelial layer, whereas invasive cancer of the cervix spreads. A system of grading and specific terminology has been devised to describe the dysplastic changes of cancer precursors. This system involves the use of the term *cervical intraepithelial neoplasia* (CIN). The CIN system grades according to extent of involvement of the epithelial thickness of the cervix; CIN grade I (mild dysplasia) involves the lower one-third of the epithelial layer and the lesion is well differentiated; CIN grade II (moderate dysplasia) involves one-third to two-thirds of the epithelial layer and is less well differentiated; and CIN grade III is an undifferentiated intraepithelial lesion with two-thirds (severe dysplasia) to full-thickness (carcinoma in situ) involvement. Once cancer has been diagnosed, the general preference is to use the International Federation of Gynecology and Obstetrics (FIGO) classification system to describe the histologic and clinical extent of the disease. The development of an internationally accepted grading system has significantly increased the data base for cervical cancer and the consistency of that data base.

The atypical cellular changes that precede frank neoplastic changes consistent with cancer of the cervix can be recognized by a number of direct and microscopic techniques, including the Papanicolaou (Pap) cytologic test, colposcopy, or cervicography. The precursor lesions can exist in a reversible form, which sometimes regresses spontaneously, or they may progress and undergo malignant change. Cancers of the cervix have a long latent period; untreated dysplasia gradually progresses to carcinoma in situ, which may remain static for 7 to 10 years before it becomes invasive.[2] After the preinvasive period, growth is rapid, and if the cancer is untreated, death follows within 2 to 5 years of the onset of symptoms.

The purpose of the Pap smear (also discussed in Chapter 5) is to detect the presence of abnormal cells on the surface of the cervix or within the endocervix. This test detects both precancerous and cancerous lesions. Although the American Cancer Society has suggested that the Pap test need not be done annually if there have been three normal tests in succession, most clinicians maintain that performing an annual test is the safest course to follow. If the woman has risk factors such as previous herpes or HPV infection, DES exposure *in utero* or a strong family history of cervical cancer, more frequent Pap smears may be recommended. There are several methods for classifying the Pap smear. One method divides the results into five classes:

Class I: Normal, or no abnormal cells

Class II: Atypical cells below the level of neoplasia (benign atypia, or inflammatory)

Class III: Abnormal cells typical of dysplasia (mild or moderate; CIN 1 or CIN 2)

Class IV: Cells consistent with cancer in situ (severe dysplasia; CIN 3)

Class V: Abnormal cells consistent with invasive squamous cell carcinoma

Pap smears are only about 80% to 90% accurate in diagnosing CIN even under optimal circumstances. Care must be taken to obtain an adequate smear from the transformation zone that includes endocervical cells, and to ensure that the cytologic examination is done by a competent laboratory. The presence of normal endometrial cells in a cervical cytologic sample during the luteal phase of the menstrual cycle or in the postmenopausal period has been associated with endometrial disease and warrants further evaluation.[10] This demonstrates that even shedding of normal cells at an inappropriate time may indicate disease.

Diagnosis of cancer requires pathologic confirmation. If a Pap smear shows atypical cells, a colposcopic study is usually done. This is a vaginal examination that is done using a colposcope, an instrument that affords a well-lighted and magnified stereoscopic view of the cervix. During colposcopy, the cervical tissue may be stained with an iodine solution (Schiller's test) or acetic acid solution to accentuate topographic or vascular changes that can differentiate normal from abnormal tissue. A biopsy sample may be obtained from suspicious areas and examined microscopically. With the availability of colposcopy, many women with abnormal Pap smears have been able to avoid cone biopsy. Cone biopsy involves the removal of a cone-shaped wedge of cervix including the entire transformation zone and at least 50% of the endocervical canal. Postoperative hemorrhage, infection, cervical stenosis, infertility, and incompetent cervix are possible sequelae that warrant avoidance of this procedure unless it is truly necessary. Diagnostic conization is indicated when a lesion is partly or completely beyond colposcopic view or colposcopically directed biopsy fails to explain the cytology.

A final diagnostic tool in areas where colposcopy is not readily available is cervicography, a noninvasive photographic technique that provides permanent objective documentation of normal and abnormal cervical patterns. Acetic acid (5%) is applied to the cervix, a cervicography camera is used to take photos, and the projected cervicogram (slide after film developing) can be sent for expert evaluation. In a recent study, the cervicogram was found to give a greater yield of CIN than Pap smear alone.[12]

Early treatment of cervical cancer involves removal of the lesion by one of various techniques. Biopsy or local cautery may be therapeutic in and of itself. Electrocautery, cryosurgery, or carbon dioxide laser therapy may be used to treat moderate or severe dysplasia that is limited to the exocervix (squamocolumnar junction clearly visible). Therapeutic conization becomes necessary if the lesion extends into the endocervical canal. Depending on the stage of involvement of the cervix, invasive cancer is treated with radiation, surgery, or both radiation and surgery. Both external beam irradiation and intracavitary cesium irradiation (insertion of a closed metal cylinder containing cesium) can be used in the treatment of cervical cancer. Intracavitary radiation is most effective when the tumor is small. The larger the tumor, the greater the reliance on external beam radiation to shrink the tumor to a size at which it can be effectively irradiated by intracavitary irradiation. Surgery can include: (1) extended hysterectomy (removal of the uterus, tubes, ovaries, and upper portion of the vagina) without pelvic lymph node dissection, (2) radical hysterectomy with pelvic lymph node dissection, or (3) pelvic exenteration (removal of all pelvic organs including the bladder, rectum, vulva, and vagina). The choice of treatment is usually influenced by the patient's age and health.

Disorders of the uterus

Endometritis

Inflammation or infection of the endometrium is an ill-defined entity that produces variable symptoms. Generally, the presence of plasma cells is required for diagnosis. Endometritis can occur as a postpartum or postabortal infection, with gonococcal or chlamydial salpingitis, following instrumentation or surgery, or secondary to the presence of an intrauterine device or tuberculosis.[13] Causative organisms, in addition to *N. gonorrhoeae*, chlamydia, and *M. tuberculosis*, include *Escherichia coli*, proteus, pseudomonas, klebsiella, bacteroides, and mycoplasma species. Abnormal vaginal bleeding, mild to severe uterine tenderness, fever, malaise, and foul-smelling discharge have been associated with endometritis, but the clinical picture is variable. Treatment involves either oral or intravenous antibiotic therapy, depending on the severity of the condition.

Endometriosis

Endometriosis is the condition in which functional endometrial tissue is found in ectopic sites outside the uterus. The site may be the ovaries, the broad ligaments, the pouch of Douglas (cul-de-sac), the pelvis, the vagina, the vulva, the perineum, or the intestines. Rarely, endometrial implants have been found in the nostrils, umbilicus, lungs, and limbs.

The cause of endometriosis is not known. There appears to have been an increase in its incidence in the developing Western countries during the past four to five decades. It is estimated that 10% to 15% of premenopausal women have some degree of endometriosis. It can be found in up to 50% of women undergoing diagnostic laparoscopy for infertility.[14] It is more common in women who have postponed childbearing. Risk factors for endometriosis may include early menarche, regular periods with shorter cycle interval (27 days or less), longer duration (greater than 7 days), heavier flow, and increased menstrual pain.[15] There are several theories that attempt to account for endometriosis. One theory suggests that menstrual blood containing fragments of endometrium is forced upward through the fallopian tubes into the peritoneal cavity. Retrograde menstruation is not an uncommon phenomenon, however, and it is unknown why endometrial cells implant and grow in some women but not in others. Another proposal is that dormant, immature cellular elements spread over a wide area during embryonic development persist into adult life and that the ensuing metaplasia accounts for the development of ectopic endometrial tissue. Yet another theory suggests that the endometrial tissue may metastasize through the lymphatics or the vascular system.

The gross pathologic changes that occur in endometriosis differ with location and duration. In the ovary, the endometrial tissue may form cysts (endometriomas filled with old blood resembling chocolate syrup [*chocolate cysts*]). Rupture of these cysts can cause peritonitis and adhesions. Elsewhere in the pelvis, the tissue may take the form of small hemorrhagic lesions called *mulberry spots* or *powder burn spots* which are surrounded by scar tissue. These ectopic implants respond to hormonal stimulation in the same way normal endometrium does, becoming proliferative, then secretory, and finally undergoing menstrual breakdown. Bleeding into the surrounding structures can cause pain and the development of significant pelvic adhesions. Extensive fibrotic tissue may occasionally mimic carcinoma and cause bowel obstruction.

Endometriosis may be difficult to diagnose because its symptoms mimic those of other pelvic disorders. Furthermore, the severity of the symptoms does not always reflect the extent of the disease. The classic triad of dysmenorrhea, dyspareunia, and infertility strongly suggest endometriosis. Accurate diagnosis can be accomplished only through laparoscopy.

The treatment modalities for endometriosis fall into three categories: (1) pain relief, (2) endometrial suppression, and (3) surgery. In young unmarried women, simple observation and antiprostaglandin analgesics may be sufficient treatment. The use of hormones to induce physiologic amenorrhea is based on the observation that pregnancy affords temporary relief by inducing atrophy of the endometrial tissue. This can be accomplished through administration of estrogen or progesterone alone, combined oral contraceptive pills, Danazol (a testosterone derivative), or long-acting gonadotropin-releasing hormone (GnRH) analogs that inhibit the pituitary gonadotropins and suppress ovulation.[16]

Surgery is the most definitive therapy for many women with endometriosis. In the past, laparoscopic use of cautery was limited to mild endometriosis without extensive adhesions. With the advent of carbon dioxide or potassium-titanyl-phosphate (KTP) lasers, in-depth treatment of endometriosis or pelvic adhesions can be accomplished via laparoscopy. Advantages of laser surgery include better hemostasis, more precision in vaporizing lesions with less damage to surrounding tissue, and better access to areas that are not well visualized or would be difficult to reach with cautery. The KTP laser is particularly useful for endometriosis because of its flexible fiberoptic delivery system, which allows tissue incision and vaporization in addition to photocoagulation, and its green beam, which makes visualization and fine focusing easier.[17] Radical treatment involves total hysterectomy and bilateral salpingo-oophorectomy (removal of tubes and ovaries) when the symptoms are unbearable or the woman's childbearing is completed. Current treatment offers relief but not cure. Recurrence of endometriosis is not uncommon regardless of the treatment (except for radical surgery). In one study, recurrence rates confirmed by surgery were 13.5% after 3 years and 40% after 5 years.[2] Pregnancy may delay but does not preclude recurrence.

Adenomyosis

Adenomyosis is the condition in which endometrial glands and stroma are found within the myometrium interspersed between the smooth muscle fibers. In contrast to endometriosis, which is usually a problem of young, infertile women, adenomyosis is generally found in multiparous women in their late thirties or forties. It is thought that events associated with repeated pregnancies, deliveries, and uterine involution may cause the endometrium to be displaced throughout the myometrium. Adenomyosis frequently coexists with uterine myomas and/or endometrial hyperplasia. Often the diagnosis of adenomyosis occurs as an incidental finding in a uterus removed for symptoms suggestive of myoma or hyperplasia.[13] Adenomyosis resolves with menopause. Hysterectomy (with preservation of the ovaries in premenopausal women) is the treatment of choice. Efforts to control this condition with pelvic irradiation or medication to suppress ovarian stimulation have been largely unsuccessful.[2]

Endometrial cancer

Endometrial cancer is the most common malignancy found within the female pelvis—occurring more than twice as often as cervical cancer. In 1988, the American Cancer Society estimated that there were 34,000 cases diagnosed and 3,000 deaths from endometrial cancer.[9] Endometrial cancer is primarily a disease of older women (peak age 55 to 65 years), suggesting that the high frequency of occurrence may reflect a demographic shift—that is, an increase in the elderly population. Estrogen stimulation has been suggested as a causative factor. A sharp rise in endometrial cancer was noted in the 1970s among middle-aged women who had received estrogen therapy for menopausal symptoms. In fact, the majority of women who develop endometrial cancer have a history consistent with exposure to abnormal hormone levels. These women often are obese, have diabetes or other evidence of endocrine disturbances, are hypertensive, have Stein-Leventhal syndrome, or have a history of previous use of sequential (estrogen for 15 to 16 days, followed by 6 to 7 days of combined estrogen and progesterone) birth control pills. The sequential birth control pills were withdrawn in the early 1970s when the association between the use of unopposed estrogen and endometrial cancer was observed. Some are mothers who took DES during pregnancy; others took estrogen for menopausal symptoms; many are nulliparous, or infertile, have had menstrual irregularities and ovulation failure, or have had breast cancer or have been treated with hormone therapy. Numerous case-control studies have demonstrated a twofold to tenfold increase in the incidence of endometrial cancer in women who have received exogenous estrogen. This risk appears to be neutralized with addition of cyclic progestin each month; and, in fact, the use of combined oral contraceptives appear to decrease the risk of developing endometrial cancer by about half.[18]

As with cervical cancer, it is believed that precancerous abnormalities of the endometrium precede endometrial cancer. These precancerous changes include endometrial hyperplasia or an abnormal pattern of growth in the cells that line the uterus. These cellular changes may be spontaneous or they may develop secondary to exposure to unopposed exogenous estrogens. Hyperplasia often causes abnormal bleeding and spotting and is usually diagnosed on dilatation and curettage (D&C), which consists of dilating the cervix and scraping the uterine cavity.

The major symptom of endometrial cancer is abnormal painless bleeding. Any postmenopausal bleeding is abnormal and warrants investigation to rule out endometrial cancer or its precursor stages. Because bleeding is such an early warning sign of the disease and because endometrial cancer tends to be rather slow-growing, particularly in its early stages, the chances of cure are good if prompt medical attention is sought. Later signs of uterine cancer may include cramping, pelvic discomfort, postcoital bleeding, lower abdominal pressure, and enlarged lymph nodes. As a screening test, the Pap smear may not be effective in detecting endometrial cancer: it is falsely negative in approximately 40% to 50% of cases. Endometrial sampling obtained by direct aspiration of the endometrial cavity is far more accurate: 80% to 90% of endometrial cancers are identified if adequate tissue is obtained. Endometrial biopsy, which can be done in the physician's office, is another method of diagnosis; D&C is the definitive procedure for diagnosis because it provides a more thorough evaluation.

Surgery and radiation therapy are the most successful methods of treatment for endometrial cancer. Combination therapy is often recommended if metastases are present. Controversy exists over which is the most appropriate form of irradiation therapy. Treatment may involve a short course of external beam or internal irradiation followed by total abdominal hysterectomy and bilateral salpingo-oophorectomy. A four-to-six-week rest period after irradiation therapy may precede surgical treatment. In cases of advanced disease, surgery may be followed by external beam irradiation or application of radium to the vaginal vault. With early diagnosis and treatment, the 5-year survival rate ranges from 85% to almost 100%. Once the cancer has metastasized to the para-aortic and abdominal lymph nodes, the survival rate decreases to less than 5%.

Leiomyomas

Leiomyomas are benign neoplasms of smooth muscle origin. They are also known as *myomas* or, colloquially, as *fibroids*. These are the most common form of pelvic tumor and are believed to occur in one out of every four or five women above the age of 35. They are seen more often and their rate of growth is more rapid in black women than in white women. Leiomyomas usually develop in the corpus of the uterus; they may be submucosal, subserosal, or intramural (Figure 37-3). Intramural fibroids are embedded within the myometrium. They are the most common type of fibroids, taking the form of a symmetrical enlargement of the nonpregnant uterus. *Subserosal* tumors are located beneath the perimetrium of the uterus. These tumors are recognized as irregular projections on the uterine surface; they may become pedunculated, displacing or impinging on other genitourinary structures and causing hydroureter or bladder problems. *Submucosal* fibroids displace endometrial tissue and are more likely to cause bleeding, necrosis, and infection than either of the other types.

Leiomyomas may be manifested as follows: they may be asymptomatic and be discovered during a routine pelvic examination, or they may cause bleeding, particularly at the time of the menstrual period. Their rate of growth is variable, but they may increase in size during pregnancy or with exogenous estrogen stimulation (oral contraceptives or menopausal estrogen replacement therapy). Interference with pregnancy is rare unless the tumor is submucosal and interferes with implantation or obstructs the cervical outlet. These tumors may outgrow their blood supply, become infarcted, and undergo degenerative changes. Most leiomyomas regress with menopause, but if bleeding, pressure on the bladder, pain, or other problems persist, hysterectomy may be required. Myomectomy (removal of just the tumors) can be done to preserve the uterus for future childbearing.

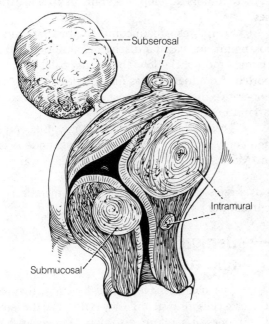

Figure 37-3 Submucosal, intramural, and subserosal leiomyomas. (*Green TH Jr: Gynecology: Essentials of Clinical Practice, 3rd ed. Boston, Little, Brown & Co, 1977*)

Cesarean section may be recommended if the uterine cavity is entered during myomectomy. If the woman is not a good surgical risk, danazol (Danocrine) or GnRH antagonists (leuprolide [Lupron]) may be used to suppress leiomyoma growth.

Disorders of the fallopian tubes and ovaries

Pelvic inflammatory disease

Pelvic inflammatory disease (PID) is an inflammation of the upper reproductive tract involving the uterus (endometritis), the fallopian tubes (salpingitis), and/or the ovaries (oophoritis). About 80% of women with acute salpingitis will have either *N. gonorrhoeae* or *C. trachomatis* identified within the reproductive tract.[19] At one time the gonococcus was thought to be the only organism responsible for non-puerperal PID. The etiology appears to be changing, however, and chlamydia, as well as other opportunistic bacteria in the Bacteroides and Peptostreptococcus groups are now involved. The organisms ascend through the endocervical canal to the endometrial cavity and then to the tubes and ovaries. The endocervical canal is slightly dilated during menstruation; thus, bacteria can gain entrance to the uterus and other pelvic structures. Once inside the upper reproductive tract, the organisms multiply rapidly in the favorable environment of the sloughing endometrium and ascend to the fallopian tube. Factors that predispose women to the development of PID include age 16 to 24, unmarried status, nulliparity, history of multiple sexual partners, and previous history of PID. Use of an intrauterine contraceptive device (IUD) has been shown to increase the risk of developing PID threefold to fivefold. However, a recent study indicates that women with only one sexual partner who are at low risk of acquiring sexually transmitted diseases have no significant risk of developing PID from use of an IUD.[20]

The symptoms of PID include lower abdominal pain, which may start just after a menstrual period, purulent cervical discharge, adnexal tenderness, and an exquisitely painful cervix. Fever (greater than 100.4°F), increased erythrocyte sedimentation rate (ESR), and an elevated white blood cell count (greater than 10,000) are often seen, even though the woman may not appear acutely ill. A newer test involves measurement of C reactive protein (CRP) in the blood. Elevated CRP is equated with inflammation.

Treatment may involve hospitalization with intravenous administration of antibiotics. Bed rest in the Fowler's position (head and knees elevated) facilitates pelvic drainage. If the condition is diagnosed early, outpatient antibiotic therapy may be sufficient. The Centers for Disease Control recommend doxycycline plus cefoxitan IV for at least 4 days followed by oral doxycycline for 10 to 14 days. Ambulatory treatment involves an initial dose of cefoxitan, amoxicillin, ampicillin, or aqueous procaine penicillin followed by 10 to 14 days of oral doxycycline.[21] Treatment is aimed at preventing complications, which can include pelvic adhesions, infertility, ectopic pregnancy, chronic abdominal pain, and tubo-ovarian abscesses. Accurate diagnosis and appropriate antibiotic therapy may decrease the severity and frequency of PID sequelae.

Ectopic pregnancy

Although pregnancy is not discussed in detail in this text, it is reasonable to mention ectopic pregnancy because it represents a true gynecologic emergency and should always be considered when a woman of reproductive age presents with the complaint of pelvic pain. Ectopic pregnancy occurs when a fertilized ovum implants outside the uterine cavity. The most common site for ectopic pregnancy is the fallopian tube. According to the Centers for Disease Control, between 1970 and 1983 the number of ectopic pregnancies increased from 17,800 to 69,600; the rate of occurrence among females aged 15 to 44 years rose from 4.5 per 1000 to 14 per 1000 reported pregnancies (live births, abortions, and ectopics).[22]

The cause of ectopic pregnancy is delayed ovum transport, which may, in turn, be caused by decreased tubal motility or distorted tubal anatomy (narrowed lumen, convolutions, or diverticuli). Factors that may predispose to the development of an ectopic pregnancy include PID, therapeutic abortion, tubal ligation or tubal reversal, previous ectopic pregnancy, infertility, and use of clomiphene citrate to induce ovulation.[23] Contraceptive failure with progestin-only birth control pills or the "morning-after pill" has also been associated with ectopic pregnancy.

The site of implantation within the tube (isthmus, ampulla, etc.) may determine the onset of symptoms and the timing of diagnosis. As the tubal pregnancy progresses, the surrounding tissue is stretched. Eventually, however, the pregnancy outgrows its blood supply at which point the pregnancy either terminates or the tube itself ruptures because it can no longer contain the growing pregnancy. Symptoms can include lower abdominal discomfort—diffuse or localized to one side—which progresses to severe pain caused by rupture, spotting syncope, referred shoulder pain from bleeding into the abdominal cavity, and amenorrhea. Physical examination usually reveals adnexal tenderness; an adnexal mass is found in only 50% of the cases. Culdocentesis (needle aspiration from the cul-de-sac) may reveal blood if rupture has occurred. Quantitative beta-hCG pregnancy tests may detect lower than normal hCG production. Pelvic ultrasound studies after 5 weeks' gestation may demonstrate an empty uterine cavity or presence of the gestational sac outside the uterus. Definitive diagnosis requires laparoscopy. Differential diagnosis for this type of pelvic pain includes ruptured ovarian cyst, threatened or incomplete abortion, PID, acute appendicitis, and degenerating fibroid.

Treatment is surgical, usually a laparotomy, with salpingostomy to remove the ectopic pregnancy if the fallopian tube has not ruptured, or salpingectomy if it has. Salpingostomy preserves fertility, but requires careful surgical technique in order to minimize the risk of recurrent ectopic pregnancies. In some cases, newer laparoscopic techniques now allow for salpingostomy without laparotomy. A recent study indicated that laparoscopic treatment of ectopic pregnancy is well tolerated by patients and more cost effective than laparotomy because of shorter convalescence and reduced postoperative analgesia.[24]

Cancer of the fallopian tube

Cancer of the fallopian tube is rare, accounting for less than 1% of all female genital tract malignancies. Fewer than 1000 cases have been reported. Diagnosis of this malignancy is extremely difficult and the disease may be well advanced when found. Most primary tubal cancers are papillary adenocarcinomas, and these tumors develop bilaterally in 40% to 50% of cases.[2]

Symptoms are uncommon, but intermittent serosanguineous vaginal discharge, abnormal vaginal bleeding, and colicky low abdominal pain have been reported. An adnexal mass may be present; however, preoperative diagnosis in most cases is leiomyoma or ovarian tumor.

Treatment is total hysterectomy, bilateral salpingo-oophorectomy and pelvic lymph node dissection. More extensive procedures may be warranted depending on the stage of the disease. The 5-year survival rates vary from 0% to 44%; if metastasis has occurred, the prognosis is poor.

Benign ovarian cysts and tumors

The ovaries have a dual function: they produce germ cells, or ova, and they synthesize the female sex hormones. Therefore, disorders of the ovaries frequently cause menstrual and fertility problems. Benign conditions of the ovaries can present as primary lesions of the ovarian structures or as secondary disorders related to hypothalamic, pituitary, or adrenal dysfunction.

Ovarian cysts

Cysts are the most common form of ovarian tumor. Many are benign. A follicular cyst is one that results from occlusion of the duct of the follicle. Each month several follicles begin to develop and are blighted at various stages of development. These follicles form cavities that fill with fluid, producing a cyst. The dominant follicle normally ruptures to release the egg (ovulation), but occasionally persists and continues growing. Likewise, a luteal cyst is a persistent cystic enlargement of the corpus luteum that is formed after ovulation and does not regress in the absence of pregnancy. Functional cysts are generally asymptomatic unless there is substantial enlargement or bleeding into the cyst. This can cause considerable discomfort, or a dull aching sensation on the affected side. The cyst may become twisted or may rupture into the intra-abdominal cavity. These cysts usually regress spontaneously.

Polycystic ovarian (Stein-Leventhal) syndrome

Ovarian dysfunction associated with infrequent or absent menses in obese infertile women was first reported in the 1930s by Stein and Leventhal, for whom the syndrome was originally named. Once thought to be relatively rare, it now appears that this clinical entity is one of the most common endocrinologic disorders among women in the reproductive years. The syndrome characterized by hirsutism, obesity, and infertility is just one manifestation of this condition. Anovulation, causing amenorrhea or irregular menses, commonly accompanies the finding of bilaterally enlarged polycystic ovaries. Whether this condition is a primary ovarian defect or a result of hypothalamic-pituitary dysfunction is still being debated. Women with polycystic ovarian disease generally have elevated LH levels with normal estrogen and FSH production. Elevated levels of testosterone, dehydroepiandrosterone sulfate (DHAS), and/or androstendione are not uncommon, and occasionally hyperprolactinemia or hypothyroidism will be present. The diagnosis can be suspected from the clinical picture and confirmed with ultrasound or laparoscopic visualization of the ovaries. The condition is usually treated by administration of the hypothalamic-pituitary-stimulating drug clomiphene citrate (Clomid) to induce ovulation. This drug is used carefully because it can induce extreme enlargement of the ovaries. If fertility is not desired, oral contraceptives can induce regular menses and prevent the development of endometrial hyperplasia due to unopposed estrogen. When medication is ineffective, laser surgery to puncture the multiple follicles can be helpful. Bilateral wedge resection is rarely performed today.

Benign ovarian tumors

Serous cystadenoma and mucinous cystadenoma are the most common benign ovarian neoplasms. Some of these adenomas, however, are considered to have low malignant potential. They are asymptomatic unless the size is sufficient to cause abdominal enlargement. Treatment is surgical oophorectomy.

Endometriomas are the chocolate cysts that develop secondary to ovarian endometriosis. (See the section on endometriosis earlier in this chapter). *Ovarian fibromas* are connective tissue tumors composed of fibrocytes and collagen. They range in size from 6 cm to 20 cm and are treated by surgical excision. *Cystic teratomas* or *dermoid cysts* are derived from primordial germ cells and are composed of varying combinations of well differentiated ectodermal, mesodermal, and endodermal elements. Not uncommonly they contain sebaceous material, hair, and/or teeth. Treatment is surgical excision.

Functioning ovarian tumors

Functioning ovarian tumors are of three types: estrogen secreting, androgen secreting, and mixed estrogen-androgen secreting. These tumors may be either benign or malignant. One such tumor, the granulosa cell tumor, is associated with excess estrogen production. When it develops during the reproductive period, the persistent and uncontrolled production of estrogen interferes with the normal menstrual cycle, causing irregular and excessive bleeding, endometrial hyperplasia, or amenorrhea and fertility problems. When it develops after menopause, it causes postmenopausal bleeding, stimulation of the glandular tissues of the breast, and other signs of renewed estrogen production. Androgen-secreting tumors (Sertoli-Leydig cell tumor or androblastoma) inhibit ovulation and estrogen production. They tend to cause hirsutism and development of masculine characteristics, such as baldness, acne, oily skin, breast atrophy, and deepening of the voice. The treatment is surgical removal of the tumor.

Ovarian cancer

Ovarian cancer is the second most common female genitourinary malignancy, and the most lethal. In 1988, 19,000 new cases of ovarian cancer were reported in the United States, two-thirds of which were in advanced stages of the disease. Most of these women die of the disease (12,000 women in 1988).[9] The incidence of ovarian cancer increases with age, being greatest between the ages of 65 and 84. Ovarian cancer is difficult to diagnose, and 60% to 70% of women have metastatic disease prior to the time of discovery. Unfortunately, there are no screening or other early methods of detection for this form of cancer. The lack of accurate diagnostic tools and previously inconsistent staging techniques have contributed to incomplete knowledge and treatment of the disease. In addition, the resistant nature of ovarian cancers significantly affects the success of treatment and thus survival. The most significant risk factor for ovarian cancer appears to be "ovulatory age"—the length of time during a woman's life when her ovarian cycle is not suppressed by pregnancy, lactation, or oral contraceptive use. The incidence of ovarian cancer is much lower in countries where women bear numerous children than in the United States.

Cancer of the ovary is complex because of the diversity of tissue types originating in the ovary. As a result of this diversity, there are a number of different types of ovarian cancers. Malignant neoplasms of the ovary can be divided into three categories: epithelial tumors, germ cell tumors, and gonadal stromal tumors. Epithelial tumors account for approximately 90% of cases.[13] These different cancers display various degrees of virulence depending on the type of tumor and degree of differentiation involved. A well-differentiated cancer of the ovary may have produced symptoms for many months and still be found operable at the time of surgery. On the other hand, a poorly differentiated tumor may have been clinically evident for only a few days but found to be widespread and inoperable. Often, no correlation exists between the duration of symptoms and the extent of the disease.

Cancers of the ovary are frequently asymptomatic, or the symptoms are so vague that the woman rarely seeks medical care until the disease is far advanced. These vague discomforts include abdominal distress, flatulence, and bloating (especially after ingesting food). These gastrointestinal manifestations may precede other symptoms by months. Many women will take antacids or bicarbonate of soda for a time before consulting a physician. The physician may also dismiss the woman's complaints as being due to other conditions, causing a further delay in diagnosis and treatment. It is not fully understood why the initial symptoms of ovarian cancer are manifested as gastrointestinal disturbances. It is thought that biochemical changes in the peritoneal fluids may irritate the bowel or that pain originating in the ovary may be referred to the abdomen and be interpreted as a gastrointestinal disturbance. Clinically evident ascites (fluid in the peritoneal cavity) is seen in about one-fourth of women with malignant ovarian tumors and is associated with worsened prognosis.

Early methods of ovarian cancer treatment consisted of homogeneous surgery, assessment of response, and subsequent chemotherapy. Current treatment methods include cytoreductive and debulking surgery to reduce the size of the tumor, followed by immediate irradiation or chemotherapy. Chemotherapy may be given prior to surgery. At the time of surgery, the uterus, fallopian tubes, ovaries, and omentum are removed; the liver, diaphragm, retroperitoneal and aortic lymph nodes, and peritoneal surface are commonly examined. Cytologic washings are commonly done to test for cancerous cells in the peritoneal fluid. The type and sequence of treatment often depend on the stage of the disease. Women with limited disease (stage Ia) do not require adjuvant treatment; women with intermediate disease (stage Ib, II) can be cured by radiotherapy following surgery; and women with advanced disease (stage III, IV) may require extensive chemotherapy. Five-year survival is 85% in women whose ovarian cancer is detected and treated early. Survival drops to 23% when the disease is advanced.[9]

Disorders of pelvic support and uterine position

The uterus and the pelvic structures are maintained in proper position by the uterosacral ligaments, the round ligaments, the broad ligament, and the cardinal ligaments. The two cardinal ligaments maintain the cervix in its normal position. The uterosacral ligaments normally hold the uterus in a forward position (Figure 37-4). The broad ligament suspends the uterus, fallopian tubes, and ovaries within the pelvis. The vagina is encased in the semirigid structure of the strong investing fascia. The muscular floor of the pelvis is a strong slinglike structure that supports the uterus, vagina, urinary bladder, and rectum (Figure 37-5).

In the female anatomy, nature is faced with the problems of supporting the pelvic viscera against the force of gravity and increases in intra-abdominal pressure associated with coughing, sneezing, defecation, laughing, and so on, while at the same time allowing for urination, defecation, and normal reproductive tract function (in particular, the delivery of a baby).

Three supporting structures are provided for the abdominal pelvic diaphragm. The bony pelvis provides support and protection for parts of the digestive tract and genitourinary structures, and the perito-

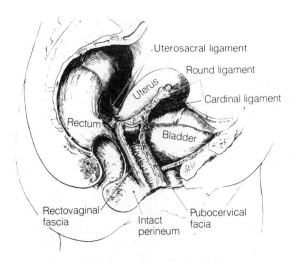

Figure 37-4 Normal support of the uterus and vagina. (*Mattingly RF: TeLinde's Operative Gynecology, 6th ed, p 39. Philadelphia, JB Lippincott, 1985*)

neum holds the pelvic viscera in place. The main support for the viscera, however, is the pelvic diaphragm, made up of muscles and connective tissue that stretch across the bones of the pelvic outlet. The openings that must exist for the urethra, the rectum, and the vagina cause an inherent weakness in the pelvic diaphragm. Congenital or acquired weakness of the pelvic diaphragm results in widening of these openings, particularly the vagina, with the possible

herniation of pelvic viscera through the pelvic floor (prolapse).

Relaxation of the pelvic outlet usually comes about because of overstretching of the perineal supporting tissues during pregnancy and childbirth. Although the tissues are stretched only during these times, there may be no difficulty until later in life, such as the fifth or sixth decade, when further loss of elasticity and muscle tone occurs. Even in a woman who has not borne children, the combination of aging and postmenopausal changes may give rise to problems related to relaxation of the pelvic support structures. The three most common conditions associated with this relaxation are cystocele, rectocele, and uterine prolapse. These may occur separately or in association with one another.

—— Cystocele

Cystocele is a herniation of the bladder into the vagina. It occurs when the normal muscle support for the bladder is weakened, so that the bladder sags below the uterus. The vaginal wall stretches and bulges downward because of the force of gravity and the pressure from coughing, lifting, straining at stool, and so on. Finally, the bladder herniates through the anterior vaginal wall, and a cystocele forms (Figure 37-6). The symptoms include an annoying bearing-down sensation, difficulty in emptying the bladder,

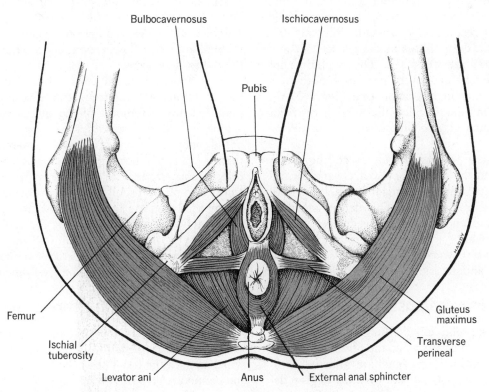

Figure 37-5 Muscles of the pelvic floor (female perineum). (*Chaffee EE, Lytle IM: Basic Physiology and Anatomy, 4th ed. Philadelphia, JB Lippincott, 1980*)

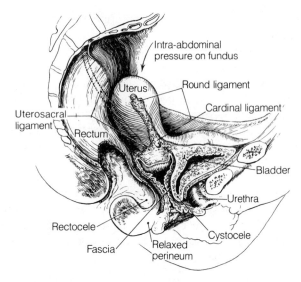

Figure 37-6 Relaxation of pelvic support structures with descent of the uterus, as well as cystocele and rectocele. (*Mattingly RF: TeLinde's Operative Gynecology, 6th ed, p 43. Philadelphia, JB Lippincott, 1985*)

frequency and urgency of urination, and cystitis. Stress incontinence may occur at times of increased abdominal pressure such as during squatting, straining, coughing, sneezing, laughing, or lifting.

Rectocele and enterocele

Rectocele is the herniation of the rectum into the vagina. It occurs when the posterior vaginal wall and underlying rectum bulge forward, ultimately protruding through the introitus as the pelvic floor and perineal muscles are weakened. The symptoms include discomfort because of the protrusion of the rectum and difficulty in defecation (see Figure 37-6). Digital pressure (splinting) on the bulging posterior wall of the vagina may become necessary for defecation.

The area between the uterosacral ligaments just posterior to the cervix may weaken and form a hernial sac into which the small bowel protrudes when the woman is standing. This defect, called an *enterocele,* may extend into the rectovaginal septum. It may be congenital or acquired through birth trauma. Enterocele can be asymptomatic or cause a dull dragging sensation and occasionally low backache.

Uterine prolapse

Uterine prolapse is the bulging of the uterus into the vagina that occurs when the primary supportive ligaments (cardinal ligaments) are stretched. Prolapse is ranked as first, second, or third degree depending on how far the uterus protrudes through the introitus. First-degree prolapse shows some descent,

but the cervix has not reached the introitus. In second-degree prolapse, the cervix or part of the uterus has passed through the introitus. The entire uterus protrudes through the vaginal opening in third-degree prolapse (procidentia).

The symptoms associated with uterine prolapse are due to irritation of the exposed mucous membranes of the cervix and vagina and the discomfort of the protruding mass. Prolapse is often accompanied by perineal relaxation, cystocele, or rectocele. Like cystocele, rectocele, and enterocele, it occurs most commonly in multiparous women, since childbearing is accompanied by injuries to pelvic structures and uterine ligaments. It may also result from pelvic tumors and neurologic conditions, such as spina bifida and diabetic neuropathy, that interrupt the innervation of pelvic muscles. A pessary may be inserted to hold the uterus in place and may stave off surgical intervention in women who want to have children or in older women for whom the surgery might pose a significant health risk.

Treatment of pelvic support disorders

Most of the disorders of pelvic relaxation require surgical correction. These are elective surgeries and are usually deferred until after the childbearing years. Often the symptoms associated with the disorders are not severe enough to warrant surgical correction. In other cases, the stress of surgery is contraindicated because of other physical disorders; this is particularly true of older women, in whom many of these disorders occur.

There are a number of surgical procedures for the conditions resulting from relaxation of pelvic support structures. Removal of the uterus through the vagina (vaginal hysterectomy) with appropriate repair of the vaginal wall (colporrhaphy) is often done when uterine prolapse is accompanied by cystocele or rectocele. A vesicourethral suspension may be done to alleviate the symptoms of stress incontinence. Finally, repair may involve abdominal hysterectomy along with anterior-posterior repair. Kegel exercises, which strengthen the pubococcygeus muscle, may be helpful in cases of mild cystocele or rectocele or after surgical repair to help maintain the improved function.

Variations in uterine position

Variations in the position of the uterus are common. Some variations are innocuous; others, which may be the result of weakness and relaxation of the perineum, give rise to various problems that compromise the structural integrity of the pelvic floor, particularly after childbirth.

Usually the uterus is flexed about 45 degrees anteriorly with the cervix positioned posteriorly and downward in the anteverted position. When the female is standing, the angle of the uterus is such that it lies practically horizontal, resting lightly on the bladder. Asymptomatic normal variations in the axis of the uterus in relation to the cervix (flexion) and physiologic displacements that arise following pregnancy or with cul-de-sac pathology include anteflexion, retroflexion, and retroversion (Figure 37-7). An anteflexed uterus is flexed forward upon itself. Retroflexion is flexion backward at the isthmus. Retroversion describes the condition in which the uterus inclines posteriorly while the cervix remains tilted forward. Simple retroversion of the uterus is the most common displacement, being found in 30% of normal women. It is usually a congenital condition caused by a short anterior vaginal wall and relaxed uterosacral ligaments; together these force the uterus to fall back into the cul-de-sac of Douglas. Retroversion can also follow certain diseases, such as endometriosis or pelvic inflammatory disease, which produce fibrous tissue adherence with retraction of the fundus posteriorly. Large leiomyomas may also cause the uterus to move into a posterior position. Dyspareunia with deep penetration or low back pain with menses can be associated with retroversion. However, most symptoms in these women are due to the associated condition (*i.e.,* adhesions, fibroids, etc.) rather than to congenital retroversion.

In summary, alterations in pelvic support frequently occur because of weaknesses and relaxation of the pelvic floor and perineum. Cystocele and rectocele involve herniation of the bladder or rectum into the

vagina. Uterine prolapse occurs when the uterus bulges into the vagina. Pelvic relaxation disorders frequently result from overstretching of the perineal supporting muscles during pregnancy and childbirth. The loss of elasticity in these structures that is a normal accompaniment of aging contributes to these problems. Variations in uterine position are common; they include anteflexion, retroflexion, and retroversion. These disorders, which are often innocuous, can be the result of a congenital shortness of the vaginal wall, the development of fibrous adhesions secondary to endometriosis or pelvic inflammatory disease, or displacement due to large uterine leiomyomas.

Menstrual disorders

Dysfunctional menstrual cycles

Although unexplained uterine bleeding can occur for many reasons, such as pregnancy, abortion, blood dyscrasias, and neoplasms, the most frequent cause in the nonpregnant female is what are commonly called dysfunctional menstrual cycles or bleeding. Dysfunctional cycles may take the form of *amenorrhea* (absence of menstruation), *hypomenorrhea* (scanty menstruation), *oligomenorrhea* (infrequent menstruation, periods more than 35 days apart), *menorrhagia* (excessive menstruation), or *metrorrhagia* (bleeding between periods). *Menometrorrhagia* is heavy bleeding both during and between menstrual periods.

Dysfunctional menstrual cycles are generally related to alterations in the hormones that support normal cyclic endometrial changes. Estrogen deprivation causes retrogression of a previously built-up endometrium and bleeding. Such bleeding is often irregular in amount and duration, the flow varying with the time and degree of estrogen stimulation, as well as the degree of estrogen withdrawal. A lack of progesterone can cause abnormal menstrual bleeding: in its absence, estrogen induces development of a much thicker endometrial layer with a richer blood supply. The absence of progesterone results from the failure of any of the developing ovarian follicles to mature to the point of ovulation with the subsequent formation of the corpus luteum and production and secretion of progesterone. Periodic bleeding episodes alternating with amenorrhea are caused by variations in the number of functioning ovarian follicles present. If a number are present and active, and if new follicles assume functional capacity, high levels of estrogen will develop, causing the endometrium to proliferate for weeks or even months. In time, however, estrogen withdrawal and bleeding will develop. This can occur for two reasons: (1) an absolute estrogen deficiency may develop when several follicles simultaneously de-

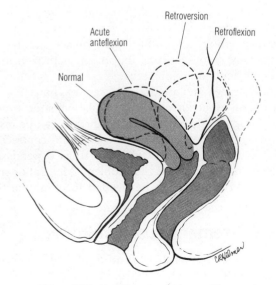

Figure 37-7 Variations in uterine position.

generate, or (2) a relative deficiency may develop as the needs of the enlarged endometrial tissue mass exceed the capabilities of the existing follicles, even though estrogen levels remain constant. Both estrogen and progesterone deficiency are associated with the absence of ovulation, hence the term *anovulatory bleeding*. Because the vasoconstriction and myometrial contractions that normally accompany menstruation are caused by progesterone, anovulatory bleeding is seldom accompanied by cramps, and the flow is frequently heavy.

Anovulatory cycles are common among adolescents during the first several years after menarche, when ovarian function is becoming established, and among perimenopausal women, whose ovarian function is beginning to decline.

Dysfunctional menstrual cycles can originate as a primary disorder of the ovaries or as a secondary defect in ovarian function related to hypothalamic-pituitary stimulation. The latter can be initiated by emotional stress, marked variation in weight (sudden gain or loss), or nonspecific endocrine or metabolic disturbances. Organic causes of irregular menstrual bleeding include endometrial polyps, submucous myoma (fibroid), blood dyscrasia, infection, endometrial cancer, polycystic ovarian disease, and pregnancy.

The treatment of dysfunctional bleeding depends on what is identified as the probable cause. A detailed history with emphasis on bleeding pattern and a physical examination should be the minimum evaluation that is done. Endocrine studies (FSH/LH ratio, prolactin, testosterone, DHAS), beta-hCG pregnancy test, endometrial biopsy, D&C with or without hysteroscopy, and progesterone withdrawal tests may be needed for diagnosis. If organic problems are ruled out and alterations in hormone levels are the primary cause, treatment may include the use of oral contraceptives, cyclic progesterone therapy, or long-acting progesterone injections.[25]

Amenorrhea

There are two types of amenorrhea—primary and secondary. Primary amenorrhea is the failure to menstruate by age 16, or by age 14 if failure to menstruate is accompanied by absence of secondary sex characteristics. Secondary amenorrhea is the cessation of menses for at least 6 months in a woman who has established normal menstrual cycles. Primary amenorrhea is usually due to gonadal dysgenesis, congenital müllerian agenesis, testicular feminization, or a hypothalamic-pituitary-ovarian axis disorder. Causes of secondary amenorrhea include ovarian, pituitary, or hypothalamic dysfunction, intrauterine adhesions (Asherman's syndrome), infections (tuberculosis, schistosomiasis), pituitary tumor, anorexia nervosa, or

strenuous physical exercise which can alter the critical body-fat to muscle ratio needed for menses to occur.[26] Diagnostic evaluation resembles that for dysfunctional uterine bleeding, with the possible addition of a computed tomographic (CT) scan to rule out a pituitary tumor. Treatment is based on correcting the underlying cause and inducing menstruation with cyclic progesterone or combined estrogen/progesterone regimens.

Dysmenorrhea

Dysmenorrhea is pain or discomfort with menstruation. Although not usually a serious medical problem, it causes some degree of monthly disability for a significant number of women. There are two forms of dysmenorrhea—primary and secondary.

Primary dysmenorrhea is menstrual pain that is not associated with a physical abnormality or pathology. It usually occurs with ovulatory menstruation beginning 6 months to 2 years after menarche. Symptoms may begin 1 to 2 days prior to menses, generally peak on the first day of flow, and subside within several hours to several days. Severe dysmenorrhea may be associated with systemic symptoms such as headache, nausea, vomiting, diarrhea, fatigue, irritability, dizziness, and syncope. The pain is typically described as dull lower abdominal aching or cramping, spasmodic or colicky in nature, often radiating to the lower back, labia majora, or upper thighs.

Secondary dysmenorrhea is menstrual pain caused by specific organic conditions such as endometriosis, uterine fibroids, adenomyosis, pelvic adhesions, intrauterine devices, or pelvic inflammatory disease. Laparoscopy is often required for diagnosis of secondary dysmenorrhea if medication for primary dysmenorrhea is ineffective.

Treatment for primary dysmenorrhea is directed at symptom control. Although analgesic agents such as aspirin and acetaminophen may relieve minor uterine cramping or low back pain, prostaglandin synthetase inhibitors such as ibuprofen, naproxen, mefanamic acid, and indomethacin are more specific for dysmenorrhea and are the treatment of choice if contraception is not a concern. Ovulation suppression and symptomatic relief of dysmenorrhea can be instituted simultaneously with the use of oral contraceptives. Relief of secondary dysmenorrhea depends on identifying the cause of the problem. Medical or surgical intervention may be needed to eliminate the problem.

Premenstrual syndrome

The premenstrual syndrome (PMS) is a distinct clinical entity characterized by a cluster of physical and psychological symptoms that are limited to 3 days to 14 days preceding menstruation and are relieved by onset of the menses. According to recent surveys, 30% to 40% of the adult female population in the United States experience some monthly symptoms that they attribute to PMS.[27] Just how many of these women have symptoms that are severe enough to warrant treatment is unknown. The incidence of PMS seems to increase with age. It is less common in women in their teens and twenties, with the highest number of women seeking help for the problem being in their mid-thirties. There is some dispute about whether PMS occurs more frequently in women who have not had children or in those who have had children. The disorder is not culturally distinct; it affects non-Westerners as well as Westerners.

The physical symptoms of PMS include painful and swollen breasts, bloating, abdominal pain, headache, and backache. Psychologically, there may be depression, anxiety, irritability, and behavioral changes. In some cases there are puzzling alterations in motor function, such as clumsiness and altered handwriting. Women with PMS may report one or several symptoms, with symptoms varying from woman to woman and from month to month in the same patient. Signs and symptoms associated with this disorders are summarized in Table 37-1.

PMS can significantly affect a woman's ability to perform at normal levels. She may lose time or function ineffectively at work. Family responsibilities and relationships may suffer. Students have been known to have lower grades during the premenstrual period. More crimes are committed by females during the premenstrual phase of the cycle, and more lives are lost to suicide during this period.

Though the causes of PMS are poorly documented, they are probably multifactorial. Like dysmenorrhea, it is only recently that PMS has become recognized as a bona fide disorder rather than merely a psychosomatic illness.

In recent years, there has been a tendency to link the disorder with endocrine imbalances such as hyperprolactinemia, estrogen excess, or alteration in estrogen-to-progesterone ratio. Prolactin concentration affects sodium and water retention, is higher in the luteal phase than the follicular phase, and can be increased by estrogens, stress, and hypoglycemia as well as by pregnancy and oral contraceptives.[27] Estrogens stimulate anxiety and nervous tension, while increased progesterone levels may produce depression. The role of hormonal factors in the etiology of PMS is supported by two well-established phenomena: first, women who have undergone a hysterectomy but not an oophorectomy may have cyclic symptoms resembling PMS; second, PMS symptoms are rare in postmenopausal women. However, research has failed to confirm these theories. Other hypotheses suggest that increased aldosterone may contribute to symptoms associated with fluid retention (headache, bloating, breast tenderness, and weight gain); that pyridoxine (vitamin B_6) deficiency may lead to estrogen excess or may decrease production of the neurotransmitters dopamine and serotonin, which in turn may contribute to PMS symptoms; or that decreased prostaglandin E_1 (PGE_1) concentrations can lead to abnormal sensitivity to prolactin, with associated fluid retention, irritability, and depression. In addition, increased appetite, binge eating, fatigue, and depression have been associated with altered endorphin activity and/or subclinical hypoglycemia.[27–29] There is also evidence that learned beliefs about menstruation can contribute to the production of PMS or at least affect the woman's response to the symptoms.

Diagnosis centers on identification of the symptom clusters by means of prospective charting for at least 3 months. A complete history and physical examination is necessary to rule out other physical causes of the symptoms. Depending on the symptom pattern, blood studies, including thyroid hormones, glucose, and prolactin assays, may be done. Psychosocial evaluation is helpful to rule out emotional illness that is merely exacerbated premenstrually.

In the past, treatment of PMS has been largely symptomatic. Attempts have been made to ef-

---

Table 37–1. Symptoms of premenstrual syndrome (PMS) by system

Body system	Symptoms
Cerebral	Irritability, anxiety, nervousness, fatigue, and exhaustion; increased physical and mental activity; lability; crying spells; depression; inability to concentrate
Gastrointestinal	Craving for sweets or salt, lower abdominal pain, bloating, nausea, vomiting, diarrhea, constipation
Vascular	Headache, edema, weakness, or fainting
Reproductive	Swelling and tenderness of the breasts, pelvic congestion, ovarian pain, altered libido
Neuromuscular	Trembling of the extremities, changes in coordination, clumsiness, backache, leg aches
General	Weight gain, insomnia, dizziness, acne

fect weight loss and reduce fluid retention through use of diuretics. Tranquilizer drugs were used to treat mood changes, and pain was treated with mild analgesics. The current treatment is still, to some extent, directed toward somatic complaints. Relief of somatic pain does not, however, totally resolve PMS suffering. The latest approach is to recommend an integrated program of personal assessment by diary, a program of regular exercise, avoidance of caffeine, and a diet low in simple sugars and high in lean proteins. Additional therapeutic regimens include vitamin or mineral supplements (particularly pyridoxine, vitamin E, and magnesium), natural progesterone supplements, bromocriptine for prolactin suppression, danazol (a synthetic androgen), spironolactone (an aldosterone antagonist and steroidogenesis inhibitor), evening primrose oil (contains linoleic acid, a precursor of prostaglandin PGE_1), or lithium for marked functional impairment from affective symptoms. Management must include education and support directed toward life-style changes. Drug therapy should be used cautiously until well-controlled studies establish criteria for use and effective treatment results. Placebo effect may account for symptom relief in a significant number of women. It is unlikely that a single cause or treatment for PMS will ever be found. Evaluation and management should focus on identifying and controlling the individual symptom clusters when possible.

In summary, menstrual disorders include dysfunctional menstrual cycles, dysmenorrhea, and premenstrual syndrome. Dysfunctional menstrual cycles occur when the hormonal support of the endometrium is altered. These cycles produce amenorrhea, oligomenorrhea, metrorrhagia, or menorrhagia. Dysmenorrhea is characterized by pain or discomfort during menses. It can occur as a primary or secondary disorder. Primary dysmenorrhea is not associated with other disorders and begins soon after menarche. Secondary dysmenorrhea is caused by a specific organic condition such as endometriosis or pelvic adhesions. It generally occurs in women with previously painless menses. Premenstrual syndrome (PMS) represents a cluster of physical and psychological symptoms that precede menstruation by a week or two. The true incidence and nature of PMS has only recently been recognized and its cause and methods for treatment are still under study.

Disorders of the breast

Most breast disease may be described as either benign or malignant. Breast tissue is never static; the breast is constantly responding to changes in hormonal, nutritional, psychological, and environmental stimuli that cause continual cellular changes. Benign breast conditions are generally nonprogressive; some forms of benign disease, however, increase the risk of malignant disease. In light of this, strict adherence to a dichotomy of benign vs. malignant disease may not always be appropriate. However, this dichotomy is useful for the sake of simplicity and clarity.

Galactorrhea

Galactorrhea is the secretion of breast milk in a nonlactating breast. Galactorrhea may result from vigorous nipple stimulation during lovemaking, exogenous hormones, internal hormonal imbalance, or local chest infection or trauma. A pituitary tumor may produce large amounts of prolactin and cause galactorrhea. Galactorrhea occurs in both men and women and is usually benign. Observation may be continued for several months prior to diagnostic hormonal screening.

Mastitis

Mastitis is an inflammation of the breast. It most frequently occurs during lactation, but may also result from other conditions.

In the lactating woman, inflammation results from an ascending infection that travels from the nipple to the ductile structures. The offending organisms originate from either the suckling infant's nasopharynx or the hands of the mother. During the early weeks of nursing, the breast is particularly vulnerable to bacterial invasion because of minor cracks and fissures that occur with vigorous suckling. Infection and inflammation cause obstruction of the ductile system; the breast area becomes hard, inflamed, and tender if not treated early. Without treatment, the area becomes walled off and may abscess, requiring incision and drainage. It is advisable for the mother to continue breast feeding during antibiotic therapy to prevent this. Mastitis is not confined to the postpartum period, however; it can occur as a result of hormonal fluctuations, tumors, trauma, or skin infection. Cyclic inflammation of the breast occurs most frequently in adolescents, who commonly have a fluctuating hormone level. Tumors may cause mastitis secondary to skin involvement or lymphatic obstruction. Local trauma or infection may develop into mastitis because of ductal blockage of trapped blood, cellular debris, or the extension of superficial inflammation.

The treatment for mastitis symptoms may include application of heat or cold, excision, aspiration, mild analgesics, antibiotics, and a supportive brassiere or breast binder.

Ductal disorders

Ductal ectasia presents in older women as a spontaneous, intermittent, usually unilateral, grayish-green nipple discharge. Palpation of the breast increases the discharge. Ectasia occurs during or after menopause and is symptomatically associated with burning, itching, pain, and a pulling sensation of the nipple and areola. The disease results in inflammation of the ducts with subsequent thickening. The treatment requires removal of the involved ductal mass.

Intraductal papillomas are benign epithelial tissue tumors that range in size from 2 mm to 5 cm. Papillomas usually present with a bloody nipple discharge. The tumor may be palpated in the areolar area. The papilloma is probed through the nipple, and the involved duct is thus removed.

Fibroadenoma and fibrocystic disease

Fibroadenoma is seen in premenopausal women (most commonly in the third and fourth decade). The clinical findings include a firm, rubbery, sharply defined round mass. On palpation the mass "slides" between the fingers and is easily movable. These masses are usually singular; only 15% are multiple or bilateral. Fibroadenoma is asymptomatic and usually found by accident. Fibroadenoma is not believed to be precancerous. The treatment involves simple excision.

Fibrocystic breast disease (mammary dysplasia) is a condition typified by the development of fibrosis and cystic tissue formation. It is the single most common disorder of the breast and accounts for 35% to 50% of the surgical procedures on the female breast. The term *fibrocystic disease* has become a catchall for breast irregularities that occur bilaterally, change cyclically, and in younger women are accompanied by dull aching pain and heaviness. Some clinicians believe that the term is overused and that the breast changes associated with this process are a result of hormonally modulated proliferative activity with incomplete resolution. This incomplete resolution may be a result of excess hormonal stimulation or hypersensitive breast epithelium.[30] On the other hand, some clinicians believe that fibrocystic disease is a part of a continuum of breast pathology related to cancer. This is particularly true when the fibrocystic disease includes epithelial hyperplasia and papillomatous or demonstrable calcifications.

Fibrocystic disease usually presents as nodular ("shotty"), granular breast masses that are more prominent and painful during the luteal or progesterone-dominant portion of the menstrual cycle. Discomfort ranges from heaviness to exquisite tenderness, depending on the degree of vascular engorgement and cystic distention. Diagnosis is made by physical examination, biopsy (either aspiration or tissue sample), and mammography. The use of mammography for diagnosis in high-risk groups under 35 years of age on a routine basis is still controversial. Mammography may be helpful in establishing the diagnosis, but increased breast tissue density in women with fibrocystic disease may make an abnormal or cancerous mass difficult to discern among the other structures.

The treatment for fibrocystic breast disease is usually symptomatic. Aspirin, mild analgesics, and local heat or cold may be recommended. Some physicians attempt to aspirate prominent or persistent cysts and send any fluid obtained to the laboratory for cytologic analysis. Women are advised to avoid foods containing the xanthines (coffee, cola, chocolate, and tea) in their daily diets, particularly premenstrually. Vitamin E may be helpful in reducing mastalgia (breast pain) and women should be encouraged to wear a good supporting brassiere. Danazol, a synthetic androgen, can be used for women with severe pain, although the potential for side effects warrants trying other methods first.

There is controversy regarding the relationship between fibrocystic disease and cancer of the breast. It appears that the catchall term "fibrocystic disease" encompasses several different disorders, some of which may have a tendency to undergo malignant changes. Nonproliferative lesions (70%) do not demonstrate added risk for cancer; proliferative lesions without atypia (26%) may have a slightly increased risk for cancer. The remaining 4% of women with "fibrocystic" disease per biopsy show proliferative lesions with atypia and have a five times increased risk of cancer.[30] Suffice it to say that any discrete mass or lump on the breast should be viewed as possible carcinoma, and malignancy should be ruled out before the conservative measures used to treat fibrocystic disease are employed.[9]

Breast cancer

Cancer of the breast is second only to lung cancer as a cause of cancer-related death in women. One in 10 women in the United States will have breast cancer in her lifetime. In 1988, breast cancer affected 135,000 American women and killed almost 42,000 women. An additional 300 deaths occurred from breast cancer in males. Risk factors for breast cancer include being female, being over age 50, having a personal or family history of breast cancer, and having had no full-term pregnancies or a first child after age 30.[9]

Almost all breast cancers (90%) are found by women themselves, often through breast self-examination. Cancer may present clinically as a mass, a puckering, nipple retraction, or an unusual discharge. Some women identify cancer when only a thickening or subtle change in breast contour is noted. The variety of symptoms and the high self-discovery rate underscore the need for regular, systematic self-examination.

Breast self-examination (BSE) should be done routinely by women over 20. Premenopausal women should conduct the examination right after the cessation of menses. This time is most appropriate in relation to the cyclic breast changes that occur in response to changes in hormone levels. Postmenopausal women and women who have had a hysterectomy should perform the examination on approximately the same day of every month. A woman can choose a day relative to her past menstrual history. Examination may conveniently be done in the shower or bath or at bedtime. The most important thing is to devise a regular, systematic, convenient, and consistent method of examination.

X-ray mammography has been shown to be the only effective screening technique for the early detection of clinically inapparent lesions. A generally slow-growing form of malignancy, breast cancer may have been present for 2 to 9 years before it reaches 1 cm, the smallest size mass normally detected by palpation. Mammography can disclose lesions as small as 1 mm, as well as clustering of calcifications that may warrant biopsy to exclude malignancy. The American Cancer Society currently recommends a baseline mammogram between 35 and 40 years of age, studies every 1 to 2 years between 40 and 49 years, and annual evaluation for women over the age of 50.

Procedures used in the diagnosis of breast cancer include physical examination, mammography, thermography, ultrasound, percutaneous needle aspiration, and excisional biopsy.[1] Breast cancer often presents as a solitary, painless, firm, fixed lesion with poorly defined borders. It can be found anywhere in the breast but is most common in the upper outer quadrant. Because of the variability in presentation, any suspicious change in breast tissue warrants further investigation. The diagnostic use of mammography enables additional definition of the clinically suspicious area (appearance, character, calcification, etc.). Placement of a wire marker under radiographic guidance can ensure accurate surgical biopsy of nonpalpable suspicious areas. Ultrasound is useful as a diagnostic adjunct to differentiate cystic from tumor tissue in women with nonspecific thickening. Biopsy provides the only definitive diagnosis of breast cancer. Thermography (temperature detection), CT mammography, and diaphanography (transillumination) are still considered experimental, since their diagnostic capabilities for breast cancer detection remain unproven. Tumors are classified histologically according to tissue characteristics and staged clinically according to tumor size, nodal involvement, and presence of metastasis. It is recommended that estrogen and progesterone receptor analysis be performed on surgical specimens. Information about the presence or absence of estrogen and progesterone receptors can be used in predicting tumor responsiveness to hormonal manipulation. High levels of both receptors improves the prognosis and increases the likelihood of remission.

At present the treatment methods for breast cancer are controversial. Treatment may include surgery, chemotherapy, radiation, and hormonal manipulation. Radical mastectomy (removal of the entire breast, underlying muscles, and all axillary nodes) has, in general, fallen into disfavor as a primary surgical therapy for breast cancer. Modified surgical techniques (mastectomy plus axillary dissection or lumpectomy) accompanied by chemotherapy or radiation have achieved outcomes comparable to radical surgical methods. Prognosis is related more to the extent of nodal involvement than to the extent of breast involvement. Greater nodal involvement requires more aggressive postsurgical treatment; therefore, many cancer specialists believe that a diagnosis of breast cancer is not complete until dissection and testing of the axillary lymph nodes has been accomplished. The 5-year survival rate for localized cancer is 90%; with nodal involvement, it is approximately 60%. Reconstructive breast surgery, done simultaneously with mastectomy or as a delayed procedure, offers improved quality of life. However, early detection is still the best bargain.

Paget's disease

Paget's disease accounts for 2% to 3% of all breast cancers. The disease presents as an eczemoid lesion localized to the nipple and areola. Paget's disease is treated locally but may indicate systemic disease. Complete examination is therefore recommended in cases of Paget's disease, including a mammogram and usually biopsy.

In summary, the breasts are subject to both benign and malignant disease. Mastitis is inflammation of the breast, occurring most frequently during lactation. Galactorrhea is an abnormal secretion of milk that may occur as a symptom of increased prolactin secretion. Both ductal ectasia and intraductal papilloma cause abnormal drainage from the nipple. Fibroadenoma and fibrocystic disease are characterized by abnormal masses in the breast that are benign.

By far the most important disease of the breast is breast cancer, which is a significant cause of death in women. At present, breast self-examination affords a woman the best protection against breast cancer. It provides the means for early detection of breast cancer and in many cases allows for early treatment and cure.

Infertility

Infertility—the inability to conceive a child after a year of unprotected intercourse—affects about 15% of couples in the United States today. *Primary infertility* refers to situations in which there has been no prior conception. *Secondary infertility* is infertility that occurs following one or more previous pregnancies. *Sterility* is the inability to father a child or, for a woman, to become pregnant because of congenital anomalies, disease, or surgical intervention. About 1% to 2% of American couples are affected by sterility.

The complexity of the process that must occur in order to achieve a pregnancy is taken very much for granted by most couples. For some couples pregnancy occurs far too easily, while for others no amount of money, hard work, love, patience, or medical resources seems to be able to bring about this amazing, desired event. Although a full discussion of the diagnosis and treatment of infertility is beyond the scope of this book, an overview of the areas where problems can occur is presented. Causes of infertility are almost equally divided between male factors (30–40%), female factors (30–40%), and combined factors (30–40%). In about 10% to 15% of infertile couples, the etiology remains unknown even after a full workup.

── Male factors

In order for pregnancy to occur, the male must be able to provide sperm in sufficient quantity, delivered to the upper end of the vagina, with adequate motility to traverse the female reproductive tract. The male contribution to this process is assessed by means of a semen analysis, which evaluates volume of semen (normally 2–5 ml), sperm density (greater than 20 million/ml), motility (greater than 50% good progressive), viability (greater than 50%), morphology (greater than 60% normal), and viscosity (full liquefaction within 20 minutes). The specimen is best collected by masturbation into a sterile container after 3 days of abstinence. Because of variability in specimens, abnormal results should lead to a repeat test before the need for treatment is presumed. *Azoospermia* is the absence of sperm; *oligospermia* refers to decreased numbers of sperm; and *asthenospermia* refers to poor motility of sperm. Tests of sperm function include a cervical mucus penetration test (postcoital test, Penetrak), sperm penetration assay (Hamster Zona Free Ovum test), and sperm antibody testing.

Causes of male infertility include varicocele, ejaculatory dysfunction, hyperprolactinemia, hypogonadotropic hypogonadism, infection, immunologic problems (sperm antibodies), obstruction, and congenital anomalies. Risk factors for sperm problems include history of mumps orchitis, cryptorchidism (undescended testes), testicular torsion, hypospadias, previous urologic surgery, infection, and exposure to known gonadotoxins.[31] Treatment depends on cause and may include surgery, medication, or the use of artificial insemination to deliver a more concentrated specimen directly to the cervical canal or uterine fundus. Artificial insemination with donor sperm can be offered if the male is sterile and this is an acceptable alternative to both husband and wife.

── Female factors

The female contribution to pregnancy is more complex, requiring production and release of a mature ovum capable of being fertilized; production of cervical mucus that assists in sperm transport and maintains sperm viability within the female reproductive tract; patent fallopian tubes with the motility potential to pick up and transfer the ovum to the uterine cavity; development of an endometrium that is suitable for the implantation and nourishment of a fertilized ovum; and a uterine cavity that allows for growth and development of a fetus. Each of these factors will be briefly discussed, along with an overview of diagnostic tests and treatment.

── Ovulatory dysfunction

In a normally menstruating female, ovulatory cycles generally begin several months to a year after menarche. Release of follicle stimulating hormone (FSH) from the pituitary causes development of several primordial follicles within the ovary. At some point a dominant follicle is selected and the remaining follicles undergo atresia. When the dominant follicle has become large enough to contain a mature ovum (16–20 mm diameter) and is producing sufficient estradiol to ensure adequate proliferation of the endometrium, production of luteinizing hormone (LH) increases—the LH surge—and the increased LH level will induce release of the ovum from within the follicle (ovulation). Following ovulation, under the influence of LH, the former follicle luteinizes and begins producing progesterone in addition to estradiol. The progesterone stimulates the development of secretory endometrium, which has the capability to nourish a fertilized ovum should one implant. The presence of progesterone after ovulation causes a rise in the woman's basal body temperature (BBT). This thermogenic property of progesterone provides the basis for the most simple, inexpensive beginning test of ovulatory function—the measurement of BBT. Women should be able to detect at least a 0.4°F rise in their basal (at rest) temperature following ovulation which should be maintained throughout the luteal phase. This biphasic temperature pattern not only demonstrates that ovulation has taken place, but where in the cycle it occurred and the length of the luteal phase. Basal temperature can be influenced by many other factors, including restless sleep, alcohol intake, drug use, fever due to illness, and change in usual rising time. However, as an initial step in the infertility investigation, it can provide useful information to direct other forms of testing.

Endometrial biopsy (removal of a sample of the endometrium during an office procedure) provides histologic evidence of secretory endometrium and the level of maturation of the lining. The luteal phase should be consistently 14 days in length, because without pregnancy and the subsequent secretion of human chorionic gonadotropin (hCG) the corpus luteum will begin to degenerate. LH is only produced by the pituitary for a period of 7 days to 10 days following the initial surge. The luteal phase of the cycle therefore is so consistent that a pathologist can tell by evaluating a section of endometrium that it is representative of a particular day of the luteal phase. The pathologist's assessment of maturation is compared to the arrival of the next menses and if a discrepancy of more than 2 days exists the woman is said to have a luteal phase defect (LPD). This diagnosis indicates that although ovulation is occurring, endometrial development is insufficient and implantation may not be possible. Pregnancy requires both fertilization and implantation. Luteal phase defect can also be suggested by an abnormal serum progesterone level 7 days after ovulation. Luteal phase defect can be treated directly with supplemental progesterone following ovulation, or with the use of clomiphene citrate to stimulate increased pituitary production of FSH and LH.

Anovulation (no ovulation) or oligo-ovulation (irregular ovulation) are other forms of ovulatory dysfunction. These problems can be identified by the tests for luteal phase defect previously described. Ovulatory problems can be primary problems of the ovary or secondary problems related to endocrine dysfunction. Therefore when disturbances in ovulation are confirmed, it is reasonable to evaluate other endocrine function before initiating treatment. If pituitary hormone (FSH, LH, prolactin) tests, thyroid studies, and tests of adrenal function (DHAS, androstendione) are normal, then ovulatory dysfunction is primary and should respond to treatment. Abnormalities in any of the other endocrine areas should be further evaluated as needed and treated appropriately. Hyperprolactinemia responds well to bromcriptine, but pituitary microadenoma may need to be ruled out first; hypothyroidism requires thyroid replacement; hyperthyroidism requires suppressive therapy and sometimes surgical intervention with thyroid replacement later; adrenal suppression can be instituted with dexamethasone—a glucocorticoid analog. Normal ovulatory function may resume without further intervention; if not, treatment can be concurrent with management of the other endocrine problem(s).

Cervical mucus problems

High preovulatory levels of estradiol stimulate the production of large amounts of clear, stretchy cervical mucus that actually aids in the transport of sperm into the uterine cavity and helps maintain an environment that keeps the sperm viable for up to 72 hours. Insufficient estrogen production (inherent or secondary to treatment with clomiphene citrate which is an anti-estrogen), cervical abnormalities from disease or invasive procedures (DES exposure, stenosis, conization), and cervical infection (chlamydia, gonorrhea, mycoplasma) can adversely affect the production of healthy cervical mucus. A postcoital test (PCT, Sims-Huhner) involves evaluation of the cervical mucus 1 to 8 hours after intercourse within the 48 hours prior to ovulation. A sample of cervical mucus is obtained using a special syringe and evaluated grossly for amount, clarity, and stretch (spinnbarkeit), and microscopically for cellularity, for number and quality of motile sperm, and for the presence of ferning after the sample has air-dried on the slide. To obtain good-quality mucus it is essential to obtain the sample within the 48 hours prior to ovulation. Tests may have to be repeated within the same cycle or in subsequent cycles to ensure appropriate timing. If inadequate estrogen effect is seen (poor-quality mucus), supplemental oral estrogen can be given in the first 9 days of the next cycle and the test can be repeated. Administration of mucolytic expectorants (1 teaspoon 4 times daily starting day 10 until ovulation is confirmed) may also improve the quality of the mucus. If mucus is good but sperm are inadequate in number or motility, further evaluation of the male may be needed. Both the male and the female should be tested for sperm antibodies when repeated postcoital tests reveal that the sperm are all dead or agglutinated. Artificial insemination with the husband's sperm may be helpful to bypass the cervical mucus. Cervical cultures for gonorrhea, chlamydia, and the mycoplasmas should be obtained with the postcoital test if they have not already been acquired. If the cultures give positive results, treatment should be instituted as needed.

Uterine cavity abnormalities

Alterations within the uterine cavity can occur secondary to DES exposure, submucous fibroids, cervical polyps, synechiae or bands of scar tissue, or congenital anomalies (bicornuate, septum, single horn, etc.). These defects may be suspected from history or pelvic examination, but require hysterosalpingography (an x-ray study in which dye is placed through the cervix to outline the uterine cavity and demonstrate tubal patency) or hysteroscopy (a study in which a lighted fiberoptic scope placed through the cervix under general anaesthesia allows direct visualization of the uterine cavity) for confirmation. Treatment is generally surgical when possible.

Tubal factors

Tubal patency is required for fertilization and can be disrupted secondary to pelvic inflammatory disease (PID), ectopic pregnancy (salpingectomy or salpingostomy), large myomas, endometriosis, pelvic adhesions, and previous tubal ligation. Hysterosalpingography can reveal the location and type of any blockage present (fimbrial, cornual, hydrosalpinx). Microsurgical repair is sometimes possible.

Even when tubal patency is demonstrated, it is possible for tubal disease to make ovum pick-up impossible. Contrary to popular belief, the ovum is not extruded directly into the fallopian tube. Rather, the tube must be free to move to engulf the ovum after release. Pelvic adhesions from previous infection, surgery, or endometriosis can interfere with the tube's mobility. Laparoscopic evaluation of the pelvis is needed for diagnosis. Laser surgery or cautery can be used for the lysis of adhesions and removal of endometriosis either through the laparoscope or, if severe, with laparotomy.

New technologies

In vitro fertilization (IVF) was developed in 1978 for women with significantly damaged or absent tubes to provide them an opportunity for pregnancy where none exists normally. The ovaries are superstimulated to produce multiple follicles using clomiphene citrate, human menopausal menotropins (Pergonal), pure FSH (Metrodin) or a combination of these drugs. Follicular maturation is monitored by means of ultrasound and assay of serum estradiol levels. When preovulatory criteria are met, an injection of hCG is given to simulate an LH surge, and 34 hours later the follicles are aspirated either laparoscopically or by one of the newer ultrasound-guided routes (transvaginal, transurethral, transvesical, or transabdominal). The follicular fluid is evaluated microscopically for the presence of ova, which, when found, are removed and placed into culture media in an incubator. The eggs are inseminated with semen from the husband that has been prepared by a wash-up technique that removes the semen, begins the capacitation process, and allows the strongest sperm to be used for fertilization. Then, 12 to 24 hours after insemination, the ova are evaluated for signs of fertilization. If signs are present, the ovum are placed back in the incubator. Finally, 48 to 72 hours after egg retrieval, the fertilized eggs are placed back into the woman's uterus by means of a transcervical catheter. Hormonal supplementation of the luteal phase is often used to increase the possibility of implantation. Clinical pregnancy rates in 1985 and 1986, as reported by the National IVF/ET registry, were 14.1% and 16.9%, respectively.[32] By mid-1988, over 3000 babies had been born worldwide using IVF technology, and future research will no doubt be focused on means of understanding and improving the implantation process. Indications for IVF have been expanded to include male factors (severe oligospermia or asthenospermia), immunologic infertility, severe endometriosis, and idiopathic or unknown infertility. There is a substantial risk of multiple births with IVF procedures.

An outgrowth of IVF technology is GIFT (gamete intra-fallopian transfer) which uses similar ovarian stimulation protocols and laparoscopic egg retrieval, and involves placing ovum and sperm directly into the fallopian tube during the same laparoscopy procedure. This procedure requires at least one patent fallopian tube and was developed primarily to try to increase the pregnancy rate in women with idiopathic infertility. The basic premise is that if a transportation problem is interfering with ovum pick-up, GIFT would solve that problem and that implantation might result more often if fertilization actually occurs within the body. Clinical pregnancy rates increased from 3 in 56 procedures in 1985 to 108 in 466 procedures in 1986.[32] The multiple birth rate with GIFT is similar to that with IVF.

In summary, infertility affects approximately 15% of couples in the United States and is often a multifactorial problem. The evaluation can be lengthy and highly stressful for the couple. Options for therapy continue to expand, but newer treatment modalities such as IVF or GIFT are expensive, and financial resources can be strained while couples seek their sometimes elusive dream of having a child.

References

1. Friedrich EG: Vulvar Disease, 2nd ed, pp 200, 130–140. Philadelphia, WB Saunders, 1983
2. Pernoll ML, Benson RC: Current Obstetric & Gynecologic Diagnosis and Treatment, pp 713, 846, 845, 851, 864, 874, 1082. Norwalk, CT, Appleton & Lange, 1987
3. Van Nagell JR, Powell DF, Gay EC: Cancer of the Vagina—Part 1. Female Patient 8(5):15, 1983
4. Manetta A, Pinto JL, Larson JE, et al: Primary invasive carcinoma of the vagina. Obstet Gynecol 72(1):77, 1988
5. Van Nagell JR, Powell DF, Gay EC: Cancer of the Vagina—Part 2. Female Patient 8(6):24, 1983
6. Robbins SL, Cotran RS, Kumar V: Pathologic Basis of Disease, 2nd ed, pp 1121. Philadelphia, WB Saunders, 1984
7. Nichols DH, Evrard JR: Ambulatory Gynecology, pp 319–322. Philadelphia, Harper & Row, 1985
8. Paavonen J, Kritchlow CW, DeRouen T, et al: Etiology of cervical inflammation. Am J Obstet Gynecol 154:556, 1986
9. American Cancer Society: Cancer Facts & Figures 1988, pp 10,11, New York, American Cancer Society, 1988
10. Nelson JH, Avarette HE, Richart RM: Dysplasia, carcinoma in situ and early invasive cervical carcinoma. Cancer Journal for Clinicians 34:306, 1984
11. Cherkis RC, Patten SF, Andrews TJ, et al: Significance of normal endometrial cells detected by cervical cytology. Obstet Gynecol 71:242, 1988
12. Tawa K, Forsythe A, et al: A comparison of Papanicolaou smear and the cervigram: Sensitivity, specificity, and cost analysis. Obstet Gynecol 71:242, 1988
13. Danforth DN, Scott JR: Obstetrics and Gynecology, 5th ed, pp 918, 1080. Philadelphia, JB Lippincott, 1986
14. Malinak LR, Wheeler JM: A practical approach to endometriosis—part 1: Diagnosis. Female Patient 10(5):39, 1985
15. Cramer DW, Wilson E, et al: The relationship of endometriosis to menstrual characteristics, smoking and exercise. JAMA 255:1904, 1986
16. Steingold KA, Cedars M, Lu JK, et al: Treatment of endometriosis with a long-acting gonadotropin-releasing hormone agonist. Obstet Gynecol 69:403, 1987
17. Daniell JF, Miller W, Tosh R: Initial evaluation of the use of potassium-titanyl-phosphate (KTP/532) laser in gynecologic laparoscopy. Fertil Steril 46(3):373, 1986
18. Centers for Disease Control Cancer and Steroid Hormone Study: Oral contraceptive use and risk of endometrial cancer. JAMA 249:1600, 1983
19. Charles D, Larsen B: Pelvic inflammatory disease: Trends and management. Female Patient 11(6):45, 1986
20. Lee NC, Rubin Gl, Borucki R: The intrauterine device and PID revisited: New results from the Women's Health Study. Obstet Gynecol 72:1, 1988
21. Centers for Disease Control: STD treatment guidelines 1985. MMWR 34, No. 4S, 1985
22. Centers for Disease Control: Ectopic pregnancy mortality 1970–1982. MMWR 36:55–52, 1987
23. Stock RJ: The changing spectrum of ectopic pregnancy. Obstet Gynecol 71:885, 1988
24. Brumsted J, Kessler C, Gibson C, et al: A comparison of laparoscopy and laparotomy for treatment of ectopic pregnancy. Obstet Gynecol 71(6):889, 1988
25. Schneider G, McDonough R, Moghissi K, et al: Dysfunctional uterine bleeding. Female Patient 11(2):22, 1986
26. Ziff RA: Amenorrhea. Female Patient 11(1):33, 1985
27. Severino SK, Anderson M, Hurt SW, et al: Premenstrual syndrome: An update. Female Patient 12(1):69, 1987
28. Lauber DW: Premenstrual syndrome. Female Patient 11(1):107, 1986
29. Fehrer TL: Chronic pain—part II: Premenstrual syndrome and breast pain. Female Patient 10(7):20, 1985
30. Hutter RVP: Goodbye to "Fibrocystic Disease." N Engl J Med 312(3):179, 1985
31. Jarow JP, Lipschultz LI: Urologic evaluation of male infertility. Contemp OB Gyn, Special Issue, Sept 87:85, 1987
32. Medical Research International. The American Fertility Society Special Interest Group: In vitro fertilization/embryo transfer in the United States: 1985 and 1986 results from the National IVF/ET Registry. Fertil Steril 49:212, 1988

Bibliography

Boyd ME: Endometriosis. Can J Surg 28:471, 1985

Bullen BA, Skrinar GS, Butins IZ, et al: Induction of menstrual disorders by strenuous exercise in untrained women. N Engl J Med 312:1349, 1985

Dmowski WP, Radwanska E, Binor Z, et al: Mild endometriosis and ovulatory dysfunction: Effect of danazol treatment on success of ovulation induction. Fertil Steril 46:784, 1986

Fayez JA, Taylor RB: Endometriosis: Staging and management. Hosp Phys 11:26, 1984

Fehrer TL: Chronic pain—part 1: Primary dysmenorrhea and cryptic pelvic pain. Female Patient 10(6):44, 1985

Gambrell RD: Abnormal uterine bleeding. Female Patient 8(6):79, 1983

Greenwood SM, Moran JJ: Chronic endometritis: Morphologic and clinical observations. Obstet Gynecol 58:176, 1981

Hansen AM, Immordino KF, Farber M: The diagnostic evaluation and therapy of secondary amenorrhea. JOGNN 3:180, 1984

Herbst AL: Diethylstilbestrol exposure—1984. N Engl J Med 311:1433, 1984

Kopans DB, Meyer JE, Sadowsky N: Breast imaging. N Engl J Med 310:960, 1984

Leis HP, Cammarata A, LaRaja R, Cruz E: Fibrocystic breast disease. Female Patient 8(5):56, 1983

Loucks A: Pelvic inflammatory disease: A review of therapy. Nurse Practitioner 10:13, 1983

Love SM, Gelman RS: Fibrocystic "disease" of the breast—a nondisease?. N Engl J Med 307:1010, 1982

Mirecki DM, Jordan VC: Steroid hormone receptors and human breast cancer. Lab Med 16:287, 1985

Molgaard CA, Golbeck AL, Gresham L: Current concepts in endometriosis. Western J Med 145(7):42, 1985

Morley GW: Cancer of the vulva. Cancer 48:597, 1981

Parazzini F, La Vecchia C, Franceschi S, et al: Risk factors for pathologically confirmed benign breast disease. Am J Epidemiol 120:115, 1984

Patterson JE: Colposcopy. JOGNN 12(1):11, 1983

Pinsonneault O, Goldstein DP: Gynecologic disorders in adolescents—part 1: pain syndromes. Female Patient 11(4):26, 1986

Pinsonneault O, Goldstein DP: Gynecologic disorders in adolescents—part 2: dysfunctional uterine bleeding and breast masses. Female Patient 11(5):30, 1986

Rico M: Breast cancer: Risk factors and etiology. Mt Sinai J Med 51:300, 1984

Riddick DH: The premenstrual syndrome. Female Patient 8(12):47, 1983

Russell KP, Drukker BH, Issacs W, et al: Breast cancer: The physician's responsibility—part 1: screening and diagnosis. Female Patient 10(9):20, 1985

Seltzer V: Pitfalls of Pap smear and colposcopy. Med Digest 2:1, 1985

Sheahan SL: Management of breast lumps. Nurse Practitioner 2:19, 1984

Soper DE, Despres B: A comparison of two antibiotic regimens for treatment of pelvic inflammatory disease. Obstet Gynecol 72:7, 1988

Vaitukaitis JL: Polycystic-ovary syndrome—what is it? N Engl J Med 309:1245, 1983

von Rueden DG, Wilson RE: Entraductal carcinoma of the breast. Surgery 158:105, 1984

Sexually Transmitted Diseases

Infections of the external genitalia
  Human papilloma virus (condylomata accuminata)
  Genital herpes
  Molluscum contagiosum
  Chancroid

Granuloma inguinale
Lymphogranuloma venereum
Vaginal infections
  Candidiasis
  Trichomonas
  Bacterial vaginosis (nonspecific vaginitis)

Vaginal/urogenital/systemic infections
  Chlamydial infections
  Gonorrhea
  Nonspecific urogenital infection
  Syphilis

Objectives

After you have studied this chapter, you should be able to meet the following objectives:

_____ Define what is meant by an *STD*.

_____ Give a reason why the reported incidences of STDs may not accurately reflect the true incidence.

_____ List common portals of entry for STDs.

_____ Name the organisms responsible for condyloma accuminata, genital herpes, molluscum contagiosum, chancroid, granuloma inguinale, lymphogranuloma venereum, candidiasis vaginal infections, trichomonas vaginal infections, bacterial vaginosis (nonspecific vaginitis), chlamydial urogenital infections, gonorrhea, nonspecific urogenital infection, and syphilis.

_____ List the STDs that pose a threat to the unborn child either *in utero* or during childbirth.

_____ State the significance of condyloma accuminata.

_____ Explain the recurrent infections in genital herpes.

_____ State the difference between wet-mount slide and culture methods of diagnosis of STDs.

_____ Compare the signs and symptoms of infections due to *Chlamydia trachomatis*, *Candida albicans*, *Trichomonas vaginalis,* and bacterial vaginosis.

_____ Compare the signs and symptoms of gonorrhea in the male and female.

_____ Describe the three stages of syphilis.

_____ State the genital and nongenital complications that can occur with chlamydial infections, gonorrhea, nonspecific urogenital infection, and syphilis.

_____ Compare the treatments for condyloma accuminata, genital herpes, molluscum contagiosum, chancroid, granuloma inguinale, lymphogranuloma venereum, vaginal candidiasis, trichomonal vaginal infections, bacterial vaginosis, chlamydial urogenital infections, gonorrhea, nonspecific urogenital infections, and syphilis.

The incidence and types of sexually transmitted diseases (STDs), as reported in the professional literature and public health statistics, are increasing. It must be recognized, however, that the incidence of disease is based on clinical reports and many STDs are either not reportable or not reported. The agents of transmission include bacteria, chlamydiae, viruses, fungi, protozoa, parasites, and unidentified microorganisms (see Chapter 9). Portals of entry include the mouth, genitalia, urinary meatus, rectum, and skin. All STDs are more common in persons with more than one sexual partner, and it is not uncommon for a person to be concurrently infected with more than one type of STD. This chapter discusses the manifestations of STDs in both men and women and has been divided into three sections: infections of the external genitalia, vaginal infections, and infections that have systemic effects as well as genitourinary manifestations.

Infections of the external genitalia

Some STDs primarily affect the mucocutaneous tissues of the external genitalia. These include human papilloma virus infection, genital herpes, molluscum contagiosum, chancroid, granuloma inguinale, and lymphogranuloma venereum.

Human papilloma virus (condylomata accuminata)

Condylomata accuminata, or genital warts, are the most common manifestation of the human papilloma virus (HPV). Although recognized for centuries, HPV-induced genital warts have become one of the fastest rising STDs of the past decade. The Centers for Disease Control (CDC) estimate that the number of visits to private physicians for genital warts increased from 169,000 in 1966 to 1 million in 1981 and to 2 million in 1983.[1,2] Reports from the United Kingdom indicate a doubling of the number of cases in the 10-year period from 1974 to 1984.[3]

The incubation period for HPV ranges from 6 weeks to 8 months. Although HPV infections are often asymptomatic, they can be detected by the presence of characteristic warty lesions. Structurally, there are four types of condylomas or warts: (1) papillous, (2) flat, (3) spiked, and (4) exophytic.[4] Papillous condylomas are soft, pink, fleshy growths of external genitalia. They are often difficult to distinguish from normal genital tissue and may require biopsy for definitive diagnosis. Until recently, papillous condylomas were the only type of condyloma recognized. The flat con-

dyloma, discovered in 1977, is the most virulent type. The flat condyloma, which is a macular, flat, granular lesion, is found most often on the cervix or introitus in women and on the frenulum or upper shaft of the penis in men. The lesions, which are frequently invisible to the naked eye, become readily apparent when the affected area is soaked with a 5% acetic acid solution. Biopsy may be required to differentiate these lesions from other hyperkeratotic or precancerous lesions. Spiked condylomas, which are less common, are small, pointed projections that are found primarily in the vagina. Exophytic or inverted condylomas grow only within the glands of the cervix and can mimic carcinoma in situ.

A relationship between HPV and genital neoplasms has become increasingly apparent over the past 10 years.[3,5,6] Currently, 46 types of HPV have been identified.[5] Several of these have been associated with genital neoplasms. Types 16 and 18 are present in over 80% of invasive squamous cell carcinomas of the cervix, vulva, and penis and in higher grades of intraepithelial neoplasms of the cervix and vulva.[3] Types 31 and 33 have been detected to a lesser degree in cervical dysplasias and neoplasms.[5] In contrast, types 6 and 11 are more often associated with benign warts and mild forms of dysplasia. It is this association with premalignant and malignant changes that has increased the concern for diagnosis and treatment of this virus.

Genital condylomas should be considered in any woman who presents with the primary complaint of vulvar pruritus or who has had an abnormal Papanicolaou (Pap) smear. Microscopic examination of a wet-mount slide preparation and cultures are used to rule out associated vaginitis. Acetic acid soaks are used prior to inspecting the vulva under magnification, and questionable areas are biopsied. Colposcopic examination of the cervix and vagina is generally advised as a follow-up measure when there is an abnormal Pap smear or when HPV lesions are identified on the vulva. The presence of koilocytes (hollow cells) on the Pap smear or pathology report is diagnostic of HPV. Because the male sexual partner may be the primary reservoir for this virus, examination of the penis using acetic acid soaks is recommended.

In the past, the primary treatment for condyloma accuminata was podophyllin 25% in tincture of benzoin. With multiple applications, this cytotoxic agent produced resolution of the lesions. However, this treatment was contraindicated in pregnancy because the medication could be absorbed systemically. Currently, the first line of treatment for vulvar, vaginal, or penile condylomas is the topical application of a 50% to 80% solution of trichloroacetic acid. This weak destructive agent produces an initial burning in the affected area, followed in several days by a sloughing of the superficial tissue. Several applications, 1 week to 2 weeks apart, may be necessary to eradicate the virus. Vulvar, vaginal, and penile condylomas may also be treated with electrocautery. Topical 5-fluorouracil (5-FU, Efudex) and laser therapy have been used successfully in the treatment of vaginal condylomas.[7] Because it can penetrate deeper than other forms of therapy, cryotherapy (freezing therapy) is the treatment of choice for cervical HPV lesions. Laser surgery can be used to remove large or widespread lesions of the cervix or lesions of the cervix that have failed to respond to other first-line methods of treatment. The results of laser treatment have been excellent, but the equipment is expensive and the method requires extensive training for safe and effective use. Interferon, either in the form of a topical application or as an intralesional injection, is under investigation as a possible form of treatment but has not as yet shown any advantage over other available forms of treatment. Sexual abstinence is necessary during any type of treatment.

Recurrence of HPV is high, occurring sometimes as early as 3 weeks to 6 weeks after treatment. Originally, it was assumed that reinfection from sexual partners was the primary cause. It is now believed that the recurrences are due to a persistent HPV infection existing in a latent state in the apparently normal tissue near the treated lesions.[2] Stress and trauma appear to be two possible factors in the reactivation of the latent virus. Extending the area of treatment for a distance of 5 mm beyond the lesion border is recommended as a method for preventing recurrences. Research may eventually lead to the prevention or eradication of this form of what appears to be a sexually transmitted neoplastic condition.

—— Genital herpes

Genital herpes is a sexually transmitted disease caused by the herpes simplex virus. Because herpes virus infection is not reportable in all states, reliable data on its true incidence and prevalence are lacking. Estimates indicate that about 270,000 to 600,000 new cases may occur each year. In a study evaluating the prevalence of genital herpes in private physician practices, it was determined that the number of physician's office visits for herpes increased tenfold between 1966 and 1981.[8]

There are five types of herpes viruses that cause infections in humans: two types of herpes simplex virus (HSV)—HSV-I, which causes cold sores, and HSV-II, which causes genital herpes; varicella-zoster virus which causes chickenpox and shingles; Epstein-Barr virus, which causes infectious mononucleosis and Burkitt's lymphoma; and the cytomegalovirus, which causes cytomegalic inclusion disease.

The herpes viruses are neurotropic: that is, they grow within neurons and share the biologic property of latency. *Latency* refers to the ability to maintain disease potential in the absence of clinical signs and symptoms. In genital herpes the virus ascends through the peripheral nerves to the sacral dorsal root ganglia (Figure 38-1). The virus can remain dormant in the dorsal root ganglia or it can reactivate, in which case the viral particles are transported back down the nerve root to the skin, where they multiply and cause a lesion to develop. During the dormant or latent period, the virus replicates in a different manner so that the immune system or available treatments have no effect on it. It is not known what reactivates the virus. It may be that the body's defense mechanisms are altered. Numerous studies have shown that host responses to infection influence initial development of the disease, severity of infection, development and maintenance of latency, and frequency of HSV recurrences.[9]

Both HSV-I and HSV-II can cause genital lesions. The herpes simplex virus is shed from active lesions and it is usually transmitted by contact with infectious lesions or genital secretions. HSV-I is often transmitted by kissing. When one has a cold sore on the mouth, HSV-I may be spread to the genital area by autoinoculation secondary to poor handwashing or through oral intercourse. HSV-II is usually transmitted by sexual contact, but can be passed to an infant during childbirth if the virus is actively being shed from the genital tract.

The incubation period for HSV is generally 2 days to 10 days. Genital HSV may present as either a

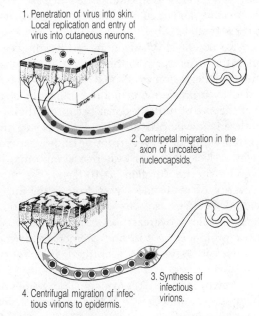

1. Penetration of virus into skin. Local replication and entry of virus into cutaneous neurons.

2. Centripetal migration in the axon of uncoated nucleocapsids.

3. Synthesis of infectious virions.

4. Centrifugal migration of infectious virions to epidermis.

Figure 38-1 Pathogenesis of primary mucocutaneous HSV infection. (*Corey L, Spear PG: Infections with herpes simplex viruses—Part 1. N Engl J Med 314:686, 1986*)

primary or a nonprimary form of infection. Primary infections are infections that occur in an person who is seronegative for antibody to HSV-I or HSV-II. Nonprimary infections refer to the clinical appearance of genital herpes in a person who is seropositive for antibodies to HSV-I or HSV-II, implying a previous asymptomatic exposure.

The initial symptoms of primary genital herpes infections include tingling, itching, and pain in the genital area followed by eruption of small pustules and vesicles. These lesions rupture on about the fifth day to form wet ulcers which are excruciatingly painful to touch and can be associated with dysuria, dyspareunia, and urinary retention. Involvement of the cervix and urethra is seen in more than 80% of women with primary infections.[10] In men, the infection can cause urethritis as well as lesions of the penis and scrotum. Rectal and perianal infections are possible with anal intercourse. Systemic symptoms associated with primary infections include fever, headache, malaise, muscle ache, and lymphadenopathy. Primary infections may be debilitating enough to require hospitalization, particularly in women. Untreated primary infections are usually self-limiting and last for about 2 weeks to 4 weeks. The symptoms usually worsen for the first 10 days to 12 days. This period is followed by a 10-day to 12-day interval during which the lesions crust over and gradually heal. Nonprimary episodes of genital herpes present with similar symptoms—albeit less severe symptoms that are usually of shorter duration and have fewer systemic manifestations. Except for the greater tendency of HSV-II to recur, the clinical manifestations of HSV-II and genital HSV-I are similar. Genital HSV-II infections are twice as likely to be reactivated, and recur 8 times to 12 times more often than genital HSV-I.[10]

Recurrent HSV infections result from reactivation of the virus stored in the dorsal root ganglia of the infected dermatomes. Actual outbreaks may be preceded by a prodrome of itching, burning, or tingling at the site of future lesions. Because individuals have already developed immune lymphocytes from the primary infection, recurrent episodes generally have fewer lesions, fewer systemic symptoms, less pain, and a shorter duration (7–10 days). Frequency and severity of recurrences vary from individual to individual. Numerous factors, including emotional stress, lack of sleep, overexertion, other infections, vigorous or prolonged coitus, and premenstrual /menstrual distress, have been identified as triggering mechanisms.

Asymptomatic disease is possible. Some individuals possess antibodies to HSV-I or HSV-II without any history of clinical disease. Asymptomatic shedding of the virus can occur from these individuals as well as those whose recurrences result in viral excretion into saliva or cervical secretions without development of overt lesions. Little is known about the frequency or quantity of asymptomatic shedding, but it appears that transmission of the disease is more likely during symptomatic periods of viral excretion.[9]

Diagnosis of genital herpes is based on the symptoms, appearance of the lesions, and identification of the virus from a Tzanck smear or cultures taken from the lesions. Depending on the laboratory, a preliminary report on cultures takes from 2 days to 5 days, and a final negative report takes from 10 days to 12 days. The stability of the virus in transport media is good for 48 hours to 72 hours, making mail transport possible. Generally, the likelihood of obtaining a positive culture decreases with each day that has elapsed after a lesion develops. The chances of obtaining a positive culture from a crusted lesion is slight, and persons suspected of having genital herpes should be instructed to have a culture within 24 hours of developing new lesions. A Tzanck smear is done by scraping a debrided lesion with a cytology spatula and smearing the exudate on a slide, allowing the slide to dry, and sending it to a laboratory for microscopic identification of multinucleated giant cells. About 50% of Tzanck smear results are falsely negative. They are, however, available in 24 hours to 48 hours, as opposed to the 2 days to 5 days required for culture tests. Newer tests for HSV-I and HSV-II include immunofluorescence assays that use monoclonal antibodies, DNA-hybridization procedures, and combined tissue-culture/immunologic detection (modified viral culture). These methods provide faster, cheaper diagnosis but require special equipment and training to perform and are less specific than viral culture techniques. These types of testing are being continually improved, however, and should be in wider use in the near future.

There is no known cure for genital herpes, and the methods of treatment are largely symptomatic. The antiviral drug Acyclovir has become a significant component of the management of genital herpes. By interfering with viral DNA replication, Acyclovir decreases the frequency of recurrences, shortens the duration of active lesions, reduces the number of new lesions formed, and decreases viral shedding in persons with primary infections. The drug is most useful in persons with depressed immune function and in those experiencing an initial outbreak. Originally available only for topical application or intravenous administration, oral Acyclovir is now the more common treatment form. Oral Acyclovir has been shown to reduce the duration of viral shedding and the healing time for recurrent lesions, but is generally not needed unless the recurrences are severe. Chronic suppressive therapy of up to 6 months duration can be used for individuals with very frequent recurrences.

Although well tolerated with few side effects, the use of Acyclovir beyond 6 months is not recommended until further studies of its long-term effects have been completed. Long-term suppressive therapy does not limit latency, and reactivation of the disease occurs after the drug is discontinued. Topical treatment with antibacterial soaps, lotions, dyes, ultrasound, and ultraviolet light have all been tried with little success. Symptomatic relief can sometimes be obtained with cool compresses (Burrow's soaks), sitz baths, topical anaesthetic agents, and oral analgesic drugs.

Good hygiene is essential to prevent secondary infection with HSV infections. Fastidious handwashing is recommended to avoid hand-to-eye spread of the infection. HSV infection of the eye is the most frequent cause of corneal blindness in the United States.[10] To prevent spread of the disease, intimate contact should be avoided until lesions are completely healed. Because up to 65% of infected newborns will die if they contract herpes infections during vaginal delivery, active infection during pregnancy may necessitate cesarean delivery. Any woman with a history of HSV should have weekly cervical cultures for HSV starting at 34 weeks' gestation to determine the need for cesarean delivery. Finally, because women with HSV-II appear to be at increased risk for developing cervical cancer, it is recommended that they obtain annual Pap smears and be alert to the development of suspicious vulvar lesions that might warrant biopsy.

Molluscum contagiosum

Molluscum contagiosum is a common viral disease of the skin that gives rise to multiple umbilicated papules. The disease is mildly contagious; it is transmitted by skin-to-skin contact, fomites, and autoinoculation. Lesions are domelike and have a dimpled appearance. A curdlike material can be expressed from the center of the lesion. Necrosis and secondary infection are possible. Diagnosis is based on the appearance of the lesion and microscopic identification of intracytoplasmic molluscum bodies. Molluscum is a benign and self-limiting disease. The goal of treatment is to prevent its spread for cosmetic reasons.[11] When indicated, treatment consists of unroofing the papule with a sterile needle or scalpel, expressing the contents of each lesion, and applying alcohol or silver nitrate to the base. Electrodesiccation, cryosurgery (freezing), or surgical biopsy are alternative treatments, but are rarely needed unless lesions are large.[11]

Chancroid

Chancroid (soft chancre) is a disease of the external genitalia and lymph nodes. The causative organism is the gram-negative bacterium *Hemophilus ducreyi*, which causes acute ulcerative lesions with profuse discharge. This disease is somewhat uncommon in the United States.[11] It is more prevalent in Southeast Asia, the West Indies, and North Africa. It is usually transmitted by sexual intercourse or through skin and mucous membrane abrasions. It is highly infectious and autoinoculation may lead to multiple chancres.

Lesions begin as a macule, progress to a pustule, and then rupture. This painful ulcer has a necrotic base and jagged edges. In contrast, the syphilitic chancre (discussed later in this chapter) is nontender and indurated. Subsequent discharge can lead to further infection of self or others. Upon physical examination, lesions and regional lymphadenopathy may be found. Secondary infection may cause significant tissue destruction. Diagnosis is confirmed through use of Gram stain and culture. The organism has shown resistance to treatment with sulfamethoxazole alone and to tetracycline. The CDC currently recommends treatment with erythromycin or an alternative regimen of sulfamethoxazole and trimethoprim.[13]

Granuloma inguinale

Granuloma inguinale (granuloma venereum) is caused by a gram-negative bacillus, the *Calymmatobacterium donovani*, which is a tiny, encapsulated, intracellular parasite. This disease is almost nonexistent in the United States. It is most frequently found in India, Brazil, the West Indies, and parts of China, Australia, and Africa. Granuloma inguinale causes ulceration of the genitalia, beginning with an innocuous papule. The papule progresses through nodular or vesicular stages until it begins to break down as pink granulomatous tissue. At this final stage, the tissue becomes thin and friable and bleeds easily. There are complaints of swelling, pain, and itching. Extensive inflammatory scarring may cause late sequelae, such as lymphatic obstruction with the development of enlarged and elephantoid external genitalia. The liver, bladder, bone, joint, lung, and bowel tissue may become involved. Genital complications include tuboovarian abscess, fistula, vaginal stenosis, and occlusion of vaginal or anal orifices. Lesions may become neoplastic. Diagnosis is made through the identification of Donovan bodies (large mononuclear cells filled with intracytoplasmic gram-negative rods) in tissue smears, biopsy samples, or culture. A 2-week to 3-week period of treatment with tetracycline, erythromycin, or gentamicin is used in treating the disorder.

Lymphogranuloma venereum

Lymphogranuloma venereum is an acute and chronic venereal disease caused by *Chlamydia trachomatis* (types L_1, L_2, P_3). The disease, although worldwide, has a low incidence outside the tropics. The majority of cases reported in the United States are in men.

The lesions of lymphogranuloma can incubate for a few days to several weeks and thereafter cause small painless papules or vesicles which may go undetected. An important characteristic of the disease is the early (1–4 weeks later) development of large, tender, and sometimes fluctuant inguinal lymph nodes called *buboes*. There may be flulike symptoms with joint pain, rash, weight loss, pneumonitis, tachycardia, splenomegaly, and proctitis. In later stages of the disease, a small percentage of persons develop elephantiasis of the external genitalia; this is due to lymphatic obstruction or fibrous strictures of the rectum or urethra caused by the inflammation and scarring. Urethral involvement may cause pyuria and dysuria. Anorectal structures may be compromised to the point of incontinence. Complications of lymphogranuloma infection may be minor or extensive, involving compromise of whole systems or progression to a cancerous state. Diagnosis is usually by means of a complement fixation test for chlamydia group antibody. High titers for this antibody differentiate this group from other chlamydial subgroups. Treatment involves 2 weeks of tetracycline or erythromycin. Surgery may be required to correct sequelae such as stricture or fistulas.

In summary, STDs that primarily affect the external genitalia include the HPV (condyloma accuminata), genital herpes (HVS-II), molluscum contagiosum, chancroid, granuloma inguinale, and lymphogranuloma venereum. The lesions of these infections occur on the external genitalia or both male and female sexual partners. Of current concern is the relationship between HPV and genital neoplasms. Genital herpes is caused by a neurotropic virus (HVS-II) that ascends through the peripheral nerves to reside in the sacral dorsal root ganglia. The herpes virus can be reactivated and produce recurrent lesions in genital structures that are supplied by the peripheral nerves of the affected ganglia. At present there is no permanent cure for herpes infections. Molluscum contagiosum is a benign and self-limiting infection that is only mildly contagious. Chancroid, granuloma inguinale, and lymphogranuloma venereum produce external genital lesions with varying degrees of inguinal lymph node involvement. These diseases are uncommon in the United States.

Vaginal infections

Candidiasis, trichomonas, and bacterial vaginosis are vaginal infections that can be sexually transmitted. Although these infections can be transmitted sexually, the male partner is usually asymptomatic.

Candidiasis

Candidiasis (also called *yeast infection, thrush,* and *moniliasis*) is the leading cause of vulvovaginitis in the United States.[12] The causative organism is a fungus in the candida family, most commonly *Candida albicans* (Figure 38-2). Other candida species, such as *C. glabrata* and *C. tropicalis*, have also been shown to cause clinical symptomatology. Additionally, 18 separate strains of *C. albicans* with varying levels of virulence have been identified.[14] These organisms are often present in healthy people without causing symptoms, and the decision of the CDC to classify candidiasis as an STD is controversial. The possibility of sexual transmission has been recognized for many years; however, candidiasis requires a favorable environment for its growth. The gastrointestinal tract also serves as a reservoir for this organism and candidiasis can develop through autoinoculation in women who are not sexually active. Although studies have documented the presence of candida on the penis of male partners of women with vulvovaginal candidiasis, few men develop balanoposthitis requiring treatment.[15]

Causes for the overgrowth of *C. albicans* include (1) antibiotic therapy, which suppresses the normal protective bacterial flora; (2) high hormone levels due to pregnancy or use of oral contraceptives, which cause an increase in vaginal glycogen stores; and (3) diabetes mellitus, which may increase the sugar levels in the vaginal mucosa, but more likely causes candidiasis because it compromises the immune system of the host.[15] Food allergies, hypothyroidism, endocrine disorders, and altered immune status have also been suggested as possible contributors to the development of vulvovaginal candidiasis.[16]

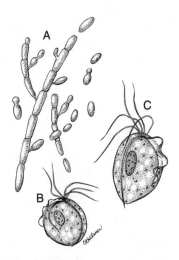

Figure 38-2 Organisms that cause vaginal infections. (**A**) *Candida albicans* (blastospores and pseudohyphae). (**B**) and (**C**) *Trichomonas vaginalis.*

In obese individuals, *Candida* may grow in skin folds underneath the breast tissue, the abdominal flap, and the inguinal folds. Vulvar pruritus, accompanied by irritation, dysuria, dyspareunia, erythema, and an odorless, thick, cheesy vaginal discharge are the predominant symptoms of the infection. Accurate diagnosis is made by identification of budding yeast filaments (hyphae) or spores on a wet mount slide using 20% potassium hydroxide (see Figure 38-2). The pH of the discharge (checked with litmus paper) is generally less than 4.5. When the wet-mount technique is negative but the clinical manifestations are suggestive of candidiasis, a culture may be necessary. Candidiasis can be confused with Döderlein cytolysis—an excess of lactobacilli—which can present with a similar clinical picture. In the case of Döderlein cytolysis, however, both wet-mount and culture techniques show only excessive lactobacilli with no yeast.

Treatment for Döderlein cytolysis involves use of a sodium bicarbonate douche two to three times a week to raise the vaginal pH and decrease the symptoms.[12] Fungicidal creams, ointments, and tablets such as clotrimazole, miconazole, butaconazole, and terconazole are effective in treating candidiasis. Gentian violet solution (1%) applied to the vagina by swabs or tampon, potassium sorbate douches, or boric acid soaks to the vulva are treatment adjuncts. Tepid sodium bicarbonate baths, clothing that allows adequate ventilation, and the application of corn starch to dry the area may increase comfort during treatment. Chronic recurrent vulvovaginal candidiasis continues to present a plague for affected women and a challenge to researchers to find a means of eradicating this nonserious but aggravating affliction.

Trichomonas

Trichomonas vaginalis is an anaerobic protozoan that can be transmitted sexually; it is shaped like a turnip and has three or four anterior flagellae (see Figure 38-2). Trichomonads can reside in the paraurethral glands of both sexes. Males harbor the organism in the urethra and prostate and are generally asymptomatic. Although 10% to 25% of women are asymptomatic, trichomonas is a common cause of vaginitis when some imbalance allows the protozoan to proliferate. This extracellular parasite feeds on the vaginal mucosa and ingests bacteria and leukocytes. The infection causes a copious frothy and malodorous discharge which is green or yellow in color. Frequently, there is erythema and edema of the affected mucosa with occasional itching and irritation. Sometimes small hemorrhagic areas, called *strawberry spots,* appear on the cervix.

Diagnosis is made microscopically by identification of the protozoan on a wet-mount slide preparation. The pH of the discharge is usually greater than 6.0. Special culture media are available for diagnosis, but are costly and not needed for diagnosis.

Because the organism resides in other urogenital structures besides the vagina, systemic treatment is recommended. The treatment of choice is metronidazole (Flagyl), an oral medication that is effective against anaerobic protozoans. Metronidazole is chemically similar to Antabuse, a drug used in treatment of alcohol addiction that causes nausea, vomiting, flushing of the skin, headache, palpitations, and lowering of the blood pressure when alcohol is ingested. Therefore alcohol should be avoided during and for 24 hours to 48 hours after treatment. Gastrointestinal disturbances and a metallic taste in the mouth are potential side effects of the drug. Metronidazole has not been proven safe in pregnancy and is used only after the first trimester for fear of potential teratogenic effects. Trichomoniasis may be alternately treated with acidification of the environment with Acijel therapeutic jelly, povidone-iodine vaginal jelly or douche, or clotrimazole vaginal suppositories. If the female is in a monogamous relationship, both sexual partners are treated simultaneously in order to decrease the incidence of recurrence. If the woman has more than one partner, abstinence during therapy and for 1 week after completion of therapy, or condoms, are recommended.

Bacterial vaginosis (nonspecific vaginitis)

Considerable controversy exists regarding the organisms responsible for a vaginal infection that produces a characteristic fishy or ammonia-smelling discharge, yet fails to produce an inflammatory response that is characteristic of most infections. A number of terms have been used to describe the nonspecific vaginitis that cannot be attributed to one of the accepted pathogenic organisms such as *Trichomonas vaginalis* or *C. albicans*. In 1955, Gardner and Dukes isolated an organism from women with this vaginitis and proposed the name *Hemophilus vaginalis,* apparently because the organism was gram-negative and required blood for growth.[17] In 1963, gram-positive isolates were found and the organism was renamed *Corynebacterium vaginale*. Because the organism did not meet all of the criteria of corynebacteria, it was renamed *Gardnerella vaginalis* in 1980, after its original discoverer, and admitted to a taxonomic genus of its own.[18] The development of a special agar on which *G. vaginalis* could be cultured led to the discovery that 40% to 70% of women harbor this organism as part of their normal vaginal flora. Further study revealed that abnormal discharge frequently contained highly motile crescent-shaped rods called mobiluncus and many more anaerobic than aerobic bacteria.[19] It has been suggested that the presence of anaerobes, which produce ammonia or amines from amino acids, favors the growth of *G. vaginalis* by raising vaginal *p*H. Because of the presence of anaerobic bacteria and the lack of an inflammatory response, a new term, *bacterial vaginosis,* was proposed.[20]

Bacterial vaginosis is thought to be sexually transmissible and may be carried asymptomatically by both the male and female. Reinfection is common and is greatly affected by vaginal *p*H in women. The predominant symptom of bacterial vaginosis is a thin grayish-white discharge that has a foul fishy odor. Burning, itching, and erythema are usually absent because the bacteria has only minimal inflammatory potential.

The diagnosis is made when at least three of the following characteristics are present: (1) homogeneous discharge, (2) production of a fishy amine odor when a 10% potassium hydroxide solution is dropped onto the secretions, (3) vaginal *p*H above 4.5 (usually 5.0 to 6.0), and (4) appearance of characteristic "clue cells" on wet-mount microscopic studies. Clue cells are squamous epithelial cells covered with masses of coccobacilli, often with large clumps of organisms floating free from the cell. Because *G. vaginalis* can be a normal vaginal flora, cultures should not be done routinely. They are of limited clinical value, since it is believed that the condition is caused by a combination of *G. vaginalis* and anaerobic bacteria.

The mere presence of *G. vaginalis* in an asymptomatic woman is not an indication for treatment. When indicated, treatment is aimed at eradicating the anaerobic component of bacterial vaginosis. The CDC recommends metronidazole, although failure rates may range from 30% to 70%. Alternative therapies include ampicillin or amoxicillin, vaginal sulfonamides, povidone preparations, and clindamycin.

In summary, candidiasis, trichomonas, and bacterial vaginosis are vaginal infections that can be spread through sexual contact. Although these infections are sexually transmitted, the male partner is usually asymptomatic. Candidiasis, also called a yeast infection, is the leading cause of vulvovaginitis in the United States. Candida can be present without producing symptoms; usually some host factor, such as altered immune status or increased sugar levels in the vaginal mucosa due to diabetes mellitus, contribute to the development of vulvovaginitis. Trichomonas is caused by an anaerobic protozoan. The infection incites the production of a copious frothy yellow-green malodorous vaginal discharge. Bacterial vaginosis is a nonspecific type of vaginal infection that produces a characteristic fishy-smelling vaginal discharge. The

infection is thought to be caused by the combined presence of *G. vaginalis* and anaerobic bacteria. The anaerobe raises the vaginal *p*H, thereby favoring the growth of *G. vaginalis*.

Vaginal/urogenital/systemic infections

Some STDs infect both genital and extragenital structures. Among the infections of this type are chlamydial infections, gonorrhea, nonspecific urogenital infection, and syphilis. Many of these infections also pose a risk to babies born to infected mothers. Some infections, such as syphilis, may be spread to the infant while *in utero*; others, such as chlamydial and gonorrheal infections, can be spread to the infant during the birth process.

Chlamydial infections

Chlamydia trachomatis is an obligate intracellular bacterial pathogen that is closely related to gram-negative bacteria. It resembles a virus in that it requires tissue culture for isolation, but like a bacteria it has both RNA and DNA and is susceptible to some antibiotics. *C. trachomatis* can be serologically subdivided into types A, B, and C—associated with trachoma; types L_1, L_2, and L_3—associated with lymphogranuloma venereum; and types D to K—associated with genital infections and their complications. The organism causes a wide variety of genitourinary infections, including nongonococcal urethritis in men and pelvic inflammatory disease in women. Chlamydia can cause significant ocular disease in the newborn; it is a leading cause of blindness in underdeveloped countries. In these countries the organism is spread primarily by flies, fomites, and nonsexual personal contact. In industrial countries, however, the organism is spread almost exclusively by sexual contact and therefore affects primarily the genitourinary structures. Although chlamydial infections are not reportable in all states, it has been estimated that the incidence is more than twice that of gonorrhea. Currently the most prevalent STD in the United States, chlamydial infections occur at an annual rate of 3 million to 10 million, according to CDC estimates.[21]

The chlamydial organism exists in two forms: (1) the elementary body, which is the infectious particle capable of entering uninfected cells; and (2) the initiator or reticulate body, which multiplies by binary fission to produce the inclusions identified in stained cells. The 48-hour growth cycle starts with attachment of the elementary body to the susceptible host cell, following which it is ingested by a process resembling

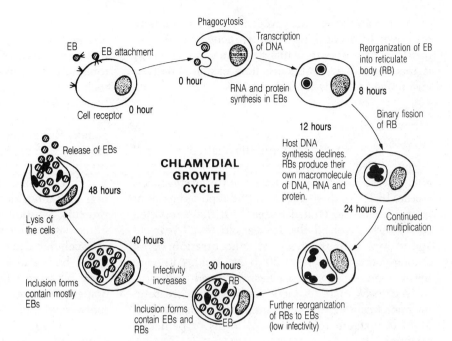

Figure 38-3 Chlamydial growth cycle. *EB,* elementary body. *RB,* reticulate body. (Thompson SE, Washington AE: *Epidemiology of sexually transmitted Chlamydia trachomatis infections. Epidemiol Rev 5:96–123, 1983*)

phagocytosis (Figure 38-3). Once within the cell, the elementary body is organized into the reticulate body, the metabolically active form of the organism, which is capable of reproduction. The reticulate body is not infectious and cannot survive outside the body. The reticulate bodies divide within the cell for up to 36 hours and then condense to form new elementary bodies, which are released when the infected cell bursts.

The signs and symptoms of chlamydial infections resemble those produced by gonorrhea. In women, chlamydial infections may cause urinary frequency, dysuria, and vaginal discharge. The most common sign is a mucopurulent cervical discharge. The cervix itself frequently hypertrophies, and becomes erythematous, edematous, and extremely friable. The organism may cause pelvic inflammatory disease, which in turn can result in infertility (11,000 women per year) or ectopic pregnancy (3,600 women per year).[21] The most significant difference between chlamydial and gonococcal salpingitis is that chlamydial infections may be asymptomatic or subclinically nonspecific. This can lead to greater fallopian tube damage as well as increase the reservoir for further chlamydial infections. Between 25% and 50% of infants born to mothers with cervical chlamydial infections develop ocular disease (inclusion conjunctivitis), and 10% to 20% develop chlamydial pneumonitis.

In men, chlamydial infections cause urethritis, including meatal erythema and tenderness, urethral discharge, dysuria, and urethral itching. Prostatitis and epididymitis with subsequent infertility may develop. The most serious complication that can de-velop with nongonococcal urethritis is Reiter's disease (see Chapter 57). In one study, two-thirds of men with untreated acute Reiter's disease were found to have a chlamydial infection of the urethra.[11]

Diagnosis of chlamydial infections takes several forms. Identification of polymorphonuclear leukocytes (PMNs) on Gram stain of male discharge or cervical discharge is presumptive evidence. The two available serologic tests can be misleading. Complement fixation tests are the most useful in diagnosing lymphogranuloma venereum. The microimmunofluorescent test is more sensitive for *C. trachomatis* types D to K, but does not distinguish among acute, chronic, or carrier states. The high rates of antichlamydial antibodies in sexually active populations renders serodiagnosis inconclusive.[11] Tissue cultures are definitive, but slow (requiring at least 3 days), costly, and not always available. Newer nonculture methods, such as direct fluorescent antibody test (DFA, Microtrak) and an enzyme-linked immunosorbent assay (ELISA-chlamydiazyme), which uses antibodies against an antigen present in the chlamydia cell wall, have been developed. These are less expensive, rapid tests requiring less sophisticated laboratory techniques, but have a lower sensitivity than culture (DFA, 90% sensitivity and 96% specificity; ELISA, 67% to 90% sensitivity and 92% to 98% specificity).[22] The positive predictive value of these tests is excellent among high-risk groups but false-positive results occur more often in populations with lower risks. The DFA test appears to be the most effective screening test available, but may require follow-up with culture if the validity of the positive result is questioned.[23]

The Centers for Disease Control recommend

use of tetracycline or doxycycline in the treatment of chlamydial infection; penicillin is ineffective. Antibiotic treatment of both sexual partners simultaneously is recommended. Abstinence from sexual activity is encouraged to facilitate cure.

Gonorrhea

Gonorrhea (colloquially called "clap," "drip," "gleet," "strain," and "whites") is a reportable disease caused by the bacterium *Neisseria gonorrhoeae*. In 1986, there were 900,868 reported cases of gonorrhea in the United States.[21] Of these reported cases, 80% involved the 15-year-old to 29-year-old age group, with the heaviest concentration being among young adults (ages 20 to 24 years). Although the incidence of gonorrhea has continued to decline since its peak in 1975, there has been an increase in infections caused by penicillinase-producing *N. gonorrhoeae* that are resistant to all forms of penicillin treatment.[24]

The gonococcus is a pyogenic (pus forming) gram-negative diplococcus that evokes inflammatory reactions characterized by purulent exudates. Humans are the only natural host for *N. gonorrhoeae*. The organism grows best in warm mucus-secreting epithelia. The portal of entry can be the genitourinary tract, eyes, oropharynx, anorectum, or skin. Transmission is usually by sexual intercourse, either heterosexual or homosexual. Autoinoculation of the organism to the conjunctiva is possible. Infants born to infected mothers can acquire the infection during passage through the birth canal and are in danger of developing gonorrheal conjunctivitis, with resultant blindness, unless treated promptly. An amniotic infection syndrome characterized by premature rupture of the membranes, premature delivery, and increased risk of infant morbidity and mortality has been recently identified as an additional complication of gonococcal infections in pregnancy.[11] Genital gonorrhea in young children should raise the possibility of sexual abuse.

The infection commonly becomes manifest 2 days to 7 days after exposure. It usually begins in the anterior urethra, accessory urethral glands, Bartholin's or Skene's glands, and the cervix. If untreated, gonorrhea spreads from its initial sites upward into the genital tract. In males, it spreads to the prostate and epididymis; in females, it commonly moves to the fallopian tubes. Pharyngitis may follow oral-genital contact.

The organism can also invade the bloodstream (disseminated gonococcal infection) causing serious sequelae such as bacteremic involvement of joint spaces, heart valves, meninges, and other body organs and tissues.[11]

Persons with gonorrhea may be asymptomatic and thus may unwittingly spread the disease to their sexual partners. Men are more likely to be symptomatic than women. In men, the initial symptoms include urethral pain and a creamy-yellow, sometimes bloody, discharge. The disorder may become chronic and affect the prostate, epididymis, and periurethral glands. Rectal infections are common in homosexual men. In women, recognizable symptoms include unusual genital or urinary discharge, dysuria, dyspareunia, pelvic pain or tenderness, unusual vaginal bleeding, including bleeding after intercourse, fever, and proctitis. Symptoms may occur or increase during or immediately after menses, since the bacterium is an intracellular diplococcus that thrives in menstrual blood but cannot survive long outside the human body. There may be infections of the uterus and development of acute or chronic infection of the fallopian tubes (salpingitis) with ultimate scarring and sterility.

Diagnosis is based on the history of sexual exposure and symptoms. It is confirmed by identification of the organism on Gram stain or culture. A Gram stain is usually an effective means of diagnosis in symptomatic males (*i.e.*, those with discharge). In women and asymptomatic men, a culture is usually preferred, since the Gram stains are often unreliable. A specimen should be collected from the appropriate site (endocervix, urethra, anal canal, or oropharynx), plated onto selective Thayer-Martin media, and placed in a CO_2 environment. *N. gonorrhoeae* is a fastidious organism with very specific nutrient and environmental needs. Optimal growth requires a *pH* of 7.4, temperature of 35.5°C, and an atmosphere containing 2% to 10% CO_2.[11] The accuracy of culture results is affected if transport is delayed or growth requirements are not available. The search for methods to provide rapid and accurate diagnosis of *N. gonorrhoeae* continues. An enzyme immunoassay for detecting gonococcal antigens (Gonozyme) is available, but has several requirements that limit its usefulness. Testing for other STDs, particularly syphilis and chlamydia, is suggested at the time of examination. Pregnant women are routinely screened at the time of their first prenatal visit; high-risk populations should have repeat cultures during the third trimester. Newborns are routinely treated with various antibacterial agents applied to the conjunctiva within an hour of birth in order to protect against undiagnosed gonorrhea as well as other diseases.

The standard treatment of gonorrhea has been with the use of injectable penicillin and oral probenecid, a drug which delays the renal excretion of penicillin. Patients allergic to penicillin were treated with oral tetracycline for 7 days instead. The current treatment recommendation to combat tetracycline- and penicillin-resistant strains of *N. gonorrhea* is ceftriaxone in a single injection.[25] In the presence of symptoms, particularly in the male partner, it is common practice to treat both partners before culture results are available because of potential loss of reproductive capacity. Persons with the disease, particularly pregnant women, should be followed with repeat cultures to determine the effectiveness of treatment. Persons with gonorrhea are instructed to refrain from intercourse or to use condoms until cultures show negative results. Because of the high rate of concomitant chlamydial infections (30% to 50%) in women with gonococcal pelvic inflammatory disease, the CDC now recommends a treatment regimen for gonorrhea that treats both infections. The combination regimen supplements the single-dose penicillin/probenecid or ceftriaxone treatment with a 7-day treatment of oral tetracycline or ampicillin/amoxicillin. Another alternative is a single dose of oral ampicillin or amoxicillin and probenecid and 7-day treatment with tetracycline. In pregnant women, erythromycin can be used as a substitute for tetracycline.[1]

Nonspecific urogenital infection

Nonspecific urogenital infection is chiefly a disease of the male urethra, but may involve the cervix, urethra, Bartholin's glands, vagina, and fallopian tubes in the female. In about 50% of cases, the disease is secondary to chlamydia infection. As discussed earlier, chlamydia is a formidable pathogen because of its long-term effects and ability to affect the newborn. This disease entity, like nonspecific vaginitis, will likely be named more specifically as the causative agents are identified. Diagnosis is made through the use of cultures. The treatment is by various antibiotic regimens and is dictated by the organism and antibiotic sensitivity.

Syphilis

Syphilis (colloquially called "lues," "old Joe," "the sore," "great poc," "las bubas," and "bad blood") is a reportable disease caused by a spirochete, *Treponema pallidum*. In the first 46 weeks of 1987, there were 31,323 new cases of syphilis reported in the United States. This represents a 32% increase over the same period in 1986 and is the highest rate of occurrence (14.7/100,000) since 1950.[26] Reasons for the reversal in the trend of decreasing incidence that characterized the previous 5 years are unknown.

The *T. pallidum* is spread by direct contact with an infectious moist lesion, usually through sexual intercourse.[1] However, bacteria-laden secretions may transfer the organism during kissing or intimate contact. Skin abrasions provide another possible portal of entry. There is rapid transplacental transmission of the organism from the mother to the fetus after 16 weeks' gestation, so that active disease in the mother during pregnancy can produce congenital syphilis in the fetus. Untreated syphilis can cause prematurity, stillbirth, and congenital defects as well as active infection in the infant. Once treated for syphilis, a pregnant woman is usually followed throughout pregnancy by repeat serum titers.

The clinical disease is divided into three stages: primary, secondary, and tertiary syphilis. The first stage, primary syphilis, is characterized by the appearance of a chancre at the site of exposure. Chancres usually appear within 3 weeks of exposure but may incubate for a week to 3 months. The primary chancre begins as a single indurated button-like papule, up to several centimeters in diameter, which erodes to create a clean-based ulcerated lesion on an elevated base. These lesions are usually painless and located at the site of sexual contact.

Primary syphilis is readily apparent in the male, where the lesion is on the penis or scrotum. Although chancres can develop on the external genitalia in females, they are more common on the vagina or cervix, and primary syphilis may therefore go untreated. There is usually an accompanying regional lymphadenopathy. The disease is very contagious at this stage, but because of the mild symptoms, it frequently goes unnoticed. The chancre usually heals within 3 to 12 weeks, with or without treatment.

The timing of the second stage of syphilis varies even more than the first, ranging in duration from 1 week to 6 months. The symptoms of a rash (especially on the palms of the hands and soles of the feet), fever, sore throat, stomatitis, nausea, loss of appetite, and inflamed eyes may come and go for a year, but usually last 3 to 6 months. Secondary manifestations may include alopecia and genital condylomata lata. Condylomata lata are elevated red-brown lesions that may ulcerate and produce a foul discharge. They range up to 2 cm to 3 cm in diameter, contain many spirochetes, and are highly contagious. Following the second stage, syphilis frequently enters a latent phase which may last the lifetime of the individual or may progress to tertiary syphilis at some point. Individuals can be infective during the first 1 to 2 years of latency.

Tertiary syphilis is a delayed response of the untreated disease. It can occur as long as 20 years after the initial infection. Only about one-third of those with untreated syphilis progress to the tertiary stage of the disease, and about one-half of these develop symptoms. About one-third undergo spontaneous cure and the remaining one-third continue to have positive serologic tests but do not develop structural lesions.[11] When syphilis does progress to the symptomatic tertiary stage, it usually takes one of three forms: (1) development of localized destructive lesions called gummas; (2) development of cardiovascular lesions; or (3) development of central nervous system lesions. The syphilitic gumma is a peculiar rubbery necrotic lesion that is caused by noninflammatory tissue necrosis. Gummas can occur singly or multiply and vary in size from microscopic lesions to large, tumorous masses. They are most commonly found in the liver, testes, and bone. Central nervous system lesions can produce dementia, blindness, or injury to the spinal cord with ataxia and sensory loss (tabes dorsalis). Cardiovascular manifestations usually result from scarring of the medial layer of the thoracic aorta with aneurysm formation (see Chapter 18). These aneurysms produce enlargement of the aortic valve ring with aortic valve insufficiency.

T. pallidum does not produce either endotoxins or exotoxins but evokes a humoral immune response that provides the basis for serologic tests. Two types of antibodies—nonspecific and specific—are produced. The nonspecific antibodies can be detected by flocculation (VDRL) tests and complement fixation (Wasserman and Kahn) tests. Because these tests are nonspecific, positive results can also occur with diseases other than syphilis. The VDRL is easy, rapid, and inexpensive and is frequently used as a screening test for syphilis. The results generally become positive 4 to 6 weeks after infection or 1 to 3 weeks after the appearance of the primary lesion. The VDRL titer is usually high during the secondary stage of the disease and becomes less during the tertiary stage. A falling titer during treatment suggests a favorable response. A specific test called the fluorescent treponemal antibody absorption (FTA-ABS) test is used as a test for specific antibodies to *T. pallidum*. FTA-ABS is used in determining whether a positive result on a nonspecific test such as the VDRL is due to syphilis.

T. pallidum cannot be cultured. Therefore, diagnosis of syphilis is based on serologic tests or dark-field microscopic examination with identification of the spirochete in specimens collected from lesions. Because the disease's incubation period may delay test sensitivity, serologic tests are usually repeated after 6 weeks when the initial test results are negative.

The treatment of choice for syphilis is penicillin. Because of the spirochetes' long generation time, effective tissue levels of penicillin must be maintained for several weeks. For this reason, long-acting injectable forms of penicillin are used. Tetracycline or erythromycin is used for treatment in persons who are sensitive to penicillin. Sexual partners should be evaluated and treated prophylactically even though they may show no sign of infection.

In summary, the vaginal/urogenital/systemic STDs—chlamydial infections, gonorrhea, nonspecific urogenital infection, and syphilis—can severely involve the genital structures and can also manifest as systemic infection. Both gonorrheal and chlamydial infections can cause a wide variety of genitourinary complications in men and women, and both can cause ocular disease and blindness in infants born to infected mothers. Nonspecific urogenital infection is primarily a disease of the male urethra, but may involve the cervix, urethra, Bartholin's glands, vagina, and fallopian tubes in the female. Syphilis is caused by a spirocete, *Treponema pallidum*. It can produce widespread systemic effects and is transferred to the fetus of infected mothers via the placenta.

References

1. Centers for Disease Control: Condyloma accuminatum—United States 1966-1981. MMWR 32(23):306, 1983
2. Ferenczy A, Silverstein S, Crum PC: Importance of latency in HPV infections. Contemp OB Gyn 11:71, 1987
3. Ferenczy A, Silverstein S, Crum PC: Genital warts, HPV, and cervical cancer. Lancet 2:1045, 1985
4. Story B: Condyloma accuminata—An epidemic with malignant potential. Physician Assistant 12:13, 1987
5. Howley PM: On human papilloma viruses. N Engl J Med 315:1089, 1986
6. Schneider A, Sawada E, Gissman L, et al: Human papillomaviruses in women with a history of abnormal Papanicolaou smears and in their male partners. Obstet Gynecol 169:555, 1987
7. Ferenczy A: Comparison of 5-FU and CO2 laser for treatment of vaginal condylomas. Obstet Gynecol 64:773, 1984
8. Becker TM, Blount HJ, Gunan ME: Genital herpes infections in private practice in the United States, 1966-1981. JAMA 111:601, 1985
9. Corey L, Spear PG: Infections with herpes simplex viruses—part 1. N Engl J Med 314:686, 1986
10. Corey L, Spear PG: Infections with herpes simplex viruses—part 2. N Engl J Med 314:749, 1986
11. Sweet RL, Gibbs RS: Infectious Diseases of the Female Genital Tract, pp 39-40,35,17-26,27-29,103-122. Baltimore, Williams & Wilkins, 1985
12. Cibley LJ, Cibley LJ: Vulvovaginitis: Current approach to diagnosis and treatment. Female Patient 11(2):41, 1986
13. Centers for Disease Control: STD treatment guidelines 1985. MMWR 34(4S), 1985
14. Robertson WH: Mycology of vulvovaginitis. Am J Obstet Gynecol 158:989, 1988
15. Sobel JB: Epidemiology and pathogenesis of recurrent vulvovaginal candidiasis. Am J Obstet Gynecol 152:924, 1985
16. Seigel J: Clinical allergies and vulvovaginitis. J Reprod Med 31:647, 1986
17. Gardner HL, Dukes CD: Haemophilus vaginalis vaginitis. Am J Obstet Gynecol 69:962, 1955

18. Jones BM: Gardnerella vaginitis. Med Lab Sci 40:53, 1983

19. Thomason JL, Schreckenberger PC, Spellacy WN, et al: Clinical and microbiological characterization of patients with nonspecific vaginosis associated with motile, curved anaerobic rods. J Infect Dis 149:814, 1984

20. Eschenback DA: Diagnosis of bacterial vaginosis (nonspecific vaginitis): Role of the laboratory. Clin Microbiol Newsletter 6:18, 1984

21. Centers for Disease Control: Summary of notifiable diseases—United States 1986 (formerly entitled Annual Summary). MMWR 35(55), 1987

22. Addiss DG, Davis JP, Katcher ML: Testing for chlamydia trachomatis: Objective criteria for recommendations for screening using nonculture techniques. Wisc Med J 86(9):25, 1987

23. Nettleman MD, Jones RB: Cost effectiveness of screening women at moderate risk for genital infections caused by chlamydial trachomatis. JAMA 260:207, 1988

24. Centers for Disease Control: Antibiotic-resistant strains of Neisseria gonorrhoeae. MMWR 36(5S), 1987

25. Abramowicz M (ed): The Medical Letter 30:5,1988

26. Centers for Disease Control: Continuing increase in infectious syphilis—United States. MMWR 37(3), 1988

Bibliography

Berg AO, Soman MP: Lower genitourinary infections in women. J Family Pract 23(1):61, 1986

Breslin E: Genital herpes simplex. Nurs Clin North Am 23:907, 1988

Britigan BE, Cohen MS, Sparling PF: Gonococcal infections: A model of molecular pathogenesis. N Engl J Med 312:1683, 1985

Brown D: Therapeutic alternatives and new treatment modalities in vulvovaginal candidiasis. J Reprod Med 31(Suppl) No 7:639, 1986

Brunham RC, Paavonen J, Stevens CE, et al: Mucopurulent cervicitis—the ignored counterpart in women of urethritis in men. N Engl J Med 311:1, 1984

Charles D, Glover DD: Antimicrobial treatment of infectious vaginopathies. Female Patient 10(3):25, 1985

Driscoll CE: Genital herpes. Female Patient 9(12):41, 1984

Fogel CI: Gonorrhea: Not a new problem but a serious one. Nurs Clin North Am 23:885, 1988

Guinan ME: Oral acyclovir for treatment and suppression of genital herpes simplex virus infection. JAMA 255:1747, 1986

Hammerschalag MR: Chlamydia trachomatis. Birth Defects 21(5):93, 1985

Lucas VA: Human papillomavirus infection: A potentially carcinogenic sexually transmitted disease (condylomata acuminata, genital warts). Nurs Clin North Am 23:917, 1988

McKay M: Identifying vulvar ulcers. Female Patient 11(3):108, 1986

McNabney WK, Barnes WG: Urethral and endocervical culturing: Gonorrhea and chlamydia. Ann Emerg Med 15(3):333, 1986

Pepper GA: Oral Acyclovir (Zovirax): Major or minor miracle? Nurse Practitioner 10(12):50, 1985

Rettig PJ: Infections due to chlamydia trachomatis from infancy to adolescence. Pediatr Infect Dis 5:449, 1986

Roddy RE: Genital herpes. Physician Assistant 7:21, 1988

Sanders LL, Harrison R, Washington AE: Treatment of sexually transmitted chlamydial infections. JAMA 255:1750, 1986

Schultz RE, Skelton HG: Value of acetic acid screening for flat condylomas in men. J Urol 139:777, 1988

Secor MC: Bacterial vaginosis. Nurs Clin North Am 23:865, 1988

Sedis A: Papilloma virus infection of female genitalia. Med Dig 4:1, 1986

Sedlacek V, Cunnane M, Carpiniello V: Colposcopy in the diagnosis of penile condyloma. Am J Obstet Gynecol 154:495, 1986

Smith LS, Lauver D: Assessment and management of vaginitis and cervicitis. Nurse Practitioner 6:34, 1986

Sohn CA, Korberly BH, Cohen AW: Treatment of vaginal infections. Female Patient 8(12):33, 1983

Sutherland JE: Vaginitis. Female Patient 9(3):103, 1984

Whalen M: Nursing management of the patient with chlamydia trachomatis infection. Nurs Clin North Am 23(4):877, 1988

Winkler B: Needed—a program to control chlamydial infections. Contemp OB Gyn 11:30, 1987

Alterations in Metabolism, Endocrine Function, and Nutrition

CHAPTER 39

Control of Gastrointestinal Function

Objectives

After you have studied this chapter, you should be able to meet the following objectives:

_____ Describe the physiologic function of the four parts of the digestive system.

_____ Describe the function of the intramural neural plexuses in control of gastrointestinal function.

_____ Differentiate between sites of tonic and rhythmic contraction in the gastrointestinal tract.

_____ Compare the effect of parasympathetic and sympathetic activity on the motility and secretory function of the gastrointestinal tract.

_____ Describe the physiology of peristalsis.

_____ List stimuli for gastrointestinal mechanoreceptors and chemoreceptors.

_____ Trace a bolus of food through the stages of swallowing.

_____ Describe at least two general disorders of gastric motility.

_____ Describe the pathology of Hirschsprung's disease.

_____ Describe the action of the internal and external sphincters in control of defecation.

_____ State the source of water and electrolytes in digestive secretions.

_____ Explain the protective function of saliva.

_____ Describe the function of the gastric secretions in the process of digestion.

_____ List three major gastrointestinal hormones and cite their function.

_____ Describe the site of gastric acid and pepsin production and secretion in the stomach.

_____ Relate the actions of aspirin and alcohol to the disruption of the integrity of the gastric mucosa.

_____ State the effect of sympathetic stimulation on mucus production by Brunner's glands.

_____ Name the secretions of the small and the large intestine.

_____ Relate the characteristics of the small intestine to its absorptive function.

_____ Explain the function of intestinal brush border enzymes.

_____ Compare the absorption of carbohydrates, fats, and proteins.

The process of digestion and absorption of nutrients requires an intact and healthy gastrointestinal tract epithelial lining that can resist the effects of its own digestive secretions. The process involves the movement of materials through the gastrointestinal tract at a rate that facilitates absorption, and it requires the presence of enzymes for the digestion and absorption of nutrients. Structurally, the gastrointestinal tract is a long, hollow tube with its lumen inside the body and its wall acting as an interface between the internal and external environments. The wall does not normally allow harmful agents to enter the body, nor does it permit body fluids and other materials to escape.

The digestive system is truly an amazing structure. In this system, enzymes and hormones are produced, vitamins are synthesized and stored, and food is dismantled and then reassembled. Catalysts and reactants play a role, and some are recycled and used again. Finally, wastes are collected and eliminated efficiently. A man-made system designed to accomplish similar functions would no doubt require miles of space, elaborate equipment, and a huge expenditure of capital. Although this chapter cannot cover gastrointestinal function in its entirety, it is designed to provide the reader with an overview that is deemed essential to an understanding of subsequent chapters.

Nutrients, vitamins, minerals, electrolytes, and water enter the body through the gastrointestinal tract. As a matter of semantics, it should be pointed out that the gastrointestinal tract is also referred to as the digestive tract, the alimentary canal, and, at times, the gut. The intestinal portion may also be called the bowel. For our purposes, the salivary glands, the liver, and the pancreas, which produce secretions that aid in digestion, are considered accessory structures.

Structure and organization of the gastrointestinal tract

In the digestive tract, food and other materials move slowly along its length as they are systematically broken down into ions and molecules that can be absorbed into the body itself. In the large intestine unabsorbed nutrients and wastes are collected for later elimination. What is important for the reader to recognize is that although the gastrointestinal tract is located within the body, it is really a long hollow tube, the lumen (hollow center) of which is an extension of the external environment. Thus, nutrients do not become part of the internal environment until they have passed through the intestinal wall and have entered the blood or lymph channels.

For simplicity and understanding, the digestive system can be divided into four parts (Figure 39-1). The *upper part*—the mouth, esophagus, and stomach—acts as an intake source and receptacle in which initial digestive processes take place. The *middle portion* consists of the small intestine—the duodenum, jejunum, and ileum. Most digestive and absorptive processes occur in the small intestine. The *lower segment*—the cecum, colon, and rectum—serves as a storage channel for the efficient elimination of waste. The *fourth part* consists of the accessory structures—the salivary glands, liver, and pancreas. These structures produce digestive secretions that help dismantle foods and regulate the use and storage of nutrients. The discussion in this chapter focuses on the first three parts of the gastrointestinal tract. The liver and pancreas are discussed in Chapter 41.

Upper gastrointestinal tract

The mouth forms the entryway into the gastrointestinal tract for food; it contains the teeth, used in the mastication of food, and the tongue and other structures needed to direct food toward the pharyngeal structures and the esophagus.

The esophagus begins at the lower end of the pharynx. It receives food from the pharynx and in the process of swallowing, a series of peristaltic contractions moves the food into the stomach. The esophagus is a muscular collapsible tube, about 25 cm (10 in) long, that lies behind the trachea. The muscular walls of the upper third of the esophagus are striated muscle; these muscle fibers are gradually replaced by smooth muscle fibers until at the lower third of the esophagus the muscle layer is entirely smooth muscle. The striated muscle of the upper esophagus is supplied by autonomic nervous system fibers that travel in the glossopharyngeal and vagus nerves and supply the smooth muscle. The upper and lower ends of the esophagus act as sphincters. The upper sphincter is formed by a thickening of the striated muscle; it prevents air from entering the esophagus during respiration. The lower sphincter, which is not identifiable anatomically, occurs at a point 1 cm to 2 cm from where the esophagus joins the stomach. The lower sphincter prevents gastric reflux into the esophagus.

The stomach is a pouchlike structure that lies in the upper part of the abdomen and serves as a food storage reservoir during the early stages of digestion. Although the luminal volume of the stomach is only about 50 ml, it can increase its volume to almost 1000 ml before intraluminal pressure begins to rise. The esophagus opens into the stomach through an opening called the cardiac orifice, so named because of its proximity to the heart. The part of the stomach that lies above and to the left of the cardiac orifice is called

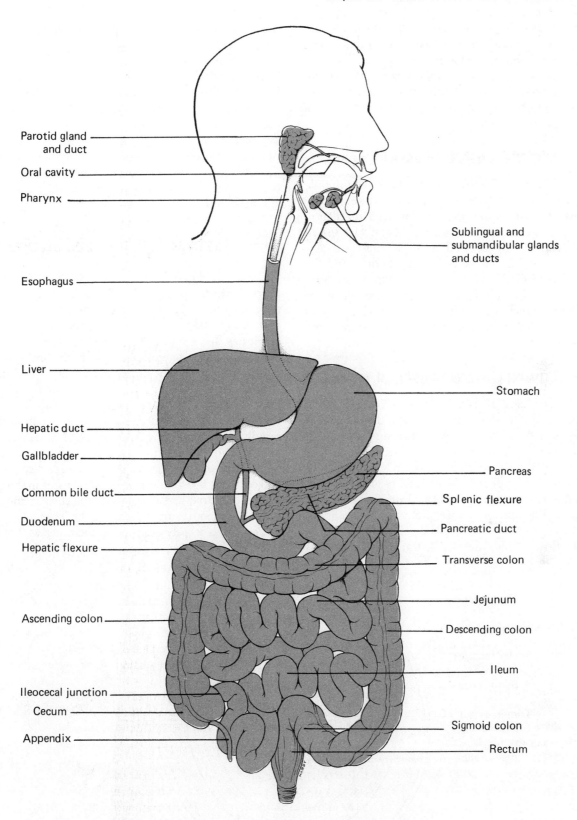

Figure 39-1 The digestive system. (*Chaffee EE, Lytle IM: Basic Physiology and Anatomy, 4th ed. Philadelphia, JB Lippincott, 1980*)

the fundus, the central portion is called the body, and the orifice encircled by a ringlike muscle that opens into the small intestine is called the pylorus. The presence of a true pyloric sphincter is controversial. Whether or not an actual sphincter is present, contractions of the smooth muscle in the pyloric area control gastric emptying.

Middle gastrointestinal tract

The small intestine, which forms the middle portion of the digestive tract, consists of three subdivisions: the duodenum, the jejunum, and the ileum. The duodenum, which is about 22 cm (10 in) in length, connects the stomach to the jejunum and contains the opening for the common bile duct and the main pancreatic duct. Bile and pancreatic juices enter the intestine through these ducts. It is in the jejunum and ileum, which are about 7 m (23 ft) in length and must be folded on themselves, that food is digested and absorbed.

Lower gastrointestinal tract

The large intestine is about 1.5 m (4.5–5 ft) in length and 6 cm to 7 cm (2.5 in) in diameter. It is divided into the cecum, colon, rectum, and anal canal. The cecum is a blind pouch that hangs down at the junction of the ileum and the colon. The ileocecal valve lies at the upper border of the cecum and prevents the return of feces from the cecum into the small intestine. The appendix arises from the cecum about 2.5 cm (1 in) from the ileocecal valve. The colon is further divided into ascending, transverse, descend-

ing, and sigmoid portions. The ascending colon extends from the cecum to the undersurface of the liver, where it turns abruptly to form the right colic (hepatic) flexure. The transverse colon crosses the upper half of the abdominal cavity from right to left and then curves sharply downward beneath the lower end of the spleen, forming the left colic (splenic) flexure. The descending colon extends the colic flexure to the rectum. The rectum extends from the sigmoid colon to the anus. The anal canal passes between the two medial borders of the levator ani muscles. Powerful sphincter muscles guard against fecal incontinence.

Gastrointestinal wall structure

The digestive tract, once it leaves the upper third of the esophagus, is essentially a five-layered tube (Figure 39-2). The inner luminal layer, or *mucosa,* is so named because its cells produce mucus that lubricates and protects the inner surface of the alimentary canal. The epithelial cells in this layer have a rapid turnover rate, being replaced every 4 to 5 days. Approximately 250 g of these cells are shed each day in the stool. Because of the regenerative capabilities of the mucosal layer, injury to this layer of tissue heals rapidly without leaving scar tissue. The *submucosal layer* is made up of connective tissue. This layer contains blood vessels, nerves, and structures responsible for secreting digestive enzymes. Movement in the gastrointestinal tract is facilitated by the *circular* and *longitudinal* smooth muscle layers. The fifth layer, the *peritoneum,* is loosely attached to the outer wall of the intestine.

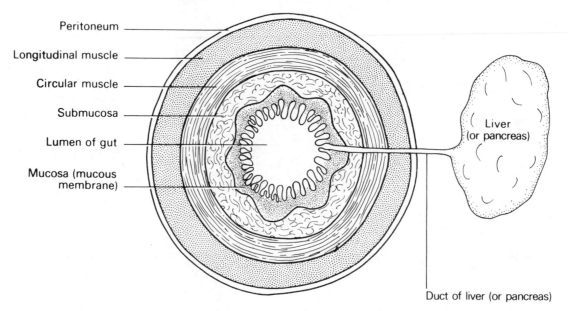

Peritoneum

Longitudinal muscle

Circular muscle

Submucosa

Lumen of gut

Mucosa (mucous membrane)

Liver (or pancreas)

Duct of liver (or pancreas)

Figure 39-2 Transverse section of the digestive system. (*Thompson JS: Core Textbook of Anatomy. Philadelphia, JB Lippincott, 1977*)

The *peritoneum* is the largest serous membrane in the body, having a surface area about equal to that of the skin. The peritoneal membrane is composed of two layers, a thin layer of squamous cells resting on a layer of connective tissue. If the squamous layer is injured because of surgery or inflammation, there is danger that adhesions (fibrous scar-tissue bands) will form, causing sections of the viscera to heal together. Unfortunately, adhesions may alter the position and movement of the abdominal viscera.

The *peritoneal cavity* is a potential space formed between what is called the *parietal peritoneum* and the *visceral peritoneum*. The parietal peritoneum comes in contact with and is loosely attached to the abdominal wall, whereas the abdominal organs are in contact with the visceral peritoneum. Thompson compares the two layers of the peritoneum to a deflated balloon.[1] If you make a fist into the balloon, the outer surface can be equated with the parietal peritoneum and the fist interfaces with the visceral peritoneum (Figure 39-3). In this case, the area within the balloon would represent the peritoneal cavity. The connective tissue layer of the peritoneum forms both the parietal and the visceral peritoneum, while the smooth squamous-cell layer of the membrane lines the cavity. The adjacent membrane layers within the peritoneal cavity are separated by a thin layer of serous fluid. This fluid prevents friction between continuously moving abdominal structures. In certain pathologic states the amount of fluid in the potential space of the peritoneal cavity is increased, causing a condition called *ascites*. The *mesentery* is a double fold of peritoneum that encloses and supports the abdominal organs (Figure 39-4). The mesentery is no more than 20 cm to 25 cm deep, about 15 cm long in the small intestine, and 7 cm long in the large intestine.

In summary, the gastrointestinal tract is a long hollow tube, the lumen of which is an extension of the external environment. The digestive tract can be divided into four parts: an upper part consisting of the mouth, esophagus, and stomach; a middle part consisting of the small intestine; a lower part consisting of the cecum, colon, and rectum; and the accessory organs consisting of the salivary glands, the liver, and the pancreas. Throughout its length, except for the mouth, throat, and upper esophagus, the gastrointestinal tract is composed of five layers: an inner mucosal layer, a submucosal layer, a layer of circular smooth muscle fibers, a layer of longitudinal smooth muscle fibers, and an outer serosal layer that forms the peritoneum and is continuous with the mesentery.

Motility

The motility of the gastrointestinal tract moves food products and fluids along its length, from mouth to anus, in a manner that facilitates digestion and absorption. Except in the pharynx and upper third of the esophagus, smooth muscle provides the contractile force for gastrointestinal motility. The rhythmic movements of the digestive tract are self-perpetuating, much like the activity of the heart, and are influenced by local, humoral (blood borne), and neural influences. The ability to initiate impulses is a property of the smooth muscle itself. Contractions occur in sheets or tubes of completely denervated muscle. Impulses are conducted from one muscle fiber to another.

The movements of the gastrointestinal tract are both tonic and rhythmic. The *tonic movements* are continuous movements that last for long periods of time—minutes or even hours. Tonic contractions occur at *sphincters*. The rhythmic movements consist of intermittent contractions that are responsible for mixing and moving food along the digestive tract. *Peristaltic movements* are rhythmic propulsive movements that occur when the smooth muscle layer constricts, forming a contractile band that forces the in-

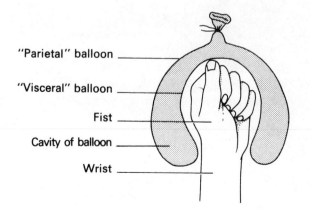

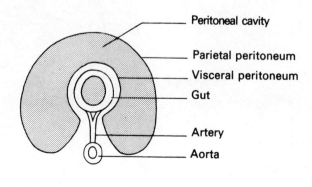

Figure 39-3 Comparison of the peritoneal cavity with a balloon. (*Thompson JS: Core Textbook of Anatomy. Philadelphia, JB Lippincott, 1977*)

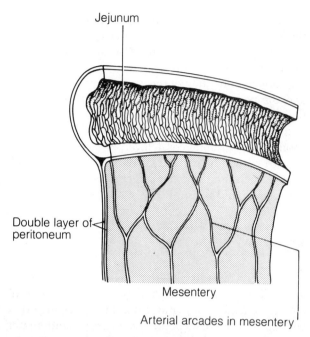

Figure 39-4 The attachment of the mesentery to the small bowel. (*Thompson JS: Core Textbook of Anatomy. Philadelphia, JB Lippincott, 1977*)

traluminal contents forward. During peristalsis the segment that lies distal to, or ahead of, the contracted portion relaxes, so that the contents move forward with ease. Normal peristalsis always moves in the direction from the mouth toward the anus.

Neural control mechanisms

The neural control of gastrointestinal tract motility involves two major plexuses, or neural networks, located within the gastrointestinal tract wall. These intramural (within the wall) plexuses extend along the length of the gastrointestinal wall. The myenteric (Auerbach's) plexus is located between the outer muscle layers, and the submucosal (Meissner's) plexus is located between the circular muscle and the submucosal layers (Figure 39-5). The activity of the neurons in the myenteric and submucosal plexuses is regulated both by local influences and by input from the autonomic nervous system. Both plexuses are aggregates of ganglionic cells, most of which receive synaptic input from the vagus nerve. The sympathetic postganglionic fibers synapse directly with the muscle fibers. The myenteric plexus primarily influences motility; whereas the submucosal plexus affects both motility and secretion. Nerve impulses initiated in one ganglionic cell spread through multiple intramural pathways, mainly in a longitudinal direction.

Nerves of the digestive tract contain many visceral afferent fibers, which can be divided into two classes: (1) those whose cell bodies are located in the nervous system and (2) those whose cell bodies are within the intramural plexuses. The first group has receptors in the mucosal epithelium and in the muscle layers; their fibers pass centrally in vagal and sympa-

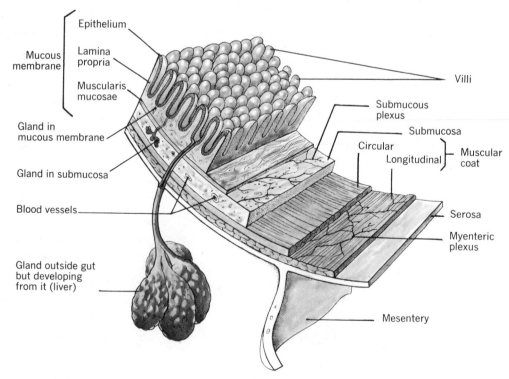

Figure 39-5 Diagram of the four main layers of the wall of the digestive tube; mucosa, submucosa, muscular, and serosa (below the diaphragm). (*Chaffee EE, Lytle IM: Basic Physiology and Anatomy, 4th ed, p 433. Philadelphia, JB Lippincott, 1980*)

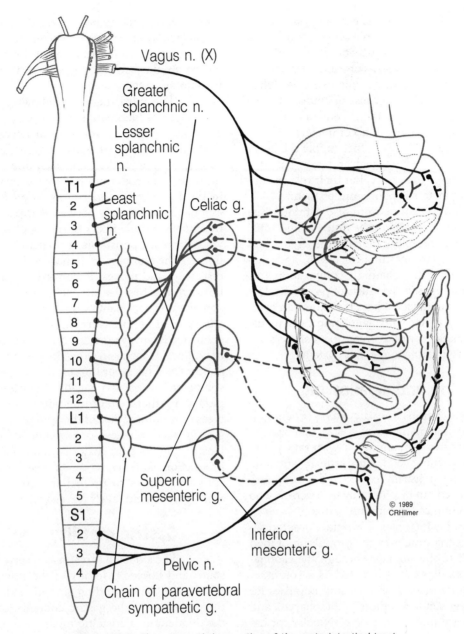

Figure 39-6 The autonomic innervation of the gastrointestinal tract.

thetic fibers. The second group exerts local control over motility by means of activity in the intramural plexus.

Efferent parasympathetic innervation to the stomach, small intestine, cecum, ascending colon, and transverse colon is by way of the vagus nerve (Figure 39-6). The rest of the colon is innervated by parasympathetic fibers in the pelvic nerve that exits from the sacral segments of the spinal cord. Preganglionic parasympathetic fibers can synapse with intramural plexus neurons or they can act directly on intestinal smooth muscle. Most parasympathetic fibers are excitatory. Numerous vagovagal reflexes, whose afferent and ef-

ferent fibers are both vagal nerves, influence motility as well as secretions of the digestive tract.

Efferent sympathetic innervation of the gastrointestinal tract is through the thoracic chain of sympathetic ganglia and the celiac, superior mesenteric, and inferior mesenteric ganglia. The sympathetic nervous system exerts several effects on gastrointestinal function. It controls the extent of mucus secretion by the mucosal glands, reduces motility by inhibiting the activity of intramural plexus neurons, enhances sphincter function, and increases the vascular smooth muscle tone of the blood vessels that supply the gastrointestinal tract. The effect of the sympathetic stimulation is to block the release of the excitatory neuromediators in the intramural plexuses, inhibiting gastrointestinal motility. Sympathetic control of gastrointestinal function is largely controlled by activity within the intramural plexuses. For example, when gastric motility is enhanced because of increased vagal activity, stimulation of sympathetic centers in the hypothalamus promptly and often completely inhibits motility. The sympathetic fibers that supply the lower esophageal, pyloric, and internal and external anal sphincters are largely excitatory, but their role in controlling these sphincters is poorly understood.[2]

Intramural plexus neurons also communicate with neurons from receptors in the mucosal and muscle layers. Mechanoreceptors monitor the stretch and distention of the gastrointestinal tract wall, and chemoreceptors monitor the chemical composition (osmolality, pH, and digestive products of protein and fat metabolism) of its contents. These receptors can communicate directly either with ganglionic cells in the intramural plexuses or with afferent fibers of the sympathetic or parasympathetic nervous system.

Chewing and swallowing

Chewing begins the digestive process; it breaks the food into particles of a size that can be swallowed, lubricates it by mixing it with saliva, and mixes starch-containing food with salivary amylase. Although chewing is usually considered a voluntary act, it can be carried out involuntarily by a person who has lost the function of the cerebral cortex.

The swallowing reflex is a rigidly ordered sequence of events that results in the propulsion of food from the mouth to the stomach through the esophagus. Although swallowing is initiated as a voluntary activity, it becomes involuntary. Sensory impulses for the reflex begin at tactile receptors in the pharynx and esophagus and are integrated in the reticular formation of the medulla and lower pons, producing the motor components of the response. Diseases that disrupt these brain centers disrupt the coordination of swallowing and predispose an individual to the risk of food and fluid lodging in the trachea and bronchi, leading to asphyxiation or aspiration pneumonia.

Swallowing consists of three phases: an oral, or voluntary phase; a pharyngeal phase; and an esophageal phase. During the oral, or voluntary, phase the bolus is collected at the back of the mouth so that the tongue can lift the food upward until it touches the posterior wall of the pharynx. At this point, the second stage of swallowing is initiated: the soft palate is pulled upward, the palatopharyngeal folds are pulled together so that food does not enter the nasopharynx; the vocal cords are pulled together, and the epiglottis is moved so that it covers the larynx; respiration is

inhibited; and the bolus is moved backward into the esophagus by constrictive movements of the pharynx. Although the striated muscles of the pharynx are involved in the second stage of swallowing, it is an involuntary stage.

The third stage of swallowing is the esophageal stage. As food enters the esophagus and stretches its walls, both local and central nervous system reflexes that initiate peristalsis are triggered. There are two types of peristalsis—primary and secondary. Primary peristalsis is controlled by the swallowing center in the brain stem and begins when food enters the esophagus. Secondary peristalsis is partially mediated by smooth muscle fibers in the esophagus and occurs when primary peristalsis is inadequate to move food through the esophagus.[3] Peristalsis begins at the site of distention and moves downward. Before the peristaltic wave reaches the stomach, the lower esophageal sphincter relaxes to allow the bolus of food to enter the stomach. The pressure in the lower esophageal sphincter is always greater than that in the stomach, an important factor in preventing the reflux of gastric contents. The opening of the lower esophageal sphincter is mediated vagally. Increased levels of the parasympathetic neuromediator acetylcholine increase the constriction of the sphincter. The hormone gastrin also increases constriction of the sphincter. Gastrin provides the major stimulus for stomach acid production, and its action on the lower esophageal sphincter serves to protect the esophageal mucosa when gastric acid levels are elevated.

Gastric motility

The stomach serves as a reservoir for ingested solids and liquids. Motility of the stomach results in the churning and grinding of solid foods and regulates the emptying of the gastric contents, or chyme, into the duodenum. Peristaltic mixing and churning contractions begin in a pacemaker area in the middle of the stomach and move toward the antrum (Figure 39-7). They occur at a frequency of 3 to 5 contractions per minute, with a duration of 2 seconds to 20 seconds. As the peristaltic wave approaches the antrum, it speeds up, and the entire terminal 5 cm to 10 cm of the antrum contracts, occluding the pyloric opening. Contraction of the antrum reverses the movement of the chyme, returning the larger particles to the body of the stomach for further churning and kneading. Because the pylorus is contracted during antral contraction, the gastric contents are emptied into the duodenum between contractions.

Although the pylorus does not contain a true anatomic sphincter, it does function as a physiologic sphincter to prevent the backflow of gastric contents and allow them to flow into the duodenum at a rate

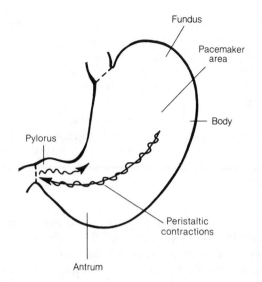

Figure 39-7 Structures of the stomach, showing the pacemaker area and the direction of chyme movement resulting from peristaltic contractions.

commensurate with the ability of the duodenum to accept them. This is important because the regurgitation of bile salts and duodenal contents can damage the antrum and lead to gastric ulcers. Likewise, the duodenum can be damaged by the rapid influx of highly acid gastric contents.

Like other parts of the gastrointestinal tract, the stomach is richly innervated by both intrinsic and extrinsic nerves. Axons from the intramural plexuses innervate the smooth muscles and glands of the stomach. Extrinsic parasympathetic innervation is provided by the vagus, and sympathetic innervation by the celiac ganglia. The emptying of the stomach is regulated by both hormonal and neural mechanisms. The hormones cholecystokinin and gastric inhibitory peptide, which are thought to control gastric emptying, are released in response to the osmolar, pH, and fatty acid composition of the chyme. Both local and central circuitry are involved in the neural control of gastric emptying. Afferent receptor fibers either synapse with the neurons in the intramural plexus or trigger intrinsic reflexes by means of the vagus or sympathetic pathways to participate in extrinsic reflexes.[3]

Disorders of gastric motility can occur when the rate is too slow or too fast (see Chapter 40). A rate that is too slow causes gastric retention. It can be caused by either obstruction or gastric atony. Obstruction can result from the formation of scar tissue following peptic ulcer. Another example of obstruction is hypertrophic pyloric stenosis. This can occur in infants with an abnormally thick muscularis layer in the terminal pylorus. Myotomy, or surgical incision of the muscular ring, is usually done to relieve the obstruction. Gastric atony can occur as a complication of

visceral neuropathies in diabetes mellitus. Surgical procedures that disrupt vagal activity can also result in gastric atony. Abnormally fast emptying occurs in the dumping syndrome, which is a consequence of certain types of gastric surgeries. This condition is characterized by the rapid dumping of highly acidic and hyperosmotic gastric secretions into the duodenum and jejunum.

Small intestine motility

The small intestine is the major site for the digestion and absorption of food; its movements are both mixing and propulsive. Regular peristaltic movements begin in the duodenum near the entry sites of the common duct and the main hepatic duct. A series of local pacemakers function to maintain the frequency of intestinal contraction. The peristaltic movements (about 12 per minute in the jejunum) become less frequent as they move further from the pylorus, becoming about 9 per minute in the ileum. The contractions produce both segmentation waves and propulsive movements through the muscles of the small intestine. With segmentation waves, slow contractions of circular muscle occlude the lumen and drive the contents forward and backward. Most of the contractions that produce segmental waves are local events involving only 1 cm to 4 cm at a time. They function mainly to mix the chyme with the digestive enzymes from the pancreas and to ensure adequate exposure of all parts of the chyme to the mucosal surface of the intestine, where absorption takes place. The frequency of segmenting activity increases after a meal. Presumably it is stimulated by receptors in the stomach and intestine, because the activity does not occur following denervation of the intestine. Propulsive movements occur with synchronized activity in a section 10 cm to 20 cm in length. They are accomplished by contraction of the proximal, or oral, portion of the intestine with the sequential relaxation of its distal, or anal, portion (Figure 39-8). Once material has been propelled to the ileocecal junction by peristaltic movement, stretching of the distal ileum produces a local reflex that relaxes the sphincter and allows fluid to squirt into the cecum.

Peristalsis

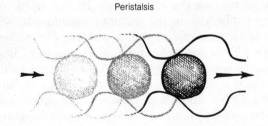

Figure 39-8 Peristaltic movements in the intestine. Areas of relaxation precede areas of contraction.

Motility disturbances of the small bowel are common, and auscultation of the abdomen can be used to assess bowel activity. Inflammatory changes increase motility. In many instances it is not certain whether changes in motility occur because of inflammation or secondary to toxins or secreted and unabsorbed materials. Delayed passage of materials in the small intestine can also be a problem. Transient interruption of intestinal motility often occurs following gastrointestinal surgery. Intubation with suction is required to remove the accumulating intestinal contents and gases until activity is resumed.

Colonic motility

As might be expected, the storage function of the *colon* dictates that movements within this section of the gut be different from those in the small intestine. Basically, movements in the colon are of two types. First are the segmental mixing movements, called *haustrations,* so named because they occur within sacculations called *haustra.* These movements produce a local digging-type action which ensures that all portions of the fecal mass are exposed to the intestinal surface. Second are the *propulsive mass movements,* in which a large segment of the colon (20 cm or more) contract as a unit, moving the fecal contents forward as a unit. Mass movements last about 30 seconds, followed by a 2 to 3 minute period of relaxation, after which another contraction occurs. A series of mass movements only lasts for 10 to 30 minutes and may only occur several times a day. Defecation is normally initiated by the mass movements. A condition called Hirschsprung's disease is characterized by a lack of neurons in the myenteric plexus in a segment of the colon. Its correction requires surgical removal of the affected segment.

Defecation

Defecation is controlled by the action of two sphincters, the *internal* and *external sphincters.* The internal sphincter is controlled by the autonomic nervous system, and the external sphincter is under the conscious control of the cerebral cortex.

The defecation reflex is integrated in the sacral segment of the spinal cord. In this reflex arc, afferent fibers from the rectum communicate with nerves in the sacral cord and with parasympathetic efferent fibers that move back to the bowel (see Figure 39-6). The efferent signals from this reflex produce increased activity along the entire length of the large bowel. Other actions associated with defecation, such as abdominal pushing movements, are simultaneously integrated in the spinal cord. To prevent involuntary defecation from occurring, the external anal sphincter is under the conscious control of the cortex. Thus, as afferent impulses arrive at the sacral cord, signaling the presence of a distended rectum, messages are transmitted to the cortex. If defecation is inappropriate, the cortex initiates impulses that constrict the external sphincter and inhibit efferent parasympathetic activity. Normally, the afferent impulses in this reflex loop fatigue easily and the urge to defecate soon dies out. At a more convenient time, contraction of the abdominal muscles compresses the contents in the large bowel, reinitiating afferent impulses to the cord.

In summary, motility of the gastrointestinal tract moves food products and fluids along its length from mouth to anus. Although the activity of gastrointestinal smooth muscle is self-propagating and can continue without input from the nervous system, its rate and strength of contractions are regulated by a network of intramural neurons that receive input from the autonomic nervous system and local receptors that monitor wall stretch and the chemical composition of its luminal contents. Parasympathetic innervation occurs by means of the vagus nerve and nerve fibers from sacral segments of the spinal cord; it serves to increase gastrointestinal motility. Sympathetic activity occurs by way of thoracolumbar output from the spinal cord, its paravertebral ganglia, and celiac, superior mesenteric, and inferior mesenteric ganglia. Sympathetic stimulation enhances sphincter function and reduces motility by inhibiting the activity of intramural plexus neurons.

Secretory function

Each day about 7000 ml of fluid is secreted into the gastrointestinal tract (Table 39-1). Only about 50 ml to 200 ml of this fluid leaves the body in the stool; the remainder is reabsorbed in the small and large intestines. These secretions are mainly water and have a sodium and potassium concentration similar to that of extracellular fluid. Because water and electrolytes for digestive tract secretions are derived from the

Table 39-1. Secretions of the gastrointestinal tract

Secretions	Amount daily (ml)
Salivary	1200
Gastric	2000
Pancreatic	1200
Biliary	700
Intestinal	2000
TOTAL	7100

extracellular fluid compartment, excessive secretion or impaired absorption can lead to extracellular fluid deficit.

Control of secretory function

The secretory activity of the gut is influenced by local, humoral, and neural influences. Neural control of gastrointestinal secretory activity is mediated through the autonomic nervous system. With secretion, as with motility, the parasympathetic nervous system increases activity, whereas sympathetic activity has an inhibitory action. Many of the local influences, including *p*H, osmolality, and chyme, consistently act as stimuli for neural and humoral mechanisms.

Gastrointestinal hormones

The gastrointestinal tract is the largest endocrine organ in the body. It produces hormones that pass from the portal circulation into the general circulation and then back to the digestive tract, where they exert their action. Among the hormones produced by the gastrointestinal tract are *gastrin*, *secretin*, and *cholecystokinin*. These hormones influence motility and the secretion of electrolytes, enzymes, and other hormones. It has been observed that gastrin also influences the growth of the exocrine pancreas and the mucosa of the stomach and small intestine. It is reported that removal of the tissue that produces gastrin results in atrophy of these structures. This atrophy can be reversed by the administration of exogenous gastrin. The gastrointestinal tract hormones and their functions are summarized in Table 39-2.

Salivary secretions

Saliva is secreted in the mouth. The salivary glands consist of the parotid, submaxillary, sublingual, and buccal glands. Saliva has three functions.

The first of these is protection and lubrication. Saliva is rich in mucus, which serves to protect the oral mucosa and to coat the food as it passes through the mouth, pharynx, and esophagus. The sublingual and buccal glands produce only mucous-type secretions. The second function of saliva is its protective antimicrobial action. The saliva not only cleanses the mouth but contains the enzyme lysozyme, which has an antibacterial action. Third, saliva contains ptyalin and amylase, which initiate the digestion of dietary starches. Of particular interest is the high potassium content in saliva—2 to 30 times that of plasma, depending on the rate of secretion. Secretions from the salivary glands are primarily regulated by the autonomic nervous system. Parasympathetic stimulation increases flow and sympathetic stimulation decreases flow. The dry mouth that accompanies anxiety attests to the effects of sympathetic activity on salivary secretions.

Mumps, or *parotitis*, is an infection of the parotid glands. Although most of us associate mumps with the contagious viral form of the disease, inflammation of the parotid glands can occur in the seriously ill person who does not receive adequate oral hygiene and who is unable to take fluids orally. Potassium iodide increases the secretory activity of the salivary glands, including the parotid glands. In a small percentage of persons, parotid swelling may occur in the course of treatment with this drug.

Gastric secretions

Three types of gastric glands in the stomach produce secretions: the cardiac, gastric, and pyloric glands. These glands are closely packed and oriented perpendicular to the mucosa, with one end opening into the surface epithelium. Both the cardiac glands (located in the vicinity of the esophageal orifice) and

Table 39-2. Major gastrointestinal hormones and their actions

Hormone	Site of secretion	Stimulus for secretion	Action
Cholecysto-kinin	Duodenum, jejunum	Amino acids	Stimulates contraction of gallbladder; stimulates secretion of pancreatic enzymes; slows gastric emptying
Gastrin	Antrum of the stomach, duodenum	Vagal stimulation; epinephrine; neutral amino acids; solutions of calcium salts, including milk; and alcohol. Secretion inhibited by acid contents in the antrum of the stomach (below *p*H 2.5)	Stimulates secretion of gastric acid and pepsinogen; increases gastric blood flow; stimulates gastric smooth muscle contraction; stimulates growth of gastric mucosa, small intestine mucosa, and exocrine pancreas
Secretin	Duodenum	Acid *p*H of chyme entering duodenum (below *p*H 3.0)	Stimulates secretion of bicarbonate-containing solution by pancreas and liver

the pyloric glands (located in the distal 4 cm to 5 cm of the antrum) produce a protective mucus. The gastric glands, which are located in the fundic area of the stomach, contain chief cells, parietal cells, mucus-producing cells, and argentaffin cells. The parietal cells produce hydrochloric acid. There are about a billion parietal cells in the stomach; together they produce and secrete about 20 mEq of hydrochloric acid in several hundred milliliters of gastric juice each hour. The chief cells secrete pepsinogen, which is rapidly converted to pepsin when exposed to the low pH of the gastric juices. Some of the argentaffin cells produce serotonin (5-hydroxytryptamine). Similar cells, located in the antrum, produce gastrin. Gastric intrinsic factor, which is produced by the parietal cells, is necessary for the absorption of vitamin B_{12}.

One of the important characteristics of the gastric mucosa is its resistance to the highly acid secretions that it produces, a property derived from the mucosa's impermeability to hydrogen ions. When the gastric mucosa is damaged by aspirin, indomethacin, ethyl alcohol, or bile salts, this impermeability is disrupted and the hydrogen ions move into the tissue. This is called breaking the mucosal barrier, and substances that alter the permeability are called barrier breakers. As the hydrogen ions accumulate in the mucosal cells, intracellular pH decreases, enzymatic reactions become impaired, and cellular structures are disrupted. The result is local ischemia, vascular stasis, hypoxia, and tissue necrosis. The mucosal surface is further protected by prostaglandins. Aspirin and indomethacin inhibit prostaglandin synthesis, which also impairs the integrity of the mucosal surface.

Both parasympathetic stimulation (via the vagus nerve) and gastrin increase gastric secretions. It has long been known that histamine increases gastric-acid secretions. Recent research and clinical use of the histamine$_2$-receptor antagonists suggest that histamine 2 (H_2) may be the final common pathway for gastric-acid production. Gastric-acid secretion and its relationship to peptic ulcer are discussed in Chapter 40.

Tests of gastric acid production

A laboratory procedure called gastric analysis is used to assess the hydrochloric acid content of gastric secretions. This procedure involves the withdrawal of samples of gastric secretions through a tube that has been inserted into the stomach. Histamine or its analog may be administered subcutaneously during the sampling procedure to stimulate acid production. When pernicious anemia is present, such stimulation fails to increase acid levels. In this case, the observed achlorhydria is said to be histamine-fast. A second means for assessing hydrochloric acid secretion is

tubeless gastric analysis. Tubeless gastric analysis is a screening test that involves the use of a cation resin dye. An acid pH of less than 3.5 is required so that the dye can be released and absorbed in the small intestine. The presence of dye in the urine is interpreted to mean that sufficient hydrochloric acid is in the stomach to maintain a pH that favors dye absorption.

Intestinal secretions

The *small intestine* both secretes digestive juices and receives secretions from the liver and pancreas (see Chapter 41). Mucus-producing glands are concentrated in the duodenum at the site where the contents from the stomach and secretions from the liver and pancreas enter. These glands, called *Brunner's glands,* serve to protect the duodenum from the acid content in the gastric chyme and from the action of the digestive enzymes. The activity of Brunner's glands is strongly influenced by autonomic factors. For example, sympathetic stimulation causes a marked decrease in mucus production, leaving this area more susceptible to irritation. Interestingly, 50% of peptic ulcers occur at this site.

In addition to mucus, the intestinal mucosa produces two other types of secretions. The first is a serous fluid (pH 6.5–7.5) secreted by specialized cells (crypts of Lieberkühn) in the intestinal mucosal layer. This fluid, which is produced at the rate of 2000 ml/day, acts as a diluent for absorption. The second type consists of surface enzymes that aid absorption. These enzymes are the peptidases—enzymes that separate amino acids—and the disaccharidases—enzymes that split sugars.

The *large intestine* usually secretes only mucus. Autonomic nervous system activity strongly influences mucus production in the bowel, as in other parts of the digestive tract. During intense parasympathetic stimulation, mucus secretion may increase to the point where the stool contains large amounts of obvious mucus. Although the bowel normally does not secrete water or electrolytes, these substances are lost in large quantities when the bowel becomes irritated or inflamed.

In summary, the secretions of the gastrointestinal tract include saliva, gastric juices, bile, and pancreatic and intestinal secretions. Each day more than 7000 ml of fluid is secreted into the digestive tract; all but 50 ml to 200 ml of this fluid is reabsorbed. Water, derived from the extracellular fluid compartment, is the major component of gastrointestinal tract secretions. Neural, humoral, and local mechanisms contribute to the control of these secretions. The parasympathetic nervous system increases secretion, whereas sympathetic activity exerts an inhibitory effect. In addition to secreting fluids containing digestive enzymes, the gastrointestinal tract produces and secretes hormones, such as gastrin, secretin, and cholecystokinin, that contribute to the control of gastrointestinal function.

Digestion and absorption

Digestion is the process of dismantling foods into their constituent parts, which are small enough to be absorbed. Digestion requires hydrolysis, enzyme cleavage, and fat emulsification. Hydrolysis is breakdown of a compound that involves a chemical reaction with water. The importance of hydrolysis to digestion is evidenced by the amount of water (7–8 liters) that is secreted into the gastrointestinal tract daily.

Absorption occurs mainly in the small intestine. The stomach is a poor absorptive structure, and only a few lipid-soluble substances, including alcohol, are absorbed from the stomach. The absorptive function of the large intestine focuses mainly on water reabsorption.

The mucosal surface of the small intestine is designed to facilitate absorption (Figure 39-9). The mucosal folds, the villi, and the microvilli in the small intestine increase its absorptive capacity 600-fold, providing a total surface area of about 250 square meters.

Absorption for the intestine is accomplished by active transport and diffusion. A number of substances require a specific transport carrier or system. For example, vitamin B_{12} is not absorbed in the absence of intrinsic factor. Transport of amino acid and glucose occurs mainly in the presence of sodium. Water is absorbed passively, obeying the usual laws of osmosis.

The small intestine is involved primarily in the digestion and absorption of nutrients. The intestinal mucosa is impermeable to most large molecules. Therefore, most proteins, fats, and carbohydrates must be broken down into smaller particles before they can be absorbed. Although some digestion of carbohydrates and proteins begins in the stomach, digestion takes place mainly in the small intestine. The hydrolysis of fats to free fatty acids and monoglycerides takes place entirely in the small intestine. The liver, with its production of bile, and the pancreas, which supplies a number of digestive enzymes, also play important roles in digestion.

The distinguishing characteristic of the small intestine is its large surface area, which in the adult is estimated to be about 4500 m^2. Anatomic features that contribute to this enlarged surface area are the circular folds that extend into the lumen of the intestine and the villi, which are fingerlike projections of mucous membrane numbering as many as 25,000, that line the entire small intestine. Each villus is covered with cells called enterocytes that contribute to the absorptive and digestive functions of the small bowel and goblet cells that provide mucus. The crypts of Lieberkühn are glandular structures that open into the spaces between the villi. The enterocytes have a life span of about 4 to 5 days, and it is believed that replacement cells differentiate from cells located in the area of the crypts. The maturing enterocytes migrate up the villus and are eventually extruded from the tip.

Each villus is equipped with an artery, vein, and lymph vessel (lacteal), which bring blood to the surface of the intestine and transport the nutrients and other materials that have passed into the blood from the lumen of the intestine (Figure 39-10). Fats rely largely on the lymphatics for absorption. This means that a decrease in blood flow to the gut (due, for example, to atherosclerosis or heart failure) may impair absorption of nutrients. Another cause of malab-

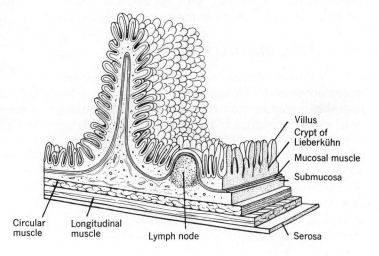

Figure 39-9 The mucous membrane of the small intestine. Note the numerous villi on a circular fold. *(Chaffee EE, Lytle IM: Basic Physiology and Anatomy, 4th ed. Philadelphia, JB Lippincott, 1980)*

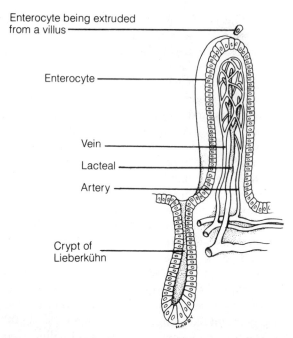

Enterocyte being extruded
from a villus

Enterocyte

Vein

Lacteal

Artery

Crypt of
Lieberkühn

Figure 39-10 A single villus from the small intestine. (Chaffee EE, Lytle IM: Basic Physiology and Anatomy, 4th ed. Philadelphia, JB Lippincott, 1980)

sorption is lymphatic obstruction resulting from lymphoma.

The enterocytes secrete a number of enzymes that aid in the digestion of carbohydrates and proteins. These enzymes are called *brush border enzymes* because they adhere to the border of the villus structures. In this way they have access to the carbohydrates and protein molecules as they come in contact with the absorptive surface of the intestine. This mechanism of secretion places the enzymes where they are needed and eliminates the need to produce enough enzymes to mix with the entire contents that fill the lumen of the small bowel. The digested molecules either diffuse through the membrane or are actively transported across the mucosal surface to enter the blood or, in the case of fatty acids, the lacteal. These molecules are then transported through the portal vein or lymphatics into the systemic circulation.

Carbohydrate absorption

Carbohydrates must be broken down into monosaccharides, or single sugars, before they can be absorbed from the small intestine. The average daily intake of carbohydrate in the American diet is about 350 g to 400 g. Starch makes up about 50% of this total, sucrose (table sugar) about 30%, lactose (milk sugar) about 6%, and maltose about 1.5%.[4] Digestion of starch begins in the mouth with the action of amylase. Pancreatic secretions also contain an amylase. As a result of the action of amylase, starch is broken down into several disaccharides, including maltose, isomal-

tose, and α-dextrins. It is the brush border enzymes that convert the disaccharides into monosaccharides that can be absorbed (Table 39-3). Sucrose yields glucose and fructose, lactose is converted to glucose and galactose, and maltose is changed to glucose. When the disaccharides are not broken down to monosaccharides, they cannot be absorbed but remain as osmotically active particles in the contents of the digestive system causing diarrhea.

Fructose is transported across the intestinal mucosa by facilitated diffusion, which does not require energy expenditure. In this case, fructose moves along a concentration gradient. Glucose and galactose, on the other hand, are transported by way of a sodium-dependent carrier system that uses adenosine triphosphate (ATP) as an energy source (Figure 39-11). Water absorption from the intestine is linked to absorption of osmotically active particles, such as glucose and sodium. It follows that an important consideration in facilitating the transport of water across the intestine (and decreasing diarrhea) following temporary disruption in bowel function is to include both sodium and glucose in the fluids that are taken. A number of carbonated soft drinks can be used for this purpose.

Lactase deficiency

The most common disaccharidase deficiency involves lactase. Although human infants have a high concentration of lactase following birth, this concentration falls rapidly in the first 4 to 5 years of life and may reach low levels in adolescence and adult life. It has been estimated that 3% to 19% of the adult white population, 70% of American blacks, and 90% of native Americans are deficient in lactase.[5] With a lactase deficiency, intolerance to milk occurs, manifested in bloating, flatulence, cramping abdominal pain, and diarrhea. These symptoms are usually relieved by avoiding lactose (milk) in the diet. Recently, yogurt has been shown to be a well-tolerated source of milk for lactase-deficient persons.[6]

Table 39–3. Enzymes used in digestion of carbohydrates

Dietary carbohydrates	Enzyme	Monosaccharides produced
Lactose	Lactase	Glucose and galactose
Sucrose	Sucrase	Fructose and glucose
Starch	Amylase	Maltose, maltotriase, and α-dextrins
maltose and maltotriose	Maltase	Glucose and glucose
α-dextrins	Isomaltase	Glucose and glucose

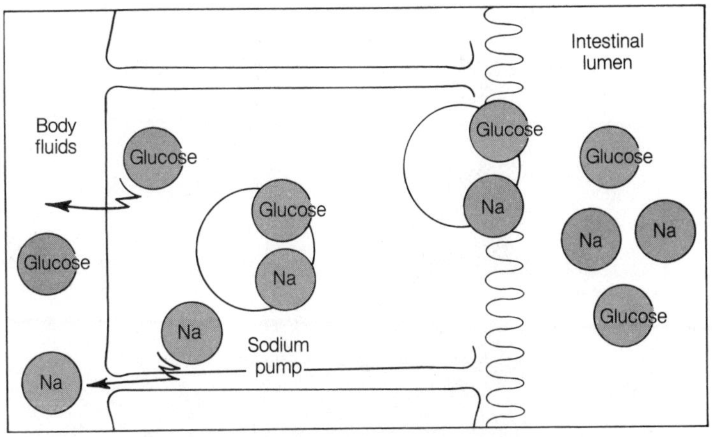

Figure 39-11 The hypothetical sodium-dependent transport system for glucose. Both sodium and glucose must attach to the transport carrier before either can be transported into the cell. The concentration of glucose builds up within the intestinal cell until a diffusion gradient develops, causing glucose to move into the body fluids. Sodium is transported out of the cell by the energy-dependent (ATP) sodium pump. This creates the gradient needed to operate the transport system.

The fact that lactase availability declines following childhood and may be rather limited in the adult may help to explain why milk is sometimes poorly tolerated following gastrointestinal tract "flu" or other disorders. One can assume that with a limited ability to produce lactase, any disruption in the regeneration of intestinal mucosa might reduce lactase levels to a point at which a temporary deficiency could occur.

Fat absorption

The average adult eats about 60 g to 100 g of fat daily, principally as triglycerides containing long-chain fatty acids. These triglycerides are broken down by pancreatic lipase. Bile salts act as a carrier system for the fatty acids and fat-soluble vitamins A, D, E, and K by forming micelles, which transport these substances to the surface of intestinal villi where they are absorbed. The major site of fat absorption is the upper jejunum. Medium-chain triglycerides, with fatty acids of lengths C-6 to C-10, are absorbed better than longer chains of fatty acids because they are more completely hydrolyzed by pancreatic lipase and they form micelles more easily. Because they are easily absorbed, medium-chain triglycerides are often used in the treatment of persons with malabsorption syndrome. The absorption of vitamins A, D, E, and K, which are fat-soluble vitamins, requires bile salts.

Fat that is not absorbed in the intestine is excreted in the stool. *Steatorrhea* is the term used to describe fatty stools. It usually indicates that there are 20 g or more of fat in a 24-hour stool sample.[2] Normally, a chemical test is done on a 72-hour stool collection, during which time the diet is restricted to 80 g to 100 g of fat per day.

Protein absorption

Proteins are broken down by pancreatic enzymes, such as trypsin, chymotrypsin, carboxypeptidase, and elastase. The amino acids are liberated either intramurally or on the surface of the villi by brush border enzymes that degrade proteins into one-, two-, and three-amino-acid particles. These amino acids are transported across the mucosal membrane in a sodium-linked process that uses ATP as an energy source.

In summary, the digestion and absorption of foodstuffs take place in the small intestine. Proteins, fats, carbohydrates, and other components of the diet are broken down into molecules that can be transported from the intestinal lumen into the body fluids.

References

1. Thompson JS: Core Textbook of Anatomy, p 292. Philadelphia, JB Lippincott, 1977
2. Davenport HW: Physiology of the Digestive Tract, 5th ed, pp 4, 229. Chicago, Year Book Medical Publishers, 1982
3. Berne RM, Levy MN: Physiology, pp 662, 671. St. Louis, CV Mosby, 1988
4. Castro GA: Digestion and absorption of specific nutrients. In Johnson LR (ed): Gastrointestinal Physiology, p 122. St. Louis, CV Mosby, 1977
5. Kosek MS: Medical genetics. In Krupp MA, Chatton MJ (eds): Medical Diagnosis and Treatment, p 1045. Los Altos, Lange Medical Publications, 1984
6. Kolars JC, Levitt MD, Motafa A, et al: Yogurt—An autodigesting source of lactose. N Engl J Med 310:1, 1984

CHAPTER 40

Alterations in Gastrointestinal Function

Objectives

After you have studied this chapter you should be able to meet the following objectives:

_____ Describe the physiologic mechanisms involved in anorexia, nausea, and vomiting.

_____ Explain the significance of melena.

_____ List the causes of esophagitis.

_____ Relate the causes of hiatal hernia to measures used in treatment of the condition.

_____ Describe the factors that contribute to the gastric mucosal barrier.

_____ Explain how aspirin disrupts the gastric mucosal barrier.

_____ Compare the causes and manifestations of acute and chronic gastritis.

_____ Describe the predisposing factors in development of peptic ulcer.

_____ Cite the three complications of peptic ulcer

_____ State the overall goals in treatment of peptic ulcer.

_____ Compare the pharmacologic actions of antacids, histamine$_2$-receptor antagonists, and mucosal protective agents as they relate to the treatment of peptic ulcer.

_____ Cite the rationale for the signs and symptoms associated with the dumping syndrome.

_____ Compare the characteristics of Crohn's disease and ulcerative colitis.

_____ List at least four systemic manifestations of inflammatory bowel disease.

_____ Characterize toxic megacolon.

_____ Relate the use of a high-fiber diet in the treatment of diverticular disease to the etiologic factors involved in the development of the condition.

_____ Describe the rationale for the symptoms associated with appendicitis.

(continued)

_____ List the risk factors associated with colorectal cancer.

_____ State the American Cancer Society screening methods for colorectal cancer.

_____ Describe the characteristics of the peritoneum that increase its vulnerability and protect it against the effects of peritonitis.

_____ State the manifestations of peritonitis.

_____ Compare the causes and manifestations of small-volume diarrhea and large-volume diarrhea.

_____ Explain why a failure to respond to the defecation urge may result in constipation.

_____ State the difference between mechanical and paralytic intestinal obstruction.

_____ Describe the manifestations of bowel obstruction.

_____ List conditions that cause malabsorption by impaired intraluminal malabsorption, mucosal malabsorption, and lymphatic obstruction.

_____ State common manifestations of the malabsorption syndrome.

Gastrointestinal disorders are not cited as the leading cause of death in the United States, nor do they receive the same publicity as heart disease and cancer. Yet, according to government reports, digestive diseases rank third in the total economic burden of illness, causing considerable human suffering, personal expenditures for treatment, lost working hours, and a drain on the nation's economy. It has been estimated that 20 million Americans, one out of every nine persons in the United States, have digestive disease. Even more important is the fact that proper nutrition or a change in health practices could prevent or minimize many of these disorders. The content of this chapter focuses on three types of gastrointestinal disorders: (1) disorders that result in alterations in the integrity of the gastrointestinal tract, (2) alterations in the digestive and absorptive functions of the gastrointestinal tract, and (3) altered motility of the gastrointestinal tract.

Manifestations of gastrointestinal tract disorders

Several signs and symptoms are common to many types of gastrointestinal disorders. These include anorexia, nausea, vomiting, and gastrointestinal bleeding. Because they occur with so many of the disorders, they are discussed separately as an introduction to the content that follows.

— Anorexia

Anorexia is loss of appetite. A number of factors influence appetite. One of these factors is hunger, which is stimulated by contractions of the empty stomach. The desire for food intake is also regulated by the hypothalamus and other associated centers in the brain. Smell plays an important role, as evidenced by the fact that appetite can be stimulated or suppressed by the smell of food. Loss of appetite is associated with emotional situations, such as fear, depres-

sion, frustration, and anxiety. Many drugs and disease states cause anorexia. In uremia, for example, the accumulation of nitrogenous wastes in the blood contributes to the development of anorexia. Anorexia is often a forerunner of nausea, and most conditions that cause nausea and vomiting also produce anorexia.

— Nausea

Nausea is an ill-defined and unpleasant subjective sensation. It is basically a conscious recognition of stimulation of the medullary vomiting center. Nausea is usually preceded by anorexia, and stimuli such as foods and drugs that cause anorexia in small doses will usually produce nausea when given in larger doses. A common cause of nausea is distention of the duodenum, or upper small intestinal tract. Nausea is frequently accompanied by autonomic responses such as watery salivation and vasoconstriction with pallor, sweating, and tachycardia. Nausea may function as an early warning signal of pathology.

— Vomiting

Vomiting is the sudden and forceful oral expulsion of the contents of the stomach. It is usually, but not always, preceded by nausea. The contents that are vomited are called vomitus.

The act of vomiting is integrated by the vomiting center, which is located in the dorsal portion of the reticular formation of the medulla near the sensory nuclei of the vagus. The act of vomiting consists of taking a deep breath, closing the airways, and producing a strong, forceful contraction of the diaphragm and abdominal muscles along with relaxation of the gastroesophageal sphincter. Respiration ceases during the act of vomiting. Vomiting may be accompanied by dizziness, light-headedness, decrease in blood pressure, and bradycardia.

The vomiting center may be stimulated directly or by impulses from the chemoreceptor trigger zone or afferent neurons of the autonomic nervous system. Many chemicals and drugs incite nausea and vomiting. These agents exert their effect by stimulating the medullary chemoreceptor trigger zone, which relays impulses to the vomiting center. The phenothiazine derivatives, such as chlorpromazine (Thorazine) and prochlorperazine (Compazine), depress vomiting caused by stimulation of the chemoreceptor trigger zone. Hypoxemia exerts a direct effect on the vomiting center, producing nausea and vomiting. This direct effect probably accounts for the vomiting that occurs during periods of decreased cardiac output, shock, environmental hypoxia, and brain ischemia caused by increased intracranial pressure. Inflammation of any of the intra-abdominal organs, including the liver, gallbladder, or urinary tract, can cause vomiting because of stimulation of the visceral afferent pathways that communicate with the vomiting center. Distention or irritation of the gastrointestinal tract also causes vomiting through stimulation of visceral afferent neurons. Vomiting, as a basic physiologic protective mechanism, limits the possibility of damage from ingested noxious agents by emptying the contents of the stomach and portions of the small intestine. Nausea and vomiting may represent a total-body response to drug therapy, including overdosage, cumulative effects, toxicity, and side effects.

Gastrointestinal tract bleeding

Bleeding from the gastrointestinal tract can be evidenced by blood that appears in either the vomitus or the feces. It can result from disease or trauma to the gastrointestinal structures, as a result of primary diseases of the blood vessels (*i.e.*, esophageal varices or hemorrhoids), or because of disorders in blood clotting.

Hematemesis

The presence of blood in the stomach is usually irritating and causes vomiting. Hematemesis refers to blood in the vomitus. It may be bright red or have a "coffee ground" appearance because of the action of the digestive enzymes.

Melena

Blood that appears in the stool may range in color from bright red to tarry black. Bright-red blood usually indicates that the bleeding is from the lower bowel. When it coats the stool, it is often the result of bleeding hemorrhoids. The word *melena* means black and refers to the passage of black and tarry stools. These stools have a characteristic odor that is not easily forgotten. The presence of tarry stools usually indicates that the source of bleeding is above the level of the ileocecal valve, although this is not always the case. With hypermotility of the gastrointestinal tract, bright-red blood may be present in the stools even though the bleeding is from the upper gastrointestinal tract. Melena can occur when as little as 100 ml of blood enter the gastrointestinal tract.[1] Furthermore, tarry stools have been shown to continue for as long as 3 days to 5 days following administration of 1000 ml to 2000 ml of blood into the gastrointestinal tract, indicating that melena is not necessarily a good sign of continued bleeding.[2] *Occult* (hidden) blood, which can only be detected by chemical means, may persist for 2 weeks to 3 weeks.[1]

Blood urea nitrogen (BUN) is frequently elevated following hematemesis or melena. This results from breakdown of the blood by the digestive enzymes and the absorption of the nitrogenous end-products into the blood. The BUN usually reaches a peak within 24 hours following the gastrointestinal hemorrhage. It does not appear when the bleeding is in the colon, because digestion does not take place at this level of the digestive system. An elevation in body temperature also usually follows gastrointestinal hemorrhage. This also occurs within 24 hours and may last for a few days to a few weeks.

In summary, many gastrointestinal tract disorders are manifested by anorexia, nausea, and vomiting. Anorexia, or loss of appetite, may occur alone or may accompany nausea and vomiting. Nausea, which is an ill-defined, unpleasant sensation, signals the stimulation of the medullary vomiting center. It often precedes vomiting and is frequently accompanied by autonomic responses such as salivation and vasoconstriction with pallor, sweating, and tachycardia. The act of vomiting, which is integrated by the vomiting center, involves the forceful oral expulsion of the gastric contents. It is a basic physiologic mechanism that rids the gastrointestinal tract of noxious agents. Disorders that disrupt the integrity of the gastrointestinal tract often cause bleeding, which can be manifested as blood in the vomitus (hematemesis) or as blood in the stool (melena).

Alterations in the integrity of the gastrointestinal tract wall

Characteristic of the gastrointestinal tract is the mucous membrane that lines its entire length from mouth to anus. This mucosal layer varies somewhat in structure, depending on its location and function. In the upper part of the digestive tract (mouth and esophagus), the mucus produced by the goblet cells acts as a lubricant to facilitate passage of food particles. In the stomach and small intestine, the mucous membrane is required to withstand the corrosive effects of hydrochloric acid and digestive enzymes. The mucosal layer in the small intestine is designed to facilitate absorption of nutrients.

The mucus-producing cells of the epithelial layer of the gastrointestinal tract have a rapid turnover rate of about 4 to 5 days. During periods of irritation or injury, this turnover rate is increased and the cells are shed at a more rapid rate. When this occurs, the rate of replacement does not always keep pace with the rate of cell loss, and the area becomes denuded, reddened, and swollen. Fortunately, the mucosal surface heals rapidly, and the area usually regenerates within a few days once the irritating stimulus has been removed. Cell regeneration is impaired, however, when the injury is extensive or prolonged. Radiation, anticancer drugs, and other factors that impair the growth of rapidly proliferating cells interfere with regeneration of the gastrointestinal mucosal lining. Treatment with anticancer agents frequently causes such side effects as stomatitis, anorexia, nausea, vomiting, and diarrhea.

Smooth muscle of the gastrointestinal tract heals by scar tissue replacement. Thus, when the injury extends into the smooth muscle layer, regeneration of both the muscularis and the mucosal layers is impaired; this renders the area more susceptible to future irritation and injury.

Esophagus

The esophagus is a tube that connects the oropharynx with the stomach. It lies posterior to the trachea and larynx and extends through the mediastinum, intersecting the diaphragm at the level of the 11th thoracic vertebra. The esophagus functions primarily as a conduit for passage of food from the pharynx to the stomach, and the structures of its walls are designed for this purpose; the smooth muscle layers provide the peristaltic movements needed to move food along its length, while the epithelial layer secretes mucus, which protects its surface and aids in lubricating food.

The act of swallowing depends on the coordinated action of the tongue and pharynx. These structures are innervated by the 5th, 9th, 10th, and 12th cranial nerves. *Dysphagia* refers to difficulty in deglutition (the act of swallowing). It can result from altered nerve function or from narrowing of the esophagus. Lesions of the central nervous system, such as a stroke, often involve the cranial nerves that control deglutition. Cancer of the esophagus and stenosis resulting from scarring reduce the size of the esophageal lumen and make swallowing difficult.

In achalasia, the lower esophageal sphincter fails to relax. Food that has been swallowed has difficulty passing into the stomach, and the esophagus

above the sphincter becomes enlarged. One or several meals may lodge in the esophagus and pass slowly into the stomach over a period of time. There is the risk of aspiration of esophageal contents into the lungs when the person lies down. Treatment is mechanical dilatation or surgical procedures to weaken the sphincter.

Esophagitis

Esophagitis refers to inflammation of the esophagus. Causative agents include chemical injury (lye, ammonia, and other caustic substances), infections, and trauma from repeated ingestion of irritating foods, such as hot liquids and spicy foods. The most common cause of esophagitis is the reflux of gastric secretions into the esophagus as the result of a hiatal hernia. Symptoms associated with esophagitis include heartburn and pain. The pain is usually located in the epigastric or retrosternal area and often radiates to the throat, shoulder, or back. As with inflammation of the mucosal layer in other parts of the gastrointestinal tract, esophagitis causes hyperemia, edema, and erosion of the luminal surface. When the damage is severe or prolonged, scarring occurs and the wall of the esophagus becomes thickened and fibrotic; this leads to difficulty in swallowing.

Hiatal hernia

A hiatal, or diaphragmatic, hernia is the herniation of the stomach through the diaphragm into the thorax. Because intra-abdominal pressure is greater than thoracic pressure, the main problem associated with a hiatal hernia is reflux of gastric secretions into the esophagus.

There are two types of hiatal hernias. The more common one is the sliding type in which the esophagogastric junction slides into the thoracic cavity when the person lies down, then moves back into the abdomen when the person assumes the upright position. The rolling, or paraesophageal, hernia is the condition in which the gastroesophageal junction remains in its normal anatomical position while the curvature of the stomach herniates through the diaphragmatic opening (Figure 40-1).

Conditions that predispose to the development of a hiatal hernia and reflux of gastric contents into the esophagus include (1) congenital or acquired weakness of the hiatal muscle, (2) conditions that increase intra-abdominal pressure (*e.g.*, obesity, pregnancy, tight-fitting clothes, and ascites), or (3) a congenital or acquired shortening of the esophagus. The latter can occur with extensive scarring of the esophagus or can result from reflex spasms.

The signs and symptoms of a hiatal hernia are

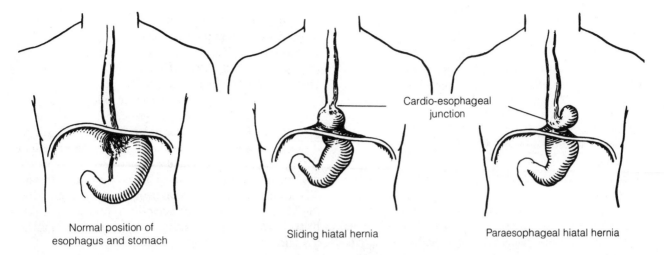

Normal position of esophagus and stomach

Cardio-esophageal junction

Sliding hiatal hernia

Paraesophageal hiatal hernia

Figure 40-1 Normal position of the esophagus and stomach and positional changes that occur with a sliding and paraesophageal hernia. (*Brunner LS, Suddarth DS: Textbook of Medical Surgical Nursing, 3rd ed. Philadelphia, JB Lippincott, 1975*)

related to the reflux of gastric contents into the esophagus. The most common manifestation is pain and heartburn, which occur about ½ hour to 1 hour following a meal. Heartburn is aggravated by any bodily position, such as the recumbent position, that increases the reflux. Often the heartburn occurs during the night. Because of its location, the pain may be confused with angina. Swelling or stenosis caused by scar tissue may cause dysphagia.

The treatment of a hiatal hernia generally focuses on conservative measures. These measures include avoidance of positions and conditions that increase gastric reflux. Frequent, small feedings are preferred to large meals because they prevent gastric distention. It is recommended that meals be eaten sitting up and that the recumbent position be avoided for several hours following a meal. Bending for long periods should be avoided, because it tends to increase intra-abdominal pressure and cause gastric reflux. Sleeping with several pillows helps to prevent reflux during the night. When esophagitis occurs, it may be necessary to institute treatment measures, such as the use of antacids, to reduce gastric secretions. Surgical treatment may become necessary when persistent gastric reflux causes damage to the esophageal wall and cannot be controlled by conservative means.

Esophageal diverticulum

A diverticulum of the esophagus is an outpouching of the esophageal wall caused by a weakness of the muscularis layer. An esophageal diverticulum tends to retain food. Complaints that the food stops before it reaches the stomach are very common, as are reports of gurgling, belching, coughing, and foul-smelling breath. Additionally, the trapped food may cause esophagitis and ulceration. Because the condition is usually progressive, correction of the defect requires surgical intervention.

Carcinoma of the esophagus

Carcinoma of the esophagus accounts for 2% of all cancer deaths in the United States. This disease is common in men over age 60.[3] It is reported that environmental factors contribute to the development of esophageal cancers. These environmental factors include (1) alterations in function that cause food or drink to remain in the esophagus for prolonged periods of time, (2) reflux esophagitis, and (3) continued exposure to irritants such as alcohol and tobacco. The incidence of esophageal cancer among heavy drinkers is 25 times greater than that of nondrinkers. In contrast to cancer of the lung, esophageal cancer is seen more frequently among pipe and cigar smokers than cigarette smokers. Unfortunately, the outlook for persons with cancer of the esophagus is particularly grim, the 5-year survival rate with radiotherapy and surgical resection being only about 5% to 10%.[3] This is because the tumor has usually spread to other areas before symptoms develop.

Stomach

The stomach is a large reservoir for the digestive tract; it lies in the upper abdomen, anterior to the pancreas, splenic vessels, and left kidney. Anteriorly, the stomach is bounded by the anterior abdominal wall and the left inferior lobe of the liver. While in the stomach, food is churned and mixed with hydrochloric acid and pepsin before being released into the small intestine.

Gastric mucosal barrier

Normally, the stomach lining is impermeable to the acid it secretes, a property that allows the stomach to contain acid and pepsin without having its wall digested. Several factors contribute to the protection of the gastric mucosa including: (1) an impermeable cell surface covering, (2) mechanisms for the selective transport of hydrogen and bicarbonate ions, and (3) the characteristics of gastric mucus.[4] These mechanisms are collectively referred to as the *gastric mucosal barrier.*

The gastric mucosal cells are covered with an impermeable hydrophobic lipid layer that prevents diffusion of ionized water-soluble molecules. Aspirin, which is unionized and lipid-soluble in acid solutions, rapidly diffuses across this lipid layer increasing mucosal permeability and destroying epithelial cells. Occult bleeding due to gastric irritation occurs in a significant number of persons who take aspirin on a regular basis (*e.g.,* as a treatment for arthritis).[3] Aspirin becomes ionized in neutral or basic solutions; therefore, buffered aspirin is less likely to penetrate the cell surface covering and cause gastric irritation. Alcohol, which is also lipid-soluble, is known to disrupt the mucosal barrier; and when aspirin and alcohol are taken in combination, as they often are, there is increased risk of gastric irritation. Bile acids also attack the lipid components of the mucosal barrier and afford the potential for gastric irritation when there is reflux of duodenal contents into the stomach.

Normally, the secretion of hydrochloric acid secretion by the parietal cells of the stomach is accompanied by secretion of bicarbonate ions. For every hydrogen ion that is secreted, a bicarbonate ion is produced and diffuses out of the cell. The bicarbonate ion serves to buffer the hydrogen ions, and, as long as bicarbonate ion production is equal to hydrogen ion secretion, mucosal injury does not occur. Changes in gastric blood flow, as in shock, tend to decrease bicarbonate production. This is particularly true in situations in which decreased blood flow is accompanied by acidosis. Aspirin and the nonsteroidal anti-inflammatory drugs (NSAIDs) such as indomethacin and ibuprofen also impair bicarbonate secretion.

The mucus that protects the gastric mucosa is of two types: water-insoluble and water-soluble.[4] Water-insoluble mucus forms a thin stable gel that adheres to the gastric mucosal surface and provides protection from the proteolytic (protein-digesting) actions of pepsin. It also forms an unstirred layer that traps bicarbonate, forming an alkaline interface between the luminal contents of the stomach and its mucosal surface. The water-insoluble mucus is washed from the mucosal surface and mixes with the luminal contents; its viscid nature makes it a lubricant that prevents mechanical damage to the mucosal surface. In addition to their effects on mucosal permeability and bicarbonate production, damaging agents such as aspirin and the NSAIDs inhibit and modify the characteristics of gastric mucus.

It is becoming increasingly evident that production of prostaglandins is an important factor in protecting the gastrointestinal mucosa from injury. The prostaglandins probably exert their effect through improved blood flow, increased bicarbonate ion secretion, and improved mucus production and characteristics. The fact that drugs such as aspirin and the NSAIDs inhibit prostaglandin synthesis probably further contributes to their ability to produce gastric irritation.

Gastritis

Acute gastritis. Acute gastritis is a transient irritation of the gastric mucosa caused by local irritants such as bacterial endotoxins, caffeine, alcohol, and aspirin. The complaints of persons with acute gastritis vary. Often, persons with aspirin-related gastritis are totally unaware of the condition or may complain only of heartburn or sour stomach. Gastritis associated with excessive alcohol consumption is a different situation: it often causes transient gastric distress, which may lead to vomiting and, in more severe situations, to bleeding and hematemesis. Gastritis caused by infectious organisms, such as the staphylococcus endotoxins, usually has an abrupt and violent onset, with gastric distress and vomiting, following the ingestion of a contaminated food source by about 5 hours. Acute gastritis is usually a self-limiting disorder; complete regeneration and healing usually occur within several days.

Chronic gastritis. Chronic gastritis is a separate entity from that of acute gastritis. This condition is characterized by progressive and irreversible atrophy of the glandular epithelium of the stomach. Atrophy of the epithelial layer involves the pepsin-producing chief cells and the acid-producing parietal cells. The parietal cells also produce intrinsic factor, which is required for vitamin B_{12} absorption. This means that both achlorhydria (lack of hydrochloric acid) and pernicious anemia occur when there is extensive atrophy of the gastric mucosa.

There appear to be two forms of chronic gastritis. The most common form is referred to as *simple atrophic gastritis.* Simple atrophic gastritis is seen most frequently in elderly persons and in heavy drinkers or cigarette smokers. A second form of the disorder, *autoimmune atrophic gastritis,* is thought to be caused by antibodies that destroy gastric mucosal cells. With the simple form of the disease there is usually only moderate impairment of acid and pepsin secretion, and vitamin B_{12} absorption remains unimpaired. This retention of acid production in a mucosal surface that has impaired defenses predisposes to peptic ulcer formation. Persons with autoimmune gastritis usually have severe impairment of acid and pepsin secretion, and about 20% of such persons have pernicious anemia.

The signs and symptoms of chronic gastritis are rather vague. Often the disorder produces no discernible symptoms. Symptoms, when they do occur, range from mild distress to complaints similar to those of peptic ulcer. In contrast to gastric ulcer pain, the discomfort associated with atrophic gastritis is not relieved by antacid therapy, nor does true gastritis pain occur during the night.

The clinical significance of atrophic gastritis resides not in its symptoms, but in its ability to produce more serious disorders—namely, pernicious anemia. Although chronic gastritis can occur without impairment of vitamin B_{12} absorption, pernicious anemia develops only in its presence. When pernicious anemia is present, there is an accompanying histamine-fast lack of hydrochloric acid.

Atrophic gastritis also predisposes to gastric ulcer, anemia, and cancer of the stomach. It has been estimated that 50% of persons with gastric ulcers have an associated chronic gastritis. A second problem that frequently occurs with chronic gastritis is a recurrent iron-deficiency anemia. The cause of this anemia is unclear, although there is evidence to suggest that a minimum level of hydrochloric acid is required for iron absorption. A more serious outcome is cancer of the stomach. Approximately 7% to 10% of persons with atrophic gastritis eventually develop gastric carcinoma.[5]

Peptic ulcers

Gastric and peptic ulcers, with their remissions and exacerbations, represent a chronic health problem. At present, 10% of the population has or will develop a peptic ulcer. As a health problem, ulcer disease accounts for 10% of hospital admissions. In terms of location, duodenal ulcers are five to ten times more common than gastric ulcers. Ulcers in the duodenum occur at any age and are frequently seen in early adulthood. Interestingly, duodenal ulcers seem to have a seasonal trend, with a higher incidence of recurrence in the spring and fall. Gastric ulcers, on the other hand, tend to affect the older age group with peak incidence in the sixth and seventh decades. Both types of ulcers affect men three to four times as frequently as they do women.

At present, there is considerable confusion regarding the terms *peptic ulcer* and *gastric ulcer*. A peptic ulcer can occur in any area of the gastrointestinal tract that is exposed to acid–pepsin secretions. For example, ulcerations in the esophagus caused by reflux of gastric secretions would be classified as a peptic ulcer. Peptic ulcers also occur in the stomach, in the duodenum, at the surgical junction where the stomach has been resected and joined to the jejunum (gastrojejunostomy), and in a Meckel's diverticulum that contains misplaced gastric tissue. A gastric ulcer, as the word implies, is an ulcer of the stomach. An ulcer of the stomach can be either a peptic gastric ulcer or a gastric ulcer associated with chronic gastritis. The remaining discussion of ulcers focuses on peptic ulcer, although the reader is reminded that not all stomach ulcers are peptic ulcers.

Predisposing factors. A peptic ulcer represents a break in the continuity of the mucosal layer. Generally speaking, it can be said that peptic ulcer formation reflects (1) an imbalance between acid and pepsin production or (2) an inability of the affected gastric mucosal barrier to resist the destructive action of these digestive agents. Seldom can ulcer development be traced to a single cause. It is more likely that both factors contribute to the development of a peptic ulcer. Nevertheless, it seems helpful, in terms of understanding ulcer development, to view these differences in causation in terms of the function that the mucosal surface affords the stomach and the duodenum.

Increased acid–pepsin production. Hydrochloric acid production is influenced by several factors, including neural and hormonal stimulation. The hormone gastrin, which is produced in the antrum of the stomach, is a potent stimulus for hydrochloric acid secretion. Increased levels of gastric acid have also been attributed to (1) increased numbers of acid–pepsin producing cells in the stomach, (2) increased sensitivity of the parietal cells to food and other stimuli (*e.g.*, both alcohol and caffeine are potent stimulators of hydrochloric acid secretion), (3) excessive vagal stimulation, and (4) impaired inhibition of gastric secretions as food moves into the intestine.

The intractable peptic ulcers observed in the *Zollinger-Ellison syndrome* are caused by a gastrin-secreting tumor of the pancreas. Normally, gastrin secretion is inhibited as food moves into the intestine. It has been postulated that this reflex inhibition of gastrin may be impaired in certain types of ulcers. For example, *Cushing's ulcer* is a special type of stress ulcer that occurs in association with severe brain injury or neurosurgery. It results from increased central stimulation of the vagus nerve, which is unresponsive to reflex mechanisms that normally control gastric secretions.

Resistance of the mucosal surface. The defenses of the mucosal surface depend on an adequate blood flow and an intact mucosal barrier. It can be assumed that any disruption in the mucosal barrier reduces these defenses and renders the mucosal surface more susceptible to the destructive effects of the hydrogen ion.

It has been suggested that a basic abnormality in persons with gastric peptic ulcers is an increased permeability of the epithelial layer of the stomach to hydrogen ions, which causes injury to the mucosal surface and reduces its resistance to further injury. It also is possible that a chronically diseased mucosal membrane is unable to secrete sufficient mucus to form an effective barrier. Reflux of bile from the intestine into the stomach has been implicated in peptic ulcer. In addition to bile, a number of drugs are recognized as "barrier breakers." Both aspirin and alcohol are known to damage this barrier.

The duodenum, which acts as a passageway for digestive enzymes and acid-laden chyme, is a common site of peptic ulcers. Brunner's glands, located between the pylorus and the site where bile and pancreatic enzymes enter the duodenum, produce a large amount of viscid mucus, which serves to protect this area. The activity of these glands is inhibited by sympathetic stimulation; this may help to explain why anxiety and stress contribute to duodenal ulcer development.

Of recent interest is the identification of a gram-negative, S-shaped bacterium, called *Campylobacter pylori,* which colonizes the mucus-secreting epithelial cells of the stomach.[6] In this location, the organism is protected from gastric acid by the overlying layer of bicarbonate-rich mucus. Because the organism will only adhere to mucus-secreting cells in the stomach, it does not usually colonize other parts of the gastrointestinal tract. The *C. pylori* has the unique capacity to interfere with the local protection of the gastric mucosa against acid. It attaches to gastric epithelium and digests the protective layer of mucus, creating areas of denuded mucosa. Since its identification in 1982, the organism has generated worldwide interest. It has been reported that up to 90% of persons with duodenal ulcer and 70% of persons with gastric ulcer have *C. pylori* infection and active chronic gastritis. Eradication of the organism can result in resolution of gastritis, with subsequent ulcer healing. At present, it is not known if *C. pylori* infection, in and of itself, can cause peptic ulcer. Some persons may have a bout of acute gastritis, but their immune system is able to eradicate the organism; others may be left with permanently damaged gastric mucosa that is susceptible to erosion and ulcer. The role, if any, that *C. pylori* plays in the development of gastritis and peptic ulcer is expected to become clearer as more definitive information becomes available.

Manifestations and complications. The clinical manifestations of uncomplicated peptic ulcer focus on discomfort and pain. The pain, which is described as burning, gnawing, or cramplike, is usually rhythmic and frequently occurs when the stomach is empty—between meals and at 1 o'clock or 2 o'clock in the morning. The pain is usually located over a small area near the midline in the epigastrium near the xiphoid and may radiate below the costal margins, into the back, or rarely, to the right shoulder. Characteristically, the pain is relieved by food or antacids. Superficial and deep epigastric tenderness and voluntary muscle guarding may occur with more extensive lesions.

A peptic ulcer can affect one or all layers of the stomach or duodenum. The ulcer may penetrate only the mucosal surface, or it may extend into the smooth muscle layers. Occasionally, an ulcer will penetrate the outer wall of the stomach or duodenum. Spontaneous remissions and exacerbations are common. Healing of the muscularis layer involves replacement with scar tissue; although the mucosal layers that cover the scarred muscle layer regenerate, the regeneration is often less than perfect, which contributes to repeated episodes of ulceration. Precipitating factors include trauma, infections, and physical or emotional stress.

The complications of peptic ulcer include hemorrhage, obstruction, and perforation. Hemorrhage is caused by bleeding from granulation tissue or from erosion of an ulcer into an artery or vein. It occurs in 10% to 15% of persons with peptic ulcer. Evidence of bleeding may consist of hematemesis or melena. Bleeding may be sudden, severe, and without warning, or it may be insidious, producing only occult (hidden) blood in the stool. Acute hemorrhage is evidenced by the sudden onset of weakness, dizziness, thirst, cold moist skin, the desire to defecate, and the passage of loose tarry or even red stools, and coffee-ground emesis. Signs of circulatory shock develop depending on the amount of blood that is lost.

Obstruction is caused by edema, spasm, or contraction of scar tissue and interference with the free passage of gastric contents through the pylorus or adjacent areas. There is a feeling of epigastric fullness and heaviness after meals; with severe obstruction, there is vomiting of undigested food. The presence of an overnight gastric residual of 50 ml of undigested food indicates obstruction.

Perforation occurs when an ulcer erodes through all the layers of the stomach or duodenum wall. With perforation, gastrointestinal contents enter the peritoneum and cause peritonitis, or penetrate adjacent structures such as the pancreas. Radiation of the pain into the back, severe night distress, inadequate pain relief from eating foods or taking antacids in persons with a long history of peptic ulcer may signify penetration. Peritonitis is discussed as a separate topic at the end of this chapter.

Diagnosis. Diagnostic procedures for peptic ulcer include history, laboratory findings, radiologic imaging, and endoscopic examination. Laboratory findings of hypochromic anemia and occult blood in the stools indicate bleeding. Gastric analysis (see Chapter 39) may be done to determine hypersecretion of gastric acids. Radiographic (x-ray) studies using a contrast media are used to detect the presence of an ulcer crater and to rule out gastric carcinoma. Gastroscopy and duodenoscopy can be used to visualize the ulcer area.

Treatment. Treatment of peptic ulcer focuses on measures to (1) decrease or neutralize the hydrochloric acid, (2) increase the resistance of the mucosal layer, and (3) promote healing.

Conservative treatment measures include (1) efforts to relieve stress and anxiety, (2) dietary management, (3) antacids, and (4) other medications that act to reduce gastric-acid secretion. Smoking has been shown to decrease the rate of ulcer healing and should be discouraged.

Although in the past the conservative treatment of peptic ulcers has usually included use of a bland diet, at present there is considerable controversy over its value. Most physicians would agree that coffee and alcoholic beverages should be avoided. Most physicians would agree, too, that the use of food as an antacid should also be avoided, because such feedings

are generally accompanied by a rebound increase in gastric acid secretion. The value of the hourly milk-and-cream regimen, which has been used for years, has also come under question. There is evidence that the calcium in milk may act as a stimulus for gastrin release and thereby increase gastric acid secretion. The use of milk and cream is also associated with an increased risk of developing the milk-alkali syndrome.

Medications used in the treatment of peptic ulcers include the selective use of antacids, mucosal protective agents, anticholinergic drugs, histamine$_2$ (H$_2$)-receptor antagonists, and sedatives or tranquilizers (Table 40-1). Anticholinergic drugs are less effective inhibitors of gastric acid secretions than antacids and H$_2$-receptor antagonists, and therefore they are usually used in combination with other methods of treatment. Sedatives and tranquilizers are individualized forms of treatment used for persons in whom stress is a large contributing factor.

Antacids. Antacids, either self-prescribed or physician-prescribed, represent a large business in the United States, with millions of dollars spent each year for these medications. Essentially four types of antacids are used to relieve gastric acidity: sodium bicarbonate, calcium carbonate, aluminum hydroxide, and magnesium hydroxide. Because *sodium bicarbonate* is water-soluble, it leaves the stomach rapidly and produces a very transient effect. It contains large amounts of sodium and tends to cause metabolic alkalosis. It is mainly used as a home remedy. *Calcium preparations* are constipating and may cause hypercalcemia and the milk-alkali syndrome. There is also evidence that oral calcium preparations increase gastric-acid secretion after their buffering effect has been utilized. *Magnesium hydroxide* is a potent antacid that acts as a

Table 40–1. Drugs used in treatment of peptic ulcer

Drug	Mechanisms of action
Anticholinergics	Block vagal stimulation of gastric acid secretion
	Decrease gastric motility, allowing antacids to remain in the stomach
Antacids	
Calcium carbonate	Neutralizes the gastric acid, but may cause rebound gastric acid secretion
	Can cause hypercalcemia associated with the milk-alkali syndrome
	Has a constipating effect
Magnesium hydroxide	Neutralizes gastric acid
	About 5% to 10% is absorbed in the intestine and may cause an increase in blood magnesium levels in persons with renal failure
	Has a laxative effect
Aluminum hydroxide	Neutralizes gastric acid; has a constipating effect
	Binds with phosphate in the intestine and can cause phosphate depletion and osteoporosis
	May also bind with other substances and drugs, increasing their excretion in the stool
H$_2$-receptor antagonists	Block histamine$_2$ receptors, inhibiting gastric acid secretion
Sedatives and tranquilizers	Relieve anxiety and tension in persons in whom this is a problem

laxative. Approximately 5% to 10% of the magnesium in this preparation is absorbed from the intestine; therefore, magnesium hydroxide should not be used in persons with renal failure, because magnesium must be excreted through the kidneys. *Aluminum hydroxide* reacts with hydrochloric acid to form aluminum chloride. It combines with phosphate in the intestine and prolonged use may lead to phosphate depletion and osteoporosis. Antacids can alter the absorption, bioavailability, and renal elimination of a number of drugs; this should be considered when antacids are administered with other medications. Many antacids contain a combination of ingredients, such as magnesium aluminum hydroxide. Antacids (aluminum hydroxide and magnesium carbonate) in combination with alginic acid (Gaviscon) tend to reduce acid reflux and are widely used in the treatment of reflux esophagitis.

H₂-receptor antagonists. Histamine is the major physiologic mediator for hydrochloric acid secretion. The H₂-receptor antagonists, cimetidine (Tagamet), ranitidine (Zantac), and famotidine (Pepcid) block gastric acid secretion stimulated by histamine, gastrin, and acetylcholine. The volume of both gastric secretion and concentration of pepsin is also reduced. These drugs are relatively well-tolerated. Central nervous system dysfunction such as slurred speech and delirium can occur in elderly persons. Cimetidine can reduce liver blood flow and interfere with the oxidative metabolism of drugs such as the warfarin-type anticoagulants, phenytoin, propranolol, chlordiazepoxide, diazepam, and theophylline. Cimeditine binds to androgen receptors and can cause gynecomastia in men and galactorrhea in women.

Mucosal protective agents. The drug sucralfate (Carafate), or aluminum sucrose sulfate, selectively binds to necrotic ulcer tissue and serves as a barrier to acid, pepsin, and bile. In addition, sucralfate may directly absorb bile salts. It is not absorbed systemically. The drug requires an acid *p*H for activation and should not be administered with antacids or a histamine₂ antagonist.

Surgical treatment. When the conservative management of peptic ulcer is ineffective, surgical intervention is often needed. Three types of surgical procedures are done: (1) subtotal gastrectomy, in which 75% to 80% of the stomach is removed and the remaining portion is attached to the jejunum; (2) truncal vagotomy and drainage, in which the vagus nerve trunks are cut and the outlet of the stomach is enlarged; and (3) truncal vagotomy and antrectomy, in which the vagus nerve trunks are cut and the distal 50% of the stomach is removed.

One of the complications following surgery for peptic ulcers is the *dumping syndrome.* It occurs to some extent in about 20% of persons who have this type of operation. It is believed to be caused by the rapid entry of hyperosmolar liquids into the intestine and is characterized by symptoms such as nausea, vomiting, diarrhea, diaphoresis, palpitations, tachycardia, light-headedness, and flushing that occur either while eating or shortly after. It is often followed (in about 2 hours) by an episode of hypoglycemia, resulting from the rapid absorption of glucose, which acts as a stimulus for insulin release by the beta cells of the pancreas. Treatment consists of limiting the diet to small, frequent feedings, which are taken without liquids and which are low in simple sugars (these are the most osmotically active parts of the diet). Symptoms usually diminish with time.

Zollinger-Ellison syndrome. The Zollinger-Ellison syndrome is a rare condition caused by a gastrin-secreting tumor. In persons with this disorder, gastric acid secretion reaches such levels that ulceration becomes inevitable. The tumors may be single or multiple; although most tumors are located in the pancreas, a few develop in the submucosa of the stomach or duodenum. About two-thirds of these tumors are malignant.[7] The increased gastric secretions cause symptoms related to peptic ulcer. Diarrhea may occur secondary to hypersecretion or as a result of inactivation of intestinal lipase and impaired fat digestion that occurs with a decrease in intestinal *p*H. The diagnosis of the Zollinger-Ellison syndrome is based on elevated serum gastrin levels and elevated basal gastric acid levels. H₂-receptor blocking drugs are used to control gastric acid secretion. Computerized tomography (CT) scan, abdominal ultrasonography, and selective angiography are used to localize the tumor. Surgical removal is indicated in situations in which the tumor is malignant and has not undergone metastasis. Gastrectomy surgery and vagotomy may be done in selected cases.

Stress ulcers. A stress ulcer, sometimes called a *Curling's ulcer,* refers to gastrointestinal ulcerations that develop in relation to major physiologic stress. These lesions occur most often in the gastric fundus and are thought to result from ischemia, tissue acidosis, and bile salts entering the stomach in critically ill persons with decreased gastrointestinal tract motility.[8,9] They are usually manifested by upper gastrointestinal tract bleeding. Persons at high risk for developing stress ulcers include those with large surface area burns, trauma, sepsis, acute respiratory distress syndrome, severe liver failure, and major surgical procedures. Monitoring and maintaining gastric *p*H >3.5 helps to prevent the development of stress ulcers. Antacids, H$_2$-receptor antagonists, and sucralfate are used in both prevention and treatment of stress ulcers. Prostaglandins have been used experimentally to promote ulcer healing.

Cancer of the stomach

Cancer of the stomach strikes approximately 24,000 persons each year and accounts for 10% of cancer deaths.[10] Although its incidence has decreased about 40% in the last 30 years, it remains the seventh leading cause of death in the United States.[10] Among the factors that increase the risk of gastric cancer are a genetic predisposition, carcinogenic factors in the diet (*e.g.*, nitrates, smoked foods), atrophic gastritis, and gastric polyps. Fifty percent of gastric cancers occur in the pyloric region or adjacent to the antrum. Compared with a benign ulcer, which has smooth margins and is concentrically shaped, gastric cancers tend to be larger, are irregularly shaped, have irregular margins, and are usually located in the greater curvature of the stomach.

Unfortunately, stomach cancers are often asymptomatic until late in their course. Symptoms, when they do occur, are usually vague and include indigestion, anorexia, weight loss, vague epigastric pain, vomiting, and an abdominal mass. Diagnosis of gastric cancer is accomplished by means of a variety of techniques, including barium x-ray studies, gastroscopy studies with biopsy, and cytologic studies (Pap smear) of gastric secretions. Cytologic studies can prove particularly useful as a routine screening test in persons with atrophic gastritis or gastric polyps.

Surgery in the form of radical subtotal gastrectomy is usually the treatment of choice. Radiation and chemotherapy have not proved particularly useful as primary treatment modalities in stomach cancer. When these methods are used, it is usually for palliative purposes or to control metastatic spread of the disease.

Small and large intestines

There are many similarities in conditions that disrupt the integrity of the small and large bowels. The wall of both the small and large intestines consists of five layers (see Figure 39-2): an outer serosal layer; a muscularis layer, which is divided into a layer of circular and a layer of longitudinal muscle fibers; a submucosal layer; and an inner mucosal layer, which lines the lumen of the intestine. Among the conditions that predispose to disruption of the integrity of the intestine are inflammatory bowel disease, diverticulitis, appendicitis, and cancer of the colon and rectum.

Inflammatory bowel disease

The term *inflammatory bowel disease* is used to designate two inflammatory gastrointestinal conditions: Crohn's disease and ulcerative colitis. The two conditions affect 200,000 to 500,000 persons in the United States, with an estimated 20,000 to 25,000 new cases each year.[11] They affect both sexes and any age group. Both diseases occur mostly between ages 15 and 20, with a secondary peak between ages 55 and 60. There is evidence to suggest that the incidence of ulcerative colitis, which is an inflammatory disorder of the rectum and colon, has reached a plateau, whereas that of Crohn's disease, which can affect either the large or small bowel, has increased steadily over the past 20 years.

The causes of both Crohn's disease and ulcerative colitis are largely unknown. The diseases appear to have a familial occurrence, which suggests a hereditary predisposition. One of the common beliefs is that hereditary factors increase the susceptibility to other etiologic factors, such as immune responses and viral infections. The Jewish population is especially susceptible to both Crohn's disease and ulcerative colitis. Although psychogenic factors may contribute to the severity and onset of both conditions, it seems unlikely that they are the primary cause.

Both Crohn's disease and ulcerative colitis are considered systemic diseases that affect organs other than the intestine. More than 100 complications have been identified in the two diseases, including erythema nodosum, arthritis, stomatitis, ankylosing spondylitis, autoimmune anemia, hypercoagulability of blood, iritis, myopericarditis, obstructive pulmonary disease, sclerosing cholangitis, and growth retardation in children.[12]

Crohn's disease. Crohn's disease is a recurrent granulomatous type of inflammatory response that can affect any area of the gastrointestinal tract from the mouth to the anus. It is a slowly progressive, relentless, and often disabling disease. The disease usually strikes in early adulthood and affects both men and women equally. Its lesions are observed most frequently in the terminal ileum or ileocecal area of the bowel. The ileum is involved in about 80% of the cases. The colon is the second most common site of involvement, and the condition may be confused with ulcerative colitis. Crohn's disease is a multisystem disease often accompanied by other manifestations, such as arthritis, gallstones, skin disorders, iritis, and keratitis.

A characteristic feature of Crohn's disease is the sharply demarcated granulomatous lesions that occur and that are surrounded by normal-appearing mucosal tissue. When the lesions are multiple, they are often referred to as skip lesions because they are interspersed between what appear to be normal segments of the bowel. All the layers of the bowel are involved, the submucosal layer being affected to the greatest extent. The surface of the inflamed bowel usually has a characteristic "cobblestone" appearance resulting from the fissures and crevices that develop and surround areas of submucosal edema. There is usually a relative sparing of the smooth muscle layers of the bowel with marked inflammatory and fibrotic changes of the submucosal layer. The bowel wall, after a time, often becomes thickened and inflexible; its appearance has been likened to a lead pipe or rubber hose. The adjacent mesentery may become inflamed, and the regional lymph nodes and channels may become enlarged. Fistulas are tubelike passages from a normal cavity or abscess that extend to a free surface of the body or another body cavity. In Crohn's disease, the inflammatory lesions may extend and penetrate the entire wall of the gut, causing abscess formation and the development of fistulous tracts. The characteristics of Crohn's disease are summarized in Table 40-2.

Clinical manifestations. The clinical course of Crohn's disease is variable; often there are periods of exacerbations and remissions, with symptoms being related to the location of the lesions. The principal symptoms include intermittent diarrhea, colicky pain (usually in the lower right quadrant), weight loss, malaise, and low-grade fever. Perianal abscesses and fistula formation are common. Their occurrence is largely due to the severity of the diarrhea, which produces ulceration of the perianal skin. As the disease progresses, there may be bleeding and malabsorption. Complications include intestinal obstruction, abdominal abscess formation, and fistula formation. The overall mortality rate is about 18%. The majority of persons with Crohn's disease eventually develop complications that require surgery.

Diagnosis and treatment. Diagnosis is usually made following x-ray studies of the gastrointestinal tract using barium as a radiopaque contrast medium. Proctosigmoidoscopy is often done to visualize the bowel and to obtain a biopsy.

Treatment methods focus on maintaining adequate nutrition, promoting healing, and preventing and treating complications. Nutritional deficiencies are common in Crohn's disease because of diarrhea, steatorrhea, and other malabsorption problems. A nutritious diet that is high in calories, vitamins, and proteins is recommended. Fats often aggravate the diarrhea, and it is generally recommended that they be avoided. Elemental diets, which are nutritionally balanced, yet are residue free and bulk free, may be given for a period of time during the acute phase of the illness. These diets are largely absorbed in the jejunum and allow the inflamed bowel to rest. Total parenteral nutrition (parenteral hyperalimentation) consists of intravenous administration of hypertonic glucose solutions to which amino acids and fats may be added. This form of nutritional therapy may be needed when food cannot be absorbed from the intestine. Because of the hypertonicity of these solutions, they must be administered through a large-diameter central vein.

In addition to nutritional therapy, sulfasalazine (Azulfidine), a poorly absorbed drug with anti-inflammatory action, and the adrenocorticosteroid hormones are frequently prescribed to treat the acute disease. Surgery is usually reserved for treatment of complications.

Table 40–2. Differentiating characteristics of Crohn's disease and ulcerative colitis

Characteristic	Crohn's disease	Ulcerative colitis
Type of inflammation	Granulomatous	Ulcerative and exudative
Level of involvement	Primarily submucosal	Primarily mucosal
Extent of involvement	Skip lesions	Continuous
Areas of involvement	Primarily ileum Secondarily colon	Primarily rectum and left colon
Diarrhea	Common	Common
Rectal bleeding	Rare	Common
Fistulas	Common	Rare
Strictures	Common	Rare
Perianal abscesses	Common	Rare
Toxic megacolon	Rare	Common
Development of cancer	Rare	Relatively common

Ulcerative colitis. Ulcerative colitis is a nonspecific inflammatory condition of the colon. It usually begins in the rectum and spreads to the left colon. It may involve the entire colon. Like Crohn's disease, the chronic form of the disease is often associated with systemic manifestations such as migratory polyarthritis, ankylosing spondylitis, uveitis, inflammatory liver disease, and various skin manifestations. There are many similarities between ulcerative colitis and Crohn's disease and, at present, it is questioned whether or not the two disorders might represent different manifestations of the same disease.

With ulcerative colitis, the inflammatory process tends to be confluent and continuous instead of skipping areas, as it does in Crohn's disease. Ulcerative colitis affects primarily the mucosal layer, although it can extend into the submucosal layer. Characteristic of the disease are the lesions that form in the crypts of Lieberkühn (see Chapter 39, Figure 39-10) in the base of the mucosal layer. The inflammatory process causes pinpoint mucosal hemorrhages to occur, which in time suppurate and develop into *crypt abscesses*. These inflammatory lesions become necrotic and ulcerate. Although the ulcerations are usually superficial, they often extend, causing large, denuded areas. As a result of the inflammatory process, the mucosal layer often develops tonguelike projections that resemble polyps and are therefore called *pseudopolyps*. Because ulcerative colitis affects the mucosal layer, bleeding is an almost constant manifestation, and bloody diarrhea is the most common complaint during the acute phase of the disease. With repeated episodes of colitis, there is thickening of the bowel wall. The pathologic features of Crohn's disease and ulcerative colitis are summarized in Table 40-2.

Clinical manifestations. Ulcerative colitis usually follows a course of remissions and exacerbations. The severity of the disease varies from mild to fulminating. Accordingly, the disease has been divided into three types depending on its severity: acute fulminating, chronic intermittent, and mild chronic. About 15% to 20% of persons with ulcerative colitis present with the *fulminating form* of the disease. This form presents with an acute episode of bloody diarrhea, fever, and acute abdominal pain. This is the most serious form of the disease, and it has been reported that as many as 35% of persons with severe attacks may die.[13] About 60% have a *mild form* of the disease, in which bleeding and diarrhea are mild and systemic signs are absent. This form of the disease can usually be managed by conservative means. The remainder of the persons with chronic ulcerative colitis have a *chronic form*, which continues after the initial attack. Compared with the milder form, usually more

of the colon surface is involved and the presence of systemic signs and complications is greater.

Diarrhea, which is the characteristic manifestation of ulcerative colitis, will vary according to the severity of the disease. There may be up to 30 to 40 bowel movements a day. Typically, the stools contain blood and mucus. Nocturnal diarrhea is usually present when daytime symptoms are severe. There may be mild abdominal cramping and incontinence of stools. Anorexia, weakness, and fatigability are common.

Complications. *Toxic megacolon* is an acute, life-threatening complication of ulcerative colitis. It is characterized by dilatation of the colon and signs of systemic toxicity. It results from extension of the inflammatory response, with involvement of neural and vascular components of the bowel. Contributing factors include use of laxatives, narcotics, and anticholinergic drugs and the presence of hypokalemia.

Cancer of the colon is one of the feared complications of ulcerative colitis. The risk of developing cancer among persons who have had the disease for 20 years is about 10% to 15%, and after 30 years the risk becomes 30%.[3]

Diagnosis and treatment. Diagnostic measures include colonoscopic examination, often with biopsy. Colon x-ray studies may be done using barium as a radiopaque contrast medium.

Measures used in treating ulcerative colitis vary with the severity of the disease. Hospitalization is required for persons with the acute, fulminating form of the disease. Sulfasalazine may be used for both short-course and long-term therapy. The adrenocorticosteroid hormones are used selectively to lessen the inflammatory response. These drugs can be given by enema or in the form of a suppository. Surgical treatment (removal of the rectum and entire colon) with the creation of an ileostomy may be required for those persons who do not respond to conservative methods of treatment.

——— Diverticular disease

Diverticulosis is a condition in which herniation of the mucosal layer of the colon occurs through the muscularis layer. Diverticular disease is very common in the United States. It is thought to affect about 30% to 50% of persons over age 60.[3] Although the disorder is very prevalent in the developed countries of the world, it is almost nonexistent in many of the African nations and other underdeveloped countries. This suggests that dietary factors (lack of fiber content), a decrease in physical activity, and poor bowel habits (in which the urge to defecate is neglected),

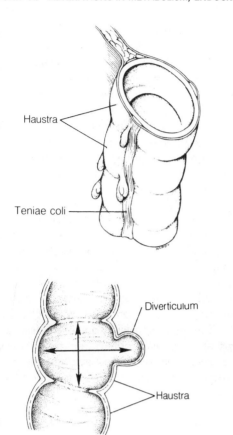

Figure 40-2 **(Top)** A portion of the sigmoid colon, showing the haustra and teniae coli; **(bottom)** a longitudinal section of the colon showing the changes that occur in diverticular disease. The muscle wall is hypertrophied, which causes the haustra to approximate during contractions of the colon. This causes a marked increase in pressure within that segment of the colon, which contributes to diverticulum formation.

along with the effects of aging, contribute to the development of the disease.

Most diverticula occur in the sigmoid colon. In the colon, the longitudinal muscle does not form a continuous layer, as it does in the small bowel. Instead there are three separate longitudinal bands of muscle called the teniae coli (Figure 40-2). It is between these longitudinal muscle bands, in the area where the blood vessels pierce the circular muscle layer to bring blood to the mucosal layer, that diverticula develop. An increase in intraluminal pressure provides the force for creating these herniations. The increase in pressure is thought to be related to the volume of the colonic contents. The more scanty the contents, the more vigorous the contractions and the greater the pressure. When the vigorous contractions continue over time, both the circular and longitudinal muscle layers hypertrophy. In many cases, the haustra (Chapter 39) may become so thick from the hypertrophy that they are approximated during contractions, causing a marked increase in the pressure within the isolated segment. According to the laws of

physics, the pressure within a tube increases as its diameter decreases. The sigmoid colon, which is the segment most vulnerable to the development of diverticula, is the segment of the colon with the narrowest diameter.

The vast majority of persons with diverticular disease remain asymptomatic. The disease is often found when x-ray studies are done for other purposes. When symptoms do occur, they are often attributed to irritable bowel syndrome or other causes. Ill-defined lower abdominal discomfort, a change in bowel habits such as diarrhea and constipation, bloating, and flatulence are often present. One of the most common complaints is pain in the lower left quadrant. When it is accompanied by other symptoms, it is often referred to as *left-sided appendicitis*. This left-sided appendicitis is often accompanied by nausea and vomiting, tenderness in the lower left quadrant, a slight fever, and elevation in white blood cell count. These symptoms usually last for several days, unless complications occur, and are usually caused by localized inflammation of the diverticulitis with perforation and development of a small localized abscess. Complications include perforation with peritonitis, hemorrhage, and bowel obstruction.

The usual treatment for diverticular disease is to prevent symptoms and complications. This includes increasing the bulk in the diet and bowel retraining so that the person has at least one bowel movement a day. According to the laws of physics, the pressure in a tube decreases as the radius increases. Thus, increasing dietary bulk also serves to decrease intraluminal pressure, the result of an increase in colonic contents and colon diameter. Surgical treatment is reserved for complications. The acute phase is treated by withholding solid food and use of a broad-spectrum antibiotic.

Appendicitis

Acute appendicitis is extremely common. It is seen most frequently in the 5-year to 30-year age group, but it can occur at any age. The appendix becomes inflamed, swollen, and gangrenous, and it eventually perforates if not treated. Although the cause of appendicitis is not known, it is thought to be related to intraluminal obstruction due to a fecalith (hard piece of stool) or twisting.

Appendicitis usually has an abrupt onset, with pain referred to the epigastric or periumbilical area. This pain is due to stretching of the appendix during the early inflammatory process. At about the same time that the pain appears, there are one or two episodes of nausea. Initially the pain is vague, but over a period of 2 hours to 12 hours it gradually increases and may become colicky in nature. When the inflammatory process has extended to involve the serosal layer of the appendix and the peritoneum, the pain becomes localized to the lower right quadrant. There is usually an elevation in temperature and a white blood cell count of over 10,000 per mm^3 with 75% or more polymorphonuclear cells. Palpation of the abdomen usually reveals a deep tenderness in the lower right quadrant, which is confined to a small area about the size of the fingertip. It is usually located at about the site of the inflamed appendix. Many times, the person with appendicitis will be able to place his or her finger directly over the tender area. Rebound tenderness, pain that occurs when pressure is applied to the area and then released, and spasm of the overlying abdominal muscles are common. Treatment consists of surgical removal of the appendix. Complications include peritonitis, localized periappendiceal abscess formation, and septicemia.

Colorectal cancer

More than 57,000 persons in the United States die each year of colorectal cancer. It is the second most common site of fatal cancer. The main drawback to successful treatment is the fact that most lesions do not produce symptoms until late in the course of the disease.

Almost all cancers of the colon and rectum are carcinomas. Of these, about 16% occur in the cecum and ascending colon, 8% in the transverse and splenic flexures, 6% in the descending colon, 20% in the sigmoid colon, and 50% in the rectum.[10]

The cause of cancer of the colon and rectum is largely unknown. Its incidence increases with age, as evidenced by the fact that 95% of persons who develop this form of cancer are over age 50. Its incidence is increased in persons with a family history of cancer, in persons with ulcerative colitis, and in those with familial multiple polyposis of the colon.

Usually, cancer of the colon and rectum is present for a long period of time before it produces symptoms. Bleeding is a highly significant early symptom, and it is usually the one that causes people to seek medical care. Other symptoms include a change in bowel habits, either diarrhea or constipation, and sometimes a sense of urgency or incomplete emptying of the bowel. Pain is usually a late symptom.

The prognosis for persons with colorectal cancer depends largely on the extent of bowel involvement and on the presence of metastasis at the time of diagnosis. This form of cancer can be divided into four categories according to the classification system by Duke. The type A tumor is limited to invasion of the mucosal and submucosal layers of the colon and has a 5-year survival rate of almost 100%. Type B tumor involves the entire wall of the colon and has a 5-year survival rate of about 54% to 67%. With type C tumor, there is invasion of the serosal layer, with involvement of the regional lymph nodes. The 5-year survival rate is approximately 23%. Type D colorectal cancer involves far-advanced metastasis.[5]

Diagnosis and treatment. Among the methods used in the diagnosis of colorectal cancers are stool occult blood tests and digital rectal examination, usually done during routine physical examinations; x-ray studies using barium (barium enema); and proctosigmoidoscopy and colonoscopy. Digital rectal examinations are most helpful in detecting neoplasms of the rectum. Rectal examination should be considered a routine part of a good physical examination. Half of all colon and rectal cancers can be detected by digital examination.[10] The American Cancer Society recommends that all asymptomatic men and women over age 50 should have a stool occult blood test and digital rectal examination done every year and a proctosigmoidoscopy examination done every 3 to 5 years after two initial negative examinations done 1 year apart as a means of early detection of colorectal cancer.[14] Persons with a positive stool occult blood test should be referred to their physicians for further study. Usually a physical examination, rectal examination, barium enema, and proctosigmoidoscopy or colonoscopy are done.

Almost all cancers of the colon and rectum bleed intermittently even though the amount of blood is small and usually not apparent in the stools. It is therefore feasible to screen for colorectal cancers using commercially prepared tests for occult blood in the stool that are now available. This method uses a guaiac-impregnated filter paper. The technique involves preparing two slides per day from different portions of the same stool for 3 days to 4 days while the patient follows a high-fiber diet that is free of meat and ascorbic acid. Although the diet is not particularly appealing, this has been shown to be a relatively reliable and inexpensive method of screening for colorectal cancer. Proctosigmoidoscopy involves examination of the rectum and sigmoid colon with a hollow, lighted tube that is inserted through the rectum. Polyps can be removed or tissue obtained for biopsy during the procedure.

Colonoscopy provides a means for direct visualization of the rectum and colon. The colonoscope consists of a flexible 4-cm glass bundle that has some 250,000 glass fibers with a lens at either end to focus and magnify the image. Light from an external source is transmitted by the fiberoptic viewing bundle. Instruments are available that afford direct examination of the sigmoid colon or the entire colon. This method is used for screening persons at high risk for developing cancer of the colon (*e.g.*, those with ulcerative colitis) and for those with symptoms. Colonoscopy is also useful for obtaining a biopsy and for removing polyps. Although this method is one of the most accurate for detecting early colorectal cancers, it is not suitable for mass screening because it is expensive and time-consuming and must be done by a person who is highly trained in the use of the instrument.

The only recognized *treatment* for cancer of the colon and rectum is surgical removal. Preoperative radiation may be used and has in some cases demonstrated increased 5-year survival rates. Postoperative adjuvant therapy with 5-fluorouracil (5-FU) has had some success. Both radiation and chemotherapy are palliative treatment methods.

—— Peritonitis

Peritonitis represents an inflammatory response of the serous membrane that lines the abdominal cavity and covers the visceral organs. It can be caused by either bacterial invasion or chemical irritation. Most commonly, enteric bacteria enter the peritoneum because of a defect in the wall of one of the abdominal organs. The most common causes of peritonitis are perforated peptic ulcer, ruptured appendix, perforated diverticulum, gangrenous bowel, pelvic inflammatory disease, and gangrenous gallbladder. Other causes are abdominal trauma and wounds. Generalized peritonitis, though no longer the overwhelming problem it once was, is still a leading cause of death following abdominal surgery.

The peritoneum has several characteristics that either increase its vulnerability to or protect it against the effects of peritonitis. One weakness of the peritoneal cavity is that it is a large, unbroken space that favors the dissemination of contaminants. For the same reason, it has a large surface that permits rapid absorption of bacterial toxins into the blood. On the other hand, the peritoneum is particularly well adapted for producing an inflammatory response as a means of controlling infection. It tends, for example, to exude a thick, sticky, and fibrinous substance that adheres to other structures, such as the mesentery and omentum, and that serves to seal off the perforated viscus and aid in localizing the process. Localization is further enhanced by sympathetic stimulation that limits intestinal motility. Although the diminished or absent peristalsis that occurs tends to give rise to associated problems, it does inhibit the movement of contaminants throughout the peritoneal cavity.

One of the most important manifestations of peritonitis is the translocation of extracellular fluid into the peritoneal cavity (through weeping or serous fluid from the inflamed peritoneum) and into the bowel as a result of bowel obstruction. Nausea and vomiting cause further losses of fluid. The fluid loss may then encourage development of hypovolemia and shock.

The onset of peritonitis may be acute, as in a ruptured appendix, or it may have a more gradual onset such as occurs in progressive inflammatory disease. Pain and tenderness are common symptoms. The pain is usually more intense over the inflamed area. The person with peritonitis usually lies very still because any movement aggravates the pain. Breathing is often shallow, in order to prevent movement of the abdominal muscles. The abdomen is usually rigid and sometimes described as boardlike, because of reflex muscle guarding. Vomiting is common. Fever, elevation in white blood cell count, tachycardia, and frequently hypotension are present. Hiccups may develop because of irritation of the phrenic nerve. Paralytic ileus occurs shortly after the onset of widespread peritonitis and is accompanied by abdominal distention. Peritonitis that progresses and if untreated leads to toxemia and shock.

Treatment measures for peritonitis are directed toward (1) preventing the extension of the inflammatory response, (2) minimizing the effects of paralytic ileus and abdominal distention, and (3) correcting the fluid and electrolyte imbalances that develop. Surgical intervention may be needed to remove an acutely inflamed appendix or to close the opening in a perforated peptic ulcer. Oral fluids are forbidden. Nasogastric suction, which entails the insertion of a tube (placed through the nose) into the stomach or intestine, is employed to decompress the bowel and relieve the abdominal distention. Fluid and electrolyte replacement is essential. These fluids are prescribed on the basis of frequent blood chemistry determinations. Antibiotics are given to combat infection. Narcotics are often needed for pain relief.

A potential complication of peritonitis is abscess formation. Should it occur, the most desirable area for drainage is into the pelvis rather than into the area under the diaphragm. Therefore, the head of the bed is often elevated about 60 degrees to 70 degrees (semi-Fowler's position) to encourage drainage of inflammatory exudate from the flank area into the pelvis.

In summary, the gastrointestinal tract is a five-layered tube that consists of an inner mucosal layer, a submucosal layer, layers of circular and longitudinal smooth muscle, and an outer serosal layer. Disruption of the integrity of its wall can occur at any level, because of numerous pathologic processes, including injury to the mucosal barrier, inflammation, structural changes, and neoplasms. The manifestations of alterations in the integrity of the digestive system depend on the process involved, the extent of the injury, and the area of the gastrointestinal tract involved.

Alterat

Th...
trointestina...
the submu...
The axons...
plexus inn...
smooth mu...
ceive impu...
cosal and r...
from the p...
systems. A...
vous systen...
whereas sy...
tivity.

Th...
—the ileo...
small intes...
the moven...
as a reser...
ml of wat...
and 15 m...
the colon...
sium is s...
amount o...
stool refle...
the colon...
American...
each day.

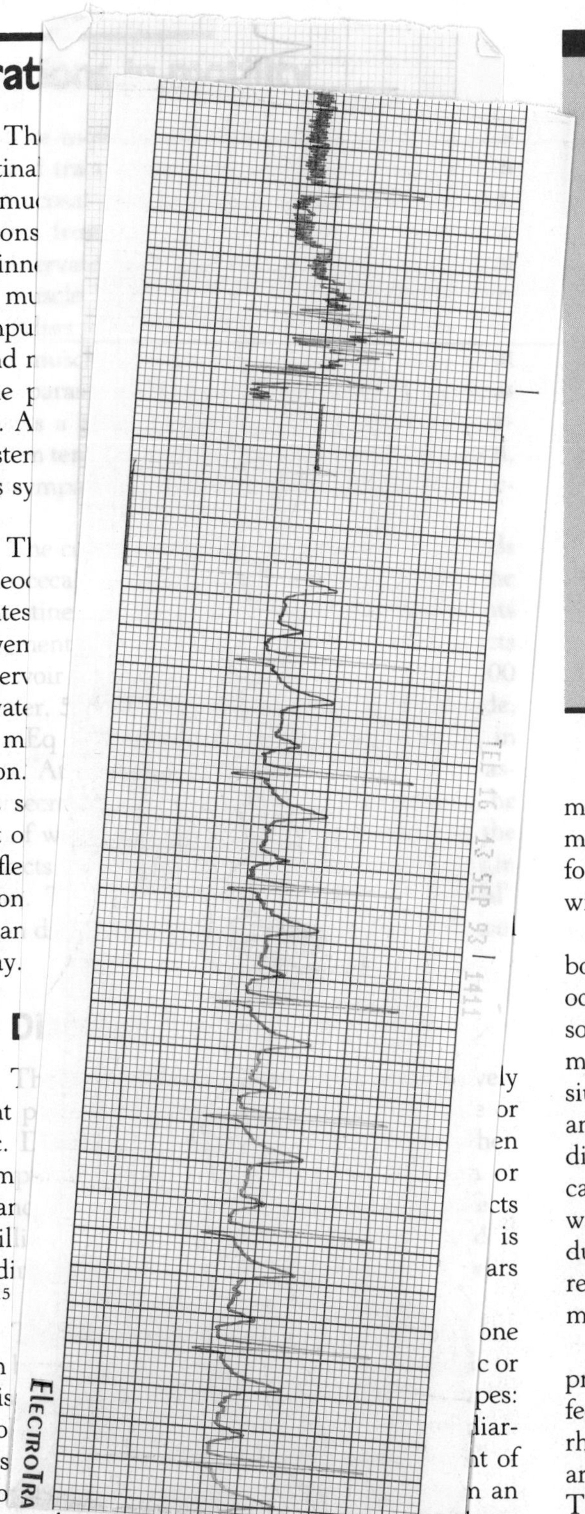

frequent...
chronic. I...
the sym...
adults ar...
500 mil...
the leadi...
of age.[15]

and can...
otherwis...
large-vo...
rhea res...
the stool...
increase in the propulsive activity of the bowel. Some
of the common causes of small- and large-volume diarrhea are summarized in Chart 40-1. Often diarrhea
is a combination of these two types.

Large-volume diarrhea

Large-volume diarrhea can be classified as
secretory or osmotic, according to the cause of the
increased water content in the feces. Water is either
pulled into the colon along an osmotic gradient (os-

Chart 40–1: Causes of large- and small-volume diarrhea

Large-volume diarrhea
Osmotic diarrhea
Saline cathartics
Dumping syndrome
Lactase deficiency
Secretory diarrhea
Failure to absorb bile salts
Fat malabsorption
Chronic laxative abuse
Carcinoid syndrome
Zollinger-Ellison syndrome
Fecal impaction
Acute infectious diarrhea
Small-volume diarrhea
Inflammatory bowel disease
Crohn's disease
Ulcerative colitis
Infectious disease
Shigellosis
Salmonellosis
Irritable colon

motic diarrhea) or is secreted into the bowel by the
mucosal cells (secretory diarrhea). The large-volume
form of diarrhea is usually a painless, watery type
without blood or pus in the stools.

In osmotic diarrhea, water is pulled into the
bowel by the hyperosmotic nature of its contents. It
occurs when osmotically active particles are not absorbed. In lactase deficiency, the lactose present in
milk cannot be broken down and absorbed. Magnesium salts, which are contained in milk of magnesia
and many antacids, are poorly absorbed and cause
diarrhea when taken in sufficient quantities. Another
cause of osmotic diarrhea is decreased transit time,
which interferes with absorption. This happens in the
dumping syndrome, which was discussed earlier in
relation to the surgical treatment of peptic ulcer. Osmotic diarrhea disappears with fasting.

Secretory diarrhea occurs when the secretory
processes of the bowel are increased. Most acute infectious diarrheas are of this type. This type of diarrhea also occurs when excess bile salts or fatty acids
are present in the gut contents as they enter the colon.
This often happens with disease processes of the
ileum, because bile salts are absorbed here. It may also
occur when bacterial overgrowth occurs in the small
bowel, which also interferes with bile absorption.
Some tumors, such as Zollinger-Ellison syndrome and
carcinoid syndrome, cause increased secretory activity
of the bowel.

Fecal impaction (the retention of hard, dried
stool in the rectum and colon) stimulates increased
secretory activity of the portion of the bowel proximal
to the impaction. In this case, the watery stool flows

around the fecal mass, representing the body's attempt to break up the mass so that it can be evacuated. This cause should be considered in any elderly or immobilized person who develops watery diarrhea. Digital examination of the rectum is done to assess for the presence of a fecal mass. In some cases, the mass may need to be removed manually with a gloved finger.

Small-volume diarrhea

Small volume diarrhea is commonly associated with acute or chronic inflammation or intrinsic disease of the colon, such as ulcerative colitis or Crohn's disease. Diarrhea with vomiting and fever suggests food poisoning, often due to staphylococcal enteroxin. Small-volume diarrhea is usually evidenced by frequency and urgency and colicky abdominal pain. It is commonly accompanied by tenesmus (painful straining at stool), fecal soiling of clothing, and awakening during the night with the urge to defecate.

Treatment

Diarrhea causes loss of fluid and electrolytes from the body. While most cases of diarrhea are self-limited and require no treatment, diarrhea can be particularly serious in infants and small children, persons with other illnesses, the elderly, and even previously healthy persons if it continues for any length of time. Fluid and electrolyte corrections are, therefore, considered to be a primary therapeutic goal in the treatment of diarrhea. Oral electrolyte replacement solutions can be given in situations of uncomplicated diarrhea that can be treated at home. Restricting oral foods and fluids may be helpful in acute diarrhea, because this decreases peristalsis. When intake is resumed following diarrhea, the diet should consist of bland foods that will not stimulate gastrointestinal motility. Cold liquids that move rapidly from the stomach to the small intestine and stimulate peristalsis should be avoided.

Drugs used in the treatment of diarrhea include camphorated tincture of opium (paregoric), diphenoxylate (Lomotil), and loperamide (Imodium), which are opium-like drugs. These drugs decrease gastrointestinal motility and stimulate water and electrolyte absorption. Adsorbents, such as kaolin and pectin, are able to adsorb undesirable constituents from solutions. These ingredients are included in many over-the-counter antidiarrheal preparations because they adsorb toxins responsible for certain types of diarrhea. Antibiotics are reserved for persons with identified enteric pathogens.

Constipation

Constipation can be defined as the infrequent passage of stools. The difficulty with this definition arises from the many individual variations of a function that are normal. In other words, what might be considered normal for one person (two or three bowel movements per week) might well be considered evidence of constipation by another.

Some common causes of constipation are failure to respond to the urge to defecate, inadequate fiber in the diet, inadequate fluid intake, weakness of the abdominal muscles, inactivity and bedrest, pregnancy, hemorrhoids, and gastrointestinal disease. Drugs such as narcotics, belladonna derivatives, diuretics, calcium, iron and aluminum hydroxide, and phosphate gels tend to cause constipation. The sudden onset of constipation may indicate serious disease (*e.g.,* one sign of cancer of the colon and rectum is a change in bowel habits).

The *treatment* of constipation is usually directed toward relieving the cause. A conscious effort should be made to respond to the defecation urge. A time should be set aside after a meal, when mass movements in the colon are most apt to occur, for a bowel movement. An adequate fluid intake and bulk in the diet should be encouraged. Moderate exercise is essential, and persons on bedrest benefit from passive and active exercises. Laxatives and enemas should be used judiciously. They should not be used on a regular basis to treat simple constipation because they interfere with the defecation reflex and may actually damage the rectal mucosa.

Intestinal obstruction

Intestinal obstruction designates an impairment of movement of intestinal contents in a cephalocaudal direction. The causes of intestinal obstruction can be categorized under two headings: mechanical and reflex paralytic (adynamic).

Mechanical obstruction can result from a number of conditions, either intrinsic or extrinsic, which encroach on the patency of the bowel lumen. These conditions include adhesions of the peritoneum, hernias, twisting of the bowel (volvulus), telescoping of the bowel (intussusception), fecal impaction, strictures, and tumors. There are three types of mechanical obstruction: simple, strangulated, and closed. With a *simple* obstruction, there is no alteration in blood supply. The term *strangulated* implies impairment of blood flow. When the bowel is obstructed on both ends, it is called a *closed* obstruction.

Reflex paralysis usually affects the small bowel. Because the ileum has the narrowest lumen, it is the most prone to obstruction. *Paralytic ileus* is seen most commonly following abdominal surgery or trauma. It occurs early in the course of peritonitis and can result from chemical irritation caused by bile, bacterial toxins, electrolyte imbalances as in hypokalemia, and vascular insufficiency.

The major effects of both types of intestinal obstruction are intestinal distention and loss of fluids and electrolytes. Gases and fluids accumulate within the area. About 7 liters to 8 liters of electrolyte-rich extracellular fluid move into the small bowel each day, and normally most of this is reabsorbed. Intestinal obstruction interferes with this reabsorption process, and a small amount of this extracellular fluid remains in the bowel or is lost in the vomitus. A loss of 7 liters to 8 liters, which represents about half of the extracellular fluid volume of an average adult, can occur in 24 hours or less following acute intestinal obstruction.

If untreated, the distention resulting from bowel obstruction tends to perpetuate itself by causing atony of the bowel and further distention. Distention is further aggravated by the accumulation of gases. About 70% of these gases are estimated to be due to swallowed air. As the process continues, the distention moves proximally, involving additional segments of bowel.

Either form of obstruction may eventually lead to strangulation, gangrenous changes, and ultimately perforation of the bowel. The increased pressure within the intestine tends to compromise mucosal blood flow, leading to necrosis and exudation of blood into the luminal fluids. This promotes rapid growth of bacteria within the obstructed bowel. Anaerobes grow rapidly in this favorable environment and produce a lethal endotoxin.

The manifestations of intestinal obstruction depend on the degree of obstruction and its duration. With acute obstruction, the onset is usually sudden and dramatic. With chronic conditions, the onset is often more gradual. The cardinal symptoms of intestinal obstruction are pain, absolute constipation, abdominal distention, and vomiting. These symptoms are common to intestinal obstruction resulting from either mechanical obstruction or paralytic ileus. Electrolyte imbalances are also common to both.

With *mechanical obstruction,* there is development of hyperperistalsis as the body attempts to move the contents of the intestine around the occluded area. This causes severe colicky pain, in contrast with the continuous pain and silent abdomen seen with paralytic ileus. With mechanical obstruction, there is also borborygmus (rumbling sounds made by propulsion of gas in the intestine), audible high-pitched peristalsis, and peristaltic rushes. Visible peristalsis may appear along the course of the distended intestine. There is extreme restlessness and conscious awareness of intestinal movements. Weakness, perspiration, and

anxiety are obvious. As the condition progresses, the vomitus may become fecal in nature and the peristaltic movements may decrease, and then disappear as the bowel fatigues.

Should *strangulation* occur, the symptoms change. The character of the pain shifts from the intermittent colicky pain caused by the hyperperistaltic movements of the intestine to a severe, unrelenting pain that is made worse by movement. Signs of *peritoneal irritation,* such as rigidity of the abdomen, become apparent. If bowel sounds had been present, they disappear because of the peritoneal irritation. Strangulation increases the risk of mortality by about 25%.

Diagnosis of intestinal obstruction is usually based on history and physical findings. Abdominal x-ray studies will reveal a gas-filled bowel.

The treatment consists of decompression of the bowel through nasogastric suction and correction of fluid and electrolyte imbalances. Strangulation and complete bowel obstruction require surgical intervention.

In summary, motility of the contents through the gastrointestinal tract relies on the activity of the myenteric plexus, which is located between the circular and longitudinal smooth muscle layers. Alterations in gastrointestinal motility can be evidenced by diarrhea, by constipation, or in acute situations by intestinal obstruction.

Malabsorption

Malabsorption is the failure to transport dietary constituents, such as fats, carbohydrates, proteins, vitamins, and minerals, from the lumen of the intestine to the extracellular fluid compartment for transport to the various parts of the body. It can selectively affect a single component, such as vitamin B_{12} or lactose, or its effects can extend to all the substances absorbed in a specific segment of the intestine. When one segment of the intestine is affected, another may compensate. For example, the ileum may compensate for malabsorption in the proximal small intestine by absorbing substantial amounts of fats, carbohydrates, and amino acids. Similarly, the colon, which normally absorbs water, sodium, chloride, and bicarbonate, can compensate for small intestine malabsorption by absorbing 50% or more of some of the end-products of bacterial carbohydrate metabolism.[16]

The conditions that impair one or more steps involved in digestion and absorption of nutrients can be divided into three broad categories: (1) intraluminal maldigestion, (2) mucosal malabsorption, and

(3) lymphatic obstruction. Intraluminal maldigestion involves a defect in processing of nutrients within the intestinal lumen. The most common causes are pancreatic insufficiency, hepatobiliary disease, and intraluminal bacterial growth. Mucosal malabsorption is caused by mucosal lesions that impair uptake and transport of available intraluminal nutrients across the mucosal surface of the intestine. They include disorders such as celiac disease, tropical sprue, and Crohn's disease. Lymphatic obstruction interferes with the transport of the products of fat digestion to the systemic circulation once they have been absorbed by the intestinal mucosa. The process can be interrupted by congenital defects, neoplasms, trauma, and selected infectious diseases.

Malabsorption syndrome

The term *syndrome* implies a common constellation of symptoms arising from multiple causes. Persons with conditions that diffusely affect the small intestine and reduce its absorptive functions share certain common features referred to as malabsorption syndrome. Among the causes of malabsorption syndrome are sprue, Crohn's disease, and resection of large segments of the small bowel.

Sprue syndromes are diseases of disturbed small intestine function characterized by impaired absorption. Celiac sprue is an intolerance to dietary gluten found in wheat, barley, and rye. There is convincing evidence that the disorder is caused by an

Table 40–3. Sites of and requirements for absorption of dietary constituents and manifestations of malabsorption

Dietary constituent	Site of absorption	Requirements	Manifestations
Water and electrolytes	Mainly small bowel	Osmotic gradient	Diarrhea Dehydration Cramps
Fat	Upper jejunum	Pancreatic lipase Bile salts Functioning lymphatic channels	Weight loss Steatorrhea Fat-soluble vitamin deficiency
Carbohydrates			
Starch	Small intestine	Amylase Maltase Isomaltase α-dextrins	Diarrhea Flatulence Abdominal discomfort
Sucrose	Small intestine	Sucrase	
Lactose	Small intestine	Lactase	
Maltose	Small intestine	Maltase	
Fructose	Small intestine	—	
Protein	Small intestine	Pancreatic enzymes (trypsin, chymotrypsin, elastin, and so forth)	Loss in muscle mass Weakness Edema
Vitamins			
A	Upper jejunum	Bile salts	Night blindness Dry eyes Corneal irritation
Folic acid	Duodenum and jejunum	Absorptive; may be impaired by some drugs (*i.e.*, anticonvulsants)	Cheilosis Glossitis Megaloblastic anemia
B_{12}	Ileum	Intrinsic factor	Glossitis Neuropathy Megaloblastic anemia
D	Upper jejunum	Bile salts	Bone pain Fractures Tetany
E	Upper jejunum	Bile salts	Uncertain
K	Upper jejunum	Bile salts	Easy bruising and bleeding
Calcium	Duodenum	Vitamin D and parathyroid hormone	Bone pain Fractures Tetany
Iron	Duodenum and jejunum	Normal *p*H (hydrochloric acid secretion)	Iron-deficiency anemia Glossitis

immunologic response to the gliadin fraction of gluten. The condition results in loss of absorptive villi from the small intestine. When the resulting lesions are extensive they may impair absorption of virtually all nutrients. In about one-third of cases, symptoms begin in childhood. The effects of celiac sprue are usually reversed after removal of all wheat, rye, barley, and oat gluten from the diet. Corn and rice products are not toxic and can be used as a substitute. In a condition called *tropical sprue,* the changes that occur in the villi resemble those seen in celiac sprue. The cause of this disorder is unclear, although administration of folic acid is known to be helpful in treatment.

Persons with intestinal malabsorption usually have symptoms directly referrable to the gastrointestinal tract that include diarrhea, steatorrhea, flatulence, bloating, abdominal pain, and cramps. Weakness, muscle wasting, weight loss, and abdominal distention are often present. Weight loss often occurs despite normal or excessive caloric intake. Steatorrhea stools contain excess fat. The fat content causes bulky, yellow-gray malodorous stools that float in the toilet and are difficult to dispose of by flushing the toilet. In a person consuming a diet containing 80 g to 100 g of fat a day, excretion of 7 g to 9 g of fat indicates steatorrhea.

Along with loss of fat in the stools, there is failure to absorb the fat-soluble vitamins. This can lead to easy bruising and bleeding (vitamin K deficiency), bone pain, predisposition to develop fractures and tetany (vitamin D and calcium deficiency), macrocytic anemia, and glossitis (folic acid deficiency). Neuropathy, atrophy of the skin, and peripheral edema may be present. Table 40-3 describes the signs and symptoms of impaired absorption of dietary constituents.

In summary, the digestion and absorption of foodstuffs take place in the small intestine. Here proteins, fats, carbohydrates, and other components of the diet are broken down into molecules that can be transported from the intestinal lumen into the body fluids. Malabsorption results when this transport system becomes impaired. It can involve a single dietary constituent or extend to involve all of the substances absorbed in a particular part of the small intestine. Malabsorption can result from disease of the small bowel and disorders that impair digestion and can (in some cases) obstruct the lymph flow by which fats are transported to the general circulation.

References

1. McBryde CM: Signs and Symptoms, p 400. Philadelphia, JB Lippincott, 1970
2. Schiff L, Stevens RJ, Shapiro N et al: Observation of oral administration of citrated blood in man. Am J Med Sci 203:409, 1942
3. Robbins SL, Kumar V: Basic Pathology, 4th ed, pp 511–512, 541, 550. Philadelphia, WB Saunders, 1987
4. Fromm D: Mechanisms involved in gastric mucosal resistance to injury. Annu Rev Med 38:119, 1987
5. Robbins SL, Cotran S, Kumar V: Pathologic Basis of Disease, 3rd ed, pp 810, 873. Philadelphia, WB Saunders, 1984
6. Marshall BJ: Peptic ulcer: An infectious disease. Hosp Pract 22 (Aug 15):87, 1987
7. Wolfe MM, Jensen RT: Zollinger-Ellison syndrome. N Engl J Med 317:1200, 1987
8. Zuckerman GR, Cort D, Schuman RB: Stress ulcer syndrome. J Intensive Care Med 3:21, 1988
9. Konopad E, Noseworthy T: Stress ulceration: A serious complication in critically ill patients. Heart Lung 17:339, 1988
10. Morton JH, Poulter CA, Pandya KJ: Alimentary tract cancer. In Rubin P (ed): Clinical Oncology, 6th ed, pp 159, 167. New York, American Cancer Society, 1983
11. Myer SA: Overview of inflammatory bowel disease. Nurs Clin North Am 19:3, 1984
12. Kirsner JB, Shorter RG: Recent developments in "nonspecific" inflammatory bowel disease. N Engl J Med 306:775, 1982
13. Janowitz HD: Chronic inflammatory disease of the intestine. In Beeson PB, McDermott W, Wyngaarden JB (eds): Cecil Textbook of Medicine, 15th ed, p 1570. Philadelphia, WB Saunders, 1979
14. Holleb AI (ed): Detecting colon and rectum cancer. CA 33(3):5, 1983
15. Bruckstein AH: Acute diarrhea. Am Family Pract 20 (Oct): 217, 1988
16. Trier JS: Intestinal malabsorption: Differentiation of cause. Hosp Pract 23 (May 13):195, 1988

Bibliography

Ballantine TVN: Appendicitis. Surg Clin North Am 6(5):1117, 1981

Binder HJ: The pathophysiology of diarrhea. Hosp Pract 19:107, 1984

Code CF: Prostaglandins and gastric ulcer. Hosp Pract 15(7):1980

Collins RH, Feldman M, Fordtran JS: Colon cancer, dysplasia, and surveillance in patients with ulcerative colitis. N Engl J Med 316:1654, 1987

Donaldson RM: Dyspepsia: The broad etiologic spectrum. Hosp Pract 22 (Sept 30):41, 1987

Drossman DA: Irritable bowel syndrome: A multifactorial disorder. Hosp Pract 23 (Sept 15):119, 1988

Dworkin HJ: Crohn's disease. Ann Intern Med 101:258, 1984

Fischer RS: Modern concepts of peptic ulcer disease: Advances in treatment. Med Times 111:111, 1983

Floch MH: Nutritional support in inflammatory bowel disease. Curr Concepts Gastroenterol 9:13, 1984

Holt KM, Isenberg JI: Peptic ulcer disease: Physiology and pathophysiology. Hosp Pract 20(1):89, 1985

Kirsner JB, Hanauer SB: Crohn's disease: The problem and its management. Hosp Pract 19(7):121, 1984

Kolars JC, Levitt MD, Aouji M et al: Yogurt—An autodigesting source of lactose. N Engl J Med 310:1, 1984

Kramer P: Dysphagia—Etiologic differentiation and therapy. Hosp Pract 23 (Mar 30):125, 1988

Lennard-Jones JE: Functional gastrointestinal disorders. N Engl J Med 308:431, 1983

Lewicki LJ, Leeson MJ: The multisystem impact on physiologic processes of inflammatory bowel disease. Nurs Clin North Am 19:71, 1984

Littman A: Lactose deficiency. Hosp Pract 22 (Jan 30):111, 1987

Myer SA: Overview of inflammatory bowel disease. Nurs Clin North Am 19:3, 1984

Newcomer AD, McGill DB: Clinical importance of lactase deficiency. N Engl J Med 310:42, 1984

Price AB, Levi J, Dolby JM et al: *Campylobacter pyloridis* in peptic ulcer disease: Microbiology, pathology, and scanning electron microscopy. Gut 26:1183, 1985

Richter JE, Castell DO: Gastroesophageal reflux. Ann Intern Med 97:93, 1982

Sanger E, Cassino T: Eating disorders. Am J Nurs 84:31, 1984

Slaughter RL: The disabled esophagus. Emerg Med 20 (Sept 15):99, 1988

Steer ML, Silen W: Diagnostic procedures in gastrointestinal hemorrhage. N Engl J Med 309:646, 1983

Vargas J: Sorting out the causes of vomiting and diarrhea. Emerg Med 20 (Feb 15):139, 1988

Wilson C: The diagnostic work-up for the patient with inflammatory bowel disease. Nurs Clin North Am 19:51, 1984

CHAPTER 41

Alterations in Function of the Hepatobiliary System and Exocrine Pancreas

Objectives

After you have studied this chapter, you should be able to meet the following objectives:

_____ Describe the anatomy of the liver.

_____ Describe the function of the liver as it relates to alcohol metabolism.

_____ Describe the enterohepatic circulation.

_____ Explain the formation and degradation of bilirubin.

_____ Compare hemolytic jaundice and obstructive jaundice with reference to their clinical manifestations.

_____ Summarize the salient features of hepatitis A and hepatitis B with which the health professional should be acquainted.

_____ Characterize postnecrotic cirrhosis and biliary cirrhosis.

_____ Summarize the three stages of alcoholic cirrhosis.

_____ Describe the clinical manifestations of alcoholic cirrhosis with reference to development of collateral channels.

_____ Explain the development of ascites in alcoholic cirrhosis.

_____ State a clinical definition of the _hepatorenal syndrome_.

_____ Explain the basis of bleeding disorders in alcoholic cirrhosis.

_____ Characterize hepatic-systemic encephalopathy.

_____ Explain the significance of the presence of serum alpha fetoprotein in an adult.

_____ Describe the physiology of the gallbladder.

_____ Describe the formation of gallstones.

_____ Compare the symptoms of acute cholecystitis with those of chronic cholecystitis.

_____ Describe the exocrine function of the pancreas.

_____ Describe the clinical manifestations of acute pancreatitis.

_____ Compare chronic calcifying pancreatitis and chronic obstructive pancreatitis.

_____ State a significant statistic relating to pancreatic cancer.

The liver, the gallbladder, and the exocrine pancreas are classified as accessory organs of the gastrointestinal tract. In addition to producing digestive secretions, both the liver and the pancreas have other important functions. The endocrine pancreas, for example, supplies the insulin and glucagon needed in cell metabolism, whereas the liver synthesizes glucose, plasma proteins, and bloodclotting factors and is responsible for the degradation and elimination of drugs and hormones, among other functions. The content of this chapter focuses on disorders of the liver, the biliary tract and gallbladder, and the exocrine pancreas.

Hepatobiliary function

The liver is the largest internal organ in the body, weighing about 1.3 kg, or 3 lb, in the adult. It is located below the diaphragm and occupies much of the right hypochondrium. The falciform ligament, which extends from the peritoneal surface of the anterior abdominal wall between the umbilicus and diaphragm, divides the liver into two lobes, a large right lobe and a small left lobe (Figure 41-1). There are two additional lobes on the visceral surface of the liver, the caudate and quadrate lobes. Except for that portion that is in the epigastric area, the liver is contained within the rib cage and in healthy persons cannot normally be palpated. The liver is surrounded by a tough fibroelastic capsule called *Glisson's capsule.*

The liver is unique among the abdominal organs in having a dual blood supply—the hepatic artery and the portal vein. About 400 ml per minute of blood enters the liver through the hepatic artery and another 1000 ml per minute enters by way of the valveless portal vein, which carries blood from the stomach, the small and the large intestines, the pancreas, and the spleen (Figure 41-2). Although the blood from the portal vein is incompletely saturated with oxygen, it supplies about 60% to 70% of the oxygen needs of the liver.[1] The venous outflow from the liver is carried by the valveless hepatic veins, which empty into the inferior vena cava just below the level of the diaphragm. The pressure difference between the hepatic vein and the portal vein is normally such that the liver stores about 200 ml to 400 ml of blood. This blood can be shifted back into the general circulation during periods of hypotension and shock. In congestive heart failure, in which the pressure within the vena cava increases, blood backs up and accumulates in the liver.

The lobules are the functional units of the liver. Each lobule is a cylindrical structure that measures about 0.8 mm to 2 mm in diameter and is several millimeters in length. There are about 50,000 to 100,000 lobules in each of the two lobes. Each lobule is composed of cellular plates of hepatic cells arranged in spokelike fashion and encircling a central vein (Figure 41-3). The central vein opens into the hepatic vein and then into the vena cava. The hepatic plates are usually two cells thick and are separated by canaliculi, which empty into the bile ducts. As bile is produced by the hepatic cells, it flows first into the canaliculi, then into the terminal bile ducts, and eventually into the one large bile duct that drains each lobe. Also, in the septa that separate the lobules are the smaller portal venules, which receive blood from the portal veins. The venules empty into the flat sinusoids that lie between the hepatic plates. Branches from the hepatic artery, which supplies the septal tissues, are also found in the intralobular septa, and blood from these arterioles empties into the sinusoids.

The venous sinusoids are lined with two types of cells: the typical endothelial cells and the Kupffer's cells. The Kupffer's cells are reticuloendothelial cells that are capable of removing and phagocytizing old and defective blood cells, bacteria, and other foreign material from the portal blood as it flows through the sinusoid. This phagocytic action removes the colon bacilli and other harmful substances that filter into the blood from the intestine.

Functions of the liver

The liver is one of the most versatile and active organs in the body. It produces bile; metabolizes hormones and drugs; synthesizes proteins, glucose, and clotting factors; stores vitamins and minerals; and converts fatty acids to ketones—and has other functions as well. In this process, the liver degrades excess nutrients and converts them into substances essential to the body. It builds carbohydrates from proteins, converts sugars to fats that can be stored, and interchanges protein molecules so that they can be used for a number of purposes. In its capacity for metabolizing drugs and hormones, the liver serves as an excretory organ. In this respect, the bile, which carries the end-products of substances metabolized by the liver, is much like the urine, which carries the body wastes filtered by the kidneys. The functions of the liver are summarized in Table 41-1. The liver's role in carbohydrate, fat, and protein metabolism is discussed in Chapters 42 and 45. The discussion in this chapter focuses on the function of the liver in alcohol metabolism, production of bile, and removal of bilirubin.

Alcohol metabolism

More than 90% of the alcohol a person drinks is metabolized by the liver. The rest is excreted through the lungs, kidneys, and skin. As a substance,

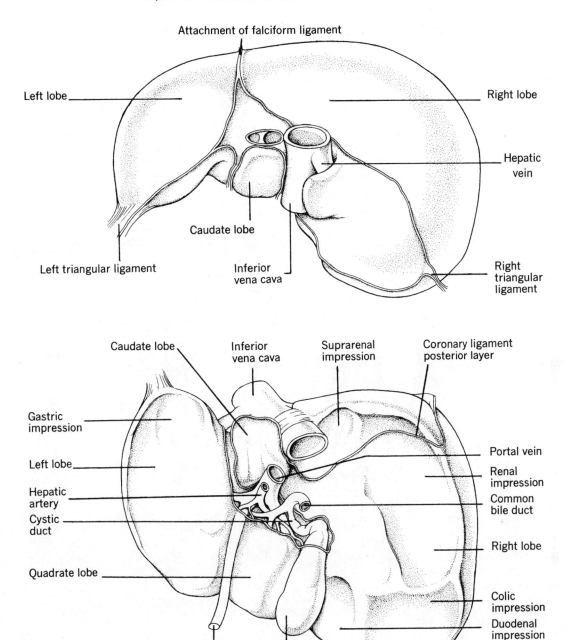

Figure 41-1 Superior posterior view (**top**) and inferior view (**bottom**) of the liver. (*Chaffee EE, Lytle IM: Basic Physiology and Anatomy, 4th ed. Philadelphia, JB Lippincott, 1980*)

alcohol fits somewhere between a food and a drug. It supplies calories but cannot be broken down or stored as protein, fat, or carbohydrate. As a food, alcohol yields 7.0 kcal/g compared with the 4.0 kcal produced by metabolism of an equal amount of carbohydrate. As a drug, it excites, hypnotizes, and then anesthetizes. (It is not a good anesthetic, however, because the euphoric stage lasts too long and the margin between the amount required for surgical anesthesia and that which will depress respiration is very narrow.)[2]

Alcohol is absorbed readily from the gastrointestinal tract, being one of the few substances that can be absorbed from the stomach. The overall metabolism of alcohol requires six oxidative steps and uses three molecules of oxygen to produce two molecules of carbon dioxide. In the process, it translocates 12 hydrogen ions and uses vital cofactors, particularly nicotinamide adenine dinucleotide (NAD), that are needed for other metabolic processes, such as gluconeogenesis. At blood levels commonly obtained by drinking, the generation of hydrogen ions by the liver often exceeds hydrogen ion elimination.[3]

The rate of alcohol metabolism is about the same for all persons, except the practicing alcoholic.

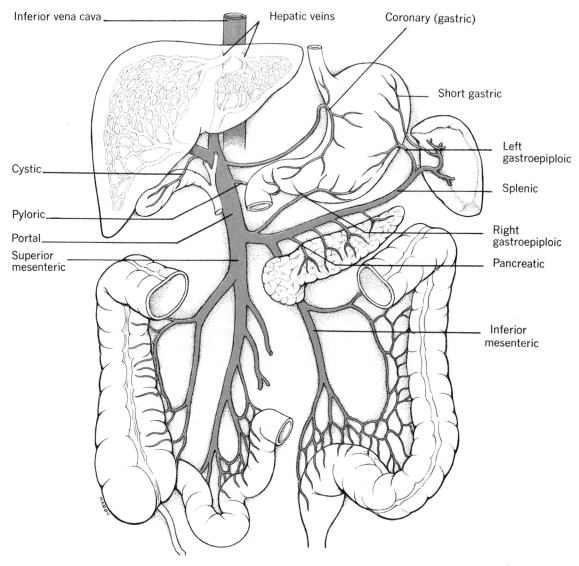

Inferior vena cava

Hepatic veins

Coronary (gastric)

Short gastric

Left gastroepiploic

Splenic

Right gastroepiploic

Pancreatic

Inferior mesenteric

Cystic

Pyloric

Portal

Superior mesenteric

Figure 41-2 The portal circulation. Blood from the gastrointestinal tract, spleen, and pancreas travels to the liver by way of the portal vein before moving into the vena cava for return to the heart. (*Chaffee EE, Lytle IM: Basic Physiology and Anatomy, 4th ed. Philadelphia, JB Lippincott, 1980*)

The rate-limiting step in the process is the availability of the enzyme alcohol dehydrogenase, which is located in the cytosol of the liver cells. The average person can metabolize about 18 g of alcohol per hour (it takes about 2 hours to metabolize one mixed drink). With prolonged and excessive ingestion of alcohol, the liver is able to almost double the rate at which alcohol is metabolized by increasing the activity of another metabolic pathway involving the microsomal system.[4] This system increases the susceptibility of heavy drinkers to the hepatotoxic effects of industrial toxins, anesthetic agents, chemical carcinogens, vitamins, and over-the-counter analgesics such as acetaminophen. Acetaminophen is generally safe when taken in recommended doses. However, a small fraction is metabolized by the microsomal system to

an active product that is highly toxic to the liver; this fraction increases with chronic alcohol use. The microsomal pathway also leads to increased production of acetaldehyde. Acetaldehyde, in turn, combines with proteins and causes injury to liver cells through antibody formation, enzyme inactivation, decreased DNA repair, and other alterations in cellular function. With cessation of drinking, the rate of alcohol metabolism by the microsomal system rapidly returns to normal.

One of the main effects of alcohol is the accumulation of fat within the liver. When alcohol is present, it becomes the preferred fuel for the liver, displacing substrates such as fatty acids, which are normally used for this purpose. Triglycerides accumulate in the liver, probably as a result of increased

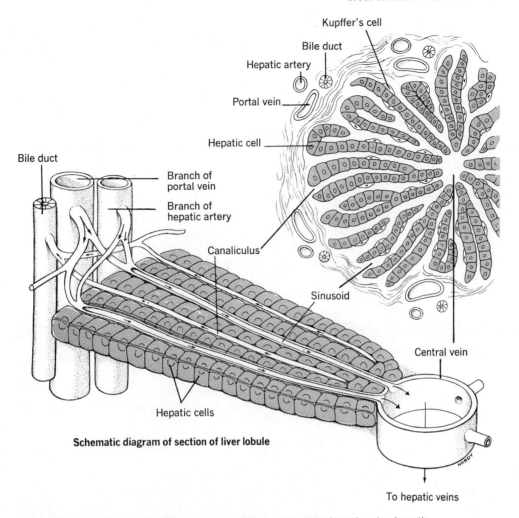

Cross section of liver lobule

Kupffer's cell

Bile duct

Hepatic artery

Portal vein

Hepatic cell

Bile duct

Branch of portal vein

Branch of hepatic artery

Canaliculus

Sinusoid

Central vein

Hepatic cells

Schematic diagram of section of liver lobule

To hepatic veins

Figure 41-3 A section of liver lobule showing the location of the hepatic veins, hepatic cells, liver sinusoids, and branches of the portal vein and hepatic artery. (*Chaffee EE, Lytle IM: Basic Physiology and Anatomy, 4th ed. Philadelphia, JB Lippincott, 1980*)

production and because of increased trapping of fatty acids within the liver cells.

Because alcohol competes for utilization of cofactors normally needed by the liver for other metabolic processes, it tends to disrupt the other functions of the liver. An altered redox state (reduction and oxidation, with accumulation of hydrogen ions) and the preferential utilization of NAD for alcohol metabolism can result in increased production and accumulation of lactic acid in the blood. The increased lactate levels tend to impair uric acid excretion by the kidney, which probably explains why excessive alcohol consumption frequently aggravates or precipitates gout. By reducing the availability of the cofactor NAD, alcohol impairs the liver's ability to form glucose from amino acids and other glucose precursors. Thus, alcohol-induced hypoglycemia and alcoholic ketoacidosis can develop when excessive alcohol ingestion occurs during periods of depleted liver glycogen stores. This

may become a particular problem for the alcoholic who has been vomiting and has not eaten for several days. Alcohol also increases the body's requirements for the B vitamins and increases urinary losses of magnesium, potassium, and zinc.

There has been considerable controversy over the interaction of diet and liver changes observed with chronic alcoholism. In fact, one of the arguments that heavy drinkers often use to justify their habit is that with proper attention to diet, they can avoid the undesirable effects of alcohol on the liver. In the past, it has been difficult to study and document the influence of nutrition on liver changes that arise with chronic alcohol abuse. However, recent animal research has demonstrated that full-blown cirrhosis of the liver can develop even when the diet is adequate.[4] This suggests that the alcohol itself plays an important role in liver injury. Studies using alcohol-fed baboons led to the discovery of alcohol-related changes in one of the enzymes of protein metabolism, gamma-glutamyl transpeptidase transferase. Serum levels of this enzyme become elevated with prolonged heavy drinking, and this enzyme test has been used in rehabilitative and industrial settings to indicate active alcoholism.[5]

Bile production

The liver produces about 600 ml to 800 ml of yellow-green bile daily. Bile contains water, bile salts, bilirubin, cholesterol, and various inorganic acids. Of these, only bile salts are important in digestion.

The liver forms about 0.5 g of bile salts daily. Bile salts are formed from cholesterol, which is either supplied by the diet or synthesized by the liver. Bile salts serve an important function in digestion: they aid in emulsifying dietary fats, and they are necessary for the formation of the micelles that transport fatty acids and fat-soluble vitamins to the surface of the intestinal mucosa for absorption. About 94% of bile salts that enter the intestine are reabsorbed into the portal circulation by an active transport process that takes place in the distal ileum. From the portal circulation, the bile salts pass into the liver where they are recycled. Normally, bile salts travel this entire circuit about 18 times before being expelled in the feces.[6] This system for recirculation of bile is called the *enterohepatic circulation.*

Bilirubin elimination

Bilirubin is the substance that gives bile its color. It is formed from senescent red blood cells. In the process of degradation, the hemoglobin from the red blood cell is broken down to form biliverdin, which is rapidly converted to free bilirubin (Figure 41-4). Free bilirubin, which is insoluble in plasma, is

Table 41–1. Functions of the liver and manifestations of altered function

Function	Manifestations of altered function
Production of bile salts	Malabsorption of fat and fat-soluble vitamins
Elimination of bilirubin	Failure to eliminate bilirubin causes elevation in serum bilirubin and jaundice
Metabolism of steroid hormones	
Estrogens and progesterone	Disturbances in gonadal function, including gynecomastia in the male
Testosterone	
Glucocorticoids	Signs of Cushing's syndrome
Aldosterone	Sodium retention and edema; hypokalemia
Metabolism of drugs	Decreased plasma binding of drugs owing to a decrease in albumin production
	Decreased removal of drugs that are metabolized by the liver
Carbohydrate metabolism	Hypoglycemia may develop when glycogenolysis and gluconeogenesis are impaired
Stores glycogen	
Synthesizes glucose from	Abnormal glucose tolerance curve may occur because of impaired uptake and release of glucose by the liver
Amino acids	
Lactic acid	
Glycerol	
Fat metabolism	
Formation of lipoproteins	Impaired synthesis of lipoproteins
Conversion of carbohydrates and proteins to fat	
Synthesis of cholesterol	
Formation of ketones from fatty acid	
Protein metabolism	
Deamination of proteins	
Formation of urea from ammonia	Elevated blood ammonia levels
Synthesis of plasma proteins	Decreased levels of plasma proteins, particularly albumin, which contributes to edema formation
Synthesis of clotting factors	Bleeding tendency
Fibrinogen	
Prothrombin	
Factors V, VII, IX, X	
Storage of minerals and vitamins	Signs of deficiency of fat-soluble and other vitamins that are stored in the liver
Filtration of blood and removal of bacteria and particulate matter by Kupffer cells	Increased exposure of the body to colon bacilli and other foreign matter

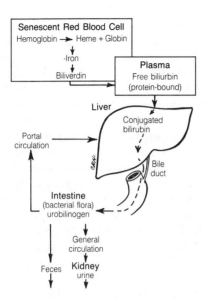

Figure 41-4 The process of bilirubin formation, circulation, and elimination.

transported in the blood attached to plasma albumin. As blood passes through the liver, bilirubin is released from the albumin-carrier molecule and absorbed by the hepatocytes. Once inside the hepatocyte, bilirubin is conjugated with either glucuronic acid or glucuronic sulfate, a process that enables the bilirubin to become soluble in bile. Conjugated bilirubin is then secreted into the canaliculi of the liver as a constituent of bile, and in this form it passes through the bile ducts into the small intestine. The bacterial flora in the intestine converts bilirubin to urobilinogen, which is highly soluble. Urobilinogen is either reabsorbed into the portal circulation or excreted in the feces. Most of the urobilinogen that is reabsorbed is returned to the liver to be reexcreted into the bile. A small amount of urobilinogen, about 5%, is reabsorbed into the general circulation and is then excreted by the kidneys.

Usually, only a small amount of bilirubin is found in the serum, the normal level of total serum bilirubin being 0.3 to 1.3 mg/dl. A simple test, the *van den Bergh test,* measures both the free and the conjugated bilirubin present in the total bilirubin. The *direct* van den Bergh test measures the conjugated bilirubin; the *indirect* test measures the free bilirubin.

Jaundice

Jaundice (icterus) is due to an abnormally high accumulation of bilirubin in the blood, as a result of which there is a yellowish discoloration to the skin and deep tissues. Jaundice develops when the plasma contains about twice the normal amount of bilirubin. Normal skin has a yellow cast, and therefore early signs of jaundice are often difficult to detect. This is

especially true in persons with dark skin. Because bilirubin has a special affinity for elastic tissue, the sclera of the eye, which contains considerable elastic fibers, is usually one of the first structures in which jaundice can be detected. The four chief causes of jaundice are (1) excessive destruction of red blood cells, (2) decreased uptake of bilirubin by the liver cells, (3) decreased conjugation of bilirubin, and (4) obstruction of bile flow, either in the canaliculi of the liver or in the intra- or extrahepatic bile ducts (Chart 41-1).

Hemolytic jaundice occurs when red blood cells are destroyed at a rate in excess of the liver's ability to remove the bilirubin from the blood. It may follow a hemolytic blood transfusion reaction or occur in diseases such as hereditary spherocytosis, in which the red cell membranes are defective (see Chapter 16), or in hemolytic disease of the newborn. Kernicterus is a condition characterized by severe neurologic symptoms that are due to high blood levels of unconjugated bilirubin; because the unconjugated bilirubin is lipid-soluble, it is able to enter nerve cells and cause brain damage. Because of the increased permeability of the blood–brain barrier in the fetus and neonate, it is a common sequela in hemolytic disease of the newborn caused by the Rh factor. Because of the availability of Rh_o immune globulin, Rh disease of the newborn is no longer a major problem. A physiologic jaundice may be seen in infants during the first week of extrauterine life and is related to the immaturity of the infant's liver and its inability to remove and conjugate sufficient amounts of bilirubin. Clinically apparent jaundice develops in about 50% of full-term and a

---

Chart 41–1:   Causes of jaundice

Excessive red blood cell destruction
　Hemolytic blood transfusion reaction
　Hereditary disorders of the red blood cell
　　Sickle cell anemia
　　Thalassemia
　　Spherocytosis
　Hemolytic disease of the newborn
Decreased uptake by the liver
　Gilbert's disease
Decreased conjugation of bilirubin
　Hepatocellular liver damage
　　Hepatitis
　　Cirrhosis
　Breast milk jaundice
Obstruction of bile flow
　Intrahepatic
　　Drug-induced cholestasis
　Extrahepatic
　　Structural disorders of the bile duct
　　Cholelithiasis
　　Tumors that obstruct bile duct
　　Liver disease

slightly higher percentage of premature infants. It usually peaks at age 3 to 4 days and resolves by the end of the first week.[7]

A condition, called *breast milk jaundice,* occurs in a small percentage of breast-fed babies. These babies have significant levels of unconjugated bilirubin, which rises progressively from the fourth day of life and reaches a maximum in 10 to 15 days. It disappears if breast-feeding is discontinued. The disorder is thought to be due to enzymes in the mother's milk that liberate free fatty acids from the constituents of the breast milk.[8] An immaturity of the infant's intestinal tract allows these fatty acids to be absorbed into the portal circulation where they travel to the liver and inhibit bilirubin conjugation. Another possible mechanism for breast milk jaundice is some factor in the milk that increases the absorption of bilirubin in the duodenum. Preheating the milk to 56°C for 15 minutes has been reported to inactivate the factors that produce the jaundice, a point that should be considered for mothers who wish to continue breast-feeding or for those administering such milk to low-birth-weight infants.

Infants at risk for developing *kernicterus* are those with : (1) clinically apparent jaundice in the first 24 hours, (2) increase in total serum bilirubin of more than 85 μmol/liter (5 mg/dl) per day, (3) total bilirubin concentration higher than 220 μmol/liter (13 mg/dl) within the first 4 days of life in term infants (4) direct serum bilirubin higher than 34 μmol/liter (2 mg/dl), and (5) visible jaundice lasting more than 1 week in full-term infants or 2 weeks in premature infants.[7] Phototherapy is used in the treatment of at-risk infants. In recent years, it has become evident that a selected spectrum of sunlight (light with wavelengths ranging from 400–500 nm) decreases neonatal jaundice. Exposure of a newborn to light in the selected wavelength acts at a depth of 2 mm from the epidermis to free the bilirubin that is bound to interstitial tissues and to change the conformation or shape of the bilirubin molecule to a more water-soluble form, which can be excreted in the stool and urine.[7] The effectiveness of the treatment is related to the area of epidermis that is exposed.

Gilbert's disease is inherited as a dominant trait and results in a reduced uptake of bilirubin. The disorder is benign and fairly common. Affected persons have no symptoms other than a slightly elevated unconjugated bilirubin, and hence jaundice. Conjugation of bilirubin is impaired whenever liver cells are damaged (hepatocellular jaundice), when transport of bilirubin into liver cells becomes deficient, or when the enzymes needed to conjugate the bile are lacking. Hepatitis and cirrhosis are the most common causes of this form of jaundice. Hepatocellular jaundice usually interferes with all phases of bilirubin metabolism—uptake, conjugation, and excretion.

Obstructive jaundice or *cholestatic jaundice* is seen when the flow of bile is obstructed. The obstruction may be of either intrahepatic or extrahepatic origin. In the *intrahepatic* form, both the conjugated and unconjugated serum bilirubin levels are abnormally high. Liver disease, drugs—especially the anesthetic halothane—oral contraceptives, estrogen, anabolic steroids, isoniazid, and chlorpromazine are all possible causative factors. *Extrahepatic cholestatic jaundice* is due to obstruction to bile flow between the liver and the intestine, with the obstruction located at any point between the junction of the right or left hepatic duct and the point where the bile duct opens into the intestine. With this form of jaundice, conjugated levels of bilirubin are elevated. Among the causes are strictures of the bile duct, gallstones, and tumors of the bile duct or the pancreas. Blood levels of bile acids are elevated in both intrahepatic and extrahepatic cholestatic jaundice. As the bile acids accumulate in the blood, pruritus develops. A history of pruritus preceding jaundice is common in obstructive jaundice of either intrahepatic or extrahepatic origin. The stools are usually clay colored because so little bile is entering the intestine, and, at the same time, the urinary bilirubin is increased. Also common to both intra- and extrahepatic jaundice is an abnormally high level of serum alkaline phosphatase. Alkaline phosphatase is produced by the liver and excreted with the bile, thus when bile flow is obstructed, the blood alkaline phosphatase becomes elevated.

Tests of liver function

The history and physical examination will, in most instances, provide clues about liver function. Diagnostic tests help to assess liver function and the extent of liver disease. A liver biopsy affords a means of examining liver tissue without necessitating surgery. Table 41-2 describes the common tests of liver function and their significance.

Functions of the gallbladder

The secretion of bile is essential for digestion of dietary fats and absorption of fats and fat-soluble vitamins from the intestine. Bile produced by the hepatocytes flows into the canaliculi, and then to the periphery of the lobules, which drain into larger ducts, until it reaches the right and left hepatic ducts. These ducts unite to form the common duct (Figure 41-5). The common duct, which is about 10 cm to 15 cm in length, descends and passes behind the pancreas and enters the descending duodenum. The pancreatic duct joins the common duct in the ampulla of Vater, which empties into the duodenum through the duodenal papilla. Muscle tissue at the junction of the papilla, called the *sphincter of Oddi,* regulates the flow of bile into the duodenum. A second sphincter (sphincter of Boyden), which is just above the point where the pancreatic duct fuses with the common duct, controls the flow of bile into this area of the common duct. When this sphincter is closed, bile moves back into the gallbladder.

The gallbladder is part of the biliary system. It is a distensible, pear-shaped muscular sac located on the ventral surface of the liver. It has a smooth muscle wall and is lined with a thin layer of absorptive cells. The cystic duct joins the gallbladder to the common duct. The function of the gallbladder is to store

Table 41-2. Tests of liver function

Type of test	Tests	Significance
Enzyme	Serum glutamic-oxaloacetic transaminase (SGOT)	Released into the serum when there is liver damage Elevated in hepatitis, cirrhosis, liver necrosis May also be elevated in myocardial infarction, skeletal muscle disease, and hematopoietic disorders
	Serum glutamic-pyruvic transaminase (SGPT)	Elevation indicates death of liver cells Elevated in hepatocellular diseae, infectious hepatitis, liver injury, and liver congestion
	Alkaline phosphatase	Rises when excretion of the enzyme is impaired because of biliary obstruction Useful in differentiating hepatocellular and obstructive jaundice
	Lactic acid dehydrogenase (LDH)	The isoenzymes LDH_1 and LDH_2 are found primarily in liver, skeletal muscle, and lung; the test is sensitive enough to detect increased fractions in infectious hepatitis before jaundice appears
	Y-glutamyl transpeptidase transferase (YGT)	The liver is the main source of this enzyme; it facilitates the transport of amino acids across the cell membrane; used to detect alcoholic liver disease and alcohol consumption
Bilirubin	Total	Measures total serum bilirubin
	Direct	Measures conjugated bilirubin (an increase usually associated with liver disease or obstruction of bile duct)
	Indirect	Measures free bilirubin (an increase usually associated with increased destruction of red blood cells)
	Icterus index	Measures the degree of jaundice by comparing the yellowness of the serum with that of a standard yellow compound
	Tests for bilirubin in urine	Usually, there is no bilirubin in urine; when present it represents conjugated bilirubin because free bilirubin that is attached cannot be filtered in the glomerulus; presence suggests liver disease or obstructive jaundice
	Urinary and fecal urobilinogen	Absence of fecal urobilinogen indicates obstruction of biliary tract An increase in fecal urobilinogen indicates excessive bilirubin production An increase in urinary urobilinogen in absence of an increased fecal urobilinogen indicates liver disease
Blood ammonia		The liver normally removes ammonia from the blood and converts it to urea; blood ammonia levels are often elevated in severe liver disease
Blood coagulation	Prothrombin time	Liver disease causes impaired synthesis of clotting factors V, VII, IX, X, prothrombin (II), and fibrinogen; prothrombin time is affected by most of these factors; the test is used to assess the risk of bleeding
Dye clearance	Sodium sulfobromophthalein (Bromsulphalein, BSP)	Liver function test, which is based on the liver's ability to remove dye from the blood
	Indocyanine green (ICG)	Also measures ability of liver to remove dye from blood (used less frequently than BSP)
Plasma proteins	Total plasma proteins	Measures total plasma proteins, including albumin, globulins, and fibrinogen
	Albumin	Albumin is decreased in cirrhosis
	Globulins	Alpha and beta globulins are increased in infectious or obstructive jaundice and decreased in liver failure, which interferes with their synthesis
Liver scan	Blood vessel structural scan	Measures the size, shape, and filling defects of the liver after intravenous injection of a radioactive substance; a radioactive detector (or scanner) outlines the liver and spleen
	Liver cell function scan ^{99m}Tc IDAs ^{131}I rose bengal	Radioactive dye is cleared from the blood by the liver; the size, shape, and filling of the liver, gallbladder, and small intestine are determined by scanning following intravenous injection of the dye (Rose bengal is seldom used because of its effect on the thyroid)
	Ultrasound	Outlines hepatobiliary structures
	Computerized tomography	Outlines hepatobiliary structures

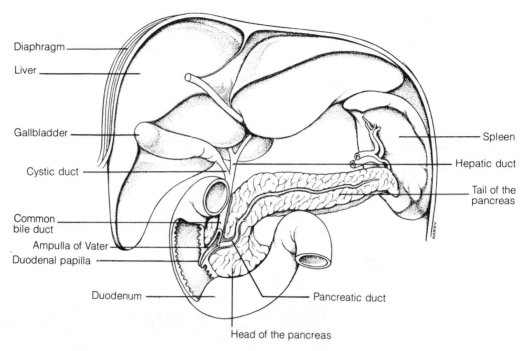

Figure 41-5 The liver and biliary system, including the gallbladder and bile ducts. (*Chaffee EE, Lytle IM: Basic Physiology and Anatomy, 4th ed. Philadelphia, JB Lippincott, 1980*)

and concentrate bile. When full, it can hold 20 ml to 50 ml of bile. Entrance of food into the intestine causes contraction of the gallbladder and relaxation of the sphincter of Oddi. The stimulus for gallbladder contraction is primarily hormonal. Products of food digestion, particularly lipids, stimulate cholecystokinin release from the mucosa of the duodenum. The role of other gastrointestinal hormones in bile release is less clearly understood. Passage of bile into the intestine is regulated largely by the pressure within the common duct. Normally, the gallbladder serves to regulate this pressure: it collects and stores bile as the gallbladder relaxes and the pressure in the common bile duct decreases and it empties into the intestine as the gallbladder contracts and causes an increase in common duct pressure. Following gallbladder surgery, the pressure in the common duct changes, causing the common duct to dilate. The flow of bile is then regulated by the sphincters in the common duct.

In summary, the hepatobiliary system consists of the liver, gallbladder, and bile ducts. The liver is the largest and, in function, one of the most versatile organs in the body. It is located between the gastrointestinal tract and the systemic circulation; venous blood from the intestine flows through the liver before it is returned to the heart. In this way, nutrients can be removed for processing and storage, and bacteria and other foreign matter can be removed by the Kupffer's

cells before the blood is returned to the systemic circulation. The liver synthesizes bile salts, fats, glucose, and plasma proteins. It metabolizes drugs and removes, conjugates, and secretes bilirubin into the bile. Jaundice occurs when bilirubin accumulates in the blood. Jaundice can occur because of excessive red blood cell destruction, failure of the liver to remove and conjugate the bilirubin, or obstructed biliary flow. The gallbladder and bile ducts serve as a passageway for the delivery of bile to the intestine, with the gallbladder storing and concentrating bile.

Alterations in liver function

Although the liver is among the organs most frequently damaged, only about 10% of hepatic tissue is required for the liver to remain functional.[1] Of the numerous pathologic processes to which the liver may be subject—including vascular disorders, inflammation, metabolic disorders, toxic injury, and neoplasms—three diseases have been selected for inclusion in this section: acute hepatitis, cirrhosis, and cancer.

Hepatitis

Hepatitis is an inflammation of the liver. It can be caused by a number of conditions including reactions to drugs and toxins (alcoholic hepatitis) and infections, such as malaria, mononucleosis, salmonellosis, and amebiasis, that cause a secondary hepatitis. One of the major infections in which the liver is the primary affected organ is viral hepatitis.

Viral hepatitis is an acute inflammatory disease usually caused by hepatitis A virus (HAV), hepatitis B virus (HBV), or other non-A, non-B virus(s) that have not as yet been elucidated. Viruses such as cytomegalovirus, herpes simplex, and rubella may be rarely implicated. About 10% of persons with hepatitis B and an even higher percentage of persons with non-A, non-B hepatitis develop chronic liver disease.

Hepatitis A

Hepatitis A, commonly called *infectious hepatitis,* is caused by a small nonenveloped RNA-containing virus. It has a brief incubation period and is usually transmitted by the fecal-oral route. Drinking contaminated milk or water and eating shellfish from infected waters are fairly common routes. At special risk are persons traveling abroad who have not previously been exposed to the virus. Institutions housing large numbers of people (usually children) are sometimes striken with an epidemic of hepatitis A. Oral behavior and lack of toilet training promote viral infection among children attending preschool day-care centers who then carry the virus home to older siblings and parents. Sexual transmission of HAV is common among homosexual men, especially those having oral-anal contact.[9] Hepatitis A is not usually transmitted by transfusion of blood or plasma derivatives, presumably because its short period of viremia usually coincides with clinical illness so that the disease is apparent and blood donations are not accepted. The Centers for Disease Control (CDC) has reported recent outbreaks of hepatitis A among drug users.[10] Between 1982 and 1986, the percentage of HAV among drug users admitted to treatment programs rose from 4% to 19%. Several possible explanations for the association between hepatitis A and drug abuse have been proposed including the use of shared needles; generally poor hygiene; or direct contamination of drugs during transport, preparation, or distribution.

Hepatitis B

Hepatitis B, often referred to as *serum hepatitis,* represents a more serious problem than hepatitis A. It has a longer incubation period and is more likely to cause serious illness and become chronic. The CDC estimates that there are more than 300,000 new cases each year and more than 1 million chronic carriers in the United States.[11] The CDC also estimates that each year in the United States there are 4,000 deaths due to hepatitis B-related cirrhosis and hepa-

tocellular carcinoma. The virus is usually transmitted through inoculation with infected blood or serum. However, the viral antigen can be found in most body secretions and can be spread by oral or sexual contact. Hepatitis B virus is highly prevalent among homosexuals and intravenous drug abusers. Mother-to-infant transmission occurs, but whether transmission occurs *in utero* or during the birth process is not known. Although the virus can be spread through transfusion or administration of blood products, routine screening methods have appreciably reduced the incidence of post-transfusion type B hepatitis.

Non-A, non-B hepatitis

Recent immunologic tests for type A and type B viruses in persons with post-transfusion hepatitis have provided evidence for the existence of one or more types of viral hepatitis—non-A, non-B hepatitis. The incidence of post-transfusion hepatitis is approximately 7% to 10%, and about 90% of these cases are caused by non-A, non-B hepatitis.[12] The carrier state for non-A, non-B hepatitis has been identified. The usual incubation period for non-A, non-B hepatitis is 7 to 8 weeks but can vary from 2 weeks to 20 weeks.

Acute hepatitis

The cellular changes that occur with hepatitis A, B, and non-A, non-B are those involving varying degrees of liver cell necrosis. The injurious effects of types A, B, and non-A, non-B hepatitis viruses are believed to arise because of an immune reaction in which the hepatitis virus in some way alters the antigenic properties of the hepatocytes. The extent of inflammation and necrosis depends on the individual immune response. The reticular framework that supports the hepatocytes is usually well preserved, except in severe cases in which varying degrees of collapse may occur. Healing occurs by regeneration of the surviving liver cells, usually without distortion of the normal architecture.

The clinical manifestations of viral hepatitis are extremely variable, ranging from asymptomatic infection without jaundice to fulminating disease (less than 1%–3%) and death in a few days. The manifestations of the disease have been divided into four phases: (1) the incubation period, (2) the prodromal or preicterus period, (3) the icterus period, and (4) the convalescent period. Table 41-3 describes the salient features of hepatitis A and B.

The incubation period ranges from weeks to months depending on the virus that is involved. The preicterus phase varies from abrupt to insidious with general malaise, myalgia, arthralgia, easy fatigability, upper respiratory symptoms, and severe anorexia out of proportion to the degree of illness. Gastrointestinal symptoms such as nausea, vomiting, and diarrhea or constipation may occur. Chills and fever may mark an abrupt onset. Upper abdominal pain may occur. In persons who smoke, there may be a distaste for smoking that parallels that of anorexia.

The icteric phase is characterized by the development of jaundice. It may follow the prodromal manifestations by 5 to 10 days or occur at the same time. The prodromal symptoms may become worse with the onset of jaundice, followed by progressive clinical improvement. Liver tenderness is common. Some persons never develop jaundice. Liver enlarge-ment (hepatomegaly) and spleen enlargement (splenomegaly) may occur.

The convalescent phase is characterized by gradual increase in sense of well-being, return of appetite, and disappearance of jaundice. The acute illness usually subsides rapidly over a 2- to 3-week period of time.

Diagnosis

Diagnosis is based on signs and symptoms. An elevation in serum bilirubin often precedes the appearance of jaundice, and enzyme tests that reflect

Table 41–3. Manifestations of viral hepatitis A and B

Features	Hepatitis A	Hepatitis B	Common manifestations
Mode of transmission	Fecal-oral route Excreted in the stool 2 weeks prior to and for 1 week after onset of clinical disease; transmitted by fecal-oral route, contaminated water, milk, shellfish Sexual transmission in homosexual men Recent outbreak among drug users	Present in the serum; transmitted by blood transfusion and blood products, needles, and other inoculation equipment; can also be transmitted by intimate sexual partners or family members; mother-to-infant transmission	
Persons at risk	Young children and persons in institutions Homosexual men and drug users	Parenteral drug abusers; persons on hemodialysis; health-care workers	
Carrier state	Not known to occur	Develops in about 5%–10% of persons who have the disease	
Incubation period	15–40 days (average, 30–38 days)*	43–160 days (average, 90 days)*	Headache Nausea Vomiting
Prodromal or preicterus period		Manifestations more severe, including Skin rash Arthralgia	3–12 days Fever Headache Epigastric distress Anorexia, nausea, vomiting Intolerance to fatty foods Diminished sense of smell Loss of taste for cigarettes Elevation of SGOT, SGPT, LDH$_1$, and LDH$_2$
Icterus period			2–6 weeks Jaundice Dark urine Clay-colored stool Elevated total bilirubin Abdominal pain and tenderness
Convalescent period			
Other		May progress to carrier state and chronicity Risk of later development of hepatocarcinoma in persons who develop chronic hepatitis	

* Richman A: Infectious hepatitis. Hosp Med 14, No 3:72, 1978

hepatocellular damage such as the serum glutamic-oxaloacetic transaminase (SGOT) and serum glutamic-pyruvic transaminase (SGPT) are elevated. Differentiation among the various viruses responsible for hepatitis requires the use of serologic markers. Specific serologic markers are available for diagnosing hepatitis A and hepatitis B, while non-A, non-B hepatitis is identified by the exclusion of A and B markers.

Prevention and treatment

The treatment of hepatitis is largely symptomatic. Bedrest, which at one time was a mainstay in treatment, has now largely been replaced with a more liberal program that permits patients to pace their own activity. Most patients will elect to limit activity because of fatigue. Dietary restrictions are usually minimal. If oral intake becomes inadequate, glucose solutions may be administered intravenously. Patients are instructed to avoid strenuous exercise and alcohol and other hepatotoxic agents.

The most effective way to prevent hepatitis is to prevent opportunities for the transmission of the virus. Because *contamination* (of blood, needles, other equipment) affords the virus ready access to the body, as previously described, the health-care worker should follow proper procedures when handling syringes and needles that have been used for drawing blood or injecting medications. Gloves should be worn when handling blood samples. Routine screening of blood donors has reduced the incidence of post-transfusion hepatitis B. There is increasing evidence, however, that other non-A, non-B viruses may be responsible for transfusion-induced hepatitis.

Gamma globulin is usually administered to close personal contacts of persons with hepatitis A. It may be advisable for persons traveling to countries where hepatitis A is endemic to receive a protective dose of gamma globulin within 2 weeks of arrival in that country and to receive booster doses if their stay is an extended one. The standard gamma globulin does not appear to afford protection against hepatitis B. However, hepatitis B immune globulin, which is not widely available, is effective if administered in a large dose within 10 days of exposure.

Two hepatitis vaccines have been developed for the prevention of hepatitis B.[12] One vaccine consists of highly purified and inactivated particles of the hepatitis B virus derived from chronic antigen carriers. The other is derived from recombinant technology. Recipients must have a negative serologic test for hepatitis B antigens. Potential candidates for the vaccine are persons at high risk for exposure to the virus, including renal dialysis patients, persons requiring repeated transfusions, male homosexuals, and newborns of hepatitis B antigen-positive mothers.

Cirrhosis

The World Health Organization (WHO) defines cirrhosis as "a diffuse process characterized by fibrosis and conversion of normal liver architecture into structurally abnormal nodules."[13] Although cirrhosis is usually associated with alcoholism, it can develop in the course of other disorders, including viral hepatitis, toxic reactions to drugs and chemicals, biliary obstruction, and cardiac disease. Cirrhosis also accompanies metabolic disorders that cause the deposition of minerals in the liver; two of these disorders are hemochromatosis (iron deposition) and Wilson's disease (copper deposition).

There are three types of cirrhosis: postnecrotic, biliary, and portal. Each of these has a different etiology; but in the end, each causes liver failure, and the ultimate outcome is much the same. Following a brief discussion of postnecrotic and biliary cirrhosis, we shall take portal (alcoholic) cirrhosis as our prototype.

Postnecrotic cirrhosis

This form of cirrhosis is characterized by the replacement of liver tissue with small to large nodules of fibrous tissue, with a resultant markedly deformed and nodular liver. Postnecrotic cirrhosis accounts for some 10% to 30% of cases of cirrhosis. It may follow viral hepatitis (type B or non-A, non-B type) or an autoimmune disease, or it may be a toxic response to drugs and other chemicals. It is a predisposing factor in hepatic cancer when it is caused by hepatitis type B.

Biliary cirrhosis

Biliary cirrhosis develops as a primary or secondary disorder that starts in the bile ducts with obstruction of bile flow (cholestasis). There is initial localized injury to biliary structures with gradual scarring and formation of bands of fibrous tissue that extend to adjacent lobular structures. Primary biliary cirrhosis accounts for about 10% of cases of cirrhosis.[1]

Primary biliary cirrhosis involves inflammation and scarring of the septal and interlobular bile ducts. The disease is seen most commonly in women 40 to 60 years of age. Abnormalities of both cell-mediated and humoral immunity suggest an autoimmune causation. It is characterized by an insidious onset and progressive scarring and destruction of liver tissue. The liver becomes enlarged and takes on a green hue due to the accumulated bile. The earliest symptoms are pruritis, followed by dark urine and pale stools. Once symptoms become clinically evident, life expectancy is about 5 years.[14] Treatment is largely symptomatic. Some success has been reported with liver transplantation (to be discussed).

Secondary biliary cirrhosis develops as the result of prolonged obstruction to bile flow. It is most commonly due to gallstones, stricture of the bile duct, or neoplasms that obstruct bile flow. Complete obstruction to outflow produces back pressure throughout the biliary system and the interlobular bile ducts are damaged as the bile becomes thick and impacted. Subtotal obstruction often leads to cholangitis and ascending infection of the biliary system. Treatment methods focus on correcting the cause of the obstruction.

Portal or alcoholic cirrhosis

Portal cirrhosis, often called *alcoholic cirrhosis* or *Laennec's cirrhosis,* is the eighth leading cause of death among adult Americans and the third leading cause of death among men 35 to 65 years of age. The most common cause of cirrhosis is excessive alcohol consumption. At least 75% of deaths attributable to alcoholism are caused by cirrhosis.[15] It is estimated that there are 10 million alcoholics in the United States. Interestingly, not all alcoholics develop cirrhosis, suggesting that other conditions such as genetic and environmental factors contribute to its occurrence. In fact, one-third of alcoholics never develop cirrhosis; in another one-third, fatty liver changes occur but not cirrhosis; the remaining one-third have cirrhosis.[16] Most deaths from alcoholic cirrhosis are attributable to liver failure, bleeding esophageal varices, or kidney failure.

Stages of development. Although the mechanism whereby alcohol exerts its toxic effects on liver structures is somewhat unclear, the changes that develop can be divided into three stages: (1) fatty changes, (2) alcoholic hepatitis, and (3) cirrhosis.

During the fatty changes stage, the liver enlarges because of excessive accumulation of fat within the liver cells. Alcohol replaces fat as a fuel for liver metabolism and impairs mitochondrial ability to oxidize fat. There is evidence that high ingestion of alcohol can cause fatty liver changes even in the presence of an adequate diet. For example, young nonalcoholic volunteers had fatty liver changes after 2 days of consuming 18 oz to 24 oz of alcohol, even though adequate carbohydrates, fats, and proteins were included in the diet.[17] The fatty changes that occur with ingestion of alcohol do not usually produce symptoms and are reversible once the alcohol intake has been discontinued.

Alcoholic hepatitis is the intermediate stage between fatty changes and cirrhosis. It is characterized by inflammation and necrosis of liver cells and thus is always serious and sometimes fatal. The necrotic lesions are generally patchy, but may involve an entire lobe. The cause is unknown. It is often seen after an abrupt increase in alcohol intake and is common in "spree" drinkers. "Ballooning" of hepatocytes and the toxic effects of the intermediates of alcohol metabolism, such as acetaldehyde, are believed to be contributory factors. This stage is usually characterized by hepatic tenderness, pain, anorexia, nausea, fever, jaundice, ascites, and liver failure; but some patients may be asymptomatic. There is a marked increase in the serum glutamic-oxaloacetic transaminase. Within 1 to 20 years, 80% of persons with alcoholic hepatitis who continue to drink will have liver changes consistent with cirrhosis.[16]

Cirrhosis is the direct result of liver injury caused by fatty changes and alcoholic hepatitis. The liver becomes yellow-orange, fatty, and diffusely scarred. Its normal structure is distorted by bands of fibrous tissue, which separate areas of regenerated cells. As the disease progresses, the liver shrinks. As normal tissue is replaced by scar tissue, blood flow through the liver is obstructed and extrahepatic shunts form, which serve as alternative routes for the return of portal blood to the heart.

Clinical manifestations

The manifestations of cirrhosis are variable, ranging from asymptomatic hepatomegaly to hepatic failure. Often there are no symptoms until the disease is far advanced; when symptoms do appear, they are vague at first, with complaints of fatigability and weight loss. At this point, the liver is often palpable and hard. Diarrhea is frequently present, although some persons may complain of constipation. There may be abdominal pain because of liver enlargement or stretching of Glisson's capsule. This pain is located in the epigastric area or in the upper right quadrant and is described as dull and aching and causing a sensation of fullness. The late manifestations of cirrhosis are related to portal hypertension and liver cell failure. Portal hypertension causes complications such as esophageal varices and ascites; in hepatocellular failure, there are decreased production of bile, plasma proteins, and blood-clotting factors and interference with removal of bilirubin, ammonia, and other substances. The manifestations of cirrhosis are discussed in the section that follows and are summarized in Table 41-4.

Portal hypertension, esophageal varices, spenomegaly, and ascites. Portal hypertension is characterized by increased resistance to flow and increased pressure in the portal venous system. Venous blood, returning to the heart from the abdominal organs, travels through the liver before entering the vena cava. The normal liver offers little resistance to portal venous flow. In cirrhosis, bands of fibrous tissue and fibrous nodules distort the architecture of the liver and increase the resistance to flow, which leads to portal hypertension. Collateral channels form between the portal and system veins as venous blood seeks alternative routes for return to the heart, the spleen becomes enlarged (splenomegaly) because of splenic vein congestion, and ascites develops as extracellular fluid accumulates in the peritoneal cavity.

With the gradual obstruction of blood flow in the liver, the pressure in the portal vein increases and large collateral channels develop between the portal and systemic veins that supply the lower rectum and esophagus and in the umbilical veins of the falciform ligament that attaches to the anterior wall of the abdomen. The presence of collaterals between the inferior and internal iliac veins may give rise to hemorrhoids. In some persons, the fetal umbilical vein is not totally obliterated; it forms a channel on the anterior abdominal wall (Figure 41-6). Dilated veins around the umbilicus are called *caput medusae*. Portopulmonary shunts may arise, causing blood to bypass the pulmonary capillaries, thereby interfering with blood oxygenation and producing cyanosis.

Clinically, the most important collateral channels are those connecting the portal and coronary veins that lead to reversal of flow and formation of thin-walled varicosities in the submucosa of the gastric fundus and esophagus (Figure 41-7). Being thin-walled, these varicosities are subject to rupture, with massive and sometimes fatal hemorrhage. Impaired hepatic synthesis of coagulation factors and decreased platelets (thrombocytopenia) due to splenomegaly may further complicate the control of esophageal bleeding. Several methods are used in the control of varicoseal bleeding including vasopressin, balloon tamponade, endoscopic injection sclerotherapy, and portosystemic shunt surgery. Vasopressin, a hormone from the posterior pituitary, produces constriction of the splanchnic arterioles and a reduction in blood flow and pressure when given intravenously. Balloon tamponade provides compression of the varices and is accomplished through the insertion of a tube with inflatable gastric and esophageal balloons. Once the tube has been inserted, the balloons are inflated (the esophageal balloon compresses the bleeding esophageal veins and the gastric balloon helps to maintain the position of the tube). During endoscopic sclerotherapy, the varices are injected with a sclerosing solution that causes obliteration of the vessel lumen.

Surgical treatment of portal hypertension consists of creating a portal–systemic shunt (an opening between the portal and a systemic vein). Although this procedure does not improve liver function, it does

Table 41–4. Manifestations of portal cirrhosis

Primary alteration in function	Manifestation
Portal hypertension	
Development of collateral vessels	Esophageal varices
	Hemorrhoids
	Caput medusae (dilated cutaneous veins around the umbilicus)
Increased pressure in the portal vein and decreased levels of serum albumin	Ascites
	Peripheral edema
Splenomegaly	Anemia
	Leukopenia
	Thrombocytopenia
Hepatorenal syndrome	Elevated serum creatinine
	Azotemia
	Oliguria
Portal–systemic shunting of blood	Hepatic-systemic encephalopathy
Hepatocellular dysfunction	
Impaired metabolism of sex hormones	Female: menstrual disorders
	Male: testicular atrophy, gynecomastia, decrease in secondary sex characteristics
	Skin disorders: vascular spiders and palmar erythema
Impaired synthesis of plasma proteins	Decreased levels of serum albumin with development of edema and ascites
	Decreased synthesis of carrier proteins for hormones and drugs
Decreased synthesis of blood-clotting factors	Bleeding tendencies
Failure to remove and conjugate bilirubin from the blood	Jaundice
Impaired bile synthesis	Malabsorption of fats and fat-soluble vitamins
Impaired metabolism of drugs cleared by the liver	Risk of drug reactions and toxicities
Impaired gluconeogenesis	Abnormal glucose tolerance
Decreased ability to convert ammonia to urea	Elevated blood ammonia levels

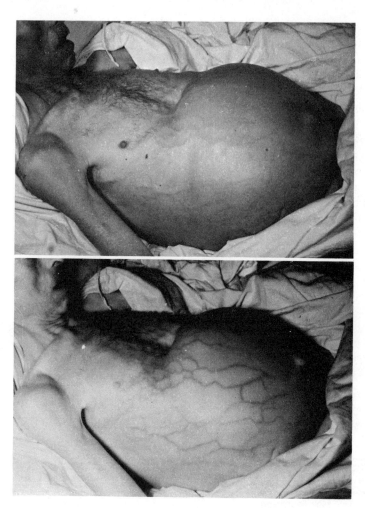

Figure 41-6 Collateral abdominal veins on the anterior abdominal wall in a patient with alcoholic liver disease as recorded by black and white photography (**top**) and infrared photography (**bottom**). (*Schiff L: Diseases of the Liver, 5th ed, p 408. Philadelphia, JB Lippincott, 1982*)

reduce the pressure within the esophageal veins and thus prevents esophageal hemorrhage. The two procedures that are done most frequently are portacaval shunt and splenorenal shunt. In a *portacaval* shunt, an opening is created between the portal vein and the vena cava. A *splenorenal* shunt involves removal of the spleen and anastomosis of the splenic vein to the left renal vein. It is often done when the spleen is enlarged, and it prevents further thrombocytopenia and leukopenia. One of the untoward sequelae that develop in some 10% of persons with a portal–systemic shunt is hepatic–systemic encephalopathy. As will be discussed, the neurologic manifestations of this disorder are believed to result from absorption of ammonia and other neurotoxic substances from the gut directly into the systemic circulation without going through the liver.

The splenomegaly observed in cirrhosis results from the shunting of blood into the splenic vein, which gives rise to such hematologic disorders as anemia, thrombocytopenia, and leukopenia.

Ascites is an accumulation of fluid within the peritoneal cavity. This fluid is a transudate of plasma, constantly being exchanged with fluid from the vascular compartment, and composed of electrolytes and albumin similar in composition to plasma. In cirrhosis, the two major factors contributing to ascites are (1) impaired synthesis of albumin by the liver, so that the plasma colloidal osmotic pressure falls, and (2) obstruction of venous flow through the liver. This obstruction causes increased accumulation of lymph, with oozing of serous fluid from the liver surface. The decreased colloidal osmotic pressure causes fluid to leak out of the capillaries in the splanchnic (visceral) circulation. Additionally, there is a rise in aldosterone, which augments retention of sodium and water by the kidneys. Among the causes postulated to be responsible for the increased aldosterone levels are an impairment of aldosterone inactivation by the liver and production by the liver of a humoral substance that stimulates aldosterone secretion. The increased aldosterone levels also result in increased elimination of potassium by the kidneys and decreased serum potassium levels. Because of the fall in serum albumin and the retention of sodium and water, peripheral edema develops, particularly in the dependent parts of the body, such as the feet.

Treatment of ascites usually focuses on dietary restriction of sodium and administration of diuretics. Water intake may also need to be restricted.

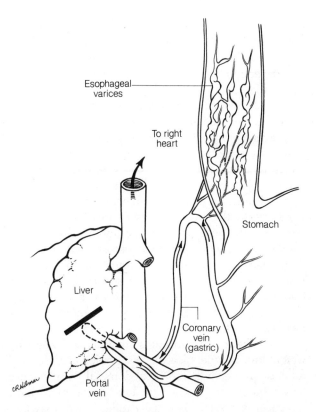

Figure 41-7 Obstruction of blood flow in the portal circulation, with portal hypertension and diversion of blood flow to other venous channels, including the gastric and esophageal veins.

To counteract the rise in aldosterone, an aldosterone-blocking diuretic along with one of the thiazide diuretics is usually prescribed. Oral potassium supplements are often given to prevent hypokalemia. Paracentesis may be done for diagnostic purposes but is seldom done to treat the ascites, because its effects are only temporary and it may cause a shift in fluid from the vascular compartment to the peritoneal cavity, along with complications such as infection and hemorrhage.

Hepatorenal syndrome. The hepatorenal syndrome refers to a functional state of renal failure sometimes seen during the terminal stages of cirrhosis and ascites. It is characterized by progressive azotemia, increased serum creatinine levels, and oliguria. Although the basic cause is not known, a decrease in renal blood flow is believed to play a part. Ultimately, when renal failure is superimposed on liver failure, azotemia and elevated levels of blood ammonia occur; this is thought to contribute to hepatic encephalopathy and coma.

A surgical procedure called the *LaVeen* continuous peritoneal–jugular shunt has been devised; the peritoneal fluid is shunted from the abdominal cavity through a one-way pressure-sensitive valve into a silicone tube that is inserted into the superior jugular vein and advanced so that the fluid empties into the superior vena cava. The procedure is reported to re-lieve refractory ascites in persons with cirrhosis and to reverse the pathophysiologic manifestations of the hepatorenal syndrome.[18]

Endocrine disorders. The liver metabolizes the sex hormones. Endocrine disorders are common accompaniments of cirrhosis, particularly disturbances in gonadal function. In women there may be menstrual irregularities (usually amenorrhea), loss of libido, and sterility. In men, the testosterone level usually falls, the testes atrophy, and loss of libido, impotence, and gynecomastia occur.

Skin disorders. Liver failure brings on numerous skin disorders. These lesions, called variously *vascular spiders, telangiectasia, spider angiomas,* and *spider nevi,* most often are seen in the upper half of the body. These lesions consist of a central pulsating arteriole from which smaller vessels radiate. (It should be kept in mind that spider angiomas may be seen in pregnancy even when liver function is normal.) *Palmar erythema* is redness of the palms, probably because of an increased blood flow resulting from higher cardiac output. Clubbing of the fingers may be seen in persons with cirrhosis. Jaundice is usually a late manifestation of liver failure.

Hematologic disorders. Anemia, thrombocytopenia, coagulation defects, and leukopenia may arise in the presence of cirrhosis. Anemia may be due to blood loss, excessive red blood cell destruction, and impaired formation of red blood cells. A folic acid deficiency may lead to severe megaloblastic anemia. Changes in the lipid composition of the red cell membrane increase hemolysis. Because factors V, VII, IX, X, prothrombin, and fibrinogen are synthesized by the liver, their decline in liver disease contributes to bleeding disorders. Malabsorption of the fat-soluble vitamin K contributes further to the impaired synthesis of these clotting factors. Often a thrombocytopenia occurs as the result of splenomegaly. Thus, the cirrhotic patient is subject to purpura, easy bruising, hematuria, and abnormal menstrual bleeding (women) and is vulnerable to bleeding from the esophagus and other segments of the gastrointestinal tract.

Hepatic–systemic encephalopathy. Hepatic–systemic encephalopathy refers to the totality of central nervous system manifestations of cirrhosis. It is characterized by neural disturbances ranging from a lack of mental alertness to confusion, coma, and convulsions. A very early sign of hepatic encephalopathy is a flapping tremor called asterixis. Loss of memory of varying degrees may occur, coupled with personality changes, such as euphoria, irritability, anxiety, and lack of concern about personal appearance and self. There may also be impairment of speech and inability to perform certain purposeful movements. The encephalopathy may progress to decerebrate rigidity and finally to a terminal deep coma.

The cause of hepatic encephalopathy is not yet known. The presence of neurotoxins, which appear in the blood because the liver has lost its detoxifying capacity, is believed to be a related factor. As has been stated, hepatic encephalopathy develops in about 10% of persons having a portal–systemic shunt.

One of the suspected neurotoxins is ammonia. One function of the liver is to convert ammonia, a by-product of protein metabolism, to urea. Ammonia is also produced in the intestine where the bacterial flora convert proteins to ammonia. The ammonia diffuses back into the portal blood and is transported to the liver where it is converted to urea before entering the general circulation. In situations in which the blood from the intestine bypasses the liver or in which the liver is unable to convert the ammonia to urea, the ammonia moves directly into the general circulation and from there to the cerebral circulation. Hence, hepatic encephalopathy may become worse following a large protein meal or gastrointestinal tract bleeding. When hypokalemic alkalosis is present, it causes increased renal production of ammonia. Narcotics and tranquilizers are poorly metabolized by the liver, and administration of these drugs may cause central nervous system depression and precipitate hepatic encephalopathy.

Fetor hepaticus refers to a characteristic musty, sweetish odor of the breath in the patient in advanced liver failure, resulting from the products of metabolism of the intestinal bacteria.

Treatment

The treatment of cirrhosis is directed toward elimination of alcohol intake; providing sufficient carbohydrate and calories to prevent protein breakdown; correcting fluid and electrolyte imbalances, particularly hypokalemia, and decreasing ammonia production in the gastrointestinal tract by limiting protein intake. A nonabsorbable antibiotic, such as neomycin, may be given to eradicate bacteria from the bowel and thus prevent this cause of ammonia production. Another drug that may be given is lactulose. It is not absorbed from the small intestine but moves directly to the large intestine where it is catabolized by the colon bacteria to small organic acids that cause production of large, loose stools with a low *p*H. The low *p*H is believed to convert ammonia to ammonium ions, which are not absorbed by the blood.[19]

Cancer of the liver

Cancers of the liver include both metastatic and primary neoplasms. Metastatic implants from primary cancers arising in areas drained by the portal vein are the most common form of neoplastic involvement of the liver. Although the metastatic lesions may produce gross distortion of liver structure, functional insufficiency is rare because sufficient intervening tissue is spared.

Primary liver tumors are relatively rare in the United States, accounting for about 2% of all cancers. The average age of onset is about 60 to 70 years.[20] There are three primary types of liver cancer—hepatocellular carcinoma, which arises from the liver cells; cholangiocarcinoma, which is a primary cancer of bile duct cells; and a mixed hepatocholangiocarcinoma.[21] Cirrhosis of the liver is present in 60% to 80% of persons with hepatocellular carcinoma. By contrast, cholangiocarcinoma has no association with cirrhosis. Three factors are thought to contribute to hepatocellular carcinoma: (1) chronic hepatitis B virus infection, (2) cirrhosis of the liver, and (3) possible hepatocarcinogens in food. Aflatoxin from moldy peanuts has been implicated.

The initial symptoms are weakness, anorexia, weight loss, fatigue, bloating, a sensation of abdominal fullness, and a dull, aching abdominal pain. Ascites, which often obscures weight loss, is common. Jaundice, if it is present, is usually mild. There may be a rapid increase in liver size and worsening of ascites in persons with preexisting cirrhosis. Usually, the liver is enlarged at the time these symptoms appear, and there is a low fever without apparent cause. Serum alpha-fetoprotein, a serum protein present in fetal life, normally is barely detectable in the serum after the age of 2 years; but it is present in some 50% to 90% of cases of hepatocarcinoma.[1]

Primary cancers of the liver are usually far advanced at the time of diagnosis; the 5-year survival rate is about 1%, and most patients die within 6 months. The treatment of choice is subtotal hepatectomy of 85% to 90% of the liver, if conditions permit.[20] The cancer is not radiosensitive. Chemotherapeutic drugs, among them methotrexate and 5-fluorouracil (5-FU) may be administered by cannula placed in the hepatic artery.

Liver transplantation

Liver transplantation is rapidly becoming a realistic form of treatment for persons with end-stage liver disease.[22,23] The introduction of cyclosporine in 1980 has markedly improved the survival rate of persons with a liver transplant. Careful selection of potential recipients and improved preoperative management have further contributed to the improved transplant results. In 1983, the National Institute of Health consensus conference concluded that liver transplantation had become a therapeutic modality, prompting many states and private insurance companies to pay for the procedure. Criteria for liver transplantation include the presence of a chronic liver disease for which all forms of therapy have failed. Conditions for which liver transplantation has been done are metabolic diseases of the liver such as Wilson's disease, primary biliary cirrhosis, alcoholic cirrhosis in persons with 1 year's abstinence or longer, chronic active hepatitis, sclerosing cholangitis, and biliary atresia in children. During the transplant procedure, the recipient liver is replaced with a donor liver and the recipient's blood vessels and bile duct are attached to the donor liver. The agents used to prevent liver transplant rejection, cyclosporine, corticosteroid drugs, and azathioprine, are the same ones used to maintain other whole-organ grafts such as heart and kidney transplants.

In summary, the liver is subject to most of the disease processes that affect other body structures, such as vascular disorders, inflammation, metabolic diseases, toxic injury, and neoplasms. Two of the most common liver diseases are hepatitis and cirrhosis. Acute viral hepatitis is caused by hepatitis A and hepatitis B viruses. Spread of hepatitis A occurs by oral-fecal transmission; it has a short incubation period and is usually followed by complete recovery. Hepatitis B has a longer incubation period and is spread through contact with contaminated blood, serum, instruments, and body secretions. Its symptoms are more severe, and it may progress to the carrier or chronic state. Cirrhosis caused by hepatitis B is associated with increased risk of hepatocarcinoma. Cirrhosis is the fourth leading cause of death in the United States. It is characterized by fibrosis and conversion of the normal hepatic architecture into structurally abnormal nodules. There are three types of cirrhosis—postnecrotic, biliary, and portal, or alcoholic cirrhosis—of which the most common is alcoholic cirrhosis. Regardless of cause, the manifestations of end-stage cirrhosis are similar and result from portal hypertension and liver cell failure. Cancers of the liver include both metastatic and primary neoplasms. Metastatic neoplasms are the most common form of liver cancer. Primary liver neoplasms are rare, accounting for only 2% of cancers, and those involving the hepatocytes or liver cells are commonly associated with cirrhosis of the liver. With the introduction of the immunosuppressant agent, cyclosporine, liver transplanation is becoming a more realistic form of treatment for end-stage liver disease.

Alterations in gallbladder function

Two very common disorders of the biliary system are *cholelithiasis* (gallstones) and *cholecystitis* (inflammation of the gallbladder). Together, these diseases affect about 15 million persons living in the United States. Close to 400,000 cholecystectomies are performed in this country each year.[24]

Composition of bile and formation of gallstones

Gallstones are due to the precipitation of substances contained in bile, mainly cholesterol and bilirubin. Bile contains bile salts, cholesterol, bilirubin, lecithin, fatty acids, and water as well as electrolytes normally found in the plasma. The cholesterol found in bile has no known function; it is assumed to be a by-product of bile salt formation, and its presence is linked to the excretory function of bile. Normally insoluble in water, cholesterol is rendered soluble by the action of bile salts, which combine with it to form micelles. In the gallbladder, water and electrolytes are absorbed from the liver bile, causing the bile to become more concentrated. Because neither lecithin nor bile salts are absorbed in the gallbladder, their concentration increases along with that of cholesterol, and, in this way, the solubility of cholesterol is maintained.

The bile of which gallstones are formed is usually supersaturated with either cholesterol or bilirubinate. The majority of gallstones, about 75%, are composed primarily of cholesterol, and the other 25% are pigment, or calcium bilirubinate, stones. Many stones have a mixed composition. Three factors contribute to the formation of gallstones: (1) abnormalities in the composition of bile, (2) stasis of bile, and (3) inflammation of the gallbladder. The formation of cholesterol stones is associated with obesity and is seen more frequently in women, especially women who have had multiple pregnancies or who are taking oral contraceptives. All of these situations cause the liver to excrete more cholesterol into the bile. Drugs such as clofibrate, which lower serum cholesterol levels, also cause increased cholesterol excretion into the bile. Malabsorption disorders stemming from ileal disease or intestinal bypass surgery, for example, tend to interfere with the absorption of bile salts, which is needed to maintain the solubility of cholesterol. Inflammation of the gallbladder alters the absorptive characteristics of the mucosal layer, allowing for excessive absorption of water and bile salts. Cholesterol gallstones are extremely common among Native Americans, which suggests that a genetic component may have a role in gallstone formation. Pigment stones containing bilirubin are seen in persons with hemolytic disease and hepatic cirrhosis.

Many persons with gallstones have no symptoms. Gallstones cause symptoms when they obstruct bile flow.[25] Small stones not more than 8 mm in diameter pass into the common duct, producing symptoms of indigestion and biliary colic. Larger stones are more likely to obstruct flow and cause jaundice.[26] The pain of biliary colic is generally abrupt in onset, increasing steadily in intensity until it reaches a climax in 30 to 60 minutes. The upper right quadrant, or epigastric area, is the usual location of the pain, often with referred pain to the back, above the waist, the right shoulder, and the right scapula or the midscapular region. A few persons will experience pain on the left side. The pain usually persists for 2 hours to 8 hours and is followed by soreness in the upper right quadrant.

Cholecystitis and cholelithiasis

Cholecystitis is inflammation of the gallbladder. It may be either acute or chronic, and both types are associated with cholelithiasis. Acute cholecystitis may be superimposed on chronic cholecystitis.

Acute cholecystitis is almost always associated with complete or partial obstruction of bile flow. It is believed that the inflammation is caused by chemical irritation from the concentrated bile, along with mucosal swelling and ischemia resulting from venous congestion and lymphatic stasis. The gallbladder is usually markedly distended. Bacterial infections may arise secondarily to the ischemia and chemical irritation. The bacteria reach the injured gallbladder through the blood, lymphatics, or bile ducts, or from adjacent organs. Among the common pathogens are staphylococci and enterococci. The wall of the gallbladder is most vulnerable to the effects of ischemia, as a result of which mucosal necrosis and sloughing occur. The process may lead to gangrenous changes and perforation of the gallbladder.

The symptoms of acute cholecystitis vary with the severity of obstruction and inflammation. It is often precipitated by a fatty meal and may be initiated with complaints of indigestion. Pain, initially similar to that of biliary colic, is characteristic of acute cholecystitis. It does not, however, subside spontaneously; it responds poorly or only temporarily to potent analgesics. When the inflammation progresses to involve the peritoneum, the pain becomes more pronounced in the right upper quadrant. The right subcostal region is tender, and there is spasm of the muscles that surround the area. Vomiting occurs in about 75% of patients, and jaundice, in some 25%. Fever and an abnormally high white blood cell count attest to the presence of inflammation. Total serum bilirubin, serum transaminase, and alkaline phosphatase are usually elevated.

The manifestations of chronic cholecystitis are more vague than those of acute cholecystitis. There may be intolerance to fatty foods, belching, and other indications of discomfort. Often there are episodes of colicky pain with obstruction of biliary flow caused by gallstones. The gallbladder, which in chronic cholecystitis usually contains stones, may be enlarged, shrunken, or of normal size. The passage of a stone into the common duct causes obstruction of bile flow and may contribute to carcinoma of the gallbladder.

Diagnosis and treatment

The current methods used in diagnosis of gallbladder disease include oral cholecystography, ultrasonography, and cholescintigraphy.[27,28] Oral cholecystography is a radiologic technique that involves the use of oral tablets containing a radiopaque contrast media that is absorbed from the gut, is excreted in the bile, and becomes concentrated in the gallbladder. The test requires a fat-free diet for 1 to 2 days before the test. The dye must be taken 10 to 14 hours before the examination; it may produce nausea and vomiting in 5% to 10% of persons and diarrhea in up to 25% of persons. Ultrasound is a widely used diagnostic method in gallbladder disease and has largely replaced the oral cholecystogram in many medical centers. The overall accuracy of ultrasound in detecting gallbladder disease is high. In addition to stones, ultrasound can detect other findings such as wall thickening, which indicates inflammation. Cholescintigraphy, also called a *gallbladder scan,* relies on the ability of the liver to extract a rapidly injected radionuclide (technetium-99m-labeled iminodiacetic acid derivative) from the blood and excrete it in the bile. Serial scanning images are obtained within several minutes of the injection of the tracer and every 10 to 15 minutes during the next hour. The gallbladder scan is highly accurate in detecting acute cholecystitis. Other methods such as computed tomographic scanning and magnetic resonance imaging are being evaluated for their possible roles in diagnosing gallbladder disease.

Gallbladder disease is usually treated by removing the gallbladder or by dissolving or fragmenting the stones.[29] The usual treatment of choice for symptomatic cholelithiasis and cholecystitis is surgical removal of the gallbladder—cholecystectomy. If the inflammation is acute, the surgery is delayed, unless complications demand immediate surgery. This allows time for the inflammatory process to subside. The gallbladder serves to store and concentrate bile; as discussed earlier in the chapter, its removal does not usually interfere with digestion.

The bile acids—chenodeoxycholic acid and ursodeoxycholic acid—have proved capable of dissolving gallstones and may be used to treat asymptomatic cholelithiasis.[29] They act by desaturating cholesterol in solution in the bile. For the treatment to be effective, the stones must be predominately cholesterol and not calcified. The treatment dissolves most stones within a year or two. Chenodeoxycholic acid is associated with elevation of low-density lipoproteins (LDL) and dose-related diarrhea and elevated liver enzymes (SGOT and SGPT). The drug is not recommended for women of childbearing years for fear they may adversely affect the fetal liver. Ursodeoxycholic acid appears to have less effect on liver enzymes and produces less diarrhea. Topical dissolution of cholelithiasis with tert-butyl ether can also be used. The procedure is carried out using a transhepatic catheter inserted under local anesthesia. This procedure, which is still experimental, is associated with risks such as bleeding and bile duct injury and is usually reserved for persons with significant disease who are not candidates for cholecystectomy.

Extracorporeal shock wave lithotripsy uses sound waves to pulverize gallstones so they can be passed through the bile duct.[30] The procedure is only suitable for radiolucent stones, because the shock waves have to be focused on each stone. Although not a common complication, stone fragments can become trapped in the bile duct. Adjunctive bile-acid therapy is often used to speed dissolution of stone fragments.[29]

—— Cancer of the gallbladder

Cancer of the gallbladder occurs in approximately 2% of persons operated on for biliary tract disease. The onset of symptoms is usually insidious and resembles cholecystitis; the diagnosis is often made unexpectedly at the time of gallbladder surgery. Because of their ability to produce chronic irritation of the gallbladder mucosa, it is believed that gallstones play a role in the development of gallbladder cancer. The 5-year survival rate is low—only about 3%.

In summary, the biliary tract serves as a passageway for the delivery of bile from the liver to the intestine. This tract consists of the bile ducts and gallbladder. The most common causes of biliary tract disease are cholelithiasis and cholecystitis. Three factors contribute to the development of gallstones: (1) abnormalities in the composition of bile, (2) stasis of bile, and (3) inflammation of the gallbladder. Cholelithiasis predisposes to obstruction of bile flow, causing biliary colic and acute or chronic cholecystitis. Cholecystectomy is usually the treatment of choice for symptomatic cholelithiasis in persons who are good surgical risks. Oral bile-acid therapy can be used to dissolve cholesterol stones, or topical dissolution of stones can be carried out through a transhepatic catheter inserted under local anesthesia. In some cases, extracorporeal shock wave lithotripsy may be used to fragment radiopaque stones so they can be eliminated through the bile duct. Cancer of the gallbladder, which has a poor 5-year survival rate, occurs in 2% of persons with biliary tract disease.

Exocrine pancreas

The pancreas lies transversely in the posterior part of the upper abdomen. The head of the pancreas is at the right of the abdomen; it rests against the curve of the duodenum in the area of the ampulla of Vater and its entrance into the duodenum. The body of the pancreas lies beneath the stomach. The tail touches the spleen. The pancreas is virtually hidden because of its posterior position. Unlike many other organs, it cannot be palpated. Because of the position of the pancreas and its large functional reserve, symptoms of disease do not usually appear until the disorder is far advanced. This is particularly true of cancer of the pancreas.

The pancreas is both an endocrine and an exocrine organ. Its function as an endocrine organ is discussed in Chapter 45. The exocrine pancreas is made up of lobules that consist of acinar cells. These cells secrete digestive enzymes into a system of microscopic ducts. These ducts are terminal branches of larger ducts that drain into the main pancreatic duct, which extends from left to right through the substance of the pancreas (see Figure 41-5). In most people, the main pancreatic duct empties into the ampulla of Vater, although in some persons it empties directly into the duodenum. The pancreatic ducts are lined with epithelial cells that secrete water and bicarbonate and thereby modify the fluid and electrolyte composition of the pancreatic secretions. The pancreatic secretions contain proteolytic enzymes that break down dietary proteins, including trypsin, chymotrypsin, carboxypolypeptidase, ribonuclease, and deoxyribonuclease. The pancreas also secretes pancreatic amylase, which breaks down starch, and lipase, which hydrolyzes neutral fats into glycerol and fatty acids. The pancreatic enzymes are secreted in the inactive form and become activated once in the intestine. This is important because the enzymes would digest the tissue of the pancreas itself were they to be secreted in the active form. The acinar cells secrete a trypsin inhibitor, which prevents trypsin activation. Because trypsin activates other proteolytic enzymes, the trypsin inhibitor prevents subsequent activation of those other enzymes. Two types of pancreatic disease are discussed in this chapter: acute and chronic pancreatitis and cancer of the pancreas.

—— Acute hemorrhagic pancreatitis

Acute pancreatitis is a severe and life-threatening disorder associated with the escape of activated pancreatic enzymes into the pancreas and surrounding tissues. These enzymes cause fat necrosis, or autodigestion, of the pancreas and produce fatty deposits in the abdominal cavity with hemorrhage from the necrotic vessels. Although a number of factors are associated with the development of acute pancreatitis, the two most important are biliary tract disease with reflux of bile into the pancreas and alcoholism. Biliary reflux is believed to activate the pancreatic enzymes within the ductile system of the pancreas. Gallstones that obstruct the common duct account for approximately 60% of nonalcoholic acute pancreatitis.[31] The precise mechanisms whereby alcohol exerts its action are largely unknown. Alcohol is known to be a potent stimulator of pancreatic secretions, and, at the same time, it often causes partial obstruction of the sphincter of Oddi. Acute pancreatitis is also associated with hyperlipidemia, hyperparathyroidism, infections (particularly viral), abdominal and surgical trauma, and drugs such as steroids and thiazide diuretics.

An important disturbance related to acute pancreatitis is the loss of a large volume of fluid into the retroperitoneal and peripancreatic spaces and the abdominal cavity. The onset is usually abrupt and dramatic, and it may follow a heavy meal or an alcoholic binge. Severe epigastric and abdominal pain often radiates to the back. The pain is aggravated when the person is lying supine; it is less severe when the person is sitting and leaning forward. Abdominal distention accompanied by hypoactive bowel sounds is common. Tachycardia; hypotension; cool, clammy skin; and fever are often evident. Signs of hypocalcemia may develop, probably as a result of the precipitation of serum calcium in the areas of fat necrosis. Mild jaundice may appear after the first 24 hours because of biliary obstruction. The serum amylase becomes elevated within the first 24 hours. Serum lipase also becomes elevated during the first 24 to 48 hours but remains elevated for 5 days to 7 days. Both enzymes remain elevated during the destructive stage of the disease and return to normal within 2 days to 5 days following the acute attack. Urinary clearance of amylase is increased. Because the serum amylase may be elevated as a result of the presence of other serious illnesses, the urinary amylase may be measured. Hyperglycemia and an elevated serum bilirubin may be present. About 5% of persons with acute pancreatitis die of the acute effects of peripheral vascular collapse. Serious complications include acute respiratory distress syndrome and acute tubular necrosis.

The treatment consists of measures directed at pain relief and restoration of lost plasma volume. Meperidine (Demerol) rather than morphine is usually given for pain relief because it causes fewer spasms of the sphincter of Oddi. Papaverine, nitroglycerin, barbiturates, or anticholinergic drugs may be given as supplements to provide smooth muscle relaxation. Oral foods and fluids are withheld, and gastric suction is instituted to treat distention of the bowel and prevent further stimulation of the secretion of pancreatic enzymes. Intravenous fluids and electrolytes are administered to replace those lost from the circulation and to combat the hypotension and shock. Intravenous colloid solutions are given to replace the fluid that has become sequestered in the abdomen and retroperitoneal space. Percutaneous peritoneal lavage has been tried as an early treatment of acute pancreatitis with encouraging results. Should a pancreatic abscess develop, it must be drained, usually through the flank. Pseudocysts that develop and persist must be treated surgically.

A *pseudocyst* is a collection of pancreatic fluid in the peritoneal cavity, enclosed in a layer of inflammatory tissue. Autodigestion or liquefaction of pancreatic tissue may be the cause. The pseudocyst is most often connected to a pancreatic duct, so that it continues to increase in mass. The symptoms depend on its location. For example, jaundice may occur when a cyst develops near the head of the pancreas close to the common duct. Pseudocysts may resolve or may require surgical intervention.

Chronic pancreatitis

Chronic pancreatitis is characterized by progressive destruction of the pancreas. It can be divided into two types: chronic calcifying pancreatitis and chronic obstructive pancreatitis. In *chronic calcifying pancreatitis,* calcified protein plugs (calculi) form in the pancreatic ducts. This form is seen most often in alcoholics. *Chronic obstructive pancreatitis* is associated with stenosis of the sphincter of Oddi. The lesions are prominent in the head of the pancreas. It is usually due to cholelithiasis and is sometimes relieved by removal of the sphincter of Oddi.

Chronic pancreatitis is manifested in episodes that are similar, albeit of lesser severity, to those of acute pancreatitis. There are persistent, recurring episodes of epigastric and upper left quadrant pain. Anorexia, nausea, vomiting, constipation, and flatulence are common. The attacks are often precipitated by alcohol abuse or overeating. Eventually, the disease progresses to the extent that both endocrine and exocrine pancreatic functions become deficient. At this point, signs of diabetes mellitus and the malabsorption syndrome become apparent. Pancreatic enzymes are given to treat the malabsorption, and the diabetes is treated with insulin. Narcotic addiction is a potential problem in persons with chronic pancreatitis.

Cancer of the pancreas

The incidence of cancer of the pancreas has almost tripled in the past 40 years.[20] At present, it is the fourth leading cause of cancer death in men and the fifth most common in women in the United States. Cancer of the pancreas is usually far advanced when diagnosed, and the 5-year survival rate is less than 9%. The cause of pancreatic cancer is unknown. Recently, an association between coffee and cancer of the pancreas was made. The relative risk associated with drinking two cups of coffee per day was 1.8 times normal; with three or more cups, it was reported to be 2.7 times normal.[32]

Cancer of the pancreas usually has an insidious onset, with symptoms of anorexia, weight loss, flatulence, and nausea. A dull, aching epigastric pain is present in about 70% to 80% of cases.[33] Overt diabetes mellitus is found in one-fifth of persons with pancreatic cancer, and almost all persons with the disease have an abnormal glucose tolerance.[33]

Because of the proximity of the pancreas to the common duct and the ampulla of Vater, cancer of the head of the pancreas tends to obstruct bile flow; this causes distention of the gallbladder and jaundice. The jaundice is frequently the presenting symptom in cancer of the head of the pancreas, and it is usually accompanied by complaints of pain and by pruritus. Cancer of the body of the pancreas generally impinges on the celiac ganglion, causing pain. The pain usually worsens with ingestion of food or with assumption of the supine position. Cancer of the tail of the pancreas has usually metastasized before symptoms appear.

Most cancers of the pancreas have metastasized by the time of diagnosis. Therefore, the treatment is usually palliative and consists of high-voltage irradiation and chemotherapy. Surgical resection of the tumor is done when the tumor is localized. The treatment results with use of single-agent or combination chemotherapy have shown steady improvement, providing some gains for survival.[20]

In summary, the pancreas is both an endocrine and an exocrine organ. Diabetes mellitus is the most common disorder of the endocrine pancreas, and it occurs independently of disease of the exocrine pancreas. The exocrine pancreas produces digestive enzymes that are secreted in an inactive form and transported to the small intestine through the main pancreatic duct, which usually empties into the ampulla of Vater and then into the duodenum through the sphincter of Oddi. The most common diseases of the exocrine pancreas are acute and chronic pancreatitis and cancer. Both acute and chronic pancreatitis are associated with biliary reflux and chronic alcoholism. Acute pancreatitis is a dramatic and life-threatening disorder in which there is autodigestion of pancreatic tissue. Chronic pancreatitis causes progressive destruction of both the endocrine and the exocrine pancreas. It is characterized by episodes of pain and epigastric distress that are similar to but less severe than that which occurs with acute pancreatitis. Cancer of the pancreas has shown a marked increase in incidence during the past 40 years. It is usually far advanced at the time of diagnosis, and as a result, the 5-year survival rate is less than 9%.

References

1. Robbins SL, Cotran RS, Kumar V: Pathologic Basis of Disease, 3rd ed, pp 884, 916, 938. Philadelphia, WB Saunders, 1984
2. Iber F: In alcoholism, the liver sets the pace. Nutrition Today 6(1):2, 1971
3. Lieber CS: Alcohol, protein metabolism, and liver injury. Gastroenterology 79(2):373, 1980
4. Lieber CS: Biochemical and molecular basis of alcohol-induced injury to liver and other tissues. N Engl J Med 319:1639, 1988
5. Lieber CS: Pathogenesis and early diagnosis of alcoholic liver injury. N Engl J Med 298(16):888, 1978
6. Guyton AC: Textbook of Medical Physiology, 7th ed, p 783. Philadelphia, WB Saunders, 1986
7. Fetus and Newborn Committee, Canadian Pediatric Society: Use of phototherapy for neonatal jaundice. Can Med Assoc J 134:1237, 1986
8. Avery GB: Neonatology, 2nd ed, p 493. Philadelphia, JB Lippincott, 1981
9. Lemon SM: Type A hepatitis. N Engl J Med 313:1059, 1985
10. Lemon SM: Hepatitis A among drug users. MMWR 37(19):297, 1988
11. Immunization Practices Advisory Committee: Update on hepatitis B prevention. MMWR 36:353, 1987
12. Knauer CM, Silverman S, Jr: Alimentary Tract and Liver. In Schroeder SA, Krupp MA, Tierney LM: Current Medical Diagnosis and Treatment, pp 398–402. Norwalk, CT, Appleton & Lange, 1987
13. Anthony PP, Ishak KG, Nayak NC et al: The morphology of cirrhosis: Definition, nomenclature, and classification. Bull WHO 55(4):522, 1977
14. Jeffries GH: Diseases of the liver. In Beeson PB, McDermott W, Wyngaarden JB (eds): Cecil Textbook of Medicine, 15th ed, pp 1639, 1670. Philadelphia, WB Saunders, 1979
15. Report to the Congress of the United States of the National Commission on Digestive Diseases, Vol 2(A), p 305, and Vol 4(2A), p 395. National Institute of Health, Public Health Service. DHEW Publication No (NIH) 79, 1984
16. Leevy CM, Kangasundororm N: Alcoholic hepatitis. Hosp Pract 13(10):115, 1978
17. Rubin E, Lieber CS: Alcohol-induced hepatic injury in nonalcoholic volunteers. N Engl J Med 278:869, 1968
18. Wapnick S, Grosberg S, Kinney M et al: LaVeen continuous peritoneal-jugular shunt. JAMA 237(2):131, 1977
19. Hardison GM: Cirrhosis—Treating the ascites and encephalopathy. Med Times 107(5):23, 1979
20. Adams JT, Poulter CA, Pondye KJ: Cancer of the digestive glands. In Rubin P (ed): Clinical Oncology, 6th ed, pp 178, 183. New York, American Cancer Society, 1983

21. Robbins SL, Kumar V: Basic Pathology, 4th ed, pp 597–599. Philadelphia, WB Saunders, 1987

22. Miller HD: Liver transplantation: Postoperative ICU care. Crit Care Nurse 8:619, 1988

23. Root RK: Liver transplantation—The first 25 years. West J Med 149:316, 1988

24. Motson RW, Way LW: Differential diagnosis of gall bladder disease. Hosp Med 13(3):26, 1977

25. Gracie WA, Ranshoff DF: The natural history of silent gallstones. N Engl J Med 307:798, 1982

26. Iber FL: Axioms on biliary tract disease. Hosp Med 15(6):52, 1979

27. Marton KI: How to image the gallbladder in suspected cholecystitis. Ann Intern Med 109:722, 1988

28. Health and Policy Committee, American College of Physicians: How to study the gallbladder. Ann Intern Med 109:752, 1988

29. Schuman BM: New weapons in the war against gallstones. Emerg Med 20(Aug 15):81, 1988

30. Mulley AG: Shock-wave lithotripsy. N Engl J Med 314:845, 1986

31. Ronson JHC: Etiologic and prognostic factors in human acute pancreatitis: A review. Am J Gastroenterol 77:633, 1982

32. MacMahon B, Yen S, Trichopoulos D et al: Coffee and cancer of the pancreas. N Engl J Med 304(11):630, 1981

33. Shroeder SA, Krupp MA, Tierney LM: Current Diagnosis and Treatment, p 424. Norwalk, CN/San Mateo, CA, Appleton & Lange, 1988

Bibliography

Buckley GB, Oshima A, Bailey RW: Pathophysiology of hepatic ischemia in cardiogenic shock. Am J Surg 151:87, 1986

Cello JP: Diagnostic approaches to jaundice. Hosp Pract 17(2):49, 1982

Cello JP, Crass RA, Grendell JH et al: Management of the patient with hemorrhaging esophageal varices. JAMA 256:1480, 1986

Fain JA, Amato-Vealey E: Acute pancreatitis: A gastrointestinal emergency. Crit Care Nurse 8(5):47, 1988

Fraser CL, Arieff AI: Hepatic encephalopathy. N Engl J Med 313:865, 1985

Gannon RB, Pickett K: Jaundice. Am J Nurs 83:404, 1983

Gerety RJ, Aronson DL: Plasma derivatives and viral hepatitis. Transfusion 22:347, 1982

Gocke DJ: Hepatitis A revisited. Ann Intern Med 105:960, 1986

Gracie WA, Ransohoff DF: The innocent gallbladder is no myth. N Engl J Med 307:798, 1982

Groszmann RJ, Atterbury CE: The pharmacologic treatment of portal hypertension. Annu Rev Med 36:81, 1985

Gurevich I: Hepatitis precautions. Am J Nurs 83:572, 1983

Hoyumpa AM Jr, Schenker S: Perspectives in hepatic encephalopathy. J Lab Clin Med 100:477, 1982

Jacobson IM, Dienstag JL: Viral hepatitis vaccines. Annu Rev Med 36:241, 1985

Levy M, Wexler MJ: Salt and water balance in liver disease. Hosp Pract 18(July):57, 1984

Lieber CS: Metabolism and metabolic effects of alcohol. Med Clin North Am 68:3, 1984

Maisels MJ: Jaundice in the newborn. Pediatr Rev 3:305, 1982

Moosa AR: Diagnostic tests and procedures in acute pancreatitis. N Engl J Med 311:639, 1984

Ranson JH: Etiologic and prognostic factors in human acute pancreatitis: A review. Am J Gastroenterol 77:633, 1982

Resnick RH: Treatment of bleeding varices: Controversy and opportunity. Hosp Pract 19(4):54A, 1984

Reynolds RB: What to do about esophageal varices. N Engl J Med 309:1575, 1983

Rocco VK, Ware A: Cirrotic ascites. Ann Intern Med 105:573, 1986

Scharschmidt BF, Goldberg HI, Schmid R: Approach to the patient with cholestatic jaundice. N Engl J Med 308:1515, 1983

Schenker S, Hoyumpa AM Jr: Pathology of hepatic encephalitis. Hosp Pract 19(9):99, 1984

Schumann D: Correction of ascites with peritoneovenous shunting: A study of clinical management. Heart Lung 12:248, 1983

Thistle JL, Cleary PA, Lachin JM et al: The natural history of cholelithiasis: The national cooperative gallstone study. Ann Intern Med 101:171, 1984

Williams RL: Drug administration in hepatic disease. N Engl J Med 309:1616, 1983

CHAPTER 42

Darlene G. Thornhill
Joan Pleuss

Alterations in Nutritional Status

Nutritional status
  Energy metabolism
    Adipose (fat) tissue
    Anabolism and catabolism
    Glucose metabolism
    Fat metabolism
    Protein metabolism
  Energy expenditure
    Metabolic rate
    Diet-induced thermogenesis
    Exercise-induced
      thermogenesis

**Nutritional needs and
  recommended daily
  allowances**
  Calories
  Proteins
  Fats
  Carbohydrates
  Vitamins
  Minerals
  Fiber
Nutritional assessment
  Diet history
  Health assessment
  Anthropometric measurements
  Laboratory studies

Overnutrition and obesity
  Causes of obesity
  Types of obesity
  Health risks associated with
    obesity
  Treatment of obesity
Undernutrition
  Malnutrition and starvation
    Malnutrition in hospitalized
      patients
  Eating disorders
    Anorexia nervosa
    Binge–purge syndrome

Objectives

After you have studied this chapter, you should be able to meet the following objectives:

_____ Define *nutritional status.*

_____ Define *calorie* and state the number of calories derived from the oxidation of 1 g of protein, fat, and carbohydrate.

_____ Describe the location and function of adipocytes in the body.

_____ Explain the difference between anabolism and catabolism.

_____ Relate the processes of glycogenolysis and gluconeogenesis to the regulation of blood glucose by the liver.

_____ Explain the process of energy substrate storage by adipocytes.

_____ Discuss the utilization of amino acids from body proteins as an energy source.

_____ Differentiate between basal metabolic rate, basal energy equivalent, diet-induced thermogenesis, exercise-induced thermogenesis, and thermogenesis in response to environmental conditions.

_____ Cite the effect of age on metabolic rate.

_____ State the purpose of the daily recommended allowance (RDA) of calories, proteins, fats, carbohydrates, vitamins, and minerals.

_____ State information for nutritional assessment that can be obtained from diet history, health assessment, body weight, skinfold and body circumference measurements, densiometry, bioelectrical impedance, computerized tomographic scans, and laboratory studies.

(continued)

_____ Compare relative body weight, the Metropolitan Life Insurance Table, and body mass index as methods for evaluating body weight in terms of undernutrition and overnutrition.

_____ Define *obesity*.

_____ Explain the difference in prevalence rates for obesity.

_____ Discuss the causes of obesity.

_____ List the health risks associated with obesity.

_____ Differentiate upper and lower body obesity and their implications in terms of health risk.

_____ Discuss the treatment of obesity as it relates to diet, behavior modification, exercise, social support, and surgical methods.

_____ Define *malnutrition* and *starvation*.

_____ List the major causes of malnutrition and starvation.

_____ State the difference between protein-calorie starvation (marasmus) and protein malnutrition (kwashiorkor).

_____ Describe how fuel sources are maintained during starvation.

_____ Explain the effect of malnutrition on muscle mass, respiratory function, acid–base balance, wound healing and immune function, bone mineralization, and the menstrual cycle in the female or testicular function in the male.

_____ State the causes of malnutrition in the hospitalized patient.

_____ Compare the eating disorders and complications associated with anorexia nervosa and the binge–purge syndrome.

"You are what you eat" is often said. To a great extent, nutrition determines how a person looks, feels, and acts. The need for adequate nutrition begins at the time of conception and continues throughout life. Nutrition provided by food or supplements in the proper proportions enables the body to maintain life, to grow both physically and intellectually, to heal and repair tissue, and, in general, to maintain the stamina necessary for well-being. The content presented in this chapter has been divided into three parts: nutritional status, overnutrition and obesity, and undernutrition.

Nutritional status

Nutritional status describes the condition of the body as it relates to the availability and utilization of nutrients. Nutrients provide the energy and materials necessary for performing the activities of daily living; for maintaining healthy skin, muscles, and other body tissues; for replacing and healing tissues; and for the effective functioning of all body systems including the immune and respiratory systems. Not only can poor nutritional status cause illness, but it can also make it impossible for the individual to recuperate from illness.

Nutrients are derived from the digestive tract through the ingestion of foods or, in some cases, through liquid feedings that are delivered directly into the gastrointestinal tract by a synthetic tube (tube feedings). The exception occurs in persons with certain illnesses in which the digestive tract is bypassed and the nutrients are infused directly into the circulatory system. Once inside the body, nutrients are used for energy or as the building blocks for tissue growth and repair. When excess nutrients are available, they frequently are stored for future use. If the required nutrients are unavailable, the body adapts by conserving and using its nutrient stores.

Energy metabolism

Energy is measured in heat units called *calories*. A calorie, spelled with a small *c* and also called a *gram calorie*, is the amount of heat or energy required to raise the temperature of 1 g of water 1°C. A *kilocalorie*, or *large calorie*, is the amount of energy needed to raise the temperature of 1 kg of water 1°C. Because a calorie is so small, kilocalories are often used in nutritional and physiologic studies. The oxidation of proteins provides 4 Kcal/g; fats, 9 Kcal/g; carbohydrates, 4 Kcal/g, and alcohol, 7 Kcal/g.

All body activities require energy whether they involve an individual cell, a single organ, or the entire body. Metabolism is the organized process through which nutrients such as carbohydrates, fats, and proteins are broken down, transformed, or otherwise converted into cellular energy. The process of metabolism is unique in that it not only allows for the continual release of energy, but it couples this energy release with physiologic functioning. For example, the energy used for muscle contraction is derived largely from energy sources that are stored in muscle cells. This energy is then released as the muscle contracts. Because most of our energy sources come from the nutrients in the food that is eaten, the ability to store energy and control its release is important.

Adipose (fat) tissue

More than 90% of body energy is stored in the adipose tissues of the body.[1] Adipocytes, or fat cells, occur either singly or in small groups in loose connective tissue. In many parts of the body, they cushion body organs such as the kidneys. In addition to isolated groups of fat cells, there are entire regions of fat tissue that are committed to fat storage. Collectively, fat cells constitute a large body organ that is metabolically very active in the uptake, synthesis, storage, and mobilization of lipids, which are the main source of fuel storage for the body. Some tissues, such as liver cells, are able to store small amounts of lipids, but when these lipids accumulate, they begin to interfere with cell function. Adipose tissue not only serves as a storage for body fuels, but it provides insulation for the body, fills body crevices, and protects body organs.

Studies of adipocytes in the laboratory have shown that fully differentiated cells do not divide. However, such cells have a long life span, and anyone born with large numbers of adipocytes runs the risk of becoming obese. Some immature adipocytes capable of division are present in postnatal life; these cells respond to estrogen stimulation and are the potential source of additional fat cells during postnatal life.[2] Fat deposition results from a proliferation of these existing immature adipocytes and can occur as a consequence of excessive caloric intake when a woman is breast-feeding or during estrogen stimulation around the time of puberty. An increase in fat cells may also occur during late adolescence and in middle-aged people who are already fat.[2]

There are two types of adipose tissue: white fat and brown fat. White fat, which despite its name is cream colored or yellow, is the prevalent form of adipose tissue in postnatal life. It constitutes 10% to 20% of body weight in adult males and 15% to 25% in adult females.[2] At body temperature, the lipid content of fat cells is present as oil. It consists of triglycerides —three molecules of fatty acids esterified to a glycerol molecule. Triglycerides, which contain no water, have the highest caloric content of all nutrients and are an efficient form of energy storage. Fat cells synthesize triglycerides, the major fat storage form, from dietary fats and carbohydrates. Insulin is required for transport of glucose into fat cells. When calorie intake is restricted for any reason, fat cell triglycerides are broken down and the resultant fatty acids and glycerol are released as energy sources.

Brown fat, as the name implies, is brown in color. It differs from white fat in terms of its thermogenic capacity or ability to produce heat. Brown fat, the site of both diet-induced thermogenesis and non-shivering thermogenesis, is found primarily in early neonatal life in humans and in animals that hibernate. It has been suggested that the presence of brown fat allows animals to eat large quantities of poor-quality diets to obtain essential nutrients, while avoiding

weight gain. The presence and role of brown fat in older children and adults is controversial at present. It has been suggested that brown fat may have a thermogenic role in humans and that the sympathetic nervous system may play a role in its activation.[3]

Anabolism and catabolism

There are two phases of metabolism—anabolism and catabolism. *Anabolism* is the phase of metabolic storage and synthesis of cell constituents. Anabolism does not provide energy for the body; rather, it requires energy. *Catabolism,* on the other hand, involves the breakdown of complex molecules into substances that can be used in the production of energy. The chemical intermediates for anabolism and catabolism are called *metabolites*—for example, lactic acid is one of the metabolites formed when glucose is broken down in the absence of oxygen.

Both anabolism and catabolism are catalyzed by *enzyme systems* located within body cells. A *substrate* is a substance on which an enzyme acts. Enzyme systems selectively transform fuel substrates into cellular energy and facilitate the use of energy in the process of assembling molecules to form energy substrates and storage forms of energy.

Because body energy cannot be stored as heat, the cellular oxidative processes that release energy are flameless and have low temperature reactions. Instead of releasing only heat—as occurs when the same fuel is burned in the environment—the free energy released from the oxidation of foods is converted to chemical energy that can be stored. The body transforms carbohydrates, fats, and proteins into the intermediary compound, adenosine triphosphate (ATP). Adenosine triphosphate is often called the energy currency of the cell because almost all body cells use ATP as their energy source (see Chapter 1). The metabolic events involved in ATP formation allow cellular energy to be stored, used, and then replenished.

Glucose metabolism

Glucose is a six-carbon molecule; it is an efficient fuel that, when metabolized in the presence of oxygen, breaks down to form carbon dioxide and water (Figure 42-1). Although many tissues and organ systems are able to use other forms of fuel, such as fatty acids and ketones, the brain and nervous system rely almost exclusively on glucose as a fuel source. The nervous system can neither store nor synthesize glucose; rather, it relies on the minute-by-minute extraction of glucose from the blood to meet its energy needs. In the fed and early fasting state, the nervous

H
|
H — C — OH
|
H — C — OH
|
H — C — OH
|
HO — C — H
|
H — C — OH
|
H — C
||
O

Glucose
(Straight Chain)

O
||
O   CH — O — C — R₁
|| |
R₂ — C — O — C   O
| ||
CH₂ — O — C — R₃

Triglyceride

H
|
R — C — COOH
|
NH₂

Amino Acid

Figure 42-1 Glucose, triglyceride, and amino acid structure. (R = fatty acid.)

system requires about 100 g to 115 g of glucose per day to meet its metabolic needs.[4,5]

The liver regulates the entry of glucose into the blood. Glucose ingested in the diet is transported from the gastrointestinal tract, through the portal vein, to the liver before it gains access to the circulatory system (Figure 42-2). The liver both stores and synthesizes glucose. When blood sugar is increased, the liver removes glucose from the blood and stores it for future use. Conversely, the liver releases its glucose stores when blood sugar drops. In this way, the liver acts as a buffer system to regulate blood sugar levels. Generally speaking, blood sugar levels reflect the difference between the amount of glucose released into the circulation by the liver and the amount of glucose removed from the blood by body cells.

Excess glucose is stored in two forms: (1) it can be converted to fatty acids and then stored in fat cells as triglycerides, or (2) it can be stored in the liver and skeletal muscle as glycogen. Small amounts of

glycogen are also stored in the skin and in some of the glandular tissues.

Glycogenolysis. Glycogenolysis, or the breakdown of glycogen, is controlled by the action of two hormones: glucagon and epinephrine. Epinephrine is more effective in stimulating glycogen breakdown in muscle. The liver, on the other hand, is more responsive to glucagon. The synthesis and degradation of glycogen are important because they help maintain blood sugar levels during periods of fasting and strenuous exercise. Only the liver, in contrast with other tissues that store glycogen, is able to release its glucose stores into the blood for use by other tissues, such as the brain and nervous system. This is because glycogen breaks down to form a phosphorylated glucose molecule. Glucose is too large, in its phosphorylated form, to pass through the cell membrane. The liver, but not skeletal muscle, has the enzyme glucose-6-phosphatase, which is needed to remove the phosphate group and to allow the glucose molecule to enter the bloodstream.

Although they are rare, a number of genetic disorders exist in which glycogen breakdown is impaired. All of these disorders result in excessive accumulation of abnormal forms of glycogen. *Von Gierke's disease* involves a genetic deficiency of glucose-6-

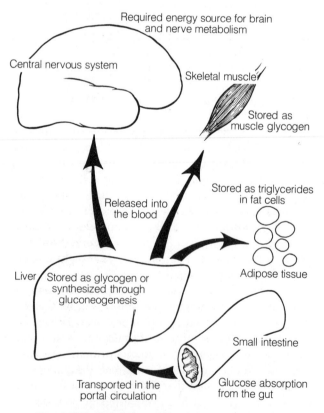

Figure 42-2 Regulation of blood glucose by the liver.

phosphatase. Children with this disease have stunted growth, liver enlargement, hypoglycemia, and hyperlipidemia resulting from mobilization of fatty acids. *McArdle's disease* is characterized by a deficiency in skeletal muscle glycogen; as a result of this deficiency, the disease causes extreme muscle weakness.

Gluconeogenesis.   The synthesis of glucose is referred to as *gluconeogenesis,* or the building of glucose from new sources. The process of gluconeogenesis converts amino acids, lactate, and glycerol into glucose. Most of the gluconeogenesis occurs in the liver. Although fatty acids can be used as fuel by many body cells, they cannot be converted to glucose.

Glucose produced through the process of gluconeogenesis is either stored in the liver as glycogen or released into the general circulation. During periods of food deprivation or when the diet is low in carbohydrates, gluconeogenesis provides the glucose that is needed to meet the metabolic needs of the brain and other glucose-dependent tissues.

Several hormones stimulate gluconeogenesis, including glucagon, glucocorticoid hormones from the adrenal cortex, and thyroid hormone.

Alcohol ingestion interferes with the liver's ability to produce glucose. This is because the metabolism of alcohol competes for the use of the same hydrogen carrier, nicotinamide-adenine dinucleotide (NAD), which is needed for glucose production. Although probably not a common occurrence, alcohol-induced hypoglycemia can occur after a period of fasting. Because glucose stimulates insulin release, this tends to occur more readily when alcohol is consumed in combination with sugar-containing mixers.

Fat metabolism

The average American diet provides 37% to 40% of calories in the form of fats. In contrast to glucose, which yields only 4 cal/g, each gram of fat yields 9 cal. Additionally, another 30% to 50% of the carbohydrates consumed in the diet are converted to triglycerides for storage.

A triglyceride contains three fatty acids linked by a glycerol molecule (see Figure 42-1). Fatty acids and triglycerides can be derived from dietary sources, they can be synthesized in the body, or they can be mobilized from fat depots. Excess carbohydrate is converted to triglyceride and is then transported by lipoproteins in the blood to adipose cells for storage. One gram of anhydrous (water-free) fat stores more than six times as much energy as one hydrated gram of glycogen. One reason weight loss is greatest at the beginning of a fast or weight-loss program is that this is when the body uses its glycogen stores. Later, when the body begins to use energy stored as triglycerides,

water losses are decreased and weight loss tends to plateau.

The mobilization of fat for use in energy production is facilitated by the action of enzymes, or lipases, that break the triglycerides into three fatty acids and a glycerol molecule. Following triglyceride breakdown, both the fatty acids and the glycerol molecule leave the fat cell and enter the circulation. Once in the circulation, many of the fatty acids are transported to the liver, where they are removed from the blood and are then either used by liver cells as a source of energy or converted to ketones.

The efficient burning of fatty acids requires a balance between carbohydrate and fat metabolism. The ratio of fatty acid and carbohydrate utilization is altered in situations that favor fat breakdown, such as diabetes mellitus and fasting. In these situations, the liver produces more ketones than it can use; this excess is then released into the bloodstream. Ketones can be an important source of energy, because even the brain adapts to the use of ketones during prolonged periods of starvation. A problem arises, however, when fat breakdown is accelerated and the production of ketones exceeds tissue utilization. Because ketone bodies are organic acids, they cause *ketoacidosis* when they are present in excessive amounts. The activation of lipases and the subsequent mobilization of fatty acids are stimulated by epinephrine, glucocorticoid hormones, growth hormones, and glucagon.

Protein metabolism

About three-fourths of body solids are proteins. Proteins are essential for the formation of all body structures, including genes, enzymes, contractile proteins in muscle, matrix of bone, and hemoglobin of red blood cells.

Amino acids are the building blocks of proteins. There are 20 amino acids present in body proteins in significant quantities. Each amino acid has an acidic group (COOH) and an amino group (NH_2) (see Figure 42-1). Unlike glucose and fatty acids, there is only a limited facility for the storage of excess amino acids in the body. Most of the stored amino acids are contained in body proteins. Amino acids in excess of those needed for protein synthesis are converted to fatty acids, ketone bodies, or glucose and are then stored or used as metabolic fuel. Each gram of protein yields 4 cal. Because fatty acids cannot be converted to glucose, the body must break down proteins and use the amino acids as a major source of substrate for gluconeogenesis during periods when metabolic needs exceed food intake. The liver has the enzymes and transfer mechanisms needed to deaminate and to convert the amino groups (NH_2) from the amino acid to urea. Thus, the breakdown or degradation of proteins and amino acids occurs primarily in the liver, which is also the site of gluconeogenesis.

Energy expenditure

The expenditure of body energy results from four mechanisms of heat production (thermogenesis): (1) basal metabolic rate (BMR) or basal energy equivalent (BEE), (2) diet-induced thermogenesis, (3) exercise-induced thermogenesis, and (4) thermogenesis in response to changes in environmental conditions. The amount of energy used varies with age, body size, rate of growth, and state of health.

Metabolic rate

The basal, or resting metabolism, refers to the chemical reactions occurring when the body is at rest. These reactions are necessary to provide energy for maintenance of normal body temperature, cardiovascular and respiratory function, muscle tone, and other essential activities of tissues and cells in the resting body. The resting metabolic rate constitutes 65% to 70% of body energy needs. The BMR can be determined by placing a person in a special chamber and measuring the total quantity of heat liberated from the body in a given period of time. Because most of the energy expended by the body is derived from oxidative reactions involving dietary nutrients, the BEE measurement can be determined indirectly by measuring oxygen utilization. The BMR and BEE are measured after 12 hours of fasting while the person is awake and at rest in a warm room. Several factors that affect BMR are age, sex, physical state, and pregnancy. A progressive decline in the normal BMR occurs with aging. Women generally have a 5% to 10% lower BMR than men because of their higher percentage of adipose tissue. The BMR decreases by 2% each new decade of life after growth has ceased (Figure 42-3).

The BEE can be estimated using the Harris-Benedict equation (Table 42-1). The Harris-Benedict equation correctly predicts the BEE for 90% of healthy adults.[6] Multiplying the BEE by a factor of 1.2 will usually adequately predict the calorie needs for maintenance of nutrition during health. A factor of 1.5 will usually provide the needed nutrients during repletion and during illnesses such as pneumonia, long-bone fractures, cancer, peritonitis, and recovery from most types of major surgery.

Diet-induced thermogenesis

The diet-induced thermogenesis, or specific dynamic action of food, describes the energy used by the body for the digestion, absorption, and assimilation of food following its ingestion. It is energy expended over and above the caloric value of the food itself. It varies from 10% to 35% depending on the type and quantity of food consumed and accounts for 6% to 10% of the total calories expended.[6] When food is eaten, the metabolic rate rises and then returns to normal within a few hours. One explanation for the thermogenic response to a meal is that it results from enhanced activity of the sympathetic nervous system and its effect on brown adipose tissue. If this is true, then decreased sympathetic activity in obese persons could account for an enhanced metabolic efficiency that allows calories to be stored rather than expended.[1]

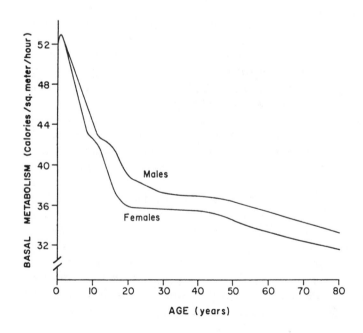

Figure 42-3 Normal basal metabolic rates at different ages for each sex. (*Guyton A: Medical Physiology, 7th ed. Philadelphia, WB Saunders, 1986*)

Exercise-induced thermogenesis

The amount of energy expended for physical activity is determined by the type of activity performed, the length of participation, and the individual's weight. Table 42-2 gives the energy expenditure for various activities.

Nutritional needs and recommended daily allowances

Nutritional status reflects the continued daily intake of nutrients over time and the deposition and utilization of these nutrients within the body. The body requires over forty nutrients on a daily basis. Several of these have had a daily recommended allowance (RDA) established. The RDA is the level of intake of essential nutrients considered to be adequate to meet the known nutrient needs of practically all healthy persons. The RDA is not the minimum requirement; it is usually two to six times the minimum daily requirement. Most persons could have 80% of the RDA in their diet and still be well nourished.

The RDA amounts are set by determining the entire range of needs, selecting the numbers at the high end, and then adding a safety factor without risking toxicity. Experts from universities and government comprise the Food and Nutrition Board of the National Research Council under the National Academy of Sciences. They continuously evaluate the current research and periodically determine and revise the RDA.[7] The latest RDA was published in 1980 (Table 42-3).

There are seventeen age and sex classifications in the RDA. It is to be used as a standard for feeding programs, school lunch programs, penal institutions, hospital and health-care facilities, and computer software used to analyze diets and recipes. The RDA is intended to be met by a variety of foods versus supplements or extensive fortification.

The United States RDA (USRDA) was established for the purpose of labeling foods. It takes the highest value of each nutrient for persons 4 years of age to adult (excluding pregnancy and lactation); therefore, the USRDA sometimes provides a margin of nutritional safety higher than the RDA.

Proteins, fats, carbohydrates, vitamins, and minerals each have their own function in providing the body with what it needs to maintain life and health. Recommended allowances have not been established for every nutrient; some are given as a safe and adequate intake while others, such as carbohydrates and fats, are expressed as a percentage of the calorie intake. The function of each of these nutrients will be presented, along with the suggested daily consumption of each.

Calories

Energy requirements will be greater during growth periods. Infants require approximately 115 Kcal/kg at birth, 105 Kcal/kg at 1 year, and 80 Kcal/kg body weight from ages 1 to 10 years. During adolescence boys require 45 Kcal/kg body weight and girls, 38 Kcal/kg body weight. During pregnancy, a woman needs an extra 300 Kcal per day above her usual requirement and during the first 3 months of breast-feeding, an additional 500 Kcal.[7] Table 42-4 gives a simple formula for determining caloric intake in healthy adults.

Proteins

Proteins are required for growth and maintenance of body tissues, enzymes and antibody formation, fluid and electrolyte balance, and nutrient transport. Proteins are composed of amino acids, nine of which are essential to the body. These are leucine, isoleucine, methionine, phenylalanine, threonine, tryptophan, valine, lysine, and histidine. The foods that provide these essential amino acids are milk, eggs, meat, fish, and poultry. These foods are referred to as complete proteins. The incomplete proteins are those that do not provide all nine essential amino acids. These include dried peas, beans, nuts, seeds, and grains. These need to be combined with each other or with complete proteins to meet the amino acid requirements. Diets that are inadequate in protein will result in kwashiorkor. If both calories and protein are inadequate, protein-calorie malnutrition occurs.

Unlike carbohydrates and fats, which are composed of hydrogen, carbon, and oxygen, proteins

---

Table 42–1. Equation for calculating basal energy expenditure (BEE)

Men

$$BEE = 66 + (13.7 \times weight\ (kg)) + (5 \times height\ (cm)) - (6.8 \times age\ (yr))$$

Women

$$BEE = 655 + (9.5 \times weight\ (kg)) + (1.7 \times height\ (cm)) - (4.7 \times age\ (yr))$$

(Krause MV, Mahan LK: Food, Nutrition and Diet Therapy. Philadelphia, WB Saunders, 1984)

Table 42–2. Energy expenditure per hour during different types of activity for a 70-kilogram man

Form of activity	Calories per hour
Sleeping	65
Awake lying still	77
Sitting at rest	100
Standing relaxed	105
Dressing and undressing	118
Tailoring	135
Typewriting rapidly	140
"Light" exercise	170
Walking slowly (2.6 miles per hour)	200
Carpentry, metal working, industrial painting	240
"Active" exercise	290
"Severe" exercise	450
Sawing wood	480
Swimming	500
Running (5.3 miles per hour)	570
"Very severe" exercise	600
Walking very fast (5.3 miles per hour)	650
Walking up stairs	1100

(Extracted from data compiled by Professor M. S. Rose. Guyton A: Medical Physiology, 7th ed. Philadelphia, WB Saunders, 1986)

contain 16% nitrogen; therefore, nitrogen excretion is an indicator of protein intake. If the amount of nitrogen taken in by way of protein is equivalent to the nitrogen excreted, the person is said to be in *nitrogen balance*. An individual is in positive nitrogen balance when the nitrogen consumed by way of protein is greater than the amount excreted. This occurs during growth, pregnancy, or healing after surgery or injury. A negative nitrogen balance often occurs during fever, illness, infection, trauma, or burns when more nitrogen is excreted than is consumed. Tissue wasting ensues.

Fats

Dietary fats are composed primarily of triglycerides (a mixture of fatty acids and glycerol). The fatty acids are either saturated (no double bonds), monounsaturated (one double bond), or polyunsaturated (two or more double bonds). The saturated fatty acids elevate blood cholesterol, while the monounsaturated and polyunsaturated fats lower blood cholesterol. Current research indicates that dietary fat should be divided equally between the three types of fatty acids.[8] Saturated fats are generally from animal

Table 42–3. Recommended daily dietary allowances,* revised 1980

	Age (yr)	Weight (kg) (lb)		Height (cm) (in)		Protein (g)	Fat-soluble vitamins			Water-	
							Vitamin A (µg R.E.)†	Vitamin D (µg)‡	Vitamin E (mg α T.E.)§	Vitamin C (mg)	Thiamin (mg)
Infants	0.0–0.5	6	13	60	24	kg × 2.2	420	10	3	35	0.3
	0.5–1.0	9	20	71	28	kg × 2.0	400	10	4	35	0.5
Children	1–3	13	29	90	35	23	400	10	5	45	0.7
	4–6	20	44	112	44	30	500	10	6	45	0.9
	7–10	28	62	132	52	34	700	10	7	45	1.2
Males	11–14	45	99	157	62	45	1000	10	8	50	1.4
	15–18	66	145	176	69	56	1000	10	10	60	1.4
	19–22	70	154	177	70	56	1000	7.5	10	60	1.5
	23–50	70	154	178	70	56	1000	5	10	60	1.4
	51+	70	154	178	70	56	1000	5	10	60	1.2
Females	11–14	46	101	157	62	46	800	10	8	50	1.1
	15–18	55	120	163	64	46	800	10	8	60	1.1
	19–22	55	120	163	64	44	800	7.5	8	60	1.1
	23–50	55	120	163	64	44	800	5	8	60	1.0
	51+	55	120	163	64	44	800	5	8	60	1.0
Pregnant						+30	+200	+5	+2	+20	+0.4
Lactating						+20	+400	+5	+3	+40	+0.5

* The allowances are intended to provide for individual variations among most normal persons as they live in the United States under usual environmental stresses. Diets should be based on a variety of common foods in order to provide other nutrients for which human requirements have been less well defined.

† Retinol equivalents. 1 Retinol equivalent = 1 µg retinol or 6 µg β carotene.

‡ As cholecalciferol. 10 µg cholecalciferol = 400 I.U. vitamin D.

§ α-tocopherol equivalents. 1 mg d-α-tocopherol = 1 α T. E.

‖ 1 N.E. (niacin equivalent) is equal to 1 mg of niacin or 60 mg of dietary tryptophan.

(Reprinted from Recommended Dietary Allowances, 9th ed, 1980, with permission of the National Academy Press, Washington, DC)

sources and remain solid at room temperature. With the exception of coconut and palm oils, unsaturated fats are found in plant oils and are usually liquid at room temperature.

Dietary fats provide energy, serve as carriers for the fat-soluble vitamins, are precursors of prostaglandins, and are a source of fatty acids. The polyunsaturated fatty acid linoleic acid is the only fatty acid that is required. A deficiency of linoleic acid will result in dermatitis. The daily requirement is 5 g or 1% to 2% of the total daily calories. Because vegetable oils are rich sources of linoleic acid, this level can easily be met.

Other than the requirement for linoleic acid, there is no specific requirement for dietary fat, provided there is adequate nutrition available for energy. Fat is the most concentrated source of energy. It is currently recommended that only 30% of the calories in the diet should come from fats. However, the typical American diet contains 37% to 40% of its calories as fat.[8]

Cholesterol is the major constituent of cell membranes and is synthesized by the body. Cholesterol metabolism and transport are discussed in Chapter 18. The daily dietary recommendation for cholesterol is 300 mg; however, many Americans have diets that contain about 600 mg.[9]

Carbohydrates

Dietary carbohydrates are composed of simple sugars, complex carbohydrates, and undigested carbohydrates (fiber). Because of their vitamin, mineral, and fiber content, it is recommended that the bulk of the carbohydrate content in the diet be in the complex form rather than as simple sugars that contain few nutrients. Sucrose (table sugar) is implicated in the development of dental caries.

There is no specific dietary requirement for carbohydrates. All of the energy requirements can be met by dietary fats and proteins. Although some tissues, such as the nervous system, require glucose as an energy source, this need can be met through the conversion of amino acids and the glycerol part of the triglyceride molecule to glucose. The fatty acids from triglycerides are converted to ketones and used for energy by other body tissues. Thus, a carbohydrate-deficient diet usually results in the loss of tissue pro-

-soluble vitamins					Minerals					
Riboflavin (mg)	Niacin (mg N.E.)‖	Vitamin B$_6$ (mg)	Folacin (μg)#	Vitamin B$_{12}$ (μg)	Calcium (mg)	Phosphorus (mg)	Magnesium (mg)	Iron (mg)	Zinc (mg)	Iodine (μg)
0.4	6	0.3	30	0.5*	360	240	50	10	3	40
0.6	8	0.6	45	1.5	540	360	70	15	5	50
0.8	9	0.9	100	2.0	800	800	150	15	10	70
1.0	11	1.3	200	2.5	800	800	200	10	10	90
1.4	16	1.6	300	3.0	800	800	250	10	10	120
1.6	18	1.8	400	3.0	1200	1200	350	18	15	150
1.7	18	2.0	400	3.0	1200	1200	400	18	15	150
1.7	19	2.2	400	3.0	800	800	350	10	15	150
1.6	18	2.2	400	3.0	800	800	350	10	15	150
1.4	16	2.2	400	3.0	800	800	350	10	15	150
1.3	15	1.8	400	3.0	1200	1200	300	18	15	150
1.3	14	2.0	400	3.0	1200	1200	300	18	15	150
1.3	14	2.0	400	3.0	800	800	300	18	15	150
1.2	13	2.0	400	3.0	800	800	300	18	15	150
1.2	13	2.0	400	3.0	800	800	300	10	15	150
+0.3	+2	+0.6	+400	+1.0	+400	+400	+150	††	+5	+25
+0.5	+5	+0.5	+100	+1.0	+400	+400	+150	††	+10	+50

The folacin allowances refer to dietary sources as determined by *Lactobacillus casei* assay after treatment with enzymes ("conjugases") to make polyglutamyl forms of the vitamin available to the test organism.

** The RDA for vitamin B$_{12}$ in infants is based on average concentration of the vitamin in human milk. The allowances after weaning are based on energy intake (as recommended by the American Academy of Pediatrics) and consideration of other factors such as intestinal absorption.

†† The increased requirement during pregnancy cannot be met by the iron content of habitual American diets nor by the existing iron stores of many women; therefore the use of 30–60 mg of supplemental iron is recommended. Iron needs during lactation are not substantially different from those of nonpregnant women, but continued supplementation of the mother for 2–3 months after parturition is advisable in order to replenish stores depleted by pregnancy.

(Designed for the maintenance of good nutrition of practically all healthy people in the U.S.A. Food and Nutrition Board, National Academy of Sciences–National Research Council)

Table 42–4. Caloric requirements based on body weight and activity level

	Sedentary	Moderate	Active
Overweight	20–25 kcal/kg	30 kcal/kg	35 kcal/kg
Normal	30 kcal/kg	35 kcal/kg	40 kcal/kg
Underweight	30 kcal/kg	40 kcal/kg	45–50 kcal/kg

(Adapted from Goodhart RS, and Shils ME: Modern nutrition in Health and Disease. 6th ed. Philadelphia, Lea and Febiger, 1980.)

teins and the development of ketosis. Because protein and fat metabolism increases the production of osmotically active metabolic wastes that must be eliminated through the kidneys, there is danger of dehydration and electrolyte imbalances. The amount of carbohydrate needed to prevent tissue wasting and ketosis is 50 to 100 g/day. In practice, the majority of the daily energy requirement should be from carbohydrate because protein is a very expensive source of calories and because it is recommended that only 30% of the calories in the diet be derived from fat. The current recommendation is that the diet should provide 50% to 60% of the calories as carbohydrates.[8] The actual intake for most Americans is closer to 45%; hence, the average American diet is too low in carbohydrates and too high in fats and proteins.

Vitamins

Vitamins are a group of organic compounds that act as catalysts in various chemical reactions. A compound cannot be classified as a vitamin unless it is shown that a deficiency of it will cause disease. Contrary to popular belief, vitamins do not provide energy directly. As catalysts they are part of the enzyme systems required for the release of energy from protein, fat, and carbohydrates. Vitamins are also necessary for the formation of red blood cells, hormones, genetic materials, and the nervous system. They are essential for normal growth and development.

There are two types of vitamins: fat-soluble and water-soluble. The four fat-soluble vitamins are vitamins A, D, E, and K. The nine required water-soluble vitamins are thiamine, riboflavin, niacin, pyridoxine, pantothenic acid, B_{12}, folic acid, biotin, and vitamin C. Because the water-soluble vitamins are excreted in the urine, it is less likely that they will become toxic to the body; but the fat-soluble vitamins are stored in the body, and they may reach toxic levels. See Table 42-5 for functions, deficiency, toxicity, and sources of vitamins.

Minerals

Minerals serve many functions. They are involved in acid–base balance and in the maintenance of osmotic pressure within body compartments. Minerals are components of vitamins, hormones, and enzymes. They maintain normal hemoglobin levels, have functions within the nervous system, and are involved in muscle contraction and skeletal development and maintenance. Minerals that are present in relatively large amounts in the body are called *macrominerals*. These include calcium, phosphorus, sodium, chloride, potassium, magnesium, and sulfur. The remainder are classified as *trace minerals;* they include iron, manganese, copper, iodine, zinc, cobalt, fluorine, and selenium. Table 42-6 lists mineral sources and functions.

Fiber

Fiber, the portion of food that cannot be digested by the human intestinal tract, increases stool bulk and facilitates bowel movements. Several studies have indicated that fiber decreases the incidence of digestive diseases and lowers blood sugar and cholesterol.[10,11]

Nutritional assessment

The nutritional status of an individual can be assessed by evaluation of the individual's dietary intake, anthropometric measurements, physical examination, and laboratory tests. The nutritional assessment can provide information regarding the adequacy of the diet, the individual's body size compared to normal ranges, and the possibility of overnutrition or undernutrition.

At present, nutritional assessment remains more of an art than a science. A global assessment obtains information about many facets of nutrition including current physical symptoms, history of acute and chronic illnesses, and a detailed physical examination. Global assessment is probably one of the most valid methods of making a nutritional diagnosis and planning nutritional care.[12,13]

Diet history

A nutritional assessment begins with evaluation of the individual's diet. This can be accomplished by recording the food consumed by actual observation or by personal recall and through the administration of a questionnaire such as a diet history. Each technique has its own shortcomings, such as the tendency to alter behavior when it is known that the behavior is being observed or reported.

Health assessment

Health assessment, including a health history and physical examination, will reveal weight changes, muscle wasting, fat stores, functional status, and nutritional status. Comparison of the individual's current weight to previous weights will identify whether the individual's weight is stable, changed drastically, or tends to fluctuate. For example, recent rapid weight loss can be a sign of cancer, a malfunctioning thyroid gland, or self-imposed starvation. A history of fluctuating weight could be associated with bulimia. Degradation of muscle, or muscle wasting, is a serious sign of malnutrition. A decrease in ability to initiate or complete activities of daily living could result from a decrease in energy caused by a poor diet, a neurologic malfunction such as multiple sclerosis, or a result of symptoms related to chronic obstructive pulmonary disease. Quality of the hair, absence of body hair, condition of gums, and skin lesions could signal a poor nutritional status.

Anthropometric measurements

Anthropometric measurements provide a means for assessing body composition, particularly fat stores and skeletal muscle; it is done by measuring height, weight, circumferences and thickness of various skinfolds. These measurements are used to determine growth patterns in children and appropriateness of current weight in adults. Body weight is the most frequently used method of assessing nutritional status; it is usually used in combination with measurements of body height to establish whether a person is underweight or overweight.

Relative weight is the actual weight divided by the desirable weight multiplied by 100. A relative weight greater than 120% is indicative of obesity. Recent changes in weight are probably a better indication of undernutrition than a low relative weight. A loss of 10% of body weight or more within a 1- to 2-month period is usually considered predictive of a poor clinical outcome in many disease states.[14]

The Metropolitan Life Insurance Table is the most widely used standard for defining levels of underweight and overweight (Table 42-7). This table, which is based on life insurance statistics relating height and weight to the likelihood of survival, provides an index of desirable weight. The upper and lower frame sizes appear to be based on the upper and lower quartiles of the population, with the medium frame representing the two middle quartiles. Using this table, obesity is defined as the condition in which body weight is greater than 30% of the weight for the specific height and frame.[14] There are some problems with the insurance table: weight ranges define lowest mortality and not necessarily ideal body weight; it is based on an ill-defined concept of frame size; it may not be representative of the United States population due to possible sampling biases; and it does not differentiate between weight gain due to increased muscle mass and weight gain due to increased fat content.

The body mass index (BMI) uses both height and weight to determine obesity. It is calculated by dividing the weight in kilograms by the height in meters squared (BMI = weight (kg)/height (m^2)). The normal BMI is 19 to 27. Persons with a BMI greater than 30 are considered obese, and those with a BMI that exceeds 40 are classified as morbidly obese.[15] The National Institute of Health (NIH) Consensus Conference on the Health Implications of Obesity has recommended the use of height and weight measurements, together with the BMI and calculations of relative weight, in defining obesity.[16]

Body weight reflects both lean body mass and adipose tissue and cannot be used as a method for describing body composition or the percentage of fat tissue present. The proper body–fat ratio is age specific. For young adults under age 30, the recommended range for males is 12% to 15% and for females, 19% to 23%. The upper limits for a 50-year-old male is 19% and for a female, about 27%.[1] During physical training, body fat usually decreases and lean body mass increases.

Several types of anthropometric measurements can be used to estimate body fat. Skinfold measurement, although difficult to perform and subject to error when used on obese individuals, can be used together with equations and tables to estimate the percentage of lean body mass and fat tissue.[17–21] Body circumferences are usually a more objective measurement and provide the information needed to calculate waist and hip ratio.[21,22]

Densitometry by underwater weighing is more accurate than either skinfold thickness or body circumference measurements in determining the percentage of body fat; however, there are limitations. It requires access to special equipment; assumes a constant density of lean body mass, which is subject to error; and necessitates an estimation of residual gas volumes in the lungs, which is often difficult.

Another method of estimating body fat is bioelectrical impedance. This method is performed by attaching electrodes at the wrist and ankle that send a harmless current through the body. The flow of the current is affected by the amount of water within the body. Because fat-free tissue contains virtually all the water and the conducting electrolytes, measurements of the resistance (impedance) to current flow can be used to estimate the percentage of body fat present. Bioelectrical impedance may become one of the most

Table 42–5. Vitamin facts

Vitamins	U.S. RDA for adults and children over age 4	Some significant sources
Fat soluble vitamins		
Vitamin A (retinol, provitamin carotenoids)	5000 IU	*Retinol:* Liver, butter, whole milk, cheese, egg yolk. *Pro-vitamin A:* carrots, leafy green vegetables, sweet potatoes, pumpkin, winter squash, apricots, cantaloupe, fortified margarine.
Vitamin D (calciferol)	400 IU	Vitamin D fortified dairy products; fortified margarine; fish oils; egg yolk. Synthesized by sunlight action on skin.
Vitamin E (tocopherol)	30 IU	Vegetable oil, margarine, shortening; green and leafy vegetables; wheat germ, whole grain products; egg yolk; butter, liver.
Water-soluble vitamins		
Vitamin C (Ascorbic acid)	60 mg	Broccoli, sweet and hot peppers, collards, brussels sprouts, strawberries, orange, kale, grapefruit, papaya, potato, mango, tangerine, spinach, tomato.
Thiamin (vitamin B_1)	1.5 mg	Pork, liver, meat; whole grains, fortified grain products; legumes; nuts.
Riboflavin (vitamin B_2)	1.7 mg	Liver; milk, yogurt, cottage cheese; meat; fortified grain products.
Niacin (nicotinamide, nicotinic acid)	20 mg	Liver, meat, poultry, fish; peanuts; fortified grain products. Synthesized from tryptophan (on the average 1 mg of niacin from 60 mg of dietary tryptophan).
Folacin (folic acid)	0.4 mg	Liver; legumes; green leafy vegetables.
Vitamin B_6 (pyridoxine, pyridoxal, pyridoxamine)	2.0 mg	Meat, poultry, fish, shellfish; green and leafy vegetables; whole grains, legumes.
Vitamin B_{12}	6.0 μg	Meat, poultry, fish, shellfish; eggs; milk and milk products.
Biotin	0.3 mg	Kidney, liver; milk; egg yolk; most fresh vegetables.
Pantothenic acid	10 mg	Liver, kidney, meats; milk; egg yolk; whole grains; legumes.

(Courtesy of the National Dairy Council®)

Some major physiologic functions	Some deficiency symptoms	Some overconsumption symptoms
Assists formation and maintenance of skin and mucous membranes, thus increasing resistance to infections. Functions in visual processes and forms visual purple. Promotes bone and tooth development.	*Mild:* Night-blindness, diarrhea, intestinal infections, impaired growth. *Severe:* Xerophthalmia.	*Mild:* Nausea, irritability, blurred vision. *Severe:* Growth retardation, enlargement of liver and spleen, loss of hair, rheumatic pain, increased pressure in skull, dermal changes.
Promotes ossification of bones and teeth, increases intestinal absorption of calcium.	Rickets in children; osteomalacia in adults, rare.	*Mild:* Nausea, weight loss, irritability. *Severe:* Mental and physical growth retardation, kidney damage, mobilization of calcium from bony tissue and deposition in soft tissues.
Functions as antioxidant protecting vitamins A and C and fatty acids from destruction; and prevents cell-membrane damage.	Almost impossible to produce without starvation; possible anemia in low-birth-weight infants.	Nontoxic under normal conditions.
Forms cementing substances, such as collagen, that hold body cells together, thus strengthening blood vessels, hastening healing of wounds and bones, and increasing resistance to infection. Aids in use of iron.	*Mild:* Bruise easily, bleeding gums. *Severe:* Scurvy.	When megadose is discontinued, deficiency symptoms may briefly appear until the body adapts. Newborns whose mothers took megadoses will show deficiency symptoms after birth until the body adapts.
Functions as part of a coenzyme to promote carbohydrate metabolism, production of ribose, a constituent of DNA and RNA. Promotes normal appetite and normal functioning of nervous system.	Impaired growth, wasting of tissues, mental confusion, low morale, edema. *Severe:* Beriberi.	None reported.
Functions as part of a coenzyme assisting cells to use oxygen for the release of energy from food. Promotes good vision and healthy skin.	Lesions of cornea, cracks at corners of mouth.	None reported.
Functions as part of a coenzyme in fat synthesis, tissue respiration, and utilization of carbohydrate for energy. Promotes healthy skin, nerves, and digestive tract. Aids digestion and fosters normal appetite.	Skin and gastrointestinal lesions, anorexia, weakness, irritability, vertigo. *Severe:* Pellagra.	None reported for nicotinamide. Flushing, headache, cramps, nausea for nicotinic acid.
Functions as part of coenzymes in amino acid and nucleoprotein metabolism. Promotes red blood cell formation.	Red tongue, diarrhea, anemia.	May obscure the existence of pernicious anemia.
Functions as part of a coenzyme involved in protein metabolism, assists in conversion of tryptophan to niacin, fatty acid metabolism, and red blood cell formation.	Irritability, muscle twitching, dermatitis near eyes, kidney stones, hypochromic anemia.	Long-term megadoses of pyridoxine may affect the peripheral nervous system resulting in loss of sensation and coordination in extremities.
Functions in coenzymes involved in nucleic acid synthesis and biologic methylation. Assists in development of normal red blood cells and maintenance of nerve tissue.	*Severe:* Pernicious anemia, neurologic disorders.	None reported.
Functions as part of a coenzyme involved in fat synthesis, amino acid metabolism, and glycogen formation.	Fatigue, depression, nausea, dermatitis, muscular pains.	None reported.
Functions as part of a coenzyme involved in energy metabolism.	Rare because found in most foods. Fatigue, sleep disturbances, nausea.	None reported.

widely available techniques for assessing body fat once its accuracy has been established.[22-24] The method is relatively inexpensive, easy to use, and portable.

Computerized tomographic (CT) scans and magnetic resonance imaging (MRI) can be used to provide quantitative pictures from which the thickness of fat can be determined. CT scan can be used to provide quantitative estimates of regional fat and give a ratio of intra-abdominal to extra-abdominal fat.[1]

Laboratory studies

Various laboratory tests on blood can aid in evaluating nutritional status. Some of the most commonly performed tests are serum albumin to assess the protein status, total lymphocyte count and delayed hypersensitivity reaction to assess cellular immunity, and creatinine–height index to assess skeletal protein. Vitamin and mineral deficiencies can be determined by measurements of their levels in blood, saliva, and other body tissues or by measuring nutrient specific chemical reactions. All of these tests are limited by

confounding factors and, therefore, need to be evaluated along with other clinical data.

In summary, nutritional status describes the condition of the body as it relates to the availability and utilization of nutrients. Nutrients provide the energy and materials necessary for performing the activities of daily living and for the growth and repair of body tissues. Metabolism is the organized process whereby nutrients such as carbohydrates, fats, and proteins are broken down, transformed, or otherwise converted to cellular energy. Glucose, fats, and amino acids from proteins serve as fuel sources for cellular metabolism. These fuel sources are ingested during meals and then stored for future use. Glucose is either stored as glycogen or converted to triglycerides in fat cells for storage. Fats are stored in adipose tissue as triglycerides. Amino acids are the building blocks of proteins, and most of the stored amino acids are contained in body proteins and as fuel sources for cellular metabolism. Energy is measured in heat units called kilocalories. The expenditure of body energy and

Table 42–6. Sources and functions of minerals

Mineral	Major sources	Functions
Calcium	Milk and milk products, fish with bones, greens	Bone formation and maintenance; tooth formation, vitamin B absorption, blood clotting, nerve and muscle function
Chloride	Table salt, meats, milk, eggs	Regulates pH of stomach, acid–base balance, osmotic pressure of extracellular fluids
Cobalt	Organ meats, meats	Aid in maturation of red blood cells (as part of B_{12} molecule)
Copper	Cereals, nuts, legumes, liver, shellfish, grapes, meats	Catalyst for hemoglobin formation, formation of elastin and collagen, energy release (cytochrome oxidase and catalase), formation of melanin, formation of phospholipids for myelin sheath of nerves
Fluoride	Fluorinated water	Strengthens bones and teeth
Iodine	Iodized salt, fish (saltwater and anadromous)	Thyroid hormone synthesis and its function in maintenance of metabolic rate
Iron	Meats, heart, liver, clams, oysters, lima beans, spinach, dates, dried nuts, enriched and whole-grain cereals	Hemoglobin synthesis, cellular energy release (cytochrome pathway), killing bacteria (myeloperoxidase)
Magnesium	Milk, green vegetables, nuts, bread, and cereals	Catalyst of many intracellular nerve impulses, retention of reactions, particularly those related to intracellular enzyme reactions; low magnesium levels produce an increase in irritability of the nervous system, vasodilatation, and cardiac dysrhythmias
Phosphorus	Meats, poultry, fish, milk and cheese, cereals, legumes, nuts	Bone formation and maintenance; essential component of nucleic acids and energy exchange forms such as adenosine triphosphate (ATP)
Potassium	Oranges, dried fruits, bananas, meats, potatoes, peanut butter, coffee	Maintenance of intracellular osmolality, acid–base balance, transmission of nerve impulses, catalyst in energy metabolism, formation of proteins, formation of glycogen
Sodium	Table salt, cured meats, meats, milk, olives	Maintenance of osmotic pressure of extracellular fluids, acid–base balance, neuromuscular function; absorption of glucose
Zinc	Whole-wheat cereals, eggs, legumes	Integral part of many enzymes including carbonic anhydrase, which facilitates combination of carbon dioxide with water in red blood cells; component of lactic dehydrogenase, important in cellular metabolism; component of many peptidases; important in digestion of proteins in gastrointestinal tract

need for metabolism are largely determined by heat production (thermogenesis) associated with: (1) the basal metabolic rate or basal energy equivalent, (2) diet-induced thermogenesis, (3) exercise-induced thermogenesis, and (4) thermogenesis in response to changes in environmental conditions.

The body requires over forty nutrients on a daily basis. Nutritional status reflects the continued daily intake of nutrients over time and the deposition and utilization of these nutrients within the body. The RDA is the recommended daily intake of essential nutrients considered to be adequate to meet the known nutritional needs of healthy persons. The RDA has seventeen age and sex classifications and includes recommendations for calories, protein, fat, carbohydrates, vitamins, and minerals. The nutritional status of an individual can be assessed by evaluation of dietary intake, anthropometric measurements, health assessment, and laboratory tests. Health assessment includes a health history and physical examination to determine weight changes, muscle wasting, fat stores, functional status, and nutritional status. Anthropometric measurements are used for assessing body composition; they include height and weight measurements and measurements (*e.g.*, skinfold thickness, body circumferences, densitometry, bioelectrical impedance, and CT scans) to determine the composition of the body in relation to lean body mass and fat tissue.

Overnutrition and obesity

"Nicotine in the lungs is invisible, alcoholism may be hidden, but the results of addiction to food...cannot be concealed. Fat on the hips is irrevocably public."[25] Obesity is a major health problem in affluent countries. Estimates of its prevalence range from 10% to 50% of the adult population.[26] These differing estimates reflect the definitions and standards used to identify the population at risk.[1] The massively obese are easy to recognize and represent only a small segment of the population—5.8% of men and 8.3% of women in the United States using the 95th percentile for the BMI.[26] Because body weight measures muscle mass as well as body fat, overweight does not necessarily indicate obesity. To be obese, a person must have an abnormally high proportion of body fat.

Causes of obesity

Obesity has been defined as an excess of body fat frequently resulting in a significant impairment of health.[15] This excess body fat is generated when the calories consumed exceed those expended through exercise and activity. Factors contributing to this imbalance are numerous and probably exist in differing combinations among obese individuals. Heredity, so-

Table 42–7. 1983 Metropolitan height and weight tables*

Men					Women				
Height					Height				
Feet	Inches	Small frame	Medium frame	Large frame	Feet	Inches	Small frame	Medium frame	Large frame
5	2	128–134	131–141	138–150	4	10	102–111	109–121	118–131
5	3	130–136	133–143	140–153	4	11	103–113	111–123	120–134
5	4	132–138	135–145	142–156	5	0	104–115	113–126	122–137
5	5	134–140	137–148	144–160	5	1	106–118	115–129	125–140
5	6	136–142	139–151	146–164	5	2	108–121	118–132	128–143
5	7	138–145	142–154	149–168	5	3	111–124	121–135	131–147
5	8	140–148	145–157	152–172	5	4	114–127	124–138	134–151
5	9	142–151	148–160	155–176	5	5	117–130	127–141	137–155
5	10	144–154	151–163	158–180	5	6	120–133	130–144	140–159
5	11	146–157	154–166	161–184	5	7	123–136	133–147	143–163
6	0	149–160	157–170	164–188	5	8	126–139	136–150	146–167
6	1	152–164	160–174	168–192	5	9	129–142	139–153	149–170
6	2	155–168	164–178	172–197	5	10	132–145	142–156	152–173
6	3	158–172	167–182	176–202	5	11	135–148	145–159	155–176
6	4	162–176	171–187	181–207	6	0	138–151	148–162	158–179

* Weights at ages 25–59 based on lowest mortality. Weight in pounds according to frame (in indoor clothing weighing 5 lb for men and 3 lb for women; shoes with 1-in heels).

(Source of basic data: 1979 Build Study. Society of Actuaries and Association of Life Insurance Medical Directors of America. 1980. Metropolitan Life Insurance Company Health and Safety Education Division. Copyright 1983 Metropolitan Life Insurance Company)

cioeconomics, culture, environmental factors, psychologic influences, and activity levels have all been implicated as causative or contributing factors in the development of obesity. Contrary to popular belief, endocrine disorders are rarely a cause of obesity.

Epidemiologic surveys indicate that the prevalence of overweight is related to social and economic conditions. The second (1976 through 1980) National Health and Nutrition Examination Survey has shown that if American women were divided into two groups according to economic status, the prevalence of obesity is much higher among those in the poverty level.[27] In contrast, men above the poverty level had a higher prevalence of overweight than men below the poverty level.

Obesity is known to run in families, suggesting a hereditary component. The question that surrounds this observation is whether the disorder arises because of genetic endowment or environmental influences. Studies of twin and adopted children have provided evidence that heredity contributes to the disorder.[28] In a large study of 3580 male and female adoptees and their biologic and adoptive parents, a strong relationship was found between the BMI of the adoptees and those of their biologic parents and a lack of correlation between the BMI of the adoptees and those of their adoptive parents.[29] The amount of internal fat is influenced by heredity more than the amount of subcutaneous fat.[28]

Although genetic factors may explain much of the individual variations in terms of excess weight, environmental influences also must be taken into account. These influences include family dietary patterns, decreased level of activity due to labor-saving devices, reliance on the automobile for transportation, and easy access to food. The obese may be greatly influenced by the availability of food, its flavor, time of day, and other cues. The composition of the diet may also be a causal factor, and the percentage of dietary fat independent of total calorie intake may play a part in the development of obesity.[30] Psychologic factors

include using food as a reward, comfort, or means of getting attention. Some individuals may overeat and use obesity as a means of avoiding threatening situations.

It is still uncertain whether obese individuals are less active or use calories more efficiently than lean persons. It has been suggested that the increased prevalence of obesity in the United States has resulted because more calories are consumed and because of modern conveniences and our more sedentary lifestyle. For example, the extension telephone saves 70 miles of walking each year—the equivalent of 2 to 3 lb of fat gain.[31] A review of the literature reveals that the obese are consistently more sedentary when compared with their normal-weight counterparts. They float more when swimming, play less tennis, and walk less per day. Even when a reasonable number of calories are consumed, fewer are expended because of inactivity.[32] A low rate of energy expenditure may contribute to the prevalence of obesity in some families.[32,33] A recent study has shown that infants who become overweight by 3 months of age have a lower energy expenditure than normal-weight infants.[34]

Types of obesity

Two types of obesity based on distribution of fat have been described: upper body obesity and lower body obesity. Upper body obesity is also referred to as *abdominal, android, or male obesity.* Lower body obesity is also known as *gluteal-femoral, gynoid, or female obesity.*[35] The obesity type is determined by dividing the waist by the hip circumference. A waist–hip ratio greater than 1.0 in men and 0.8 in women indicates upper body obesity (Figure 42-4). Research suggests that fat distribution may be a more important factor for morbidity and mortality than overweight or obesity.[1]

Upper body obesity is characterized by larger fat cells and is typically more predominant in men than women.[36] CT scans have shown that these indi-

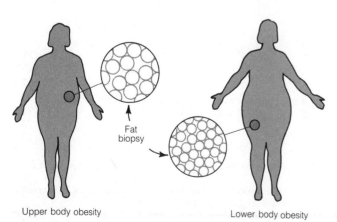

Fat
biopsy

Upper body obesity

Lower body obesity

Figure 42-4 Distribution of body fat and size of fat cells in persons with upper and lower body obesity. (Courtesy of Ahmed Kissebah, MD, PhD, Medical College of Wisconsin, Milwaukee, Wisconsin)

viduals have a greater ratio of intra-abdominal fat to subcutaneous fat.[37] Women are more likely to have a greater ratio of gluteal-femoral obesity because of increased number of fat cells in this region. Triglycerides accumulate more readily in the gluteal-femoral adipocytes than in the abdominal fat cells. However, the abdominal cells are more lipolytically active. This places persons with upper body obesity at greater risk for ischemic heart disease, stroke, and death independent of total body fat. They also tend to exhibit hypertension, elevated levels of triglycerides and decreased levels of high density lipoproteins, hyperinsulinemia and diabetes mellitus, gallbladder disease, menstrual irregularities, and infertility.[37–42]

In terms of weight reduction, some studies have shown that persons with upper body obesity are easier to treat than those with lower body obesity. Other studies have shown no difference in terms of success with weight-reduction programs between the two types of obesity.[43–48]

Health risks associated with obesity

Social ostracism and isolation are not the only complications of obesity. Obese individuals are more likely to develop high blood pressure, hyperlipidemia, cardiovascular disease, glucose intolerance, insulin resistance, diabetes, infertility, and cancer of the endometrium, breast, prostate, and colon.[49] Obese women between 20 and 30 years of age have a sixfold increase in the risk of gallbladder disease; by age 60 years, nearly one-third of obese women can expect to develop gallbladder disease.[49] In massively obese men, there may be a decrease in free testosterone.[50] Obese women often show less regularity in menstrual cycles, greater frequency of menstrual abnormalities, and infertility problems.[51]

The increased weight associated with obesity stresses the bones and joints, increasing the likelihood of arthritis. Because some drugs are lipophilic and exhibit increased distribution in fat tissue, the administration of these drugs, including some anesthetic agents, can be more dangerous in obese persons.[52] If surgery is required, the obese person heals slower than the same age nonobese person.

It is only with morbid obesity that respiratory function is usually impaired. Sleep apnea and respiratory impairment are prevalent in the morbidly obese population (see Chapter 26). Other respiratory derangements include increased oxygen need to supply the increased body mass, increased respiratory rate to compensate for the resistance offered by chest and body fat, and decreased ventilation to the lower lungs.[53]

Treatment of obesity

Studies have shown that weight reduction in obese individuals is beneficial to health. Data from the Framingham study showed a 10% reduction in weight for men was associated with a fall in serum glucose of 2.5 mg/dl, a fall in serum cholesterol of 11.3 mg/dl, a fall in systolic blood pressure of 6.6 mmHg, and a fall in uric acid of 0.33 mg/dl.[54] For each 10% reduction in body weight in men, these data predict an anticipated 20% decrease in coronary heart disease. Two factors that determine the need for treatment to produce weight loss are the health risk associated with total body fatness and the distribution of body fat. Persons with a BMI of 25 to 30 kg/m² have a low risk of health problems, those with a BMI of 30 to 35 kg/m² have a moderate risk, and those with a BMI above 40 kg/m² have a high risk.[55] The higher the proportion of upper body fat, the greater the risk of health problems. The risk of obesity is increased in persons who are less than 40 years of age, who are of the male sex, or who have associated health problems such as diabetes mellitus, hypertension, or hyperlipidemia.

There is no single effective treatment for obesity. Treatment methods include nutritionally adequate weight-loss diets, behavior modification, exercise, social support, and, in situations of morbid obesity, surgical methods. With conventional techniques, 20% of participants lose 20 lb (9.1 kg) and maintain that loss over 2 years, while only 5% lose 40 lb (18.2 kg).[56] Obviously, the success rate is very discouraging. Some factors have been shown to be predictors of better outcomes. Close care provider–client contact and length of that contact appear to be more important than the specific features of the weight-loss program. Careful client selection is necessary in order to include only those persons who are sufficiently motivated.[57] This decreases frustration for the caregiver and the client and increases the likelihood of success. In addition, individuals who have better self-concepts, exercise more, and have greater social support are usually more successful in losing weight.

Weight-loss diets should have a reduced fat content and contain more complex carbohydrates with an emphasis on a wide variety of unprocessed foods. Increasing the fiber content of the diet decreases caloric density, allowing a larger volume of food. Empty calories, such as fat, sucrose, and alcohol, should be limited. Diets that advocate large amounts of protein or fat or eating one food at a time provide no advantage and may even be harmful. A decrease of 500 to 1000 cal from maintenance will usually produce a 1- to 2-lb (.5- to .9-kg) weight loss per week.

Behavior modification has proven successful for achieving and maintaining weight loss and has also reported the lowest attrition rates. However, the average loss of any behavioral program reported in the literature is 1 lb per week, with 16 lb being the average total achieved.

Because many individuals need to lose a great deal more than 16 lb, newer forms of treatment have evolved. Very low-calorie diets are often used for severely obese individuals in conjunction with behavior modification techniques. The very low-calorie diets usually contain 400 cal to 500 cal of a liquid protein fortified with electrolytes and vitamins. Weight loss averages 2 lb to 4 lb (.9 kg to 1.8 kg) per week. Because of the severe calorie restriction, these diets require medical supervision and frequent laboratory testing. Side effects include fatigue, orthostatic hypotension, and fluid and electrolyte disorders. Because severe calorie restriction is undesirable for pregnant and lactating women, these diets are contraindicated for that group, as well as for children, who still require protein for growth.

Exercise is an important part of a weight-loss program. It increases energy expenditure and helps preserve lean body tissue during weight loss. Exercise may also help to prevent the compensatory decrease in metabolic rate occurring with a reduction in calories that often makes weight loss difficult.[58] However, there is a high dropout rate from exercise programs. Many overweight persons feel self-conscious, and some types of activities may prove to be uncomfortable or painful. For this reason, many weight-loss programs encourage walking for 10 to 15 minutes three to four times a week. The effect of this simple prescription may have long-lasting effects and may encourage other forms of exercise. Recommendations such as using the stairs versus the elevator and walking instead of using the car for short distances are encouraged. More strenuous types of exercise may require cardiovascular screening for establishing risk and developing an individualized exercise program.

The surgical treatment for obesity is usually reserved for the extremely overweight (more than 100 lb or 45 kg). Gastric surgeries intended to limit food intake but maintain normal digestion and absorption have proven to be relatively safe and effective.[58] Two types of gastric surgeries, gastric bypass and gastroplasty, are currently used for treating obesity.[55] Gastric bypass procedures establish a direct connection between the stomach and the small intestine. In one procedure, the stomach immediately adjacent to the esophagus is connected by way of a loop of intestine to the jejunum closing the larger portion of the stomach so that the stomach contents bypass part of the upper intestine. The smaller upper portion of the stomach is designed to hold 50 ml to 60 ml of food, causing a feeling of fullness with a small amount of food. Gastroplasty procedures are designed to reduce the size of the stomach and consist of banding or wrapping procedures. Complications of gastric surgeries can include anemia due to iron and vitamin B_{12} deficiency, as well as thiamine deficiency and its associated neuropathy. The use of intestinal bypass surgeries has largely been abandoned because of the high incidence of serious complications such as wound infections, pulmonary emboli, serious fluid and electrolyte disorders, liver disease, severe diarrhea, and malnutrition.[58]

In summary, obesity is defined as excess body fat resulting from consumption of calories in excess of those expended for exercise and activities. Heredity, socioeconomics, culture, environmental factors, psychologic influences, and activity levels have been implicated as causative factors in the development of obesity. The health risks associated with obesity include hyperlipidemia and cardiovascular disease including hypertension; insulin resistance, glucose intolerance, and diabetes mellitus; menstrual irregularities and infertility; cancer of the endometrium, breast, prostate, and colon; and gallbladder disease. There are two types of obesity—upper body and lower body obesity. Upper body obesity is associated with a higher incidence of complications. The treatment of obesity focuses on adequate weight-loss diets; behavior modification; exercise; social support; and, in situations of marked obesity, surgical methods.

Undernutrition

Undernutrition ranges from the selective deficiency of a single nutrient to starvation in which there is deprivation of all ingested nutrients. Undernutrition can result from willful eating behaviors as in anorexia nervosa and the binge–purge syndrome, lack of food availability, or health problems that impair food intake and decrease its absorption and utilization. There is general agreement that malnutrition is the most widespread cause of morbidity and mortality throughout the world. In the United States, poverty, homelessness, and hunger promote malnutrition among all age groups. Weight loss and malnutrition are common during illness, recovery from trauma, and hospitalization.

Malnutrition and starvation

Malnutrition and starvation are conditions in which a person does not receive or is unable to use an adequate amount of calories and nutrients for body function. There is a wide range of causes of starvation. Some causes are willful (*e.g.*, the person with anorexia nervosa who does not consume enough food to maintain weight and health). Persons who are unable to absorb their food, such as those with Crohn's disease, are also at risk. Most cases of food deprivation result in semi- or partial starvation. Malnutrition can occur in persons with chronic obstructive lung disease when their air hunger interferes with their ability to eat; eventually the resultant malnutrition further complicates their respiratory status and food consumption. Studies indicate that 30% to 40% of persons with chronic lung disease are significantly undernourished as determined by body weight and anthropometric estimates of body fat and muscle mass.[59,60]

In malnutrition and starvation, the amount of food consumed and absorbed is drastically reduced. Most of the literature on starvation and malnutrition has dealt with infants and children of underdeveloped countries. The classic approach to the study of this population commonly divides cases into marasmus and kwashiorkor, with intermediate cases of marasmic kwashiorkor combining certain features of each condition.[61] Marasmus is characterized by progressive wasting due to inadequate food intake that is equally deficient in calories and protein. The child with marasmus has a wasted appearance with stunted growth and loss of subcutaneous fat, but with relatively normal skin, hair, liver function, and affect.[61] Kwashiorkor results from a protein deficiency. The term *kwashiorkor* comes from the African word meaning *the disease suffered by the displaced child*, because the condition develops soon after a child is displaced from the breast and placed on a starchy gruel feeding following the arrival of a new baby. The child with kwashiorkor is characterized by edema, desquamating skin, discolored hair, hepatic enlargement, anorexia, and extreme apathy.[61]

Depending on the prestarvation state, the metabolic events of starvation permit life to continue for months without caloric intake. In healthy, normally fed persons, there is fuel enough to last for more than 80 days, assuming utilization of 2,000 Kcal/day; about 85% of these calories are stored in fat tissue, 14% in body proteins, and 1% in stored carbohydrate sources.[4] Despite the limited carbohydrate stores, which are depleted within 12 to 24 hours without food, a continuing supply of glucose is essential for survival. The central nervous system uses about 115 g of glucose a day, and red blood cells, bone marrow, kidneys, and peripheral nervous system use another 36 g of glucose.[4] One of the critical adaptive mechanisms in starvation is the production of new glucose (gluconeogenesis). The liver uses glycerol, lactate, and amino acids in the synthesis of glucose. The glycerol skeleton, obtained from triglycerides released from fat cells, plays a significant role in glucose synthesis. The predominant fuel for other tissues is fatty acids and ketones. For this reason, a state of ketosis is common during starvation.

Proteins have vital enzymatic and structural functions, and the body avoids using them as a fuel source until the late stages of starvation. Eventually, protein wasting ensues, with substantial weight loss, the most well-known and easily recognized sign of starvation. This weight loss is caused by loss of lean body tissue and fat along with diuresis. The importance of protein conservation to survival has been demonstrated in animal studies, in which a premorbid increase in nitrogen excretion due to protein utilization heralded the final stages of starvation.[4] Death from starvation occurs when one-third to one-half of the body's protein is lost rather than from hypoglycemia.[4]

Daily weight loss can range from 1 lb to several pounds depending on the stage of starvation.[4] Wound healing is poor, and the body is unable to fight off infection because of multiple immunologic malfunctions throughout the body.[5] The muscles used for breathing become weakened and respiratory function becomes compromised as muscle proteins are used as a fuel source. A reduction in respiratory function has many implications, especially for persons with burns, trauma, infection, chronic respiratory disease, or persons who are being mechanically ventilated because of respiratory failure.[62,63]

Although intellectual functioning remains intact despite the ketosis that occurs during starvation, depression and emotional lability are common. There is a diminished appetite and decreased desire for fluids due to altered hypothalamic function that occurs with ketosis. A marked decrease in libido is observed with starvation. The female experiences anovulation and amenorrhea, while the male experiences decreased testicular function.[5] The kidney does not go untouched by starvation. Calcium and phosphate are excreted as bone is dissolved; and uric acid is retained, which can cause gout.[4]

Malnutrition in hospitalized patients

Malnutrition is much more prevalent in hospitalized patients than previously estimated. It has been estimated to occur in 30% to 50% of hospitalized persons, despite socioeconomic status or illness experienced.[64] This malnutrition increases morbidity, mortality, incidence of complications, and length of hospital stay.

Individuals may enter the hospital in a malnourished state. This malnutrition may be caused by poverty, inadequate food storage and preparation facilities, addiction to drugs or alcohol, adherence to fad diets, or even poorly fitting dentures. Furthermore, the hospitalized patient often finds eating a healthful diet difficult; they often have restrictions on food and water intake in preparation for tests and surgery. Pain, medications, special diets, and stress can decrease appetite. Even when the patient is well enough to eat, eating alone in a room where unpleasant treatments may be given is not conducive to eating.

Although hospitalized patients may appear to need fewer calories because they are on bedrest, their actual need for caloric intake may be higher because of other energy expenditures. For example, more calories are expended during fever when the metabolic rate is increased. There may also be an increased need for protein to support tissue repair following trauma or surgery.

Two types of malnutrition occur in the hospitalized patient: protein-calorie malnutrition and protein malnutrition.[65] Protein-calorie malnutrition is indicated when there is an unplanned weight loss of 10% in less than 2 weeks. It is characterized by loss of fat stores and muscle atrophy. Appetite is diminished, and diarrhea is a common complaint. There is little or no edema with protein-calorie malnutrition. Protein malnutrition is characterized by depressed visceral and endogenous protein synthesis. Plasma protein levels, particularly albumin, are decreased; this results in a decreased plasma colloidal pressure and development of edema (see Chapter 28). A hallmark of protein malnutrition is general apathy.[65] There may be an expression of appetite, yet often the foods that are eaten are high in carbohydrate and low in protein.

Cachexia is a state in which a person who is malnourished has marked wasting of body mass. The malnutrition that frequently accompanies heart failure is known as cardiac cachexia.[66] It is thought that this cachexia is caused by a decrease in the quality and quantity of food ingested, abnormal metabolism, and loss of nutrients by way of stool and urine. Decreased food intake could easily be influenced by the difficulty experienced in breathing, which is much more pronounced during eating. In addition, vascular congestion could influence stomach emptying and intestinal motility, causing abdominal distress. Medications used to manage congestive heart failure can also cause a decreased appetite (anorexia) or actually deplete the body of needed minerals. The fact that the person with heart disease seems to lose weight quicker than a person experiencing starvation suggests that more than just a decrease in the quality and quantity of food is taking place. A hypermetabolic state seems to be in process. More energy is expended to accomplish the respiratory work needed for survival.[66]

Eating disorders

An eating disorder is a gross disturbance in eating behavior that jeopardizes a person's physical and psychologic health. Eating disorders develop despite a normally functioning gastrointestinal tract and appetite. Anorexia nervosa and the binge–purge syndrome are chronic problems in which there is a preoccupation with food, eating, and weight loss.

Anorexia nervosa

Anorexia nervosa was first described in the scientific literature over a hundred years ago by Sir William Gull.[67] Anorexia nervosa is a self-starvation syndrome in which a person willingly loses an excessive amount of weight (20% or more of original body weight), exhibits muscle wasting, suffers from disturbances in body image, and experiences unreasonable fears about becoming obese. In actuality, the term *anorexia*, meaning loss of appetite, is a misnomer because hunger is actually felt; but, in this case, it is denied.

Anorexia nervosa is more prevalent in young women than men. The disorder typically begins in teenage women who are either obese or perceive themselves as being obese. An interest in weight reduction becomes an obsession with severely restricted caloric intake and, frequently, excessive physical exercise.

Many organ systems are affected by the malnutrition that occurs in persons with anorexia nervosa. The severity of the abnormalities tends to be related to the degree of malnutrition and reversed with refeeding. The most frequent complication of anorexia is amenorrhea and loss of secondary sex characteristics with decreased levels of estrogen, which can eventually lead to osteoporosis. Constipation, cold intolerance and failure to shiver in the cold, bradycardia, hypotension, decreased heart size, electrocardiographic changes, blood abnormalities, and dry skin with lanugo (increased amounts of fine hair) are common. Unexpected sudden deaths have been reported; the risk appears to increase as weight drops to less than 35% to 40% of ideal weight. It is believed that these deaths are due to myocardial degeneration and heart failure rather than heart dysrhythmias.[68]

The most exasperating aspect of the treatment of anorexia is the inability of the anorexic to recognize that there is a problem. Because anorexia is a form of starvation, it can lead to death if left untreated. Research suggests that anorexics can achieve a weight gain by way of treatment, although they may not reach ideal weight.[68] Frequently their abnormal eating pattern of avoiding high-calorie foods continues. There is no preferred single form of treatment. Psychologic interventions are often helpful.

The binge–purge syndrome

The binge–purge syndrome is an eating disorder that encompasses an array of distinctive behaviors, feelings, and thoughts. Bulimia, a term that literally means ox hunger, is characterized by secretive episodes or binges of eating large quantities of easily consumed high-caloric foods, such as doughnuts or ice cream. There are also periods of severe food restriction by way of dieting or fasting and purging to prevent weight gain. The purging behaviors that accompany binge eating distinguish bulimarexia from bulimia. Purging behaviors include self-induced vomiting, diuretic-induced diuresis, and laxative-induced diarrhea. Vomiting can be induced through the use of ipecac or self-stimulation of the gag reflex. Diuretics are used to reduce weight by increasing urinary excretion. An excessive intake of sorbitol-containing foods or abuse of laxatives causes weight loss through diarrhea.

Persons who experience the binge–purge syndrome are usually women in their late teens through the mid-thirties. Their weights may fluctuate but not to the dangerously low levels seen in individuals with anorexia nervosa. The thoughts and feelings of persons with bulimia or bulimarexia range from fear of not being able to stop eating to a concern about gaining too much weight. They also experience feelings of sadness, anger, guilt, shame, and low self-esteem.

The complications of the binge–purge syndrome include those resulting from overeating, self-induced vomiting, and cathartic and diuretic abuse.[69] Among the complications of self-induced vomiting are dental disorders, esophagitis, fluid and electrolyte disorders, and parotitis. Dental abnormalities, such as sensitive teeth, increased dental caries, and periodontal disease, occur with frequent self-induced vomiting. This is because the frequent presence of vomitus with its high-acid content causes tooth enamel to dissolve. Esophagitis, dysphagia, and esophageal strictures are also common. With frequent vomiting, there is often reflux of gastric contents into the lower esophagus due to relaxation of the lower esophageal sphincter. Vomiting may lead to aspiration pneumonia, especially in intoxicated or debilitated persons. Potassium, chloride, and hydrogen are lost in the vomitus, and frequent vomiting also predisposes to metabolic alkalosis with hypokalemia (see Chapters 27 and 29). An unexplained physical response to bulimarexia is the development of benign, painless parotid gland enlargement.

Use of emetic drugs and cathartics is associated with problems of drug overdose and abuse. Excessive doses of syrup of ipecac, which is sometimes used to induce vomiting, can produce serious cardiac disorders including conduction defects, dysrhythmias, and myocarditis. Chronic laxative use disrupts intestinal motility and normal bowel habits and causes higher stool electrolyte concentrations—the most frequent complication of potassium deficiency.

The primary goal of therapy for the binge–purge syndrome is to establish a regular healthful eating pattern. Unlike those who suffer from anorexia nervosa, the person with bulimia or bulimarexia is upset by the behaviors practiced and the thoughts and feelings experienced and is more willing to accept help. Persons with bulimia or bulimarexia who have been successfully treated for their eating disorder have reported that making meal plans, eating a balanced diet of three regular meals a day, avoiding high sugar foods and other binge foods, recording food intake, recording binge/vomit episodes, exercising regularly, finding alternative activities, and avoiding alcohol and drugs are helpful in maintaining their more healthful eating behaviors post-treatment.[70]

In summary, undernutrition can range from a selective deficiency of a single nutrient to starvation in which there is a deprivation of all ingested nutrients. Malnutrition and starvation are among the most widespread causes of morbidity and mortality in the world. The body adapts to starvation through the use of fat stores and glucose synthesis to supply the energy needs of the central nervous system. Malnutrition is common during illness, recovery from trauma, and hospitalization. The effects of malnutrition and starvation on body function are widespread. They include loss of muscle mass, impaired wound healing, impaired immunologic function, decreased appetite, loss of calcium and phosphate from bone, anovulation and amenorrhea in women, and decreased testicular function in men. A reduction in respiratory muscle function that occurs with starvation has many implications for persons with lung disease, infection, and trauma. Anorexia nervosa and the binge–purge syndrome are eating disorders that result in malnutrition. In anorexia nervosa, distorted attitudes about eating lead to serious weight loss and malnutrition. Bulimia is characterized by binge eating; bulimarexia is characterized by binge eating and purging with self-induced vomiting and use of laxatives or diuretics.

References

1. Bray GA, Gray DS: Obesity. Part 1—Pathogenesis. West J Med 149:429, 1988
2. Cormack DH: Ham's Histology, 9th ed, pp 181, 183. Philadelphia, JB Lippincott, 1987
3. Timms-Hagen J: Thermogenesis in brown adipose tissue as an energy buffer. N Engl J Med 311:1549, 1984
4. Sauded K, Felig P: The metabolic events of starvation. Am J Med 60:117, 1976
5. Cahill CF Jr: Starvation in man. Clin Endocrinol Metab 5(2):405, 1976
6. Krause MW, Mahan LK: Food, Nutrition and Diet Therapy. Philadelphia, WB Saunders, 1984
7. Committee on Dietary Allowances, Food Nutrition Board: Recommended Dietary Allowances, 9th ed. National Academy of Sciences—National Research Council. Washington DC, National Academy Press, 1980

8. Report of the National Cholesterol Education Program Expert Panel on Detection, Evaluation, and Treatment of High Blood Cholesterol in Adults. Arch Intern Med 148:36, 1988

9. USDA, USDHHS: Nutrition and your health: Dietary guidelines for Americans, 2nd ed. Home and Gar Bull No 232, Washington DC, USDA/USDHHS, Aug 1985

10. Schneeman BO: Dietary fiber: Comments on interpreting recent research. J Am Diet Assoc 87:1163, 1987

11. Trowell H: Physiologic role of dietary fiber: A ten year review. Contemp Nutr 11(7):1, 1986

12. Grant JP: Nutritional assessment in clinical practice. Nutr Clin Prac vol 1:3, 1986

13. Baker JP, Detsky AS, Wesson DE et al: Nutritional assessment: A comparison of clinical judgement and objective measures. N Engl J Med 306:969, 1982

14. Blackburn GL: Guest editorial. Top Clin Nutr 2:1, 1987

15. Blackburn GL: Obesity and weight loss. Top Clin Nutr 2:viii, 1987

16. Burton BT, Foster WR, Hirsh J et al: Health implications of obesity. An NIH Consensus Development Conference. Int J Obes 9:155, 1985

17. Johnson FE: Relationship between body composition and anthropometry. Hum Biol 54:221, 1982

18. Lohman TG: Skinfolds and body density and their relationship to body fatness: A review. Am J Clin Nutr 46:537, 1987

19. Womersley J, Durnin JVGA: A comparison of skinfold method with extent of 'overweight' and various weight–height relationships in the assessment of obesity. Br J Nutr 38:271, 1977

20. Mueller WH, Wear ML, Hanis CL et al: Body circumferences as alternatives to skinfold measurements of body fat distribution in Mexican-Americans. Int J Obes 11:309, 1986

21. Fanelli MT, Kuzmarski RJ, Hirsch M: Estimation of body fat from ultrasound measurements of subcutaneous fat and circumferences in obese women. Int J Obes 12:125, 1988

22. Lukaski HC, Bolonchuk WW, Hall CB: Validation of tetrapolar bioelectrical impedance method to assess body composition. J Appl Physiol 60:1327, 1986

23. Segal KR, VanLoan M, Fitzergerald PI: Lean body mass estimation by bioelectrical impedance analysis: A four-site cross-validation study. Am J Clin Nutr 47:7, 1988

24. Coh SH: How valid are bioelectrical impedance measurements of body composition studies? Am J Clin Nutr 42:889, 1985

25. Epstein LH, Wing RR, Voloski A: Childhood obesity. Pediatr Clin North Am 32(Apr):2, 1985

26. Bray GA: Overweight is risking fate. Ann NY Acad Sci 499:14, 1987

27. Plan and operation of the National Health and Nutrition Examination Survey, 1976–1980. DDHS Publication (PHS) 81–1317, Vital and Health Statistics, Series 1, No 15. National Center for Health Statistics, Hyattsville, MD, 1981

28. Bouchard C, Perusse L, LeBlanc C et al: Inheritance and the amount and distribution of body fat. Int J Obes 12:205, 1988

29. Stunkard AJ, Throkild IA, Sorenson T et al: An adoption study of human obesity. N Engl J Med 314:193, 1986

30. Romieu I, Willett WC, Stamfler MJ et al: Energy intake and other determinants of human body fat. Am J Nutr 47:406, 1988

31. Ruvissin E, Lillioja A, Knowler WC et al: Reduced rate of energy expenditure for body-weight gain. N Engl J Med 318:467, 1988

32. Stern JS; Is obesity a disease of inactivity? In Stunkard AJ, Stellar E (eds): Eating and Its Disorders. New York, Raven Press, 1984

33. Bogardus C, Lillioja S, Ravussin E et al: Familial dependence of the resting metabolic rate. N Engl J Med 315:96, 1987

34. Roberts SB, Savage J, Coward W et al: Energy expenditure and intake in infants born to lean and overweight mothers. N Engl J Med 318:461, 1988

35. Bistrian BR: The medical treatment of obesity. Arch Intern Med 141:429, 1981

36. Krotkiewski M, Bjorntorp P, Sjostrom P: Impact of obesity on metabolism in men and women. J Clin Invest 72:1150, 1983

37. Ashwell M, Cole TJ, Dixon AK: Obesity: New insight into the anthropometric classification of fat distribution shown by computed tomography. Br J Med 290:1692, 1985

38. Bjorntorp P: Adipose tissue in obesity. In Hirsch J, Van Itallie TB (eds): Recent Advances in Obesity Research, 4th ed, p 163. London, John Libby, 1985

39. Kissebah AK, Vydelingum N, Murray R et al: Relationship of body fat distribution to metabolic consequences of obesity. J Clin Endocrinol Metab 54:254, 1982

40. Kalkhoff RK, Hartz AH, Rupley D et al: Relationship of body fat distribution to blood pressure, carbohydrate tolerance, and plasma lipids in healthy obese women. J Lab Clin Med 102:621, 1983

41. Sparrow D, Borkan GA, Gerzof SF et al: Relationship of fat distribution to glucose tolerance. Diabetes 35:411, 1986

42. Ohlson LO, Larsson B, Svardsudd K: The influence of body fat distribution on the incidence of diabetes mellitus. Diabetes 34:1055, 1985

43. Wadden TA, Stunkard AJ, Johnston FE et al: Body fat distribution in adult obese women. II. Changes in fat distribution accompanying weight reduction. Am J Clin Nutr 47:229, 1988

44. den Besten C, Vansant G, Westrate JA et al: Resting metabolic rate and diet-induced thermogenesis in abdominal and gluteal-femoral women before and after weight reduction. Am J Clin Nutr 47:840, 1988

45. Krotkiewski M, Sjostrom L, Bjorntorp P et al: Adipose tissue cellularity in relation to prognosis for weight reduction. Int J Obes 1:395, 1975

46. Vansant G, den Besten C, Westrate J et al: Body fat distribution and the prognosis for weight reduction: Preliminary observations. Int J Obes 12:133, 1988

47. Brownell KD: The psychology and physiology of obesity: Implications for screening and treatment. J Am Diet Assoc 84:406, 1984

48. Kissebah AK, Freedman DS, Peiris AN: Health risks of obesity. Med Clin North Am, 73(1):111, 1989

49. Hartz AJ, Rupley DC, Rimm AA: The association of girth measurements with disease in 32,856 women. Am J Epidemiol 119:71, 1984

50. Kley HK, Solbach HG, McKinnan JC et al: Testosterone decrease and estrogen increase in male patients with obesity. Acta Endocrinol 91:553, 1979

51. Hartz AJ, Barboriak PN, Wong A et al: The association

of obesity with infertility and associated menstrual abnormalities in women. Int J Obes 3:57, 1979

52. Abernethy DR, Greenblatt DJ: Drug disposition in humans: An update. Clin Pharmacokinetics 11:199, 1986
53. Wittels EH: Obesity and hormonal factors in sleep and sleep apnea. Med Clin North Am 69:6, 1985
54. Ashley FW Jr, Kannel WB: Relation of weight change to changes in atherosclerotic traits: The Framingham Study. J Chron Dis 27:103, 1974
55. Bray GA, Gray DS: Obesity. Part II—Treatment. West J Med 149:555, 1988
56. Leiter LA: Obesity: Overview of pathogenesis and treatment. Can J Phys Pharm 64:824, 1986
57. Brownell K: Obesity: Understanding and treating a serious, prevalent, and refractory disorder. J Consult Clin Psych 50:820, 1982
58. Ackerman S: The management of obesity. Hosp Pract 18:117, 1983
59. Braun SR, Keim NL, Dixon RM et al: The prevalence and determinants of nutritional changes in chronic obstructive lung disease. Chest 86:559, 1984
60. Hunter AMB, Carey MA, Larsh HW: The nutritional status of patients with chronic obstructive lung disease. Am Rev Respir Dis 124:376, 1981
61. Kinney JM, Weisman C: Forms of malnutrition in stressed and unstressed patients. Clin Chest Med 7:19, 1986
62. Dudely DF: Malnutrition and respiratory muscles. Clin Chest Med 7:91, 1986
63. Openbrier DR, Covey M: Ineffective breathing pattern related to malnutrition. Nurs Clin North Am 22:225, 1987
64. Mullen JL: Consequences of malnutrition in the surgical patient. Surg Clin North Am 61(June):3, 1981
65. Dougherty S: The malnourished respiratory patient. Crit Care Nurse 8:13, 1988
66. Pittman JG, Cohen P: The pathogenesis of cardiac cachexia. N Engl J Med 271:403, 1964
67. Gull WW: Anorexia nervosa. Trans Clin Soc London 7:22, 1974
68. Drossman DA: Anorexia nervosa: A comprehensive approach. Adv Intern Med 28:339, 1983
69. Halmi KA, Falk JR, Schwartz E: Binge-eating and vomiting: A survey of a college population. Psychol Med 11:695, 1981
70. Gannon MA, Mitchell JE: Subjective evaluation of treatment by patients treated for bulimia. J Am Diet Assoc 86:4, 1986

Bibliography

—— Nutritional status

Harper AE: Transitions in health status: Implications for dietary recommendations. Am J Nutr 45:1094, 1987
Owen OE: Resting metabolic requirements of men and women. Mayo Clin Proc 63:503, 1988
Schneider EL, Yining EM, Hadley EC: Recommended dietary allowances and the health of the elderly. N Engl J Med 314:157, 1986
Strain GW: Nutrition, brain function and behavior. Psychiatr Clin North Am 4:253, 1981
Titchenal CA: Exercise and food intake: What is the relationship? Sports Med 6:135, 1988

Truswell AS: Evolution of dietary recommendations, goals, and guidelines. Am J Clin Nutr 45:1060, 1987

—— Overnutrition and obesity

Bennett W: Dietary treatments of obesity. Ann NY Acad Sci 499:250, 1986
Dietz WH: Childhood obesity. Ann NY Acad Sci 499:47, 1986
Felig P: Very-low-calorie protein diets. N Engl J Med 310:589, 1984
Hagan RD: Benefits of aerobic conditioning and diet for overweight adults. Sports Med 5:144, 1988
Hirssch J, Leibel RL: New light on obesity. N Engl J Med 318:509, 1988
Jequier E: Energy utilization in human obesity. Ann NY Acad Sci 499:73, 1986
Kannel WB, Garrison RJ, Wilson PWF: Obesity and nutrition in elderly diabetic patients. Am J Med 80(Suppl 5A):22, 1986
Mackenzie M: Obesity as failure in the American culture. Obesity Bariatric Med 5:49, 1976
Seidel JC, Deurenber P, Hautvast JGAJ: Obesity and fat distribution in relation to health—Current insights and recommendations. World Rev Nutr Diet 50:57, 1987
Simopoulos AP: Characteristics of obesity: An overview. Ann NY Acad Sci 499:4, 1986

—— Undernutrition

Anderson AE: Anorexia nervosa: Who are you? Where are you? Mayo Clin Proc 63:511, 1988
Apelgren K, Rombeau JL, Twomey PL et al: Comparison of nutritional indices and outcome in critically ill patients. Crit Care Med 10:305, 1982
Barrocas A, Webb GL, Webb WR: Nutritional considerations in the critically ill. South Med J 75:848, 1982
Bessey PG, Custer MD: Nutritional support in surgical care. Ala J Med Sci 24:158, 1987
Halmi KA: Anorexia nervosa and bulimia. Annu Rev Med 38:373, 1987
Harris RT: Bulimarexia and related serious eating disorders with medical complications. Ann Intern Med 99:800, 1983
Herzog DB: Eating disorders. N Engl J Med 313:295, 1985
Kirkley BG: Bulimia: Clinical characteristics, development, and etiology. J Am Diet Assoc 86:468, 1986
Legaspi A, Roberts JP, Horowitz GD et al: Effect of starvation and total parenteral nutrition on electrolyte homeostasis in man. J Parenter Enteral Nutr 12:109 1988
Michel L, Serrano A, Malt RA: Nutritional support of hospitalized patients. N Engl J Med 304:1147, 1981
Ohlrich ES: Pitfalls in the care of patients with anorexia nervosa and bulimia. Semin Adolesc Med 2:81, 1986
Oster JR: The binge–purge syndrome: A common albeit unappreciated cause of acid–base and fluid-electrolyte disturbances. South Med J 80:58, 1987
Salmond S: Recognizing protein-calorie malnutrition. Crit Care Update 9:5, 1982
Story M: Nutritional management and dietary treatment of bulimia. J Am Diet Assoc 86:517, 1986
Walsh TB: The endocrinology of anorexia nervosa. Psychiatr Clin North Am 3:299, 1980
Waterlow JC: Kwashiorkor revisited: The pathogenesis of oedema in kwashiorkor and its significance. Trans R Soc Trop Med Hyg 78:436, 1984

Mechanisms of Endocrine Control

Objectives

After you have studied this chapter, you should be able to meet the following objectives:

_____ Compare the classic endocrine system with the diffuse endocrine system.

_____ Define *hormone function*.

_____ State a difference between the synthesis of protein hormones and that of steroid hormones.

_____ Describe four mechanisms of hormone delivery to target cells.

_____ State three ways in which hormones are inactivated or metabolized.

_____ State the function of a hormone receptor.

_____ Describe two alterations in hormone receptors that could be used to explain changes in hormone action.

_____ State the difference between fixed hormone receptor interactions and mobile hormone receptor interactions.

_____ Describe the role of the hypothalamus in regulating pituitary control of endocrine function.

_____ State the major difference between positive and negative feedback control mechanisms.

_____ Compare endocrine hypofunction and endocrine hyperfunction.

_____ Describe the radioimmunoassay method of measuring hormone levels.

The endocrine system is involved in all of the integrative aspects of life, including growth, sex differentiation, metabolism, and adaptation to an ever-changing environment. This chapter focuses on general aspects of endocrine function, organization of the endocrine system, hormone receptors and hormone actions, and regulation of hormone levels.

The endocrine system

Hormones

Hormones are generally thought of as *chemical messengers* that are transported in body fluids. Although the endocrine system was once thought to consist solely of discrete *endocrine glands* and their hormones, termed the *classic endocrine system,* it is now known that a number of other chemical messengers modulate the body processes.

Hormones of the classic endocrine system are synthesized by endocrine glands, secreted into the bloodstream, and then transported to distant sites, or target cells, where they exert their action. The neurotransmitters (neurohormones), such as the catecholamines (epinephrine, norepinephrine, and dopamine), are also chemical mediators that are synthesized by nerve cells and released from nerve endings.

A number of hormonal peptides have now been identified; these peptides are produced by what is sometimes referred to as the *diffuse endocrine system.*

Unlike the well-defined glands of the classic endocrine system, the diffuse endocrine system is dispersed throughout various organs and cells and is intermingled with nonendocrine cells.[1] A great deal of mystery still surrounds these hormonal peptides. A number of them have been found in both brain and peripheral tissues, and their wide range of actions suggests that they act locally in a number of ways, depending on the tissues that they serve. Perhaps the most interesting of these peptides are the endorphins and enkephalins (see Chapter 47).

Structural classification

Hormones have diverse structures ranging from single modified amino acids (epinephrine and thyroxine), polypeptides (growth hormone and insulin), and glycoproteins (follicle-stimulating hormone and luteinizing hormone) to lipids (steroid hormones such as cortisol). Chart 43-1 presents a listing of hormones according to structure.

Function

Hormones do not initiate reactions; rather they are modulators of body and cellular responses. Most hormones are present in the blood at all times —but in greater or lesser amounts depending on the needs of the body. Hormones can produce either a generalized or a localized effect. For example, thyrotropin acts selectively on the thyroid gland, whereas

Chart 43–1: Classes of hormones based on structure			
Peptides and proteins		**Steroids**	**Amines**
Glycoprotein	*Polypeptides*		
Follicle-stimulating hormone (FSH)	Adrenocorticotropic hormone (ACTH)	Aldosterone	Epinephrine
Human chorionic gonadotropin (HCG)	Angiotensin	Cortisol	Norepinephrine
Luteinizing hormone (LH)	Calcitonin	Estradiol	Thyroxine (T_4)
Thyroid-stimulating hormone (TSH)	Cholecystokinin	Progesterone	Triiodothyronine (T_3)
	Erythropoietin	Testosterone	
	Gastrin	Vitamin D	
	Glucagon		
	Growth hormone		
	Insulin		
	Insulin-like growth peptides (somatomedins)		
	Melanocyte-stimulating hormone (MSH)		
	Nerve growth factor		
	Oxytocin		
	Parathyroid hormone		
	Prolactin		
	Relaxin		
	Secretin		
	Somatostatin		
	Vasopressin (ADH)		

(Greenspan FS, Forsham PH: Basic and Clinical Endocrinology, p 1. Los Altos, CA, Lange Medical Publications, 1983)

epinephrine affects the function of many body systems. Table 43-1 lists the major functions and sources of body hormones. These hormones are discussed more fully in other sections of the text.

—— Synthesis

The mechanisms for hormone synthesis vary with hormone structure. Protein and peptide hormones are synthesized and stored in granules or vesicles within the cytoplasm of the cell until secretion is required. The lipid-soluble steroid hormones are released as they are synthesized.

Protein and peptide hormones are synthesized in the rough endoplasmic reticulum in a manner similar to the synthesis of other proteins (see Chapter 1). The appropriate amino acid sequence is dictated by messenger RNAs from the nucleus. Usually synthesis involves the production of a prehormone, which is modified by the addition of peptides or sugar units. These prehormones often contain extra peptide units that ensure proper folding of the molecule and insertion of essential linkages. If extra amino acids are present, as in insulin, the hormone is called a *prohormone*. Following synthesis and sequestration in the endoplasmic reticulum, the protein and peptide hormones move into the Golgi complex where they are packaged in granules or vesicles. It is in the Golgi complex that prohormones are converted into hormones.

Steroid hormones are synthesized within the smooth endoplasmic reticulum, and steroid-secreting cells can be identified by their large amounts of smooth endoplasmic reticulum. Certain steroids serve as precursors for the production of other hormones. In the adrenal cortex, for example, progesterone and other steroid intermediates are enzymatically con-

Table 43–1. Functional classification of hormones

Function	Hormone	Major source
Control of water and electrolyte metabolism	Aldosterone	Adrenal cortex
	Antidiuretic hormone (ADH)	Posterior pituitary
	Calcitonin	C cells, thyroid
	Parathyroid hormone	Parathyroid
	Angiotensin	Kidney
Control of gastrointestinal function	Cholecystokinin	Gastrointestinal tract
	Gastrin	Gastrointestinal tract
	Secretin	Gastrointestinal tract
Regulation of energy, metabolism, and growth	Glucagon	α cells, pancreatic islets
	Insulin	β cells, pancreatic islets
	Growth hormone	Anterior pituitary
	Somatomedin	Liver
	Somatostatin	Hypothalamus, CNS, pancreatic islets
	Thyroid hormones	Thyroid gland
Neurotransmitters	Dopamine	CNS
	Epinephrine	Adrenal medulla
	Norepinephrine	Adrenal medulla and nervous system
Reproductive function	Chorionic gonadotropins	Placenta
	Estrogens	Ovary
	Oxytocin	Posterior pituitary
	Progesterone	Ovary
	Prolactin	Anterior pituitary
	Testosterone	Testes
Stress and control of inflammation	Glucocorticoids	Adrenal cortex
Tropic hormones (regulation of other hormone levels)	Adrenocorticotropic hormone (ACTH)	Anterior pituitary
	Follicle-stimulating hormone (FSH)	Anterior pituitary
	Luteinizing hormone (LH)	Anterior pituitary
	Thyroid-stimulating hormone (TSH)	Anterior pituitary

verted into either aldosterone, cortisol, or androgens (see Chapter 44).

Transport

Hormones are delivered from cells of the endocrine gland to target cells by one of four mechanisms: (1) blood-borne delivery in which hormones that are synthesized by classic endocrine glands are released into the bloodstream; (2) neurocrine, in which the neuron contacts its target cells by axonal extensions, such as those that connect the hypothalamus with the posterior pituitary gland; (3) neuroendocrine, in which hormones, such as epinephrine, are released from neurons into the bloodstream; and (4) paracrine, in which the released chemical messenger diffuses to its target cell through the interstitial fluid, such as occurs in the diffuse endocrine system.[2]

Hormones that are released into the bloodstream circulate either as free molecules or as hormones attached to transport carriers. Peptide hormones and protein hormones generally circulate unbound in the blood. Steroid hormones and thyroid hormone are carried by specific proteins synthesized in the liver. The extent of carrier binding influences the rate at which hormones leave the blood and enter the cells. The half-life of a hormone—the time it takes for the body to reduce the concentration of the hormone by one-half—is positively correlated with its percentage of protein binding. Thyroxine, which is more than 99% protein bound, has a half-life of 6 days. Aldosterone, which is only 15% bound, has a half-life of only 25 minutes.[3] Drugs that compete with a hormone for binding with the transport carrier molecules increase hormone action by increasing the availability of the active unbound hormone. For example, aspirin competes with thyroid hormone for binding to transport proteins; this can produce serious effects during thyroid crisis, when affected persons are already suffering from the effects of excessive hormone levels.

Metabolism

Hormones secreted by endocrine cells must be continuously inactivated to prevent their accumulation. Both intracellular and extracellular mechanisms participate in the termination of hormone function. Some hormones are enzymatically inactivated at receptor sites where they exert their action. Peptide hormones have a short life span and are inactivated by enzymes that split peptide bonds. They are inactivated mainly in the liver and kidneys. As was previously mentioned, steroid hormones are bound to protein carriers for transport and are inactive in the bound state. Their activity depends on the availability of transport hormones. Unbound adrenal and gonadal steroid hormones are conjugated in the liver, which renders them inactive, and then excreted in the bile or urine. Thyroid hormones are also transported by carrier molecules. The free hormone is rendered inactive by the removal of amino acids (deamination) in the tissues and is also conjugated in the liver and eliminated in the bile.

Rate of reaction

Hormones react at different rates. The neurotransmitters, such as epinephrine, have a reaction time of milliseconds. Thyroid hormone, on the other hand, requires days for its effect to occur. Hormones are continually being metabolized or inactivated and removed from the body.

Mechanisms of action

Hormones exert their action by binding to specific receptor sites located on the surfaces of the target cells. The function of these receptors is to recognize a specific hormone and translate the hormonal signal into a cellular response. The structure of these receptors varies in a manner that allows target cells to respond to one hormone and not to others. For example, receptors in the thyroid are specific for the thyroid-stimulating hormone, whereas receptors on the gonads respond to the gonadotropic hormones.

The response of a target cell to the action of a hormone will vary with the *number* of receptors present and with the *affinity* of these receptors for hormone binding. A variety of factors influence the number of receptors that are present on target cells and their affinity for hormone binding (Figure 43-1).

There are generally 2,000 to 10,000 hormone receptor molecules per cell.[3] The number of hormone receptors on a cell may be altered for any of several reasons. Antibodies may destroy the receptor proteins. Sustained levels of excess hormone may decrease the number of receptors per cell in a process called *down regulation*. This acts to modify the effect of chronic exposure to a given hormone. In some instances, the reverse effect occurs, and an increase in hormone levels appears to recruit its own receptors (*up regulation*), increasing the sensitivity of the cell to the hormone. Obesity has been shown to cause a decrease in the number of insulin receptors that are present on fat cells, and it is speculated that this may influence impaired glucose tolerance in the obese noninsulin-dependent diabetic. On the other hand, it has been shown that the oral hypoglycemic drugs, the sulfonylureas, cause an increase in the number of insulin receptors on body cells.

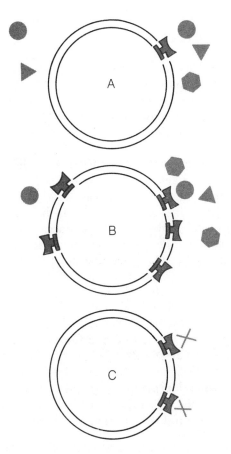

Figure 43-1 (**A**) The role of cell-surface receptors in mediating the action of hormones. Hormone action is affected by (**B**) the number of receptors that are present and by (**C**) the affinity of these receptors for hormone binding.

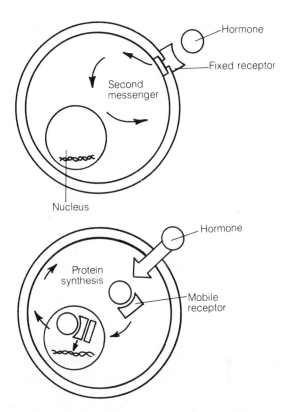

Figure 43-2 The two types of hormone–receptor interactions: the fixed membrane receptor, **top,** and the intracellular mobile receptor, **bottom.**

The affinity of receptors for binding hormones is also affected by a number of conditions. For example, the pH of the body fluids plays an important role in the affinity of insulin receptors. In ketoacidosis, the lowering of the pH from 7.4 to 7.0 reduces insulin binding by about one-half.[4]

Hormone–receptor interactions go about the process of modulating cell activity in two ways. One type of response occurs with the peptide hormones, which circulate in the blood in their free state. These hormones interact with fixed membrane receptors in a manner that incites the release of a *second messenger* (usually cyclic AMP), which in turn activates a series of enzyme reactions that serve to alter cell function (Figure 43-2). Glucagon, for example, incites glycogen breakdown by way of the second messenger system.

A second type of receptor mechanism is involved in mediating the action of hormones, such as the steroid and the thyroid hormones, which are transported in body fluids attached to carrier proteins (Figure 43-2). These hormones, being lipid-soluble, pass freely through the cell membrane and then attach to an intracellular *mobile receptor* in the cytoplasm of the cell. This hormone–receptor complex moves through the cytoplasm, becomes activated, and enters the nucleus where it causes activation or repression of gene activity with subsequent production of messenger RNA and protein synthesis. Chart 43-2 lists hormones that act by the two types of receptors.

Chart 43–2: Hormone–receptor interactions

Fixed messenger interactions

Glucagon
Insulin
Epinephrine
Parathyroid hormone
Thyroid-stimulating hormone
Adrenocorticotropic hormone
Follicle-stimulating hormone
Luteinizing hormone
Antidiuretic hormone
Secretin

Mobile hormone–receptor–nuclear interactions

Estrogen
Testosterone
Progesterone
Adrenal cortical hormones
Thyroid hormone

—— Control of hormone levels

Hormone secretion varies widely over a 24-hour period. Some hormones, such as growth hormone and adrenocorticotropic hormone (ACTH), have diurnal fluctuations that vary with the sleep–awakening cycle. Others, such as the female sex hormones, are secreted in a complicated cyclic manner. The levels of hormones like insulin and antidiuretic hormone (ADH) are regulated by the amount of organic and inorganic substances present in the body. The levels of many of the hormones are regulated by feedback mechanisms that involve the hypothalamic–pituitary–target cell system.

—— Hypothalamic–pituitary regulation

Because the integration of body function relies on input from both the nervous system and the endocrine system, it seems logical that input from the nervous system would participate in the regulation of hormone levels. In this respect, the hypothalamus and the pituitary (hypophysis) act as an integrative link between the central nervous system and the many endocrine-mediated functions of the body. These two structures are connected by blood flow in the hypophyseal portal system, which begins in the hypothalamus and drains into the anterior pituitary gland, and by the nerve axons that connect the supraoptic and paraventricular nuclei of the hypothalamus with the posterior pituitary gland (Figure 43-3). Embryologically, the anterior pituitary gland developed from glandular tissue and the posterior pituitary developed from neural tissue.

The endocrine hypothalamus. The synthesis and release of anterior pituitary hormones are largely regulated by the action of releasing or inhibiting hormones from the hypothalamus, which is the coordinating center of the brain for endocrine, behavioral, and autonomic nervous system function. It is at the level of the hypothalamus that emotion, pain, body temperature, and other neural input are communicated to the endocrine system. The posterior pituitary hormones, ADH and oxytocin, are synthesized in the cell bodies of the nerve axons that travel to the posterior pituitary. The release and function of ADH are discussed in Chapter 27.

Anterior pituitary gland. The pituitary gland has been called the "master gland" because its hormones control the function of a number of target

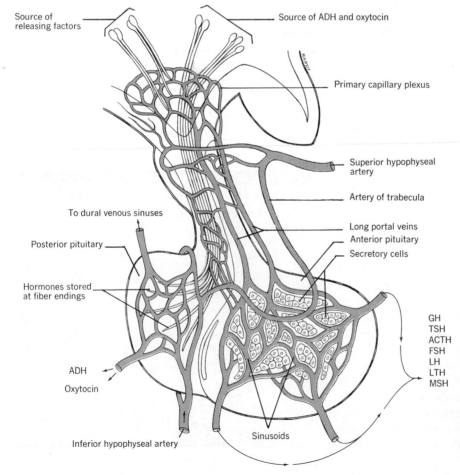

Source of releasing factors

Source of ADH and oxytocin

Primary capillary plexus

Superior hypophyseal artery

Artery of trabecula

Long portal veins
Anterior pituitary
Secretory cells

To dural venous sinuses

Posterior pituitary

Hormones stored at fiber endings

ADH

Oxytocin

Inferior hypophyseal artery

Sinusoids

GH
TSH
ACTH
FSH
LH
LTH
MSH

Figure 43-3 The hypothalamus and the anterior and posterior pituitary. Hypothalamus releasing or inhibiting hormones are transported to the anterior pituitary by way of the portal vessels. ADH and oxytocin are produced by nerve cells in the supraoptic and paraventricular nuclei of the hypothalamus and then transported through the nerve axon to the posterior pituitary where they are released into the circulation. *(Chaffee EE, Greisheimer EM: Basic Physiology and Anatomy, 3rd ed. Philadelphia, JB Lippincott, 1974)*

glands or cells. Hormones produced by the anterior pituitary control body growth and metabolism (growth hormone), function of the thyroid gland (thyroid-stimulating hormone), glucocorticoid hormone levels (adrenocorticotropic hormone), function of the gonads (follicle-stimulating and luteinizing hormones), and breast growth and milk production (prolactin). Melanocyte-stimulating hormone, which controls pigmentation of the skin, is produced by the pars intermedia of the pituitary.

Feedback mechanisms

The level of many of the hormones in the body is regulated by negative feedback mechanisms. The function of this type of system is similar to that of the thermostat in a heating system. In the endocrine system, sensors detect a change in the hormone level and adjust hormone secretion so that body levels are maintained within an appropriate range. When the sensors detect a decrease in hormone levels, they initiate changes that cause an increase in hormone production; and when hormone levels rise above the set point of the system, the sensors cause hormone production and release to decrease. For example, an increase in thyroid hormone is detected by sensors in the hypothalamus or anterior pituitary gland, and this causes a reduction in the secretion of thyroid-stimulating hormone with a subsequent decrease in the output of thyroid hormone from the thyroid gland. The feedback loops for the hypothalamic–pituitary feedback mechanisms are illustrated in Figure 43-4. Exogenous forms of hormones (given as drug preparations) can influence the normal feedback control of hormone production and release. One of the most common examples of this influence occurs with the administration of the adrenal cortical hormones, which causes suppression of the hypothalamic–pituitary–target cell system that regulates the production of these hormones.

Although the levels of most hormones are regulated by negative feedback mechanisms, a small number are under positive feedback control in which rising levels of a hormone cause another gland to release a hormone that is stimulating to the first. There must, however, be a mechanism for shutting off the release of the first hormone, or its production would continue unabated. An example of such a system is that of the female ovarian hormone estradiol. Increased estradiol production during the follicular stage of the menstrual cycle produces increased gonadotropin (FSH) production by the anterior pituitary gland. This stimulates further increases in estradiol levels until the demise of the follicle, which is the source of estradiol, results in a fall in gonadotropin levels.

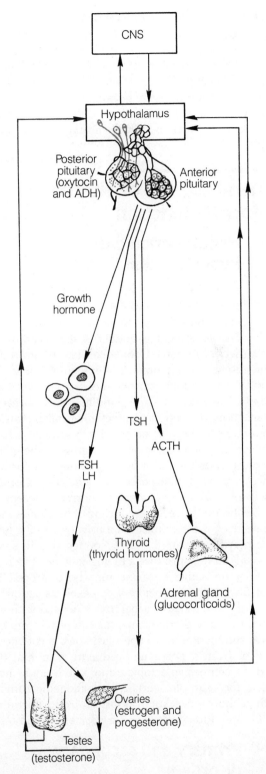

Figure 43-4 Control of hormone production by hypothalamic-pituitary–target cell feedback mechanism. Hormone levels from the target glands regulate the release of hormones from the anterior pituitary by means of a negative feedback system.

In summary, the endocrine system acts as a communications system that uses chemical messengers, or hormones, for the transmission of information from cell to cell and from organ to organ. Hormones act at the level of the cell membrane, which has surface receptors that are specific for the different types of hormones. Many of the endocrine glands are under the regulatory control of other parts of the endocrine system. The hypothalamus and the pituitary gland form a complex integrative network that joins the nervous system and the endocrine system; this central network controls the output from many of the other glands in the body.

General aspects of altered endocrine function

Hypofunction and hyperfunction

Disturbances of endocrine function can usually be divided into two categories: hypofunction and hyperfunction.

Hypofunction of an endocrine gland can occur for a variety of reasons. Congenital defects can result in the absence or impaired development of the gland or the absence of an enzyme needed for hormone synthesis. Destruction of the gland may occur because of disruption in blood flow, infection or inflammation, autoimmune responses, or neoplastic growth. There may be a decline in function with aging, or the gland may atrophy as the result of drug therapy or for unknown reasons. Some endocrine-deficient states are associated with receptor defects: hormone receptors may be absent; the receptor binding of hormones may be defective; or the cellular responsiveness to the hormone may be impaired. It is suspected that in some cases a gland may produce a biologically inactive hormone, or an active hormone may be destroyed by circulating antibodies before it can exert its action.

Hyperfunction is generally associated with excessive hormone production. This can result from excessive stimulation and hyperplasia of the endocrine gland or from a hormone-producing tumor of the gland. Sometimes an ectopic tumor will produce hormones; for example, certain bronchogenic tumors produce hormones such as antidiuretic hormone (ADH) and adrenocorticotropic hormone (ACTH).

Primary and secondary disorders

Endocrine disorders can generally be divided into two groups—primary and secondary. *Primary defects* in endocrine function originate within the target gland responsible for producing the hormone. In *secondary disorders* of endocrine function, the target gland is essentially normal, but its function is altered by defective levels of stimulating hormones or releasing factors from the hypothalamic–pituitary system. For example, adrenalectomy produces a primary deficiency of adrenal corticosteroid hormones. Removal or destruction of the pituitary gland, on the other hand, eliminates ACTH stimulation of the adrenal cortex and brings about a secondary deficiency.

Diagnostic methods

There are a number of techniques for assessing endocrine function and hormone levels. One technique measures the effect of a hormone on body function. Measurement of blood glucose, for example, reflects insulin levels and is an indirect method of assessing insulin availability. Another technique, the *bioassay,* measures the effect of a hormone on animal function. A bioassay can be done using the intact animal or a portion of tissue from the animal. At one time, female rats or male frogs were used to test women's urine for the presence of human chorionic gonadotropin, which is produced by the placenta during pregnancy. Today, the most widely used technique for measuring hormone levels is the *radioimmunoassay.* This method uses a radiolabeled form of the hormone and a hormone antibody that has been prepared by injecting an appropriate animal with a purified form of the hormone. The unlabeled hormone in the sample being tested competes with the radiolabeled hormone for attachment to the binding sites of the antibody. Measurement of the radiolabeled hormone–antibody complex then provides a means of arriving at a measure of hormone level in the sample. Because hormone binding is competitive, the amount of radiolabeled hormone–antibody complex that is formed will decrease as the amount of unlabeled hormone in the sample is increased.

In summary, endocrine disorders are the result of hypo- or hyperfunction of an endocrine gland. They can occur as a primary defect in hormone production by a target gland or as a secondary disorder resulting from a defect in the hypothalamic–pituitary system that controls a target gland's function. Laboratory tests that measure hormone levels or assess the effect of a hormone on body function (*e.g.,* assessment of insulin function through blood sugar levels) are used in the diagnosis of endocrine disorders.

References

1. Polak JM, Path MRC, Bloom SR: Neuropeptides of the gut: A newly discovered major control system. World J Surg 3:393, 1979
2. Hadeley ME: Endocrinology, p 32. Englewood Cliffs, NJ, Prentice-Hall, 1984
3. Berne RM, Levy MN: Physiology, 2nd ed, pp 825, 832–833. St Louis, CV Mosby, 1988
4. Kahn CR: Probing receptor activity in cell control. Patient Care 13(1):84, 1984

Linda S. Hurwitz
Carol Mattson Porth

CHAPTER 44

Alterations in Endocrine Control of Growth and Metabolism

Objectives

After you have studied this chapter, you should be able to meet the following objectives:

_____ State the general functions of growth hormone and the somatomedins.

_____ State the effects of a deficiency in growth hormone.

_____ Define *short stature*.

_____ Define *constitutional short stature*.

_____ State the mechanisms of short stature in hypothyroidism, poorly controlled diabetes mellitus, treatment with adrenal glucocorticosteroid hormones, malnutrition, and psychosocial dwarfism.

_____ List three causes of tall stature.

_____ Explain why children with isosexual precocious puberty are tall-statured as children, but short-statured as adults.

_____ Describe the conditions predisposing to acromegaly.

_____ Explain the potential relationship between growth hormone and diabetes.

_____ Describe the synthesis of thyroid hormones.

_____ Describe the hypothalamic–pituitary–thyroid feedback system.

_____ Explain why blood cholesterol levels are decreased in hyperthyroidism.

_____ State the relationship between cardiovascular function and thyroid function.

_____ Describe the general effects of thyroid hormone on the muscular system.

(continued)

_____ Name three tests of thyroid function.

_____ List the signs and symptoms of hyperthyroidism the health professional should be able to recognize.

_____ State the manifestations of thyroid storm.

_____ State the triad of conditions that constitute Graves' disease.

_____ Describe the effects of congenital hypothyroidism.

_____ Describe the manifestations of the condition known as myxedema.

_____ State the underlying cause of the adrenogenital syndrome.

_____ State the role of the adrenal sex hormones and the mineralocorticoids.

_____ Explain the regulation of the glucocorticoids by negative feedback mechanisms.

_____ Explain the influence of cortisol on body metabolism.

_____ Describe the action of cortisol on inflammation.

_____ State the purpose of the 24-hour urine specimen with reference to adrenal cortical function.

_____ State the underlying cause or causes of Cushing's syndrome.

_____ Describe the clinical manifestations of Cushing's syndrome.

_____ Explain the underlying pathology that is present in Addison's disease.

_____ Compare the manifestations of Addison's disease with those of secondary adrenal insufficiency.

_____ Describe the overall treatment of adrenal insufficiency.

The endocrine system affects all aspects of body function, including growth and development, body appearance, and metabolism. In terms of body image, it is the endocrine system that determines the size, shape, texture, and sexual characteristics of the body. In this chapter, disorders of growth and growth hormone (GH) and alterations in thyroid and adrenocortical function will be discussed.

Growth and growth hormone disorders

A number of hormones are essential for normal body growth. Pituitary growth hormone, one of the most important hormones, produces its growth effects through a group of polypeptide hormones called somatomedins. Insulin, thyroid hormone, and androgens are also essential for normal growth and maturation. In addition to its actions on carbohydrate and fat metabolism, insulin plays an essential role in growth processes. Children with diabetes, particularly those with poor control, often fail to grow normally even though GH levels are normal. When levels of thyroid hormone are lower than normal, bone growth and epiphyseal closure are delayed. Androgens such as testosterone and dihydrotestosterone exert anabolic growth effects through their actions on protein synthesis. Glucocorticoids, at excessive levels, are inhibitory to growth, apparently because of their antagonistic effect on GH secretion.

___ Growth hormone

Growth hormone (GH), also called *somatotropin,* is a 191-amino-acid polypeptide hormone synthesized and secreted by special cells in the anterior pituitary called somatotropes. For many years it was thought that GH was produced primarily during periods of growth. However, this has proved to be incorrect, because the rate of GH production in adults is almost as great as in children. It is now known that GH is not only necessary for growth, but also contributes to the regulation of metabolic functions.[1,2] All aspects of cartilage growth are stimulated by GH; one of the most striking effects of GH is on linear bone growth resulting from its action on the epiphyseal cartilage plates of long bones. Other tissues share the metabolic response to GH. The width of bone increases because of enhanced periosteal growth; visceral and endocrine organs, skeletal and cardiac muscle, skin, and connective tissue all undergo increased growth in response to GH. In many instances, the increased growth of visceral and endocrine organs is accompanied by enhanced functional capacity. For example, increased growth of cardiac muscle is accompanied by an increase in cardiac output. Aside from its effects on growth, GH facilitates the rate of protein synthesis by all of the cells of the body; it enhances fatty acid mobilization and increases the utilization of fatty acids for fuel; and it maintains or increases blood glucose levels by decreasing the utilization of glucose for fuel. Growth hormone has an initial effect of increasing insulin levels. However, the predominant effect of prolonged GH excess is to increase glucose levels despite an insulin increase. This occurs because GH induces a resistance to insulin in the peripheral tissues, thereby inhibiting the uptake of glucose by muscle and adipose tissues.

Many of the effects of GH depend on a family of peptides called *somatomedins,* which are produced by the liver. Growth hormone cannot directly produce bone growth; instead it acts indirectly by causing the liver to produce the somatomedins. These peptides, in turn, act on cartilage and bone to promote their growth. At least four different somatomedins have been identified. In addition to their effects on growth, laboratory experiments suggest that the different somatomedins also influence the metabolic functions of GH.

Growth hormone is carried unbound in the plasma and has a half-life of about 20 to 50 minutes. The secretion of GH is regulated by two hypothalamic hormones: growth hormone releasing factor (GH-RH) and growth hormone release inhibiting hormone, also called *somatostatin.* Somatostatin is also produced by delta cells in the islets of Langerhans in the pancreas where it influences glucagon and insulin release. These hypothalamic influences are tightly regulated by neural, metabolic, and hormonal factors. The secretion of GH fluctuates over a 24-hour period with peak levels occurring 1 to 4 hours after onset of sleep (during sleep stages 3 and 4). The nocturnal sleep bursts, which account for 70% of daily GH secretion, are greater in children than adults.[3] Growth hormone secretion is stimulated by hypoglycemia, fasting, starvation, increased blood levels of amino acids (particularly arginine), and stress conditions such as trauma, excitement and emotional stress, and heavy exercise. Growth hormone is inhibited by increased glucose levels, free fatty acid release, cortisol, and obesity. Impairment of secretion, leading to growth retardation, is not uncommon in children with severe emotional deprivation.

—— Short stature

Short stature is a condition in which the attained height is well below the fifth percentile or linear growth is below normal for age and sex. Short stature, or growth retardation, has a variety of causes, including abnormalities such as Turner's syndrome (see Chapter 4), GH deficiency, hypothyroidism, and panhypopituitarism. Other conditions known to cause short stature include protein-calorie malnutrition, chronic diseases such as renal failure and poorly controlled diabetes mellitus, certain therapies such as exogenous corticosteroid administration, and malabsorption syndromes. Emotional disturbances can lead to functional endocrine disorders causing psychoso-

---

Chart 44–1:   Causes of short stature

Variants of normal
  Genetic short stature
  Constitutional short stature

Endocrine disorders
  Growth hormone deficiency
    Primary growth hormone deficiency
      Idiopathic growth hormone deficiency
      Pituitary agenesis
    Secondary growth hormone deficiency
      Hypothalamic–pituitary tumors
      Postcranial radiation
      Head injuries
      Brain infections
      Hydrocephalus
      Biologically inactive growth hormone production
  Hypothyroidism
  Diabetes mellitus in poor control
  Glucocorticoid excess
    Endogenous (Cushing's disease)
    Exogenous glucocorticoid drug treatment

Chronic illness
Malnutrition
  Nutritional deprivation
  Malabsorption syndrome

Functional endocrine disorders
  Psychosocial dwarfism

Chromosomal disorders
  Turner's syndrome

---

cial dwarfism. The causes of short stature are summarized in Chart 44-1.

Two forms of short stature, genetic short stature and constitutional short stature, are not disease states but variations from population norms. Genetically short children tend to have a height close to the mean height of their parents. *Constitutional short stature* is a term used to describe children (particularly boys) who have moderately short stature, thin build, delayed skeletal and sexual maturation, and absence of other causes of decreased growth.

Catch-up growth is a term used to describe an abnormally high growth rate that occurs as a child approaches normal height for age. It occurs after the initiation of therapy for GH deficiency and hypothyroidism and the correction of chronic diseases.

Psychosocial dwarfism involves a functional hypopituitarism and is seen in some emotionally deprived children. These children usually present with poor growth, potbelly, and poor eating and drinking habits. Typically, there is a history of disturbed family relationships in which the child has been severely neglected or disciplined. Often the neglect is confined to one child in the family. Growth hormone function usually returns to normal after the child is removed from the home. The diagnosis depends on improvement in behavior and catch-up growth. Family therapy is usually indicated, and foster care may be necessary.

Accurate measurement of height is an extremely important part of the physical examination of children. Completion of the developmental history and growth charts is essential. Growth curves and growth velocity studies are also needed. Diagnosis of short stature is not made on a single measurement but is based on actual height as well as velocity of growth and parental height. Children are considered short-statured when their height and linear growth velocity are below normal for their age and sex. Genetically short children generally have a well-proportioned stature.

The diagnostic procedures for short stature include tests to rule out nonendocrine causes. If the cause is hormonal, extensive hormonal testing procedures are initiated. Usually both GH and somatomedin levels are determined. Tests can be performed using insulin (to induce hypoglycemia), levodopa, and arginine, all of which stimulate and evaluate GH reserve. If a prompt rise in GH is realized, the child is considered normal. Radiologic films are used to assess bone age, which is most often delayed. The size and shape of the sella turcica (depression in the sphenoid bone that contains the pituitary gland) are studied to determine if a pituitary tumor exists. Once the cause of short stature has been determined, treatment can be initiated.

Growth hormone deficiency

There are several forms of growth hormone deficiency. Children with idiopathic growth hormone deficiency lack GH releasing factor but have adequate somatotropes, whereas children with pituitary tumors or agenesis of the pituitary lack somatotropes. The term *panhypopituitarism* refers to conditions that cause a deficiency of all of the anterior pituitary hormones. In a rare condition called Laron's dwarfism, growth hormone levels are normal or elevated but there is a hereditary defect in somatomedin production.

When short stature is caused by a GH deficiency, GH replacement therapy is the treatment of choice. Growth hormone is species specific, and only primate GH is effective in humans. Growth hormone is now produced by recombinant DNA (rDNA) technology and is no longer in limited supply. Previously, human growth hormone (HGH) was derived solely from human cadavers; and treatment of one child required from one and one-half to two human pituitary glands a week. In 1985, the National Hormone and Pituitary Program halted the distribution of

human pituitary-derived growth hormone in the United States after receiving reports that three persons died of Creutzfeldt-Jakob disease. The disease, which is caused by a neurotropic virus, was thought to be transmitted by cadaver GH preparations. Growth hormone produced by the recombinant DNA method is a 192-amino-acid molecule that contains all 191 amino acids of HGH plus an additional methionyl molecule. For this reason, the rDNA-derived hormone is commonly called *methionyl-HGH*. Clinical trials of methionyl-HGH were begun in the United States in 1981, and the product is now available for clinical use. Clinical trials for four other forms of GH are being conducted in the United States.[4] Methionyl-HGH is administered subcutaneously three times weekly during the period of active growth. Clinical studies are also being conducted on children with constitutional short stature and Turner's syndrome. It is still too early to predict the outcome of treatment for these children. There are concerns over misuse of the drug to produce additional growth in children with normal GH function who are of near-normal height. Guidelines for use of the hormone are being established.[5] Methods for synthesis of human growth hormone releasing factor have recently been developed, and it has become available for use in clinical research.[6]

Tall stature

Just as there are children who are short for their age and sex, there are also children who are tall for their age and sex. Normal variants of tall stature include genetic tall stature and constitutional tall stature. As with short stature, children with exceptionally tall parents tend to be taller than children with short parents. The term *constitutional tall stature* is used to describe a child who is taller than his or her peers and is growing at a velocity that is within the normal range for bone age. Other causes of tall stature are genetic or chromosomal disorders such as Marfan's syndrome or XYY syndrome (see Chapter 4). Endocrine causes of tall stature include excessive growth hormone, sexual precocity because of early onset of estrogen and androgen secretion, and thyrotoxicosis. With sexual precocity, linear growth during childhood is increased but stature in adulthood is decreased because of premature epiphyseal closure.

Exceptionally tall children (genetic tall stature and constitutional tall stature) can be treated with sex hormones (estrogens in girls and testosterone in boys) to effect early epiphyseal closure. Such treatment is undertaken only after full consideration of the risks involved. To be effective, such treatment must be instituted 3 to 4 years before epiphyseal fusion.

Isosexual precocious puberty

Precocious sexual development may be idiopathic or may be caused by gonadal, adrenal, or hypothalamic tumors. Isosexual precocious puberty is defined as early activation of the hypothalamic–pituitary–gonadal axis, resulting in the development of appropriate sexual characteristics and fertility.[7,8] Sexual development is considered precocious and warrants investigation when it occurs before 8 years of age for girls and before 10 years of age for boys. In girls, about 90% of cases are idiopathic. In boys, about 40% to 60% are related to central nervous system disease.

Diagnosis of precocious puberty is based on physical findings of early thelarche (beginning of breast development), adrenarche (beginning of augmented adrenal androgen production), and menarche (beginning of menstrual function). Radiologic findings may indicate advanced bone age. Individuals with precocious puberty are usually tall for their age as children, but are short as adults because of the early closure of the epiphyses. The most common sign in boys is early genital enlargement.

Depending on the cause of precocious puberty, the treatment may involve surgery, medication, or no treatment. In females, medroxyprogesterone can be given to arrest menstruation in the very young child. Parents often need education, support, and anticipatory guidance in dealing with their feelings and the child's physical needs and in relating to a child that appears older than his or her years.

Growth hormone excess

Growth hormone excess occurring before puberty and before the fusion of the epiphyses of the long bones has occurred results in gigantism. When GH excess occurs in adulthood or after the epiphyses of the long bones have fused, a condition known as acromegaly develops.

Gigantism

Excessive secretion of GH by somatotrope adenomas causes gigantism in the prepubertal child. It occurs when the epiphyses are not fused and high levels of somatomedins stimulate excessive skeletal growth. Fortunately, the condition is now very rare because of early recognition and treatment of the adenoma.

Acromegaly

Acromegaly is a chronic and debilitating disorder of body growth and metabolic derangements in the adult caused by excess levels of GH. Most cases of acromegaly (about 95%) are caused by pituitary adenoma. The disorder usually has an insidious onset, and presenting symptoms are often present for a considerable period of time before a diagnosis is made. Early manifestations include excessive sweating with an unpleasant odor, oily skin, heat intolerance, moderate weight gain, muscle weakness and fatigue, menstrual irregularities, and decreased libido. Hypertension is relatively common. Paresthesias may develop because of nerve entrapment and compression caused by excess soft tissue and accumulation of subcutaneous fluid. Virtually every organ of the body is increased in size. Enlargement of the heart and accelerated atherosclerosis may lead to an early death.

When the production of excessive GH occurs after the epiphyses of the long bones have closed, as in the adult, the person cannot grow taller; but the soft tissues continue to grow. Enlargement of the small bones of the hands and feet and in the membranous bones of the face and skull results in a pronounced enlargement of the hands and feet, a broad and bulbous nose, a protruding lower jaw, and a slanting forehead (Figure 44-1). The teeth become splayed, causing a disturbed bite and difficulty in chewing. The cartilaginous structures in the larynx and respiratory tract also become enlarged, resulting in a deepening of the voice and tendency to develop bronchitis. Vertebral changes often lead to kyphosis, or hunchback. Bone overgrowth often leads to arthralgias and degenerative arthritis of the spine, hips, and knees.

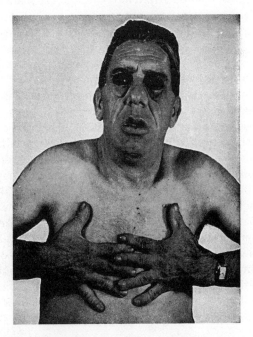

Figure 44-1 Acromegaly, showing protrusion of the lower jaw, heavy lips, and "spade" hands. (*Chaffee EE, Lytle IM: Basic Physiology and Anatomy, 4th ed, p 527. Philadelphia, JB Lippincott, 1980*)

The metabolic effects of excess levels of GH include alterations in fat and carbohydrate metabolism. Increased levels of GH have a diabetogenic effect. Insulin antagonism leads to abnormal glucose tolerance, and increased mobilization of fatty acids predisposes to ketoacidosis. The increase in blood sugar stimulates the beta cells of the pancreas to produce additional insulin. Growth hormone also has a direct stimulatory effect on beta cells.[1] Long-term elevation of GH results in overstimulation of the beta cells, literally causing them to "burn out," which predisposes to development of diabetes mellitus. Impaired glucose tolerance or frank diabetes is present in up to 68% of persons with acromegaly.[9]

The pituitary gland is located in the pituitary fossa of the sphenoid bone (sella turcica), which lies directly below the optic nerve. Almost all persons with acromegaly have a recognizable adenohypophyseal tumor.[10] Enlargement of the pituitary gland eventually causes erosion of the surrounding bone, and because of its location, this can lead to headaches, visual field defects resulting from compression of the optic nerve, and cranial nerve palsies (III, IV, VI). Compression of other pituitary structures can cause secondary hypothyroidism, hypogonadism, and adrenal insufficiency.

The diagnosis of acromegaly is facilitated by the typical features of the disorder (enlargement of the hands and feet and coarsening of facial features). Laboratory tests to detect elevated levels of GH not suppressed by a glucose load are used to confirm the diagnosis. Computerized tomography (CT scans) and nuclear magnetic resonance imaging may be done to detect and localize the pituitary lesions. Because most of the effects of GH are mediated by the somatomedins, somatomedin–C (SM-C) levels may provide information related to disease activity.

The goals of treatment in acromegaly are the rapid normalization of GH to prevent or reverse progression of the disorder; prevention or reversal of the pressure effects of the tumor on structures surrounding the sella turcica; and preservation or restoration of normal pituitary function.[9] Pituitary tumors can be removed surgically using the transsphenoidal approach, or their size can be reduced with irradiation. Dopamine agonists normally raise GH levels. Bromocriptine, a long-acting dopamine antagonist, has been used with some success in the medical management of acromegaly. However, high doses are often required, and side effects may be troublesome. Of recent interest is the development of a somatostatin analogue that could be used to suppress GH production.[11,12]

In summary, a number of hormones are essential for normal body growth and maturation, including growth hormone, insulin, thyroid hormone, and androgens. Growth hormone exerts its growth effects through a group of polypeptide hormones called somatomedins. Growth hormone also exerts an effect on metabolism and is excreted in the adult as well as in the child. Its metabolic effects include a decrease in peripheral utilization of carbohydrates and an increased mobilization and utilization of fatty acids. In children, alterations in growth include short stature, isosexual precocious puberty, and tall stature. Short stature is a condition in which the attained height is well below the fifth percentile or the linear growth velocity is below normal for a child's age or sex. Short stature can occur as a variant of normal growth (genetic short stature or constitutional short stature) or as the result of endocrine disorders, chronic illness, malnutrition, emotional disturbances, or chromosomal disorders. Short stature resulting from GH deficiency can now be treated with human growth hormone preparations. Isosexual precocious puberty defines a condition of early activation of hypothalamic–pituitary–gonadal axis (before 8 years of age in girls and 10 years of age in boys) resulting in the development of appropriate sexual characteristics and fertility. It causes tall stature during childhood but results in short stature in adulthood because of the early closure of the epiphyses. Tall stature describes the condition in which children are tall for their age and sex. It can occur as a variant of normal growth (genetic tall stature or constitutional tall stature) or as the result of a chromosomal abnormality or GH excess. Growth hormone excess in adults results in acromegaly, which involves proliferation of bone, cartilage, and soft tissue along with the metabolic effects of excessive hormone levels.

Thyroid disorders

The thyroid gland is a shield-shaped structure located immediately below the larynx in the anterior middle portion of the neck. The thyroid gland is composed of a large number of tiny saclike structures called follicles (Figure 44-2). These are the functional cells of the thyroid. Each follicle is formed by a single layer of epithelial (follicular) cells and is filled with a secretory substance called colloid, which consists largely of a glycoprotein–iodine complex, thyroglobulin.

Control of thyroid function

The thyroglobulin that fills the thyroid follicles is a large glycoprotein molecule that contains 140 tyrosine amino acids. In the process of thyroid synthesis, iodine is attached to these tyrosine amino acids. Both thyroglobulin and iodide (I^-) are secreted into the colloid of the follicle by the follicular cells.

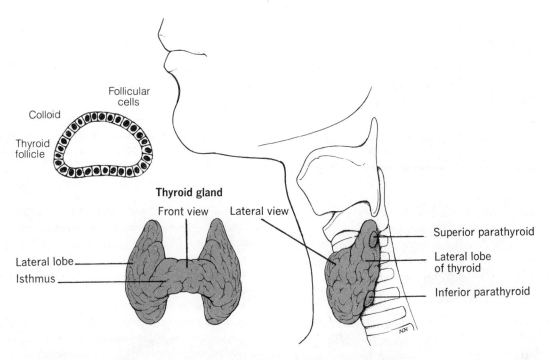

Figure 44-2 The thyroid gland and the follicular structure. (*Chaffee EE, Lytle IM: Basic Physiology and Anatomy, 4th ed, p 434. Philadelphia, JB Lippincott, 1980*)

The thyroid is remarkably efficient in its utilization of iodine. A daily absorption of 100 μg to 200 μg of dietary iodine is sufficient to form normal quantities of thyroid hormone. In the process of removing iodine from the blood and storing it for future use, iodine is pumped into the follicular cells against a concentration gradient. As a result, the concentration of iodide within the normal thyroid gland is about 40 times that in the blood. Once inside the follicle, most of the iodide is oxidized by the enzyme peroxidase in a reaction that facilitates combination with a tyrosine molecule to form *monoiodotyrosine* and then *diiodotyrosine* (Figure 44-3). In time, two diiodotyrosine residues become coupled to form *thyroxine* (T_4); or a monoiodotyrosine and a diiodotyrosine become coupled to form *triiodothyronine* (T_3). Only T_4 (90%) and T_3 (10%) are secreted into the circulation. Thyroid hormones are bound to thyroid-binding globulin and other plasma proteins for transport in the blood. There is evidence that T_3 is the active form of the hormone and that T_4 is converted to T_3 before it becomes active.

The secretion of thyroid hormone is regulated by the hypothalamic–pituitary–thyroid feedback system (Figure 44-4). In this system, thyrotropin-releasing hormone (TRH), which is produced by the hypothalamus, controls the release of thyroid-stimulating hormone (TSH) from the anterior pituitary gland. TSH increases the overall activity of the thyroid gland by (1) increasing the thyroglobulin breakdown and

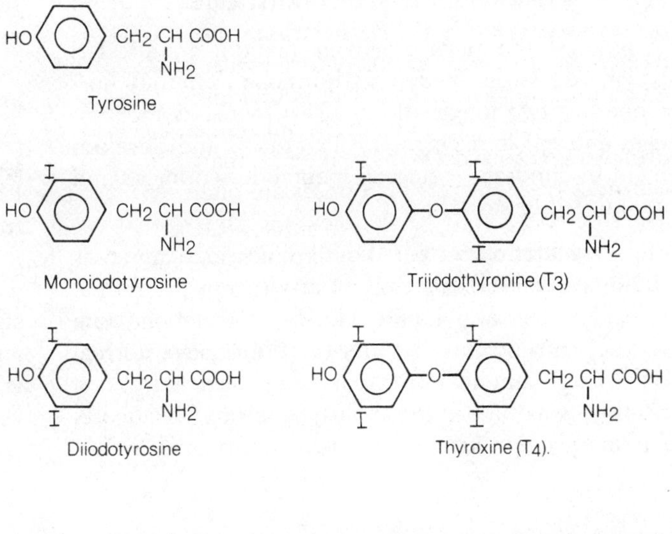

Figure 44-3 Chemistry of thyroid hormone production.

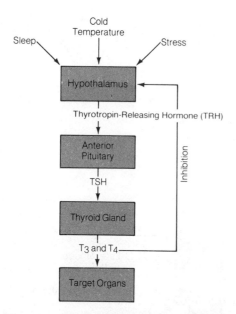

Figure 44-4 The hypothalamic–pituitary–thyroid feedback system, which regulates the body levels of thyroid hormone.

release of thyroid hormone from follicles into the bloodstream, (2) activating the iodide pump, (3) increasing the oxidation of iodide and coupling of iodide to tyrosine, and (4) increasing the number of follicle cells and the size of the follicles. The effect of TSH on the release of thyroid hormones occurs within about 30 minutes, whereas the other effects require days or weeks. Increased levels of thyroid hormone act in the feedback mechanism by inhibiting TRH. High levels of iodide cause a temporary decrease in thyroid activity that lasts for several weeks, probably through a direct inhibition of TSH on the thyroid. Lugol's solution, which is an iodide preparation, is sometimes given to hyperthyroid patients in preparation for surgery as a means of decreasing thyroid function. Cold exposure is one of the strongest stimuli for increased thyroid hormone production and is probably mediated through TRH from the hypothalamus.

Actions of thyroid hormone

All the major organs in the body are affected by altered levels of thyroid hormone. Thyroid hormone has two major effects: (1) it increases metabolism and (2) it is necessary for growth and development in children, including mental development and attainment of sexual maturity.

Metabolic rate. Thyroid hormone increases the metabolism of all body tissues except the retina, spleen, testes, and lungs. The basal metabolic rate (BMR) can increase by 60% to 100% above normal when large amounts of thyroxine are secreted.[1] As a result of this higher metabolism, the rate of glucose, fat, and protein utilization increases. Lipids are mobi-

lized from adipose tissue, and the catabolism of cholesterol by the liver is increased. As a result, blood levels of cholesterol are decreased in hyperthyroidism and increased in hypothyroidism. Muscle proteins are broken down and used as fuel, probably accounting for some of the muscle fatigue that occurs with hyperthyroidism. The absorption of glucose from the gastrointestinal tract is increased. Because vitamins are essential parts of metabolic enzymes and coenzymes, an increase in metabolic rate "speeds up the use" of vitamins and tends to cause vitamin deficiency.

Cardiovascular function. Cardiovascular and respiratory functions are strongly affected by thyroid function. With an increase in metabolism, there is a rise in oxygen consumption and production of metabolic end-products with an accompanying increase in vasodilatation. Blood flow to the skin, in particular, is augmented as a means of dissipating the body heat that results from the higher metabolism. Blood volume, cardiac output, and ventilation are all increased as a means of maintaining blood flow and oxygen delivery to body tissues. Heart rate and cardiac contractility are enhanced as a means of maintaining the needed cardiac output. Blood pressure, on the other hand, is apt to change very little, because the increase in vasodilatation tends to offset the increase in cardiac output.

Gastrointestinal tract function. Thyroid hormone enhances gastrointestinal function with an increase in both motility and production of gastrointestinal secretions. An increase in appetite and food intake accompanies the higher metabolic rate. At the same time, weight loss occurs because of the increased utilization of calories.

Neuromuscular effects. Thyroid hormone produces marked effects on muscle function and tone. Slight elevations in hormone levels cause skeletal muscles to react more vigorously, and a drop in hormone levels causes muscles to react more sluggishly. In the hyperthyroid state, a fine muscle tremor is present. The cause of this tremor is unknown, but it may represent an increased sensitivity of the neural synapses in the spinal cord that control muscle tone.

In the infant, thyroid hormone is necessary for normal brain development. The hormone enhances cerebration; in the hyperstate, it causes extreme nervousness, anxiety, and difficulty in sleeping.

Evidence suggests a strong interaction between thyroid hormone and the sympathetic nervous system. As will be discussed later, many of the signs and symptoms of hyperthyroidism suggest overactivity of the sympathetic division of the autonomic nervous system, for example, tachycardia, palpitations, and sweating. In addition, tremor, restlessness, anxiety, and diarrhea may reflect autonomic nervous system imbalances. Drugs that block sympathetic activity have proved to be valuable adjuncts in the treatment of hyperthyroidism because of their ability to relieve some of these undesirable symptoms.

Tests of thyroid function

There are various tests that aid in diagnosing thyroid disorders. Direct measures of T_3, T_4, TSH, and thyroid-binding globulin have been made available through radioimmunoassay methods. The resin uptake test for T_3 measures the unsaturated binding sites of the thyroid hormones. Measurement of either T_3 or T_4 by radioimmunoassay plus T_3 resin uptake can be used to provide an estimate of free T_3 or T_4. Abnormalities of thyroid-binding globulin (TBG) can be detected through direct measurement of TBG. The *TSH* test differentiates primary and secondary thyroid disorders. The radioactive iodine uptake test measures the ability of the thyroid gland to remove and concentrate iodine from the blood. The *TRH stimulation test* is used to differentiate between hypothalamic and pituitary causes of secondary hypothyroidism. A test dose of TRH is given, and serum levels of TSH are measured. The thyroid scan detects thyroid nodules and active thyroid tissue. Ultrasonography can be used to differentiate between cystic and solid thyroid lesions. Protein-bound iodine (PBI) measures the organic iodine that is bound to plasma proteins. This test is easily influenced by medications that contain iodine and by conditions that affect binding of thyroid hormone; therefore, it is not used as frequently as it was in the past.

The basal metabolic rate (BMR) is an indirect measure of thyroid function, and it, too, has been largely replaced by more accurate and quantitative tests. The photomotogram is a test that measures the speed of relaxation of the Achilles tendon. This test is done with the person kneeling on a chair with the foot positioned in such a way as to interrupt a photoelectric light beam. In this way, a timer is initiated when the Achilles tendon is tapped with a reflex hammer and is stopped when the foot returns to its normal position. The reflex time is increased in hypothyroidism and decreased in hyperthyroidism.

Alterations in thyroid function

An alteration in thyroid function can represent either a hypofunctional or a hyperfunctional state. The manifestations of these two altered states are summarized in Table 44-1. Disorders of the thyroid may represent a congenital defect in thyroid development

Table 44–1. Manifestations of hypothyroid and hyperthyroid states

Level of organization	Hypostate	Hyperstate
Basal metabolic rate	Decreased	Increased
Sensitivity to catecholamines	Decreased	Increased
General features	Myxedematous features	Exophthalmos
	Deep voice	Lid lag
	Impaired growth (child)	Decreased blinking
Blood cholesterol levels	Increased	Decreased
General behavior	Mental retardation (infant)	Restlessness, irritability, anxiety
	Mental and physical sluggishness	Hyperkinesis
	Somnolence	Wakefulness
Cardiovascular function	Decreased cardiac output	Increased cardiac output
	Bradycardia	Tachycardia and palpitations
Gastrointestinal function	Constipation	Diarrhea
	Decreased appetite	Increased appetite
Respiratory function	Hypoventilation	Dyspnea
Muscle tone and reflexes	Decreased	Increased, with tremor and fibrillatory twitching
Temperature tolerance	Cold intolerance	Heat intolerance
Skin and hair	Decreased sweating	Increased sweating
	Coarse and dry skin and hair	Thin and silky skin and hair
Weight	Gain	Loss

or they may develop later in life, with a gradual or a sudden onset.

Goiter is an increase in the size of the thyroid gland. It can occur in hypothyroid, euthyroid, and hyperthyroid states. Goiters may be diffuse, involving the entire gland without evidence or nodularity, or they may contain nodules. Diffuse goiters usually become nodular. Goiters may be toxic, producing signs of extreme hyperthyroidism, or *thyrotoxicosis,* or they may be nontoxic. Diffuse nontoxic and multinodular goiters are the result of compensatory hypertrophy and hyperplasia of follicular epithelium secondary to some derangement that impairs thyroid hormone output. The degree of thyroid enlargement is usually proportional to the extent and duration of thyroid deficiency. The increased thyroid mass usually achieves a normal, or *euthyroid,* state eventually. Multinodular goiters produce the largest thyroid enlargements and are often associated with thyrotoxicosis. When sufficiently enlarged they may compress the esophagus and trachea, causing difficulty in swallowing, a choking sensation, and inspiratory stridor. Such lesions may also compress the superior vena cava, producing distention of the veins of the neck and upper extremities, edema of the eyelids and conjunctiva, and syncope with coughing.

Hypothyroidism

Hypothyroidism can occur as a congenital or an acquired defect. The absence of thyroid function at birth is called *cretinism.* When the condition occurs later in life it is called *myxedema.* Currently the term *cretin* hardly seems appropriate for describing the normally developing infant in whom replacement thyroid hormone therapy was instituted shortly after birth.

Congenital hypothyroidism

Congenital hypothyroidism is perhaps one of the most common causes of preventable mental retardation. It affects about 1 out of 4000 infants. Hypothyroidism in the infant may result from a congenital lack of the thyroid gland or from abnormal biosynthesis of thyroid hormone or deficient TSH secretion. With congenital lack of the thyroid gland, the infant usually appears normal and functions normally at birth because hormones have been supplied *in utero* by the mother.

Thyroid hormone is essential for normal brain development and growth, almost half of which occurs during the first 6 months of life. If untreated, congenital hypothyroidism causes mental retardation and impairment of growth. Long-term studies show that closely monitored thyroxine supplementation

begun in the first 6 weeks of life results in normal intelligence.[13,14] However, if treatment is delayed to between 3 months and 7 months, 85% of these infants will have definite retardation.[15] Fortunately, neonatal screening tests have been instituted to detect congenital hypothyroidism during early infancy. Screening is usually done in the hospital nursery between the first and the fifth days of life. In this test, a drop of blood is taken from the infant's heel and analyzed for T_4 and TSH.

Myxedema (acquired hypothyroidism)

When hypothyroidism occurs in older children or adults it is called *myxedema.* The term myxedema implies the presence of a nonpitting mucus-type edema caused by an accumulation of a hydrophilic mucopolysaccharide substance in the connective tissues throughout the body. The hypothyroid state may be mild, with only a few signs and symptoms, or it may progress to a life-threatening condition called *myxedematous coma.* It can result from destruction or dysfunction of the thyroid gland (primary hypothyroidism) or as a secondary disorder caused by impaired hypothalamic or pituitary function.

Primary hypothyroidism is much more common than secondary hypothyroidism. It may result from thyroidectomy (surgical removal) or ablation of the gland with radiation. Certain goitrogenic agents, such as lithium carbonate (used in the treatment of manic-depressive states) and the antithyroid drugs propylthiouracil and methimazole in continuous dosage, can block hormone synthesis and produce hypothyroidism with goiter. Large amounts of iodine (ingestion of kelp tablets or iodide-containing cough syrups or administration of iodide-containing radiographic contrast media) can also block thyroid hormone production and cause goiter, particularly in persons with autoimmune thyroid disease. Iodine deficiency, which can cause goiter and hypothyroidism, is rare in the United States because of the widespread use of iodized salt and other iodide sources.

Probably the most common cause of hypothyroidism is Hashimoto's thyroiditis, an autoimmune disorder in which the thyroid gland may be totally destroyed by an immunologic process. It is the major cause of goiter and hypothyroidism in children. Hashimoto's thyroiditis is predominantly a disease of women, with a female-to-male ratio of 10:1.[17] The course of the disease varies. At the onset, only a goiter may be present. In time, hypothyroidism usually becomes evident. Although the disorder generally causes hypothyroidism, a hyperthyroid state may develop midcourse in the disease. The transient hyperthyroid state is due to leakage of preformed thyroid hormone from damaged cells of the gland.

Myxedema affects almost all of the organ systems in the body. The manifestations of the disorder are largely related to two factors: (1) the hypometabolic state resulting from thyroid hormone deficiency and (2) myxedematous involvement of body tissues. Although the myxedema is most obvious in the face and other superficial parts, it also affects many of the body organs and is responsible for many of the manifestations of the hypothyroid state (Figure 44-5).

The hypometabolic state associated with myxedema is characterized by a gradual onset of weakness and fatigue, a tendency to gain weight despite a loss in appetite, and cold intolerance. As the condition progresses, the skin becomes dry and rough and acquires a pale yellowish cast, which is due primarily to carotene deposition, and the hair becomes coarse and brittle. There is loss of the lateral one-third of the eyebrows. Gastrointestinal motility is decreased, giving rise to constipation, flatulence, and abdominal distention. Nervous system involvement is manifested in mental dullness, lethargy, and impaired memory.

As a result of fluid accumulation, the face takes on a characteristic puffy look, especially around the eyes. The tongue is enlarged, and the voice is hoarse and husky. Myxedematous fluid can collect in the interstitial spaces of almost any organ system. Pericardial or pleural effusion may develop. Mucopolysaccharide deposits in the heart cause generalized cardiac dilatation, bradycardia, and other signs of altered cardiac function. The signs and symptoms of hypothyroidism are summarized in Table 44-1.

Diagnosis of hypothyroidism is based on history, physical examination, and laboratory tests. A low serum T_4, low resin T_3, and elevated TSH are characteristic of primary hypothyroidism. The tests for antithyroid antibodies may be done when Hashimoto's thyroiditis is suspected. In secondary hypothyroidism, a TRH stimulation test is helpful in differentiating between pituitary and hypothalamic disease. Hypothyroidism is treated by replacement therapy with purified thyroid hormones obtained from domestic animals such as cows, pigs, and sheep, or with synthetic preparations.

Myxedematous coma

Myxedematous coma is a life-threatening end-stage expression of hypothyroidism. It is characterized by coma, hypothermia, cardiovascular collapse, hypoventilation, and severe metabolic disorders that include hyponatremia, hypoglycemia, and lactic acidosis. It occurs most often in the elderly and is seldom seen in persons under age 50.[18] The fact that it occurs more frequently in winter months suggests that cold exposure may be a precipitating factor. The severely hypothyroid person is unable to metabolize sedatives, analgesics, and anesthetic drugs, and these agents may precipitate coma.

Hyperthyroidism

Hyperthyroidism, or *thyrotoxicosis,* results from excessive delivery of thyroid hormone to the peripheral tissue. It is seen most frequently in women 20 to 40 years of age. It is commonly associated with hyperplasia of the thyroid gland, multinodular goiter, and adenoma of the thyroid. Occasionally it develops as the result of the ingestion of an overdose of thyroid hormone. When the condition is accompanied by exophthalmos (bulging of the eyeballs) and goiter, it is called Graves' disease. Thyroid crisis, or storm, is an acutely exaggerated manifestation of the hyperthyroid state.

Many of the manifestations of hyperthyroidism are related to the increase in oxygen consumption and increased utilization of metabolic fuels associated with the hypermetabolic state as well as the increase in sympathetic nervous system activity that occurs. The fact that many of the signs and symptoms of hyperthyroidism resemble those of excessive sympathetic activity suggests that the thyroid hormone may heighten the sensitivity of the body to the catecholamines or that thyroid hormone itself may act as a pseudocatecholamine. With the hypermetabolic state, there are

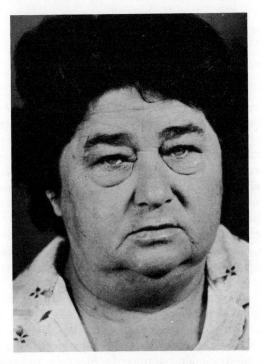

Figure 44-5 Patient with myxedema. *(Courtesy of Dr. Herbert Langford. From Guyton A: Medical Physiology, 6th ed, p 941. Philadelphia, WB Saunders, 1981. Reprinted by permission.)*

frequent complaints of nervousness, irritability, and fatigability. Weight loss is common despite a large appetite. Other manifestations include tachycardia, palpitations, shortness of breath, excessive sweating, and heat intolerance. The person appears restless and has a fine muscle tremor. Even in persons without exophthalmos there is an abnormal retraction of the eyelids and infrequent blinking so that they appear to be staring. The hair and skin are usually thin and have a silky appearance. The signs and symptoms of hyperthyroidism are summarized in Table 44-1.

The treatment of hyperthyroidism is directed toward reducing the level of thyroid hormone. This can be accomplished through surgical removal of part or all of the thyroid gland, eradication of the gland with radioactive iodine, or the use of drugs that decrease thyroid function and thereby the effect of the thyroid hormone on the peripheral tissues. The beta-adrenergic blocking drug propranolol is often administered to block the effects of the hyperthyroid state on sympathetic nervous system function. It is given in conjunction with other antithyroid drugs such as propylthiouracil and methimazole. These drugs prevent the thyroid gland from converting iodine to its organic (hormonal) form in the thyroid and block the conversion of T_4 to T_3 in the tissues. *Lugol's solution* (iodide) may be given to depress the thyroid gland in preparation for surgery. Unfortunately, this action is short-lived, and, in a few weeks, the symptoms reappear and may be intensified.

Graves' disease

Graves' disease is a state of hyperthyroidism, goiter, and exophthalmos. The cause of Graves' disease and the development of the exophthalmos, which results from edema and cellular infiltration of the orbital structures and muscle, is poorly understood. Current evidence suggests that it is an immune disorder characterized by abnormal stimulation of the thyroid gland by thyroid-stimulating antibodies that act through the normal TSH receptors. The exophthalmos is thought to result from an exophthalmos-producing factor whose action is enhanced by antibodies. The ophthalmopathy of Graves' disease can cause severe eye problems, including paralysis of the extraocular muscles, involvement of the optic nerve with some visual loss, and corneal ulceration because the lids do not close over the protruding eyeball. The exophthalmos usually tends to stabilize following treatment of the hyperthyroidism. Unfortunately, not all of the ocular changes are reversible. Figure 44-6 depicts a woman with Graves' disease.

Thyroid storm

Thyroid storm (crisis) is an extreme and life-threatening form of thyrotoxicosis, rarely seen today because of improved diagnosis and treatment

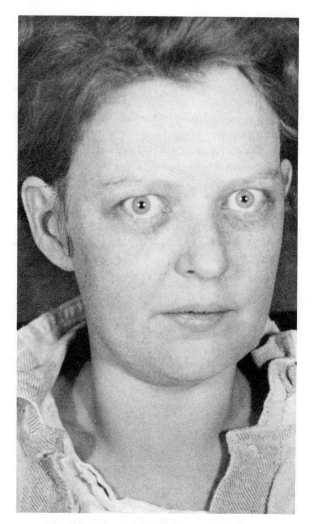

Figure 44-6 Woman with Graves' disease. Note the exophthalmos and enlarged thyroid gland. (*Chaffee EE, Lytle IM: Basic Physiology and Anatomy, 4th ed. Philadelphia, JB Lippincott, 1980*)

methods. When it does occur, it is seen most often in undiagnosed cases or in persons with hyperthyroidism who have not been adequately treated. It is often precipitated by stress, such as an infection (usually respiratory), by diabetic ketoacidosis, by physical or emotional trauma, or by manipulation of a hyperactive thyroid gland during thyroidectomy. Thyroid storm is manifested by a very high fever, extreme cardiovascular effects (tachycardia, congestive failure, and angina), and severe central nervous system effects (agitation, restlessness, and delirium). The mortality rate is high.

Thyroid storm requires rapid diagnosis and implementation of treatment. Peripheral cooling is initiated with cold packs and a cooling mattress. For cooling to be effective, the shivering response must be prevented. General supportive measures to replace fluids, glucose, and electrolytes are essential during the hypermetabolic state. A beta-adrenergic blocking drug, such as propranolol, is given to block the undesirable effects of thyroxin on cardiovascular function. Glucocorticoids are used to correct the relative adrenal insufficiency resulting from the stress imposed by the hyperthyroid state and to inhibit the peripheral conversion of T_4 to T_3. Propylthiouracil or methimazole may be given to block thyroid synthesis. Drugs that deplete the peripheral stores of catecholamines (*e.g.*, reserpine or guanethidine) may be given in addition to beta-adrenergic blocking drugs.[19,20] A saturated solution of potassium iodide is used to inhibit thyroid hormone release. Lithium also inhibits thyroid hormone release and is used for persons who are iodine-sensitive.

In summary, thyroid hormones play a role in the metabolic process of almost all body cells and are necessary for normal physical and mental growth in the infant and small child. Alterations in thyroid function can present as either a hypostate or a hyperstate. Hypothyroidism can occur as either a congenital or an acquired defect. When it is present at birth, it is called cretinism; when it occurs later in life, it is termed myxedema. Congenital hypothyroidism leads to mental retardation and impaired physical growth unless treatment is initiated during the first months of life. Hypothyroidism leads to a decrease in metabolic rate and an accumulation of a mucopolysaccharide substance within the intercellular spaces; this substance attracts water and causes a mucus-type of edema called myxedema. Hyperthyroidism causes an increase in metabolic rate and alterations in body function similar to those produced by enhanced sympathetic nervous system activity. Graves' disease is characterized by the triad of hyperthyroidism, goiter, and exophthalmos.

Disorders of adrenal cortical function

—— Control of adrenal cortical function

The adrenal glands are small, bilateral structures that weigh about 5 g each and lie retroperitoneally at the apex of each kidney (Figure 44-7). The medulla, or inner, portion of the gland secretes epinephrine and norepinephrine and is an extension of the sympathetic nervous system. The cortex forms the bulk of the adrenal gland and is responsible for secreting three types of hormones: the glucocorticoids, the mineralocorticoids, and the adrenal sex hormones. Because the sympathetic nervous system secretes catecholamines, adrenal medullary function is not essential for life, but adrenal cortical function is. The total

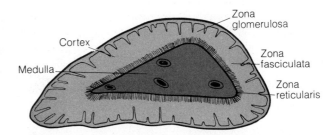

Figure 44-7 The adrenal gland, showing the medulla and the three layers of the cortex. The zona glomerulosa is the outer layer of the cortex and is primarily responsible for mineralocorticoid production. The middle layer, the zona fasciculata, and the inner layer, the zona reticularis, produce the glucocorticoids and the adrenal sex hormones.

loss of adrenal cortical function is fatal in 3 to 10 days if untreated.[1] This section of the chapter describes the synthesis and function of the adrenal cortical hormones and the effects of adrenal cortical insufficiency and excess.

—— Biosynthesis of adrenal cortical hormones

More than 30 hormones are produced by the adrenal gland. Of these hormones, aldosterone is the principal mineralocorticoid, cortisol (hydrocortisone) is the major glucocorticoid, and androgens are the chief sex hormones. All of the adrenal cortical hormones have a similar structure in that all are steroids and are synthesized from acetate and cholesterol; thus, the glucocorticoid drugs are often called steroids. Each of the steps involved in the synthesis of the various hormones requires a specific enzyme (Figure 44-8). The secretion of both the glucocorticoids and the adrenal androgens are controlled by adrenocorticotropic hormone (ACTH) secreted by the anterior pituitary gland.

—— Adrenal sex hormones

The adrenal sex hormones are synthesized primarily by the zona reticularis and the zona fasciculata of the cortex (see Figure 44-7). These sex hormones probably exert little effect on normal sexual function. There is evidence, however, that the adrenal sex hormones contribute to the pubertal growth of body hair, particularly pubic and axillary hair in women. They may also play a role in the steroid hormone economy of the pregnant woman and the fetal-placental unit.[21]

—— Mineralocorticoids

The mineralocorticoids play an essential role in regulating potassium and sodium levels and water balance. They are produced in the zona glomerulosa, the outer layer of cells of the adrenal cortex. Aldoste-

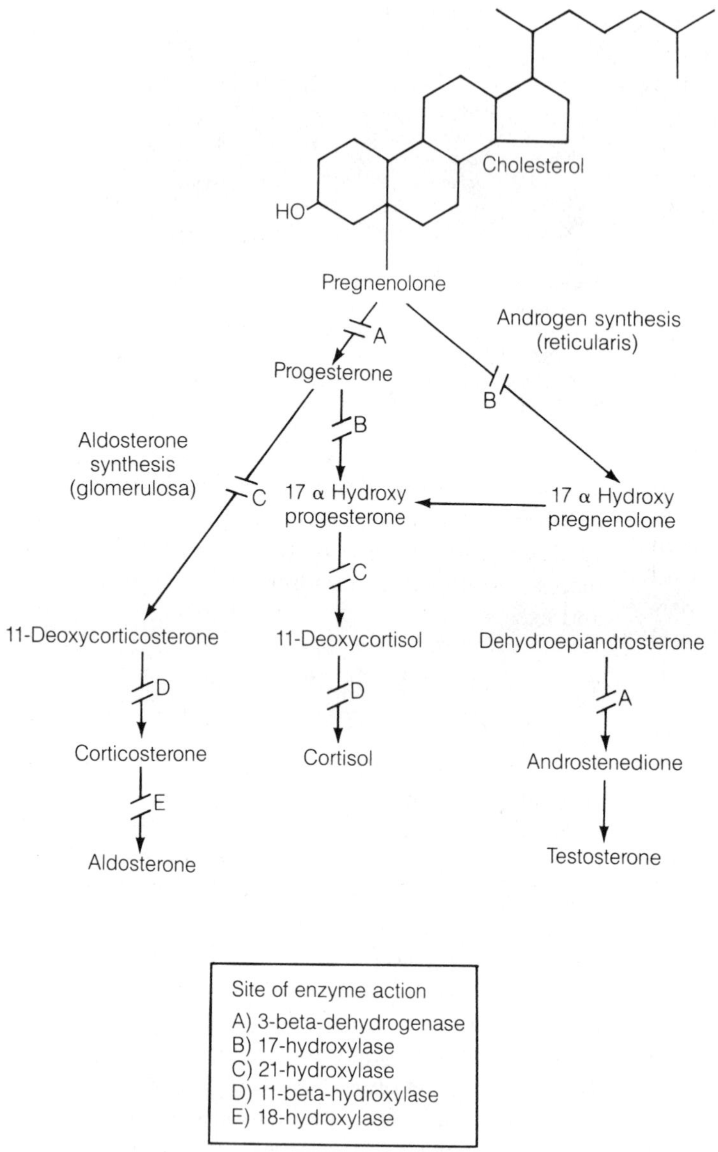

Site of enzyme action

A) 3-beta-dehydrogenase
B) 17-hydroxylase
C) 21-hydroxylase
D) 11-beta-hydroxylase
E) 18-hydroxylase

Figure 44-8 Predominant biosynthetic pathways of the adrenal cortex. Critical enzymes in the biosynthetic process include 11-beta-hydroxylase and 21-hydroxylase. A deficiency in one of these enzymes blocks the synthesis of these hormones dependent on that enzyme and routes the precursors into alternative pathways.

rone is regulated by the renin–angiotensin mechanism and by blood levels of potassium. ACTH is relatively unimportant in the day-to-day regulation of aldosterone. Increased levels of aldosterone promote sodium retention by the distal tubules of the kidney while increasing urinary losses of potassium. The influence of aldosterone on fluid and electrolyte balance is discussed in Chapter 27.

—— Glucocorticoids

The glucocorticoid hormones are synthesized in the zona fasciculata and the zona reticularis. The blood levels of these hormones are regulated by negative feedback mechanisms of the hypothalamic–pituitary–adrenal (HPA) system (Figure 44-9). In the same manner that other pituitary hormones are controlled by releasing factors from the hypothalamus, the corticotropin-releasing factor (CRF) is important in controlling the release of ACTH. Cortisol levels, in turn, increase as ACTH levels rise. There is considerable diurnal variation in ACTH levels, which reach their peak in the early morning (around 6 AM to 8 AM) and decline as the day progresses. As will be discussed later, one of the earliest signs of Cushing's syndrome is loss of this diurnal variation. Increased plasma cortisol levels act in a negative feedback manner on receptors in the hypothalamus to decrease CRF and on the anterior pituitary to decrease ACTH. The stimulation of hypothalamic receptors and the release of CRF serve to integrate neural influences with the function of the adrenal cortex.

The glucocorticoids perform a necessary function in response to stress and are essential for survival. When produced as part of the stress response, these hormones aid in regulating the meta-

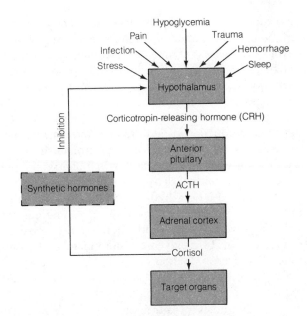

Figure 44-9 The hypothalamic–pituitary–adrenal (HPA) feedback system that regulates glucocorticoid (cortisol) levels. Cortisol release is regulated by ACTH. Stress exerts its effects on cortisol release through the HPA system and the corticotropin-releasing factor (CRF), which controls the release of ACTH from the anterior pituitary gland. Increased cortisol levels incite a negative feedback inhibition of ACTH release. Pharmacologic doses of synthetic steroids inhibit ACTH release by way of the hypothalamic CRF.

bolic functions of the body and in controlling the inflammatory response. The actions of cortisol are summarized in Table 44-2. The reader will note that many of the anti-inflammatory actions attributed to cortisol result from the administration of pharmacologic levels of the hormone.

Metabolic effects. Cortisol stimulates glucose production by the liver, promotes protein breakdown, and causes mobilization of fatty acids. As body proteins are broken down, amino acids are mobilized and transported to the liver, where they are used in the production of glucose. The mobilization of fatty acids serves to convert cell metabolism from the utilization of glucose for energy to the utilization of fatty acids instead.

As glucose production by the liver rises and peripheral glucose utilization falls, there is moderate insulin resistance. In diabetics and persons who are diabetes-prone, this has the effect of raising the blood sugar.

Psychic effects. The glucocorticoid hormones appear to be involved either directly or indirectly in emotional behaviors. Receptors for these hormones have been identified in brain tissue, which suggests that they play a role in the regulation of behavior.[22] It has been noted that persons treated with adrenal cortical hormones have displayed behavior ranging from mildly aberrant to psychotic.

Anti-inflammatory effects. Large quantities of cortisol are required for an effective anti-inflammatory action. This is achieved by the administration of pharmacologic doses of synthetic cortisol. The increased cortisol blocks inflammation at an early stage by decreasing capillary permeability and stabilizing the lysosomal membranes so that inflammatory mediators are not released. Cortisol suppresses the immune response by reducing antibody and cell-mediated immunity. With this lessened inflammation comes a reduction in fever. During the healing phase, cortisol suppresses fibroblast activity and thereby lessens scar formation. A recently described attribute of cortisol is its ability to inhibit prostaglandin synthesis, which may account in large part for its anti-inflammatory actions.[21]

Suppression of adrenal function

A highly significant aspect of long-term therapy with pharmacologic preparations of the adrenal cortical hormones is adrenal insufficiency on withdrawal of the drugs. The deficiency is due to suppression of the HPA system. Chronic suppression causes atrophy of the entire system, and abrupt withdrawal of drugs can cause acute adrenal insufficiency. Furthermore, recovery to a state of normal adrenal function may be prolonged, requiring up to 12 months.[21]

Tests of adrenal function

There are a number of diagnostic tests by which adrenal cortical function and the hypothalamic–pituitary axis may be evaluated. Blood levels of cortisol and ACTH can be measured using radioimmunoassay methods. A 24-hour urine specimen measures the excretion of 17-ketosteroids, 17-ketogenic steroids, and 17-hydroxycorticosteroids. These metabolic end-products of the adrenal hormones and the male androgens provide information about alterations in the biosynthesis of the adrenal cortical hormones. Suppression and stimulation tests afford a means of assessing the state of the hypothalamic–pituitary–adrenal feedback system. For example, a test dose of ACTH may be given to assess the response of the adrenal cortex to pituitary stimulation. Similarly, administration of dexamethasone (a synthetic glucocorticoid drug) provides a means of measuring negative feedback suppression of ACTH. Adrenal tumors and ectopic ACTH-producing tumors are generally unresponsive to ACTH suppression by dexamethasone. Metyrapone (Metopirone) blocks the final step in cortisol synthesis, producing 11-dehydroxycortisol, which does not inhibit ACTH. This test measures the ability of the pituitary to release ACTH.

Congenital adrenal hyperplasia (adrenogenital syndrome)

Congenital adrenal hyperplasia (CAH) describes a congenital disorder caused by an autosomal recessive trait in which a deficiency exists in any of the five enzymes necessary for the synthesis of cortisol. A common characteristic of all types is a defect in the synthesis of cortisol that results in increased levels of ACTH and adrenal hyperplasia. The increased levels of ACTH overstimulate the pathways of steroid hormone production, particularly those involving the production of adrenal androgens. Mineralocorticoids may be produced in excessive or insufficient amounts, depending on the precise enzyme deficiency. Both males and females are affected. Males are seldom diagnosed at birth, unless they have enlarged genitalia or lose salt and manifest adrenal crisis; in female infants, an increase in androgens is responsible for creating the virilization syndrome of ambiguous genitalia.

The two most common enzyme deficiencies are the 21-hydroxylase and 11-beta-hydroxylase deficiencies. The clinical manifestations of both deficiencies are largely determined by the functional properties of the steroid intermediates and the completeness of the block in the cortisol pathway.

A spectrum of 21-hydroxylase deficiency states exists, which ranges from simple virilizing CAH to a complete salt-losing enzyme deficiency. Simple virilizing CAH impairs the synthesis of cortisol, and steroid synthesis is shunted to androgen production. Persons with these deficiencies usually produce sufficient aldosterone or aldosterone intermediates to prevent signs and symptoms of mineralocorticoid deficiency. The salt-losing form is accompanied by deficient production of aldosterone and its intermediates. This results in fluid and electrolyte disorders after the fifth day of life, including hyponatremia, hyperkalemia, vomiting, dehydration, and shock.

The 11-beta-hydroxylase deficiency also manifests a spectrum of clinical severity. There is not only excessive androgen production but also impaired conversion of 11-deoxycorticosterone to corticosterone. The overproduction of 11-deoxycorticosterone, which has mineralocorticoid activity, is responsible for the hypertension that accompanies this deficiency.

Diagnosis of adrenogenital syndrome depends on the precise biochemical evaluation of metabolites in the cortisol pathway as well as on clinical signs and symptoms. The signs and symptoms of the salt-losing form of 21-hydroxylase deficiency include dehydration, shock, vomiting, decreased sodium levels, and increased potassium levels. In both 11-beta-hydroxylase and 21-hydroxylase deficiencies, virilization of the female genitalia is evident. In the female, one may see an enlarged clitoris, fused labia,

Table 44–2. Actions of cortisol

Major influence	Effect on body
Glucose metabolism	Stimulates gluconeogenesis
	Decreases glucose utilization by the tissues
Protein metabolism	Increases breakdown of proteins
	Increases plasma protein levels
Fat metabolism	Increases mobilization of fatty acids
	Increases utilization of fatty acids
Anti-inflammatory action (pharmacologic levels)	Stabilizes lysosomal membranes of the inflammatory cells, preventing the release of inflammatory mediators
	Decreases capillary permeability to prevent inflammatory edema
	Depresses phagocytosis by white blood cells to reduce the release of inflammatory mediators
	Suppresses the immune response
	Causes atrophy of lymphoid tissue
	Decreases eosinophils
	Decreases antibody formation
	Decreases the development of cell-mediated immunity
	Reduces fever
	Inhibits fibroblast activity
Psychic effect	Tends to contribute to emotional stability
Permissive effect	Facilitates the response of the tissues to humoral and neural influences, such as that of the catecholamines, during trauma and extreme stress

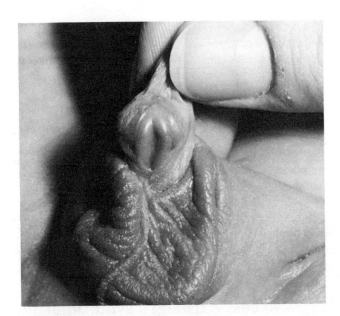

Figure 44-10 Female infant with congenital adrenal hyperplasia demonstrating virilization of the genitalia. Note the enlarged clitoris and the fused labia, which resembles a scrotal sac. (*Hurwitz LS: Nursing implications of selected endocrine disorders. Nurs Clin North Am 15(3):528, 1980. Reprinted with permission.*)

and urogenital sinus (Figure 44-10). Males may have no outward features that are noticeable at birth. In both males and females, other secondary sex characteristics are normal, and fertility is unaffected if appropriate therapy is instituted.

Medical treatment of adrenogenital syndrome includes oral or parenteral cortisol replacement. Deoxycorticosterone acetate (DOCA) pellets may be implanted in the skin of the scapula as a mineralocorticoid replacement. Fludrocortisone acetate may also be given to children who are salt losers. Depending on the degree of virilization, reconstructive surgery during the first 2 years of life is indicated to reduce the size of the clitoris, separate the labia, and exteriorize the vagina. Surgery has provided excellent results and does not impair sexual function.

─── Adrenal insufficiency

There are two forms of adrenal insufficiency: primary and secondary. Primary adrenal insufficiency, or Addison's disease, is due to the destruction of the adrenal gland. Secondary adrenal insufficiency is due to a disorder of the HPA system.

─── Primary adrenal insufficiency (Addison's disease)

In 1855, Thomas Addison, an English physician, provided the first detailed clinical description of primary adrenal insufficiency. Addison's disease is a relatively rare disorder in which all the layers of the adrenal cortex are destroyed. Most often the underlying problem is idiopathic adrenal atrophy, which probably has an autoimmune basis. Tuberculosis is an infrequent cause, as is amyloidosis, or a fungal infection (particularly histoplasmosis). Bilateral adrenalectomy, sometimes done in the past for breast cancer, is an obvious cause of primary adrenal insufficiency.

Addison's disease, like insulin-dependent diabetes mellitus, is a chronic metabolic disorder that requires lifetime hormone replacement therapy. The adrenal cortex has a large reserve capacity, and the manifestations of adrenal insufficiency do not usually become apparent until about 90% of the gland has been destroyed.[17] These manifestations are primarily related to (1) hyperpigmentation resulting from elevated ACTH levels, (2) mineralocorticoid deficiency, and (3) glucocorticoid deficiency. Although lack of the adrenal androgens exerts few effects in men because the testes produce these hormones, women will have sparse axillary and pubic hair. The manifestations of adrenal insufficiency are summarized in Table 44-3.

Hyperpigmentation. In Addison's disease, ACTH levels are elevated in response to the fall in cortisol. At this point, it is important to note that the amino acid sequence of ACTH is strikingly similar to that of melanocyte-stimulating hormone (MSH); thus, hyperpigmentation is seen in about 98% of persons with Addison's disease and is helpful in distinguishing the primary and secondary forms. The skin looks bronzed or suntanned in both exposed and unexposed areas, and the normal creases and pressure points tend to become especially dark. The gums and oral mucous membranes may become bluish black in color. This hyperpigmentation becomes more pronounced during periods of stress.

Mineralocorticoid deficiency. Mineralocorticoid deficiency causes increased urinary losses of sodium, chloride, and water along with decreased excretion of potassium. The result is hyponatremia, loss of extracellular fluid, decreased cardiac output, and hyperkalemia. There may be an abnormal appetite for salt. Orthostatic hypotension is common. Dehydration, weakness, and fatigue are often present as early symptoms. If loss of sodium and water is extreme, cardiovascular collapse and shock will ensue.

Glucocorticoid deficiency. Because of a lack of glucocorticoids, the patient has poor tolerance to stress. This deficiency causes hypoglycemia, lethargy, weakness, fever, and gastrointestinal symptoms such as anorexia, nausea, vomiting, and weight loss.

Secondary adrenal insufficiency

Secondary adrenal insufficiency can occur as the result of hypopituitarism or because the pituitary gland has been surgically removed. However, a far more common cause than either of these is the rapid withdrawal of glucocorticoids that have been administered therapeutically. These drugs suppress the HPA system, with resulting adrenal cortical atrophy and lack of cortisol. It is important to note that this suppression continues long after drug therapy has been discontinued and could be critical during periods of stress or when surgery is done. It has been suggested that a person receiving pharmacologic doses of the glucocorticoids for more than 1 to 4 weeks may have suppression of the HPA system for up to a year after the drugs have been discontinued.[23]

Acute adrenal crisis

Acute adrenal crisis is a life-threatening situation. If Addison's disease is the underlying problem, exposure to even a minor illness or stress can precipitate nausea, vomiting, muscular weakness, hypotension, dehydration, and vascular collapse. The onset of adrenal crisis may be sudden, or it may progress over a period of several days. The symptoms may also occur suddenly in children with salt-losing forms of the adrenogenital syndrome. Massive bilateral adrenal hemorrhage causes an acute fulminating form of adrenal insufficiency. Hemorrhage can be caused by meningococcal septicemia (called *Waterhouse-Friderichsen syndrome*), adrenal trauma, anti-coagulant therapy, adrenal vein thrombosis, or adrenal metastases.

Adrenal insufficiency is treated with replacement glucocorticoid therapy. In acute adrenal insufficiency, cortisol is given intravenously followed by rapid infusion of saline and glucose. The day-to-day regulation of the chronic phase of Addison's disease is usually accomplished with oral cortisol, and higher doses are given during periods of stress. Because these patients are likely to have episodes of hyponatremia and hypoglycemia, they need to have a regular schedule for meals and exercise.

Glucocorticoid hormone excess (Cushing's syndrome)

Cushing's syndrome is characterized by a chronic elevation in glucocorticoid (and adrenal androgen) hormones. Because the condition is most frequently caused by increased ACTH production, the mineralocorticoids are usually not involved in the syndrome.

Cushing's syndrome can result from either overproduction of hormones by the body or long-term therapy with one of the potent pharmacologic prepa-

Table 44–3. Manifestations of adrenal cortical insufficiency and excess

Parameter	Adrenal cortical insufficiency	Glucocorticoid excess
Electrolytes	Hyponatremia* Hyperkalemia*	Hypokalemia
Fluids	Dehydration* (elevated BUN, others)	Edema
Blood pressure	Hypotension* Shock* Orthostatic hypotension	Hypertension
Musculoskeletal	Muscle weakness* Fatigue*	Muscle wasting Fatigue
Hair and skin	Skin pigmentation Loss of hair (axillary and pubic)	Easy bruisability Hirsutism, acne, and striae (abdomen and thighs)
Inflammatory response	Low resistance to trauma, infection, and stress	Decrease in eosinophils Lymphocytopenia
Gastrointestinal	Nausea, vomiting* Abdominal pain*	Possible gastrointestinal bleeding
Glucose metabolism	Hypoglycemia*	Impaired glucose tolerance Glycosuria Elevated blood sugar
Emotional	Depression and irritability	Emotional lability to psychosis
Other	Menstrual irregularity Decreased axillary and pubic hair in women	Oligomenorrhea Impotence in the male Centripetal obesity (moon face and buffalo hump)

* Present in acute adrenal insufficiency.

rations of glucocorticoids (*iatrogenic Cushing's syndrome*). Three important forms of Cushing's syndrome result from excess glucocorticoid production by the body. One is a *pituitary form,* which results from excessive production of ACTH by a tumor of the pituitary gland; it accounts for about two-thirds of the disease cases, and because this form of the disease was the one originally described by Cushing, it is called Cushing's disease. The other forms of excess glucocorticoid levels are referred to as Cushing's syndrome.* The second form is the *adrenal form,* caused by an adrenal tumor. The third is the *ectopic* Cushing's, due to an ACTH-producing tumor such as occurs in some bronchogenic cancers.

The major manifestations of Cushing's syndrome represent an exaggeration of the normal effects of cortisol. Altered fat metabolism causes a peculiar deposition of fat characterized by a protruding abdomen; subclavicular fat pads or "buffalo hump" on the back; and a round, plethoric "moon face." There is muscle weakness, and the extremities are thin because of protein breakdown and muscle wasting. In advanced cases, the skin over the forearms and legs becomes thin, having the appearance of parchment. Purple striae (stretch marks), from stretching of the catabolically weakened skin and subcutaneous tissues, are distributed on the abdomen and hips. Osteoporosis results from destruction of bone proteins and alterations in calcium metabolism. With osteoporosis there may be back pain, compression fractures of the vertebrae, and rib fractures. As calcium is mobilized from bone, renal calculi may develop. Derangements in glucose metabolism are found in some 90% of patients, with clinically overt diabetes mellitus occurring in about 20%.[17] The glucocorticoids possess mineralocorticoid properties; this causes hypokalemia as a result of excessive potassium excretion and hypertension resulting from sodium retention. Inflammatory and immune responses are inhibited, resulting in increased susceptibility to infection. Cortisol increases gastric acid secretion, and this may provoke gastric ulceration and bleeding. An accompanying increase in androgen levels causes hirsutism, mild acne, and menstrual irregularities in women.

Excess levels of the glucocorticoids may give rise to extreme emotional lability, ranging from mild euphoria and absence of normal fatigue to grossly psychotic behavior. The manifestations of glucocorticoid excess are summarized in Table 44-3.

Diagnosis of Cushing's syndrome depends on the finding of elevated plasma levels of cortisol. As was mentioned, one of the prominent features of Cushing's syndrome is loss of the diurnal pattern of cortisol secretion. Therefore, cortisol determinations are often made on three blood samples: one taken in the morning, one in late afternoon or early evening, and a third drawn the following morning after a midnight dose of dexamethasone. Measurement of plasma ACTH, 24-hour urinary 17-ketosteroids, 17-ketogenic steroids, and 17-hydroxycorticosteroids, and suppression or stimulation tests of the HPA system are often made. Skull x-ray films and intravenous pyelograms, which outline the shadows of the kidneys and adrenal glands, may be done. Computerized tomograms (CT) afford a means for locating adrenal or pituitary tumors.

The *treatment* of Cushing's syndrome, whether by surgery, irradiation, or drugs, is largely determined by the etiology. Adrenalectomy may be done if an adrenal tumor is present. With the recent development of the transsphenoidal approach for removal of a pituitary tumor using microsurgical techniques, surgical treatment today is far more efficient than in the past. In children and in adults with mild clinical symptoms, cobalt radiation is often the preferred method for treating pituitary Cushing's. One drawback of radiation therapy is the long time lag (18 months in some cases) before complete remission occurs.[24] An adrenolytic agent, such as mitotane, that produces adrenal atrophy and interferes with biosynthetic pathways may be used in the treatment of persons with inoperable tumors, persons whose tumors have not been fully treated, or persons in whom irradiation has not yet taken effect.

In summary, the adrenal cortex produces three types of hormones: mineralocorticoids, glucocorticoids, and adrenal sex hormones. The mineralocorticoids along with the renin–angiotensin mechanism aid in controlling body levels of sodium and potassium. The glucocorticoids have anti-inflammatory actions and aid in regulating glucose, protein, and fat metabolism during periods of stress. These hormones are under the control of the hypothalamic–pituitary–adrenal (HPA) system. The adrenal sex hormones exert little effect on the day-to-day control of body function, but probably contribute to the development of body hair in women. The adrenal genital syndrome describes a genetic defect in the cortisol pathway resulting from a deficiency of one of the enzymes needed for its synthesis. Depending on the enzyme involved, the disorder causes virilization of female infants and, in some instances, fluid and electrolyte disturbances because of impaired mineralocorticoid synthesis. Chronic adrenal insufficiency is called Addison's disease. It can be caused by destruction of the adrenal gland or by dysfunction of the HPA system. Adrenal insufficiency requires replacement

---

* In this text the term Cushing's syndrome designates both Cushing's disease and Cushing's syndrome.

therapy with cortical hormones. Acute adrenal insufficiency is a life-threatening situation. Cushing's syndrome exists when the glucocorticoid level is abnormally high. This syndrome may be a result of pharmacologic doses of cortisol, a pituitary or adrenal tumor, or an ectopic tumor that produces ACTH. The clinical manifestations of Cushing's syndrome reflect the very high level of cortisol that is present.

References

1. Guyton A: Medical Physiology, 7th ed, pp 887–891, 901, 911 Philadelphia, WB Saunders, 1986
2. Berne RM, Levy MN: Physiology, 2nd ed, pp 915–921. St Louis, CV Mosby, 1988
3. Findling JW, Tyrell BJ: Anterior pituitary and somatomedins: 1. Anterior pituitary. In Greenspan FS, Forsham PH: Basic and Clinical Endocrinology, p 45. Los Altos, Lange Medical Publishers, 1983
4. Bercu BB: Growth hormone treatment and the short child: To treat or not to treat? J Pediatr 110:991, 1987
5. Underwood LE: Report on the conference on uses and possible abuses of biosynthetic human growth hormone. N Engl J Med 311:606, 1984
6. Thorner MO, Reschke J, Chitwood J et al: Acceleration of growth in two children treated with human growth hormone-releasing factor. N Engl J Med 312:4, 1985
7. Tichy AM, Malasanos LG: The physiological role of hormones in puberty. Am J Matern Child Nurs 1:384, 1976
8. Williams RH (ed): Textbook of Endocrinology. Philadelphia, WB Saunders, 1974
9. Karpf DB, Braunstein GD: Current concepts in acromegaly: Etiology, diagnosis, and treatment. Compr Ther 12(1):22, 1986
10. Daughaday WH, Cryer P: Growth hormone hypersection and acromegaly. Hosp Pract 13(8):76, 1978
11. Bloom SR: Acromegaly. Am Med J 82(Suppl 5B):88, 1987
12. Daughaday W: A new treatment for an old disease. N Engl J Med 313:1604, 1985
13. Glorieux J, Dussault JH, Morissette J et al: Follow-up at ages 5 and 7 years on mental development in children with hypothyroidism detected in the Quebec Screening Program. J Pediatr 107:913, 1985
14. New England Congenital Hypothyroid Collaborative: Neonatal hypothyroid screening: Status of patients at 6 years of age. J Pediatr 107:915, 1985
15. Klein AH, Meltzer S, Kenney F et al: Improved prognosis in congenital hypothyroidism treated before age three months. J Pediatr 81:912, 1972
16. Fisher D: Screening for congenital hypothyroidism. Hosp Pract 12(12):77, 1977
17. Robbins SL, Cotran RS, Kumar V: Pathologic Basis of Disease, 3rd ed, pp 1207, 1235, 1238. Philadelphia, WB Saunders, 1984
18. Meek JC: Myxedema coma. Crit Care Q 3:131, 1980
19. Evanelisti JT, Thorpe CJ: Thyroid storm—A nursing crisis. Heart Lung 12:184, 1983
20. Howton JC: Thyroid storm presenting as coma. Ann Emerg Med 17:343, 1988
21. Tepperman J: Metabolic and Endocrine Physiology, 4th ed, pp 173, 187, 189. Chicago, Year Book Medical Publishers, 1980
22. McEwan BS: Influences of the adrenocortical hormone on pituitary and brain function. Monogr Endocrinol 12:467, 1978
23. Axelrod L: Glucocorticoid therapy. Medicine 55(1):49, 1976
24. Gold EM: Cushing's syndrome. Hosp Pract 14(6):75, 1979

Bibliography

Aron DC: Cushing's syndrome: Current concepts in diagnosis and treatment. Compr Ther 13(12):37, 1987

Burke CW: Adrenocortical insufficiency. Clin Endocrinol Metab 14:947, 1985

Chopra IJ, Solomon DH: Pathogenesis of hyperthyroidism. Annu Rev Med 34:267, 1983

Cooper DS: Antithyroid drugs. N Engl J Med 311:1353, 1984

Frazer T, Gavin JR, Daughaday WH et al: Growth-hormone dependent growth failure. J Pediatr 101:12, 1982

Gabrilove JL, Krakoff LR: Diagnosis and pathophysiology of Cushing's syndrome. Compr Ther 12(1):17, 1986

Gavin LA: The diagnostic dilemmas of hyperthyroxinemia and hypothyroxinemia. Adv Intern Med 33:185, 1988

Gorman G: Ophthalmopathy of Graves' disease. N Engl J Med 308:453, 1983

Hardy J: Cushing's disease some 50 years later. Can J Neurol Sci 9:375, 1982

Hintz RL, Rosenfeld RG: Clinical uses of synthetic growth hormone. Hosp Pract 18(10):115, 1983

Howlett TA, Rees LH, Besser GM: Cushing's syndrome. Clin Endocrinol Metab 14:911, 1985

Hurley JR: Thyroid disease in the elderly. Med Clin North Am 67:497, 1983

Hurwitz LS: Nursing implications of selected pediatric endocrine disorders. Nurs Clin North Am 15(3):525, 1980

Jackson IMD: Thyrotropin-releasing hormone. N Engl J Med 306:145, 1982

Larsen PR: Thyroid–pituitary interaction. N Engl J Med 306:23, 1982

Leigh H, Kramer SI: The psychiatric manifestations of endocrine disease. Adv Intern Med 29:413, 1984

Mazzaferri EL: Thyrotoxicosis. Postgrad Med 73(4):85, 1983

McClung MR, Greer MA: Treatment of hyperthyroidism. Annu Rev Med 31:385, 1980

Mininberg DT, Levine LS, New MI: Current concepts in congenital adrenal hyperplasia. Ann Pathol 17(Part 2):179, 1982

Nasr H: Endocrine disorders in the elderly. Med Clin North Am 67(2):481, 1983

Rush DR, Hamburger SC: Endocrine metabolic emergencies. South Med J 77:220, 1984

Sakiyama R: Common thyroid disorders. Am Family Pract 38(1):227, 1988

Sawin CT, Herman T, Molitch ME et al: Aging and the thyroid. Am J Med 75:206, 1983

Smith LH, Rapoport B: The ophthalmopathy of Graves' disease. West J Med 142:532, 1985

Strakosch C, Wenzel B, Row VV et al: Immunology of autoimmune thyroid disease. N Engl J Med 307:1499, 1983

Styne DM, Grumbach MM, Kaplan SL et al: Treatment of Cushing's disease in childhood and adolescence with transsphenoidal microadenomectomy. N Engl J Med 310:889, 1984

Utiger RD: Beta-adrenergic-antagonist therapy for hyperthyroid Graves' disease. N Engl J Med 310:1597, 1984

Vliet GV, Styne DM, Kaplan SL et al: Growth hormone treatment of short stature. N Engl J Med 309:1016, 1983

Wass JAH, Laws ER Jr, Randall RV et al: The treatment of acromegaly. Clin Endocrinol Metab 15(3):683, 1986

Whitehead EM, Shalet SM, Davies D et al: Pituitary gigantism: A disabling condition. Clin Endocrinol 17:271, 1982

Diabetes Mellitus

Objectives

After you have studied this chapter, you should be able to meet the following objectives:

_____ State the sequence of events in insulin production.

_____ Describe the actions of insulin with reference to glucose, fats, and proteins.

_____ Compare the actions of insulin with those of glucagon.

_____ Describe the role of epinephrine in glycogenolysis.

_____ Explain the relationship between growth hormone and glucose tolerance.

_____ Explain the role of the adrenal cortical hormones in gluconeogenesis.

_____ Give a clinical description of diabetes mellitus.

_____ List the distinguishing characteristics of insulin-dependent diabetes mellitus (IDDM) and noninsulin-dependent diabetes mellitus (NIDDM).

_____ Explain why IDDM predisposes to the development of ketoacidosis whereas NIDDM does not.

_____ List three causes of secondary diabetes.

_____ Cite at least three indications for the use of glucose tolerance tests during pregnancy.

_____ Describe the suspected role of two environmental factors in the etiology of diabetes mellitus.

_____ Describe the possible relationship between obesity and the development of NIDDM.

_____ Describe the clinical manifestations of hypoglycemia that the health professional should be able to recognize.

_____ Cite the possible differences in symptoms of an insulin reaction in young and in elderly persons.

(continued)

_____ Describe measures used in the treatment of an insulin reaction.

_____ Describe the clinical manifestations of diabetic ketoacidosis and their physiologic significance.

_____ Explain how "hypoglycemia begets hyperglycemia."

_____ Describe the clinical condition resulting from the hyperosmolar state.

_____ Cite a common characteristic of tissues that are affected by the chronic complications of diabetes.

_____ Relate the possible mechanisms of the sorbitol pathway, formation of abnormal glycoproteins, and problems with tissue oxygenation to diabetes and the development of the chronic complications of the disease.

_____ Describe the pathologic changes that may occur with diabetic peripheral neuropathies.

_____ Describe the pathology underlying diabetic retinopathy.

_____ Describe the vascular complications that may occur with diabetes mellitus.

_____ Explain the relationship between diabetes mellitus and infection.

_____ State the purpose of the glucose tolerance test.

_____ List the advantages of self blood glucose monitoring.

_____ Explain the purpose of measuring the level of glycosylated hemoglobin in the blood.

_____ Describe the difference between the wash test and the dry test for self blood glucose monitoring.

_____ Name and describe two types of urinary tests for glucose.

_____ Describe the three "polys" that characterize diabetes mellitus.

_____ List five principles for diet management in persons with diabetes.

_____ Explain the difference between the free, weighed, and exchange methods for diabetic diets.

_____ Explain the advantages of high-fiber diets and complex carbohydrates in the dietary management of diabetes.

_____ State the actions of the oral hypoglycemic agents in terms of the lowering of blood sugar.

_____ Name and describe the three types (according to duration of action) of insulin.

_____ Cite the advantages of human insulin versus pork or beef insulin.

_____ Explain how continuous subcutaneous insulin infusion systems function.

_____ Describe the present obstacles to the use of artificial pancreas and pancreas transplants.

_____ Explain why exercise is beneficial to diabetics.

_____ Explain the differences in blood sugar regulation during exercise in the nondiabetic person and the person with insulin-dependent diabetes, and relate this to the increased risk for development of hypoglycemia in the person with diabetes during exercise.

Diabetes mellitus is a chronic alteration in health that currently affects more than 12 million persons in the United States. Diabetes affects persons in all age groups and from all walks of life. Among both young and old, diabetes increases the risk of vascular problems, blindness, peripheral neuropathies, and kidney disease. Diabetes increases the risk of maternal complications during pregnancy, and infants of diabetic mothers have a greater than normal incidence of congenital anomalies; they are also more prone to develop neonatal complications, such as respiratory distress syndrome and hypoglycemia.

The term *diabetes mellitus* means "the running through of sugar." In spite of its recent increase, the disease did not originate in the 20th century. Reports of the disorder can be traced back to the 1st century A.D. when Aretaeus the Cappadocian described the disorder as a chronic affection that was characterized by intense thirst and voluminous honey-sweet urine—"the melting down of flesh into urine."[1] It was the discovery of insulin by Banting and Best in 1921 that transformed the once-fatal disease into a chronic health problem.

Diabetes can be defined as a disorder of carbohydrate, protein, and fat metabolism resulting from an imbalance between insulin availability and insulin need. It can represent an absolute insulin deficiency, the impaired release of insulin by the pancreatic beta cells, the presence of inadequate or defective insulin receptors, or the production of insulin that is inactive or destroyed before it can carry out its action. The person with uncontrolled diabetes is unable to transport glucose into fat and muscle cells; and as a result, the body cells are starved and breakdown of fat and protein is increased.

Hormonal control of blood sugar

The body uses glucose, fatty acids, and other substrates as fuel to satisfy its energy needs. Although the respiratory and circulatory systems combine efforts to furnish the body with oxygen needed for metabolic purposes, it is the liver, in concert with the pancreatic hormones insulin and glucagon, that control the body's fuel supply. Secretion of both insulin and glucagon is regulated by blood glucose levels. Insulin is released in response to an increase in blood sugar, and glucagon, to a decrease in blood sugar. Both insulin and glucagon are transported from the pancreas, through the portal circulation, to the liver where they exert an almost instantaneous effect on blood glucose levels.

Glucose is an optional fuel for tissues such as muscle, adipose tissue, and the liver that can use fatty acids and other fuel substrates for energy. The brain, however, relies exclusively on glucose for its energy needs. Because the brain can neither synthesize nor store more than a few minutes' supply of glucose, normal cerebral function requires a continuous supply from the circulation. Severe and prolonged hypoglycemia can cause brain death, and even moderate hypoglycemia can result in substantial brain dysfunction.[2] Consequently, the body maintains a system of counterregulatory mechanisms to counteract hypoglycemia-producing situations and, thus, ensure brain function and survival. The physiologic mechanisms that prevent or correct hypoglycemia include the actions of the counterregulatory hormones: glucagon, the catecholamines, growth hormone, and the glucocorticoids.

Insulin

Insulin is produced by the pancreatic cells in the islets of Langerhans. The active form of the hormone is composed of two polypeptide chains—an A chain and a B chain (Figure 45-1). Before 1967, it was assumed that each chain was formed separately and then joined. It is now known that the chains emerge with the appropriate linkage required for biologic activity from a single chain called *proinsulin*. In converting proinsulin to insulin, enzymes in the beta cell cleave proinsulin at specific sites to form two substances, active *insulin* and a *C-peptide* chain (the link that served to join the A and B chains before they were separated). Both active insulin and the C-peptide chain are released simultaneously from the beta cell (Figure 45-2). The C-peptide chains can be measured, and this measurement can be used to study beta-cell activity. For example, injected insulin in the mature-onset diabetic would provide few, if any, C-peptide chains, whereas insulin secreted by the beta cells would be accompanied by secretion of C-peptide chains.

Insulin secreted by the beta cells enters the portal circulation and travels directly to the liver where about 50% is either utilized or degraded. Once it has been released into the general circulation, insulin has a half-life of about 15 minutes. This is because circulating insulin is rapidly bound to peripheral tissues or is destroyed by the liver or kidneys. There is much similarity in the structure of insulin among the different species; this has permitted the use of insulin extracted from beef and pork sources in the treatment of human diabetes mellitus.

The actions of insulin are threefold: (1) it provides for glucose storage, (2) it prevents fat breakdown, and (3) it increases protein synthesis. Although several hormones are known to increase blood sugar, insulin is the only hormone that is currently known to have a direct effect in lowering blood sugar. The actions of insulin are summarized in Chart 45-1.

Insulin lowers blood sugar by facilitating its transport into skeletal muscle and adipose tissue. Although liver cells do not require insulin for glucose transport, a rise in insulin levels does cause an increase in hepatic uptake of glucose, presumably by increasing the intracellular trapping of glucose

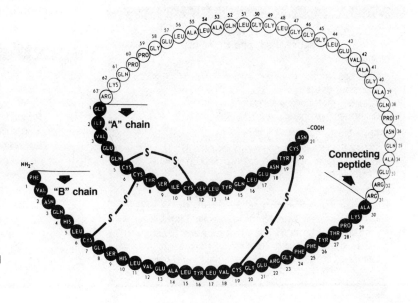

Figure 45-1 Amino-acid sequence of porcine proinsulin showing the A chain, the B chain, and the C-peptide link. (*Shaw WN, Chance RE: Diabetes 17(12):738, 1968*)

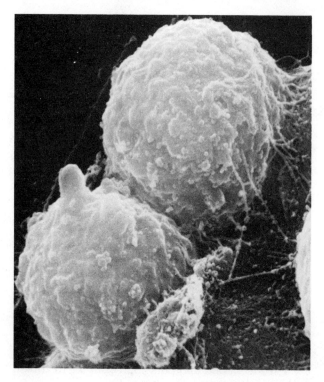

Figure 45-2 A scanning electron micrograph of an insulin-secreting beta cell from the islets of Langerhans in the pancreas. (*Courtesy of Kenneth Siegesmund, Ph.D., Anatomy Department, Medical College of Wisconsin*)

through the attachment of a phosphate group. Insulin also decreases the breakdown of glucose and fat stores and stimulates both glycogen and triglyceride synthesis. In relation to body proteins, insulin both inhibits protein breakdown and increases protein synthesis. When sufficient glucose and insulin are present, protein breakdown is inhibited because the body is able to use glucose and fatty acids as a fuel source. Insulin also increases the active transport of amino acids into body cells and accelerates protein synthesis within the cell. In the child and the adolescent, insulin is needed for normal growth and development.

Insulin release is regulated by blood glucose levels, increasing as blood sugar levels rise and decreasing when blood sugar declines. Serum insulin levels begin to rise within minutes after a meal, reach a peak in about 30 minutes, and then return to baseline levels within 3 hours. Between periods of food intake, insulin levels remain low and sources of stored glucose and amino acids are mobilized to supply the energy needs of glucose-dependent tissues. The glucose tolerance test, which is described later in this chapter, uses a glucose challenge as an indirect measure of the body's ability to secrete insulin and to remove glucose from the blood.

Glucagon

Glucagon is a small protein molecule produced by the pancreatic alpha cells of the islets of Langerhans. Like insulin, glucagon travels by way of the portal vein to the liver where it exerts its main action.

The actions of glucagon are diametrically opposed to those of insulin. Glucagon stimulates glycogenolysis and gluconeogenesis, increases lipolysis, and enhances the breakdown of proteins. The actions of glucagon are summarized in Chart 45-2.

It has been suggested that abnormalities in glucagon secretion contribute to the elevation in blood sugar observed in diabetes mellitus. Unger suggested that it is the ratio of insulin to glucagon, rather than the absolute amount of either hormone, that determines blood sugar levels.[3] According to theory, glucagon secretion is unopposed in the diabetic because of the lack of insulin, which therefore leads to increased production of glucose by the liver.

Chart 45–1: Actions of insulin on glucose, fats, and proteins

Glucose
Increases glucose transport into skeletal muscle and adipose tissue
Increases glycogen synthesis
Decreases gluconeogenesis

Fats
Increases glucose transport into fat cells
Increases fatty acid transport into adipose cells
Increases triglyceride synthesis

Proteins
Increases active transport of amino acids into cells
Increases protein synthesis by accelerating translation of RNA by ribosomes and increases transcription of DNA in the nucleus to form increased amounts of RNA
Decreases protein breakdown by enhancing the use of glucose and fatty acids as a fuel source

---

Chart 45–2: Actions of glucagon on glucose, fats, and proteins

Glucose
Promotes the breakdown of glycogen into glucose-6-phosphate
Increases gluconeogenesis

Fats
Enhances lipolysis in adipose tissue, liberating glycerol for use in gluconeogenesis

Proteins
Increases breakdown of proteins into amino acids for use in gluconeogenesis
Increases transport of amino acids in hepatic cells
Increases conversion of amino acids into glucose precursors

Catecholamines

The catecholamines, epinephrine and norepinephrine, help maintain blood sugar levels during periods of stress. The actions of epinephrine are summarized in Chart 45-3. Epinephrine inhibits insulin release and promotes glycogenolysis by stimulating the conversion of muscle and liver glycogen to glucose. It is important to recall that muscle glycogen cannot be released into the blood; nevertheless, the mobilization of these stores for muscle use conserves blood sugar for use by other tissues such as the brain and the nervous system. During periods of exercise and other types of stress, epinephrine inhibits insulin release from the beta cells and thereby decreases the movement of glucose into muscle cells. The catecholamines also increase lipase activity and thereby cause increased mobilization of fatty acids; this also serves to conserve glucose. The blood sugar-elevating effect of epinephrine is an important homeostatic mechanism in hypoglycemia.

Growth hormone

Growth hormone has many specific metabolic effects. It increases protein synthesis in all cells of the body, mobilizes fatty acids from adipose tissue, and antagonizes the effects of insulin. Growth hormone produces a decrease in both cellular uptake and utilization of glucose, thereby producing an increase in blood sugar, sometimes to as high as 50% to 100% of normal.[4] In turn, this increase in blood sugar increases the stimulus for insulin secretion by the beta cells. The secretion of growth hormone is normally inhibited by insulin and increased levels of blood glucose. During periods of fasting when both blood glucose levels and insulin secretion fall, growth hormone levels increase. Exercise, such as running and cycling, and various stresses including anesthesia, fever, and trauma produce an increase in growth hormone levels.

A chronic hypersecretion of growth hormone, as occurs in acromegaly (see Chapter 44), can lead to glucose intolerance and development of diabetes mellitus. In persons who already have diabetes, moderate elevations in growth hormone that occur during periods of poor control can themselves produce the entire spectrum of metabolic abnormalities associated with poor regulation, despite optimized insulin treatment.[5]

Glucocorticoid hormones

The glucocorticoids exhibit an important effect in increasing blood glucose. They are synthesized in the adrenal cortex along with other corticosteroid hormones. There are several steroid hormones with glucocorticoid activity; the most important of these is cortisol, which accounts for about 95% of all glucocorticoid activity.[4]

The glucocorticoid hormones are critical to survival during periods of fasting and starvation. They stimulate gluconeogenesis by the liver, sometimes producing a sixfold to tenfold increase in hepatic glucose production. These hormones also cause a moderate decrease in tissue utilization of glucose. In predisposed individuals, the prolonged elevation of glucocorticoid hormones can lead to hyperglycemia and the development of diabetes mellitus. In persons with diabetes, even transient increases in cortisol can complicate control.

Cortisol levels increase during periods of stress such as that produced by infection, pain, trauma and surgery, prolonged and strenuous exercise, and acute anxiety. Hypoglycemia is a potent stimulus for cortisol secretion. The control of cortisol secretion is discussed in Chapter 44.

In summary, energy metabolism is controlled by a number of hormones, including insulin, glucagon, epinephrine, growth hormone, and the glucocorticoids. Of these hormones, only insulin has the effect of lowering blood sugar. Insulin's blood-lowering action results from its ability to increase the transport of glucose into body cells and to decrease hepatic production and release of glucose into the bloodstream. Other hormones—glucagon, epinephrine, growth hormone, and the glucocorticoids—serve to maintain or increase blood sugar. Glucagon and epinephrine promote glycogenolysis. Glucagon and the glucocorticoids increase gluconeogenesis. Growth hormone decreases the peripheral utilization of glucose. Whereas insulin has the effect of decreasing lipolysis and utilization of fats as a fuel source, both glucagon and epinephrine increase fat utilization.

Classification and etiology

Although diabetes mellitus is clearly a disorder of insulin availability, it is probably not a single disease. A classification system that divides diabetes into insulin-dependent and noninsulin-dependent

---

Chart 45–3: Actions of epinephrine on metabolism

Mobilizes glycogen stores
Decreases movement of glucose into body cells
Inhibits insulin release from beta cells
Mobilizes fatty acids from adipose tissue

forms was developed by an international workshop sponsored by the National Diabetes Data Group of NIH (Table 45-1).[6] The system has been endorsed by the American Diabetes Association. Included in the classification system is a category for gestational diabetes (diabetes that develops during pregnancy), impaired glucose tolerance (abnormal glucose tolerance test without other signs of diabetes), and a secondary form of diabetes caused by other conditions (e.g., Cushing's syndrome).

—— Type I insulin-dependent diabetes mellitus

Type I or insulin-dependent diabetes mellitus (IDDM) is characterized by an absolute insulin deficiency state. This type of diabetes, formerly called juvenile diabetes, occurs more commonly in juveniles but can occur at any age. IDDM is a catabolic dis-

order characterized by an elevation in blood sugar and a breakdown of both body fats and proteins. One of the actions of insulin is the inhibition of lipolysis (fat breakdown) and the release of free fatty acids from fat cells. In the absence of insulin, ketosis develops when these fatty acids are released from fat cells and converted to ketones in the liver. Because of their absolute lack of insulin, persons with type I diabetes mellitus are particularly prone to develop ketoacidosis. All persons with IDDM require exogenous insulin replacement to reverse the catabolic state, control blood sugar levels, and prevent ketosis. Because of their reliance on exogenous insulin, persons with IDDM may experience marked alterations in blood sugar—a condition referred to as *labile diabetes*.

It has been suggested that IDDM results from a genetic predisposition (diabetogenic genes), a hypothetical triggering event involving an environmental agent (viral infection or chemical toxin) that serves to

Table 45–1. Classification of diabetes and glucose intolerance states

Classification	Former terminology	Characteristics
Diabetes mellitus (DM)		
Type I		
Insulin-dependent diabetes mellitus (IDDM)	Juvenile-onset diabetes	Persons in this subclass are dependent on injected insulin Ketosis prone
Type II		

Noninsulin-dependent diabetes mellitus (NIDDM)
  1. Nonobese NIDDM
  2. Obese NIDDM (60%–90%)
	Adult-onset, maturity-onset diabetes	Persons in this subclass are not insulin dependent, but they may use insulin
		Not ketosis prone
		Frequently obese

Other types		

Pancreatic disease
  Hormonal
  Drug- or chemical-induced insulin receptor abnormalities
  Certain genetic defects
  Other types
	Secondary diabetes	Presence of diabetes and associated condition

Impaired glucose tolerance (IGT)		
Nonobese IGT	Asymptomatic, chemical, subclinical, borderline, latent diabetes	Based on nondiagnostic fasting glucose levels and glucose tolerance test between normal and diabetic
Obese IGT IGT associated with other conditions, including (1) pancreatic disease, (2) hormonal, (3) drug or chemical, (4) insulin-receptor abnormalities, or (5) genetic syndromes		
Gestational diabetes mellitus (GDM)	Gestational diabetes	Glucose intolerance that developed during pregnancy Increased risk of perinatal complications Increased risk of developing diabetes within 5–10 years after parturition

(Adapted from National Diabetes Data Group: Classification and diagnosis of diabetes mellitus and other categories of glucose intolerance. Diabetes 28:1042, 1979. Reprinted with permission of the American Diabetic Association.)

incite an immune response, and immunologically mediated beta cell destruction.[7,8] Much recent evidence has focused on the major histocompatibility complex (MHC) genes that code the human leukocyte antigens (HLA) found on the surface of body cells (see Chapter 11). One group of HLA, coded by the class II MHC immune response genes, regulate immune cell interactions. There is a strong association between two of the antigens (DR3 and DR4) coded by these immune response genes and IDDM. Thus, it appears that what is inherited as part of the HLA genotype in IDDM is a susceptibility to an abnormal immune response that affects beta cells. Islet-cell antibodies have been found in as many as 60% to 95% of newly diagnosed persons with IDDM and in persons who later develop the disease.[7,8] In addition to the MHC genes, an insulin gene relating beta-cell replication and function has been identified on chromosome 11.

Because of the immune characteristics, IDDM is thought to be triggered by environmental factors such as viruses or chemical agents in genetically predisposed persons. An underlying genetic defect on chromosome 11 relating beta-cell replication and regeneration may predispose to beta-cell failure, or specific HLA genes may predispose to the development of antibodies that destroy beta cells. Viruses are known to cause diabetes in animals, and several studies suggest that a virus may trigger the onset of diabetes in humans. The onset of IDDM has been observed to rise in late summer and winter; this corresponds with the prevalence of common viral infections in the community.[9,10] Mumps,[11] coxsackievirus-group B, type A,[12] and congenital rubella[13,14] have all been associated with the development of IDDM. Among the suspected chemical toxins are the nitrosamines, which are sometimes found in smoked and cured meats. The nitrosamines are related to streptozocin, which is used to induce diabetes in experimental animals, and to the rat poison, Vacor, which can produce diabetes when ingested by humans.[15]

The fact that IDDM is thought to result from an interaction between genetic and environmental factors has led to research into methods directed at prevention and early control of the disease. These methods include the identification of genetically susceptible persons and early intervention in newly diagnosed persons with IDDM. Following the diagnosis of IDDM, there is often a short period of beta-cell regeneration called the *honeymoon period* during which symptoms of diabetes disappear and insulin injections are not needed. Immune interventions designed to interrupt the destruction of beta cells during the so-called honeymoon period are being investigated with hopes of finding a way for preventing complete and irreversible beta-cell failure.

Type II noninsulin-dependent diabetes mellitus

Noninsulin-dependent diabetes mellitus (NIDDM), formerly known as maturity-onset diabetes, describes a condition of fasting hyperglycemia that occurs despite the availability of insulin. NIDDM is a nonketotic form of diabetes, it is not associated with HLA markers or inset-cell antibodies, and persons with the disease are usually not dependent on insulin to sustain life. Persons with NIDDM are usually older, they are frequently overweight, and they have fewer problems with control than persons with IDDM. Insulin levels in persons with NIDDM are usually sufficient to prevent lipolysis and the development of ketosis but are inadequate to lower blood sugar by effecting the transport of glucose into fat cells. The metabolic abnormalities that contribute to the hyperglycemia that occurs in NIDDM include impaired insulin secretion, peripheral insulin resistance, and increased hepatic glucose production. Two subgroups of NIDDM are currently distinguished by the presence or absence of obesity.

Most persons with NIDDM (80%) are overweight.[15] The type of obesity, as well as the presence of obesity, are important considerations in the development of NIDDM. Research has shown that persons with upper body obesity are at greater risk for developing NIDDM than persons with lower body obesity (see Chapter 42).[15–18] Obese persons have been shown to have increased resistance to the action of insulin and impaired suppression of glucose production by the liver, resulting in both hyperglycemia and hyperinsulinemia (Figure 45-3). The increased insulin resistance has been attributed to either a decreased number of insulin receptors in the peripheral adipose tissues or to the impairment of insulin receptor function. In addition to insulin resistance, there is an accompanying impairment of insulin release from beta cells in response to glucose. Insulin resistance and beta-cell function usually improve with weight loss, to the extent that many persons with NIDDM can be managed with a weight-reduction program and exercise.

A second type of NIDDM occurs in nonobese persons. These persons have an absent or blunted early insulin response to glucose. Included in this subgroup are younger persons with a strongly positive family history suggesting autosomal dominant transmission. Persons with the nonobese type of NIDDM usually respond well to the oral hypoglycemic agents.

Other types

In other types of diabetes, formerly known as secondary diabetes, the relationship between the etio-

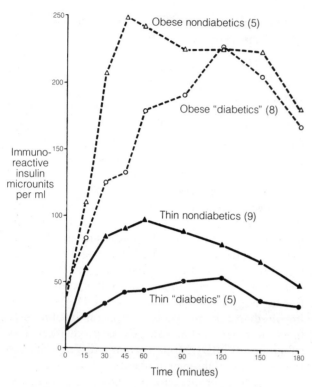

Figure 45-3 The mean absolute insulin responses in thin and obese diabetic subjects during a 3-hour (100-g) oral glucose tolerance curve. (*Bagdade JD, Biermann EL, Porter D: The significance of basal insulin levels in evaluation of the insulin response to glucose in diabetic and nondiabetic subjects. J Clin Invest 46(10):1553, 1967*)

logic agent and glucose intolerance is known. Diabetes can occur secondary to pancreatic disease or the removal of pancreatic tissue; endocrine diseases, such as acromegaly; Cushing's syndrome; or pheochromocytoma. Endocrine disorders that produce hyperglycemia do so by either increasing the hepatic production of glucose or decreasing the cellular utilization of glucose.

Several diuretics—thiazides, furosemide, and ethacrynic acid—tend to elevate blood sugar. These diuretics increase potassium loss, which is thought to impair insulin release. Other drugs known to cause hyperglycemia include the following: diazoxide, glucocorticoids, levodopa, oral contraceptives, sympathomimetics, phenothiazines, phenytoin, and total parenteral nutrition (hyperalimentation). Drug-related increases in blood sugar are usually reversed once the drug has been discontinued.

Impaired glucose tolerance

The diagnosis *impaired glucose tolerance* describes an individual with plasma glucose levels between those considered normal and those considered diabetic. Calorie restriction and weight reduction are important for overweight persons in this class.

Gestational diabetes

Gestational diabetes refers to glucose intolerance of varying degree that occurs during pregnancy. Indications for the use of glucose tolerance tests during pregnancy are a family history of diabetes, glycosuria, a history of stillbirth or spontaneous abortion, the presence of fetal anomalies in previous pregnancy, a previous large or heavy-for-date baby, obesity in the mother, advanced maternal age, or five or more pregnancies. The presence of more than one of these risk factors is particularly indicative of increased risk. Diagnosis and careful medical management are essential because these women are at higher risk for complications of pregnancy, mortality, and fetal abnormalities. Fetal abnormalities include macrosomatia (large body size), hypoglycemia, hypocalcemia, polycythemia, and hyperbilirubinemia. Some states now require glucose tolerance tests in pregnancy at designated weeks of gestation, usually between the 24th and 28th weeks.

Treatment of gestational diabetes includes close observation of mother and fetus. Maternal fasting and postprandial blood-glucose levels should be measured regularly. Fetal surveillance depends on the degree of risk for the fetus. The frequency of growth measurements and determinations of fetal distress depends on available technology and gestational age. All women with gestational diabetes mellitus require nutritional guidance. If dietary management alone does not achieve a fasting blood glucose level of ≤105 mg/dl or a 2-hour postprandial blood glucose of ≤120 mg/dl, insulin therapy may be indicated. Oral hypoglycemic agents are not recommended in pregnancy. Self blood glucose monitoring is essential because urine glucose monitoring in pregnancy is not acceptable practice today.

Women with gestational diabetes are at increased risk of developing diabetes 5 to 10 years after delivery. After pregnancy, the woman should be reclassified as either a person with diabetes mellitus or one with impaired glucose tolerance. In most women, glucose tolerance returns to normal, and a classification of previously abnormal glucose tolerance is made.[6]

In summary, diabetes mellitus is a disorder of carbohydrate, protein, and fat metabolism resulting from an imbalance between insulin availability and insulin need. The disease can be classified as insulin-dependent diabetes mellitus (IDDM), in which there is an absolute insulin deficiency, or noninsulin-dependent diabetes mellitus (NIDDM), in which there is a lack of insulin availability or effectiveness. At present, the etiology of IDDM and NIDDM is unknown. Other types of diabetes include secondary forms of carbohydrate intolerance, which occur secondary to some other condition, such as pancreatic disorders, which destroy beta cells, or endocrine diseases such as Cushing's syndrome, which causes increased production of glucose by the liver and decreased utilization of glucose by the tissues. Gestational diabetes develops during pregnancy, and although glucose tolerance often returns to normal after childbirth, it indicates increased risk of developing diabetes.

Manifestations

Diabetes mellitus may have a rapid or insidious onset. In IDDM, signs and symptoms are often acute and of sudden origin. On the other hand, NIDDM often develops more insidiously; its presence may be detected during a routine medical examination or when a patient seeks medical care for other reasons.

The most commonly identified signs and symptoms of diabetes are often referred to as the three "polys"—*polyuria* (excessive urination), *polydipsia* (excessive thirst), and *polyphagia* (excessive hunger). These three symptoms are closely related to the hyperglycemia (elevated blood sugar) and glycosuria (sugar in the urine) that are present in diabetes. Glucose is a small, osmotically active molecule. When blood sugar is sufficiently elevated, the amount of glucose filtered by the glomeruli of the kidney will exceed the amount that can be reabsorbed by the renal tubules; this results in *glycosuria* and large accompanying losses of water in the urine. Thirst results from intracellular dehydration that occurs as blood sugar levels rise and water is pulled out of body cells, including those in the thirst center. Cellular dehydration also causes dryness of the mouth. This early symptom may be easily overlooked in NIDDM, in which there is a gradual increase in blood sugar without accompanying signs of ketoacidosis. Polyphagia is usually not present in persons with NIDDM. In IDDM, it probably results from cellular starvation and the depletion of cellular stores of carbohydrates, fats, and proteins.

Weight loss, despite normal or increased appetite, is a common occurrence in the person with uncontrolled IDDM. The cause of weight loss is twofold. First, loss of body fluids results from osmotic diuresis. Vomiting may exaggerate the fluid loss in ketoacidosis. Second, body tissue is lost because the lack of insulin forces the body to use its fat stores and cellular proteins as sources of energy. In terms of weight loss, there is often a marked difference between NIDDM and IDDM. Weight loss is a frequent phenomenon in the person with uncontrolled IDDM, whereas the individual with uncomplicated NIDDM often has problems with obesity.

Other signs and symptoms of hyperglycemia include recurrent blurring of vision, fatigue, paresthesias, and skin infections. In NIDDM, these are often the symptoms that prompt a person to seek medical treatment. Blurred vision develops as the lens and retina are exposed to hyperosmolar fluids. Lowered plasma volume produces weakness and fatigue. Paresthesias reflect a temporary dysfunction of the peripheral sensory nerves; they are more common in persons presenting with subacute IDDM. Chronic skin infections are common in NIDDM. Both hyperglycemia and glycosuria favor the growth of yeast organisms. Pruritus and vulvovaginitis resulting from candidal infections are common initial complaints in women with diabetes.

Acute complications

Three major acute complications of diabetes are ketoacidosis, nonketotic hyperosmolar coma, and hypoglycemia. The body responds to acute changes in physiologic functioning with a series of predictable compensatory responses. The acute complications of diabetes are no exception.

Diabetic ketoacidosis

Ketoacidosis occurs when ketone production by the liver exceeds cellular utilization and renal excretion. In persons with type I IDDM, lack of insulin leads to mobilization of fatty acids and subsequent increase in ketone production.

Compared with an insulin reaction (to be discussed), diabetic ketoacidosis is usually slower in onset and recovery is more prolonged. There is usually a history of a day or two of polyuria and polydipsia, nausea and vomiting, and marked fatigue with eventual stupor that can progress to coma. Blood sugar levels are elevated (ranging from 250 mg/dl to values greater than 1000 mg/dl), and urine sugar is greater than 2% to 5% with blood glucose levels above 240 mg/dl. Plasma *p*H and bicarbonate are decreased, and urine tests for acetone (Acetest or Ketostix) are positive. Serum potassium is often normal or elevated, despite total potassium depletion resulting from protracted polyuria and vomiting. The signs and symptoms of ketoacidosis are summarized in Chart 45-4.

There are two major metabolic derangements in diabetic ketoacidosis, *hyperglycemia* and *metabolic acidosis*. The hyperglycemia leads to osmotic diuresis, dehydration, and a critical loss of electrolytes. The metabolic acidosis is caused by the excess ketoacids that require buffering by the bicarbonate ion; this

---

Chart 45-4: Signs and symptoms of diabetic ketoacidosis

Onset—(1-24 hours)
Laboratory findings
    Blood sugar greater than 250 mg/100 ml
    Urine sugar greater than 2%
    Ketonemia and presence of ketones in the urine
    Decreased plasma pH (less than 7.3) and bicarbonate
        (less than 24 mEq)
Dehydration due to hyperglycemia
    Warm, dry skin
    Dry mucous membranes
    Tachycardia
    Weak, thready pulse
    Acute weight loss
    Hypotension
Ketoacidosis
    Anorexia, nausea, and vomiting
    Odor of ketones on the breath
    Depression of the central nervous system
        Lethargy and fatigue
        Stupor
        Coma
    Abdominal pain
Compensatory responses
    Rapid, deep respirations (Kussmaul's respiration)

---

leads to a marked decrease in serum bicarbonate levels. The breath has a characteristic fruity smell because of the presence of the volatile ketoacids. A number of signs and symptoms that occur in diabetic ketoacidosis are related to compensatory mechanisms. The heart rate increases as the body compensates for a decrease in blood volume, and the rate and depth of respiration increase (Kussmaul's respiration) as the body attempts to prevent further decreases in pH. Metabolic acidosis and its treatment are discussed in Chapter 29.

Diabetic ketoacidosis is seen most frequently in the insulin-dependent diabetic. It can occur at the onset of the disease, often before the disease has been diagnosed. For example, a mother may bring a child into the hospital with reports of lethargy, vomiting, and abdominal pain, unaware that the child has diabetes. Stress tends to increase the release of gluconeogenic hormones and predisposes the person to the development of ketoacidosis. Consequently, the development of ketoacidosis is often preceded by physical or emotional stress, for example, infection, pregnancy, or extreme anxiety.

The treatment of diabetic ketoacidosis focuses on correcting the fluid and electrolyte imbalances and returning blood pH to normal. Usually this is accomplished through the administration of insulin and intravenous fluid and electrolyte replacement solutions. Because insulin resistance accompanies severe acidosis, the current practice is to use smaller doses of insulin (usually added to the intravenous solution)

than were used in the past. Frequent monitoring of laboratory tests of serum electrolytes is used as a guide for fluid and electrolyte replacement. It is important to replace fluid and electrolytes and correct pH before bringing the blood glucose to a normal level. Too rapid a drop in blood sugar may cause hypoglycemic symptoms and cerebral edema. A sudden change in osmolality of the extracellular fluid occurs when blood sugar is lowered rapidly, and this can cause cerebral edema. Serum potassium levels often fall as acidosis is corrected and extracellular potassium moves into the intracellular compartment; at this time it may be necessary to add potassium to the intravenous infusion. The identification and treatment of the underlying cause, such as infection, are also important.

Hyperosmolar nonketotic coma

Hyperosmolar hyperglycemic nonketotic (HHNK) coma is characterized by plasma osmolarity of 350 mOsm/liter or more, blood sugar in excess of 600 mg per 100 ml of blood, the absence of ketoacidosis, and depression of the sensorium.[19]

Hyperosmolar coma may occur in a variety of conditions, including NIDDM, acute pancreatitis, severe infections, myocardial infarction, and treatment with oral or parenteral hyperalimentation solutions. Two factors appear to contribute to the hyperglycemia that precipitates the condition: an increased resistance to the effects of insulin and an excessive carbohydrate intake.

In hyperosmolar states, the increased serum osmolarity has the effect of pulling water out of body cells, including brain cells. The most prominent manifestations are dehydration, neurologic signs and symptoms, polyuria, and thirst (Chart 45-5). One patient is reported to have consumed 9 quarts of skim

---

Chart 45-5: Signs and symptoms of hyperosmolar coma

Onset—insidious; 24 hours to 2 weeks
Laboratory findings
    Blood sugar greater than 600 mg/100 ml
    Serum osmolarity 350 mOsm/liter or greater
Severe dehydration
    Dry skin and mucous membranes
    Extreme thirst
Neurologic manifestations
    Depressed sensorium lethargy to coma
    Neurologic deficits
        Positive Babinski's sign
        Paresis or paralysis
        Sensory impairment
        Hyperthermia
        Hemianopia
    Seizures

milk in a single day. The neurologic signs include grand mal seizures, hemiparesis, Babinski's reflexes, aphasia, muscle fasciculations, hyperthermia, hemianopia, nystagmus, visual hallucinations, and others.[20] Blood glucose levels of 4800 mg per 100 ml of blood have been reported. The onset of hyperosmolar coma is often insidious; and because it occurs most frequently in older persons, it may be mistaken for a stroke.

Treatment of hyperosmolar coma requires judicious medical observation and care. This is because water moves back into brain cells during treatment, posing a threat of cerebral edema. Extensive potassium losses, which have also occurred during the diuretic phase of the disorder, require correction. Because of the problems encountered in the treatment and the serious nature of the disease conditions that cause hyperosmolar coma, the prognosis for this disorder is less favorable than that for ketoacidosis; the mortality rate has been reported to be 40% to 70%.[20]

Hypoglycemia

Hypoglycemia, or an insulin reaction, usually occurs in insulin-treated diabetics. It occurs when blood sugar falls below 50 mg per 100 ml of blood and is characterized by sudden onset and rapid progression (Chart 45-6). The signs and symptoms of hypoglycemia can be divided into two categories: those caused by altered cerebral function and those related to activation of the autonomic nervous system. Because the brain relies on blood glucose as its main energy source, hypoglycemia causes behaviors related to altered cerebral function. Headache, difficulty in problem solving, disturbed or altered behavior, coma, and convulsions are common. At the onset of the hypoglycemic episode, activation of the parasympathetic nervous system causes hunger. The initial parasympathetic response is followed by activation of the sympathetic nervous system; this causes anxiety, tachycardia, sweating, and constriction of the skin vessels (the skin is cool and clammy). Although persons respond differently in insulin reaction, each person usually has the same individual pattern of response during each insulin reaction. For this reason, it is helpful if this response pattern can be identified during the early stages of treatment in the person with insulin-dependent diabetes.

The signs and symptoms of hypoglycemia are more variable in children and in the elderly. Elderly persons may not display the typical autonomic responses associated with hypoglycemia but frequently develop signs of impaired function of the central nervous system, including mental confusion and bizarre behavior. Some medications, such as beta-adrenergic blocking drugs, interfere with the symptomatic response normally seen in hypoglycemia.

Many factors tend to precipitate insulin reaction in the person with insulin-dependent diabetes: error in insulin dose, failure to eat, increased exercise, decreased insulin need following removal of a stress situation, change in insulin site. Alcohol tends to decrease liver gluconeogenesis, and the person with diabehavior. Some medications, such as beta-adrenergic blocking drugs, interfere with the symptomatic response normally seen in hypoglycemia.

The most effective treatment of an insulin reaction is the immediate ingestion of a concentrated carbohydrate source, such as sugar, honey, candy, or orange juice. Alternative methods for increasing blood sugar may be required when the diabetic is unconscious or unable to swallow. Glucagon may be given intravenously, intramuscularly, or subcutaneously. The liver contains only a limited amount of glycogen (about 75 g); glucagon will be ineffective in persons whose glycogen stores have been depleted. It is therefore recommended that glucagon be given only once and not repeated. Repeating the dose may cause vomiting, which will worsen the situation. A small amount of honey or glucose gel (available in most pharmacies) can be inserted into the buccal pouch (under the tongue) in situations in which swallowing is impaired. Monosaccharides such as glucose or fructose, which can be absorbed directly into the bloodstream, work

---

Chart 45–6: Signs and symptoms of insulin reaction*

Onset—sudden
Laboratory findings
    Blood sugar less than 50 mg/100 ml
Impaired cerebral function (due to decreased glucose availability for brain metabolism)
    Feeling of vagueness
    Headache
    Difficulty in problem solving
    Slurred speech
    Impaired motor function
    Change in emotional behavior
    Convulsions
    Coma
Compensatory autonomic nervous system responses
    Parasympathetic responses
        Hunger
        Nausea
        Hypotension
        Bradycardia
    Sympathetic responses
        Anxiety
        Sweating
        Vasoconstriction of skin vessels (skin is pale and cool)
        Tachycardia

*There is a wide variation in manifestation of signs and symptoms among individuals, that is, not every person with diabetes will have all or even most of the symptoms.

best for this purpose. It is important not to overtreat hypoglycemia so as to cause hyperglycemia. Usually treatment consists of an initial administration of about 10 g glucose, which can be repeated as necessary. Complex carbohydrates may be administered once the acute reaction has been controlled (see section entitled "Diabetic Diet"). In gestational diabetes, milk is recommended to treat hypoglycemia. This use of a complex sugar prevents rebound hyperglycemia, which can be harmful to the fetus. In situations of severe, life-threatening hypoglycemia, it may be necessary to administer glucose (20–50 ml of a 50% solution) intravenously.

Somogyi phenomenon

The Somogyi phenomenon describes a cycle of insulin-induced posthypoglycemic episodes. In 1924, Joslin and his associates noted that hypoglycemia was associated with alternate episodes of hyperglycemia.[21] It was not until 1959, however, that Somogyi presented the results of his 20 years of studies, which confirmed the observation that "hypoglycemia begets hyperglycemia."[22] In a person with diabetes, insulin-induced hypoglycemia produces a compensatory increase in blood levels of catecholamines, glucagon, cortisol, and growth hormone. These counter-regulatory hormones cause blood sugar to become elevated and produce some degree of insulin resistance. A vicious circle begins when the increase in blood sugar and insulin resistance are treated with larger insulin doses. Often the hypoglycemic episode occurs during the night or at a time when it is not recognized, rendering the diagnosis of the phenomenon more difficult. Figure 45-4 illustrates the events that occur with the Somogyi phenomenon.

Recent research suggests that even rather mild insulin-associated hypoglycemia, which may be asymptomatic, can cause hyperglycemia in IDDM through the recruitment of counterregulatory mechanisms, although the insulin action does not wane. A concomitant waning of the effect of insulin (end of the duration of action), when it occurs, exacerbates posthypoglycemic hyperglycemia and accelerates its development. It was suggested that these research findings may explain the labile nature of the disease in some persons with diabetes. Measures to prevent hypoglycemia and the subsequent activation of counter-regulatory mechanisms include a redistribution of dietary carbohydrates and an alteration in insulin dose or method of administration.[23]

Chronic complications

The chronic complications of diabetes include neuropathies, nephropathies, and other vascular lesions. Interestingly, these disorders occur in the insulin-independent tissues of the body—those tissues that do not require insulin for glucose entry into the cell. This probably means that intracellular glucose concentrations in these tissues approach or equal those in the blood.

Theories of pathogenesis

The interest among researchers in explaining the causes and development of chronic lesions in the person with diabetes has led to a number of theories. Several of these theories have been summarized to prepare the reader for understanding specific chronic complications.

Polyol pathway. A polyol is an organic compound that contains three or more hydroxyl groups. The polyol pathway refers to the intracellular mechanisms responsible for changing the number of hydroxyl units on a sugar. In the sorbitol pathway, glucose is first transformed to sorbitol, and then to fructose. Although glucose is readily converted to sorbitol, the rate at which sorbitol can be converted to fructose and then metabolized is limited. Sorbitol is osmotically active, and it has been hypothesized that the presence of excess intracellular amounts may alter cell function in those tissues that use this pathway.

Formation of abnormal glycoproteins. Glycoproteins, or what might be termed sugar proteins, are normal components of the basement membrane in smaller blood vessels and capillaries. It has been suggested that the increased intracellular concentration of glucose associated with uncontrolled blood sugar levels in diabetes favors the formation of abnormal glycoproteins. These abnormal glycoproteins are thought to produce structural defects in the basement membrane of these vessels.

Problems with tissue oxygenation. Proponents of the tissue oxygenation theories suggest that many of the chronic complications of diabetes arise because of a decrease in oxygen delivery in the small

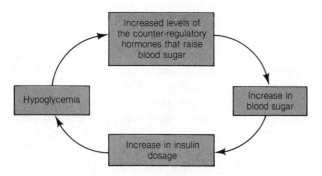

Figure 45-4 The cycle of events that occur with the Somogyi phenomenon.

vessels of the microcirculation. Among the factors believed to contribute to this inadequate oxygen delivery is a defect in red cell function that interferes with the release of oxygen from the hemoglobin molecule. In support of this theory is the finding of a twofold to threefold increase in glycosylated hemoglobin ($HbA_{1a} + HbA_{1b} + HbA_{1c}$) in persons with diabetes. In glycosylated hemoglobin, a glycoprotein is substituted for valine in the beta chain, causing a high affinity for oxygen.[24] There is a reported decline in red cell 2,3-diphosphoglycerate (2,3-DPG) during the acidotic and recovery phases of diabetic ketoacidosis. The glycolytic intermediate 2,3-DPG reduces the hemoglobin affinity for oxygen. Both an increase in glycosylated hemoglobin and a decrease in 2,3-DPG tend to increase the hemoglobin's affinity for oxygen, and less oxygen is released for tissue use.

Peripheral neuropathies

Although the incidence of peripheral neuropathies is known to be high among people with diabetes, it is difficult to document exactly how many persons are affected by these disorders. This is because of the diversity in clinical manifestations and because the condition is often far advanced before it is recognized.

Two types of pathologic changes have been observed in connection with diabetic peripheral neuropathies. The first is a thickening of the walls of the nutrient vessels that supply the nerve, leading to the assumption that vessel ischemia plays a major role in the development of these neural changes. The second and more recent finding has been a segmental demyelinization process that affects the Schwann cell. This demyelinization process is accompanied by a slowing of nerve conduction. Recent research on the sorbitol pathway suggests that the formation and accumulation of sorbitol within Schwann cells may lead to injury and impair nerve conduction.

It now appears that the diabetic peripheral neuropathies are not a single entity. The clinical manifestations of these disorders vary with the location of the lesion(s). Although there are several methods for classifying the diabetic peripheral neuropathies, a simplified system divides them into somatic and autonomic disturbances (Chart 45-7).

In addition to the actual discomforts associated with the loss of sensory or motor function, lesions in either the somatic or peripheral nervous system predispose the person with diabetes to additional complications. Loss of feeling, touch, and position sense increases the risk of falling. Impairment of temperature and pain sensation increases the risk of serious burns and injuries to the feet. Defects in vasomotor reflexes can lead to dizziness and syncope when

---

Chart 45–7: Classification of diabetic peripheral neuropathies

Somatic

Polyneuropathies (bilateral sensory)
  Paresthesias, including numbness and tingling
  Impaired pain, temperature, light touch, two-point discrimination, and vibratory sensation
  Decreased ankle and knee-jerk reflexes
Mononeuropathies
  Involvement of a mixed nerve trunk that includes loss of sensation, pain, and motor weakness
Amyotrophy
  Associated with muscle weakness, wasting, and severe pain of muscles in the pelvic girdle and thigh

Autonomic

Impaired vasomotor function
  Postural hypotension
Impaired gastrointestinal function
  Gastric atony
  Diarrhea, often postprandial and nocturnal
Impaired genitourinary function
  Paralytic bladder
  Incomplete voiding
  Impotence
  Retrograde ejaculation
Cranial nerve involvement
  Extraocular nerve paralysis
  Impaired pupillary responses
  Impaired special senses

---

the person moves from the supine to the standing position. Incomplete emptying of the bladder due to vesicle dysfunction predisposes the person to urinary stasis and bladder infection and increases the risk of renal complications (see Chapter 33).

In the male, disruption of sensory and autonomic nervous system function can cause impotence. Diabetes is the leading physiologic cause of impotence, and it occurs in both IDDM and NIDDM. Of the 5 million men with diabetes in the United States, 30% to 60% suffer from impotence.[25]

Nephropathies

The person with diabetes is predisposed to several types of renal disease, including pyelonephritis and nephropathies. Pyelonephritis occurs in the nondiabetic person as well as in the diabetic (discussed in Chapter 31). Nephropathies refer to chronic renal vascular complications and are a common cause of death in long-term diabetic patients.

The basement membrane of the glomerulus is composed of complex glycoproteins. It has been suggested that the increased intracellular concentration of glucose in the person with diabetes contributes to the formation of abnormal glycoproteins and glycoprotein linkage in the basement membrane of the glomerulus. Kimmelstiel-Wilson syndrome is a form of glomerulosclerosis that involves the development of nodular lesions in the glomerular capillary of the kidney causing impaired blood flow with progressive loss of kidney function and eventual renal failure. Kimmelstiel-Wilson lesions are thought to occur only in people with diabetes. Diffuse glomerulosclerosis, which is a linear thickening of the glomerular membrane, is found in both diabetes and nondiabetics. Changes in the basement membrane in Kimmelstiel-Wilson syndrome and diffuse glomerulosclerosis allow plasma proteins to escape in the urine, causing proteinuria, the development of hypoproteinemia (decreased levels of plasma proteins), and edema.

Retinopathies

Diabetes is the leading cause of acquired blindness in the United States. Although the person with diabetes is at increased risk for developing cataracts and glaucoma, retinopathy is the most common pattern of disease in the eye. It has been estimated that 20% to 50% of persons with diabetes may have retinopathy, and 10% of those may be at risk for visual loss.[26]

There are two types of diabetic retinopathy: (1) background, or nonproliferative, retinopathy and (2) proliferative retinopathy (Figure 45-5). Nonproliferative, or background, retinopathy is characterized by microaneurysms, or fusiform outpouchings, that protrude from one side of the capillary. These microaneurysms form weakened spots in the capillary wall that tend to leak fluid or to rupture, giving rise to retinal edema and hemorrhage. Hard waxy exudates form as pockets of protein and lipids leak through the wall of the weakened capillary. Usually old hemorrhages and exudate are constantly reabsorbed as new hemorrhages are formed. The retinopathies are discussed further in Chapter 51.

Proliferative retinopathy differs from background retinopathy in that new blood vessels (neovascularization) develop on the surface of the retina and extend into the area between the retina and vitreous. These new vessels, like the background microaneurysms, are very fragile and tend to rupture easily. When hemorrhage occurs, blood from these lesions flows into the vitreous, obstructing the flow of light from the lens to the retina. As the condition progresses, scar tissue and adhesions develop between the vitreous and the retina. When the scar tissue contracts, it can cause vitreous hemorrhage or retinal detachment.

The retinal vessels can be viewed by means of an ophthalmoscope. This allows for early diagnosis and follow-up observation of retinal lesions. The intravenous injection of fluorescein dye provides a method for outlining the retinal vasculature and detecting sites of obstruction and leakage. Normally, the retinal capillary endothelial cells are tightly joined, so that the dye does not escape into the vitreous.

Methods used in the treatment of diabetic retinopathy include the destruction and scarring of the proliferative lesions with photocoagulation. The diabetic retinopathy study demonstrated that panretinal photocoagulation may delay or prevent visual loss in

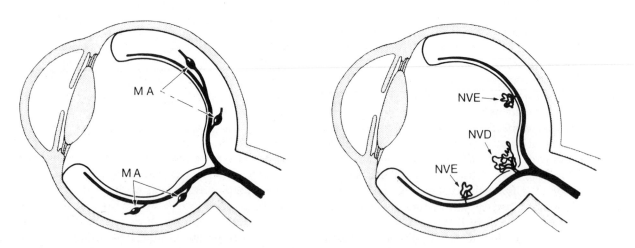

Figure 45-5 Nonproliferative and proliferative lesions in retinopathy of the person with diabetes. *Background retinopathy:* In background diabetic retinopathy, the blood vessel changes are contained within the retina. The microaneurysms (*MA*) are shown schematically within the substance of the retina. *Proliferative retinopathy:* In proliferative diabetic retinopathy, new vessel formation breaks through the surface of the retina to grow into the vitreous cavity. When the vessels are near the optic nerve or disk area, they are termed neovascularization of the disk; when the new vessel formation occurs elsewhere in the retina away from the disk, it is referred to as neovascularization elsewhere. (*Copyright 1978 by the American Diabetes Association, Inc. Reprinted from Diabetes Forecast by permission.*)

more than 50% of eyes with proliferative retinopathy.[27] Removal and replacement of the vitreous with a clear replacement solution (vitrectomy) may be used in those situations in which vitreal hemorrhage has caused blindness.

Vascular complications

There is little doubt that diabetes contributes to disease of both the microcirculation and the macrocirculation. Diabetic involvement of the small vessels in the retina is an example of disease of the microcirculation. It is also known that people with diabetes are at risk for developing lesions of vessels in the macrocirculation, including the coronaries, cerebral vessels, and peripheral arteries.

There is much controversy about the cause(s) of vascular pathology in diabetes. Among the factors thought to contribute to the increased prevalence of atherosclerosis in people with diabetes are hypertension, hyperlipidemia, increased platelet adhesiveness, other alterations in blood coagulation factors, and accumulation of sorbitol within the walls of the larger vessels.

Studies suggest that diabetes is an important risk factor in the development of heart disease, including coronary artery disease, and other forms of myocardial dysfunction.[27] Autonomic innervation of the heart may also become impaired in the person with diabetes. With impaired autonomic function, the heart rate response to many stresses is lessened.

Vascular disorders also affect the cerebral circulation. Evidence suggests that cerebral artery atherosclerosis develops earlier and is more extensive in people with diabetes than in nondiabetic persons.

The effects of the disease on vessels in the lower extremities is evidenced by an increased frequency of peripheral vascular insufficiency and intermittent claudication in people with diabetes compared with nondiabetic persons. Impairment of the peripheral vascular circulation may become severe enough to cause ulceration, infection, and eventually gangrene of the feet. Persons with diabetes are at least 15 times more likely to suffer amputation than those without diabetes. Among persons with diabetes, about 20% of hospital admissions are for foot problems.[27]

In persons with diabetes, lesions of the feet represent both the effects of vascular insufficiency and sensory neuropathy. Persons with sensory neuropathies have impaired pain sensation and are often unaware of the constant trauma to the feet caused by poorly fitting shoes, improper weight bearing, pebbles in the shoes, or infections such as athlete's foot. Common sites of trauma are the back of the heel, the plantar metatarsal area, or the great toe where weight is borne during walking. Motor neuropathy with weakness of the intrinsic muscles of the foot may result in increased weight bearing over the metatarsal heads. Because of the constant risk of foot problems, it is important that persons with diabetes wear proper fitting shoes and inspect their feet daily, looking for blisters, open sores, or fungal infection (athlete's foot) between the toes. If their eyesight is poor, a family member should do this for them. In the event that a lesion is detected, prompt medical attention is needed to prevent serious complications. Smoking should be avoided because it causes vasoconstriction and contributes to vascular disease. Because cold produces vasoconstriction, proper foot coverings should be used to keep the feet warm and dry. With autonomic neuropathy the skin tends to become dry and crack; if this occurs, a hydrous lanolin preparation should be applied two or three times a day.[28] Toenails should be cut straight across to prevent ingrown toenails. The toenails are often thickened and deformed, requiring the services of a podiatrist.

Infections

Although not specifically either an acute or a chronic complication, infections are common concerns of the person with diabetes. Certain types of infections occur with increased frequency in persons with diabetes: soft tissue infections of the extremities, osteomyelitis, urinary tract infections and pyelonephritis, candidal infections of skin and mucous surfaces, and tuberculosis. At present, there is a question whether or not the problem seems more prevalent because the infections are more serious in people with diabetes.

There are several known causes for the suboptimal response to infection in the person with diabetes. One is the presence of chronic complications, such as vascular disease and neuropathies; the other is the presence of hyperglycemia and altered neutrophil function. Sensory deficits may cause the person with diabetes to ignore minor trauma and infection, and vascular disease may impair circulation and delivery of blood cells and other substances needed to produce an adequate inflammatory response and effect healing. Pyelonephritis and urinary tract infections are relatively common in the person with diabetes, and it has been suggested that these infections may bear some relationship to the presence of a neurogenic bladder or nephrosclerotic changes in the kidney. Hyperglycemia and glycosuria may influence the growth of microorganisms and increase the severity of the infection. Recently, it has been shown that chemotaxis and phagocytosis are impaired in neutrophils that have been exposed to increased concentrations of glucose.

In summary, diabetes mellitus is a chronic disease characterized by a state of insulin deficiency. This insulin deficiency can be absolute, as in insulin-dependent diabetes mellitus, or it can be relative, as in noninsulin-dependent diabetes. The metabolic disturbances associated with diabetes affect almost every system in the body. The acute complications include diabetic ketoacidosis, hypoglycemia, and, in the person with noninsulin-dependent diabetes, hyperosmolar, hyperglycemic nonketotic coma. The chronic complications of diabetes affect the noninsulin-dependent tissues, including the retina, blood vessels, kidney, and peripheral nervous system.

Diagnosis and management

There are various tests that measure blood and urine glucose levels. These tests are used to screen for diabetes and to follow the progress of persons with known diabetes. Tests that measure insulin levels usually involve the use of radioimmunoassay techniques. The treatment plan for diabetes usually involves diet, hypoglycemic agents, and exercise. Weight loss and dietary management may be sufficient to control blood sugar levels in persons with NIDDM. The continuous insulin pump has provided an alternative method for insulin administration, and pancreas transplants are being studied as a possible future treatment for diabetes.

—— Blood tests

—— Glucose tolerance test

The glucose tolerance test is an important screening test for diabetes. The test measures the body's ability to store glucose by removing it from the blood. Using blood sugar levels, the test measures the response to a given amount of concentrated glucose at selected intervals, usually ½, 1, 1½, 2, and 3 hours (urine glucose may also be measured at these times). Insulin levels, as well as proinsulin and C-peptide levels, may also be measured at these intervals. In the normal individual, blood sugars will return to normal within 3 hours after ingestion of a glucose load, in which case it can be assumed that sufficient insulin is present to allow glucose to leave the blood and enter body cells. Because the person with diabetes lacks the ability to respond to an increase in blood glucose by releasing adequate insulin to facilitate storage, blood sugar levels not only rise above those observed in normal persons but remain elevated for longer periods of time (Figure 45-6). The glucose tolerance test is a useful diagnostic measure for detecting subclinical forms of diabetes—the stage of the disease in which

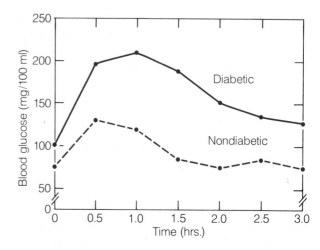

Figure 45-6 Results of a glucose tolerance test for diabetics and nondiabetics. Blood samples are usually taken at half-hour intervals following ingestion of a glucose solution containing 1.75 g of glucose per kilogram of body weight. The test may be modified for use as a screening tool.

the fasting blood sugar may still be normal and other obvious signs of diabetes are not yet detectable. A variation of the glucose tolerance test is the cortisone glucose tolerance test. The administration of cortisone challenges the body's ability to metabolize glucose. Another form of the glucose tolerance test is used for screening purposes; this form of the test involves sampling blood sugar 2 hours following a glucose challenge.

—— Fasting blood sugar test

Fasting blood sugars measure blood sugar levels after food has been withheld for a period of 8 to 12 hours.

—— Capillary blood tests and self blood glucose monitoring

Technologic advances have provided the means for self blood glucose determination using a drop of capillary blood. This method has not only provided health professionals with a rapid and economical method for monitoring blood glucose but has given people with diabetes a means of maintaining near-normal blood glucose levels through self glucose monitoring techniques.[29] These methods use a drop of capillary blood obtained by pricking the finger with a special needle or small lancet. The drop of blood is placed on a reagent strip, and glucose levels are determined. New lancet types (e.g., Autolet with a Monolet lancet) have made the technique virtually painless.

Several methods of self glucose monitoring are available, and new products are continually being developed. There are currently two types of reagent strip methods: a wash test and a dry test. Wash tests, such as Dextrostix and Visidex I, use a drop of blood on the reagent strip that is washed off with distilled water. After waiting a prescribed period of time, the result (in milligrams per deciliter) can be read by using either a color chart or an electronic meter. In the dry test method, the sample of blood is obtained in the same way, but the reagent strip is blotted with a cotton ball or cotton-tipped applicator. Tests such as Chem-strip BG, Visidex II, and Glucoscan GM use the dry method. As with the wash test results, the results of this test are read using a color chart or meter (Accu-check or Glucoscan). The ease, accuracy, and convenience of self blood glucose monitoring techniques have made urine testing a second choice in monitoring glucose levels. Urine tests provide only a reflection of blood glucose levels, whereas capillary blood glucose monitoring methods provide actual blood glucose levels. Self blood glucose monitoring has become a part of the standard care plan for people with labile or brittle diabetes and those on continuous subcutaneous insulin infusion and for pregnant women with diabetes mellitus. It is recommended for persons with both type I and type II diabetes mellitus who wish to maintain normal blood sugar levels. Capillary blood glucose monitoring is also the method of choice for testing and treating patients with diabetic ketoacidosis.

Glycosylated hemoglobin

This test measures the amount of glycosylated hemoglobin (hemoglobin into which glucose has been incorporated) present in the blood. Normally hemoglobin does not contain glucose when it is manufactured and released from the bone marrow. During its 120-day life span in the red blood cell, 5% to 8% of the hemoglobin A_1 normally becomes glycosylated to form glycohemoglobin A_{1a}. In diabetes with hyperglycemia, the increase in glycohemoglobin is usually caused by an increase in hemoglobin A_{1c}. A hemoglobin A_{1c} value of 11% to 15% indicates poor control over time. Because glucose entry into the red blood cell is not insulin dependent, the rate at which glucose becomes attached to the hemoglobin molecule depends on blood sugar. Glycosylation is essentially irreversible; hence, the level of glycosylated hemoglobin present in the blood provides an index of blood sugar levels over the previous 2 months or more.

Urine tests

Two types of tests are used to measure glucose content in the urine—copper reduction and glucose oxidase tests. Clinitest uses a copper-reduction reagent that is responsive to a number of substances. Consequently, Clinitest may give false-positive results. The glucose oxidase tests (Tes-Tape, Clinistix, and Diastix) contain an enzyme that specifically reacts with glucose. Certain substances, such as urine ketones, interfere with color changes in the glucose oxidase tests and in some situations may produce a false-negative result. The glucose oxidase tests are very sensitive to small amounts of glucose and are usually not recommended for use in children. The actual amount of glucose (milligram percent or milligrams/100 ml urine), represented by the results of the various tests as 1+, 2+, 3+, and 4+, also varies. For example, a 2+ result with Clinitest is representative of ¾ mg% glucose; with Diastix, it represents ½ mg% glucose; and with TesTape, ¼ mg%. Because many factors affect the accuracy of both types of urine tests, the reader is referred to other literature sources, including the package insert that comes with the urine testing reagent. The pharmacist is a valuable resource when the effect of a specific drug on urine testing methods is under consideration.

Diabetic diet

Diet therapy is usually prescribed to meet the specific needs of each person with diabetes. Goals and principles of diet therapy differ between type I and type II diabetes as well as between lean and obese persons.

A task force of the American Diabetes Association met in 1986 to develop nutritional recommendations and principles for persons with diabetes mellitus. These recommendations are similar to those of the American Heart Association, the American Cancer Society, the Nutritional Committee for Recommendations for Children with Diabetes of the American Academy of Pediatrics, and the 1985 U.S. Dietary Guidelines.[30] The task force recommended that: (1) calories should be prescribed to achieve and maintain a desirable weight with additional allocation of calories to provide for growth and metabolic needs in children and pregnant or lactating women, (2) carbohydrates should be liberalized, ideally up to 55% to 65% of the total calories, and individualized, with the amount depending on blood sugar, lipid levels, and individual eating patterns, (3) the recommended dietary allowance (RDA) for protein of 0.8 g/kg of body weight for adults should be used and modified if needed, and (4) total fat should compromise less than 30% of the diet and cholesterol should be less than 300 mg/day.

In the obese person with type II diabetes, the principles of diet therapy are different. Dietary interventions are directed toward weight reduction, improvement in blood glucose and lipid levels, and consistency in day-to-day nutrient intake. These interventions include: (1) well-balanced and nutritious meals, (2) control of calories for weight loss and achievement of ideal body weight, (3) control of monosaccharides in the diet, and (4) distribution of carbohydrate, protein, and fat according to individual desires and need for weight management.

Several methods of dietary control can be used. One method is the free diet, which essentially allows the person eat in a method that is satisfying but avoids concentrated sugars. A complete diet history should be taken before this method is suggested. This method may be acceptable for persons who have already established therapeutic eating habits. A second method involves weighing food. This method is difficult for many people but may be useful for those who are having difficulty in portion control.

The third and most frequently prescribed meal plan is the exchange system.[31] In this system, foods are divided into six categories. Each food in a particular category (in the amount designated) has an equivalent amount of carbohydrate, protein, and fat. The six exchange categories are milk, meats, fruits, breads or grains, vegetables, and fats. The foods within each category are interchangeable in the prescribed amounts. For example, in the fruit list, one-half cup of orange juice can be exchanged for one-fourth cup of grape juice or half a grapefruit. In the meat group, one egg can be exchanged for 1 oz of cheese or 1 oz of chicken. Fats are included based on whether or not the meat choices are lean, medium, or high in fat content. Polyunsaturated fats are encouraged to avoid problems with hyperlipidemia. The exchange system is easy to learn and provides a highly nutritious well-balanced diet.

Recently there has been much controversy over high-fiber and carbohydrate content in the diabetic diet. It is believed that high-fiber, complex-carbohydrate diets prevent large fluctuations in blood glucose levels, thereby providing better glucose control. For some persons with diabetes, pasta provides better glucose control curves than potatoes; rice may provide better control curves than bread. These concepts are particularly important during pregnancy, in which the goal is to maintain glucose levels between 60 mg/dl and 120 mg/dl. Even mild hyperglycemia has been shown to be detrimental to the fetus; increased episodes of hyperglycemia have been shown to cause significant increases in congenital anomalies. The recommendation that pregnant women with diabetes avoid monosaccharides and include high-fiber complex carbohydrates in their diets is now widely accepted. In some instances, milk and other complex carbohydrate sources are used to treat hypoglycemia for the primary purpose of avoiding counterregulatory responses.

In addition to improved glycemic response, other benefits of fiber may include lowering of low-density lipoprotein cholesterol and total cholesterol and improving the satiety of a meal. The best fiber to achieve this is the soluble fiber variety of foods that include legumes, oat bran, barley, and fruits. The insoluble variety, which is most effective for relief of constipation, includes wheat bran and whole grains. A practical goal of fiber intake should be 40 g/day to achieve beneficial effects.

Two-thirds of adults who have diabetes also have hypertension. For this reason, reducing daily sodium is desirable. The American Heart Association and the American Diabetes Association suggest a daily intake of 3000 mg. This can be achieved by choosing foods naturally low in sodium and by modifying cooking habits to use less salt. Given the complications and risks presented to persons with diabetes, the low-sodium diet may be useful in preventing complications.

Sucrose (common table sugar) should be limited not because of its glycemic response, but because its long-term effects coupled with increased lipid levels may lead to cardiovascular disease. In addition, sucrose is considered an empty-calorie food. Moderate use of an alternative low-calorie sweetener by persons with diabetes is acceptable. Excessive use of any food is not without adverse effects.

The American Diabetes Association provides literature with more detailed information on diet therapy and patient education. Included is the method of calculating individual meal plans. Nutritionists are valuable resources to the nurse, physician, and patient and should be included in diet management.

Hypoglycemic agents and therapy

There are two forms of hypoglycemic agents—the oral sulfonylureas and injectable insulin. Phenformin, a previously used oral hypoglycemic agent, was discontinued from general use in the United States in 1977 following a directive from the U.S. Department of Health, Education, and Welfare. This was because of a very toxic side effect, lactic acidosis.

Sulfonylureas

The sulfonylureas are thought to cause the release of insulin from the pancreas and to increase insulin binding and the number of insulin receptors. This means that these agents are effective only when some residual beta-cell function remains. They cannot be substituted for insulin in the person with insulin-dependent diabetes who has an absolute insulin deficiency. Both first- and second-generation sulfonylurea preparations are now available. The second-generation compounds are considered to be more potent than the first-generation agents. Glipizide is the new-

Table 45–2. Sulfonylurea preparations: half-life and duration of action

Sulfonylurea preparations	Half-life (hr)	Duration of action (hr)
First generation		
Tolbutamide (Orinase)	4–6	6–12
Tolazamide (Tolinase)	7	10–14
Acetohexamide (Dymelor)	5–7	12–14
Chlorpropamide (Diabinese)	36	Up to 60
Second generation		
Glyburide (Micronase)	10	24
Glipizide (Glucotrol)	4	≤24

est of the second-generation drugs. This compound appears to be the most potent secretagogue of its generation, both for first-phase insulin secretion and in long-term sustained stimulation.[32] These preparations differ in dose and duration of action (Table 45-2). Because the sulfonylureas increase the rate at which glucose is removed from the blood, it is important to recognize that these drugs can cause hypoglycemic reactions.

—— Insulin

Insulin-dependent diabetes requires treatment with insulin. Insulin is destroyed in the gastrointestinal tract and must be administered by injection. All insulin is measured in units, the international unit of insulin being defined as the amount of insulin required to lower the blood sugar of a fasting 2-kg rabbit from 145 mg to 120 mg/100 ml blood. Insulin preparations are categorized according to onset, peak, and duration of action. There are three principal types of insulin: short, intermediate, and long acting (Table 45-3). Insulin is supplied in U40, U100, and U500 (units per milliliter) strengths, with U100 being the most common. Insulin regimens using two or three daily injections of regular insulin or regular mixed with intermediate-acting insulin are being used more often. These regimens provide a blood glucose level that is within a more normal physiologic range than that provided by the once-a-day injection.

In the last 10 years, many companies have entered the insulin-manufacturing market. To date, 46 different types of insulin preparation are available.[33] After much research, human insulin has also become available. The current manufacture of human insulin uses recombinant DNA.[34] Because of this manufacturing method, human insulin is slightly more expensive than beef/pork mixtures or pure beef insulin but less expensive than pure pork insulin. Beef insulin differs from human insulin by three amino acids, and pork insulin differs from human insulin by one amino acid. Many people with diabetes develop antibodies to beef and pork insulin. The use of human insulin has the potential for eliminating these problems. However, a change from pork or beef to human insulin should be carefully monitored because hypoglycemia can occur from an increased receptivity to the human insulin.

Table 45–3. Insulin: activity peak and duration of action

Type of preparation	Activity peak (hr)	Duration (hr)
Rapid-acting		
Insulin injection (regular, crystalline zinc, Actrapid, Humulin-R, Velosulin)	½–3	5–7
Prompt insulin zinc suspension (Semilente, Semitard)	1–4	12–16
Intermediate-acting		
Isophane insulin suspension (NPH, Humulin-N, Protophane)	8–12	18–24
Insulin zinc suspension (Lente, Monotard, Lentard, Insulatard)	8–12	18–24
Combination of rapid-acting and intermediate-acting		
Insulin injection plus isophane insulin suspension (Mixtard 30:70)	½–3	18–24
Long-acting		
Protamine zinc insulin suspension (PZI)	8–16	24–36
Insulin zinc suspension extended (Ultralente, Ultratard)	8–16	24–36

Continuous subcutaneous insulin infusion

Recent technologic advances have provided the means for improving control of diabetes through the use of continuous subcutaneous insulin infusion (CSII).[35,36] The method closely simulates the normal pattern of insulin secretion by the body. A basal insulin level is maintained, and bolus doses of regular insulin are delivered prior to meals. Multiple split-dose insulin injection management can also achieve this level of control. The choice of management is determined by the person with diabetes.

The CSII technique involves the subcutaneous insertion of a small needle into the abdomen. Tubing from the needle is connected to a syringe, which is set into a small infusion pump worn on a belt or in a jacket pocket. The computer-operated pump then delivers a set basal amount of insulin. In addition to the basal amount delivered by the pump, a bolus amount of insulin may be delivered when needed by pushing a button. Self blood glucose monitoring is a necessity when using this method of management. Each basal and bolus dose is determined individually and programmed into the computer of the infusion pump. Only those persons who are highly motivated to do frequent blood glucose tests and to make daily insulin adjustments are candidates for this method of injection.

Examples of CSII pumps are the CPI, Minimed, and Autosyringe. Because this method is no longer considered experimental, many health insurance companies cover the cost. Although the pump's safety has been proven, strict attention must be paid to signs of hypoglycemia. People with diabetes who do not sense hypoglycemia or whose counterregulatory response is impaired are not candidates for the CSII technique.

Artificial pancreas

Some institutions use the artificial pancreas (Biostator) to regulate persons with diabetes who have extremely labile glucose levels or to study patients for new methods of glucose control. The artificial pancreas is a large machine that senses blood glucose levels and delivers the correct amount of insulin by means of computer analysis. Glucose levels can be documented as frequently as every 10 seconds, and insulin can be delivered at regular intervals. Two intravenous lines are maintained, one for glucose sampling and the other for insulin delivery. Approximately 2 ml of blood are removed every hour for glucose determination. Therefore, children must be monitored frequently for blood losses if they are on the machine. As the artificial pancreas maintains blood glucose levels in a preestablished range, graphs are recorded and printed by the computer. Calculations are then produced that aid in glucose management after the person is disconnected from the machine and returns to normal activity. Although the artificial pancreas is large, research is being done to miniaturize the entire system so that it can be used for the management of persons with diabetes outside the hospital environment.

Pancreas transplantation

Pancreas transplantation is being performed with increased frequency and success rate for the treatment of diabetes. Islet cell transplants have proven largely unsuccessful in terms of establishing a permanent insulin-independent normoglycemic state, and at this time pancreas transplantation is the only practical method of total endocrine replacement therapy for persons with diabetes. When successful, pancreas transplants can restore carbohydrate metabolism to normal or nearly normal. Between 1966 and 1986, 852 pancreas transplants were performed in the United States.[37] Since 1983, overall graft survival rates have been greater than 40%.[37] The indications for pancreas transplant are early nephropathy, progressive retinopathy, neuropathy, or extreme difficulty with diabetic management. Persons with pancreas transplants require immunosuppression, usually a combination of cyclosporin, azathioprine, and prednisone, to prevent transplant rejection.[38,39] The procedure is often done on persons who need a kidney transplant and require immunosuppression for that purpose.[38]

A variety of transplant methods have been used and are classified according to whether a whole pancreas or segment of the pancreas is used and according to the technique used for management of the pancreatic duct (occlusion or drainage). For segmental transplant procedures, the body and tail of the pancreas (approximately 50%) are removed from the donor.[38] The segmental approach allows pancreatic grafts from living related donors. Donors who have normal glucose tolerance levels prior to partial pancreatectomy are usually normal following donation. Cadaver donors are used for entire pancreas transplants. The pancreatic graft is placed intraperitoneally, and provision for drainage of pancreatic exocrine secretions is established by anastomosis of the pancreatic duct to either the intestine or the urinary system (ureter or bladder) of the recipient. Duct ligation was done in early transplant cases, but this method is infrequently used with present methods of transplantation.[38]

As with kidney transplantation, pancreas transplants are not lifesaving procedures. However, they do afford the potential for significantly improving the quality of life. For the present, the most serious problem is the requirement for immunosuppression and the need for diagnosis and treatment of rejection.

Exercise

Exercise has long been credited with improving glucose tolerance and decreasing blood lipid levels. So important is exercise in the management of diabetes that a planned program of regular exercise is usually considered to be an integral part of the therapeutic regimen for every person with diabetes.

During short-term exercise, the uptake of glucose into the exercising muscle increases 7-fold to 20-fold. Blood levels of insulin tend to regulate glucose release by the liver. In the nondiabetic person, exercise is accompanied by an adrenergically induced decrease in insulin release from the beta cells and an increased breakdown of liver glycogen stores with the release of glucose into the bloodstream. When exercise is prolonged for more than 2 hours, the exercising muscles obtain the greater amount of their energy from fatty acids, and glucose release from the liver is derived from gluconeogenesis.

In the person with IDDM, the beneficial effects of exercise are accompanied by an increased risk of hypoglycemia. The reasons for a decrease in blood sugar levels during exercise in persons with IDDM are twofold. First, there is often an increased absorption of insulin from the insulin injection site. This increased absorption is more pronounced when insulin is injected into the subcutaneous tissue of the exercised muscle, but it seems to occur even when insulin is injected into other body areas. Second, because the person with IDDM cannot reduce blood insulin levels, glucose release by the liver is reduced. However, for the person with IDDM who exercises during periods of poor control (when blood glucose levels are elevated and ketonemia is present), control of the diabetes will usually deteriorate further, and blood sugar and ketone levels will rise to higher levels. This is because the liver has already begun to produce glucose and ketones because of a preexisting insulin deficiency, and the additional stress of exercise causes a further increase.

In some persons with IDDM, the symptoms of hypoglycemia occur many hours after cessation of exercise. This may be because subsequent insulin doses (in persons using multiple daily insulin injections) are not adjusted to accommodate the exercise-induced decrease in blood sugars. The cause of hypoglycemia in persons who do not administer a second insulin dose is unclear. It may be related to the fact that skeletal muscles increase their uptake of glucose following exercise as a means of replenishing their glycogen stores or that the liver and skeletal muscles are more sensitive to insulin during this period of time. Persons with IDDM should be aware that delayed hypoglycemia may occur following exercise and that there may be a need to alter either their insulin dose and/or their carbohydrate intake.

Although of benefit to persons with diabetes, exercise must be weighed on the risk–benefit scale. For patients with complications, vigorous exercise can be harmful and can cause eye hemorrhage as well as other problems. If poorly controlled, exercise can cause a further deterioration in blood glucose levels. Because most sporadic exercise has only transient benefits, a regular exercise or training program is the most beneficial. It is not only better for cardiovascular conditioning, but can maintain a muscle–fat ratio that enhances peripheral insulin receptivity.

In summary, the diagnosis of diabetes mellitus is based on clinical signs of the disease, including the presence of glucose in the urine and the blood. The glucose tolerance test is an important screening method for diabetes. It involves the body's response to a given amount of concentrated glucose, using blood sugar levels. In persons with insulin-dependent diabetes, the self-use of capillary glucose testing provides a means of maintaining near-normal blood sugar levels through frequent monitoring of blood glucose and adjustment of insulin dosage. Urine sugars provide an indirect method of monitoring glucose levels and may also be used in the management of diabetes. Glycosylation involves the attachment of glucose to the hemoglobin molecule; it is an irreversible process. The measurement of glycosylated hemoglobin provides an index of blood sugar levels over several months. The treatment of diabetes includes diet, exercise, and, in many cases, the use of a hypoglycemic agent. Dietary management focuses on maintaining a well-balanced diet, controlling calories to achieve and maintain an optimum weight, and regulating the distribution of carbohydrates, proteins, and fats. Two types of hypoglycemic agents are used in the management of diabetes: injectable insulin and the oral sulfonylurea drugs. Type I diabetes requires treatment with injectable insulin. The sulfonylurea agents increase insulin release from the pancreas, the number of insulin receptors, and the binding of insulin to these receptors. These drugs require a functioning pancreas and may be used in the treatment of noninsulin-dependent diabetes mellitus. Exercise improves glucose tolerance and reduces blood lipid levels. The presence of insulin in the blood impairs glucose release by the liver. Blood levels of injected insulin cannot be controlled by physiologic feedback mechanisms; therefore, the beneficial effects of exercise in persons with insulin-dependent diabetes are accompanied by an increased risk of hypoglycemia.

References

1. Waif SO (ed): Diabetes Mellitus. Indianapolis, Eli Lilly, 1980

2. Cryor PE, Gerich JE: Glucose counterregulation, hypoglycemia, and intensive insulin therapy in diabetes mellitus. N Engl J Med 313:232, 1985

3. Unger RH: The essential role of glucagon in pathogenesis of diabetes mellitus. Lancet 1:14, 1985

4. Guyton A: Medical Physiology, 7th ed, pp 888, 910. Philadelphia, WB Saunders, 1986

5. Press M, Tamborlane WV, Sherwin RS: Importance of raised growth hormone levels in mediating the metabolic derangements of diabetes. N Engl J Med 310:810, 1984

6. National Diabetes Data Group: Classification and diagnosis of diabetes mellitus and other categories of glucose intolerance. Diabetes 28:1039, 1979

7. Eisenbarth GS: Type I diabetes mellitus: A chronic autoimmune disease. N Engl J Med 314:1360, 1986

8. Skyler JS, Rabinovitch A: Etiology and pathogenesis of insulin dependent diabetes mellitus. Pediatr Ann 16:682, 1987

9. Gamble DR, Taylor KW: Seasonal incidence of diabetes mellitus. Br Med J 3:631, 1969

10. MacMillan DR, Kotoyan M, Zeidner D et al: Seasonal variations in the onset of diabetes in children. Pediatrics 59:113, 1977

11. Sulz HA, Hart BA, Zielezny M et al: Is mumps virus an etiologic factor in juvenile diabetes mellitus? Preliminary report. J Pediatr 86:654, 1975

12. Yoon JW, Onodera T, Jensen AB et al: Virus-induced diabetes mellitus, XI. Replication of Coxsackie B 3 virus in human pancreatic beta cell cultures. Diabetes 27:778, 1978

13. Johnson GM, Tudor RB: Diabetes mellitus and congenital rubella infection. Am J Dis Child 120:453, 1970

14. Plotkin SA, Kaye R: Diabetes mellitus and congenital rubella. Pediatrics 46:450, 1970

15. Tuomilehto J, Wolf E: Primary prevention of diabetes. Diabetes Care 10:238, 1987

16. Karam JH: Therapeutic dilemmas in type II diabetes mellitus—Improving and maintaining B-cell and insulin sensitivity. West J Med 148:685, 1988

17. Kissebah AH, Vydelingum N, Murray M et al: Relation of body fat distribution to metabolic complications of obesity. J Clin Endocrinol Metab 54:254, 1982

18. Kalkoff RK, Hartz AH, Rupley D et al: Relationship of body fat distribution to blood pressure, carbohydrate tolerance, and plasma lipids in healthy obese women. J Lab Clin Med 102:621, 1983

19. Whitehouse FW: Two minutes with diabetes: "My patient is not responding and is very dehydrated." Med Times 101:35, 1970

20. Podolsky S: Hyperosmolar nonketotic coma in the elderly diabetic. Med Clin North Am 62(4):816, 1978

21. Joslin EP, Gray H, Root HL: Insulin in hospital and home. J Metabol Res 2:651, 1924

22. Somogyi M: Exacerbation of diabetes in excess insulin action. Am J Med 26:169, 1957

23. Bolli GB, Gotterman IS, Campbell PJ: Glucose counterregulation and waning of insulin in the Somogyi phenomenon (posthypoglycemic hyperglycemia). N Engl J Med 311:1214, 1984

24. Ditzel J, Standl E: The problem of tissue oxygenation in diabetes mellitus. Acta Med Scand (Suppl 578):49, 1975

25. Carlin BW: Impotence and diabetes. Metabolism 37:19, 1988

26. Centers for Disease Control: Screening for diabetic eye disease—Mississippi. MMWR 32(12):157, 1983

27. Browner WS: Preventable complications of diabetes mellitus. West J Med 145:701, 1986

28. LoGerfo FW, Coffman JD: Vascular and microvascular disease of the foot in diabetes. N Engl J Med 311:1615, 1984

29. Skyler JS: Patient self-monitoring of blood glucose. Clin Diabetes 1(4):12, 1983

30. American Diabetes Association: Nutritional recommendations and principles for individuals with diabetes mellitus: 1986. Diabetes Care 10:126, 1987

31. American Diabetes Association: Exchange Lists for Meal Planning. New York, 1976

32. Shuman CR: Glipizide: An overview. Am J Med 74:55, 1983

33. Karam JH, Etzwiler DD: Insulins: Overview and outlook. Clin Diabetes 1(4):1, 1983

34. Skyler JS (ed): Symposium on human insulin of recombinant DNA origin. Diabetes Care 5(Suppl 2):1, 1982

35. Felig P, Bergman M: Insulin pump treatment of diabetes. JAMA 250:1045, 1983

36. American Diabetes Association (Policy Statement): Indications for use of continuous insulin delivery systems and self-measurement of blood glucose. Diabetes Care 5:140, 1982

37. Sutherland DER, Moudry KC: Clinical pancreas and islet transplantation. Transplant Proc 19:113, 1987

38. Sutherland DER, Moudry KC: Pancreas transplant registry report. Transplant Proc 19:5, 1987

39. Sutherland DER, Goetz FC, Najarian JS: Current status of transplantation of the pancreas. Adv Surg 20:303, 1987

Bibliography

American Diabetes Association (Position Statement): Gestational diabetes mellitus. Diabetes Care 9(4):430, 1986

American Diabetes Association (Consensus Statement): Self-monitoring of blood glucose. Diabetes Care 10(1):75, 1987

Anderson JW: Dietary fiber and diabetes: A comprehensive review and practical application. J Am Diet Assoc 87:1189, 1987

Ashbury AK: Understanding diabetic neuropathy. N Engl J Med 319:577, 1988

Ashbury AK, Porte D (cochair): Consensus statement: Report and recommendations of the San Antonio Conference on Diabetic Neuropathy. Diabetes 37:1000, 1988

Bantle JP: The dietary treatment of diabetes mellitus. Med Clin North Am 72:1285, 1988

Bays HE, Pfeifer MA: Peripheral diabetic neuropathy. Med Clin North Am 72:1439, 1988

Bolli GB, Dimitriadis GD, Pehling BA et al: Abnormal glucose counterregulation after subcutaneous insulin in insulin-dependent diabetes mellitus. N Engl J Med 310:1706, 1984

Cahill GF: Hyperglycemic hyperosmolar coma. J Am Geriatr Soc 31:103, 1983

Duck SD, Wyatt DT: Factors associated with brain herniation in the treatment of diabetic ketoacidosis. J Pediatr 113:10, 1988

Ferner RE: Oral hypoglycemic agents. Med Clin North Am 72:1323, 1988

Foster DW, McGarry JD: The metabolic derangements and treatment of diabetic ketoacidosis. N Engl J Med 309:159, 1983

Freinkel N, Dooley SL, Metzker BE: Care of the pregnant woman with insulin-dependent diabetes mellitus. N Engl J Med 31:96, 1985

Fulop M: The treatment of severely uncontrolled diabetes mellitus. Adv Intern Med 29:327, 1984

Goldstein DE: Is glycosylated hemoglobin clinically useful? N Engl J Med 310:384, 1984

Greene D: The pathogenesis and prevention of diabetic neuropathy and nephropathy. Metabolism 37(Suppl 1):25, 1988

Gulan M, Gotteman IS, Zinman B: Biosynthetic human insulin improves postprandial glucose excursions in type I diabetes. Ann Intern Med 107:506, 1987

Horton ES: Exercise and diabetes mellitus. Med Clin North Am 72:1301, 1988

Kahn CR: Insulin resistance. N Engl J Med 315:252, 1986

Kitabchi AE, Fisher JN, Matteri R: The use of continuous insulin delivery systems in treatment of diabetes mellitus. Adv Intern Med 28:49, 1983

Kitabchi AE, Murphy MB: Diabetic ketoacidosis and hyperosmolar hyperglycemic nonketotic coma. Med Clin North Am 72:1545, 1988

Klein R: Recent developments in the understanding and management of diabetic retinopathy. Med Clin North Am 72:1415, 1988

Krane EJ, Rockhoff MA, Wallman JK et al: Subclinical brain swelling in children during treatment of diabetic ketoacidosis. N Engl J Med 312:1147, 1985

Kreisberg RA: Aging, glucose metabolism, and diabetes: Current concepts. Geriatrics 42:67, 1987

Kroc Collaborative Study: Blood glucose control and the evolution of diabetic retinopathy and albuminuria. N Engl J Med 311:365, 1984

Martin DB: Type II diabetes. N Engl J Med 314:1314, 1986

Mogensen CE, Christensen CK: Predicting diabetic nephropathy in insulin-dependent patients. N Engl J Med 311:89, 1984

Moller DE, Flier JS: Problems with insulin resistance. Hosp Pract 23(Oct 30):83, 1988

Powers MA (ed): American Diabetes Association, Inc., and The American Diabetic Association: Nutrition guide for professionals: Diabetes education and meal planning. New York, American Diabetes Association, 1988

Rayfield EJ, Ault MJ, Keusch GT: Infection and diabetes: The case of glucose control. Am J Med 72:439, 1982

Robbins DC, Tager HS, Rubenstein AH: Biologic and clinical importance of proinsulin. N Engl J Med 310:1165, 1984

Roberts M: Diabetes and stress: A type A connection. Psychology Today 21(July):22, 1987

Rosenbloom AL: Primary and subspecialty care of diabetes mellitus in children and youth. Med Clin North Am 31(1):107, 1984

Ruderman NB, Schneider S: Exercise and the insulin-dependent diabetic. Hosp Pract 21(May 30):41, 1986

Skyler JS: Insulin pharmacology. Med Clin North Am 72:1337, 1988

Skyler JS: Why control blood glucose. Pediatr Ann 16:713, 1987

Stolar MW: Atherosclerosis in diabetes: The role of hyperinsulinemia. Metabolism 37(2):1, 1988

Symposium on Human Insulin. Diabetes Care 6(Suppl 1) (March/April): (entire issue) 1983

Ward GM: The insulin receptor concept and its relation to the treatment of diabetes. Drugs 33:156, 1987

Webb SM, Castaner MF: Glucose counterregulation in diabetic autonomic neuropathy. Clin Physiol 7:66, 1987

Wood FC, Bierman EL: Is diet the cornerstone in management of diabetes. N Engl J Med 315:1224, 1986

Alterations in Neuromuscular Function

Robin L. Curtis

CHAPTER 46

Organization and Control of Neural Function

Organization of the nervous system
 Hierarchy of control
 Central and peripheral nervous systems
 Soma and viscera
 Terminology

Segmental organization of the nervous system
 Cell columns
 Longitudinal tracts
Nervous tissue cells
 Neurons
 Supporting cells
 Metabolic requirements

Nerve cell communication
 Impulse generation and conduction
 Synaptic transmission
 Messenger molecules

Objectives

After you have studied this chapter, you should be able to meet the following objectives:

_____ State the difference between the CNS and PNS.

_____ Cite the significance of the hierarchy of control levels of the CNS.

_____ Use the segmental approach to explain the development of the nervous system and the organization of the postembryonic nervous system.

_____ Explain the difference between the viscera and the soma of a body segment.

_____ State the origin and destination of nerve fibers contained in the dorsal and ventral roots.

_____ Define ganglia, cell column, and tract.

_____ State the type of structures that are innervated by general somatic afferent, general visceral afferent, special sensory afferent, general visceral efferent, special visceral efferent, and general somatic efferent neurons.

_____ State the function of association neurons in the nervous system.

_____ Name and describe the anatomy of the three parts of a neuron.

_____ State the function of the supporting cells of the nervous system.

_____ Describe the function of Schwann's cells with reference to the node of Ranvier.

_____ State the function of the myelin sheath.

_____ Define conductance.

_____ Describe the interaction of the presynaptic and postsynaptic terminals.

_____ Explain the occurrence of both spatial and temporal summation.

_____ State the difference in structure of the three types of neurotransmitters: amino acids, monoamines, and neuropeptides.

_____ Briefly describe how neurotransmitters are synthesized, stored, released, and inactivated.

_____ Describe current thinking on how alterations in neurotransmitter release or action can alter body function.

The nervous system, in coordination with the endocrine system, provides the means by which cell and tissue functions are integrated into a solitary, surviving organism. It controls skeletal muscle movement and helps to regulate cardiac and visceral smooth muscle activity. The nervous system makes possible the reception, integration, and perception of sensory information; it provides for memory and problem solving; and it facilitates adjustment to an ever-changing external environment. No part of the nervous system functions separately from other parts; and in the human, who is a thinking and feeling creature, the effects of emotion can exert a strong influence on both neural and hormonal control of body function. On the other hand, alterations in both neural and endocrine function (particularly at the biochemical level) can exert a strong influence on psychologic behavior.

This chapter is divided into three parts: the organization of the nervous system, nervous tissue cells, and neuronal communication.

Organization of the nervous system

Hierarchy of control

The development of the nervous system can be traced far back into evolutionary history. In the course of its development, newer functional features and greater complexity resulted from the modification and enlargement of more primitive structures. In a moving organism, rapid reaction to environmental danger, to potential food sources, or to a sexual partner was required for the survival of the species. Thus, the front, or rostral, end of the central nervous system became specialized as a means of sensing the external environment and controlling reactions to it. In time, the ancient organization, which is largely retained in the spinal cord segments, was expanded in the forward segments of the nervous system. Of these, the most forward have undergone the most radical modification and have developed into the forebrain: the diencephalon and the cerebral hemispheres. The dominance of the front end of the central nervous system is reflected in a hierarchy of control levels—brain stem over spinal cord, forebrain over brain stem. Because the newer functions were added onto the outside of older functional systems and because the newer functions became concentrated at the rostral end of the nervous system, they are much more vulnerable to injury. These three principles—(1) no part of the nervous system functions independently of the other parts, (2) newer systems control older systems, and (3) the newer systems are more vulnerable to injury—form a basis for understanding many of the manifestations that occur when the nervous system suffers injury or disease.

The central and peripheral nervous systems

The nervous system can be divided into two parts—the central nervous system (CNS) and the peripheral nervous system (PNS). The CNS consists of the brain and spinal cord, which is located within the protected confines of the axial skeleton (cranium and spinal column). The PNS is located outside these structures. The basic design of the nervous system provides for the concentration of computational and control functions within the CNS. In this design, the PNS functions as an input–output system for relaying input to the CNS and for transmitting output messages that control effector organs, such as muscles and glands.

The functioning cells of the nervous system are called *neurons.* Neurons have branching cytoplasm-filled processes, the dendrites and the axons, which project from the cell body and are unique to the nervous system. The axonal processes are particularly designed for rapid communication with other neurons and the many body structures that are innervated by the nervous system. Afferent, or sensory, neurons transmit information from the PNS to the CNS. Efferent, or motor neurons, carry information away from the CNS. Interspersed between the afferent and efferent neurons is a network of interconnecting neurons that serve to modulate and control the body's response to changes in the internal and external environments. These interconnecting networks facilitate the establishment of response patterns and allow for storage of information on which learning and memory are based. Complex neural networks provide the means for subjective experiences, such as perception and emotion. These also provide for intelligence, judgment, and anticipation of events.

The soma and viscera

On cross section, the body is organized into a soma and a viscera (Figure 46-1). The soma, or body wall, includes all of the structures derived from the embryonic ectoderm, such as the epidermis of the skin and the CNS. A migrating ectodermal derivative called the *neural crest* is the source of many cell types, including the pigment cells of the dermis and afferent and autonomic ganglion neurons of the PNS. The mesodermal connective tissues of the soma include the dermis of the skin, skeletal muscle, bone, and the outer lining of the body cavity (somatic pleura and somatic peritoneum). *For the nervous system,* all of the

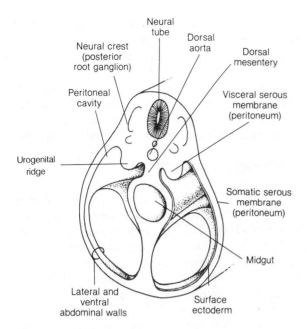

Figure 46-1 Cross section of a human embryo, illustrating the development of somatic and visceral structures.

more internal structures constitute the viscera, including the great vessels derived from the intermediate mesoderm, the urinary system, and the gonadal structures. The viscera also includes the inner lining of the body cavities, such as the visceral pleura and peritoneum, and the mesodermal tissues that surround the entoderm-lined gut and its derivative organs (lungs, liver, and pancreas).

There are both somatic and visceral nerves. The *somatic nerves* innervate the skeletal muscle and the smooth muscle and glands of the skin and body wall. The *visceral nerves* supply the visceral organs of the body, transmitting information through the autonomic nerves in the PNS to control the smooth and cardiac muscle as well as the glands of the visceral organs. This visceral system is largely of reflex, or involuntary, function.

Terminology

One aspect of understanding the nervous system has to do with orientation of the nervous system in relation to the body. Structures that are located toward the front of the body are described as being in an *anterior* or *ventral* position and those that are located toward the back are *posterior* or *dorsal*. The term *superior* indicates upper, and *inferior* indicates lower. The term *cephalic*, which also means head end, is sometimes used to indicate a superior position and *caudal*, an inferior position. Another important term is the Latin word *rostrum* (beak); it refers to the front end in the embryo and to the region of the nose and mouth in postembryonic life. Other terms that are used to describe the position of nervous system structures are

medial, which means near the middle, and *lateral*, which means toward the side or furthest from the middle. A *proximal* structure is one that is located nearest the trunk, and a *distal* structure is one that is located furthest from the trunk. An *afferent* nerve fiber is one that conveys information toward the CNS, and an *efferent* nerve fiber is one that conveys information away from the CNS.

Segmental organization of the nervous system

Throughout life, the organization of the nervous system retains many patterns that were established during early embryonic life. It is this early pattern of organization that is presented as a framework for understanding the nervous system.

The CNS begins its development as a hollow tube of surface ectoderm that closes and sinks below the skin surface along the longitudinal axis of the embryo. The cephalic portion of the tube becomes the brain, and the more caudal part becomes the spinal cord. In the process of development, the basic organizational pattern of the body is that of a longitudinal series of segments, each repeating the same fundamental pattern (Figure 46-2). Although the early mus-

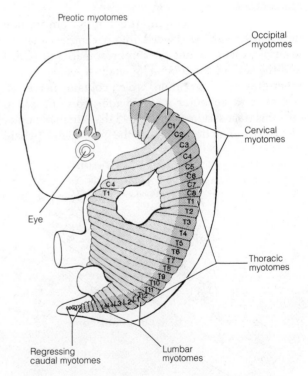

Figure 46-2 The developing muscular system in a 6-week-old embryo. The segmental muscle masses, or myotomes, which give rise to most skeletal muscles, reflect the basic segmental organization of the body and head. Efferent cranial nerves innervating the myotomes of the head are as follows: preotic myotomes (nerves III, IV, and VI), and the occipital myotomes (XII). (*Moore KL: The Developing Human, 2nd ed, p 317. Philadelphia, WB Saunders, 1977*)

cular, skeletal, vascular, and excretory systems and the nerves that supply these somatic and visceral structures have the same segmental pattern, it is the nervous system that most clearly retains this organization in the adult. The CNS and its associated peripheral nerves are thus made up of 43 or so segments, 33 of which form the spinal cord and spinal nerves, and 10, the brain and its cranial nerves (Figure 46-3).

Each segment of the CNS is accompanied by two pairs (one member of a pair on each side) of bundled nerve fibers, or *roots:* a ventral pair and a dorsal pair. Ganglia are collections of nerve cells. The paired dorsal roots interconnect a pair of *dorsal root ganglia* and their corresponding CNS segment. These ganglia contain the afferent nerve cell bodies, each of which has two axon-like processes—one which ends in a peripheral receptor and the other that enters the central neural segment. The axon-like process that enters the central neural segment communicates with a neuron called an *input association (IA) neuron.* Somatic afferents transmit information from the soma to somatic IA neurons, and visceral afferents transmit information from the viscera to visceral IA neurons. The paired ventral roots of each segment are bundles of axons that provide efferent (motor) output to effector sites such as muscle and glandular cells of the body segment.

On cross section, the hollow embryonic neural tube can be divided into a central canal, or ventricle, that contains the cerebrospinal fluid (CSF) and the wall of the tube. The latter develops into an inner gray cellular portion, which contains nerve cell bodies, and an outer white matter portion, which contains tract systems of the CNS that are made up of nerve cells. The dorsal half of the gray matter (where

the sensory IA neurons that communicate with the dorsal roots are located) is called the *dorsal horn.* The ventral portion, or *ventral horn,* contains efferent neurons that communicate by way of the ventral roots with effector cells of the body segment. Many of the CNS neurons develop axons that grow longitudinally as tract systems that intercommunicate between neighboring and distal segments of the neural tube.

Cell columns

The complexity of the organizational structure of the nervous system is somewhat simplified by a pattern in which PNS and CNS neurons are repeated as parallel cell columns running lengthwise along the nervous system. In this organizational pattern, afferent neurons, dorsal horn cells, ventral horn cells, and autonomic ganglion neurons are organized as a series of 12 cell columns. A box of 24 colored beverage straws (2 sets of 12 different colors) can be used as an analogy to represent the cell columns. In this model, each lateral half of the nervous system (right and left sides) is represented in mirror fashion by one set of 12 colored straws. If these straws were cut crosswise (equivalent to a transverse section through the nervous system) at several places along their length, the spatial relationship between these straws would be repeated in each section.

The 12 pairs of cell columns can be further grouped according to their location in the PNS: four in the dorsal ganglia that contain sensory neurons; one that contains peripheral autonomic ganglia and their CNS components; four in the dorsal horn that contain the sensory IA neurons; and three in the ventral horn that contain motor neurons. Each column of dorsal root ganglia projects to its particular column of IA neurons in the dorsal horn. The IA neurons distribute afferent information to local reflex circuitry and more rostal and elaborate segments of the CNS. The ventral roots contain both output association (OA) neurons and lower motor neurons (LMNs). The lower motor neurons provide the final circuitry for organizing efferent nerve activity. The efferent neurons send their axons into the body to innervate skeletal, smooth, or cardiac muscle, and glandular cells.

Between the input association neurons and the output association neurons are chains of small internuncial neurons, which are arranged in complex circuits. The internuncial neurons provide the discreteness, appropriateness, and intelligence of responses to stimuli. Most of the billions of CNS cells in the spinal cord and brain gray matter are internuncial neurons.

The effectiveness of a CNS-mediated response to changed environmental conditions depends on the functional integrity of the neurons and effector

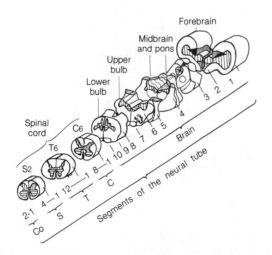

Figure 46-3 The adult human CNS. The dorsal (*vertical hatching*) and ventral (*horizontal hatching*) horns of the gray matter are surrounded by the white matter that contains the longitudinal tracts. Numbers indicate segmental divisions of the neural tube. (*Adapted from Elliott HC: Neuroanatomy. Philadelphia, JB Lippincott, 1969*)

cells in the particular sequence called a *reflex*. A reflex is a highly predictable relationship between a stimulus and a response. It is mediated by the transmission of receptor-derived action potentials in the afferent neurons that stimulate activity in a network of CNS association neurons of the dorsal or ventral gray matter leading to action potentials in efferent neurons. These efferents, in turn, stimulate effector responses in structures such as skeletal, smooth, or cardiac muscle and glands. The activity of these effectors constitutes the reflex response.

Four columns of afferent (sensory) neurons in the dorsal root ganglia directly innervate four corresponding columns of input association neurons in the dorsal horn. These are categorized as special and general afferents. Special somatic afferent fibers are concerned with internal sensory information such as joint and tendon sensation (proprioception). The general somatic afferents innervate the skin and other somatic structures; they respond to stimuli such as those that produce pressure or pain. The general somatic afferent IA column cells relay the sensory information to protective and other reflex circuits and also project the information to the forebrain where it is perceived as painful, warm, cold, and such. The special somatic afferent IA column cells relay their information to local reflexes concerned with posture and movement. These neurons also relay information to the cerebellum, contributing to coordination of movement, and to the forebrain, contributing to experience. Afferents innervating the labyrinth and derived auditory end organs of the inner ear also belong to the special soma category.

General visceral afferent neurons innervate visceral structures such as the gastrointestinal tract and urinary bladder; they project to the general visceral IA column, which relays to vital reflex circuits and sends information to the forebrain regarding visceral sensations of stomach fullness, bladder pressure, sexual experience, and others. Special visceral afferent cells innervate specialized gut-related receptors, such as the taste buds and receptors of the olfactory mucosa. Their central processes communicate with special sensory input association column neurons that project to reflex circuits to produce salivation, chewing, swallowing, and other responses. The forebrain projection fibers from these association cells provide for the sensations of taste (gustation) and smell (olfaction).

The ventral horn contains three separate longitudinal cell columns, each containing OA and efferent neurons: general visceral efferent, branchial efferent, and general somite efferent cell. The OA neurons coordinate and integrate the function of the efferent cells of its column. General visceral efferent neurons transmit the efferent output of the autonomic nervous system and are called *preganglionic neurons*. Their axons project through the segmental ventral roots to innervate smooth and cardiac muscle and glandular cells of the body, most of which are in the viscera. The general visceral efferent cells of the autonomic nervous system are structurally and functionally divided into the sympathetic and parasympathetic nervous system (discussed in Chapter 48). Branchial efferent neurons innervate the branchial arch skeletal muscles: the muscles of mastication, facial expression, head turning, and muscles of the pharynx and larynx. The general somite efferent column neurons supply the somite-derived muscles of the body and head, which include the skeletal muscles of the body, limbs, tongue, and extrinsic eye muscles.

Longitudinal tracts

The gray matter of the cell columns in the CNS is surrounded by bundles of myelinated and unmyelinated axons (white matter) that travel longitudinally along the length of the neural axis. This white matter can be divided into three layers—an inner, a middle, and an outer layer (Figure 46-4). The inner, or *archi*, layer contains short fibers that project for a maximum of about five segments before reentering the gray matter. The middle, or *paleo*, layer projects six or more segments. Both the archi and the paleo layer fibers have many branches, or *collaterals*, that enter the gray matter of intervening segments. The outer, or *neo*, layer contains large-diameter axons that can

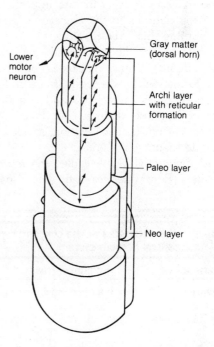

Figure 46-4 The three concentric subdivisions of the tract systems of the white matter. Migration of neurons into the archi layer converts it into the reticular formation of the white matter.

travel the entire length of the nervous system (Table 46-1). The term *suprasegmental* refers to higher levels of the CNS, such as the brain stem and cerebrum and structures above a given CNS segment. Both paleo- and neo-level fibers have suprasegmental projections.

The longitudinal layers are arranged in bundles, or fiber tracts, which contain axons that have the same destination, origin, and function. These longitudinal tracts are named systematically to reflect their origin and destination, the site of origin being named first and the site of destination second. For example, the *spinothalamic tract* originates in the *spinal* cord and terminates in the *thalamus*. The *corticospinal* tract originates in the cerebral *cortex* and ends in the *spinal* cord.

Inner layer. The inner layer of white matter contains the axons of neurons of the gray matter that interconnect with neighboring segments of the nervous system. The axons of this layer permit the pool of motor neurons of several segments to work together as a functional unit. They also allow the afferent neurons of one segment to trigger reflexes that activate motor units in neighboring as well as the same segments. In terms of evolution, this is the oldest of the three layers, and, thus, it is sometimes referred to as the archi-level layer. It is the first of the longitudinal layers to become functional, and it appears to be limited to reflex types of movements. Reflex movements of the fetus (quickening) that begin during the fifth month of intrauterine life involve the inner archi-level layer.

The inner layer of the white matter differs from the other two layers in one important aspect. Many of the neurons in the embryonic gray matter migrate out into this layer, resulting in a rich mixture of neurons and local fibers called the *reticular formation*. The circuitry of most reflexes is contained in the reticular formation. In the brain stem, the reticular formation becomes quite large and contains major portions of vital reflexes, such as those controlling respiration, cardiovascular function, swallowing, and vomiting, to mention a few.

A functional system called the *reticular activation system* (RAS) operates in the lateral portions of the reticular formation of the medulla, pons, and especially the midbrain. The convergence of information from all sensory modalities, including those of the somesthetic, auditory, visual, and visceral afferent nerves, bombards the neurons of this system. The RAS has both descending and ascending portions. The descending portion communicates with all spinal segmental levels through higher-level reticulospinal tracts and serves to facilitate many of the cord-level reflexes. For example, it speeds up reaction time and stabilizes postural reflexes. The ascending portion, sometimes called the *centroencephalic system,* accelerates brain activity, particularly thalamic and cortical activity. This is reflected by the appearance of awake brain-wave patterns. Thus, sudden stimuli not only result in protective and attentive postures but also increased awareness.

Middle layer. The middle layer of the white matter contains most of the major fiber tract systems required for sensation and movement. It contains the spinoreticular and spinothalamic tracts. This system consists of larger-diameter and longer suprasegmental fibers, which ascend to the brain stem and are largely functional at birth. In terms of evolutionary development, these tracts are quite old, and, therefore, this layer is sometimes called the paleo layer. It facilitates many of the primitive functions, such as the "auditory startle reflex," which occurs in response to loud noises. This reflex consists of turning the head and body toward the sound, dilating the pupils of the eyes, catching of the breath, and quickening of the pulse.

Outer layer. The outer layer of the tract systems is the newest of the three layers in terms of evolutionary development, and, hence, is sometimes called the neo layer. It becomes functional at about the second year of life, and it contains the pathways needed for bladder training. Myelination of the neo-layer suprasegmental tracts, which include many of those required for the most delicate coordination and skill, is not complete until sometime around the 10th to the 12th year of life. This includes the development of tracts needed for fine manipulative skills, such as

Table 46–1. Characteristics of the concentric subdivisions of the longitudinal tracts in the white matter of the central nervous system

Characteristics	Archi-level tracts	Paleo-level tracts	Neo-level tracts
Segmental span	Intersegmental (less than five segments)	Suprasegmental (five or more segments)	Suprasegmental
Number of synapses	Multisynaptic	Multisynaptic but fewer than archi-level tracts	Monosynaptic with target structures
Conduction velocity	Very slow	Fast	Fastest
Examples of functional systems	Flexor withdrawal reflex circuitry	Spinothalamic tracts	Corticospinal tracts

the finger–thumb coordination required for the use of many tools and the toe movements needed for acrobatics. Being the newest to evolve and being on the outside of the brain and spinal cord, these tracts are the most vulnerable to injury. When these outer tracts are damaged, the paleo and archi tracts often remain functional, and rehabilitation methods can result in quite effective use of the older systems. Delicacy and refinement may be gone, but basic function remains. For example, a very important outer system, or neosystem, the corticospinal system, permits the fine manipulative control required for writing. If this is lost, paleo-level systems remaining intact permit the grasping and holding of objects. Thus, the hand can still be used to perform its basic functions.

Collateral communication pathways. Axons in the archi and paleo layers characteristically possess many collateral branches, which move into the gray cell columns or synapse with the reticular formation as the axon passes each succeeding CNS segment. Should a major axon be destroyed at some point along its course, these collaterals provide multisynaptic alternative pathways that bypass the local damage. Neo-level tracts do not possess these collaterals but are instead highly discrete as to the target neurons with which they communicate. Because of their discreteness, damage to the neo tracts causes permanent loss of function. Damage to the archi or paleo systems, on the other hand, is usually followed by slow return of function, presumably through the use of these collateral connections. For example, the surgical section of pathways carrying pain impulses (spinothalamic paleo-level tracts) can be used for temporary relief of intractable pain. The pain experience usually returns after some weeks or months. When it does return, it is often poorly localized and sometimes more unpleasant than it was initially. Consequently, this surgical procedure, which is called a tractotomy, is usually reserved for persons who are not expected to survive for longer than a few months.

In summary, the nervous system can be divided into two parts: the CNS and the PNS. The CNS develops from the ectoderm of the early embryo by formation of a hollow tube that closes and sinks below the surface of its longitudinal axis. The cavity of the tube forms the ventricles of the brain and spinal canal, and the side wall develops to form the brain stem and spinal cord. The brain stem and spinal cord are subdivided into the dorsal horn, which contains neurons that receive and process incoming or afferent information, and the ventral horn, which contains efferent motor neurons that handle the final stages of output processing.

The segmental pattern of early embryonic development is retained in the fully developed nervous system. Each one of the 43 or more body segments is interconnected to corresponding CNS or neural tube segments by segmental afferent and efferent neurons. Afferent neurons enter the CNS by way of the dorsal root ganglia and the dorsal roots. Afferent neurons of the dorsal root ganglia are of four types: general somatic afferent, special somatic afferent, general visceral afferent, and special visceral afferent. Each of these afferent neurons synapse with their appropriate input association neurons in the cell columns of the dorsal horn (*e.g.*, general somatic afferents synapse with neurons in the general somatic afferent IA cell column). Efferent fibers from motoneurons in the ventral horn exit the CNS in the ventral roots. General somatic efferent neurons are LMNs that innervate somite-derived skeletal muscles, and general visceral efferent neurons are preganglionic fibers that synapse with postganglionic fibers that innervate visceral structures. This general pattern of afferent and efferent neurons, which is generally repeated in each segment of the body, forms parallel cell columns running lengthwise through the CNS and PNS.

Longitudinal communication between CNS segments is provided by neurons that send the axons into nearby segments by means of the innermost layer of the white matter, the ancient archi-level system of fibers. These cells provide for coordination between neighboring segments. Neurons have invaded this layer, and the mix of these cells and axons, called the reticular formation, is the location of much of the important reflex circuitry of the spinal cord and the brain stem. Paleo-level tracts, which are located outside this layer, provide the longitudinal communication between more distant segments of the nervous system; this layer includes most of the important ascending and descending tracts. The recently evolved neo-level systems, which become functional during infancy and childhood, travel on the outside of the white matter and provide the means for very delicate and discriminative function. The outside position of the neo tracts, as well as their lack of collateral and redundant pathways, makes them the most vulnerable to injury.

Nervous tissue cells

Nervous tissue contains two types of cells—neurons and supporting cells. The neurons are the functional cells of the nervous system. Neurons exhibit membrane excitability and conductivity and secrete neuromediators and hormones, such as epinephrine and antidiuretic hormone. The *supporting cells,* such as Schwann's cells in the PNS and the glial cells in the CNS, function to *protect* the nervous system and *supply* metabolic support for the neurons.

Neurons

To understand the brain and nervous system, it is necessary to understand how neurons are constructed, how they work, and how they communicate with one another. The human brain consists of several trillion cells, each of which must communicate with several thousand others. The average nerve cell ranges in size from 2/100 mm to 4/100 mm, and a synapse measures no more than 1/1000 mm.[1]

Neurons have three distinct parts—the cell body and its cytoplasm-filled processes, the dendrites, and the axons (Figure 46-5). These processes form the functional connections, or synapses, with other nerve cells, with receptor cells, or with effector cells.

The *cell body*, or *soma*, contains a large, vesicular nucleus, one or more distinct nucleoli, and a well-developed endoplasmic reticulum with ribosomes. The nucleus has the same DNA code content that is present in other cells of the body. The nucleoli, which are composed of both DNA and RNA, are associated with protein synthesis. There are large masses of ribosomes, which are prominent in many neurons. These acidic RNA masses, which are involved in protein synthesis, stain as dark *Nissl* bodies with basic histologic stains (see Figure 46-5).

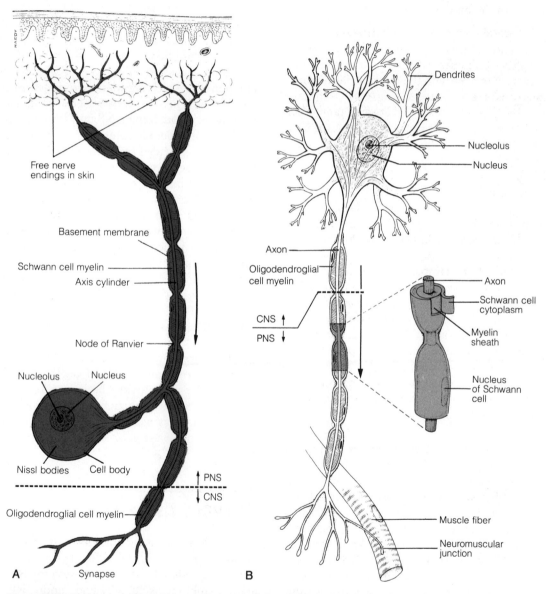

Figure 46-5 (**A**) A typical afferent neuron that carries information from surface receptors (in this case the skin) to the CNS. The cell body and axons are in the PNS, while the central axon penetrates into the CNS wherein myelin is provided by oligodendroglial cells. (**B**) Myelinated efferent neuron with axon entering the PNS to innervate skeletal muscle cells. (*Chaffee EE, Lytle IM: Basic Physiology and Anatomy, 4th ed. Philadelphia, JB Lippincott, 1980*)

The *dendrites* (treelike) are multiple, branched extensions of the nerve cell body; they are the main source through which neurons receive information and conduct information *toward* the cell body. The dendrites and cell body are studded with synaptic terminals from axons and dendrites of other neurons (Figure 46-6).

The *axon* is a long efferent process that projects from the cell body and carries impulses away from the cell. There is usually only one axon to a nerve cell. Most axons undergo multiple branching, resulting in many axonal terminals. The cytoplasm of the cell body extends to fill both the dendrites and the axon (see Figure 46-5). There are no Nissl bodies in the *axon hillock,* which is the point where the axon leaves the cell body. The proteins and other materials that are used by the axon are synthesized in the cell body and then flow down the axon through its cytoplasm.

The cell body of the neuron is equipped for a high level of metabolic activity. This is necessary because the cell body must synthesize the cytoplasmic and membrane constituents required to maintain the function of the axon and its terminals. Some of these axons extend for a distance of 1 m to 1.5 m and have a volume that is sometimes 200 to 500 times greater than the cell body itself. Two axonal transport systems, one slow and one rapid, move molecules from the cell body through the cytoplasm of the axon to its terminals. Replacement and nutrient molecules are slowly forced out of the cell body and down the axon as they are synthesized, moving at the rate of about 1 μm/day. Other molecules, such as some of the neurosecretory granules or their precursors, are transported by a rapid energy-dependent active transport system, moving at the rate of about 400 μm/day. In many instances, membrane-bound vesicles containing neurosecretory granules (neurotransmitters, neuromodulators, or neurohormones) are moved to the axon synaptic terminals by the active transport process. For example, rapid axonal transport carries antidiuretic hormones and oxytocin from hypothalamic neurons through their axons to the posterior pituitary where the hormones are released into the blood. A reverse rapid axonal transport system serves to move materials including target cell messenger molecules from axonal terminals back to the cell body.

Supporting cells

Supporting cells of the nervous system, Schwann's cells of the PNS and the several types of glial cells of the CNS, provide the neurons with protection and metabolic support. The supporting cells segregate the neurons into isolated metabolic compartments, which are required for normal neural function. Together with the tightly joined endothelial cells of the capillaries in the CNS, these supporting cells may contribute to what is called the blood–brain barrier. This term is used to emphasize the impermeability of the nervous system to large and potentially harmful molecules. In addition, the many-layered myelin wrappings of Schwann's cells of the PNS and the oligodendroglia of the CNS provide the myelin sheath

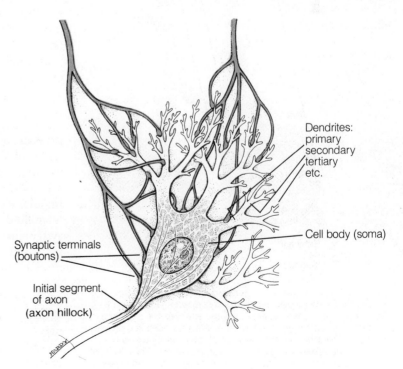

Figure 46-6 Synaptic terminals in contact with the dendrites and cell body of an efferent neuron. (*Chaffee EE, Lytle IM: Basic Physiology and Anatomy, 4th ed. Philadelphia, JB Lippincott, 1980*)

segments that serve to increase the velocity of nerve impulse conduction in axons having larger diameters.

Normally, the nerve cell bodies in the PNS are collected into *ganglia,* such as the dorsal root and autonomic ganglia. Each of the cell bodies and processes of the peripheral nerves is surrounded, or enclosed, in cellular sheaths of supporting cells. The cells that surround the ganglion cells are called *satellite cells.* The satellite cells secrete a basement membrane that apparently protects the cell body from the diffusion of large molecules. Collagen, secreted by fibroblasts, protects the nerve from mechanical forces. Thus, in the PNS, all parts of a neuron and its supporting cells are surrounded by a covering called the *endoneurial sheath,* which is made up of continuous basement membrane surrounded by layers of collagen. The presence of the endoneurial sheath is essential to the regeneration of peripheral axon. Finally, the entire ganglion is protected by a heavy collagenous layer, which also surrounds the large bundles of neural processes in the PNS, called the epineurial sheath.

The processes of the larger nerves, the axons of both the afferent and efferent neurons, are surrounded by the cell membrane and cytoplasm of Schwann's cells, which are close relatives of the satel-

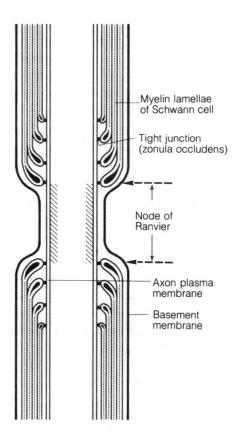

Figure 46-8 Schematic drawing of a longitudinal section through a node of a myelinated axon of the PNS. Sealed junctions between myelin lamellae of the Schwann cell and the axon plasma membrane seal in the intracellular fluids within the internodal region. Extracellular fluids of the PNS communicate directly with the bare axon at the node. In the CNS, there is no basement membrane in the internode and nodal regions.

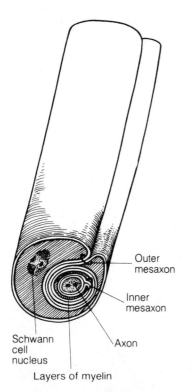

Figure 46-7 The Schwann cell migrates down a larger axon to a bare region, and then settles down and encloses the axon in a fold of its plasma membrane. It then rotates around and around, wrapping the axon in many layers of plasma membrane, with most of the Schwann cell cytoplasm squeezed out. The resultant thick, multiple-layered coating around the axon is called myelin.

lite cells. The Schwann's cell surrounds the nerve process and then twists many times in jelly-roll fashion (Figure 46-7). Schwann's cells line up along the neuronal process, and each of these cells, in turn, forms its own discrete myelin segment. The end of each myelin segment attaches to the cell membrane of the axon by means of sealed junctions. Successive Schwann's cells are separated by short extracellular fluid gaps called the *nodes of Ranvier,* where the myelin is missing. The nodes of Ranvier serve to increase nerve conduction by allowing the impulse to jump from node to node in a process called *saltatory conduction.* In this way, the impulse can travel more rapidly through the extracellular fluid than it could if it were required to move systematically along the entire nerve process. This increased conduction velocity greatly reduces reaction time, or time between the application of a stimulus and the subsequent motor response. The short reaction time that occurs when there is a rapid conduction velocity is of particular importance in peripheral nerves with long distances (sometimes 1–2 m) for conduction between the CNS and distal effector organs (Figure 46-8).

In addition to its role in increasing conduction velocity, the myelin sheath aids in nourishing the neuronal process. Because there are essentially no glycogen stores within the cytoplasm of the neuron, the major source of energy is derived from the supporting cells, in this case the myelin sheath, or from the vascular system at the nodes of Ranvier. In some pathologic conditions, such as multiple sclerosis in the CNS and Guillain–Barré syndrome in the PNS, the myelin may degenerate or be destroyed, leaving a section of bare axonal process, which eventually dies unless remyelinization takes place. Thus, the metabolic intervention of the supporting cells is essential for the long-term survival of the neuron and its processes.

Each of the end-to-end series of Schwann's cells is enclosed within a continuous tube of basement membrane, which is surrounded by a multilayered collagen-rich tubular *endoneurial tube* (Figure 46-9). These endoneurial tubes are bundled together with blood vessels and lymphatics into nerve *fascicles,* which are surrounded by a collagenous *perineurial sheath.* Usually, several fascicles are further surrounded by the heavy, protective *epineurial sheath* of the peripheral nerve. The protective layers that surround the peripheral nerve processes are continuous with the connective tissue capsule of the sensory endings and the connective tissue that surrounds the effector structures, such as the skeletal muscle cell. Centrally, the connective tissue layers continue along the dorsal and ventral roots of the nerve and fuse with the meninges that surround the spinal cord and brain. The endoneurial tube does not penetrate the CNS. The absence of these tubular collagenous structures is thought to be a major factor in the less effective axonal regeneration that occurs within the CNS compared with the PNS.

The supporting cells of the CNS consist of the oligodendroglia, astroglia, microglia, and the ependymal cells. The *oligodendroglial cells* form the myelin for the CNS. Instead of forming a myelin covering for a single axon, these cells reach out with several processes, each wrapping around and forming a multilayered myelin segment around several different axons (Figure 46-10). The coverings of the nerve axons in the CNS also function in speeding the velocity of nerve conduction in a manner similar to that of the peripheral myelinated fibers. Myelin has a high lipid content, which gives it a *whitish* color, and, thus, the name *white matter* is given to the masses of myelinated fibers of the spinal cord and brain.

A second type of glial cell, the *astroglia,* is particularly prominent in the gray matter, or more central portion of the brain. These large cells have many processes, some reaching to the surface of the capillaries, others reaching to the surface of the nerve cells, and still others filling most of the intercellular space of the CNS (see Figure 46-10). The astrocytic linkage between the blood vessels and the neurons may provide a transport mechanism for the exchange of oxygen, carbon dioxide, metabolites, and so on. The astrocytes are capable of filling their cytoplasm with microfibrils, and masses of these cells form the special type of scar tissue called *gliosis* that develops in the CNS when brain tissue is destroyed.

A third type of glial cell, the *microglia,* is a phagocytic cell that is available for cleaning up debris following cellular damage, infection, or cell death. The *ependymal* cells form the lining of the neural tube cavity, the ventricular system. In some areas, these cells combine with a rich vascular network to form the choroid plexus where production of the cerebrospinal fluid (CSF) takes place.

Metabolic requirements

Nervous tissue has a high need for metabolic energy. Although the brain amounts to only 2% of the body's weight, it consumes 20% of its oxygen. Despite this high need, the brain cannot store oxygen nor can

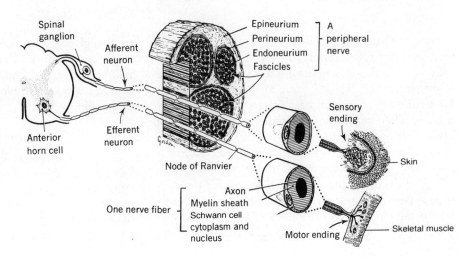

Figure 46-9 Peripheral nerve sheaths. The heavy connective tissue epineurium sheathes the whole nerve trunk. The perineurium sheathes bundles of axons or fasciculi. A large fasciculus is enlarged and cut away to illustrate internal structure as are two smaller fasciculi at the bottom of the diagram. The innermost connective tissue layer, the endoneurium, is made up of several layers of connective tissue fibers and fibrocytes that surround each individual fiber or myelinated axon. Unmyelinated fibers are not visible at this magnification. (*Chaffee EE, Lytle IM: Basic Physiology and Anatomy, 4th ed. Philadelphia, JB Lippincott, 1980*)

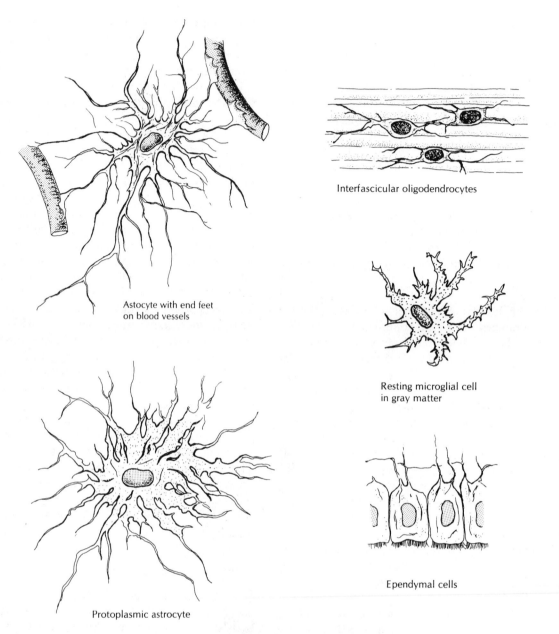

Astocyte with end feet
on blood vessels

Interfascicular oligodendrocytes

Resting microglial cell
in gray matter

Ependymal cells

Protoplasmic astrocyte

Figure 46-10 Neuroglial cells of the central nervous system. *(Barr ML, Kiernan JA: The Human Nervous System: An Anatomical Viewpoint, 5th ed, p 28. Philadelphia, JB Lippincott, 1988)*

it engage in anaerobic metabolism. An interruption in the blood or oxygen supply to the brain leads to clinically observable signs and symptoms. In the absence of oxygen, brain cells continue to function for about 10 seconds. Unconsciousness occurs almost simultaneously when cardiac arrest occurs, and the death of brain cells begins within 4 to 6 minutes. Interruption of blood flow also leads to the accumulation of metabolic by-products that are toxic to neural tissue.

Glucose is the major fuel source for the nervous system, yet the nervous system has no provisions for storing glucose. Unlike muscle cells, it has no glycogen stores and must rely on glucose from the blood or the glycogen stores of supporting cells. Persons receiving insulin for diabetes may experience signs of neural dysfunction and unconsciousness (insulin reaction or shock) when blood glucose drops as a result of an insulin excess.

In summary, nervous tissue is composed of two types of cells, neurons and supporting cells. Neurons are composed of three parts: a cell body, which controls cell activity; the dendrites, which conduct information toward the cell body; and the axon, which carries impulses from the cell body. The supporting cells consist of Schwann's cells of the PNS and the glial cells of the CNS. The supporting cells protect and provide metabolic support for the neurons and aid in segregating them into isolated compartments, which is necessary for normal neuronal function. The function of the nervous system demands a high amount of metabolic energy. Glucose is the major fuel for the nervous system, and, although the brain comprises only 2% of body weight, it consumes 20% of its oxygen supply. In general, neurons exemplify the principle that the more specialized the function of a cell type, the less its ability to regenerate.

Nerve cell communication

Neurons are classified as excitable tissue. This means that they are able to initiate and conduct electrical impulses. Basic to an understanding of nerve function is an appreciation of the events that occur during the excitation and initiation of an action potential in a nerve or muscle cell (see Chapter 1). The discussion in this chapter focuses on action potentials that occur in nerves; many of the same types of phenomena occur in other types of excitable tissue, such as muscle.

—— Impulse generation and conduction

An impulse, or action potential, represents the lateral, or lengthwise, movement of electrical charge along the cell membrane. This phenomenon is based on the rapid flow, sometimes called *conductance,* of charged ions through the membrane in a progressive manner along the length of the neuron's axon. In excitable tissue, ions such as sodium, potassium, chloride, and calcium carry the electrical charges that are involved in the initiation and transmission of such impulses.

During the depolarization process, the neuronal membrane becomes selectively permeable to the sodium ion and the rapid inflow of sodium ions produces local currents that travel through the adjacent cell membrane and this, in turn, causes the sodium channels in this part of the membrane to open, and depolarization occurs. Thus, the impulse moves progressively along the nerve, depolarizing the membrane ahead of the action potential. The impulse is conducted longitudinally along the membrane from one part of the axon to other parts. In unmyelinated fibers, this sequence of events moves the impulse progressively along the axon. Conduction in myelinated fibers follows a similar pattern, but because of the high resistance in the myelinated segments, the current

flow jumps from node to node (saltatory conduction) as was described earlier. This is a more rapid process, and myelinated axons conduct up to 50 times faster than unmyelinated fibers.

—— Synaptic transmission

Neurons communicate with neighboring neurons or other target cells by one of two methods: ionic passage between cells (*electrical synapse*) or by neurosecretion (*chemical synapse*). The function of neurons can be closely linked by opposition of their cell membranes in a *gap junction* where submicroscopic channels between the cells permit the passage of sodium and potassium ions with the result that an action potential can pass directly and quickly from one cell to another. Gap junctions can communicate in either direction. Thus they may couple the two cells into a close functional relationship in circuits where this is required.

The more common mechanism by which neurons communicate with other neurons or target cells is the chemical synapse in which messenger molecules are secreted near selective receptor molecules on the membrane of a target cell. Because there is a secreting cell surface, a space between the cells, and a receiving surface of the target cell, the chemical synapse is both a slower communicating mechanism and a one-way communication link. The synapse consists of special presynaptic and postsynaptic membrane structures. The synaptic cleft separates the pre- and postsynaptic membranes. The presynaptic terminal secretes one and often several chemical messenger molecules (neurotransmitters, neuromodulators, and trophic factors) into the synaptic cleft. The most rapid acting of these neuromediators, the neurotransmitters, *diffuse* into and unite with receptors on the postsynaptic membrane, and this causes either excitation or inhibition of the postsynaptic neuron by producing hypopolarization or hyperpolarization of the postsynaptic membrane, respectively (Figure 46-11). Hypolarization increases nerve excitability by bringing the membrane potential closer to threshold potential so that a smaller stimulus is needed to cause the nerve to fire. Hyperpolarization has the opposite effect. It increases the stimuli needed for depolarization and renders the nerve less excitable.

A neuron's cell body and dendrites are covered by thousands of synapses, any or many of which can be active at any moment in time. Because of this rich synaptic capability, each neuron resembles a little integrator in which there are many circuits of neurons that interact with each other. It is the complexity of these interactions that gives the system its intelligence in terms of the subtle integrations involved in producing behavioral responses, and that makes the predic-

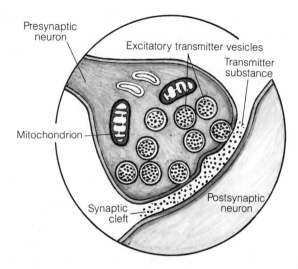

Figure 46-11 Synapse, showing the pre- and postsynaptic neuron. (*Chaffee EE, Lytle IM: Basic Physiology and Anatomy, 4th ed. Philadelphia, JB Lippincott, 1980*)

tion of stimulus–response relationships somewhat hazardous in the absence of a millisecond-to-millisecond knowledge of the excitatory and inhibitory activity that takes place on the surfaces of each neuron in a functional circuit. It is amazing, with billions of these little integrators capable of becoming involved in such a response, that predictions are possible at all. It is even more astounding that the basic microcircuitry involved in the nervous system is reproduced reliably during the development of each new organism.

There are several types of synapses. Axonic terminals of an afferent neuron can develop in close apposition to the dendrites (*axodendritic synapse*), to the cell body (*axosomatic synapse*), or to the axon (*axoaxonic synapse*) of a CNS neuron. The mechanism of communication between the *presynaptic* axonic terminal and the *postsynaptic* neuron is similar in all three types of synapses. In all three, the action potential sweeps into the axonic terminals of the afferent neuron and triggers rapid secretion of neurotransmitter molecules from the axonic, or presynaptic, surface. Conversion of action potentials into secretion is called *coupling*, and, although it is not completely understood, it is believed that the release of calcium ions is involved.

Many CNS neurons possess thousands of synapses on their dendritic or somatic surfaces. The combination of the neurotransmitter with the receptor sites can produce either excitation or inhibition. When the combination of a neurotransmitter with a receptor site causes partial depolarization of the postsynaptic membrane, it is called an *excitatory postsynaptic potential (EPSP)*. In other synapses, the combination of a transmitter with a receptor site is inhibitory in the sense that the combination of the transmitter with the receptor site causes the local nerve membrane to

become hyperpolarized and less excitable. Then it is called an *inhibitory postsynaptic potential (IPSP)*.

An action potential does not begin in the membrane adjacent to the synapse. Instead it begins in the initial segment of the axon, the *axon hillock*, which is more excitable than the rest of the nerve. The local currents resulting from any one EPSP (sometimes called a *generator potential*) are usually insufficient to pass threshold and cause depolarization of the axon's initial segment. However, if several EPSPs occur simultaneously, the area of depolarization can become large enough and the currents at the initial segment can become strong enough to exceed the threshold potential and initiate a conducted action potential. This summation of depolarized areas is called *spatial summation*. The EPSPs can also summate and cause an action potential if they come in close temporal (time) relation to each other. This temporal aspect of the occurrence of two or more EPSPs is called *temporal summation*.

IPSPs can also undergo spatial and temporal summation with each other and with EPSPs, reducing the effectiveness of the latter by a roughly algebraic summation. If the sum of EPSPs and IPSPs keeps the depolarization at the initial segment below threshold levels, the generation of an action potential does not occur.

The spatial and temporal summation required in the distribution and timing of synaptic activity serves as a sensitive and very complicated switch requiring just the right combination of incoming activity before the cell releases its own message in the form of the action potential. The frequency of action potentials in the axon, on the other hand, is an all-or-none language (digital language), which can vary only as to the presence or absence of such impulses and their frequency.

Messenger molecules

Neurotransmitters are the chemical messenger molecules of the nervous system. The process of neurotransmission involves the synthesis, storage, and release of a neurotransmitter; the reaction of the neurotransmitter with a receptor; and termination of the receptor action. The recent development of new research methods including staining techniques and use of radiolabeled antibodies have allowed scientists to study and gain answers in each of these areas.

Both the nervous system and the endocrine system use chemicals as messengers. As more information is obtained about the chemical messengers of both systems, the distinction between the nervous system and the endocrine system becomes somewhat blurred. Many neurons, such as those in the adrenal cortex, secrete transmitters that are released into the bloodstream; and it has been found that other neurons possess receptor sites for hormones. On the other hand, many hormones have turned out to be neurotransmitters. Vasopressin, a peptide hormone that is released from the posterior pituitary gland, is also a neurotransmitter for nerve cells in the hypothalamus. Today, more than a dozen of these cell-to-cell messengers are known to be capable of relaying signals in either the nervous system or in the endocrine system.[2]

Neurotransmitters are synthesized in the cytoplasm of the axon terminal. The synthesis of transmitters may require one or more enzyme-catalyzed steps (one for acetylcholine and three for norepinephrine). The various types of neurons are limited in terms of the type of transmitter they can synthesize by their enzyme systems. The suffix *-ergic* and the name of the transmitter produced is often used to classify neurons. Accordingly, a dopaminergic neuron is one that produces dopamine. After synthesis, the transmitter molecules are stored in the axon terminal in tiny membrane-bound sacs called *synaptic vesicles*. There may be thousands of vesicles in a single terminal, each containing 10,000 to 100,000 molecules of transmitter. The vesicle protects transmitters from enzyme destruction within the nerve terminal.

The arrival of an impulse at a nerve terminal causes a large number of transmitter molecules to be released into the synaptic space. Neurotransmitters exert their actions through specific proteins, called *receptors,* embedded in the postsynaptic membrane. These receptors are tailored precisely to match the size and shape of the transmitter. In each case, the interaction between a transmitter and receptor results in a specific physiologic response. The action of a transmitter is determined by the type of receptor it binds to. For example, acetylcholine is excitatory when it is released at a myoneural junction, and it is inhibitory when it is released at the sinoatrial node in the heart. Receptors are named according to the type of neurotransmitter they interact with. For example, the term *cholinergic receptor* is used to indicate a receptor that binds acetylcholine. Some neuromediators act as modulators of neural action rather than initiators.

Rapid removal of a transmitter, once it has exerted its effects on the postsynaptic membrane, is necessary to maintain precise control of neural transmission. A transmitter that has been released can undergo one of three fates. It can be broken down into inactive substances by enzymes, it can be taken back up into the presynaptic neuron in a process called *reuptake,* or it can diffuse away into the intercellular fluid until its concentration is too low to influence postsynaptic excitability. Acetylcholine, for example, is rapidly broken down by acetylcholinesterase into acetic acid and choline, with the choline being taken back into the presynaptic neuron for reuse in acetylcholine synthesis. The catecholamines, on the other hand, are largely taken back into the neuron in an unchanged form for reuse. The catecholamines can also be degraded by enzymes in the synaptic space or by enzymes that are present in the nerve terminals.

Neurotransmitters tend to be small molecules that incorporate a positively charged nitrogen atom; they include amino acids, peptides, and monoamines. Amino acids are the building blocks of proteins and are present in body fluids. Peptides are low-molecular molecules that yield two or more amino acids on hydrolysis. They include substance P, vasopressin, and the endorphins and enkephalins. Monoamines are an amine molecule containing one amino group (NH_2). Serotonin, dopamine, norepinephrine, and epinephrine are monoamines that are synthesized from amino acids. Fortunately, the nervous system is protected by the blood–brain barrier from circulating amino acids and other molecules that could act in an unregulated manner as neuromediators.

There is still much to be learned about the role of certain amino acids and peptides as neurotransmitters. For example, several amino acids (glutamic acid and aspartic acid) appear to exert powerful excitatory effects on synaptic transmission. Glycine, another amino acid, is known to have strong inhibitory effects. One of the most common inhibitory transmitters is gamma-aminobutyric acid (GABA). This amino acid is unique in that it is synthesized almost exclusively in the brain and spinal cord. It has been established that almost one-third of all synapses use GABA.[2] With the inclusion of amino acids as neurotransmitters comes the puzzling aspect that the same amino acid can function as both a neurotransmitter and as a building block for protein synthesis.

It was not until the mid-1970s that it became known that peptides could act as neurotransmitters.[3] Some of the newest and most exciting of the neuropeptides are the endorphins, enkephalins, and substance P, which appear to be involved in pain sensation. The endorphins and enkephalins, which have been described as the body's own morphine, undoubtedly contribute to a decrease in pain perception and feeling of well-being (see Chapter 47). Substance P, a chain of 11 amino acids, is present in a number of neuronal pathways in the brain and primary sensory fibers in the peripheral nervous system. Because substance P excites spinal neurons that respond to painful stimuli, it has been suggested the substance is involved in transmitting painful information from the periphery to the CNS.[4]

The actions of most neurotransmitters are localized in specific clusters of neurons with axons that project to highly specific brain regions. As more is learned about the location and mechanism of action of the various neurotransmitters, it has become increasingly apparent that many disease conditions have their origin in altered neurotransmitter responses. In some cases, there is evidence of degeneration or dysfunction of the neurons producing the neuromediator; in others, there is an apparent alteration in the postsynaptic response to the neuromediator. For example, the neurons containing dopamine are concentrated in regions of the midbrain known as the *substantia nigra* and *ventral tegmentum*. Many of these dopamine-containing neurons project their axons to areas of the forebrain that are thought to be involved in regulation of emotional behavior. Other dopamine fibers terminate in regions near the middle of the brain called the *corpus striatum*. These latter fibers seem to play an essential role in the performance of complex motor movements. Degeneration of the dopamine fibers in this area of the brain leads to the tremors and rigidity that are characteristic of Parkinson's disease. Some forms of mental illness, such as schizophrenia, are thought to involve abnormal release or responses to neurotransmitters in the brain. Pharmacologic methods of supplying neurotransmitters (as in Parkinson's disease) or modifying their actions (as in the case of psychoactive drugs) are used to treat some of these disorders. Undoubtedly, more specific treatment methods will become available as more is learned about the transmission of neural information.

Other classes of messenger molecules are often secreted by axon terminals in addition to or instead of neurotransmitters. Neuromodulator molecules apparently react with postsynaptic receptors to produce slower and longer lasting changes in membrane excitability. This has the effect of making the action of the faster acting neurotransmitter molecules more or less effective. Some of the peptide molecules may fall into the modulator category. Neurohumoral mediators reach the target cell through the blood stream and produce an even slower action than the neuromodulators. Neurotrophic factors are required to maintain the long term survival of the postsynaptic cell and are secreted by axon terminals independent of an action potential. Examples include motoneuron to muscle cell trophic factors and neuron to neuron trophic factors in sequential chains of CNS sensory systems. Trophic factors from the target cell that can enter the axon terminal and are essential to the long term survival of the presynaptic neuron have also been demonstrated. Target cell to neuron trophic factors probably have great significance in establishment of specific neural connections during normal embryonic development.

In summary, neurons, which are able to generate and conduct impulses, are classified as excitable tissue. Neurotransmitters are chemical messengers that serve to control neural function; they selectively cause either excitation or inhibition of action potentials. A synapse is a one-way communication link between neurons; it has both presynaptic and postsynaptic components. Neurotransmitters released from the presynaptic terminals of one neuron diffuse across the synaptic cleft and unite with receptors in the postsynaptic surface of another neuron as a means of communicating information between the two neurons. Thus, a neuron integrates ongoing synaptic activity, resulting in the production or nonproduction of an action potential. Once initiated, an action potential travels rapidly along the cell's axon to trigger transmitter release for synaptic communication with the next neuron in the circuit. This combination of integration of excitatory and inhibitory synaptic activity and rapid communication of impulses permits the complex functioning that is characteristic of the nervous system. Axon terminals often secrete other messenger molecules in addition to or instead of neurotransmitters. These have slower and longer lasting postsynaptic effects and include neuromodulators, neurohormones, and neurotrophic factors. Target cells also secrete trophic factors required for the long term survival of the innervating neuron.

References

1. Report on Convulsive and Neuromuscular Disorders to the National Advisory Neurological and Communicative Disorders and Stroke Council, p 103. National Institute of Health, National Institute on Communicative Disorders and Stroke, US Department of Health, Education, and Welfare, Public Health Service, NIH Publication No 79–1913.
2. Bloom FE: Neuropeptides. Sci Am 245(10):148, 1981
3. Iverson LL: The chemistry of the brain. Sci Am 241(9):134, 1979
4. Snyder SH: The molecular basis for communication between cells. Sci Am 253(4):132, 1985

Bibliography

Stevens S: The neuron. Sci Am 241(9):54, 1979
Wurtman RJ: Nutrients that modify brain behavior. Sci Am 246(4):50, 1982

CHAPTER 47

Sheila M. Curtis
Robin L. Curtis

Somatosensory Function and Pain

Objectives

After you have studied this chapter, you should be able to meet the following objectives:

_____ Name the three somatosensory modalities.

_____ Define *proprioception* and *kinesthesia*.

_____ Explain what is meant by a sensory unit.

_____ Trace the pathway of an impulse originating in a somatosensory receptor.

_____ State the significance of the dermatomes in a neurologic examination.

_____ Name the reflex that causes the skin surface to be moved away from a noxious stimulus.

_____ Cite the determinant of sensory acuity.

_____ Contrast the role of rapid-adapting and slow-adapting afferents in maintaining posture.

_____ Compare the discriminative pathway with the anterolateral pathway, and explain the clinical usefulness of this distinction.

_____ Describe the sensory homunculus in the cerebral cortex.

_____ Outline the procedure for clinical assessment of somatosensory function, citing the aspects of sensory function being tested.

_____ Differentiate between the specificity and pattern theories of pain.

_____ Explain the gate control theory of pain.

(continued)

_____ Describe the function of nociceptors in response to pain information.

_____ State the difference between the A-delta and C-fiber neurons in the transmission of pain information.

_____ Trace the transmission of pain signals with reference to the neospinothalamic, paleospinothalamic, and reticulospinal pathways.

_____ Describe the function of endogenous analgesic mechanisms as they relate to transmission of pain information.

_____ Give examples of visceral, cutaneous, and somatic pain.

_____ Differentiate acute pain from chronic pain.

_____ Describe the mechanisms of referred pain, and list the common sites of referral for cardiac and other types of visceral pain.

_____ Compare pain threshold and pain tolerance.

_____ Explain the psychosocial and cultural factors that influence a person's response to pain.

_____ Cite common physiologic manifestations of pain.

_____ State how the pain response may differ in children and elderly persons.

_____ Define _hypesthesia, hyperesthesia, hyperalgesia, dysesthesia, paresthesia, anesthesia, hyperpathia, analgesia,_ and _hypoalgesia._

_____ Give examples of alterations in sensitivity to pain or its perception that may place the affected person at risk.

_____ Differentiate between the causes of tension-type headaches and migraine headaches and their treatments.

_____ List at least five foods commonly associated with occurrence of migraine headaches.

_____ Cite the most common cause of temporomandibular joint (TMJ) pain.

_____ Describe the cause and characteristics of trigeminal neuralgia and postherpetic neuralgia.

_____ Cite a possible mechanism of phantom-limb pain.

_____ State the mechanisms whereby non-narcotic and narcotic analgesic, tricyclic antidepressant, and anticonvulsive drugs relieve pain.

_____ Describe the proposed mechanisms of pain relief associated with the use of heat, cold, and transcutaneous electrical nerve stimulation.

_____ Compare the methods used in acupuncture and acupressure.

_____ Relate the concept of imagery to pain relief.

_____ Define _biofeedback._

_____ Describe the advantages of a multidisciplinary approach to the treatment of pain disorders.

Sensory mechanisms provide a continuous stream of information about the seeming realities of the person, the outside world, and the interactions between the two. The term _somesthesia_ (body + sensation) is used to describe a person's awareness of their body. The somatosensory component of the nervous system provides an awareness of body sensations such as touch, temperature, and pain, which are different from the special senses such as vision, hearing, smell, and taste. This chapter is divided into two parts—the first describes the organization and control of somatosensory function, and the second focuses on pain as a somatosensory modality.

Organization and control of somatosensory function

Somatosensory experience can be divided into _modalities,_ a term used for qualitative, subjective distinctions between sensations such as _touch, heat,_ and _pain._ Such experiences require the function of both sensory receptors and forebrain structures in the thalamus and cerebral cortex. The sensory receptors for somatosensory function consist of discrete nerve endings in the skin and other body tissues, with the exception of bone structures beneath, the periosteum, and of the brain itself. Between 2 and 3 million sensory neurons deliver a steady stream of action potentials as a code representing the status of their sensory endings. Only a very small proportion of this information reaches awareness; most provides input essential for a myriad of reflex and automatic mechanisms that keep us alive and manage our functioning.

Somesthesia can be subdivided with reference to the location of the sensory nerve endings. Cutaneous modalities include touch (tactile) and more complex sensations of itch and tickle; temperature (warm to hot and cool to cold); and pain including the bright, sharp type, and the dull, stinging, burning, aching type. In deeper structures of the body wall and the limbs, afferent nerve endings supply the deep connective tissues, joint capsules, ligaments, muscles, tendons, periosteum of bone, and blood vessel walls. Some of these sensory endings provide the basis for the coordination of movement and contribute to the experience of body, head, and limb position (_proprioception_) and of movement (_kinesthesia_). When stimulated at a frequency high enough to be associated with tissue damage, these afferents also send a message that is interpreted as pain.

Somesthetic innervation patterns

The innervation of the body, including the head, retains a basic segmental organizational pattern that was established during embryonic development. Thirty-three spinal (segmental) nerves provide sensory and motor innervation of the body wall, the limbs, and the viscera (see Chapter 46). Sensory input to each spinal cord segment is provided by afferent sensory neurons with cell bodies in the dorsal root ganglia. A *sensory unit* consists of a single dorsal root ganglion neuron, its receptive terminals in a small region of the periphery, and its central axon, which synapses with a dorsal horn association neuron. The receptive endings of the peripheral sensory neurons supply the skin, fascial sheets, muscles, tendons, joint capsules, periosteum, marrow cavities, and parietal lining of the body cavities. Action potentials originating from any of the many receptive endings of an afferent neuron are conducted through the dorsal root into the spinal cord association cell columns. The afferent neuron, in a sense, cannot distinguish among information coming from its various peripheral terminals. If the applied stimulus results in an action potential in any terminal branch, the impulse is transmitted to the dorsal horn association cells in the central nervous system (CNS).

Peripheral distribution of the sensory neurons (dermatomes)

Each segment of the body, with few exceptions, contains a pair of dorsal root ganglia within which the general sensory afferent neurons innervating the body wall, or soma, of that segment live. Between 30,000 and 50,000 afferent neuron cell bodies reside in each of the paired dorsal root ganglia of each segment; their central axons project to the corresponding spinal segment through the dorsal roots.[1] Segmental innervation of head segments follows this same pattern by means of cranial nerves.

The region of the body wall that is supplied by a single pair of dorsal root ganglia is called a *dermatome*. These nerve-innervated strips occur in a regular sequence moving upward from the second coccygeal segment through the cervical segments, reflecting the basic segmental organization of the body and the nervous system (Figure 47-1). The dermatome map is used for detecting the level and extent of sensory defects resulting from segmental nerve or spinal cord damage.

In the peripheral nervous system, fusion between neighboring spinal nerves in structures called *plexuses* results in an overlapping of sensory innervation from neighboring dermatomes. The spinal nerves from the upper limbs fuse in the brachial plexus, and those from the lower limbs fuse in the lumbosacral plexus. This overlapping system provides a built-in protection, so that damage to one or two adjacent dorsal roots does not result in a complete loss of sensory input from that segment or segments. Partial loss of sensory innervation results in reduced ability for discrete localization within a sensory field.

Central distribution of sensory input

Sensory systems are organized as a serial succession of neurons consisting of: (1) first-order (primary) afferent neurons that transmit sensory information from the periphery; (2) second-order (secondary) CNS association neurons that communicate with various reflex networks and sensory pathways that travel directly to the thalamus; and (3) third-order (tertiary) neurons that relay information from the thalamus to the cerebral cortex.[2] Many interneurons process and modify the sensory information at the level of the second- and third-order neurons, and myriads more participate before coordinated and appropriate learned-movement responses occur. The number of participating neurons increases exponentially from the primary through the secondary and the secondary through the tertiary levels. By providing multiple parallel projections along with mechanisms for filtering, amplifying, and modulating information, this expansion of neurons serves as a safety feature.

Sensory input from primary neuron receptors is distributed to one or more dorsal horn input association cell columns, each of which has a characteristic pattern of central projection. The function of these input association column neurons is to relay afferent signals to: (1) local reflex circuits, providing rapid, lower motoneuron responses; (2) more rostral parts of the reflex hierarchy, permitting more complex, organized response patterns; (3) the reticular activating system, contributing to general wakefulness of forebrain systems; and (4) the thalamus, where sensation and perceptive functions begin.

One function of the second-order association cells is to relay afferent information into reflex circuits. If a skin receptor on the finger, which responds to increased temperature, is stimulated by skin contact with a hot object, a series of events takes place (Figure 47-2). First, the heat produces local changes in the receptors that are converted to action potentials. The action potentials are then transmitted through the peripheral nerve to the cell body in the dorsal root ganglion, and from there through its axon into the spinal cord segment. In the spinal cord segment, association

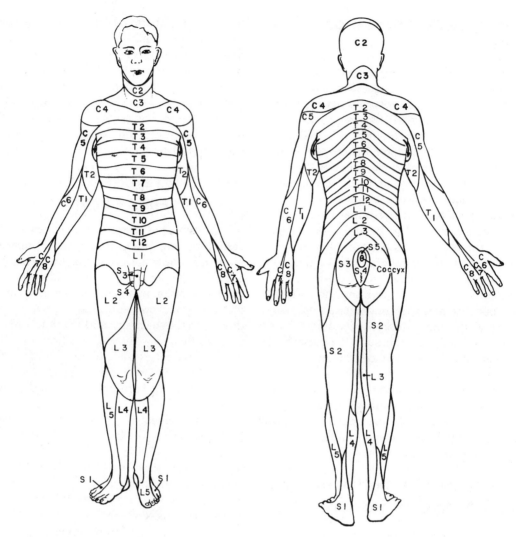

Figure 47-1 Cutaneous distribution of spinal nerves (dermatomes). (*Barr M: The Human Nervous System, p 253. New York, Harper & Row, 1979*)

neurons can trigger an action potential in a lower motoneuron resulting in skeletal muscle contraction and movement of the skin surface away from the stimulus. This protective reflex is called the *flexor-withdrawal reflex*.

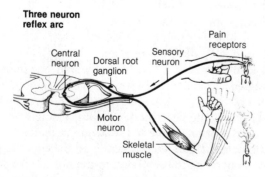

Figure 47-2 The flexor–withdrawal reflex. (*Adapted from Chaffee EE, Lytle IM: Basic Physiology and Anatomy, 4th ed, p 240. Philadelphia, JB Lippincott, 1980*)

Somesthetic input association column neurons of the dorsal horn distribute the afferent signals to different reflex circuits—pain and temperature to the flexor-withdrawal circuit and deep pressure to a stepping reflex circuit. All of the somesthetic input signals are projected by other association neurons to higher levels of the nervous system as necessary input for more complex reflex patterns. The same information that triggered the spinal cord flexor-withdrawal reflex is projected by spinoreticular fibers to other reflexes at the brain stem level, where the circuitry for catching the breath, a sudden rise in heart rate, and other responses such as vocalization occur. At a higher level of control, for instance, projections of the spinoreticular fibers to midbrain circuits allow the regaining of position when balance is lost. This illustrates the concept of the *hierarchy of reflexes* in which the same afferent information contributes to more and more complex reaction patterns, each at a progressively more rostral location in the CNS that controls the various components organized at lower levels.

Input to the thalamus can be distributed to the lateral or intermediate nuclei. The lateral nuclei project to the sensory cortex where meaning and the perceptive aspects of somatosensory experience are integrated. The intermediate nuclei project to the limbic system where many of the emotional aspects of sensation are mediated. The intermediate nuclei are also capable of contributing a crude, poorly localizable sensation to the opposite side of the body. The thalamus, in the absence of the cortex, provides an awareness of pain but it has no meaning.

Stimulus discrimination

Discrimination of the location of a stimulus is called *acuity* and is based on the sensory field within a dermatome innervated by an afferent neuron. High acuity (*i.e.,* the ability to make fine discriminations of location) requires high density of innervation by afferent neurons. For example, acuity is high on the thumb, but lower on the back of the hand. High acuity also requires a projection system through the nervous system to the forebrain that preserves distinctions between activity in neighboring sensory fields.

Afferent neurons differ as to the intensity of the applied physical or chemical energy at which they begin to fire. This *afferent threshold* is usually lower than the *subjective sensation threshold,* the intensity at which the stimulus is first experienced. For highly developed discriminative systems, under ideal conditions, these thresholds may correspond closely. However, many factors such as attitude, attention, and emotion can greatly elevate the subjective threshold. Once the subjective threshold is reached, the intensity of the experienced sensation is based on the rate of impulse generation in the afferent neuron, which, in turn, is related to the stimulus intensity (amount of physical or chemical stimulus energy) applied. Equal subjective intensity increases are related to exponential increases in physical stimulus energy. This relationship holds true for all sensory systems, including the somesthetic system, and is based on characteristics of the receptor endings.

Some afferent neurons maintain a more or less steady rate of firing to a continuous stimulus. This is true for afferents from muscle, tendons, and joints, where continuous feedback information is necessary for maintaining posture. These slow-adapting afferent neurons contrast with rapid-adapting afferent neurons, which signal only the onset, sudden change, and conclusion of a stimulus. Rapid-adapting afferent neurons are required to signal moving, brief, or vibrating stimuli.

The qualitative aspects of different types of stimuli are based on the differential sensitivity of the terminals of different afferent neurons. This provides the basis for characterizing subjective differences between types of stimulus energy, the *sensory modalities.* Some afferent neurons are particularly sensitive to increased skin temperature, and these signals are interpreted as warm or hot. Others are particularly sensitive to slight indentations of the skin, and their signals are interpreted as touch. Cool versus cold, sharp versus dull pain, delicate touch versus deep pressure, and joint movement versus joint position are all based on a different population of afferent neurons or on central integration of several modalities occurring at the same time. For example, the sensation of itch results from a combination of pain and touch, and the sensation of tickle requires a gentle, moving tactile stimulus over cool skin.

Ascending pathways

Somesthetic afferents transmit the sensations of vibration and fine touch, as well as the more crude sensations of pain and temperature. For these sensations, the input association cell columns in the dorsal horn of the spinal cord are the indirect source of spinoreticular projections to the reticular activating system. The spinoreticular projections are the basis for increased wakefulness or awareness following strong somesthetic stimulation and for the generalized startle reaction that occurs with sudden and intense somesthetic stimuli. The responses of the reticular activating system include postural as well as autonomic nervous system responses, such as a rise in blood pressure and heart rate, dilation of the pupils, and the pale moist skin that results from constriction of the cutaneous blood vessels and activation of sweat glands. In addition, the sensory association cell columns relay afferent information to the forebrain, where sensation and perception occur. Two parallel pathways, the dorsal column discriminative pathway and the anterolateral pathway, reach the thalamic level of sensation, each taking a different route. The discriminative pathway provides for rapid transmission of information relating fine touch and pressure, vibration, and position sense. The anterolateral system provides for slower transmission of pain, thermal sensations, crude touch and pressure, and tickle and itch sensations.

Discriminative pathway

The rapid-transmission discriminative pathway to the thalamus and cerebral cortex involves primary afferent axons that travel up the dorsal columns of the spinal cord white matter and synapse with highly evolved somesthetic input association neurons in the medulla. Second-order neurons provide a fur-

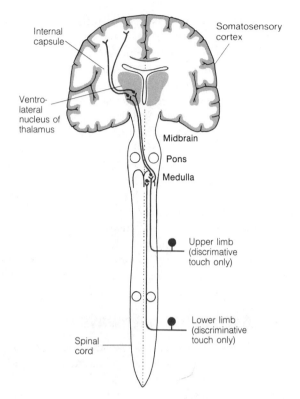

Figure 47-3 The discriminative pathway, an ascending system for rapid transmission of sensations relating joint movement (kinesthesis), body position (proprioception), vibration, and delicate touch. Primary afferents travel up the dorsal columns of the spinal cord white matter and synapse with somesthetic input association neurons in the medulla. Secondary neurons project through the brainstem to the thalamus and synapse with tertiary neurons, which relay the information to the primary somesthetic cortex on the opposite side of the brain.

ther large-diameter projection through the brain stem without collateral branches (Figure 47-3). This discriminative pathway transmits accurate localization and delicate intensity discriminative information to the opposite side of the brain (see Figure 47-3). There, third-order neurons relay information to the primary somesthetic cerebral cortex. Sensory information arriving at the thalamus by this route is discretely localizable and delicately analyzable in terms of intensity grades. This pathway is highly dependent on parietal cortical function and has little projection into the intermediate thalamic nuclei. This is the only pathway taken by sensations of joint movement (kinesthesia), body position (proprioception), vibration, and delicate, discriminative touch, such as is required to differentiate correctly between touching skin at two neighboring points (two-point discrimination) versus only one point.

The discriminative pathway uses only three neurons to transmit information from a sensory receptor to the somesthetic strip of parietal cerebral cortex of the opposite side: (1) the primary sensory neuron that projects its central axon to the dorsal column nuclei; (2) the dorsal column neuron that sends its axon through a rapid conducting tract, the *medial lemniscus,* that crosses at the base of the medulla and travels to the thalamus on the opposite side of the brain where basic sensation begins; and (3) the thalamic neuron that projects its axon to the primary sensory cortex, site of discriminative sensation.

Sensory cortex

The sensory cortex is located in the parietal lobe, which lies behind the central sulcus and above the lateral sulcus (Figure 47-4). The strip of parietal cortex that borders the central sulcus is called the *primary sensory cortex* because it receives primary sensory information by way of direct projections from the lateral nuclei of the thalamus. A distorted map of the body and head surface, called a *homunculus,* reflects the density of cortical neurons devoted to sensory input from afferents in corresponding periphery areas. As depicted in Figure 47-5, much more cortical surface is devoted to areas of the body such as the thumb, forefinger, lips, and tongue where fine touch and pressure are essential for function. The cortical area devoted to body surface area correlates with the density of afferent innervation in that area.

Parallel to and just behind the primary somesthetic cortex (toward the occipital cortex) lies the parietal association areas, which are required to transform the raw material of sensation into meaningful learned perception. Most of the *perceptive* aspects of body sensation, or somesthesia, require the function of this parietal association cortex. Thalamic association nuclei are also involved. The perceptive aspect, or meaningfulness, of a stimulus pattern involves the integration of present sensation with past learning. For instance, your past learning plus present tactile sensation give you the perception of sitting on a soft chair rather than on a hard bicycle seat. One of the important functions of the discriminative pathway is to inte-

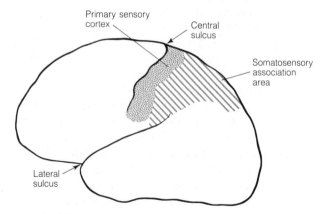

Figure 47-4 The primary somesthetic and association somatosensory cortex.

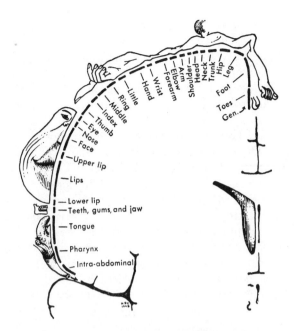

Figure 47-5 The homunculus as determined by stimulation studies on the human cortex during surgery. (*Penfield E, Rasmussen T: The Cerebral Cortex of Man. New York, Macmillan, 1955. Copyright © by Macmillan Publishing Co., Inc., renewed 1978 by Theodore Rasmussen*)

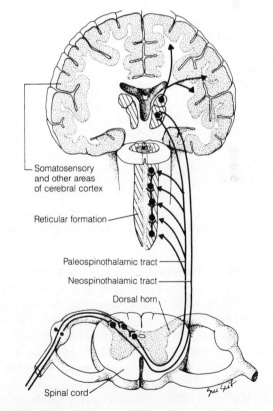

grate the input from multiple receptors. The sense of shape and size of an object in the absence of visualization, called *stereognosis*, is based on precise afferent information from muscle, tendon, and joint receptors. A screwdriver has a different shape from a knife, not only in the texture of its parts (tactile sensibility), but also in its shape based on the relative position of the fingers as they are moved over the object (proprioception). This complex, interpretive perception requires not only that the discriminative system must be functioning optimally, but also that higher order parietal association cortex processing and prior learning must have occurred.

If the discriminative somesthetic pathway is functional, but the parietal associational cortex has become discretely damaged, the person can correctly describe the object but does not recognize that it is, indeed, a screwdriver. This deficit is called *astereognosis*. If the somesthetic, but not the parietal association cortex, is irritated by a growing tumor or by meningeal scar tissue, hallucinations of a "strange tingling sensation" or of "something moving over the skin" are experienced. These are usually unpleasant and without any meaning. This abnormal neural firing may cause an "aura" (sensory seizure), which can then progress to a generalized tonic-clonic seizure. Cortical lesions from cerebrovascular accidents or growing tumors usually destroy large areas, affecting both the somesthetic and parietal associational cortex. Damage to the somesthetic cortex on the nondominant (usually right) side of the brain can produce a

condition called the *hemineglect syndrome* in which the entire left side of the body is ignored as if it does not exist as part of the self (see Chapter 50). This syndrome is less evident after lesions of the same region on the dominant side.

Anterolateral pathway

The anterolateral or spinothalamic pathway consists of bilateral multisynaptic slow-conducting tracts that transmit sensory signals that do not require discrete localization of signal source or discrimination of fine gradations in intensity (Figure 47-6). This slow-conducting system is sometimes called the *paleospinothalamic tract* indicating that it is phylogenetically older than the neospinothalamic discriminative system. The anterolateral fibers originate in the dorsal horns where the dorsal root neurons enter the spinal cord; they cross in the anterior commissure, within the few segments of origin, to the opposite anterolateral white column where they ascend upward toward the

Figure 47-6 The neospinothalamic and paleospinothalamic subdivisions of the anterolateral sensory pathway. The neospinothalamic tract runs to the thalamic nuclei and has fibers that project to the somatosensory cortex. The paleospinothalamic tract sends collaterals to the reticular formation and other structures, from which further fibers project to the thalamus. These fibers influence the hypothalamus and limbic system, as well as the cerebral cortex. (*Rodman MJ, Smith DW: Pharmacology and Drug Therapy in Nursing, 2nd ed, p 263. Philadelphia, JB Lippincott, 1979*)

brain. The anterolateral system carries the sensations of crude touch, temperature, and pain.

Tactile sensation. In addition to the discriminative pathway, tactile sensibility uses a primitive and crude alternative relay to the thalamus. The afferent axons carrying tactile information up the dorsal columns have many branches or collaterals, and some of these synapse in the dorsal horn near the level of dorsal root entry. After several synapses, axons are projected up *both sides* of the anterolateral aspect of the spinal cord to the thalamus. From there, some projections travel to the somesthetic cortex, especially of the side opposite the stimulus. Few fibers travel all the way to the thalamus. Most synapse on reticular formation neurons, which send their axons on toward the thalamus. Because of these multiple routes, total destruction of the pathway rarely occurs. The lateral nuclei of the thalamus receiving this information are capable of contributing a crude, poorly localized sensation from the opposite side of the body.

The only time this crude alternative system becomes essential is when the discriminative pathway is damaged. Then, in spite of projection to the somatesthetic cortex of anterolateral system information, only a poorly localizable, high threshold sense of touch remains. Such persons lose all kinesthesia, proprioception, and two-point discrimination. They can detect touch stimuli to one versus the other hand, but more force must be delivered to the skin.

The anterolateral pathway also projects into the intermediate nuclei of the thalamus, which have close connections with the limbic cortical systems. This circuitry that gives touch its affective or emotional aspects (*e.g.*, the particular unpleasantness of heavy pressure and the peculiar pleasantness of the tickling and gentle rubbing of the skin). The anterolateral pathway is multisynaptic and, therefore, slow and crudely graded.

Thermal sensation. Dorsal root ganglion afferents with receptive endings in the skin for warm-hot or for cool-cold send their central axons into the segmental dorsal horn of the spinal cord. Cranial nerves innervating the face and inside of the mouth send their axons to equivalent nuclei of the brain stem. Thermal information is projected to the forebrain through the multisynaptic, slow-conducting anterolateral *paleospinothalamic* system of the *opposite side*. Thalamic and cortical somesthetic regions for temperature are mixed with those for tactile sensibility. Connections through the medial thalamus into the limbic system are associated with the high emotional content of thermal sensation. The ascending information for temperature sensation does not use the discriminative path.

Conduction of thermal information through peripheral nerves is quite slow compared with the rapid tactile afferents. If a person places a foot in a tub of hot water, the tactile sensation of the water on the skin occurs well in advance of the burning sensation. The anterolateral thermal projection system is also quite slow compared to the discriminative tactile pathway. Thus, the foot has been withdrawn from the hot water by the flexor-withdrawal reflex well before the excessive heat is perceived by centers in the forebrain. Local anesthetic agents block the small diameter afferents carrying thermal sensory information before blocking the large diameter axons carrying discriminative touch information. Absence of thermal sensitivity (athermia) resulting from partial peripheral nerve block, or from damage to the anterolateral system, is not experienced as a loss of hot and cold sensations. The affected area will not become numb until all tactile information has been blocked from reaching the thalamus and cortex.

Clinical assessment of somesthetic function

Clinically, neurologic assessment of somesthetic function can be done by testing the integrity of spinal segmental nerves. A pinpoint pressed against the skin of the sole of the foot that results in a flexor-withdrawal reflex and a complaint of pain confirms the functional integrity of the afferent terminals in the skin, the entire pathway through the peripheral nerves of the foot, leg, and thigh to the sacral (S1) dorsal root ganglion, and through the dorsal root into the spinal cord segment. It confirms that the somesthetic input association cells receiving this information are functioning and that the reflex circuitry of the cord segments (L5 to S2) are functioning. Further, the lower motoneurons of the L4 to S1 ventral horn can be considered operational, and their axons through the ventral roots, the mixed peripheral nerve, and the muscle nerve to the muscles producing the withdrawal response can be considered intact and functional. The communication between the lower motoneuron and the muscle cells is functional, and these muscles have normal responsiveness and strength. All of this information is obtained in a fraction of a second by pressing the pinpoint and observing the quick reflex response. Testing is done at each segmental level, or dermatome, moving upward along the body and neck from coccygeal segments through the high cervical levels to test the functional integrity of all of the spinal nerves. Similar dermatomes cover the face and scalp; and these, although innervated by cranial segmental nerves, are tested in the same manner.

The experienced examiner who observes a normal flexor-withdrawal reflex rules out peripheral nerve disease, disorders of the dorsal root and ganglion, diseases of the myoneural junction, and severe muscle diseases. Normal reflex function also indicates that many major descending CNS tract systems are functioning within normal limits. If the person reports the pinprick sensation and identifies its location accurately, then many ascending systems through much of the spinal cord and brain are also functioning normally, as are basic intellect and speech mechanisms.

The integrity of the discriminative (dorsal column-medial lemniscus) versus the anterolateral tactile pathways is tested with the person's eyes closed by gently brushing the skin with a wisp of cotton, by touching an area with two versus one pencil points, by touching corresponding parts of the body on each side simultaneously or in random sequence, and by passively bending the person's finger one way, then another, in random order. If only the anterolateral pathway is functional, the tactile threshold will be markedly elevated, two-point discrimination and proprioception will be missing entirely, and the patient will have difficulty discriminating which side of the body received stimulation.

In summary, the somatosensory component of the nervous system provides an awareness of body sensations such as touch, temperature, and pain. Afferent neurons of the dorsal root ganglia innervate a corresponding segment of the body as general soma afferent (somatesthetic) neurons. A sensory unit consists of a single dorsal root ganglion afferent neuron, its terminals in a small region of the periphery , and its central axon that terminates on dorsal horn association neurons. The soma innervated by somatesthetic afferent neurons of one set of dorsal root ganglia is called a dermatome. By means of a multisynaptic circuit, pressure stimuli sufficiently strong to cause tissue damage trigger a highly predictable flexor-withdrawal reflex by activating a lower motoneuron innervated skeletal muscle contraction. Somatesthetic afferents transmit the discriminative sensations of vibration and delicate touch, as well as the more crude sensations of pain and temperature.

The tactile system can be considered the basic somatesthetic system. Loss of temperature or of pain sensitivity leaves the person with no awareness of deficiency; however, if the tactile system is lost, total anesthesia (numbness) of the involved body part results. The tactile system uses two anatomically separated pathways to relay touch information to the opposite side of the forebrain—the dorsal column discriminative pathway and the anterolateral pathway. Both pathways cross to the opposite side of the nervous system. The discriminative pathway crosses at the base of the medulla, and the anterolateral pathway crosses within the first few segments of entering the cord. Normal delicate touch, vibration, position, and movement sensations use the discriminative, two-neuron pathway to reach the thalamus where tertiary relay occurs to the primary somesthetic strip of parietal cortex. The anterolateral pathway consists of bilateral multisynaptic slow-conducting tracts that preserve crude tactile sensation even when there is considerable damage to the spinal cord. In contrast to the tactile system, temperature sensations of "warm-hot" and "cool-cold" result from skin thermal afferents, which project to the thalamus and cortex only through the anterolateral system of the opposite side. Presentation of the ipsilateral dorsal column (discriminate touch) system and/or the contralateral temperature projection systems permits diagnostic analysis of the level and extent of damage in spinal cord lesions.

Pain

Pain is a complex and personal phenomenon. It involves not only anatomical structures and physiologic behaviors but psychologic, social, cultural, and cognitive factors as well. It has been demonstrated repeatedly that learning is an important factor in a person's response to painful stimuli. Pain can be a prepotent or overwhelming experience, often disruptive to customary behavior. When severe, pain demands and directs all of one's attention.

Pain is probably the most common symptom that motivates a person to seek professional help. Indeed, it sends sufferers to the physician's office more often, and with greater speed, than any other symptom. Its location, radiation, duration, and severity give important clues to its etiology. In spite of its unpleasantness, pain can serve a useful purpose, because it warns of impending tissue injury, and causes the person to seek relief. For example, an inflamed appendix could progress in severity, rupture, and even cause death were it not for the warning afforded by the pain. Pain may also be an indication of depression or dependency. It may also be used for secondary gain, either consciously or unconsciously.

Definitions

What is pain? What is its purpose? Is it of any use? Does it help or harm? Scientific disciplines have attempted to answer these and other questions about pain. The many definitions of pain flowing from these efforts serve to highlight its complex nature. Yet, in the face of intense interest about pain and research on it, we still have much to learn about this very human, very common experience. The puzzle of pain persists.

Historically, pain has often been looked on as a punishment or a means of atonement. The term itself—Greek *poine*; Latin *poena*; French *peine*—means punishment. Some Western cultures have viewed pain as something to be avoided at all costs. Aristotle regarded pain as the antithesis of pleasure, whereas Freud discussed the pleasure principle in relation to the avoidance of pain. It is impossible to really separate the pain sensation from emotion, because the sensation itself is only a part, and perhaps not even the main part, of the total pain experience. Responses to pain are patterned according to the norms of the person's cultural group. Zborowski, in his studies of Italian and Jewish women, found that both groups had low levels of pain tolerance and complained loudly when in pain. Interestingly, this behavior occurred for different reasons. The Italian women were relatively satisfied once their pain was relieved, whereas the Jewish women pursued the matter further, demanding to know its meaning.[3]

Sternbach described pain as "an abstract concept that refers to (1) a personal, private sensation of hurt; (2) a harmful stimulus which signals current and impending tissue damage; (3) a pattern of responses which operate to protect the organism from harm."[4] Useful as this definition is, it fails to describe all facets of the experience called pain.

Margo McCaffery, a nurse in private practice with more than 20 years of experience in the management of pain, has provided one of the most clinically useful definitions to date. She states, "Pain is whatever the experiencing person says it is, existing whenever he says it does."[5] Clinically, there are advantages to this definition. It is broad enough to cover the client's expression of pain, verbal or nonverbal; but, perhaps more important, it indicates that the client is believed, which is critical to developing the trust relationship so important in managing pain. Merskey believes that if pain is accepted as a psychologic phenomenon with physiologic correlates, rather than vice versa, some clinical problems can be prevented (*i.e.*, the patient will not be considered a malingerer or a liar if no objective cause for the pain can be found).[6]

Scientifically, pain has been viewed within the context of nociception. Nociception is associated with tissue damage (Latin *nocere*, "to injure"). Researchers have used the flexor-withdrawal reflex (*i.e.*, withdrawal of the hand away from a nociceptive stimulus) to describe pain. Such stimuli include pressure from a sharp object, application of a metal object heated to approximately 10°C or more above or cooled approximately 10°C or more below skin temperature, or a strong electrical current applied to the skin. Nociceptive stimuli are those that occur at or close to an intensity that causes tissue damage; therefore, they can be objectively defined. It is the subjective report of the experience accompanying nociceptive stimuli, using words such as unpleasant, hurtful, or painful, that has proven difficult to quantify. In addition to triggering withdrawal reflexes, nociceptive stimuli are actively avoided and function as negative reinforcers for learning. The flexor-withdrawal reflex can be inhibited through learning, through cultural pressure, and even through distraction.

Pain mechanisms and responses

The mechanisms of pain are many and complex. There are peripheral nerve fibers and their receptor endings that monitor the stimuli for pain, the spinal cord circuitry that processes pain information, the pathways that project pain information to the brain, the thalamus and cortex that integrate and modulate pain, and finally the subjective reaction to pain.

Pain theories

Traditionally, two theories have been offered to explain the physiologic basis for painful experience. The first, the *specificity theory*, regards pain as a separate sensory modality evoked by the activity of specific receptors that transmit information to pain centers or regions in the forebrain where pain is experienced. The second theory includes a group of theories collectively referred to as *pattern theory*. It proposes that pain receptors share endings or pathways with other sensory modalities but that different patterns of activity (spatial or temporal) of the same neurons can be used to signal painful and nonpainful stimuli. For example, light touch applied to the skin would produce the sensation of touch through low-frequency firing of the receptor; intense pressure would produce pain through high-frequency firing of the same receptor. Both theories focus on the neurophysiologic basis of pain, and both probably apply. Specific nociceptive afferents have been identified. In addition, almost all afferents, if driven at a very high frequency, can be experienced as painful. But these theories fail to address the motivational-cognitive, cultural, and affective components of pain.

The gate control theory, which was originally proposed by Melzack and Wall in 1965, was a modification of specificity theory to meet the challenges proposed by the pattern theories. This theory postulated the presence of neural gating mechanisms at the segmental spinal level to account for interactions between pain and other sensory modalities.[7] The gate control theory proposes a spinal cord level network of transmitting (t) cells and internuncial neurons that can inhibit the t cells to form a segmental level gating mechanism that can block projection of pain information to the brain.

According to the gate control theory, the internuncial fibers involved in the gating mechanism are activated by large-diameter faster-propagating fibers that carry touch (tactile) information. Thus, the simultaneous firing of the large-diameter touch fibers can block the transmission of impulses from the small-diameter myelinated and unmyelinated pain fibers. Pain therapists have long known that pain intensity can be temporarily reduced during active tactile stimulation. For example, repeated sweeping of a soft-bristled brush on the skin (brushing) over or near a painful area can sometimes result in pain reduction for several minutes to several hours.

Pain modulation is now known to be a much more complex phenomenon than that proposed by the original gate control theory. Tactile information is transmitted by small-, as well as large-diameter, fibers. Also, major interactions between sensory modalities, including the gating phenomenon, occur at several levels of the CNS rostral to the input segment. Perhaps the most puzzling aspect of brushing and other locally applied stimuli that can block the experience of pain is the relatively long-lasting effects (minutes, hours) of such treatments. This prolonged effect has been very difficult to explain on the basis of specificity theories, including the gate control theory. Other extremely important factors include endogenous opioids and their receptors at both the segmental and brain stem levels, descending feedback modulation, altered sensitivity, learning, and culture. In spite of this, the Melzack and Wall theory has served a useful purpose. It excited interest in pain, and stimulated research and clinical activity related to the pain-modulating systems.

Pain receptors and pathways

Receptors that have pain as their lowest intensity threshold stimulus are known as pain receptors. Structurally, the receptors of the peripheral pain fibers are free nerve endings. These receptors are widely distributed in the skin, dental pulp, some internal organs, periosteum, and meninges. Considerable controversy remains regarding the production of pain by the overstimulation of other receptors, such as those for temperature and pressure. The available evidence seems to support the idea that cellular destruction leads to the release of pain-producing substances. Extracts from damaged tissue produce pain when injected into normal skin. Bradykinin is one of the most potent examples; it causes pain when extremely low

doses are injected intra-arterially or intraperitoneally. It is broken down relatively rapidly and, therefore, may be involved primarily in acute pain. Other substances that have been implicated in producing pain are substance P, acetylcholine, and histamine. Prostaglandins may increase the sensitivity of pain receptors by enhancing bradykinin's pain-provoking effect.[8] The effectiveness of these compounds in provoking nociceptive reflexes and the experience of pain suggests that pain afferents are, at least in part, chemoreceptors.[8]

The peripheral branches of the afferent fibers that transmit pain information to the spinal cord form two subpopulations. The population of smaller nonmyelinated types of fibers are referred to as C fibers. These are the smallest of all peripheral fibers; they transmit impulses at the rate of 0.5 m to 2 m per second. A second population consists of the small myelinated A-delta fibers, which have considerably greater conduction velocities, transmitting impulses at a rate of 5 m to 30 m per second. The axons of A-delta and C-fiber neurons travel through the dorsal root to the dorsal horn of the spinal cord where they ascend and descend one or two segments, projecting collaterals into the dorsal horn association columns of these segments. Activated circuits of the association columns communicate with four categories of circuitry: (1) the segmental level flexor-withdrawal reflex, (2) the reticular activating system, (3) the forebrain limbic system, and (4) the thalamus and cortex. The local cord level flexor-withdrawal reflex is designed to remove endangered tissue from a damaging stimulus.

From the dorsal horn, axons of association projection neurons cross through the anterior commissure within a few segments of entering the spinal cord to the opposite side and then ascend upward to the brain in the anterolateral sensory pathway. There are three subdivisions in the anterolateral pathway: the neospinothalamic, the paleospinothalamic, and the spinoreticular systems (see Figure 47-6). The A-delta afferent fibers project, after a single spinal level synapse, through the moderately rapid neospinothalamic pathway to the thalamus. The fibers in the neospinothalamic tract are mainly associated with the spatial and temporal aspects of sharp, bright, or fast pain. Projections of this system to the parietal somesthetic area probably provide the precise location of first pain. Small unmyelinated C-fiber afferents, which are concerned with diffuse, dull, aching, and unpleasant pain, travel through the slower conducting multisynaptic paleospinothalamic tract. This system terminates in several thalamic regions including the intralaminar nuclei, which project to the limbic cortex, and is associated with the emotional aspects of pain.

The spinoreticular system projects bilaterally to the reticular formation of the brain stem. This system, in conjunction with the collaterals of the paleospinothalamic system, facilitates avoidance reflexes at all levels. It also contributes to an increase in the electroencephalographic (EEG) activity associated with alertness and indirectly influences hypothalamic functions associated with sudden alertness, such as increased heart rate and blood pressure. This may explain the tremendous arousal effects of certain pain stimuli.

Pain perception

The basic sensation of hurtfulness, or pain, occurs at the level of the thalamus. In the neospinothalamic system, interconnections between the lateral thalamus and the somatosensory cortex are necessary to add precision and discrimination to the pain sensation. Association areas of the parietal cortex are essential to the perception, or learned meaningfulness, of the pain experience. For example, if a mosquito bites a person's index finger on the left hand and only the thalamus is functional, the person will complain of pain somewhere on the hand. With the primary sensory cortex functional, the person can localize the pain to the precise area on the index finger. The association cortex, on the other hand, is necessary in order to interpret the buzzing and the sensation that preceded the pain as being related to a mosquito bite. The paleospinothalamic system projects diffusely from the intralaminar nuclei of the thalamus to large areas of the limbic cortex. These connections are probably associated with the hurtfulness as well as the mood-altering and attention-narrowing effect of pain.

Endogenous analgesic mechanisms

One of the exciting advances in the understanding of pain has been the recent elucidation of neuroanatomical pathways that arise in the midbrain and brain stem, descend to the spinal cord, and function in the modulation of ascending pain impulses. One such pathway begins in an area of the midbrain called the *periaqueductal gray (PAG)* region. Four years after the introduction of the gate control theory, it was found that focal stimulation of the midbrain PAG regions produced a state of analgesia. The resultant analgesia lasted for many hours and was sufficient to permit abdominal surgery, although levels of consciousness and reactions to auditory and visual stimuli remained unaffected. A few years later, opiate receptors were found to be highly concentrated in this and other regions of the CNS where electrical stimulation produced analgesia. Because of these findings, the PAG area of the midbrain is often referred to as the *endogenous analgesia center.*

Recent studies have shown that the endogenous analgesia center receives input from widespread areas of the CNS including the cerebral cortex, hypothalamus, brain stem reticular formation, and the spinal cord by way of the paleospinothalamic and neospinothalamic tracts. This region is intimately connected to the limbic system, which is associated with emotional experience. The neurons of the endogenous analgesia center have axons that descend into the nucleus raphe magnus in the rostral medulla. The axons of neurons in this medullary pain center project to the dorsal horn of the spinal cord where they terminate in the same layers as the entering primary pain fibers (Figure 47-7). Stimulation of the medullary nuclei is thought to inhibit pain transmission by dorsal horn projection neurons.[9] There is also evidence of noradrenergic neurons that can inhibit transmission of pain impulses at the level of the spinal cord. Studies indicate that the rostral pons has noradrenergic neurons with axons that project to the medullary nuclei and to the dorsal horn cells of the spinal cord.[9a] The discovery that norepinephrine can block pain transmission had led to studies directed at the combined administration of narcotics and clonidine (a central acting alpha-adrenergic agonist) for pain relief.

The opioids are morphine-like substances that are manufactured in many regions of the CNS, including the pituitary gland. The discovery of morphine receptors led to a search for natural body substances capable of interacting with these receptors. The natural ligands, or binding molecules, for these opiate receptors are the endogenous opioid peptides (the endorphins and enkephalins), which were discovered in 1975. New therapeutic approaches to the treatment of pain were envisioned when (1) it was discovered that these peptides exert inhibitory modulation of pain transmission and (2) the release of endogenous opioids following CNS stimulation was correlated with patient reports of pain relief. Endorphins are found primarily in the amygdala, limbic system, hypothalamic–pituitary axis, and other brain stem structures. The enkephalins are found primarily in short interneurons in the PAG of the midbrain, limbic system, basal ganglia, hypothalamus, and spinal cord dorsal horn. These morphine-like substances tend to mimic the peripheral and central effects of morphine and central effects of other opiate drugs.

Since the discovery of the opioids, other neuromodulators for pain have been identified. Serotonin has been implicated as a neuromodulator in the NRM medullary nuclei that project to the spinal cord. It has been shown that tricyclic antidepressant compounds, such as amitriptyline, have analgesic properties independent of their antidepressant effects. These drugs, which enhance the effects of serotonin by blocking its presynaptic uptake, have been found to be effective in the management of certain types of chronic pain.[10,11] Substance P, another neuropeptide, is an

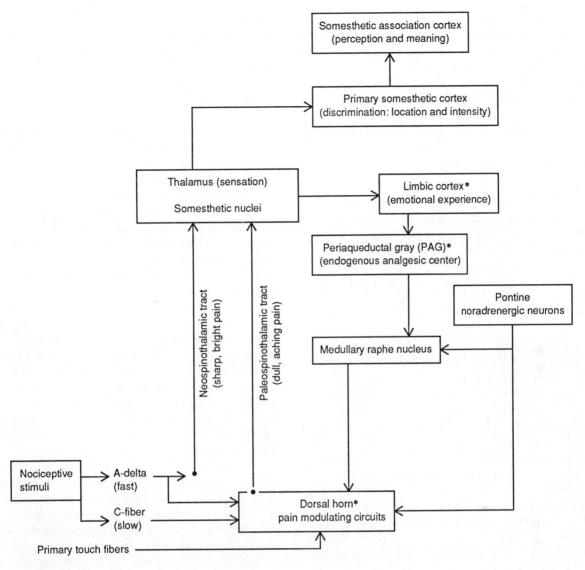

Figure 47-7 Primary pain pathways. The transmission of incoming nociceptive impulses is modulated by dorsal horn circuitry that receives inhibitory input from peripheral touch receptors and from descending pathways involving the periaqueductal endogenous analgesic center in the midbrain, the pontine noradrenergic neurons, and the raphe nucleus in the medulla.

11-amino acid peptide that is widely distributed throughout the nervous system. Considerable research data support the role of substance P as a transmitter substance used by unmyelinated C-fiber afferents related to nociception and slow pain.[12] There is some evidence that enkephalins and other opioid peptides modulate pain at the spinal level by inhibiting the release of substance P.

Fast pain versus slow pain

Two qualitatively differentiated types of pain can be readily appreciated—fast pain and slow pain. Fast pain is a short, well-localized sensation; it starts and stops abruptly when the stimulus is instituted or stopped. Examples are a pinprick or strong pinch. Fast pain has its origin in the free nerve endings of myelinated A-delta axons located in the skin that respond to strong mechanical pressure and high temperature. It is associated with the flexor-withdrawal reflex and with the sensation of bright, sharp pain experience. Slow pain is experienced as a throbbing, burning, or aching sensation. It has its origin in the free nerve endings of the very slow conducting unmyelinated C fibers. The slow pain receptors have chemoreceptor properties and respond to compounds liberated as a result of tissue damage from excessive mechanical, chemical, and cold or hot stimuli. These two fiber conduction groups of afferents partially explain the two components of pain. The farther the stimulus is from the brain, the more time separates the fast and slow components.

Classification

The types of pain can be classified according to source, duration, objective signs, and referral.

Source

The sources of pain are commonly divided into four general categories: cutaneous, deep somatic, visceral pain, and functional or psychogenic. Cutaneous pain arises from superficial structures, such as the skin and subcutaneous tissues. A paper cut on the finger is an example of easily localized superficial, or cutaneous, pain. It tends to be a sharp, bright pain with a burning quality and may be either abrupt or slow in onset. It can be localized accurately and may be distributed along the dermatomes. Because there is an overlap of nerve fiber distribution between the dermatomes, the boundaries of pain frequently are not as clear-cut as the dermatonal diagrams indicate.

A second type of pain is related to the deep somatic structures, such as the periosteum, muscles, tendons, joints, and blood vessels. Deep somatic pain tends to be more diffuse than cutaneous pain. Various stimuli, such as strong pressure exerted on bone, ischemia to a muscle, or tissue damage, can produce deep somatic pain. This is the type of pain one experiences from a sprained ankle. Radiation of pain from the original site of injury can occur. For example, damage to a nerve root can cause the person to experience pain radiating along its fiber distribution.

A third type of pain, called *visceral,* or *splanchnic,* pain, originates in the viscera. Common examples of visceral pain are renal colic, pain due to cholecystitis, pain associated with acute appendicitis, and ulcer pain. Although the viscera are diffusely and richly innervated, cutting or burning of viscera, as opposed to similar noxious stimuli applied to cutaneous or superficial structures, is unlikely to cause pain. Instead, strong abnormal contractions of the gastrointestinal system, distention, or ischemia affecting the walls of the viscera can induce severe pain. Anyone who has suffered from either severe gastrointestinal distress or ureteral colic can readily attest to the misery involved. We are most accustomed to thinking of visceral pain as emanating from the abdominal cavity. However, visceral pain tends to be diffuse, especially in early stages.

Visceral pain is transmitted by small unmyelinated pain fibers that travel within the nerves of the autonomic system and project to visceral input associ-

ation neurons of the cord or brain stem. Besides sending projections to the forebrain, these input association neurons also project into visceral reflex circuits. Consequently, visceral pain is often accompanied by autonomic responses such as nausea, vomiting, sweating, pallor, and possibly shock. Pain from the lower end of the esophagus and below the midtransverse colon tends to travel the course of cranial nerves IX and X and the parasympathetic nerves entering the sacral region of the spinal cord. Pain fibers entering the thoracolumbar region of the spinal cord travel the course of the sympathetic nerves.

Unlike organic or somatogenic pain, which originates in the body, or soma, functional or psychogenic pain is attributed to the psyche or emotions. In both situations, the physical sensation of pain is the same. The person may be unaware that the origin of the pain is emotional and may experience it as if the pain were truly originating from an organic disorder. Many persons who suffer from pain of psychogenic origin have had developmental difficulties during adolescence. It is important to note that persons with pain usually experience both its physical and its emotional aspects. It is difficult to conceive of pain as being either purely organic or purely functional. McCaffery's statement that "pain is whatever the experiencing persons says it is and exists whenever he says it does" is particularly applicable here.[5]

Positive placebo reactors (those who experience pain relief from such measures as pills containing inert or ineffective substances) may be found among those suffering from organic or functional pain. In the past there was no adequate explanation for the behavior of positive placebo reactors, and, in fact, such persons were often regarded as malingerers. Research has demonstrated the importance of higher central nervous system control over sensory input. The discovery of the endogenous modulators of pain, such as the endorphins and enkephalins, suggests that placebos may trigger the release of pain-modulating substances, which cause the pain to diminish. (See the section entitled "Placebo Response" later in this chapter.)

Duration

Pain can also be classified according to duration and characterized as acute or chronic pain. The pain research of the past 25 years has emphasized the importance of differentiating acute pain from chronic pain and dealing with them separately. This is because they differ from each other in etiology, mechanisms, pathophysiology, and function, and because the diagnosis of and therapy for each are distinctive (Table 47-1).

Acute pain is usually defined as pain of less than 6 months' duration. It consists of unpleasant sensory, perceptual, and emotional components with associated somatic, autonomic, psychologic, and behavioral responses. Acute pain is caused by noxious, or tissue-damaging stimuli; and its purpose is to serve as a protective, or warning, system. Besides alerting the person to the existence of actual or impending tissue damage, it prompts a search for professional help. The pain's location, intensity, duration, and radiation, as well as those factors that aggravate or relieve it, are essential diagnostic clues. Unlike chronic pain, it is extremely rare for acute pain to be due to psychologic factors alone. Acute pain is often accompanied by anxiety, which usually disappears when the pain is relieved.

Chronic pain is defined as pain of 6 months' duration or longer. The pain may be continuous (*e.g.,* arthritis) or intermittent (*e.g.,* angina or intermittent claudication). Unlike acute pain, persistent chronic pain usually serves no useful function. To the contrary, it imposes physiologic, psychologic, family, and economic stresses and may exhaust the resources of a person. In contrast to acute pain, psychologic and environmental influences may play an important role in the development of behaviors associated with chronic pain. Chronic pain is often associated with depression and despair rather than anxiety. Amazingly, this depression is often relieved spontaneously when the pain is removed.

It is extremely important to appreciate that persons suffering chronic pain may not exhibit the somatic, autonomic, or affective behaviors associated with acute pain. One reason for this is that the stress response cannot be maintained for long periods of time. Then, too, certain behaviors viewed as acceptable in patients with severe but short-lived pain would not be expected or considered appropriate in the chronic situation. With chronic pain, it is important to heed the person's own description of the pain because the expected psychophysiologic responses may or may not be present.

One proposed classification of chronic pain divides the affected persons into two broad groups according to life expectancy (brief versus normal). This classification assumes clinical importance primarily if a decision must be reached concerning long-term use of narcotics for pain relief.

Referral

Referred pain is that pain perceived at a site different from its point of origin but innervated by the same spinal segment. Pain originating in the abdominal or thoracic viscera tends to be diffuse and poorly localized and is often perceived at a site far removed from the affected area. For example, the pain associated with myocardial infarction is often referred to the left arm, neck, and chest.

Referred pain may arise alone or concurrent with pain located at the origin of the noxious stimuli. Although the term *referred* is usually applied to pain originating in the viscera and experienced as if originating from the body wall, it may also be applied to

Table 47–1. Characteristics of acute and chronic pain

Characteristic	Acute pain	Chronic pain
Onset	Recent	Continuous or intermittent
Duration	Short duration	6 months or more
Autonomic responses	Consistent with sympathetic fight or flight response*	Absence of autonomic responses
	Increased heart rate	
	Increased stroke volume	
	Increased blood pressure	
	Increased pupillary dilation	
	Increased muscle tension	
	Decreased gut motility	
	Decreased salivary flow (dry mouth)	
Psychologic component	Associated anxiety	Increased irritability
		Associated depression
		Somatic preoccupation
		Withdrawal from outside interests
		Decreased strength of relationships
Other types of response		Decreased sleep
		Decreased libido
		Appetite changes

* Responses are approximately proportional to intensity of the stimulus.

pain arising from somatic structures. An example would be pain referred to the chest wall due to nociceptive stimulation of the diaphragm, which receives somatic innervation from the intercostal nerves.

An understanding of pain reference is of great value in diagnosing illness because afferent neurons from visceral or deep somatic tissue enter the spinal cord at the same level as those from the cutaneous areas to which the pain is referred (see Figure 47-8 for sites of referred pain).

The sites of referred pain are determined during the development of the organ systems in the embryo. Let us say that a person has peritonitis but complains of pain in the shoulder. Internally, there is irritation or inflammation of the central diaphragm. In the embryo, the diaphragm originates in the neck, and

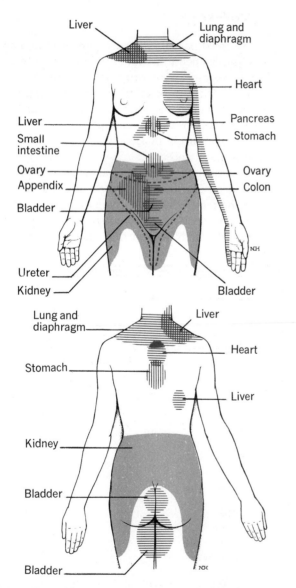

Figure 47-8 Areas of referred pain: **(Top)**, anterior view; **(bottom)** posterior view. (Chaffee EE, Lytle IM: Basic Physiology and Anatomy, 4th ed, p 266. Philadelphia, JB Lippincott, 1980)

its central portion is innervated by the phrenic nerve, which enters the cord at the level of fifth to seventh cervical segment (C5 to C7). As the fetus develops, the diaphragm descends to its adult position between the thoracic and abdominal cavities, innervated by the phrenic nerve. Therefore, fibers entering the spinal cord at the C5 to C7 level carry information from the neck area as well as from the diaphragm, and the diaphragmatic pain is interpreted by the forebrain as originating from the neck area.

Although the *visceral* pleura, pericardium, and peritoneum are said to be relatively free of pain fibers, the *parietal* pleura, pericardium, and peritoneum do react to nociceptive stimuli. Visceral inflammation can involve parietal and somatic structures, and this, in turn, may give rise to diffuse local or referred pain. For example, irritation of the parietal peritoneum resulting from appendicitis often gives rise to pain directly over the inflamed area in the lower right quadrant. Also, such stimuli can evoke pain referred to the umbilical area.

Another type of pain is *muscular spasm*, or *guarding*, when somatic structures are involved. Guarding is a protective-reflex rigidity, and its purpose is to protect the affected body parts (*e.g.*, an abscessed appendix or a sprained muscle). This protective guarding may give rise to pain of muscle ischemia causing both local and referred pain.

Pain from the viscera may be localized only with difficulty. There are several explanations for this. First, innervation of visceral organs is very poorly represented at the forebrain (perception) levels. A second possible explanation is that the brain does not easily learn to localize sensations originating in organs that are only imprecisely visualized. For example, a cut on the third finger of the right hand can be readily seen, identified, and localized, whereas an inflamed internal organ can be localized only vaguely. A third explanation is that sensory information from thoracic and abdominal viscera can travel by two pathways to the central nervous system. The first route is called the *visceral*, or *true visceral, pathway*. According to this hypothesis, the pain information travels with the fibers of the autonomic nervous system that only enter the spinal cord in the T1 to T12 and S1 to S4 segments. Therefore, the pain is felt at a site on the surface of the body distant to the pain locus.

The second route, the parietal pathway, which is somatic, is not usually considered to be a pathway for visceral pain, but may be the pain route with inflammation of the parietal pleura, pericardium, and peritoneum. Sensations traveling along this pathway can be localized directly over the affected part, a common example being pain in the right lower quadrant associated with an inflamed appendix.

It is always possible that referred pain can be

one consequence of an anatomical anomaly. Therefore, the reader should be aware of the referral phenomenon when trying to identify the source of pain. Although pain may be the stimulus that prompts the person to seek professional help, a careful history and examination are necessary to assess the problem correctly. It should be remembered that pain is almost always a warning that pathophysiologic processes are occurring in the source organ, whether correctly localized by the person or not. All hypotheses explaining the referral phenomenon propose that confusion occurs in forebrain interpretation of the actual location of the pain source, often with learned referral to a familiar body part or region or to the site of previously experienced chronic pain.[13] If pain referral is present, the phenomenon should be explained to the patient.

Reactions to pain

Reactions to pain are affected by pain threshold and tolerance. Although the terms are often used interchangeably, pain threshold and pain tolerance are not the same entity. The former is more closely associated with nociceptive (*i.e.,* tissue damaging) stimuli, whereas the latter relates more to the total pain experience. Separation and identification of the role of each of these concepts continue to pose fundamental problems for the pain management team, as well as pain researchers.

Pain threshold

Pain threshold is usually defined as the least intense stimulus that will cause pain. Although pain threshold is still controversial, it is generally accepted that the threshold is similar in most persons, particularly under controlled experimental conditions. For example, on exposure to heat of increasing intensity, most people state that the sensation of heat converts to pain at approximately 45°C.

Pain tolerance

Pain tolerance is usually defined as the maximum intensity or duration of pain that a person is willing to endure—the point beyond which the person wants something done about the pain. Tolerance is not necessarily indicative of the severity of pain. Psychologic, familial, cultural, and environmental factors significantly influence the intensity of pain a person is willing to tolerate.

Physical reactions

Physical reactions to pain may be manifested by biting the lips, clenching the teeth, and facial expressions, such as frowning or wrinkling the brows.

Protective body movements can be both involuntary and voluntary. The previously mentioned flexor-withdrawal reaction, which moves the body part away from the pain source, is involuntary. Voluntary movements, such as changes in posture and relaxation exercises, often relieve discomfort.

Physiologic responses

Physiologic responses to pain involve activation of the sympathetic nervous system, which evokes the "fight or flight" response, with catecholamine release from the adrenal medulla. What happens is this: as blood is shifted from nonvital to vital parts of the body, the vessels of the skin and the abdominal viscera (spleen, kidneys, and intestine) constrict, while those of the heart, skeletal muscles, lungs, and brain dilate. The face becomes pallid, and the pupils become dilated. Respirations, heart rate, and strength of cardiac contraction increase. Muscle tension rises, and energy stores are mobilized to supply the body with glucose. A relative decline in parasympathetic activity may result in a loss of appetite, nausea, and vomiting. Gastrointestinal motility and digestive gland secretion also diminish. After a period of time, a parasympathetic rebound response occurs and the heart rate, blood pressure, and respiratory rate may fall below the pre-pain level. This is likely when pain is intense but of short duration.

Pain that persists or is repetitive results in adaptative responses, with observable decreases in sympathetic activity. Pain receptors show little if any adaptation. On the contrary, reactions to long-term pain tend to be centrally mediated. With time, physiologic and psychologic coping mechanisms evolve, but these behavioral responses do not necessarily indicate pain relief. The person may merely be too fatigued to respond.

Occasionally, pain is associated with neurogenic shock (see Chapter 23) due to inhibition of the medullary vasomotor center with decreased vasomotor tone. This mechanism is not well understood; it is believed that it might cause circulatory collapse, despite the presence of sympathetic activity.

During rapid eye movement (REM) sleep, the EEG activity becomes desynchronized and the sympathetic nervous system becomes activated (see Chapter 26). Certain disorders in which pain predominates, such as angina and ulcer, appear to be exacerbated during this stage of sleep.

Psychosocial reactions

Psychosocial reactions to pain are deeply influenced by the same factors that affect pain tolerance, including past experiences with pain. A verbally competent person may be able to describe accurately the location, duration, and intensity of the pain, as well as his or her ability or willingness to tolerate it. A change in the tone of voice may be as revealing as the words spoken. Previous personal and family experiences with certain diseases, such as cancer, can significantly affect the degree of fear, anxiety, and depression associated with pain and, consequently, the person's reaction to it.

Pain that necessitates absence from work will probably be of greater importance to one who is paid an hourly wage than to one who has ample health insurance and sick time available.

Vocalizations comprise a group of responses such as crying, groaning, grunting, and gasping. Their frequency, loudness, and duration can assume greater significance in situations where the person is either too young or too confused to be verbally competent. These manifestations are particularly important in young children and elderly persons.

Cultural and environmental factors may also play a role in pain perception. For example, a person who values stoicism is unlikely to cry out in public when subjected to painful stimuli, whereas this may be an accepted response for someone of another culture.

Pain can provide reassurance. In one study, the members of a group of men, matched as to injuries, gave very different responses depending on the circumstances of their wounding.[14] Trauma inflicted on the battlefield evoked denial of pain and refusal of medication; the same types of injuries inflicted on civilians evoked complaints of pain and requests for pain relief. These striking differences have been attributed to the emotional state at the time of injury as well as the significance each person attached to the injuries. For the soldier, being wounded may have afforded a face-saving escape from unpleasant, life-threatening situations. It meant being transported to a relatively safe environment, perhaps even home. But a civilian with the same type of injury may have felt that life-style as well as income was threatened.

Age factors

Pain is multidimensional, and each person is affected differently. When the problems of pain are addressed, elderly persons and children may require special attention compared with young or middle-aged adults.

The literature regarding pain in elderly persons is sparse, and more studies are needed. Several aspects require particular attention.[15] Elderly persons often receive inappropriate dosages of medications because of tissue changes resulting from the normal aging process. Abrupt hospitalization may cause dis-

orientation, decreased exercise, loss of control over one's life, inability to express pain, and regression. Depression and fear of death may also cause special problems. Degenerative changes can result in intermittent or continuous chronic pain. These problems must be considered when dealing with pain in elderly persons.

One startling finding has been that children, unlike adults, are often permitted to suffer intense postoperative pain even when pain medication has been ordered and is available. The factors resulting in this behavior on the part of caregivers need to be investigated and addressed. Some of these factors include inappropriate beliefs that (1) children suffer less intense pain because of their immature nervous systems, (2) children recover quickly, (3) children should not have narcotics because they may become addicted, (4) respiratory depression is a particular threat, (5) children are unable to identify where they hurt, and (6) the nurse who uses the needle will get negative feedback.[16]

Circumcision, heel lancing, and other noxious stimuli to preterm and full-term neonates result in physiologic changes. These include cardiorespiratory effects such as marked increases in heart rate and blood pressure, large changes in transcutaneous partial pressure of oxygen, and increased palmar sweating. Hormonal and metabolic changes include increased plasma-renin activity and increased plasma levels of epinephrine, norepinephrine, and cortisol. Marked hormonal changes associated with surgery under light anesthesia result in severe stress reactions and increased postoperative morbidity and mortality. Evidence is now mounting that use of anesthetics for surgery in the neonate is not only recommended as effective, but as necessary to prevent pathologic stress reactions.

In their well-referenced paper, Anand and Hickey discuss their own work and a number of other studies related to pain and its control in the neonate.[17] These same authors identify behavioral changes indicative of pain in newborns subjected to circumcision without anesthesia. They warn that the persistence of certain of these responses implies a greater capacity for memory than is commonly assumed. They suggest that memory of these experiences associated with pain and stress may disrupt normal adaptation of the newborn.

Pain in the human fetus and neonate presents special problems because it is often assumed that they suffer less intensely, or not at all, due to the immaturity of their nervous systems. Considerable research evidence now suggests that by late gestation, pain pathways, cortical and subcortical pain centers, and neurochemical systems associated with pain transmission and modulation are developed and functional.[18]

As with systems associated with pain perception in the adult, the neuropeptides and endogenous opioid systems also seem to be involved in the neonate. Endogenous opioids are released by the human fetus at birth and in response to fetal and neonatal distress.[19] Beta-endorphin plasma concentrations increase with difficult births, and evidence suggests birth asphyxia may be a potent stimulus to the release of these endogenous opioids.[20,21] Newborns with apnea of prematurity also demonstrate marked increases in cerebrospinal fluid levels of beta-endorphin, as do infants with pain or infants who require invasive procedures for their treatment.[22,23] Because these levels are 10,000 times less than those required to produce analgesia in the adult, they are not likely to be high enough to decrease analgesic or anesthetic requirements.[24,25]

In children, complex relationships may occur between previous threats or experiences with pain and their current response. Like adults, children appear to be better able to cope with pain when they are informed about what is happening to them and are helped to develop appropriate coping strategies. Doll play, a variety of sensory inputs, films, and videotapes may help them cope. Distraction, hypnosis, guided-relaxation imagery, and various other techniques can be used effectively, depending on the child's age. Children who have an inaccurate understanding of what is happening to them may develop fantasies of mutilation, become extremely anxious, and doubt their ability to cope. Realistic reassurance measures that promote their sense of control and coping abilities are recommended.[5,16] The child's developmental level, position in the family, and understanding of what happened or is happening, and why, are only a few of the variables that need study.

—— Alterations in pain sensitivity and perception

Sensitivity to pain varies among persons, as well as in the same person, under different conditions and in different parts of the body. Irritation, mild hypoxia, and mild compression of a peripheral nerve often result in hyperexcitability of the sensory nerve fibers or cell bodies. This is experienced as unpleasant hypersensitivity (*hyperesthesia*), or increased painfulness (*hyperalgesia*). Spontaneous, unpleasant sensations called *paresthesias* occur with more severe irritation (*e.g.,* the "pins-and-needles" sensation that follows temporary compression of a peripheral nerve). The general term *dysesthesia* is given to distortions (usually unpleasant) of somesthetic sensation that often accompany partial loss of sensory innervation. *Hyperpathia* is a syndrome in which a painful stimulus results in a prolonged unpleasant experience, especially upon repetitive stimulus application. This pain

can be explosive and radiates through a peripheral nerve distribution.[26] It is associated with pathologic changes in peripheral nerves, such as localized hypoxia. More severe pathology can result in reduced or lost tactile (*hypesthesia, anesthesia*), temperature (*hypothermia, athermia*), and pain sensation (*hypoalgesia*). *Analgesia* is a lack of pain without loss of consciousness.

Pain may occur with or without an apparently adequate stimulus; on the other hand, even in the presence of an adequate noxious stimulus, pain may be absent. Most familiar to us is pain following adequate stimulation. For example, a hand touched by a flame will be quickly withdrawn. The interesting feature of this reaction, known as *local sign,* is that the hand is moved away from the painful stimulus in whichever direction is appropriate—up, down, or either side, as demanded by the situation. In each such situation, the response serves to remove the limb or other body part from the noxious stimulus. Responses that outlast the stimulus are characteristic of polysynaptic, multisegmental spinal reflexes.

Allodynia (Greek *allo,* "other" and *odynia,* "painful") is the term used for the puzzling phenomenon of pain that follows a non-noxious stimulus to apparently normal skin. This term is intended to refer to instances where otherwise normal tissues may be abnormally innervated or may be referral sites for other loci that give rise to pain with non-noxious stimuli.[27,28] It may be that an area is hypersensitive because of inflammation or another cause, and a normally subthreshold stimulus is sufficient to trigger the sensation of pain. This response is thought to be chemically mediated, possibly the result of tissue damage in the surrounding area. *Trigger points* that are fired off by light tactile stimulation to a highly localized point on the skin or mucous membrane can repeatedly produce immediate intense pain at that site or elsewhere. *Myofascial trigger points* are foci of exquisite tenderness found in many muscles and can be responsible for pain projected to sites remote from the points of tenderness.[29,30] These trigger points cause reproducible myofascial pain syndromes in specific muscles. According to recent reports, these pain syndromes are the major source of pain in clients at chronic pain treatment centers.[30] One recent report indicated that 85% of 233 consecutive admissions to one comprehensive pain center were assigned a primary organic diagnosis of myofascial pain syndrome.[31] The diagnosis of myofascial pain is frequently overlooked and, as a consequence, inadequately treated.[32] Trigger points are widely distributed in the back of the head and neck and in the lumbar and thoracic regions.[27]

The inability to sense pain may result in trauma, infection, even loss of a body part or parts.

Inherited insensitivity to pain may take the form of congenital indifference or congenital insensitivity to pain. In the former, transmission of nerve impulses appears normal but appreciation of painful stimuli at higher levels appears to be absent. In the latter, a peripheral nerve defect apparently exists such that transmission of painful nerve impulses does not result in perception of pain. Whatever the cause, persons who lack the ability to perceive pain are at constant risk of tissue damage because pain is not serving its protective function.

Persons with diabetes mellitus may develop neurologic deficits, most commonly in the nerves that supply the feet. As a consequence, these persons may lack sensation and the ability to perceive pain in the feet—which explains why persons with diabetes are cautioned about the necessity of meticulous foot care to prevent trauma. In other disease processes, pain pathways may be accidentally or deliberately destroyed to prevent noxious stimuli from relaying messages to the brain.

Head pain

Headache

Headache is discussed here because it is a type of pain that is recognized almost universally. Although headache is extremely common, its cause is frequently not known. There are many types of headache, the most common of which are tension-type (muscle contraction) headache and migraine headache. Hypertension, as well as traction on intracranial pain-sensitive structures by tumors, subdural hemorrhages, or the weight of the brain after CSF removal can also induce headaches. Depression can result in headache and is a frequently overlooked cause in children. Other causes of headaches include systemic infections with fever, convulsive states, and hypoxic conditions such as cyanotic heart disease and severe asthma. It is estimated that 50% to 90% of adult Americans experience headache at some time, at a cost of millions of workdays lost and billions of dollars spent on headache relief.[32] Physicians estimate that at least 20% of the complaints they receive are related to headache.[33] Bille's study revealed that 40% of children have experienced headache by 7 years of age, and 75% by the age of 15.[34]

Although it is always difficult to classify and define diseases, the field of pain related to headache presents particular problems. The absence of laboratory tests, which could serve as diagnostic criteria for any of the primary headache forms, reflects the paucity of physiologic data available. There are typical and pure forms of headache, but transitional forms also occur and these cause confusion. Over time a person may have more than one form of headache, and those they have may undergo not only quantitative but also qualitative changes. Therefore, a new system has been developed that classifies headaches, rather than persons. A person may have more than one form of headache, however, each particular headache can fit only one set of diagnostic criteria.

Until 1988, most current headache classifications were derived from a 1962 publication of the Ad Hoc Committee on the Classification of Headache.[35] In 1988, the first edition of The Classification and Diagnostic Criteria for Headache Disorders, Cranial Neuralgias, and Facial Pain prepared by the Headache Classification Committee of the International Headache Society was published, along with ten General Rules considered essential to the correct use of this new system.[36] The new classification system is constructed in an hierarchical manner with up to four digits, and there are operational diagnostic criteria for all headache disorders. Routine diagnoses are expected at the one- or two-digit level. Diagnoses to the fourth digit are expected at specialized diagnostic and treatment centers. Although the primary purpose for development of this classification system was research, the operational diagnostic criteria are expected to influence the diagnosis and treatment of headaches. The chosen criteria for a particular diagnosis represent a compromise between sensitivity and specificity and are expected to help clarify some of the problems of the 1962 classification system. The major classifications of the new system are given in Chart 47-1. Subclassifications to the second digit are included for migraine and tension-type headaches because these are the two most commonly encountered types of headaches in clinical practice.

Tension-type headache. Under the new classification system, the various muscle contraction and psychogenic headaches are called tension-type headaches. The most common form of headache in adults and adolescents is the tension headache resulting from sustained contraction of the muscles of the neck and scalp.[37] Contraction of these muscles causes pressure on nerves in the area, and it can also constrict blood vessels at the base of the neck. When these mechanisms increase pressure, waste products (e.g., lactic acid) also accumulate, causing more pain. The usual source of this tensing of muscles is an unconscious reaction to stress. However, any activity that requires the head to be held in one position, such as typing, repairing jewelry, or using a microscope, can cause muscle contraction headache. Even sleeping in a cold room or with the neck in an inappropriate or strained position can cause a tension headache.

Prevention and treatment are best approached by identifying and removing precipitating factors. This can include such measures as sleeping in a warm room, wearing a scarf to avoid muscle spasms when exposed to the cold, and using a small pillow under the neck for sleeping. Proper eye care, light, and posture during reading, as well as exercising the neck and shoulders frequently, should lower the incidence of muscle spasms. Sleep, deep relaxation exercises, and massage of sore or tense muscles can help to decrease or eliminate painful headaches. Biofeedback (to be discussed) may be used in the treatment of tension headache. Use of medication can often be decreased or eliminated by successfully employing one or more of the above alternative approaches to pain relief.

Migraine headache. Migraine headache is a disorder characterized by paroxysmal attacks of intense head pain, with vasoconstriction followed by vasodilatation, or normal blood flow followed by hyperemia. Throbbing unilateral pain, photophobia, anorexia, and nausea with vomiting frequently accompany these headaches. Such neurologic deficits as hemiparesis and hemisensory defects may sometimes be noted. Migraine headache affects between 12 million and 16 million Americans. It occurs in all age groups, even in young infants. Incidence according to sex is equal in young children, but in adolescents and adults, it occurs 3 to 10 times more frequently in females than males. In some cases it can be associated with certain days in the menstrual cycle. In 70% to 80% of cases, there is a positive family history.[34]

In contrast to the 1962 headache classification system,[35] which included migraine headaches in the vascular headache classification, the 1988 system has added a separate classification for migraine headaches.[36] This is in accord with recent research findings that have demonstrated a probable neurogenic etiology to this type of headache.

The two major types of migraine are called *migraine without aura* (formerly referred to as common migraine) and *migraine with aura* (formerly called classic or classical migraine). An aura is a complex of focal neurologic symptoms that initiates or accompanies a migraine headache attack. It is indicative of focal cerebral dysfunction and typically lasts 20 to 30 minutes.[36] Alterations in sensory or motor function can occur. A typical visual aura can consist of flashing lights, blind spots, double vision, or hallucinations. These symptoms are consistent with foci of cerebral ischemia, and, therefore, changes in oxygen availability. Pain receptors are sensitive to this diminution in oxygen. Premonitory symptoms (formerly called prodromal symptoms) can occur a day or two before a migraine (with or without aura). These can include symptoms of hyper- or hypoactivity, craving for certain foods, depression, repetitive yawning, and other atypical symptoms.[36]

Chart 47–1:   Classification and diagnostic criteria for headache disorders, cranial neuralgias, and facial pain

1. Migraine
    1.1 Migraine without aura
    1.2 Migraine with aura
    1.3 Ophthalmoplegic migraine
    1.4 Retinal migraine
    1.5 Childhood periodic syndromes that may be precursors to or associated with migraine
    1.6 Complications with migraine
    1.7 Migrainous disorder not fulfilling above criteria
2. Tension-type headache
    2.1 Episodic tension-type headache
    2.2 Chronic tension-type headache
    2.3 Headache of the tension-type not fulfilling the above criteria
3. Cluster headache and chronic paroxysmal hemicrania
4. Miscellaneous headaches unassociated with structural lesion
5. Headache associated with head trauma
6. Headache associated with vascular disorders
7. Headache associated with nonvascular intracranial disorders
8. Headache associated with substances or their withdrawal
9. Headache associated with noncephalic infection
10. Headache associated with metabolic disorder
11. Headache or facial pain associated with disorder of cranium, neck, eyes, ears, nose, sinuses, teeth, mouth or other facial or cranial structures
12. Cranial neuralgias, nerve trunk pain, and deafferentation pain
13. Headache not classifiable

(Adapted from Oleson J: Classification and diagnostic criteria for headache disorders, cranial neuralgias and facial pain. Cephalgia 8(Suppl 7):13–19, 1988)

Migraine headache sufferers are advised to moderate caffeine intake and to avoid large fluctuations in estrogen levels by eliminating oral contraceptives and postmenopausal hormones. Reducing psychologic and environmental stresses can also decrease the precipitation of attacks. Dietary changes include avoiding tyramine-containing foods, cured meats, and monosodium glutamate (Chart 47-2). Smoke-filled rooms and hypoglycemia, whether early morning or fast induced, can increase migraine attacks.

When dietary and life-style changes and nonpharmacologic approaches, such as biofeedback and relaxation techniques, fail to achieve relief, medications may be necessary. The goal is prevention because it is much more effective than treatment. Administration of ergotamine tartrate at the onset of symptoms is effective in the majority of cases including adults, adolescents, and children over 10 years of age. This drug should not be used in pregnancy due to its oxytocic effect. Tolfenamic acid, a prostaglandin E antagonist, is a new and effective medication and may result in fewer side effects than ergotamine. This drug is still being investigated and is not advised for children. Other drugs used for preventive therapy are propranolol (a beta-adrenergic blocker), anticonvulsants, and amitriptyline. The latter is frequently used for treating childhood depression that presents as headache. Clonidine, cyproheptadine, and methysergide are also used, although methysergide is not recommended for children. Midrin is a good substitute for ergotamine; it contains a mild vasoconstrictor, sedative, and acetaminophen. Other drugs used are monoamine oxidase (MAO) inhibitors, platelet antagonists, steroidal and nonsteroidal anti-inflammatory drugs.

Temporomandibular joint pain

Temporomandibular joint (TMJ) syndrome is now known to be one of the major causes of headaches. It is usually caused by an imbalance in the joint movement due to poor bite; bruxism (teeth grinding); or joint problems such as inflammation, trauma, or degenerative changes. The pain is almost always referred. Headache associated with this syndrome is common in both adults and children and can cause chronic pain problems. Treatment of TMJ pain is aimed at correcting the problem, and in some cases this may be difficult.

Causalgia

Causalgia is an extremely painful condition that follows sudden and violent deformation of peripheral nerves. This problem is often initiated in combat due to nerve damage by high-velocity missiles (*e.g.*, bullets or metal fragments). The nerve is typically damaged, but not severed. The classic syndrome was described by Mitchell in 1864 for men sustaining gunshot wounds to the extremities.[37a] The median and sciatic nerves are most commonly affected. The pain is characteristically burning and can be elicited with the slightest movement or touch to the affected area. It is excruciating, and even clothing or puffs of air are sufficient to set it off in severe cases. It can be exacerbated by emotional upsets or any increased peripheral sympathetic nerve stimulation. Sympathetic components are part of all variations of causalgia. These are characterized by vascular and trophic (nutritive) changes to the skin, soft tissue, and bone. Reflex sympathetic dystrophy is a disorder of the sympathetic nervous system characterized by rubor or pallor, sweating or dryness, edema, pain, or skin atrophy (see Chapter 48).

Treatment by sympathetic blockade is usually successful and may be the reason this condition is considered a dysautonomia (*i.e.*, a dysfunction of the autonomic nervous system). In some cases, electrical stimulation of the large myelinated fibers innervating the area from which the pain arises is effective. Controversy remains regarding the mechanisms involved in these pain relief measures. The long-term use of

---

Chart 47–2: Foods that cause migraine headache

Tyramine-containing foods
- Red wine
- Strong or aged cheese
- Smoked herring
- Chicken livers
- Canned figs
- Broad bean pods

Sodium nitrate–containing cured meats
- Bacon
- Hot dogs
- Salami

Fruits
- Avocados
- Bananas
- Citrus fruits

Dairy products
- Yogurt
- Sour cream

Baked goods
- Fresh bread
- Coffee cake
- Doughnuts

Other
- Monosodium glutamate
- Chocolate
- Nuts, peanut butter
- Fermented, pickled, and marinated foods
- Onions

narcotics is discouraged due to the danger of addiction. Effective treatment is imperative to prevent invalidism and, in severe cases, suicide.

Neuralgia

Neuralgia is characterized by severe, brief, often repetitiously occurring attacks of lightning-like or throbbing pain. It occurs along the distribution of a spinal or cranial nerve and is usually precipitated by stimulation of the cutaneous region supplied by that nerve.

Trigeminal neuralgia

Trigeminal neuralgia, or *tic douloureux,* is one of the most common and severe neuralgias. It is manifested by facial tics or grimaces. It is characterized by stabbing, paroxysmal attacks of pain usually limited to the unilateral sensory distribution of one or more branches of the trigeminal nerve, most often the maxillary division. Victims describe the pain as excruciating. It may be triggered by light touch, eating, swallowing, shaving, talking, chewing gum, washing the face, sneezing, or no apparent reason. Stimulation of small-diameter afferent fibers is more effective in provoking attacks than cold, warm, or noxious stimuli. Abnormalities of facial sensation are not likely between attacks. Neurologic deficits are rare as they are in neuralgias of cranial nerves VII, IX, and X.

The drug carbamazepine (Tegretol), which is a tricyclic compound, may be used to control the pain of trigeminal neuralgia and may delay or eliminate the need for surgery. Surgical release of vessels, dural structures, or scar tissue surrounding the semilunar ganglion or root in the middle cranial fossa often eliminates the symptoms. If not, transection or blocking peripheral branches of cranial nerve V produces loss of all sensation, including pain. A more satisfactory treatment is section of the descending spinal tract of nerve V in the brain stem. This may be effective because it removes background inflow of impulses on which spontaneous attacks depend. Dissociation of facial sensation occurs in that pain and temperature disappear, but there is only a slight decrease in tactile activity. This neurosurgical procedure provided evidence that the nucleus caudalis of the trigeminal complex is necessary for the transmission of facial pain. There remains considerable controversy regarding the pathophysiology of trigeminal neuralgia.

Postherpetic neuralgia

The pain associated with postherpetic neuralgia (herpes zoster, or shingles) follows recovery from an infection of the dorsal root ganglia and corresponding areas of innervation by the herpes zoster virus (see Chapter 8). Postherpetic neuralgia most often affects the thoracic spinal nerves. The ophthalmic division of the trigeminal nerve, which innervates the upper face and eye, is the cranial nerve most often affected.

Herpes zoster is due to the same herpes virus that causes varicella (chickenpox) and is thought to represent a localized recurrent infection by the varicella virus that has remained latent in the dorsal root ganglia since the initial attack of chickenpox. Reactivation of viral replication is associated with a decline in immunity, such as that which occurs with aging. During the acute attack of herpes zoster, the reactivated virus travels centrifugally from the ganglia to the skin of the corresponding dermatomes causing a localized vesicular eruption and hyperpathia (abnormally exaggerated subjective response to pain). In the acute infection, proportionately more of the large nerve fibers tend to be destroyed. Regenerated fibers appear to have smaller diameters. Older patients tend to have pain, dysesthesia, and hyperesthesia after the acute phase; these are increased by minor stimuli. Because there is a relative loss of large fibers with age, elderly persons tend to be particularly prone to suffering due to the shift in the proportion of large- to small-diameter nerve fibers.

Postherpetic neuralgia is extremely distressing and is most efficaciously treated early (*i.e.,* in the first 3 months) before the condition becomes established. High doses of systemic corticosteroids and oral acylovir (a drug that inhibits herpesvirus DNA replication) may reduce the incidence of postherpetic neuralgia when used early in the disease.[38] The administration of pharmacologic doses of vitamin E (d-alpha tocopherol acetate) may be used.[38] Although the mechanism of action is unclear, vitamin E therapy has been shown to prevent the progression of some types of neurologic lesions. A tricyclic antidepressant drug such as amitriptyline may be used for pain relief. Regional nerve blockade (stellate ganglion, epidural, local infiltration, or peripheral nerve) has been used with limited success.[38]

Phantom-limb pain

This type of neurologic pain follows amputation of a limb or part of a limb. At first, it is characterized by sensations of tingling, heat and cold, or heaviness. The pain that follows is burning, shooting, or crushing. It may disappear spontaneously or persist for many years. The basic mechanisms involved remain controversial. One theory is that abnormal sensory input secondary to limb amputation or trauma alters the pattern of information processing in the central nervous system. A closed self-exciting neuronal loop in the posterior horn of the spinal cord is postulated to send impulses to the brain, resulting in pain. Even the slightest irritation to the amputated limb area can initiate this cycle. In some persons, neuromas form near the regenerating end of a nerve. It is known that when a peripheral nerve is cut, the scar tissue that forms becomes a barrier to regenerating outgrowth of the axon. Often the growing axon becomes trapped in the scar tissue, forming a tangled growth (neuroma) of small diameter axons, including both primary nociceptive afferents and sympathetic efferents.

These afferents show increased sensitivity to innocuous mechanical stimuli and to sympathetic activity and circulating catecholamines. The absence of the inhibitory effects of the large-diameter fibers may also contribute to the pain problem.

Treatment has been accomplished by the use of sympathetic blocks, transcutaneous electrical nerve stimulation of the large myelinated afferents innervating the area, and relaxation training.[39] Controversy continues as to the precise mechanisms responsible for the usefulness of these methods. Many of the complications following limb amputation can be alleviated by immediate fitting of a prosthesis and conscientious stump care. Stump care includes bandaging to support the remaining muscles, protect the soft tissues, and prevent the formation of edematous fluids. Care must be taken to prevent infection. After the amputation wound has healed, the stump must be shrunk and shaped into a conical form to permit the correct fitting of a prosthesis. This is done by the proper application of elastic bandages or devices. The reader is referred to a specialty text for more complete information on stump care.

Assessment of pain

The relief and management of pain require careful assessment to consider the cause of the pain, evaluate its severity, and determine the type of pain that is present. As with other disease states, it is preferable to eliminate the cause rather than treat the symptoms. Even if the cause cannot be eliminated, measures to relieve the painful state are often more successful when the origin of the discomfort is known. A careful history will often provide information about triggering factors (injury, infection, or disease) and site of nociception (peripheral receptor or visceral organ). Observation of facial expression and posture may provide additional information about the severity and component responses to pain. For example, alterations in normal posture such as limping may increase the spread of pain to neighboring myotomes with progressive complaints such as stiffness and soreness that is worsened by activity or cold. It is not uncommon for someone who has hobbled around on a leg cast to develop back pain.

Unlike many other bodily responses such as temperature and blood pressure, the degree or severity of pain cannot be measured objectively. To overcome this problem, various methods have been developed for quantifying the severity of pain in a given person. Among the methods used for pain measurement are the numerical value and visual analog scale, the verbal descriptor scales, physiologic/behavioral measures, and multidimensional measures such as the two-component scale and the McGill pain questionnaire.[40] Because of the personal nature of pain, most pain instruments are more useful in evaluating individual versus group responses to pain.

The numeric value and visual analog scales ask a person to give a numeric value to their pain, with zero representing no pain and ten representing the most intense pain imaginable. The visual analog scale uses a straight line, often 10 cm in length, which represents a continuum of pain intensity. The person is asked to choose a point on the continuum that represents his or her present state of pain intensity. Verbal descriptor scales consist of three to five numerically ranked choices of words such as none, slight, mild, moderate, or severe. The word that is chosen is used to determine the intensity of pain on an ordinal scale.

The physiologic/behavioral measures incorporate the observation of physiologic and behavorial variables into the pain assessment tool. For example, Hanken and McDowell designed a multidimensional rating scale that uses six variables to measure pain: (1) attention directed toward the pain, (2) anxiety, (3) verbal statement of the degree of pain, (4) skeletal muscle response, (5) characteristics of the respirations, and (6) amount of perspiration.[41] Johnson and Rice developed an instrument that measured two components of pain experience: (1) the physical sensation component and (2) the reactive component.[42] The physical sensation of pain was rated on a scale of 0 to 100, and the distress caused by the pain was rated on a scale labeled slightly distressing, mildly distressing, moderately distressing, and just bearable.

The McGill questionnaire (Figure 47-9) measures both the physiologic and psychologic dimensions of pain.[43,44] The instrument is divided into four parts. The first part uses a drawing of the body on which the person indicates the location of pain. The second part uses 20 lists of words to describe the sensory, affective, evaluative, and other qualities of pain, with the selected words being given a numeric score (e.g., words implying the least pain are assigned a value of 1 and next a value of 2, and so on). The third part asks the person to select words such as brief, momentary, and constant to describe the pattern of pain. The fourth part of the instrument evaluates the present pain intensity (PPI) on a scale of 0 to 5.

McGill Pain Questionnaire

Patient's Name ______ Date ______ Time ______ am/pm

PRI: S ______ (1-10) A ______ (11-15) E ______ (16) M ______ (17-20) PRI(T) ______ (1-20) PPI ______

1 FLICKERING, QUIVERING, PULSING, THROBBING, BEATING, POUNDING
2 JUMPING, FLASHING, SHOOTING
3 PRICKING, BORING, DRILLING, STABBING, LANCINATING
4 SHARP, CUTTING, LACERATING
5 PINCHING, PRESSING, GNAWING, CRAMPING, CRUSHING
6 TUGGING, PULLING, WRENCHING
7 HOT, BURNING, SCALDING, SEARING
8 TINGLING, ITCHY, SMARTING, STINGING
9 DULL, SORE, HURTING, ACHING, HEAVY
10 TENDER, TAUT, RASPING, SPLITTING
11 TIRING, EXHAUSTING
12 SICKENING, SUFFOCATING
13 FEARFUL, FRIGHTFUL, TERRIFYING
14 PUNISHING, GRUELLING, CRUEL, VICIOUS, KILLING
15 WRETCHED, BLINDING
16 ANNOYING, TROUBLESOME, MISERABLE, INTENSE, UNBEARABLE
17 SPREADING, RADIATING, PENETRATING, PIERCING
18 TIGHT, NUMB, DRAWING, SQUEEZING, TEARING
19 COOL, COLD, FREEZING
20 NAGGING, NAUSEATING, AGONIZING, DREADFUL, TORTURING

PPI
0 NO PAIN
1 MILD
2 DISCOMFORTING
3 DISTRESSING
4 HORRIBLE
5 EXCRUCIATING

BRIEF	RHYTHMIC	CONTINUOUS
MOMENTARY	PERIODIC	STEADY
TRANSIENT	INTERMITTENT	CONSTANT

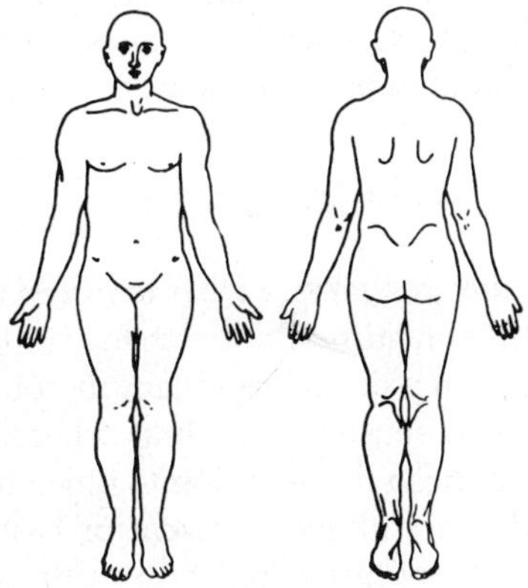

E = EXTERNAL
I = INTERNAL

COMMENTS:

Figure 47-9 McGill pain questionnaire. The pain rating index (PRI) is the sum of rank values for the 20 words: S, sensory; A, affective; E, evaluative; M, miscellaneous; PRI(T), total. *(Cousins MJ, Bridenbaugh PO: Neural Blockade in Clinical Anesthesia and Management of Pain, 2nd ed., p 853. Philadelphia, JB Lippincott, 1988)*

Treatment of pain

The treatment of pain may employ a number of methods including stimulation-induced analgesia, psychologic techniques, pharmacologic treatment, and surgical intervention. Often a multidisciplinary approach is used. The decision about which approach should be tried is based on the duration, characteristics, cause, and mechanisms of pain, if known; the age and social responsibilities of the person; the prognosis; any previous therapy; and psychologic considerations.

Ideally, removal of the sources of noxious

stimuli, including anything that causes exacerbation, would be effective in relieving pain. When this not possible, attempts are made to moderate the reaction to pain. Distraction, imagery, relaxation therapy, biofeedback, and heat and cold have all been found useful in some cases. Focal electrical stimulation of periaqueductal gray area (PAG) in the midbrain has been shown to decrease pain in the specific body area represented. Drug therapy can include pharmacologic agonists or antagonists working at opioidergic or serotoninergic synapses. Anti-inflammatory and vasoconstrictive agents, antidepressant and antianxiety drugs, and sometimes anticonvulsant drugs have been used successfully. If none of these approaches are effective, then it may be necessary to interrupt pain pathways by such methods as spinal blocks, use of local anesthetics, or surgical interruption of pain fiber tracts.

Psychologic techniques

Distraction and imagery. Distraction (*i.e.,* focusing one's attention on stimuli other than painful stimuli) is often helpful in pain management. It could be considered a type of sensory shielding whereby attention to pain is sacrificed for attention to objective or physical stimuli that are already present or easily obtained. Examples are counting, repeating phrases or poems, engaging in activities that require concentration such as projects, activities, work, conversation, describing slides or pictures, and rhythmic breathing. Television, adventure movies, music, and humor can also provide diversion. It is often a mistake to assume that a person who appears to be able to cope with pain by the use of distraction does not have pain. This person should not be punished for his or her efforts by withholding of appropriate medications.[5]

Imagery consists of using one's imagination to develop a mental picture—a visual image. In pain management, therapeutic guided imagery (goal-directed imaging) is used. It can be employed in conjunction with relaxation techniques, biofeedback, and other management methods to develop sensory images that can decrease the perceived intensity of pain. It can also be used to lessen anxiety and reduce muscle tension.

Biofeedback. Biofeedback is a method used to provide feedback to a person concerning the current status of some body function (*e.g.,* finger temperature, temporal artery pulsation, blood pressure, or muscle tension). It is a process of learning designed to make the person aware of certain of his or her own body functions for the purpose of modifying these functions at a conscious level (see Chapter 6). Interest in this treatment modality rose with the possibility of using biofeedback in the management of migraine and tension headaches, or for other pain that had a muscle tension component.

Heat and cold

Both heat and cold are used in the treatment of pain. Each of the temperature modalities has its advantages and advocates. The type of thermal modality used depends on the type of pain being treated, and, in many cases, personal preference.

Heat. Historically, heat has proven to be a very useful method for relieving pain. Some of the earliest sources of therapeutic heat were heated stones, sand, oils, and water, or simply the radiant heat from the sun or a fire.[45] Currently, application is achieved through a number of methods such as immersion in hot water, hot packs, electrically heated pads, infrared rays, and shortwave diathermy.

Care must be taken not to use excessive heat. When excessive heat is used, the heat itself becomes a noxious stimulus, which results in the perception of pain. More importantly, this can be regarded as a warning signal of impending tissue damage and an indication that removal of the heat source is essential to avoid a burn.

Heat dilates blood vessels and increases local blood flow, it can influence the transmission of pain impulses, and it increases collagen extensibility.[46] Overall, an increase in local circulation can reduce the level of nociceptive stimulation by reducing local ischemia caused by muscle spasm or tension, it can increase the removal of metabolites and inflammatory mediators that act as nociceptive stimuli, and it can help to reduce swelling and relieve pressure on local nociceptive endings. Heat is carried to the posterior horn of the spinal cord in the large-diameter myelinated fibers and may exert its effect by "closing the pain gate" to the predominantly small-diameter fibers.[45] It may also produce the release of endogenous opioids through placebo-type mechanisms. Often, limitation in the range of movement is the result of muscle shortening. Heat has been shown to alter the collagen fibers in ligaments, tendons, and joint structures so that they are more easily extended and can be stretched further before the nociceptive endings are stimulated. Thus, heat is often applied prior to therapy aimed at stretching joint structures and increasing range of motion.

Cold. Like heat, application of cold has been shown to produce a dramatic reduction in the level of pain that some persons perceive. Ice forms the major source of cold application to the body. When placed on the skin, heat is conducted to the ice-exposed surface from the deeper tissues; as a result, there is a rapid cooling of the superficial tissues of up to

15°C within 2 to 5 minutes.[46] The deeper tissues are not cooled as much and take longer to cool—it can take up to 20 minutes to develop a temperature drop of 5°C, longer if there is a thick subcutaneous fat layer.

Cold exerts its effect on pain through both circulatory and neural mechanisms. The initial response to local application of cold is sudden local vasoconstriction. This initial vasoconstriction is followed by alternating periods of vasodilatation and vasoconstriction during which the body "hunts" for its normal level of blood flow to prevent local tissue damage. This gives rise to the so-called *Lewis hunting reaction* whereby the circulation to the cooled area undergoes alternating periods of pallor due to ischemia and flushing due to hypermia.[47] The vasoconstriction is caused by local stimulation of sympathetic fibers and direct cooling of blood vessels and the hyperemia by local autoregulatory mechanisms. In situations of acute injury, cold is used to produce vasoconstriction and prevent extravasation of blood into the tissues; pain relief results from decreased swelling and stimulation of nociceptive endings. The vasodilatation that follows can be useful in removing substances that stimulate nociceptive endings.

Cold can also have a marked and dramatic effect on chronic pain that results from muscle spasm that causes an accumulation of metabolites within the muscle. For example, the severe pain of joint inflammation suffered by persons with rheumatoid arthritis is often appreciably reduced with application of the ice. In terms of pain modulation, the sensation of cold can be carried to the posterior horn of the spinal cord by way of large-diameter fibers and influence the closing of the pain gate. The application of ice can be considered a noxious stimulus and, as such, can influence the release of endogenous opioids from the periaqueductal gray area (PAG).

Stimulation-induced analgesia

Chapman has called the early 1970s the "stimulation-induced analgesia" period of investigation.[48] Electrical stimulation, which includes electrical acupuncture and transcutaneous electrical nerve stimulation, may gradually increase the pain threshold to almost double.[48] Stimulation-induced analgesia is one of the oldest known methods of pain relief. Historical references to the use of electricity to decrease or control pain date back to the year 46 A.D. when a Roman physician, Scribonius Largus, described how the stimulus from the electric eel was able to provide pain relief for headache and gout.[49]

Transcutaneous electrical nerve stimulation. Transcutaneous electrical nerve stimulation (TENS) refers to the transmission of electrical energy across the surface of the skin to the nervous system. TENS units have been developed that are convenient, easily transported, and relatively economical to use. Most are about the size of a transistor radio or cigarette package. These battery-operated units deliver a measurable amount of current to a target site.

The system usually consists of three parts: a pair of electrodes, lead wires, and a stimulator. The electrical stimulation is delivered in a pulsed waveform that can be varied in terms of pulse amplitude, pulse width, and pulse rate. The type of stimulation used varies with the type of pain being treated. Electrode placement is determined by the physiologic pathways and an understanding of the pain mechanisms involved. They may be placed on either side of a painful area, over an affected dermatome, over an affected peripheral nerve where it is most superficial, or over a nerve trunk. For example, the electrodes are commonly placed medial and lateral to the incision when treating postoperative pain.

There is probably no one explanation for the physiologic effects of TENS. Each specific type of stimulator may have different sites of action and, thus, may be explained by more than one theory.[50] The gate control theory has been proposed as one possible mechanism.[51] According to this theory, pain information is transmitted by small-diameter A-delta and C fibers. Large-diameter afferent A fibers, as well as small-diameter fibers, carry tactile information mediating touch, pressure, and kinesthesia. Transcutaneous electrical nerve stimulators function on the basis of preferentially firing off impulses in the large fibers carrying nonpainful information. According to the gate control theory, increased activity in these large fibers closes the gate to block or modulate transmission of painful information to the forebrain. A second possible explanation is that high-frequency stimulation (50–60 Hz), produced by some units, simply acts as a counterirritant.[52] A third possible explanation is that stimulators that produce strong rhythmic contractions may act through the release of endogenous analgesics such as the endorphins and enkephalins.[53] A fourth explanation, probably the best explanation for quick analgesia with brief, intense stimulation, is that of a conduction block.[54]

TENS has the advantage that it is noninvasive, is easily regulated by the person or health professional, and is quite effective in some forms of acute and chronic pain. Its use can be taught preoperatively, affording a reduction in both hospital days and postoperative analgesic medication.

Acupuncture. The practice of acupuncture consists of achieving a therapeutic effect by introducing needles into specific points on the surface of the body. There are charts available that describe the points used to relieve pain at certain anatomical sites in the body. Sometimes palpation is used. It is usually useful to stimulate points that are not normally painful but which become so when symptoms are present. The practice of acupuncture dates back thousands of years to ancient China when the stimulation was achieved by using "needles" made of bone, stone, or bamboo. Interest in acupuncture peaked in the 1970s as communication between the Eastern and Western medical communities became established and reports of complete surgical analgesia by use of acupuncture alone reached the Western world. However, later findings indicated that complete analgesia is unlikely. The Chinese are practicing electroacupuncture, in which electrical impulses are passed through the needles. Heat may also be applied to the needles, resulting in heat penetration to the depth of the needle. Various theories of how acupuncture achieves analgesia have been proposed, including the gate control theory and stimulation of endogenous opioid release. Pain relief from acupuncture and electroacupuncture has been shown to be reversible by the morphine antagonist naloxone.[55] Inconsistencies in some experimental results indicate that future experimental work is needed.[56,57]

Acupressure is the means of stimulating acupressure points without using needles. It is particularly popular in Japan where it is called Shiatsu (*shi* meaning finger and *atsu* meaning pressure).[50] Pressure may be applied with a finger or thumb, or any blunt instrument. Many techniques are used, including massaging in a circular motion for between 3 and 5 minutes, pressing inward toward the center of the body and releasing three times, or vibrating the point with fingertip pressure.

Pharmacologic treatment

The use of drugs to control pain is only one aspect of the overall program for pain relief. These agents have been used for many years to relieve pain of short duration, enabling the person to achieve mobility, for example, after surgery, when exercises such as coughing and deep breathing may be required.

An analgesic drug is defined as a medication that acts on the nervous system to decrease or eliminate pain without inducing loss of consciousness. In general, analgesic drugs have no powerful curative effects. Analgesics are categorized as narcotic or nonnarcotic, addictive or nonaddictive, prescriptive or over-the-counter, strong or weak, and peripherally or centrally acting. The ideal analgesic would be potent yet nonaddicting and would have few side effects. It would be effective, yet would not alter the state of awareness. Tolerance would not occur. Finally, it would not be expensive.

Non-narcotic oral analgesics. Aspirin, or acetylsalicylic acid, is an example of a non-narcotic, nonaddictive, over-the-counter analgesic drug.

Aspirin acts both centrally and peripherally to block the transmission of pain impulses. Aspirin also has antipyretic and anti-inflammatory properties, and, like steroids, it is known to inhibit prostaglandins, which make the nerves more sensitive to chemicals such as bradykinin. It does have the well-known side effect of bleeding due to local and systemic effects. Locally, it causes irritation of the gastrointestinal tract; systemically, it causes prolonged bleeding time by inhibiting platelet aggregation. The latter effect may last for several days, so regular daily doses should be avoided at least 1 week prior to surgery. Severe liver disease, vitamin K deficiency, hypoprothrombinemia, or any type of bleeding disorder, like hemophilia, can be a contraindication to the use of aspirin in some persons.

Acetaminophen (Tylenol) may be an effective alternative to aspirin in some persons. Although equivalent to aspirin as an effective analgesic and antipyretic agent, it differs by its lack of anti-inflammatory properties. It lacks platelet-inhibiting properties and does not cause gastric bleeding. The drug can cause liver damage. Children under 5 years of age appear to be less susceptible to this hepatotoxicity. Because there is controversy regarding prolonged use or large doses, the drug should be used with caution.

Another group of drugs with aspirin-like properties are the nonsteroidal anti-inflammatory drugs (NSAIDS). The NSAIDS include ibuprofen (Motrin, Rufen), naproxen (Anaprox, Naprosyn), fenoprofen (Nalfon), and indomethacin (Indocin). These drugs act mainly through the inhibition of prostaglandin synthesis. They decrease the sensitivity of blood vessels to bradykinin and histamine, affect lymphokine production from T-lymphocytes, reverse vasodilatation, and decrease the release of inflammatory mediators from granulocytes, mast cells, and basophils. To varying degrees, all of the NSAIDS are inhibitors of prothrombin synthesis; all are analgesic, anti-inflammatory, and antipyretic; and all inhibit platelet aggregation. They are all gastric irritants, but to a lesser extent than aspirin. Nephrotoxicity has also been observed. In addition to their use in rheumatoid and osteoarthritis, the NSAIDS (ibuprofen and naproxen) have proved useful in primary dysmenorrhea.

Narcotic analgesics. The term *narcotic*, or *opioid*, is used to refer to a group of drugs, natural or synthetic, with morphine-like actions. The older term *opiate* was used to designate drugs derived from opium—morphine, codeine, and many other semisynthetic congeners of morphine. The pain-relieving (analgesic) and psychopharmacolgic properties of morphine have been known for centuries. However, the discovery that the brain contains its own (endogenous) analgesic, morphine-like chemicals, which comprise a group of peptides known as endorphins, is very recent. Three distinct families of opioid peptides have been identified thus far: the *enkephalins,* the *endorphins,* and the *dynorphins.* Dynorphin appears to be the most potent of these peptides.[58] Each family of opioid peptides is derived from a genetically distinct precursor molecule (*e.g.,* proenkephalin, proendorphin, and prodynorphin). Each of these precursors contains a number of biologically active peptides, both opioid and nonopioid. The precursor molecules are found not only in the central nervous system, but in blood and various other tissues.

The opioids exert their action through opioid receptors. Several types of opioid receptors have been identified at various sites in the central and peripheral nervous systems. These receptors are particularly concentrated in areas of the brain where the enkephalins have also been found to be localized. Research has indicated that there are at least four and possibly more major categories of opioid receptors in the CNS. These receptors have been designated as *mu, kappa, delta,* and *sigma* receptors.[58] To add to the complexity, there are probably subtypes within each category. For example, two types of mu receptors have been identified—mu_1 and mu_2. Both endogenous and exogenous opioids bind to these receptors. Mu receptors seem to be more important at supraspinal sites, and sigma and kappa receptors seem to be more important at the spinal level. Analgesia has been associated with both mu and kappa receptors, while dysphoria and psychometric effects have been associated with sigma receptors. Delta receptors are thought to be involved in affective responses.[58] The narcotic antagonists bind selectively to mu receptors. As more information becomes available regarding the opioids and their receptors, it seems likely that pain medications can be developed that act selectively at certain receptor sites, thus providing more effective pain control, while producing fewer side effects and affording less danger of addiction. For example, there is evidence to suggest that mu_1 receptors are involved in analgesia but not in respiratory depression.[59] If this is true, it might be possible to develop opioid drugs that produce effective analgesia but not undesirable side effects such as respiratory depression.

The term *tolerance* implies a decreased responsiveness to a drug that occurs with continued administration. The development of tolerance and physical dependence with repeated use is a characteristic of opioid drugs, and the potential for developing psychologic dependence on the drugs is one of the major limitations to their clinical use. There are three classes of narcotic drugs: agonists, antagonists, and agonist-antagonists. The morphine-like agonists bind to discrete opioid receptors and cause analgesia. They include morphine, hydromorphone (Dilaudid), methadone (Dolophine), levorphanol (Levo-Dromoran), oxymorphone (Numorphan), heroin, meper-

idine (Demerol), and codeine. The narcotic antagonists, such as naloxone (Narcan), are drugs that bind to opioid receptors but block the action of morphine-like agonists and do not have analgesic properties of their own. Naloxone can reverse the effects of morphine immediately and is frequently used in the treatment of narcotic overdose. The mixed agonist–antagonist drugs produce analgesia in nontolerant persons but will produce withdrawal in persons tolerant to morphine-like drugs. The mixed agonist–antagonist drugs include pentazocine (Talwin), nalbuphine (Nubain), butorphanol (Stadol). All of the agonist opioid drugs can produce significant respiratory depression by inhibiting brain stem respiratory mechanisms, and all can suppress the cough reflex. Another side effect common to narcotic analgesics is constipation. Tolerance develops to the respiratory depression and cough suppression, but not to the constipation. The agonist–antagonist drugs usually produce sedation in addition to analgesia when given in therapeutic doses. Severe respiratory depression may be less common with agonist–antagonist analgesics than with pure agonist drugs.

The narcotics are indicated for relief of pain that cannot be relieved with less effective agents such as the non-narcotic analgesic drugs. When used for temporary relief of severe pain such as that occurring postoperatively, there is much evidence that narcotics given routinely before the pain becomes extreme are far more effective than those administered in a sporadic manner; patients seem to require fewer doses and are better able to resume regular activities earlier. Narcotics are also used for treatment of pain in persons with limited life expectancy. Because there is often undue concern about the possibility of addiction, many chronic pain sufferers with a short life expectancy receive inadequate pain relief. Many pain experts agree that it is quite appropriate to provide the level of narcotic necessary to relieve the severe, intractable pain of persons whose life expectancy is very limited. Oral medications are preferable to injection; tolerance is usually minimal after a few weeks. Addiction is not considered a problem in cancer patients.

In persons with cancer pain, morphine remains the most useful strong narcotic. The World Health Organization (WHO) has requested that oral morphine be part of the essential drug list and made available throughout the world as the drug of choice.[60] Oral forms of morphine are well absorbed from the gastrointestinal tract and have a half-life of about 2.5 hours and a duration of action of 4 to 6 hours. Liquid forms of the drug are usually given at 4-hour intervals to maintain an adequate blood level for analgesia, while minimizing the potential for toxic side effects.[61] A controlled-release tablet form of the drug, morphine sulfate pentahydrate (MS Contin), is available. The controlled-release tablets are designed to maintain a steady level of analgesia over a 12-hour period, allowing the patient to have long periods of rest and sleep through the night.

A newly developed approach to opioid administration is the use of continuous infusion pumps. Infusion pumps can be used to deliver narcotics by way of the subcutaneous or intravenous route on a continuous or demand basis.[61,62] Continuous subcutaneous narcotic infusion can be accomplished using a portable infusion pump attached to a small butterfly needle inserted into the subcutaneous tissues. Continuous intravenous infusion of narcotics is also used, but this method presents problems with adjusting the infusion rate to meet changing dose requirements. An alternate approach, patient-controlled analgesia (PCA), has proved effective for relieving postoperative pain and for pain management in persons with cancer.[63] This system consists of a microprocessor-controlled infusion pump that delivers the opioid drug through an intravenous cannula. A pushbutton on the system enables persons to deliver their own narcotic dose as needed. A lock-out system, which prevents overdosing, is programmed into the system.

The administration of narcotics into the intrathecal or epidural spaces for the relief of acute and chronic pain has recently gained popularity in clinical practice.[64] The procedure requires the introduction of a catheter into the epidural or intrathecal space by an anesthesiologist or other physician trained in the technique. With this method, every precaution must be taken that no drugs or solutions are given that could damage the spinal cord. This method offers the advantage of providing effective analgesia while minimizing the central depressant effects common to systemic narcotic administration. The intrathecal or epidural administration route is particularly effective in persons who have had surgery and in whom respiratory function is already compromised (e.g., chest trauma, respiratory insufficiency, or obesity). The procedure is also used for chronic pain such as that associated with cancer or long-term debilitating diseases. This type of pain control is based on the finding of opioid receptors in the cell bodies of the primary afferent neurons in the dorsal root ganglia and in the dorsal horn cells of the spinal cord that are involved in pain transmission.

Tricyclic antidepressants. The fact that the pain-suppression system has nonendorphin synapses raises the possibility that potent centrally acting nonopiate drugs may be useful in relieving pain. Serotonin has been shown to play an important role in producing analgesia. The tricyclic antidepressant drugs that block the removal of serotonin from the synaptic cleft (imipramine, amitriptyline, and doxepin) have been shown to produce pain relief in some persons. The drugs are particularly useful in some chronic painful conditions such as postherpetic neuralgia.

Anticonvulsant drugs. Certain anticonvulsant drugs such as carbamazepine (Tegretol) and phenytoin (Dilantin) have specific analgesic effects that are effective in some pain conditions. These drugs, which suppress spontaneous neuronal firing, are particularly useful in the management of pain that occurs following nerve injury.

Placebo response. An interesting phenomenon that deserves comment is the placebo response (Latin, "I will please"). A placebo is an inert substance. At one time "placebo reactors" were thought to be malingerers or to have psychogenic or functional pain that was more imaginary than real. Newer research indicates that most persons are, to a greater or lesser degree, placebo reactors.

The analgesic effect of the placebo was postulated to be mediated by the release of endogenous opioids when it was discovered that naloxone reversed its effects in patients with postoperative dental pain.[64] Response to the placebo, like that to opiates, appears to be more effective for moderate or severe pain. There is some evidence to suggest that a certain pain intensity must be reached before the endogenous opioid-mediated analgesic system can be activated.[65] Naloxone has been found to enhance the effect of placebos in some instances. Some postulate that two separate mechanisms may be responsible for the observation that there are positive and negative placebo reactions.[66] Further research regarding the properties of the endogenous analgesic system is needed to clarify these observations.

Placebos are not recommended as a test to determine if pain is imaginary or real, mild or severe, nor are they recommended as a means of assessing other physiologic or psychologic reactions, such as changes in blood pressure, respiration, heart rate, gastrointestinal activity, or temperature.

Surgical intervention

Surgery for severe intractable pain of either peripheral or central origin has met with some success. It can be used to remove the cause or block the transmission of pain. Persons with phantom-limb pain, severe neuralgia, inoperable cancer of certain types, or causalgia sometimes suffer so intensively that they consider suicide as their only means of escape. In these extreme cases, surgery may be the only remaining treatment that seems to offer relief from the agony. Nevertheless, surgical methods to relieve pain are usually considered a last resort because damage to nerve cell bodies is irreversible. In addition, a penalty is paid due to damage to other systems, predisposing the patient to other problems. Although severed axons may regenerate, full recovery is highly unlikely. After a few weeks or months, the pain often returns and may be more disturbing than the condition for which the surgery was done. Regenerating nerve fibers may give rise to dysesthesias (extremely uncomfortable sensations); but, if survival time is short, surgery may be warranted. However, in some cases, such as removal of a tumor pressing on nerve fibers or removal of an inflamed appendix, pain is completely relieved.

Surgery to block the transmission of pain signals along peripheral or central pathways may be successful. Peripherally, nerve section (neurotomy) or section of a dorsal root ganglion (rhizotomy) is not uncommon; some success has been reported for this type of surgery, particularly in trigeminal neuralgia.

At the spinal cord level, cordotomy (severing of the anterolateral quadrant of the cord) and tractotomy (interruption of the lateral spinothalamic tract) may require very deep incisions into the cord to give adequate relief. With such deep incision, bladder function may be affected. The success of these types of surgery depends on the source of pain and the cord level involved. Electrical stimulation or pharmacologic agents, or both, are often used either to determine the appropriate surgical site or to eliminate the need for surgery.

Hypophysectomy, the removal of the pituitary gland, has an interesting history. It was done originally in efforts to prevent metastasis in certain hormone dependent malignancies, including some breast cancers. It was found, rather unexpectedly, that the pain was often immediately and totally relieved. It is now most likely to be employed to relieve intractable pain due to disseminated cancer of the prostate or breast which cannot be controlled by morphine or more localized means. The mechanism of pain relief is not yet understood. It is particularly mysterious because the pituitary is a rich source of endogenous opioids.

Multidisciplinary approach

The notion of a multidisciplinary approach to complex chronic pain problems was first put into practice more than 30 years ago. It has been found to be particularly effective. Today, a number of pain clinics have been established. This team approach uses the knowledge and expertise of many health professionals to diagnose and manage complex types of pain. Besides being useful clinically, the team approach is effective in both teaching and in collaborative research. The acute pain model assumes an objective cause that can be treated and diminished or eliminated within a short time, but unfortunately, the most perplexing difficulties are those relating to chronic pain. This approach has demonstrated its value in addressing many of the chronic pain problems from the physical, physiologic, and psychosocial aspects simultaneously.

In summary, pain is an elusive and complex phenomenon; it is a symptom common to many illnesses. Pain is a highly individualized experience that is shaped by a person's culture and previous life experiences, and, thus, it is very difficult to measure. Traditionally there have been two principal theories of pain; specificity and pattern theories. However, neither theory accounts for the motivational–cognitive, cultural, and affective components of pain. Pain can be classified according to source, duration, objective signs, and areas of referral. Reactions to pain, which are affected by pain threshold, pain tolerance, and age factors, are manifested through physical reactions, physiologic responses, and psychosocial reactions.

Pain and pain disorders are universal experiences. Headache is so common, it is experienced by 75% of the population by the age of 15. Pain may occur with or without an adequate stimulus; or it may be absent in the presence of an adequate stimulus—either of which describes a pain disorder. There may be analgesia (lack of pain without loss of consciousness), hyperalgesia (increased sensitivity to pain), hypoalgesia (decreased sensitivity to pain), or hyperpathia (an unpleasant and prolonged response to pain).

Pain can be either acute or chronic; the latter is particularly difficult to manage. Controversy continues as to whether chronic pain should be viewed as a physiologic phenomenon with psychologic correlates or as a psychologic phenomenon with physiologic correlates. A growing body of data suggests that the latter definition may eliminate many of the chronic pain management problems.

Current treatment modalities include use of physical, psychologic, pharmacologic, neurosurgical, and stimulation-induced analgesic methods, singly or in combination. The last 4 to 5 years have seen a tremendous increase in the available information related to the endogenous opioid analgesic systems. This information has answered some previous questions and raised many more that need to be explored.

It is becoming apparent that even with chronic pain, the most effective approach is early treatment or even prevention. Once pain is present, the greatest success in the management of problems related to assessment and appropriate effective treatment is achieved with the use of multidisciplinary teams.

References

1. Bkinkov SM: The Human Brain in Figures and Tables, p 57. New York, Plenum Press, 1968
2. Martin JH: Anatomic substrates for somatic sensation. In Kandel ER, Schwartz JH (eds): Principles of Neuroscience, 2nd ed, pp 301–315. New York, Elsevier, 1985
3. Zborowski M: Cultural components in response to pain. J Soc Issues 8:16, 1952

4. Sternbach R (ed): The Psychology of Pain. New York, Raven Press, 1978

5. McCaffery M: Nursing Management of the Patient with Pain, 2nd ed. Philadelphia, JB Lippincott, 1979

6. Merskey H: Pain and personality. In Sternbach RA (ed): The Psychology of Pain, pp 123–124. New York, Raven Press, 1978

7. Melzack R, Wall PD: Pain mechanisms: A new theory. Science 150:971, 1965

8. Ottoson D: Physiology of the Nervous System, pp 462–463. New York, Oxford University Press, 1983

9. Kelly DD: Central representation of pain and analgesia. In Kandel ER, Schwartz JH (eds): Principles of Neuroscience, pp 331–342. New York, Elsevier, 1985

9a. Basabaum AI: Cytochemical studies of the neural circuitry underlying pain and pain control. Acta Neurochir 38(suppl):5, 1987

10. Payne RP: Anatomy, physiology, and neuropharmacology of cancer pain. Med Clin North Am 71(2):153, 1987

11. Fields HL: Neurophysiology of pain and pain modulation. Am J Med (Sept):2, 1984

12. Saria A: The role of substance P and other neuropeptides in transmission of pain. Acta Neurochir [Suppl] 38:33, 1987

13. Henry JA, Montuschi E: Cardiac pain referred to site of previously experienced somatic pain. Br Med J 2:1605, 1978

14. Beecher HK: Nature of significance of wound to pain experienced. JAMA 161:1609, 1956

15. Wachter-Shikora NL: The elderly patient in pain and the acute care setting. Nurs Clin North Am 18(2):395, 1983

16. Beecher HK: Measurement of Subjective Responses. New York, Oxford University Press, 1959

17. Anand KJS, Hickey PR: Pain and its effects in the human neonate and fetus. N Engl J Med 317(21):1321, November 19, 1987

18. Gilles FJ, Shankle W, Dooling EC: Myelinated tracts: Growth patterns. In Gilles FH, Leviton A, Dooling EC (eds): The Developing Human Brain: Growth and Epidemiologic Neuropathology, pp 117–183. Boston, John Wright, 1983

19. Gautray JP, Jolivet A, Vielh JP et al: Presence of immunoassayable b-endorphin in human amnionic fluid: Elevation in cases of fetal distress. Am J Obstet Gynecol 129:211, 1977

20. Puolakka J, Kauppila A, Leppaluoto J et al: Elevated beta-endorphin immunoreactivity in umbilical cord blood after complicated delivery. Acta Obstet Gynecol Scand 61:513, 1982

21. Wardlaw SL, Stark RI, Baxi L et al: Plasma beta-endorphin and beta-lipotropin in the human fetus at delivery: Correlation with arterial pH and pO_2. J Clin Endocrinol Metab 49:888, 1979

22. Orlowski JP: Cerebrospinal fluid endorphins and the infant apnea syndrome. Pediatrics 78:233, 1986

23. Sankaran K, Hindmarsh KW, Watson VG: Plasma beta-endorphin concentration in infants with apneic spells. Am J Perinatol 1:331, 1984

24. Lerman J, Robinson S, Willis MM: Anesthetic requirements for halothane in young children 0–1 month and 1–6 months of age. Anesthesiology 59:421, 1983

25. Foley KM, Kourides IA, Inturrisi CE et al: Beta-endorphin: Analgesic and hormonal effects in humans. Proc Natl Acad Sci USA 76:5377, 1979

26. Merskey H, Albe-Fessard JJ, Bonica JJ et al: Pain terms: A list with definitions and notes on usage: Recommended by the IASP Subcommittee on Taxonomy. Pain 6:249, 1979

27. Mehta M: Current views on non-invasive methods in pain relief. In Swerdlow M (ed): The Therapy of Pain, 2nd ed, pp 115. Boston, MTP Press, 1986

28. Travell JG, Rinzer SH: The myofascial genesis of pain. Postgrad Med 11:425, 1952

29. Travell JG: Basis for the multiple uses of local block of somatic trigger areas (procaine infiltration and ethylene chloride spray). Mississippi Valley Med J 7:113, 1949

30. Simons DG: Appendix: Myofascial pain syndromes due to trigger points. In Osterweis M, Kleinman A, Mechanic D (eds): In Pain and Disability: Clinical, Behavioral, and Public Policy Perspectives, pp 285–292. Washington, DC, National Academic Press, 1987

31. Fishbain AA, Goldberg M, Meagher BR et al: Male and female chronic pain patients categorized by DSM-III psychiatric diagnostic criteria. Pain 26:181, 1986

32. The Interagency Committee on New Therapies for Pain and Discomfort: Report of the White House, IV-38. National Institute of Health, Education and Welfare, May 1979

33. Diamond S: In Kahn AP: Headaches, p 4. Chicago, Contemporary Books, 1983

34. Bille B: Migraine in school children. Acta Paediatr Scand 51(Suppl 136):1, 1962

35. Friedman AP (Chr): Ad Hoc Committee on the Classification of Headache: Classification of Headache. Arch Neurol 6:173–176, 1962

36. Olesen J (Chair): Headache Classification Committee of the International Headache Society. The Classification and Diagnostic Criteria for Headache Disorders, Cranial Neuralgias, and Facial Pain. Cephalalgia 8(Suppl 7):1–96, 1988

37. Diamond S, Delessio DJ: The Practicing Physician's Approach to Headache, 2nd ed, p 1. Baltimore, Williams and Wilkins, 1978

37a. Hitchcocke KE: Current views on the role of neurosurgery for pain relief, p 187. In Swerdlow M (ed): The Therapy of Pain, ed 2. Norwell MA, MTP Press, 1986

38. Rees RB, Odom RB: Skin and appendages. In Schroeder SA, Krupp MA, Tierney LM (eds): Current Medical Diagnosis and Treatment, pp 71–72. Norwalk, CT, Appleton & Lange, 1988

39. Mannheimer JS, Lampe GN: Clinical Transcutaneous Electrical Nerve Stimulation. Philadelphia, FA Davis, 1984

40. McGuire DB: The measurement of clinical pain. Nurs Res 33:152, 1984

41. Hanken A, McDowell W: Development of a rating scale to measure pain. In Newton M, Hunt W, McDowell W et al (eds): A Study of Nurse Action in Relief of Pain. Columbus, Ohio State University School of Nursing, 1964

42. Johnson JE, Rice VH: Sensory and distress components of pain: Implications for the study of clinical pain. Nurs Res 23:203, 1974

43. McGuire DB: Assessment of pain in cancer patients using the McGill Pain Questionnaire. Oncol Nurs Forum 11(6):32, 1984

44. Melzack R: The McGill Pain Questionnaire: Major properties and scoring methods. Pain 22:1, 1975

45. Licht S: History of therapeutic heat and cold. In Lehman

JF (ed): Therapeutic Heat and Cold, 3rd ed. Baltimore, Williams and Wilkins, 1984

46. Nigel PP: Heat and cold. In Wells PE, Frampton V, Bowsher D: Pain Management in Physical Therapy, pp 169–180. Norwalk, CT, Appleton & Lange, 1988

47. Keating W: Cold vasodilatation after adrenalin. J Physiol 159:101, 1961

48. Chapman CR: Contribution of research on acupuncture and transcutaneous electrical stimulation to the understanding of pain mechanisms and pain relief. In Roland F, Beers J, Bassett EG: Mechanisms of Pain and Analgesic Compounds, pp 7–183. New York, Raven Press, 1979

49. Hymes A: A review of the historical area of electricity. In Mannheimer JS, Lampe GN (eds): Clinical Transcutaneous Electrical Stimulation, p 1. Philadelphia, FA Davis, 1984

50. Michel TH (ed): International Perspectives in Physical Therapy, pp 96–97, 129–130. Edinburgh, Churchill Livingstone, 1985

51. Wolf SL: Neurophysiologic mechanisms of pain modulation: Relevance to TENS. In Mannheimer JS, Lampe GN (eds): Clinical Transcutaneous Electrical Stimulation, p 41. Philadelphia, FA Davis, 1984

52. Anderson SA: Pain control by sensory stimulation. In Bonica JJ (ed): Advances in Pain Research and Therapy, p 569. New York, Raven Press, 1979

53. Ignelzi RJ, Nyquist JK: Excitability changes in peripheral nerve fibers after repetitive electrical stimulation: Implications for pain modulation. J Neurosurg 51:824, 1979

54. Sjolund BH, Terenius L, Erickson MBE: Increased cerebro-spinal fluid levels of endorphin after electroacupuncture. Acta Physiol Scand 100:382, 1977

55. Sherman JE, Liebeskind JC: An endorphinergic centrifugal substrate of pain modulation: Recent findings, current concepts and complexities. In Bonica JJ (ed): Pain. New York, Raven Press, 1980

56. Buchsbaum MS, Davis GC, Bunney WE Jr: Naloxone alters pain perception and somatosensory evoked potentials in normal subjects. Nature 270:620, 1977

57. Chapman CR, Benedetti C: Analgesia following transcutaneous electrical stimulation and its partial reversal by a narcotic antagonist. Life Sci 21:7401, 1977

58. Jaffe JH, Martin WR: Opioid analgesics and antagonists, In Gilman AG, Goodman LS, Rall TW et al: Goodman and Gilman's The Pharmacological Basis of Therapeutics, 7th ed, pp 491–495. New York, Macmillan, 1985

59. Pasternak GW: Multiple morphine and enkephalin receptors and the relief of pain. JAMA 259:1362, 1988

60. Swerdlow M, Stjernward J: Cancer pain relief—An urgent problem. World Health Forum 3:325–330, 1982

61. Foley KM, Inturrisi CE: Analgesic therapy in cancer pain: Principles and practice. Med Clin North Am 71:207, 1987

62. Dennis EMP: An ambulatory infusion pump for pain control: A nursing approach to home care. Cancer Nurs 7(Aug):309, 1984

63. Fields HL, Levine JD: Pain—Mechanisms and management. West J Med 141:347, 1984

64. Lieb RA, Hurtig JB: Epidural and intrathecal narcotics for pain management. Heart Lung 14:164, 1985

65. Levine JD, Gordon NC, Fields HL: The mechanism of placebo analgesia. Lancet 2:654, 1978

66. Levine JD, Gordon, NC, Fields HL: Naloxone dose dependently produces analgesia and hyperalgesia in postoperative pain. Nature 278:740–741, 1979

Bibliography

Abu-Saad H: Assessing children's responses to pain. Pain 19:163–171, 1984

Aronoff GM (ed): Evaluation and Treatment of Chronic Pain. Baltimore, Urban & Schwarzenberg, 1985

Barber J, Adrian C (eds): Psychological Approaches to the Management of Pain. New York, Brunner/Mazel, 1982

Basbaum AI: Cytochemical studies of the neural circuitry underlying pain and pain control. Acta Neurochir [Suppl] 8:5–15, 1987

Besson J-M, Chaouch A: Peripheral and spinal mechanisms of nociception. Physiol Reviews 67(1):67–186, January 1987

Boyd DB, Merskey H, Nielson JS: The pain clinic: An approach to the problem of chronic pain. In Smith WL, Merskey H, Gross SC (eds): Pain: Meaning and Management. New York, SP Medical & Scientific Books, 1980

Brenner JI, Berman MA: Chestpain in childhood and adolescence. J Adolesc Health Care (Review) 3(4):271–276, January 1983

Brogden RN: Non-steroidal anti-inflammatory analgesics other than salicylates. Drugs 32(Suppl 4):27, 1986

Cervero F, Tattersall JEH: Somatic and sensory integration in the thoracic spinal cord. Prog Brain Res 67:189, 1986

Cobb SC: Teaching relaxation techniques to cancer patients. Cancer Nursing 4:157–161, April 1984

Dahl JB, Daugaar HV, Larsen P et al: Patient-controlled analgesia: A controlled trial. Acta Anaesthesiol Scand 31:744–747, 1987

Davis GC: Endorphins and pain (Review). Psychiatr Clin North Am 6(3):473–487, September 1983

DeLander GE, Hopkins CJ: Spinal adenosine modulates descending antinociceptive pathways stimulated by morphine. J Pharm Exp Ther 239:88–93, 1986

Diamond S: Headaches: Common but not ordinary. Part I. Migraine. Emerg Med 16:32–42, July 15, 1984

Donovan M: Cancer pain...you can help! Nurs Clin North Am 17(4):713–728, December 1982

Farkash AE, Portenoy RK: The pharmacological management of chronic pain in the paraplegic patient. J Am Parapleg Soc 9:3–4, July-October 1986

Fitz RD: Therapeutic traction: A review of neurological principles and physical applications. J Manipulative Physiol Ther 7(1):39–49, March 1984

Foley KM (Chair): Report of the Commission on the Evaluation of Pain. Washington, DC, Superintendent of Documents, US Government Printing Office, 1987

Foley KM: The treatment of pain in the patient with cancer. CA 36:4:194–215, July/August 1986

Fox GS: Epidural morphine for postoperative analgesia. Can J Surg 31(1):14–15, 1988

Graves DA, Foster TS, Batenhorst RL et al: Patient-controlled analgesia. Ann Intern Med 99(3):360–366, September 1983

Hawley DD: Postoperative pain in children: Misconceptions, descriptions, and interventions. Pediatr Nurs 16(1):10–14, February 1984

Herz A: Opiates, opioids and their receptors in the modulation of pain. Acta Neurochir [Suppl] 38:36–40, 1987

Janig W: Neuronal mechanisms of pain with special emphasis on visceral and deep somatic pain. Acta Neurochir [Suppl] 38:16–32, 1987

Johnson JA, Repp EC: Nonpharmacologic pain management in arthritis. Nurs Clin North Am 19(4):583–591, 1984

Kaplan RM, Metzger G, Jablecki C: Brief cognitive and relaxation training increases tolerance for a painful clinical electromyographic examination. Psychosom Med 45:2:155, 1983

Katz J, Melzack R: Referred sensations in chronic pain patients. Pain 28:51–59, 1987

Larson SJ: Surgical treatment of pain in patients with spinal cord injury. J Am Parapleg Soc 9(3–4):51–52, July-October 1986

Lasagna L: The management of pain. Drugs 32(Suppl 4):1–7, 1986

Levine JD, Gordon NC: Pain in prelingual children and its evaluation by pain-induced vocalizations. Pain 14(2):85–93, October 1982

Lewit K, Simons DG: Myofascial pain: Relief by post-isometric relaxation. Arch Phys Med Rehabil 65:452–456, August 1984

Manders KL: Integrated approach to the management of pain: A National Institutes of Health Consensus Report Synopsis. Indiana Medicine 79(12):1053–1055, December 1986

McGuire DB: Selecting an instrument to measure cancer-related pain. Oncol Nurs Forum 11(6):85, 1984

McQuay H: Central analgesics. Acta Neurochir [Suppl] 38:41–43, 1987

Meinhart NT, McCaffery M: Pain, A Nursing Approach to Assessment and Analgesia. Norwalk, CT, Appleton-Century-Crofts, 1983

Neri M, Agazzani E: Aging and right-left asymmetry in experimental pain measurement. Pain 19:43–48, 1984

Pearce S: A review of cognitive-behavioral methods for the treatment of chronic pain. J Psychosom Res 27(5):431–440, 1983

Pearson J, Brandeis L, Cuello AC: Depletion of substance P-containing axons in substantia gelatinosa of patients with diminished pain sensitivity. Nature 295:61–63, 1982

Perlman SL: Modern techniques of pain management. West J Med 148:54, 1988

Porges P: Local anesthetics in the treatment of chronic pain (Review). Recent Results Cancer Res 89:127–136, 1984

Procacci P, Zoppi M, Maresca M: Clinical approach to visceral sensation. Prog Brain Res 67:21–28, 1986

Ray A, Khanna SK, Bhattacharya M et al: Modulation of analgesic and anti-inflammatory effects of aspirin. Indian J Med Res 86:264–268, August 1987

Sanford PR, Barry DT: Acute somatic pain can refer to sites of chronic abdominal pain. Arch Phys Med Rehab 69:532–533, July 1988

Swerdlow M (ed): The Therapy of Pain, 2nd ed. Boston, MTP Press, 1986

Warga C: Pain's gatekeeper. Psychology Today 21(8):51–56, August 1987

Willer JC, Bergeret S, De Broucker T et al: Low dose epidural morphine does not affect non-nociceptive spinal reflexes in patients with postoperative pain. Pain 32:9–14, 1988

Willis WD: Visceral inputs to sensory pathways in the spinal cord. Prog Brain Res 67:207–225, 1986

Woolsey RM: Chronic pain following spinal cord injury. J Am Parapleg Soc 9(3–4):39–41, July-October 1986

Woolsey RM: Symposium on pain in spinal cord injured patients—An overview. J Am Parapleg Soc 9(3–4):27–28, July-October 1986

Yaksh TL: Spinal opiate analgesia: Characteristics and principles of action. Pain 11:293–346, 1981

Young PA: The anatomy of the spinal cord pain paths: A review. J Am Parapleg Soc 9(3–4):28–38, July-October 1986

Normal and Altered Autonomic Nervous System Function

Organization and control of autonomic nervous system (ANS) function
Visceral afferent pathways
Autonomic efferent pathways
  Sympathetic nervous system
  Parasympathetic nervous system
Central integrative pathways

Neurotransmission
  Acetylcholine and cholinergic receptors
  Catecholamines and adrenergic receptors
Alterations in ANS function
  Organ and system dysfuncton
    Vision
    Skin and thermal regulation
    Circulatory function
    Pheochromocytoma
    Gastrointestinal function
    Metabolic function
    Sexual function

Disorders of peripheral ANS function
  Denervation hypersensitivity
Disorders of central ANS function
  Progressive autonomic failure
Diagnostic methods

Objectives

After you have studied this chapter, you should be able to meet the following objectives:

_____ Compare the sensory and motor components of the autonomic nervous system (ANS) with those of the somatic nervous system.

_____ Describe major sources of afferent input to the ANS.

_____ Compare the characteristics of CNS outflow, general effector functions, and neurotransmission for the sympathetic and parasympathetic nervous systems.

_____ Describe the synthesis, reuptake, and metabolism of catecholamines.

_____ Describe the synthesis and metabolism of acetylcholine.

_____ Differentiate the main locations of $beta_1$ and $beta_2$ receptors.

_____ Differentiate the locations of muscarinic and nicotinic receptors.

_____ Compare the general features of effector function produced by interruption of somatic motor neuron and an autonomic motor neuron.

_____ State the effect of interruption of ANS innervation on the eye and vision; the skin and thermal regulation; the circulatory system and control of blood flow and blood pressure; gastrointestinal system and gastrointestinal function; metabolic functions; and sexual function.

_____ State the pathology associated with a pheochromocytoma.

_____ List the possible manifestations of autonomic peripheral neuropathies.

_____ Describe the condition called progressive autonomic failure.

_____ Describe at least three diagnostic methods of assessing autonomic function.

The ability to maintain homeostasis and perform the activities of daily living in an ever-changing physical environment is largely vested in the autonomic nervous system (ANS). The ANS functions at the subconscious level and is involved in regulating, adjusting, and coordinating vital visceral functions such as blood pressure and blood flow, body temperature, respiration, digestion, metabolism, and elimination. Common synonyms for the ANS are the *involuntary nervous system* and *vegetative nervous system*. The ANS is strongly affected by emotional influences and is involved in many of the expressive aspects of behavior. Blushing, pallor, palpitations of the heart, clammy hands, and dry mouth are several emotional expressions that are mediated through the ANS. Of recent interest has been the use of biofeedback and relaxation exercises for modifying the subconscious functions of the ANS.

For purposes of organization, this chapter has been divided into two parts: (1) the organization and control of ANS function, and (2) disorders of ANS function. Additional content on ANS function as it relates to specific alterations in body function is integrated into other chapters of the book.

Organization and control of autonomic nervous system (ANS) function

The nervous system can be conceptually divided into the somatic and autonomic nervous systems. The somatic nervous system, with its sensory and motor components, provides contact with the external world and regulation of behaviors directed toward interacting with the external environment. The autonomic nervous system functions by responding to stimuli from within the body and by maintaining the constancy of the internal environment. Although the nervous system can be conceptually divided, the distinction between the somatic and autonomic nervous systems becomes blurred when the higher levels of integrated responses are considered. Indeed, almost all somatic reflexes have a visceral component and vice versa. For example, the response to cold stimulates contraction of the piloerector skin muscles (goose bumps) by way of the ANS, and contraction of the voluntary muscles (shivering), which is controlled by the somatic nervous system. Exposure to a bright light produces avoidance movements (somatic) as well as constriction of the pupils (ANS).

As with the somatic nervous system, the ANS is represented in both the central nervous system (CNS) and the peripheral nervous system (PNS).

Traditionally, the ANS has been defined as a general efferent system innervating visceral organs. The efferent outflow from the ANS is divided between its two divisions—the sympathetic nervous system and parasympathetic nervous system. The afferent input to the ANS is provided by visceral afferent neurons, generally not considered to be part of the ANS.

The functions of the sympathetic nervous system include maintaining body temperature and adjusting blood flow and blood pressure to meet the changing needs of the body that occur with activities of daily living, such as moving from the supine to the standing position. The sympathoadrenal system can also discharge as a unit when there is a critical threat to the integrity of the individual—the fight or flight response. During a stress situation, the heart rate accelerates; the blood pressure rises; blood flow shifts from the skin and gastrointestinal tract to the skeletal muscles and brain; blood sugar increases; the bronchioles and pupils dilate; the sphincters of the stomach, intestine, and internal urethra constrict; and the rate of secretion of exocrine glands that are involved in digestion diminishes. Emergency situations often require vasoconstriction and shunting of blood away from the skin and into the muscles and brain, a mechanism that provides for a reduction in blood flow should a wound occur and preservation of vital functions needed for survival. Sympathetic function is often summarized as catabolic in that its actions predominate during periods of pronounced energy expenditure, such as when survival is threatened.

In contrast to the sympathetic nervous system, the functions of the parasympathetic nervous system are concerned with conservation of energy, resource replenishment and storage (anabolism), and maintenance of organ function during periods of minimal activity. The parasympathetic nervous system slows heart rate, stimulates gastrointestinal function and related glandular secretion, promotes bowel and bladder elimination, and contracts the pupil, protecting the retina from excessive light during periods when visual function is not vital to survival.

The two divisions of the ANS are generally viewed as having opposite and antagonistic actions (*i.e.,* if one activates, the other inhibits a function). Exception are functions, such as sweating and regulation of arteriolar blood vessel diameter, that are controlled by a single division of the ANS, in this case the sympathetic nervous system. Both the sympathetic and parasympathetic nervous systems are continually active. The effect of this continual or basal (baseline) activity is referred to as *tone*. The tone of an effector organ or system can be increased or decreased and is usually regulated by a single division of the ANS. For example, vascular smooth muscle tone is controlled by the sympathetic nervous system. Increased sympathetic activity produces local vasoconstriction due to increased vascular smooth muscle tone, and decreased activity results in vasodilatation due to decreased tone. In structures such as the SA node and AV node of the heart, which are innervated by both divisions of the ANS, one division predominates in controlling tone. In this case the tonically active parasympathetic nervous system exerts a constraining or braking effect on heart rate, and when parasympathetic outflow is withdrawn, similar to releasing a brake, heart rate increases. The increase in heart rate that occurs with vagal withdrawal can be further augmented by sympathetic stimulation. Table 48-1 describes the responses of effector organs to sympathetic and parasympathetic impulses.

Visceral afferent pathways

Sensory information from the viscera is conveyed to the CNS by way of visceral afferent fibers. Both the parasympathetic and sympathetic peripheral nerves have fibers that carry visceral afferent and sensation information (about 80% of vagal fibers are sensory afferent fibers that supply the heart, lungs, and other viscera). The general visceral afferent fibers are involved in the mediation of vasomotor, respiratory, and viscerosomatic reflexes and interrelated visceral activities, such as gastrointestinal functioning and bladder emptying. In addition, they carry information concerning visceral sensations such as discomfort and pain.

The receptors of the *general visceral afferent* neurons monitor conditions of the internal environment, such as the chemical composition of body fluids and the pressure and stretch of internal organs. Some visceral afferents terminate in specialized chemoreceptors, such as those of the carotid and aortic bodies that monitor blood pH, oxygen (PO_2), and carbon dioxide (PCO_2). The pressure-sensitive baroreceptor endings in the carotid sinus and aorta sense changes in blood pressure. General visceral afferent receptors in the mucosal, smooth muscle, and connective tissue of the gastrointestinal tract monitor smooth muscle stretch and changes in the composition of the gastrointestinal contents. Distention of the bowel can stimulate increased motility, and the presence of microbial growth products can stimulate sensory receptors and cause diarrhea. The pharynx, trachea, bronchi, and lungs are richly innervated by visceral afferent endings. These endings provide the afferent input for the sneezing and cough reflexes.

Some general visceral afferent fibers join sympathetic nerves such as the splanchnic nerve, while others from the same viscera travel in parasympathetic nerves, such as the vagus and the pelvic nerves. The cell bodies for the visceral afferents are located in the ganglia of the facial (VII), glossopharyngeal (IX), and vagus (X) cranial nerves; the thoracic and upper lumbar dorsal root ganglia; and the dorsal root ganglia of sacral levels 2, 3, and 4. The central axons of the afferent neurons enter the dorsal horn gray matter or its equivalent in the brain stem and synapse with association neurons (interneurons) of the same or neighboring segments. The association neurons use multisynaptic pathways that project to: (1) local reflex circuits, (2) centers in the brain stem that contribute to the hierarchic control mechanisms of visceral reflexes, and (3) the thalamus and other higher centers where visceral sensations are perceived and integrated into cognitive and emotional responses. Spinal interneurons frequently receive convergent input from both somatic and visceral efferent fibers. These convergent pathways are thought to contribute to the referred pain that occurs with visceral pathology such as the referred pain in the left arm that often occurs with myocardial infarction.

General visceral sensation afferents monitor visceral sensations such as feelings of hunger, fullness of the bladder and rectum, sensations that originate in the sexual organs during coitus, and visceral pain.[1] Visceral afferent information reaches the sensation level in an area of the thalamus that has projections to a small area of the parietal sensory cortex. Visceral pain, which is discussed in Chapter 47, can arise from a common visceral sensation. For example, fullness of the bladder is perceived as the need to micturate. If it is inconvenient to empty the bladder, the sensation becomes stronger and more unpleasant. During severe urinary retention, as occurs with outflow obstruction, the sensation becomes exceedingly painful. At the point when visceral sensations become unpleasant and painful, autonomic effector responses often manifest themselves. Distention of the gut to the point that the sensation of nausea occurs is often accompanied by increased heart rate and sweating. Because the intermediate thalamic nuclei that receive visceral signals communicate with the limbic system, visceral sensation can have a very strong emotional component. For example, sensations of fullness, pressure, and visceral pain, and those associated with deep structure stimulation during voiding, defecation, and sexual activity can have strong emotional components.

Autonomic efferent pathways

The outflow of both divisions of the ANS follow a two-neuron pathway. The first motoneuron, called the *preganglionic neuron,* lies in a motor cell column in the ventral horn of the spinal cord or its equivalent location in the brain stem and is located in the CNS. The second motoneuron, called the *post-*

Table 48-1. Responses of effector organs to autonomic nerve impulses

Effector organs	Adrenergic impulses		Cholinergic impulses
	Receptor type†	Responses†	Responses†
Eye			
Radial muscle, iris	α_1	Contraction (mydriasis) ++	—
Sphincter muscle, iris		—	Contraction (miosis) +++
Ciliary muscle	β	Relaxation for far vision +	Contraction for near vision +++
Heart			
S-A node	β_1	Increase in heart rate ++	Decrease in heart rate; vagal arrest +++
Atria	β_1	Increase in contractility and conduction velocity ++	Decrease in contractility, and shortened action-potential duration ++
A-V node	β_1	Increase in automaticity and conduction velocity ++	Decrease in conduction velocity; A-V block +++
His-Purkinje system	β_1	Increase in automaticity and conduction velocity +++	Little effect
Ventricles	β_1	Increase in contractility, conduction velocity, automaticity, and rate of idioventricular pacemakers +++	Slight decrease in contractility claimed by some
Arterioles			
Coronary	$\alpha; \beta_2$	Constriction +; dilatation§ ++	Dilatation ±
Skin and mucosa	α	Constriction +++	Dilatation‖
Skeletal muscle	$\alpha; \beta_2$	Constriction ++; dilatation§# ++	Dilatation** +
Cerebral	α	Constriction (slight)	Dilatation‖
Pulmonary	$\alpha; \beta_2$	Constriction +; dilatation§	Dilatation‖
Abdominal viscera	$\alpha; \beta_2$	Constriction +++; dilatation# +	—
Salivary glands	α	Constriction +++	Dilatation ++
Renal	$\alpha_1; \beta_1, \beta_2$	Constriction +++; dilatation# +	—
Veins (systemic)	$\alpha_1; \beta_2$	Constriction ++; dilatation ++	—
Lung			
Tracheal and bronchial muscle	β_2	Relaxation +	Contraction ++
Bronchial glands	$\alpha_1; \beta_2$	Decreased secretion; increased secretion	Stimulation +++
Stomach			
Motility and tone	$\alpha_2; \beta_2$	Decrease (usually)†† +	Increase +++
Sphincters	α	Contraction (usually) +	Relaxation (usually) +
Secretion		Inhibition (?)	Stimulation +++
Intestine			
Motility and tone	$\alpha_1; \beta_1, \beta_2$	Decrease†† +	Increase +++
Sphincters	α	Contraction (usually) +	Relaxation (usually) +
Secretion		Inhibition (?)	Stimulation ++
Gallbladder and ducts	β_2	Relaxation +	Contraction +
Kidney	β_1	Renin secretion ++	—
Urinary bladder			
Detrusor	β	Relaxation (usually) +	Contraction +++
Trigone and sphincter	α	Contraction ++	Relaxation ++
Ureter			
Motility and tone	α	Increase	Increase (?)
Uterus	$\alpha; \beta_2$	Pregnant: contraction (α); relaxation (β_2). Nonpregnant: relaxation (β_2)	Variable‡‡
Sex organs, male	α	Ejaculation +++	Erection +++
Skin			
Pilomotor muscles	α	Contraction ++	—
Sweat glands	α	Localized secretion§§ +	Generalized secretion +++

Table 48-1. Responses of effector organs to autonomic nerve impulses (continued)

| Effector organs | Adrenergic impulses | | Cholinergic impulses |
	Receptor type†	Responses‡	Responses‡
Spleen capsule	α; β_2	Contraction +++; relaxation +	—
Adrenal medulla		—	Secretion of epinephrine and norepinephrine (nicotinic effect)
Skeletal muscle	β_2	Increased contractility; glycogenolysis; K^+ uptake	—
Liver	α; β_2	Glycogenolysis and gluconeogenesis +++	Glycogen synthesis +
Pancreas			
Acini	α	Decreased secretion +	Secretion ++
Islets (β cells)	α_2	Decreased secretion +++	—
	β_2	Increased secretion +	—
Fat cells	α; β_1	Lipolysis +++	—
Salivary glands	α_1	Potassium and water secretion +	Potassium and water secretion +++
	β	Amylase secretion +	
Lacrimal glands		—	Secretion +++
Nasopharyngeal glands		—	Secretion ++
Pineal gland	β	Melatonin synthesis	—
Posterior pituitary	β_1	Antidiuretic hormone secretion	—

† Where a designation of subtype is not provided, the nature of the subtype has not been determined unequivocally.

‡ Responses are designated 1+ to 3+ to provide an approximate indication of the importance of adrenergic and cholinergic nerve activity in the control of the various organs and functions listed.

§ Dilatation predominates *in situ* due to metabolic autoregulatory phenomena.

‖ Cholinergic vasodilatation at these sites is of questionable physiologic significance.

Over the usual concentration range of physiologically released, circulating epinephrine, β-receptor response (vasodilatation) predominates in blood vessels of skeletal muscle and liver; α-receptor response (vasoconstriction), in blood vessels of other abdominal viscera. The renal and mesenteric vessels also contain specific dopaminergic receptors, activation of which causes dilatation.

** Sympathetic cholinergic system causes vasodilatation in skeletal muscle, but this is not involved in most physiologic responses.

†† It has been proposed that adrenergic fibers terminate at inhibitory β receptors on smooth muscle fibers, and at inhibitory α receptors on parasympathetic cholinergic (excitatory) ganglion cells of Auerbach's plexus.

‡‡ Depends on stage of menstrual cycle, amount of circulating estrogen and progesterone, and other factors.

§§ Palms of hands and some other sites ("adrenergic sweating").

(Gilman AG, Goodman LS, Rall TW et al: Goodman and Gilman's The Pharmacological Basis of Therapeutics, 7th ed. New York, Macmillan, 1985)

ganglionic neuron, synapses with a preganglionic neuron in an autonomic ganglion and is located in the PNS. The two divisions of the ANS differ in terms of location of preganglionic cell bodies, relative length of preganglionic fibers, general function, nature of peripheral responses, and pre· and postganglionic neuromediators (Table 48-2). This two-neuron outflow pathway and the interneurons in the autonomic ganglia that add further modulation to ANS function are features distinctly different from the arrangement in somatic motor innervation.

Most visceral organs are innervated by both sympathetic and parasympathetic fibers. Exception are structures, such as blood vessels and sweat glands, that have input from only one division of the ANS. The fibers of the sympathetic nervous system are distributed to effectors throughout the body, and, as a result, sympathetic actions tend to be more diffuse than those of the parasympathetic nervous system in which there is a more localized distribution of fibers. The preganglionic fibers of the sympathetic nervous

system may traverse a considerable distance and pass through several ganglia before finally synapsing with postganglionic neurons, and their terminals make contact with a large number of postganglionic fibers. In some ganglia, the ratio of preganglionic to postganglionic cells may be 1:20; because of this, the effects of sympathetic stimulation are diffuse.[2] In addition, there is considerable overlap, so that one ganglion may be supplied by several preganglionic fibers. In contrast to the sympathetic nervous system, the parasympathetic nervous system has its postganglionic neurons located very near or within the organ of innervation, and the ratio of pre- to postganglionic communication is often 1:1 so that its effects are much more circumscribed.[2]

The sympathetic nervous system

The preganglionic fibers of the sympathetic nervous system are in the thoracic and upper lumbar segments of the spinal cord, and this part of the ANS is also called the *thoracolumbar division*. These pre-ganglionic neurons, which are located primarily in the ventral horn intermediolateral cell columns, are largely myelinated and relatively short. The post-ganglionic neurons of the sympathetic nervous system are located in either the paravertebral ganglia of the sympathetic chains that lie on either side of the verte-bral column or in prevertebral sympathetic ganglia such as the celiac ganglia (Figure 48-1). In addition to postganglionic efferent neurons, the sympathetic gan-glia contain neurons of the internuncial, short-axon type, similar to those associated with complex cir-cuitry in the brain and spinal cord. Many of these appear to inhibit, while others modulate preganglionic to postganglionic transmission. The full significance of these modulating circuits remains under investiga-tion.

The axons of the preganglionic neurons leave the spinal cord by way of the ventral root of the spinal nerve and travel by way of nerve branches called *white rami* to the paravertebral ganglia (Figure 48-2). Within the sympathetic chain of ganglia, pregangli-onic fibers may synapse with neurons of the ganglion it enters; pass up or down the chain and synapse with one or more ganglia, or it may pass through the chain and move outward through a splanchnic nerve to ter-minate in one of the prevertebral ganglia (celiac, supe-rior mesenteric, or inferior mesenteric) that are scat-tered along the dorsal aorta and its branches. Preganglionic fibers from the thoracic segments of the cord pass upward to form the cervical chain. Post-ganglionic sympathetic axons of the cervical and lower lumbosacral chain ganglia spread further through nerve plexuses along continuations of the great arter-ies. Thus, cranial structures, particularly blood ves-sels, are innervated by the spread of postganglionic axons along the internal and carotid arteries into the face and the cranial cavity. The sympathetic fibers from T1 generally pass up the sympathetic chain into the head; those from T2 pass into the neck; those from T1 to T5 to the heart: those from T3, T4, T5, and T6 to the thoracic viscera; those from T7, T8, T9, T10, and T11 to the abdominal viscera; and those from T12, L1, L2, and L3 to the kidneys and pelvic organs.[3] Many of the preganglionic fibers from the fifth to the last thoracolumbar segment pass through the paravertebral ganglia to continue as the splanchnic nerves. Most of these fibers do not synapse until they reach the celiac ganglion; others pass to the adrenal medulla. The adrenal medulla, which is part of the sympathetic nervous system, contains postganglionic sympathetic neurons that secrete sympathetic neuro-transmitters directly into the bloodstream.

Some of the postganglionic fibers from the paravertebral ganglia re-enter the segmental nerve through unmyelinated branches called *gray rami* and are then distributed to all parts of the body wall in the spinal nerve branches. These fibers innervate the sweat glands, piloerector muscles of the hair follicles, all of the blood vessels of the skin and skeletal muscles, and the CNS itself.

The parasympathetic nervous system

The preganglionic fibers of the parasympa-thetic nervous system, also referred to as the *craniosa-cral division* of the ANS, originate in the brain stem cranial nerves and sacral segments of the spinal cord (Figure 48-3). The central regions of origin are the

---

Table 48–2. Characteristics of the sympathetic and parasympathetic nervous systems

Characteristic	Sympathetic outflow	Parasympathetic outflow
Location of preganglionic cell bodies	Thoracic 1–12, lumbar 1 and 2	Cranial nerves: III, VII (intermedius), IX, X; sacral segments 2, 3, and 4
Relative length of preganglionic fibers	Short—to paravertebral chain of ganglia or to aortic prevertebral of ganglia	Long—to ganglion cells near or in the innervated organ
General function	Catabolic—mobilizes resources in anticipation of challenge for survival (preparation for "fight-or-flight" response)	Anabolic—concerned with conservation, renewal, and storage of resources
Nature of peripheral response	Generalized	Localized
Transmitter between preganglionic terminals and postganglionic neurons	Acetylcholine (ACh)	ACh
Transmitter of postganglionic neuron	ACh (sweat glands and skeletal muscle vasodilator fibers); norepinephrine (NE) (most synapses); NE and epinephrine (secreted by adrenal gland)	ACh

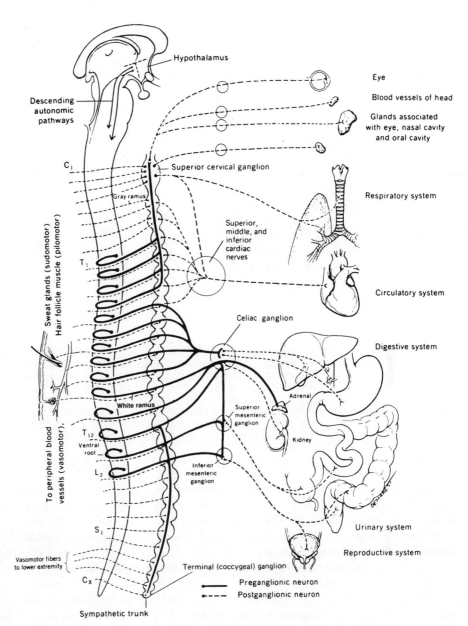

Figure 48-1 Diagrammatic representation of the sympathetic division of the autonomic nervous system. (*Noback CR, Demarest RJ: The Nervous System—Introduction and Review, 2nd ed. New York, McGraw-Hill, 1977*)

midbrain, pons, medulla oblongata, and the sacral part of the spinal cord. The midbrain outflow passes through the oculomotor (III) cranial nerve to the ciliary ganglia that lies in the orbit behind the eye; it supplies the pupillary sphincter muscle of the eye and the ciliary muscles that control lens thickness for accommodation. Pontine outflow comes from preganglionic fibers of the facial (VII) nerve, which synapse in the submandibular ganglia, supplying the submandibular and sublinguinal glands, and the pterygopalatine ganglia, supplying the lacrimal and nasal glands. The medullary outflow develops from cranial nerves VII, IX, and X. Fibers in the glossopharyngeal (IX) nerve synapse in the otic ganglia, which supply the parotid salivary glands. About 75% of parasympathetic efferent fibers are carried in the vagus (X) nerve.

The vagus nerve provides parasympathetic innervation for the heart, trachea and lungs, esophagus, stomach, small intestine and proximal half of the colon, liver, gallbladder, pancreas, kidneys, and upper portions of the ureters.

The sacral preganglionic axons leave the S2 to S4 segmental nerves by gathering into the pelvic nerves, also called the *nervi erigentes*. The pelvic nerves leave the sacral plexus on each side of the cord and distribute their peripheral fibers to the bladder, uterus, urethra, prostate, distal portion of the transverse colon, descending colon and rectum. The sacral parasympathetic fibers also supply the external genitalia to facilitate sexual function.

With the exception of cranial nerves III, VII, and IX that synapse in discrete ganglia, the long para-

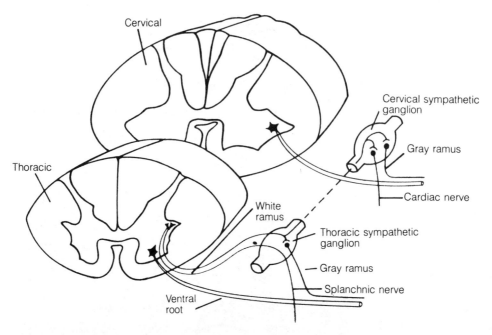

Figure 48-2 Autonomic elements of the spinal nerves. In the thoracolumbar region, each ventral nerve root carries a contingent of efferent sympathetic fibers. These pass to the neighboring sympathetic trunk as a white ramus. Some of the fibers synapse in ganglia of corresponding levels, but others emerge from the trunk without synapsing. Fibers emerge from the ganglia to pass to plexuses or to rejoin the nerves as gray rami passing to peripheral or meningeal structures. In the cervical and sacral regions, the ventral roots give off no white rami. Fibers from other levels synapse in the ganglia, however, and secondary fibers pass off as gray rami to join the nerve trunks. (*Elliott HC: Neuroanatomy. Philadelphia, JB Lippincott, 1969*)

sympathetic preganglionic fibers pass uninterrupted to short postganglionic fibers located in the organ wall. In the walls of these organs, postganglionic neurons send axons to smooth muscle and glandular cells that modulate their functions.

The gastrointestinal tract has its own intrinsic network of ganglionic cells located between the smooth muscle layers, called the *enteric* (intramural) *plexus,* that controls local peristaltic movements. This network of parasympathetic postganglionic neurons and interneurons runs from the upper portion of the esophagus to the internal anal sphincter. Local afferent sensory neurons respond to mechanical and chemical stimuli and communicate these influences to motor fibers in the enteric plexus. The number of neurons in the enteric neural network (10^8) is so large that it approximates that of the spinal cord.[4] It is thought that this enteric nervous system is capable of independent function without control from CNS fibers.[4] The CNS has a modulating role, by way of preganglionic innervation of the plexus, converting local peristalsis to longer distance movements, thereby speeding the transit of intestinal contents.

Central integrative pathways

Local reflex circuits interrelating visceral afferent and autonomic efferent activity are integrated into a hierarchic control system in the spinal cord and brain stem. Progressively greater complexity in the responses and greater precision in their control occur at each higher level of the nervous system. As mentioned earlier, most visceral reflexes contain contributions from the lower motoneurons that innervate skeletal muscles as part of their response patterns. The distinction between purely visceral and somatic reflex hierarchies becomes less and less meaningful at the higher levels of hierarchic control and behavioral integration.

For most autonomic-mediated functions, the hypothalamus serves as the major control center. The hypothalamus, which has connections with the cerebral cortex, the limbic system, and the pituitary gland, is in a prime position to receive, integrate, and transmit information to other areas of the nervous system. The neurons concerned with thermoregulation, thirst, and feeding behaviors are found in the hypothalamus. The hypothalamus is also the site for integrating neuroendocrine function. Hypothalamic releasing and inhibiting hormones control the secretion of anterior pituitary hormones (thyroid-stimulating hormone, adrenocorticotropic hormone, growth hormone, luteinizing hormone and follicle-stimulating hormone, and prolactin). The supraoptic nuclei of the hypothalamus are involved in water metabolism through synthesis of antidiuretic hormone (ADH) and its release from the posterior pituitary gland (see Chapter 27). Oxytocin, which

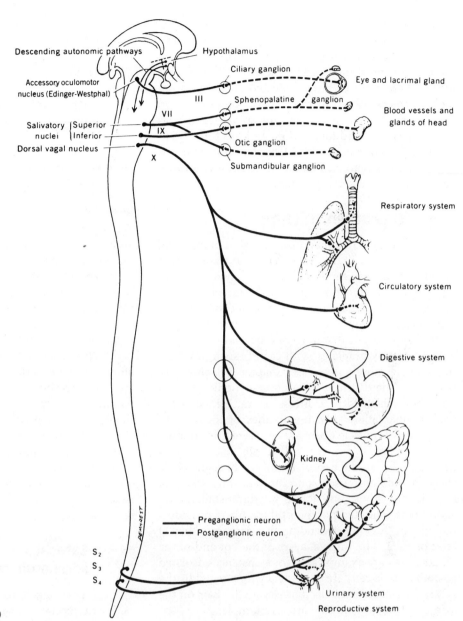

Figure 48-3 Diagrammatic representation of the parasympathetic division of the autonomic nervous system. (*Noback CR, Demarest RJ: The Nervous System—Introduction and Review, 2nd ed. New York, McGraw-Hill, 1977*)

causes contraction of the pregnant uterus and milk letdown during breast-feeding, is synthesized in the hypothalamus and released from the posterior pituitary gland in a manner similar to that of ADH.

Organization of many life-support reflexes occurs in the reticular formation of the medulla and pons. These areas of reflex circuitry, often called *centers,* produce complex combinations of autonomic and somatic efferent functions required for the respiration, gag, cough, sneeze, swallow, and vomit reflexes, as well as the more purely autonomic control of the cardiovascular system. At the hypothalamic level, these reflexes are integrated into more general response patterns such as rage, defensive behavior, eating, drinking, voiding, and sexual function. Forebrain and especially limbic system control of these behaviors involves inhibiting or facilitating release of the re-

sponse patterns according to social pressures during general emotion-provoking situations.

Reflex adjustments of cardiovascular and respiratory function occur at the level of the brain stem. A prominent example is the carotid sinus baroreflex. Increased blood pressure in the carotid sinus increases the discharge from afferent fibers that travel by way of the ninth cranial nerve to cardiovascular centers in the brain stem. These centers increase the activity of descending efferent vagal fibers that slow heart rate, while inhibiting sympathetic fibers that increase heart rate and blood vessel tone. One of the striking features of ANS function is the rapidity and intensity with which it can change visceral function. Within 3 to 5 seconds it can increase heart rate to about twice its resting level. Bronchial smooth muscle tone is largely controlled by way of parasympathetic fibers carried in the vagus nerve. These nerves produce mild to moderate constriction of the bronchioles (see Chapter 24).

Other important ANS reflexes are located at the level of the spinal cord. As with other spinal reflexes, these reflexes are modulated by input from higher centers. When there is loss of communication between the higher centers and the spinal reflexes, as occurs in spinal cord injury, these reflexes function in an unregulated manner (see Chapter 49). There is uncontrolled sweating, vasomotor instability, and reflex bowel and bladder function.

Neurotransmission

The generation and transmission of impulses in the ANS occur in the same manner as transmission in other neurons (see Chapter 46). There are self-propagating action potentials with transmission of impulses across synapses and other tissue junctions by way of neurohumoral transmitters. However, the somatic motoneurons that innervate skeletal muscles divide into many branches, with each branch innervating a single muscle fiber (see Chapter 49); this is in contrast to the distribution of postganglionic fibers of the ANS, which form a diffuse neural plexus at the site of innervation. The membranes of the cells of many smooth muscle fibers are connected by conductive protoplasmic bridges, called *gap junctions,* that permit rapid conduction of impulses through whole sheets of smooth muscle, often in repeating waves of contraction. Thus, autonomic neurotransmitters released near a limited portion of these fibers provide a modulating function extending to a large number of effector cells. The muscle layers of the gut and of the bladder wall are examples. In some instances, isolated smooth muscle cells are individually innervated by the ANS; the piloerector cells that elevate the hair on the skin during cold exposure are an example.

The main neurotransmitters of the autonomic nervous system are acetylcholine and the catecholamines, epinephrine and norepinephrine. Acetylcholine is released at all of the sites of preganglionic transmission in the autonomic ganglia of both sympathetic and parasympathetic nerve fibers and at the sites of postganglionic transmission in parasympathetic nerve endings. It is also released at sympathetic nerve endings that innervate the sweat glands and cholinergic vasodilator fibers found in skeletal muscle. Norepinephrine is released at most sympathetic nerve endings. The adrenal medulla, which is an extension of the sympathetic nervous system, produces epinephrine along with small fractions of norepinephrine. Dopamine, which is an intermediate compound in the synthesis of norepinephrine, also acts as a neurotransmitter. It is the principal inhibitory transmitter of internuncial neurons in the sympathetic ganglia. It

also has vasodilator effects on renal, splanchnic, and coronary blood vessels when given intravenously and is sometimes used in the treatment of shock (see Chapter 23).

Acetylcholine and cholinergic receptors

Acetylcholine is synthesized in the terminal endings of cholinergic fibers from choline and acetyl coenzyme A (acetyl CoA). Once acetylcholine is secreted by the cholinergic nerve endings, it is rapidly broken down by the enzyme acetylcholinesterase. The choline molecule is transported back into the nerve ending where it is used again in the synthesis of acetylcholine. Receptors that respond to acetylcholine are called *cholinergic receptors.* There are two types of cholinergic receptors: muscarinic and nicotinic. Muscarinic receptors are present in cholinergic postganglionic fibers of the autonomic nervous system. Nicotinic receptors are found in autonomic ganglia and the end-plates of skeletal muscle. Acetylcholine has excitatory effects on both muscarinic and nicotinic receptors; yet in the heart and lower esophageal sphincter, it has an inhibitory effect. Recent evidence indicates that there are different types of muscarinic receptors.

The drug atropine is a antimuscarinic or muscarinic cholinergic-blocking drug that prevents the action of acetylcholine at both excitatory and inhibitory muscarinic receptor sites. Because it is a muscarinic-blocking drug, it exerts little effect at nicotinic receptor sites.

Catecholamines and adrenergic receptors

The catecholamines, which include norepinephrine, epinephrine, and dopamine, are synthesized in the axoplasm of sympathetic nerve terminal endings from the amino acid tyrosine (Figure 48-4). In the process of catecholamine synthesis, tyrosine is hydroxylated (has a hydroxyl group added) to form DOPA, DOPA is decarboxylated (has a carboxyl group removed) to form dopamine, and dopamine is hydroxylated to form norepinephrine. In the adrenal gland, an additional step occurs during which norepinephrine is methylated (a methyl group is added) to form epinephrine. Epinephrine is also called *adrenalin,* and sympathetic neurons, *adrenergic* neurons. Each of the steps in neurotransmitter synthesis requires a different enzyme, and the type of neurotransmitter that is produced depends on the type of enzymes that are available in a nerve terminal. For example, the postganglionic sympathetic neurons that supply blood vessels synthesize norepinephrine, whereas postganglionic neurons in the adrenal me-

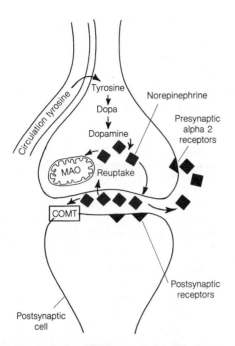

Figure 48-4 Synthesis, reuptake, and metabolism of norepinephrine. Presynaptic alpha$_2$ receptors control norepinephrine release in the central nervous system.

dulla produce both epinephrine or norepinephrine. Epinephrine accounts for about 80% of the catecholamines released from the adrenal gland. The synthesis of epinephrine by the adrenal medulla is influenced by the glucocorticoid secretion from the adrenal cortex. These hormones are transported, by way of a intra-adrenal vascular network, from the adrenal cortex to the adrenal medulla where they cause the sympathetic neurons to increase their production of epinephrine by way of increased enzyme activity.[2] Thus, any stress situation sufficient to evoke increased levels of glucocorticoids also increases epinephrine levels.

As the catecholamines are synthesized, they are stored in vesicles. The final step of norepinephrine synthesis occurs in these vesicles. During an action potential, the neurotransmitter molecules are released from the storage vesicles. The storage vesicles not only provide a means for concentrated storage of the catecholamines but they also protect them from the cytoplasmic enzymes that degrade the neurotransmitter.

In addition to neuronal synthesis, there is a second major mechanism for replenishment of norepinephrine in sympathetic nerve terminals. This mechanism consists of the active recapture or reuptake of the released neurotransmitter into the nerve terminal. From 50% to 80% of the norepinephrine that is released during an action potential is removed from the synaptic area by an active reuptake process.[3] This process not only terminates the action of the neuro-

transmitter but also allows it to be reused by the neuron. The remainder of the released catecholamines either diffuse into the surrounding tissue fluids or are degraded by two special enzymes: catechol-O-methyltransferase (COMT), which is diffusely present in all tissues, and monoamine oxidase (MAO), which is found in the nerve endings themselves.[3] Some drugs, such as the tricyclic antidepressants, are thought to increase the level of catecholamines at the site of nerve endings in the brain by blocking the reuptake process. Others, such as the MAO inhibitors, decrease the enzymatic degradation of the neurotransmitters and, thus, increase their levels.

The catecholamines can cause either excitation or inhibition of smooth muscle contraction, depending on the site, dose, and type of receptor present. Norepinephrine has potent excitatory activity and low inhibitory activity. Isoproterenol exhibits the reverse pattern of action. Epinephrine is potent as both an excitatory agent and as an inhibitory agent. The excitatory or inhibitory responses of organs to neurotransmitters are mediated by interaction with special structures in the cell membrane called *receptors*. The receptors in sympathetic neurons are called *adrenergic receptors*. In 1948, Ahlquist proposed the terms alpha and beta for the receptor sites where catecholamines produce their excitatory (alpha) and inhibitory (beta) effects.[5]

In vascular smooth muscle, excitation of alpha receptors causes vasoconstriction, and excitation of beta receptors causes vasodilatation. Both endogenous and exogenously administered norepinephrine produce marked vasoconstriction of the blood vessels in the skin, kidneys, and splanchnic circulation that are supplied with alpha receptors. Beta receptors are most prevalent in the heart, the blood vessels of skeletal muscle, and the bronchioles. Blood vessels in skeletal muscle have both alpha and beta receptors. In these vessels, high levels of norepinephrine produce vasoconstriction; low levels produce vasodilatation. The low levels are thought to have a diluting effect on norepinephrine levels in the arteries of these blood vessels so that the beta effect predominates.[6] In vessels with few receptors such as those that supply the brain, norepinephrine has little effect.

Alpha-adrenergic receptors have been further subdivided into alpha$_1$ and alpha$_2$ receptors, and beta-adrenergic receptors, into beta$_1$ and beta$_2$ receptors. Beta$_1$ receptors are found primarily in the heart and can be selectively blocked by beta$_1$ receptor blockers. Beta$_2$ receptors are found in the bronchioles and in other sites that have beta-mediated functions. Alpha$_1$ receptors are found primarily in postsynaptic effector sites; they mediate responses in vascular smooth muscle. Alpha$_2$ receptors are mainly located presynaptically and can inhibit the release of norepinephrine from sympathetic nerve terminals. Alpha$_2$ receptors are abundant in the central nervous system and are thought to influence the central control of blood pressure. Table 48-1 lists the receptor type and effector responses of the various organs that are innervated by the ANS.

The various classes of adrenergic receptors provide a mechanism by which the same adrenergic neurotransmitter can have many discretely different effects on differing effector cells. This mechanism also permits neurotransmitters carried in the bloodstream, whether from neuroendocrine secretion by the adrenal gland or from subcutaneous or intravenous administered drugs, to produce the same effects.

The catecholamines that are produced and released from sympathetic nerve endings are referred to as *endogenous neuromediators*. Sympathetic nerve endings can also be activated by *exogenous* forms of these neuromediators, which reach the nerve endings by way of the bloodstream after being injected into the body or being administered by mouth. These drugs mimic the action of the neuromediators and are said to have a *sympathomimetic* action. Other drugs can selectively block the receptor sites on the neurons and temporarily prevent the neurotransmitter from exerting its action.

In summary, the ANS regulates, adjusts, and coordinates the visceral functions of the body. The ANS, which is divided into the sympathetic and parasympathetic systems, is an efferent system. It receives its afferent input from visceral afferent neurons. The ANS has both CNS and PNS components. The outflow of both the sympathetic and parasympathetic nervous system follows a two-neuron pathway, which consists of a preganglionic neuron located within the CNS and a postganglionic neuron located outside the CNS. Sympathetic fibers leave the CNS at the thoracolumbar level, and the parasympathetic fibers leave at the craniosacral level. In general, the sympathetic and parasympathetic nervous systems have opposing effects on visceral function—if one excites, the other inhibits. The hypothalamus serves as the major control center for most ANS functions; local reflex circuits interrelating visceral afferent and autonomic efferent activity are integrated in a hierarchic control system in the spinal cord and brain stem.

The main neurotransmitters for the ANS are acetylcholine and the catecholamines—epinephrine and norepinephrine. Acetylcholine is the transmitter for all preganglionic neurons, for postganglionic parasympathetic neurons, and for selected postganglionic sympathetic neurons. The catecholamines are the neurotransmitters for most postganglionic sympathetic neurons. The neurotransmitters exert their target action through specialized cell surface receptors—cholinergic receptors that bind acetylcholine and adrenergic receptors that bind the catecholamines. The cholinergic receptors are divided into nicotinic and muscarinic receptors, and adrenergic receptors are divided into alpha and beta receptors.

Alterations in ANS function

Disorders of ANS function rarely occur as a separate disease. Because the control of the internal environment is vested in the ANS, most conditions that threaten the physiologic or psychologic integrity of the individual are accompanied by changes in ANS function.

The manifestations of altered ANS function are quite different from disorders of the somatic nervous system. When motoneurons are interrupted, the skeletal muscles they innervate are completely paralyzed. In contrast, the smooth muscle and other tissues that are innervated by the ANS usually have some level of spontaneous activity, and it is the control over this spontaneous activity that is lost when ANS innervation is disrupted. For example, the heart will continue to beat when all innervation from the ANS is removed. This has been repeatedly demonstrated in heart transplant procedures in which the cardiac innervation is severed. Likewise, the peristaltic movement of the gastrointestinal tract continues, despite loss of ANS innervation in spinal cord injury, although modified so that transit time may become altered.

Organ and system dysfunction

Disorders of the ANS can be manifested as dysfunction of a single body organ or system or as a dysfunction of multiple organ systems. Disturbances in function of a single organ system can result from disorders of either central or peripheral ANS function. These disorders may occur singly or as a symptom of an accompanying disease condition.

Vision

Three functions of the eye are controlled by the ANS: pupil size, lens thickness, and lacrimation or tearing. Sympathetic activity causes pupil dilatation by contraction of the radial muscle of the iris. This enhances visual acuity by increasing the amount of light that enters the eye. The parasympathetic nervous system controls the circular muscles of the iris and causes pupil constriction; it is reflexly stimulated when excess light enters the eye.

Adjustment of lens thickness, used for focusing on near objects (called *accommodation*), is controlled almost entirely by the parasympathetic division of the ANS. At rest, the lens is normally held in a flattened shape by the tension (from the sclera) on its radial suspensory ligaments. Thus, the resting eye is in focus for distant objects (see Chapter 51). Parasympathetic excitation results in contraction of the ciliary muscle; this releases the tension and allows the lens to assume a more convex or thickened shape, which brings near objects into focus. Atropine, a cholinergic blocking drug, is sometimes used to facilitate thorough inspection of the retina and optic disc during an ophthalmoscopic eye examination. When instilled into the conjunctival sac, the drug diffuses into the iris and ciliary body and blocks signal transmission at parasympathetic synapses with a resultant paralysis of lens accommodation and pupillary enlargement. Usually homoatropine, which is less potent and has a shorter duration of action than atropine, is used.

Tearing or lacrimation is controlled by the parasympathetic nervous system; it is increased with local irritation and reflex stimulation. Emotional reactions that involve crying are undoubtedly mediated by way of input from the cortex and limbic systems.

Horner's syndrome. Horner's syndrome is a disorder of sympathetic function that causes a drooping of the upper eyelid (ptosis), backward displacement of the eye into the orbit (enophthalmos), a fixed and constricted pupil, and generalized vascular dilatation and loss of sweating over the affected half of the face. Postganglionic neurons of the superior cervical ganglion follow the internal carotid artery and then the ophthalmic artery into the orbit to innervate the blood vessels of the face, the dilator muscles of the iris, and the tarsal muscles of the eyelid. Horner's syndrome is usually caused by damage to the sympathetic chain, the superior cervical ganglion, or the internal carotid artery. The most common causes are mediastinal tumors, particularly bronchiogenic carcinoma, Hodgkin's disease, and metastatic tumors. Other causes are surgical or accidental trauma to the neck and CNS conditions, such as occlusion of the posterior inferior cerebellar artery and multiple sclerosis. Hemisection or transection of the cervical spine interrupts descending control of sympathetic outflow causing ipsilateral (hemisection) or bilateral (transection) Horner's syndrome. This is called *central Horner's syndrome*.

Tonic pupil (Adie's syndrome). Tonic pupil is characterized by a pupil that is initially larger than normal and responds poorly to light. The disorder results from damage to the ciliary ganglion that contains the PNS postganglionic fibers and aberrant regeneration of its nerve fibers. The affected pupil usually remains larger than normal for 2 to 6 months and then becomes smaller than the normal one.[7] The reduction in pupil size is thought to be caused by an aberrant regeneration process in which fibers that normally control accommodation grow to innervate the affected pupillary sphincter muscles. The neuronal drive associated with normal ciliary function then constricts the pupil by way of the aberrant nerves to give a small pupil. The initial changes in accommodation resolve as the ciliary fibers regenerate.

Argyll Robertson pupil. In the condition called Argyll Robertson pupil, the pupil does not respond to light but is capable of accommodation. The condition is usually bilateral and is characterized by small (1–2 mm) and irregular-shaped pupils. The pupils do not dilate to atropine. In the past, the most common cause of the Argyll Robertson pupil was CNS syphilis. At present, other causes include diabetes mellitus, degenerative disorders, and tumors of the midbrain. The sites of the CNS lesion usually are not known.

Skin and thermal regulation

The sweat glands of the skin, the piloerector muscles, and the skin blood vessels are all controlled by the sympathetic nervous system. All of these mechanisms are involved in temperature regulation (see Chapter 7). Contraction of the pilomotor muscles causes "goose bumps" when the skin is exposed to a cold environment. This slightly reduces the surface area for heat loss. Skin blood flow regulates the conduction of heat from internal body structures to the skin where heat can be released into the external environment. Skin blood vessels dilate when there is a need to dissipate body heat and constrict when there is a need to conserve body heat. Skin blood flow also decreases when there is a need to divert blood flow to vital centers such as occurs with circulatory shock.

Unlike most sympathetically innervated organs, the sweat glands have cholinergic rather than adrenergic receptors. Because adrenergic receptors respond to both neural stimulation and humoral sources of catecholamines, the fact that sweat glands have cholinergic receptors allows them to be active during fever and exposure to hot weather when sympathetic outflow to skin vessels is reduced as a means of maintaining vasodilatation. The sweat glands and skin vessels are also innervated by separate efferent neurons; thus, the two functions are sorted out by CNS mechanisms as well.

Sweating disorders may take the form of increased sweating above normal to a given stimulus (hyperhidrosis) or absent or decreased sweating (anhidrosis).

Hyperhidrosis, particularly of the hands and feet, can be a social embarrassment and can occur without pathology. It is often associated with emotional reactions. It can also be caused by endocrine disorders such as hyperthyroidism, acromegaly, or pheochromocytoma (to be discussed). Recurring and transient periods of hyperhidrosis accompanied by vasomotor instability often accompany hormonal changes that occur during menopause. Localized cutaneous areas of sweating may occur following injury to a peripheral nerve that carries both afferent and efferent fibers. It is often accompanied by severe pain (causalgia) along the course of the nerve (discussed in Chapter 47). It is most common after injury to the median or sciatic nerves. Sweating may occur as part of an isolated spinal cord reflex that is provoked by bladder distention or other sensory stimuli in persons with spinal cord transection.

Anhidrosis can result from impaired sympathetic innervation of sweat glands, degeneration of sweat glands, or decreased sensitivity of the sweat glands to acetylcholine. Persons with diabetic neuropathy involving sympathetic pathways often show signs of anhidrosis over the lower extremities and trunk. There may be hyperhidrosis of the face and neck and drenching nocturnal sweats independent of a hypoglycemic event.[8] Another unusual feature of diabetic neuropathy is severe facial sweating at mealtimes. The presence of abnormal sweating patterns in diabetes should suggest the possibility of peripheral neuropathy and should be considered when sweating is used as an indicator of a hypoglycemic event.

Impairment of sweating and vasodilatation occurs in persons with cervical cord injuries. Such persons may become vulnerable to the effects of environmental heat and to hyperpyrexia during infection.

Sweating may be impaired in elderly persons due to degenerative changes in the sweat glands and to changes in sweat gland sensitivity to acetylcholine. A reduction in sweating capability is thought to be one of the factors that contribute to the increased incidence of heat stroke in elderly persons during a heat wave.[8]

Circulatory function

The heart is innervated by both divisions of the ANS. The sympathetic nervous system innervates both the sinoatrial (SA) and the atrioventricular (AV) nodes as well as the ventricles; it increases both heart rate and force of ventricular contraction. The parasympathetic innervation of the heart, by way of the vagus, is largely restricted to the SA and AV nodes; its effect is to slow heart rate. The resistance of the peripheral blood vessels, which is a major determinant of blood pressure and flow, is largely controlled by the sympathetic nervous system. Most blood vessels, especially those of the abdominal viscera and skin, constrict when there is increased sympathetic activity. These blood vessels normally constrict and divert the flow of blood to the vital organs such as the heart and brain during times of need.

The cardiovascular system assumes a pivotal role in homeostasis by adjusting the blood supply to the various organs in relation to need. The circulation to the brain and other vital centers is largely controlled by autonomically mediated circulatory reflexes that match pressure and flow to the needs of the individual tissue beds. When going from the supine to the standing position, for example, cerebral blood flow is protected by the baroreceptor reflex. This reflex incorporates pressure-sensitive receptors in the carotid sinus and aorta, cardiovascular regulatory centers in the brain stem, and autonomic effector responses that alter heart rate and total peripheral resistance to meet the changing demands of the circulatory system and to maintain blood flow to vital centers. Volume receptors control total blood volume and are the circulatory system's protection against inadequate filling of the vascular compartment. Disorders of circulatory function occur when the autonomic reflexes that control cardiovascular function are exaggerated, deficient, or inappropriate. They include such disorders as cardiac dysrhythmias and abnormal blood pressure responses to normal activities of daily living.

Orthostatic hypotension represents an abnormal drop in blood pressure that occurs with assumption of the upright position. It may result from an impaired vasoconstrictor response and peripheral pooling of blood with a temporary lack of blood flow to the brain.

Fainting or syncope refers to a transient loss of consciousness resulting from inadequate cerebral blood flow. It is usually preceded by sweating, pallor, blurring of vision, dizziness, and nausea. Fainting may have an abrupt onset, with an initial increase in sympathetic activity leading to increased heart rate and vascular resistance. The initial sympathetic response is very brief and is followed by a sudden drop in heart rate, a decrease in vascular resistance, a profound fall in blood pressure and cerebral blood flow, and loss of consciousness.[9] Fainting occurs more commonly in persons who are in the upright position, and assumption of the supine position during a faint usually results in a return of consciousness. Factors that predispose to fainting include a reduction in venous return to the heart resulting from orthostatic or postural stress, blood loss, or an increased intrathoracic pressure due to performance of Valsalva's maneuver.[10] The risk of syncope is increased in a hot environment due to vasodilatation and loss of extracellular fluid volume caused by sweating. Emotional fainting can occur as the result of reduced vasoconstrictor outflow and increased vasodilator outflow from CNS centers that influence blood vessel tone. Most normal individuals can precipitate presyncopal conditions, particularly in hot weather, when they hyperventilate and produce cerebral vasoconstriction secondary to decreased cerebral carbon dioxide levels. Assumption of the standing position or standing without moving the legs to promote venous return contributes to the presyncopal condition.[9] Immobility and prolonged bedrest lead to a decrease in vascular volume and deconditioning of vascular smooth muscle and the skeletal muscle pumps that return blood to the heart. Thus, dizziness and the potential for fainting are common following immobility or bedrest.

Micturition syncope can occur immediately following bladder emptying. Loss of consciousness is abrupt, and recovery is rapid and complete. A full bladder tends to cause vasoconstriction, a condition that does not usually produce hypertension because it is counteracted by the baroreceptor reflex. It has been suggested that syncope occurs when the constricted vessels suddenly dilate. It is more common in males, probably because the standing position contributes to pooling of blood in the extremities. The reflex effects of bladder distention on circulation are much more pronounced in paraplegic persons with cord injuries above T6.

The baroreceptor reflex is less efficient in many elderly persons, and this may contribute to syncope and falls.[11,12] This is particularly true when multiple stresses are placed on the circulation. These stresses include sudden assumption of the standing position from either the seated or supine position, vasodilatation due to a warm room or bed, a full bladder, use of medications that impair autonomic function, and decreased vascular volume due to inadequate fluid intake or use of diuretics. Orthostatic hypotension is further discussed in Chapter 19.

Postprandial hypotension is a decrease in blood pressure that occurs following a meal. It has been shown that insulin release has a depressant effect on baroreflex function.[13] Consequently, the consumption of a meal that is high in carbohydrate content, with the subsequent release of insulin, has the potential for producing a postprandial decrease in blood pressure. This aspect of autonomic function has many practical implications for persons who already have disorders of ANS function such as the elderly or persons who have had a stroke. Several studies have shown a significant reduction of postprandial blood pressure in elderly persons.[13–15] In persons who have had a stroke, autoregulation of the cerebral vessels in the affected area is lost; slight orthostatic falls in blood pressure following carbohydrate ingestion have the potential of further compromising blood flow to the area. Therefore, ingestion of small, low-carbohydrate meals and afterwards avoidance of positions that produce orthostatic hypotension are suggested as a means of minimizing brain ischemia.

Pheochromocytoma

A pheochromocytoma is a tumor of chromaffin tissue (tissue containing sympathetic nerve cells that stain with chromium salts) found in the adrenal medulla; but it can arise in other sites where there is chromaffin tissue, such as the sympathetic ganglia. Although only 0.1% to 0.2% of persons with hypertension have an underlying pheochromocytoma, the disorder can cause lethal hypertensive crises; and 8% to 10% of the tumors are malignant.[16]

Like adrenal medullary cells, the tumor cells of a pheochromocytoma produce and secrete the catecholamines epinephrine and norepinephrine. Thus, the hypertension is the result of massive release of these catecholamines. Often their release is paroxysmal, occurring several times a month to several times a day and lasting for one minute to several hours. The most frequent symptoms, in addition to hypertension, are headache, sweating, and tachycardia. Nervousness, tremor, pallor of the face, weakness, fatigue, and weight loss occur less frequently. Often there is marked variability in blood pressure between episodes. Several tests are available to differentiate this type of hypertension from other types. One of the most commonly used diagnostic methods is the determination of 24-hour levels of urinary catecholamines and their metabolites, including vanillylmandelic acid (VMA). Once the presence of a pheochromocytoma has been established, the tumor needs to be located. Computerized tomographic (CT) scans are often used for this purpose. Surgical removal of operable tumors is curative.[16]

Gastrointestinal function

Normal digestive function requires both digestive secretions and motility. The parasympathetic nervous system has the major control of the salivary gland activity. The sympathetic nervous system controls blood flow in the mouth and related structures, including the salivary glands. Its effect on salivation is probably indirect, by way of vasoconstriction of the salivary gland arterioles, resulting in reduced extracellular fluid delivery, and, thus, increasing the viscosity of the salivary secretions, experienced as a dry mouth. The muscarinic anticholinergic drug atropine blocks parasympathetic activity and, thus, produces a dry mouth. If the parasympathetic innervation of the salivary gland is interrupted, the gland ceases to secrete saliva. If only one gland is affected, a dry mouth may not pose a problem and swallowing may not be affected.

The gastrointestinal tract has its own set of nerves known as the intramural, or enteric, plexus. Both sympathetic and parasympathetic stimulation can affect gastrointestinal tract motility (see Chapter 39). Parasympathetic activity increases the activity of the gastrointestinal tract, and sympathetic activity decreases the activity. Alterations in intramural plexus function can result in problems with swallowing or movement of food through the gastrointestinal tract.

Achalasia. Achalasia (cardiospasm) involves a failure of relaxation of the lower esophagus and is thought to result from abnormal parasympathetic innervation. In advanced cases, there is absence or degeneration of the ganglion cells in the intramural plexus. The main symptom is difficulty swallowing, with weight loss and vomiting occurring in some people.

Hirschsprung's disease. Hirschsprung's disease, also called *congenital megacolon,* is a congenital absence of autonomic ganglion cells from the intramural plexus of the colon. The ganglia are absent from the anorectal junction, in most cases from the rectum, and sometimes from sections of the sigmoid colon.[17] Constipation is present from birth. There is a delay in the initial passing of meconium; the rectum is usually empty and the rest of the colon is distended. Vomiting usually follows. In some cases, there are alternating periods of obstruction and sudden passage of diarrheal stools. Complications include fluid and electrolyte disturbances and perforation of the distended bowel. The treatment for this condition is surgical resection of the affected portion of the colon.

Metabolic function

Sympathetic stimulation also has metabolic functions: it inhibits insulin release from beta cells in the pancreas, it increases glucose release from the liver, and it increases lipolysis. All of these functions result in increased availability of blood glucose or of its lipid precursors, which supports increased skeletal muscle and brain function required during the fight or flight response. The hypothalamus is thought to play an important role in appetite, satiety, and hunger. There is increasing evidence that the autonomic nervous system contributes to feeding patterns and weight gain. In animal studies, for example, decreased sympathetic activity leads to excess energy storage in fat cells by means of decreased lipolysis (fat breakdown) and increased lipogenesis (fat generation).[18] Recent studies have shown an association between percentage of body fat and responses to tests of ANS function.[19]

Sexual function

In the male, sexual function requires erection and emission-ejaculation. Erection involves vascular engorgement of the spongelike erectile tissue in the corpora cavernosa and corpora spongiosum that results from arterial dilatation and venous constriction. This is primarily a parasympathetic function and requires sacral outflow by way of the pelvic nerves. Parasympathetic impulses, in addition to promoting erection, cause the urethral glands and the bulbourethral glands to secrete mucus. This mucus flows through the urethra and aids in lubrication. Emission consists of expulsion of semen into the posterior urethra and reflex closure of the internal sphincter of the bladder to prevent reflux of secretions into the bladder. Both expulsion of semen into the posterior urethra and closure of the internal sphincter depend on sympathetic impulses that leave the cord at the lower thoracic and upper lumbar regions. The afferent neurons that trigger emission run in the pudendal and pelvic nerves to the sacral cord and with the sympathetic fibers to the thoracolumbar cord. Ejection of semen from the anterior urethra (ejaculation) depends on the rhythmic contractions of the bulbocavernous and ischiocavernous muscles supplied by the somatic pudendal nerve. The entire period of emission and ejaculation is called the male orgasm.

Both erection and emission-ejaculation are largely reflex in nature. Erection can occur despite partial or complete lesions above the level of the sacral cord. Afferent impulses resulting from stimulation of the genitalia or perineum are transmitted through the pudendal nerve to the sacral cord, and efferent parasympathetic impulses from the same segments reach the corpora cavernosa and spongiosum leading to vasodilation and congestion. In some cases, persistent erection (priapism) may occur. For emission-ejaculation to occur, the lower thoracic and upper lumbar sympathetic connections must be intact.

Impotence (failure of erection) can result from any disorder that affects sacral parasympathetic function including injury, polyneuropathy, and multiple sclerosis. Emission-ejaculation can be inhibited by drugs that act directly on the sympathetic nervous system (*e.g.,* antihypertensive drugs and many tranquilizers). Impotence and problems with emission-ejaculation may occur in men who suffer from diabetic autonomic neuropathy. Ejection of semen from the urethra is controlled by the somatic pudendal nerve and does not occur in men with lower motor neuron lesions of this nerve.

Fertility may also be impaired in men with partial loss of ANS function due to lesions of the spinal cord above the lumbar or sacral segments. Even if they are able to ejaculate, sperm counts show few motile sperms in the ejaculate. The cause of the decreased sperm count is unknown, but it is thought that impairment of temperature regulation in the scrotum may be a contributing factor.

In women, disorders of ANS function interfere with orgasm. This occurs with lesions of the cauda equina and spinal cord. There is no evidence that ovulation or menstruation is affected. Delivery of a baby can occur after spinal cord transection or interruption of sympathetic nerve supply. After spinal cord transection, labor may occur without the mother knowing that labor has begun and may be accompanied by autonomic hyperreflexia.

Disorders of peripheral ANS function

Disorders of the peripheral autonomic nervous system may occur in isolation, as in acute and subacute autonomic neuropathies, or in association with a generalized peripheral neuropathy as in Guillain-Barré syndrome (see Chapter 49). The peripheral neuropathies most likely to cause severe ANS dysfunction are those in which small myelinated and unmyelinated fibers are damaged in baroreflex afferents, the afferents to the heart, and the afferent pathways to the mesenteric blood vessels.[20]

Autonomic neuropathy is common in diabetes mellitus, and clinical features include impaired sweating, postural hypotension, impaired control of heart rate, diarrhea, impaired esophageal and gastric motility, impotence, and sphincter and pupillary disturbances of the eye. Long-term alcohol abuse can lead to alcohol-induced neuropathy. Degeneration of both the vagus and sympathetic neurons occur in severe cases. Disturbances of esophageal motility in chronic alcoholics with peripheral neuropathies may be a manifestation of damage to the vagus nerve. Peripheral neuropathies with associated autonomic manifestations may result from the toxic effects of exposure to heavy metals such as thallium, arsenic, organic solvent, and other chemicals. Other disease conditions that can affect the peripheral ANS are chronic renal failure, rheumatoid arthritis, systemic lupus erythematosus, and mixed connective tissue disorders.

Denervation hypersensitivity

When autonomically innervated smooth muscle is deprived of its innervation, it becomes extremely sensitive to its neurotransmitters. During the first week or so after sympathetic or parasympathetic nerve injury, the innervated organ becomes more and more sensitive to circulating neurotransmitters. This is called *denervation hypersensitivity*. The mechanisms

of the hypersensitivity are not completely understood. The number of receptors on the postsynaptic membrane are increased when acetylcholine or norepinephrine are no longer released from the neuron. This is called *upregulation* and is caused by genetic mechanisms that are responsible for replacing the receptors. The increased number of receptors produces an increased response to neurotransmitters that circulate in the blood—whether they are from endogenous sources such as the adrenal gland, or from exogenous sources, such as medications.

Disorders of central ANS function

The most common pathologies of disturbed autonomic function of CNS origin are degeneration of the intermediolateral cell columns (progressive autonomic failure) or diseases that cause damage to the descending pathways that synapse with the intermediolateral column cells (spinal cord tumors, cerebrovascular accidents, brain stem tumors, multiple sclerosis, or Parkinson's disease).[20]

Progressive autonomic failure

A condition called progressive autonomic failure is a degenerative disorder of the central and peripheral autonomic nervous systems. It can occur as a primary disorder (idiopathic autonomic insufficiency) or as a secondary disorder associated with other diseases such as Parkinson's disease and Wernicke's encephalopathy (see Chapter 53), spinal cord injury (see Chapter 49), and stroke (see Chapter 50).

Idiopathic autonomic insufficiency is a disorder of unknown cause. The condition is more common in males and usually strikes during middle age. The disorder may occur as an uncomplicated progressive autonomic failure, or it may be complicated by parkinsonian features or multisystem atrophy. In males, impotence is an early symptom, and manifestations of sphincter disturbances such as urinary hesitancy, urgency, and incontinence are common. Loss of sweating ability is characteristic. These early signs, which may go unrecognized, are followed by orthostatic hypotension—a hallmark of the disorder. Postural hypotension may be manifested by dizziness and weakness after standing or walking. There may be sudden drop attacks, but more often there is a gradual fading of consciousness over a half minute or so while the person is walking or standing. A neckache radiating to the occipital region of the skull and shoulders often precedes the actual loss of consciousness. Sometimes there are transient visual disturbances, scotomata, positive hallucinations, or tunnel vision.[21] The visual disturbances may be particularly troubling when the person is standing or walking. Symptoms are often worse in the morning, after meals, and in hot weather or other conditions that predispose to an unfavorable redistribution of blood volume. Persons treated with bedrest for hypotension may develop persistent recumbent hypertension, mainly due to loss of baroreflex function.[22]

The prognosis is better for persons with uncomplicated idiopathic autonomic insufficiency; in these persons, postural hypotension, impairment of sweating, and disturbances of heart rate and blood pressure may be the only manifestations. In persons in whom the condition is complicated by parkinsonian features, there is facial immobility, bradykinesia, tremor, and rigidity. Multisystem failure (sometimes called the Shy-Drager syndrome) is characterized by progressive pyramidal, bulbar, extrapyramidal, and cerebellar deterioration; iris atrophy; Horner's syndrome; and other ocular disturbances. There may also be a laryngeal stridor during sleep, sudden inspiratory gasps, sleep apnea, and cluster breathing, as well as other disturbances of respiration. The presence of parkinsonian features or multisystem atrophy is associated with a much poorer outcome, with death occurring in 4 to 8 years.[20]

The most troubling aspect of progressive autonomic failure is orthostatic hypotension. Treatment measures, including drug therapy, are used to increase blood volume, vasomotor tone, or both.[22] Treatment is complicated by the fact that the supine position tends

Table 48–3. Tests of autonomic nervous system (ANS) function

Test	Normal response	Part of the ANS tested
Graded postural stress (a tilt table is used; heart rate and blood pressure are monitored)	Fall in pulse pressure (decrease in systolic and increase in diastolic pressures) and increased rate at high levels of tilt	Sympathetic vasoconstriction at low levels of tilt; arterial baroreceptors at high levels tilt
Heart rate to standing	Increase heart rate to about 15th beat with slowing to about 30th beat; then stabilizes	Baroreflex afferents; parasympathetic withdrawal of the vagal heart rate response (immediate); peripheral sympathetic vasoconstriction (stabilization of heart rate)
Isometric handgrip (a handgrip device is used; contraction is maintained at a given percentage of maximum contraction for 5 min)	Increase in systolic and diastolic pressure	Input from central CNS command and metabolic or mechanical changes in contracting muscle; sympathetic vasoconstrictor response
Valsalva test (done by blowing into a mouthpiece for 15 seconds; heart rate is monitored during and immediately following the strain). Intra-arterial blood pressure may also be monitored	Rise in phase II (end of strain) and phase IV slowing (5–20 second post strain) of heart rate	Baroreflex afferents; sympathetic increase in heart rate and vasoconstriction; vagal slowing of heart rate
Respiratory sinus arrhythmia—heart rate variation with respiration (heart rate is measured during normal or forced breathing and the difference between inspiratory and expiratory rate calculated)	Heart rate increases during inspiration and decreases during expiration	Pulmonary receptors in the lung; vagal efferent control of heart rate
Cold pressor test (hand immersed in cold or ice water for 1 to 2 min)	Increase in blood pressure	Afferent pain and temperature receptors; sympathetic vasoconstrictor response
Emotional stress (mental arithmetic, loud noise, confusing instructions for task, and so forth)	Increase in blood pressure; decrease in skin blood flow	Input from the cortex; sympathetic vasomotor response
Sweat tests (done by applying radiant heat to body)	Sweat is detected with chemicals that change color when wet	Pattern of sweating can be observed. Postganglionic lesions can be distinguished from preganglionic lesions with iontophoresis or injection of a cholinergic drug into the skin
Pupillary innervation (instillation of adrenergic or cholinergic drugs into the conjunctival sac)	Appropriate constriction or dilatation	Postganglionic control of autonomic innervation of pupil

to produce hypertension. Elevation of the head of the bed at night is usually advocated for this reason.[22] Tights, a tightly fitting elastic support garment that compresses the vessels in the legs and lower abdomen, may be used to control symptoms by decreasing the amount of blood that can be pooled in the abdomen and legs. In severe cases, antigravity suits may be used. Unfortunately, these support devices are restricting and uncomfortable, particularly in hot weather. The mineralocorticoid drug 9-a Fluorocortisol and sodium chloride may be used to increase blood volume. Oral sympathomimetic drugs (*e.g.*, ephedrine, phenylephrine) may be prescribed for persons with severe symptoms. Beta-adrenergic blocking drugs have been used to prevent possible beta-agonist-induced vasodilatation. Caffeine has a pressor effect and may be useful in preventing postprandial decreases in blood pressure.

—— Diagnostic methods

The integrity and function of the autonomic nervous system are usually assessed through the use of tests that stress selected autonomic reflexes. These tests include the blood pressure and heart rate response to a change in posture (tilt test or free standing), respiration (respiratory sinus arrhythmia), isometric (handgrip) exercise, Valsalva test, cold pressor test, and mental stress. Plasma catecholamines and catecholamine metabolites in the urine can be measured. Pupillary innervation can be assessed using various autonomic drugs. These tests are summarized in Table 48-3.

In summary, disorders of the ANS can affect a single organ or system and can result in diseases that affect either central or peripheral ANS function. The visceral structures that are innervated by the ANS usually have some level of spontaneous activity and it is modulation of this spontaneous activity that is lost when ANS function is interrupted. Alterations in ANS function can alter the ability of the eye to control pupil size, lens focus, accommodation, and tearing; the function of the sweat glands, piloerector muscles, and blood vessels of the skin; the ability of the circulatory system to maintain blood flow and blood pressure; the motility and release of digestive secretion by the gastrointestinal tract; the control of metabolic functions; and sexual functioning. Disorders of the peripheral ANS may occur in isolation as acute or subacute neuropathies or in association with generalized peripheral neuropathies. Autonomic neuropathy is common in diabetes mellitus. Progressive autonomic failure describes a degenerative disorder of the central and peripheral ANS.

References

1. Procacci P, Zoppi M, Maresca M: Clinical approach to visceral sensation. Prog Brain Res 67:21, 1986
2. Gilman AG, Goodman LS, Rall TW et al: The Pharmacological Basis of Therapeutics, 7th ed, p 84. New York, Macmillan, 1985
3. Guyton A: Medical Physiology, 7th ed, pp 687, 689. Philadelphia, WB Saunders, 1986
4. Appenzeller O: The Autonomic Nervous System, 3rd ed, p 276. New York, Elsevier, 1982
5. Alquist RP: A study of the adrenotropic receptors. Am J Physiol 153:586, 1948
6. Schmitt RF, Thews G: Human Physiology, p 115. New York, Springer-Verlag, 1983
7. Smith SA: Pupillary function in autonomic failure. In Bannister R (ed): Autonomic Failure, 2nd ed, pp 396–397. New York, Oxford Medical Publications, 1988
8. Collins KJ: Autonomic control of sweat glands and disorders of sweating. In Bannister R: Autonomic Failure, 2nd ed, pp 748–765. New York, Oxford Medical Publications, 1988
9. Porth CJ, Bamrah VS, Tristani FE et al: The Valsalva maneuver: Mechanisms and clinical implications. Heart Lung 13:507, 1984
10. Hainsworth R: Fainting. In Bannister R (ed): Autonomic Failure, 2nd ed, pp 142–158. New York, Oxford Medical Publications, 1988
11. Weiner WJ, Nora LM, Glantz RH: Elderly inpatients: Postural reflex impairment. Neurology (Cleveland) 34:945, 1984
12. Smith SA, Fasler JJ: Age-related changes in autonomic function: Relationship with postural hypotension. Age Ageing 12:206, 1983
13. Lipsitz LA, Fullerton KJ: Postprandial blood pressure reduction in healthy elderly. J Am Geriatr Soc 34:267, 1986
14. Fagan TC, Conrad KA, Mar JH et al: Effects of meals on hemodynamics: Implications for antihypertensive drug studies. Clin Pharmacol Ther 39:255, 1986
15. deMey C, Enterling D, Brendel E: Postprandial changes in supine and erect heart rate, systemic blood pressure and renin activity in normal subjects. Eur J Pharm 32:471, 1987
16. Bravo EL, Gifford RW: Pheochromocytoma: Diagnosis, localization, and management. N Engl J Med 311(20):1298, 1984
17. Robbins SL, Kumar V: Basic Pathology, p 540. Philadephia, WB Saunders, 1987
18. Bray GA, York DA: Hypothalamic and genetic obesity in experimental animals: And autonomic and endocrine hypothesis. Physiol Rev 59:719, 1979
19. Peterson HR, Rothchild M, Weinber CR: Body fat and activity of the autonomic nervous system. N Engl J Med 318(17): 1077, 1988
20. McLeod JG, Tuck RR: Disorders of the autonomic nervous system: Part I. Pathology and clinical features. Ann Neurol 21:419, 1987
21. Bannister R: Autonomic failure: Symptoms. In Bannister R (ed): Autonomic Failure, 2nd ed, p 267–288. New York, Oxford Medical Publications, 1988

22. McLeod JG, Tuckk RR: Disorders of the autonomic nervous system: Part II. Investigation and treatment. Ann Neurol 21:519, 1987

Bibliography

Bradshaw MJ, Edwards RTM: Postural hypotension—Pathophysiology and management. Q J Med 60:643, 1986

Bray GA: Autonomic and endocrine factors in the regulation of energy balance. Fed Proc 45(5):1404, 1986

Colan RV, Snead OC, Oh Sj et al: Acute autonomic and sensory neuropathy. Ann Neurol 8:441, 1980

Henrich WL: Autonomic insufficiency. Arch Intern Med 142:339, 1982

Kaijser L, Sachs C: Autonomic cardiovascular responses in old age. Clin Physiol 5:347, 1985

Onrot J, Goldberg MR, Biagioni I et al: Hemodynamic and humoral effects of caffiene in autonomic failure. N Engl J Med 313:549, 1985

Onrot J, Goldberg MR, Hollister AS et al: Management of chronic orthostatic hypotension. Am J Med 80:454, 1986

Robertson D, Wade D, Robertson RM: Postprandial alterations in cardiovascular hemodynamics and autonomic dysfunctional states. Am J Cardiol 48:1048, 1981

Wallin BG, Stjernberg L: Sympathetic activity in man after spinal cord injury. Brain 107:183, 1984

Warfield CA: The sympathetic dystrophies. Hosp Pract 19(5):52c, 1984

Ziegler MG: Postural hypotension. Annu Rev Med 31:239, 1980

Ziegler MG, Lake CR, Kopin IJ: The sympathetic nervous system defect in primary orthostatic hypotension. N Engl J Med 296:293, 1977

Sylvia Eichner
Robin L. Curtis

CHAPTER 49

Alterations in Motor Function

Objectives

After you have studied this chapter, you should be able to meet the following objectives:

_____ Trace a voluntary muscle movement from its initiation in the supplementary motor cortex, through the basal ganglia, cerebellum, brain stem circuits, spinal cord circuits, to the lower motoneuron (LMN) and myoneural junction; and state the contribution of each of these neural components.

_____ Define the function of the following muscle types: _extensors, flexors, adductors, abductors, rotators, agonists, antagonists,_ and _synergists._

_____ Describe the longitudinal and transverse organization of the spinal cord.

_____ Define _motor unit,_ and explain why this is the smallest unit of motor function.

_____ Compare the functions of the dorsal and ventral horns of the spinal cord.

_____ Explain why a lumbar puncture is performed below the level of the third lumbar vertebrae.

(continued)

_____ Relate the function of the stretch reflex and muscle tone.

_____ Compare the myotatic, reverse myotactic, and flexor-withdrawal reflexes.

_____ State the contributions of the primary motor cortex, the premotor area, and the supplementary motor cortex to motor function.

_____ Describe the functions of the pyramidal versus extrapyramidal systems.

_____ Explain the causes of muscle atrophy.

_____ Describe the pathology associated with Duchenne muscular dystrophy.

_____ Relate the clinical manifestations of myasthenia gravis to its etiology.

_____ Trace the steps in regeneration of an injured peripheral nerve.

_____ Describe the manifestation of peripheral nerve root injury due to a ruptured intervertebral disk.

_____ Compare the cause and manifestations of peripheral mononeuropathies with peripheral polyneuropathies.

_____ Explain why eliciting the deep tendon reflexes (DTRs) at specific segmental levels provides a rapid means of clinical assessment of the PNS and the functional integrity of the spinal cord.

_____ Define paresis, paralysis, monoparesis, hemiparesis, diparesis, paraparesis, and quadriparesis.

_____ Compare the manifestations of upper motoneuron (UMN) and lower motoneuron (LMN) injury.

_____ Describe the neural mechanisms involved in clonus.

_____ Describe the common motor deficits that occur with stroke.

_____ Describe the function of the cerebellum in motor function, and relate it to the cerebellar ataxia and tremor.

_____ State the alterations in motor control that occur with chorea, athetosis, hemiballismus, and tremor.

_____ Briefly state the mechanisms of neural injury in spinal cord injury (SCI).

_____ Relate the function of higher neural centers to muscle spasms that occur following recovery from SCI.

_____ Describe the events that culminate in spinal shock.

_____ Relate the effects of altered ventilation and communication function to level of injury in SCI.

_____ Describe the alterations in autonomic nervous system function that occur following SCI according to level of injury.

_____ Explain the occurrence of hypertension following SCI.

_____ Explain the effects of sensorimotor dysfunction that occurs following SCI on skin integrity, development of edema, pain, and deep vein thrombosis.

_____ Describe the alterations in bowel, bladder, and sexual function that occur with SCI, according to level of injury.

_____ Use the concepts of health stabilization, life-style modification, and community integration to explain the continuum of care for a person with SCI.

Effective motor function requires not only that muscles move but also that the mechanics of their movement be programmed in a manner that provides for smooth and coordinated movement. In some cases, purposeless and disruptive movements can be almost as disabling as the relative or complete absence of movement. This chapter is organized into four sections: control of motor function, alterations in function of the neuromuscular unit, alterations in pyramidal versus extrapyramidal function, and spinal cord injury. Although motor function relies on continuous input from sensory neurons, the focus of this chapter is on the efferent output that controls movement. Spinal cord injury is presented as an example of a condition that affects multiple motor systems.

Control of motor function

Movement begins *in utero* at about 21 weeks gestation with the quickening of the fetus, and the capability for some coordinated movement is present at birth. Maturation of the spinal cord and brain circuitry during the first year or two of life allows the child to defy the force of gravity and learn to sit, then stand, and in rapid sequence master the skills of walking, running, jumping, and climbing.

Motor function, whether it involves walking, running, or precise finger movements, requires both movement and maintenance of posture. Posture can be described as the active muscular resistance to the displacement of the body by gravity or acceleration.[1] The two functions are intricately related, and it is virtually impossible to successfully perform one without the other. Purposeful movement of the hands and feet is accomplished only by first placing the body and the arm or leg in a stable posture and appropriate position.

The structures that control posture and movement are located throughout the neuromuscular system. The system consists of the neuromuscular unit, which includes the motoneurons, the myoneural junction, and the muscle fibers; the spinal cord, which contains the basic reflex circuitry for posture and movement; the descending pathways from the brain stem circuits, the cerebellum, basal ganglia, and the motor cortex (Figure 49-1). Delicate, skillful, intentional movement of distal and especially flexor muscles of the limbs and the speech apparatus is initiated and controlled from the frontal motor regions of cerebral cortex. These areas receive information from the somesthetic thalamus and cortex, and, indirectly, from the cerebellum and basal ganglia. Programming of and ongoing direction of skilled movement require the functions of the premotor areas of the cerebral cortex. Descending axons from the motor cortex project to the spinal cord; there they indirectly innervate lower motoneurons (LMNs) that supply the muscle fibers. Accurate and smoothly coordinated movement requires the participation of the brain stem reticular formation for basic movement patterns and basal ganglia circuits, which provide the supporting and additional automatic movement sequences that give gracefulness to skilled activity. The cerebellum provides continuous, smooth trajectory correcting adjustments. The entire motor system depends on optimally facilitated motor units on a background of stretch reflex and vestibular system input to maintain stable postural support.

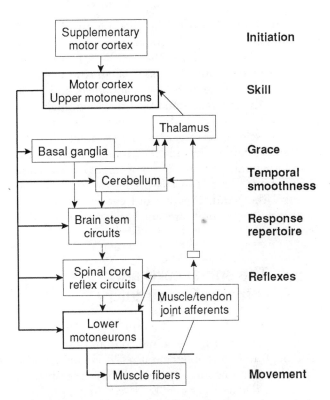

Figure 49-1 Functional diagram of neural pathways for control of motor function.

Functional organization of muscle groups

Skeletal muscle is composed of muscle cells, or fibers, which contain the interacting actin and myosin filaments that generate the contractile force required for movement (see Chapter 1). In terms of function, muscles can be classified as *extensors,* muscles that increase the angle of a joint, or *flexors,* muscles that decrease the angle of a joint. In the legs, groups of extensor muscles work together to resist gravity and function to maintain the upright posture and provide locomotion power. In general, flexor muscle groups assist gravity, participate in withdrawal reflexes, and provide the more delicate aspects of manipulation. Other muscle groups act roughly in pairs: *adductors* versus *abductors,* which move a part toward or away from the midline of the body; *rotators,* which work in pairs to rotate a part of the limb, the trunk, or the head around each part's longitudinal axis. Many muscles participate in more than one of these functions. Coordinated movement requires the action of two or more muscle groups—*agonists,* which promote a movement; *antagonists,* which oppose it; and *synergists,* which assist the agonist muscles by stabilizing a joint or contributing additional force to the movement. Some simple types of movement require only a burst of energy from an agonist muscle group. Other types of movements, such as self-terminated actions, require a smooth sequence of movements: agonist, antagonist,

and, finally, agonist to stop the movement. Agonist and antagonist contractions are programmed by higher brain centers to fit the situation. Simple movements are programmed before they start so that the movement proceeds from start to finish without modification. Self-terminated movements are more complex and are programmed to start and are then modified as they proceed.

The neuromuscular unit

The neurons that control motor function are referred to as *motoneurons* or sometimes as *alpha motoneurons.* A motor unit consists of one motoneuron and the group of muscle fibers it innervates within a muscle. All muscles contain thousands of muscle fibers and are innervated by many—often many hundred—motor units. The alpha motoneurons supplying a motor unit are located in the ventral horn of the spinal cord and are called lower motoneurons (LMNs). The synapse between an LMN and the muscle fibers of a motor unit is called the *neuromuscular junction, myoneural junction,* or *motor end-plate.* The motor unit functions as a single unit. If an action potential is generated in the LMN, then, by way of the neuromuscular junction, all the muscle cells in the motor unit will fire simultaneously. Upper motoneurons (UMNs), which exert control over LMNs, project from the motor strip in the cerebral cortex to the ventral horn and are fully contained within the CNS.

Axons of the LMNs exit the spinal cord at each segment to innervate skeletal muscle cells, including those of the limbs, back, abdomen, and chest. Each LMN undergoes multiple branching, making it possible for a single LMN to innervate from 10 to 2000 muscle cells. In general, large muscles—those containing hundreds and thousands of muscle cells and providing gross motor movement—have large motor units. This is in sharp contrast to those that control the hand, tongue, and eye movements in which the motor units are small and permit very discrete control.

The spinal cord and spinal reflex circuitry

All of the basic circuitry needed for movement is contained in the spinal cord and brain stem. Although the basic interneural reflex circuitry of the spinal cord is anatomically fixed, the mode of function is governed to a great extent by descending input from higher centers.

In the adult, the spinal cord is located in the upper two-thirds of the spinal canal of the vertebral column (Figure 49-2). It extends from the foramen magnum at the base of the skull to a cone-shaped termination, the conus medullaris, which is usually located at the level of the first or second lumbar vertebra in the adult. From this point, the dorsal and ventral roots angle downward from the cord, forming what is called the *cauda equina,* or horse's tail. The filum terminale, which is composed of nonneural tissues and the *pia mater,* continues caudally and attaches to the second sacral vertebra.

The location of the spinal cord in relation to the vertebral column results in a disparity between the positions of each succeeding cord segment and the exit of its dorsal and ventral nerve roots through the corresponding intervertebral foramina (Figure 49-3). This disparity becomes more pronounced at the more caudal levels. The arachnoid and its enclosed subarachnoid space, which is filled with cerebrospinal fluid (CSF), do not close down on the filum terminale until they reach the second sacral vertebra. This results in the formation of a pocket of CSF, the dural *cisterna spinalis,* which extends from about the second lumbar vertebra to the second sacral vertebra. Because there is an abundant supply of spinal fluid and the spinal cord does not extend this far, the area is often used for sampling the CSF. A procedure called a spinal tap, or puncture, can be done by inserting a special type of needle into the dural sac at the level of L3 and L4. The spinal roots, which are covered with pia

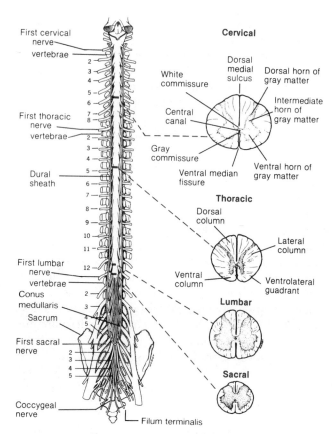

Figure 49-2 The spinal cord within the vertebral canal. The spinal canal and meninges have been opened. The spinal nerves and vertebrae are numbered on the left. Cross (transverse) sections with regional variations in gray matter and increasing proportions of white matter as the cord is ascended appear on the right. (*Modified from Chaffee EE, Lytle IM: Basic Physiology and Anatomy, 4th ed. Philadelphia, JB Lippincott, 1980*)

mater, are in relatively little danger of trauma from the needle used for this purpose.

Longitudinal organization

The peripheral nerves that carry information to and from the spinal cord are called spinal nerves. There are 32 or more pairs of spinal nerves (8 cervical, 12 thoracic, 5 lumbar, 5 sacral, and 2 or more coccygeal); each pair is named for the segment of the spinal cord from which it exits. Because the first cervical (C1) spinal nerve exits the spinal cord just above the first cervical vertebra, the nerve is given the number of the bony vertebra just below it. The numbering was changed for all lower levels, however. Thus, an extra cervical nerve, the C8 nerve, exits above the T1 vertebra, and each subsequent nerve is numbered for the vertebra just above its point of exit (Figure 49-3).

Segmental spinal nerves

Each spinal cord segment communicates with its corresponding body segment through the paired segmental spinal nerves (Figure 49-4). Each spinal

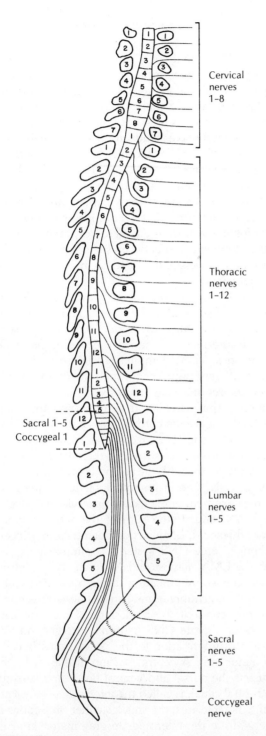

Figure 49-3 Relation of segments of the spinal cord and spinal nerves to the vertebral column. (*Barr ML, Kiernan JA: The Human Nervous System: An Anatomical Viewpoint, 5th ed, p 65. Philadelphia, JB Lippincott, 1988*)

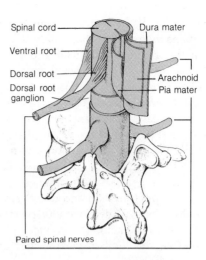

Figure 49-4 Spinal cord and meninges. (*Chaffee EE, Lytle IM: Basic Physiology and Anatomy, 4th ed, p 234. Philadelphia, JB Lippincott, 1980*)

eral surface of the cord (the ventral root), carrying the axons of efferent neurons into the periphery. These two roots fuse at the intervertebral foramen, forming the mixed spinal nerve—mixed because it has both afferent and efferent axons.

After emerging from the vertebral column, the mixed spinal nerve divides into two branches: a small dorsal primary ramus and a larger ventral primary ramus (Figure 49-5). The thoracic and upper lumbar spinal nerves also give rise to a third branch (the ramus communicans) that contains sympathetic axons supplying the blood vessels, the genitourinary system, and the gastrointestinal system. The dorsal ramus contains sensory fibers from the skin and motor

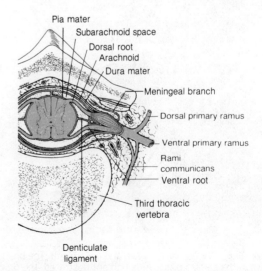

Figure 49-5 Cross section of vertebral column at the level of the third thoracic vertebra, showing the meninges, the spinal cord, and the origin of a spinal nerve and its branches or rami. (*Modified from Chaffee EE, Lytle IM: Basic Physiology and Anatomy, 4th ed, p 235. Philadelphia, JB Lippincott, 1980*)

nerve, along with blood vessels that supply the spinal cord, enters the spinal canal through an intervertebral foramen where it divides into two branches, or roots, one of which enters the dorsolateral surface of the cord (the dorsal root), carrying the axons of afferent neurons into the CNS. The other leaves the ventrolat-

fibers to muscles of the back. The anterior primary ramus contains motor fibers that innervate the skeletal muscles of the anterior body wall and the legs and arms.

The spinal nerves do not go directly to skin and muscle fibers; instead, they form complicated nerve networks called *plexuses*. A plexus is a site of intermixing nerve branches. A number of spinal nerves enter a plexus and interconnect with other spinal nerves before exiting from the plexus. The nerves that emerge from a plexus form smaller and smaller branches that supply the skin and muscles of the various parts of the body. There are four plexuses of the peripheral nervous system: the cervical plexus, the brachial plexus, the lumbar plexus, and the sacral plexus (Figure 49-6).

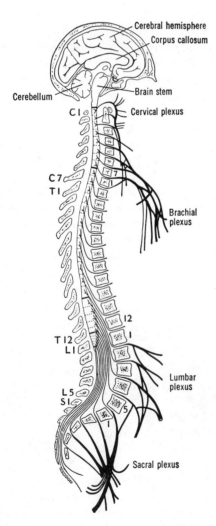

Figure 49-6 Drawing of the brain and cord in situ. The brain is shown in the median plane. Although not illustrated, the first cervical vertebra articulates with the base of the skull. The letters along the vertebral column indicate cervical, thoracic, lumbar, and sacral. Note that the cord ends at the upper border of the second lumbar vertebra. (*Gardner E: Fundamentals of Neurology, 2nd ed, p 35. Philadelphia, WB Saunders, 1975*)

Transverse organization

The spinal cord is oval or rounded on transverse section. The internal gray matter has the appearance of a butterfly or letter H (see Figure 49-5). Some of the neurons that make up the gray matter of the cord have processes or axons that leave the cord, enter the peripheral nerves, and supply tissues such as autonomic ganglia or skeletal muscles. Other neurons in the gray portion of the cord are concerned with input or reflex mechanisms and are called *internuncial neurons* or *interneurons* (see Chapter 46). The white matter of the cord that surrounds the gray matter contains nerve fiber tracts or descending axons that transmit information between segments of the cord or from higher levels of the CNS, such as the brain stem or cerebrum.

The extensions of the gray matter that form the letter H are called the horns. Those that extend posteriorly are called the *dorsal horns,* and those that extend anteriorly are called the *ventral horns.* The dorsal horns contain input association neurons that receive afferent impulses through the dorsal roots and other interconnecting neurons. The ventral horns contain output association neurons and the efferent LMNs that leave the cord by way of the ventral roots.

The spinal cord contains many small internuncial neurons that surround the efferent motoneurons and synapse with the cell body or dendrites of the efferent cells. Action potentials of these internuncial neurons exert either excitatory or inhibitory effects on the LMN, and, if the sum of the action potentials passes threshold, LMN action potentials are triggered. Although some CNS systems communicate directly with the LMN, almost all LMN activity is controlled by systems communicating through excitatory or inhibitory internuncial neurons. These internuncial neurons represent the final stage of communication between elaborate CNS neuronal circuits and transmission of information to the skeletal muscle cells of the motor unit. A central portion of the cord, which connects the dorsal and ventral horns and surrounds the central canal, is called the *intermediate gray matter.* In the thoracic area, the small, slender projections that emerge from the intermediate gray matter are called the *intermediolateral columns of the horns.* These columns contain the visceral output association neurons and the efferent neurons of the sympathetic nervous system.

The amount of gray matter present in the cord is largely determined by the amount of tissue innervated by a given segment of the cord (see Figure 49-2). Larger amounts of gray matter are present in the lower lumbar and upper sacral segments, which supply the lower extremities, and in cervical segment 5 to thoracic segment 1, which supply the upper limbs. The volume of white matter in the spinal cord also increases progressively toward the brain because more and more ascending fibers are added and because the number of descending axons is greater.

Spinal reflexes

A reflex provides a highly reliable relationship between a stimulus and a motor response. Its anatomical basis consists of an afferent neuron, the connection or synapse with CNS neurons that communicate with the effector neuron, and the effector neuron that innervates a muscle or organ. Reflexes are essentially "wired in" to the CNS in that normally they are always ready to function; with training, most reflexes can be modulated to become parts of more complicated movements. A reflex may involve neurons within a single cord segment (segmental reflexes), several or many segments (intersegmental reflexes), or structures in the brain (suprasegmental reflexes). Two important types of spinal motor reflexes are discussed in this chapter: the myotatic reflex and the flexor-withdrawal reflex. Autonomic reflexes, which control visceral function, are discussed in Chapter 48.

Myotatic reflex. The *myotatic,* or stretch reflex, transmits proprioception information to the CNS on the length and tension of skeletal muscles, tendons, and joints. There are two types of proprioceptors: muscle spindle receptors and Golgi tendon organs.

Most skeletal muscles contain large numbers of specialized stretch receptors, called *muscle spindles,* that transmit information on muscle length (Figure 49-7). These encapsulated receptor organs are scattered throughout the muscle substance. They contain miniature skeletal muscle fibers surrounded at their middle by helical receptive terminals (annulospiral endings) of large diameter afferent neurons (Group Ia). The muscle spindles are attached in parallel to the connective tissue within the skeletal muscle so that stretching a muscle stretches the spindle fibers and increases the rate of impulse generation of its Ia afferent neurons.

Axons of Ia spindle afferent neurons enter the spinal cord through the dorsal root and have several branches, including one that terminates mainly in the segment of entry and one that ascends the dorsal column of the cord to the medulla of the brain stem. The *segmental branch* makes a connection, among several others, that passes directly to the anterior gray matter and establishes monosynaptic contact with each of the LMNs that have motor units in the muscle containing the spindle source of input. This single synapse or monosynaptic connection is the only known instance of direct afferent-to-efferent neuron reflex in the nervous system.

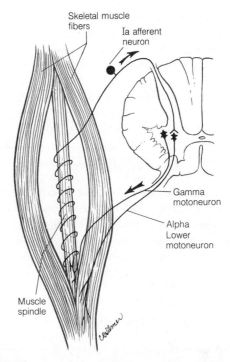

Figure 49-7 Schematic diagram of Ia spindle afferent, alpha and gamma efferent innervation which provides the basis for the stretch reflex.

When a muscle begins to be lengthened, the spindle is stretched; this causes the afferent spindle fibers to increase their rate of firing and produce an opposing muscle contraction through monosynaptic contact with the LMNs that supply the muscle. Another segmental branch communicates with motor units in antagonistic muscles; inhibition of these muscle units assists further in opposing muscle stretch. The opposite effects occur when a muscle is suddenly shortened. The monosynaptic pathway starts or stops firing with almost no delay, and the stretch reflex is over in a fraction of a second. Branches of the Ia axon ascend the spinal cord, sending collateral branches into the dorsal horn of the adjacent segments influencing reflex function at each level. The intersegmental reflexes are particularly important in coordinating hand, leg, neck, and limb movements. The ascending fibers ultimately provide information about muscle length to the cerebellum and cerebral cortex. Descending motor systems can also inhibit or modulate the reflex, making the muscle available for use as a part of programmed movement.

The sensitivity of the spindle fibers is controlled by small efferent gamma motoneurons that are part of the spindle unit. The gamma motoneurons, which differ from alpha motoneurons that innervate fibers of a skeletal muscle, do not produce whole muscle contraction; instead, they control the length of the tiny muscle fibers within the muscle spindle around which the annulospiral endings are wound.

The CNS control of these spindle fibers, by way of the gamma motoneurons, can adjust the sensitivity of the Ia impulse rate and, thus, of the stretch reflex. The gamma efferent motoneurons are strongly influenced by descending output from the brain stem reticular system, the cerebellum, and the basal ganglia. The central control of spindle fiber sensitivity is required to monitor and predict the sequence of muscle contractions needed to move a limb from a fixed starting position through an active range of movement.

The *Golgi tendon organs* are highly sensitive stretch receptors located in muscle tendons. Instead of being attached in parallel with the muscle, the Golgi tendon organs are connected in series with a muscle and register the ongoing force developed in a tendon. In this way, a change in muscle tension is detected rather than a change length. By acting as constant monitors of tension, the inhibitory effect of the musculotendinous spindles provide protection against muscle or tendon damage due to excessive pull and tension.

Muscle tone is the tendency of muscles to reflexly oppose movement around a joint. High tone results in stability of posture, and low tone results in looseness or floppiness of a limb. Tone regulation must be ongoing if one is to stabilize joints so that controlled movement can occur around other joints. The myotatic, or stretch, reflex provides the basis for the maintenance of normal muscle tone and stabilizes joint position and posture. A joint rotation will stretch one or more flexor, extensor, or rotator muscles, and this is immediately opposed by contraction of the stretched muscle. The greater the passive stretch, the greater the strength of muscle contraction opposing the stretch. The stretch reflex, which has rapid dynamic (rate of change) components and slow static (steady state) components, is continuously available to all muscles in the body, neck, and head. This reflex stabilizes posture against gravitational pull or against any other force that tends to move bones around joints.

The *inverse myotatic reflex* is initiated by the Golgi tendon organs. In this circuit, the afferent sensory fibers for the tendon terminate on spinal interneurons that inhibit homonymous (from the same muscle) and synergistic motoneurons, including those acting at other joints. The reflex, which is most prominent in the antigravity muscles, relaxes the muscle in response to tension created by its contraction. This is in contrast to the lower threshold myotatic reflex in which stimulation of the spindle fibers incites contraction—hence the name *inverse myotatic reflex*. The inverse myotatic reflex also has a cross-component. If, for example, the inverse myotatic reflex produced relaxation of the quadriceps in one leg, the cross-component would produce contraction in the quadriceps of

the other leg. The inverse myotatic reflex provides postural stability to ambulatory movements. For example, when the inverse myotatic reflex produces relaxation of antigravity muscles (with flexion) of one leg as we walk, the cross-component produces contraction and extension of the opposite leg.

In persons with spastic paralysis (to be discussed), the inverse myotatic reflex becomes hyperactive and produces what is called the *clasp-knife reaction*. If one were to flex passively the lower limb of such a person at the knee, increasing resistance would be encountered. This resistance would continue to increase until, at some point, it would abruptly cease and the leg could then be passively flexed. Similar signs are seen in spastic upper limbs.

Flexor-withdrawal reflex. Spinal level reflexes provide the "bricks" that are used by higher brain centers to build complex motor movements. Other than the myotatic and inverse myotatic reflex, most spinal reflexes are entirely polysynaptic and require several segments of the spinal cord to function at a more complex organizational level. They involve automatic integration of many muscle groups into the response, modifying local stretch reflex excitability in the process. The *flexor-withdrawal reflex* is stimulated by any tissue threatening or damaging stimulus and quickly moves the body part away from the offending stimulus (usually by flexing a limb part). When the sole of the foot receives firm pressure stimulation, the *extensor-thrust* reflex pattern results in forceful extension, providing stable body support in basic standing patterns (see Chapter 47). Alternate *stepping* between opposite limbs during walking and running also involves all four limbs and the entire length of the spinal cord. This is retained as the swinging of the arms in normal human walking and running. Other spinal level reflexes include reflex relaxation of the external anal and urethral sphincters during defecation and urination and coordinated contraction of intercostal, diaphragmatic, back, and shoulder muscles during the inspiratory part of the respiratory cycle. Intact neuronal circuitry and normal-range excitability of these reflexes are required for brain stem and forebrain motor control to operate properly.

Motor function of the brain stem

Normally one doesn't have to consciously control the muscle activity that allows one to stand erect despite the force of gravity. Instead, input from brain stem structures subconsciously influences reflex mechanisms of the spinal cord and allows maintenance of body posture, pacing of steps, and recovery of posture when balance is disrupted.

The anatomical components of the brain stem

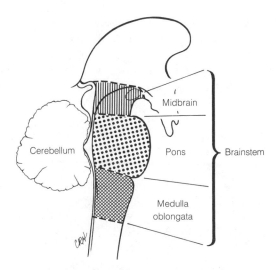

Figure 49-8 Brain stem structures.

are the medulla, pons, and midbrain (Figure 49-8). At its caudal end, the brain stem is continuous with the spinal cord and, at its rostral end, it is continuous with the diencephalon that is bounded by the cerebral hemispheres. The motor centers of the brain stem are the red nucleus, lateral vestibular nucleus, superior colliculus, and certain parts of the reticular formation.

The brain stem centers are located between the higher motor centers and the spinal cord and form part of the descending control systems that influence the motor component of spinal cord and cranial nerve reflexes. The lateral vestibular nucleus gives rise to an uncrossed tract, which projects to the ventral horn of the spinal cord; it is excitatory to extensor motor neurons and inhibits flexor neurons. For example, when the head and body begin to tilt to one side, the tilt is opposed by vestibular reflex contraction of the neck flexors of the opposite side and of limb extensor muscles of the same side, maintaining a stable head and body posture. Input from the labyrinth (see Chapter 52) is concerned with bending, rotation, and linear acceleration or deceleration.

The reticular formation in the pons and medulla gives rise to two reticulospinal tracts: (1) the medullary fibers, which excite flexor neurons and inhibit extensor motoneurons and (2) the pontine fibers, which excite extensors and inhibit flexors. Interplay between these descending tract systems modifies the excitability of spinal reflexes to produce complex motor movements, such as coordination of walking and running movements, and righting reflexes, which maintain or re-establish body and head positions. Many fundamental automatic movement patterns are provided by the brain stem's reticular formation circuitry including respiratory movements, sneezing and coughing, and chewing and swallowing. The brain stem also contains circuitry for coordination of auto-

nomic and somatic motor functions such as shivering and vomiting. Damage to brain stem motor areas often results in death because of the fundamental importance of these life-sustaining responses.

The cerebellum

The cerebellum is located in the posterior fossa of cranium superior to the pons (see Figure 49-8). It is separated from the cerebral hemispheres by a fold of dura mater, the tentorium cerebelli. The cerebellum consists of a small unpaired median portion, called the *vermis,* and two large lateral masses, the cerebellar hemispheres. In contrast to the brain stem with its external white matter and internal gray nuclei, the cerebellum, like the cerebrum, has an outer cortex of gray matter and a core of white matter. A series of nuclei are embedded deep in the white matter. Axons from cells of the cortex and association fibers of the nuclei connect cortex to cortex communication, cortex to nuclei communication, and vice versa. Projection fibers from the nuclei relay information to many regions, particularly to the motor cortex by means of a thalamic relay.

The temporal synergistic functions of the cerebellum participate in all movement of limbs, trunk, head, larynx, and eyes, whether the movement is part of a voluntary movement or of a highly learned semi-automatic or automatic movement. During highly skilled movements, the motor cortex sends signals to the cerebellum, informing it about the movement that is to be performed. The cerebellum makes continuous adjustments, resulting in smoothness of movement, particularly during the delicate maneuvers. Highly skillful movement requires extensive motor training, and there is considerable evidence that many of these learned movement patterns involve cerebellar circuits.

The cerebellum receives sensory input from the vestibular system, eyes, ears, skin, muscles, joints, and tendons that monitor movement. It is the main central target for proprioceptive information. The sensory input from a given area of the body arrives at the same area in the cerebellum as input from the motor cortex that controls the motor units in that body area. In this way, the cerebellum is able to assess continuously the status of each body part—position, rate of movement, and forces, such as gravity, that are opposing movement. The cerebellum compares what is actually happening with what is intended to happen; it then transmits appropriate corrective signals back to the motor system, instructing it to increase or decrease the activity of certain muscle groups and regulating their contractions so that smooth and accurate movements are performed.

One of the functions of the cerebellum is the dampening of muscle movement. All body movements are basically pendular (swinging to and fro). As movement begins, momentum develops and must be overcome before movement can be stopped. Because of momentum, all movements have a tendency to overshoot if they are not dampened. In the intact cerebellum, subconscious signals stop movement precisely at the intended point. In providing for this type of control, the cerebellum predicts the future position of moving parts of the body; the rapidity with which the limb is moving, as well as the projected time for the course of movement, is detected from incoming proprioceptive signals. This allows the cerebellum to inhibit agonist muscles and excite antagonist muscles when movement approaches the point of intention.

The basal ganglia

The basal ganglia are the several large masses of neurons that lie on either side of the thalamus and surround the internal capsule. The term *corpus striatum* (striped body) is sometimes used interchangeably with basal ganglia. The major components of the basal ganglia are the caudate (tailed) nucleus, the putamen, and the globus pallidus (pale body). The globus pallidus and putamen make up the lentiform nucleus. As with the motor cortex, the nuclei on the left side control movement on the right side of the body, and vice versa. Circuits interconnecting the premotor cortex and supplementary motor cortex, the basal ganglia, and parts of the thalamus provide associated movements that accompany highly skilled behaviors. The basal ganglia provide gracefulness to the performance as well as the supportive background for highly skilled movements. An intact and functional basal ganglia provide the swinging of the arms during walking and running and the follow-through movements that accompany throwing a ball or swinging a club. Parkinson's disease involves dysfunction of the basal ganglia, which results in abnormal movements.

The motor cortex

The motor cortex is located in the posterior part of the frontal lobe. It consists of the primary, premotor, and supplementary motor cortex. The primary motor cortex (area 4) is located on the rostral surface and adjacent portions of the central sulcus (see Figure 50-6). The premotor area (area 6) lies immediately rostral to the primary motor cortex. The neurons in the primary motor cortex are arranged in a somatotopic array or distorted map of the body (motor homunculus [Figure 49-9]). The distorted body map represents the neurons that control voluntary movement of a particular body part. The body parts that require the greatest dexterity have the greatest cortical areas devoted to them. Over one-half of the primary

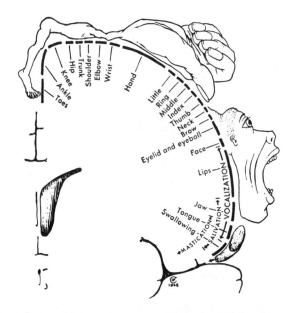

Figure 49-9 Representation of the relative extent of motor cortical area 4 devoted to muscles of the various body regions. Medial surface is at the left, lateral fissure is at the right with pharyngeal and laryngeal muscle representation extending toward the insula. *(Penfield E, Rasmussen T: The Cerebral Cortex in Man: A Clinical Study of Localization of Function. New York, Macmillan, 1968)*

motor cortex is concerned with controlling the muscles of the hands and muscles of speech.[2] The supplementary motor cortex is found in the part of area 6 that lies on the medial surface of the hemisphere.

The primary motor cortex is very thick. It contains many layers of pyramid-shaped output neurons that project to the cortex of the opposite side, to the premotor cortex, to the somesthetic strip of the parietal cortex that is located on the other side of the central sulcus, to the basal ganglia, and to the thalamus on the same side of the brain. The large pyramidal cells located in the fifth layer project to the brain stem and spinal cord. These UMNs send their axons through the subcortical white matter and the internal capsule to the deep surface of the brain stem, through the ventral bulge of the pons, to the ventral surface of the medulla where they form a ridge or pyramid. At the junction between the medulla and cervical spinal cord, 80% or more of the UMN axons cross the midline (decussate) to form the lateral *corticospinal tract* or pyramidal tract in the lateral white matter of the spinal cord. This tract extends throughout the spinal cord, with roughly 50% of its fibers terminating in the cervical segments, 20% in the thoracic segments, and 30% in the lumbosacral segments.[3] Most of the remaining uncrossed fibers travel down the ventral column of the cord, mainly to cervical levels, where they cross and innervate contralateral LMNs.

The premotor area sends some fibers into the corticospinal tract but mainly innervates the primary motor strip. The premotor cortex is richly interconnected with the thalamus and with higher-order associative cortical areas. Complex manipulative movement, as well as larger movement patterns of whole limbs and limb girdles, is initially organized in the associating cortical areas before projecting to the motor cortex. Thus, the primary motor cortex is mainly a first-order level of descending projection necessary for precise movement. Discrete lesions within the primary motor cortex result in profound weakness or paralysis in specific muscle groups of the opposite side. Lesions restricted to the premotor cortex result in weakness or paralysis of the larger limb girdle muscles.

On the medial surface of the hemisphere in the premotor region, a *supplementary motor region* contains representation of all parts of the body. The supplementary cortex is intimately involved in the initiation of planned delicate skillful movement. Bilateral lesions result in long-lasting loss (akinesia) of movements involving both hands or both feet and can result in long-term loss of speech (mutism).

Monosynaptic innervation of LMNs by UMNs only occurs for the most distal muscles involved with delicate manipulative skills (*e.g.,* those of the hands and fingers, tongue, mouth, and pharynx). For LMNs of other muscles, the connection is multisynaptic and less discrete. As the UMN axons pass along their long pathways, collateral branches move out and innervate regions of the basal ganglia, the thalamus, the brain stem, and nuclei that project into the cerebellum. The primary motor cortex receives input from thalamic regions that transmit feedback information from the cerebellum, the basal ganglia, and the somatesthetic projection nuclei. The primary sensory cortex, particularly the part receiving and analyzing proprioceptive afferent information, also projects to the motor cortex.

The pyramidal versus extrapyramidal systems

By convention, motor tracts are classified as belonging to one of two motor systems: pyramidal and extrapyramidal systems. The so-called pyramidal system consists of the motor pathways originating in the motor cortex and terminating in the brain stem (corticobulbar fibers) and the spinal cord (corticospinal fibers). The corticospinal fibers traverse the ventral surface of the medulla in a bundle called the *pyramid* before decussating (crossing to the opposite side) at the medulla–spinal cord junction; hence the name *pyramidal system.* Other fibers from the cortex project to the cerebellum and basal ganglia before they descend and innervate motoneurons. These fibers do not decussate in the pyramids, hence the name *extrapyra-*

midal. The pyramidal and extrapyramidal systems have different effects on muscle tone. The pyramidal system is largely excitatory; it provides control of delicate muscle movement. The extrapyramidal system provides the more crude, background supportive movement patterns. In terms of actual function, the pyramidal and extrapyramidal systems do not function independent of each other. The concept of two separate systems is helpful, however, in understanding motor function. Table 49-1 summarizes the characteristics of the pyramidal and extrapyramidal motor systems.

In summary, motor function involves the neuromuscular unit, spinal cord circuitry, brain stem neurons, the cerebellum, the basal ganglia, and the motor cortex. A motor unit consists of one LMN and the group of muscle fibers it innervates within the muscle. Stretch receptors provide muscle tone by means of the stretch reflex. The basic reflex circuitry controlling muscle function is located in the spinal cord. Brain stem circuits contribute basic movement patterns, the cerebellum provides temporal smoothness to movement, and the basal ganglia provides gracefulness. Upper motoneurons, which provide delicate control over LMNs, project from the motor strip in the cerebral cortex to the ventral horn. The UMNs in the motor cortex send their axons through the subcortical white matter, and internal capsule and the deep surface of the brain stem, to the ventral surface to the opposite side of the medulla where they form a pyramid before crossing the midline to form the lateral corticospinal tract in the spinal cord.

Disorders of the neuromuscular unit

Skeletal muscle disorders

Disorders of skeletal muscle groups involve both atrophy and dystrophy. *Atrophy* describes a shrinkage, death, or disappearance of muscle cells secondary to some type of nerve injury or disease. *Muscular dystrophy* is a primary disorder of muscle tissue and is characterized by defect in the muscle fibers.

Muscle atrophy

Maintenance of muscle strength requires relatively frequent movements against resistance. Reduced use results in muscle atrophy, which is characterized by a reduction in the diameter of the muscle fibers due to a loss of protein filaments. When a normally innervated muscle is not used for long periods of time, the muscle cells shrink in diameter, and although the muscle cells do not die, they become weakened. This is called *disuse atrophy* and occurs with conditions such as immobilization and chronic illness.

The most extreme examples of muscle atrophy, however, are found in disorders that deprive muscles of their innervation. This is called *denervation atrophy*. During early embryonic development, outgrowing skeletal nerves innervate partially mature muscle cells. If the developing muscle cells are not innervated, they will not mature and will eventually die. In the process of innervation, randomly contracting muscle cells become enslaved by the innervating neurons, and from then on, the muscle cell contracts only when stimulated by that particular neuron. If the LMN dies or its axon is destroyed, the skeletal muscle cell is again free of neural domination. When this happens, it begins to have temporary spontaneous contractions (called *fibrillations*) of its own. It also begins to lose its contractile proteins and, after several months, if not reinnervated, will degenerate.

If a peripheral motor neuron is crushed and its endoneurial tube remains intact, regenerating axons can grow down the connective tissue tube to

Table 49–1. Characteristics of pyramidal and extrapyramidal motor control

Feature	Pyramidal	Extrapyramidal		Peripheral
Nomenclature	(1) Voluntary motor pathway (2) Upper motor neuron (UMN) pathway (3) Corticospinal pathway	(1) Involuntary motor pathway (2) Extracorticospinal		(1) Final common pathway (2) Lower motor neuron (LMN) pathway
Location	From the Betz cells of the frontal lobe motor strip to the anterior horn cell of the spinal cord	Motor cortex with projections into basal ganglia, and communication with the reticular formation	Cerebellum	From the ventral horn cells of the spinal cord to the neuromuscular junction
Function	Initiates and transmits impulses for highly skilled voluntary movement to spinal cord	(1) Inhibits muscle tone throughout the body (2) Initiates and regulates associated or background movement patterns	(1) Coordinate movements by monitoring and making adjustments in motor activity elicited by other parts of the nervous system (2) Dampen muscle movement	Transmits impulses from the spinal cord to skeletal muscles
Disruption	Muscle weakness; loss of fine manipulative skills; hyperactive reflexes and spastic paralysis on the contralateral side—hemiplegia	Muscle rigidity and incoordination Loss of discrete movement Abnormal postures and automatic movements	Incoordination, intention tremors, ataxia, overshooting; inability to progress in orderly sequence from one movement to another	Hypoactive reflexes and paresis or flaccid paralysis, usually monoplegia. Destruction results in denervation atrophy followed by muscle cell degeneration and muscle wasting
Extent of damage	Small amount of damage in important area (*e.g.,* internal capsule) causes extensive decrease in function	If part of basal ganglia is left intact, gross postural and "fixed" movements can still be performed; widespread damage leads to muscle rigidity throughout the body	Depends on the extent of damage to the cerebellum	Extensive damage (several levels) before function is significantly decreased

(Courtesy of Mary Wierenga, R.N., Ph.D., School of Nursing, University of Wisconsin-Milwaukee)

reinnervate the muscle cell. If the nerve is cut, however, scar tissue between the cut ends of the endoneurial tube reduces the likelihood of axonic reinnervation by the original axon, and muscle cell loss is likely to occur. If some intact LMN axons remain within the muscle, nearby denervated muscle cells apparently emit what is called a *trophic signal*, probably a chemical messenger, that signals intact axons to sprout and send outgrowing collaterals into the denervated area and recapture control of some of the denervated muscle fibers. The degree of axonic regeneration that occurs after injury to an LMN depends on the amount of scar tissue that develops at the site of injury and how quickly reinnervation occurs. If reinnervation occurs after the muscle cell has degenerated, no recovery is possible. Thus, peripheral nerve section usually results in some loss of muscle cell function, which is experienced as weakness. Collateral sprout reinnervation results in enlarged motor units and, therefore, a reduction in the discreteness of muscle control following recovery.

Muscular dystrophy

Muscular dystrophy is a term applied to a number of genetic disorders that produce progressive deterioration of skeletal muscles because of mixed muscle cell hypertrophy, atrophy, and necrosis. They are primary diseases of muscle tissue and probably do not involve the nervous system. As the muscle undergoes necrosis, fat and connective tissue replace the muscle fibers, which increases muscle size and results in muscle weakness. The increase in muscle size resulting from connective tissue infiltration is called *pseudohypertrophy*. The muscle weakness is insidious in onset but continually progressive, varying with the type of disorder.

The most common form of the disease is Duchenne's muscular dystrophy, which has an incidence of about 3 per 100,000. Duchenne's muscular dystrophy is inherited as a recessive single gene defect on the X chromosome and, hence, is transmitted from the mother to her male offspring. A spontaneous (mutation) form may occur in females. Another form of dystrophy, Becker's muscular dystrophy, is similarly X-linked, but has its onset later in childhood or adolescence and has a slower course. In Duchenne's muscular dystrophy, the postural muscles of the hip and shoulder are affected first and the child usually performs normally until around 3 years of age when frequent falling begins to occur. Wheelchairs are usually needed at a mean age of 9.5 years.[4] Death due to respiratory and cardiac muscle involvement usually occurs in young adulthood. About 70% of deaths result from respiratory causes alone.[4] Observation of the child's voluntary movement and a complete family history provide important diagnostic data for the disease. Muscle biopsy, which shows fat in the muscle tissues, electromyograms, and serum levels of the enzyme creatine phosphokinase (CPK), which leaks out of damaged muscle fibers, can be used to confirm the diagnosis. Gene probes are being developed that can be used for carrier detection and prenatal diagnosis.[5]

To date, there is no cure for any of the muscular dystrophies. Although there has been exciting research advances toward identifying the gene and gene product involved in Duchenne's muscular dystrophy,[6,7] new cases continue to occur. Imbalances between agonist and antagonist muscles lead to abnormal postures and the development of contractures and joint immobility. Management of the disease is directed toward maintaining ambulation and preventing deformities. Passive stretching, correct or counter posturing, and splints help to prevent deformities. Precautions should be taken to avoid respiratory infections.

Disorders of the myoneural junction

The transmission of impulses at the myoneural junction is mediated by the release of the neurotransmitter *acetylcholine* (ACh) from the axon terminals. Acetylcholine binds to specific receptors in the end-plate region of the muscle fiber surface to cause muscle contraction. Studies suggest that there are over a million binding sites per motor end-plate.[1]

Acetylcholine is active in the myoneural junction for only a brief period of time during which an action potential is generated in the innervated muscle cell. Some of the transmitter diffuses out of the synapse, and the remaining transmitter is rapidly inactivated by an enzyme called *acetylcholinesterase*. This enzyme splits the ACh molecule into choline and acetic acid. The choline is transported back into the nerve terminal and reused in the synthesis of acetylcholine. The rapid inactivation of acetylcholine at the myoneural junction allows for repeated muscle contractions and, thus, gradations of contractile force.

A number of drugs and agents can alter neuromuscular function by changing the release, inactivation, or receptor binding of ACh. Curare acts on the postjunctional membrane of the motor end-plate to prevent the depolarizing effect of the neurotransmitter. Blocking of neuromuscular transmission by curare-type drugs is used during many types of surgical procedures to facilitate relaxation of involved musculature. Physostigmine and neostigmine inhibit acetylcholinesterase and allow acetylcholine released from the motoneuron to accumulate. These drugs are used in the treatment of myasthenia gravis (to be discussed). Toxins from the botulism organism produce paralysis by blocking acetylcholine release. Spores from the botulism organism may be found in soil-grown foods that are not cooked at temperatures of at least 100°C in home-canning procedures. The organophosphates (*e.g.*, malathion and parathion) that are used in some insecticides bind acetylcholinesterase. They produce excessive and prolonged ACh action with depolarization block of cholinergic receptors, including those of the myoneural junction. Other organophosphate compounds were developed as nerve gases during World War I with similar and, if absorbed in high concentrations, lethal effects due to loss of respiratory muscle function.

—— Myasthenia gravis

Myasthenia gravis is a disorder of transmission at the myoneural junction that affects communication between the motoneuron and the innervated muscle cell. The incidence of myasthenia gravis is about 1 in 10,000 to 1 in 40,000 persons in the United States.[8] The disease may occur at any age, but the peak incidence of onset is between 20 and 30 years and is about three times more common in women than men. A small second peak occurs in later life and affects men more often than women. The disorder appears transiently and lasts for days to weeks in about 10% of infants born to mothers with myasthenia gravis.

Myasthenia gravis is thought to result from a decrease in ACh receptor sites at the myoneural junction that leads to decreased muscle function. Evidence indicates that the reduction in ACh receptors results from an autoimmune response. Recent research has demonstrated the presence of an ACh receptor antibody in 85% of persons with myasthenia gravis.[9] This receptor antibody is thought to cause receptor degradation and inhibition of receptor synthesis. The exact mechanism that triggers the autoimmune response is unknown but is thought to be related to abnormal T-lymphocyte characteristics (see Chapter 11). About 75% of persons with myasthenia gravis also have thymic abnormalities, either a thyoma (thymus tumor) or thymic hyperplasia (increased thymus weight due to increased number of thymus cells).[10]

The primary clinical manifestations of myasthenia are weakness of the eye muscles, with ptosis (drooping of the upper eyelids) and diplopia caused by weakness of the extraocular muscles. Neuromuscular and eyelid weakness can be checked following instructions to have a person firmly close his or her eyes. Normally eyelashes are not seen with firm eye closure. In persons with myasthenia gravis, the eyelid muscles are weakened and the eyelashes often remain visible.[11] Extraocular muscle weakness can be tested by having the person maintain an upward gaze for 2 to 3 minutes while observations for eye muscle fatigue are being made.

The clinical course varies. The disease may progress from ocular muscle weakness to generalized weakness, including respiratory weakness. Chewing and swallowing may be difficult, and persons with the disease often choose to eat soft puddings and cereals rather than meats and hard fruit. Masticatory weakness can be checked by having the person repetitively open and close the jaw against resistance.[11] Weakness in limb movement is usually more pronounced in proximal than in distal parts of the extremity, so that climbing stairs and lifting objects are difficult. As the disease progresses, the muscles of the lower face are affected, causing speech impairment. When this happens, the person often supports the chin with one hand to assist in speaking. In most people, symptoms are least evident when arising in the morning, but grow worse with effort and as the day proceeds. General muscle weakness can be assessed by having the person continuously maintain a position such as holding the arms overhead or extending the fingers.

Cranial nerve weakness and progressive muscle fatigue after exertion without sensory symptoms, changes in consciousness, or autonomic dysfunction are early signs of myasthenia gravis. Because the disease is relatively uncommon, it frequently goes undiagnosed until generalized weakness occurs. The diagnosis is based on the Tensilon (edrophonium chloride) test, during which edrophonium, a short-acting acetylcholinesterase inhibitor, is administered intravenously. The drug has the effect of decreasing the breakdown of ACh at the myoneural junction by the enzyme acetylcholinesterase. When weakness is due to myasthenia gravis, a dramatic transitory improvement in muscle function occurs. Another diagnostic method is to assay the titer ACh receptor antibodies circulating in the blood.

A recent advance in diagnostic methods for myasthenia gravis is the single-fiber electromyography, which is available in many medical centers. The technique involves recording the action potential from two or more muscle fibers within a muscle unit. This method can diagnose myasthenia gravis in 95% of cases.[11]

Treatment methods include use of pharmacologic agents, management of myasthenic crisis, thymectomy, and plasmapheresis. Pharmacologic treatment with anticholinesterase drugs inhibits the hydrolysis of ACh at the myoneural junction by acetylcholinesterase. Pyridostigmine (Mestinon) and neostigmine (Prostigmin) are the drugs of choice. Corticosteroid drugs, which suppress the immune response, are used in cases of a poor response to anticholinesterase drugs and thymectomy. Immunosuppressant drugs may also be used, often in combination with plasmapheresis.

Thymectomy, or surgical removal of the thymus, may be used as a treatment for myasthenia gravis. Because the mechanism whereby surgery exerts its effect is unknown, the treatment is controversial. Currently, thymectomy is performed in persons with thymoma, regardless of age, and in persons 50 to 60 years of age or older with recent onset of moderate disease. Plasmapheresis, a procedure in which the plasma with the IgG fraction is separated and removed from the person's blood, is a recent treatment method yielding variable results. Usually six to eight treatments are needed to bring about a transient improvement.

Persons with myasthenia gravis may develop a sudden exacerbation of symptoms and weakness known as *myasthenia crisis*. This usually occurs during a period of stress, such as infection, emotional upset, pregnancy, alcohol ingestion, cold, or following surgery. Many times, no primary cause can be identified. However, myasthenic crisis resulting from the need for more medication is virtually indistinguishable from cholinergic crisis resulting from too much medication. In the case of too much medication, cholinergic crisis is often accompanied by nausea, vomiting, pallor, sweating, salivation, colic, diarrhea, miosis, or bradycardia due to the muscarinic effects of the anticholinesterase drugs. Whatever the cause, prompt medical treatment is needed. To determine whether the crisis was precipitated by the disease process or by cholinergic drugs, the Tensilon test is used. If the crisis is myasthenic, the symptoms will improve. Provision for respiratory support should be available in either case.

Peripheral nerve disorders

The peripheral nervous system (PNS) consists of the motor and sensory nerves of the cranial and spinal nerves, the peripheral parts of the autonomic nervous system, and peripheral ganglia. A peripheral neuropathy is any primary disorder of the peripheral nerves. The result is usually muscle weakness, with or without atrophy, and/or sensory changes. The disorder can involve a single nerve (mononeuropathy) or multiple nerves (polyneuropathy).

Unlike the nerves of the CNS, peripheral nerves are fairly strong and resilient. This is because they contain a series of connective tissue sheaths that enclose their nerve fibers.[12] An outer fibrous sheath called the *epineurium* surrounds the moderate- to large-sized nerves; inside, a sheath called the *perineurium* invests each bundle of nerve fibers; and then,

within each bundle, a delicate sheath of connective tissue known as the *endoneurium* surrounds each individual nerve fiber (see Chapter 46, Figure 46-9). Small peripheral nerves lack the epineurial covering. Within its endoneurial sheath, each nerve fiber is invested by a segmented sheath of Schwann's cells. The Schwann's cells produce the myelin sheath that surrounds the peripheral nerves. Each Schwann's cell, however, can only myelinate one segment of a single axon—the one that it covers—so that myelination of an entire axon requires the participation of a long line of these cells.[12]

Peripheral nerve injury and repair

Neurons exemplify the general principle that the more specialized the function of a cell type, the less able it is to regenerate. In neurons, cell division ceases by the time of birth, and from then on the cell body of a neuron is unable to divide and replace itself. Although the entire neuron cannot be replaced, it is often possible for the dendritic and axon cell processes to regenerate as long as the cell body remains viable.

When a peripheral nerve is destroyed by a crushing force or by a cut that penetrates the nerve, the portion of the nerve fiber that is separated from the cell body rapidly undergoes degenerative changes, while the central stump and cell body of the nerve are often able to survive (Figure 49-10). Because the cell body synthesizes the material required for nourishing and maintaining the axon, it is likely that the loss of these materials results in the degeneration of the separated portion of the nerve fibers.

Following injury, the Schwann cells that are distal to the site of damage are also able to survive, but their myelin degenerates in a process called *Wallerian degeneration*. The Schwann cells assist other phagocytic cells in the area in the cleanup of the debris caused by the degenerating axon and myelin. As they remove the debris, the Schwann cells multiply and fill the empty endoneurial tube. At this point, nothing further happens, unless a regenerating nerve fiber penetrates into the endoneurial tube, in which case, the Schwann cells reform the myelin segments around the fiber.

Meanwhile, the cell body of the neuron responds to the loss of part of its nerve fiber by shifting into a phase of greatly increased protein and lipid synthesis. It does this by dispersing the masses of ribosomes, which stain as Nissl granules. They cease to be stainable and disappear in a process called *chromatolysis*. In the process, the nucleus moves away from the axonal side of the cell body, as though displaced by the active synthetic apparatus of the cells. These changes reach their height within about 10 days of

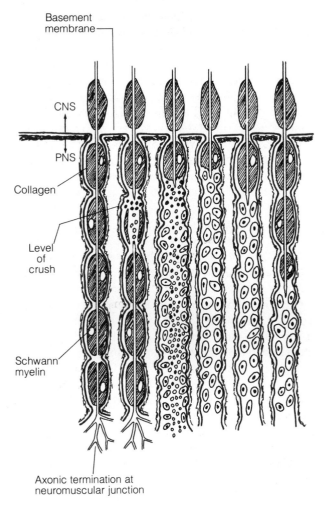

Basement
membrane

CNS

PNS

Collagen

Level
of
crush

Schwann
myelin

Axonic termination at
neuromuscular junction

Figure 49-10 Sequential stages in efferent axon degeneration and regeneration within its endoneural tube, following peripheral nerve crush injury.

injury and continue until regrowth of the nerve fiber ceases.

In the process of regeneration, the injured nerve fiber develops one or more new branches from the proximal nerve stump, which grow into the developing scar tissue. If a crushing injury has occurred and the endoneurial tube is intact through the trauma area, the outgrowing fiber will grow back down this tube to the structure that was originally innervated by the neuron. If, however, the injury involves the severing of a nerve, then the outgrowing branch must come in contact with its original endoneurial tube if it is to be reunited with its original target structure. The rate of outgrowth of regenerating nerve fibers is about 1 mm to 2 mm per day, so that the recovery of conduction to a target structure depends on not only regrowth into the appropriate endoneurial tube but also on the distance involved. It can take weeks or months for the regrowing fiber to reach the end organ and communicative function to be re-established. Further time is required for the Schwann cells to form new myelin

segments and for the axon to recover its original diameter and conduction velocity.

The successful regeneration of a nerve fiber in the PNS depends on many factors. If a nerve fiber is destroyed relatively close to the neuronal cell body, the chances are that the nerve cell will die, and, if it does, it will not be replaced. If a crushing type of injury has occurred, partial or often full recovery of function occurs. A cutting type trauma to a nerve is an entirely different matter. Connective scar tissue forms rapidly at the wound site, and, when it does, only the most rapidly regenerating axonal branches are able to get through to the intact distal endoneurial tubes. A number of scar-inhibiting agents have been used in an effort to reduce this hazard but have met with only moderate success. In another attempt to improve nerve regeneration, various types of tubular implants have been placed to fill longer gaps in the endoneurial tube.

Perhaps the most difficult problem is the alignment of the proximal and distal endoneurial tubes so that regenerating fiber can return down its former tube and innervate its former organ. This problem is similar to realigning a large telephone cable that has been cut so that all the wires are reconnected exactly as before the separation. Microscopic alignment of the cut edges during microsurgical repair results in improved success. An efferent nerve fiber that formerly innervated a skeletal muscle will regrow down an endoneurial tube formerly occupied by an afferent fiber, will reach the former sensory area, and then its cell body will eventually die. A sensory fiber that grows down an endoneurial tube that connects with a skeletal muscle fiber will undergo the same fate. If, however, these fibers grow down endoneurial tubes that innervate the appropriate type of target organ, reinnervation and function may return, even though the fibers have changed places. Under the best of conditions, a 10% regeneration to the appropriate organ is considered a success once a peripheral nerve has been severed. Even so, considerable function will return with that amount of innervation.

Peripheral nerve root injury: Ruptured intervertebral disk

The intervertebral disk is considered the most critical component of the load-bearing structures of the spinal column. The structural components of the disk make it capable of absorbing shock and changing shape while allowing movement.[12] The intervertebral disk can become dysfunctional due to trauma or the effects of aging. This results in movement between the articulating vertebral segments and the loss of the elastic properties of the disk itself. With aging or dysfunction, the nucleus pulposus (inner portion of the disk) can be squeezed out of place and herniate

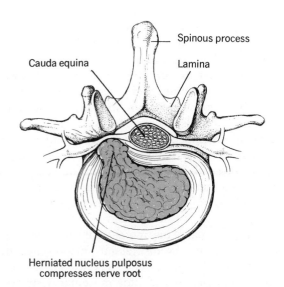

Cauda equina

Spinous process

Lamina

Herniated nucleus pulposus
compresses nerve root

Figure 49-11 A ruptured intervertebral disk. The soft central portion of the disk is protruding into the vertebral canal, where it exerts pressure on a spinal nerve root. (*Chaffee EE, Lytle IM: Basic Physiology and Anatomy, 4th ed, p 103. Philadelphia, JB Lippincott, 1980*)

through the annulus fibrosus (outer portion of the disk), a condition referred to as a herniated, or slipped disk (Figure 49-11). When this happens, the nucleus pulposus usually moves laterally or dorsally, causing irritation or crushing of a nerve root or the spinal cord. This irritation causes spontaneous firing of the sensory afferents and severe pain along the peripheral distribution of the nerve. Crushing damage to the dorsal roots results in reduction or loss of sensation, and crushing of the ventral roots produces muscle weakness. The signs and symptoms of a slipped disk are localized to the area of the body innervated by the nerve roots.

The level at which a slipped disk occurs is important. Usually it occurs at the lower levels of the lumbar spine where both the mass being supported and the bending of the vertebral column are greatest. When the injury occurs in this area, only the cauda equina will be irritated or crushed. Because these elongated dorsal and ventral roots contain endoneurial tubes of connective tissue, regeneration of the nerve fibers is likely. However, several weeks or months are required for full recovery to occur because of the distance to the innervated muscle or skin of the lower limbs. A slipped disk pressing into the spinal canal at higher levels can destroy the ventral white matter or can completely transect the cord. Here, regeneration is unlikely, and the paralysis and anesthesia of the caudal body regions may be permanent.

Mononeuropathies

Mononeuropathies are usually caused by localized conditions such as trauma, compression, or infections, that affect a single spinal nerve, plexus, or peripheral nerve trunk. Fractured bones may lacerate or compress nerves; excessively tight tourniquets may injure nerves directly or produce ischemic injury; and infections such as herpes zoster may affect a single segmental afferent nerve distribution. Recovery of nerve function is usually complete following compression lesions and incomplete or faulty following nerve transection.

Carpal tunnel syndrome. Carpal tunnel syndrome is an example of a compression-type mononeuropathy that is relatively common. It is caused by compression of the median nerve as it travels with the flexor tendons through a canal made by the carpal bones and transverse carpal ligament. The condition can be caused by a variety of conditions that produce either a reduction in the capacity of the carpal tunnel (bony or ligament changes) or increase in the volume of the tunnel contents (*e.g.,* inflammation of the tendons, synovial swelling, or tumors).[13] Carpal tunnel syndrome can be a feature of many systemic diseases such as rheumatoid arthritis, hyperthyroidism, acromegaly, and diabetes mellitus. The condition can result from wrist injury; it can occur during pregnancy and use of birth control drugs; and it is seen in persons with repetitive use of the wrist (flexion–extension movements and stress associated with pinching and gripping motions). One cause of carpal tunnel syndrome is the hand motions used by supermarket checkers.[14,15]

Carpal tunnel syndrome is characterized by pain, paresthesia, and numbness of the thumb and first two-and-a-half digits of the hand; pain in the wrist and hand, both worsening at night; atrophy of abductor pollicis muscle; and weakness in precision grip. All of these abnormalities may contribute to clumsiness of fine motor activity. Diagnosis is usually based on hypoesthesia confined to median nerve distribution, a positive Tinel's sign, and positive Phalen's sign. Tinel's sign describes the development of a tingling sensation radiating into the palm of the hand that is elicited by light percussion over the median nerve at the wrist. The Phalen test is performed by having the person hold the wrist in complete flexion for about a minute; if numbness and paresthesia along the median nerve are reproduced or exaggerated, the test is considered to be positive.[16] Electromyography and nerve conduction studies are often done to confirm the diagnosis and rule out other causes of the disorder. Treatment includes rest and splinting. The use of splints may be confined to nighttime use. In cases in which splinting is ineffective, corticosteroids may be injected into the carpal tunnel to reduce inflammation and swelling. Surgical intervention consists of operative division of the volar carpal ligaments as a means of relieving pressure on the medial nerve.

—— Polyneuropathies

Polyneuropathies lead to symmetric sensory, motor, or mixed sensorimotor deficits. The condition is characterized by demyelination or axonal degeneration of peripheral nerves. Typically, the longest axons are involved first, with symptoms beginning in the distal part of the extremities. If the autonomic nervous system is involved, there may be postural hypotension, constipation, and impotence. Polyneuropathies can result from immune mechanisms (Guillain-Barré syndrome), toxic agents (arsenic polyneuropathy, lead polyneuropathy, alcoholic polyneuropathy), and metabolic diseases (diabetes mellitus and uremia). Different causes tend to affect axons of different diameters and to affect sensory, motor, or autonomic neurons to different degrees.

Guillain-Barré syndrome. Guillain-Barré syndrome is a subacute polyneuropathy. The manifestations of the disease involve an infiltration of mononuclear cells around the capillaries of the peripheral neurons, edema of the endoneurial compartment, and demyelination of ventral spinal roots. The annual incidence of Guillain-Barré ranges from 0.6 to 1.9 cases per 100,000 population. About 85% of persons with the disease achieve a spontaneous recovery.

The cause of Guillain-Barré syndrome is unknown. In more than 50% of the cases, an upper respiratory or gastrointestinal disorder occurs 1 to 4 weeks before the onset of the neurologic manifestations. About 25% of persons with the disease have antibodies to either cytomegalovirus or Epstein-Barr virus. Other infectious agents include parainfluenza 2, measles, mumps, and hepatitis A and B viruses, as well as *Mycoplasma pneumoniae*, *Salmonella typhi*, and *Chlamydia psittaci*. A widely studied outbreak of the disorder followed the swine flu vaccination program of 1976–77.[17] It has been suggested that an altered immune response to peripheral nerve antigens contributes to the development of the disorder.

The disorder is characterized by progressive ascending muscle weakness of the limbs, producing a symmetric flaccid paralysis. Symptoms of paresthesia and numbness often accompany the loss of motor function. The rate of disease progression varies, and there may be disproportionate involvement of either the upper or lower extremities. Paralysis may progress to involve the respiratory muscles; about 20% of persons with the disorder require ventilatory assistance.[18] Autonomic nervous system involvement that causes postural hypotension, arrhythmias, facial flushing, abnormalities of sweating, and urinary retention is common.

Guillain-Barré syndrome is usually a medical emergency. There may be a rapid development of ventilatory failure and autonomic disturbances that threaten circulatory function. Treatment includes support of vital functions and prevention of complications such as skin breakdown and thrombophlebitis. Recent clinical trials have shown the effectiveness of plasmapheresis in decreasing morbidity and shortening the course of the disease. Treatment is most effective if initiated early in the course of the disease. Use of corticosteroid therapy is controversial.

In summary, the motor unit consists of the lower motoneuron, the myoneural junction, and the skeletal muscle that the nerve innervates. Disorders of the neuromuscular unit include muscular dystrophy, myasthenia gravis, and peripheral nerve disorders. Muscular dystrophy is a term used to describe a number of disorders that produce progressive deterioration of skeletal muscle. Muscle necrosis with fat and connective tissue replacement is seen. The disease usually affects children. One form, Duchenne's muscular dystrophy, is inherited as a sex-linked trait and transmitted by the mother to her offspring. Myasthenia gravis is a disorder of the myoneural junction, most likely resulting from a deficiency of functional acetylcholine receptors, which causes weakness of the skeletal muscles. Because the disease affects the myoneural junction, there is no loss of sensory function. The most common manifestations are weakness of the eye muscles with ptosis and diplopia. Weakness of the jaw muscles can make chewing and swallowing difficult. Usually the proximal muscles and extremities are involved, making it difficult to climb stairs and lift objects. Myasthenia crisis, which involves a sudden and transient weakness, may occur and necessitate mechanical ventilatory assistance. Disorders of peripheral nerves include mononeuropathies and polyneuropathies. Mononeuropathies involve a single spinal nerve, plexus, or peripheral nerve trunk. Carpal tunnel syndrome, a mononeuropathy, is caused by compression of the medial nerve that passes through the carpal tunnel in the wrist. Polyneuropathies produce symmetric sensory, motor, and mixed sensorimotor deficits. A number of conditions, including immune mechanisms, toxic agents, and metabolic disorders, are implicated as causative agents in polyneuropathies. Guillain-Barré syndrome is a subacute polyneuropathy of uncertain etiology. It causes progressive ascending motor, sensory, and autonomic nervous system manifestations. Respiratory involvement may occur and necessitate mechanical ventilation. A spontaneous recovery occurs in about 85% of persons with Guillain-Barré syndrome.

Alterations in muscle tone and motor power

Disorders of motor function include weakness and paralysis, which result from lesions in the voluntary motor pathways including the UMNs of the corticospinal and corticobulbar tracts or the LMNs that leave the CNS and travel by way of the peripheral nerve to the muscle. Muscle tone, which is a necessary component of muscle movement, is a function of the muscle spindle (myotatic) system and the extrapyramidal system, which monitors and buffers input to the LMNs by way of the UMNs.

Alterations in muscle tone

Disorders of skeletal muscle tone are characteristic of many nervous system pathologies. Any interruption of the myotatic reflex circuit by peripheral nerve injury, pathology of the neuromuscular junction and of skeletal muscle fibers, damage to the corticospinal system, injury to the spinal cord, or spinal nerve root results in disturbance of muscle tone. As explained earlier in the chapter, muscle tone is defined as resistance to passive movement around a joint. It may be described as less than normal (*hypotonia*), absent (*flaccidity*), or excessive (*hypertonia, rigidity, spasticity,* or *tetany*). The latter three terms are extremes of hypertonia that include other distinguishing features.

Clinically, the muscle tone is evaluated by asking a person to relax while supporting the limb except at the joint being investigated. The distal part of the extremity is then moved passively around the joint. Normally there is mild resistance to movement. A method for assessing muscle stretch excitability is to tap the tendon of a muscle briskly with a reflex hammer, which is normally immediately followed by a sudden contraction or *muscle jerk* (Figure 49-12). Here the stretch reflex has been "tricked" by the sudden tug on the tendon. A synchronous burst of Ia nerve activity from the many spindles in the muscle results in essentially simultaneous firing of a large number of LMN units. The stretch reflex was tricked into responding, as though the muscle had been suddenly stretched. These muscle jerk reflexes are called *deep tendon reflexes* (DTRs). They are usually checked at the wrists, elbows, knees, and Achilles tendons.

The DTRs can provide a great amount of information in a brief period of time. A normal range DTR indicates that (1) the afferent peripheral process in the peripheral muscle and nerves is normal; (2) the dorsal root ganglion function is normal; (3) the dorsal root function is normal; and (4) the dorsal, intermediate, and ventral horns are functioning appropriately,

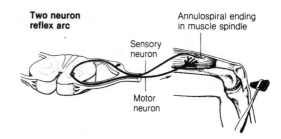

Figure 49-12 Testing the stretch reflex with a reflex hammer. (*Adapted from Chaffee EE, Lytle IM: Basic Physiology and Anatomy, 4th ed, p 240. Philadelphia, JB Lippincott, 1980*)

as are the ventral root and lower motor neuron cell body and axon. It also means that (5) the neuromuscular synapse is functioning normally; (6) the muscle fibers are capable of normal contraction; and (7) suprasegmental input is normal. Using this method of assessment, it is possible to test the function of many spinal nerves and spinal cord segments and some of the cranial nerves and brain stem segments in a short time. If abnormality of excitability is detected, further tests are required to determine the nature and location of the pathologic process.

Paresis and paralysis

The word *plegia* is Greek for a blow, a stroke, a paralysis. Terms used to describe the extent and anatomical location of motor damage are *paralysis,* meaning loss of movement, and *paresis,* implying weakness or incomplete loss of muscle function. *Monoparesis* or *monoplegia* results from the destruction of pyramidal innervation of one limb; *hemiparesis or hemiplegia,* both limbs on one side; *diparesis/diplegia* or *paraparesis/paraplegia,* both upper or lower limbs; and *quadriparesis/quadriplegia,* all four limbs. Paresis or paralysis can be further categorized to upper motor neuron origin or lower motor neuron origin.

Upper motoneuron lesions

A UMN lesion can involve the motor cortex, the internal capsule, or other brain structures through which the corticospinal tract descends, or the spinal cord. When the lesion is above the level of the pyramids at the caudal end of the brain stem, paralysis will affect structures on the opposite side of the body. In UMN disorders involving injury to the T12 level or above, there is an immediate profound weakness and loss of fine skilled voluntary limb movement, reduced bowel and bladder control, and diminished sexual functioning, followed by an exaggeration of muscle tone. With UMN lesions, the LMN spinal reflexes remain intact while communication and control from higher brain centers are lost. The normal pull of gravity against the weight of the body may initiate stretch reflexes. Because the descending inhibitory influence accompanying the UMN tracts is no longer intact, the reflex contractions are uninhibited. The resultant extreme hypertonicity is often called *spasticity* or *spastic paralysis*. The spasticity is often greatest in the flexor muscles of the upper limbs and extensor muscles of the lower limbs. Sometimes a lesion of the pyramidal tract is not severe enough to cause total paralysis, but produces a relatively minor degree of weakness. In this case, the finer and more skilled movements are most severely impaired. Spasticity is manifested by increased resistance to passive movement of a joint in which the initial resistance to movement quickly fades away.

Clonus is rhythmic, repeated contraction in response to the sudden stretch of a muscle that has been maintained by gentle pressure. It is seen in hypertonia associated with UMN lesions. It is caused by an oscillating stimulation of the muscle spindles that occurs when the spindle fibers are activated by an initial muscle stretch. This results in reflex contraction of the muscle and unloading of the spindle fibers with decreased afferent activity. The reduced spindle fiber activity causes the muscle to relax, which again causes the spindle fiber to be stretched, and the cycle starts over.

Lower motoneuron lesions

In contrast to UMN lesions in which the spinal reflexes remain intact, LMN disorders disrupt communication between the muscle and all neural input from spinal cord reflexes, including the stretch reflex, which maintains muscle tone.

Infection or irritation of the cell body of the LMN or its axon can lead to hyperexcitability, which causes spontaneous contractions of the muscle units. These can be observed as a twitching and squirming on the muscle surface, a condition called *fasciculations*. Toxic agents, such as the tetanus toxin (*Clostridium tetani*), produce extreme hyperexcitability of the LMN, which results in continuous firing at maximum rate. The resultant sustained contraction of the muscles is called *tetany*. Tetany of muscles on both sides of a joint produces immobility or tetanic paralysis. When the poliomyelitis virus attacks an LMN, it first irritates the LMN causing fasciculations to occur. These fasciculations are often followed by neuronal death. Weakness and severe muscle wasting of denervation atrophy results. If muscles are totally denervated, total weakness, called *flaccid paralysis,* occurs.

With complete LMN lesions, the muscles of the limbs, bowel, bladder, and genital areas become atonic; and it is impossible to elicit contraction by stretching the tendons. One of the outstanding features of lower motoneuron lesions is the profound development of muscle atrophy. Damage to the LMNs with or without spinal cord damage may be called *peripheral nerve injury* and may occur at any level of the spinal cord (*e.g.,* C7 peripheral nerve injury will lead to LMN hand weakness only). All segments below the level of injury that have intact LMNs will manifest UMN signs. Usually injury to the spinal cord at the T12 level or below results in LMN injury and flaccid paralysis to all areas below the level of injury. This is because the spinal cord ends at the T12–L1 level and from this level the spinal roots of the LMNs continue caudally in the vertebral column.

Alterations in motor function associated with stroke

Damage to the corticospinal system is a common component of stroke because the system passes through much of the internal capsule, a common target of cerebrovascular accidents. Also it is a very long tract system and, therefore, is vulnerable at many locations. Further, damage to the system has profound consequences to functions that are uniquely human —fine manipulative skills of the fingers and of the speech apparatus. Severe damage to the fibers controlling digital manipulation results in profound and permanent weakness of the small hand muscles with total loss of finger–thumb opposition and independent control of individual fingers. The hand can still be moved as a whole, and crude grasping and holding of items return after a recovery period. If the lower limb is affected, other signs of corticospinal damage include the loss of certain superficial abdominal reflexes and the appearance of a dorsiflexion (especially of the big toe) and splaying of the toes on stimulation of the sole of the foot, called the *Babinski's sign.*

During the third through eighth week after corticospinal damage, muscle tone gradually increases and eventually reaches an excessive level accompanied by other signs of hyperactive stretch reflexes such as clonus and exaggerated DTRs. The resultant *spastic paralysis* in the upper limb is selective for the in-rotators of the shoulder, flexors of the elbow, supinators of the forearm, and flexors of the fingers. Motor units in these muscles are particularly innervated by the UMNs. As a result, the classic spastic posture for the upper limb is a very stiffly held, flexed forearm rotated against the chest with the fingers curled tightly over the thumb and hand turned upward. Spasticity of the lower limb particularly affects the adductor extensors of the hip and extensors of the knee so that the gait of a fully developed spastic leg is stiff-legged with no movement at the knee and with the foot adducted (toes turned in toward the midline).

There are two major theories as to the cause of this slow developing but permanent spasticity. The older theory is that the pyramidal tract also contains fibers delivering inhibition to the segmental stretch reflexes. With interruption of the pyramidal tract, this inhibition is lost and extremely hyperactive muscle tone results.[19] A more recent theory suggests that the loss of UMN synapses on spinal segmental neurons is followed by outgrowth or plastic replacement of the denuded synapses by the segmental stretch afferents.[20] This would result in greatly increased facilitory power of the stretch reflexes. The only LMNs affected would be those that before were directly or indirectly innervated by UMNs. This theory recognizes the malleability of CNS synaptic relationships, which has been well demonstrated during maturation[21] and in other adult CNS systems.[22] At present, no decisive data support either theory, and both mechanisms may contribute. The slow onset of spasticity favors the plasticity or outgrowth theory, however.

In spite of various exercise and movement routines, the loss of strength and of fine manipulative movement apparently cannot be prevented. Attempts to slow and prevent the gradually developing spasticity have had some success, giving promise that at least this crippling aspect of corticospinal damage eventually might become preventable. Stroke is discussed further in Chapter 50.

In summary, alterations in musculoskeletal function include weakness resulting from lesions of voluntary UMN pathways of the corticobulbar and corticospinal tracts and the LMN of the peripheral nerves. Muscle tone is maintained through the combined function of the muscle spindle system and the extrapyramidal system that monitors and buffers UMN innervation of the LMNs. Hypotonia is a condition of less than normal muscle tone, and hypertonia or spasticity is a condition of excessive tone. Paresis refers to weakness in muscle function, and paralysis refers to a loss of muscle movement. UMN lesions produce spastic paralysis, and LMN lesions produce flaccid paralysis. Damage to the UMNs of the corticospinal and corticobulbar tracts is a common component of stroke.

Alterations in movement coordination and abnormal movements

Increased muscle tone or abnormal muscle movements are usually due to involvement of the extrapyramidal system. The extrapyramidal system arises from the motor cortex and is routed indirectly through the brain, with projections to the basal ganglia and cerebellum. From the basal ganglia and cerebellum, the fibers communicate with the next level of control, the reticular formation in the brain stem. The extrapyramidal system is usually considered a functional rather than an anatomical unit because of its many projections. In contrast with the direct route of the corticospinal or pyramidal tract, the extrapyramidal tract reaches the spinal cord only after many detours and indirect routing.

Disorders of cerebellar function

The functions of the cerebellum, or "little brain," are essential for smooth, coordinated, skillful movement. The cerebellum influences both voluntary and automatic aspects of movement. It does not initiate activity, but it is responsible for the temporal smoothness of correlated muscle action throughout the body. Because its function is to enhance cerebral cortical (pyramidal) motor function, the cerebellum is often classified as part of the extrapyramidal system.

The signs of cerebellar dysfunction can be grouped into three classes: vestibulo-cerebellar, cerebellar ataxia or decomposition of movement, and cerebellar tremor. These disorders occur on the side of cerebellar damage, whether by congenital defect, vascular accident, or growing tumor. The abnormality of movement occurs whether the eyes are open or closed. Thus, visual monitoring of movement cannot compensate for cerebellar defects.

Damage to the part of the cerebellum associated with the vestibular system leads to difficulty or inability to maintain a steady posture of the trunk, which normally requires constant readjusting movements. This is seen as an unsteadiness of the trunk, called *trunkal ataxia,* and it can be so severe that standing is not possible. The ability to fix the eyes on a target can also be affected. Constant conjugate readjustment of eye position (*nystagmus*) results, making reading extremely difficult, especially when the eyes are deviated toward the side of cerebellar damage.

Cerebellar ataxia and tremor are different aspects of defects in the smooth, continuously correcting functions. Cerebellar dystaxia or, if severe, ataxia, includes a *decomposition of movement:* each succeeding component of a complex movement occurs separately instead of being blended into a smoothly proceeding action. Because ethanol specifically affects cerebellar function, persons who are inebriated often walk with a staggering and unsteady gait. Rapid alternating movements such as supination–pronation–supination of the hands is jerky and performed slowly (dysdiadochokinesia). Reaching to touch a target breaks down into small sequential components, each going too far, followed by overcorrection. The finger moves jerkily toward the target, misses, corrects in the other direction, and misses again until, finally, the target is reached. This is called *over-and-under reaching,* and the general term is *dysmetria.*

Cerebellar tremor is a rhythmic back-and-forth movement of a finger or toe that worsens as the target is approached. The tremor results from the inability of the damaged cerebellar system to maintain ongoing fixation of a body part and to make smooth, continuous corrections in the trajectory of the movement; overcorrection occurs, first in one direction and then the other. Often the tremor of an arm or leg can be detected during the beginning of an intended movement, and, thus, the common term for cerebellar tremor is *intention tremor.* Cerebellar function as it relates to tremor can be assessed by asking a person to touch one heel to the opposite knee, to gently move the toes along the back of the opposite shin, or to move the hand so as to touch the nose with a finger.

Cerebellar function can also affect the motor skills of chewing and swallowing (dysphagia) and of speech (dysarthria). Normal speech requires smooth control of respiratory muscles and highly coordinated control of the laryngeal, lip, and tongue muscles. Cerebellar dysarthria is characterized by slow, slurred speech of continuously varying loudness. Rehabilitative efforts directed by speech therapists include learning to slow the rate of speech and to compensate as much as possible through the use of less-affected muscles.

—— Disorders of the basal ganglia

Disorders of the basal ganglia comprise a complex group of motor disturbances characterized by involuntary movements, alterations in muscle tone, and disturbances in body posture. The basal ganglia contribute *gracefulness* to cortically initiated and controlled skilled movements. The basal ganglia receive indirect input from the cerebellum and from all sensory systems including vision, and direct input from the motor cortex. The basal ganglia appear to organize the basic movement patterns into more complex patterns and to *release* them when commanded by the motor cortex. Many aspects of movement of the trunk, shoulder or hip girdles, and proximal parts of the limbs are automatic (*e.g.,* the swinging of the arms during walking and running or the follow-through of a throwing movement). The coordination and precision with which these movements are performed can be improved through learning and practice. Not everyone, however, can become an accomplished ballerina or gymnast. The basic repertoire of these fundamental complex movement patterns is built into brain stem

circuitry that is under gene control, and individual differences limit the extent to which learning and practice can enhance their accomplishment.

The globus pallidus is the site where basic movement patterns are generated. The globus pallidus is normally under constant inhibition by the caudate, putamen, and subthalamic nuclei. This inhibition is removed (*disinhibited*) by the motor cortex when a particular motor sequence is required as a part of a skilled sequence. Damage to this area of the basal ganglia results in extremely reduced movement (bradykinesia or hypokinesia). There is a loss of the automatic movements of the opposite side of the body, such as swinging of the arms when walking. The affected limbs can be passively placed in any position, even a very unusual one, and that position may be held for long time periods. On the other hand, if the globus pallidus is functionally intact and inhibitory control by caudate, putamen, or subthalamic nuclei are removed, constant movements (*hyperkinesia*) result. These movements, which include tremor, hemiballismus, chorea, and athetosis, cannot be intentionally controlled and are, thus, called *involuntary movements.*

Tremor is an involuntary alternating rhythmic contraction of opposing muscle groups. It is usually fairly uniform in frequency and amplitude. Tremor of extrapyramidal origin is usually increased during rest and diminished during voluntary activities. *The parkinsonian syndrome* (see Chapter 53) results in hypokinesis, tremor of body parts when they are not being used for skillful purposes. Certain tremors are considered physiologic—they are transient and occur with unusual experiences in normal people. They may be related to fatigue, emotional stress, or environmental conditions, such as shivering that occurs with cold exposure. Toxic tremors are produced by endogenous toxic states such as thyrotoxicosis.

The term *ballismus* originated from a Greek word meaning *to jump around. Hemiballismus* involves a constant, violent flinging movement of one arm or leg that may occur in elderly persons as the result of a small stroke that involves the subthalamic nucleus on the opposite side of the body. The movements may disappear only during deep sleep, but getting to sleep with this continuous violent movement can be most difficult.

The caudate and putamen are inhibitory to movements that are driven by the globus pallidus. Localized damage to these structures can result in slow twisting, wormlike movements of the face, leg, arm, or wrist and fingers as if using a screwdriver. These movements, called *athetoid,* result from continuous and prolonged contraction of both agonist and antagonist muscle groups. These movements are normal, smooth useful movements, except that they occur continuously in nonrhythmic, often irregular sequence.

Choreiform movements, which are quick and jerky but also coordinated and graceful, involve the face, tongue, swallowing muscles, and distal arm or leg. Choreiform movements are accentuated by movement and environmental stimulation; they often interfere with normal voluntary activities. The lesions causing the movements are principally located in the caudate and lentiform nuclei (*e.g.,* globus pallidus; putamen). The word *chorea* originated from the Greek word meaning *to dance*. There may be grimacing movements of the face, raising of the eyebrows, rolling of the eyes, and curling, protrusion, and withdrawal of the tongue. In the limbs, the movements are largely peripheral; there may be *piano-playing* flexion, extension movements of the fingers, elevations and depressions of the shoulders. The limb movements disappear during sleep. Movements of the face or limbs may occur alone or, as is more common, in combination.

Sydenham's chorea, sometimes called St. Vitus' dance, can occur in children during rheumatic fever. It is usually a self-limited disorder and leaves no permanent signs. *Huntington's chorea* is a hereditary (autosomal dominant) disease of sometimes late onset, appearing in middle maturity. It is a chronic and progressive degenerative disorder involving the basal ganglia, with progressive widespread destruction in the cerebral cortex. After onset, the chorea and an accompanying mental deterioration progress toward death over a period of about 15 years. The condition appears to be caused by a progressive loss of the inhibitory GABA-ergic neurons and small acetylcholine neurons in the caudate and putamen (see Chapter 53).

The term *dystonia* refers to the abnormal maintenance of a posture resulting from a twisting, turning movement that involves the limbs, neck, or trunk. In some disorders of movement, simultaneous opposing movements can result in paralysis or nonmovement. Long-sustained simultaneous hypertonia across a joint can result in degenerative changes and permanent fixation in unusual postures. *Spasmodic torticollis,* the most common type of dystonia, affects the muscles of the neck and shoulder. The condition, which is caused by bilateral and simultaneous contraction of the neck and shoulder muscles, results in the unilateral head turning or head extension, sometimes limiting rotation. Often elevations of the shoulder accompany the spasmodic movements of the head and neck. Eventually, immobility of the cervical vertebrae can lead to degenerative fixation in the twisted posture. Torsional spasm involving the trunk can also occur.

The "extrapyramidal" signs in all of these conditions intensify during highly emotional situations. When skilled movement is required, such as attempting to get out of a bus, to make change, or to write, apparently the defect can be partially overridden by motor cortical function. For instance, if a mildly affected person with the parkinsonian syndrome is carrying an open newspaper and attending to something else, arm and hand tremor can be severe. But the moment that person begins to read, the tremor decreases or is lost. However, people with movement disorders are very self-conscious, and, if people start to stare, the emotional aspect often results in an intensification of the tremor.

In summary, alterations in coordination of muscle movements and abnormal muscle movements result from disorders of the cerebellum and basal ganglia. The function of the cerebellum is essential for smooth coordinated movements. Cerebellar disorders include vestibulo-cerebellar dysfunction, cerebellar ataxia, and cerebellar tremor. The basal ganglia supply the aspect of gracefulness to muscle movement. Disorders of the basal ganglia are characterized by involuntary movements, alterations in muscle tone, and disturbances in posture. These disorders include tremor, hemiballismus, chorea, and athetosis.

Spinal cord injury

Traumatic spinal cord injury (SCI) may occur with or without damage to the spinal column. The spinal column and its components, however, are the main protector of the spinal cord from stress and injury. Currently, there are 200,000 or more persons living with spinal cord injury (SCI).[23] Nationally, there are approximately 15,000 to 20,000 spinal injuries that result in paralysis each year. The most frequent cause of spinal cord injury is motor vehicle accidents, followed by falls, violence, sports injuries, and other types of injuries, which include attempted suicide and occupational injuries. Of sports-related injuries, 66% are due to diving.

The average age for SCI is between 16 years and 30 years, with 19 years being the most frequent age.[23] As age increases, the etiology of injury changes, with falls becoming the most frequent cause. Males sustain SCI at a rate four times higher than that of females. This may be because males are involved in more high-risk activities. Alcohol and drugs have been cited as contributing factors in an increasing number of cases.

—— The spinal column

The spinal column, which is located in the posterior midline of the body, begins at the base of the skull and ends at the coccyx, or "tailbone." There are 34 to 37 individual vertebral bodies, or vertebrae, that make up the spinal column: 7 cervical, 12 thoracic, 5 lumbar, 5 fused sacral, and 3 to 5 fused coccygeal. Each vertebra in the vertebral column shares common characteristics (*e.g.,* each consists of an anterior portion, or body, and a posterior portion, called the *vertebral* or *neural arch;* Figure 49-13). The vertebral arch is composed of two pedicles, two laminae, a spinous process, and four articular processes.

The design of the vertebra is to provide bony protection for the cord by forming a vertebral foramen or spinal canal. The cervical vertebrae also have transverse foramen within the transverse processes that form a passageway for the vertebral artery, vertebral vein, and sympathetic nerves. The size and function of the vertebrae are directly related to their specific location in the spinal column. Generally, vertebral bodies increase in size to bear additional weight as they descend along the spinal column. The width of the spinal canal varies at different levels also. The atlas (C1) and the axis (C2) are formed in a manner that allows for flexion, extension, and rotation of the head. The intermediate-sized thoracic vertebrae are heart-shaped and limited in movement. They also possess tubercles for rib attachment. Each vertebra articulates with the next above and below by means of articular processes bearing facet, sliding synovial joints. These provide some support as well as major limitation of movement. They also can be a frequent source of back pain. The design of the lumbar spine allows for powerful flexion and some extension; these lumbar vertebrae are large and heavy to accommodate the attachment of lower limb muscles.

The bony structure of the closely approximated vertebrae provides good protection for the spinal cord, nerve roots, and posterior root ganglia. Major support and protection for the spinal cord are provided by this column of vertebral bodies, along with the fibrocartilaginous intervertebral disks and strong bands of fibers known as ligaments. Intervertebral disks contain a firm gelatinous structure called the nucleus pulposus, which gives substance to the disk. The nucleus pulposus is surrounded by a layer of fibrocartilage called the annulus fibrosus. The vertebral disks are held in place by strong ligaments. The two major longitudinal ligaments extend from the axis (C2) to the sacrum on the anterior and posterior surfaces of the vertebral bodies and disks. Other fibrous connective tissue ligaments that attach at various sites between the parts of neighboring vertebrae also support and limit movement of the spinal column, thereby protecting the spinal cord.

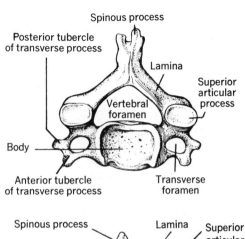

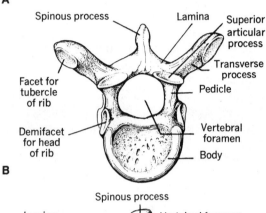

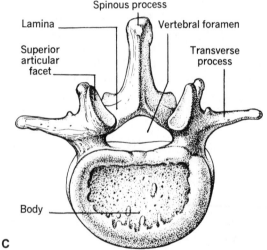

Figure 49-13 Views of three types of vertebrae. **A,** Fourth cervical vertebra, superior aspect. **B,** Sixth thoracic vertebra, superior aspect. **C,** Third lumbar vertebra, superior aspect. (*Chaffee EE, Greisheimer EM: Basic Physiology and Anatomy. Philadelphia, JB Lippincott, 1974*)

When the ligaments are damaged, the spine is considered unstable. In an unstable spine, further unguarded movement of the spinal column could result in compression or overstretching of neural tissue; whereas, in a stable spine, further movement of the spinal column will not impinge on the spinal cord. Most traumatic injuries to the spinal column render it unstable, warranting precautionary measures such as immobilization with collars and back boards and limiting the movement of persons at risk or with known spinal cord injury. Other stabilizing forces are the rib cage, superficial and deep-trunk muscles, and the normal curvatures of the spine at the cervical (anteriorly convex), thoracic (concave), lumbar (convex), and pelvic (concave) levels.

Mechanisms of injury

Injury to the vertebral column

Injury to the vertebral column is caused by motion or trauma to the spinal column; it is related to the amount and direction of motion, the force causing the motion, and the actual damage due to these factors. The amount of motion that is possible in the spine is determined by the size of the intervertebral disks. The direction of motion is determined by the facet joints. The orientation of the facet joint surface varies from region to region.[24] Flexion injuries occur when there is forward or lateral bending of the spinal column that exceeds the limits of normal movement. Typical flexion injuries result, for example, when in a motor vehicle accident the head is hyperextended then thrown forward or when the head is struck from behind during a fall with the back of the head as the point of impact. Flexion with rotation as concurrent forces where the vertebral bodies are twisted or turned on each other is a potent mechanism of injury as well.

Extension injuries occur when there is excessive forced bending (hyperextension) of the spine backward. A typical extension injury involves a fall in which the chin or face is the point of impact, causing hyperextension of the neck.

Injuries of forward and lateral flexion, rotation, and extension occur more commonly in the cervical spine than in any other area. The majority of cervical flexion and extension injuries occur between C4 and C6. Limitations imposed by the ribs, spinous processes, and joint capsules in the thoracic spine region make it less flexible than the cervical spine. While all motions are possible, flexion and extension are greater in the lower thoracic spine than in the upper thoracic spine due to changes in facet orientation, and rotation is more limited in the lower thoracic spine.

A compression injury causing the vertebral bones to shatter, squash, or even burst, occurs when there is spinal loading from a high velocity blow to the top of the head or landing forcefully on one's feet (Figure 49-14). This typically occurs at the cervical level (*e.g.*, diving injuries) or in the thoracolumbar area (*e.g.*, falling from a distance and landing on the feet). The spine becomes increasingly stiffer and more inflexible from the lower thoracic area through the lumbar area. The exact location of increased stiffness and inflexibility may vary among individuals and may range from T7 to L4. This area is, therefore, subject to mechanical failure and accounts for a high number of spine injuries in the thoracolumbar junction.

Injury to the spinal cord

A fracture can occur at any part of the bony vertebrae, causing fragmentation of the bone. It most often involves the pedicle, lamina, or processes (facets). The injury may occur when bone fragments become lodged in the spinal canal or cord itself and compress the cord. Dislocation/subluxation (partial dislocation) injury causes the vertebral bodies to be-

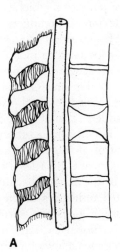 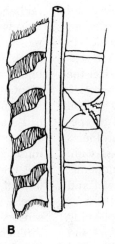 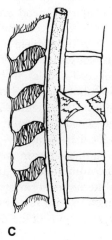

A **B** **C**

Figure 49-14 Progressive degrees of compression fracture. **A,** Severe compression fracture showing the biconcave profile produced by the adjacent discs. **B,** A more severe degree of fracture. A vertical fracture has joined the deformed, concave end-plates. The anterior body fragment is comminuted and displaced anteriorly. **C,** A more severe degree of compression fracture. The posterior body fragment is now comminuted and displaced posteriorly into the spinal canal. Neural damage may occur. The neural arch is intact. This spine is stable. (*Rockwood CA, Green DP: Fractures. Philadelphia, JB Lippincott, 1977*)

come displaced. Normally, the vertebral bodies rest on top of one another, separated by the intervertebral disks and held in alignment by ligaments. Disruption of the ligaments allows for shifting or dislocation of the anatomical alignment of the vertebrae and can cause compression and overstretching of neural tissue.

The blood flow to the spinal cord is supplied by three sources: the anterior spinal artery, which provides the main blood supply for the anterior two-thirds of the spinal cord; the posterior spinal arteries, which provide the main blood supply for the posterior one-third of the cord; and the radicular arteries, which supply the outer circumference of the cord at various levels. Interruption of blood flow to the cord can cause permanent damage.

Contusions of the cord occur when the cord is jarred in the spinal canal. This movement of the cord results in hemorrhage and edema. As cord tissue swells, blood flow can be disrupted and oxygen deprivation can cause necrosis of neural tissue. Lacerations occur when there is cutting or tearing of the spinal cord. This causes injury to nerve tissue with associated bleeding and edema. Gunshot and knife wounds to the spinal cord are common types of laceration injuries.

The severity of bony injury or radiographic findings may not always correspond with the extent of neurologic damage. Also, the location of bony injury may not coincide with the clinical findings of motor and sensory deficits (e.g., C6 compression fracture with motor and sensory level of functioning at C7, or C4, C5).

—— Alterations in function

Alterations in body function that result from spinal cord injury depend on the level of injury and the amount of cord involvement. Because of variations that occur with incomplete injuries, the discussion in this section focuses on complete (total motor and sensory) spinal cord injuries. Table 49-2 summarizes the functional abilities by level of injury. The myotome and dermatome (see Figure 47-1) charts show skeletal muscle and sensory areas of skin innervated by specific spinal cord segments. The physical problems discussed in this chapter are those associated with: ventilation/communication, function of the autonomic nervous system, sensorimotor integrity, bowel and bladder function, and sexual function.

Dysfunctions of the nervous system following SCI cover varying degrees of sensorimotor loss and altered reflex activity based on the level of injury and extent of cord damage. Paraplegia, as described earlier, refers to paralysis of the lower portion of the body, which includes the legs and may include the trunk. Anatomically, paraplegia occurs with injury to the second thoracic cord segment and below. Quadriplegia refers to paralysis of the lower portions of the body with partial or complete paralysis of the arms and hands. Injury to the first thoracic cord segment or above results in quadriplegia. Functional distinctions in quadriplegia may be considered in two categories: respiratory and motor function for mobility and self-care needs.

In the recent past, a more mobile society, along with advances in on-site emergency services and skilled maintenance of health care, have led to the emergence of two subgroups of quadriplegia: respiratory quadriplegia and respiratory pentaplegia. The diaphragm is innervated primarily by the C3 to C5 spinal nerves. Respiratory quadriplegia occurs with a C2 to C3 functional level injury. With this level of injury, there is full sensation of the head and upper neck, with some control of neck muscles. Partial preservation of the accessory respiratory muscles may enable independent ventilation for limited periods of time. Respiratory pentaplegia occurs with injuries at the C1 level. With this level of injury, there is little or no neck and face sensation or neck muscle control, and there is no potential for developing independent spontaneous ventilation, even for a short period of time.

Motor function in cervical injuries ranges from complete dependence to independence with or without assistance devices in activities of mobility and self-care. The functional levels of cervical injury relate to C5, C6, C7, and C8 innervation. At the C5 level, deltoid and biceps function is spared, allowing full head, neck, and diaphragm control with good shoulder strength and full elbow flexion. At the C6 level, wrist dorsiflexion by way of the wrist extensors is functional, allowing for tenodesis, which is the natural bending inward or flexion of the fingers when the wrist is extended or bent backward. Tenodesis is a key movement because it can be used to pick up objects when finger movement is absent. A functional C7 injury allows full elbow flexion and extension, wrist plantar flexion and some finger control. At the C8 level, finger flexion is added. Thoracic cord injuries (T1 to T12) allow for full upper extremity control with limited to full control of intercostal and trunk muscles and balance. Injury at the T1 level allows for full fine motor control of the finger. Because of the lack of specific functional indicators at the thoracic levels, the level of injury is usually determined by sensory level testing. Functional capacity in the L1 through L5 nerve innervations allows for hip flexors, hip abductors (L1 to L3), movement of the knees (L2 to L5), and ankle dorsiflexion (L4 to L5). Sacral (S1 to S5) innervation allows for full leg, foot, and ankle control, as well as innervation of perineal musculature for bowel, bladder, and sexual function.

Altered reflex activity in spinal cord injury is essentially determined by UMN and LMN lesions. Generally, any injury to the cord at the T12 level or above is considered an UMN injury. Injuries below the T12 level are considered LMN injuries. However, injuries near the T12 level can result in mixed UMN/ LMN deficits (*e.g.,* flaccid paralysis of the bladder with spastic urethral sphincter).

With cord injury, the extent of neural deficit at each anatomical level is determined by whether the injury is complete or incomplete. Complete spinal cord injury is characterized by a lack of any movement or sensation below the level of the injury. This means, for instance, that in a person with a diagnosed complete C5 injury, the function of the C5 nerve roots and cord segment will be intact, while the function of the C6 roots and cord segment and below will not be functional. Complete spinal cord injury can result

Table 49–2. Functional abilities by level of cord injury

Injury level	Segmental sensorimotor function	Dressing, eating	Elimination	Mobility*
C1	Little or no sensation or control of head and neck. No diaphragm control. Requires continuous ventilation	Dependent	Dependent	Limited. Voice or sip-N-puff controlled electric wheelchair
C2 to C3	Head and neck sensation; some neck control. Independent of mechanical ventilation for short periods	Dependent	Dependent	Same as for C1
C4	Good head and neck sensation and motor control; some shoulder elevation; diaphragm movement	Dependent; may be able to eat with adaptive sling	Dependent	Limited to voice, mouth, head, chin, or shoulder-controlled electric chair
C5	Full head and neck control; shoulder strength; elbow flexion	Independent with assistance	Maximal assistance	Electric or modified manual wheel chair, needs transfer assistance
C6	Fully innervated shoulder; wrist extension or dorsiflexion	Independent and/or with minimal assistance	Independent and/or with minimal assistance	Independent in transfers and wheel chair independently
C7 to C8	Full elbow extension; wrist plantar flexion; some finger control	Independent	Independent	Independent; manual wheelchair
T1 to T5	Full hand and finger control; use of intercostal and thoracic muscles	Independent	Independent	Independent; manual wheelchair
T6 to T10	Abdominal muscle control, partial to good balance with trunk muscles	Independent	Independent	Independent; manual wheelchair
T11 to L5	Hip flexors, hip abductors (L1–3); knee extension (L2–4); knee flexion and ankle dorsiflexion (L4–5)	Independent	Independent	Short distance to full ambulation with assistance
S1 to S5	Full leg, foot and ankle control; innervation of perineal muscles for bowel, bladder, and sexual function (S2–4)	Independent	Normal to impaired bowel and bladder function	Ambulate independent with or without assistance

* Assistance refers to adaptive equipment, set up, or physical assistance.

from severance of the cord, disruption of nerve fibers although they remain intact, or interruption of total blood supply to that cord segment. However, complete severance of the cord is rarely seen. Incomplete spinal cord injury occurs when there is any sparing of movement and/or sensation below the level of injury. The level of incomplete lesions can be determined by the presenting clinical symptoms, which reflect the predominant area of the cord that is involved. A condition called *central cord syndrome* occurs when injury is predominantly in the central gray or white matter of the cord. Because the corticospinal tract fibers are organized with those controlling the arms being located more centrally and those controlling the legs located more laterally, some external axonal transmission remains intact if central cord syndrome occurs. Therefore, motor and sensory function of the upper extremities may be affected, but the lower extremities may not be affected, or they may be affected to a lesser degree. Bowel, bladder, and sexual functions are usually affected to varying degrees, paralleling the degree of lower extremity involvement. This syndrome usually occurs in the cervical cord, rendering the lesion a UMN with spastic paralysis. Central cord damage is more frequent in elderly persons with narrowing or stenotic changes in the spinal canal related to arthritis or persons in any age group with congenital spinal stenosis.

Anterior artery or *anterior cord syndrome* is usually caused by damage due to infarction of the anterior spinal artery resulting in damage to the anterior two-thirds of the cord. The deficits result in loss of motor function provided by the corticospinal tracts as well as loss of pain and temperature sensation caused by damage to the lateral spinothalamic tracts. The posterior one-third of the cord is relatively unaffected, preserving position, vibration, and touch sense.

A condition called *Brown-Sequard syndrome* results from damage to a hemisection of the anterior and posterior cord. The effect is a loss of voluntary motor function from the corticospinal tract and loss of discriminative touch, vibration, and proprioception on the ipsilateral side of the body and contralateral loss of pain and temperature from the lateral spinothalamic tracts.

Conus medullaris syndrome involves damage to the conus medullaris or the end of the spinal cord at the L1 to L2 vertebral level. Functional deficits resulting from this type of injury usually result in LMN or flaccid bowel, bladder, and sexual function. Motor function in the legs and feet may be impaired without significant sensory impairment. Damage below the L3 vertebra level usually results in LMN and sensory neuron damage known as *cauda equina syndrome*. Functional deficits present as varying patterns of asymmetric flaccid paralysis, sensory impairment, and

pain. *Sacral sparing* results when the radicular arteries supplying the outer circumference of the cord are spared. This allows for sacral sensation in an otherwise paralyzed person.

Spinal shock

Spinal shock or neurogenic shock is the term used to describe the transient state of areflexia that occurs immediately following cord transection. It involves the motor pathways, and the manifestations are flaccid paralysis, lack of tendon reflexes and autonomic function, regardless of whether the level of lesion will eventually produce spastic (UMN) or flaccid (LMN) paralysis. The basic mechanisms accounting for the transient spinal shock are unknown. Spinal shock may last for minutes, hours, days, or weeks after which isolated spinal-cord activity returns. Usually, if reflex function returns by the time the person reaches the hospital, the neuromuscular changes are reversible. This kind of reversible spinal shock may occur in football-type injuries where jarring of the spinal cord within the canal produces a concussion-like phenomenon in which there is temporary loss of movement and reflexes followed by full recovery within days.

In persons in whom high level paraplegia or quadriplegia persists, hypotension and bradycardia may become critical, but manageable, problems. Circulatory function is impaired by a loss of sympathetic control of heart rate, peripheral vascular resistance and lack of muscle tone in paralyzed limbs resulting in sluggish circulating blood flow and venous return. The resulting bradycardia and hypotension can usually be managed with slow fluid resuscitation and body positioning that facilitates venous return. Spinal shock and true hemorrhagic shock (hypotension and tachycardia) must be differentiated and treated accordingly. Spinal shock is usually self-limiting, and the return of reflexes in UMN lesions usually occurs in a caudal-rostral direction with the first returning reflexes being those in the sacral area (rectal sphincter contraction) followed by those of the lumbar area (the lower extremities). However, bradycardia and hypotension may persist and become asymptomatic normal parameters. The length of time that it takes to adjust to the altered circulatory status is variable and may take as long as a year.

Ventilation/communication

Ventilation requires movement of both the expiratory and inspiratory muscles, all of which receive innervation from the spinal cord. The main muscle of ventilation, the diaphragm, is innervated by segments C3 to C5. The intercostal muscles, located between the ribs, are innervated by spinal segments

T1 through T7. These muscles function in elevating the rib cage and are needed for coughing and deep breathing. The major muscles of expiration are the abdominal muscles, which receive their innervation from levels T6 to T12. By forcing the abdominal viscera against the diaphragm, the muscles exert pressure on the diaphragm and return the thoracic cage to its resting position. Coughing and deep breathing, which are vital to the removal of mucus and foreign particles from the respiratory tract, are facilitated by the elevation of the rib cage and expansion of the anteroposterior and lateral dimensions of the chest wall, followed by strong respiratory muscle contraction forcing air out of the lungs.

While the ability to inhale and exhale may be preserved at various levels of spinal cord injury, functional deficits in ventilation are most apparent in the quality of the breathing cycle and the ability to oxygenate tissues, give off carbon dioxide, and mobilize secretions. As described earlier, cord injuries involving C1 to C3 result in lack of respiratory effort and will require assisted ventilation. Although C3 to C5 injury allows for partial or full diaphragmatic function, ventilation will be diminished due to loss of intercostal muscle function, resulting in shallow breaths and a weak cough. Below C5 level, as less intercostal and abdominal musculature is affected, the ability to take a deep breath and cough is less impaired. Maintenance therapy consists of muscle training to strengthen existing muscles for endurance and mobilizing secretions.

With assisted ventilation, whether continuous or intermittent, ensuring adequate communication of needs is also essential. There are several ways of ensuring communication of needs with use of verbal or nonverbal communication systems. Verbal approaches may consist of fenestrated tracheal tubes to provide air flow and vibration of the vocal cords, talking tracheostomy tubes, diaphragmatic pacing, electrolarynx-type devices, and mechanical ventilation with an air leak. Nonverbal communication techniques include boards or cards displaying the person's most frequently used words, computerized scanning programs, and mouth-stick control devices.

Autonomic nervous system function

Spinal cord injury not only interrupts the function of the somatic nerves that control skeletal muscle function, but it also interrupts visceral afferent input and autonomic outflow from below the site of injury, parasympathetic outflow from the cranial and sacral segments of the spinal cord, and sympathetic outflow from the thoracic and lumbar segments. Interruption of autonomic outflow results in continued function above the level of injury, while the spinal and autonomic reflexes below the level of injury are uncontrolled.

The autonomic regulation of circulatory function and thermoregulation present the most severe problems in SCI. The higher the level of injury and the greater the body surface area affected, the more profound the effects on circulation and thermoregulation. Persons with injury at the T6 level or above will experience problems in regulating vasomotor tone; those with injuries below the T6 level usually have sufficient sympathetic function to maintain adequate vasomotor function. The level of injury and its corresponding problems may vary among persons and situations, and some dysfunctional effects may be seen at levels below T6. With lower lumbar and sacral injuries, sympathetic function remains essentially unaltered (see Chapter 48).

Vasovagal response. The vagus (X) nerve normally exerts a continuous inhibitory effect on heart rate. Vagal stimulation that causes a marked bradycardia by way of an intact cervical outflow portion of the vagus nerve is called the vasovagal response. Visceral afferent input to the vagal centers in the brain stem of persons with quadriplegia or high-level paraplegia can produce marked bradycardia when unchecked by a dysfunctional sympathetic nervous system. Severe bradycardia and even asystole can result when the vasovagal response is elicited by deep endotracheal suctioning or rapid position change. Preventive measures, such as hyperoxygenation prior to, during, and following suctioning, are advised. Rapid position changes should be avoided or anticipated, and anticholinergic drugs should be immediately available to counteract severe episodes of bradycardia.

Autonomic hyperreflexia. Following spinal cord injury, the spinal reflex circuits are largely isolated from the rest of the central nervous system. Afferent somatic and visceral sensory input that enters the spinal cord through intact segmental nerves is unaffected. Likewise, the efferent outflow from intact reflex centers below the site of injury is largely unaffected. However, the transmission of ascending sensory input to higher centers and descending motor control output from higher centers is blocked at the site of injury. Thus, what are lacking are the regulation and integration of reflex function by higher autonomic and motor control centers in the brain and brain stem. Usually persons with injuries at the T6 level or below have sufficient sympathetic outflow to control visceral reflexes.

In persons with T6 injuries and above, the baroreflex response is disturbed. The aortic and carotid sinus baroreceptors and afferent input to the cardiovascular centers in the brain stem, as well as the parasympathetic cranial output that controls heart rate, remain intact. However, the efferent loop that exits the CNS by way of the thoracic spinal nerves and controls peripheral vascular resistance becomes nonfunctional. When stimulated, the sympathetic reflexes controlling peripheral vascular resistance function in an unregulated manner, and severe hypertension can occur. As blood pressure rises, the uncoordinated baroreflex response produces a vagal slowing of heart rate—the result can be unchecked hypertension accompanied by a severe baroreflex-mediated bradycardia.

The terms *autonomic dysreflexia* or *autonomic hyperreflexia* refer to an acute episode of exaggerated sympathetic reflex responses that occur in persons with spinal cord injury. It is usually characterized by severe hypertension ranging as high as 300/160 mmHg, bradycardia, and headache ranging from dull to severe and pounding.[25] Below the level of injury, the reflex response stimulates major sympathetic outflow tracts resulting in vasospasm, hypertension, skin pallor, and gooseflesh that represents the piloerector response. Continued hypertension produces a baroreflex-mediated vagal slowing of heart rate to bradycardia levels. Above the level of the lesion, the sympathetic vasomotor response results in arterial vasodilatation, headache, flushed skin, nasal stuffiness, profuse sweating, and anxiety.

The dysreflexic response is usually initiated by stimuli that would normally cause pain or discomfort in the abdominal or pelvic region. They include visceral distention (full bladder or rectum), stimulation of pain receptors (such as occurs with pressure, ingrown toenails, dressing changes, diagnostic or operative procedures), and visceral contractions, such as ejaculation, bladder spasms, or uterine contractions. In approximately 80% of cases, the dysreflexic response results from a full bladder.[25]

Autonomic dysreflexia is a clinical emergency, and without prompt and adequate treatment, convulsions, loss of consciousness, and even death can occur. The major components of treatment include monitoring blood pressure while removing or correcting the initiating cause or stimulus. The person should be placed in an upright position, and all support hose or binders should be removed to promote venous pooling of blood and reduce venous return, thereby decreasing blood pressure. If the stimuli have been removed or the stimuli cannot be identified and the upright position established but the blood pressure remains elevated, drugs that block autonomic function are administered.

Postural hypotension. Postural or orthostatic hypotension usually occurs in persons with T4 to T6 injuries and above related to the interruption of sympathetic innervation to blood vessels in the extremities and abdomen. Pooling of blood, along with gravitational forces, impairs venous return to the heart, and there is a subsequent decrease in cardiac output when the person is placed in an upright position. This usually occurs when the person is placed in the seated position in bed or transferred from the bed to the wheelchair. The signs of orthostatic hypotension include dizziness, pallor, excessive sweating above the level of the lesion, complaints of blurred vision, and possibly fainting. Because of the disruption in autonomic function at the time of injury, the blood pressure and heart rate may already be low, but asymptomatic. Postural hypotension is usually prevented by slow changes in position and devices to promote venous return.

Body temperature regulation. As the autonomic control of circulatory function, the sympathetic nervous system is most influential in maintaining temperature homeostasis. The central mechanisms for thermoregulation are located in the hypothalamus. In response to cold, the hypothalamus stimulates vasoconstrictor responses in peripheral blood vessels, particularly those of the skin. This results in decreased loss of body heat to the external environment, thereby maintaining heated circulation to vital internal organs. Increased heat production results from increased metabolism, voluntary activity, or shivering. Shivering can almost double the heat production of the body. In order to reduce heat, hypothalamic-stimulated mechanisms produce vasodilatation of skin blood vessels to dissipate heat and sweating to increase evaporative heat losses.

Following spinal cord injury, the communication between the thermoregulatory centers in the hypothalamus and the sympathetic effector responses below the level of injury are disrupted—the ability to control blood vessel responses that conserve or dissipate heat is lost as are the abilities to sweat and shiver. The higher the level of injury is, the greater the disturbance in thermoregulation. In quadriplegia and high paraplegia, there are few defenses against changes in the environmental temperature and body temperature tends to assume the temperature of the external environment, a condition known as *poikilothermy*. Persons with lower level injuries will have varying degrees of thermoregulation. Disturbances in thermoregulation are chronic and may cause continual loss of body heat. Treatment consists of education in the adjustment of clothing and awareness of how environmental temperatures affect the person's ability to accommodate these changes.

Edema

Edema following spinal cord injury is related to decreased peripheral vascular resistance, areflexia or decreased tone in paralyzed limbs, and immobility that causes increased venous pressure and abnormal pooling of blood in the abdomen, lower limbs, and upper extremities. Orthostatic or dependent edema in the dependent body parts is usually relieved by positioning to overcome gravitational forces or compression devices (such as support stockings and binders) that encourage venous return.

Deep vein thrombosis

Deep vein thrombosis (DVT), as a complication of spinal cord injury, occurs with about the same prevalence (15%) as in the postoperative population.[26,27] Although it is seen more frequently in the postacute phase of spinal cord injury, it often has its origin during the events surrounding the initial injury. Impairment of vasomotor tone, initial loss of muscle tone, trauma to the vein wall, hypercoagulability, and immobility predispose to sluggish venous blood flow and the risk of DVT. Preventable measures include assessment for risk and presence of DVT and measures to prevent venous pooling of blood.

Sensorimotor integrity

Following the period of spinal shock, isolated spinal reflex activity and muscle tone that is not under the control of higher centers return. In an upper motoneuron (UMN) injury, this may result in hypertonia and spasticity of skeletal muscles below the level of injury, where the normal communication pathways to higher centers for voluntary motor control have been interrupted by the spinal cord lesion. These spastic movements are involuntary versus voluntary, a distinction that needs to be explained to both the spinal cord injured person and his or her family members. Spastic movements, which occur below the level of injury, can be tonic (sustained tone) or clonic (intermittent) and are usually heightened initially postinjury, reaching a peak in about 2 years, and then gradually diminishing.

These movements occur in most spinal injuries above the T12 level where the reflex arc is preserved. In T12 or below injuries, the reflex response itself is damaged at the cord or spinal nerve level preventing spasticity. Spasticity in and of itself is not detrimental to the spinal cord injured person and may even facilitate maintenance of muscle tone to prevent muscle wasting, improve venous return, and aid in mobility. Spasms become detrimental, however, when they impair safety and the ability to make functional gains in mobility and activities of daily living, such as feeding, dressing, and toileting, as well as vocational and avocational interests. Spasms may also cause trauma to bones and tissues leading to joint contractures and skin breakdown. Spasms may occur in flexion or extension patterns.

Treatment includes trying to break the spasm when it interferes with activities by promoting the opposite movement. For example, if an extensor spasm of the hand occurs, an attempt to flex the hand with moderate pressure is used to oppose the spasm. Because the stimuli that precipitate spasms vary from person to person, careful assessment needs to be done to identify the factors that precipitate spasm in each person. Passive range-of-motion exercises to stretch spastic muscles should be done at least twice a day, avoiding stimuli that elicit spasm or, in cases where spasm cannot be avoided, preparing the person for the spastic response. The stimuli for reflex muscle spasm arise from somatic or visceral afferent pathways that enter the cord below the level of injury. The most common of these stimuli are: bladder infection, stone, or fistula; bowel distention or impaction; pressure area or irritations of the skin; and infections. Antispasmodic medications may be warranted and need to be carefully monitored for effectiveness.

Skin. The entire surface of the skin is innervated by cranial or spinal nerves organized into dermatomes showing cutaneous distribution (see Chapter 47). The central and autonomic nervous systems also play a vital role in skin function. Impulses from the peripheral nervous system carry sensory information to the brain and receive information for motor control and reflex activity at each dermatome. Through the control of vasomotor and sweat gland activity, the autonomic nervous system influences skin condition by providing adequate circulation, excretion of body fluids, and temperature regulation. The lack of sensory warning mechanisms and voluntary motor ability below the level of injury coupled with circulatory changes place the spinal cord injured person at major risk for disruption of skin integrity. Significant factors associated with disruption of skin integrity are: pressure, shearing forces, and localized trauma and skin irritation. Relieving pressure, allowing adequate circulation to the skin, and skin inspection are primary ways of maintaining skin integrity. Of all the complications following spinal cord injury, skin breakdown is the most preventable.

Pain. Chronic pain following SCI is a diverse and unpredictable experience that, for some people, can be severe.[28-30] Pain varies in etiology and nature depending on the type and extent of SCI. It is more common among persons with paraplegia compared to persons with quadriplegia.[30] Three types of pain have been described by persons with SCI: central and visceral pain, mechanical pain, and radicular pain.[30,31]

Central pain is a diffuse burning sensation that is experienced in body parts below the level of injury and is aggravated by touch and movement. It is associated with incomplete lesions of the spinal cord and is attributed to CNS mechanisms, possibly an abnormal firing of deafferented input association or projection neurons. Visceral pain involves a poorly localized, burning discomfort of the abdomen and pelvis. It is often related to some intra-abdominal event such as bladder distention or urinary tract infection. It is thought that the etiology of visceral pain may be similar to that of central pain. Mechanical or fracture pain consists of a deep-seated aching sensation over or around the site of spinal fracture. It is thought to result from alterations in normal weight and stress-bearing mechanisms that result in stretching or compression of pain-sensitive structures. Radicular (spinal nerve root) pain presents as an aching or shooting type of pain that radiates into a more or less well-defined nerve root distribution affecting the arm, leg, or trunk. Although the pain occurs in its severest form in partial SCI lesions, it is also seen in transected cauda equina lesions. The cause of radicular pain in SCI is obscure but may result from compression or injury of nerve roots by a herniated nucleus pulposus, a fracture fragment, or a dislocated veretebra or neuronal hyperexcitability due to local ischemia.

The management of chronic pain in a person with SCI begins with assessment measures to determine the type of pain that is present and, if possible, the underlying mechanisms. Transcutaneous electrical nerve stimulation (TENS) and the tricyclic antidepressant drugs (*e.g.,* amitriptyline, doxepin, and imipramine) have proved useful in treating central pain.[31] Mechanical pain is often treated with nonsteroidal anti-inflammatory drugs (NSAID) and physical therapy.[31] Anticonvulsant drugs (carbamazepine and phenytoin) are often effective in relieving radicular pain.[31] The mechanisms of drug action and specifics of chronic pain management are discussed in Chapter 47.

Bowel and bladder function

Among the most devastating consequences of spinal cord injury is the loss of bowel and bladder function. Loss of these functions are apparent immediately postinjury and require a great deal of time, expense, materials, and human energy for management. Micturition, or the act of voiding, can be described as the sequence of events involving sensory input that occurs with bladder filling, activation of the spinal reflex voiding center, stimulation and provision of cerebral control, and progression and termination of actual voiding.[32] While the anatomy and function of the kidneys or production of urine is not greatly altered following spinal cord injury, almost all persons with spinal cord injury experience some loss of blad-

der function. Therefore, management must be directed toward functional improvement of the voiding problem itself.

The neural control of bladder function is supplied by sympathetic nerve fibers that allow for relaxation of the detrusor muscle during bladder filling (T1 to L2), parasympathetic nerve fibers that supply the reflex voiding center (S2 to S4), the motoneurons that travel in the pelvic nerve and supply the external urethral sphincter (S2 to S4), and the micturition center in the brain stem (see Chapter 33). The micturition center coordinates the activity of the detrusor muscle and the external sphincter by way of input from ascending spinal pathways and descending pathways from higher voluntary control centers in the cortex. Following resolution of spinal shock, which renders the bladder areflexic, bladder dysfunction is manifested by disruption of neural pathways between the bladder and the reflex voiding center (lower motoneuron lesion) or between the reflex voiding center and higher brain centers for communication and coordinated sphincter control (upper motoneuron lesion). Persons with UMN or spastic bladders lack awareness of bladder filling (storage) and voluntary control of voiding (evacuation). In LMN or flaccid bladder dysfunction, lack of awareness of bladder filling and lack of bladder tone render the person unable to void voluntarily or involuntarily. Of specific importance to optimal bladder function is the storage and evacuation of urine under low pressure to prevent damage to the bladder and urethra and, more importantly, to the kidneys.

Normally, the low-pressure urine storage mechanism is achieved through sympathetic inhibition of detrusor muscle contractile activity coordinated with increased urethral closing pressure until the reflex voiding threshold is reached. At threshold, the stretched detrusor muscle elicits a parasympathetic response inducing urethral smooth muscle relaxation along with balanced bladder contraction until complete emptying is achieved. After spinal cord injury, involuntary voiding reflexes (UMN) may be elicited during filling along with higher level external sphincter response, which may lead to incontinence and prevent full emptying of the bladder. These reflexes usually occur at high volumes. In LMN injury, there is no bladder function other than storage or external sphincter response leading to retention with overflow and leakage of urine. This loss of control of bladder emptying not only influences the quality of a person's life, but also carries with it a lifetime threat of severe renal problems.

The principal goals of bladder management are to provide low-pressure drainage to the urinary bladder and prevent complications with consideration for the person's physical life-style, potential for cooperation, and support from family and community. Management techniques for neurogenic bladder dysfunctions consist of methods of continuous or intermittent drainage, external collection, and manual techniques (*e.g.*, Crede's maneuver, Valsalva's maneuver, or bladder tapping).

Bowel elimination in spinal cord injury is also a coordinated effort involving the intrinsic nerve supply (intramural plexus) to the large intestine, autonomic nervous system, and, similar to voiding, central nervous system innervation. Intrinsic control of the bowel is supplied by networks of nerve fibers in the bowel wall that respond to fecal distention with increased peristalsis. Parasympathetic innervation from the vagus nerve and the S2 to S4 cord segments, or the defecation reflex center, affects the colon, rectum, and internal and external sphincters. Sympathetic innervation from T6 through L3 segments affects the same area. Parasympathetic effects are seen in increased motility and peristalsis, relaxed sphincter tone, increased gastrointestinal secretions, maintenance of smooth muscle tone; while sympathetic activity provides the antagonistic control to the parasympathetic effects.

Defecation is controlled by communications between the brain, the defecation center (S2 to S4), and the external anal sphincter. After spinal cord injury, UMN damage can occur when injury to the cord is sustained above the S2 to S4 cord segments. The person acquires spastic functioning of the defecation reflex with involuntary control of the external sphincter. Lower motoneuron injury occurs with damage to the cord at the defecation reflex center or between the S2 to S4 segments and the external sphincters. This causes flaccid functioning of the defecation reflex and loss of anal sphincter tone. Even though intrinsic contractile responses are intact, without the defecation reflex, peristaltic movements are ineffective in evacuating stool.

The goal of bowel management following spinal cord injury is to establish complete evacuations, which minimize incontinence and complications and afford dignity and independence to the person. The principal methods of bowel management include measures such as a high-fluid and high-fiber diet, mobility at the highest level that is possible, medications, consistent timing of evacuation, privacy and positioning, and techniques such as digital stimulation and Valsalva's maneuver.

Sexual function

While the physical act of sex itself may change with SCI, the ability to enjoy a caring relationship with another person remains and often takes on greater importance than prior to injury.

Spinal cord injury at any level abolishes communication pathways between the genital and higher centers. Erotic and emotional feelings and thoughts, however, may still be experienced in areas above the level of injury, especially when the mouth and neck are stimulated. Extragenital circulatory, musculoskeletal, and respiratory responses such as increased heart rate, breathing, and muscle tone that are mediated by centers above the level of injury may occur.

Sexual function, as in bladder and bowel control, is mediated by the S2 to S4 segments of the spinal cord. The genital sexual response in SCI, which is manifested by an erection in men and vaginal lubrication in women, may be initiated by mental or touch stimuli depending on the level of injury. The T11 to L2 cord segments have been identified as the mental-stimuli sexual response area where autonomic nerve pathways in communication with the cortex leave the cord and innervate the genitalia. The S2 to S4 cord segments have been identified as the sexual-touch reflex center. In a T10 or above SCI (UMN lesion), reflex sexual response to genital touch may occur freely. However, a sexual response to mental stimuli (T11 to L2) will not occur due to the spinal lesion blocking the communication pathway. In an injury at T12 or below (LMN), the sexual reflex center may be damaged and there may be no response to touch. Therefore, cord damage below the T12 segment may result in sexual arousal by mental stimuli. For persons with lesions between L2 to S1, sexual response to mental or touch stimuli may occur. In men, lack of erectile ability or inability to experience penile sensations or orgasm is not a reliable indicator of fertility, which should be evaluated by an expert. In women, fertility is parallel to menses; usually it is delayed 3 months to 5 months after injury. There are hazards to pregnancy, labor, and birth control devices relative to SCI that require understanding, but need not be prohibitive. The severity of injury is not the most important determining factor in the outcome of sexual well-being. Satisfaction is most often the result of good sexual communication and shared intimacy and is independent of orgasm.

The spinal cord continuum of care

The spinal cord continuum of care begins the moment of injury and ensues throughout the life span. While it is not in the scope of this text to address the psychosocial issues surrounding SCI, one cannot deal with the physical problems without encountering the emotional and behavioral effects. Some aspects of SCI may be predictable, however, there are many factors that influence the outcome. One approach to life with

SCI may be with relation to concepts of health stabilization or restoration of physical function, life-style modification or integration of physical deficits with premorbid life-style and postinjury status, and community integration or independent functioning and socialization in the community (Table 49-3). Rather than stages, or phases, of recovery and rehabilitation in SCI, it may be thought of as a perpetual cycle that the person enters and re-enters at any point along the life span. As aspects of one area change, so do the others in response to the needs of the person in establishing a mind and body wellness equilibrium. Health stabilization concerns surround the restoration of physical function, whether due to acute or chronic changes, as well as the psychosocial mechanisms necessary to deal with the situation on a short-term basis. Life-style modification deals with incorporating the changes in physical function with developmental tasks and cognitive exploration of beliefs and values regarding health, wellness, disability, self, and others. Community integration focuses on applying life-style modifications for independent living in realistic situations. The impact of physical disability in unstructured and unpredictable situations provides for the ultimate challenge in socialization and independent functioning.

The future of spinal cord injury

Prevention of SCI is of paramount importance. In the meantime, the major questions revolve around the optimal care for persons who sustain spinal cord injury. The issues relate to the methods of management that allow for the best chance of preserving neurologic function and preventing complications. It is now known that the spinal cord not only suffers immediate physical effects from trauma, but also secondary pathologic processes such as ischemia and edema. Decreased blood flow and edema lead to small vessel compression; decreased oxygenation of tissue; release of vasoactive substances such as norepinephrine, dopamine, and serotonin; and damage to cell membranes affecting maintenance of cellular sodium and potassium levels. A substantial amount of research is being directed toward developing methods to arrest and reverse these damaging effects. Using devices to produce hypothermia and thus decrease the metabolic needs of the cord and to supply oxygen to the damaged cord through the use of hyperbaric oxygen are two methods being studied. Medications to stabilize the capillary endothelial membrane, maintain intracellular potassium, and preserve lysosomal and membrane-bound isoenzymes have also been investigated with controversial results.

In general, adequate immobilization immediately following injury is a necessary and effective treatment. Immediate surgery remains controversial. Up to this time, it has not been found to produce better outcomes or return of function.[33] The principal disadvantage is that immediate surgery is traumatizing to an already traumatized cord and, in fact, may cloud other injuries or complications. Early surgical treatment procedures of the spine are aimed at internal skeletal stabilization so that early mobilization and rehabilitation may occur. Other mechanical research involves functional electrical stimulation to reactivate paralyzed systems, nerve regeneration, and tissue-bridge implants to provide support for regenerating CNS axons across a damaged area. Until a cure is found, prevention in the form of health promotion, early diagnosis, and prompt intervention and rehabilitation to prevent further complications and restore optimal functioning is essential.

In summary, SCI is a disabling neurologic condition most commonly caused by motor vehicle accidents, falls, and sports injuries. It occurs most frequently in males and people under 30 years of age. SCI is caused by abnormal motion or trauma to the spinal column; it includes injuries caused by excessive forward and lateral flexion, rotation, and extension of the spinal column. Dysfunctions of the nervous system following SCI cover varying degrees of sensorimotor

Table 49-3. The spinal cord continuum of care

Health stabilization	Life-style education	Community integration
Ventilation/communication function	Self care	Physical barriers
Autonomic nervous system regulation	Mobility	Equipment needs
Bowel and bladder control		Home care availability
Sensorimotor integrity		Professional health-care availability
Psychosocial impact	Psychosocial barriers	Psychosocial balance
	Developmental/cognitive level	Community re-entry
	Values/beliefs	Support systems
	Self concept/sexuality	Role adjustment
	Client/family education	

loss and altered reflex activity based on the level of injury and extent of cord damage. Dependent on the level of injury, the physical problems of SCI include spinal shock; ventilation/communication problems; autonomic nervous system dysfunction that predisposes to the vasovagal response, autonomic hyperreflexia, impaired body temperature regulation, and postural hypotension; altered sensorimotor integrity that contributes to uncontrolled muscle spasms, altered pain responses, and threat to skin integrity; impaired muscle pump and venous innervation leading to edema of dependent areas of the body and risk of deep vein thrombosis; alterations in bowel and bladder elimination; and impaired sexual function. The treatment of SCI involves a continuum of care that begins at the moment of injury and ensues throughout the life span. The continuum of care incorporates health stabilization or restoration of physical function, life-style modification or integration of physical deficits with premorbid life-style and postinjury status, and community integration or independent functioning and socialization in the community. SCI research focuses on prevention of injury, preservation of neurologic function, and prevention of complications.

References

1. Berne RM, Levy MN: Physiology, 2nd ed, pp 244, 51. St Louis, CV Mosby, 1988
2. Guyton A: Medical Physiology, 7th ed, p 633. Philadelphia, WB Saunders, 1986
3. Noback CR, Demarest RJ: The Human Nervous System, 3rd ed, p 197. New York, McGraw-Hill, 1981
4. Smith PEM, Calverley PMA, Edwards RHT et al: Practical problems in the respiratory care of patients with muscular dystrophy. N Engl J Med 316:1197, 1987
5. Bartlett RJ, Pericak-Vance MA, Koh J et al: Duchenne muscular dystrophy: High frequency of deletions. Neurology 38:1, 1988
6. Slater CR: The missing link in DMD? Nature 330:693, 1987
7. Webster C, Silberstein L, Hays AR et al: Fast muscle fibers are preferentially affected in Duchenne muscular dystrophy. Cell 52:503, 1988
8. Lindstrom JM, Keesey JC, Mulder DG: Myasthenia gravis—Current concepts. West J Med 142:797, 1985
9. Vincent A: Acetylcholine receptors and myasthenia gravis. Clin Endocrinol Metab 12:57, 1983
10. Robbins SL, Kumar V: Basic Pathology, 4th ed, pp 720–721. Philadelphia, WB Saunders, 1987
11. Sellman MS, Mayer RF: Weakness and 'tiredness': When to suspect myasthenia gravis. Geriatrics 40(1):92, 1985
12. Cormack DH: Ham's Histology, 9th ed, pp 335, 373–374. Philadelphia, JB Lippincott, 1987
13. Hodgkins ML, Grady D: Carpal tunnel syndrome. West J Med 148:217, 1988
14. Margolis W, Krause JF: The prevalence of carpal tunnel syndrome in female supermarket checkers. J Occup Med 29:953, 1987
15. Barnhardt S, Rosinstock L: Carpal tunnel in grocery checkers. West J Med 147:37, 1987
16. Bowens BA: Carpal tunnel syndrome. J Neurosurg Nurs 19:129, 1981
17. Prydun M: Guillain-Barré syndrome. J Neurosurg Nurs 15:27, 1983
18. Ferner R, Barnet M, Hughes RAC: Management of Guillain-Barré syndrome. Br Hosp Med 2:525, 1987
19. Magoun HW, Rhines R: An inhibitory mechanism in the bulbar reticular formation. J Neurophysiol 9:165–171, 1946
20. McCouch GP, Austin GM, Liu C-N et al: Sprouting as a cause of spasticity. J Neurophysiol 21:205, 1958
21. Mariani, J, Delhaye-Bouchaud N: Elimination of functional synapses during development of the nervous system. NIPS 2:93, 1987
22. Lund RD: Development and Plasticity of the Brain. New York, Oxford University Press, 1978
23. National Spinal Cord Injury Statistical Center: Spinal Cord Injury Fact Sheet. Birmingham, University of Alabama, 1987
24. Buchanan L, Nawoczensk DA: Spinal Cord Injury: Concepts and Management Approaches. Baltimore, Williams and Wilkins, 1987
25. Chui L, Bhatt K: Autonomic dysreflexia. Rehab Nurs (Mar-Apr): 16, 1983
26. Casas ER, Sanchez MP, Arias CR et al: Prophylaxis of venous thrombosis and pulmonary embolism in patients with acute traumatic spinal cord lesions. Paraplegia 14:178, 1976
27. Brach BB, Moser DM, Cedar L et al: Venous thrombosis in acute spinal cord paralysis. J Trauma 17:289, 1977
28. Waibrod H, Hansen D, Gerbershagen HU: Chronic pain in paraplegia. Neurosurgery 15:933, 1984
29. Nepomuceno C, Fine PR, Richards JS et al: Pain in patients with spinal cord injury. Arch Phys Med Rehab 60:605, 1979
30. Woolsey RM: Chronic pain following spinal cord injury. Paraplegia 19(3 & 4):27, 1986
31. Farkash AE, Portenoy RK: The pharmacologic management of chronic pain in the paraplegic patient. Paraplegia 19(3 & 4):41, 1986
32. Zedjlik CM: Management of Spinal Cord Injury, p 271. California, Wadsworth Sciences Division, 1983
33. Maiman DJ, Larson SJ, Benzel EC: Neurological improvement associated with late decompression of the thoracolumbar spinal cord. Neurosurgery 14:302, 1984

Bibliography

Adelstein W, Watson P: Cervical spine injuries. J Neurosurg Nurs 15(2):65, 1983

Berk PA: Dyskinesias: Nursing care and surgical intervention. J Neurosurg Nurs 14(1):23, 1982

Black K: Spinal cord injuries. Top Acute Care Trauma Rehab 1:1, 1987

Carew, TJ: Posture and locomotion. In Kandel ER, Schwartz JH (eds): Principles of Neural Science, 2nd ed, pp 478–486. New York, Elsevier, 1981

Chan CW: Some techniques for relief of spasticity and their physiological basis. Physio Can 38(2):85, 1986

Dudas S, Stevens KA: Central cord injury: Implications for nursing. J Neurosurg Nurs 16(2):84, 1984

Erickson RP: Autonomic hyperreflexia: Pathophysiology and medical management. Arch Phys Med Rehab 61:431, 1980

FitzGerald MJT: Neuroanatomy: Basic and Applied. Philadelphia, Bailliere Tindall, 1985

Ghetz C: Voluntary movement. In Kandel ER, Schwartz JH (eds) Principles of Neural Science, 2nd ed, pp 487–501. New York, Elsevier, 1981

Goddard LR: Sexuality and spinal cord injury. J Neurosci Nurs 20:240, 1988

Kaslow RA, Sullivan-Bolyai JZ, Holman RC et al: Risk factors for Guillain-Barré syndrome. Neurology 37:685, 1987

Klawans HL: Chorea. Can J Neurol Sci 14:536, 1987

McGeer PL, McGeer EF, Itagaki S et al: Anatomy and physiology of the basal ganglia. Can J Neurol Sci 14:363, 1987

Merrit JL: Management of spasticity in spinal cord injury. Mayo Clin Proc 56:614, 1981

Pettibone KA: Management of spasticity in spinal cord injury: Nursing concerns. J Neurosci Nurs 20:217, 1988

Pollard JD: A critical review of therapies in acute and chronic inflammatory demyelinating polyneuropathies. Muscle Nerve 10:214, 1987

Rice GPA: Pharmacotherapy of spasticity: Some theoretical and practical considerations. Can J Neurol Sci 14:510, 1987

Ruby EB: Advanced Neurological and Neurosurgical Nursing. St Louis, CV Mosby, 1984

Walton JN: Brain's Diseases of the Nervous System, 3rd ed. New York, Oxford University Press

Disorders of Brain Function

Objectives

After you have studied this chapter, you should be able to meet the following objectives:

_____ Describe the organization of the brain on the basis of embryonic development.

_____ Describe the location and functions of the forebrain, midbrain, pons, cerebellum, and medulla.

_____ Cite the origin of cranial nerves XII, XI, X, IX, VIII, VII, VI, V, IV, and III.

_____ Describe the function of the cranial nerves XII, XI, X, IX, VIII, VII, VI, V, IV, and III, and relate to manifestations of altered function that occur with injury or disease.

_____ State the characteristics of the dominant and nondominant hemispheres of the brain.

_____ Describe the location of the frontal, parietal, temporal, occipital, and limbic lobes of the cerebral cortex, and state their general classes of function.

_____ Name the layers of the meninges.

_____ Trace the circulation of the cerebral spinal fluid (CSF).

_____ State the contribution of the internal carotid arteries, the vertebral arteries, and the circle of Willis to the cerebral circulation.

(continued)

_____ Trace the two major sources of blood flow to the cerebral circulation and distinguish the differential effects of ischemia on these supplies.

_____ List the major arteries supplying the cerebral cortex and explain why the middle cerebral artery has particular clinical importance.

_____ Explain the autoregulation of cerebral blood flow.

_____ Describe the central nervous system ischemic response.

_____ State the purpose of the blood–brain barrier.

_____ Differentiate between cerebral hypoxia and cerebral ischemia.

_____ Describe the no-reflow phenomenon as it relates to the cerebral circulation.

_____ Define cerebral vascular accident.

_____ Characterize transient ischemic attacks.

_____ Describe the subclavian steal syndrome.

_____ Compare thrombotic strokes, embolic strokes, lacunar infarct strokes, and stroke due to an intracerebral hemorrhage.

_____ Describe the progression of motor deficits that occurs as a result of stroke.

_____ Compare the manifestations of expressive, receptive, fluent, and nonfluent aphasia.

_____ Describe the characteristics of the denial or hemiattention syndrome.

_____ Cite the most common cause of subarachnoid hemorrhage.

_____ State the complications associated with subarachnoid hemorrhage.

_____ Describe the compensatory mechanisms used to prevent large changes in intracranial pressure (ICP) from occurring when there are changes in brain, blood, and CSF volume.

_____ Describe methods for assessing or monitoring changes in ICP.

_____ Compare the causes of communicating and noncommunicating hydrocephalus.

_____ Differentiate between cytotoxic and vasogenic cerebral edema.

_____ Explain the causes of tentorial herniation of the brain and its consequences.

_____ Describe the effects of contrecoup injury.

_____ Compare the symptoms of concussion with those of contusion.

_____ List the constellation of symptoms involved in the postconcussion syndrome.

_____ Differentiate among the location, manifestations, and morbidity associated with epidural, subdural, and intracerebral hematoma.

_____ List the sequence of events that occur with meningitis.

_____ Describe the symptoms of encephalitis.

_____ Relate the activity of the bulboreticular facilatory area to level of consciousness.

_____ Define conscious, confusion, lethargy, obtundation, stupor, and coma.

_____ Trace the progression of symptoms from consciousness to unconsciousness.

_____ State the Harvard criteria of irreversible coma.

_____ Explain the difference between the terms seizure activity and epileptic seizure.

_____ State four or more causes of seizures other than epilepsy.

_____ Differentiate between the origin of seizure activity in partial and generalized forms of epilepsy.

_____ Define clonic and tonic as they relate to seizure activity.

_____ Compare the manifestations of simple partial seizures and complex partial seizures and those of minor motor seizures and major motor seizures.

_____ Describe the precautions to be followed in prescribing anticonvulsant drugs.

_____ Characterize status epilepticus.

The brain is protected from external forces because it is located in the rigid confines of the skull and cushioned by the cerebral spinal fluid. Its internal environment and electrical circuitry are maintained by the blood–brain barrier, and its metabolic needs are protected by regulatory mechanisms that ensure its blood supply. Despite these many protections, the brain is extremely vulnerable to injury from ischemia, trauma, tumors, degenerative processes, and metabolic derangements. Although these same conditions may affect other parts of the body, the distribution and location of function in the brain render it particularly vulnerable to focal lesions. Disturbance in function of a small area of the brain, for example, can severely compromise specific functions such as speech, vision, and the ability to move a particular side of the body.

By contrast, two-thirds of the kidney mass can be destroyed without seriously compromising renal function.

The content in this chapter has been organized into six sections: (1) brain structure and function, (2) alterations in cerebral blood flow, (3) increased intracranial pressure, (4) head injury and infection, (5) altered levels of consciousness, and (6) seizure disorders.

Brain structure and function

The brain is the center for control of meaningful activity. It provides us with a conscious awareness of our surroundings and the ability to feel, hear, see, taste, and smell the world around us; to direct and plan our movements; to speak and interact with people we come in contact with; and to remember previous experiences and use that memory as a basis for decision making. Without the function of higher brain centers, the body functions at a vegetative level.

The brain can be divided into three parts: the forebrain, which forms the two cerebral hemispheres, the thalamus and the hypothalamus; the midbrain; and the hindbrain, which is divided into the pons, cerebellum, and medulla.

An important concept to keep in mind is that the more rostral, recently elaborated parts of the neural tube gain dominance, or control, over regions and functions at lower levels. They do not replace the more ancient circuitry but merely dominate it. Thus, following damage to the more vulnerable parts of the forebrain, a brain stem organism remains capable of respiration and survival if environmental temperature is regulated and if nutrition and other aspects of care are provided. However, all aspects of intellectual function, including experience, perception, and memory, are usually lost.

Development of the brain

The structure and organization of the brain usually become clearer when considered in the context of embryonic development. In the process of development, the more rostral part of the embryonic neural tube—approximately ten segments—undergoes extensive modification and enlargement to form the brain (Figure 50-1). In the early embryo, three swellings, or primary vesicles, develop, subdividing

these ten segments into the prosencephalon (forebrain), which contains the first two segments; the metencephalon, or midbrain, which develops from segment 3; and the rhombencephalon, or hindbrain, which develops from segments 4 to 10 (Figure 50-2). The ten brain segments represent modifications of the spinal cord level neural tube and are often called, collectively, *the brain stem.* The term does not include later developed outgrowths—the cerebral hemispheres, the optic nerve and retina, and the cerebellum.

The central canal of the prosencephalon develops two pairs of lateral outpouchings, which carry the neural tube with them: (1) the optic cup, which becomes the optic nerve and retina, and (2) the telencephalic vesicles, which become the cerebral hemispheres with their enlarged cerebrospinal fluid-filled cavities, the first and second, or lateral, ventricles. The remaining neural tube of these three segments is called the diencephalon ("between brain"); it develops into the thalamus and hypothalamus. The neurohypophysis (posterior pituitary) grows as a midline ventral outgrowth at the junctions of segments 1 and 2. A dorsal outgrowth, the pineal body, develops between segments 2 and 3, the diencephalic–mesencephalic junction.

The ventral half of the neural tube gray matter, the basal lamina, becomes the output oriented horn of the spinal cord and brain stem, including the hypothalamus. Most of the brain, as seen grossly, represents tremendous enlargements, outpouchings, outgrowths, and cortex formation derived from the alar lamina, which in the spinal cord is the source of the dorsal horns.

Both the central and peripheral nervous systems differentiate very early in embryonic life and hold a critical position in providing a necessary stimulus for differentiation of many other body tissues, particularly the skeletal muscles. By the end of the third month of gestation, the gross structure of the brain and spinal cord is established. The remaining period of intrauterine growth involves increases in cell number of both neurons and glial cells to a final neural-to-glial ratio of about 1:20 synaptic relationships that develop during this period and provide the basic circuitry required for subsequent mature neural function. Axon overgrowth of the major tract systems and the myelination of most of these occur during this vulnerable period. A phenomenal increase in brain weight occurs during the 3- to 5-month period of intrauterine life. At birth, the average brain weighs about 300 g, approximately 12.5% of total body weight. During postuterine life, brain growth continues, but at a decreasing rate, while body growth continues at an increasing rate. As a result, the adult human brain weight (1450–1500 g in the male, and

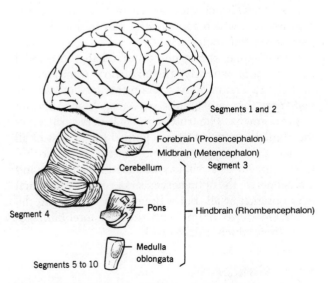

Segments 1 and 2

Forebrain (Prosencephalon)

Midbrain (Metencephalon)

Cerebellum

Segment 3

Segment 4

Pons

Hindbrain (Rhombencephalon)

Medulla
oblongata

Segments 5 to 10

Figure 50-1 The segments of the forebrain, midbrain, and hindbrain. (*Modified from Chaffee EE, Lytle IM: Basic Physiology and Anatomy, 4th ed, p 203. Philadelphia, JB Lippincott, 1980*)

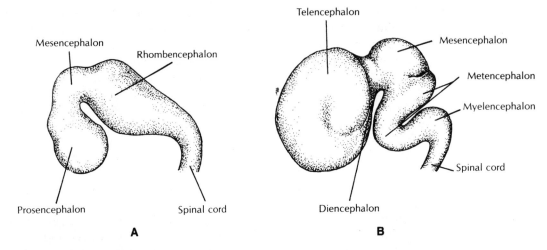

Figure 50-2 **A**, Primary brain vesicles (fifth week). **B**, Secondary brain vesicles (seventh week). The diencephalon is partly hidden by the expanding telencephalon, which develops into the cerebral hemispheres. (*Barr ML, Kiernan JA: The Human Nervous System: An Anatomical Viewpoint, 5th ed, p 5. Philadelphia, JB Lippincott, 1988*)

1200–1300 g in the female) is about five times that at birth and yet is only about 2.4% of total body weight. Maximum brain weight is reached between ages 20 and 29 and is then followed by a gradual decrease in weight with advancing years.

During the latter two-thirds of intrauterine life, the cerebral cortex increases its volume relative to that of deeper structures; this is achieved by a greatly increased surface area, which occurs with increasing development of the number and depth of infoldings. The adult cerebral cortex, with its many infoldings, or grooves, is equivalent to an area of about 160,000 mm^2 and contains about 16.5 billion neurons.[1] The most recently enlarged parts of the neocortex develop later in postnatal life, particularly the portions of the frontal, parietal, and temporal cortex that grow out and cover the insula. The cerebellar cortex also undergoes a tremendous increase in area during the latter half of embryonic life and infancy, achieving an area of 84,000 mm^2, again with the development of many deep sulci and narrow gyri. The cerebellar cortex of the adult contains approximately 100 billion neurons.

The third neural tube segment, which forms the midbrain, retains its basic spinal segment-like organization. Segment 4 of the rhombencephalon becomes much enlarged and flattened laterally, giving the fourth ventricle its rhomboid shape. This segment, called the *metencephalon,* or pons, also grows up and over the fourth ventricle and is a major contributor to the function of the fully developed cerebellum.

The remaining segments, 5 through 10, become the medulla oblongata, with the widened fourth ventricle narrowing to form a central canal, which continues through the spinal cord segments. The most rostral segment (5) of the medulla fuses with the pons

and is often called the caudal pons. It also contributes to the caudal part of the cerebellum. The junction of segment 10 of the brain stem with the cervical spinal segments occurs at the foramen magnum, the large opening in the skull through which the neural tube passes.

Each of these brain segments, except for segment 2, retains some portion of the basic segmental organization of the nervous system. The evolutionary development of the brain is reflected in the cranial nerves and upper cervical segmental nerves because the original pattern was for many branches to occur directly from the neural tube, each containing a particular component, or functional grouping, of axons. Thus, one segment would have paired branches to body muscles and another set of visceral structures, and so on. The classic pattern of the spinal nerve organization, which consists of a pair of dorsal and a pair of ventral roots, is a more recent evolutionary development that has not occurred in the cranial nerves. Consequently, the arbitrary numbered 1 through 12 cranial nerves retain the ancient pattern, and more than one cranial nerve can branch from a single segment. The truly segmental nerve pattern of the cranial nerves is further clouded by the loss of all branches from segment 2 and most of the branches from segment 1. It should be noted that the second cranial nerve, the optic nerve, is not really a segmental nerve branch at all, but a brain tract connecting the retina (modified brain) with the first forebrain segment from which it developed.

─── Hindbrain

The hindbrain (medulla and pons) is a distorted, enlarged, and elaborated version of the spinal cord. It contains the neuronal circuits required for the basic breathing, eating, and locomotive functions required for survival. It is surrounded on the outside by the long tract systems that interconnect the forebrain with lower parts of the CNS (see Figure 50-1).

—— Medulla

The medulla oblongata represents the caudal five segments of the brain part of the neural tube, and, thus, the cranial nerve branches entering and leaving it have similar functions, as do the spinal segmental nerves. The ventral horn area in the medulla is quite small, but the dorsal horn is enlarged, processing a great amount of the information pouring through the cranial nerves. The segmental peripheral nerve components of the medulla can be divided into those that leave the neural tube ventromedially (hypoglossal and abducent cranial nerves) and those that exit dorsolaterally (vagus, spinal accessory, glossopharyngeal, and vestibulocochlear cranial nerves). Because the signs and symptoms of pathology reflect the spatial segregation of brain stem components, neurologic syndromes resulting from trauma, tumors, aneurysms, and cerebrovascular accidents are often classified as ventral or dorsolateral syndromes.

The lower motoneurons (LMNs) of the lower segments of the medulla supply the extrinsic and intrinsic muscles of the tongue by means of the *hypoglossal (XII) cranial nerve.* Damage to the hypoglossal nerve results in partial or total denervation and, therefore, weakness or paralysis of tongue muscles. When the tongue is protruded, it deviates toward the damaged and therefore weak side because of the greater protrusion strength on the normal side. The axons of the hypoglossal nerve leave the medulla adjacent to two long, longitudinal ridges along the medial undersurface of the medulla called the pyramids. The pyramids contain the corticospinal axons that provide for fine manipulative control for the spinal LMNs. Lesions of the ventral surface of the caudal medulla result in the syndrome of alternating *hypoglossal hemiplegia,* characterized by signs of ipsilateral (same side) denervation of the tongue and contralateral (opposite side) weakness or paralysis of both the upper and lower extremities.

The *vagus nerve (X)* has both afferent sensory and efferent motor fibers that innervate the gastrointestinal tract (from the laryngeal pharynx to the midtranserve colon), the heart, and the lungs; the pharyngeal taste buds (special visceral afferents) and muscles of the pharynx and larynx. The fibers carried in the vagus are responsible for both afferent and an important efferent innervation of these structures and therefore for initiation of many essential reflexes and for many normal functions. For example, 80% of the

fibers of the vagus are afferents, some of which are involved in initiated vomiting and hiccup reflexes and in ongoing feedback during swallowing and speech. The unilateral loss of vagal function results in slowed gastrointestinal motility, a permanently husky voice, and deviation of the uvula away from the damaged side. Bilateral loss of vagal function seriously damages reflex maintenance of cardiovascular and respiratory reflexes. Swallowing becomes difficult and in some cases paralysis of laryngeal structures causes life-threatening airway obstruction. Endotracheal intubation or tracheostomy is then necessary to prevent asphyxia.

The powerful head-turning muscle, the sternocleidomastoid, and the trapezius muscle, which elevates the shoulders, are innervated by the *spinal assessory (XI)* cranial nerve with LMNs in the upper four cervical spine segments. Lateral rootlets from these segmental levels combine and enter the cranial cavity through the foramen magnum and then exit through the jugular foramen with cranial nerves (IX) and (X). Loss of spinal accessory nerve function results in drooping of the shoulder on the damaged side and weakness when turning the head to the opposite side.

The dorsolateral *glossopharyngeal (IX)* cranial nerve contains the same components as the vagus nerve, but for a more rostral segment of the gastrointestinal tract and the pharynx. This nerve provides the special sensory innervation of the taste buds of the oral pharynx and the back of the tongue; the afferent innervation of the oral pharynx and the baroreceptors of the carotid sinus; the efferent innervation for the otic ganglion, which controls the salivary function of the parotid gland; and the efferent innervation of the stylopharyngeal muscle of the pharynx. This cranial nerve is seldom damaged, but when it is, anesthesia of the ipsilateral oral pharynx and dry mouth because of reduced salivation occur.

The *vestibulocochlear (VIII)* cranial nerve, formerly called the auditory nerve, is attached laterally at the junction of the medulla oblongata and the pons. It consists of two distinct fiber divisions, both of which are purely sensory: (1) the cochlear division, which arises from cell bodies in the cochlea in the inner ear and transmits impulses related to the sense of hearing, and (2) the vestibular division, which arises from two ganglia which innervate cell bodies in utricle, saccule, and semicircular canals and transmits impulses related to head position and movement of the body through space. Injury to the cochlear division results in tinnitus or nerve deafness versus conduction deafness; injury to the vestibular division leads to vertigo, nystagmus, and some postular instability.

In the most rostral segment of the medulla, LMNs send their axons out ventrally on either side of the pyramids and then forward into the orbit through the *abducent (VI) cranial nerves* to innervate the lateral rectus muscles of the eyes. As the name indicates, the abducent nerves abduct the eye (lateral and outward rotation); peripheral damage to them results in weakness or loss of eye abduction medial strabismus.

The facial nerve (VII) and its intermediate component (the intermedius) contain both afferent and efferent components. The intermedius nerves innervate the nasopharynx and taste buds of the palate, the forward two-thirds of the tongue, the submandibular and sublinguinal salivary glands, the lacrimal glands, and mucous membranes of the nose and roof of the mouth. Loss of this branch of the facial nerve can lead to eye dryness with risk of corneal scarring and blindness. Frequent irrigation of the conjunctival sac with an artificial tear solution is necessary. The LMNs of the facial nerve innervate the muscles that control head movements and facial expression: wrinkling of the brow, wiggling of the ears, movement of the scalp, and forceful closure of the eyes, nose, and lips. Unilateral loss of facial nerve function results in flaccid paralysis of the muscles of one-half of the head, a condition called *Bell's palsy*. The facial nerve passes through a bony canal at the back of the middle ear cavity. Bell's palsy has been attributed to inflammatory reactions involving the facial nerve in or near this bony canal. Because such injuries result from pressure caused by edematous tissue, the integrity of the endoneurial tube is retained and regeneration with full recovery of all muscles generally occurs within a period of several months.

Pons

The pons, or bridge, develops from the fourth neural tube segment. The central canal of the spinal cord, which is greatly enlarged in the pons and rostral medulla, forms the fourth ventricle (Figure 50-3). An enlarged area on the ventral surface of the pons contains the pontine nuclei, which receive information from all parts of the cerebral cortex. The axons of these neurons form a massive bundle that swings around the lateral side of the fourth ventricle to enter the cerebellum. The reticular formation of the pons is large and contains the circuitry for masticating food and manipulating the jaws during speech. The trigeminal (V) and facial (VII) cranial nerves have their origin in the pons.

The *trigeminal (V) cranial nerve,* which has sensory and motor subdivisions, exits the brain stem laterally on the forward surface of the pons. The trigeminal is the main sensory nerve conveying the modalities of pain, temperature, touch, and proprioception to the superficial and deep regions of the face. The regions innervated include the skin of the anterior scalp and face, the conjunctiva and orbit, the meninges, the paranasal sinuses, and the mouth, including the teeth and the anterior two-thirds of the tongue. The LMNs of the trigeminal nerve innervate skeletal muscles that are involved with mastication, which also contribute to swallowing and speech, movements of the soft palate, and tension of the tympanic membrane. The latter apparently has a protective reflex

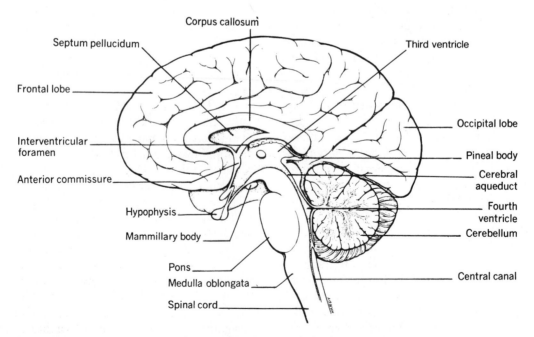

Figure 50-3 Midsagittal section of the brain. (*Chaffee EE, Lytle IM: Basic Physiology and Anatomy, 4th ed, p 214. Philadelphia, JB Lippincott, 1980*)

function, dampening movement of the middle ear ossicles during high intensity sound.

Cerebellum

The cerebellum, or "little brain," is located above the fourth ventricle. Similar to a complicated computer system, the cerebellum serves to interrelate visual, auditory, somatesthetic, and vestibular information with ongoing motor activity so that highly skilled movement can be smoothly performed. Functions of the cerebellum are discussed in Chapter 49.

Midbrain

The midbrain develops from the third segment of the neural tube and its organization is similar to that of a spinal segment. The central canal is re-established as the cerebral aqueduct, interconnecting the fourth ventricle with the third ventricle (see Figure 50-3). The oculomotor (III) and trochlear (IV) cranial nerves are located in the midbrain.

Massive fiber bundles of the cerebral peduncles pass from the forebrain to the pons along the ventral surface of the midbrain. On the dorsal surface, four "little hills," the superior and inferior colliculi, are areas of cortical formation. The inferior colliculus is involved in directional turning and, to some extent, the experiencing of the direction of sound sources. The superior colliculus is an essential part of the reflex mechanisms that control eye movements when the visual environment is being surveyed.

The central gray matter contains the LMNs that innervate most of the skeletal muscles that move the optic globe about and raise the eyelids. These axons leave the midbrain through the *oculomotor (III)* cranial nerve. This nerve also contains axons that control pupillary constriction and ciliary muscle focusing of the lens. Damage to the ventrally exiting cranial nerve III and to the adjacent cerebral peduncle, which includes the corticospinal axon system on one side, results in paralysis of eye movement combined with contralateral hemiplegia (discussed in Chapter 51).

A small compact group of cells in the ventral part of the central gray matter contains the LMNs that innervate the superior oblique eye muscles that tilt the upper part of the eye toward the face when it is abducted, or turned outward, and tilt it downward and toward the face when the eye is adducted, or turned inward. These axons emerge dorsolaterally and caudally as the *trochlear (IV)* cranial nerve and decussate (cross over) in the medulla before exiting the brain stem. Lesions involving the trochlear cranial nerve are unusual. The diplopia or double vision re-

sulting from such lesions is vertical and effects downward gaze to the opposite side. Walking downstairs becomes particularly difficult.

Forebrain

The forebrain is the most rostral part of the brain; it consists of the telencephalon or "end-brain," and the diencephalon or "between-brain." The diencephalon forms the core of the forebrain, and the telencephalon forms the cerebral hemispheres.

Diencephalon

The two forwardmost brain segments form an enlarged dorsal horn-ventral horn structure with a narrow, deep, enlarged central canal—the third ventricle—separating the two sides. This region is called the *diencephalon.* The dorsal horn part of the diencephalon is the thalamus and subthalamus, and the ventral horn part is the hypothalamus (Figure 50-4).

The dorsal part of the diencephalon, the thalamus, is the location of mechanisms that make experience possible. The thalamus consists of two large egg-shaped masses, one on either side of the third ventricle. The thalamus is divided into several major parts, and each part is divided into distinct nuclei, which are the major relay stations for information going to and from the cerebral cortex. All sensory pathways, except those for smell, have direct projec-

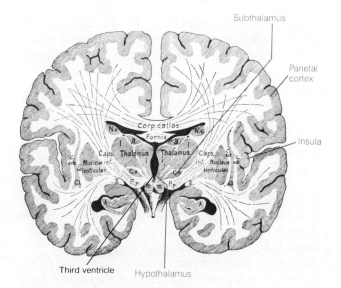

Figure 50-4 Frontal section of the brain passing through the third ventricle showing the thalamus, subthalamus, hypothalamus, internal capsule (*caps int.*), external capsule (*c. ext.*), corpus callosum (*corp. callos.*), basal ganglia (caudate nucleus [*c.s.*], *lenticular nucleus*), insula, and parietal cortex. (*Modified from Villiger E, Addison WHF [eds]: Brain and Spinal Cord. Philadelphia, JB Lippincott, 1931*)

tions to thalamic nuclei, which, in turn convey the information to restricted areas of the sensory cortex. The coordination and integration of peripheral sensory stimuli occur within the thalamus and there is some crude interpretation of highly emotion-laden auditory experiences that not only occur, but can be remembered. Thus, a person can come out of a deep coma and remember a considerable amount of what was said at the bedside. The thalamus also plays a role in relaying critical information regarding motor activities to and from selected areas of the motor cortex. Two neuronal circuits that are significant in this regard are: (1) the pathway from the cerebral cortex to the pons and cerebellum and then, by way of the thalamus, back to the motor cortex, and (2) the feedback circuit that travels from the cortex to the basal ganglia, then to the thalamus, and from the thalamus back to the cortex. Through its connections with the ascending reticular activating system, the thalamus processes neural influences that are basic to cortical excitatory rhythms (those recorded on the electroencephalogram) that are essential to sleep–wakefulness cycles and to the process of attending to stimuli. In addition to their cortical connections, the thalamic nuclei have connections with each other and with neighboring nonthalamic brain structures such as the limbic system. Through their connections with the limbic system, some thalamic nuclei are involved in the relationship between stimuli and their emotional responses. The subthalamus contains movement control systems related to the basal ganglia (see Chapter 49).

The ventral horn portion of the diencephalon is the hypothalamus, which borders the third ventricle and includes a ventral extension, the neurohypophysis (posterior pituitary). The hypothalamus is the area of master-level integration of homeostatic control of the body's internal environment. Maintenance of blood gas concentration, water balance, food consumption, and major aspects of endocrine (see Chapter 44) and autonomic nervous system control (see Chapter 48) require hypothalamic function.

The internal capsule is a broad band of projection fibers that lies between the thalamus medially and the basal ganglia laterally (see Figure 50-4). The internal capsule contains all of the fibers that interconnect the cerebral cortex with deeper structures including the basal ganglia, thalamus, midbrain, pons, medulla, and spinal cord. Lesions of the internal capsule cause serious impairment because many important connections are concentrated in a small area.

Cerebral hemispheres

The two cerebral hemispheres are lateral outgrowths of the diencephalon. The hemispheres contain the lateral ventricles (ventricles I and II), which are interconnected with the third ventricle of the diencephalon by a small opening, called the interventricular foramen (of Monro).

The hemispheres are separated by the heavy longitudinal fold of dura mater (tough mother), called the *falx cerebri,* which attaches to the forward-most floor of the cranial cavity and extends occipitally to fuse with a roughly horizontal fold of dura, the *tentorium cerebelli.* The falx cerebri carries the inferior sagittal venous sinus in its lower edge and the superior sagittal sinus at its junction with the outer dural lining of the cranial cavity. The corpus callosum is a massive commissure, or bridge, of myelinated axons interconnecting the cerebral cortex of the two sides of the brain. Two smaller commissures, the anterior and posterior commissures, connect the two sides of the more specialized regions of the cerebrum and diencephalon.

A section through the cerebral hemispheres will reveal a surface of cerebral cortex, a subcortical layer of white matter made up of masses of myelinated axons, and deep masses of gray matter, the basal ganglia (caudate, putamen, globus pallidus), which border the internal, lateral ventricle.

The surfaces of the hemispheres are lateral (side), medial (area between the two sides of the brain), and basal (underside). The cerebral cortex exposed to view from the side is the recently evolved layered cortex. The surface of the hemispheres contains many ridges and grooves. The ridge between two grooves is called a *gyrus,* and the groove is called a *sulcus.* The cerebral cortex is arbitrarily divided into lobes named after the bones that cover them: the frontal, parietal, temporal, and occipital lobes (Figure 50-5).

Cerebral dominance refers to the fact that control of certain learned forms of behavior is exerted primarily by one of the two cerebral hemispheres. Handedness, perception of language, performance of speech, and appreciation of spatial relationships are primarily expressions of one or the other hemispheres.[2] By convention, speech is usually used to designate the dominant hemisphere. The dominant hemisphere has a major role in verbal and analytic abilities, and the nondominant hemisphere has a major role in nonverbal and artistic abilities. In most persons, even left-handed persons, the left hemisphere is the dominant hemisphere for speech. Although it is assumed that the dominance of speech and handedness are assigned to the same hemisphere, this is not always the case.

The interhemispheric communication pathways are largely undeveloped at birth. The communication pathways between the two hemispheres increase with age and are fairly well developed by the second or third year of life. Cerebral dominance

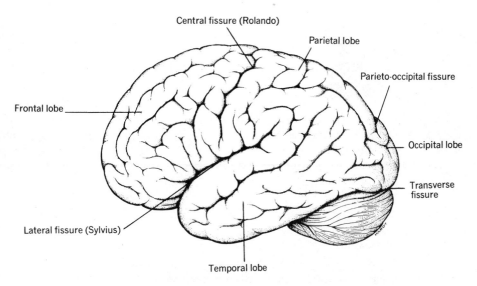

Figure 50-5 Lateral aspect of the left cerebral and cerebellar hemispheres.

probably develops gradually throughout childhood. This explains why a child with a injury to the normally dominant hemisphere can be trained to become left-handed and proficient in speech; whereas, an older person with similar deficits finds such learning difficult or impossible.

Frontal lobe. The frontal lobe extends from the frontal pole to the central sulcus and is separated from the temporal lobe by the lateral sulcus. The frontal lobe can be subdivided rostrally into the frontal pole and laterally into the superior, middle, and inferior gyri, which continue on the undersurface over the eyes as the orbital cortex. The precentral gyrus (area 4), adjacent to the central sulcus, is the primary motor cortex (see Figure 50-5). The frontal cortex just rostral to the precentral gyrus is called the *premotor* or *motor associated cortex* (areas 8, 6). This area is involved in the organization of more complex, learned movement patterns and damage results in dyspraxia or apraxia. Such patients can manipulate a screwdriver, for instance, but cannot use it to loosen a screw.

The regions of the frontal lobe and in front of the association motor cortex are called the premotor frontal cortices. These areas are associated with the medial thalamic nuclei, which are also related to the limbic system. In general terms, the prefrontal cortex appears to be involved in the anticipation and prediction of the consequences of behavior. This "future-oriented" region is particularly depressed by many drugs including alcohol.

Parietal lobe. The parietal lobe of the cerebrum lies behind the central sulcus (the post central gyrus) and above the lateral sulcus. The strip of cortex bordering the central sulcus is called the primary somatosensory cortex (areas 3, 1, 2) because it receives very discrete sensory information from the lateral nuclei of the thalamus (Figure 50-6). Just behind the primary sensory cortex is a region of somesthetic association cortex (areas 5, 7), which is interconnected with thalamic nuclei and with the primary sensory cortex. This region is necessary to appreciate perception or meaningfulness of sensory information. The somesthetic functions of the sensory cortex are discussed in Chapter 47.

Temporal lobe. The temporal lobe lies below the lateral sulcus and merges with the parietal and occipital lobes (see Figure 50-5). It has a polar region and three primary gyri: superior, middle, and inferior. It is separated from the limbic areas on the ventral surface by the collateral or rhinal sulcus. The primary auditory cortex (area 41) involves the part of the superior temporal gyrus that extends into the lateral sulcus (see Figure 50-6). This area is particularly important for fine discrimination from sound entering the opposite ear. The more exposed part of the superior temporal gyrus involves the auditory association or perception area (area 22). The gnostic aspects of hearing (*e.g.*, the meaningfulness of a certain sound pattern, such as that of water dripping) require the function of this area. The remaining portion of the temporal cortex has a less well-defined function but is apparently important in long-term memory recall. Irritation or stimulation can result in vivid hallucinations of long-past events.

The cortices of the frontal, parietal, and temporal lobes surrounding the older cortex of the *insula*, located deep in the lateral fissure, represent the most recently evolved parts of the cerebral cortex. These areas contain primary and association functions for motor control and somesthesias for the lips and tongue

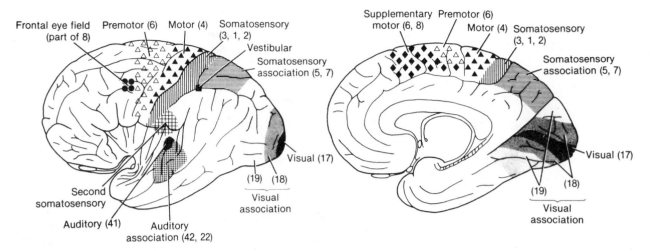

Figure 50-6 Motor and sensory areas of the cerebral cortex. The lateral view (**left**) of the left (dominant) side is drawn as though the lateral sulcus had been pried open, exposing the insula. The diagram on the **right** represents the areas in a brain that has been sectioned in the median plane. (*Reproduced by permission from Nolte J: The Human Brain. St Louis, CV Mosby, 1981*)

and for audition; thus, they are particularly involved in speech mechanisms, which will be discussed later.

Occipital lobe. The occipital lobe is located posterior to the temporal and parietal lobes and is only arbitrarily separated from them. The medial surface of the occipital lobe contains a deep sulcus extending from the limbic lobe to the occipital pole, the *calcarine sulcus,* which contains the primary visual cortex (area 17). Stimulation of this cortex causes the experiencing of bright lights near the visual field. Destruction results in a condition called *cortical blindness* in which the affected person can see nothing, yet has normal visual reflexes to bright lights and moving objects. Just superior and inferior and extending onto the lateral side of the occipital pole is the association cortex for vision (areas 18 and 19). This area is closely connected with the primary visual cortex and with complex nuclei of the thalamus. The integrity of the association cortex is required for gnostic visual function—the meaningfulness of visual experience.

The neocortical areas of the parietal lobe, between the somesthetic and the visual cortices, have a function in interrelating the texture, or "feel," of an object with its visual image. Between the auditory and visual association areas, the parieto-occipital region is necessary for interrelating the sound and image of an object or person.

Limbic lobe. The medial aspect of the cerebrum is organized as three concentric bands of cortex, the limbic lobe, surrounding the interconnection between the lateral and third ventricle (the interventricular foramen). The innermost band just above and below the cut surface of the corpus callosum is folded out of sight but is an ancient, three-layered cortex ending as the hippocampus in the temporal lobe. Just

outside the folded area is a band of transitional cortex, which includes the cingulate and the parahippocampal gyri (Figure 50-7). The neocortex, influencing limbic function, includes the orbital cortex on the underside of the frontal lobe. Outside this is the neocortex of the hemisphere merging into the more specific areas briefly described earlier. This limbic lobe has intimate connections with the medial nuclei and the intralaminar nuclei of the thalamus, with the deep nuclei of the cerebrum (amygdaloid nuclei, septal nuclei) and with the hypothalamus. In general, this region of the brain is involved in emotional experience and in the control of emotion-related behavior. Stimulation of specific areas in this system can lead to feelings of dread, high anxiety, or exquisite pleasure.

Meninges

Inside the skull and vertebral column, the brain and spinal cord are loosely suspended and protected by several connective tissue sheaths called the meninges (Figure 50-8). The surfaces of the spinal cord, brain, and segmental nerves are covered with a delicate connective tissue layer called the *pia mater* (delicate mother). The surface blood vessels and those that penetrate the brain and spinal cord are encased in this protective tissue layer. A second very delicate, nonvascular, and waterproof layer, called the *arachnoid* because of its spider-web appearance, encloses the entire CNS (Figure 50-9). The cerebrospinal fluid (CSF) is contained within the subarachnoid space. Immediately outside the arachnoid is a continuous sheath of strong connective tissue, the *dura mater* (tough mother), which provides the major protection for the brain and spinal cord. The cranial dura often splits into two layers, and the outer layer serves as the

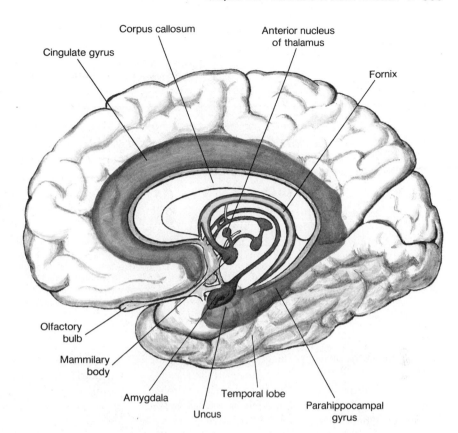

Figure 50-7 The limbic system. This includes the limbic cortex (cingulate gyrus, parahippocampal gyrus, uncus) and associated subcortical structures (thalamus, hypothalmus, amygdala). (*Chaffee EE, Lytle IM: Basic Physiology and Anatomy, 4th ed, p 211. Philadelphia, JB Lippincott, 1980*)

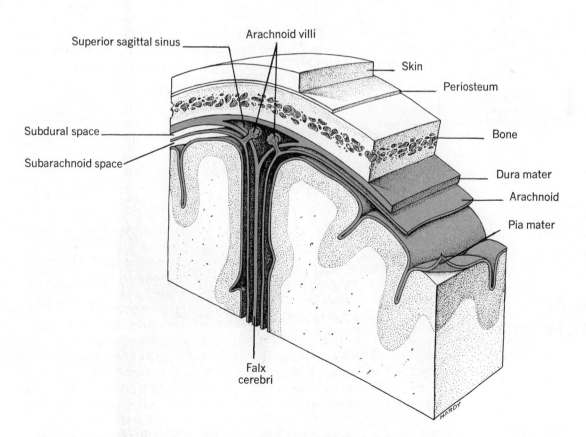

Figure 50-8 The cranial meninges. Arachnoid villi shown within the superior sagittal sinus are one site of cerebrospinal fluid absorption into the blood. (*Chaffee EE, Lytle IM: Basic Physiology and Anatomy, 4th ed. Philadelphia, JB Lippincott, 1980*)

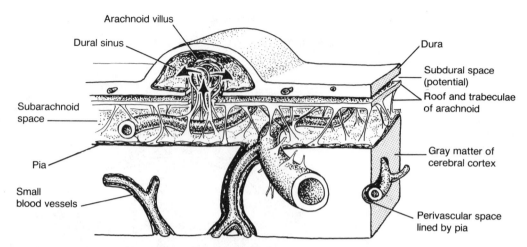

Figure 50-9 Schematic diagram of the three connective tissue membranes (pia, arachnoid, and dura) comprising the meninges of the central nervous system. Cerebrospinal fluid is resorbed by way of the arachnoid villi projecting into the dural sinuses, as indicated by arrows. (*After Weed; from Cormack DH: Ham's Histology, 9th ed, p 367. Philadelphia, JB Lippincott, 1987*)

periosteum of the inner surface of the skull (Figure 50-10).

The inner layer of the dura forms two folds. The first, a longitudinal fold, the *falx cerebri*, separates the cerebral hemispheres and fuses with a second transverse fold, called the *tentorium cerebelli*. The latter acts as a hammock, supporting the occipital lobes above the cerebellum. The tentorium forms a tough septum, which divides the cranial cavity into the anterior and middle fossae, and contains the cerebral hemispheres and a posterior fossa, which lies inferior to it and contains the brain stem and cerebellum. The tentorium attaches to the petrous portion of the temporal bone and the dorsum sellae of the cranial floor, with a semicircular gap, or *incisura*, formed at the midline to permit the midbrain to pass forward from the posterior fossa. The resultant compartmentalization of the cranial cavity is the basis for the commonly used terms *supratentorial*—above the tentorium—and *infratentorial*—below the tentorium. The cerebral

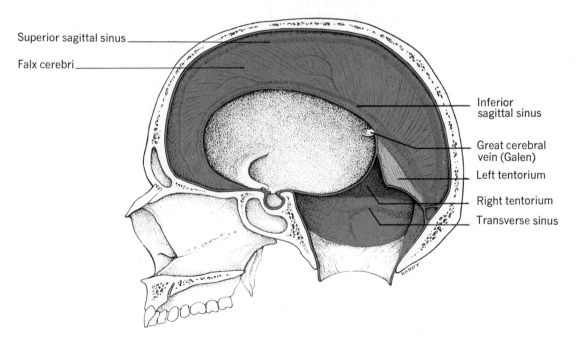

Figure 50-10 Cranial dura mater. The skull is open to show the falx cerebri and the right and left portions of the tentorium cerebelli as well as some of the cranial venous sinuses. (*Chaffee EE, Lytle IM: Basic Physiology and Anatomy, 4th ed, p 219. Philadelphia, JB Lippincott, 1980*)

hemispheres and the diencephalon are supratentorial structures, and the pons, cerebellum, and medulla are infratentorial. The strong folds of the inner dura, the tentorium and falx cerebri, normally support and protect the brain, which floats in the CSF within the enclosed space. During extreme trauma, however, the sharp edges of these folds can damage the brain as it floats inside the cranium. Space-occupying lesions such as enlarging tumors or hematomas can squeeze the brain against these edges or through the small openings of the tentorium, the incisura (herniation). As a result, brain tissue can be compressed, contused, or destroyed, often with permanent deficits (to be discussed).

Ventricular system and cerebrospinal fluid

The linings of the embryonic neural tube undergo multiple foldings in several areas to develop into structures called the *choroid plexuses,* which are present in the ventricular system and which secrete the CSF (Figure 50-11). Although about 500 ml of CSF are secreted each day, the total volume in the ventricular system and spinal canal is only about 150 ml, so that the CSF is completely replaced about three times a day.

The CSF produced in the ventricles must flow through the interventricular foramen, the third ventricle, the cerebral aqueduct, and the midbrain and fourth ventricle to escape from the neural tube. Three other openings, or *foramina,* allow the CSF to flow into the subarachnoid space. Two of these, the *foramina of Luschka,* are located at the lateral corners of the fourth ventricle. The third, the medial *foramen of Magendie,* is located in the midline at the caudal end of the fourth ventricle. About 30% of the CSF passes down into the subarachnoid space that surrounds the spinal cord, mainly on its dorsal surface, and moves back up to the cranial cavity along its ventral surface.

Reabsorption of the CSF into the vascular system occurs along the sides of the superior sagittal

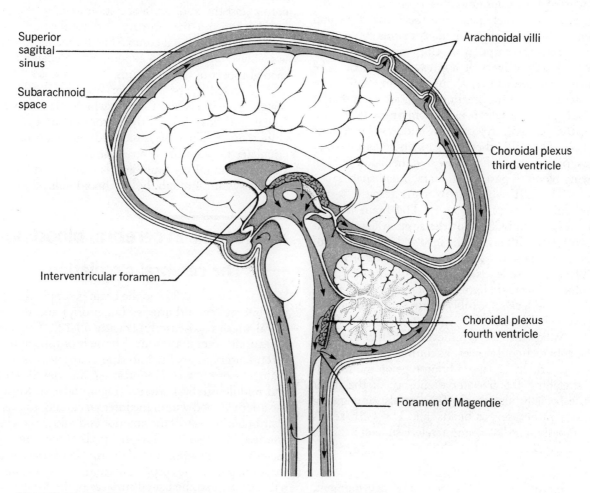

Figure 50-11 The flow of cerebrospinal fluid from the time of its formation from blood in the choroid plexuses until its return to the blood in the superior sagittal sinus. (Note: Plexuses in the lateral ventricles are not illustrated.) (*Chaffee EE, Lytle IM: Basic Physiology and Anatomy, 4th ed, p 221. Philadelphia, JB Lippincott, 1980*)

Table 50–1. Composition of cerebrospinal fluid compared with plasma

Substance	Plasma	Cerebrospinal fluid
Protein mg/dl	7500.00	20.00
Na^+ mEq/liter	145.00	141.00
CL^- mEq/liter	101.00	124.00
K^+ mEq/liter	4.50	2.90
HCO^- mEq/l	25.00	24.00
pH	7.4	7.32
Glucose mg/dl	92.00	61.00

sinus in the anterior and middle fossae. To reach this area, the CSF must pass along the sides of the medulla and pons, and then through the tentorial incisura that surrounds the midbrain. The major part of the flow continues along the sides of the hypothalamus to the region of the optic chiasma and then laterally and superiorly along the lateral fissure and over the parietal cortex to the superior sagittal sinus region. Here the waterproof arachnoid has protuberances, the *arachnoid villi,* which penetrate the inner dura and venous walls of the superior sagittal sinus.

The reabsorption of CSF into the vascular system occurs by way of a pressure gradient. The normal CSF pressure is about 150 mm H_2O. The microstructures of the arachnoid villi are such that, if the CSF pressure falls below approximately 50 mm H_2O, the passageways collapse and reverse flow is blocked. The villi, therefore, function as one-way valves, permitting CSF outflow into the blood but not allowing blood to pass into the arachnoid spaces.

The CSF is similar in many respects to the extracellular fluid (Table 50-1). The brain literally floats in CSF, and CSF provides support for the ventricular system. It may also be involved in a number of other functions and control mechanisms. For example, blood glucose levels are reflected in the CSF, and hypothalamic centers have been shown to respond to these glucose levels, possibly contributing to hunger and eating behaviors.

When the CSF is removed from the ventricles or the subarachnoid spaces, as during a spinal puncture, the partially collapsed brain tugs on the meninges, stretching the free nerve endings of the inner dura, especially along its major vessels, and giving rise to a rather severe headache. The CSF refills fairly rapidly, and headache rarely lasts more than a day or so.

In summary, in the process of development, the most rostral part of the embryonic neural tube develops to form the brain. The brain can be divided into three parts: the hindbrain, midbrain, and forebrain. The hindbrain, consisting of the medulla oblongata and pons, contains the neuronal circuits required for eating, breathing, and locomotive functions required for survival. Cranial nerves XII, XI, X, IX, VIII, VII, VI, and V are located in the hindbrain. The midbrain contains cranial nerves III and IV. The forebrain is the most rostral part of the brain; it consists of the diencephalon and the telencephalon. The dorsal horn part of the diencephalon is the thalamus and subthalamus, and the ventral horn part is the hypothalamus. The cerebral hemispheres are the lateral outgrowths of the diencephalon. One of the hemispheres is the dominant hemisphere; it has a major role in verbal, spatial, and analytic abilities, and the nondominant hemisphere has a major role in nonverbal and artistic abilities. The cerebral hemispheres are arbitrarily divided into lobes, the frontal, parietal, temporal, and occipital lobes, named after the bones of the skull that cover them. The premotor area and primary motor cortex are located in the frontal lobe; the primary sensory cortex and somesthetic association cortex, in the partial cortex; the primary auditory cortex and the auditory association area, in the temporal lobe; and the primary and association visual cortex, in the occipital cortex. The limbic lobe, which is involved with emotion experience, is located in the medial aspect of the cerebrum. The brain is enclosed and protected by the pia mater, arachnoid, and dura mater. The protective CSF in which the brain and spinal cord float, isolates them from minor and moderate trauma. The CSF is secreted into the ventricles, circulates through the ventricular system, passes outside to surround the brain and is reabsorbed into the venous system through the arachnoid villi.

Alterations in cerebral blood flow

The cerebral circulation

The blood flow to the brain is supplied by the two internal carotid arteries (anteriorly) and the vertebral arteries (posteriorly) (Figure 50-12). The internal carotid artery, a terminal branch of the common carotid artery, branches into several arteries: the ophthalmic, posterior communicating, anterior cerebral, and middle cerebral arteries (Figure 50-13). Most of the arterial blood within the internal carotid arteries is distributed by way of the anterior and middle cerebral arteries. The rostral and medial parts of the cerebrum including the anterior half of the thalamus, the corpus striatum, part of the corpus callosum, part of the internal capsule, and the lateral surfaces of the frontal and parietal lobes, are supplied by the anterior cerebral arteries. The posterior cerebral arteries supply the remaining portions of the temporal and occipital lobes.

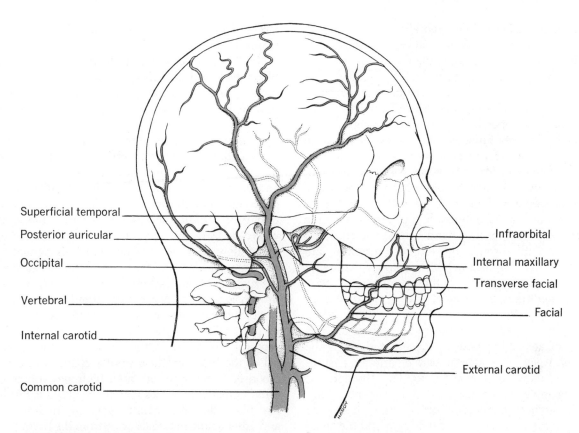

Figure 50-12 Branches of the right external carotid artery. The internal carotid artery ascends to the base of the brain. The right vertebral artery is also shown as it ascends through the transverse foramina of the cervical vertebrae. (*Chaffee EE, Lytle IM: Basic Physiology and Anatomy, 4th ed, p 338. Philadelphia, JB Lippincott, 1980*)

The middle cerebral artery passes laterally, supplying the insula, and then emerges on the lateral cortical surface, supplying the inferior frontal gyrus, the motor and premotor frontal cortex concerned with delicate face and hand control. It is the major vascular source for the primary and association somesthetic cortex for the face and hand and the superior temporal gyrus with the primary and association auditory cortex. It also is a major source of supply for the genu and the posterior limb of the internal capsule and much of the

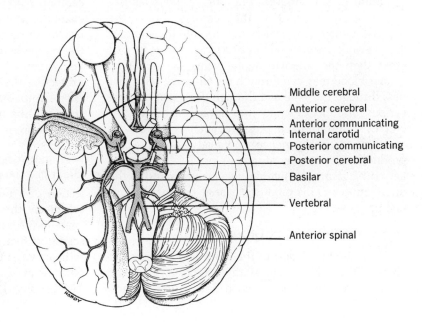

Figure 50-13 The circle of Willis as seen at the base of a brain removed from the skull. (*Chaffee EE, Lytle IM: Basic Physiology and Anatomy, 4th ed, p 852. Philadelphia, JB Lippincott, 1980*)

basal ganglia. The middle cerebral artery is, functionally, a continuation of the internal carotid, and emboli of the internal carotid most frequently become lodged in branches of the middle cerebral. Consequences of ischemia of these areas are perhaps the most devastating, resulting in damage to the fine manipulative skills of the face or upper limb and to both receptive and expressive speech functions. Occlusion of the local branches of the artery result in more restricted deficits.

The two vertebral arteries arise from the subclavian artery and enter the foramina in the transverse spinal processes at the level of the sixth cervical spine and continue upward through the foramina of the upper six vertebrae; they wind behind the atlas and enter the skull through the foramen magnum and unite to form the basilar artery. Branches of the basilar and vertebrate arteries supply the medulla, pons, cerebellum, midbrain, and caudal part of the diencephalon.

The internal carotid and vertebral arteries communicate at the base of the brain through the *circle of Willis;* this anastomosis of arteries ensures continued circulation should blood flow through one of the main vessels be disrupted. There are no significant anastomotic connections other than in these large cerebral vessels at the base of the brain and the small capillary channels within 1 cm of the arterial circle. Occlusions of adjacent or terminal arteries from the large cerebral vessels may result in neural damage because the anastomotic connections may not be adequate to allow blood to reach the ischemic area in sufficient quantity and with sufficient rapidity to meet the high metabolic needs of the occluded area.

The cerebral blood is drained by two sets of veins: the deep, or great, cerebral venous system and the superficial venous system; both systems empty into the dural venous sinuses. The dural venous sinuses return blood and CSF to the heart by way of the internal jugular vein, which empties into the superior vena cava. Venous blood has alternative routes for exit other than the internal jugular veins; for example, venous blood may exit through the emissary veins that pass through the skull and through veins that traverse various foramina to empty into extracranial veins. Increases in intrathoracic pressure, such as occur with coughing or performance of Valsalva's maneuver, produce a rise in central venous pressure that is reflected back into the internal jugular veins and to the dural sinuses. This produces a brief rise in intracranial pressure.

Regulation of blood flow

The blood flow to the brain is maintained at about 750 ml/min or one-sixth of the resting cardiac output. The regulation of blood flow to the brain is largely controlled by autoregulatory or local mechanisms that respond to the metabolic needs of the brain. The autoregulation (self-regulation) of cerebral blood flow is very efficient within a mean arterial blood pressure range of about 60 mmHg to 160 mmHg. In persons with hypertension, this autoregulatory range shifts to a higher level.

At least three different metabolic factors have been shown to affect cerebral brain flow: carbon dioxide concentration, hydrogen ion concentration, and oxygen concentration. Increased carbon dioxide concentration and increased hydrogen ion concentration produce an increase in cerebral blood flow; whereas decreased oxygen concentration increases blood flow. Carbon dioxide, which is converted to carbonic acid in body fluids, exerts its effect through the hydrogen ion. Carbon dioxide, by way of the hydrogen ion, provides a potent stimulus for control of cerebral blood flow—a doubling of the carbon dioxide pressure (PCO_2) in the blood results in a doubling of cerebral blood flow. Other substances that alter the pH of the brain produce similar changes in cerebral blood flow. Because increased hydrogen ion concentration greatly depresses neural activity, it is fortunate that blood flow increases to wash the hydrogen ions and other acidic materials away from the brain tissue.[3]

The cerebral blood vessels are innervated by the sympathetic nervous system, and research indicates that these vessels can respond to sympathetic stimulation. Under normal physiologic conditions, however, the sympathetic nervous system exerts little effect on cerebral blood flow. This is because local regulatory mechanisms are so powerful that they compensate almost entirely for the effects of sympathetic stimulation. However, in situations where there is a failure of local mechanisms, sympathetic control of cerebral blood pressure becomes very important. For example, when the arterial pressure rises to very high levels during strenuous exercise or other conditions, the sympathetic nervous system constricts the large- and intermediate-sized blood vessels as a means of protecting the smaller, more easily damaged vessels. Also, sympathetic reflexes are believed to cause vasospasm in the intermediate and large arteries in some types of brain damage, such as rupture of a cerebral aneurysm.

Several methods can be used to study cerebral blood flow. A brain scan involves the intravenous injection of a radioactive isotope that is able to move selectively through the blood–brain barrier of damaged tissue as compared to normal tissue. Special scanning methods are used to detect the increased radioactivity in the damaged areas of the brain. Two other types of radioisotope imaging, positron emission tomography (PET) and single-photon emission computed tomography (SPECT), are used to study the distribution of blood flow and metabolic activity of the brain. Both methods involve the detection of photons emitted from radionuclides. The radionuclides used for these two tests are very short-lived (minutes), and they emit radioactive energy as they move through the circulation. These forms of imaging may be used for studying the effect of cerebral activity on cerebral blood flow, localizing the site of epileptic seizure origin, and determining brain damage following a stroke.

Blood–brain barrier

The blood–brain barrier segregates the brain from substances in the blood that perfuse other tissues in the body. Many of these substances, such as hormones, amino acids, and the potassium ion, influence the firing of nerve cells; if the brain were exposed to such materials, uncontrolled nervous system activity might result.

The blood–brain barrier depends on the unique characteristics of the brain capillaries.[4,5] The endothelial cells of brain capillaries are joined by continuous tight junctions that prevent passage of unwanted materials. In addition to the endothelial cell junctions, the brain capillaries are almost completely surrounded by processes of supporting cells of the brain, called astrocytes. While excluding unwanted materials, the blood–brain barrier is able to recognize essential nutrients and transport them into the brain. Reverse transport systems remove materials from the brain. Large molecules such as proteins and peptides are largely excluded from crossing the blood–brain barrier. Acute cerebral lesions, such as trauma and infection, increase the permeability of the blood–brain barrier and alter brain concentrations of proteins, water, and electrolytes.

The blood–brain barrier prevents many drugs from entering the brain. Most highly water soluble compounds are excluded from the brain, while those that are lipid soluble cross the lipid layers of the blood–brain barrier with ease. Some drugs, such as the antibiotic chloramphenicol, are highly lipid soluble and, therefore, enter the brain readily. Other medications, such as penicillin, have a low solubility in lipids and enter the brain slowly, if at all. Alcohol, nicotine, and heroin are very lipid soluble and rapidly enter the brain to affect feelings and behavior, which helps to explain why these compounds are abused. Some substances which enter the capillary endothelium are converted by metabolic processes to a chemical form incapable of moving into the brain. One such substance is L-dopa, a precursor of dopamine that readily enters the endothelium; once there, some of it is modified by enzymes into dopamine, a form that does not cross the blood–brain barrier.[5]

Hypoxic and ischemic injury

Although the brain makes up only 2% of the body weight, it receives one-sixth of the resting cardiac output and accounts for 20% of the oxygen consumption.[6] It follows that deprivation of oxygen or blood flow can have a deleterious effect on brain structures. By definition, hypoxia denotes a deprivation of oxygen with maintained blood flow; ischemia, a situation of greatly reduced or interrupted blood flow. Hypoxia is usually seen in conditions such as exposure to reduced atmospheric pressure, carbon monoxide poisoning, severe anemia, and failure to oxygenate the blood. Because hypoxia results from decreased oxygen levels in the blood, it produces a generalized depressant effect on the brain. Ischemia can be focal as in stroke or global as in cardiac arrest. Ischemic encephalopathy occurs in circumstances of severe systemic hypotension or cardiac arrest when problems with resuscitation have occurred.

The cellular pathophysiology of hypoxia and ischemia are quite different, and the brain tends to have a very different sensitivity to the two conditions. Contrary to popular belief, hypoxia is fairly well tolerated. Neurons are capable of substantial anaerobic metabolism and fairly tolerant of pure hypoxia; it commonly produces euphoria, listlessness, drowsiness, and impaired problem solving. Unconsciousness and convulsions may occur when hypoxia is sudden and severe. However, the effects of severe hypoxia (anoxia) on brain function are seldom seen because the condition rapidly leads to cardiac arrest and ischemia.

In contrast to hypoxia, neurons are poorly tolerant of ischemia. Unconsciousness occurs within seconds of complete cessation of blood flow as in cardiac arrest. If circulation is restored immediately, consciousness will be quickly regained. However, if blood flow is not promptly restored, severe pathologic changes take place. Energy sources, glucose and glycogen, are exhausted in 2 to 3 minutes and cellular adenosine triphosphate (ATP), in 4 to 5 minutes. When ischemia is sufficiently severe or prolonged, infarction or death of all the cellular elements of the brain occurs.

An exception to the time frame above is the circumstances of cold-water drowning in which the person, especially a child, is submerged in cold water for longer than 10 minutes.[7] Hypothermia develops and causes a reduction in the cerebral metabolic requirements for oxygen; it subsequently serves as a protective mechanism for the neurons. In this case, recovery can be rapid and remarkable. Resuscitation efforts should not be discontinued precipitously.

Unfortunately, brain injury caused by ischemia does not cease once circulation is restored. Damage to cells and blood vessels can prevent adequate blood flow from occurring. This is called the *no-reflow phenomenon* and is thought to be due to alterations in the blood vessel lumen, vasospasm, and increased blood viscosity. It has been suggested that the tissues surrounding the blood vessels swell as their energy-dependent sodium–potassium membrane pump fails. Swelling occurs as fluid follows sodium into the cell. The endothelial cells of the blood vessels probably swell for the same reason. Vasospasm and calcium both act on the cerebral vessels to prevent flow from occurring. During ischemia, calcium tends to accumulate in the neurons and has been shown to cause a decrease in ATP production. These calcium ions also contribute to the change in membrane potential that promotes contraction of smooth muscle and vasospasm. Calcium-channel blocking drugs have been used to prevent this from occurring and have opened new areas of research. Sludging of blood occurs during the period of no flow or low flow and results in increased blood viscosity. Frequently hemodilution is carried out to combat this problem.

Hypermetabolism due to increased circulating catecholamines has been implicated as a contributing factor in reperfusion damage. Catecholamine release results in an increased cerebral metabolic rate and increased need for all energy-producing substrates, which the damaged brain is unable to maintain. Treatment is aimed at providing oxygen to the troubled brain and decreasing the metabolic rate through the use of barbiturates.[8]

Another area of recent interest in reperfusion injury is free oxygen radicals that are liberated from partially damaged tissue or from blood once blood flow has been restored. Free radicals are highly reactive chemical species that combine with and injure cerebrovascular endothelium; they also impair the vessel's ability to respond to carbon dioxide by increasing blood flow.

Because injured brain cells are operating with impaired metabolic machinery following an ischemic event, they are more vulnerable to injury should repeated episodes of ischemia occur. This explains why there is increased morbidity after repeated episodes of hypotension following circulatory arrest or multiple ischemic events.

The neurologic deficits that result from ischemic brain injury vary widely. If the period of non-flow/low flow is minimal, there is usually minimal to nonexistent neurologic damage. When the period is extensive or resuscitation is lengthy, the early neurologic picture is that of fixed and dilated pupils, abnormal motor posturing, and coma.[9] If the brain recovers, there is gradual improvement in neurologic status, although cognitive defects usually persist and can prevent a return to preischemic functioning level. Due to advancement in technology and experience of emergency medical personnel, individuals are surviving ischemic events with increasing frequency, but neurologic recovery has not paralleled these advances. The increasing numbers of disabled or vegetative survivors make research and treatment in this area critical.

Cerebral vascular accident (stroke)

The terms *cerebral vascular accident (CVA)* and *stroke* are used to designate focal neurologic deficits resulting from compromised blood flow. In the United States, stroke remains the third leading cause of death, despite a general decline in incidence over the past 30 years. This decline cannot be traced to a single factor, but it is probably due to early identification and treatment of risk factors such as hypertension. Various definitions have been used to classify stroke. These include transient ischemic attack, thrombotic stroke, lacunar infarctions, cerebral embolism, and intracerebral hemorrhage. Of these various subtypes, atherosclerotic (thrombotic) and lacunar strokes account for about 66% of cases, cerebral embolism for 5% to 14%, and intracerebral and subarachnoid hemorrhage (to be discussed later) for the remaining 14% to 20%.[10]

Among the risk factors for stroke are hypertension, atherosclosis, and alcohol abuse. Alcohol can contribute to stroke in several ways: (1) induction of cardiac arrhythmias and defects in ventricular wall motion that lead to cerebral embolism, (2) induction of hypertension, (3) enhancement of blood coagulation disorders, and (4) reduction of cerebral blood flow.[11] A recent cause of stroke has been cocaine. Cardiovascular events begin soon after cocaine use and include increased blood pressure, heart rate, body temperature, and metabolic rate. Cocaine also causes vasospasm and enhances the platelet response. The reported ages of persons with cocaine stroke have ranged from newborn (maternal cocaine used) to 48 years of age. Both ischemic and hemorrhagic strokes have been reported. The mechanisms of cocaine-related stroke vary. In some persons, stroke was associated with hemorrhage from aneurysms or arteriovenous malformations; and in other cases, it was associated with thrombotic lesions.[12,13,13a]

Transient ischemic attacks

Transient ischemic attacks (TIAs) are characterized by focal ischemic cerebral neurologic deficits that last for less than 24 hours (usually less than 1–2 hours). The causes of TIAs, which are sometimes called "angina of the brain," include atherosclerotic disease of cerebral vessels and emboli. TIAs are important because they precede a stroke in many cases. Diagnosis may permit surgical or medical intervention and, thus, prevent extensive damage. Overall, the risk of a stroke is greatest in the first month following a TIA. About one out of four persons who have a TIA will have another one shortly after the first.

The signs and symptoms of TIA depend on the cerebral vessel that is involved. There is often numbness and mild weakness of contralateral body structures. The forearm, hand, and angle of the mouth are commonly affected areas with middle cerebral involvement. Brief global aphasia may occur in transient ischemia of the left hemisphere. There may be transient visual disturbances such as graying-out, blurring, or fogging of vision if the posterior cerebral artery is affected.

Treatment of TIA depends on the type and the location of the ischemia-producing lesion. After numerous studies, it is now generally accepted that a small daily dose of aspirin results in a 25% to 30% reduction in stroke after TIA.[14] It has been shown that other platelet antiaggregates (sulfinpyrazone or dipyridamole) are no more effective than aspirin. Anticoagulants, such as warfarin, are not recommended because of the risk of hemorrhage. In some cases, ischemia may be due to focal loss of cerebral autoregulation, and blood flow to the area of the brain involved can be particularly sensitive to any rise or fall in blood pressure. Dehydration and relative hypotension should be avoided. In persons with hypertension, the judicious use of medication to lower blood pressure may be indicated. However, care must be taken to avoid rapid decreases in blood pressure or hypotensive episodes.[15] Surgical treatment using endarterectomy (arterial surgery to remove atherosclerotic plaque) may be used for persons with ulcerative carotid lesions. The use of a surgical procedure called an *extracranial–intracranial bypass operation* remains controversial. This procedure involves the redirecting of blood flow from an artery in the scalp through the cranium into the arteries that supply the brain. This usually involves anastomosing the superficial temporal artery that supplies the brain with the middle cerebral artery.[16]

Subclavian steal is a phenomenon in which there is transient cerebral ischemia as blood flows in a reverse direction from the vertebral artery into the vessels of the arm, stealing blood from the basilar artery and the circle of Willis. This usually occurs when the arm is exercised and the subclavian artery becomes occluded near its origin. Its symptoms include dizziness, lightheadedness, and syncope; the radial pulse is absent or diminished; and there is usually a 20 mmHg or more difference in blood pressure between the affected and unaffected arms. Although relatively rare, accounting for only 4% of all cerebrovascular diseases and 17% of extracranial carotid disorders, subclavian steal should be considered when there are complaints of dizziness and lightheadedness.[17] With the vascular surgery that is now available to redirect the blood flow, the prognosis for recovery is excellent.

Thrombotic stroke

Thrombi are the most common cause of stroke. Thrombi usually occur in atherosclerotic blood vessels. In the cerebral circulation, atherosclerotic plaques are found most commonly at arterial bifurcations. Common sites include larger vessels of the brain, notably the junctions of the internal carotid origin, vertebral arteries, and the junction of the basilar and vertebral arteries. Ischemia occurs from vessel obstruction due to thrombosis or disruption of an atherosclerotic plaque. Atherosclerotic thrombosis usually occurs gradually over several days during which the CNS symptomatology may plateau and then deteriorate further. In most cases, only one region supplied by a single cerebral artery is affected. Usually, thrombotic strokes are seen in older people and are frequently accompanied by evidence of arteriosclerotic heart disease. The thrombotic stroke is not associated with activity and may occur in a person at rest. Consciousness may or may not be lost, and improvement may be rapid.

In contrast to transient ischemic attack, a neurologic deficit that continues to progress or worsen over a period of 1 or 2 days is called a *stroke-in-evolution*. It is a gradually evolving stroke occurring in a person with a history of TIAs and is most likely due to thrombosis. A *completed stroke* describes the condition in which there has been maximum neurologic deficit, the person's condition has stabilized or is improving, and there is residual neurologic damage. Recovery may take place over days, weeks, or months, and may be only partial.

Embolic stroke

An embolic stroke is caused by a moving blood clot. It usually affects the smaller cerebral vessels, often at bifurcations. The most frequent site of embolic strokes is the middle cerebral artery distribution. Although most cerebral emboli originate in a thrombus in the left heart, they may also originate in an atherosclerotic plaque in the carotid arteries. The embolus travels quickly to the brain and becomes lodged in a small artery through which it cannot pass. Therefore, embolic stroke usually has a sudden onset with immediate maximum deficit.

Various cardiac conditions predispose to formation of emboli that produce embolic stroke including rheumatic heart disease, atrial fibrillation, recent myocardial infarction, ventricular aneurysm, and bacterial endocarditis. Recent advances in the diagnosis and treatment of heart disease can be expected to alter favorably the incidence of embolic stroke.

Lacunar infarcts

Lacunar infarcts are small (1.5–2.0 cm) to very small (3–4 mm) infarcts located in the deeper noncortical parts of the brain or in the brain stem. They result from occlusion of the smaller penetrating branches of large cerebral arteries—commonly, the middle cerebral, posterior cerebral and less commonly, anterior cerebral, vertebral, or basilar arteries. In the process of healing, lacunar infarcts leave behind a small cavity, or lacuna. The cause of the infarct is a degenerative disease of small cerebral arteries that occurs in persons with hypertension that is different from the atherosclerotic lesions seen in the larger cerebral arteries. Because of their size and location, lacunar infarcts do not usually cause deficits such as aphasia, apractic agnosia of the minor hemisphere, homonymous hemianopia, isolated memory impairment, stupor, coma, loss of consciousness, or seizures. Instead, they often produce pure motor or sensory deficits.

Intracerebral hemorrhage

The most frequently fatal stroke is rupture of the vessel wall—intracerebral hemorrhage. With rupture of a blood vessel, hemorrhage into the brain substance or subarachnoid space occurs, resulting in edema, compression of the brain contents, or spasm of the adjacent blood vessels. The most common predisposing factor is hypertension. Other causes of hemorrhage are aneurysm, trauma, erosion of the vessels by tumors, vascular malformations, and blood dyscrasias. A cerebral hemorrhage occurs suddenly, usually when the person is active. The person may complain of a severe headache and stiff neck (nuchal rigidity), the result of blood entering the cerebrospinal fluid (CSF). Focal symptoms depend on which vessel is involved. There is usually contralateral hemiplegia, with initial flaccidity progressing to spasticity. The hemorrhage and resultant edema exert great pressure on the brain substance, and the clinical course progresses rapidly to coma and frequently to death.

Manifestations of stroke

The specific manifestations of stroke are determined by the cerebral artery that is affected and by the area of brain tissue that is supplied by that vessel

(Table 50-2). The manifestations may include loss of consciousness, motor impairment, sensory deficits, agnosias, visual disturbances, aphasia, and the hemineglect syndrome. When the patient regains consciousness (if consciousness was lost), characteristically there will be contralateral hemiplegia, with either a speech disturbance or a spatial-perceptual deficit depending on which side of the brain is affected, and possibly incontinence.

Motor deficits

Initially following a stroke affecting the posterior limb of the internal capsule, there is profound weakness, characterized by a decrease in or absence of normal muscle tone. There is a tendency toward foot drop, outward rotation of the leg, and dependent edema in the affected extremities. Putting the extremities through passive range-of-motion exercises helps to maintain the joint function and to prevent edema, shoulder subluxation (incomplete dislocation), and muscle atrophy. The smooth sequential movement of the exercises may also help to re-establish motor patterns.

Early motor recovery (usually 3–8 weeks) is seen with the beginning of spasticity—the resistance of muscle groups to passive stretch, with an increase of muscle tone. Spasticity follows the decline in cerebral edema and the initial flaccidity, because inhibition of muscle tone from the basal ganglia is reduced. With spasticity, the flexor muscles are usually more strongly affected in the upper extremities; the extensor muscles are more strongly affected in the lower extremities.[18] Involuntary muscle contractions are manifested in shoulder adduction, forearm pronation, finger flexion, and knee and hip extension. If spasticity has not appeared within 6 weeks (maximally within 3 months), function will probably not return to that extremity. Passive range-of-motion exercises should be continued, and positioning should be directed toward keeping all the joints in functional position.

Aphasia

Aphasia is a general term that encompasses varying degrees of inability to comprehend, integrate, and express language. It is estimated to be present in 40% of persons with stroke.[19] The most common cause is a vascular lesion of the middle cerebral artery of the dominant hemisphere; the left hemisphere being dominant in about 90% of the population.

Aphasia is most accurately described as a disorder of language abilities rather than a speech disorder. The term *language* implies a higher level integrative function that includes perception, integration, and formulation of verbal stimuli; whereas, a speech disorder is essentially a neuromuscular problem. For example, a person with dysarthria—an imperfect articulation of speech—still can retain some language ability.

Two categories are usually used when describing aphasia: expressive and receptive. Motor, or expressive, aphasia is the loss of the ability to express thoughts and ideas in speech or writing. The person with expressive aphasia may be able, with difficulty, to utter two or three words, usually words having an emotional overlay. Automatic speech and social phrases are usually easier to articulate. Although comprehension is usually intact, in speech some words may be omitted or inappropriate words may be used (*e.g.*, "weathery winter"). Jargon aphasia is the utterance of nonexistent words, which the person is unable to recognize as such and believes to be correct and appropriate. Receptive, or sensory, aphasia is the inability to comprehend written or spoken words. Receptive aphasia is also called *Wernicke's aphasia* or auditory aphasia.

Some persons manifest elements of both expressive and receptive aphasia, called mixed aphasias. When all language ability is lost—both receptive and expressive—the aphasia is said to be global or total. Most aphasias are partial, however, and a thorough speech evaluation is essential to determine the type and extent of aphasia and the therapy needed.

One of the most common characteristics of aphasia is distorted spontaneous or conversational speech, which is usually classified as fluent (many) or nonfluent (few) words. Although the terms fluent and nonfluent have been in use for years, they have recently been reemphasized. Fluency refers to the characteristics of speech and not to content or ability to comprehend. Fluent output requires little or no effort, is articulate, and is of increased quantity. It is rambling and wordy, yet meaningless—what is sometimes called empty speech. There are three categories of fluent aphasia: Wernicke's, anomic, and conduction aphasia.[19] Wernecke's aphasia is characterized by an inability to comprehend the speech, reading, and writing not only of other persons but also of oneself. Anomic aphasia is speech that is nearly normal, but in which the person has difficulty selecting appropriate words. Inappropriate word use in the presence of good comprehension is called conduction aphasia. Conduction aphasia is due to destruction of the fiber system interconnecting Wernicke's and Broca's areas, under the insula.

Nonfluent aphasia presents opposite problems: poor articulation, poor modulation, dysarthria,

Table 50–2. Signs and symptoms of stroke by involved cerebral artery

Cerebral artery	Brain area involved	Signs and symptoms*
Anterior cerebral	None if proximal to patent anterior communicating artery; infarction of the medial aspect of one frontal lobe if lesion is distal to communicating artery; bilateral frontal infarction if flow in other anterior cerebral artery is inadequate.	Paralysis of contralateral foot or leg; impaired gait; paresis contralateral arm; contralateral sensory loss over toes, foot, and leg; problems making decisions or performing acts voluntarily; lack of spontaneity, easily distracted; slowness of thought; aphasia dependent on the hemisphere involved; urinary incontinence
Middle cerebral	Massive infarction of most of lateral hemisphere and deeper structures of frontal, parietal, and temporal lobes; internal capsule; basal ganglia	Contralateral hemiplegia (face and arm); contralateral sensory impairment; aphasia; homonymous heminanopsia; altered consciousness (confusion to coma); inability to turn eyes toward paralyzed side; denial of paralyzed side or limb (hemiattention); possible acalculia, alexia, finger agnosia and left–right confusion; vasomotor paresis and instability
Posterior cerebral	Occipital lobe; anterior and medial portion of temporal lobe	Homonymous hemianopsia and other visual defects such as color blindness, loss of central vision, and visual hallucinations; memory deficits, perseveration (repeated performance of same verbal or motor response)
	Thalamus involvement	Loss of all sensory modalities; spontaneous pain; intentional tremor; mild hemiparesis; aphasia
	Cerebral peduncle involvement	Oculomotor nerve palsy with contralateral hemiplegia
Basilar and vertebral	Cerebellum and brain stem	Visual disturbances such as diplopia, ataxia, vertigo, dysphagia, dysphonia

* Dependent on hemisphere involved.

and sparse output of words with considerable effort and limited to short phrases or single words. The words are substantive and have considerable meaning. Nonfluent aphasia may also be Broca's aphasia. If the aphasia-producing lesion affects the frontal and parietal speech areas, a mixed or global aphasia may result, with problems of nonfluent aphasia and the comprehension difficulties of Wernicke's aphasia.

There is a correlation between the anatomical location of cerebral damage and the aphasia syndrome, which was recognized by Broca and Wernicke more than a century ago. Although exceptions exist, most persons with nonfluent aphasia have lesions rostral to the central fissure, known as anterior Broca's aphasia; people with fluent aphasia have a lesion posterior to the fissure known as posterior Wernicke's aphasia.[20]

Denial or hemiattention

Because of an inability to analyze and interpret incoming sensory information due to the disruptive lesion of the brain and the internal production of abnormal signals, a high percentage of persons with stroke have a form of denial of illness and a denial of one-half of their own body and environment on that side of the body (hemiattention).[21] Importantly, such persons are unaware of the deficit. For example, a person with left hemiplegia may raise the right arm when asked; but when asked to raise the left arm, respond by saying, "I just did." Spatial orientation is often impaired and there is difficulty localizing stimuli, their own limbs, and objects in space. Affected persons may totally disregard stimuli coming from the involved side of the body, even though they can see and hear. The affected side of the body may go unattended and ungroomed (hemineglect). It is not uncommon for a person to only wash or shave the unaffected side, but not the affected side, of the body. When asked to draw a picture of themselves, these persons often draw a person with only one arm and leg. The condition is more common in persons with strokes that affect the nondominant side of the brain, usually the right hemisphere, which is more involved with spatial orientation, body image, and inductive modes of reasoning.

Diagnosis and treatment

Accurate diagnosis of stroke is based on a complete history and thorough physical and neurologic examination. A careful history, including TIAs, their rapidity of onset and focal symptoms, as well as those of any other diseases that may be present, will help to determine the type of stroke that is involved. CT scans and MRI have also become important tools

in diagnosing stroke and in differentiating cerebral hemorrhage and intracranial lesions that mimic stroke.[22] Arteriography may be used to demonstrate the site of the vascular abnormality and afford visualization of most intracranial vascular areas. The use of PET makes it possible to define the location and size of strokes by providing data on cerebral blood flow and volume and brain cell metabolism.

The treatment of stroke is largely symptomatic. The main goals are prevention of complications and treatment of any underlying disease. There is some controversy over whether or not effort should be made to lower the blood pressure after a stroke. A chief consideration is to maintain oxygenation of brain tissue, and the possibility exists that a rapid fall in blood pressure could compromise blood flow and oxygenation. There is also controversy over the use of anticoagulants as a means of preventing further occlusion. Anticoagulants represent a double-edged sword because they could precipitate hemorrhage. Small daily doses of aspirin are of benefit in preventing further strokes in persons with TIAs and mild stroke.[23] Surgical attempts at restoring blood supply to the brain focus on removing any clots from the carotid or vertebral arteries or bypassing occluded vessels.

Symptomatic treatment is aimed at preventing complications and promoting the fullest possible recovery of function. During the acute phase, proper positioning and range-of-motion exercises are essential. Early rehabilitation efforts include all members of the rehabilitation team—physician, nurse, speech therapist, physical therapist, and occupational therapist, and the family.

Cerebral aneurysms and subarachnoid hemorrhage

The arachnoid is a fine weblike and waterproof mesh of connective tissue strands that lies between the dura mater and the pia mater that surrounds the brain and spinal cord. The subarachnoid space is filled with CSF, which enters from the ventricles and is reabsorbed into the venous system via arachnoid protruberances (arachnoid villa) through the inner dura. The circle of Willis is formed by the anastomosis of the medium-sized arterial branches that course in the pia mater adjacent to the subarachnoid space (see Figure 50-12). These vessels have a well-developed internal elastic layer but lack external elastic support.

An aneurysm is a localized weakness in the muscular wall of an arterial vessel. Most cerebral aneurysms are small saccular aneurysms called *berry aneurysms*. The most common cause of subarachnoid hemorrhage is cerebral aneurysm, which occurs at the junctions of the vessels of the circle of Willis and is responsible for 80% of the approximately 26,000 cases of subarachnoid hemorrhage that occur each year.[24] Cerebral aneurysms are seen most frequently between the ages of 30 and 60 years and are rarely seen in children. A history of hypertension may be present. Aneurysms occur more frequently in females and have been associated with contraceptive drugs, cigarette smoking, and cocaine abuse.[13a,25]

Two theories regarding the pathogenesis of aneurysm formation have been proposed. One proposes a developmental defect in the vessel wall; the other proposes degeneration of the vessel wall due to conditions such as atherosclerosis, hypertension, and situations of abnormal blood flow.[26a] Aneurysms frequently occur at the site of vessel bifurcations. Once an aneurysm has begun to form in a vessel, it does not recede; instead, most increase in size and produce weakening of the vessel wall, often to the extent that only a thin fibrous vessel wall remains. Aneurysm progression depends on many factors, including blood pressure and flow phenomenon. Rupture of aneurysms is not inevitable; intact aneurysms are frequently found at autopsy as an incidental finding.[6] Once an aneurysm ruptures, tissue pressure usually causes a clot to form and bleeding is short-lived.[24] The clot robs the brain of intracranial space, causing compression and distortion of neural tissue.

The signs and symptoms of subarachnoid hemorrhage include headache, nuchal rigidity (neck stiffness), and photophobia. If severe, alteration in level of consciousness will occur. The bleeding into the subarachnoid space causes meningeal irritation or a chemical meningitis with the resulting signs of headache and nuchal rigidity. The distinguishing feature of the disorder is the headache, which is frequently described as "the worst headache of my life." The optic nerves are ensheathed in meninges, and meningeal irritation causes photophobia. Occasionally nausea and vomiting will accompany the presenting symptoms. In other cases, there may be no focal neurologic findings. In cases of severe bleeding, the headache may be accompanied by collapse and loss of consciousness. Dependent on the course of the bleeding, the headache subsides slowly over a matter of days. Hypertension is a frequent finding and may be the result of the hemorrhage. Electrocardiographic changes may occur because of massive autonomic nervous system discharge followed by increased levels of circulating catecholamines. A giant aneurysm may present as a space-occupying lesion. In many instances, more than one aneurysm will be confirmed on arteriography, in which case, the aneurysm that has ruptured is determined by clinical signs.

The deficits that can result as complications of aneurysm rupture make this entity a major health problem. These complications include rebleeding, vasospasm, and hydrocephalus. Rebleeding and vasospasm are the most severe and most difficult to treat. Rebleeding, which has its highest incidence on the first day, results in further and usually catastrophic neurologic deficits.[26] Rebleeding from an aneurysm that has been surgically repaired is that of the normal population or approximately 1%.

Vasospasm is a dreaded complication of aneurysmal bleeding. The condition is difficult to treat and is associated with a high incidence of morbidity and mortality. Although the description of aneurysm-associated vasospasm is relatively uniform, its proposed mechanisms are controversial.[27] Usually the condition develops 4 to 12 days after aneurysm rupture and involves a focal narrowing of the cerebral artery or arteries that can be visualized on arteriography. Clinically, there is a gradual deterioration in neurologic status as blood supply to the brain in the region of the spasm is decreased; this can usually be differentiated from the rapid deterioration seen in rebleeding. Vasospasm can often be predicted by the amount of blood seen in the basal cisterns on CT scan. Vasospasm is treated by maintaining adequate cerebral perfusion pressure by way of increased intravascular volume in an attempt to increase or maintain vessel patency. There is risk of rebleeding from this therapy. Early surgery may provide some protection from vasospasm.

Another complication of aneurysm rupture is the development of hydrocephalus. It is thought to result from obstruction of the arachnoid villi of the CSF system, which are responsible for reabsorption of CSF. The lysis of blood in the subarachnoid space causes the protein content of the CSF to increase, thereby preventing diffusion of CSF across the arachnoid villi, plugging the system, and resulting hydrocephalus. Occasionally, hydrocephalus can be medically managed by the use of osmotic diuretics, but if neurologic deterioration is significant, surgical placement of a shunt is indicated. Hydrocephalus is diagnosed by serial CT scans and increasing size of the ventricles and clinical signs of increased intracranial pressure (to be discussed).

The diagnosis of subarachnoid hemorrhage is made by clinical presentation, lumbar puncture, CT scan, and arteriogram. Lumbar puncture will show blood in the cerebral spinal fluid. This must be distinguished from trauma that occurs during the spinal tap. In order to distinguish between the two sources of blood, the spinal fluid is centrifuged. Blood from subarachnoid hemorrhage will have undergone hemolysis.[28] The CT scan will show blood in the basilar cisterns and around the cerebral convexities. The arteriography is the definitive diagnostic tool for presence and location of the aneurysm. Arteriography involves the injection of a contrast media into an artery so that vessel can be visualized using fluoroscopic or x-ray methods and defects, such as vasospasm, can be detected. Frequently, subarachnoid hemorrhage of unknown etiology may be due to an aneurysm not seen because of vasospasm. These individuals need to be followed at regular intervals to determine the presence or absence of aneurysm once vasospasm has subsided.

The course of treatment after aneurysm rupture depends on the extent of neurologic deficit. Persons with less severe deficits (with or without headache and no neurologic deficits) may undergo cerebral arteriography and early surgery, usually within 24 hours. A procedure called *clipping* is often used in which a silver clip is inserted and tightened around the neck of the aneurysm. It appears that this procedure offers protection from rebleeding and other complications. Persons with more severe neurologic deficits (*e.g.,* stupor or coma and presence of neurologic deficits) are managed medically for approximately 10 days in an effort to improve their clinical status, and may then undergo arteriography and surgery. No more than half of persons with subarachnoid hemorrhage survive until surgery, but of those who do survive, over 75% regain their previous level of activity.[27]

In summary, blood flow to the brain is supplied by the two internal carotid arteries and the two vertebral arteries and drained by two sets of veins: the deep cerebral venous system and the superficial venous system. The blood–brain barrier protects the brain from substances in the blood that would disrupt brain function. Cerebral vascular accident, or stroke, is a sudden severe deficit in neurologic function caused by a decrease in the blood supply to areas of the brain. It is the third leading cause of death in the United States and a major cause of disability. Uncontrolled hypertension is a significant risk factor for the development of stroke. Stroke can result from hemorrhage, embolus, or thrombus. The effects of stroke depend on the location of the blood vessel that is involved and can include motor, sensory, and speech manifestations. Treatment is primarily symptomatic, involving the combined efforts of the health-care professionals in the rehabilitation team, the patient, and the family. A subarachnoid hemorrhage involves bleeding into the arachnoid space. Most subarachnoid hemorrhages are the result of a ruptured cerebral aneurysm. Fifty percent of people with subarachnoid hemorrhage do not survive the initial hemorrhage. Presenting symptoms include headache, nuchal rigidity, photophobia, and nausea. Complications include rebleeding, vasospasm, and hydrocephalus. Current treatment includes maintaining medical stability, preventing complications, and early surgery, usually within the first 24 hours.

Alterations in cerebral volumes and pressures

Intracranial pressure is the pressure within the cranial cavity. The standard measurement is that pressure within the lateral ventricles. The cranial cavity contains blood (about 10%), brain tissue (about 80%), and CSF (about 10%) within the rigid confines of a nonexpandable skull. Each of these three volumes contributes to the intracranial pressure (ICP), which normally is maintained within a range of 50 mm H_2O to 200 mm H_2O (4–15 mmHg). The volumes of each of these components can vary slightly without causing marked changes in intracranial pressure. This is because small increases in the volume of one component can be compensated for by a decrease in the volume of one or both of the other two components. This is termed the *Monro-Kellie hypothesis*. Normal fluctuations in intracranial pressure occur with respiratory movements and activities of daily living such as straining, coughing, and sneezing.

Abnormal variation in intracranial volume with subsequent changes in ICP can be caused by a volume change in any of the three intracranial components. For example, an increase in tissue volume can result from a brain tumor, brain edema, or bleeding into brain tissue. An increase in blood volume develops when there is vasodilatation of cerebral vessels or obstruction of venous outflow. Excess production, decreased absorption, or obstructed circulation of CSF affords the potential for an increase in the CSF component. When the change in volume is due to a brain tumor, it tends to occur slowly and is usually localized to the immediate area, whereas the increase resulting from head injury usually develops rapidly.

Of the three intracranial substances, CSF and blood volume are the most able to compensate for changes in ICP; tissue volume is relatively restricted in its ability to undergo change. Initial increases in ICP are buffered by both a translocation of CSF to the spinal subarachnoid space and increased reabsorption of CSF. The rate of CSF production by the choroid plexuses of the third and fourth ventricles is relatively constant. However, the rate of reabsorption and removal is controlled by the pressure difference between the CSF in the subarachnoid space and the blood in the dural sinuses. Because changes in ICP produce an increase in CSF pressures without increasing dural sinus pressures, reabsorption of CSF is increased. Intracranial blood volume is determined by the cerebral blood flow, the resistance of the cerebral blood vessels to flow, and the cerebral perfusion pressure. The cerebral vascular resistance refers to the resistance across the blood vessels in the brain; it increases with vessel constriction and decreases with vessel dilatation. As explained earlier, increases in P_{CO_2} produce vasodilatation of cerebral blood vessels and rapid and significant changes in cerebral blood flow.

The impact of increases in blood, brain tissue, or CSF volumes on ICP varies among individuals and depends on the amount of increase that occurs, the effectiveness of compensatory mechanisms, and cerebral elasticity and plasticity. Brain structures are plastic (easily molded) and elastic (resistant to deformation). Plasticity is the more prominent characteristic and, therefore, more vulnerable to change. The blood vessels provide the major elastic component, and brain tissue provides the major plastic component. The ICP remains normal as long as the increase in volume does not exceed the CSF or blood volume that is displaced.[29] The compensation of the brain tissue is determined by the cerebral elastance or its reciprocal compliance (ICP = elastance × volume). When elastance is high, even small increases in volume increase the ICP to dangerous levels (Figure 50-14). When the CSF and blood can no longer compensate for the increased volume and the excess space in the cranial cavity is filled, the ICP rises sharply and may result in cerebral hypoxia or brain shift.

The cerebral perfusion pressure (CPP) is the difference between the mean arterial blood pressure (MABP) and the intracranial pressure (CPP = MABP − ICP). The cerebral perfusion pressure is determined by the pressure gradient between the internal carotid artery and the subarachnoid veins, which, in turn, reflect cerebral vascular resistance and cerebral blood flow. Both the MABP and ICP are frequently monitored in persons with brain conditions that increase ICP and impair brain perfusion. Normal CPP ranges from 60 mmHg to 80 mmHg. Neuronal death occurs at levels below 50 mmHg. When the

pressure in the cranial cavity approaches or exceeds the mean systemic arterial pressure, tissue perfusion becomes inadequate, cellular hypoxia results, and, if maintained, neuronal death may occur. The highly specialized cortical neurons are the most sensitive to oxygen deficit; therefore, a decrease in the level of consciousness is one of the earliest and most reliable signs of increased intracranial pressure. The increasing cellular hypoxia leads to general neurologic deterioration. The level of consciousness may deteriorate from alertness through confusion, lethargy, obtundation, stupor, and coma.

One of the late reflexes seen with marked increase in intracranial pressure is the CNS ischemic response, which is triggered by ischemia of the vasomotor center in the brain stem. Neurons in the vasomotor center respond directly to ischemia by producing a marked increase in mean arterial blood pressure, sometimes to levels as high as 270 mmHg and is accompanied by a widening of the pulse pressure and a reflex slowing of the heart rate. This triad of signs, sometimes called the *Cushing reflex* (or response), is an important but late indicator of increased intracranial pressure. It results from a severely increased intracranial pressure that compresses the blood flow to the brain stem. If the increase in blood pressure initiated by the CNS ischemic reflex is greater than the pressure surrounding the compressed vessels, blood flow will be re-established. The ischemic reaction is a last ditch effort by the nervous system to maintain the cerebral circulation. The Cushing reflex is seldom seen in modern clinical settings since the advent of intracranial pressure monitoring.

Manifestations and assessment methods

Changes in ICP can be assessed through direct or indirect methods. Indirect methods assess physiologic parameters such as blood pressure, heart rate, pupillary response, and changes in level of consciousness that change with increases in ICP. Direct measurements for continuous monitoring of ICP have emerged over the past three decades and are available in many acute-care settings.

Other indirect methods include radiologic studies such as computerized tomography (CT scan) and magnetic resonance imaging (MRI). CT scans detect changes in the position of brain structures and provide indirect evidence of changes in ICP. The introduction of CT scanning to emergency neurologic care has had a significant impact on the speed of diagnosis of neurologic injury. MRI will also indicate shifting of brain structures. The technique uses a magnetic field to align atomic nuclei along their axis of rotation. When the magnetic field is discontinued, the atoms emit energy as they return to their original

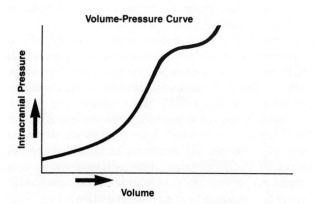

Volume-Pressure Curve

Intracranial Pressure

Volume

Figure 50-14 Changes in intracranial pressure. The initial, gradually sloping section of the curve indicates the effects of compensation. The steep portion of the curve signifies that even small increases in volume will exponentially increase the pressure because compensatory mechanisms are exhausted. At very high pressures, the curve flattens out momentarily, before again increasing its slope. (*Pollack-Latham CL: Intracranial pressure monitoring. Part 1: Physiologic principles. Crit Care Nurse 7(5):40, 1987*)

position. By using special tomographic computing techniques a tissue image can be obtained. MRI has been useful in degenerative neurologic disease and detection of small brain tumors. It is not useful in an emergency because all metal objects must be removed from the scanning area, a difficult task with intravenous fluids, traction, and ventilator equipment.

Sophisticated bedside methods for direct monitoring of ICP are now available. The bedside monitoring methods can provide continuous information about volume–pressure relationships, cerebral compliance, pulse pressure, pressure waves, and cerebral perfusion pressure. The current methods of measuring ICP use one of three types of sensors: an intraventricular polyethylene catheter that is inserted into the anterior horn of the lateral ventricle on the nondominant hemisphere, a subarachnoid screw (a hollow screw and transducer wick) that is implanted into the subarachnoid space, and an epidural fiberoptic sensor that is implanted into the epidural space (Figure 50-15). An advantage of the the epidural fiberoptic sensor is that there is no need to penetrate the brain and subarachnoid space, and consequently there is less danger of infection or uncontrolled loss of CSF fluid.

The ICP waveforms that are seen during pressure monitoring are the result of systolic and diastolic arterial pressures that are transmitted through the viscoelastic brain tissues and CSF and look similar to a dampened arterial pressure wave. There are three types of intracranial pressure waves: A, B, and C waves. The A waves, now called plateau waves, are the most important and are only seen in advanced stages of ICP. B waves also result from pathologic conditions and can be premonitory to A waves. B waves are usually observed at ICP levels of 15 mmHg

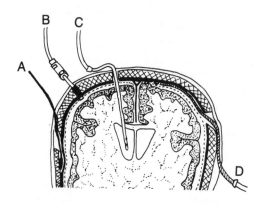

Figure 50-15 Coronal section of brain showing placement of several ICP monitoring devices: *A,* epidural fiberoptic sensor; *B,* Richmond subarachnoid screw; *C,* intraventricular catheter; and *D,* subdural cup catheter. (*Reprinted with permission of the publisher from Mortara RW: Intracranial pressure monitoring in the emergency setting. Medical Instrumentation 16[4]:197–198, 1982. Copyright 1982 by the Association for the Advancement of Medical Instrumentation, Arlington, VA*)

to 40 mmHg and are due to fluctuations in cerebral blood flow.[30] C waves relate to normal changes in arterial blood pressure and have no known clinical significance. They occur every 4 to 8 minutes and increase fluid pressure and intracranial pressure by as much as 20 mmHg.

Hydrocephalus

One form of increased volume in the cranial cavity is hydrocephalus, which is defined as an abnormal increase in CSF volume within any part or all of the ventricular system. The two causes of hydrocephalus are decreased absorption or overproduction of CSF. Decreased absorption can result from a block in the CSF pathway to the arachnoid villi or a failure of the villi to transfer the CSF to the venous system. An obstruction to CSF flow can be caused by congenital malformations, infections, or tumors encroaching on the ventricular system. This is sometimes called *noncommunicating* or *obstructive hydrocephalus* because the flow within the ventricular system is obstructed from reaching the arachnoid villi. Impaired transfer of CSF from the villi to the venous system is sometimes called *communicating hydrocephalus* because the CSF pathways are open and communicate with the arachnoid villi. Communicating hydrocephalus can occur if too few villi are formed, if postinfective (meningitis) scarring occludes them, or if the villi become obstructed with fragments of blood or infectious debris. Adenomata of the choroid plexus can cause an overproduction of CSF. This form of hydrocephalus is much less common than that resulting from decreased absorption of CSF.

The signs of ICP elevation associated with hydrocephalus depend on the type of hydrocephalus, the age of onset, and the extent of pressure rise. When hydrocephalus occurs in infants and small children before the sutures of the skull have fused, head enlargement is a prominent manifestation. Head enlargement does not occur in adults, and increases in ICP depend on whether the condition developed rapidly or slowly. Acute hydrocephalus is usually manifested by increased ICP. Slowly developing hydrocephalus is less apt to produce an increase in ICP, but may produce deficits such as progressive dementia and gait changes. CT scans are used to diagnose all types of hydrocephalus. The usual treatment is a shunting procedure, which provides an alternative route for return of CSF to the circulation.

Cerebral edema

Cerebral edema, or brain swelling, is an increase in tissue volume secondary to abnormal fluid accumulation. There are two types of brain edema:

vasogenic and cytotoxic.[31] Vasogenic edema results from an increase in the extracellular fluid that surrounds brain cells. Cytotoxic edema involves the actual swelling of brain cells themselves. Brain edema may or may not produce an increase in intracranial pressure. The impact of brain edema depends on the brain's compensatory mechanisms and the extent of the swelling.

Vasogenic edema occurs in conditions such as tumors, prolonged ischemia, infectious processes (*e.g.*, meningitis) that impair function of the blood–brain barrier and allow transfer of water and protein into the interstitial space. When brain injury occurs, the blood–brain barrier is disrupted and increased permeability occurs. There is almost free diffusion across the capillary membranes. Vasogenic edema occurs primarily in the white matter of the brain, possibly because the white matter is more compliant than the gray matter and offers less resistance to flow. Vasogenic edema can displace a cerebral hemisphere and can be responsible for various types of herniation. The functional manifestations of vasogenic edema include focal neurologic deficits, disturbances in consciousness, and severe intracranial hypertension.

In cytotoxic edema, all of the cellular elements of the brain swell (neurons, glia, and endothelial cells). Cytotoxic edema results from hypo-osmotic states such as water intoxication or severe ischemia that impairs the function of the sodium–potassium membrane pump, which causes rapid accumulation of sodium within the cell followed by water moving along the osmotic gradient. Cytotoxic edema occurs in both white and gray matter of the brain. Major changes in cerebral function, such as stupor and coma, occur with cytotoxic edema. The edema associated with ischemia may be severe enough to produce cerebral infarction with necrosis of brain tissue.

Arterial occlusion usually produces both vasogenic and cytogenic edema. Although edema is viewed as a pathologic process, it does not necessarily disrupt brain function unless it results in an increase in intracranial pressure. The localized edema surrounding a brain tumor often responds to corticosteroid therapy; but these drugs have little effect on the generalized edema that develops rapidly in trauma. The mechanism of action of the corticosteroid drugs in treatment of cerebral edema is unknown, but in therapeutic doses they seem to stabilize cell membranes and scavenge free radicals.

—— Brain herniation

The cranial cavity is divided into compartments by two main folds in the dura mater: the falx cerebri and the tentorium cerebelli. The falx cerebri is a central longitudinal fold that partially separates the two hemispheres. The tentorium cerebelli separates the cerebrum from the cerebellum and brain stem.

Brain herniation is the displacement of brain tissue under the tough dural folds of the falx cerebri or through tentorium cerebelli. A rising intracranial pressure created by increased volume causes displacement of the cerebral tissue toward a less-dense area. There are different types of herniation syndromes, based on the area of the brain that has herniated and the structure under which it has been pushed (Figure 50-16). They are commonly divided into two broad categories, supratentorial and infratentorial, based on whether they are located above or below the tentorium.

There are three major patterns of supratentorial herniation: cingulate or across the falx, uncal or lateral, and central or transtentorial. Cingulate herniation involves the displacement of the cingulate gyrus and hemisphere beneath sharp edges of the falx cerebri to the other side of the brain. The most common form of supratentorial herniation is uncal herniation in which a lateral mass pushes the brain tissue centrally and forces the medial aspect of the temporal lobe (uncus) under the edge of the tentorial incisura, into the posterior fossa, initially causing pressure on the oculomotor or third cranial nerve, which controls pupillary constriction. This pressure results in an ipsilateral or contralateral (due to pressure transmitted to the opposite side) pupillary dilatation. Central or bilateral herniation of the uncus through the tentorial notch results from a generalized increase in the pressure of the supratentorial compartment, which causes a downward displacement of supratentorial structures. This interferes with the reticular activating system. As a result, central herniations are first evidenced by changes in the level of consciousness.

Infratentorial herniation results from in-

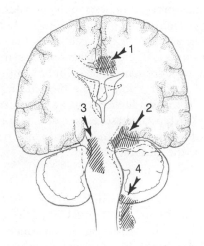

Figure 50-16 Brain herniations: *1*, cingulate or across the falx; *2*, uncal or lateral; *3*, central or transtentorial; and *4*, infratentorial.

creased pressure in the infratentorial compartment. It often progress rapidly and can cause death because it is likely to involve the lower brain stem centers that control vital functions. Herniation may occur either superiorly through the tentorial incisura or inferiorly through the foramen magnum. Upward displacement of brain tissue can cause blockage of the aqueduct of Sylvius and lead to hydrocephalus and coma. Downward displacement of the midbrain through the tentorial notch or the cerebellar tonsils through the foramen magnum can interfere with medullary functioning and cause cardiac or respiratory arrest. In cases of pre-existing intracranial pressure, herniation may occur when pressure is released from below, such as in a lumbar puncture. If the CSF pathway is blocked and fluid cannot leave the ventricles, the volume will expand, as will the downward displacement through the tentorial notch. The expanding volume will cause all function at a given level to cease as destruction progresses in a rostral–caudal direction. The result of this displacement is brain stem ischemia and hemorrhage extending from the diencephalon to the pons. If the lesion expands rapidly, displacement and obstruction occur quickly, leading to irreversible infarction and hemorrhage.

Each herniation syndrome has distinguishing features in the early phases, but as forced downward displacement on the pons and medulla continues, clinical signs become similar. In the early stages, central herniation is manifested by a clouding of consciousness with bilaterally small pupils with a small range of constriction. The clouding of consciousness is due to pressure on the reticular activating system (RAS) in the upper midbrain, which is responsible for wakefulness. Lateral or uncal herniation produces an initial pupillary dilatation with sluggish or no reaction to light. Consciousness may be unimpaired because the RAS has not as yet been affected. Deterioration, however, may proceed rather rapidly—making it important to recognize the distinguishing early features of lateral herniations. As both central and lateral herniations progress, there will be changes in motor strength and coordination of voluntary movements because of compression of the descending motor pathways. As the condition progresses, the respiratory rate decreases, blood pressure rises, and the heart rate slows. Body temperature may or may not rise. The end result is the Cushing reflex.

In summary, the contents of the cranial cavity consist of brain tissue, blood, and CSF. The collective volumes of these three intracranial components determine ICP. A variation in volume of any of these three components can cause the ICP to rise, affecting cerebral function. Compensatory mechanisms protect the brain from small variations in the volume of any of these three components. Large variations, however, exceed the compensatory mechanisms and may lead to hypoxia, brain herniation, and death. Among the causes of ICP are hydrocephalus and head injury. Hydrocephalus represents an abnormal increase in CSF volume within a part or all of the ventricular system. It is caused by overproduction of CSF or obstruction of its flow through the ventricular system. Brain edema represents an increase in tissue volume secondary to abnormal fluid accumulation. There are two types of brain edema: vasogenic, which results from an increase in extracellular fluid, and cytotoxic, which involves the actual swelling of brain cells. Brain herniation is the displacement of brain tissue under the tough dural folds of the falx cerebri or past the tentorium cerebelli. Brain herniation is commonly divided into two broad categories, supratentorial and infratentorial, based on location of the herniation.

Head injury and infection

The brain is enclosed within the protective confines of the rigid bony skull. Although the skull affords protection for the tissues of the CNS, it also provides the potential for development of ischemic and traumatic injuries. This is because the skull cannot expand to accommodate the increase in volume that occurs when there is swelling or bleeding within the confines of the skull. The bony structures themselves can cause injury to the nervous system. Fractures of the skull can compress sections of the nervous system, or they can splinter and cause penetrating wounds.

One of the most serious types of direct injury is skull fracture. Skull fractures can be divided into three groups: simple, depressed, and basilar. A *simple linear* skull fracture is a break in the continuity of bone. Multiple linear skull fractures can cause splintering and crushing of bone. When bone fragments are embedded into the brain tissue, the fracture is said to be *depressed*. A fracture of the bones that form the base of the skull is called a basilar skull fracture.

Usually radiologic examination is needed to confirm the presence and extent of a skull fracture. This is important because of the possible damage to the underlying tissues. A frequent complication of basilar skull fractures is leakage of CSF from the nose (rhinorrhea) or ear (otorrhea); this occurs because of the proximity of the base of the skull to the nose and ear. There may be lacerations to the vessels of the dura, with resultant intracranial bleeding. Damage to the cranial nerves may also result from basilar skull fractures if the fracture is in the vicinity of the foramina from which the cranial nerves exit the skull. The effects of traumatic brain injuries can be divided into two categories: primary effects, in which damage is due to impact, and secondary injuries, in which damage results from the subsequent brain swelling, intracranial hematomas, infection, cerebral hypoxia, and ischemia. Because secondary injuries follow rapidly, usually within hours of direct injury, it is often difficult to distinguish them from the damage done by the primary injury. The distinction between primary or direct and secondary injuries is crucial, however, because the main objective of treatment is to prevent or minimize secondary brain injury.

Primary injuries include concussion and contusion. Even if there is no break in the skull, a blow to the head can cause severe and diffuse brain damage. Such closed injury can be classified (1) as mild, moderate, or severe, or (2) as a concussion or contusion.

In mild head injury, there may be momentary loss of consciousness without demonstrable neurologic symptoms or residual damage, except for possible residual amnesia. Microscopic changes can usually be detected in the neurons and glia within hours of injury. *Concussion* is defined as a momentary interruption of brain function with or without loss of consciousness. Although recovery usually takes place within 24 hours, mild symptoms, such as headache, irritability, insomnia, and poor concentration and memory may persist for months. This is known as the postconcussion syndrome. Because these complaints are vague and subjective, they are sometimes regarded as being of psychologic origin. Recent findings, however, support the belief in an organic basis for the postconcussion symptoms. Postconcussion syndrome can have a significant effect on activities of daily living and return to employment. Persons with postconcussion syndrome may need cognitive retraining for severe level disabilities.

Moderate head injury is characterized by a longer period of unconsciousness and may be associated with neurologic manifestations, such as hemiparesis, aphasia, and cranial nerve palsy. In this type of injury, many small hemorrhages and some swelling of brain tissue occur. Frequently, a contusion or bruising of brain tissue is visualized on CT scan, whereas a concussion cannot be visualized.

In severe head injury, there is cerebral contusion and tearing and shearing of brain structures. It is often accompanied by neurologic deficits such as hemiplegia. Severe head injuries often occur with injury to other parts of the body such as the extremities, chest, and abdomen. Extravasation of blood may occur; if the contusion is severe, the blood may accumulate as in intracranial hemorrhage. Similarly, when laceration of the brain directly under the area of injury occurs, especially if the skull is fractured, hemorrhage may be sufficiently extensive to form a hematoma.

Contusions are often distributed along the rough, irregular inner surface of the brain and are more likely to occur in the frontal or temporal lobes, resulting in cognitive and motor deficits.

Although the skull and CSF provide protection for the brain, they can also contribute to trauma of this nature. A form of brain injury that can cause concussion or contusion due to bouncing of the brain in the closed confines of the rigid skull is called a *coup/contrecoup injury* (Figure 50-17). In this mechanism of injury, the brain is thrown against the same side of the skull (coup) in one continuous motion, which causes damage immediately below the site of impact. The brain then rebounds and strikes the opposite side of the skull (contrecoup), which causes injury in regions of the brain opposite the side of impact. This occurs because the brain floats freely in the CSF, while the brain stem is stable. As the brain strikes the rough surface of the cranial vault, brain tissue, blood vessels, nerve tracts, and other structures are bruised and torn.

Persons with this type of injury can remain minimally responsive to their environment and have a normal CT scan. They may develop a chronic vegetative state characterized by sleep–wake cycles and alertness but no cognitive awareness of self and environment. This state may be caused by torquing motion on the brain stem disrupting the tracts of the reticular activating system and causing widely scattered shearing of axons. This shearing can only be visualized microscopically. Although neurons do not regenerate, research has shown that axons regenerate and nearby undamaged axons will sprout and grow into new terminals.[31] The effects of this phenomenon remain unknown.

The significance of secondary injuries depends on the extent of damage caused by the primary injury. Certain secondary injuries have been discussed

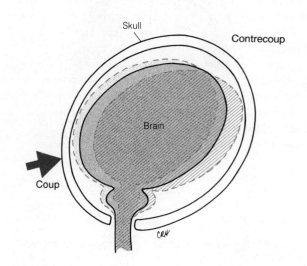

Figure 50-17 Movement of the brain in coup/contrecoup injury.

such as increased intracranial pressure, cerebral edema, and brain herniation. In addition, hematoma can result from shearing of a blood vessel, which also causes contusion. Intracerebral hematomas can be caused by trauma and can result in increased intracranial pressure, which may proceed to herniation of cranial contents through the tentorial notch.

Epidural hematoma

Epidural hematomas are usually caused by a severe head injury in which the skull is fractured. An epidural (extradural) hematoma is one that develops between the skull and the dura, outside the dura (Figure 50-18). It is usually due to a tear in the middle meningeal artery, which is located under the thin temporal bone, and, because the bleeding is arterial in origin, rapid compression of the brain occurs. Epidural hematoma is more common in a young person because the dura is not so firmly attached to the skull surface as it is in an older person; as a consequence, the dura can be easily stripped away from the inner surface of the skull, allowing the hematoma to form.[32]

Typically, a person with an epidural hematoma presents the following picture: a history of head injury, a brief period of unconsciousness followed by a lucid period in which consciousness is regained, followed by rapid progression to unconsciousness. The lucid interval is not always present, but when it is, it is of great diagnostic value. With rapidly developing unconsciousness, there are focal symptoms related to the area of the brain involved. These symptoms can include ipsilateral (same side) pupil dilatation and contralateral (opposite side) hemiparesis. If the hema-

toma is not removed, the condition progresses, with increased intracranial pressure, tentorial herniation, and finally death.

Subdural hematoma

A subdural hematoma develops in the area between the dura and the arachnoid (subdural space) and is the result of a tear in the arachnoid that allows blood from the small bridging veins that connect veins on the surface of the cortex (in the pia mater) to the dural sinuses: superior as well as inferior sagittal sinuses. These veins pass through the CSF, then through the arachnoid and dura. They are readily snapped in head injury, when the brain moves suddenly in relation to the cranium (see Figure 50-18). Bleeding can occur between the dura and arachnoid (subdural hematoma) or into the subarachnoid space and the CSF. It develops more slowly than an epidural hematoma because the tear is in the venous system, whereas epidural hematomas are arterial. Subdural hematomas are classified as acute, subacute, or chronic. Symptoms of acute hematoma are seen within 24 hours of the injury, whereas subacute hematoma does not produce symptoms until 2 to 10 days following injury. Symptoms of chronic subdural hematoma may not arise until several weeks after the injury. These classifications are based partially on pathologic considerations.

Acute subdural hematomas progress rapidly and carry a high mortality because of the severe secondary injuries related to edema and increased intracranial pressure. The high mortality rate has been associated with uncontrolled intracranial pressure increase, loss of consciousness, decerebrate posturing, and delay in surgical removal of the hematoma.[32] The clinical picture is similar to that of epidural hematoma except that there is usually no lucid interval. In subacute hematoma, there may be a period of improvement in the level of consciousness and neurologic symptoms, only to be followed by deterioration if the hematoma is not removed.

Symptoms of chronic subdural hematoma develop weeks after a head injury, so much later, in fact, that the person may not remember having had a head injury. This is especially true of older persons with fragile vessels and whose brain has shrunk away from the dura. Seepage of blood into the subdural space may occur very slowly. Because the blood in the subdural space is not absorbed, fibroblastic activity begins and the hematoma becomes encapsulated. Within this encapsulated area, the cells are slowly lysed and a fluid with a high osmotic pressure is formed. This creates an osmotic gradient with fluid from the surrounding subarachnoid space being

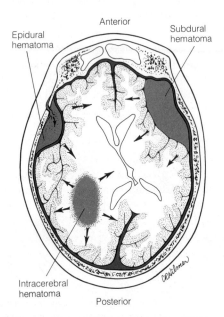

Anterior

Epidural hematoma

Subdural hematoma

Intracerebral hematoma

Posterior

Figure 50-18 Location of epidural, subdural, and intracerebral hematomas.

pulled into the area; in turn, the mass increases in size, exerting pressure on the cranial contents. In some instances, the clinical picture is less defined, the most prominent symptom being a decreasing level of consciousness indicated by drowsiness, confusion, and apathy. Headache may also be present. Morbidity and mortality are highest with subdural hematoma as compared with epidural and intracerebral hematoma.

Intracerebral hematoma

Intracerebral hematoma can also result from head injury. This type of bleeding occurs in the brain tissue itself. Blood often leaks into the CSF causing the same problems as a bridging vein bleed, only the phenomenon is more rapid because of the arterial origin. The severe motion that the brain undergoes can cause bleeding within brain tissue or a contusion can coalesce into a hematoma (see Figure 50-18). Intracerebral hematoma occurs more frequently in older people and alcoholics whose brain vessels are more friable. Intracerebral hematomas can occur in any lobe of the brain, but are seen most frequently in the frontal or temporal lobes. There can be one hematoma or many.

The signs and symptoms produced by an intracerebral hematoma depend on its size and location within the brain. Signs of increased intracranial pressure can be manifested if the hematoma is large and encroaching on vital structures. A hematoma in the temporal lobe can be dangerous because of the potential for lateral herniation.[33]

Treatment of an intracerebral hematoma can be medical or surgical. If someone has a large hematoma with a rapidly deteriorating neurologic condition, surgery to evacuate the clot is generally indicated. Surgery may not be needed in someone who is neurologically stable despite neurologic deficits; in this case, the hematoma may resolve much like a contusion.

Infections

Infections of the CNS may be classified according to the structure involved: the meninges—meningitis; the brain parenchyma—encephalitis; the spinal cord—myelitis; the brain and spinal cord—encephalomyelitis. They may also be classified by the type of invading organism: bacterial, viral, or other. In general, the pathogens enter the CNS through the bloodstream by crossing the blood–brain barrier or by direct invasion through skull fracture, a bullet hole, or, more rarely, contamination during surgery or lumbar puncture.

Meningitis

Meningitis is an infection of the pia mater, the arachnoid, and the subarachnoid space. Usually the inflammation is caused by an infection, but chemical meningitis may also occur. There are two types of acute infectious meningitis: acute pyogenic meningitis (usually bacterial) and acute lymphocytic (generally viral) meningitis.[34,35]

The most common pyogenic infectious agents are *Hemophilus influenzae, Neisseria meningitidis,* and *Streptococcus pneumoniae.* The *H. influenzae* form occurs most frequently in children under 5 years of age and accounts for 70% of all cases.[36] Meningococcus, which is often found as normal flora in the upper respiratory tract is the second most frequent causative agent. Meningococcus meningitis occurs in children and young adults. The very young and the very old are at most risk for pneumococcus meningitis. Risk factors associated with contracting meningitis include head trauma with basilar skull fractures, otitis media, sinusitis or mastoiditis, neurosurgery, dermal sinus tracts, systemic sepsis, or an immunocompromised host.

The most common symptoms of acute pyogenic meningitis are fever and chills; headache; back, abdominal, and extremity pains; and nausea and vomiting. Meningeal signs such as those seen in subarachnoid hemorrhage can also be present (*i.e.,* photophobia and nuchal rigidity). Two assessment techniques can help determine whether or not meningeal irritation is present. Kernig's sign is resistance to extension of the leg while the patient is lying with the hip flexed at a right angle. Brudzinski's sign is seen when forcible flexion of the neck results in flexion of the hip and knee. These signs are caused by stretching of the inflamed meninges in these postures, particularly where it tags down at the foramen magnum. Stretching of the inflamed meninges is extremely painful; hence, the resistance to stretching. A petechial rash is found in most persons with meningococcal meningitis. These petechiae may vary from pinhead size to large ecchymoses or even areas of skin gangrene that sloughs if the person survives. Other types of meningitis may also produce a petechial rash. Persons infected with *H. influenzae* and pneumococcus may present with obtundation and seizures, whereas those with meningococcus are apt to present with bizarre behaviors.[35,37] A spinal tap yields a cloudy and purulent CSF under increased pressure. The CSF typically contains large numbers of polymorphonuclear white blood cells (up to 90,000 per mm^3), increased protein content, and reduced sugar content. Bacteria can be seen on smear and can be easily cultured with appropriate media.[34]

Arthritis, cranial nerve damage (especially the

eighth nerve, with resulting deafness), and hydrocephalus may occur as complications of pyogenic meningitis. As the pathogens enter the subarachnoid space, they cause inflammation, characterized by a cloudy, purulent exudate. Thrombophebitis of the bridging veins and dural sinuses may develop, followed by congestion and infarction in the surrounding tissues. Ultimately, the meninges thicken and adhesions form. These adhesions may impinge on the cranial nerves, giving rise to cranial nerve palsies, or may impair the outflow of CSF, causing hydrocephalus.

Viral meningitis presents in much the same way as bacterial meningitis, but the course is less severe and the CSF findings are markedly different—there are lymphocytes in the fluid rather than polymorphonuclear cells, the protein elevation is only moderately elevated, and the sugar content is usually normal. The acute viral meningitides are self-limiting and usually require only symptomatic treatment. Viral meningitis can be caused by many different viruses including mumps, coxsackie, Epstein-Barr virus, and herpes simplex type II. In many cases, the virus cannot be identified.

CSF analysis will confirm or rule out meningitis and will often identify the organism. Other observations should include (1) the presence of infection, (2) alterations in behavior or level of consciousness, and (3) neurologic symptoms. Treatment depends on the etiologic agent. In bacterial meningitis, prompt therapy is essential to prevent death and minimize serious sequelae. Persons who have been exposed to someone with meningococcal meningitis should be treated prophylactically.

Encephalitis

Generalized infection of the parenchyma of the brain or spinal cord is almost always caused by a virus. The infection takes one of these forms: (1) inflammation caused by direct invasion, in encephalitis, (2) a postinfectious noninflammatory process, in Reye's syndrome, (3) a postinfectious inflammatory process, in encephalomyelitis, and (4) a slow-growing infection that has a prolonged incubation period and runs a chronic course.[36]

The pathologic picture of encephalitis includes local necrotizing hemorrhage, which ultimately becomes generalized, with prominent edema. There is progressive degeneration of nerve cell bodies. The histologic picture, though rather general, demonstrates some specific characteristics; for example, the poliovirus selectively destroys the cells of the anterior horn of the spinal cord.[5]

Encephalitis, like meningitis, is characterized by fever, headache, and nuchal rigidity. In addition, a wide range of neurologic disturbances are present,

such as lethargy, disorientation, seizures, dysphagias, focal paralysis, delirium, and coma. The nervous system is subject to invasion by many viruses, such as arbovirus, poliovirus, and rabies virus. The mode of transmission may be the bite of a mosquito (arbovirus), rabid animal (rabies virus), or ingestion (poliovirus). A common cause of encephalitis in the United States is herpes simplex virus. Diagnosis of encephalitis is made by clinical history and presenting symptoms, in addition to the traditional CSF studies.

In summary, although the skull and the CSF provide protection for the brain, they can also contribute to brain injury through compression and bone splinters that occur with skull fracture and contrecoup injuries. Head injuries may be due to either penetration or impact, each type affecting the brain and supporting structures in different ways. Head injuries can be classified as direct, resulting from the immediate effects of injury, skull fracture, concussion, or contusion; or as secondary, resulting from edema or hemorrhage and infection. Secondary injury may result from epidural, subdural, or intracerebral hematoma formation. Infections of the CNS may be classified according to the structures involved (meningitis, encephalitis) or the type of organism causing the infection. The damage caused by infection may predispose to hydrocephalus, seizures, or other neurologic defects.

Altered levels of consciousness and brain death

Consciousness is a condition in which the individual is fully responsive to stimuli and demonstrates awareness of the environment. Arousal from sleep, wakefulness, and the ability to respond to stimuli rely on an intact reticular activating system (RAS) in the brain stem. Cognition and the ability to respond to the environment rely on an intact cerebral cortex. Therefore, altered forms of consciousness can result from dysfunction or interruption along the pathways of the reticular system. This brain stem system projects downward to the spinal cord and upward to the diencephalon.

The RAS is a diffuse, primitive system of interlacing nerve cells and fibers. It is driven by input from all the sensory systems which account for the arousal caused by stimuli such as a loud noise or stamping of the feet. The *bulboreticular facilitatory area* is located in the uppermost lateral parts of the medulla, and all of the pons, mesencephalon, and diencephalon. The facilitatory area is intrinsically active. There are two positive feedback loops: (1) to the cerebral cortex and back to the reticular formation and (2) to the peripheral muscles and back to the reticular formation through the spinal cord. If no inhibitory signals are being transmitted from other parts of the body, continuous nerve impulses will be transmitted both downward to the motor areas of the cord and upward toward the brain, producing immediate marked activation of the cerebral cortex (arousal). Stimulation of the facilitatory area causes an increase in muscle tone in localized areas or throughout the body. Thus, once the RAS becomes activated, the feedback impulses from both the cerebral cortex and the periphery maintain excitation. After prolonged wakefulness, the neurons in the RAS gradually become less excitable. When this happens, neuronal mechanisms give way to lower-level functioning and sleep.

—— Rostral–caudal progression of coma

Consciousness is an awareness of self and environment. It exists on two continua: normal wakefulness to sleep, and pathologic wakefulness to coma. Table 50-3 defines terms commonly used in describing the unconscious state. A person's level of consciousness can vary due to the extent of injury, medical stability, fever, and pain-producing stimuli.

Deterioration of brain function usually follows a rostral to caudal progression, which is observed as the brain initially compensates for the injury and

Table 50–3.	Terms used in description of unconscious states
Term	**Characteristics**
Consciousness	Alertness, orientation to person, place, and time; normal speech, voluntary movement; oculomotor activity
Confusion	Alteration in perception of stimuli; disorientation to time, first, and then to place, and eventually to person; shortened attention span
Lethargy	Orientation to person, place, and time; slow vocalization; decreased motor and oculomotor activity
Obtundation	Awakening in response to stimulation; continuous stimulation needed for arousal; eyes usually closed
Stupor	Vocalization only in response to stimuli that cause pain; markedly decreased spontaneous movement; eyes closed
Coma	No vocalization; posturing and respirations dependent on level; no spontaneous eye movement; brain stem reflexes intact

(Courtesy of Mary Wierenga, R.N., Ph.D., School of Nursing, University of Wisconsin-Milwaukee)

subsequently decompensates with the loss of autoregulation and cerebral perfusion. The hemispheres are most susceptible to damage, hence the most frequent sign of brain dysfunction is altered level of consciousness and change in behavior. As brain structures in the diencephalon, midbrain, pons, and medulla are affected, additional motor and pupillary signs become evident. Hemodynamic and respiratory instability are the last signs to occur because their regulatory centers are located low in the medulla. The specific signs that accompany this progressive deterioration are outlined in Table 50-4.

Disruptions affecting the diencephalon, midbrain, pons, and medulla usually cause a predictable pattern of change in level of consciousness. The highest level of consciousness is seen in an alert person who is oriented to person, place, and time and is totally aware of the surroundings. The first symptoms of diminution in level of consciousness are decreased concentration, agitation, dullness, and lethargy. With further deterioration, the person becomes obtunded and may respond only to vigorous shaking. Early respiratory changes include yawning and sighing with progression to Cheyne-Stokes breathing (see Chapter 24). These signs are indicative of bilateral hemisphere damage with danger of tentorial herniation. Although the pupils may respond briskly to light, the full range of eye movements is seen only when the head is passively rotated from side to side (oculocephalic reflex, or "doll's eyes" maneuver) or when the caloric test (injection of hot or cold water into the ear canal) is done to elicit nystagmus. In the "doll's eye" test, the eyes move in the direction of rotation rather than rolling in the opposite direction, as occurs normally. There is some combative movement as well as purposeful movement in response to pain. As coma progresses, the bulboreticular facilitatory area becomes more active as fewer inhibitory signals descend from the basal ganglia and cerebral cortex. This results in a condition called *decorticate posturing,* which is characterized by flexion of the upper extremities and extension of the lower extremities.

With progression continuing in rostral–caudal direction, the midbrain becomes involved. Respirations change from Cheyne-Stokes breathing to neurogenic hyperventilation in which the frequency of ventilation may exceed 40 breaths per minute because of uninhibited stimulation of both the inspiratory and expiratory centers. The pupils become fixed in midposition and no longer respond to stimuli. Muscle excitability increases, producing a condition called *decerebrate posturing,* in which the arms are rigid and extended with the palms of the hands turned away from the body.

As coma advances to involve the pons, the pupils remain in midposition and fixed, and the decerebrate posturing continues. Breathing comes apneustic, with sighs evident in midinspiration and with prolonged inspiration and expiration because of excessive stimulation of the respiratory center.

With medullary involvement, the pupils remain fixed in midposition. Respiration become atatic (*i.e.*, totally uncoordinated and irregular). Apnea may occur because of the loss of responsiveness to carbon dioxide stimulation. Complete ventilatory assistance should be considered for any person with atactic breathing. Because the medulla has bulboreticular neurons but not facilitatory neurons, the hyperexcitability that gave rise to decorticate and decerebrate posturing disappears, giving way to flaccidity.

In progressive brain deterioration, the patient's neurologic capabilities appear to fall off in stepwise fashion. Similarly, as neurologic function returns, there appears to be stepwise progress to higher levels of consciousness. An assessment tool called the *Glasgow Coma Scale* is often used to describe levels of coma. This scale uses three aspects of neurologic function, eye-opening, verbal, and motor response, to arrive at a numeric score that represents the level of coma.[38,39]

—— Brain death

With advances in scientific knowledge and technology that have provided the means for artificially maintaining ventilatory and circulatory function, the definition of death has had to be re-examined. In 1968, criteria for irreversible coma were published by a Harvard Medical School Ad Hoc Committee.[40] The criteria included the following: (1) unresponsiveness, (2) no spontaneous respiration for a period of 3 minutes without assistance, (3) absence of CNS reflexes and ocular movements and presence of fixed, dilated pupils, (4) flat EEG for at least 10 minutes, (5) the same findings during a repeat examination 24 hours later, and (6) no evidence of hypothermia or CNS depressants that may alter these findings.

Since 1968, several other criteria have been proposed that modify the Harvard criteria. All have as their fundamental assumption the irreversibility of coma and the absence of responsiveness and respirations. Some complex movement processes at the spinal level may remain with complete brain destruction; therefore, all criteria rely on observation of coma, apnea, cranial nerve reflexes, and the absence of brain stem reflexes. However, it should not be overlooked that there are legal and moral aspects of brain death, which must be taken into consideration.

Diagnostic tests that determine the functional conduction of impulses in the brain include the brain stem auditory-evoked response (BAER) and the somatosensory-evoked response (SSER). Recently these evoked responses have been used in determining the prognosis in brain injury and brain death.[41] With these tests, a waveform is produced when a stimulus is presented to the brain stem auditory tracts by way of earphones, or somatosensory CNS tracts by way of electrode placement to the median nerve or peroneal nerve. Computer circuitry and impulse averaging produce the waveform that is repeatable much like an ECG. Normal waveforms indicate normal impulse conduction in the brain stem (BAER) and cortex (SSER). When neurologic injury occurs, the waveform is altered and damage can be localized but not pinpointed.

In summary, consciousness is a state of awareness of self and environment. It exists on two continua: a normal continuum of wakefulness and sleep and a pathologic continuum of wakefulness and coma. Consciousness depends on the normal functioning of the reticular activating system. Coma can be metabolic, supratentorial, or tentorial in origin. It usually follows a rostral–caudal progression with characteristic changes in levels of consciousness, pupillary response, muscle tone, and respiratory activity occurring as the diencephalon through the medulla are affected.

Table 50-4. Rostral–caudal progression of coma

Area involved	Levels of consciousness	Pupils	Muscle tone	Respiration
Diencephalon (thalamus/ hypothalamus)	Decreased concentration, agitation, dullness, lethargy Obtundation	Respond to light briskly Full range of eye movements only on "doll's eyes" or caloric test	Some purposeful movement in response to pain; combative movement Decorticate	Yawning and sighing → Cheyne-Stokes
Midbrain	Stupor → coma	Midposition fixed (MPF)	Decerebrate	Neurogenic hyperventilation
Pons	Coma	MPF	Decerebrate	Apneustic
Medulla	Coma	MPF	Flaccid	Atactic

(Courtesy of Mary Wierenga, R.N., Ph.D., School of Nursing, University of Wisconsin-Milwaukee)

Seizure disorders

A seizure can be defined as a spontaneous, uncontrolled paroxysmal, transitory discharge of neurons in the brain. This uncontrolled activity causes symptoms based on the location of the involved area —bizarre muscle movements, strange sensations and perception, and loss of consciousness.

A seizure is not a disease but a symptom of an underlying disorder. Seizures may be caused by almost all serious illnesses or injuries affecting the brain, including congenital deformities, vascular lesions, head injury, drug or alcohol abuse, infections, and tumors. Seizures that recur spontaneously without a reversible cause are called epileptic seizures. Although seizures are commonly associated with epilepsy, the two are not necessarily the same. For example, metabolic abnormalities are the major cause of pathologic conditions that give rise to epileptic seizures and that are reversible. Examples include electrolyte imbalances, hypoglycemia, hypoxia, hypocalcemia, and alkalosis. Toxemia of pregnancy, water intoxication, uremia, and CNS infections such as meningitis may precipitate a seizure. The rapid withdrawal of sedative-hypnotic drugs, such as alcohol or barbiturates, is another cause of seizures.[42] In children, a high fever (temperature over 104°F) may precipitate a seizure. In fact, everyone has a seizure threshold, which, when exceeded, can result in seizure activity. Whether or not seizure activity occurs depends on the seizure threshold and the extent to which it is altered by a pathologic condition.

Many theories have been proposed to explain the initiation of the abnormal brain activity that occurs with seizures. Seizures may be caused by alterations in membrane permeability or in the distribution of ions across the neuronal cell membranes. Another cause may be decreased inhibition of cortical or thalamic neuron activity. Neurotransmitter imbalances such as an acetylcholine excess or GABA (an inhibitory neurotransmitter) deficiency have been proposed as a cause.

Epilepsy

Recurrence of seizures without evidence of a reversible metabolic cause is called *epilepsy*. Epileptic and nonepileptic seizures have the same pathology during the event—both result from excessive discharge of cerebral neurons. Epilepsy is the second most prevalent neurologic disorder. Two million Americans, 1 out of every 100 people, have epilepsy.[43] There are two types of epilepsy: primary epilepsy, also called idiopathic epilepsy, which does not have a known cause, and secondary epilepsy, or structurally induced epilepsy, which has a known cause.

The age of onset can be a clue to the type or cause of seizure. Seizures first occurring between the ages of 2 and 18 years with no known cause may be due to the vulnerability of the developing nervous system to seizure activity.[44] Genetic predisposition as a possible cause of idiopathic seizures is currently being investigated. After 20 years of age, seizures are usually due to structural damage, trauma, tumor, or stroke.

In secondary epilepsy, seizures result from cerebral scarring due to head injury, cerebral vascular accident, infection, degenerative CNS disease, or recurrent childhood febrile seizures. Head injury is one of the main causes of seizures. Approximately 10% of persons with acute head injury may have seizures, probably because of bleeding, edema, and neuronal damage.[45] The likelihood of post-traumatic seizures depends on the severity of the underlying injury or disease, whether or not unconsciousness was present, and whether or not the dura was penetrated.

Classification

Although a knowledge of the etiology is important, seizure management is usually directed toward identifying the seizure type and controlling seizure occurrence. In 1969, a classification system was developed by the International League Against Epilepsy. This system combined clinical and electroencephalographic (EEG) manifestations to describe seizure activity.[45] This classification system was prompted by the need for more accurate diagnosis and quantification of seizure activity for use with new and more specific types of medications. A revision of the original classification was proposed in 1981 that allows for description of seizure progression, which helped to improve the accuracy of diagnosis (Chart 50-1).[46] As technology advances and the knowledge of medications and their effects on the various types of seizures is increased, the classification system will probably continue to be redefined.

There are two main classifications of seizures, depending on whether a part of the brain (partial) or the whole brain (generalized) is initially involved. Partial seizures have evidence of a local onset, whereas generalized seizures do not exhibit a local onset.

Partial seizures. Partial seizures are classified as simple partial, complex partial, and partial seizures secondarily generalized. Partial seizures are classified primarily on whether consciousness, defined as awareness or responsiveness to the environment, is impaired. Seizures are classified as simple partial seizures when consciousness is not impaired. If consciousness is impaired, the seizure is classified as a

Chart 50-1: Classification of epileptic seizures

Partial seizures

Simple partial seizures (no impairment of consciousness)
  Motor symptoms
  Sensory symptoms
  Autonomic signs
  Psychic symptoms
Complex partial seizures (impairment of consciousness)
  Simple partial onset followed by impaired
    consciousness
  Impairment of consciousness at onset
Partial seizures evolving to secondarily generalized
    seizures
  Simple partial leading to generalized seizures
  Complex partial leading to generalized seizures
  Simple partial leading to generalized seizures
Unclassified seizures
  Classification not possible due to inadequate or
    incomplete data

Generalized seizures

Absence seizures (true petit mal)
Atonic seizures
Myoclonic seizures
Clonic seizures
Tonic
Tonic-clonic seizures

(Adapted from Commission on Classification and Terminology
of the International League Against Epilepsy. Epilepsia 22:489, 1981)

complex partial seizure. One of the problems with the 1969 classification system was that it failed to account for seizure progression. Simple partial seizures may exist alone or may progress to complex partial seizures or to generalized tonic-clonic seizures.

Simple partial seizures. Simple partial seizures usually involve only one hemisphere and are not accompanied by loss of consciousness or responsiveness. These seizures have also been referred to as elementary partial seizures, partial seizures with elementary symptomatology, or focal seizures. The 1981 Commission on Classification and Terminology of the International League Against Epilepsy has classified simple partial seizures according to (1) motor signs, (2) sensory symptoms, (3) autonomic manifestations, and (4) psychic symptoms. The observed clinical signs and symptoms depend on the area of the brain where the abnormal neuronal discharge is taking place. If the motor area of the brain is involved, the earliest symptom is motor movement corresponding to the location of onset on the contralateral side of the body. The motor movement may remain localized or may spread to other cortical areas with sequential involvement of body parts in an epileptic type "march," known as a Jacksonian seizure. If the sensory portion of the brain is involved, there may be no observable clinical manifestations. Sensory symptoms correlating with the location of seizure activity on the contralat-

eral side of the brain may involve somatic sensory disturbance (tingling, and crawling sensations) or special sensory disturbance (visual, auditory, gustatory, or olfactory phenomenon). When abnormal cortical discharge stimulates the autonomic nervous system, flushing, tachycardia, diaphoresis, hypotension or hypertension, or pupillary changes may be evident.

The term *prodrome* or *aura* has traditionally meant a sensory warning sign of impending seizure activity or the onset of seizure that affected persons could describe because they were conscious. It is now thought that the aura itself is part of the seizure.[44] Because consciousness is maintained and only a small portion of the brain is involved, an aura is a simple partial seizure. Simple partial seizures may progress to complex partial seizures or generalized tonic-clonic seizures that result in unconsciousness. Therefore, the aura in simple partial seizure may, in fact, be a warning sign of impending complex partial seizures.

Complex partial seizures. Complex partial seizures involve impairment of consciousness and often arise from the temporal lobe. The seizure begins in a localized area, but may rapidly progress to both hemispheres. These seizures also may be referred to as temporal lobe seizures or psychomotor seizures. Complex partial seizures are often accompanied by automatisms. Automatisms are repetitive nonpurposeful activity such as lip-smacking, grimacing, patting or continually rubbing clothing. Confusion during the postictal (following a seizure) state is common. Hallucinations and illusionary experiences such as *déjà vu* (familiarity with unfamiliar events or environments) or *jamais vu* (unfamiliarity with a known environment) have been reported. There may be overwhelming fear, uncontrolled forced thinking or flood of ideas, and feelings of detachment and depersonalization. A person with partial seizure is sometimes misunderstood and believed to require hospitalization for a psychiatric disorder.

Generalized epilepsy. Seizures are classified as primary and generalized when the first EEG and clinical changes indicate involvement of both cerebral hemispheres. The clinical symptoms include unconsciousness and involve varying bilateral degrees of symmetric motor responses without indication of localization to one hemisphere. These seizures include absence (petit mal), akinetic, myoclonic, and major motor or tonic-clonic (grand mal) seizures.

Although absence seizures have been characterized as a blank stare, motionlessness, and unresponsiveness, motion occurs in about 90% of absence seizures. This motion takes the form of automatisms such as lip-smacking, mild clonic motion usually in the eyelids, increased or decreased postural tone, and autonomic phenomena. There is often a brief loss of contact with the environment. The seizure usually lasts only a few seconds, and then the person is able to resume normal activity immediately. The manifestations are often so subtle that they may pass unnoticed. Absence seizures typically occur only in children and either cease in adulthood or evolve into generalized major motor seizures, especially if absence occurred in childhood. In akinetic or atonic seizures, there is a sudden split-second loss of muscle tone leading to a slackening of the jaw, drooping of the limb, or falling to the ground. These seizures are also known as *drop attacks.*

The major motor or convulsive seizures include myoclonic, tonic, clonic, and tonic-clonic seizures. A myoclonic seizure involves bilateral jerking of muscles, either generalized or confined to the face, trunk, or one or more extremities. Tonic seizures are characterized by a rigid, violent contraction of the muscles fixing the limbs in a strained position. Clonic seizures consist of repeated contractions and relaxations of the major muscle groups.

The tonic-clonic seizure, formerly called a *grand mal seizure,* is the most common major motor seizure. Frequently a person has a vague warning (probably a simple partial seizure) and experiences a sharp tonic contraction of the muscles with extension of the extremities and immediate loss of consciousness. Incontinence of bladder and bowels is common. Cyanosis may occur from contraction of airway and respiratory muscles. The tonic phase is followed by the clonic phase, which involves rhythmic bilateral contraction and relaxation of the extremities. At the end of the clonic phase, the person remains unconscious until the reticular activating system begins to function again. This is termed the *postictal phase.* The tonic-clonic phases last approximately 60 seconds to 90 seconds.

The prevalence of primary tonic-clonic seizures has probably been overestimated; most tonic-clonic seizures are probably secondary generalized partial seizures or less dramatic seizures (absence).[44] The tonic-clonic seizure is the only type of seizure activity (primarily from drug or alcohol withdrawal) that occurs in about 10% of persons with seizures.

Unclassified seizures. Unclassified seizures are those seizures that cannot be placed in one of the above categories. These seizures are observed in the neonatal and infancy period of life. Determination of whether the seizure is focal or generalized is not possible. Unclassified seizures are difficult to control with medication.

Diagnosis and treatment

The diagnosis of epilepsy is based on a thorough history and neurologic examination, including a full description of the seizure. The physical examination helps rule out any metabolic disease that could precipitate seizures. Skull x-rays and CT or MRI scans are used to identify structural defects. One of the most useful diagnostic tests is the electroencephalogram, which is used to record changes in the brain's electrical activity. It is used to support the clinical diagnosis of epilepsy, to provide a guide for prognosis, and to assist in classifying the seizure disorder.

The first rule of treatment is to protect the person from injury during a seizure; the next is to treat any underlying disease. Persons with epilepsy should be advised to avoid situations that could be dangerous or life-threatening if seizures should occur. Treatment of the underlying disorder may reduce the frequency of seizures. Once the underlying disease is treated, the aim of treatment is to bring the seizures under control

Table 50–5. Anticonvulsant medications

Drug	Types of seizures	Side effects	Half-life (hr)	Steady state level (days)
Carbamazepine (Tegretol)	Partial, tonic-clonic	Blood dyscrasias, leukopenia, aplastic anemia	12	3–4
Phenytoin (Dilantin)	Partial, tonic-clonic	Hirsutism, gingival hyperplasia, coarsening of features, teratogenic potential	24	5–10
Ethosuximide (Zarontin)	Absence, generalized	Relatively free of side effects	40	5–10
Valproate (Depakene)	Generalized, absence	Hepatitis, weight gain, hair loss, fine tremor, drug interaction, gastrointestinal irritation	8	2–4
Phenobarbital	Tonic-clonic	Drowsiness, irritability	50–150	14–21
Primidone (Mysoline)	Tonic-clonic, simple partial, complex partial	Drowsiness, ataxia, behavior changes	12	4–7
Clonazepam (Clonopin)	Absence	Drowsiness, double vision, behavior changes	18	?

with the least possible disruption in life-style and minimum side effects from medication. With proper drug management, 60% to 80% of persons with epilepsy can obtain good seizure control.[47] During the last 20 years, the therapy for epilepsy has changed drastically due to the improved classification system, the ability to measure serum anticonvulsant levels, and the availability of potent new anticonvulsant drugs.

Anticonvulsant medications. Whenever possible, a single drug should be used in epilepsy therapy. This eliminates drug interactions and additive side effects. Among the drugs used in treatment of epilepsy are carbamazepine, phenytoin, ethosuximide, valproate, phenobarbital, primidone, and clonazepam.[48] Carbamazepine and phenytoin are the drugs of choice in partial seizures. They are also used for tonic-clonic seizures secondary to partial seizures. Ethosuximide is the drug of choice for absence seizures, but is not effective for tonic-clonic seizures progressed from partial seizures. Valproate is helpful for people with many of the minor motor seizures and tonic-clonic seizures. Valproate and ethosuximide can be used together. Phenobarbital is used for tonic-clonic seizures as is primidone. In addition, primidone is prescribed for simple and complex partial seizures. Absence and myoclonic seizures can be treated with clonazepam. Atonic seizures are highly resistant to therapy. Table 50-5 lists the drugs commonly used in the treatment of seizures, their side effects, half-life, and time to steady-state levels.

Determining the proper dose of the anticonvulsant drug(s) is often a long and tedious process, which can become very frustrating to the person with epilepsy. Consistency in taking the medication is essential. Anticonvulsant drugs should never be discontinued abruptly; rather, the dose should be decreased slowly to prevent seizure recurrence.

The most frequent cause of recurrent seizures is patient noncompliance with drug regimens.[48] Ongoing education and support are extremely important in the management of seizures. The psychosocial implications of a diagnosis of epilepsy continue to have a large impact on those affected with the disorder.

Other therapy. Although surgical therapy has limited use in the treatment of epilepsy, surgical removal of a single isolated cortical lesion is sometimes indicated if a single lesion can be identified and removed without leaving a neurologic deficit and seizures have not been controlled with adequate trials of anticonvulsant drugs. Corpus callostomy, another procedure used in the treatment of intractable seizures, involves sectioning or separating the fibers of the corpus callosum to prevent spread of a unilateral seizure to a generalized seizure. Indications for this type of surgery include drop attacks with second-degree generalization that occur several times a week and cause repeated injury despite adequate drug levels. The number of persons who can benefit from this type of surgical procedure is small, and the goal is to reduce the seizures, not eliminate them.

Status epilepticus

Seizures that do not stop spontaneously or occur in succession without recovery are called *status epilepticus*. There are as many types of status epilepticus as there are types of seizures. Tonic-clonic status epilepticus is a medical emergency and, if not promptly treated, may lead to respiratory failure and death.

The main cause of status epilepticus in persons with epilepsy is noncompliance with medication therapy, and in a person with no history of epilepsy it is neurologic or systemic disease. If status epilepticus is due to neurologic or systemic disease, the cause needs to be identified and treated immediately because the seizures will probably not respond until the underlying cause has been corrected. When status epilepticus is the result of discontinuing medication, the drug regimen should be reinstituted as soon as possible. The prognosis is related to the underlying cause more than to the seizures themselves.

In summary, seizures are caused by spontaneous, uncontrolled, paroxysmal, transitory discharge from cortical centers in the brain. Seizures may occur as a reversible symptom of another disease condition or as a recurrent condition called epilepsy. Epileptic seizures are classified as partial or generalized seizures. Partial seizures have evidence of local onset, beginning in one hemisphere. They include simple partial seizures, in which consciousness is not lost, and complex partial partial seizures, which begin in one hemisphere but progress to involve both. Generalized seizures involve both hemispheres and include unconsciousness and rapidly occurring widespread bilateral symmetric motor responses. They include minor motor seizures such as absence, akinetic seizures, and major motor or grand mal seizures. Control of seizures is the primary goal of treatment and is accomplished with anticonvulsant medications. Anticonvulsant medications interact with each other and need to be monitored closely when more than one drug is used.

References

1. Blinkov SM, Glezer II: The Human Brain in Figures and Tables, p 201. New York, Basic Books, 1968
2. Noback CR, Demarest RJ: The Human Nervous System, pp 518–520. McGraw-Hill, 1981

3. Guyton A: Textbook of Medical Physiology, 7th ed, p 339. Philadelphia, WB Saunders, 1986

4. Bradbury MWB: The blood–brain barrier. Circ Res 57(2):214, 1985

5. Goldstein GW, Betz AL: The blood–brain barrier. Sci Am 255(3):74, 1986

6. Robbins SL, Cotran RS, Kumar V: Pathologic Basis of Disease 2nd ed, pp 1385, 1388, 1393. Philadelphia, WB Saunders, 1987

7. Martin TG: Drowning and near drowning. Hosp Med 22(7):53, 1986

8. Hunter C: Cardiopulmonary cerebral resuscitation: Nursing interventions. Crit Care Nurse 7(3):46, 1987

9. Neatherlin JS, Brillhardt B: Glasgow coma scores in the patient post cardiopulmonary resuscitation. J Neurosci Nurs 20(2):104, 1988

10. Dyken ML, Wolf PA, Barnett HJM et al: Risk factors in stroke. A statement for physicians by the subcommittee on risk factors and stroke of the Stroke Council. Stroke 15:1105, 1984

11. Gorelick PB: Alcohol and stroke. Curr Concepts Cerebrovasc Dis 21(5):21, 1986

12. Levine SR, Welch KMA: Cocaine and stroke. Curr Concepts Cerebrovasc Dis 22(5):25, 1987

13. Levine SR, Welch KMA: The neurologic impact of cocaine abuse. Emerg Med 20:99, 1988

13a. Wojack JC, Flamm ES: Intracranial hemorrhage and cocaine abuse. Stroke 18:712, 1987

14. Grotta JC: Current medical and surgical therapy for cerebrovascular accident. N Engl J Med 317(24):1505, 1987

15. Rothrock JF: Clinical evaluation and management of transient ischemic attacks. West J Med 146:452, 1987

16. Mitchel S, Yates RR: Extracranial–intracranial bypass surgery. J Neurosci Nurs 17(5):288, 1985

17. DeLaria GA, Javid H: Evaluating subclavian steal syndrome. Consultant 20(2):88, 1980

18. Bobath B: Adult Hemiplegia: Evaluation and Treatment, 2nd ed. London, William Heinemann Medical Books, 1978

19. Palmer EP: Language dysfunction in cerebrovascular disease. Primary Care 6(4):827, 1979

20. Holland AL: Treatment of aphasia following stroke. Stroke 14(2):5, 1979

21. Ruskin AP: Understanding stroke and its rehabilitation. Curr Concepts Cerebrovasc Dis 17(6):27, 1982

22. Campbell JK: Use of computerized tomography and radionuclide scan in stroke. Stroke 12(3):11, 1977

23. Gent M: Single studies and overview analyses: Is aspirin of value in cerebral ischemia? Stroke 18(3):541, 1987

24. Crowell RM: Aneurysm and arteriovenous malformations. Neurol Clin 3(2):291, 1985

25. Petitti DB, Wingerd J: Use of oral contraceptives, cigarette smoking and risk of subarachnoid hemorrhage. Lancet 2:234, 1978

26. Jane JA, Cassel NF, Torner JC et al: The natural history of aneurysms and arteriovenous malformations. J Neurosurg 62(3):321, 1985

26a. Ferguson GG: Physical factors in initiation, growth, and rupture of human intracranial aneurysms. J Neurosurg 37:666, 1972

27. Mitchel SK, Yates RR: Cerebral vasospasm: Theoretical causes, medical management, and nursing implications. J Neurosci Nurs 18:315, 1986

28. Adams RD, Victor M: Principles of Neurology, 3rd ed. New York, McGraw-Hill, 1981

29. Langfitt TW, Weinstein JD, Kassell NF: Cerebral vasomotorparalysis produced by intracranial hypertension. Neurology (Minneapolis) 15:622, 1965

30. Sayama I, Auer LM: Oscillating cerebral blood volume: The origin of B-waves. In Ischii S, Nagai H, Brock M (eds): Intracranial Pressure V. Berlin, Springer-Verlag, 1983

31. Fishman RA: Brain edema. N Engl J Med 293(14):706, 1975

32. Cotman CW, Nieto-Sampedro M: Progress in facilitating the recovery of function after central nervous system trauma. Ann NY Acad Sci 457:83, 1985

33. Mauldin R, Coleman L: Intracerebral herniation. J Neurosurg Nurs 15(6):287, 1983

34. Robbins SL, Cotran RS, Kumar V: Pathologic Basis of Disease, 3rd ed, pp 1378–1379. Philadelphia, WB Saunders, 1984

35. Weinstein L: Bacterial meningitis: Specific etiologic diagnosis on the basis of distinctive epidemiologic, pathogenetic, and clinical features. Med Clin North Am 69(2):219, 1985

36. Gold R: Bacterial meningitis—1982. Am J Med 75(1B):98, 1983

37. Pendergast V: Bacterial meningitis update. J Neurosci Nurs 19(2):95, 1987

38. Ingersoll GL, Leyden DB: The Glasgow Coma Scale for patients with head injuries. Crit Care Nurs 7(5):26, 1987

39. Knight RL: The Glasgow Coma Scale: Ten years later. Crit Care Nurs 6(3):65, 1986

40. Black PM: Criteria of brain death. Review and comparison. Postgrad Med 57(2):69, 1975

41. Hummelgard AB, Martin EM, Singer ER: Prognostic value of brainstem auditory evoked potentials in head trauma. J Neurosurg Nurs 16(4):181, 1984

42. Hawken M: Seizures: Etiology, classification, intervention. J Neurosurg Nurs 11(3):166, 1979

43. US Department of Health and Human Services: Epilepsy: Hope through Research. Public Health Services, National Institute of Health, Superintendent of Documents, Washington, DC, US Government Printing Office, NIH Publication No 81–167, 1981

44. Porter RJ: Epilepsy: 100 Elementary Principles. Philadelphia, WB Saunders, 1984

45. Gastault H: Clinical and electroencephalographic classification of epileptic seizures. Epilepsia 11:102, 1970

46. Commission on Classification and Terminology of the International League Against Epilepsy: Proposal for revised clinical and electroencephalographic classification of epileptic seizures. Epilepsia 22:489, 1981

47. Barry K, Teixerira S: The role of the nurse in the diagnostic classification and management of epileptic seizures. J Neurosurg Nurs 15(4):243, 1983

48. Santilli N, Sierzant TL: Advances in treatment of epilepsy. J Neurosci Nurs 19(3):141, 1987

Bibliography

—— Alterations in cerebral blood flow

Becker DP: Brain cellular injury and recovery—Horizons improving medical therapies in stroke and trauma. West J Med 148:670, 1988

Chase M, Whelan-Decker E: Nursing management of a patient with subarachnoid hemorrhage. J Neurosci Nurs 16(1):23, 1984

Cohen LG, Hallet M: Noninvasive mapping of motor cortex. Neurology 38:904, 1988

DeWitt LD, Wechsler LR: Transcranial doppler. Stroke 19(7):915, 1988

DeWitt LD, Weschler LR: Transcranial doppler. Stroke 22:31, 1987

Dobkin BH: Management of transient ischemic attacks. Hosp Pract 22(Mar 15):113, 1987

Fisher CM: Lacunar strokes and infarcts: A review. Neurology (NY) 32:871, 1982

Fode NC: Subarachnoid hemorrhage from ruptured intracranial aneurysm. Am J Nurs 88:673, 1988

Foulkes MA, Wolf PA, Price TR et al: The stroke data bank: Design, methods, and baseline characteristics. Stroke 19:547, 1988

Gillum RF: Stroke in blacks. Stroke 19(1):1, 1988

Gorelick PB: Cerebrovascular disease: Pathophysiology and diagnosis. Nurs Clin North Am 21(2):275, 1986

Helgason CM: Blood glucose and stroke. Stroke 19(8):1049, 1988

Huang PS: Cerebral vascular disease: Update. Del Med J 59(1):13, 1987

Jackson LO: Cerebral spasm after an intracranial aneurysmal subarachnoid hemorrhage: A nursing perspective. Heart Lung 15(1):14, 1986

Kassel NF, Saski T, Colahan ART et al: Cerebral vasospasm following aneurysmal subarachnoid hemorrhage. Stroke 16:562, 1985

Kasuya A, Holm K: Pharmacologic approach to stroke management. Nurs Clin North Am 21(2):289, 1986

Kristler JP, Ropper AH, Herzog RC: Therapy of ischemic vascular disease due to atherothromboses. N Engl J Med (Parts I and II) 311:27, 1984

Little N, Ratcheson RA, Tarlov E: Think subarachnoid hemorrhage. Patient Care 22(121):4, 1988

Miller E, Williams S: Alterations in cerebral perfusion: Clinical concept or nursing diagnosis. J Neurosci Nurs 19:183, 1987

Mori E, Tabuchi M, Yoshida T et al: Intracarotid urokinase with thromboembolic occlusion of the middle cerebral artery. Stroke 19:802, 1988

Pimental PA: Alterations in communication: Aspects of aphasia, dysarthria, and right hemisphere syndrome in the stroke patient. Nurs Clin North Am 21(2):321, 1986

Rothrock JF: Clinical evaluation and management of transient ischemic attacks. West J Med 146:452, 1987

Weisber LA: Diagnostic classifications of stroke, especially lacunes. Stroke 19(9):1071, 1988

—— Increased intracranial pressure

Cascino GD: Neurophysiologic monitoring in the intensive care unit. J Intensive Care Med 3:215, 1988

Morrison CAM: Brain herniation syndromes. Crit Care Nurs 7(5):34, 1987

Pollack-Latham C: Intracranial pressure monitoring: Parts I and II. Crit Care Nurs 7(5, 6):40, 1987

Scwiry B, Giffin JP, Cottrell JE: Intracranial hypertension: Physiology, pathophysiology and management. J Am Assoc Nurse Anesth 52(3):264, 1984

—— Head injury and brain infection

Becker DP (moderator): Brain cellular injury and recovery— Horizons for improving medical therapies in stroke and trauma. West Med J 148:670, 1988

Bricolo A, Turaxxi S, Alexandre A et al: Decerebrate rigidity in acute head injury. J Neurosurg 47:680, 1977

Connolly R, Zewe GE: Update: Head injuries. J Neurosci Nurs 13(4):195, 1981

Ferido T, Habel M: Spasticity in head trauma and CVA patients: Etiology and management. J Neurosci Nurs 20(1):17, 1988

Hall JW, Speilman G, Gennarelli TA: Auditory evoked responses in acute head injury. J Neurosurg Nurs 14:225, 1982

Henneman EA: Brain resuscitation. Heart Lung 15(1):3, 1986

Hinkle J: Care of patients with minor head injury. J Neurosci Nurs 20(1):8, 1988

Jorden RC: Pathophysiology of brain injury. Crit Care Q 5(4):1, 1983

Little NE: Postconcussion syndrome—What is it. Emerg Med 20(8):30, 1988

Palmer M, Wyness MA: Positioning and handling: Important considerations in care of the severely head-injured patient. J Neurosci Nurs 20:42, 1988

Vulcan BM: Acute bacterial meningitis in infancy and childhood. Crit Care Nurs 7(5):53, 1987

Yanko J: Head injuries. J Neurosci Nurs 16(6):173, 1984

—— Seizure disorders

Berkovic SF, Andermann F, Anderman E et al: Concepts of absence epilepsies: Views and reviews. Neurology 37:993, 1987

Berkovic SF, Andermann F, Carpenter S et al: Progressive myoclonus epilepsies: Specific causes and diagnosis. N Engl J Med 315(5):296, 1986

Bradford HF, Patterson DW: Current views of the pathobiochemistry of epilepsy. Mol Aspects Med 9(2):119, 1987

DeVroom HL, Considine EP: Advances in the localization of epileptic loci for surgical resection. J Neurosci Nurs 19(2):77, 1987

Engel J (Moderator): UCLA Conference: Recent developments in diagnosis and therapy in epilepsy. Ann Intern Med 97:584, 1982

Evans OB, Hanson RR, Snead CO: The primary generalized epilepsies in children. Semin Neurol 8(1):12, 1988

Snead OC: Epilepsy in children: A practical approach. Semin Neurol 8(1):24, 1988

Talwar D, Sher PK: The partial epilepsies of childhood. Semin Neurol 8(1):1, 1988

Alterations in Vision

Objectives

After you have studied this chapter, you should be able to meet the following objectives:

_____ List the three layers of the eyeball.

_____ Differentiate between exophthalmos and proptosis.

_____ Describe the normal characteristics of the lateral and medial canthi.

_____ Cite the difference between marginal blepharitis, a hordeolum, and a chalazion.

_____ Describe eyelid changes that occur with entropion and ectropion.

_____ Explain how the strength of the orbicularis oculi can be tested.

_____ Compare symptoms associated with the red eye caused by conjunctivitis, corneal irritation, acute glaucoma, subconjunctival hemorrhage, and blepharitis.

_____ List at least four causes of dry eye.

_____ Describe the appearance of corneal edema.

(continued)

_____ List the symptoms of keratitis.

_____ Explain the mechanism of pupillary constriction and dilatation.

_____ Compare closed-angle and open-angle glaucoma.

_____ Define *refraction* and *accommodation*.

_____ Describe the visual changes that occur with cataract.

_____ Describe the function of the retina and its photoreceptors.

_____ Differentiate between retinal structures supplied by the choroid capillaries and those supplied by the retinal arteries.

_____ State the value of the funduscopic examination of the eye using the ophthalmoscope.

_____ State the cause of color blindness.

_____ Relate the phagocytic function of the retinal pigment epithelium to the development of retinitis pigmentosa.

_____ Describe the pathogenesis of background and proliferative diabetic retinopathy and their mechanisms of visual impairment.

_____ Explain the pathology and visual changes associated with macular degeneration.

_____ Discuss the cause of retinal detachment.

_____ Trace the pathways of the nasal and temporal retina from the optic nerve to the primary visual cortex.

_____ Define *scotoma* and discuss its significance.

_____ Describe a method for testing the visual field.

_____ Name the six extraocular muscles and their cranial nerves.

_____ Define *smooth pursuit, saccadic, vestibular, vergence,* and *tremor eye movements*.

_____ Describe two causes of strabismus.

_____ Explain the difference between paralytic and nonparalytic strabismus.

_____ Explain the need for early diagnosis and treatment of strabismus in infants and small children.

_____ Define *amblyopia* and explain its pathogenesis.

Nearly 11.5 million persons in the United States—1 in every 19—suffer from some degree of visual impairment. Of these, 12% are unable to see well enough to read ordinary newsprint, even with the aid of glasses, and another 4% are classified as legally blind.[1] More than 50% of blind people are over age 65, and the majority of these are over 85 years of age. Alterations in vision can result from disorders of the eyeball and supporting structures, intraocular pressure, optics and lens function, vitreous and retinal function, visual pathways and cortical function, and eye movements.

The eye and supporting structures

The optic globe, or eyeball, is a remarkably mobile, nearly spherical structure contained within a pyramid-like cavity of the skull called the *orbit* (Figure 51-1). The eyeball consists of an outer supporting fibrous layer (sclera), a vascular layer (uveal tract), and a neural layer (retina). The interior is filled with transparent media (the aqueous and vitreous humors), which allow the penetration and transmission of light to photoreceptors in the retina. The exposed surface of the eye is protected by the eyelid, a skin flap that provides a means for shutting out most light and pattern vision. Tears bathe its surface, protecting the eye from irritation by foreign objects, preventing friction between the eye and the lid, and maintaining the hydration of the cornea. Two eyes on the same horizontal plane, with extraocular muscles for directional rotation of the eyeball, provide different images of the same objects and the basis for depth perception of near objects.

Orbit

The orbit is a pyramidal cavity with walls formed by the union of seven cranial and facial bones: the frontal, maxillary, zygomatic, lacrimal, sphenoid, ethmoid, and palatine bones (Figure 51-2). The superior surface of the maxillary bone forms the main floor of the orbit. Tumors of the nasal antrum may invade the orbit and cause the eyeball to protrude. The superior maxillary, lacrimal, and ethmoid bones form the medial wall of the orbit. This wall is very thin, and infections of the ethmoid sinus may invade the orbit. The lateral wall is triangular in shape; it is formed anteriorly by zygomatic bone and posteriorly by sphenoid bone. It is the thickest wall, particularly at the orbital margin where the wall is most apt to be exposed to trauma. The apex of the orbital pyramid, located in the posterior medial part of the orbit, is pierced by an opening called the *optic foramen,* through which the optic nerve, ophthalmic artery, and sympathetic nerves from the carotid plexus pass. A larger opening, the superior orbital fissure, permits passage of branches of cranial nerves III, IV, V (ophthalmic division), and VI (ophthalmic division). These provide motor innervation of the extrinsic and intrinsic eye muscles and provide sensory innervation

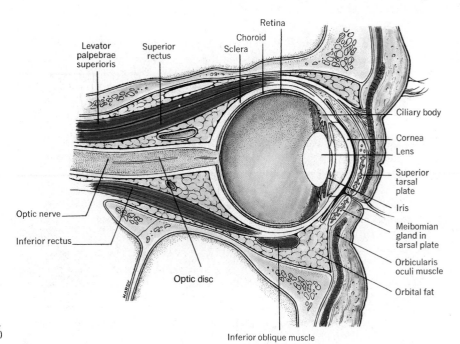

Figure 51-1 The eye and its appendages, lateral view. (*Chaffee EE, Lytle IM: Basic Anatomy and Physiology, 4th ed. Philadelphia, JB Lippincott, 1980*)

of the orbit and its contents. The eyeball occupies only the anterior one-fifth of the orbit; the remainder is filled with muscles, nerves, the lacrimal glands, and adipose tissue that supports the normal position of the optic globe. A layer of fascia known as Tenon's capsule surrounds the globe of the eye from the cornea to the posterior segment and separates the eye from the orbital fat.

Because the walls of the orbit are rigid, any space-occupying lesion results in protrusion of the eyeball, a condition called *exophthalmos*. When the eyelid also protrudes, the condition is known as *prop-*

tosis. Exophthalmos is associated with endocrine disorders of pituitary or hypothalamic origin. It is commonly seen in persons with hyperthyroidism (see Chapter 44). The condition causes a delay in lid closure (lid lag) and, in severe cases, an inability of the lids to close completely, resulting in exposure and drying of the cornea. Because the optic nerve has sufficient length within the orbit, protrusion greater than 5 mm is required before nerve damage occurs.

Enophthalmos, or deeply sunken eyes, may be an individual characteristic, but it also occurs with severe loss of orbital fat during malnutrition and starvation. Severe developmental defects during the first month of fetal life can result in the absence of one or both optic globes (*anophthalmos*), and growth defects during the last 3 months of gestation can result in abnormally small eyes (*microphthalmos*).

— Eyelids

The eyelids are called the *palpebrae*, and the oval space between the upper and lower lids is the *palpebral fissure.* The angle where the upper and lower lids meet is referred to as a *canthus;* the lateral canthus is the outer, or temporal, angle and the medial canthus is the inner, or nasal, angle (Figure 51-3). A line through the lateral and medial canthi defines the angle of the palpebral fissure and is usually horizontal. In children with Down's syndrome, this line slants upward laterally, giving the child a Mongolian appearance (see Chapter 4). A fold of skin, the *epicanthic fold,* covers the medial canthus and is characteristic of the Asian race as well as persons with certain chromo-

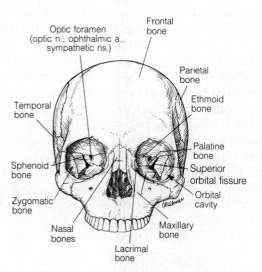

Figure 51-2 Anterior view of the skull showing the orbital cavity and optic foramen that form an opening for the optic nerve, blood vessels (*e.g.,* ophthalmic artery), and sympathetic nerves that supply the eye.

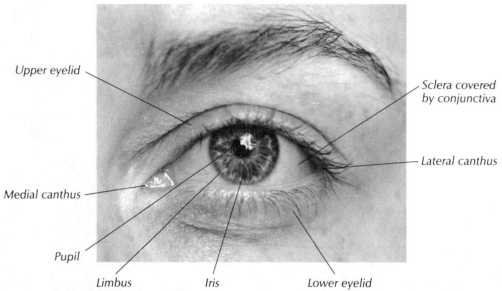

Figure 51-3 Right eye. (Bates B: A Guide to Physical Examination and History Taking, 4th ed, p 147. Philadelphia, JB Lippincott, 1987)

somal abnormalities. The spacing between the two orbits is highly variable. The term *hypertelorism* is used if they are spaced abnormally far apart, and *hypotelorism,* if they are abnormally close together.

In each lid, a tarsus, or plate of dense connective tissue, gives the lid its shape (see Figure 51-1). Each tarsus contains modified sebaceous glands (meibomian glands), the ducts of which open onto the eyelid margins. The sebaceous secretions enable airtight closure of the lids and prevent rapid evaporation of tears.

Eyelid inflammation

Marginal blepharitis, or inflammation of the eyelids, is the most common disorder of the eyelids. There are two main types: seborrheic and staphylococcal. The chief symptoms are irritation, burning, redness, and itching of the eyelid margins. The seborrheic form is usually associated with seborrhea (dandruff) of the scalp or brows. Treatment includes careful cleansing with a wet applicator or clean washcloth to remove the scales. A nonirritating baby shampoo can be used. When the disorder is associated with a microbial infection, an antibiotic ointment is prescribed.

A *hordeolum (stye)* is caused by infection of the sebaceous glands of the eyelid and can be either internal or external. The main symptoms are pain, redness, and swelling. The treatment is similar to that for abscesses in other parts of the body: heat in the form of warm compresses is applied, and antibiotic ointment may be used. Incision or expression of the infectious contents of the abscess may be necessary. A *chalazion* is a small nodule that is formed due to fatty

degeneration of a hordeolum. It is treated by surgical excision.

The two striated muscles that provide movement of the eyelids are the levator palpebrae and the orbicularis oculi. The levator palpebrae, which is innervated by the oculomotor (III) cranial nerve, raises the upper lid. The orbicularis oculi, which is supplied by the facial (VII) cranial nerve, closes the lid. The palpebral portion of this muscle is used for gentle closure, and the orbital portion is used for forcible closure of the lids.

Normally the edges of the eyelids are in such a position that the palpebral conjunctiva that lines the eyelids is not exposed and the eyelashes do not rub against the cornea. Turning in of the lid is called *entropion*. It is usually caused by scarring of the palpebral conjunctiva or degeneration of the fascial attachments to the lower lid that occurs with aging. Turning inward of the eyelashes causes corneal irritation. *Ectropion* refers to eversion of the lower lid. The condition is usually bilateral and caused by relaxation of the orbicularis oculi muscle because of seventh nerve weakness or the aging process. Ectropion causes tearing and ocular irritation and may lead to inflammation of the cornea. Both entropion and ectropion can be treated surgically. Electrocautery penetration of the lid conjunctiva can also be used to treat mild forms of ectropion. Contraction of the scar tissue that follows tends to draw the lid up to its normal position.

Eyelid weakness

Drooping of the upper lid is called *ptosis.* It can result from weakness of the muscle that elevates the upper lid (levator palpebrae superioris) or of the circular ring of muscles (orbicularis oculi) that forcefully close the palpebral fissure. Weakness of this muscle causes not ptosis, but open eyelid. Severe weakness or flaccidity of the muscles can result from damage to the innervating cranial nerves or to the nerves' central nuclei in the midbrain and the caudal pons.

The facial (VII) cranial nerve reaches the orbicularis oculi after exiting the skull under the parotid gland and then traveling deep to the skin across the face. Thus, trauma to the zygomatic and buccal branches of the facial nerve with a resultant ptosis is relatively common. Weakness of the orbicularis oculi is tested by placement of the examiner's fingers on the muscular sphincter ring while the eye is open and then asking the person to close the eye. Movement of the eyelid is also affected in a condition called *Bell's palsy*, which involves paralysis of muscles on one side of the face because of a lesion of the facial nerve or its nucleus in the caudal pons.

Damage to the oculomotor nerve is much less common than damage to the facial nerve because the oculomotor nerve is protected by the skull throughout its path. However, ptosis resulting from third cranial nerve injury can occur in midbrain stroke and basal skull fractures and from tumors located deep in the orbit or in the cavernous sinus. Drooping of the eyelids because of generalized weakness of the extraocular muscles occurs in some forms of muscular dystrophy and is an early and common intermittent manifestation of myasthenia gravis (see Chapter 49).

—— Conjunctiva

The inner surface of the eyelid is lined with a thin layer of mucous membrane, the palpebra conjunctiva. The conjunctiva folds back at the fornix (reflexion of the conjunctiva from the eyelid to eyeball) and covers the optic globe to the junction of the cornea and sclera. When the eyes are closed, the conjunctiva lines the closed conjunctival sac. The conjunctiva is extremely sensitive to irritation and inflammation. The lining of the upper lid is innervated by the ophthalmic division (V1) of the trigeminal (V) cranial nerve and that of the lower lid, by the maxillary division (V2) of the same nerve.

—— Conjunctivitis

Conjunctivitis, or inflammation of the conjunctiva, (sometimes called redeye or pinkeye) is one of the most common forms of eye disease. It varies in severity from mild hyperemia with tearing (hay fever conjunctivitis) to a severe necrotizing process (membranous conjunctivitis). Conjunctivitis may result from infection, allergens, chemical agents, physical irritants, or radiant energy. Infections may extend from areas adjacent to the conjunctiva or may be blood-borne, such as in measles or chickenpox.

The main symptoms of conjunctivitis are redness of the eye, ocular discomfort or foreign body sensation, gritty or burning sensation, and tearing. Severe pain suggests corneal rather than conjunctival disease. Itching is common in allergic conditions. A discharge, or exudate, may be present with all types of conjunctivitis. It is usually watery when the conjunctivitis is caused by allergy, foreign body, or viral infection and mucopurulent in the presence of bacterial or fungal infection. A characteristic of many forms of conjunctivitis is papillary hypertrophy. This occurs because the conjunctiva is bound to the tarsus by fine fibrils. As a result, inflammation that develops between the fibrils causes the conjunctiva to be elevated in mounds called *papillae*. When the papillae are small, the conjunctiva has a smooth, velvety appearance. A red papillary conjunctivitis suggests bacterial or chlamydial conjunctivitis. In allergic conjunctivitis, the papillae often become flat-topped, polygonal, and milky in color and have a cobblestone appearance. Edema of the conjunctiva is called *chemosis*.

Allergic conjunctivitis. Allergic conjunctivitis (hay fever) is a common disorder associated with exposure to allergens such as pollen. It causes bilateral tearing, itching, and redness of the eyes. The treatment includes the use of cold compresses, antihistamines, and vasoconstrictor eyedrops. The local application of corticosteroids may be used on a short-term basis.

Bacterial conjunctivitis. Common agents of bacterial conjunctivitis are *Streptococcus pneumoniae*, *Staphylococcus aureus*, *Neisseria gonorrhoeae*, *Neisseria meningitidis*, and *Hemophilus influenzae*. All of these organisms produce a copious purulent discharge. The eyelids are sticky, and there may be excoriation of the lid margins. There is usually no pain or blurring of vision. Treatment may include local application of antibiotics. The disease is usually self-limiting, lasting about 10 days to 14 days if untreated.

Viral conjunctivitis. One of the most common causes of viral conjunctivitis is adenovirus type 3, which is usually associated with pharyngitis, fever, and malaise. It causes generalized hyperemia, copious tearing, and minimal exudate. Children are affected more often than adults. Contaminated swimming pools are common sources of infection. There is no specific treatment for this type of viral conjunctivitis; it usually lasts 7 days to 14 days.

Herpes simplex virus conjunctivitis is characterized by unilateral infection, irritation, mucoid discharge, pain, and mild photophobia. Herpetic vesicles may develop on the eyelids and lid margins. Although the infection is usually caused by the type 1 herpes virus, it can also be caused by the type 2 virus. It is often associated with herpes simplex virus keratitis, in which the cornea shows discrete epithelial lesions. Local corticosteroid preparations increase the activity of the herpes simplex virus, apparently by enhancing the destructive effect of collagenase on the collagen of the cornea. Therefore, the use of these medications should be avoided in persons suspected of having herpes simplex conjunctivitis or keratitis.

Chlamydial conjunctivitis. Inclusion conjunctivitis is usually a benign suppurative conjunctivitis transmitted by the *Chlamydia trachomatis* group that causes venereal infections (see Chapter 38). It is spread by contaminated genital secretions and occurs in newborns of mothers having *C. trachomatis* birth canal infections. It can also be contracted through swimming in unchlorinated pools. The incubation period varies from 5 days to 12 days, and the disease may last for several months if untreated. The infection is usually treated with systemic erythromycin and topical tetracycline ointment.

A more serious form of infection is caused by a different group of *C. trachomatis*. This form of chlamydial infection not only affects the conjunctiva, but also causes ulceration and scarring of the cornea. It is the leading cause of blindness in many poorly developed countries with dry and sandy regions. In the United States, the infection is largely confined to the American Indians of the Southwest. It is transmitted by direct human contact, contaminated particles (fomites), and flies.

Diagnosis. Because a red eye may be the sign of several eye conditions, conjunctivitis must be differentiated from conjunctival injection, ciliary injection, glaucoma, subconjunctival hemorrhage, and blepharitis. The major causes of red eyes and their diagnostic features are described in Table 51-1. The diagnosis of conjunctivitis is based on history, physical examination, and microscopic and culture studies to identify the cause. Infectious diseases are often bilateral and involve other family members. Unilateral disease suggests irritant sources, such as foreign bodies or chemical irritation.

⸻ Lacrimal apparatus

The lacrimal gland is the source of the serous secretions called tears. This gland lies in the orbit, superior and lateral to the eyeball (Figure 51-4). Approximately 12 small ducts connect the tear gland to the superior conjunctival fornix. Tears, which contain about 98% water, 1.5% sodium chloride, and the antibacterial enzyme lysozyme, are essential to the main-

tenance of vision because of their lubricant and possibly antibacterial properties. Lubrication between the two layers of conjunctiva permits comfortable eye and lid movement.

A reddish elevation, the lacrimal caruncle, is in the medial canthus. Minute openings, the lacrimal puncta, in the edge of the lids just above and below the caruncle, are the entrances of the superior and inferior canaliculi, which permit entrance of tears into the lacrimal sac and nasolacrimal duct (tear duct). The nasolacrimal duct empties into the nasal cavity.

⸻ Dry eyes

The thin layer of tears that covers the cornea is essential in preventing drying and damage of the outer layer of the cornea. Tear film is from glands in the eyelid as well as the lacrimal gland. The tear film is composed of three layers: (1) the superficial lipid layer, derived from the sebaceous glands and thought to retard evaporation of the aqueous layer, (2) the aqueous layer, secreted by the lacrimal glands, and (3) the mucinous layer that overlies the cornea and epithelial cells.[2] Because the epithelial cell membranes are relatively hydrophobic and cannot be wetted by aqueous solutions alone, the mucinous layer plays an essential role in wetting these surfaces. Periodic blinking of the eyes is needed to maintain a continuous tear film over the ocular surface. Disruption of any of the tear film components or of the blinking action of the eyelids can lead to the breakup of the tear film and dry spots on the cornea. A number of conditions cause reduced function of the lacrimal glands. With aging, the lacrimal glands tend to diminish their secretion, and as a result, many older persons awaken from a night's sleep with highly irritated eyes. Dry eyes also result from loss of reflex lacrimal gland secretion due to congenital defects, infection, irradiation, damage to the parasympathetic innervation of the gland, and medications such as antihistamines, beta-adrenergic blocking drugs, and anticholinergic drugs (atropine and scopolamine). The wearing of contact lenses tends to contribute to eye dryness through decreased blinking.

Sjögren's syndrome is a systemic disorder in which there is lymphocytic and plasma cell infiltration of the lacrimal and parotid glands. The disorder is associated with diminished salivary and lacrimal secretions (sicca complex), resulting in keratoconjunctivitis sicca and xerostomia (dry mouth). The syndrome occurs mainly in women near menopause and is often associated with connective tissue disorders such as rheumatoid arthritis.

Persons with dry eyes complain of dry or gritty sensation in the eye, burning, itching, inability to produce tears, photosensitivity, redness, pain, and

Table 51–1. Red eyes

	Conjunctival injection	Ciliary injection	Acute glaucoma	Subconjunctival hemorrhage	Blepharitis
Appearance					
Process	Dilatation of the conjunctival vessels	Dilatation of branches of the anterior ciliary artery, which supply the iris and related structures	Dilatation of branches of the anterior ciliary artery; may also show some conjunctival vessel dilatation	Blood outside the vessels between the conjunctiva and sclera	Inflammation of the eyelids
Location of redness	Peripheral vessels of the conjunctiva, fading toward the iris	Central deeper vessels around the iris	Central deeper vessels around the iris; may also be peripheral	A homogeneous red patch, usually in an exposed part of the bulbar conjunctiva	Lid margins
Appearance of vessels	Irregularly branched	May radiate regularly or appear as a diffuse flush around the iris	Radiating regularly around the iris; peripherally may be irregularly branching	Vessels themselves not visible	Conjunctival and ciliary vessels normal unless there is associated disease
Color	Vessels bright red	Vessels more violet or rose-colored	Vessels around iris violet or rose-colored	Patch is bright red, fading with time to yellow	Lid margins red, may have yellowish scales
Movability	Conjunctival vessels can be moved against the globe by pressure on the lower lid	Dilated vessels are deeper; cannot be moved by lid pressure	Dilated vessels around the iris are deep; cannot be moved by lid pressure	Not movable	Not relevant
Pupil size and shape	Normal	Normal or small and irregular	Dilated, often oval, seen through a steamy cornea	Normal	Normal
Visual acuity	Not affected	Decreased	Decreased	Not affected	Not affected
Significance	Superficial conjunctival condition, as from irritation, infection, allergy, vasodilators	Disorder of cornea or inner eye. Requires prompt evaluation	Sudden increase in intraocular pressure because of blocked drainage from the anterior chamber; an ocular emergency	Often none; may result from trauma, sudden increase in venous pressure (e.g., cough), bleeding disorder	Often associated with seborrhea, staphylococcal infections

(Bates B: A Guide to Physical Examination, 3rd ed. Philadelphia, JB Lippincott, 1983)

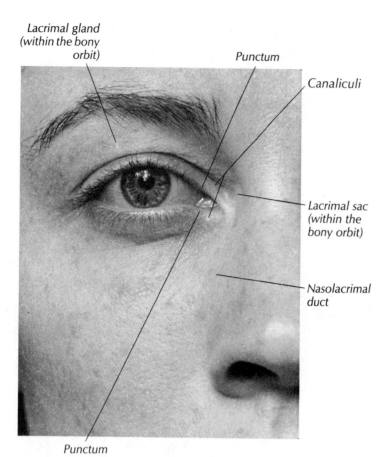

Lacrimal gland
(within the bony
orbit)

Punctum

Canaliculi

Lacrimal sac
(within the
bony orbit)

Nasolacrimal
duct

Punctum

Figure 51-4 Lacrimal apparatus. (Bates B: A Guide to Physical Examination and History Taking, 4th ed, p 148. Philadelphia, JB Lippincott, 1987)

difficulty in moving the eyelids. Dry eyes and the absence of tears can cause keratinization of the cornea and conjunctival epithelium. In severe cases, corneal ulcerations can occur. Consequent corneal scarring can cause blindness.

Assessment of tear formation can be done using the Schirmer filter paper test. With this test, a 35-mm by 5.0-mm strip of filter paper (Iso-Sol strips) is folded and placed in the lower conjunctival sac of both eyes for 5 minutes. Generally, tear formation is considered normal if the portion of the paper that is moistened measures 15 mm or more.

The treatment of dry eyes includes frequent instillation of artificial tear solutions into the conjunctival sac. Recently, a slow-released artificial tear insert (Lacrisert) has been made available. The insert, which contains hydroxypropyl cellulose, is inserted into the inferior conjunctival cul-de-sac. Water is pulled into the insert from the capillaries, and a hydroxypropyl cellulose tear solution is released over a 12-hour period.

Dacryocystitis

Dacryocystitis is an infection of the lacrimal sac. It occurs most often in infants or in persons over 40 years of age. It is usually unilateral and most often

occurs secondary to obstruction of the nasolacrimal duct. Often the cause of the obstruction is unknown, although there may be a history of severe trauma to the midface. The symptoms include tearing and discharge, pain, swelling, and tenderness. The treatment includes application of heat (warm compresses) and antibiotic therapy. In chronic forms of the disorder, surgical repair of the tear duct may be necessary. In infants, dacryocystitis is usually due to failure of the nasolacrimal ducts to open spontaneously before birth. When one of the ducts fail to open, a secondary dacryocystitis may develop. These infants are usually treated with gentle massage of the tear sac, instillation of antibiotic drops into the conjunctival sac, and if that fails, probing of the tear duct.

Sclera and cornea

The optic globe, or eyeball, is a spherical structure (Figure 51-5). The globe has three layers, each of which is further subdivided. The outer layer of the eyeball consists of a tough, opaque, white fibrous layer called the sclera. Its strong yet elastic properties maintain the shape of the globe. The sclera is homologous to the dermis of the facial skin and is continuous except for a number of tiny holes at the optic disk, the

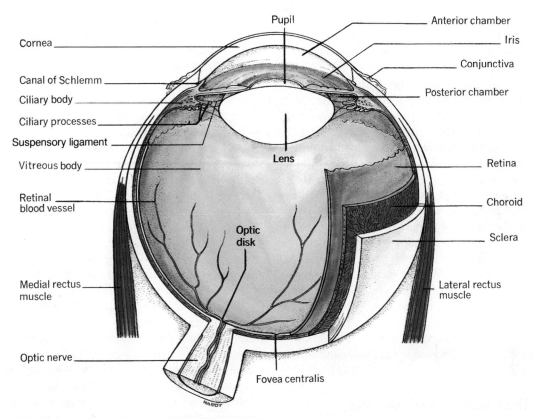

Figure 51-5 Transverse section of the eyeball. (*Chaffee EE, Lytle IM: Basic Physiology and Anatomy, 4th ed, p 775. Philadelphia, JB Lippincott, 1980*)

lamina cribrosa sclerae through which the optic nerve axons exit the retina. In jaundice, the sclera appears yellow because of staining from excessive levels of circulating bilirubin. The tough sclera is continuous with the extension of the cranial dura mater that surrounds and protects the optic nerve. In an inherited collagen disease known as *osteogenesis imperfecta* (see Chapter 56), the sclera is quite thin, and the pigmented choroid shows through, providing a bluish cast to the sclera. Subconjunctival hemorrhage frequently is associated with even light trauma to the head or optic globe.

At the anterior part of the eyeball, the scleral structure becomes the transparent cornea. The point at which the cornea joins the sclera is called the *limbus* (see Figure 51-3). Because light passes from air into the liquid and solid transparent media of the eye at the corneal surface, the major part of refraction (bending) of light rays and focusing occurs at this point. The cornea has three layers: an extremely thin outer epithelial layer, which is continuous with the ocular conjunctiva, a middle stromal layer called the *substantia propria,* and an inner endothelial layer that lies adjacent to the aqueous humor of the anterior chamber. The thick substantia propria constitutes 90% of the cornea; its anterior condensation (Bowman's mem-

brane) is attached to the basement membrane of the epithelial layer. Descemet's membrane, the basement membrane of the endothelium, separates the endothelium from the stromal layer. The substantia propria is composed of regularly arranged collagen bundles embedded in a mucopolysaccharide matrix. The regular organization of the collagen fibers, which makes the substantia propria transparent, is necessary for light transmission. Hydration within a limited range is necessary to maintain the spacing of the collagen fibers and transparency. The cornea is avascular and derives its nutrient and oxygen supply by means of diffusion from blood vessels of the adjacent sclera, from the aqueous humor at its deep surface, and from tears. The corneal epithelium is heavily innervated by sensory neurons. Epithelial damage causes discomfort that ranges from a foreign body sensation and burning of the eyes to severe stabbing or knifelike incapacitating pain. Reflex lacrimation is common.

Trauma that causes abrasions of the cornea can be extremely painful, but, if minor, the abrasions usually heal in a few days. The epithelial layer is capable of regeneration, and small defects heal without scarring. If the stroma is damaged, healing occurs more slowly and the danger of infection is increased. Injuries to Bowman's membrane and the stromal layer heal with scar formation and permanent opacification. Opacities of the cornea impair the transmission of light. A minor scar can severely distort vision because it disturbs the refractive surface.

The integrity of both the epithelium and the endothelium is necessary to maintain the cornea in its relatively dehydrated state. Damage to either structure leads to edema and loss of transparency. Among the causes of corneal edema are prolonged and uninterrupted wearing of hard contact lenses, which can deprive the epithelium of oxygen, disrupting its integrity. The edema disappears spontaneously when the cornea comes in contact with the atmosphere. Corneal edema also occurs when there is a sudden rise in intraocular pressure. If intraocular pressure rises rapidly above 50 mmHg, as in acute glaucoma, subendothelial edema develops. With corneal edema, the cornea appears dull, uneven, and hazy. A decrease in visual acuity and iridescent vision (rainbows around lights) occur. Iridescent vision results from epithelial and subepithelial edema, which splits white light into its component parts with blue in the center and red on the outside.

Abnormal corneal deposits

The cornea is frequently the site of deposition of abnormal metabolic products. In hypercalcemia, calcium salts can precipitate within the cornea, producing a cloudy band keratopathy. Cystine crystals are deposited in cystinosis, cholesterol esters in hypercholesterolemia, and a golden ring of copper in hepatolenticular degeneration due to Wilson's disease (called a Kayser-Fleischer ring). Pharmacologic agents, such as chloroquine, can result in crystal deposits in the cornea. In arcus senilis, a grayish white infiltrate occurs at the periphery of the cornea. It represents an extracellular lipid infiltration and is seen in most persons over 60 years of age.

Keratitis

Keratitis refers to inflammation of the cornea. It can be caused by infections, hypersensitivity reactions, ischemia, defects in tearing, trauma, and interruption in sensory innervation, such as occurs with local anesthesia. Keratitis can be divided into two types: ulcerative, in which part of the epithelium, stroma, or both are destroyed, and nonulcerative, in which all the layers of the epithelium are affected by the inflammation but the epithelium remains intact. Causes of ulcerative keratitis include infectious agents such as those causing conjunctivitis (*e.g.*, staphylococcus, pneumococcus, chlamydia, and herpesvirus), exposure trauma and misuse of contact lens. Exposure trauma may be due to deformities of the lid, paralysis of the lid muscles, or severe exophthalmos. Mooren's ulcer is a chronic, painful, indolent ulcer that occurs in the absence of infection. It is usually seen in older persons and may affect both eyes. Nonulcerative keratitis is associated with a number of diseases, including syphilis, tuberculosis, and lupus erythematosus. It may also result from a viral infection entering through a small defect in the cornea.

Symptoms of keratitis include photophobia, discomfort, and lacrimation. The discomfort may range from foreign body sensation to severe pain. Defective vision results from the changes in transparency and curvature of the cornea that occur. If ulceration is present, it will stain green when a drop of fluorescein dye is instilled. Generally, peripheral involvement of the cornea is related to the same disorders that affect the conjunctiva (discussed earlier).

Advances in ophthalmologic surgery now permit corneal transplantation using a cadaver cornea. Unlike kidney or heart transplant procedures, which are associated with considerable risk of rejection of the transplanted organ, the use of cadaver corneas entails minimal danger of rejection, because this tissue is not exposed to the vascular and, therefore, immunologic defense system. Instead, the success of this type of transplant operation depends on the prevention of scar tissue formation, which would limit the transparency of the transplanted cornea.

Uveal tract

The middle vascular layer, or uveal tract, of the eye includes the choroid, the ciliary body, and the iris (see Figures 51-1 and 51-5). The uveal tract is an incomplete ball with gaps at the pupil and at the optic disk, where it is continuous with the arachnoid and pial layers surrounding the optic nerve. The choroid is rich in dispersed melanocytes, which function to prevent the diffusion of light through the wall of the optic globe. The pigment of these cells absorbs light within the eyeball and light that penetrates the retina. The light absorptive function prevents the scattering of light and is important for visual acuity, particularly with high background illumination levels.

The ciliary body is an anterior continuation of the choroid layer. It has both smooth muscle and secretory functions. Its smooth muscle function contributes to alteration in lens shape, and its secretory function, to production of aqueous humor.

The iris is an adjustable diaphragm that permits alteration in pupil size and in the amount of light entering the eye. The pupillary diameter can be varied from approximately 2 mm to 8 mm. The posterior surface of the iris is formed by a two-layer epithelium continuous with those layers covering the ciliary body. The anterior layer contains the dilator, or radial mus-

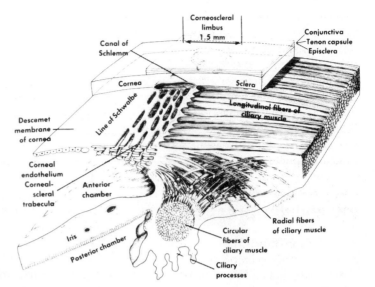

Figure 51-6 Schematic construction of the ciliary body and angle recess in humans. Anteriorly the area is covered by the cornea and posteriorly by the sclera, which contains the canal of Schlemm. The termination of the corneal endothelium is marked by the line of Schwalbe. The ciliary muscle consists of longitudinal fibers, which are mainly parallel to the sclera; radial fibers, which are intermediate; and a circular muscle, which is most internal. The cornealscleral trabecula provide a filtering area between the anterior chamber angle and the canal of Schlemm. (*Redrawn from Von Mollendorf W, Bargmann W [eds]: Handbuch der mikroskopischen Anatomie des Menschen, Berlin, Springer-Verlag, 1964. From Newell FW: Ophthalmology: Principles and Concepts, 5th ed. St Louis, CV Mosby, 1982*)

cles, of the iris (Figure 51-6). Just anterior to these muscles is the loose, highly vascular connective tissue stroma. Embedded in this layer are concentric rings of smooth muscle cells that compose the sphincter muscle of the pupil. The anteriormost layer of the iris forms a highly irregular anterior surface and contains many fibroblasts and melanocytes. Eye color differences result from the density of the pigment. The amount of pigment decreases from dark brown eyes through shades of brown and gray to blue.

Several mutations affect the pigment of the uveal tract, including albinism. Albinism is a genetic (autosomal recessive trait) deficiency of tyrosinase, which is necessary for the synthesis of melanin by the melanocytes. Classic albinism is termed tyrosine-negative albinism, and the affected individual has white hair, pink skin, and light blue eyes. In these individuals, excessive light penetrates the unpigmented iris and to some extent the anterior sclera and unpigmented choroid. Their photoreceptors are flooded with excess light, and visual acuity is markedly reduced. In addition, excess stimulation of the photoreceptors at normal or high illumination levels is experienced as painful (photophobia). Tryosine-positive albinism results from the genetic defects in which a reduced but variable amount of tyrosine is synthesized by the pigment cells. Hair and skin color vary among these persons. Reduced choroid and iris pigment results in variable acuity and photophobic abnormalities. A third type of hereditary defect involves the absence of pigment in the choroid and iris with normal pigmentation elsewhere. This is called ocular albinism and results from a chromosomal abnormality of the X chromosome. Other hereditary syndromes include reduced or absent choroid and iris pigment, as in phenylketonuria. Persons with tyrosine-negative albinism or ocular albinism usually have continuous

back-and-forth excursion eye movements (physiologic nystagmus), which makes reading difficult.

Uveitis

Inflammation of the entire uveal tract is termed uveitis. One of the serious consequences of the condition can be the involvement of the underlying retina. Parasitic invasion of the choroid can result in local atrophic changes that usually involve the retina; examples include toxoplasmosis and histoplasmosis. Sarcoid deposition in the form of small nodules results in irregularities of the underlying retinal surface.

In summary, the optic globe, or eyeball, is protected posteriorly by the bony structures of the orbit and anteriorly by the eyelids. It is continuously bathed by a protective layer of tears. Protrusion of the eyes is called exophthalmos, and the condition of deeply sunken eyes is called enophthalmos. The eyelids are called the palpebrae. Marginal blepharitis is the most common disorder of the eyelids. It is commonly caused by a staphylococcal infection or seborrhea (dandruff). The term ptosis refers to a drooping of the upper lid. It can be caused by injury to the facial (VII) or oculomotor (III) cranial nerves. The conjunctiva lines the inner surface of the eyelids and covers the optic globe to the junction of the cornea and sclera. Conjunctivitis (also called redeye or pinkeye) is a common eye disorder. It is important to differentiate between redness caused by conjunctivitis and that caused by more serious eye disorders, such as acute glaucoma or corneal lesions. Tears protect the cornea from drying and irritation. Impaired tear production or conditions that prevent blinking and the spread of tears produce drying of the eyes and predispose them to corneal irritation and injury. Trauma or disease that involves the stromal layer of the cornea heals with scar formation and permanent opacification. These opacities interfere with the transmission of light and may impair vision. The uveal tract is the middle vascular layer of the eye. It contains melanocytes that prevent diffusion of light through the wall of the optic globe. Inflammation of the uveal tract (uveitis) can affect visual acuity; albinism, an inherited pigment defect, can cause photophobia.

Intraocular pressure

The fluid-filled anterior and posterior chambers of the anterior segment of the eye are divided by the iris and the closely adjacent lens into the posterior and anterior chambers, the pupil forming the only passageway between the two chambers (Figure 51-7). The posterior chamber, which is the smaller chamber, is restricted by the gellike vitreous humor that fills the remaining space within the cavity of the globe.

The transparent aqueous humor, which fills the space between the cornea and lens, is secreted by the ciliary epithelium in the posterior chamber. The secreted aqueous humor flows slowly through the thin passageway between the lens and the iris and is then reabsorbed by a specialized region at the iridic angle. At the iridocorneal angle, the aqueous humor normally passes through a porous trabeculated region of the sclera (see Figure 51-6) that permits entry into a circular venous ring called *Schlemm's canal* and from

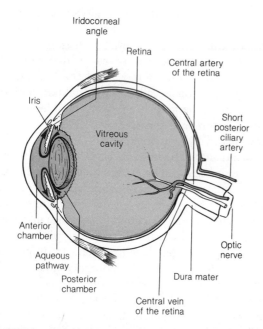

Figure 51-7 Anterior and posterior chambers of the eye. Arrows indicate the pathway of aqueous flow.

there into the anterior ciliary veins. The anterior ciliary veins continue into the choroid and enter the ophthalmic veins at the back of the eye.

The aqueous humor helps to maintain the intraocular pressure and metabolism of the lens and posterior cornea. The interior pressure of the eye must exceed that of the atmosphere to prevent the eyeball from collapsing. In addition, the aqueous humor serves a nutritive function for the lens and the posterior surface of the cornea. It contains a low protein concentration and a high concentration of ascorbic acid, glucose, and amino acids. It also mediates the exchange of respiratory gases.

The hydrostatic pressure of the aqueous humor results from a balance of several factors: (1) the rate of secretion, (2) the resistance to flow through the narrow opening between the lens and iris at the entrance into the anterior chamber, and (3) the resistance to resorption at the trabeculated region of the sclera at the iridocorneal angle. Normally the rate of aqueous production is equal to the rate of aqueous outflow, so that the intraocular pressure is maintained within a normal range of 12 mmHg to 21 mmHg. Abnormalities in the balance between these factors leads to increased pressure in the aqueous humor, a disease complex called *glaucoma*.

The secretion of aqueous humor is an active process that continues regardless of the pressure in the secreted fluid. The secretory activity of the ciliary epithelium requires the enzyme *carbonic anhydrase,* and medical management of excessive aqueous production often includes the use of the carbonic anhydrase inhibitor acetazolamide (Diamox). Rarely is increased intraocular pressure due to the overproduction of aqueous humor; instead, it usually results from interference with outflow anywhere along the outflow pathway (pupil, trabecular meshwork, or Schlemm's canal). Congenital deformities of the trabecular meshwork, clogging of the meshwork with cellular debris from various intraocular pathologies, and adhesions of the peripheral iris to the trabecular meshwork can all result in increased intraocular pressure. As intraocular pressure rises because of impaired outflow, the Schlemm's canal is compressed, causing a further reduction in aqueous outflow.

── Glaucoma

Glaucoma includes a group of conditions that cause a rise in intraocular pressure that if left untreated, increases sufficiently to cause ischemia and degeneration of the optic nerve, leading to progressive blindness. An initial gradual loss of peripheral vision (Figure 51-8) is followed by loss of central vision. Glaucoma can occur in any age group but is most prevalent in the elderly. It accounts for 13% of all

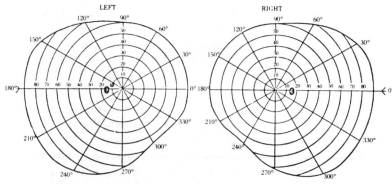

THE FIELD OF VISION (peripheral vision) with both eyes is 180° recorded on these charts.

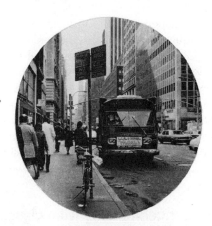

NORMAL VISION A person with normal or 20/20 vision sees this street scene.

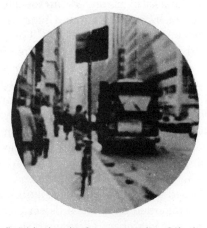

CATARACT diminished acuity from an opacity of the lens. The field of vision is unaffected. There is no scotoma, but the person has an overall haziness of the view, particularly in glaring light conditions.

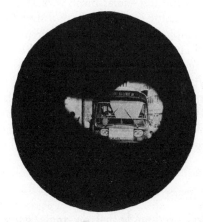

GLAUCOMA Advanced glaucoma involves loss of peripheral vision but the individual still retains most of his central vision.

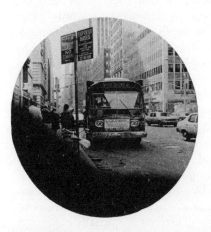

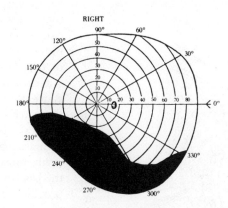

RETINAL DETACHMENT shown here in the active stage. There are many causes for detachment, but the hole or tear allows fluid to lift the retina from its normal position. This elevated retina causes a field or vision defect, seen as a dark shadow in the peripheral field. It may be above, or below as illustrated.

Figure 51-8 Photographs representing the eye diseases, done as if the camera were the right eye. The accompanying visual-field chart showing the area of visual loss also represents the right eye. (*Photo courtesy The Lighthouse, The New York Association for the Blind*)

cases of blindness and affects about 2% of people over 40 years of age.[1] The condition is often asymptomatic, and a significant loss of peripheral vision may occur before medical attention is sought, emphasizing the need for routine screening measurement of intraocular pressure in persons over age 40.

Glaucoma is commonly classified as closed-angle (narrow-angle) or open-angle (wide-angle) glaucoma depending on the location of the compromised aqueous humor circulation and resorption. Glaucoma may occur as a congenital or an acquired condition, and it may present as a primary or secondary disorder. Primary glaucoma occurs without evidence of preexisting ocular or systemic disease. Secondary glaucoma can result from inflammatory processes that affect the eye, tumors or blood cells from trauma producing hemorrhage that obstruct the outflow of aqueous humor, or hemorrhage caused by trauma.

Congenital (infantile) glaucoma

Congenital glaucoma is caused by a disorder in which the anterior chamber retains its fetal configuration, with the trabecular meshwork attached to the root of the iris, or is covered with a membrane. The earliest symptoms are excessive lacrimation and photophobia. Affected infants tend to be fussy, have poor eating habits, and rub their eyes frequently. Diffuse edema of the cornea is usually present, giving the eye a grayish white appearance. Chronic elevation of the intraocular pressure before the age of 3 years causes enlargement of the entire globe (buphthalmos). Early surgical treatment is necessary to prevent blindness.

Closed-angle glaucoma

In closed-angle (narrow-angle) glaucoma, the anterior chamber is narrow, and outflow becomes impaired when the iris thickens as the result of pupil dilatation (Figure 51-9). As the iris thickens, it re-

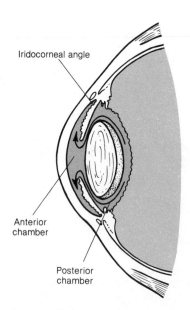

Figure 51-9 Narrow anterior chamber and iridocorneal angle in closed-angle (narrow-angle) glaucoma.

stricts the circulation pathway between the base of the iris and the sclera, reducing or eliminating access to the angle where aqueous reabsorption occurs. Approximately 5% to 10% of all cases of glaucoma fall into this category.

The symptoms of closed-angle glaucoma are related to sudden intermittent increases in intraocular pressure. These occur after prolonged periods in the dark, emotional upset, and other conditions that cause extensive and prolonged pupil dilatation. Administration of pharmacologic agents such as atropine, which cause pupillary dilatation (mydriasis), can also precipitate an acute episode of increased intraocular pressure in persons with the potential for closed-angle glaucoma. Attacks of increased intraocular pressure are manifested by ocular pain and blurred or iridescent vision caused by corneal edema. The pupil may be enlarged and fixed. The symptoms are often spontaneously relieved by sleep and conditions that promote pupillary constriction. With repeated or prolonged attacks, the eye becomes reddened, and edema of the cornea may develop, giving the eye a hazy appearance. A unilateral, often excruciating, headache is common. Nausea and vomiting may be present, causing the headache to be confused with migraine.

Closed-angle glaucoma usually occurs as the result of an inherited anatomical defect that causes a shallow anterior chamber. This defect is exaggerated by the anterior displacement of the peripheral iris that occurs in older persons because of the increase in lens size that occurs with aging. Some persons with a congenitally narrow anterior chamber never develop symptoms, and others develop symptoms only when they are elderly. The depth of the anterior chamber can be evaluated by transillumination or by a technique called *gonioscopy* (to be discussed later). Because of the dangers of vision loss, persons with narrow anterior chambers should be warned about the significance of blurred vision, halos, and ocular pain should these symptoms occur.

The treatment of closed-angle glaucoma is primarily by surgical intervention. Removing the iris (iridectomy) or cutting a window through the base of the iris (iridotomy) by surgical incision or laser beam provides relief. The anatomical abnormalities responsible for closed-angle glaucoma are usually expressed bilaterally, but progression may not be symmetric.

Open-angle glaucoma

With open-angle glaucoma, an abnormal increase in intraocular pressure occurs in the absence of an obstruction between the trabecular meshwork and the anterior chamber. Instead, it usually occurs because of an abnormality of the trabecular meshwork that impairs the flow of aqueous humor between the anterior chamber and Schlemm's canal. Open-angle glaucoma tends to manifest itself after age 35 and is the most common type of glaucoma, accounting for approximately 90% of all cases. The condition is usually asymptomatic, and chronic, causing progressive loss of visual field unless it is appropriately treated. Because it is usually asymptomatic, routine screening tonometry is the best means of detecting the disorder. In some persons, the use of moderate amounts of topical corticosteroid medications can cause an increase in intraocular pressure. Sensitive persons may also sustain an increase in intraocular pressure with the use of systemic corticosteroid drugs.

In contrast to closed-angle glaucoma, which can be treated surgically, open-angle glaucoma is usually treated medically. Among the drugs used in the treatment of open-angle glaucoma are miotics (drugs that cause pupillary constriction). These drugs increase the efficiency of the outflow channels, although the exact mechanism of their effect is unknown. Pilocarpine, a cholinergic-stimulating drug, is often used for this purpose. Other drugs that are used in the treatment of open-angle glaucoma are epinephrine, timolol, (Timoptic), and acetazolamide (Diamox). Epinephrine, an adrenergic neuromediator with both alpha and beta effects, reduces aqueous production by means of beta-receptor mechanisms (probably secondary to vasoconstriction in the ciliary processes) and increases aqueous outflow by means of alpha-receptor mechanisms. Timolol, a beta-adrenergic blocking drug, presumably lowers intraocular pressure by reducing aqueous production. Acetazolamide, a carbonic anhydrase inhibitor, reduces the secretion of aqueous humor by the ciliary epithelium. With the exception of acetazolamide, most drugs that are used in the treatment of glaucoma are applied topically.

When a reduction in intraocular pressure cannot be maintained through pharmacologic methods, surgical treatment may become necessary. Until recently, the main surgical treatment for open-angle glaucoma was a filtering procedure in which an opening is created between the anterior chamber and the subconjunctival space. A new argon laser technique, in which about 100 spots are applied 360 degrees around the trabecular meshwork, has now been developed.[3] The microburns resulting from the laser treatment scar rather than penetrate the trabecular meshwork, a process that is thought to enlarge the outflow channels by increasing the tension exerted on the trabecular meshwork. In another type of procedure, photocoagulation of the ciliary processes (cyclocryotherapy) may be used to destroy the ciliary epithelium and reduce aqueous humor production.

Diagnostic methods

Among the methods used in detecting and evaluating glaucoma are measurement of intraocular pressure, ophthalmoscopy, perimetry, transillumination technique, and gonioscopy. Perimetry, a technique used to assess visual field loss, is discussed in the section on visual pathways.

Intraocular pressure measurements. Intraocular pressure measurements are made indirectly by means of an instrument called a tonometer. There are two types of tonometers: a contact tonometer, an instrument that is placed on the anesthetized eye, and a noncontact tonometer, in which an air pulse is used. The Schiotz' tonometer (Figure 51-10) is an indentation tonometer that measures the amount of corneal deformation produced by a given force. The noncontact tonometer flattens the cornea with an air blast, increasing the amount of light that is reflected from the cornea. The time required for complete flattening of the cornea is measured electronically and used as a measure of intraocular pressure. Although a single high measurement of intraocular pressure (24–32 mmHg) is suggestive of glaucoma, repeated measurements are needed before a definite diagnosis can be made.[4]

Ophthalmoscopy. Increased intraocular pressure causes damage to optic nerve structures (optic disk) that can be recognized on ophthalmoscopic examination. The normal optic disk has a centrally placed depression called the *optic cup*. With progressive atrophy of axons caused by glaucoma, pallor of the optic disk develops, and the size and depth of the optic cup increase. Regular ophthalmoscopic ex-

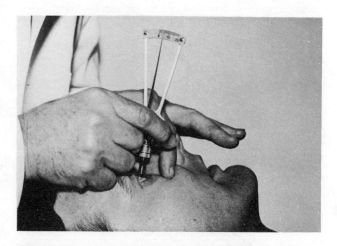

Figure 51-10 After a local anesthetic is instilled into the eye, the Schiotz tonometer is gently rested on the eyeball; the indicator measures in millimeters of mercury the ocular tension. *(Courtesy of F. H. Roy, M.D. From Brunner LS, Suddarth DS: Textbook of Medical-Surgical Nursing, 5th ed, Philadelphia, JB Lippincott, 1984)*

amination is important for detecting eye changes that occur with glaucoma, because changes in the optic cup precede the visual field loss.

Gonioscopy and transillumination. Gonioscopy and transillumination are used to assess anterior chamber depth. Gonioscopy uses a special contact lens and either mirrors or prisms so that the angle of the anterior chamber can be seen and measured. The transillumination requires only a penlight. The light source is held at the temporal side of the eye and directed horizontally across the iris.[5] In persons with a normal-sized anterior chamber, the light passes through the anterior chamber to illuminate both halves of the iris. In contrast, in a person with a narrow anterior chamber, only the half of the iris adjacent to the light source is illuminated (Figure 51-11).

In summary, glaucoma is one of the leading causes of blindness in the United States. It is characterized by conditions that cause an increase in intraocular pressure, which, if untreated, can lead to atrophy of the optic disk and progressive blindness. The aqueous humor is formed by the ciliary epithelium in the posterior chamber and flows through the pupil to the angle formed by the cornea and the iris. Here it filters through the trabecular meshwork and enters Schlemm's canal for return to the venous circulation. Glaucoma results from the impeded outflow of aqueous humor from the anterior chamber of the eye. There are two major forms of glaucoma: closed-angle and open-angle. Closed-angle glaucoma is caused by a narrow anterior chamber and blockage of the outflow channels at the angle formed by the iris and the cornea. This occurs when the iris becomes thickened during pupillary dilatation. In open-angle glaucoma microscopic obstruction of the trabecular meshwork

occurs. Open-angle glaucoma is usually asymptomatic, and considerable loss of the visual field often occurs before medical treatment is sought. Routine screening tonometry provides the means for early detection of glaucoma before vision loss has occurred.

Optics and lens function

The function of the eye is to transform light energy into nerve signals that can be transmitted to the brain for interpretation. Optically, the eye is similar to a camera. It contains a lens system, an aperture for controlling light exposure (the pupil), and a retina that corresponds to the film.

Refraction

When light passes from one medium to another, its velocity is either decreased or increased, and the direction of light movement is changed. The bending of light at an angulated surface is called *refraction*. When light rays pass through the center of a lens, their direction is not changed; however, rays passing laterally through a lens are bent (Figure 51-12). Usually, the refractive power of a lens is described as the distance (in meters) from its surface, at which the rays come into focus (focal length), or as the reciprocal of this distance (diopters). For example, a lens that brings an object into focus at 0.5 meters has a refractive power of 2 diopters ($0.5/1.0 = 2.0$). With a fixed power lens, the closer an object is to the lens, the further behind the lens the focus point will be. The closer the object, the stronger as well as the more perfect the focusing system must be.

In the eye, the major refraction of light begins at the convex corneal surface. Further refraction

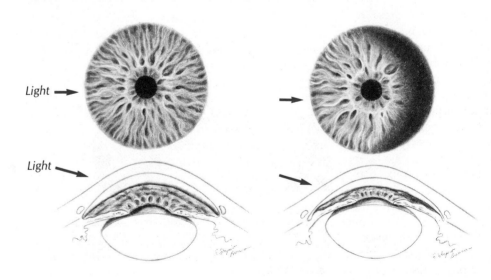

Light →

Light →

Figure 51-11 Transillumination of the iris. In the eye with a normal anterior chamber, the iris is evenly illuminated by light shining obliquely into the anterior chamber. In the eye with a narrow anterior chamber, the iris is unevenly illuminated and shadowed. (*Bates B: A Guide to Physical Examination and History Taking, 4th ed. Philadelphia, JB Lippincott, 1987*)

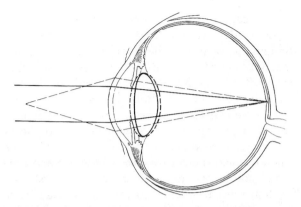

Figure 51-12 Accommodation. The solid lines represent rays of light from a distant object, and the dotted lines represent rays from a near object. The lens is flatter for the former and more convex for the latter. In each case the rays of light are brought to a focus on the retina. (*Chaffee EE, Lytle IM: Basic Physiology and Anatomy, 4th ed. Philadelphia, JB Lippincott, 1980*)

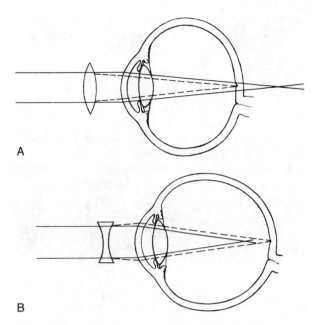

Figure 51-13 A, Hyperopia: corrected by a biconvex lens, as shown by the dotted lines; **B,** myopia: corrected by a biconcave lens, shown by the dotted lines. (*Chaffee EE, Lytle IM: Basic Physiology and Anatomy, 4th ed. Philadelphia, JB Lippincott, 1980*)

occurs as light moves from the posterior corneal surface to the aqueous humor, from the aqueous humor to the anterior lens surface, and from the posterior lens surface to the vitreous humor. In the eye, the focusing surface, the retina, is at a fixed distance from the lens; thus, adjustability in the refractive power of the lens is needed to keep the image of close objects in sharp focus on the retina. This is called *accommodation.* The adjustable lens shape and the adjustable pupillary opening must be under the control of a feedback system that makes these adjustments while evaluating image sharpness. All of this is accomplished by accommodation and pupillary reflexes under the control of the visual acuity evaluation centers in the primary visual and association cortex. These areas provide feedback control of the lens shape and, therefore, of vision clarity.

A perfectly shaped optic globe and cornea result in optimal visual acuity, that is, a sharp image in focus at all points on the retinal surface in the posterior part, or fundus, of the eye (emmetropia). Unfortunately, individual differences in the formation and growth of the eyeball and cornea frequently result in inappropriate image focal formation. For distant vision, if the optic globe is too short, the image is focused posterior to (in back of) the retina. This is called *hyperopia,* or *farsightedness* (Figure 51-13). In such cases, the accommodative changes of the lens cannot bring near objects into focus. This type of defect is corrected by appropriate biconvex lenses. If an infinitely distant target is focused anterior to (in front of) the retina, the eyeball is too long. This condition is called *myopia,* or *nearsightedness* (see Figure 51-13). It can be corrected with an appropriate biconcave lens. Radial keratotomy, a form of refractive corneal surgery, can be performed to correct the de-

fect. This surgical procedure involves the use of radial incisions to alter the corneal curvature.

Nonuniform curvature of the horizontal plane, in contrast with the vertical plane, of the refractive transparent media, usually of the cornea, is called *astigmatism* and must be corrected by a compensatory lens. Spherical aberration involves a cornea with a nonspherical surface. Lens correction can be made for this defect as well.

Accommodation

The lens is an avascular transparent biconvex body, whose posterior side is more convex than the anterior side. It measures about 9 mm to 10 mm in the transverse diameter and about 4 mm in the anteroposterior diameter. A thin, homogeneous, and highly elastic carbohydrate-containing lens capsule is attached to the surrounding ciliary body by delicate suspensory radial ligaments called *zonules,* which hold the lens in place (Figure 51-14). In providing for a change in lens shape, the tough and elastic sclera acts as a bow, and the zonule and lens capsule act as the bow string. Thus, the lens capsule is normally under tension, and the lens is flattened. Some of the smooth muscle fibers of the ciliary body are oriented parallel to the scleral surface and insert more anteriorly at the scleral–corneal junction. Many of the fibers are oriented radially as a sphincter around the eyeball (see Figure 51-6). Contraction of the muscle fibers of the

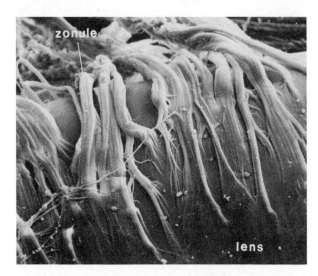

Figure 51-14 Scanning micrograph of a portion of the zonule, attached to the periphery of the lens, from a monkey's eye. Note the large bundles of fibers attached to the capsule of the lens below. (*Courtesy of P. Basu. From Ham AW, Cormack DH: Histology, 8th ed. Philadelphia, JB Lippincott, 1979*)

ciliary body results in a bending-in of the anterior sclera, relieving the tension on the zonules and thus on the lens capsule. Under these conditions, the rather elastic lens assumes a nearly spherical shape. Altering the normally flat lens shape to a more spherical shape increases the focusing power of the lens and has the effect of bringing the focused image of a near object forward to the retinal surface.

Accommodation is the process whereby a clear image is maintained as the gaze is shifted from a far to a near object. It requires convergence of the eyes, pupillary constriction, and thickening of the lens through contraction of the ciliary muscle. Accommodation is under the control of the parasympathetic oculomotor (III) cranial nerve. The cell bodies of this nerve are contained in the oculomotor nuclear complex located in the midbrain, and its preganglionic axons synapse with postganglionic neurons of the ciliary ganglion in the orbit (Figure 51-15). The postganglionic axons enter the back of the eye and travel in the choroid layer to the ciliary muscle fibers. Visual function must be present to evaluate and adjust the clarity of the image. Thus, accommodation depends on the functional integrity of the entire visual system, including the forebrain and midbrain circuitry. Accommodation does not occur during sleep. An absolutely blind person cannot accommodate, nor can a person in coma.

When a refractive defect of the corneal surface does not permit the formation of a sharp image, the accommodative reflex continues the unsuccessful attempts of ciliary muscle contraction to alter the lens shape. The discomfort or pain associated with continuous muscle contraction is experienced as eye strain.

Paralysis of the ciliary muscle, and thus of accommodation, is called *cycloplegia*. Pharmacologic paralysis is sometimes necessary to facilitate ophthalmoscope examination of the fundus of the eye, especially in small children who are unable to hold a steady fixation during the examination. The lens shape is totally under the control of the pretectal region and the parasympathetic pathway by way of the

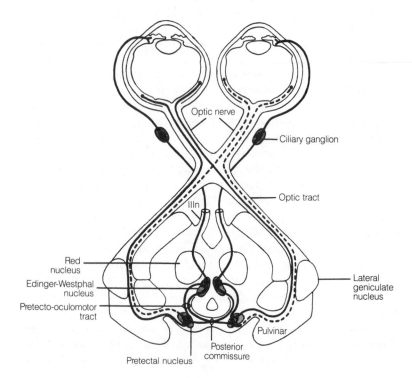

Figure 51-15 Diagram of the path of the pupillary light reflex. (*Reproduced, with permission, from Walsh FB, Hoyt WF: Clinical Neuro-ophthalmology, 3rd ed, vol 1. Baltimore, Williams & Wilkins, © 1969*)

oculomotor nerve to the ciliary muscle. Accommodation is lost with the destruction of this pathway.

The lens consists of transparent fibers arranged in concentric layers, of which the external layers are the newest and softest. There is no loss of lens fibers with aging. Instead, additional fibers are added to the outermost portion of the lens. As the lens ages, it thickens and its fibers become less elastic, so that the range of focus or accomodation is diminished to the point where reading glasses become necessary for near vision. This is called *presbyopia*.

—— Pupillary reflexes

The pupillary reflex, which controls the size of the pupillary opening, is controlled by the autonomic nervous system. The sphincter muscle that produces pupillary constriction is innervated by postganglionic parasympathetic neurons of the ciliary ganglion and other scattered ganglion cells between the scleral and choroid layers (see Figure 51-15). The oculomotor (III) cranial nerve, located in the midbrain, provides the preganglionic innervation for these parasympathetic axons. Innervation for the dilator muscle is derived from thoracic sympathetic preganglionic neurons that send axons along the sympathetic chain to innervate the postganglionic neurons in the superior cervical ganglion. The postganglionic neurons send axons along the internal carotid and ophthalmic arteries to the posterior surface of the optic globe. These axons travel between the scleral and choroid layers to reach the dilator muscles of the iris. The pupillary reflex is controlled by a region in the midbrain called the pretectum. The pretectal areas on each side of the brain are interconnected, accounting for the binocular aspect of the light reflex. These areas project axons to nuclei of the midbrain called the *Edinger-Westphal nuclei*. These nuclei contain the parasympathetic preganglionic neurons, which innervate the ciliary ganglion and thus control the sphincters of the iris. Midbrain level evaluation with feedback control provides an automatic brightness control mechanism. The functional importance of this reflex mechanism is its rapidity, compared with the very slow light- and dark-adaptive retinal mechanism.

Normal function of the pupillary reflex mechanism is tested by shining a bright light into one eye of the person being tested. A rapid constriction of the pupil exposed to light should occur (direct light reflex, or direct pupillary reflex). Because the reflex is normally bilateral, the contralateral pupil should also be constricted (consensual light reflex, or consensual pupillary reflex). By shining the light first into one eye and then into the other eye and noting the response of both pupils, considerable information can be gathered about the function of the central nervous system circuitry.

The circuitry of the light reflex is partially separated from the main visual pathway. This is illustrated by the fact that the pupillary reflex remains unaffected when lesions to the optic radiations or the visual cortex occur. The cortically blind person retains direct and consensual light reflexes. The light reflex also functions under light anesthetic levels and is used to evaluate the depth of anesthesia. When the reflex is lost, the anesthesia level is approaching that which will depress the respiratory reflexes as well.

The function of the sympathetic and parasympathetic control of the iris (and pupillary size) is differentially affected by many pharmacologic agents. The integrity of the dual control of pupillary diameter is somewhat vulnerable to trauma, tumor enlargement, or vascular disease. Careful attention to inappropriate or unequal pupil diameters is diagnostically important. Reflex pupillary dilatation occurs more quickly in lightly pigmented eyes than in dark eyes. Damage to the oculomotor nucleus or nerve not only eliminates innervation of many of the extraocular muscles and the levator muscle of the upper lid but also results in permanent pupillary dilation (*mydriasis*) in the affected eye. Persons with mydriasis experience discomfort in normal or brightly lit environments because of loss of pupillary constriction in the affected eye. Lesions affecting descending brain control of sympathetic outflow which passes through the cervical spinal cord, ascending sympathetic preganglionic axons of the sympathetic ganglia, or sympathetic postganglionic axonal plexus in the wall of the carotid artery, can interrupt the sympathetic control of the iris dilator muscle, resulting in permanent pupillary constriction (*miosis*). Tumors of the orbit that compress structures behind the eye can eliminate all pupillary reflexes, usually before destroying the optic nerve. Inequality in pupillary size is called *anisocoria*.

Bilateral pupillary constriction is characteristic of opiate usage. Bilateral pupillary dilation, being a sympathetic system function, is a part of general sympathetic activation, such as occurs during intense emotional responses associated with anger or fear. Unilateral pupillary dilation can be stimulated by a pinch to the lateral side of the neck, called the ciliospinal reflex. Pupillary dilation results when topical parasympathetic blocking agents such as atropine or homatropine are applied and sympathetic pupillodilatory function is left unopposed. These medications are used by ophthalmologists to facilitate the examination of the transparent media and fundus of the eye. As was previously mentioned, pupillary dilatation can increase the resistance to the flow of aqueous humor between the iris and lens, precipitating an increase in intraocular pressure in closed-angle glaucoma. Miotic drugs such as pilocarpine have the opposite effect, facilitating aqueous humor circulation.

Cataract

A cataract is a lens opacity that interferes with the transmission of light to the retina. It has been estimated that 5 million to 10 million persons in the United States are visually disabled because of cataracts.[1] A number of factors contribute to the development of cataracts, including genetic defects, environmental and metabolic influences, viruses, injury, and aging. Although there is no accepted method of classification, most cataracts can be described as congenital, senile, traumatic, or secondary to systemic or ocular disease.

Congenital cataract

A congenital cataract is one that is present at birth. Among the causes of congenital cataracts are genetic defects, toxic environmental agents, and viruses such as rubella. Maternal rubella during the first trimester can cause congenital cataract. Exposure of the embryo to ionizing radiation levels as low as 50 rads, such as occurs during barium enema or fluoroscopy, can induce congenital cataract. Cataracts and other developmental defects of the ocular apparatus depend both on the total dose and the embryonic stage at the time of exposure. During the last trimester of fetal life, genetic or environmental malformation of the superficial lens fibers can occur. Most congenital cataracts are not progressive and are not dense enough to cause significant visual impairment. However, if the cataracts are bilateral, and significant opacity is present, lens extraction should be done on one eye by age 2 months, to permit the development of vision and prevent nystagmus. If the surgery is successful, the other eye should be done soon after.

Traumatic cataract

Traumatic cataracts are most often caused by foreign body injury to the lens or blunt trauma to the eye. Foreign body injury that interrupts the lens capsule allows aqueous and vitreous humor to enter the lens and initiate cataract formation. Other causes of traumatic cataract are overexposure to heat (glassblower's cataract) or to ionizing radiation. The radiation dose necessary to cause a cataract varies with the amount and type of energy; younger lenses are most vulnerable.

Senile cataract

With aging, both the nucleus and the cortex of the lens enlarge as new fibers are formed in the cortical zones of the lens. In the nucleus the old fibers become more compressed and dehydrated. In addition, metabolic changes occur. Lens proteins become more insoluble, and concentrations of calcium, sodium, potassium, and phosphate increase. During the early stages of cataract formation, a yellow pigment and vacuoles accumulate in the lens fibers. Unfolding of protein molecules, cross-linking of sulfhydryl groups, and conversion of soluble to insoluble proteins, leading to the loss of lens transparency, occur.

Cataracts due to metabolic and toxic agents

Disorders of carbohydrate metabolism are the most common metabolic causes of cataract. Normally, glucose enters lens cells by diffusion and is then reduced to sorbitol (an alcohol) by the intracellular enzyme aldose reductase. Sorbitol diffuses out of the lens fibers very slowly, creating an osmotic gradient for the entry of water. In uncontrolled diabetes mellitus, the entry of water into the lens fibers accelerates with increased production of osmotically active sorbitol. The lens fibers swell and change their refractive properties, causing myopic changes and blurring of vision. The condition is slowly reversible unless it is long-standing, in which case lens fiber destruction and permanent cataracts occur. The sugar galactose exerts the same effect in persons with galactosemia.

Cataract can result from a number of drugs. Dinitrophenol, a drug widely used for weight reduction during the 1930s, triparanol, chlorpromazine, and the adrenocorticosteroid drugs have all been implicated as causative agents in cataract formation. Busulfan, a cancer treatment drug, has been clearly linked to cataract formation. Frequent examination of lens transparency should accompany the use of these and any other substances with cataract-forming effects.

Signs and symptoms

The chief symptom of cataract is a gradual decline in visual acuity (see Figure 51-8). Vision for far and near objects decreases. Dilation of the pupil in dim light improves vision. With nuclear cataracts (those involving the lens nucleus), the refractive power of the anterior segment often increases to produce an acquired myopia. Thus, persons with hyperopia may experience a second sight or improved reading acuity until increasing opacity reduces acuity. Central lens opacities may divide the visual axis and cause an optical defect in which two or more blurred images are seen. On ophthalmoscopic examination, cataracts may appear as a gross opacity filling the pupillary aperture or as an opacity silhouetted against the red background of the fundus.

Treatment

A partially opaque lens is termed an *immature cataract,* and a totally opaque lens is a *mature cataract.* Following the mature stage, leakage of protein from the degenerated cells results in shrinkage, and the lens is called *hypermature.* The treatment consists of surgical removal of the cataract (cataract extraction). Surgical removal is indicated when the opacity has advanced to the stage at which it produces a visual defect that interferes with normal activities or when the cataract threatens to cause other eye problems such as secondary glaucoma or uveitis. The absence of the lens is called *aphakia.* Following surgery to remove the lens, the loss of the refractive role of the lens can be compensated for by thick convex lenses, contact lenses, or an intraocular lens implant that is inserted during lens extraction. It has been estimated that 600,000 cataract extractions are performed annually in the United States.[6]

In summary, the refractive properties of the eye depend on the size and shape of the eyeball and the cornea and on the focusing abilities of the lens. In terms of visual function, refraction refers to the ability to focus an image on the retina. Errors in refraction occur when the visual image is not focused on the retina because of individual differences in the size or shape of the eyeball or cornea. In hyperopia, or farsightedness, the image falls in back of the retina. In myopia, or nearsightedness, the image falls in front of the retina. Because the focusing power of the eyeball and cornea is fixed, it is the lens that provides the means for the focusing of near images on the retina. The lens is a transparent and avascular biconvex structure suspended behind the iris and between the anterior chamber and the vitreous body that aids in visual focus. It is enclosed in an elastic capsule and attached to the ciliary body suspensory ligament. When the ciliary muscle contracts, the ligament relaxes and the lens becomes more nearly spherical, enabling the eye to focus on objects that are nearer to the eye. Relaxation of the ciliary muscle allows the eye to focus on distant objects. This mechanism is called accommodation and is controlled by the autonomic nervous system. Stimulation of the parasympathetic nervous system contracts the ciliary muscle and increases refractive power. With aging, the lens thickens and loses its ability to focus on near objects, a condition called presbyopia. A cataract is a lens opacity. It can occur as the result of congenital influences, metabolic disturbances, infection, injury, and aging. The most common type of cataract is the senile cataract that occurs with aging. The treatment for a totally opaque or mature cataract is surgical extraction. An intraocular lens implant may be inserted during the surgical procedure to replace the lens that has been removed; otherwise, thick convex lenses or contact lenses are used to compensate for the loss of lens function.

Vitreous and retinal function

The posterior segment, which constitutes five-sixths of the eyeball, contains the transparent vitreous humor and the neural retina. It is this interior part of the posterior chamber, called the *fundus,* that is visualized through the pupil with an ophthalmoscope.

Vitreous humor

The vitreous humor is a colorless, structureless gel that fills the posterior segment of the eye. It consists of about 99% water, some salts, glycoproteins, and dispersed collagen fibrils. The vitreous is attached to the ciliary body and the peripheral retina in the region of the ora serrata and to the periphery of the optic disk.

The vitreous is a biologic gel. Disease, aging, and injury can disturb the factors that maintain water in suspension, causing liquefaction to occur. With the loss of gel structure, fine fibers, membranes, and cellular debris develop. When this occurs, floaters (images) can often be noticed as these substances move within the vitreous cavity during head movement. In disease, blood vessels may grow from the surface of the retina or optic disk onto the posterior surface of the vitreous, and blood may fill the vitreous cavity.

The removal and replacement of the vitreous with a balanced saline solution (vitrectomy) can restore sight in some persons with vitreous opacities resulting from hemorrhage or vitreoretinal membrane formations that cause legal blindness. In this procedure, a small probe with a cutting tip is used to remove the opaque vitreous and membranes. The procedure is difficult and requires complex instrumentation. It is of no value if the retina is not functional.

Retina

The function of the retina is to receive visual images, partially analyze them, and transmit this modified information to the brain. Disorders of the retina and its function include (1) congenital photoreceptor abnormalities such as color blindness, (2) disturbances in blood vessels such as vascular retinopathies with hemorrhage and the development of opacities, (3) separation of the pigment and sensory layers of the retina (retinal detachment), (4) derangements of the pigment epithelium (retinitis pigmentosa), and (5) abnormalities of Bruch's membrane and choroid (macular degeneration). The retina has no pain fibers; therefore, most diseases of the retina are painless and do not cause redness of the eye.

The retina is composed of two parts: an outer pigmented layer and an inner neural layer. The neural retina covers the inner aspect of the posterior two-thirds of the eyeball. Posteriorly, the retina is continuous with the optic nerve; anteriorly, the neural retina ends a short distance behind the ciliary body in a wavy border called the *ora serrata*.

The single pigment layer is separated from the vascular portion of the choroid by a thin layer of elastic tissue (Bruch's membrane), which contains collagen fibrils in its superficial and deep portions. The cells of the pigmented layer receive their nourishment by diffusion from the choroid vessels. Its tight junctions (and those of the retinal blood vessels) provide the blood–retina barrier. The neural retina is composed of three layers of neurons: a posterior layer of photoreceptors, a middle layer of bipolar and ganglion cells that communicate with the photoreceptors, and a superficial marginal layer containing the axons of the ganglion cells as they collect and leave the eye by way of the optic nerve (Figure 51-16). The interneurons, the horizontal and amacrine cells, have cell bodies in the bipolar layer, and they play an important role in modulating retinal function. Light must pass through the transparent inner layers of the sensory retina before it reaches the photoreceptors.

Photoreceptors

There are two types of photoreceptors: rods, capable of black–white discrimination, and cones, capable of color discrimination. Both types of photoreceptors are thin, elongated, mitochondria-filled cells with a single highly modified cilium (Figure 51-17). The cilium has a very short base, or inner segment, and a highly modified outer segment. The plasma membrane of the outer segment is highly folded to form membranous disks (rods) or conical shapes (cones) containing visual pigment. These disks are continuously synthesized at the base of the outer seg-

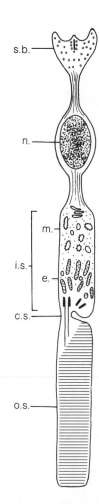

Figure 51-17 Retinal rod, showing its component parts and the distribution of its organelles. Its outer segment (o.s.) contains the disks. The connecting structure between the outer and inner segments is labeled c.s. The inner segment is labeled i.s. In the outermost part of this there is a basal body, from which a modified cilium extends into the inner part of the outer segment. The inner segment is described as consisting of two parts, the ellipsoid portion (e) and the myoid portion (m). The former contains abundant mitochondria. The myoid portion contains rER, free ribosomes, and Golgi saccules. Farther in, the cell is constricted until it bulges to surround the nucleus (n). It then narrows again and ends in an expansion called the synaptic body (s.b.) because here the photoreceptor synapses with other nerve cells. (*Courtesy of R. Young. From Ham AW, Cormack DH: Histology, 8th ed. Philadelphia, JB Lippincott, 1979*)

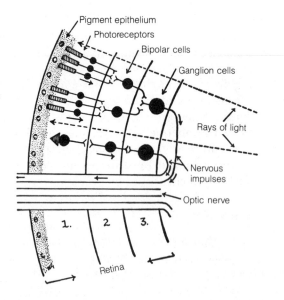

Figure 51-16 Basic arrangement of the three orders of neurons in the nervous portion of the retina. Note that light rays and nerve impulses travel in opposite directions through the retina. (*From Ham AW, Cormack DH: Histology, 8th ed. Philadelphia, JB Lippincott, 1979*)

ment and shed at the distal end. The discarded membranes are phagocytized by the retinal pigment cells. If this phagocytosis is disrupted, as in retinitis pigmentosa, the sensory retina degenerates.

Rods. Photoreception involves the transduction of light energy into an altered ionic membrane potential of the rod cell. Light passing through the eye penetrates the nearly transparent neural elements to produce decomposition of the photochemical substance (visual pigment) called *rhodopsin* in the outer segment of the rod. Light that is not trapped by a rhodopsin molecule is absorbed by either the retinal pigment melanin or the more superficial choroid melanin. Rhodopsin consists of a protein (opsin) and a vitamin A-derived pigment called *retinal pigment*. During light stimulation, rhodopsin is broken down into its component parts (opsin and retinal), and retinal is converted into vitamin A. The reconstitution of rhodopsin occurs during total darkness; vitamin A is transformed into retinal, and then opsin and retinal combine to form rhodopsin. Because there are considerable stores of vitamin A in the retinal pigment cells and in the liver, a vitamin A deficiency must exist for weeks or months to have an impact on the photoreceptive process. Reduced sensitivity to light, a symptom of vitamin A deficiency, first affects night vision and is quickly reversed by injection or ingestion of the vitamin.

A pattern of light on the retina falls on a massive array of photoreceptors. These photoreceptors communicate with bipolar and other interneurons before action potentials in ganglion cells relay the message to the brain. For rods, this microcircuitry involves the convergence of signals from many rods on a single ganglion cell. This arrangement maximizes spatial summation and the detection of stimulated (light versus dark) receptors. Rod-based vision is particularly sensitive to detecting light, and especially moving light stimuli at the expense of clear pattern discrimination. Thus, rod vision is particularly adapted for night and low-level illumination.

Dark adaptation is the process by which rod sensitivity increases to the optimum level. This requires approximately ½ hour in total or near-total darkness and involves only rod receptor (black-and-white) vision. During daylight, or high-intensity bombardment, the concentration of vitamin A increases and the concentration of the photopigment retinal decreases. During dark adaptation, increased synthesis of retinal from vitamin A results in a higher concentration of rhodopsin available to capture the light energy.

Cones and color sensitivity. Cone receptors that are selectively sensitive to different wavelengths of light provide the basis for color vision. Three types of cones, or cone-color systems, respond to the more blue, green, and red portions of the visible electromagnetic spectrum. This selectivity is due to the presence of one of three color-sensitive molecules to which the photochemical substance (visual pigment) is bound. The decomposition and reconstitution of the cone visual pigments is believed to be similar to that of the rods. The color a person senses depends on which set of cones or combination of sets of cones is stimulated in a given image.

Color vision vastly increases the richness of visual experience. The subjective experience of color can be analyzed according to three aspects: hue, saturation, and brightness. Hue is the experience of pure color. It is related to the proportion of involvement of each of the primary cone-color systems. Approximately 200 gradations of color dimension can be discriminated. Saturation refers to the purity of the color as contrasted with the amount of gray mixed with the color. The same red can be weak or strong (more saturated). Brightness experience refers to the total amount of light received from an object in relation to its background. Increased brightness turns brown into orange. Approximately 500 steps of brightness can be discriminated for each saturation of each hue. Brightness is shared by the black–white rod system with gradations from black through grays to whites.

Cones do not have the dark adaptation of rods. Consequently, the dark-adapted eye is a rod receptor eye with only black–gray–white experience (*scotopic vision*). The light-adapted eye (*photopic vision*) adds the capacity for color discrimination. Rhodopsin has its maximum sensitivity in the blue–green region of the spectrum. If red lenses are worn in daylight, only the red cones (and green cones to some extent) are in use; the rods (and blue cones) are essentially in the dark, and dark-adaptation proceeds. This method is used by military and night-duty airport control tower personnel to allow adaptation to take place before they go on duty in the dark.

Color blindness. Color blindness is a misnomer for a condition in which individuals appear to confuse, mismatch, or experience reduced acuity for color discrimination. Such people are often unaware of their defect until challenged by problems resulting from difficulties in discriminating a red from a green traffic light or mismatches of colors in an art class. Most often the result of genetic factors, the deficit can result from defective function of one or more of the three color-cone mechanisms. The deficiency is most often partial but can be complete. Rarely are two of the color mechanisms missing. When this does occur, usually red and green are missing. Extremely rare are persons with no color mechanisms. For such people, the world is experienced entirely as black, gray, and white.

The genetically color-blind person has never experienced the full range of normal color vision and is unaware of what he or she is missing. Color discrimination is necessary for everyday living, and color-blind people, knowingly or unknowingly, make color discriminations based on other criteria, such as brightness or position. For example, the red light of a traffic signal is always the upper light, and the green is the lower light. The color-blind individual gets into trouble when brightness differences are minimal and discrimination must be based on hue and saturation qualities.

The genes responsible for color blindness affect receptor mechanisms rather than central acuity. The gene for red and green mechanisms is sex-linked (on the X chromosomes), resulting in a much higher incidence among males of red, green, or red-green color blindness. The gene affecting the blue mechanism is autosomal. Acquired color defects are more complex but tend to follow a general rule: disease of the more peripheral retina affects blue discrimination, and disease of the more central retina affects red and green discrimination. This is because there are no blue cones in the central fovea.

The simplest test for color discrimination defects employs pseudoisochromatic plates that use numbers or letters buried in a matrix of colored dots. These plates are arranged so that common color-blindness defects result in misreading of the number or letter. Proper testing conditions require good lighting and the use of a control plate interpretable by the most color-blind individuals, in order to eliminate inability to read as a confounding factor.

Macula and fovea

A minute area in the center of the retina, called the macula, is especially capable of acute and detailed vision. This area is composed entirely of cones. In the central portion of the macula, the *fovea centralis*, the blood vessels and innermost layers are displaced to one side instead of resting on top of the cones. This allows light to pass unimpeded to the cones without passing through several layers of retina. The density of cones drops off rapidly away from the fovea. There are no rods in the fovea, but their density increases as the cones decrease in density toward the periphery of the retina. Many cones are connected on a one-to-one basis with ganglion cells. In addition, retinal microcircuitry for cones emphasizes the detection of edges. This type of circuitry favors high acuity. A concentration of acuity favoring cones at the fovea supports the use of this part of the retina for fine analysis of focused central vision.

Retinal blood supply

The blood supply for the retina is derived from two sources: the choriocapillaries of the choroid and the branches of the central retinal artery. The nutritional needs of the retina, including oxygen supply to the pigment cells and rods and cones, involve diffusion from blood vessels in the choroid. Because the choriocapillaries provide the only blood supply for the fovea centralis, detachment of this part of the sensory retina from the pigment epithelium causes irreparable visual loss. The bipolar, horizontal, amacrine, and ganglionic cells as well as the ganglion cell axons that gather at the disk are supplied by the branches of the retinal artery. The central artery of the retina is a branch of the ophthalmic artery. It enters the globe through the optic disk. Branches of the artery radiate over the entire retina, except for the central fovea, which is surrounded but is not crossed by arterial branches. The retinal veins follow a distribution parallel to the arterial branches and bring venous blood to the central vein of the retina, which exits the back of the eye through the optic disk. Funduscopic examination of the eye with an ophthalmoscope provides an opportunity to examine the retinal blood vessels as well as other aspects of the retina (Figure 51-18). Because the retina is an extension of the brain and the blood vessels are, to a considerable extent, representative of brain blood vessels, the ophthalmoscopic examination of the fundus of the eye provides an opportunity for the study and diagnosis of metabolic and vascular diseases of the brain, as well as pathologic processes that are specific to the retina itself.

The functioning of the retina, like that of other cellular portions of the central nervous system, is highly dependent on an oxygen supply from the vascular system. One of the earliest signs of decreased perfusion pressure in the head region is a graying-out or blackout of vision, which usually precedes loss of consciousness. This can occur with a large increase in intrathoracic pressure (*e.g.*, straining during defecation), which interferes with the return of venous blood to the heart, with systemic hypotension, and often during sudden postural movements under conditions of decreased vascular adaptability.

Ischemia of the retina occurs under general circulatory collapse. If a person survives cardiopulmonary arrest, for instance, permanent decreased visual acuity can occur as a result of edema and the ischemic death of retinal neurons. This is followed by primary optic nerve atrophy proportional to the extent of ganglionic cell death. The ophthalmic artery, the source of the central artery of the retina, takes its origin from the internal carotid artery. Intermittent retinal ischemia can accompany internal carotid or common ca-

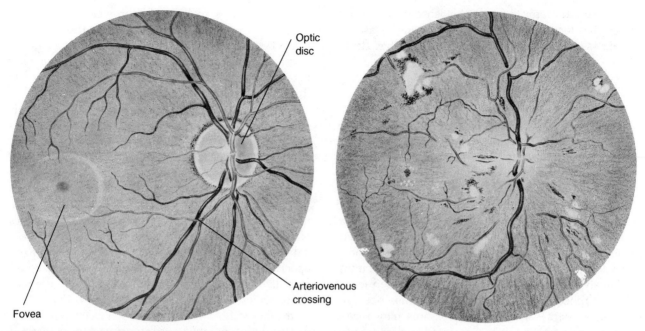

Figure 51-18 Fundus of the eye as seen in retinal examination with an ophthalmoscope: (**left**) normal fundus; (**right**) pathologic fundus. The macula is not evident, but one can see flame-shaped hemorrhages and interrupted arteriovenous crossings. (*Chaffee EE, Lytle IM: Basic Physiology and Anatomy, 4th ed. Philadelphia, JB Lippincott, 1980*)

rotid stenosis. In addition to ipsilateral intermittent blindness, contralateral hemiplegia or sensory deficits may accompany the episodes, depending on the competency of the circle of Willis in providing the brain with alternative arterial support. Treatment with anticoagulants or surgical endarterectomy may provide relief. Arteritis of the ophthalmic and central artery occurs more frequently in aged persons; if severe, it can result in occlusive disease and permanent visual deficits.

Papilledema

The central retinal artery enters the eye through the optic *papilla* in the center of the optic nerve. The central vein of the retina follows the same path. The entrance and exit of the central artery and veins of the retina through the tough scleral tissue at the optic papilla can be compromised by any condition causing persistent increased intracranial pressure. The most common of these conditions are cerebral tumors, subdural hematomas, hydrocephalus, and malignant hypertension. The thin-walled, low-pressure veins are the first to collapse, with the consequent backup and slowing of arterial blood flow. Under these conditions, capillary permeability increases, and leakage of fluid results in edema of the optic papilla, called papilledema. The interior surface of the papilla is normally cup-shaped and can be evaluated through

an ophthalmoscope. With papilledema, sometimes called *choked disk,* the optic cup is distorted by protrusion into the interior of the eye. Because this sign does not occur until the intracranial pressure is significantly elevated, compression damage to the optic nerve fibers passing through the lamina cribrosa may have begun. Thus, as a warning sign, papilledema occurs quite late. Unresolved papilledema will result in the destruction of the optic nerve axons and blindness.

Retrolental fibroplasia

Retrolental fibroplasia is a bilateral retinal disease of premature infants who must be given high concentrations of oxygen during the first 10 days of life to sustain life. Vascularization of the retina begins during the fourth month of gestation and moves from the optic nerve toward the ora serrata. The nasal periphery is completely vascularized by the eighth month, and the temporal periphery, only after full-term birth. During the period of blood vessel immaturity, the vessels respond to an increase in oxygen tension by vasoconstriction, obliteration, and suspension of normal vessel growth. This is followed by dilatation of the vessels that are present and growth of new vessels and supporting tissue (fibrovascular proliferation) into the vitreous. The disease often progresses rapidly to blindness. However, in many cases partial or complete regression may occur in one or both eyes. In some babies, photocoagulation of the ridge that forms between the vascular and avascular retina may be beneficial. Once blindness has developed, no treatment will restore sight.

Vascular retinopathies

Vascular disorders of the retina result in microaneurysms, neovascularization, hemorrhage, and formation of retinal opacities. *Microaneurysms* are outpouchings of the retinal vasculature. On ophthalmoscopic examination they appear as minute unchanging red dots associated with blood vessels. They tend to leak plasma and are often surrounded by edema, which gives the retina a hazy appearance. Microaneurysms can be identified with certainty using fluorescein angiography (the fluorescein dye is injected intravenously and the retinal vessels are subsequently photographed using a special ophthalmoscope and fundus camera). The microaneurysms may bleed. Areas of hemorrhage and edema tend to clear spontaneously; however, they reduce visual acuity if they encroach on the macula and cause degeneration before they are absorbed.

Neovascularization involves the formation of new blood vessels. They can develop from the choriocapillaries, extending between the pigment layer and the sensory layer, or from the retinal veins, extending between the sensory retina and the vitreous cavity and sometimes into the vitreous. These new blood vessels are fragile, leak protein, and tend to bleed. Neovascularization occurs in a number of conditions that impair retinal circulation, including stasis because of hyperviscosity of blood or decreased flow, vascular occlusion, sickle cell disease, sarcoidosis, diabetes mellitus, and retinopathy of prematurity (retrolental fibroplasia). The cause of new blood vessel formation is uncertain. The stimulus is presumably a diffusible factor that is released during impaired perfusion or oxygenation of retinal tissue. The vitreous humor is thought to contain a substance that normally inhibits neovascularization, and this factor is, apparently suppressed under conditions in which the new blood vessels invade the vitreous cavity.

Hemorrhage can be preretinal, intraretinal, or subretinal. Preretinal hemorrhages occur between the retina and the vitreous. These hemorrhages tend to be large because the blood vessels are only loosely restricted; they may be associated with a subarachnoid or subdural hemorrhage and are usually regarded as a serious manifestation of the disorder. They usually reabsorb without complications unless they penetrate into the vitreous. Intraretinal hemorrhages occur because of abnormalities of the retinal vessels, diseases of the blood, increased pressure within the retinal vessels, or vitreous traction on the vessel. Systemic causes include diabetes mellitus, hypertension, and blood dyscrasias. Subretinal hemorrhages are those that develop between the choroid and pigment layer of the retina. A common cause of subretinal hemorrhage is neovascularization. Photocoagulation may be used to treat microaneurysms and neovascularization.

Light normally passes through the transparent inner portions of the sensory retina before reaching the photoreceptors. *Opacities* such as hemorrhages, exudate, cotton-wool patches, edema, and tissue proliferation produce a localized loss of transparency that can be observed with the use of an ophthalmoscope. *Exudates* are opacities resulting from inflammatory processes. The development of exudates often results in the destruction of the underlying retinal pigment and choroid layer. *Deposits* are localized opacities consisting of lipid-laden macrophages or accumulated cellular debris. *Cotton-wool patches* are retinal opacities with hazy, irregular outlines. They occur in the nerve fiber layer and contain cell organelles. Cotton-wool patches are associated with retinal trauma, severe anemia, papilledema, and diabetic retinopathy.

Atherosclerosis of retinal vessels. In atherosclerosis, the lumen of the arterioles becomes narrowed. As a result, the retinal arteries become tortuous and narrowed. At sites where the arteries cross and compress veins, the red cell column of the vein appears distended. Exudate accumulates on arteriolar walls as plaque or cytoid bodies. Deep and superficial hemorrhages are common. Atheromatous plaques of the central artery are associated with danger of stasis, thrombi of the central veins, and occlusion.

Retinal artery occlusion. Complete occlusion of the central artery of the retina results in sudden unilateral blindness (anopsia). This is an uncommon disorder of older persons and is most often due to embolism or atherosclerosis. Because the retina has a dual blood supply, the survival of retinal structures is possible if blood flow can be reestablished within 2 hours.[2] If blood flow is not restored, the infarcted retina swells and opacifies. Because the receptors of the central fovea are supplied with blood from the choroid, they survive; a cherry-red spot (healthy fovea) is seen surrounded by the pale white opacified retina. Although the nerve fibers of the optic disks are adequately supplied by the choroid, the disk becomes pale because of the death of the optic fibers (optic atrophy) following the death of their ganglionic cells.

Occlusions of branches of the central artery, called branch arterial occlusions, are essentially retinal strokes. These occur mainly as a result of emboli and local infarction in the neural retina. The opacification that follows is often slowly resolved, and retinal transparency is restored. Local blind spots (scotomas) occur, however, because of the destruction of local elements of the retina. Loss of the axons of destroyed ganglion cells results in some optic nerve atrophy.

Central retinal vein occlusion. Occlusion of the central retinal vein results in venous dilatation, stasis, and reduced flow through the retinal veins. It is usually monocular and causes rapid deterioration of visual acuity. Superficial and deep hemorrhages throughout the retina follow, because of the increased capillary wall fragility resulting from the decreased venous outflow as well as lack of arterial inflow.

Among the causes of central retinal vein obstruction are hypertension, diabetes mellitus, and conditions such as sickle cell anemia, which slow the venous blood flow. The reduction in blood flow results in neovascularization with fibrovascular invasion of the space between the retina and the vitreous humor. In addition to obstructing normal visual function, the new vessels are fragile and prone to hemorrhage. Escaped blood may fill the space between the retina and vitreous, producing the appearance of a sudden veil over the visual field. The blood can find its way into the aqueous humor (hemorrhagic glaucoma). Photocoagulation of the spreading new blood vessels with high-intensity light or laser beam is used to prevent blindness and eye pain. As the hemorrhage is resolved, degenerating blood products can produce contraction of the vitreous and formation of fibrous tissue within it, causing tears and detachment of the retina.

Much more common are local vein occlusions with regional and focal capillary microhemorrhages that produce the same but more restricted pathologic effects. These microhemorrhages result in the formation of rings of yellow exudate composed of lipid and lipoprotein blood-breakdown products. Microhemorrhages deep in the neural retina are somewhat restricted by the vertical organization of the neural elements and result in dot hemorrhages. Microhemorrhages in the layer of ganglionic cell axon bundles result in cotton-wool spots.

Diabetic retinopathy. One of the complications of diabetes mellitus is the greatly increased fragility of the retinal capillaries (see Chapter 45). Diabetic retinopathy is the third leading cause of new blindness, for all ages, in the United States. It ranks first as the cause of new blindness in persons between the ages of 20 and 74 years.[1] Diabetic retinopathy can be divided into two types: background and proliferative. Background retinopathy is confined to the retina. It involves thickening of the retinal capillary walls and microaneurysm formation. Ruptured capillaries cause small intraretinal hemorrhages, and microinfarcts may cause cotton-wool exudates. A sensation of glare (because of the scattering of light) is a common complaint.

Some diabetics with background retinopathy develop neovascularization on the back of the vitreous (proliferative retinopathy). New vessels with delicate supporting tissue grow from the retina. When this happens, the retina is still attached to the vitreous, and the neovascular tissue adheres to the posterior vitreous, forming a contractile vascular membrane. Repeated bleeding into the vitreous results from contraction of the vascular membrane, accompanied by retinal tears, detachment, and progressive blindness. Photocoagulation provides the only major direct treatment modality for the neovascularization that leads to microhemorrhage. It destroys not only the proliferating vessels, but also the ischemic retina, and therefore reduces the stimulus for further neovascularization. Vitrectomy has proved effective in removing vitreous hemorrhage and severing vitreoretinal membranes that develop.

Hypertensive retinopathy. Longstanding systemic hypertension results in the compensatory thickening of arteriolar walls, which effectively reduces capillary perfusion pressure. Ordinarily, retinal blood vessels are transparent and are seen as a red line; in venules, the red cells resemble a string of boxcars. On ophthalmoscopy, arteries appear paler than veins because they *have thicker* walls. The thickened arterioles in chronic hypertension become opaque and have a copperwiring appearance. Edema, microaneurysms, intraretinal hemorrhages, exudates, and cotton-wool spots are all observed. Malignant hypertension involves swelling of the optic disk as a result of the local edema produced by escaped fluid. If the condition is permitted to progress long enough, serious visual deficits result.

Sudden increases in blood pressure do not permit the protective thickening of arteriolar walls, and hemorrhage is likely to occur. Trauma to the optic globe or the head, sudden high blood pressure in eclampsia, and some types of renal disease are characteristically accompanied by edema of the retina and optic disk as well as an increased likelihood of hemorrhage.

Macular degeneration

Macular degeneration is characterized by destructive changes of the yellow pigmented area surrounding the central fovea (the macula) resulting from vascular disorders. It is the leading cause of blindness in persons over 75 and of new blindness among persons over age 65 years.[1] Macular degeneration is characterized by the loss of central vision, usually in both eyes. The person may find it difficult to see at long distances (*e.g.*, in driving), to do close work (*e.g.*, reading), to see faces clearly, or to distinguish colors. However, the person may not be severely incapacitated because the peripheral retinal function usually remains intact. With the help of low-vision aids, persons can usually continue their normal activities.

The most common causes of macular degeneration are neovascularization and sclerosis of the choriocapillaries. Although rare, macular degeneration can occur as a hereditary condition in young people and sometimes in adults. With neovascularization there is growth of new vessels in the potential space between Bruch's membrane and the basement membrane of the pigment epithelium. It usually occurs in the posterior pole of the retina in areas where there is an abnormality of Bruch's membrane because of senile degeneration, choroidal scars, or high degree of myopia. The new vessels cause serous and hemorrhagic detachment of the pigment epithelium and loss of vision. Sclerosis of the choriocapillaries, with irregular thickening of Bruch's membrane, is a frequent finding in the elderly. Loss of central vision may result from atrophy of the pigment epithelium, serous detachment, or development of new vessels with subsequent bleeding.

Retinal detachment

Retinal detachment involves the separation of the sensory retina from the pigment epithelium (Figure 51-19). It occurs when traction on the inner sensory layer or a tear in this layer allows fluid, usually vitreous, to accumulate between the two layers. Retinal detachment that occurs secondary to breaks in the sensory layer of the retina is termed rhegmatogenous detachment (*rhegma* in Greek meaning "rent" or "hole"). The vitreous is normally adherent to the retina at the optic disk, macula, and periphery of the retina. When the vitreous shrinks, it separates from the retina at the posterior pole of the eye (posterior vitreous detachment); but at the periphery, the vitreous pulls on the attached retina, which can lead to tearing of the retina. Sometimes flashing lights (photopsias) are experienced when this occurs. Vitreous fluid can then enter the tear and contribute to further the separation of the retina from its overlying pigment layer. Myopia and aphakia are two of the most common predisposing factors. Detachment may also occur secondary to the presence of exudates that separate the two retinal layers. Exudative detachment may occur secondary to intraocular inflammations, intraocular tumors, or certain systemic diseases. Inflammatory processes include posterior scleritis, uveitis, or parasitic invasion.

Detachment of the neural retina from the retinal pigment layer (retinal detachment) separates the receptors from their major blood supply, the choroid. If detachment continues for some time, permanent destruction and therefore blindness of that part of the retina will occur. The bipolar and ganglion cells will survive because their blood supply, by way of the retinal arteries, remains intact. Without receptors, however, there is no visual function.

The primary symptom of retinal detachment is loss of vision. There is no pain. Because the process begins in the periphery and spreads circumferentially and posteriorly, initial visual disturbances may involve only one quadrant of the visual field. Large peripheral detachments may be present without involvement of the macula, so that visual acuity remains unaffected. The tendency, however, is for detachments to enlarge until all of the retina is detached.

Diagnosis is based on the ophthalmoscopic appearance of the retina. Treatment is aimed at closing retinal tears and reattaching the retina. Small tears may be closed using cryotherapy (freezing) or photocoagulation (laser). Rhegmatogenous detachment usually requires surgical treatment. One method, called scleral buckling, involves forcing infolds of the sclera so as to oppose the separated pigment and retinal layers (Figure 51-20). Another approach is used in severe cases. After the eyeball at the flat part of the ciliary body is surgically entered, the vitreous and retina are manipulated with instruments. When approximation of the two layers is accomplished, tiny laser beam burns are made so that subsequent scar formation will weld the layers together.

Retinitis pigmentosa

Retinitis pigmentosa is a group of hereditary diseases that cause slow degenerative changes in the retinal receptors. Slow destruction of the rods occurs,

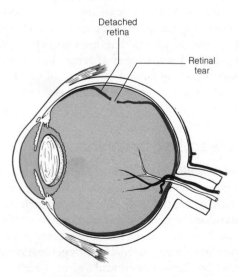

Detached retina

Retinal tear

Figure 51-19 Detached retina.

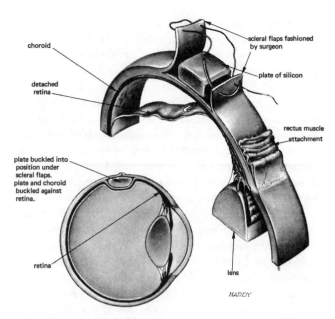

choroid

detached retina

plate buckled into position under scleral flaps. plate and choroid buckled against retina.

retina

scleral flaps fashioned by surgeon

plate of silicon

rectus muscle attachment

lens

HARDY

Figure 51-20 Scleral buckling for detached retina (Ethicon, Inc.). (*Brunner LS, Suddarth DS: Textbook of Medical-Surgical Nursing, 6th ed. JB Lippincott, 1988*)

progressing from the peripheral to the central regions of the retina. Based on research with animal models, the probable mechanism of the disorder is a defect in phagocytic mechanisms of the pigment cells that cause membrane debris to accumulate and destroy the photoreceptors. The destruction results in dark lines and areas in which the pigment of the retinal pigment layer is unmasked by receptor loss. Night blindness, the first symptom of the disorder, often begins in early youth, with gross visual handicap occurring in the middle or advanced years. At present there is no effective treatment for this group of hereditary diseases.

Tests of retinal function

The diagnosis of retinal disease is based on history, tests of visual acuity, refraction, visual field tests, color vision tests, and often fluorescein angiography. Electroretinography (ERG) can be used to measure the electrical activity of the retina in response to a flash of light. The recorded ERG represents the difference in electrical potential between an electrode placed in a corneal contact lens and one placed on the forehead. The test can be used to evaluate retinal function in persons with an opaque lens or vitreous body. The electro-oculogram (EOG) records the electrical potentials between the front of the eye and the retina in the back of the eye. It is recorded from two electrodes, one placed above and the other lateral to the eye. The EOG measures eye movement and is frequently used in sleep studies.

In summary, the retina covers the inner aspect of the posterior two-thirds of the eyeball and is continuous with the optic nerve. It contains the neural receptors for vision, and it is here that light energy of different frequencies and intensities is converted to graded action potentials and transmitted to visual centers in the brain. The retina is composed of an outer pigmented layer, which prevents the scattering of light stimuli and contains the enzymes for the synthesis of visual pigments. There are two types of photoreceptors: rods, capable of black-and-white discrimination, and cones, capable of color discrimination. Both rods and cones contain visual pigments. With exposure to light energy within a particular frequency, the visual pigment decomposes, causing nerve excitation. There is a maximal density of cones in an area of the posterior retina called the macula. The fovea centralis, the area of highest acuity, has no rods and contains the highest concentration of cones. The rods, which sense maximal spatial relationships, have their highest density toward the periphery of the eye. The photoreceptors normally shed portions of their outer segments. These segments are phagocytized by cells in the pigment epithelium. Failure of phagocytosis, as in retinitis pigmentosa, results in degeneration of the pigment layer and blindness. The retina receives its blood from two sources: the choriocapillaries, which supply the pigment layer and the outer portion of the sensory retina adjacent to the choroid, and the branches of the retinal artery, which supply the inner half of the retina. The retinal blood vessels are normally apparent through the ophthalmoscope. Disorders of retinal vessels can result from a number of local and systemic disorders, including diabetes mellitus, hypertension, sickle cell anemia, and vascular changes associated with aging. They cause vision loss through changes that result in hemorrhage, the production of opacities, and separation of the pigment epithelium and sensory retina. Other retinal pathologies that can result in partial or total blindness include separation (detachment) of retinal layers and hereditary degeneration of photoreceptors (retinitis pigmentosa).

Visual pathways and cortical centers

Full visual function requires normally developed brain-related functions of photoreception, visual sensation, and perception. These functions depend on the integrity of the retinal circuitry, optic nerve, forebrain, and midbrain.

Optic pathways

Visual information is carried to the brain by the axons of the retinal ganglion cells forming the optic nerve. Surrounded by pia mater, CSF, arachnoid, and dura mater, the optic nerve represents an outgrowth of the brain rather than a peripheral nerve. The optic nerve extends from the back of the optic globe through the orbit and the optic foramen, into the middle fossa, and on to the optic chiasm at the base of the brain—a distance of 40 mm to 50 mm in the adult (Figure 51-21). Axons from the nasal half of the retina remain medial and those from the temporal retina remain lateral in the optic nerve.

The two optic nerves meet and fuse at the optic chiasm, located on the ventral and most rostral end of the brain stem, just in front of the infundibular stalk and pituitary gland. In the chiasm, axons from the nasal retina of the opposite side and axons from the temporal retina on the same side are organized to form the optic tracts. Thus, one optic tract contains fibers from both eyes that are transmitting information from the same visual field. The fibers of the optic tracts move laterally around the cerebral peduncles to synapse in the lateral geniculate nucleus (LGN) of the thalamus and from there pass through the optic radiation to the primary visual cortex in the calcarine area of the occipital lobe. The LGN receives input from the visual cortex, oculomotor centers in the brain stem,

and the brain stem reticular formation. It is thought to modify the pattern and strength of the retinal input. Axons from cells located in the lateral geniculate form the optic radiations that travel to the visual cortex. The pattern for information transmission that was established in the optic tract is retained in the optic radiations. For example, the axons from the right visual field, represented by the nasal retina of the right eye and the left temporal retina of the left eye, are united at the chiasm and continue through the left optic tract and left optic radiation to the left visual cortex, where visual experience is first perceived. The left primary visual cortex thus receives two representations of the right visual field. The left LGN and the left primary visual cortex retain physical separation of information from the left and right representations of the right visual field. At the cortical level, interaction between these slightly disparate representations occurs and provides the basis for the sensation of depth in the near visual field.

Visual cortex

The primary visual cortex (area 17) is located in the calcarine fissure of the occipital lobe; it is at this level that visual sensation is first experienced (Figure 51-22). The immediately neighboring associational visual cortex (areas 18 and 19), together with their thalamic nuclei, must be functional for added meaningfulness of visual perception. This higher-order aspect of the visual experience depends on previous learning.

Approximately 1 million retinal ganglion cell axons pass through the optic nerve and tract to reach the LGN in the thalamus, and more than 100 million geniculate neuron axons provide the input to the billions of neurons in the visual cortex. Here the spatial representation of the visual field is retained in a distorted retinal map. The proportion of cells of the LGN and of the primary visual area devoted to analysis of the central visual field is greatly expanded, compared with that of the peripheral retina. From 80% to 90% of the cellular mass and area of the primary visual cortex is concerned with central vision. This accounts for the greatly increased visual acuity of central vision, not only at the retina but also at all levels of the visual pathway.

Circuitry in both the primary visual cortex and the associational visual areas is extremely discrete with respect to the location of retinal stimulation. For example, specific neurons respond to the moving edge of a particular inclination, specific colors, or familiar shapes.

This fine-grained organization of the visual cortex with functionally separate and multiple representations of the same visual field provides the major

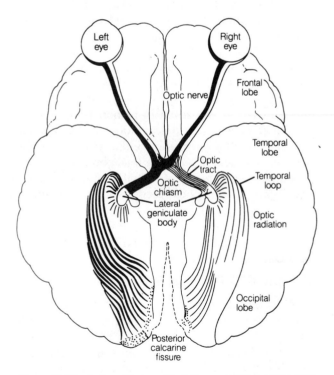

Figure 51-21 Optic pathways. All of the nasal fibers of the right and left eye decussate (cross) at the optic chiasm. (*Newell FW: Ophthalmology: Principles and Concepts, 5th ed. St Louis CV Mosby, 1982*)

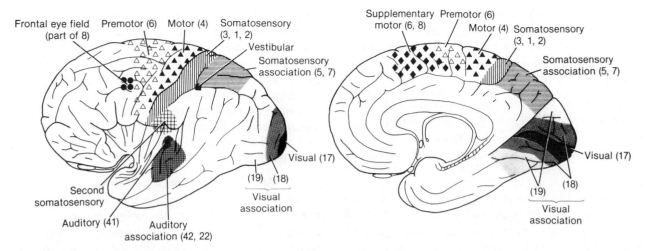

Figure 51-22 Lateral view of the cortex with the lateral sulcus pried open to expose the insula (**left**) and medial view of the cortex (**right**), illustrating the location of the visual, visual association, auditory, and auditory association areas. (*Nolte J: The Human Brain, p 271. St Louis, CV Mosby, 1981. Reproduced with permission.*)

basis for visual sensation and perception. Because of this discrete circuitry, lesions of the visual cortex must be large to be detected clinically.

A flash of light delivered to the retina will evoke potentials that can be measured and recorded by placing electrodes on the scalp over the occipital lobes. The waves of the evoked potentials, called pattern-reversed-evoked potentials or visual-evoked potentials, have proven to be a useful tool for clinical evaluation of the functional integrity of the successive levels of the visual pathway.

Visual fields

The visual field refers to that area that is visible during fixation of vision in one direction. Because the visual system is organized with reference to the visual fields rather than to direct measures of neural function, the terminology for normal and abnormal visual characteristics is usually based on visual field orientation.

Most of the visual field is binocular, or seen by both eyes. This binocular field is subdivided into central and peripheral portions. The central portion provides high visual acuity and corresponds to the field focused on the central fovea; the peripheral and surrounding portion provides the capacity to detect objects, particularly moving objects. Beyond the visual field shared by both eyes, the left lateral periphery of the visual field is seen exclusively by the left nasal retina, and the right peripheral field, by the right nasal retina.

As with a camera, the simple lens system of the eye inverts the image of the external world on each retina. The right and left sides of the visual field are also reversed. The right binocular visual field is seen by the left retinal halves of each eye: the nasal half of the right eye and the temporal half of the left eye.

Once the level of the retina is reached, the nervous system plays a consistent game. The upper half of the visual field is received by the lower half of the retinas of both eyes, and the representations of this upper half of the field are carried in the lower half of each optic nerve to synapse in the lower half of the LGN of each side of the brain. Neurons in this part of the LGN send their axons through the inferior half of the optic radiation which loops into the temporal lobe to the lower half of the primary visual cortex on each side of the brain.

Because of the lateral separation of the two eyes, the visual field as viewed by the two eyes results in a slightly different view of the world by each eye, called *binocular disparity*. Disparity between the laterally displaced images seen by the two eyes provides a powerful source of three-dimensional depth perception for objects within a distance of 30 m. Beyond that distance, the difference in the two images becomes insignificant, and depth perception is based on other cues such as the superimposition of the image of near objects over that of far objects, or the relatively faster movement of near objects than of far objects.

Visual field defects

Visual field defects occur as a result of damage to the visual pathways or the visual cortex. Visual field testing or perimetry is used to identify defects and determine the location of lesions. The periphery of the opposite visual field is represented on the medial surface and in the depths of a deep medial calcarine sulcus of the occipital cortex (area 17). The central, high acuity part of the visual half field extends somewhat over the occipital pole. The visual association cortex surrounds the primary cortex on the superior, lateral, and inferior occipital lobe. This area is required for complex analysis and learned meaningfulness of visual stimuli.

Retinal defects. All of us possess a hole, or scotoma, in our visual field of which we are unaware. Because the optic disc, where the optic nerve fibers exit the retina, does not contain photoreceptors, a corresponding location in the visual field constitutes a blind spot. Local retinal damage caused by small vascular accidents (retinal stroke) and other localized pathology can produce additional blind spots. As with the normal blind spot, persons are not usually aware of the existence of scotomata in their visual fields unless they encounter problems seeing objects in certain restricted parts of the visual field.

Absences near or in the center of the bilateral visual field can be annoying and even disastrous. Although the hole is not recognized as such, the person finds that a part of a printed page appears or disappears depending on where the fixation point is held. Most persons learn to position their eyes so as to use the remaining central foveal vision for high-acuity tasks. Defects in the peripheral visual field, including the monocular peripheral fields, are less annoying but potentially more dangerous. Often the person is unaware of the defect and, when walking or driving an automobile, does not see cars or bicyclists until their image reaches the functional visual field—sometimes too late to avert an accident. With careful education, a person can learn to shift the gaze constantly in such a

way as to obtain visual coverage of important parts of the visual field. If the damage is at the retinal or optic nerve level, only the monocular field of the damaged eye becomes a problem. A lesion affecting the central foveal vision of one eye can result in complaints of eye strain during reading and other close work, because only one eye is really being used. Localized damage to the optic tracts, LGN, optic radiation, or primary visual cortex will affect corresponding parts of the visual fields of both eyes.

Disorders of the optic pathways. The visual pathway extends from the front to the back of the head. It is much like a telephone line between distant points in that damage at any point along the pathway results in functional defects (Figure 51-23). Among the disorders that can interrupt the visual pathway are vascular lesions, trauma, and tumors. For example, normal visual system function depends on vascular adequacy in the ophthalmic artery and its branches; the central artery of the retina; the anterior and middle cerebral arteries, which supply the intracranial optic nerve, chiasm, and optic tracts; and the posterior cerebral artery, which supplies the lateral geniculate, optic radiation, and visual cortex. In turn, adequacy of the posterior cerebral artery function depends on that of the vertebral and basilar arteries that supply the brain stem. Vascular insufficiency in any one of these arterial systems can seriously affect vision. Examination of the visual system function is of particular diagnostic use because lesions at various points along the pathway have characteristic symptoms that assist in the localization of pathology.

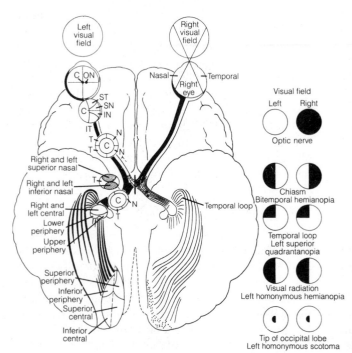

Figure 51-23 Typical visual field defects that occur with damage to different regions of the optic pathways. Visual fields are diagrammed to reflect the source of the light that stimulates the retina. C = central, ON = optic nerve, ST = superior temporal, IT = inferior temporal, SN = superior nasal, IN = inferior nasal, T = temporal, N = nasal. Light from the temporal side stimulates the nasal portion of the retina, light from above stimulates the lower portion, and so on. Thus, the visual field defect caused by a lesion affecting fibers arising from the nasal half of the retina is diagrammed as a temporal field defect. (*Newell FW: Ophthalmology: Principles and Concepts, 5th ed. St Louis, CV Mosby, 1982*)

Visual field defects of each eye and of the two eyes together are useful in localizing lesions affecting the system. Blindness in one eye is termed *anopia*. If half of the visual field for one eye is lost, the defect is termed *hemianopia*; loss of a quarter field is called *quadrantanopia*. Enlarging pituitary tumors can produce longitudinal damage through the optic chiasm with loss of the medial fibers of the optic nerve representing both nasal retinas and thus, both temporal visual half-fields. Loss of the temporal or peripheral visual fields on both sides results in a narrow binocular field, commonly called *tunnel vision*. The loss of different half-fields in the two eyes is called a *heteronymous* loss, and the abnormality is called *heteronymous hemianopia*. Destruction of one or both lateral halves of the chiasm is not uncommon with multiple aneurysms of the circle of Willis. Here the function of the left or both temporal retinas occurs, and the nasal fields of the left or of both eyes are lost. The loss of the nasal fields of both eyes is called *bitemporal heteronymous anopia*. With both eyes open, the person with bilateral defects still has the full binocular visual field.

Loss of the optic tract, lateral geniculate, full optic radiation, or complete visual cortex on one side results in loss of the corresponding visual half-fields in each eye. *Homonymous* means the same for both eyes. In left-side lesions, the right visual field is lost for each eye and is called *complete right homonymous hemianopia*. Partial injury to the left optic tract, LGN, or optic radiation can result in the loss of a quarter of the visual field, again the same for both eyes. This is called *homonymous quadrantanopia* and, depending on the lesion, it can involve the upper (superior) or lower (inferior) fields. Because the optic radiation fibers for the superior quarter of the visual field traverse the temporal lobe, superior quadrantanopia is more common. The LGN, optic radiation, and visual cortex all receive their major blood supply from the posterior cerebral artery; thus, unilateral occlusion of this artery results in complete loss of the opposite field (homonymous hemianopia). Bilateral occlusion of these arteries results in total cortical blindness.

Disorders of the visual cortex. Discrete damage in the binocular portion of the primary visual cortex can also result in scotomas in the corresponding visual fields. If the visual loss is in the central high-acuity part of the field, severe loss of visual acuity and pattern discrimination occurs. The central, high acuity portion of the visual field is located at the occipital pole. This region can be momentarily compressed against the occipital bone (contrecoup) upon severe trauma to the frontal part of the cranium. Mechanical trauma to the cortex results in firing of neurons, experienced as flashes of light or "seeing stars." Destruction of the polar visual cortex causes severe loss of visual acuity and pattern discrimination. Such damage is permanent and cannot be corrected with lens.

The bilateral loss of the entire primary visual cortex, called *cortical blindness,* eliminates all visual experience. Some suggestion remains that crude analysis of visual stimulation exists on reflex levels. Eye-orienting and head-orienting responses to bright moving lights, pupillary reflexes, and blinking at sudden bright light are retained even though vision has been lost. Extensive damage to the visual association cortex (areas 18, 19) that surrounds an intact primary visual cortex results in a loss of the learned meaningfulness of visual images (visual agnosia). The patient can see the patterns of color, shapes, and movement, but can no longer recognize formerly meaningful stimuli. Familiar objects can be described but not named or reacted to meaningfully. However, if other sensory modalities (hearing, touch, *etc.*) can be applied, full recognition occurs. Thus, this disorder represents a problem of recognition rather than intellect.

Testing of visual fields

Crude testing of the binocular visual field and the visual field of each individual eye (monocular vision) can be accomplished without specialized equipment. In the confrontation method, the examiner stands or sits 2 feet to 3 feet in front of the person to be tested and instructs the person to focus on an object such as a penlight with one eye closed. The object is moved from the center toward the periphery of the person's visual field and from the periphery toward the center, and the person is instructed to report the presence or absence of the object. By moving the object through the vertical, horizontal, and oblique aspects of the visual field, a crude estimate can be made of the visual field. If the test object is kept midway between the examiner and the person being tested, the examiner can close the corresponding eye and compare the person's monocular vision with his or her own. Large field defects can be estimated by the confrontation method, and it may be the only way for testing young children and uncooperative adults. Rapidly presenting the examiner's fingers toward the eyes and observing for a reflex blink to the threat is sometimes the only way to detect a visual field deficit in someone with decreased consciousness.

Accurate determination of the presence, size, and shape of smaller holes, or scotomata, in the visual field of a particular eye can be demonstrated by the ophthalmologist only through the use of a method known as *perimetry*. This is done by having the person look with one eye toward a central spot directly in front of the eye while the head is stabilized by a chin rest or bite board. A small dot of light or a colored object is moved back and forth in all areas of the visual field. The person reports whether or not the stimulus is visible and, if a colored stimulus is used, what the perceived color is. A hemispherical support is used to control and standardize the movement of the test object, and a plot of radial coordinates of the visual field is made (see Figure 51-8). Perimetry provides a means of determining alterations from normal and, with repeated testing, a way of following the progress of the disease or treatment.

In summary, visual information is carried to the brain by axons of the retinal ganglion cells forming the optic nerve. The two optic nerves meet and fuse in the optic chiasm. The axons of each nasal retina cross in the chiasm and join the uncrossed fibers of the temporal retina of the opposite eye in the optic tract. From the optic chiasm, the crossed fibers of the nasal retina of one eye and the uncrossed temporal fibers of the other eye pass to the LGN and then to the primary visual cortex, which is located in the calcarine fissure of the occipital lobe. Damage to the visual pathways or visual cortex leads to visual field defects that can be identified through visual field testing or perimetry and used to determine the lesion's location. Damage to the visual association cortex can result in seeing an object, but with loss of learned recognition (visual agnosia).

Eye movements

Normal vision is dependent on the coordinated action of the entire visual system as well as a number of central control systems. It is through these mechanisms that an object is simultaneously imaged on the fovea of both eyes and perceived as a single image. Strabismus and amblyopia are two disorders that affect this highly integrated system.

Extrinsic eye muscles

Each eyeball can rotate around its vertical axis (lateral or medial rotation in which the pupil moves away from or toward the nose), its horizontal left–right axis (vertical elevation or depression in which the pupil moves up or down), and its longitudinal horizontal axis (intorsion or extorsion in which the top of the pupil moves toward or away from the nose).

Six extrinsic muscles (four rectus and two oblique) control the movement of each eye (Figure 51-24). The four rectus muscles are named according to where they insert into the sclera on the medial, lateral, inferior, and superior surfaces of the eye. The two oblique muscles insert on the lateral posterior quadrant of the eyeball: the superior oblique on the upper surface and the inferior oblique on the lower.

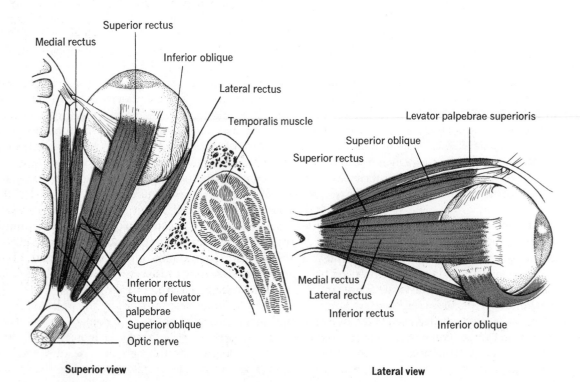

Figure 51-24 Extrinsic muscles of the right eye: (**left**) viewed from above within the orbital cavity; (**right**) lateral view. (*Chaffee EE, Lytle IM: Basic Anatomy and Physiology, 4th ed. Philadelphia, JB Lippincott, 1980*)

Each of the three sets of muscles in each eye is reciprocally innervated so that one muscle relaxes when the other contracts. The medial and lateral recti contract reciprocally to move the eye from side to side; the superior and inferior recti contract to move the eye up and down. The oblique muscles rotate the eye around its optic axis. Although the origins and insertions of the extrinsic eye muscles would seem to make their role in eye movement predictable, their function is somewhat complex. This is because the muscles insert into a rotatable eyeball.

Inserting approximately on the horizontal plane, the antagonistic medial and lateral recti rotate the eye medially (adduction) or laterally (abduction). When the optical axes of the two eyes are parallel, these muscles provide horizontal conjugate (paired) gaze. Convergence (moving toward a common point) and divergence (moving away from a common point) of the optical axes of the eyes result from the differential contraction of the recti muscles accompanied by coordinated inhibition of the antagonistic muscles. The phrase *being yoked together* is often used to describe such direct antagonism between eye muscles.

The actions of the superior and inferior recti are more complex. Their predominant action is the elevation and depression of the eyeball, usually a conjugate movement. Because of their medial orbit origin, both muscles contribute to medial rotation. In addition, each contributes to some extent to intorsion (superior rectus) and extorsion (inferior rectus). Major functions of the oblique muscles is the extorsion (the inferior oblique pulls the inferior surface of the eyeball medially) and the intorsion (the superior oblique pulls the superior surface of the eyeball medially) of the optic globe. These muscles function as antagonists for rotation around the longitudinal axis of the eye. Because of the insertion position posterior to the equator of the eyeball, the superior oblique pulls the upward-pointed eye downward, assisting the function of the inferior rectus. The inferior oblique, similarly, pulls upward a downward-pointed eye, assisting the superior rectus. When the eye is strongly medially deviated, the oblique muscles function almost entirely as elevator and depressor muscles.

The extraocular muscles are innervated by three cranial nerves: the trochlear (IV) innervates the superior oblique, the abducens (VI) innervates the lateral rectus, and the oculomotor (III) innervates the remaining four muscles. The medial longitudinal fasciculus (MLF) connects the nuclei of these cranial nerves. This important tract system transmits impulses that coordinate conjugate movements of the eye. Eye movements are further influenced by input from control centers in the frontal cortex (frontal premotor area), the visual association area, and the superior colliculus, a midbrain optic reflex center that is concerned with eye movements. Strong signals are also transmitted into the oculomotor system from the vestibular nuclei by way of the MLF (to be discussed later).

Eye movements and gaze

Conjugate movements are those in which the optical axes of the two eyes are kept parallel, sharing the same visual field. *Gaze* refers to the act of looking steadily in one direction. Eye movements can be categorized into five classes of movement: smooth pursuit, saccadic, vestibular, vergence, and tremor. Smooth pursuit (object following), saccadic (position correcting), and vestibular (nystagmus) movements involve conjugate coordination. *Vergence* (divergence and convergence) movements involve coordinated movements of the eyes in opposite directions. A *tremor* refers to involuntary rhythmic oscillatory (quivering) movements. Small-range optical tremor is a normal and useful independent function of each eye. Eye movements are important motor capabilities that are integrated into vestibular, auditory, and visual reflex and learned functions.

Smooth pursuit movements

Smooth pursuit movements are tracking movements that serve to maintain an object at a fixed point in the center of the visual fields of both eyes. The object may be moving and the eyes following it, or the object may be stationary and the head of the observer moving. Voluntary pursuit movements are tested by asking the person to follow a finger or another object as it is moved smoothly through the visual field. Successful conjugate tracking requires a functional optic system communicating to the superior colliculus and to the primary visual cortex. The communication from the primary visual cortex to the superior colliculus must also be functional.

Normal eye posture is a conjugate gaze directed straight forward with the head held in a forward-looking posture. Smooth pursuit movements normally begin from this position. In fact, holding a strongly deviated gaze becomes tiring within about 30 seconds, and most people will make head and body rotation adjustments to bring the eyes to a central position within that time period.

Saccadic movements

Saccadic eye movements are sudden, jerky conjugate movements that quickly change the fixation point. During reading, the fixation pattern involves a focus on a word or short series of words and then a sudden jump of the eyes to a new fixation point on the next word or phrase. These shifts in fixation points are saccadic movements. The neural circuitry that makes coordinated saccadic movements possible remains under study, but certain areas of the midbrain reticular formation are essential for these movements. Saccadic movements are quick readjustments of the binocular fixation point that must occur to accomplish a change in fixation. This readjustment occurs while searching the visual environment. Changes in fixation point must be accomplished quickly in order to provide the person with a new, stable part of the visual field on which to focus. No sensation of blur is experienced during the period of rapid eye movement, although the mechanism by which the blurred vision is eliminated is not understood.

The visual startle reaction in which the eyes are quickly turned in the direction of a sudden and intense visual stimulus entering the periphery of the visual field, is saccadic movement initiated by the optic system. This reflex occurs in the absence of the cortical portion of the visual system (cortical blindness). The auditory startle reaction (startle reflex) involves rapid saccadic movements in the direction of a sudden auditory stimulus. It is present in the neonate and in persons with impaired cortical auditory apparatus.

The frontal eye fields of the premotor cortex are of critical importance for voluntary saccadic movements such as reading. If this frontal premotor area is not functional, a person can describe objects in the visual field but cannot voluntarily search the visual environment.

Vergence movements

Convergence of the optical axes of the two eyes is an automatic aspect of changing binocular fixation from a distant to a close fixation point. This readjustment of the position of each eye in relation to the other accompanies changes in ciliary muscle activity that affect the lens shape and pupillary dilation that exposes more of the lens refractive surface. All of these adjustments function to permit a closer and sharper binocular retinal image and are included in the function of accommodation. Convergence can occur smoothly as a pursuit-like, continuous adjustment when a moving object approaches the observer. Convergence can also occur as a saccadic movement when fixation is changed from a distant to a near object, or vice versa. Divergence occurs when a fixated object recedes in the visual field. The convergence–divergence aspect of accommodation requires a functional visual cortex and intact projection to the pretectal area and to the parasympathetic efferent neurons of the oculomotor nerve. A region of the midbrain reticular

formation near the oculomotor nuclei must also be functional for convergence to occur. Master control is by the depth perception mechanism of the occipital visual association cortex. Voluntary convergence is achieved by altering the fixation point to one close to the eyes, requiring participation of the frontal eye fields.

Optic tremor

Without special equipment, the very fine continuous tremor of each eye is difficult to detect. This tremor is attributed to the inequality in the number of motor units active in opposing extraocular muscles at any moment. Because of the great amplification factor between the minute shifts in eye position relative to the large shifts in a distant fixation point, one might expect eye tremor to be a serious impediment to acuity. Yet, the visual system functions rapidly enough to keep up with these minute shifts in fixation; if the tremor were eliminated, the visual image would quickly fade away through adaptation of the individual cone receptors. The function of the tremor is to keep the retinal image moving over the receptor array so that it is constantly encountering recovered or unadapted receptors.

Horizontal gaze

Lateral conjugate gaze is accomplished through a reflex mechanism involving the medulla, pons, and midbrain, which contain the sixth, fourth, and third cranial nerve nuclei. Lateral rotation of an eye results from the increased activity of the sixth-nerve-innervated lateral rectus muscle accompanied by the corresponding reduced activity of the third-nerve-innervated medial rectus muscle. Synergists of the medial rectus, the third-nerve-innervated superior and inferior recti, also must be inhibited. Communication between the sixth nerve and third nerve nuclei must be rapid and precise. Conjugate (bilateral) side-to-side eye movement involves lateral rotation of one eye and medial rotation of the other. This requires close coordination between the sixth nerve nucleus of one side and the third nerve nucleus of the other. Further, smooth movement in conjugate gaze requires continuous variation in the contractional tone in synergists as well as in opposing eye muscles throughout the full range of dual eye rotation.

Reflex coordination of lateral gaze involves a longitudinal tract system of the brain stem, the medial longitudinal fasciculus (MLF), that interconnects the lower motor neurons of the sixth and third cranial nerves. A region in the reticular formation near the sixth nerve nucleus, called the pontine gaze center, controls this highly coordinated reflex mechanism.

Destruction of the lateral gaze control region on one side results in ipsilateral gaze palsy, that is, there is lateral gaze to the contralateral side but not to the affected side. Interruption of the MLF on one side between the sixth and third nerve nuclei, called internuclear ophthalmoplegia which occurs in multiple sclerosis, results in abnormality of the contralateral lateral gaze: the eye on the affected side fails to adduct (cranial nerve III) when the contralateral eye abducts (cranial nerve VI). Bilateral destruction of the MLF results in loss of adduction during lateral gaze to either side. A visual target moving smoothly in the horizontal plane is followed by this conjugate gaze mechanism through the intervention of the superior colliculus, which communicates directly with this gaze center through tectobulbar fibers. Conjugate following of a bright, smoothly moving target occurs automatically, even in the absence of a functional visual cortex. In deep coma, for instance, the presence of visual following indicates that the brain stem, including the midbrain, remains functional. Voluntary control of conjugate following of a horizontally moving object in the visual field requires the function of the primary and associational visual cortices that project axons to the superior colliculus.

When a lateral conjugate following movement exceeds the range of eye rotation, head rotation is often added. The MLF extends down to cervical spinal levels; descending control from the horizontal gaze center by way of this tract is exerted on the spinal accessory and other cervical-level lower motoneurons. By this means the powerful head-turning muscles, the sternocleidomastoid, and other cervical muscles are smoothly brought into play. The major function of the MLF is the coordination circuitry of the lateral gaze mechanism.

Vertical gaze

Vertical gaze, or the upward and downward rotation of an eye, involves four extraocular muscles. The third-nerve-innervated superior rectus and inferior oblique work in concert to rotate the eye upward with coordinated inhibition of the inferior rectus (III) cranial nerve and superior oblique (IV) cranial nerve. Conjugate vertical gaze, upward or downward, with parallel optical axes of the two eyes is coordinated by a vertical gaze center located in the midbrain deep to the rostral end of the MLF. Communication between this center and the innervational nuclei does not use the MLF. Instead, another major longitudinal tract system, the central tegmental fasciculus (CTF), provides longitudinal communication.

Torsional conjugate eye movements

Conjugate twisting, or torsion, of the two eyes occurs when the head is tipped to one side. Exact, appropriate countertorsion of the two eyes serves to preserve a stable visual field in spite of minor head movements. A torsion gaze center, or control region, in the reticular formation of the brain stem has yet to be clearly localized.

Conjugate gaze control is extremely precise, and the central circuits providing this capability are quite complex. The superior colliculus, the midbrain vertical and medullary horizontal gaze centers, and the cerebellum, which add temporal smoothness to these coordinated movements, are all involved.

Disorders of eye movement

Strabismus

Strabismus, or squint, refers to any abnormality of eye coordination that results in loss of binocular eye alignment and focus of a visual image on corresponding points of the two retinas. In standard terminology, the disorders of eye movement are described according to the direction of movement. *Esotropia* refers to medial deviation; *exotropia*, to lateral deviation; *hypertropia*, to upward deviation; *hypotropia*, to downward deviation; and *cyclotropia*, to torsional deviation. The term *concomitance* refers to equal deviation in all directions of gaze. A nonconcomitant strabismus is one that varies with the direction of gaze. Strabismus may be divided into (1) paralytic (nonconcomitant) forms, in which there is weakness or paralysis of one or more of the extraocular muscles, or (2) nonparalytic (concomitant), in which there is no primary muscle impairment. Strabismus is termed *intermittent*, or *periodic*, when there are periods in which the eyes are parallel. It is *monocular* when the same eye always deviates and the fellow eye fixates.

Paralytic strabismus. Paralytic strabismus results from paresis (weakness) or plegia (paralysis) of one or more of the extraocular muscles. When the normal eye fixates, the affected eye is in the position of primary deviation. In the case of esotropia, there is weakness of one of the lateral rectus muscles, usually the result of palsy of the abducens (VI) cranial nerve. When the affected eye fixates, the unaffected eye is in a position of secondary deviation. The secondary deviation of the unaffected eye is greater than the primary deviation of the affected eye. This is because the affected eye requires an excess of innervational impulse to maintain fixation; the excess impulses also are distributed to the unaffected eye (Hering's law of equal innervation), causing overaction of its muscles.[2]

Paralytic strabismus is uncommon in children but accounts for nearly all cases of adult strabismus; it can be caused by a number of conditions. Paralytic strabismus is most commonly seen in adults who have had cerebral vascular accidents and may also occur as the first sign of a tumor or inflammatory condition involving the central nervous system. One type of muscular dystrophy exerts its effects on the extraocular muscles. Initially eye movements in all directions are weak, with later progression to bilateral optic immobility. Weakness of eye movement and lid elevation is often the first evidence of myasthenia gravis. The pathway of the oculomotor (III), trochlear (IV), and abducens (VI) cranial nerves through the cavernous sinus and the back of the orbit make them vulnerable to basal skull fracture and tumors of the cavernous sinus (cavernous sinus syndrome) or orbit (orbital syndrome). In infants, paralytic strabismus can be caused by birth injuries affecting either the extraocular muscles or the cranial nerves supplying these muscles. It can also result from congenital anomalies of the muscles. In general, paralytic strabismus in an adult with previously normal binocular vision causes diplopia (double vision). This does not occur in persons who have never developed binocular vision.

Nonparalytic strabismus. In nonparalytic strabismus there is no extraocular muscle weakness or paralysis, and the angle of deviation is always the same in all fields of gaze. With persistent deviation, secondary abnormalities may develop because of overaction or underaction of the muscles in some fields of gaze. Nonparalytic esotropia is the most common type of strabismus. The disorder may be accommodative, nonaccommodative, or a combination of the two. Accommodative strabismus is caused by disorders such as uncorrected hyperopia, in which the esotropia occurs with accommodation. The onset of this type of esotropia characteristically occurs at between 18 months and 4 years of age (because the accommodation is not well developed until that time). The disorder is most often monocular but may be alternating. About 50% of the cases of esotropia fall into this category. The causes of nonaccommodative strabismus are obscure. The disorder may be related to faulty muscle insertion, fascial abnormalities, or faulty innervation. There is evidence that idiopathic strabismus may have a genetic basis; siblings may have similar disorders.

Diagnosis and treatment. Examination by a qualified practitioner is indicated in any infant whose eyes are not aligned at all times during waking hours after 6 months of age.[2] Diagnostic measures emphasize two major areas: (1) ocular deviation and (2) visual acuity. Rapid assessment of extraocular muscle function is accomplished by three methods. First, in a somewhat darkened room and with the child staring straight ahead, a penlight is pointed at the midpoint between the two eyes, and a bright dot of reflected light can be seen on the cornea of each eye. With normal eye alignment, the reflected light should appear at the same spot on the cornea of each eye. Nonparallelism of the two eyes indicates muscle imbalance because of weakness or paralysis of the deviant eye. With the second method, the person is asked to follow the movement of a small object (a pencil point or lighted penlight) as it is moved through the extremes of what are called the six cardinal positions of gaze. In extreme lateral gaze, normal subjects can show a few quick beats of a jerky or nystagmoid movement (to be discussed). Nystagmoid movement is abnormal if it is prolonged or present in any other eye posture. The third method (called the cover–uncover test) eliminates binocular fusion as a factor in maintaining parallelism between the eyes. The examiner looks at the patient and estimates which eye is used for fixation. The patient's attention is directed toward a fixation object such as a small picture or tongue blade. A light should not be used because it may not stimulate accommodation. If a mild weakness is present, the eye with blocked vision will drift into a resting position, the extent of which depends on the relative strength of the muscles. The eye should snap back when the card is removed. The test is always done for both near and far fixation. Visual acuity is evaluated to obtain a comparison of the two eyes. An illiterate E chart (or similar test chart) can be used for young children.

Treatment of strabismus is directed toward the development of normal visual acuity, the correction of the deviation, and superimposition of the retinal images to provide binocular vision. Both nonsurgical and surgical methods can be used. In children, early treatment is important; the ideal age to begin is 6 months. Nonsurgical treatment includes occlusive patching, pleoptics, and prism glasses. Occlusive patching (alternating between the affected and the unaffected eye) may be used to prevent loss of vision in one eye. Prism glasses compensate for an abnormal alignment of an optic globe. Long-acting miotics in weak strengths (echothiophate iodide solution, Phospholine, or isoflurophate ointment, Floropryl) may be used in treating accommodative esotropia. In young children, these drugs can be used instead of glasses. They act by altering the accommodative convergence relationship in a favorable manner so that fusion is maintained despite accommodation. Miosis also allows for clearer vision with less accommodation in both near and far vision. Surgical procedures may be used to strengthen a muscle or weaken a muscle by altering its length or attachment site.

—— Amblyopia

Amblyopia describes a condition of diminished vision (uncorrectable by lenses) in which no detectable organic lesion of the eye is present. This condition is sometimes referred to as *lazy eye*. It is caused by visual deprivation (conditions such as cataracts) or abnormal binocular interactions (strabismus or anisometropia) during visual immaturity. Normal development of the thalamic and cortical circuitry necessary for binocular visual perception requires simultaneous binocular use of each fovea during a critical period of time early in life (0 to 5 years).[2] In infants with monocular cataracts, this time is before 4 months of age. In conditions causing abnormal binocular interactions, one image is suppressed to provide clearer vision. In esotropia, vision of the deviated eye is suppressed to prevent diplopia. A similar situation exists in anisometropia in which the refractive indexes of the two eyes are different. Even though the eyes are correctly aligned, they are unable to focus together and the image of one eye is suppressed. In experimental animals, monocular deprivation results in reduced synaptic density in the LGN and the primary visual cortical areas that process input from the affected eye or eyes.

The reversibility of amblyopia depends on the maturity of the visual system at the time of onset and the duration of the abnormal experience. If esotropia is involved, some persons will alternate eyes and not experience diplopia. With late-adolescent or adult onset, this habit pattern must be unlearned after correction.

Peripheral vision is less affected than central foveal vision in amblyopia. Suppression becomes more evident with high illumination and high contrast. It is as if the affected eye did not possess central vision and the person learns to fixate with the nonfoveal retina. If bilateral congenital blindness or near blindness (*e.g.,* cataracts) occurs and remains uncorrected during infancy and early childhood, the person will remain without pattern vision and will have only overall field brightness and color discrimination. This is essentially bilateral amblyopia.

Treatment.   The treatment of children with the potential for developing amblyopia must be instituted well before the age of 6 to avoid the suppression phenomenon. Surgery for congenital cataracts and ptosis should be done early. Severe refractive errors should be corrected. In strabismus, alternately blocking vision in one eye and then the other forces the child to use both eyes for form discrimination. The duration of occlusion of vision in the good eye must be short and closely monitored, or deprivation amblyopia can develop in the good eye as well. Although amblyopia is not likely to occur after the age of 8 or 9, plasticity in central circuitry is evident even in adulthood. For example, after refractive correction for longstanding astigmatism in adults, visual acuity improves slowly, requiring several months to reach normal levels.

In summary, normal vision depends on coordinated movement of the two eyes. Eye movements depend on the action of six extraocular muscles (four recti and two oblique) and their cranial (III, IV, and VI) nerve innervation. Conjugate eye movements are those in which the optical axes of the two eyes are kept parallel, sharing the same visual field. There are five types of eye movements: smooth pursuit (tracking movements), saccadic (position correcting), vestibular (nystagmus), vergence (divergence and convergence), and tremor (fine movements). Lateral gaze is used in viewing lateral objects. It involves the coordinated movements of the extraocular muscles and their cranial nerve nuclei, the MLF tract of the brain stem, and the pontine lateral gaze center. Unilateral destruction of the pontine gaze center results in ipsilateral gaze paralysis. Vertical gaze facilitates looking upward and downward. It is controlled by the action of the extraocular muscles and their cranial nerve nuclei, the central tegmental fasciculus pathway, and the midbrain vertical gaze center.

Disorders of eye movements include strabismus, or squint, and amblyopia. Strabismus refers to abnormalities in the coordination of eye movements with loss of binocular eye alignment and focus of a visual image on corresponding parts of the two retinas. Esotropia refers to medial deviation; exotropia, to lateral deviation; hypertropia, to upward deviation; hypotropia, to downward deviation; and cyclotropia, to torsional deviation. Paralytic strabismus is caused by weakness or paralysis of the extraocular muscles. Nonparalytic strabismus results from the inappropriate length or insertion of the extraocular muscles or from accommodation disorders. Amblyopia (lazy eye) is a condition of diminished vision that cannot be corrected by lenses and one in which no detectable organic lesion in the eye can be observed. It results from inadequately developed CNS circuitry because of visual deprivation (cataracts) or abnormal binocular interactions (strabismus or anisometropia) during the period of visual immaturity.

References

1. National Society to Prevent Blindness: Vision Problems in the U.S. New York, 1980
2. Vaughan D, Asbury T: General Ophthalmology, 10th ed, pp 52, 139. Los Altos, CA, Lange Medical Publications, 1982

3. Wise JB: Long-term control of adult open-angle glaucoma by argon laser treatment. Ophthalmology 88:197, 1981

4. Newell FW: Ophthalmology, 5th ed, pp 341. St Louis, CV Mosby, 1982

5. Bresler MJ, Hoffman RS: Prevention of iatrogenic acute narrow-angle glaucoma. Ann Emerg Med 10:535, 1981

6. Schwab IR, Armstrong MA, Friedman GD et al: Cataract extraction: Risk factors in a health maintenance organization population under 60 years of age. Arch Ophthalmol 106:1062, 1988

Bibliography

Baylor DA: How photoreceptors respond to light. Sci Am 256(4):40, 1987

Birnbaum MH: Clinical management of myopia. Am J Optom Physiol Opt 58:554, 1981

Calhoun JH: Cataracts in children. Pediatr Clin North Am 30(6):1061, 1983

Capino DG, Leibowitz HM: Age-related macular degeneration. Hosp Pract 23(Mar 30):23, 1988

Chew E, Morin JD: Glaucoma in children. Pediatr Clin North Am 30(6):1043, 1983

Cobo M: Ocular herpes simplex infections. Mayo Clin Proc 63:1154, 1988

Gitschlag G, Scott WE: Strabismus, ambylopia, and dyslexia. Prim Care 9:661, 1982

Grant WM, Burke JF: Why do some people go blind with glaucoma? Am Acad Opthalmol 89:991, 1982

Greenwald MJ: Visual development in infancy and childhood. Pediatr Clin North Am 30(6):977, 1983

Hamrick S, Meredith LL: Therapeutic ultrasound. AORN J 47:950, 1988

Helms HA: New considerations in the treatment of cataracts. Ala J Med Sci 24:62, 1987

Hitchings RA: Glaucoma. Practitioner 232:171, 1988

Koretz JF, Handelman GH: How the human eye focuses. Sci Am 259(1):92, 1988

Lerman S: Ocular phototoxicity. N Engl J Med 319:1475, 1988

Liesegang TJ: Cataracts and cataract operations (subject review). Parts 1 and 2. Mayo Clin Proc 59:556, 1984

Lindstrom RL: Advances in corneal transplantation. N Engl J Med 15:57, 1986

Marcus DF, Bovino JA: Retinal detachment. JAMA 247:873, 1982

Meltzer MA: Diagnosis of eyelid and periorbital abnormalities. Hosp Pract 20(9):67, 1984

Nelson LB: Diagnosis and management of strabismus and amblyopia. Pediatr Clin North Am 30(6):1003, 1983

Nirkankari VS, Katzen LE, Richards RD et al: Prospective clinical study of radial keratotomy. Am Acad Opthalmol 89:677, 1982

Resler MM, Tumulty G: Glaucoma update. Am J Nurs 83:752, 1983

Richards RD: Glaucoma. Am Family Pract 35:212, 1987

Riordan P, Pascoe PT, Vaughan DG: Refractive change in hyperglycemia: Hyperopia, not myopia: Br J Opthalmol 66:500, 1982

Roper-Hall M J: Cataract: A world problem. Ophthalmic Surg 19:393, 1988

Ruttum MS, Nelson DB, Wamser MJ: Detection of congenital cataracts and other ocular opacities. Pediatrics 79:814, 1987

Stryer L: The molecules of visual excitation. Sci Am 257(1):42, 1987

Teisch SA: Retinal manifestations of vascular diseases. Hosp Pract 20(8):69, 1984

White GL, Thiese SM, Lundergan MK: Contact lens care and complications. Am Family Pract 37:187, 1988

Wittenberg S: Solar radiation and the eye: A review of knowledge relevant to eye care. Am J Optom Physiol Opt 63:676, 1986

CHAPTER 52

Robin L. Curtis
Sheila M. Curtis

Alterations in Hearing and Vestibular Function

Objectives

After you have studied this chapter, you should be able to meet the following objectives:

_____ List the structures of the external, middle, and inner ear, and cite their function.

_____ Cite the impact of damage to Wernicke's area in the brain.

_____ Describe the symptoms of impacted cerumen.

_____ Relate the functions of the eustachian tube to the development of otitis media.

_____ Explain why infants and small children are more prone to develop otitis media.

_____ List three common symptoms of otitis media.

_____ Describe the disease process that occurs with otosclerosis, and relate this to the hearing loss that occurs.

_____ Differentiate between conductive and sensorineural hearing loss.

_____ List at least three drug groups that have potential ototoxicity.

_____ Explain the function of the vestibular system.

_____ Describe normal nystagmus eye movements.

_____ List the symptoms of motion sickness.

_____ Describe the pathology associated with Meniere's syndrome.

The ears are paired organs that are responsible for hearing and maintenance of equilibrium and effective posture (vestibular function). The ear consists of an external ear, middle, and inner ear. The external and middle ear function in capturing, transmitting, and amplifying sound. The inner ear contains the receptive organs that are selectively stimulated by either sound waves (hearing) or head position and motion (vestibular function).

Hearing

Hearing is a specialized sense that provides the ability to perceive vibration of sound waves. The compression waves that produce sound have both frequency and intensity. *Frequency* indicates the rate of change with time (cycles per second [cps] or hertz [Hz]). Most people cannot hear compression waves that have a frequency higher than 20,000 Hz. Waves of higher frequency are called ultrasonic waves, meaning that they are above the audible range. In the audible frequency range, the subjective experience correlated with sonic frequency is the pitch of a sound. Waves below 20 Hz to 30 Hz are experienced as a rattle or drum beat rather than a tone. The ear is most sensitive to waves in the frequency range of 1000–3000 Hz. Wave intensity is represented by either amplitude or units of sound pressure. By convention, the *intensity* (in power units, or ergs per square centimeter) of a sound is expressed as the ratio of intensities between the sound and a reference value. A tenfold increase in sound pressure is called a *bel*, after Alexander Graham Bell. This representation is often too crude to be of use; the most often used unit is the decibel, or one-tenth of a bel. In the normal sonic environment, approximately 1 decibel of increased intensity (loudness) can be detected. The region of audible speech sounds falls between 42 decibels and 70 decibels.

Auditory system

The ear receives sound waves, distinguishes their frequency, translates this information into nerve impulses, and transmits them to the central nervous system. The auditory system can be divided into five parts: the external ear, the middle ear, the inner ear, auditory brain stem pathways, and the primary and associational auditory cortex of the brain's temporal lobe.

External ear

The external ear is called the *pinna*, or *auricle*. It is supported by elastic cartilage and shaped like a funnel. The funnel shape concentrates high-frequency sound entering from the lateral-forward direction into the *external acoustic meatus,* or *ear canal* (Figure 52-1). The shape also helps prevent front–back confusion of sound sources. The anterior portion of the pinna and external ear canal are innervated by branches of the mandibular division of the trigeminal (V) cranial nerve. The posterior portions, including the back of the external ear as well as the posterior wall of the ear canal, are innervated by auricular branches of the facial (VII), glossopharyngeal (IX), and vagus (X) cranial nerves. Because of the vagal innervation, the insertion of a speculum or an otoscope into the external ear canal can stimulate coughing or vomiting reflexes, particularly in small children.

The external ear canal extends from the auricle to the tympanic membrane, or eardrum. Its outer two-thirds is supported by elastic cartilage, and its inner one-third, by the tympanic bone. It is somewhat S-shaped and acts as a resonator, amplifying frequencies around 3500 Hz. A thin layer of skin containing fine hairs, sebaceous glands, and ceruminous glands line the ear canal. The ceruminous glands secrete cerumen or earwax, which has certain antimicrobial properties and is thought to serve a protective function.

Tympanic membrane

The tympanic membrane (or eardrum), which separates the external ear from the middle ear, has three layers: (1) an outer layer of thin skin continuous with the lining of the external acoustic meatus, (2) a middle layer of tough collagenous fibers mixed with fibrocytes and some elastic fibers, and (3) an inner epithelial layer continuous with the lining of the middle ear. It is attached in a manner that allows it to vibrate freely when audible sound waves enter the external auditory canal. When viewed through an otoscope, the tympanic membrane appears as a shallow, almost circular cone pointing inward toward its apex, the umbo (Figure 52-2). The landmarks include the lightened stripe over the handle of the malleus, the umbo at the end of the handle, the pars tensa, which constitutes most of the drum, and the pars flaccida, the small area above the malleus attachment. Light is usually reflected from the pars tensa at approximately the 4 o'clock position. Normally, the tympanic membrane is semitransparent, and a small whitish cord, which traverses the middle ear from back to front, can be seen just under its upper edge. This is the corda tympani, a branch of the intermedius component of the facial (VII) cranial nerve.

Middle ear and eustachian tube

The middle ear is a tiny cavity, roughly the shape of a red blood cell set on edge, located in the petrous (stony) temporal bone. Its lateral wall is

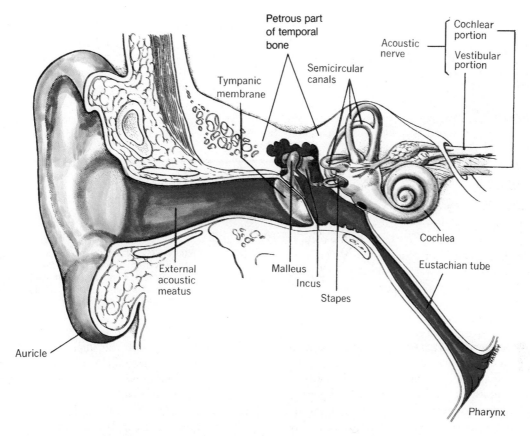

Figure 52-1 The ear: external, middle, and internal subdivisions. (*Chaffee EE, Lytle IM: Basic Physiology and Anatomy, 4th ed. Philadelphia, JB Lippincott, 1980*)

formed by the tympanic membrane, and its medial wall is formed by the bone dividing the middle and inner ear. Two tissue-covered openings in the medial wall, the oval and the round windows, provide for the transmission of sound waves between the air-filled middle ear and the fluid-filled inner ear. Posteriorly the middle ear is continuous with small air pockets in the temporal bone called *mastoid air spaces* or *cells* (Figure 52-3). In early life, these air spaces are filled with hematopoietic tissue. Replacement of hematopoi-

etic tissue with air sacs begins during the third year of life and is completed at puberty.

There is a gap in the bone between the anterior and medial walls for a canal, called the *eustachian tube,* or *auditory tube,* which connects with the naso-pharynx (see Figure 52-3). The middle ear is filled with the air that reaches it from the nasopharynx by way of the auditory tube; it is lined with a mucous membrane that is continuous with the pharynx and mastoid air cells. Infections from the nasopharynx can

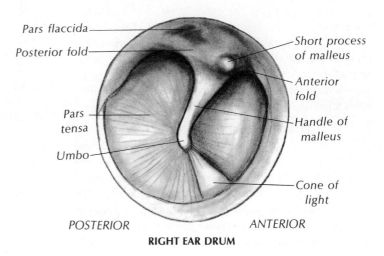

Figure 52-2 Right eardrum. (*Bates B: A Guide to Physical Examination, 3rd ed. Philadelphia, JB Lippincott, 1983*)

RIGHT EAR DRUM

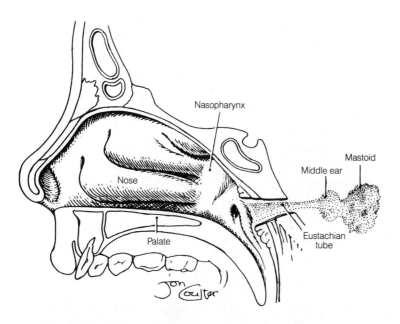

Figure 52-3 Nasopharynx-eustachian tube-mastoid air cell system. (*Bluestone CD: Recent advances in pathogenesis, diagnosis, and management of otitis media. Pediatr Clin North Am 28(4):36, 1981. Reproduced with permission*)

travel from the nasopharynx along the mucous membrane of the auditory tube to the middle ear, causing otitis media. Near the opening of the auditory tube, the columnar epithelial lining changes to the pseudostratified cilated-columnar surface of the pharynx, which contains occasional mucus-secreting cells. Hypertrophy of the mucus-secreting cells contributes to the mucoid secretions that develop during certain types of otitis media.

The auditory tube, which connects the middle ear with the nasopharynx, serves three basic functions: (1) ventilation of the middle ear, along with equalization of middle ear and ambient pressures, (2) protection of the middle ear from unwanted nasopharyngeal sound waves and secretions, and (3) drainage of middle ear secretions into the nasopharynx.[1] The nasopharyngeal entrance to the auditory tube, which is usually closed, is opened by the action of the tensor veli palatini muscles (Figure 52-4). Stimulation occurs as a part of the swallowing and yawning reflexes and provides the mechanism for equalizing the pressure of the middle ear with that of the atmosphere. This equalization ensures that the pressures on both sides of the tympanic membrane are the same, so that sound transmission is not reduced and rupture does not result from sudden changes in external pressure, such as occurs during plane travel.

Ossicles. Three tiny bones, the auditory ossicles, are suspended from the roof of the middle ear cavity and connect the tympanic membrane with the oval window. They are connected by synovial joints and are covered with the epithelial lining of the cavity. The *malleus* (hammer) has its handle firmly fixed to the upper half of the tympanic membrane. The head of the malleus articulates with the *incus* (anvil), which,

in turn, articulates with the *stapes* (stirrup), which is inserted and sealed into the oval window by an annular ligament. The ossicles are arranged so that their lever movements transmit vibrations from the tympanic membrane to the oval window and from there to the fluid in the inner ear. It is the piston-like action of the stapes footplate that sets up compression waves in the inner ear fluid. Air and liquid offer different degrees of impedance (resistance) to the transmission of sound waves. Therefore, the bones of the middle ear serve as impedance-matching devices between the low

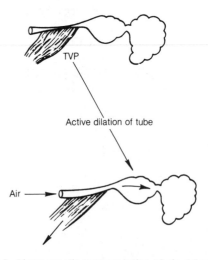

Figure 52-4 Diagrammatic representation of physiologic pressure regulation of the middle ear by the active opening of the eustachian tube by the tensor veli palatini muscle (*TVP*). An alternative mechanism is by gradient-activated opening of the eustachian tube. (*Bluestone CD: Recent advances in the pathogenesis, diagnosis, and management of otitis media. Pediatr Clin North Am 28(4):727, 1981. Reproduced with permission*)

impedance of the air and the high impedance of the cochlear fluid. This matching is accomplished by (1) concentrating the pressure from the large area of the tympanic membrane (43–55 mm^2) to the small area of the oval window (about 3 mm^2) and (2) amplifying the air-transmitted sound waves into the force required to set up compression waves in the fluid of the inner ear. The latter is accomplished by the ossicular lever system, which increases the pressures from the tympanic membrane to the oval window.

Two tiny skeletal muscles, the *tensor tympani* and the *stapedius,* support the ossicles. The tensor tympani is positioned in the roof of the auditory tube and inserts on the base of the malleus handle. The functional role of this muscle is in dispute. The stapedius muscle alters the movement of the stapes, reducing the displacement of fluid in the inner ear. Reflex contraction of this muscle by means of the facial nerve, the stapedial reflex, provides a protective mechanism for the delicate inner ear structures when high-intensity sound occurs.

Inner ear

The inner ear contains a labyrinth or system of intercommunicating channels and the receptors for hearing and position sense. The outer bony wall of the inner ear, the bony labyrinth, encloses a thin-walled, membranous duct system, the membranous labyrinth (Figure 52-5). Two separate fluids are found in the inner ear. A fluid called the *perilymph* separates the bony labyrinth from the membranous labyrinth, and one called the *endolymph* fills the membranous labyrinth. The bony labyrinth is divided into three compartments: the cochlea, the vestibule, and the semicircular canals. The cochlea, which contains the auditory receptors, is a bony tube shaped like a snail shell that winds around a central bone column called the modiolus. The utricle, saccule, and semicircular canals contain the receptors for head position sense and are discussed later in the chapter.

The membranous cochlear duct is a triangular-shaped structure that completely stretches across the cochlear canal, separating it into two parallel tubes, each containing perilymph: the scala vestibuli and the scala tympani (Figure 52-6). One side of the cochlear duct, the basilar membrane, stretches under tension laterally from the modiolus to an elastic spiral ligament. The second side, the vestibular (Reissner's membrane), is a delicate layer of squamous epithelial cells. The third side consists of a well-vascularized epithelium, the stria vascularis, that is the source of endolymph. The cochlear duct separates the scala vestibuli and the scala tympani from the base of the cochlea throughout its two and one-half spiral turns to its apex. An opening at the apex, called the helico-

trema, permits fluid waves to move between the two scalae. Sound waves, delivered by the stapes footplate to the perilymph, travel throughout the fluid of the inner ear, including up to the scala vestibuli, to the apex of the cochlea. The fluid pressure wave results in compensatory displacements of the round window, compressing the air of the middle ear cavity and auditory canal.

Perched on the basilar membrane and extending along its entire length is an elaborate arrangement of columnar epithelium called the organ of Corti. Continuous rows of hair cells, separated into inner and outer rows, can be found within the cell arrangement. The cells have hairlike cilia that protrude through openings in an overlying supporting reticular membrane into the endolymph of the cochlear duct. A gelatinous mass, the tectorial membrane, extends from the medial side of the duct to enclose the cilia of the outer hair cells. Vibrations of the organ of Corti cause the hairs to be bent against the fixed tectorial membrane. Each hair cell is supplied by a nerve fiber, some by more than one. It is the bending of the hair fibers that transform (transduce) sound energy, which thus far has been mechanical, into membrane potential changes, transmitter release, and stimulation of nerve endings. It is generally agreed that the inner rows of hair cells, transducing different frequencies, are arranged sequentially with those transducing the higher tones located on the lower (basal) end of the cochlear duct, and those transducing lower tones located near its apex. Thus, selective destruction of hair cells in a particular segment of the cochlea can lead to hearing loss of particular tones. The outer rows of hair cells appear to provide the signals upon which the experience of sound loudness is based.

Neural pathways

Afferent fibers from the organ of Corti have their cell bodies in the spiral ganglion in the central portion of the cochlea. Nerve fibers from the spiral ganglion (vestibulocochlear, or auditory, nerve [VIII]) travel to the cochlear nuclei located in the pons (Figure 52-7). Many of the secondary nerve fibers from the cochlear nuclei pass to the opposite side of the pons. These secondary fibers may project to cell groups called the trapezoid, the superior olivary nucleus, or rostrally toward the inferior colliculus of the midbrain. Ipsilateral projections and interconnections between the nuclei of the two sides occur throughout the central auditory system. Consequently, impulses from either ear are transmitted through the auditory pathways to both sides of the brain stem.

A number of reflexes, initiated by sound stim-

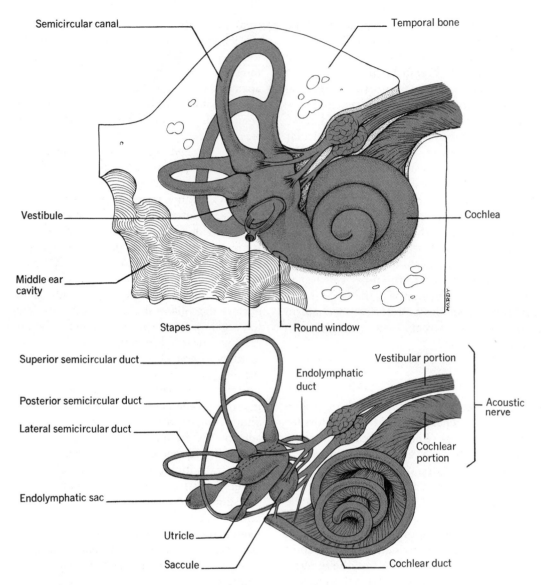

Figure 52-5 (**Top**) Diagram of the bony labyrinth; (**bottom**) the membranous labyrinth as seen when removed from the bony labyrinth. (*Chaffee EE, Lytle IM: Basic Anatomy and Physiology, 4th ed. Philadelphia, JB Lippincott, 1980*)

uli, are integrated in the central auditory pathways. The superior olivary nucleus is involved in basic auditory reflexes, including the stapedial and tensor tympani reflexes. A comparison of impulses from the two sides, which provides the basis for spatial localization of a sound source, occurs at the level of the inferior colliculus. Superior colliculus function is required for auditory startle reflexes, which include rapid saccadic eye movements and turning of the head and body toward the sound source. The superior olivary nucleus, which has extensive connections with the brain stem respiratory and cardiovascular centers, integrates the heart rate, blood pressure, and respiratory changes that occur with the auditory startle reflex.

From the inferior colliculus, the auditory pathway passes to the medial geniculate nucleus of the thalamus, where all the fibers synapse. Considerable evidence supports the capability of this level of organization to provide crude auditory experience, including crude tone and intensity discrimination as well as the directionality of a sound source. From the medial geniculate nucleus, the auditory tract spreads by way of the auditory radiation to the primary auditory cortex (area 41) located mainly in the superior temporal gyrus and insula (see Figure 50-6). The auditory association cortex (areas 42 and 22) borders the primary cortex on the superior temporal gyrus. This area and its associated high-order thalamic nuclei are necessary for auditory gnosis or the meaningfulness of sound to occur. Past experience, as well as precise analysis of momentary auditory information, is integrated during this process.

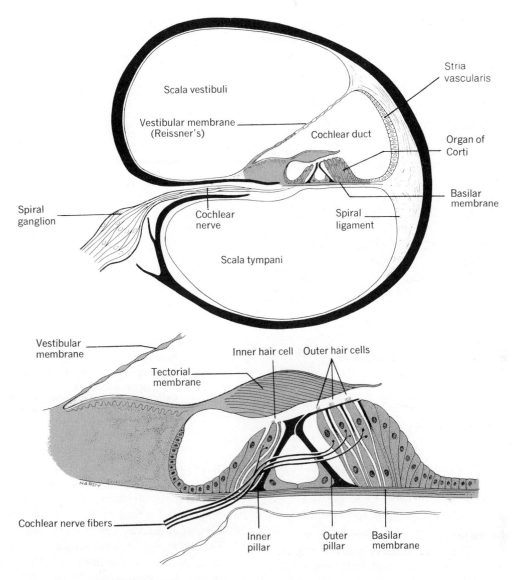

Figure 52-6 (Top) Drawing of a portion of the cochlea. Note the relation of the cochlear duct to the scalae, vestibuli and tympani. **(Bottom)** The spiral organ of Corti has been removed from the cochlear duct and greatly enlarged. *(Chaffee EE, Lytle IM: Basic Physiology and Anatomy, 4th ed. Philadelphia, JB Lippincott, 1980)*

Disorders of auditory function

Hearing loss may be the most common physical disability suffered by people in the United States. It has been estimated that approximately 8% of the population suffer some hearing loss, and approximately 3% have a disabling hearing loss.[2]

Alterations in external ear function

The external ear conducts sound waves to the tympanic membrane. The function of the external ear is disturbed when sound transmission is obstructed by excessive amounts of accumulated cerumen or inflammation of the external ear (otitis externa).

Impacted cerumen. Although the cerumen (earwax) produced by the glands of the ear canal normally dries up and leaves the ear, it can accumulate causing narrowing of the canal. Repeated unskilled attempts to remove the wax may pack it more deeply into the ear canal. Usually, impacted earwax produces no symptoms until the canal becomes completely occluded, at which point a feeling of fullness, deafness, tinnitus, or coughing because of vagal stimulation develops. On otoscopic examination a mass of yellow, brown, or black wax is visualized.

Removal of earwax can often be accomplished through the otoscope using a dull-ring curet. If this is not possible, the wax may be dislodged using a large syringe or dental irrigating device to produce a

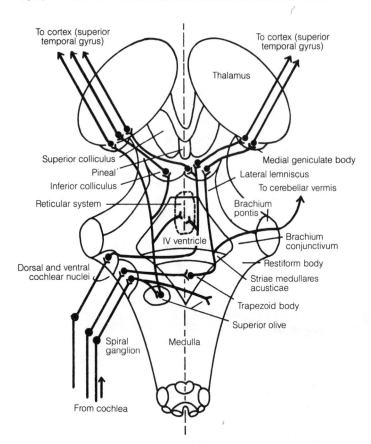

Figure 52-7 Simplified diagram of main auditory pathways superimposed on a dorsal view of the brain stem. Cerebellum and cerebral cortex removed. *(Reproduced with permission from Ganong W: Review of Medical Physiology, 7th ed. Los Altos, CA, Lange, 1975)*

water stream. A few drops of baby shampoo, baby oil, or hydrogen peroxide can be instilled into the ear for several days prior to irrigation to soften the wax. Commercial products are available and effective.

Otitis externa. Otitis externa may vary in severity from a mild eczematoid dermatitis to severe cellulitis. It can be caused by infectious agents or materials contained in earphones or earrings (contact dermatitis). Infections of the external ear are usually bacterial in origin, with occasional secondary infection by fungi. Predisposing factors include moisture in the ear canal following swimming (swimmer's ear) or bathing, trauma resulting from scratching or attempts to clean the ear, and allergic dermatitis. External otitis is usually accompanied by redness, scaliness, narrowing of the canal because of swelling, itching, and pain. Inflammation of the pinna or canal makes movement of the auricle painful. There may be watery or purulent drainage and intermittent deafness. Treatment methods include the use of topical antibiotic ointments, eardrops, and topical corticosteroids to reduce inflammation.

Alterations in middle ear function

Otitis media. Otitis media, or inflammation of the middle ear, may occur in any age group, although children are most commonly affected; it is the most common diagnosis made by physicians who care

for children. It has been estimated that approximately $2 billion is spent annually on medical and surgical treatment of the disorder.[1] This figure includes the expenses of the estimated 1 million children who receive tympanostomy tubes each year and for the 60,000 children who have tonsillectomies and adenoidectomies annually, many of which are performed to prevent otitis media.

Otitis media can be acute, subacute, or chronic. It may or may not be infectious in origin and may or may not be associated with effusion (collection of fluid and exudate). Infants and small children are at the highest risk for developing it, the peak prevalence occurring between 6 and 36 months. There are two reasons for the increased risk in infants and small children: (1) the auditory tube is shorter, more horizontal, and wider in this age group than in older children and adults, and (2) infection can spread more easily through the canal of the infant who spends most of the day lying in bed. Bottle-fed babies have a higher incidence of otitis media than breast-fed babies, probably because bottle-fed babies are held in a more horizontal position during feeding, and swallowing while in the horizontal position facilitates the reflux of milk into the middle ear. Breast-feeding also provides for the transfer of protective maternal antibodies to the infant. The incidence of otitis media is higher among children with craniofacial anomalies (cleft palate and Down's syndrome), Alaskan natives (Eskimos), and Native Americans.

Abnormalities of the auditory tube are important factors in the pathogenesis of middle ear infections. Two major types of auditory tube dysfunction contribute to otitis media: obstruction and abnormal patency (Figure 52-8). Obstruction can be either mechanical or functional. Functional obstruction results from the persistent collapse of the auditory tube because of a lack of tubal stiffness or an abnormal muscular opening mechanism. It is common in infants and small children because the amount and stiffness of the cartilage supporting the auditory tube are less than in older children and adults. Also, age-related changes in the craniofacial base tend to render the muscle responsible for opening the auditory tube less efficient in this age group. Mechanical obstruction can be either intrinsic or extrinsic, the most common obstruction being caused by intrinsic swelling resulting from upper respiratory tract infection or allergy. Extrinsic obstruction can result from the enlargement of adenoid tissue or a tumor. With obstruction, air in the middle ear is absorbed, causing a negative pressure and the transudation of serous fluid into the middle ear.

The abnormally patent tube either does not close or does not close completely. In children, air and secretions may be pumped into the auditory tube during nose blowing and crying. Organisms or foreign material from the nasopharynx incite an inflammatory response (see Chapter 10) with exudate, leukocytosis, and hypertrophy of the mucous glands in the eustachian tube and mucous membrane lining the middle ear.

Acute otitis media. Acute otitis media is characterized by either a suppurative (purulent or pus-containing) or serous (serum-type) exudate. Most cases of otitis media follow an upper respiratory tract infection that has been present for several days. *Streptococcus pneumoniae* and *Hemophilus influenzae* are the most frequently isolated organisms.

Acute suppurative otitis media is characterized by otalgia (earache), fever (up to 104°F), and hearing loss. Occasionally there may be rhinorrhea, vomiting, and diarrhea. Pain usually increases as purulent exudate accumulates behind the tympanic membrane (ear drum). An infant may cry and rub the infected ear, while an older child will complain of sharp or severe pain in the ear. If the tympanic membrane ruptures because of excessive pressure, the pain will be relieved, and a purulent drainage will be present in the external ear canal.

Acute serous otitis media may also occur following a viral disease, with an allergy, or following sudden changes in atmospheric pressure. If air cannot pass back through the auditory tube upon descent during an airplane flight, hearing loss and discomfort will develop. This occurs most commonly in those who travel while suffering from an upper respiratory infection. Yawning, swallowing, and chewing gum seem to facilitate the opening of the auditory tube, which equalizes air in the middle ear. Signs of acute serous otitis media include conductive hearing loss, eardrum retraction, and fluid level or air bubbles visible through the tympanic membrane.

Recurrent otitis media. Recurrent otitis media can occur as an acute episode of otitis media along with almost every respiratory tract infection. Most of the children with recurrrent otitis media respond well to treatment and have fewer recurrences with advancing age. However, some children have persistent middle ear effusion with superimposed recurrent episodes of acute otitis media.

Chronic otitis media. Otitis media that persists beyond 3 months is usually considered chronic.[2] Chronic otitis media can occur with or without effusion. Chronic suppurative otitis media is most common in those who have suffered ear problems during early childhood. With the chronic infection, permanent perforation of the tympanic membrane often occurs. Ear ossicles may be destroyed, and chronic changes can occur in the mucosa of the ear. The chronic condition is frequently exacerbated by upper respiratory infections.

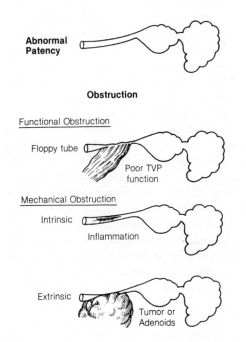

Abnormal Patency

Obstruction

Functional Obstruction

Floppy tube

Poor TVP function

Mechanical Obstruction

Intrinsic

Inflammation

Extrinsic

Tumor or Adenoids

Figure 52-8 Pathophysiology of the eustachian tube. (*Bluestone CD: Recent advances in pathogenesis, diagnosis, and management of otitis media. Pediatr Clin North Am 28(4):737, 1981. Reproduced with permission*)

Diagnosis and treatment. Diagnosis of otitis media is often made by otoscopic examination of the tympanic membrane. A bulging, lusterless eardrum with subsequent obliteration of the bony landmarks and cone of light are observed. Gentle movement of the pinna can help distinguish otitis media from otitis externa. This maneuver does not produce pain in purulent otitis media but causes severe discomfort in otitis externa. A culture of middle ear effusion fluid is used for verifying the presence and type of microorganism present. A needle can be inserted through the inferior part of the tympanic membrane to obtain a specimen of effusion fluid, or a culture can be made of the drainage present in the external ear canal when the tympanic membrane has perforated.

Use of the pneumatic otoscope permits the introduction of air into the canal for the purpose of determining tympanic membrane flexibility. The movement of this membrane is decreased in some cases of acute otitis media and absent in chronic middle ear infection. Tympanometry is an important advance in the identification of middle ear disease. A tympanogram is obtained by inserting a small probe into the external auditory canal; a tone of fixed characteristics is then presented through the probe, and the mobility of the tympanic membrane is measured electronically while the external canal pressure is artificially varied.

The treatment of otitis media includes the use of appropriate antibiotic therapy. Oral ampicillin or amoxicillin is commonly prescribed. Additional supportive therapy, including analgesics, antipyretics, and local heat may be indicated. A myringotomy (surgical incision of the tympanic membrane) may be done to relieve pressure on the eardrum, reduce pain and hearing loss, and prevent the ragged opening that can follow spontaneous rupture of the eardrum. The use of antihistamines and decongestants is controversial. They are usually of most benefit to children with serous otitis media of an allergic origin.

Tympanostomy tubes may be used in the treatment of children with recurrent or chronic otitis media. Insertion of the tubes is one of the most commonly performed surgical procedures in the United States; however, the long-term benefits are controversial. Placement of the tubes is usually performed under general anesthesia. The ears of children with the tubes must be kept out of water. Spontaneous extrusion of the tubes usually occurs after 5.5 months to 7 months.[3,4] The side effects include recurrent otorrhea, persistent perforation, scarring and atrophy of the eardrum, and cholesteatoma.

Complications. Complications of otitis media are not common, but they can follow inadequate treatment. The most common are those associated with the aural (ear) cavity and surrounding temporal bone. Intracranial complications are rare but are the most serious complications.

One of the most common complications of otitis media is persistent conductive hearing loss. Fluid may be present in the middle ear for weeks or months after an acute bout of otitis media. This may impair hearing and affect the child's learning of language skills. Fortunately, hearing loss that is associated with fluid collection usually resolves when the effusion clears. Permanent hearing loss may occur as the result of damage to the tympanic membrane or other middle ear structures.

Adhesive otitis media involves an abnormal healing reaction to an inflamed middle ear. It produces irreversible thickening of the mucous membranes and may cause impaired movement of the ossicles and, possibly, conductive hearing loss. Tympanosclerosis involves the formation of whitish plaques and nodular deposits on the submucosal surface of the tympanic membrane with possible adherence of the ossicles and conductive hearing loss. Perforation of the eardrum occurs most often following acute otitis media; although it usually heals spontaneously, tympanoplasty may be necessary.

A cholesteatoma is a saclike mass containing a silvery white debris of keratin, which is shed by the squamous epithelial lining of the eardrum. As the lining of the epithelium sheds and desquamates, the lesion expands and erodes the surrounding tissues. The lesion, which is associated with chronic middle ear infection, is insidiously progressive, and erosion may involve the temporal bone, causing intracranial complications. The treatment involves microsurgical techniques to remove the cholesteatoma material.

The mastoid antrum and air cells constitute a portion of the temporal bone and may become inflamed as an extension of an acute or chronic otitis media. Because of the use of antibiotics, acute mastoiditis (a complication of acute otitis media) is unusual. If it does occur, there is necrosis of the mastoid process and destruction of the bony intercellular matrix, which are visible by x-ray examination. Mastoid tenderness and drainage of exudate through a perforated tympanic membrane can occur. Chronic mastoiditis can develop as the result of chronic middle ear infection. The usefulness of antibiotics for this condition is limited. Mastoid or middle ear surgery, along with other medical treatment, may be indicated.

Intracranial complications, although rare, can develop if the infection spreads through vascular channels, by direct extension, or through preformed pathways such as the round window. These complications are seen more often with chronic suppurative otitis media and mastoiditis. They include meningitis, focal encephalitis, brain abscess, lateral sinus thrombophlebitis or thrombosis, labyrinthitis, or facial nerve paralysis. Any child who develops persistent headache, tinnitus (ringing in the ear), stiff neck, or visual or other neurologic symptoms should be investigated for possible intracranial complications.

Otosclerosis. Otosclerosis is a familial, autosomal-dominant disorder that causes conductive deafness, sensorineural hearing loss, and tinnitus. It is a disorder of the otic capsule, which becomes the petrous part of the temporal bone that surrounds the inner ear. Otosclerosis may begin at any time in life but usually does not appear until after puberty, most frequently between the ages of 20 and 30 years. There is an increase in the disease process during pregnancy.

In otosclerosis, the disease process begins with resorption of bone in one or more foci. During active bone resorption, the bone structure appears spongy and softer than normal (osteospongiosis). The resorbed bone is replaced by an overgrowth of new, hard sclerotic bone. The process is slowly progressive, involving more areas of the temporal bone, especially in front of and posterior to the stapes footplate. As it invades the footplate, the pathologic bone increasingly immobilizes the stapes, reducing the transmission of sound. Pressure of otosclerotic bone on inner ear structures or the eighth nerve may contribute to the development of tinnitus, sensorineural hearing loss, and vertigo.

The symptoms of otosclerosis involve an insidious hearing loss. Initially, one is unable to hear a whisper or someone speaking at a distance. In the earliest stages, the bone conduction by which the person's own voice is heard remains relatively unaffected. Therefore, the person's own voice sounds unusually loud and the sound of chewing becomes intensified. Because of bone conduction, these people can usually hear fairly well on the telephone, which provides an amplified signal. Also, they often are able to hear better in a noisy environment, probably because the masking effect of background noise causes people to speak louder.

The treatment of otosclerosis can be either medical or surgical. A carefully selected well-fitting hearing aid may allow a person with conductive deafness to lead a normal life. Sodium fluoride has been used in the medical treatment of osteospongiosis. Because much of the conductive hearing loss associated with otosclerosis is due to stapedial fixation, the surgical treatment involves stapedectomy with stapedial reconstruction using either the patient's own stapes or a stapedial prosthesis. The argon laser beam may be used in the surgical procedure.

Abnormalities of central auditory pathways

The auditory pathways in the brain involve intercommunication between the two sides of the head at many levels. As a result, strokes, tumors, abscesses, and other focal abnormalities rarely produce more than a mild reduction in auditory acuity on the side opposite the lesion. However, when it comes to the intelligibility of auditory language, lateral dominance becomes very important. On the dominant side, usually the left side, the more medial and dorsal portion of the associational auditory cortex is of crucial importance. This area is called *Wernicke's area*, and damage here is associated with auditory receptive aphasia (an agnosia of speech). Persons with damage to this area of the brain can speak intelligibly and can read normally but are unable to understand the meaning of major aspects of audible speech.

Irritative foci affecting the auditory radiation or the primary auditory cortex can produce roaring or clicking sounds, which appear to come from the auditory environment of the opposite side (auditory hallucinations). Focal seizures originating in or near the auditory cortex are often immediately preceded by the perception of ringing or other sounds preceded by a prodrome (aura). Damage to the auditory association cortex, especially if bilateral, results in deficiencies of sound recognition and memory (auditory agnosia). If the damage is in the dominant hemisphere, speech recognition can be affected (sensory aphasia).

Disorders of internal ear function and deafness

More than 13 million people in the United States have some hearing impairment. Of these persons, 6 million are seriously handicapped, and more than 1.7 million are totally deaf.[5] There are many causes of hearing loss or deafness. Most fit into the categories of conductive, sensorineural (perceptive), or mixed deficiencies involving a combination of conductive and sensorineural function deficiencies of the same ear.

Conductive hearing loss. Conductive hearing deficit occurs with external ear or middle ear disorders such as impacted cerumen, perforation of the tympanic membrane, fluid or pus in the middle ear, or ossicle fusion. A partial hearing loss can occur if sonic stimuli are not adequately transmitted to the inner ear through the external acoustic meatus (auditory canal), the tympanic membrane (eardrum), the middle ear, and the chain of ossicles.

Sensorineural hearing loss. Sensorineural, or perceptive, hearing loss can occur when disorders affect the inner ear, the auditory nerve, or the auditory pathways of the brain. With this type of deafness, sound waves are conducted to the inner ear, but abnormalities of the cochlear apparatus or auditory nerve decrease or distort the transfer of information to the brain. Spontaneous ringing of the ears accompanies cochlear nerve irritation. Abnormal function resulting from damage or malformation of the central auditory pathways and circuitry is included in this category. Sensorineural hearing loss may be congenital as a result of birth trauma, maternal rubella, or malformations of the inner ear. Trauma to the inner ear, vascular disorders with hemorrhage or thrombosis of vessels that supply the middle ear, can also cause sensorineural deafness. Other causes of sensorineural deafness are infections and drugs.

Environmentally induced deafness can occur through direct exposure to excessively intense sound, as in the workplace or at a concert. This type of deafness was once called "boilermaker's deafness" because of the intense reverberating sound to which riveters were exposed when putting together boiler tanks. Noise pollution is often characterized by high-intensity sounds of a specific frequency that cause corresponding damage to the organ of Corti.

Deafness or some degree of hearing impairment is the most common serious complication of bacterial meningitis in infants and children. It has been reported that sensorineural deafness complicates bacterial meningitis in 10% of cases and is most likely to follow *S. pneumoniae* meningitis.[6]

Drugs that damage inner ear structures are labeled ototoxic. Vestibular symptoms of ototoxicity include light-headedness, giddiness, and dizziness; if severe, cochlear symptoms can consist of tinnitus or hearing loss. The hearing loss is sensorineural and may be bilateral or unilateral, transient or permanent. Several classes of drugs have been identified as having ototoxic potentials: aminoglycoside antibiotics and other basic antibiotics with similar ototoxic potential, antimalarial drugs, loop diuretics, and salicylates. In addition to these drug groups, many other drug groups have been implicated in causing ototoxicity. The risk of ototoxicity depends on the total dose of the drug and its concentration in the bloodstream. The risk is increased in persons with impaired kidney functioning and in those previously or currently treated with another potentially ototoxic drug. Table 52-1 lists drugs with the potential for producing ototoxicity.

Old age hearing loss. Hearing loss is a common disability in the elderly. It has been estimated that 30% of people over age 65 and 50% of people over 85 years of age have significant hearing handicaps.[5] Decreased acuity begins in early adulthood and progresses for as long as the individual lives.[7] This contrasts with other sensory losses in the aged that tend to reach a plateau in functional deficit. High-frequency sounds are affected more than low-frequency sounds. Males are affected earlier and experience a greater loss than females. Individuals also experience what is called phonetic regression, or a word-discrimi-

Table 52-1. Major ototoxic drugs

Drug	Auditory function	Vestibular function
Aminoglycoside antibiotics		
Amikacin	+	0
Gentamicin	+	+
Kanamycin	+	+
Neomycin	+	+
Streptomycin	+	+
Tobramycin	+	+
Other antibiotics		
Colistin (topical middle ear)	0	+
Erythromycin (intravenous)	+*	0
Minocycline	0	+
Polymyxin B (topical middle ear)	0	+
Vancomycin	+	0
Antimalarial drugs		
Chloroquine and quinine	+*	0
Loop diuretics		
Ethacrynic acid	+	+
Furosemide	+*	0
Bumetanide	+*	0
Salicylates (aspirin)	+*	0
Cisplatin	+	0

* Effects are rarely permanent.
+ = yes; 0 = no

nation loss, which interferes with normal communication.

Hearing tests. To estimate hearing, each ear is tested separately. Specific procedures used to assess hearing in the infant and small child depend on the age and developmental level (details of procedures can be found in texts on physical assessment).

The ability to hear is tested by occluding first one ear and then the other. The examiner stands 1 foot to 2 feet away and whispers numbers in the direction of the unoccluded ear. Care is taken to prevent lipreading. A ticking watch may also be used, but this only tests the higher frequencies.

Audiogram. The audiogram is an important method of analyzing a person's hearing. It requires highly specialized sound production and control equipment. Pure tones of controlled intensity are delivered, usually to one ear at a time, and the minimum intensity needed for hearing to be experienced is plotted as a function of frequency. The Békésy method permits the subject to test himself or herself. The equipment generates continuous pure tones that decrease in intensity as long as the subject presses a button. When the subject releases the button, the equipment then increases the intensity until the button is pressed again. The frequency spectrum is tested by continuous advancement.

Tests of conduction versus sensorineural deafness.

If a hearing loss is present, conduction deafness must be distinguished from sensorineural deafness. A tuning fork of 1024 Hz is used to test hearing for two reasons: (1) it tests within the range of human speech (400–5000 Hz), and (2) it does not confuse sound with palpable vibration. The tuning fork is tapped on the handle to set it into light vibration.

Weber's test.

Weber's test evaluates bone conduction by the lateralization of sound. The test is performed by placing the base of a lightly vibrating tuning fork on the middle of the forehead or at the vertex of the patient's head. It can also be placed on the upper (maxillary) incisor teeth. The person is then asked to determine whether sound is heard better in one ear than in the other. With conductive deafness, the bone-conducted sound is heard more loudly and clearly on the side with the conduction deficit because the inner ear structures are functional and remain undisturbed by extraneous environmental sounds.

Rinne test.

The Rinne test compares air and bone conduction of sound. The test is done by placing the base of the lightly vibrating tuning fork on the mastoid process until the sound is no longer heard. The vibrating fork is then quickly placed near the external auditory meatus of the ear to be tested. If the sound is louder when the tuning fork is placed in front of the ear, hearing is normal, or there is no sensorineural component. If the sound is louder when the tuning fork is placed over the mastoid process, conduction hearing loss is indicated. If the sound is heard the same in both places, a mixed hearing loss is possible.

Brain stem-evoked responses.

In recent years, a noninvasive method has been developed that permits functional evaluation of certain defined parts of the central auditory pathways. Scalp electrodes and high-gain amplifiers are required to produce a record of the electrical wave activity elicited during repeated acoustic stimulations of either or both ears. Certain of the early waves come from discrete portions of the pons and midbrain auditory pathways, and localized damage can to some extent be correlated with specific sensorineural abnormalities. This method is called the brain stem-evoked response (BSER), and it has advanced from the research laboratory to fairly widespread use in the neurology and otolaryngology clinics.

Treatment of deafness.

Conduction deafness can be corrected through the use of electrical amplification methods (hearing aids). Hearing aids deliver sound stimuli directly to the skull bones with sufficient added power to, in turn, directly vibrate the inner ear apparatus. This method bypasses the middle ear conduction apparatus. Amplification is of no assistance with sensorineural hearing loss. With sensorineural deficit, a hearing aid serves only to increase the intensity of a signal experienced as distorted. In mixed hearing loss, amplification can provide improvement only for the conduction problems that are part of the syndrome. Although most standard tests for auditory acuity use pure tone stimuli, intelligibility of sound stimuli is not necessarily correlated with pure tone loss. Damage to the very important communicative function of auditory language produces a social isolation that is potentially very damaging to a person's mental attitude and motivation for rehabilitation.

Recently, surgically implantable cochlear prostheses for the profoundly deaf have been developed. A number of auditory prostheses have been produced that use electrodes implanted outside or within the cochlea or in the modiolus. A cochlear prosthesis, as presently developed, does not provide normal hearing. Rather, it provides perception of background noises. For example, the cochlear prosthesis allows the person to hear footsteps and become aware that someone is speaking, so that lipreading can be used. It also allows for recognition of protective sounds, such as the sound of an automobile approaching, the sound of a fire alarm, and the opening and closing of doors. Improvements have been made that increase the quality of speech recognition. The method has promise except for those few pathologic conditions in which total labyrinthine destruction or total cochlear nerve degeneration has occurred.

In summary, hearing is a specialized sense whose external stimulus is the vibration of sound waves. The ear receives the sound waves, distinguishes their frequencies, translates this information into nerve impulses, and transmits these to the central nervous system. The auditory system consists of the external ear, middle ear, inner ear, auditory pathways, and central auditory cortex. Among the disorders of the auditory system are infections of the external and middle ear, otosclerosis, and conduction and sensorineural deafness. Otitis externa is an inflammatory process of the external ear. The middle ear is a tiny air-filled cavity located in the temporal bone. The auditory tube connects the middle ear to the nasopharynx and allows for equalization of pressure between the middle ear and the atmosphere. Infections can travel from the nasopharynx to the middle ear along the auditory tube causing otitis media, or inflammation of the middle ear. The auditory tube is shorter and more horizontal in infants and young children, and infections of the middle ear are a common problem in these age groups. Otitis media can be acute, subacute, or chronic. The most common form, acute suppurative otitis media, usually follows an upper respiratory tract infection. It is characterized by otalgia, fever, and hearing loss. The effusion that accompanies otitis media can persist for weeks or months, interfering with hearing and impairing speech development. Otosclerosis is a familial disorder of the otic capsule. It causes bone resorption followed by excessive replacement with sclerotic bone. The disorder eventually causes immobilization of the stapes and conduction deafness. Deafness, or hearing loss, can develop as the result of a number of auditory disorders. Deafness can be conductive, sensorineural, or mixed. Conduction deafness occurs when transmission of sound waves from the external to the inner ear is impaired. Sensorineural deafness can involve cochlear structures of the inner ear or the neural pathways that transmit auditory stimuli.

Vestibular function

The vestibular receptive organs, which are located in the inner ear, and their central nervous system connections contribute to the reflex activity necessary for effective posture and movement in a physical world governed by momentum and a gravitational field. Because the vestibular apparatus is part of the inner ear and is thus located in the head, it is head motion and acceleration that are sensed. The vestibular system serves two general and related functions: (1) it maintains body balance in the presence of forces acting on the head through postural reflexes, and (2) it maintains the steady position of visual objects in spite of marked changes in head position through vestibulo-ocular reflexes.

—— Vestibular system

The peripheral apparatus of the vestibular system lies embedded in the petrous portion of the temporal bone, adjacent to and continuous with the cochlea of the auditory system. All of the vestibular structures are contained in bony canals called the bony labyrinth. A membranous labyrinth that has the same shape as the bony labyrinth is fitted into the bony canals. The area immediately surrounding the membranous labyrinth is filled with perilymph, in which the membranous labyrinth floats. The composition of the perilymph is very similar to that of the cerebral spinal fluid (CSF), and a tubular perilymphatic duct connects the perilymph fluid with the CSF in the subarachnoid space of the posterior fossa. The membranous labyrinth is filled with endolymph. A small-diameter tubular extension, the endolymphatic sac, connects this system with the subdural space near the jugular foramen, providing an exit for the slowly circulating endolymph into the lymphatic system. The endolymph has a high potassium concentration and is similar to intracellular fluid.

The vestibular apparatus is divided into five prominent divisions: three semicircular ducts, a utricle, and a saccule (see Figure 52-5). The receptors of these structures are differentiated into the angular acceleration–deceleration receptors of the semicircular canals and the linear acceleration–deceleration and static gravitational receptors of the utricle and saccule. The utricle and saccule are two widened membranous sacs within the bony vestibule. The utricle connects the ends of each semicircular duct. The saccule communicates with the utricle through a small duct and with the cochlear duct of the auditory apparatus through the ductus reuniens.

There are small patches of tall columnar hairlike ciliated epithelial cells in the floor of the utricle (utricular macula), in the side wall of the saccule (saccular macula), at the base of each semicircular duct (cristae), and along the floor of the cochlear duct (organ of Corti; see Figure 52-6). Each hair cell has several microvilli and one true cilium called a kinocilium. Ganglion cells, homologous with dorsal root ganglion cells, form three afferent ganglia: the superior vestibular ganglion, which innervates the hair cells of the utricular macula and the cristae of the superior and horizontal semicircular ducts; the inferior vestibular ganglion, which innervates the saccular macula and the cristae of the inferior semicircular duct; and the spiral (or acoustic) ganglion, which innervates the cochlear duct. The central axons of these ganglion cells become the superior and inferior vestibular nerves and the cochlear auditory nerve. They are often collectively called the eighth cranial nerve, and they enter the side of the nearby medullary–pontine junction of the brain stem. The axons of the vestibular nerves terminate in the four vestibular nuclei (superior, lateral, medial, and inferior vestibular nuclei).

—— Semicircular ducts

The three semicircular ducts, each about two-thirds of a circle, are arranged at right angles to each other, with the horizontal duct tilted at approximately 12 degrees above the normal horizontal plane of the head (see Figure 52-5). The horizontal ducts of the two sides of the head are in the same plane and the superior duct of one side is parallel with the inferior duct of the other side. At the junction of each semicircular duct and the utricle, an enlargement of each semicircular duct, called an *ampulla*, contains the hair cell sensory surface raised into a crest, or crista, at right angles to the duct. The stereocilia of each hair cell extend into a flexible gelatinous mass, the cupula, which essentially closes off fluid flow through the semicircular ducts. When the head begins to rotate around the axis of a semicircular duct (*i.e.*, undergoes angular acceleration), the momentum of the endolymph causes an increase in pressure to be applied to one side of the cupula. This is similar to the lagging behind of the water in a glass that is suddenly rotated, except that the endolymph cannot flow past the cupula and instead applies a differential pressure to its two sides, bending it and the cilia of the hair cells. This results in a reduced membrane potential across the hair cell plasma membrane when the hair is bent toward the microvilli and an increased membrane potential when the hair cell is bent in the opposite direction. Impulses from the cristae are transmitted by the vestibular part of the vestibulocochlear (VIII) cranial nerve to the vestibular nuclei of the caudal pons.

Maximal stimulation of the afferents of a semicircular duct results when rotation of the head occurs exactly in the plane of the membranous duct. Because of the orientation of the three semicircular ducts, angular accelerations of the head will always result in action potentials in at least one and usually more than one of the vestibular nerve branches to the three cristae. If the angular acceleration reduces to a steady angular velocity, friction between the endolymph and the duct wall gradually results in, first, a reduction of pressure and then a loss of differential pressure on the two sides of the cupula—a form of sensory adaptation. Upon the sudden reduction or cessation of head rotation, the momentum of the endolymph will apply pressure on the cupula from the opposite direction. Thus, the semicircular duct system provides a mechanism for signaling to the CNS the direction and rate of accelerations and decelerations in head rotation.

Utricle and saccule

The hair cell surface (macula) of the utricle is oriented approximately in the horizontal plane. The macula of the saccule is oriented in the vertical plane. In both instances, the stereocilia of the hair cells extend into a gelatinous mass within the endolymph. Myriad microscopic crystals of calcium carbonate and calcium phosphate, called *otoliths,* are embedded in this gelatinous material, adding considerably to its total mass. The gelatinous mass with its otoliths is called the otolithic membrane. When the head is tilted, the gelatinous mass shifts its position because of the pull of the gravitational field bending the stereocilia of the macular hair cells. Although each hair cell becomes hyperpolarized or hypopolarized depending on the direction in which the cilia are bending, the hair cells are oriented in all directions, making these sense organs sensitive to static or changing head position in relation to the gravitational field. The central connections from the maculae provide the mechanism by which head, body, and eye postural adjustments occur in response to tilting the head and by which a stable visual fixation point ("optic grasp" of the visual field), as well as postural support of a stable head position, is maintained. Projections to the forebrain provide the basis for sensations of head tilt away from the horizontal plane.

In addition to this rather static tilt reception function, the utricle and saccule provide the organism with linear acceleration and deceleration reception. When the head is accelerated in linear fashion, such as the initial or terminal phase of an elevator ride or during automobile acceleration or deceleration, differential movement between the head and the otolithic membranes provides the basis for reflex compensatory bracing of neck, trunk, and limbs. They also provide the input data on which the air-righting reflexes are based. A cat dropped from an upside-down position lands on its feet and will do so even if blindfolded. Most vestibular reflexes, including air righting, are functional at birth. If a newborn is supported in the prone position, and the support is momentarily (and with great care) removed, the trunk is extended and all four limbs are extended as falling begins. In the supine position, the trunk is flexed and the limbs are flexed as the fall progresses. On the other hand, the head-on-body vestibular reflexes of the infant are not sufficiently operational during the first 6 weeks or so after birth to maintain head posture. This is why the newborn's head must be supported when the newborn is lifted in the supine position to prevent extreme cervical flexure and possible damage to the cervical segmental nerves.

Central nervous system connections

The nerve fibers from the vestibular receptors travel in the vestibular portion of the vestibulocochlear (VIII) cranial nerve (see Figure 52-5) to the superior, medial, lateral, and inferior vestibular nuclei located at the junction of the medulla and pons. In addition, some of the afferent fibers travel to the ipsilateral cerebellar cortex and a deep cerebellar nucleus called the *fastigial nucleus.* The part of the cerebellum receiving vestibular input is called the *archicerebellum,* or the *flocculonodular lobe.* On the output side, cells in the fastigial nucleus receiving afferent terminals and terminals from cortical neurons send their axons back to the vestibular nuclei of the same and opposite sides of the brain stem.

A fiber tract called the *medial longitudinal fasciculus* (MLF) extends from the midbrain to the upper part of the spinal cord; it lies close to the medial plane and interconnects the vestibular nuclei with motor nuclei, particularly those of cranial nerves III, IV, VI, and XI. In addition to complex internal circuitry, neurons from the vestibular nuclei project into the nearby reticular formation and provide powerful control on postural reflexes of the eyes, head, body, and limbs. Projections occur to the pons lateral gaze control center, to the vertical and torsional gaze control regions, to the sixth cranial nerve nuclei, to the MLF, to the fourth and third nerve nuclei, and to cervical-level lower motoneurons innervating the sternocleidomastoid and other neck muscles that control head turning and posture. The MLF projections primarily control horizontal or lateral turning and gaze. In addition, extensive projections into and through the reticular formation follow the central tegmental fasciculus (CTF) pathway controlling the vertical and rotatory (torsion) gaze reflexes.

Eye movement reflexes

Vestibular control of conjugate eye posture can be understood in terms of complex reflex bilateral (conjugate) eye movements that preserve eye fixation on stable objects in the visual field. The term *nystagmus* is used to describe vestibular-controlled eye movements that occur in response to angular and rotational movements of the head. As one begins to sway or fall, such visual stability is essential to successful recovery attempts. Thus, as the body and head begin rotation, the eyes in conjugate fashion move in exactly the opposite direction, maintaining the previous fixation point. This is called the slow phase of nystagmus. If the rotation continues beyond the range of lateral eye movement, a very quick (rapid nystagmus) conjugate eye correction (saccadic return) occurs as if to obtain a new stable fixation point, and then the slow phase continues again. This nystagmus pattern continues as long as angular acceleration continues. When a steady rotational velocity is reached, compensatory nystagmus movements gradually wane as the disparity between the movement of endolymph and the semicircular duct wall is lost, as the pressure on the two sides of the cupula is equalized.

Clinically, the direction of this nystagmus pattern is named for the fast, or saccadic, phase. The reflex circuitry is in very precise control of motor units in the nuclei innervating the extrinsic muscles of the eye by way of cranial nerves III, IV, and VI. In fact, the precision of nystagmus movements is as great in persons with eyes closed and in the congenitally blind as it is in normal-sighted persons. If the eyes are not allowed to move, or if stimulation is strong, the head will also move in nystagmoid fashion as a result of vestibular control of the sternocleidomastoid muscles by cranial nerve XI.

Vestibular-driven nystagmus can occur in any plane. Beginning rotation of the head around a transverse axis in head-over-heels fashion is accompanied by compensatory nystagmus, which has its slow, smooth-pursuit phase in the upward direction and its fast phase in the direction of rotation. Starting rotation around the frontal–occipital axis (*i.e.*, head tilting to

the side) is accompanied by compensatory slow-phase torsion eye movements, twisting in the direction opposite to the rotation. The saccadic phase will be in the direction of body rotation. In each instance, nystagmus can be understood in terms of repeated attempts to grasp stable fixed visual fields as the head rotates, with a quick correction to a new, stable fixation point.

Nystagmus can be classified in terms of the direction of eye movement: horizontal, vertical, rotatory, or mixed. Nystagmus derived from a sense organ or vestibular nerve is of the slow phase–fast phase or jerky type described previously. Nystagmus resulting from CNS pathology usually has equal slow and fast rates in each direction, called pendular nystagmus.

If the visual environment is rotated or appears to rotate past a person with a normally functioning visual system, even though the head remains in a fixed position, a fixation point is selected and a smooth pursuit movement will rotate the eyes to the limit of the binocular field. At this point, a saccadic correction quickly moves the eyes back to a new fixation point, and the pursuit will occur again. This visually induced, or optokinetic, nystagmus and the associated vertigo are experienced when a moving object such as a car or train moves past the visual field. The phenomenon demonstrates the ability of visual stimuli to overpower the vestibular end organs' signals that the head is indeed stable in relation to gravitational and inertial forces.

Thalamic and cortical projections

Some of the neurons of the vestibular nuclei project their axons rostrally to the ventrolateral nuclei of the thalamus. In addition to the intrathalamic circuitry, thalamic projections go to the primary vestibular cortex near the somesthetic area of the parietal lobe. These thalamic and cortical projections provide the basis for the subjective experiences of position in space, of rotation, and of vertigo that accompany the onset or sudden cessation of head rotation. Vertigo is often experienced as a result of toxic conditions, such as alcohol toxicity, or of infective conditions. During such episodes, nystagmus is observed.

Severe damage to the forebrain or to the brain stem rostral to the pons often results in loss of rostral control of these static vestibular reflexes. If the patient's head is moved from side to side or up and down, the eyes retain a stable fixation point. Thus, the eyes move in conjugate gaze much as those of a doll with counterweighted eyes. This phenomenon, called "doll's eyes," demonstrates the always-present vestibular static reflexes without forebrain interference or suppression. If doll's eyes are present, brain stem function at the level of the pons is considered intact (in a comatose person). These static vestibular reflexes are to be contrasted with rapid or dynamic vestibular reflexes (nystagmus and the linear acceleration and deceleration reflexes).

Postural reflexes

Sudden changes in balance or orientation, such as falling to the right or left or backward or forward, result in powerful reflexes needed to maintain equilibrium and posture.

The descending portion of the MLF, essentially a medial vestibulospinal tract, continues at least into thoracic cord levels and provides vestibular control of the muscle tone of axial mucles, including the dorsal back muscles. A rapid-conducting lateral vestibulospinal tract descends the spinal cord to provide powerful vestibular control of the lower motoneurons of the upper and lower limbs. As the head begins to tip (*i.e.,* rotate) on the neck or as a part of general body tipping, the vestibular system activates the appropriate extensor muscles of the neck, trunk, and limbs, opposing the direction of the tilt. These powerful reflex adjustments in muscle tone assist in maintaining stable head and, therefore, body postural support during static posture and during passive or active movement.

All of the vestibular nuclei receive input from the cerebellum as well as the vestibular nerve. The cerebellar connections of the vestibular system are necessary for adjustments of temporally smooth, coordinated movements to ongoing head movement, tilt, or angular acceleration. For instance, accurate grasping can occur during a fall, indicating cerebellar adjustments based on vestibular information during the performance of a smooth, accurate movement.

Vestibular reflexes are quite powerful, and considerable learning is required to inhibit or greatly modify them, as is necessary for acrobatic pilots, divers, and gymnasts. Dancers and skaters who engage in rapid spinning movements also learn to use or at least partially inhibit these reflexes.

Alterations in vestibular function

Disorders of vestibular function are characterized by a condition called vertigo, in which a hallucination of motion occurs; that is, either the person is stationary and the environment is in motion (objective vertigo), or the person is in motion and the environment is stationary (subjective vertigo). Vertigo should be differentiated from dizziness, which is characterized by light-headedness, fainting, and unsteadiness. Abnormal nystagmus, tinnitus, and hearing loss are other common manifestations of vestibular dysfunc-

tion, as are autonomic manifestations such as perspiration, nausea, and vomiting. Disorders of vestibular function can be either peripheral (involving the labyrinth) or central (involving the vestibular connections).

Spontaneous nystagmus that occurs without head movement or visual stimuli is always pathologic. It seems to appear more readily and more severely when fatigue is present and, to some extent, can be influenced by psychologic factors. Nystagmus derived from the central nervous system, in contrast with peripheral end organ or eighth cranial nerve sources, is rarely accompanied by vertigo. If present, the vertigo is of mild intensity.

Disorders of peripheral vestibular function

Motion sickness. One of the most common alterations of vestibular function is motion sickness. It is caused by repeated rhythmic stimulation of the vestibular system, such as is encountered in car, air, or boat travel. Vertigo, malaise, nausea, and vomiting are the principal symptoms. Autonomic signs, including lowered blood pressure, tachycardia, and excessive sweating, may occur. Antimotion sickness drugs are often used to ameliorate these symptoms. Motion sickness usually decreases in severity with repeated exposure.

Vestibular system injury or irritation. The inner ear is vulnerable to injury caused by fracture of the petrous portion of the temporal bones; infection of nearby structures, including the middle ear and meninges, and blood-borne toxins and infections. Damage to the vestibular system can occur as a side effect of certain drugs or from allergic reactions to foods. The aminoglycosides (*e.g.,* streptomycin and gentamicin) have a specific toxic affinity for the vestibular portion of the inner ear. Shellfish seem to be the most common food allergen producing vertigo. Alcohol can also cause transient episodes of vertigo.

Severe irritation or damage of the vestibular end organs or nerves results in severe balance disorders reflected by instability of posture, dystaxia, and falling accompanied by vertigo. With irritation, falling is away from the affected side; and with destruction, it is toward the affected side. Adaptation to asymmetric stimulation occurs within a few days, after which the signs and symptoms diminish and are eventually lost. Following recovery, there is usually a slightly reduced acuity for tilt, and the person walks with a somewhat broadened base to improve postural stability. The neurologic basis for this adaptation to unilateral loss of vestibular input is not understood. Following adaptation to the loss of vestibular input from one side, the loss of function of the opposite vestibular apparatus produces signs and symptoms identical to those resulting from unilateral rather than bilateral loss. Within weeks, adaptation is again sufficient for locomotion and even for driving a car. Such a person relies very heavily on visual and proprioceptive input and has severe orientational difficulty in the dark, particularly when traversing uneven terrain.

Meniere's syndrome. Meniere's syndrome is a disorder of vestibular function caused by an overaccumulation of endolymph, also called endolymphatic hydrops. It is characterized by fluctuating episodes of tinnitus, feelings of ear fullness, and violent rotary vertigo that often renders the person unable to sit or walk. There is a need to lie quietly with the head fixed in a comfortable position, avoiding all head movements that aggravate the vertigo. Symptoms referable to the autonomic nervous system, including pallor, sweating, nausea, and vomiting, are usually present. The more severe the attack is, the more prominent the autonomic manifestations. A fluctuating hearing loss occurs, and initially there is a return to normal after the episode subsides; but as the disease progresses, it becomes more severe and permanent. Meniere's syndrome is usually unilateral, and because the sense of hearing is bilateral, persons with the disorder are often not aware of the full extent of their hearing loss.

A number of conditions, such as allergy, adrenal–pituitary insufficiency, trauma, and hypothyroidism, can cause Meniere's syndrome. The most common form of the disease is an idiopathic form thought to be caused by a single viral injury to the fluid transport system of the inner ear.

Methods used in the diagnosis of Meniere's syndrome include audiograms, vestibular testing by electronystagmography, and petrous pyramid x-rays. Administration of hyperosmolar substances, such as glycerin and urea, often produces acute temporary hearing improvement in persons with Meniere's syndrome and is sometimes used as a diagnostic measure of endolymphatic hydrops. The diuretic furosemide may also be used for this purpose.

The treatment of Meniere's syndrome can be either medical or surgical. Medical treatment consists primarily of bedrest, sedation, and antiemetic and antimotion-sickness drugs. Use of a low-salt diet and diuretic therapy may be useful in decreasing the frequency of attacks. Surgical treatment is indicated in persons who do not benefit from medical treatment. Surgical methods include an endolymphatic–subarachnoid shunt in which excess endolymph from the inner ear is diverted into the subarachnoid space. Surgical labyrinthine destruction can be used to eliminate vertigo. This procedure is reserved for persons with severe deafness of the involved ear, in which the disease is unilateral and of more than 2 years' dura-

tion. An otic–perotic shunt (cochleosacculotomy) can be performed through the external auditory canal and round window. Cryosurgery involves the application of intense cold to the lateral semicircular canal. This procedure either reduces the sensitivity of the vestibular apparatus or creates a fistula in the membranous labyrinth, causing a shunt between the endolymph and the perilymph. Vestibular nerve resection may also be done.

Disorders of central vestibular function

Abnormal nystagmus and vertigo can occur as a result of central nervous system pathology. Compression of the vestibular nuclei by cerebellar tumors invading the fourth ventricle results in progressively severe signs and symptoms. In addition to abnormal nystagmus and vertigo, vomiting, and broad-base and dystaxic gait become progressively more evident. Some drugs (e.g., anticonvulsants) can also cause abnormal nystagmus. Centrally derived nystagmus usually has equal excursion in both directions (pendular). Congenital and lifelong nystagmus abnormalities are not uncommon, often occurring as part of a number of hereditary syndromes. It can also accompany other motor defects in cerebral palsy and degenerative syndromes such as multiple sclerosis. Abnormal nystagmus can make reading and other tasks requiring precise eye positional control very difficult. When assessing for minimal nystagmus changes in possible brain damage, the patient is asked to fixate on the tester's finger; the tester then moves it laterally within the patient's visual field. At the most extreme limit of lateral deviation, ipsilateral nystagmoid eye flutter enduring longer than three beats and nystagmus upon eye deviation in any other plane indicate hyperexcitability of the vestibular reflex systems.

Diagnostic methods

Diagnosis of vestibular disorders is based on a description of the symptoms, a history of trauma or exposure to agents that are destructive to vestibular structures, and physical examination. Tests of eye movements (nystagmus) and muscle control of balance and equilibrium are often used.

Tests of postrotational nystagmus. If the head is suddenly slowed or stopped from a steady angular velocity of rotation, the same sequence of reflex conjugate eye movements occurs, but in the opposite direction. Because it is easier to observe a person's responses following the cessation of rotation than it is for the observer to rotate with the person, the postrotational nystagmus is usually used to study the adequacy of vestibular reflexes. A rotatable chair

(Bárány chair), much like a barber's chair, is used for this purpose. The person being tested is strapped into the chair with the head positioned so that the plane of one pair of semicircular ducts is in the horizontal plane (plane of rotation). The person is then rotated until a steady rate of rotation is achieved. The chair is suddenly stopped, and the ensuing reflex postrotational nystagmus and the compensatory movements of the body and limbs are observed. Each of the three primary planes of the ducts can be tested in turn, the corresponding semicircular ducts of both sides being tested simultaneously. Unilateral defects are not clearly detected by this method. After the rotation in the Bárány chair is stopped, the person being tested is asked to point toward a fixed visual target. The pointing arm will drift past the target; this is called *past-pointing*. Because of the danger of injury associated with the powerful vestibular reflexes of the body and limbs, only trained personnel should perform the Bárány chair tests.

Caloric stimulation. A more commonly performed test of vestibular reflexes involves irrigation of the external meatus of one ear with warm (40°C) or cold (25°C) water. The resulting changes in temperature, as conducted through the petrous portion of the temporal bone, set up convection currents in the otic fluid that mimic the effects of angular acceleration. Maximal stimulation occurs in the semicircular duct that is vertical during irrigation, and the corresponding nystagmoid eye movements can be assessed. An advantage of the caloric stimulation method is the ability to test the vestibular apparatus on one side at a time.

Electronystagmography. The caloric test for evaluating nystagmoid eye movements is based on subjective observation and, therefore, is subject to error. A more precise and objective diagnostic method of evaluating nystagmus is through the use of electronystagmography (ENG). With this method, the standard caloric stimulus is delivered to the ear canal, and the duration and velocity of eye movements are recorded using electrodes in a manner similar to electrocardiography. Electrodes are placed lateral to the outer canthus of each eye and above and below each eye. A ground electrode is placed on the forehead.

Romberg test. The Romberg test is used to demonstrate disorders of static vestibular function. The person being tested is requested to stand with feet together and arms extended forward so that the degree of sway and arm stability can be noted. The person is then asked to close his or her eyes. When visual clues are removed, postural stability is based on proprioceptive sensation from the joints, muscles, and tendons and from static vestibular reception. Deficiency in vestibular static input will be indicated by greatly

increased sway and a tendency for the arms to drift toward the side of deficiency.

If vestibular input is severely deficient, the subject will fall toward the deficient side. Care must be taken, because defects of proprioceptive projection to the forebrain will also result in some arm drift and postural instability toward the deficient side. Only if two-point discrimination and vibratory sensation from the lower and upper limbs are bilaterally normal can the deficiency be attributed to the vestibular system.

Antivertigo drugs

Among the methods used to treat vertigo are the antivertigo or antimotion-sickness drugs. Drugs used in the treatment of vertigo include anticholinergic drugs (scopolamine, atropine), monoaminergic drugs (amphetamine, ephedrine), and antihistamines (meclizine [Antivert]), cyclizine [Marezine], dimenhydrinate [Dramamine], promethazine [Phenergan]. Animal studies have documented that drugs with anticholinergic or monoaminergic activity diminish the excitability of neurons in the vestibular nucleus.[8] Although the antihistamines have long been used in treating vertigo, little is known about their mechanism of action. However, most of these drugs have some anticholinergic activity, and some also enhance sympathetic activity by blocking the reuptake of monoamines at the synaptic nerve terminals.[8] A transdermal scopolamine preparation (Transderm-V) has recently become available for use in treating motion sickness. The medication is prepared on slow-release microporous polypropylene membrane contained in a patch that can be placed behind the ear. A small dose of the drug is released slowly and absorbed over a 3-day period. This method of drug delivery has proven effective in preventing motion sickness with minimal side effects. To be effective, however, the patch must be in place for several hours before exposure to motion.

In summary, the vestibular system plays an essential role in the equilibrium sense, which is closely integrated with visual and proprioceptive (position) senses. The receptors for the vestibular system, which are located in the semicircular ducts of the inner ear, respond to changes in linear and angular acceleration of the head. The vestibular nerve fibers travel in the vestibulocochlear (VIII) cranial nerve to the vestibular nuclei located at the junction of the medulla and pons. Some of the fibers pass through the nuclei to the cerebellum. The cerebellar connections are necessary for temporally smooth, coordinated movements during ongoing head movements, tilt, and angular acceleration. The vestibular nuclei also connect with the nuclei of the oculomotor (III), trochlear (IV), and abducens (VI) cranial nerves. Vestibular control of conjugate eye movements serves to preserve eye fixation on stable objects in the visual field during head movement. The term nystagmus is used to describe vestibular-controlled eye movements that occur in response to angular and rotational movements of the head. Neurons of the vestibular nuclei also project to the thalamus, to the temporal cortex, and to the somatesthetic area of the parietal cortex. The thalamic and cortical projections provide the basis for the subjective experiences of position in space and of rotation and vertigo. Disorders of the vestibular system include motion sickness and Meniere's syndrome. Meniere's syndrome, which is caused by an overaccumulation of endolymph, is characterized by severe disabling episodes of tinnitus, feelings of ear fullness, and violent rotary vertigo. The diagnosis of vestibular disorders is based on a description of the symptoms, a history of trauma or exposure to agents destructive to vestibular structures, and tests of eye movements (nystagmus) and muscle control of balance and equilibrium. Among the methods used in the treatment of vertigo that accompanies vestibular disorders are the antivertigo, or antimotion-sickness, drugs. These drugs act by diminishing the excitability of neurons in the vestibular nucleus.

References

1. Bluestone CD: Otitis media in children: To treat or not to treat. N Engl J Med 306:1399, 1982
2. Senturia BH, Bluestone CD, Paradise JL et al: Report of the Ad Hoc Committee on Definition and Classification of Otitis Media and Otitis Media with Effusion. Ann Otolaryngol 89(Suppl):3, 1980
3. Barfold C, Roborg J: Secretory otitis media: Long-term observations after treatment with grommets. Arch Otolaryngol 106:553, 1980
4. Al-Sheikhle ARJ: Secretory otitis media in children. (A retrospective study of 249). J Laryngol Otol 94:1117, 1980
5. Meyerhoff WL: Diagnosis and Management of Hearing Loss, p 1. Philadelphia, WB Saunders, 1984
6. Dodge PR, Hallowell D, Feigin RD et al: Prospective evaluation of hearing impairment as a sequela of acute bacterial meningitis. N Engl J Med 311:879, 1984
7. Brown RD, Wood CD: Vestibular pharmacology. Trends Pharmacol Sci (Feb):150, 1980
8. Baloh RW: The dizzy patient. Postgrad Med 73:317, 1983

Bibliography

—— Hearing

Balkany TJ: An overview of electronic cochlear prosthesis: Clinical and research considerations. Otolaryngol Clin North Am 16(1):209, 1983

Bentzen O: Otosclerosis, a universal disease. Adv Otorhinolaryngol 29:151, 1983

Bluestone CD: Recent advances in the pathogenesis, diagnosis, and management of otitis media. Pediatr Clin North Am 28(4):727, 1981

Bluestone CD, Fria TJ, Arjona SK et al: Controversies in screening for middle ear disease and hearing loss in children. Pediatrics 77:57, 1986.

Bluestone CD, Klein JO, Paradise JL et al: Workshop on effects of otitis media in the child. Pediatrics 71:639, 1983

Brondbo K, Hawke M, Abel SM et al: The natural history of otosclerosis. J Otolaryngol 13:164, 1983

Callahan CW, Lazoritz S: Otitis media and language development. Am Fam Pract 37:186, 1988

Cantekin E, Phillips DC, Doyle WJ et al: Gas absorption in the middle ear. Ann Otolaryngol 89(Suppl):71, 1980

Causse JB, Causse JR: Minimizing cochlear loss during and after stapedectomy. Otolaryngol Clin North Am 15(4):813, 1982

Crawford LV, Goode RL, Grundfast KM et al: Otitis media: Selecting the therapy. Patient Care (Sept):108, 1983

D'Alonzo BJ, Cantor AB: Ototoxicity: Etiology and issues. J Fam Pract 16:489, 1983

DiChara E: A sound method for testing children's hearing. Am J Nurs 84:1104, 1984

Dobie RA: Noise-induced hearing loss: The family physician's role. Am Fam Pract 36:141, 1987

Dodge PR, Davis H, Feigin RD et al: Prospective evaluation of hearing impairment as a sequela of acute bacterial meningitis. N Engl J Med 311:869, 1984

Ecliachar I, Joachims HZ, Goldsher M et al: Assessment of long-term middle ear ventilation. Acta Otolaryngol 96:105, 1983

Farmer HS: A guide to treatment of external otitis. Am Fam Pract 21:96, 1980

Feigin RD: Otitis media: Closing the information gap. N Engl J Med 306:1417, 1982

Fireman P: Newer concepts in otitis media. Hosp Pract 22(11A):85, 1987.

Herzon FS: Tympanostomy tubes. Arch Otolaryngol 106:645, 1980

Hinojosa R, Lindsay JR: Profound deafness. J Otolaryngol 106:193, 1980

Human Communication and Its Disorder. NINDS Monograph No 10. DHEW Publication No (NIH) 76–1090, 1970

Magnuson B, Falk B: Eustachian tube malfunction and middle ear disease in new perspective. J Otolaryngol 12:187, 1983

Paparella MM, Goycoolea MV, Meyerhoff WL: Inner ear pathology and otitis media—A review. Ann Otolaryngol 89(Suppl):249, 1980

Paradise JL: Otitis media during early life: How hazardous to development? A critical review of the evidence. Pediatrics 68:869, 1981

Paradise JL: On classifying otitis media as suppurative or nonsuppurative, with a suggested clinical schema. J Pediatrics 111:948, 1987

Rubin W: Diagnosis: Noise and hearing loss. Hosp Med 19(5):77, 1983

Shea JJ: Otosclerosis and tinnitus. J Laryngol Otol 4(Suppl):149, 1981

Singh RP: Anatomy of Hearing and Speech. New York, Oxford University Press, 1980

Spellman FA: The cochlear prosthesis: A review of the design and evaluation of electrode implants for the profoundly deaf. CRC Crit Rev Biomed Eng 8(5):223, 1982

Square R, Cooper JC, Hearne EM et al: Eustachian tube function. Arch Otolaryngol 108:567, 1982

Sutton D: Cochlear pathology: Hazards of long-term implants. Arch Otolaryngol 110:164, 1984

Teele DW, Klein JO, Rosner BA: Epidemiology of otitis media in children. Ann Otolaryngol 89(Suppl):5, 1980

—— Vestibular function

Baldwin RL: The dizzy patient. Hosp Pract 19(10):151, 1984

Brooks GB: Meniere's disease: A practical approach. Drugs 25:77, 1983

Condi JK: Types and causes of nystagmus in the neurosurgical patient. J Neurosurg Nurs 15(2):56, 1983

Dix MR: Positional nystagmus of the central type and its neural mechanisms. Acta Otolaryngol 95:585, 1983

Gussen R: Vascular mechanisms in Meniere's disease. Arch Otolaryngol 108:544, 1982

Mohr D: The syndrome of paroxysmal positional vertigo—A review. West J Med 145:645, 1986

Pulec JL: Meniere's syndrome. Hosp Med 19(6):81, 1981

Schmidt PH: Pathophysiology of Meniere attack: Facts and theories. Acta Otolaryngol 95:417, 1983

Shea JJ: Intracochlear shunt. Otolaryngol Clin North Am 16(1):293, 1983

Tonndorf J: Vestibular signs and symptoms in Meniere's disorder: Mechanical consideration. Acta Otolaryngol 95:431, 1983

Wall CW III, Black FO: Postural stability and rotational tests: Their effectiveness for screening dizzy patients. Acta Otolaryngol 95:235, 1983

Wolfson RJ, Silverstein H, Marlowe FI et al: Vertigo. Clin Symposia 33(6): 1981

CHAPTER 53

Degenerative, Demyelinating, and Neoplastic Disorders of the Nervous System

Degenerative brain disorders
  Dementias
    Alzheimer's disease
    Multi-infarct dementia
    Pick's disease
    Creutzfeldt-Jakob's disease
    Wernicke-Korsakoff's syndrome
    Huntington's disease

Parkinson's disease and parkinsonism
  Etiology
  Manifestations
  Treatment

Demyelinating diseases
  Multiple sclerosis
    Pathophysiology
    Etiology
    Manifestations and clinical course
    Diagnosis
    Treatment
  Brain tumors
    Manifestations
    Diagnosis and treatment

Objectives

After you have studied this chapter, you should be able to meet the following objectives:

_____ State the criteria for a diagnosis of dementia.

_____ Compare the etiologies associated with Alzheimer's disease, multi-infarct dementia, Pick's disease, Creutzfeldt-Jakob disease, the Wernicke-Korsakoff's syndrome, and Huntington's disease.

_____ Describe the changes in brain tissue that occur with Alzheimer's disease.

_____ Explain how a diagnosis of Alzheimer's disease is arrived at.

_____ Use the three stages of Alzheimer's disease to describe its progress.

_____ State the reason for banning persons who have received human-derived growth hormone from blood, tissue, and organ donation.

_____ Cite the difference between Wernicke's disease and the Korsakoff's component of the Wernicke-Korsakoff's syndrome.

_____ State the pros and cons for the presymptomatic use of genetic testing for Huntington's disease.

_____ Compare the causes of the primary and secondary forms of parkinsonism.

_____ Explain the symptoms of Parkinson's disease with reference to the extrapyramidal system.

_____ Differentiate between the actions of anticholinergic drugs and dopamine agonists in controlling the symptoms of Parkinson's disease.

_____ Explain the significance of demyelinization and plaque formation in multiple sclerosis.

_____ Describe the manifestations of multiple sclerosis.

_____ List the current methods used in treatment of multiple sclerosis.

_____ List the major categories of brain tumors.

_____ Interpret the meaning of benign and malignant as it relates to brain tumors.

_____ Describe the general manifestations of brain tumors.

_____ List the methods used in diagnosis of brain tumors.

_____ State the three methods of treatment for brain tumors.

There are several types of brain disorders that produce progressive deterioration of function. These include degenerative brain disorders such as dementia and parkinsonism and demyelinating diseases such as multiple sclerosis. Brain tumors are neoplasms that arise from central nervous system (CNS) tissues or as metastases from tumors outside the CNS. Although some brain tumors are successfully treated, many produce progressive destruction of brain tissue.

Degenerative brain disorders

Degenerative brain disorders are diseases that selectively affect one or more functional systems of neurons while leaving others intact. They generally produce symmetrical and progressive involvement of the CNS, affect similar areas of the brain, and produce similar clinical syndromes.[1] Thus degenerative disorders affecting the cortex tend to produce dementias and those affecting the basal ganglia, extrapyramidal movement disorders.

Dementias

Dementia is a syndrome of intellectual deterioration severe enough to interfere with occupational or social performance. It involves disturbances in memory, language use, perception, and motor skills, and in the ability to learn necessary skills, solve problems, think abstractly, and make judgments. Chart 53-1 describes the characteristics of dementia as presented in the Diagnostic and Statistical Manual for Mental Disorders (DSM-III-R).[2] Depression is the most common treatable illness that may masquerade as dementia and needs to be ruled out when a diagnosis of dementia is considered. This is important because cognitive functioning usually returns to baseline levels when depression is treated. Dementia can be caused by any disorder that permanently damages large association areas of the cerebral hemispheres, including Alzheimer's disease, multi-infarct dementia, Pick's disease, Creutzfeldt-Jakob disease, Wernicke-Korsakoff syndrome, and Huntington's chorea.

Alzheimer's disease

Dementia of the Alzheimer's type occurs in middle or late life and accounts for 50% to 70% of all cases of dementia. The disorder affects 1.5 to 2 million Americans and may be the fourth leading cause of death in the United States.[3] The risk of developing Alzheimer's disease increases with age. Approximately 4% of persons over age 65 years have Alzheimer's disease. By age 80, prevalence reaches 20%. As the elderly population in the United States con-

---

Chart 53–1: Diagnostic criteria for dementia

A. Demonstrable evidence of impairment in short-term and long-term memory. Impairment of short-term memory (inability to learn new information) may be indicated by inability to remember three objects after 5 minutes. Long-term memory impairment (inability to remember information that was known in the past) may be indicated by inability to remember personal information (*e.g.,* what happened yesterday, place, occupation) or facts of common knowledge (*e.g.,* past presidents, well-known dates).

B. At least one of the following:
   (1) impairment in abstract thinking, as indicated by inability to find similarities and differences between related words, difficulty in defining words and concepts, and other similar tasks.
   (2) impaired judgment, as indicated by inability to make reasonable plans to deal with interpersonal, family, and job-related problems and issues
   (3) other disturbances of higher cortical function, such as aphasia (disorder of language), apraxia (inability to carry out motor activities despite intact comprehension and motor function), agnosia (failure to recognize and identify objects despite intact sensory function), and "constructual difficulty" (*e.g.,* inability to copy three-dimensional figures, assemble blocks, or arrange sticks in specific designs)
   (4) personality change (*i.e.,* alteration or accentuation of premorbid traits)

C. The disturbance in A and B significantly interferes with work or usual social activities or relationship with others.

D. The disturbance does not occur exclusively during the course of delirium.

---

tinues to increase, the number of persons with Alzheimer's-type dementia can also be expected to increase.

Pathophysiology. Alzheimer's disease is characterized by cortical atrophy and loss of neurons, the presence of neurofibrillary tangles, neuritic plaques, granulovacuolar degeneration, and cerebrovascular amyloid. The neurofibrillary tangles, found within the cytoplasm of abnormal neurons, consist of fibrous proteins that are wound around each other in a helical fashion. These tangles are resistant to chemical or enzymatic breakdown and so they persist in brain tissue long after the neuron in which they arose has died and disappeared. The neuritic plaques are patches or flat areas composed of clusters of degenerating nerve terminals, both dendritic and axonic. The granulovacuolar bodies consist of intraneural cytoplasmic vacuoles. Granulovacuolar degeneration brings about a progressive decline in nerve function, eventually leading to death of the nerve cell. Amyloid is a starchy material; it is found in and around blood vessels and is a component of the neuritic plaques.

Hippocampal function, in particular, may be compromised by the pathologic changes that occur in Alzheimer's disease. The hippocampus is crucial to information processing, acquisition of new memories, and retrieval of old memories. The development of neurofibrillary tangles in the endorhinal cortex and superior portion of the hippocampal gyrus interferes with cortical input and output, thereby isolating the hippocampus from the remainder of the cortex and rendering it functionless.[4]

Neurochemically, Alzheimer's disease has been associated with a decrease in the level of choline acetyltransferase activity in the cortex and hippocampus. This enzyme is required for the synthesis of acetylcholine, a neurotransmitter that is associated with memory. The reduction in choline acetyltransferase is quantitatively related to the numbers of neuritic plaques and severity of dementia. Evidence supporting the role of acetylcholine in Alzheimer's disease comes from studies using scopolamine, a drug that blocks muscarinic cholinergic receptors. Memory deficits similar to those found in normal elderly persons have been induced in healthy young persons through the administration of scopolamine.[5] Furthermore these deficits were reversed by administering physostigmine, a drug that prevents acetylcholine breakdown and thereby enhances its action. Unfortunately, attempts to increase brain levels of acetylcholine or its precursors in persons with Alzheimer's disease have been unsuccessful. Initial trials using choline and lecithin, the precursors of acetylcholine, have failed to demonstrate any improvement in memory. Physostigmine has produced some improvement in a few patients. However, the drug has limited usefulness because of its potentially toxic side effects and short half-life (about 2 hours).[6]

Etiology.   The etiology of Alzheimer's disease is unknown. Several hypotheses have been proposed, but as yet none has been able to explain the neuronal changes that occur with Alzheimer's disease. It is quite possible that Alzheimer's disease is really a group of related disorders with different etiologies. Recently, investigators have begun to identify subgroups of persons with the disorder, characterized by factors such as age of onset, family history, and environmental factors. The detection of abnormal proteins in the brain lesions of persons with Alzheimer's disease has provided further areas for research.

Because the disease was first recognized among relatively young persons, it was originally thought that there were two separate types of Alzheimer's disease: a presenile type, affecting persons under 65 years of age, and a senile type, affecting persons over 65 years of age. It is now known that the biochemical and pathologic changes are the same regardless of age. However, it is not known if the etiologies for the two age groups are the same.

In a small percentage of persons with Alzheimer's disease, the disorder appears to have an autosomal dominant inheritance. Families have been identified in which which there are 10 or more members, representing 4 or 5 generations, who have developed dementia of the Alzheimer's type.[4] Furthermore, there are strong similarities between the brain changes that occur in persons with Alzheimer's disease and those that occur in older persons (*i.e.*, 40 years of age or older) with Down's syndrome (see Chapter 4). Brain changes in persons with both disorders show the same pattern of neurofibrillary tangles and degenerative changes, suggesting that a defective gene on chromosome 21 may be involved in the inherited form of Alzheimer's disease.[7]

Environmental agents that are implicated in the development of Alzheimer's disease include trauma, exposure to metals, and viral agents or other infections. Repeated head trauma such as occurs in boxers can cause a condition called *dementia pugilistica*. Although the relationship between head trauma and the development of Alzheimer's disease is uncertain, there are many similarities between the pathologic changes that occur in dementia pugilistica and those that occur in Alzheimer's disease. Aluminum and silicon, presumably in the form of aluminum silicates, have been found in the core of the neuritic plaques, but it is not yet clear how this compound is formed or what role it plays, if any, in the development of Alzheimer's disease.[6] There is no evidence that exposure to exogenous forms of aluminum, as in aluminum-containing antacids, increases the risk of Alzheimer's; thus, a direct relationship between exogenous aluminum and aluminum deposits in the brains of persons with Alzheimer's has not been established. The search for link between a viral or infectious pathogen and the development of Alzheimer's disease derives from the discovery that several dementing diseases, including Creutzfeldt-Jakob disease, are caused by infectious agents.

An abnormal protein called *A68* has been found in brain tissue and cerebrospinal fluid from people with Alzheimer's disease.[8] It has been suggested that this protein contributes to the formation of other abnormal proteins, such as those that make up the neurofibrillary tangles and neuritic plaques. The molecular structure of the abnormal proteins found in the brain lesions of persons with Alzheimer's disease is being investigated. Once that has been accomplished, the identification of the genes involved in the synthesis of these proteins is expected to follow. If any of the genes turn out to be unique, then a genetic, toxic, or viral pathogenesis may be established.[8]

Manifestation. Alzheimer's-type dementia follows an insidious and progressive course. Major symptoms include loss of memory, disorientation, impaired abstract thinking and impulse control, and changes in personality and affect.[9] Three stages of Alzheimer's dementia have been identified, each characterized by progressive degenerative changes (Chart 53-2).

Stage 1, which may last for 2 to 4 years, is characterized by a subjective memory deficit that is often difficult to differentiate from the normal forgetfulness that occurs in the elderly. While most elderly forget unimportant events and details, persons with Alzheimer's disease randomly forget important and unimportant details. They forget where things are placed, get lost easily, and have trouble remembering appointments. Both recent and remote memory are affected. Mild changes in personality such as a flat affect, lack of spontaneity, and loss of a previous sense of humor occur during this stage.

As the disease progresses, the person with Alzheimer's disease enters the second or confusional stage of dementia. This stage may last several years and is marked by a more global impairment of cognitive functioning. During this stage there are changes in higher cortical functioning needed for language, spatial relationships, and problem solving. Depression may occur in persons who are aware of their deficits. There is extreme confusion, disorientation, lack of insight, and inability to carry out the activities of daily living. Personal hygiene is neglected and language becomes becomes impaired due to difficulty in remembering and retrieving words. Wandering, especially in the late afternoon or early evening, becomes a problem. The *sundown syndrome,* which is characterized by confusion, restlessness, agitation, and wandering, may become a daily occurrence late in the afternoon. Some persons may become hostile and abusive toward family members.

Stage 3 is the terminal stage. It is usually relatively short (1–2 years) in comparison to the other stages, but has been known to last for as long as 10 years.[9] The person becomes incontinent, apathetic, and unable to recognize family or friends. It is usually during this stage that the sufferer is institutionalized.

Diagnosis and treatment. Alzheimer's disease is essentially a diagnosis of exclusion. There are no peripheral biochemical markers or tests for the disease. The diagnosis can be confirmed only by microscopic examination of tissue obtained from a cerebral biopsy or at autopsy. At present the diagnosis is based on clinical findings. Criteria for the clinical diagnosis of Alzheimer's disease have been established by a work group under the auspices of the Department of Health and Human Services Task Force on Alzheimer's Disease.[10] A diagnosis of Alzheimer's disease requires the presence of dementia established by clinical examination and documented by results of a Mini-mental status test, Blessed dementia test, or similar examination that yield evidence of deficits in two or more areas of cognition and progressive worsening of memory or other cognitive functions. Brain imaging, either computed tomography (CT scan) or magnetic resonance imaging (MRI), is done to rule out other brain disease. Metabolic screening should be done for known reversible causes of dementia such as vitamin B_{12} deficiency, thyroid dysfunction, and electrolyte imbalance. A diagnostic accuracy of 80% can be achieved on the basis of clinical examination alone, and laboratory tests to exclude other disorders increase the accuracy to 90%.[6]

There is no specific treatment for Alzheimer's dementia. Drugs are used primarily to control depression, agitation, or sleep disorders. Two major goals of care are the maintenance of the person's socialization and provision of support for the family. Reminiscence group therapy has been found useful in maintaining socialization and establishing group relationships. Self-help groups that provide support for family and friends have become available, with support from the Alzheimer's Disease and Related Disorders Association. Day-care and respite centers are available in many areas to provide relief for caregivers.

Chart 53–2: Stages of Alzheimer's disease

Stage 1

Memory loss
Lack of spontaneity
Subtle personality changes
Disorientation to time and date

Stage 2

Impaired cognition and abstract thinking
Restlessness and agitation
Wandering, "sundown"
Inability to carry out activities of daily living
Impaired judgment
Inappropriate social behavior
Lack of insight, abstract thinking
Repetitive behavior
Voracious appetite

Stage 3

Emaciation—indifference to food
Inability to communicate
Urinary and fecal incontinence
Seizures

(Matteson MA, McConnell ES: Gerontological Nursing, p 251. Philadelphia, JB Lippincott, 1988)

Multi-infarct dementia

Dementia associated with cerebral vascular disease does not result directly from atherosclerosis, but rather from infarction due to multiple emboli that disseminate throughout the brain—hence the name multi-infarct dementia. About 20% to 25% of dementias are vascular in origin, and the incidence is closely associated with hypertension.[9] Other contributing factors are arrhythmias, myocardial infarction, peripheral vascular disease, diabetes mellitus, and smoking. The usual onset is between ages 55 and 70 years. The disease differs from Alzheimer's in its presentation and tissue pathology. The onset may be gradual or abrupt and there may be focal neurologic symptoms related to local areas of infarction.

Pick's disease

Pick's disease is a rare form of dementia characterized by atrophy of the frontal, temporal, and parietal lobes of the brain. The neurons in the affected areas contain cytoplasmic inclusions called Pick bodies.

The average age at onset of Pick's disease is 54 years. The disease is more common in women than men. Behavioral manifestations may be noted earlier than memory deficits, taking the form of a striking absence of concern and care, a loss of initiative, echolalia (automatic repetition of anything said to the person), hypotonia, and incontinence. The course of the disease is relentless, with death ensuing within 2 to 10 years. The immediate cause of death generally is infection.

Creutzfeldt-Jakob's disease

Creutzfeldt-Jakob's disease is a rare transmissible form of dementia, thought to be caused by an infective protein agent called a *prion*. The pathogen is resistant to chemical and physical methods commonly used for sterilizing medical and surgical equipment. The disease has reportedly been transmitted through corneal transplants and human growth hormone obtained from cadavers. The National Hormone and Pituitary Program halted the distribution of human-pituitary hormone in 1985 after reports that three young persons who had received the hormone had died of Creutzfeldt-Jakob disease.[11] Because of the uncertainty and dangers surrounding the transmission of Creutzfeldt-Jakob disease, it has been recommended that persons who received human-derived growth hormone refrain from blood, tissue, or organ donation.[12]

Creutzfeldt-Jakob disease causes degeneration of the pyramidal and extrapyramidal systems and is most readily distinguished by its rapid course. Affected persons are usually demented within 6 months of onset. The disease is uniformly fatal, with death often occurring within 7 months.[1] The early symptoms consist of abnormalities in personality and vi-

sual/spatial coordination. Extreme dementia and myoclonus follow as the the disease progresses.

Wernicke-Korsakoff's syndrome

Wernicke-Korsakoff's syndrome is due to chronic alcoholism. Wernicke's disease is characterized by weakness and paralysis of the extraocular muscles, nystagmus, ataxia, and confusion. Signs of peripheral neuropathy may be present. The person has an unsteady gait and complains of diplopia. There may be signs attributable to alcohol withdrawal—delirium, confusion, hallucinations, and others. It is generally agreed that this disorder is caused by a deficiency of thiamine (vitamin B_1), and many of the symptoms are reversed when nutrition is improved with supplemental thiamine.

The Korsakoff component of the syndrome involves severe impairment of recent memory. There is often difficulty in dealing with abstractions, and the person's capacity to learn is defective. Confabulation (the recitation of imaginary experiences to fill in gaps in memory) is probably the most distinctive feature of the disease. Polyneuritis is also common. Unlike Wernicke's disease, Korsakoff's psychosis does not improve significantly with treatment.

Huntington's disease

Huntington's disease is a rare hereditary disorder characterized by chronic progressive chorea, psychological changes, and dementia. Although the disease is inherited as an autosomal dominant disorder, symptoms do not usually develop until after 30 years of age.[13] By the time the disease has been diagnosed, the person has often passed the gene on to his or her children.

Huntington's disease produces localized death of brain cells. The first and most severely affected neurons are the caudate nucleus and putamen of the basal ganglia. The neurochemical changes that occur with the disease are complex. The neurotransmitter gamma-aminobutyric acid (GABA) is an inhibitory neurotransmitter in the basal ganglia. Post-mortem studies have shown a decrease of GABA and GABA receptors in the basal ganglia of persons dying of Huntington's disease. It has also been shown that the levels of acetylcholine, an excitatory neurotransmitter in the basal ganglia, are reduced in persons with Huntington's disease. At the same time, the dopaminergic pathway of the nigrostrial system, which is affected in parkinsonism (discussed later in this chapter), is preserved in Huntington's disease, suggesting that an imbalance in dopamine and acetylcholine may contribute to manifestations of the disease.

Depression and personality changes are the most common early psychological manifestations; memory loss is often accompanied by impulsive behavior, moodiness, antisocial behavior, and a tendency to emotional outbursts.[13] Other early signs of the disease are lack of initiative, loss of spontaneity, and inability to concentrate. Fidgetiness or restlessness may represent early signs of dyskinesia followed by choreiform and some dystonic posturing (see Chapter 49). Eventually, progressive rigidity and akinesia (rather than chorea) develop in association with dementia.

There is no cure for Huntington's disease. The treatment is largely symptomatic. Drugs may be used to treat the dyskinesias and behavioral disturbances.

In recent years the study of the genetics of Huntington's disease has led to the discovery that the gene for the disease is located on chromosome 4.[13] The discovery of a marker probe for the gene locus has raised the possibility of predictive testing for the disease. The testing procedure requires obtaining DNA samples from the person at risk and several relatives to determine which member of the gene pair travels with marker probe for the Huntington's gene in a particular family. DNA for determining the genotype can be obtained from the blood of a consenting person, from amniotic fluid, or from frozen brain tissue from a diseased person.[13] Presymptomatic testing raises many ethical questions, including that of providing a person with knowledge that he or she is carrying a gene that will eventually lead to prolonged physical and mental deterioration.

Parkinson's disease and parkinsonism

Parkinsonism is a degenerative disorder of basal ganglia function that results in variable combinations of slowness of movement (bradykinesia), increased muscle tonus (rigidity), tremor, and impaired automatic postural responses.

The basal ganglia, a group of deep cerebral nuclei, include the caudate nucleus and putamen (collectively called the *striatum*), the globus pallidus, the subthalamic nucleus, and the substantia nigra (see Chapter 49). The caudate nucleus and putamen function together to initiate and regulate gross intentional movements of the body. To accomplish this function, the striatal structures transmit impulses into the globus pallidus and then by way of the thalamus to the motor cortex, in particular the premotor and supplementary motor cortex.[14] A dopaminergic pathway, the nigrostriatal pathway, connects the substantia nigra to the striatum. It is assumed that this pathway is inhibitory to the striatal neurons that communicate with the motor cortex via the thalamic nuclei. The striatum also contains many cholinergic interneurons that functionally oppose the dopaminergic input.

The movement disorders associated with parkinsonism result primarily from a defect in the nigrostriatal pathway. Destruction of neurons in the substantia nigra causes this tract to degenerate, and as a result the dopamine that is normally secreted in the striatum is no longer present. The neurons that secrete acetylcholine remain functional and in the absence of dopamine become overactive, thus contributing to the motor symptoms that are characteristic of parkinsonism.[14]

Etiology. The alterations in motor function that characterize parkinsonism are seen in many different toxic and disease states. The most common form of parkinsonism is idiopathic Parkinson's disease (paralysis agitans), named after James Parkinson, who first described the disorder in 1817. The disease usually begins after age 50 years; most cases are diagnosed in the sixth and seventh decade of life. Parkinsonism can also develop as a postencephalitic syndrome, as a side effect of therapy with antipsychotic drugs that block dopamine receptors, as a toxic reaction to a chemical agent, or as an outcome of severe carbon monoxide poisoning. Symptoms of parkinsonism may also accompany conditions such as cerebral vascular disease, neoplasms, or degenerative neurologic diseases that structurally damage the nigrostriatal pathway.

Postencephalitic parkinsonism was a particular problem in the 1930s and 1940s, as a result of an outbreak of lethargic encephalitis (sleeping sickness) that occurred in 1914 to 1918.[15] Drug-induced parkinsonism can follow the taking of antipsychotic drugs in high doses (*e.g.,* phenothiazines and butyrophenones). These drugs block dopamine receptors and dopamine output by the cells of the substantia nigra. Of recent interest was the development of parkinsonism in a group of individuals who had attempted to make a narcotic drug and instead synthesized a compound called *MPTP* (1-methyl-4-phenyl-1,2,3,6-tetrahydropyridine).[16–18] This compound selectively destroys the dopaminergic neurons of the substantia nigra. This incident has led to investigations into the role of toxins, both those that are produced by the body as a part of metabolic processes and those that enter the body from outside sources, in the pathogenesis of Parkinson's disease.

Manifestations. Parkinson's disease often begins insidiously with weakness and tremor. Tremor of the distal segments of the limbs is an early symptom; it usually occurs at rest and involves a rhythmic alternating flexion and contraction of the muscles that produces the appearance of pill-rolling movements. The tremor is gradually followed by rigidity, which is most evident on passive joint movement, and involves jerky cogwheel type movements that require considerable energy to perform. Flexion contractions may occur as a result of the rigidity. In addition, there is slowness in initiating (bradykinesia) movements and difficulty in sudden unexpected stopping of voluntary movements and loss of unconscious associative movements. People with Parkinson's disease have difficulty initiating walking. When they walk, they lean forward with their head bent and take small, shuffling steps without swinging their arms, tend to move faster and faster, and stop only with difficulty.

As the disease progresses, the facial expression becomes stiff and masklike. There is loss of eye-blinking and failure to express emotion. The person may drool because of difficulty in moving the saliva to the back of the mouth and swallowing it. The speech is slow, monotonous, without modulation, and poorly articulated.

Because the basal ganglia also influence the autonomic nervous system, persons with Parkinson's disease often have excessive and uncontrolled sweating, sebaceous secretion, and salivation. Autonomic symptoms such as constipation, urinary incontinence, and lacrimation may also be present.

Dementia is an important feature associated with Parkinson's disease. It occurs in approximately 40% of persons with the disease and seems to occur independent of drug therapy.[19] The mental state of some persons with Parkinson's disease may be indistinguishable from that seen in Alzheimer's disease.[20] It has been suggested that many of the brain changes in both diseases may be due to degeneration of acetyl-choline-containing neurons in a region of the brain called the *nucleus basalis of Maynert,* which is the main source of cholinergic innervation of the cerebral cortex.[21] Persons with Parkinson's disease also have other neurochemical disturbances that might account for some of the features of dementia.

There are several stages in the progression of Parkinson's disease. The symptoms are usually noted first on one side of the body and progress to bilateral involvement, with early postural changes beginning 1 to 2 years after onset. The tremor often begins in one or both hands and then becomes generalized. Postural changes and gait disturbances continue to become more pronounced until the person has significant disability and requires constant care.

Treatment. The treatment of parkinsonism consists mainly of drug therapy and general supportive measures to provide emotional support and encouragement to continue as much physical activity as possible. Physical therapy and speech therapy are often helpful. The quality of life can often be improved by the provision of simple aids to activities of daily living, such as rails placed in strategic parts of the home and special table cutlery with large handles. Neural transplantation of autologous (self) adrenal medullary tissue into the basal ganglia has been performed experimentally.[21,22] However, it is still too early to determine if this procedure will become a viable treatment option for persons with parkinsonism.

Drug therapy. Antiparkinsonism drugs act in one of two ways: (1) to increase the functional ability of the underactive dopaminergic system, or (2) to reduce the excessive influence of excitatory cholinergic neurons on the extrapyramidal tract. The first group includes levodopa and Sinemet, amantadine (Symmetrel), and bromocriptine (Parlodel). Dopamine does not cross the blood–brain barrier. Administration of levodopa, a precursor of dopamine that does cross the blood–brain barrier, has yielded significant improvement in clinical symptoms of Parkinson's disease. The second group of drugs are the anticholinergic drugs. Because dopamine transmission is disrupted in Parkinson's disease, there is a preponderance of cholinergic activity, which is decreased with anticholinergic drugs.

Drugs that increase dopamine. The evidence of decreased dopamine levels in the striatum in Parkinson's disease led to the administration of large doses of L-dopa (L-dihydroxyphenylalanine) or the synthetic compound levodopa, which is absorbed from the intestinal tract, crosses the blood-brain barrier, and is converted to dopamine by centrally acting dopa decarboxylase. Unfortunately, only a small percentage of (1–3%) of administered levodopa actually enters the brain unaltered; the rest is metabolized outside the brain, predominantly by decarboxylation to dopamine, which cannot cross the blood–brain barrier.[23] This means that large doses of levodopa are needed when the drug is used alone, and this leads to many side effects. However, when levodopa is given in combination with a dopa decarboxylase inhibitor (carbidopa) that does not cross the blood–brain barrier, the peripheral metabolism of levodopa is reduced, plasma levels of levodopa are higher, plasma half-life is longer, more dopa is available for the entry into the brain, and a smaller dose is needed.

Sinemet is a preparation containing levodopa and carbidopa. Individuals are started on very small doses of Sinemet and the dose is gradually increased until therapeutic levels are reached. Some of the side effects of levodopa may be relatively mild when the drug is given in combination with carbidopa to reduce its extracerebral metabolism. Side effects such as nausea and vomiting, cardiac dysrhythmias, and postural hypotension are considerably reduced when Sinemet is used. Dyskinesias occur in about 80% of persons receiving levodopa for long periods and appears to be dose-related.[24] Other adverse effects of levodopa include depression, restlessness, somnolence, confusion, hallucinations, nightmares, changes in mood, and other changes in behavior or personality that occur later in the course of treatment and become more common with time. Dyskinesias and behavioral side effects are more common in persons receiving levodopa in combination with carbidopa rather than levodopa alone, presumably because higher levels are reached in the brain.

A later complication of levodopa treatment is the "on-off phenomenon," in which frequent abrupt and unpredictable fluctuations in motor performance occur during the day. These fluctuations include periods of dyskinesias (the "on" response) and periods of marked bradykinesia (the "off" response). Some fluctuations are due to the timing of drug administration, in which the "on" response coincides with peak drug levels and the "off" response with low drug levels.[24]

Amantadine (Symmetrel) acts by augmenting release of dopamine from the remaining intact dopaminergic terminals in the nigrostriatal pathway of persons with Parkinson's disease. It is used to treat persons with mild symptoms, but no disability. Bromocriptine (Parlodel) acts directly to stimulate dopamine receptors. It is used as adjunctive therapy in Parkinson's disease. It is often used for persons who have become refractory to L-dopa or have developed an on-off phenomenon.

Anticholinergic drugs. Prior to the discovery of levodopa, anticholinergic drugs were the mainstay of treatment for parkinsonism. Today, anticholinergic drugs are used primarily in mild cases or when levodopa is not tolerated. Treatment is started with a small dose of one preparation and the dose increased until benefit occurs or side effects develop. If treatment is ineffective, the drug is gradually withdrawn and another preparation tried. Ethopropazine (Parsidol) is probably the most helpful drug in this group for relieving tremor.[27] Other anticholinergic drugs are benztropine (Cogentin), biperiden (Akineton), chlorphenoxamine (Phenoxene), cycrimine (Pagitane), Orphenadrine (Disipal, Norflex), procyclidine (Kemadrin), and trihexyphenidyl (Artane).[27] The anticholinergic drugs lessen the tremors and rigidity and afford some improvement of function. However, their potency seems to decrease over time and increasing the dosage merely increases side effects such as blurred vision, dry mouth, bowel and bladder problems, and some mental changes.

In summary, degenerative diseases are disorders that selectively affect one or more functional systems of neurons, while leaving others intact. Dementia is a degenerative syndrome in which intellectual deterioration is severe enough to interfere with occupational and social performance. Dementia can be caused by any disorder that permanently damages large association areas of the cerebral hemispheres, including Alzheimer's disease, multi-infarct dementia, Pick's disease, Creutzfeldt-Jakob disease, and Huntington's disease. Multi-infarct dementia is associated with vascular disease, and Pick's disease with atrophy of the frontal and temporal lobes. Creutzfeldt-Jakob disease is a rare transmissible form of dementia. Wernicke-Korsakoff's syndrome is due to chronic alcoholism. Huntington's disease is a rare hereditary disorder characterized by chronic progressive chorea, psychological change, and dementia. By far the most common cause of dementia (50% to 70%) is Alzheimer's disease. The condition is a major health problem among the elderly. It is characterized by cortical atrophy and loss of neurons, the presence of neuritic plaques, granulovacuolar degeneration, and cerebrovascular amyloid. The disease follows an insidious and progressive course that begins with memory impairment and terminates in inability to recognize family or friends and loss of bodily functions.

Parkinson's disease is a disorder of the basal ganglia that results in variable combinations of bradykinesia, rigidity, tremor, and impaired automatic postural responses to position and movement. The striatal structures of the basal ganglia modulates the excitatory input that travels from the thalamus to the motor cortex, particularly the premotor cortex and supplementary motor cortex. Parkinsonism is characterized by a defect in the nigrostriatal pathway and a resultant decrease in dopamine levels in the striatum. The striatum also contains many cholinergic interneurons that normally oppose the dopaminergic input. In the absence of dopamine, these neurons become overactive, causing the motor symptoms that are characteristic of parkinsonism. Treatment consists of medications to increase brain dopamine levels or to decrease acetylcholine with anticholinergic agents.

Demyelinating diseases

The loss of myelin sheaths with relative preservation of the demyelinated nerve axons is characteristic of a group of neurologic disorders called *demyelinating diseases.* The most common of these is multiple sclerosis.

In the central nervous system (CNS), myelin is formed by the oligodendrocytes, chiefly those lying between the nerve fibers and the white matter. This function is equivalent to that of the Schwann cells in the peripheral nervous system (see Chapter 46). The properties of the myelin sheath—high electrical resistance and low capacitance—permit it to function as an electrical insulator. Small uninsulated junctures, called the *nodes of Ranvier,* exist between the cells of the myelin sheath. Impulses jump from node to node, thus speeding conduction of impulses and reducing the metabolic work required to maintain the ionic gradients necessary for neural conduction.

The process of myelination of the CNS begins early in the fourth month of fetal life. It is incomplete at birth and some fibers continue to become myelinated during the first year of life.[28] The total amount of myelin increases from birth to maturity. Although myelin is relatively stable, there is continual removal and replacement of individual components. Studies indicate that the myelin formed early in life is the most stable and that newly formed myelin is more easily broken down and replaced.[29] There are two major myelin proteins, proteolipid protein and basic protein, that are incorporated in the myelin sheath and are involved in the replacement process. Myelin enzymes, capable of degrading myelin proteins, have been identified. These enzymes may be involved in normal catabolic processes and could have a role in some forms of demyelination.[29]

Demyelinated nerve fibers display a variety of conduction abnormalities ranging from decreased conduction velocity to conduction blocks. In the demyelinated fiber, conduction velocity is decreased so that the threshold is reached very slowly or not at all.[30]

Multiple sclerosis

Multiple sclerosis is a major cause of neurologic disability among young and middle-aged adults. The disease is rarely diagnosed in persons under age 15 or over 55 years, with a peak incidence of onset around the age of 30.[31] Estimates of the total number of cases of multiple sclerosis in the United States range from 123,000 to 250,000. In approximately 60% of the cases, the disease is characterized by exacerbations and remissions over many years from several different sites in the CNS. Initially, there is normal or near-normal neurologic function between exacerbations. As the disease progresses, there is less improvement between exacerbations and increasing neurologic dysfunction.

Pathophysiology

Multiple sclerosis is characterized by demyelination in the white matter of the brain (usually periventricular), brain stem, or spinal cord. Sharp-edged demyelinated patches, ranging from 1 mm to 4 cm, are macroscopically visible throughout the white matter of the central nervous system.[32] These lesions, which represent the end result of acute myelin breakdown, are called *plaques.* Oligodendrocytes (see Chapter 46) are decreased in number and may be absent, especially in older lesions. The sequence of myelin breakdown is not well understood although it is known that the lesions contain small amounts of myelin basic proteins, increased amounts of proteolytic enzymes, macrophages, lymphocytes, and plasma cells. Acute, subacute, and chronic sclerotic lesions are scattered throughout the CNS.

The recent use of MRI has shown that the lesions of multiple sclerosis may occur in two stages: a first stage that involves the sequential development of small inflammatory lesions and a second stage during which the lesions extend and consolidate and during which both demyelination and gliosis (scar tissue development) occur.[33] It is not known whether the inflammatory process, present during the first stage, is directed against the myelin or against the oligodendrocytes. Remyelination of the nervous system was considered to be impossible until a few years ago. Recent evidence has shown that remyelination can occur in the CNS if the process that initiated the demyelination is halted before the oligodendrocyte dies.[29]

Etiology

The cause of multiple sclerosis remains unknown. Geographic distribution and migration studies suggest an environmental influence. The disease is more prevalent in the colder northern latitudes; it is more common in the northern Atlantic states, the Great Lakes region, and the Pacific Northwest than in the southern parts of the United States. Other high-incidence areas include northern Europe, Great Britain, southern Australia, and New Zealand. Migration studies have shown that persons who move from a high-risk area tend to retain the risk of their birthplace if they move after age 15 or adopt the risk of their new home if they migrate as children.[1]

There is also a family tendency in some cases of multiple sclerosis, suggesting a genetic influence on susceptibility. However, studies of monozygotic twins have found that the second twin develops the disease only in 30% of cases, suggesting that an exogenous or environmental trigger such as an infectious agent is required to produce the disease.[30] There is also a strong association between multiple sclerosis and certain HLA antigens (see Chapter 11).[1]

Many believe that the disease has an immunologic basis, but this has not been confirmed. The demyelination process in multiple sclerosis is marked by prominent lymphocytic invasion in the lesion. Both T_4 helper cells and T_8 suppressor cells are present. In some persons a sharp decline in the suppressor T-cell population in the blood accompanies exacerbations of the disease.[1]

Manifestations and clinical course

The interruption of neural conduction in the demyelinated nerves is manifested by a variety of symptoms depending on the location and duration of the lesion. Areas commonly affected by multiple sclerosis are the optic chiasm, optic nerves, brain stem, cerebellum, the corticospinal tracts, and posterior cell columns of the spinal cord. Typically, an otherwise healthy person suffers an acute or subacute episode of paresthesias, optic neuritis (visual clouding or loss of vision in part of the visual field with pain on movement of the globe), diplopia, or paralysis. Paresthesias are evidenced as numbness and tingling on the face or involved extremities. Lhermitte's symptom is an electric-shock–like tingling down the back and onto the legs that is produced by flexion of the neck. Other common symptoms are abnormal gait, bladder dysfunction, vertigo, nystagmus, and speech disturbance. The symptoms are usually painless, last for several days to weeks, and then completely or partially resolve. After a period of normal or relatively normal function, new symptoms appear. Psychological manifestations, such as mood swings, may represent a psychological reaction to the nature of the disease or, more likely, involvement of the white matter of the cerebral cortex. Depression, euphoria, inattentiveness, apathy, forgetfulness, and loss of memory may occur.

Small increases in body temperature can temporarily worsen existing neurologic deficits in persons with multiple sclerosis by producing a block of impulse conduction in demyelinated nerve fibers. This observation forms the basis for the hot bath test, which is sometimes used to aid in the diagnosis of multiple sclerosis.[34] The test is performed by having the person recline in a whirlpool or hot bath. The water level is adjusted so that both axillae are submerged and the temperature of the water is raised to 110°F while neurologic function is monitored. If new neurologic deficits are observed, the test is terminated and the water is cooled to reverse the conduction block and its attendant symptoms. Prolonged neurologic sequelae have been observed in persons with multiple sclerosis following unintentional exposure to high environmental temperatures such as those encountered in a hot tub or while sunbathing.[35,36]

A small percentage of people develop an acute form of multiple sclerosis that progresses rapidly with incomplete remissions of short duration. This form of multiple sclerosis can be fatal within a few months or years. There is also a benign form of the disease that has a few mild exacerbations followed by complete recovery. In the benign form, a person remains relatively asymptomatic without neurologic dysfunction for many years. There may also be a subclinical form of the disease, since demyelination has been observed in asymptomatic persons on autopsy.[32] Because of the varied clinical courses of multiple sclerosis, persons in whom the disease is recently diagnosed have some justification for optimism.

Diagnosis

The diagnosis of multiple sclerosis is difficult because there is no specific laboratory test for the disease, manifestations are variable, and there may be lengthy delays between the first appearance of symptoms and recurrence. A definite diagnosis of multiple sclerosis requires evidence of two attacks and clinical findings consistent with two separate lesions or clinical evidence of one lesion and paraclinical (*e.g.,* MRI or CT scans) evidence of a second lesion.[37] The attacks must each last a minimum of 24 hours, be separated by a period of at least 1 month, and be unexplained by other mechanisms.[37]

Although no laboratory test can be used to diagnose multiple sclerosis, examination of the cerebrospinal fluid (CSF) is helpful. A large percentage of patients with multiple sclerosis have elevated IgG levels and some have oligoclonal patterns (discrete electrophoretic bands) even with normal IgG levels. There may also be a mild increase in total protein or lymphocytes in the CSF. These tests can be altered in a variety of inflammatory neurologic disorders and are not specific for multiple sclerosis.

Recently, electrophysiologic evaluations (evoked potential studies) and CT scans have aided in the identification and documentation of lesions; but they still do not provide information about the cause of the lesions. MRI studies can detect the multiplicity of lesions even when CT scans are normal. A computer-assisted method of MRI has been developed that measures lesion size. Many new areas of myelin abnormality are asymptomatic. Serial MRI studies can be done to detect asymptomatic lesions, monitor the progress of existing lesions, and evaluate the effectiveness of treatment.

Treatment

The variety of symptoms, unpredictable course, and lack of specific diagnostic methods have made the evaluation and treatment of multiple sclerosis difficult. Persons who are minimally affected by the disorder require no specific treatment. Corticotropin (ACTH) and corticosteroids can shorten the duration of an acute attack. Long-term administration does not, however, appear to alter the course of the disease and may have harmful side effects. Several studies have indicated that intensive immunosuppressive therapy with intravenous cyclophosphamide may help arrest the chronic progressive course of active multiple sclerosis. Plasmapheresis has proved beneficial in some cases.

The primary treatment of multiple sclerosis is symptomatic. Pharmacologic treatment may include (1) dantrolene (Dantrium), baclofen (Lioresal), or diazepam (Valium) for spasticity; (2) cholinergic drugs for bladder problems; and (3) antidepressant drugs for depression. The person should be encouraged to live as healthy a life-style as possible, including good nutrition and adequate rest and relaxation. Physical therapy may help maintain muscle tone. Every effort should be made to avoid excessive fatigue, physical deterioration, emotional stress, and extremes of environmental temperature, which may precipitate exacerbation of the disease.

In summary, multiple sclerosis is an example of a demyelinating disease in which there is a slowly progressive breakdown of myelin and formation of plaques, but sparing of the axis cylinder of the neuron. The cause of multiple sclerosis remains unknown. Geographic distributions and migration studies suggest an environmental influence. Interruption of neural conduction in multiple sclerosis is manifested by a variety of disabling signs and symptoms that depend on the neurons that are affected. The most common symptoms are paresthesias, optic neuritis, and motor weakness. The disease is usually characterized by exacerbations and remissions. Initially, near-normal function returns between exacerbations. The variety of symptoms, course of the disease, and lack of specific diagnostic tests make diagnosis and treatment of the disease difficult. At present treatment is largely symptomatic.

Brain tumors

Brain tumors account for 2% of all cancer deaths. The American Cancer Society reports that there are over 14,000 new cases and over 10,000 deaths from brain and CNS cancers each year.[38] Another 67,000 patients (18% of all cancer patients) develop metastases to the brain from other sites.[39] In children, brain tumors are second only to leukemia as a cause of death from cancer and kill about 1600 children and young adults annually.

Brain tumors can arise from any structure within the cranial cavity. Most begin in brain tissue (neurons or neuroglia), but the pituitary, the pineal

region, and the meninges are also sites of tumor development. Furthermore, the brain can be the site for metastatic spread of cancers that arise outside the nervous system. Primary intracranial neoplasms (those arising within the intracranial cavity) can be classified according to site of origin and histologic type (Chart 53-3). Benign vs malignant has its own meaning when it relates to brain tumors. In most neoplasms, the term *malignant* is used to describe the lack of cell differentiation, the invasive nature of the tumor, and its ability to metastasize. In the brain, however, even a well-differentiated and histologically benign tumor may grow and cause death because of its location.

The neuroglial tumors make up 50% of all primary brain tumors in adults. They occur most commonly in the cerebrum, most frequently in persons between 40 and 60 years of age. Collectively, the neoplasms of astrocyte origin are the most common type of primary brain tumor in the adult; they fall into three clinicopathologic groups: (1) astrocytomas, including glioblastoma multiforme, (2) brain stem glioma, and (3) pilocyte astrocytoma.[1] Astrocytomas are graded from I to IV, with grade I comprising well-differentiated astrocytes and grade IV comprising poorly differentiated and pleomorphic cells (see Chapter 5). The term *glioblastoma multiforme* is commonly used as a synonym for highly malignant forms of astrocytoma, namely grades III and IV. Brain stem gliomas occur in the first two decades of life and make up about 20% of brain tumors in this age group.[1] Pilocytic astrocytomas are distinguished from other astrocytomas by their cellular appearance and their benign behavior. Typically, they occur in children

---

Chart 53–3: Types of primary brain tumors

Tumors of neuroglial cells
 Astrocytoma
  Glioblastoma multiforme
  Brain stem glioma
  Pilocyte astrocytoma
 Oligodendroglioma
 Ependymoma
 Mixed gliomas

Tumors of primitive brain cells
 Medulloblastoma

Tumors of neurons
 Neuroblastoma
 Ganglion cell tumors

Tumors arising from supporting tissues
 Meningioma and tumors of related tissue

Pineal tumors

Pituitary tumors

Developmental tumors
 Hemangioblastoma and tumors of blood vessel origin
 Craniopharyngiomas

and young adults and are usually located in the cerebellum, but can also be found in the floor and walls of the third ventricle, the optic chiasm and nerves, and occasionally in the cerebral hemispheres. Oligodendrogliomas comprise about 5% of glial tumors; they are most common in middle life and are found in the cerebral hemispheres.[1] Ependymomas are derived from the single layer of epithelium that lines the ventricles and spinal canal. Although they can occur at any age, they are most likely to occur in the first two decades of life and most frequently affect the fourth ventricle; they constitute 5% to 10% of brain tumors in this age group.[1] The spinal cord is the most common site for ependymomas in middle life.

Meningiomas develop from the meningothelial cells of the arachnoid and are thus outside the brain. They comprise about 20% of primary brain tumors and generally have their onset in the middle or later years of life.[1] Meningiomas are slow-growing, well-circumscribed, and often highly vascular tumors. They are usually benign and complete removal is possible if the tumor does not involve vital structures. Pituitary adenomas comprise 12% to 14% of brain tumors; they are usually nonmalignant.[1] Medulloblastomas, which consist of primitive, undifferentiated neuronal cells, make up 30% of primary brain tumors in children.[1] Craniopharyngiomas are composed of cells derived from the embryonic notochord and are tumors of children and young adults. They commonly occur in the midline of the nervous system and are highly invasive, making surgical removal difficult or impossible.

The cause of brain tumors is unknown. Childhood tumors are considered to be developmental in origin. Although a number of chemical and viral agents can cause brain tumors in laboratory animals, there is no evidence that these agents cause brain cancer in humans.

—— ## Manifestations

Intracranial tumors give rise to focal disturbances in brain function and increased intracranial pressure. Focal disturbances occur because of brain compression, tumor infiltration, disturbances in blood flow, and brain edema. Alterations in brain function due to focal lesions, increased intracranial pressure, and cerebral edema are discussed in Chapter 50.

Tumors may be located intra-axially (within brain tissue) or extra-axially (outside brain tissue). Disturbances in brain function are generally greatest with fast-growing, infiltrative, intra-axial tumors because of compression, infiltration, and necrosis of brain tissue. Extra-axial tumors, such as meningiomas, may reach a large size without producing signs and symptoms. Cysts may form within tumors and contribute to brain compression. Cerebral edema develops around brain tumors, is usually of the vasogenic type, and is characterized by increased brain water and expanded extracellular fluid. The edema is thought to result from increased permeability of tumor capillary endothelial cells.

Because the volume of the intracranial cavity is fixed, brain tumors cause generalized intracranial pressure when they reach sufficient size. Tumors can obstruct the flow of cerebral spinal fluid in the ventricular cavities and produce hydrocephalic dilatation of the proximal ventricles and atrophy of the cerebral hemispheres. Complete compensation of ventricular volumes can occur with very slow growing tumors, but with rapidly growing tumors increased intracranial pressure becomes an early sign. Depending on the location of the tumor, brain displacement and herniation of the uncus or cerebellum may occur (see Chapter 50).

The clinical manifestations of brain tumors depend on the size and location of the tumor. General signs and symptoms include headache, nausea and vomiting, mental changes, papilledema and visual disturbances, alterations in sensory and motor function, and seizures.

The brain itself is insensitive to pain. The headache that accompanies brain tumors results from compression or distortion of pain-sensitive dural or vascular structures. It may be felt on the same side of the head as the tumor, but is more commonly diffuse in nature. In the early stages, the headache, which is caused by irritation, compression, and traction on the dural sinuses or blood vessels, is mild and occurs in the morning when the person awakens. It usually disappears when the person has been up for a short time. The headache becomes more constant as the tumor enlarges and is often worsened by coughing, bending, or sudden movements of the head.

Vomiting occurs with or without preceding nausea and is a common symptom of increased intracranial pressure and brain stem compression. Direct stimulation of the vomiting center, which is located in the medulla, may contribute to the vomiting that occurs with brain tumors. The vomiting is often projectile in nature. Vomiting due to a brain tumor is usually unrelated to meals and is often, but not always, associated with headache.

Papilledema (edema of the optic disk) results from increased intracranial pressure and obstruction of the cerebral spinal fluid pathways. It is associated with decreased visual acuity, diplopia, and deficits in the visual fields. Visual defects associated with papilledema are often the reason that persons with brain tumor seek medical care.

Personality and mental changes are common with brain tumors. Persons with brain tumor are often irritable initially and later become quiet and apathetic. They may become forgetful, seem preoccupied, and appear to be psychologically depressed. Because of the mental changes, a psychiatric consultation may be sought before a diagnosis of brain tumor is made.

Focal signs and symptoms are determined by the location of the tumor. Tumors arising in the frontal lobe may grow to large size, produce an increase in intracranial pressure, and cause signs of generalized brain dysfunction before focal signs are present. On the other hand, tumors that impinge on the visual system cause visual loss or visual field defects long before generalized signs develop. Certain areas of the brain have a relatively low threshold for seizure activity; tumors arising in relatively silent areas of the brain may produce focal epileptogenic discharges. Temporal lobe tumors often produce seizures as their first symptom. Hallucinations of smell or hearing as well as déjà vu phenomenon are common focal manifestations of temporal lobe tumors. Brain stem tumors commonly produce upper and lower motor neuron signs, such as weakness of facial muscles and ocular palsies that occur with or without involvement of sensory or long motor tracts. Cerebellar tumors often cause ataxia of gait.

—— Diagnosis and treatment

Diagnostic procedures for brain tumor include physical and neurologic examinations, visual field and funduscopic examination, CT scans and MRI, skull x-rays, technetium pertechnetate brain scans, electroencephalography, and cerebral angiography. Physical examination is used to assess motor and sensory function. Since the visual pathways travel through many areas of the cerebral lobes, detection of visual field defects can provide information about the location of tumors. A funduscopic examination is done to determine the presence of papilledema. CT scans have become the screening procedure of choice for diagnosing and localizing brain tumors as well as other intracranial masses. MRI scans may be diagnostic when a clinically suspected tumor is not detected by CT scanning. Skull x-rays are used to detect calcified areas within a neoplasm or erosion of skull structures due to tumors. Brain tumors tend to disrupt the blood–brain barrier; as a result the uptake of the radioactive isotope used in a brain scan is increased within a tumor. About 75% of persons with a brain tumor have an abnormal electroencephalogram; in some cases, the results of the test can be used to localize the tumor. Cerebral angiography can be used to locate a tumor and visualize its vascular supply, information that is important when planning surgery.

The three general methods for treatment of brain tumors are surgery, radiation, and chemotherapy.[40] The initial treatment of most brain tumors is surgical excision. Removal may be limited by the location of the tumor and its invasiveness. Most malignant brain tumors respond to external irradiation. Radiation can increase longevity and, at times, can allay symptoms when tumors recur. The treatment dose depends on the tumor's histologic type and radioresponsiveness, and on the anatomic site and the level of tolerance of the surrounding tissue. The use of chemotherapy for brain tumors is still being investigated.

In summary, brain tumors account for 2% of all cancer deaths and are the second most common type of cancer in children. Brain tumors can arise primarily from intracranial structures, and in addition tumors from other parts of the body often metastasize to the brain. Primary brain tumors can arise from any structure within the cranial cavity. Most begin in brain tissue, but the pituitary, the pineal region, and the meninges are also sites of tumor development. Brain tumors give rise to focal disturbances in brain function and increased intracranial pressure. Focal disturbances result from brain compression, tumor infiltration, disturbances in blood flow, and cerebral edema. The clinical manifestations of brain tumor depend on the size and location of the tumor. General signs and symptoms include headache, nausea and vomiting, mental changes, papilledema and visual disturbances, alterations in motor and sensory function, and seizures. Diagnostic tests include physical examination, visual field testing and funduscopic examination, CT scans, MRI studies, skull x-rays, brain scans, electroencephalography, and cerebral angiography. Treatment includes surgery, radiation, and chemotherapy.

References

1. Robbins SL, Kumar V: Basic Pathology, 4th ed, pp 746, 733, 749–750. Philadelphia, WB Saunders, 1987
2. American Psychiatric Association: Diagnostic and Statistical Manual of Mental Disorders, 3rd ed, rev. Washington, DC, American Psychiatric Association, 1987
3. Kwentus JA, Hart R, Lingon W, et al: Alzheimer's disease. Am J Med 81:91, 1986
4. Hyman BT, Van Hoesen GW, Kromer I, et al: Understanding the memory loss in Alzheimer's disease. Am J Alzheimer's Care and Related Disorders 1:18, 1986
5. Hasan MK, Baker DJ: Alzheimer's disease: Recent advances. West Virginia Med J 83:427, 1987
6. Katzman R: Alzheimer's disease. N Engl J Med 314:964, 1986
7. Karlinsky H: Alzheimer's disease in Down's syndrome. J Am Geriatrics Soc 34:728, 1986
8. Candy JC, Edwardson JA, Klinowski J, et al: Co-localization of aluminum and silicon in senile plaques: Implications for the neurochemical pathology of Alzheimer's disease. In Traber, Gispen WH (ed): Senile Dementia of the Alzheimer Type, pp 183–197. Berlin, Springer-Verlag, 1985
9. Matteson MA, McConnell ES: Gerontological Nursing, pp 249–254. Philadelphia, JB Lippincott, 1988

10. McKhann G, Drachman D, Folstein M, et al: Clinical diagnosis of Alzheimer's disease: Report of the NINCDS-ADRDA Work Group under the Auspices of the Department of Health and Human Services Task Force on Alzheimer's Disease. Neurology 34:939, 1984
11. Brown P, Gajdusek C, Gibbs CJ, et al: Potential epidemic of Creutzfeldt-Jakob disease from human growth hormone therapy. N Engl J Med 313:728, 1985
12. Rappaport EB: Iatrogenic Creutzfeldt-Jakob disease. Neurology 37:1520, 1987
13. Martin JB: Huntington's disease: Pathogenesis and management. N Engl J Med 315:1267, 1987
14. Guyton A: Medical Physiology 7th ed, p 626. Philadelphia, WB Saunders, 1986
15. Robbins SL, Cotran RS, Kumar V: Pathologic Basis of Disease 3rd ed, p 1417. Philadelphia, WB Saunders, 1984
16. Ballard PA, Tetreed JW, Langston JW: Permanent human parkinsonism due to 1-methyl-4-phenyl 1,2,3,6-tetrahydropydrine (MPTP): Seven cases. Neurology 35:949, 1985
17. Langston JW: MPTP: Insights into the etiology of Parkinson's disease. Eur Neurol 26 (Suppl 1):2, 1987
18. Lewin R: Parkinson's disease: An environmental cause? Science 229:257, 1985
19. Cummings T: The dementia of Parkinson's disease. Eur Neurol 28 (Suppl 1):15, 1988
20. Hakim AM, Mathieson G: Dementia in Parkinson disease: A neuropathologic study. Neurology (Minneap) 29:1209, 1979
21. Whitehouse PJ, Hedreen JC, White CL, et al: Basal forebrain neurons in the dementia of Parkinson's disease. Ann Neurol 13:243, 1983
22. Backlund EO, Granberg PO, Hamberger B, et al: Transplantation of adrenal medullary tissue to striatum in parkinsonism. J Neurosurg 62:169, 1985
23. Merz B: Adrenal-to-brain transplants improve the prognosis for Parkinson's disease. JAMA 257:2691, 1987
24. Katzung BG: Basic and Clinical Pharmacology, p 306–309. Norwalk, CT, Appleton & Lange, 1987
25. Lang AE, Blair RDG: Parkinson's disease in 1984: An update. Can Med Assoc J 131:1031, 1984
26. Nutt JG, Woodward WR, Hammerstad JP: The "on-off" phenomenon in Parkinson's disease. N Engl J Med 310:483, 1984
27. Aminoff MJ: Nervous system. In Schroeder SA, Krupp MA, Tierney LM: Current Medical Diagnosis & Treatment, p 596. Norwalk CT, Appleton & Lange, 1988
28. Cormack DH: Ham's Histology, 9th ed, pp 344–345. Philadelphia, JB Lippincott, 1987
29. Norton WT: Recent advances in myelin biochemistry. Ann New York Acad Sci 70:5–10, 1984
30. Gonzalez-Scarano F, Spellman RS, Nathanson N: Epidemiology. In McDonald WE, Silberg DH: Multiple Sclerosis, pp 37–55. Boston, Butterworth, 1986
31. Waxman SG: Membranes, myelin and the pathophysiology of multiple sclerosis. N Engl J Med, 306:1529, 1982
32. McFarlin DE, McFarland HF: Multiple sclerosis. N Engl J Med 307:1183, 1982
33. Paty DW: Multiple sclerosis: Assessment of disease progression and effects of treatment. Can J Neurol 14:518, 1987
34. Davis FA: The hot tub test in multiple sclerosis. pp 44–48 In Poser DW, Scheinber L, McDonald WI, Ebers GC: The diagnosis of multiple sclerosis. New York, Thieme-Stratton, 1984
35. Berger JR, Sheremata WA: Persistent neurological deficit precipitated by hot bath test in multiple sclerosis. JAMA 249:171, 1983
36. Berger JR, Sheremata WA: Letter to the editor. JAMA 253:203, 1985
37. Poser C, Paty D, Scheinber L, et al: New diagnostic criteria for multiple sclerosis. Ann Neurol 13:227, 1983
38. American Cancer Society. Cancer Facts & Figures—1988. New York, American Cancer Society, 1988
39. Hickey J: The Clinical Practice of Neurological and Neurosurgical Nursing, pp 327–345. Philadelphia, JB Lippincott, 1981
40. McDonald JV, Salazar OM, Rubin P, et al: Central nervous system tumors. In Rubin P (ed): Clinical Oncology 6th ed, pp 267–272. New York, American Cancer Society, 1983

Bibliography

Rivera VM: Multiple sclerosis. Is the mystery beginning to unfold. Postgrad Med 79:217, 1986

Conneally PM: Huntington's disease. Genetics and epidemiology. Am J Hum Genet 36:506, 1984

Davies P: Neurochemical studies: An update on Alzheimer's disease. J Clin Psych 49, no 5 (Suppl):23, 1988

Davis L: Huntington's disease: Clues to the culprit. Sci News 130 (Oct 11):229, 1986

Davis L, Mohs RC: Cholinergic drugs in Alzheimer's disease. N Engl J Med 315:1286, 1986

Edwards DD: Still stalking MS. Sci News 132 (Oct 10):234, 1987

Delgado JM, Billo JM: Care of the patient with Parkinson's disease: Surgical and nursing interventions. J Neurosci Nurs 20:142, 1988

Glickstein JK: Therapeutic interventions in Alzheimer's disease. Rockville, MD, Aspen, 1988

Langstonal JW: Parkinson's disease: Current view. Am J Fam Pract 35:201, 1987

Larner AJ: Aetiological role of viruses in multiple sclerosis: A review. J Royal Soc Med 79:412, 1986

Lees AJ: L-dopa treatment and Parkinson's disease. Q J Med 59:230, 1986

Levine J: Do they really want to know? A new test confounds potential Huntington's disease victims. Time 128 (Oct 20):80, 1986

Poser CM: Pathogenesis of multiple sclerosis: A critical reappraisal. Acta Neuropathologica 71:1, 1986

Sayetta RB: Theories of the etiology of multiple sclerosis: A critical review. J Clin Lab Immunol 21(2):55, 1986

Schoenberg BS: Environmental risk factors for Parkinson's disease: The epidemiologic evidence. Can J Neurol Sci 14:407, 1987

Yanagisawa N: Pathophysiology of involuntary movements in Parkinson's disease. Eur Neurol 26:30, 1987

Stern Y, Mayeux R, Sano M, et al: Predictors of disease course in patients with probable Alzheimer's disease. Neurology 37:1649, 1987

Weinshenker BG, Ebers GC: The natural history of multiple sclerosis. Can J Neurol Sci 14:255, 1987

Wurtman RJ: Alzheimer's disease. Sci Am 252:62, 1985

Alterations in Skeletal Support and Movement

CHAPTER 54

Structure and Function of the Skeletal System

Characteristics of skeletal tissue
  Bone
    Types of bone
    Bone cells
    Classification of bones
    Bone marrow
    Periosteum and endosteum

Cartilage
Tendons and ligaments
Joints and articulations
  Synarthroses
  Amphiarthroses

Diarthroses
  Synovium and synovial fluid
  Articular cartilage
  Blood supply
  Innervation
  Bursae
  Intra-articular menisci

Objectives

After you have studied this chapter, you should be able to meet the following objectives:

_____ List the common components of bone, cartilage, and the dense connective tissue of ligaments and tendons.

_____ Compare the properties of the intercellular collagen and elastic fibers of skeletal tissue.

_____ Name and state the function of the four types of bone cells.

_____ Draw a long bone, and label the diaphysis, epiphysis, and metaphysis.

_____ State the location and function of the periosteum and the endosteum.

_____ Compare bone and cartilage in terms of their structure and function.

_____ Cite the characteristics and name at least one location of elastic cartilage, hyaline cartilage, and fibrocartilage.

_____ Define a *tendon* and a *ligament*.

_____ Name the three kinds of joints, and give one example of each type.

_____ Describe the source of blood supply to a diarthrodial joint.

_____ Explain why pain is often experienced in all the joints of an extremity when only a single joint is affected by a disease process.

_____ Describe the structure and function of a bursa.

_____ Explain the pathology associated with a torn meniscus of the knee.

Without the skeletal system, movement in the external environment would not be possible. The bones of the skeletal system serve as a framework for the attachment of muscles, tendons, and ligaments. The skeletal system protects and maintains soft tissues in their proper position, provides stability for the body, and maintains the body's shape. The bones act as a storage reservoir for calcium, and the central cavity of some bones contains the hematopoietic connective tissue in which blood cells are formed.

The skeletal system consists of the axial and appendicular skeleton (Figure 54-1). The axial skeleton, which is composed of the bones of the skull, thorax, and vertebral column, forms the axis of the body. The appendicular skeleton consists of the bones of the upper and lower extremities, including the shoulder and hip. For our purposes, the skeletal system is considered to include the bones and cartilage of the axial and appendicular skeleton as well as the connective tissue structures (ligaments and tendons) that connect the bones and join muscles to bone.

Characteristics of skeletal tissue

The tissues found in bones, cartilage, tendons, and ligaments have many things in common. Each of these connective tissue types consists of living cells, nonliving intercellular protein fibers, and an amorphous, or shapeless, ground substance. The tissue cells are responsible for secreting and maintaining the intercellular substances in which they are housed. These substances provide the structural characteristics of the tissue. For example, the intercellular matrix of bone is impregnated with calcium salts, providing the hardness that is characteristic of this tissue.

Two main types of intercellular fibers are found in skeletal tissue: collagenous and elastic. Collagen is an inelastic and insoluble fibrous protein. Because of its molecular configuration, collagen has great tensile strength; the breaking point of collagenous fibers found in human tendons is reached with a force of several hundred kilograms per square centimeter.[1] Fresh collagen is colorless, and tissues that contain large numbers of collagenous fibers generally appear white. It is the collagen fibers in tendons and ligaments that give these structures their white color. Elastin is the major component of elastic fibers that allows them to stretch several times their length and rapidly return to their original shape when the tension is released. Ligaments and structures that must undergo repeated stretching contain a high proportion of elastic fibers.

Bone

Bone is connective tissue in which the intercellular matrix has been impregnated with inorganic calcium salts so that it has great tensile and compressible strength but is light enough to be moved by coordinated muscle contractions. The intercellular matrix is composed of two types of substances—organic matter and inorganic salts. The organic matter, including bone cells, blood vessels, and nerves, constitutes about one-third of the dry weight of bone; the inorganic salts make up the other two-thirds.

The organic matter consists primarily of collagen fibers embedded in an amorphous ground substance. The inorganic matter consists of hydroxyapatite, an insoluble macrocrystalline structure of calcium phosphate salts, and small amounts of calcium carbonate and calcium fluoride. Bone may also take up lead and other heavy metals, thereby removing these toxic substances from the circulation. This can be viewed as a protective mechanism. The antibiotic tetracycline drugs are readily bound to calcium deposited in newly formed bones and teeth. When tetracycline is given during pregnancy, it can be deposited in the teeth of the fetus, causing discoloration and deformity. Similar changes can occur if the drug is given for long periods to children under 6 years of age.

Types of bone

There are two types of mature bones, cancellous and compact bone (Figure 54-2). Both types are formed in layers and are therefore called lamellar bone. Cancellous, or spongy, bone is found in the interior of bones and is composed of trabeculae, or spicules, of bone, which form a lattice-like pattern. These lattice-like structures are lined with osteogenic cells and filled with either red or yellow bone marrow. Cancellous bone is relatively light, yet its structure is such that it has considerable tensile strength and weight-bearing properties. Compact (cortical) bone has a densely packed calcified intercellular matrix that makes it more rigid than cancellous bone. The relative quantity of compact and cancellous bone varies in different types of bones throughout the body and in different parts of the same bone, depending on the need for strength and lightness. Compact bone is the major component of tubular bones. It is also found along the lines of stress on long bones and forms an outer protective shell on other bones.

Bone cells

Four types of bone cells participate in the formation and maintenance of bone tissue: (1) osteo-

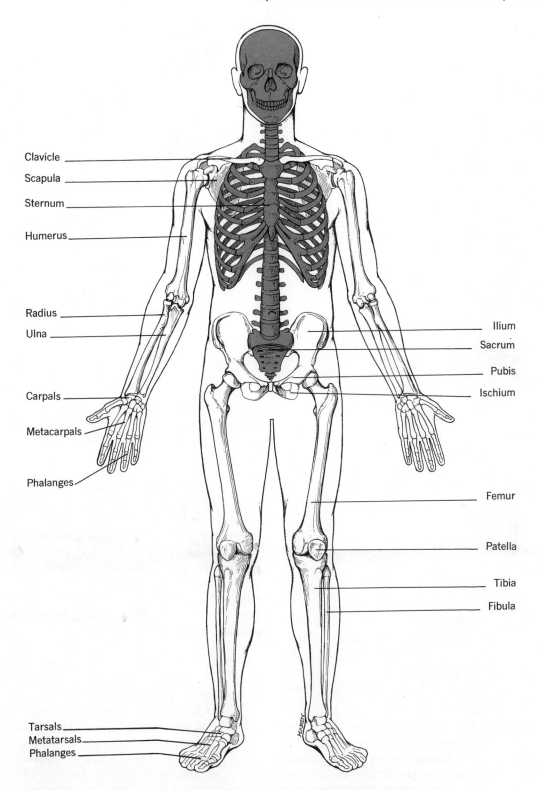

Clavicle

Scapula

Sternum

Humerus

Radius

Ulna

Carpals

Metacarpals

Phalanges

Ilium

Sacrum

Pubis

Ischium

Femur

Patella

Tibia

Fibula

Tarsals
Metatarsals
Phalanges

Figure 54-1 The skeleton. The bones of the head and the trunk that form the axial skeleton are shown in color, and those of the extremities forming the appendicular skeleton are uncolored. (*Chaffee EE, Lytle IM: Basic Physiology and Anatomy, 4th ed. Philadelphia, JB Lippincott, 1980*)

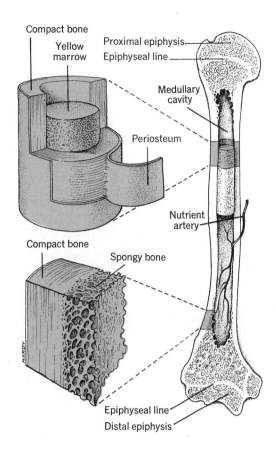

Figure 54-2 A long bone shown in longitudinal section. (*Chaffee EE, Lytle IM: Basic Physiology and Anatomy, 4th ed. Philadelphia, JB Lippincott, 1980*)

Table 54-1. Function of bone cells

Type of bone cell	Function
Osteogenic cells	Undifferentiated cells that differentiate into osteoblasts. They are found in the periosteum, endosteum, and epiphyseal growth plate of growing bones.
Osteoblasts	Bone-building cells that synthesize and secrete the organic matrix of bone. Osteoblasts also participate in the calcification of the organic matrix.
Osteocytes	Mature bone cells that function in the maintenance of bone matrix. Osteocytes also play an active role in releasing calcium into the blood.
Osteoclasts	Bone cells responsible for the resorption of bone matrix and the release of calcium and phosphate from bone.

genic cells, (2) osteoblasts, (3) osteocytes, and (4) osteoclasts (Table 54-1).

Osteogenic cells. The undifferentiated osteogenic cells are found in the periosteum, endosteum, and epiphyseal plate of growing bone. These cells differentiate into osteoblasts and are active during normal growth; they may also be activated in adult life during healing of fractures and other injuries. Osteogenic cells also participate in the continual replacement of worn-out bone tissue.

Osteoblasts. The osteoblasts, or bone-building cells, are responsible for the formation of the bone matrix. Bone formation occurs in two stages: ossification and calcification. Ossification involves the formation of osteoid, or prebone. Calcification of bone involves the deposition of calcium salts in the osteoid tissue. The osteoblasts synthesize collagen and other proteins that make up osteoid tissue. They also participate in the calcification process of the osteoid tissue, probably by controlling the availability of calcium and

phosphate. Osteoblasts secrete the enzyme alkaline phosphatase, which is thought to act locally in bone tissue to raise calcium and phosphate levels to the point at which precipitation occurs. The activity of the osteoblasts undoubtedly contributes to the rise in serum levels of alkaline phosphatase that follows bone injury and fractures.

Osteocytes. The osteocytes are mature bone cells that are actively involved in maintaining the bony matrix. Death of the osteocytes results in the resorption of this matrix. The osteocytes lie in a small lake filled with extracellular fluid, called a *lacuna,* and are surrounded by a calcified intercellular matrix (Figure 54-3). Extracellular fluid-filled passageways permeate the calcified matrix and connect with the lacunae of adjacent osteocytes. These passageways are called *canaliculi.* Because diffusion does not occur through the calcified matrix of bone, the canaliculi serve as communicating channels for the exchange of nutrients and metabolites between the osteocytes and the blood vessels on the surface of the bone layer.

The osteocytes, together with their intercellular matrix, are arranged in layers, or lamellae. In compact bone, 4 to 20 lamellae are arranged concentrically around a central haversian canal, which runs essentially parallel to the long axis of the bone. Each of these units is called a *haversian system,* or *osteon.* The haversian canals contain blood vessels that carry nutrients and wastes to and from the canaliculi (Figure 54-4). The blood vessels from the periosteum enter the bone through tiny openings called *Volkmann's canals* and then connect with the haversian systems.

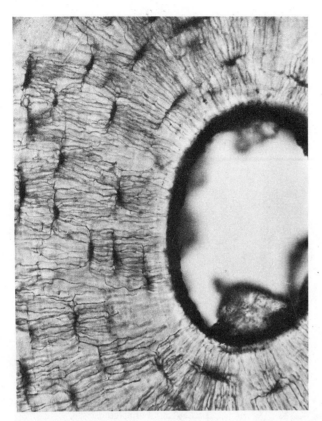

Figure 54-3 Photomicrograph of a ground bone section. The lacunae in which osteocytes reside appear as dark flattened ovals. The fine lines (canaliculi) connect the lacunae to each other and to the canal on the right. In life, this canal contained blood vessels that supplied interstitial fluid to the canaliculi. (*Reprinted from Ham's, Cormack DH: Histology, 9th ed, p 278. Philadelphia, JB Lippincott, 1987*)

Cancellous bone is also composed of lamellae, but its trabeculae are usually not penetrated by blood vessels. Instead, the bone cells of cancellous bone are nourished by diffusion from the endosteal surface through canaliculi, which interconnect their lacunae and extend to the bone surface.

Osteoclasts. Osteoclasts are bone cells that function in the resorption of bone, removing both the mineral content and the organic matrix. Unlike the osteoblasts, which originate in osteogenic cells, the osteoclasts are formed by the fusion of blood-derived monocytes. Although the mechanism of osteoclast formation and activation remains elusive, it is known that parathyroid hormone increases the number and resorptive function of the osteoclasts. Calcitonin, on the other hand, is thought to reduce the number and resorptive function of the osteoclasts. The mechanism whereby osteoclasts exert their resorptive effect on bone is also unclear. These cells may secrete an acid that removes calcium from the bone matrix, thus releasing the collagenic fibers for digestion by either osteoclasts or mononuclear cells.

Classification of bones

Bones are classified, on the basis of their shape, as (1) long bones, (2) short bones, (3) flat bones, and (4) irregular bones. Long bones are found in the upper and lower extremities. Short bones are irregularly shaped bones located in the ankle and the wrist. Except for their surface, which is compact bone, these bones are spongy throughout. Flat bones are composed of a layer of spongy bone between two layers of compact bone. They are found in areas such as the skull and rib cage, where extensive protection of underlying structures is needed or, as in the scapula, where a broad surface for muscle attachment must be provided. Irregular bones, because of their shapes, cannot be classified in any of the previous groups. This group includes such bones as the vertebrae and the bones of the jaw.

A typical long bone has a shaft, or diaphysis, and two ends, called epiphyses. Long bones are usually narrow in the midportion and broad at the ends so that the weight they bear can be distributed over a wider surface. The shaft of a long bone is formed mainly of compact bone roughly hollowed out to form a marrow-filled medullary canal. The ends of long bones are covered with articular cartilage that rests on a bony plate, the subchondral bone.

In growing bones the part of the bone shaft that funnels out as it approaches the epiphysis is called the metaphysis (Figure 54-5). It is composed of bony trabeculae that have cores of cartilage. In the child, the epiphysis is separated from the metaphysis by the cartilaginous growth plate. After puberty, the metaphysis and epiphysis merge, and the growth plate is obliterated.

Bone marrow

Bone marrow occupies the medullary cavities of the long bones throughout the skeleton and the cavities of cancellous bone in the vertebrae, ribs, sternum, and flat bones of the pelvis. The cellular composition of the bone marrow varies with both age and skeletal location. Red bone marrow contains developing red blood cells and is the site of blood cell formation. Yellow bone marrow is composed largely of adipose cells. At birth, nearly all of the marrow is red and hematopoietically active. As the need for red blood cell production decreases during postnatal growth, red marrow is gradually replaced with yellow bone marrow in most of the bones. In the adult, red marrow persists in the vertebrae, ribs, sternum, and ilia.

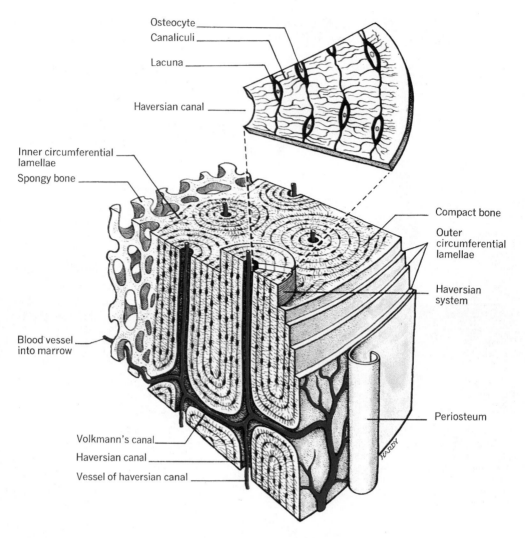

Figure 54-4 Haversian systems as seen in a wedge of compact bone tissue. The periosteum has been peeled back to show a blood vessel entering one of Volkmann's canals. (*Upper right*) Osteocytes lying within lacunae; canaliculi permit interstitial fluid to reach each lacuna. (*Chaffee EE, Lytle IM: Basic Physiology and Anatomy, 4th ed. Philadelphia, JB Lippincott, 1980*)

Periosteum and endosteum

Bones are covered, except at their articular ends, by a membrane called the periosteum (see Figure 54-2). The periosteum has an outer fibrous layer and an inner layer that contains the osteogenic cells needed for bone growth and development. The periosteum contains blood vessels and acts as an anchorage point for vessels as they enter and leave the bone. The endosteum is the membrane that lines the spaces of spongy bone, the marrow cavities, and the haversian canals of compact bone. It is composed mainly of osteogenic cells. These osteogenic cells contribute to the growth and remodeling of bone and are necessary for bone repair.

Cartilage

Cartilage is a firm but flexible type of connective tissue consisting of cells and intercellular fibers embedded in an amorphous gel-like material. It has a smooth and resilient surface and a weight-bearing capacity exceeded only by that of bone.

Cartilage is essential for growth both before and after birth. It is able to undergo rapid growth while maintaining a considerable degree of stiffness. In the embryo, most of the axial and appendicular skeleton is formed first as a cartilage model and is then replaced by bone. In postnatal life, cartilage continues to play an essential role in the growth of long bones and persists as articular cartilage in the adult.

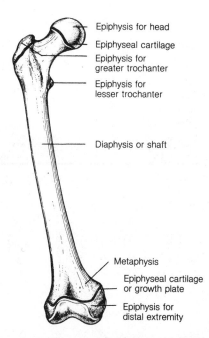

Epiphysis for head
Epiphyseal cartilage
Epiphysis for greater trochanter
Epiphysis for lesser trochanter

Diaphysis or shaft

Metaphysis
Epiphyseal cartilage or growth plate
Epiphysis for distal extremity

Figure 54-5 A femur, showing epiphyseal cartilages for the head, metaphysis, trochanters, and distal end of the bone. (*Adapted from Chaffee EE, Lytle IM: Basic Physiology and Anatomy, 4th ed. Philadelphia, JB Lippincott, 1980*)

There are three types of cartilage: elastic cartilage, hyaline cartilage, and fibrocartilage. *Elastic cartilage* contains some elastin in its intercellular substance. It is found in areas, such as the ear, where some flexibility is important. Pure cartilage is called *hyaline cartilage* (from the Greek, meaning·glass) and is pearly white. It is the type of cartilage seen on the articulating ends of fresh soup bones found in the supermarket. *Fibrocartilage* has characteristics that are intermediate between dense connective tissue and hyaline cartilage. It is found in the intervertebral disks, in areas where tendons are connected to bone, and in the symphysis pubis.

Hyaline cartilage is the most abundant type of cartilage. It forms much of the cartilage of the fetal skeleton. In the adult, hyaline cartilage forms the costal cartilages, which join the ribs to the sternum and vertebrae, many of the cartilages of the respiratory tract, the articular cartilages, and the epiphyseal plates.

Cartilage cells, which are called *chondrocytes*, are located in lacunae. These lacunae are surrounded by an uncalcified gel-like intercellular matrix of collagen fibers and ground substance. Cartilage is devoid of blood vessels and nerves. The free surfaces of most hyaline cartilage, with the exception of articular cartilage, is covered by a layer of fibrous connective tissue called the *perichondrium*.

It has been estimated that about 65% to 80% of the wet weight of cartilage is water held in its gel structure.[2] Because cartilage has no blood vessels, this tissue fluid allows for the diffusion of gases, nutrients, and wastes between the chondrocytes and blood vessels outside the cartilage. Diffusion cannot take place if the cartilage matrix becomes impregnated with calcium salts. Therefore, cartilage dies if it becomes calcified.

Tendons and ligaments

In the skeletal system, tendons and ligaments are dense connective tissue structures that connect muscles and bones. Tendons connect muscles to bone, and ligaments connect the movable bones of joints. Tendons can appear as cordlike structures or as flattened sheets, called aponeuroses, such as in the abdominal muscles.

The dense connective tissue found in tendons and ligaments has a limited blood supply and is composed largely of intercellular bundles of collagen fibers arranged in the same direction and plane. This type of connective tissue provides great tensile strength and can withstand tremendous pulls in the direction of fiber alignment. At the sites where tendons or ligaments are inserted into cartilage or bone, a gradual transition from pure dense connective tissue to either bone or cartilage occurs. In cartilage this transitional tissue is called fibrocartilage.

Tendons that might rub against bone or other friction-generating surfaces are enclosed in double-layered sheaths. An outer connective tissue tube is attached to the structures surrounding the tendon, and an inner sheath encloses the tendon and is attached to it. The space between the inner and outer sheath is filled with a fluid similar to synovial fluid.

In summary, skeletal tissue includes bone, cartilage, ligaments, and tendons. These skeletal structures are composed of similar tissue types; each has living cells and nonliving intercellular fibers and ground substance that is secreted by the cells. The characteristics of the various skeletal tissue types are determined by the intercellular matrix. In bone, this matrix is impregnated with calcium salts to provide hardness and strength. There are four types of bone cells: osteocytes, or mature bone cells; osteoblasts, or bone-building cells; osteoclasts, which function in bone resorption; and osteogenic cells, which differentiate into osteoblasts. A typical long bone has a shaft, or diaphysis, and two ends called epiphyses. Densely packed compact bone forms the outer shell of a bone, and lattice-like cancellous bone forms the interior.

Cartilage is a firm, flexible type of skeletal tissue that is essential for growth both before and after birth. There are three types of cartilage: elastic, hyaline, and fibrocartilage. Hyaline cartilage, which is the most abundant type, forms the costal cartilages that join the ribs to the sternum and vertebrae, many of the cartilages of the respiratory tract, and the articular cartilages. Tendons and ligaments are dense connective skeletal tissue that connect muscles and bones. Tendons connect muscles to bones and ligaments connect the movable bones of joints.

Joints and articulations

Articulations, or joints, are areas where two or more bones meet. The term *arthro* is the affix used to designate a joint. For example, *arthrology* is the study of joints and *arthroplasty* is the repair of a joint. There are three classes of joints, based on movement and the type of tissue present in the joint: synarthroses, amphiarthroses, and diarthroses (Figure 54-6).

Synarthroses

Synarthroses are immovable joints in which the surfaces of the bones come in direct contact with each other and are fastened together by fibrous tissue, cartilage, or bone. The bones of the skull are joined by synarthroses.

Amphiarthroses

Amphiarthroses are slightly movable joints connected by cartilage. There are two types of amphiarthrotic joints: symphyses, which are connected by fibrocartilage disks, and synchondroses, which have cartilages that are eventually replaced by bone. The symphysis pubis of the pelvis and the bodies of the vertebrae that are joined by intervertebral disks are examples of symphysis articulations. The normal process of bone elongation in bones with epiphyses involves synchondrosis between the end and the shaft of the bone. After growth is completed, the synchondroses become ossified.

Diarthroses

Diarthrodial joints (synovial joints) are freely movable joints. Most joints in the body are of this type. Although they are classified as freely movable, their movement actually ranges from almost none (sacroil-

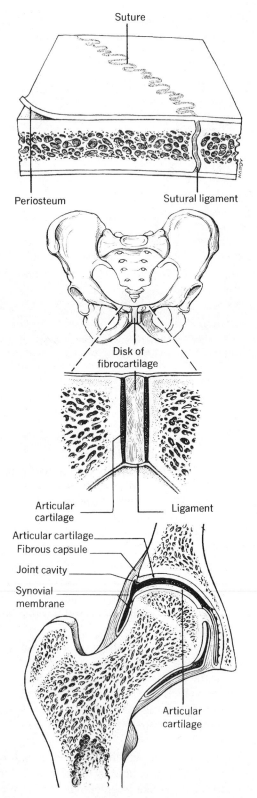

Figure 54-6 Three types of joints. (**Top**) Synarthrosis, which is joined by a fibrous suture ligament; (**center**) amphiarthrosis, symphysis type, which is joined by a disk of fibrocartilage; (**bottom**) diarthrosis, or synovial joint, in which bones are joined by ligaments and a fibrous joint capsule. (*Chaffee EE, Lytle IM: Basic Physiology and Anatomy, 4th ed. Philadelphia, JB Lippincott, 1980*)

iac joint) to simple hinge movement (interphalangeal joint), to movement in many planes (shoulder or hip joint). The bony surfaces of these joints are covered with thin layers of articular cartilage, and the cartilaginous surfaces of these joints slide past each other during movement. As discussed in Chapter 57, diarthrodial joints are the joints most frequently affected by rheumatic disorders.

In a diarthrodial joint the articulating ends of the bones are not connected directly but are indirectly linked by a strong fibrous capsule (joint capsule) that surrounds the joint and is continuous with the periosteum. This capsule supports the joint and helps to hold the bones in place. Additional support may be provided by ligaments that extend between the bones of the joint. The joint capsule consists of two layers: an outer fibrous layer and an inner membrane, the synovium. The synovium surrounds the tendons that pass through the joints as well as the free margins of other intra-articular structures such as ligaments and menisci. The synovium forms folds that surround the margins of articulations but do not cover the weight-bearing articular cartilage. These folds permit stretching of the synovium so that movement can occur without tissue damage.

Synovium and synovial fluid

The synovium secretes a slippery synovial fluid with the consistency of egg white. This fluid acts as a lubricant and facilitates the movement of the articulating surfaces of the joint. Normal synovial fluid is clear, is colorless or pale yellow, does not clot, and contains fewer than 100 cells/mm³. The cells are predominantly mononuclear cells derived from the synovium. The composition of the synovial fluid is altered in many inflammatory and pathologic joint disorders. Aspiration and examination of the synovial fluid plays an important role in the diagnosis of joint diseases.

Articular cartilage

The articular cartilage is an example of hyaline cartilage and is unique in that its free surface is not covered with perichondrium. It has only a peripheral rim of perichondrium, and calcification of the portion of cartilage abutting the bone may limit or preclude diffusion from blood vessels supplying the subchondral bone. Articular cartilage is apparently nourished by the diffusion of substances contained in the synovial fluid bathing the cartilage. Regeneration of most cartilage is slow; it is accomplished primarily by growth that requires the activity of perichondrium cells. In articular cartilage, which has no perichondrium, superficial injuries heal very slowly.[3]

Blood supply

The blood supply to a joint arises from blood vessels that enter the subchondral bone at or near the attachment of the joint capsule and form an arterial circle around the joint. The synovial membrane has a rich blood supply, and constituents of plasma diffuse rapidly between these vessels and the joint cavity. Because many of the capillaries are near the surface of the synovium, blood may escape into the synovial fluid following relatively minor injuries.[2] Healing and repair of the synovial membrane is usually rapid and complete. This is important because synovial tissue is injured in many surgical procedures that involve the joint.

Innervation

The nerve supply to joints is provided by the same nerve trunks that supply the muscles that move the joints. These nerve trunks also supply the skin over the joints. As a rule, each joint of an extremity is innervated by all the peripheral nerves that cross the articulation; this accounts for the referral of pain from one joint to another.[4] For example, hip pain may be perceived as pain in the knee.

The tendons and ligaments of the joint capsule are sensitive to position and movement, particularly stretching and twisting. These structures are supplied by the large sensory nerve fibers that form proprioceptor endings (see Chapter 49). The proprioceptors function reflexively to adjust the tension of the muscles that support the joint and are particularly important in maintaining muscular support for the joint. For example, when a weight is lifted, there is a proprioceptor-mediated reflex contraction and relaxation of appropriate muscle groups to support the joint and protect the joint capsule and other joint structures. Loss of proprioception and reflex control of muscular support leads to destructive changes in the joint.

The synovial membrane is innervated only by autonomic fibers that control blood flow. It is relatively free of pain fibers, as is evidenced by the fact that surgical procedures on the joint are often done under local anesthesia. The joint capsule and the ligaments of joints have pain receptors; these receptors are more easily stimulated by stretching and twisting than the other joint structures. Pain arising from the capsule tends to be diffuse and poorly localized.

Bursae

In some diarthrotic joints, the synovial membrane forms closed sacs that are not part of the joint. These sacs, called *bursae,* contain synovial fluid. Their purpose is to prevent friction on a tendon. Bursae are

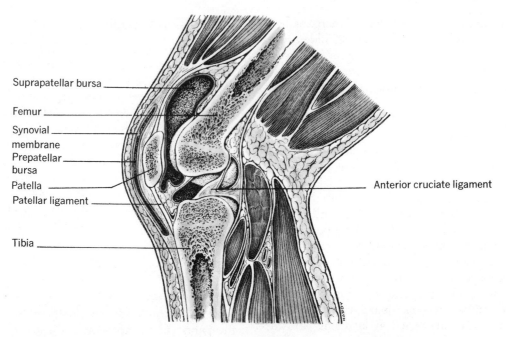

Figure 54-7 Sagittal section of knee joint, showing prepatellar and suprapatellar bursae. (*Chaffee EE, Lytle IM: Basic Physiology and Anatomy, 4th ed. Philadelphia, JB Lippincott, 1980*)

present in areas where pressure is exerted because of close approximation of joint structures (Figure 54-7). Such conditions occur when tendons are deflected over bone or where skin must move freely over bony tissue. Bursae may become injured or inflamed, causing discomfort, swelling, and limitation in movement of the involved area. A bunion is an inflamed bursa of the metatarsophalangeal joint of the great toe.

Intra-articular menisci

Intra-articular menisci are fibrocartilage structures that develop from portions of the articular disk that occupied the space between articular cartilage surfaces during fetal development. Menisci may extend partway through the joint and have a free inner border (as at the lateral and medial articular surfaces of the knee), or they may extend through the joint, separating it into two separate cavities (as in the sternoclavicular joint). The menisci of the knee joint may be torn as the result of an injury. The detached portion may interfere with joint motion and cause recurring pain and locking or giving way of the joint. When this happens, the injured structure is often removed surgically. Following removal, a new structure sometimes grows in from the fibrous capsule of the joint. The new meniscus is almost a complete duplicate of the old except that it is made up of dense connective

tissue rather than the fibrocartilage of the original structure.

In summary, articulations, or joints, are areas where two or more bones meet. Synarthroses are immovable joints in which bones are joined together by fibrous tissue, cartilage, or bone. Amphiarthroses are slightly movable joints connected by cartilage. Most joints in the body are diarthrodial, or synovial, joints, which are freely movable. The surfaces of these joints are covered with a thin layer of articular cartilage. The articulating ends of bones in a diarthrodial joint are linked by the fibrous joint capsule. The joint capsule consists of two layers: an outer fibrous layer and an inner membrane, the synovium. A slippery fluid called the synovial fluid, which is secreted by the synovium and is present in the joint capsule, acts as a lubricant and facilitates movement of the joint's articulating surfaces. Bursae, which are closed sacs containing synovial fluid, prevent friction in areas where tendons are deflected over bone or where skin must move freely over bony tissue. Menisci are fibrocartilaginous structures that develop from portions of the articular disk that occupied the space between the articular cartilage during fetal development. The menisci may have a free inner border, or they may extend through the joint, separating it into two cavities. The menisci in the knee joint may be torn as a result of injury.

References

1. Bloom W, Faucett DW: A Textbook of Histology, p 160. Philadelphia, WB Saunders, 1975

2. Cormack DH: Ham's Histology, 9th ed, pp 271, 333, 333. Philadelphia, JB Lippincott, 1987

3. Hooker H: Histology of cartilage and synovium. In Wilson FC (ed): The Musculoskeletal System: Basic Processes and Disorders, 2nd ed, p 213. Philadelphia, JB Lippincott, 1980

4. Rodman GP, Schumacker HR (eds): Primer on Rheumatic Diseases, 8th ed, p 15. Atlanta GA, Arthritis Foundation, 1983

Alterations in Skeletal Function: Trauma and Infection

Objectives

After you have studied this chapter, you should be able to meet the following objectives:

_____ Describe the physical agents responsible for soft tissue trauma.

_____ Name the three types of soft tissue injuries.

_____ Compare muscle strains and ligamentous sprains.

_____ Describe the healing process of soft tissue injuries.

_____ State three causes of joint dislocation.

_____ Name three causes of fractures.

_____ Differentiate between open and closed fractures.

_____ List the signs and symptoms of a fracture.

_____ Describe the fracture healing process.

_____ Relate individual and local factors to the healing process in bone.

_____ Differentiate between internal and external fixation methods used in the treatment of fractures.

_____ Explain the importance of immobilization for fracture healing.

_____ Define *traction*.

_____ Cite the five goals of traction.

_____ Name the three types of traction.

_____ Explain how traction provides a pulling force.

_____ Explain why muscle and joint function should be maintained during fracture healing.

_____ Describe the pathogenesis of the compartment syndrome.

_____ Explain the origin and development of fat embolization.

_____ Differentiate between the early complications of fractures and later complications of fracture healing.

_____ Explain the implications of bone infection.

_____ Describe how an acute form of osteomyelitis becomes chronic.

The musculoskeletal system includes the bones, joints, and muscles of the body together with associated structures such as ligaments and tendons. This system, which constitutes more than 70% of the body, is subject to a large number of disorders. These disorders affect people in all age groups and walks of life, causing pain, disability, and deformity. The discussion in this chapter focuses on trauma and infections of skeletal structures.

Injury and trauma of musculoskeletal structures

Trauma, which commonly includes injury to musculoskeletal structures, is the third leading cause of death in the United States. A broad spectrum of injuries result from numerous physical forces. Injuries to the musculoskeletal system include blunt tissue trauma, disruption of tendons and ligaments, and fractures of bony structures.

Many of the external physical agents that cause injury to the musculoskeletal system are typical of a particular environmental setting, activity, or age group. In the home, common accidents include tripping over cords or falling on wet floors. In sports injuries, an athlete's conditioning, protection, and movement often determine the outcome of trauma-producing events. Specific injuries are associated with particular sports, such as tennis elbow, jogger's heel, and injuries to tendons, cartilage, and ligaments seen in contact sports. Trauma resulting from high-speed motor accidents is now ranked as the number one killer of adults under the age of 35. Motorcycle accidents are especially common in young men, with fractures of the distal tibia, midshaft femur, and radius occurring most often. There are increasing numbers of musculoskeletal injuries in children using off-road vehicles, especially boys who live in rural areas.

The elderly are at particular risk for injuries caused by falls. Impaired hearing and sight, dizziness, and unsteadiness of gait contribute to falls in the older person. Falls in the elderly are often compounded by osteoporosis, or bone atrophy, which makes fractures more likely. Fractures of the vertebrae, proximal humerus, and hip are particularly common in this age group. Adrenocorticosteroid medications used for the treatment of diseases such as asthma and rheumatoid arthritis can lead to decreased bone density. Fractures of the ribs and vertebrae are common types of fractures associated with bone loss in these persons.

Soft tissue injury

Most skeletal injuries are accompanied by soft tissue injuries. These injuries include contusions, hematomas, and lacerations. They are discussed here because of their association with skeletal injuries.

A *contusion* is an injury to soft tissue that results from direct trauma and is usually caused by striking a body part against a hard object. With a contusion, the skin overlying the injury remains intact. Initially the area becomes ecchymotic (black and blue) because of local hemorrhage; later the discoloration gradually changes to brown and then to yellow as the blood is reabsorbed.

A large area of local hemorrhage is called a *hematoma* (blood tumor). Hematomas cause pain as blood accumulates and exerts pressure on nerve endings. The pain increases with movement or when pressure is applied to the area. The pain and swelling of a hematoma takes longer to subside than that accompanying a contusion. A hematoma may become infected because of bacterial growth. Unlike a contusion, which does not drain, a hematoma may eventually split the skin because of increased pressures and subsequently produce drainage.

The treatment for both a contusion and a hematoma consists of elevating the affected part and applying cold for the first 24 hours to reduce the bleeding into the area. A hematoma may need to be aspirated. After the first 24 hours, heat or cold should be applied intermittently for periods of 20 minutes at a time.

A *laceration* is an injury in which the skin is torn or its continuity is disrupted. The seriousness of a laceration depends on the size and depth of the wound and on whether there is contamination from the object that caused the injury. Puncture wounds from nails or rusted material may result in the growth of very toxic bacteria, leading to gas gangrene or tetanus.

Lacerations are usually treated by wound closure, which is done once the area is sufficiently cleansed; the closed wound is then covered with a sterile dressing. It is important to minimize contamination of the wound and to control bleeding. Contaminated wounds and open fractures are copiously irrigated and debrided, and the skin is usually left open to heal in order to prevent the development of an anaerobic infection or a sinus tract.

Strains and sprains

Tendons and ligaments, which connect bones and muscles, can be severed by cutting injuries or damaged by forcible twisting or stretching. A *strain* is a stretching injury to a muscle or a musculotendinous unit caused by mechanical overloading. This type of injury may result from either an unusual muscle contraction or an excessive forcible stretch. Although there is usually no external evidence of a specific injury, pain, stiffness, and swelling are present. The most common sites for muscle strain are the lower back and the cervical region of the spine. The elbow and the shoulder are also supported by musculotendinous units that are subject to strains. Foot strain is associated with the weight-bearing stresses of the feet; it may be caused by inadequate muscular and ligamentous support, overweight, or excessive exercise such as standing, walking, or running.

A *sprain,* which involves the ligamentous structures surrounding the joint, resembles a strain, but the pain and swelling subside more slowly (Figure 55-1). It is usually caused by abnormal or excessive movement of the joint. With a sprain the ligaments may be incompletely torn or, as in a severe sprain, completely torn or ruptured. The signs of sprain are pain, rapid swelling, heat, disability, discoloration, and limitation of function. Any joint may be sprained, but the ankle joint is most commonly involved. Most ankle sprains occur when the foot is turned inward under a person, forcing the ankle into inversion beyond the structural limits. Other common sites of sprain are the knee and elbow (on the ulnar side). As with a strain, the soft tissue injury that occurs with a sprain is not evident on x-ray. Occasionally, however, a chip of bone is evident when the entire ligament, including part of its bony attachment, has been ruptured or torn from the bone.

Healing of the dense connective tissues in

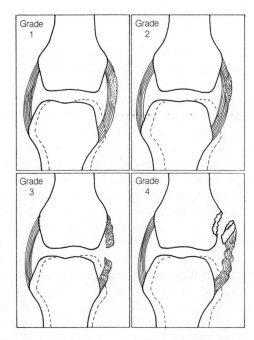

Figure 55-1 Degrees of sprain on the medial side of the right knee: grade 1, mild sprain of the medial collateral ligament; grade 2, moderate sprain with hematoma formation; grade 3, severe sprain with total disruption of the ligament; and grade 4, severe sprain with avulsion of the medial femoral condyle at the insertion of the medial collateral ligament. *(Adapted from Spickler LL: Knee injuries of the athlete. Orthop Nurs 2(5):12–13, 1983)*

tendons and ligaments is similar to that of other soft tissues. If properly treated, injuries usually heal with the restoration of the original tensile strength. Repair is accomplished by fibroblasts from the inner tendon sheath or, if the tendon has no sheath, from the loose connective tissue that surrounds the tendon. Capillaries infiltrate the injured area during the initial healing process and supply the fibroblasts with the materials they need to produce large amounts of collagen. Formation of the long collagen bundles begins within 4 to 5 days, and although tensile strength increases steadily thereafter, it is not sufficient to permit strong tendon pulls for 4 to 5 weeks.[1] During the first 3 weeks, there is a danger that muscle contraction will pull the injured ends apart; should this occur, the tendon will heal in the lengthened position. There is also a danger that adhesions will develop in areas where tendons pass through fibrous channels, such as in the distal palm of the hands, rendering the tendon useless.

The treatment of muscle strains and ligamentous sprains is similar in several ways. For an injured extremity, elevation of the part followed by local application of cold may be sufficient. Compression, accomplished through the use of adhesive wraps or a removable splint, helps reduce swelling and provides support. A cast is applied for severe sprains, especially those severe enough to warrant surgical repair. Immobilization for a muscle strain is continued until the pain and swelling have subsided. In a sprain, the affected joint is immobilized for several weeks. Immobilization may be followed by graded active exercises. Early diagnosis, treatment, and rehabilitation are essential in preventing chronic ligamentous instability.

In the lumbar and cervical spine regions, muscle strains are more common than sprains. For these strains, treatment usually consists of bed rest, traction, application of heat, and massage. Occasionally cold may be substituted during the first 24 hours to reduce pain and swelling of the affected area. Exercises, correct posture, and good body mechanics help to reduce the risk of reinjury.

Dislocations

Dislocation of a joint is the loss of articulation of the bone ends within the joint capsule caused by displacement or separation of the bone end from its position in the joint. It usually follows a severe trauma that disrupts the holding ligaments. Dislocations are seen most often in the shoulder and acromioclavicular joints, occasionally in the hip, and rarely in the knee. A *subluxation* is a partial dislocation in which the bone ends within the joint are still in partial contact with each other.

Dislocations can be congenital, traumatic, or pathologic. Congenital dislocations occur in the hip and knee. Traumatic dislocations occur after falls, blows, or rotational injuries. For example, car accidents often cause dislocations of the hip and accompanying acetabular fractures because the direction of impact. In the shoulder and patella, dislocations may become recurrent, especially in athletes. They recur with the same motion but require less and less force each time. Pathologic dislocation in the hip is a late complication of infection, rheumatoid arthritis, paralysis, and neuromuscular diseases. Dislocations of the phalangeal joints are not serious and are usually reduced by manipulation. Less common sites of dislocation, seen mainly in young adults, are the wrist and midtarsal region. They are usually the result of violent force.

Diagnosis of a dislocation is made by physical examination and confirmed by x-ray. The symptoms are pain, deformity, and limited movement. With recurrent dislocations, the person often senses the impending dislocation and may have a look of apprehension when range of joint motion is tested.

The treatment depends on the site, mechanism of injury, and associated injuries such as fractures. Dislocations that do not reduce spontaneously usually require manipulation or surgical repair. Various surgical procedures can also be used to prevent redislocation of the patella, shoulder, or acromioclavicular joints. Immobilization is necessary for several weeks following reduction of a dislocation; this allows for healing of the joint structures. In dislocations affecting the knee, alternatives to surgery are isometric quadriceps-strengthening exercises and a temporary brace. Surgical procedures, such as joint replacement, may be necessary in certain pathologic dislocations.

Recurrent subluxation and dislocation of the patella are common injuries in young adults. They account for about 10% of all athletic injuries and are more common in females. Sports such as skiing or tennis may cause stress on the patella. These sports involve external rotation of the foot and lower leg with knee flexion, a position that exerts rotational stresses on the knee. There is often a sensation of the patella "popping out" when the dislocation occurs. Other complaints include the knee giving out, swelling, crepitus, stiffness, and loss of range of motion. Congenital knee variations are predisposing factors. Treatment can be difficult, but nonsurgical methods are used first. They include immobilization with the knee extended, bracing, administration of salicylates, and isometric quadriceps-strengthening exercises. Surgical intervention is often necessary.

Chondromalacia

Chondromalacia, or softening of the articular cartilage, is seen most commonly on the undersurface of the patella and occurs most frequently in young adults. It can be the result of recurrent subluxation of the patella or overuse in strenuous athletic activities. Patients with this disorder typically complain of pain, particularly when climbing stairs or sitting with the knees bent. Occasionally there is weakness of the knee. The treatment consists of rest, isometric exercises, and application of ice after exercise. Part of the patella may be surgically removed in severe cases. In less severe cases the soft portion is shaved, using a saw inserted through an arthroscope.

Loose bodies

Loose bodies are small pieces of bone or cartilage inside the joint. These can be the result of trauma to the joint or may occur when cartilage has worn away from the articular surface, causing a part of the surface bone to die. When this happens, a piece of bone separates and becomes free-floating. The symptoms are painful catching and locking of the joint. Loose bodies are commonly seen in the knee, elbow, hip, and ankle. The loose body repeatedly gets caught in the crevice of a joint, pinching the underlying healthy cartilage; unless the loose body is removed, it may cause osteoarthritis and restricted movement. The treatment consists of removal using operative arthroscopy.

Fractures

Normal bone can withstand considerable compression and shearing forces and, to a lesser extent, tension forces. A fracture is any break in the continuity of bone that occurs when more stress is placed on the bone than it is able to absorb. Grouped according to their etiology, fractures can be divided into three major categories: (1) fractures caused by sudden injury, (2) fatigue or stress fractures, and (3) pathologic fractures. The most common fractures are those resulting from sudden injury. The force causing the fracture may be direct, such as a fall or blow, or indirect, such as a massive muscle contraction or trauma transmitted along the bone. For example, the head of the radius or clavicle can be fractured by the indirect forces that result from falling on an outstretched hand. A fatigue, or stress, fracture results from repeated wear on a bone. This type of fracture most commonly occurs in the metatarsal bones as a result of marching or running. A pathologic fracture occurs in bones that are already weakened by disease or tumors. Fractures of this type may occur spontaneously with little or no stress. The underlying disease state can be local, as with infections, cysts, or tumors, or it can be generalized, as in osteoporosis, Paget's disease, or disseminated tumors.

Classification

Fractures are usually classified according to (1) type, (2) location, and (3) direction of the fracture line (Figure 55-2).

Types.   The type of fracture is determined by its communication with the external environment, the degree of break in continuity of the bone, and the character of the fracture pieces. A fracture can be classified as either open or closed. When the bone fragments have broken through the skin, the fracture is called an *open* or *compound fracture.* Open fractures are often complicated by infection, osteomyelitis, delayed union, or nonunion. In a *closed fracture* there is no communication with the outside skin.

The degree of a fracture is described in terms of a partial or complete break in the continuity of bone. A *greenstick fracture,* which is seen in children, is an example of a partial break in bone continuity and resembles the kind seen when a young sapling is broken. This kind of break occurs because children's bones, especially until about age 10, are more resilient than the bones of adults.

A fracture is also described by the character of the fracture pieces. A *comminuted fracture* has more than two pieces. A *compression fracture,* such as occurs in the vertebral body, involves two bones that are crushed or squeezed together. A fracture is called *impacted* when the fracture fragments are wedged to-

gether. This type usually occurs in the humerus and is often less serious and generally treated without surgery.

Pattern.   The direction of the trauma or mechanism of injury produces a certain configuration or pattern of fracture. *Reduction* is the restoration of a fractured bone to its normal anatomic position. The pattern of a fracture indicates the nature of the trauma and provides information about the easiest method for reduction. Transverse fractures are caused by simple angulatory forces. A spiral fracture results from a twisting motion, or torque. A transverse fracture is not likely to become displaced or lose its position after it is reduced. On the other hand, spiral, oblique, and comminuted fractures are often unstable and may change position following reduction.

Location.   A long bone is divided into three parts: proximal, midshaft, and distal (see Figure 55-2). A fracture of the long bone is described in relation to its position in the bone. Other descriptions are used when the fracture affects the head or neck of a bone, involves a joint, or is near a prominence such as a condyle or malleolus.

Signs and symptoms.   The signs and symptoms of a fracture include pain, tenderness at the site of bone disruption, swelling, loss of function, deformity of the affected part, and abnormal mobility. The deformity varies according to the type of force applied, the area of the bone involved, the type of fracture produced, and the strength and balance of the surrounding muscles. In long bones, three types of deformities—angulation, shortening, and rotation—are seen. Severely angulated fracture fragments may be felt at the fracture site and often push up against the soft tissue to cause a tenting effect on the skin. Bending forces and unequal muscle pulls cause angulation. Shortening of the extremity occurs as the bone fragments slide and override each other because of the pull of the muscles on the long axis of the extremity (Figure 55-3). Rotational deformity occurs when the fracture fragments rotate out of their normal longitudinal axis; this can result from rotational strain produced by the fracture or unequal pull by the muscles that are attached to the fracture fragments. A crepitus or grating sound may be heard as the bone fragments

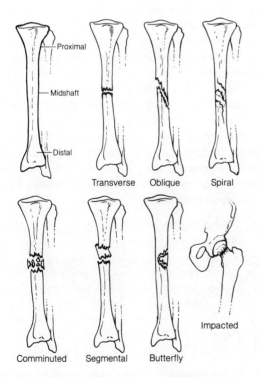

Figure 55-2 Classification of fractures. Fractures are classified according to location (proximal, midshaft, or distal), the direction of fracture line (transverse, oblique, spiral), and type (comminuted, segmental, butterfly, or impacted).

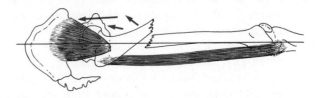

Figure 55-3 Displacement and overriding of fracture fragments of a long bone (femur) caused by severe muscle spasm.

Table 55–1. Blood loss from fractures of different bones

Involved bone site	Average blood loss (ml)
Radius and ulna	150
Humerus	200–300
Tibia and fibula	500
Femur	500–1000
Pelvis (unilateral)	1000–1500
Pelvis (bilateral)	2000–3000

rub against each other. In the case of an open fracture, there is bleeding from the wound where the bone protrudes. Blood losses that occur with different fractures are described in Table 55-1. Blood loss from a pelvic fracture or multiple long bone fractures can cause hypovolemic shock in a trauma victim (see Chapter 23).

Shortly after the fracture has occurred, nerve function at the fracture site may be temporarily lost. The area may become numb and the surrounding muscles flaccid. This condition has been termed *local shock*. During this period, which may last for a few minutes to half an hour, fractured bones may be reduced with little or no pain. Following this brief period, pain sensation returns, and with it muscle spasms and contractions of the surrounding muscles.

─── Healing

Bone healing occurs in a manner similar to soft tissue healing. It is, however, a more complex process and takes longer. Although the exact mechanisms of bone healing are open to controversy, five stages of the healing process have been identified: (1) hematoma formation, (2) cellular proliferation, (3) callus formation, (4) ossification, and (5) consolidation and remodeling (Figure 55-4). The degree of response during each of these stages is in direct proportion to the extent of trauma.

Hematoma formation. Hematoma formation occurs during the first 48 hours to 72 hours following fracture. It develops as blood from torn vessels in the bone fragments and surrounding soft tissue leaks between and around the fragments of the fractured bone. As a result of hematoma formation, clotting factors remain in the injured area to initiate the formation of a fibrin meshwork, which serves as a framework for the ingrowth of fibroblasts and new capillary buds. Granulation tissue, the result of fibroblasts and new capillaries, gradually invades and replaces the clot. When a large hematoma develops, healing is delayed because macrophages, platelets, oxygen, and nutrients for callus formation are prevented from entering the area.

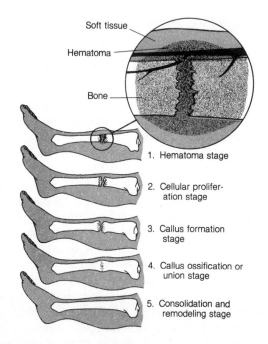

1. Hematoma stage
2. Cellular proliferation stage
3. Callus formation stage
4. Callus ossification or union stage
5. Consolidation and remodeling stage

Figure 55-4 Healing of a fracture. During hematoma formation (*1*), a locally formed clot serves as a fibrin meshwork for subsequent cellular invasion. Cellular proliferation (*2*) involves the invasion of the hematoma area by fibroblastic and endothelial cells. During callus formation (*3*), osteoblasts enter the area and produce the osteoid matrix. Callus formation is followed by union (*4*). The remodeling of the healed fracture is the last stage of the healing process (*5*).

Cellular proliferation. Three layers of bone structure are involved in the cellular proliferation that occurs during bone healing following a fracture: the periosteum or outer covering of the bone; the endosteum or inner covering; and the medullary canal, which contains the bone marrow. During this process the osteoblasts, or bone-forming cells, multiply and differentiate into a fibrocartilaginous callus. The fibrocartilaginous callus is softer and more flexible than callus. Cellular proliferation begins distal to the fracture, where there is a greater supply of blood. After a few days, a fibrocartilage "collar" becomes evident around the fracture site. The collar edges on either side of the fracture eventually unite to form a bridge, which connects the bone fragments.

Callus formation. During the early stage of callus formation the fracture becomes "sticky" as osteoblasts continue to move in and through the fibrin bridge to help keep it firm. Cartilage forms at the level of the fracture, where there is less circulation. In areas of the bone with muscle insertion, periosteal circulation is better, bringing in the nutrients necessary to bridge the callus. The bone calcifies as mineral salts are deposited. This stage occurs in 3 to 4 weeks.

Ossification. Ossification involves the final laying down of bone. This is the stage at which the fracture has been bridged and the fracture fragments are firmly united. Mature bone replaces the callus, and the excess callus is gradually resorbed by the osteoclasts (cells that resorb bone). The fracture site now feels firm and immovable and appears united on x-ray. At this point, it is safe to remove the cast.

Remodeling. Remodeling involves resorption of the excess bony callus that develops within the marrow space and encircling the external aspect of the fracture site. The remodeling process is directed by mechanical stress and direction of weight bearing. It continues according to Wolff's law—bone responds to mechanical stress by becoming thicker and stronger in relation to its function.

Healing time. Healing time depends on the site of the fracture, the condition of the fracture fragments, hematoma formation, and other local and host factors. In general, fractures of long bones, displaced fractures, and fractures with less surface area heal slower. Function usually returns within 6 months after union is complete. However, return to complete function may take longer.

Factors affecting healing. The factors that influence bone healing are local factors and those specific to the patient. Local factors include (1) the nature of the injury or the severity of the trauma, including fracture displacement and edema; (2) the degree of bridge formation that develops during bone healing; (3) the amount of bone loss (*e.g.*, it may be too great for the healing to bridge the gap); (4) the type of bone that is injured (*e.g.*, cancellous bone heals faster than cortical bone); (5) the degree of immobilization that is achieved (movement disrupts the fibrin bridge and cartilage forms instead of bone); (6) local infection, which retards or prevents healing; (7) local malignancy, which must be treated before healing can proceed; (8) bone necrosis, which prevents blood flow into the fracture site; and (9) intra-articular fractures (those through a joint), which may heal more slowly and may eventually produce arthritis. Individual factors that may delay bone healing are the patient's age, current medications, debilitating diseases, such as diabetes and rheumatoid arthritis, local stress around the fracture site, circulatory problems, coagulation disorders, and poor nutrition.

—— Diagnosis and treatment

A *splint* is a device for immobilizing the movable fragments of a fracture. When a fracture is suspected, the injured part should always be splinted before it is moved. This is essential for preventing further injury.

Diagnosis is the first step in the care of fractures and is based on history and physical manifestations. X-ray examination is used to confirm the diagnosis and direct the treatment. The ease of diagnosis varies with the location and severity of the fracture. In the trauma patient, the presence of other more serious injuries may make diagnosis more difficult. A thorough history includes the mechanism, time, and place of the injury, first recognition of symptoms, and any treatment initiated. A complete history is important because a delay in seeking treatment or weight bearing on a fracture may have caused further injury or displacement of the fracture.

Treatment of fractures depends on the general condition of the patient, the presence of associated injuries, the location of the fracture, its displacement, and whether the fracture is open or closed. There are three objectives for treatment of fractures: (1) reduction of the fracture, (2) immobilization, and (3) preservation and restoration of the function of the injured part.

Reduction. Reduction of a fracture is directed toward replacing the bone fragments to as near a normal anatomic position as possible. This can be accomplished by closed manipulation or surgical (open) reduction. Closed manipulation uses methods such as manual pressure and traction. Fractures are held in reduction by external or internal fixation devices. Surgical reduction involves the use of various types of hardware to accomplish internal fixation of the fracture fragments (Figure 55-5). Primary closure of crush injuries in the extremities is delayed until tissue viability is determined. The wound is first debrided and immobilized with an external fixation device. Reconstruction is done later using cancellous bone grafts, microvascular composite tissue grafts, or via tissue regeneration with distraction devices.[2]

Immobilization. Immobilization prevents movement of the injured parts and is the single most important element in obtaining union of the fracture

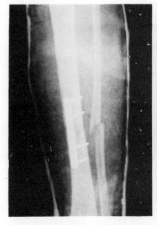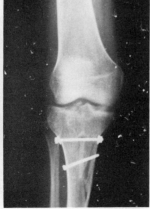

Figure 55-5 (Left) Internal fixation of the tibia with compression plate. **(Right)** Internal fixation of an intra-articular fracture of the upper tibia with a screw and bolt. (*Farrell J: Illustrated Guide to Orthopedic Nursing, 2nd ed. Philadelphia, JB Lippincott, 1982*)

fragments. Immobilization can be accomplished through the use of external devices, such as splints, casts, external fixation devices, or traction, or by means of internal fixation devices inserted during surgical reduction of the fracture.

Splints. Splints are made from many different materials. Metal splints or air splints may be used during transport to a health care facility as a temporary measure until the fracture has been reduced and another form of immobilization instituted. Plaster of Paris splints, which are molded to fit the extremity, work well. Splinting should be done if there is any suspicion of a fracture because motion of the fracture site can cause pain, bleeding, more soft tissue damage, and nerve or blood vessel compression. If the fracture has sharp fragments, movement can cause perforation of the skin and conversion of a closed fracture into an open one. When a splint is applied to an extremity, it should extend from the joint above the fracture site to the joint below it.

Casts. Casts (plaster or synthetic material) are commonly used to immobilize fractures of the extremities. They are often applied with a joint in partial flexion to prevent rotation of the fracture fragments. Without this flexion, the extremity, which is essentially a cylinder, tends to rotate within the cylindrical structure of the cast.

The application of a cast brings the risk of impaired circulation to the extremity because of blood vessel compression. A cast applied shortly after a fracture may not be large enough to accommodate the swelling that inevitably occurs in the hours that follow. Therefore, after a cast is applied, the peripheral circulation must be observed carefully until this danger has passed. Should the circulation become inadequate, the parts that are exposed at the distal end of the cast (*e.g.,* the toes with a leg cast and the fingers with an arm cast) usually become cold and cyanotic or pale. An increase in pain may occur initially, followed by paresthesia (tingling or abnormal sensation) or anesthesia as the sensory neurons that supply the area are affected. There will be a decrease in the amplitude or absence of the pulse in areas where the arteries can be palpated. Capillary refill time, which is assessed by applying pressure to the fingernail and then observing the rate of blood return, is prolonged to greater than 3 seconds. This condition demands immediate measures, such as splitting the cast, to restore the circulation and prevent permanent damage to the extremity. A casted extremity should always be elevated above the level of the heart for the first 24 hours to minimize swelling.

External fixation devices. With external fixation devices, pins or screws are inserted directly into the bone above and below the fracture site. They are

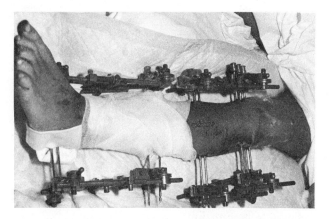

Figure 55-6 Hoffman device (a form of external fixation) applied to a 19-year-old male with compound comminuted fractures of the tibia and fibula. Note the demarcation of the toes due to vascular insufficiency.

then secured to a metal frame and adjusted to align the fracture. The Hoffman device (Figure 55-6) is often used for this purpose. Meticulous care is needed at the pin sites to prevent infection. This method of treatment is used primarily for open fractures, infections such as osteomyelitis and septic joints, unstable closed fractures, and limb lengthening. Limb lengthening devices are being used for traumatic losses of bone and soft tissue. These devices create a continuous distractive force that activates regeneration in bone, soft tissue, nerves, and blood vessels.

Traction. Another method for achieving immobility and maintaining reduction is *traction.* Traction is a pulling force applied to an extremity or part of the body while a counterforce, or countertraction, pulls in the opposite direction. Countertraction is usually exerted by the body's weight on the bed. Traction is used to maintain alignment of the fracture fragments and reduce muscle spasm.

Effective traction prevents movement of the fracture site. Fractures caused by trauma are associated with muscle injury and spasm. These muscle contractions cause overriding and displacement of the bone fragments, particularly when the fractures affect long bones. The five goals of traction therapy are to (1) correct and maintain the skeletal alignment of either entire bones or joints; (2) reduce pressure on a joint surface; (3) correct, lessen, or prevent deformities such as contractures and dislocations; (4) decrease muscle spasm; and (5) immobilize a part in order to promote healing. Traction may be used as a temporary measure prior to surgery or as a primary treatment method.

There are three types of traction: manual traction, skin traction, and skeletal traction (Figure 55-7). *Manual traction* consists of a steady, firm pull that is exerted by the hands. It is a temporary measure used to manipulate a fracture during closed reduction,

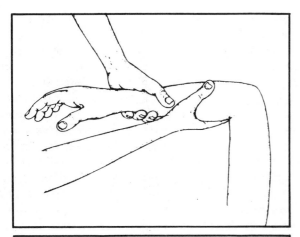

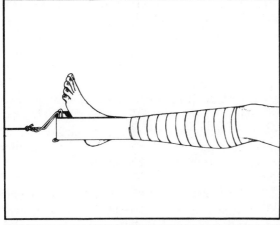

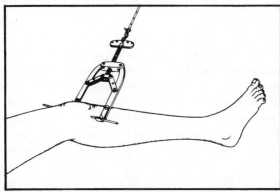

Figure 55-7 Three types of traction. **(Top)** Manual traction, in which the hands are used to exert a pulling force on the bone to be realigned; **(middle)** skin traction, in which strips of tape or some type of commercial skin traction strips are applied directly to the skin; **(bottom)** skeletal traction, in which the traction force is applied directly to the bone using pins, wires, or screws. *(Courtesy of Zimmer, Inc., Warsaw, Indiana)*

for support of a neck injury during transport when cervical-spine fracture is suspected, or for reduction of a dislocated joint.

Skin traction is a pulling force applied to the skin and soft tissue. It is accomplished by strips of adhesive, flannel, or foam secured to the injured part. Skin traction is used to treat strains (cervical and pelvic traction), hip dislocation (Bryant's or Buck's ex-

tension traction), and femoral fractures in children (Russell traction) and as a temporary or primary treatment for hip fractures (Buck's extension traction).

Skeletal traction is a pulling force applied directly to the bone. Pins, wires, or tongs are inserted through the skin and subcutaneous tissue into the bone distal to the fracture site. Muscles, tendons, arteries, and nerves are identified during the insertion process so that they are not penetrated. Pins are not inserted into joints or open areas. Skeletal traction provides an excellent pull. It can be used for long periods and with large amounts of weight. It is commonly used for fractures of the femur, the humerus, and the cervical spine (Crutchfield tongs applied to the skull). Skeletal traction is also used in maintaining alignment of fractures that are casted and in certain types of reconstructive foot surgery.

Pin tract infection is a complication of skeletal traction. Pin insertion sites should be inspected daily for redness, drainage, and shifting of the traction device. Larger pins need to be cleansed daily with hydrogen peroxide or an antibiotic solution.

Three forces always operate with traction: (1) the pull of the traction itself, (2) countertraction, and (3) friction. Because these are vector forces, they have both magnitude and direction. The forces are calculated by using weights to create a pull on different lengths of rope between pulleys of different angles. The number of pulleys used in the traction set-up affects the total pulling force: for example, two pulleys in the line of pull double the pulling force of the weight. Ropes are secured to the traction device and weight hanger. The ropes should be free of friction and hang unimpeded in the pulley grooves, while the weights attached to the pulling ropes should hang freely and not be removed unless traction is intermittent. Weights are prescribed according to the site of the fracture, the strength of the muscle mass, and the age and weight of the patient. The weight used with skin traction is 10 lb or less. Skeletal traction may require more weight.

The angles of traction are determined by the placement of bars on the bedframe holding the pulleys and the position of the affected body part. The resultant line of pull should be along the axis of the bone.

Preservation and restoration of function.
During the period of immobilization required for fracture healing, the preservation and restoration of function of muscles and joints is an ongoing process in the unaffected as well as the affected extremities. Exercises designed to preserve function, maintain muscle strength, and reduce joint stiffness should be started early. Active range of motion, in which the individual moves the extremity, is done on unaffected extremities; and isometric, or muscle-tensing, exercises are

done on the affected extremities. In some instances, an electrical muscle stimulator is applied directly to the skin to stimulate isometric muscle contraction as a means of preventing disuse atrophy. After the fracture has healed, a program of physical therapy may be necessary. However, the most important factor in restoring function is the person's own active exercises.

Muscles tend to atrophy during immobilization because of lack of use. Joints stiffen as muscles and tendons contract and shorten. The degree of muscle atrophy and joint stiffness depends on several factors. In adults, the degree of atrophy and muscle stiffness are directly related to the length of immobilization, with longer periods of immobility resulting in greater stiffness. Children have a natural tendency to move on their own, and this movement maintains muscle and joint function. Therefore, they usually have less atrophy and recover sooner once the source of immobilization has been removed. Associated soft tissue injury, infection, and preexisting joint disease increase the risk of stiffness. Even though limbs are immobilized in a functional position, casts are removed as soon as fracture healing has taken place.

Complications

The complications of fractures can be divided into two groups: (1) early complications associated with loss of skeletal continuity, injury from bone fragments, pressure due to swelling and hemorrhage, or development of fat emboli, and (2) complications associated with fracture healing. The early complications of fractures depend on the severity of the fracture and the area of the body that is involved. For example, bone fragments from a skull fracture may cause injury to brain tissue, or multiple rib fractures may lead to a flail chest and respiratory insufficiency. With flail chest, the chest wall on the fractured side becomes so unstable that it may move in the opposite direction as the patient breathes (*i.e.*, in during inspiration and out during expiration).

Compartment syndrome. Compartment syndrome is a compression of nerves and blood vessels that can follow a fracture or crush injury. In this condition, excessive swelling around the site of injury results in increased pressure (30 mmHg or more) within a closed compartment. This increase in pressure occurs because fascia, which covers and separates muscles, is inelastic and unable to compensate for the extreme swelling. The condition causes severe pain because of passive stretching of soft tissue and skin. Nerve compression may cause changes in sensation, paresthesias such as burning or tingling, diminished reflexes, and eventually loss of motor function. Compression of blood vessels may cause muscle ischemia and loss of function. Muscles and nerves may be per-

manently damaged if the pressure is not relieved. In contrast to ischemia caused by a tight bandage or cast, in the compartment syndrome the peripheral pulses are normal. The compartment syndrome is more common with crushing injuries, in closed fractures, and when external compression of a limb produces a tourniquet effect. Treatment is directed at reducing the compression of blood vessels and nerves. Constrictive dressings and casts are loosened, and the involved area is elevated. Intracompartmental pressure is often monitored, either with needle injection or continuous measurements. Normal intracompartmental pressure is about 6 mmHg. A fasciotomy, or transection of the fascia that is restricting the muscle compartment, may be required when the pressure in the area rises above 30 mm Hg, which is roughly equal to the perfusion pressure in the capillary beds. Irreversible nerve and muscle damage can be avoided if the fasciotomy is done within 24 hours of the onset of clinical symptoms for compartment pressures of 40 mmHg or less.[3] Compartment syndrome may also occur with prolonged pressure on the limbs, as in surgery or with exercise. Exercise-related compartment syndrome is most seen as a chronic condition commonly referred to as shin splints.

Fat emboli. Fat emboli result from the presence of intracellular fat globules in the lung parenchyma and peripheral circulation after a long-bone fracture or other major trauma. There are two theories about the origin of fat emboli. One theory is that fat globules are released from the bone marrow or subcutaneous tissue at the fracture site into the venous system through torn veins.[4] The second theory postulates that the fat emboli develop intravascularly secondary to an alteration in lipid stability caused by increased release of tissue lipases, catecholamines, glucagon, or other steroid hormones in response to the stress of injury.[5]

Fat embolism syndrome (FES) describes a respiratory deficiency state caused by decreased alveolar diffusion of oxygen due to fat embolism. Three degrees of severity are seen: subclinical, overt clinical, and fulminating. While the subclinical and overt clinical forms of FES respond well to treatment, the fulminating form is often fatal. There are three possible outcomes when fat emboli enter the pulmonary circulation: (1) small emboli can mold to vessel caliber, pass through the lung, and then enter the systemic circulation, where they are either trapped in the tissues or eliminated through the kidney; (2) the fat particles can be broken down by alveolar cells and eliminated through sputum; and (3) there can be local lipolysis with release of free fatty acid.[6] Free fatty acids cause direct injury to the alveolar capillary membrane, which leads to hemorrhagic interstitial pneumonitis with disruption of surfactant production and development of the adult respiratory distress syndrome. In addition, the fat globules become coated with platelets, causing a thrombocytopenia. Serotonin released by the sequestered platelets causes bronchospasm and vasodilatation.

Clinically, the incidence of fat embolization is related to fractures of bones containing the most marrow—that is, long bones and the bones of the pelvis. Initial symptoms begin to develop within a few hours to 3 to 4 days after injury and do not appear beyond 1 week following the injury. The first symptoms include a subtle change in behavior and signs of disorientation due to the presence of emboli in the cerebral circulation combined with respiratory depression. There may be complaints of substernal chest pain and dyspnea accompanied by tachycardia and a low-grade fever. Diaphoresis, pallor, and cyanosis become evident as respiratory function deteriorates. A petechial rash that does not blanch with pressure often occurs 2 to 3 days after the injury. This rash is usually found on the anterior chest, axillae, neck, and shoulders. It may also appear on the soft palate and conjunctiva. The rash is thought to be related to embolization of the skin capillaries or thrombocytopenia.

An important part of the treatment of fat emboli is early diagnosis. Arterial blood gases should be assayed immediately upon recognition of clinical manifestations. In a person suspected of having FES, a sustained arterial oxygen tension (PO_2) of less than 60 mmHg, an arterial carbon dioxide tension (PCO_2) of more than 55 mmHg, or a blood pH of less than 7.3 is diagnostic.[7] Treatment is directed toward correcting hypoxemia and maintaining adequate fluid balance. Mechanical ventilation may be required. Corticosteroid drugs are administered to decrease the inflammatory response of lung tissues, decrease the edema, stabilize the lipid membranes to reduce lipolysis, and combat the bronchospasm. Corticosteroids are also given prophylactically to high-risk persons. The only preventative approach to FES is early stabilization of the fracture.

Impaired healing. *Union* of a fracture has occurred when the fracture is solid enough to withstand normal stresses and it is clinically and radiologically safe to remove the external fixation. In children, fractures generally heal within 4 to 6 weeks; in adolescents, they heal within 6 to 8 weeks; and in adults, they heal within 10 to 18 weeks.

Delayed union is the failure of a fracture to unite within the normal time period (*e.g.*, 20 weeks for a fracture of the tibia or femur in an adult). The treatment for delayed union consists in determining and correcting the cause of the delay. *Malunion* is healing with deformity, angulation, or rotation that is visible on x-ray. It is usually treated by surgery. *Non-*union* is failure to produce union and cessation of the processes of bone repair. It is characterized by mobility of the fracture site and pain on weight bearing. Muscle atrophy and loss of range of motion may also be present. Nonunion is usually established 6 to 12 months after the time of the fracture. The complications of fracture healing are summarized in Table 55-2.

Treatment methods for impaired bone healing include surgical interventions, bracing, or electrical stimulation of the bone ends. Electrical stimulation is thought to stimulate the osteoblasts to lay down a network of bone. Three types of commercial bone growth stimulators are available: a noninvasive model, which is placed outside the cast; a seminoninvasive model, in which pins are inserted around the fracture site; and a totally implantable type, in which a cathode coil is wound around the bone at the fracture site and is operated by a battery pack implanted under the skin. Figure 55-8 depicts a noninvasive type of electrical stimulator.

In summary, many external physical agents can cause trauma to the musculoskeletal system. There are particular factors that can place an individual at greater risk for injury. Some soft tissue injuries such as contusions, hematomas, and lacerations are relatively minor and easily treated. Muscle strains and ligamentous sprains are caused by mechanical overload on the connective tissue. They heal more slowly than the minor soft tissue injuries and require some degree of immobilization. Healing of soft tissue begins within 4 to 5 days of the injury and is primarily the function of fibroblasts, which produce collagen. Joint dislocation is caused by trauma to the supporting structures. Repeated trauma to the joint can cause articular softening (chondromalacia) or the separation of small pieces of bone or cartilage, called loose bodies, within the joint.

Fractures occur when more stress is placed on a bone than the bone can absorb. The nature of the stress determines the type of fracture and the character of the resulting bone fragments. Healing of fractures is a complex process that takes place in five stages: hematoma formation, cellular proliferation, callus formation, ossification, and consolidation and remodeling. For satisfactory healing to take place, the affected bone has to be reduced and immobilized. This is accomplished by either a surgically implanted internal fixation device or devices such as splints, casts, or traction or external fixation apparatus. The complications associated with fractures can occur early when damage to soft tissue, blood vessels, and nerves is present or later when the healing process is interrupted. Local factors related to the healing environment and the individual's general physical condition affect the healing process.

Bone infections

Bone infections are difficult to treat and eradicate. Their effects can be devastating; they can cause pain, disability, and deformity. Chronic bone infections may drain for years because of a sinus tract. This occurs when a passageway develops from an abscess or cavity within the bone to an opening through the skin.

Iatrogenic bone infections

Iatrogenic bone infections are those inadvertently brought about by surgery or other treatment. These infections include complications of pin tract infection in skeletal traction, sepsis (infected) joints in joint replacement surgery, and wound infection following any surgery. Measures to prevent these infections include: (1) preparation of the skin to reduce bacterial growth prior to surgery or insertion of traction devices or wires; (2) strict operating room protocols, including disinfection of the operative site and a wide surrounding field with draping to prevent egress of the patient's and operating room personnel's flora into the area; (3) prophylactic use of antibiotics; and (4) maintenance of sterile technique after surgery when working with drainage tubes and dressing changes. Because of the danger of infection, orthopaedic wounds are kept covered with a sterile dressing until they are closed.

Osteomyelitis

Osteomyelitis represents an acute or chronic pyogenic infection of the bone. The term *osteo* refers to bone and *myelo* to the marrow cavity, both of which are involved in this disease. Osteomyelitis can be caused by hematogenous (through the bloodstream) seeding, direct extension, or direct contamination of an open fracture or wound. In most cases, *Staphylococcus aureus* is the infecting organism.[8]

The most common cause of osteomyelitis is the direct contamination of bone from an open wound. It may be the result of an open fracture, a gunshot wound, or a puncture wound. Inadequate debridement, introduction of foreign material into the wound, and extensive tissue injury increase the bone's susceptibility to infection. If the infection is not sufficiently treated, the acute infection may become chronic. Osteomyelitis may also occur as a complication of surgery, such as in the sternum following open heart surgery or in extremities after bone allograft or total joint replacement.

Acute hematogenous osteomyelitis

Acute hematogenous osteomyelitis is almost always limited to those under 21 years of age. It affects, in order of frequency, the femur, tibia, humerus, and radius.[8] The condition usually manifests itself as an acute febrile systemic illness of 48 hours or less duration accompanied by the signs of local bone involvement. Although the incidence of the acute form

Table 55–2. Complications of fracture healing

Complication	Manifestations	Contributing factors
Delayed union	Failure of fracture to heal within predicted time as determined by x-ray	Large displaced fracture Inadequate immobilization Large hematoma Infection at fracture site Excessive loss of bone Inadequate circulation
Malunion	Deformity at fracture site Deformity or angulation on x-ray	Inadequate reduction Malalignment of fracture at time of immobilization
Nonunion	Failure of bone to heal before the process of bone repair stops Evidence on x-ray Motion at fracture site Pain on weight bearing	Inadequate reduction Mobility at fracture site Severe trauma Bone fragment separation Soft tissue between bone fragments Infection Extensive loss of bone Inadequate circulation Malignancy Bone necrosis Noncompliance with restrictions

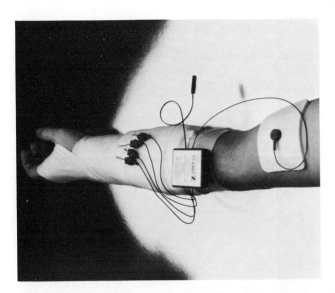

Figure 55-8 One type of electrical stimulator used in the treatment of nonunion *(Zimmer, Inc., Warsaw, Indiana. From Farrell J: Illustrated Guide to Orthopedic Nursing, 2nd ed. Philadelphia, JB Lippincott, 1982)*

of osteomyelitis has declined, there is an apparent increase in the subacute form.[9] Subacute osteomyelitis has an insidious onset in which symptoms are typically present for 2 weeks or more before diagnosis. The infection generally begins in the metaphysis of the bone where the nutrient artery channels terminate and the blood flow is sluggish. Because of the bone's rigid structure, there is little room for swelling, and the pus that forms finds its way to the surface of the bone to form a subperiosteal abscess. The blood supply to the bone may become obstructed by septic thrombi, in which case the ischemic bone becomes necrotic. It then separates from the viable surrounding bone to form a fragment of bone known as a sequestrum (Figure 55-9).

In children, acute hematogenous osteomyelitis is usually preceded by staphylococcal or streptococcal infections of the skin, sinuses, teeth, or middle ear. There is a history of trauma in one-third of the cases; the trauma apparently reduces the bone's ability to respond to infection. Intravenous drug users are at risk for infections with streptococcus and pseudomonas.

The signs and symptoms of acute hematogenous osteomyelitis are those of bacteremia accompanied by symptoms referable to the site of the bone lesion. There is often pain on movement of the affected extremity, loss of movement, and local tenderness followed by heat and swelling. X-ray studies may appear normal initially, but they will show evidence of periosteal elevation and increased osteoclastic activity once an abscess has formed. Changes will be evident on a bone scan 10 to 14 days before any radiographic changes are seen.

In the adult, hematogenous osteomyelitis usually affects the axial skeleton and the irregular bones in the wrist and ankle. It is most common in debilitated patients and in those with a history of chronic skin infections, chronic urinary tract infections, and intravenous drug use.

The treatment of acute osteomyelitis begins with identification of the causative organism through blood cultures, aspiration cultures, and Gram stains. Antibiotics are first given intravenously and then orally. The amount of rest needed by the affected limb and pain control measures used are based on symptomatology. Debridement and surgical drainage may also be necessary.

Chronic osteomyelitis

Chronic osteomyelitis has long been recognized as a disease. The incidence, however, has decreased in the last century because of improvements in surgical techniques and antibiotic therapy. Chronic osteomyelitis includes all inflammatory processes in the bone, excluding those in rheumatic diseases, that are caused by microorganisms. It may be the result of delayed or inadequate treatment of acute hematogenous osteomyelitis or osteomyelitis caused by direct contamination of bone. Acute osteomyelitis is considered to have become chronic when either the infection persists beyond 6 to 8 weeks or when the acute process has been adequately treated and is expected to resolve. Chronic osteomyelitis can persist for years; it may appear spontaneously, after a minor trauma, or when resistance is lowered. The hallmark feature of chronic osteomyelitis is the presence of infected dead bone, a sequestrum, that has separated from the living bone. A sheath of new bone, called the involucrum, forms around the dead bone. Radiologic techniques such as x-rays, bone scans, and sinograms are used to identify the infected site. Chronic osteomyelitis or infection around a total joint prosthesis can be difficult to diagnose because the classic signs of infection are not apparent and the blood leukocyte count may not be elevated. A subclinical infection may be present for years. Bone scans, although not specific, are used to rule out other conditions including malignancy.

Treatment

The treatment of bone infections begins with wound cultures to identify the microorganism and its sensitivity to antibiotic therapy. This is followed by surgery to remove foreign bodies (*e.g.*, metal plates or screws) or sequestra and by long-term antibiotic therapy. Wounds may be left open and packed or closed with a continuous wound-irrigation system being left in place for several days to several weeks after surgery. The irrigation system consists of an antibiotic or sodium chloride solution that is flushed directly into the

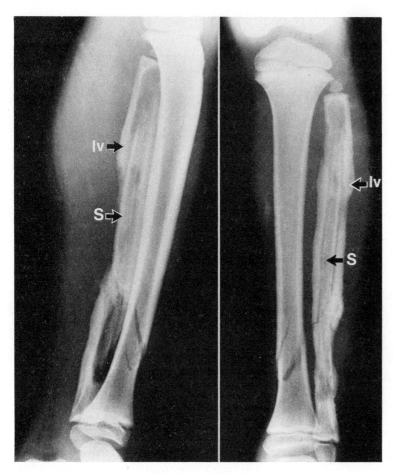

Figure 55-9 Hematogenous osteomyelitis of the fibula of 3 months' duration. The entire shaft has been deprived of its blood supply and has become a sequestrum (*S*) surrounded by new immature bone, involucrum (*Iv*). Pathologic fractures are present in the lower tibia and fibula. (*Wilson FC: The Musculoskeletal System: Basic Processes and Disorders, 2nd ed, p 150. Philadelphia, JB Lippincott, 1980*)

site of the infection and suctioned out by means of a closed drainage system. Immobilization of the affected part is usually necessary, with restriction of weight bearing on a lower extremity.

Hyperbaric oxygenation. Chronic refractory osteomyelitis that has been resistant to other forms of treatment may be treated with hyperbaric oxygenation. Hyperbaric oxygenation, which is the intermittent, short-term administration of 100% oxygen at a pressure above normal atmospheric pressure, increases tissue oxygenation and vascularity and reduces edema by releasing pressure on the capillary bed. The improvement in local vascularity enhances bone and soft tissue healing and produces a bacteriocidal effect by facilitating the host's leukocyte defense response. The increased oxygen also creates a favorable environment for the removal of bony debris and remnants of the infectious process by osteoclasts. Hyperbaric oxygenation is known to increase the rate of granulation tissue formation but has not been proved effective in all forms of osteomyelitis. It is thought to be best utilized for anaerobic infections. Not all hospitals and medical centers have facilities for hyperbaric oxygenation treatment.

Tuberculosis

Tuberculosis can spread from one part of the body, such as the lungs or occasionally the lymph nodes, to the bones and joints. It is caused by *Mycobacterium tuberculosis*. The disease is localized and progressively destructive. In about 50% of cases it affects the vertebrae, but it is also frequently seen in the hip and knee. The disease is characterized by bone destruction and abscess formation. Local symptoms include pain, immobility, and muscle atrophy; joint swelling, mild fever, and leukocytosis may also be present. Diagnosis is confirmed by a positive culture. The most important part of the treatment is antituberculosis drug therapy. Because of improved methods to prevent and treat tuberculosis, its incidence had diminished in recent decades. However, the incidence is now on the rise again: in 1986 there was an increase of 2.5%, the first substantial rise since 1952.[10] Unfortunately, however, the diagnosis of tuberculosis in the bones and joints may still be missed.

In summary, bone infections occur because of either the direct or the indirect invasion of the skeletal circulation by microorganisms, most commonly the bacterium *Staphylococcus aureus*. Osteomyelitis, or infection of the bone and marrow, can be an acute or chronic disease. Acute osteomyelitis is seen most often as a result of the direct contamination of bone by a foreign object. Chronic osteomyelitis is a long-term process that can recur spontaneously at any time throughout a person's life. The incidence of all types of bone infection has been dramatically reduced since the advent of antibiotic therapy.

References

1. Wright PH, Brashear HR: The local response to trauma. In Wilson FC (ed): The Musculoskeletal System: Basic Processes and Disorders, 2nd ed, p 264. Philadelphia, JB Lippincott, 1980
2. Martini Z, Castaman E: Tissue regeneration in the reconstruction of lost bone and soft tissue in the limbs: A preliminary report. Br J Plast Surg 40:142, 1987
3. Rorabeck CH: The treatment of compartment syndromes of the leg. J Bone Joint Surg 66(B):93, 1984
4. Oh WH, Mital MA: Fat embolism: Current concepts of pathogenesis, diagnosis, and treatment. Orthop Clin North Am 9:767, 1976
5. Maylan JA, Evenson MA: Diagnosis and treatment of fat embolism. Annu Rev Med 28:885, 1979
6. Oldman GL, Weise W. Fat embolism. Ariz Med 36:885, 1979
7. Lindeque BGP, Schoeman HS, Dommisse GF, et al: Fat embolism and the fat embolism syndrome. J Bone Joint? 1:128, 1987
8. Robins Sl, Cotran RS: Pathologic Basis of Disease. Philadelphia, WB Saunders, 1984
9. Jones NS, Anderson DJ, Stiles PJ: Osteomyelitis in a general hospital. J Bone Joint Surg 69(B):779, 1987
10. Tuberculosis, Final Data–United States, 1986. MMWR 36:817, 1988

Bibliography

Adinhoff AD, Hollister JR: Steroid induced fractures and bone loss in patients with asthma. N Engl J Med 309:265, 1983

Aronson DD, Singer RM, Higgins RF: Skeletal traction for fractures of the femoral shaft in children. J Bone Joint Surg 69(A) 9:1435, 1987

Blockey NJ: Chronic osteomyelitis: An unusual variant. J Bone and Joint Surg 65(B):120, 1983

Bolton ME: Hyperbaric oxygen therapy. Am J Nurs 81:1199, 1981

Chan KM, Tham KT, Chiu HS, et al: Post-traumatic fat embolism: Its clinical and subclinical presentations. J Trauma 24:5, 1984

Christianson F: Closed wound irrigation in orthopedics. Orthop Nurs Assoc J 6:359, 1979

Cole WG, Dalziel RE, Leitl J: Treatment of acute osteomyelitis in childhood. J Bone Joint Surg 64(A):218, 1982

Farrell J: Orthopedic pain: What does it mean? Am J Nurs 84:466, 1984

Gamron RB: Taking the pressure off compartment syndrome. Am J Nurs 88:1076, 1988

Gill KP, La Flamme D: External fixation: The erector sets of orthopedic nursing. Can Nurs 80:29, 1984

Hoshowsky VM: Chronic lateral ligament instability of the ankle. Orthop Nurs 7(3):33, 1988

Johnson J: Respiratory complications of orthopedic injuries. Orthop Nurs 5(1):24, 1986

Kilcoyne RF et al: Acute osteomyelitis of the lower extremity. Nurs Mirror 155:7, 1982

Kuska BM: Acute onset compartment syndrome. J Emerg Nurs 8:75, 1982

Lavine LS, Grodzinsky AJ: Electrical stimulation repair of bone. J Bone Joint Surg 69(A):626, 1987

Lupien AE: Head off compartment syndrome before it's too late. RN:39, 1980

Lynden JC, Spielman FJ: Bilateral compartment syndrome following prolonged surgery in the lithotomy position. Anesthesiology 60:236, 1984

Merritt K: Factors increasing the risk of infection in patients with open fracture. J Trauma 28:823, 1988

Miller MC: Nursing care of the patient with external fixation therapy. Orthop Nurs 12(1):11, 1980

Moorey BF, Dunn JM, Heimbach RD, Davis J: Hyperbaric oxygen and chronic osteomyelitis. Clin Orthop Rel Res 144:121, 1979

Nade S: Acute hematogenous osteomyelitis in infancy and childhood. J Bone Joint Surg 65(B):109, 1983

Osborne LJ, DiGiacomo I: Traction: A review with nursing diagnoses and interventions. Orthop Nurs 6(4):14, 1987

Patterson DC, Lewis GN, Cass CA: Treatment of delayed union and nonunion with implanted direct current stimulator. Clin Orthop Rel Res 140:117, 1980

Pyper A, Black GB: Orthopedic injuries in children associated with use of off-road vehicles. J Bone Joint Surg 70(A):275, 1988

Rorabeck CH, Bourne RB, Fowler PJ: The surgical treatment of exertional compartment syndrome in athletes. J Bone Joint Surg 65(A):1245, 1983

Searls K et al: External fixation: General principles patient care. Crit Care Q 6:45, 1983

Septimus EJ, Musher DM: Osteomyelitis: Recent clinical and laboratory aspects. Orthop Clin North Am 10:347, 1979

Sisk TD: General principles and techniques of external skeletal fixation. Clin Orthop Rel Res 180:96, 1983

Sugarman B, Young EJ: Infected implants and infection control. Asepsis 9(4):14, 1987

Taylor JF: Osteomyelitis: The acute form. Nurs Times 72:486, 1976

Taylor JF: Osteomyelitis: The chronic form. Nurs Times 72:535, 1976

Valerz JM: Surgical implants: Orthopedic devices. AORN 37:1341, 1983

Wald ER: Risk factors in osteomyelitis. Am J Med 78 (suppl B): 206, 1985

CHAPTER 56

Kathleen E. Gunta

Alterations in Skeletal Function: Congenital Disorders, Metabolic Bone Disease, and Neoplasms

Objectives

After you have studied this chapter you should be able to meet the following objectives:

_____ Differentiate between the processes of endochondral and intramembranous ossification that occur during embryonic development.

_____ Describe the function of the epiphysis in skeletal growth.

_____ Cite at least three factors that can affect epiphyseal growth.

_____ Explain how an infant's limbs differ from those of an adult.

_____ Define *femoral anteversion*.

_____ Differentiate between toeing-in and internal tibial torsion.

_____ Define *genu varum* and *genu valgum*.

_____ Name one treatment for flatfeet.

_____ Identify two childhood diseases that are classified as osteochondroses.

_____ Describe the pathology of Legg–Calvé–Perthes disease.

_____ List the symptoms of Osgood–Schlatter disease.

_____ Explain why it is important to treat a slipped capital femoral epiphyseal as soon as it is diagnosed.

_____ Cite the incidence of scoliosis.

_____ List the cardinal signs of scoliosis that serve as a basis for school screening programs.

_____ Contrast the conservative and surgical treatments of scoliosis.

_____ Describe the physical appearance of an infant with congenital dislocation of the hip.

_____ Give the recommended schedule for clinical examination to detect congenital hip dislocation.

(continued)

_____ Explain the treatment for a newborn with club-foot.

_____ List the problems that occur because of defective tissue synthesis in osteogenesis imperfecta.

_____ Name the three factors that are responsible for maintaining the equilibrium of bone tissue.

_____ Compare structural remodeling of bone with internal remodeling.

_____ Cite the functions of parathyroid hormone, vitamin D, and calcitonin in bone metabolism.

_____ Trace the activation of vitamin D in the body.

_____ Define the term *osteopenia*.

_____ Describe the primary features of osteoporotic bone.

_____ Cite the sex, race, and age groups of persons most frequently affected by osteoporosis.

_____ List three factors that contribute to the development of osteoporosis.

_____ Describe the action of fluoride in the treatment of osteoporosis.

_____ Contrast osteomalacia, rickets, and osteoporosis.

_____ Relate vitamin D deficiency to the inadequate mineralization of bone that occurs in osteomalacia and rickets.

_____ Describe the appearance of bone affected by Paget's disease (osteitis deformans).

_____ List the clinical manifestations of Paget's disease.

_____ Differentiate between the properties of benign and malignant bone tumors.

_____ Name the three major symptoms of bone cancer.

_____ Describe the population primarily affected by osteogenic sarcoma.

_____ Contrast osteogenic sarcoma and chondrosarcoma.

_____ List the primary sites of tumors that frequently metastasize to the bone.

_____ Explain why metastasis to the bone frequently occurs without involving other organs.

_____ State the three primary goals for treatment of metastatic bone disease.

During childhood, skeletal structures grow in both length and diameter and sustain a large increase in bone mass. The term *modeling* refers to the formation of the macroscopic skeleton, which ceases at maturity (age 18 to 20 years). Bone remodeling functions to replace existing bone and occurs in both children and adults. It involves both resorption and formation of bone. With aging, bone resorption and formation are no longer perfectly coupled, and there is loss of bone. Alterations in musculoskeletal structure and function may develop as a result of normal growth and developmental processes or as a result of impairment of skeletal development due to hereditary or congenital influences. Other skeletal disorders can occur later in life as a result of metabolic disorders or neoplastic growth.

Alterations in skeletal growth and development

—— Bone growth and remodeling

—— Embryonic development

The skeletal system develops from the mesoderm, the thin middle layer of embryonic tissue, by two different ossification processes: endochondral or intramembranous ossification. Endochondral ossification involves ossification of a cartilaginous bone model. Intramembranous ossification occurs where there is no preexisting cartilage model. In the skull, it involves ossification of the loose layer of mesenchymal tissue that fills the space between the brain and the skin.

Development of the vertebrae of the axial skeleton begins at about the fourth week in the embryo; during the ninth week, ossification begins with the appearance of ossification centers in the lower thoracic and upper lumbar vertebrae. The limb buds of the appendicular skeleton make their appearance late in the fourth week. The hand pads are present on day 33, and the finger rays are evident on day 41 of embryonic development.[1]

—— Bone growth in childhood

During the first two decades of life, the skeleton undergoes general overall growth. The long bones of the skeleton, which grow at a relatively rapid rate, are provided with a specialized structure called the epiphyseal growth plate. As long bones grow in length, the deeper layers of cartilage cells in the growth plate multiply and enlarge, pushing the articular cartilage further away from the metaphysis and diaphysis of the bone. As this happens, the mature and enlarged cartilage cells at the metaphyseal end of the plate become metabolically inactive and are replaced by bone cells (Figure 56-1). This process allows bone growth to proceed without changing the shape of the bone or causing disruption of the articular cartilage. The cells in the growth plate stop dividing at puberty, at which time the epiphysis and metaphysis fuse.

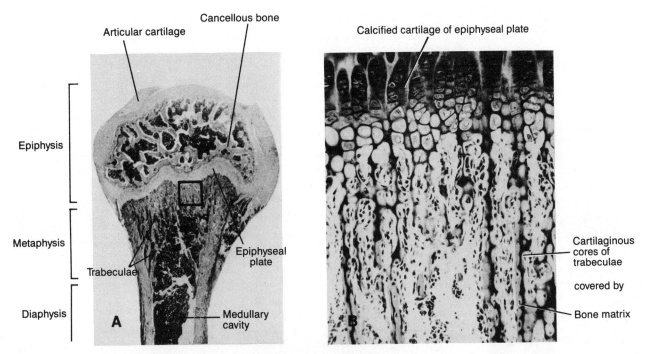

Figure 56-1 **(A)** Low-power photomicrograph of one end of a growing long bone (rat). Osteogenesis has now spread from the epiphyseal center of ossification so that only the articular cartilage above and the epiphyseal disk below remain cartilaginous. On the diaphyseal side of the epiphyseal plate (disk), metaphyseal trabeculae extend down into the diaphysis. **(B)** Medium-power photomicrograph of the area indicated in **A,** showing trabeculae on the diaphyseal side of the epiphyseal plate (disk). These have cores of calcified cartilage on which bone has been deposited. The cartilaginous cores of the trabeculae were formerly partitions between columns of chondrocytes in the epiphyseal plate (disk). (*Cormack DH: Ham's Histology, 9th ed, p 299. Philadelphia, JB Lippincott, 1987*)

A number of factors can influence the growth of cells in the epiphyseal growth plate. Epiphyseal separation can occur in children as the result of accidents. The separation usually occurs in the zone of the mature enlarged cartilage cells, which is the weakest part of the growth plate. The blood vessels that nourish the epiphysis, which pass through the growth plate, are ruptured when the growth plate separates. This can cause cessation of growth and a shortened extremity.

The growth plate is also sensitive to nutritional and metabolic changes. Scurvy (vitamin C deficiency) impairs the formation of the organic matrix of bone, causing slowing of growth at the epiphyseal plate and cessation of diaphyseal growth. In rickets (vitamin D deficiency) calcification of the newly developed bone on the metaphyseal side of the growth plate is impaired. Thyroid and growth hormones are both required for normal growth. Alterations in these and other hormones can affect growth (see Chapter 44).

Growth in the diameter of bones occurs by oppositional growth of new bone on the surface of existing bone along with an accompanying resorption of bone on the endosteal surface; in this manner the shape of the bone is maintained. Figure 56-2 illus-

trates how bone is deposited and resorbed during structural remodeling at the ends of growing long bones. As a bone grows in diameter, concentric rings are added to the bone surface, much as rings are added to a tree trunk: these rings form the lamellar structure of mature bone. Osteocytes, which develop from osteoblasts, become buried in the rings. Haversian channels form as periosteal vessels running along the long axis become surrounded by bone.

Alterations occurring during normal growth periods

Infants and children undergo changes in muscle tone and joint motion during growth and development. These changes usually cause few problems and are corrected during normal growth processes. The normal folded position of the fetus *in utero* causes physiologic flexion contractures of the hips and a froglike appearance of the lower extremities. The hips are externally rotated and the patellae point outward, while the feet appear to point forward because of the internal pulling force of the tibiae. During the first year of life the lower extremities begin to straighten out in preparation for walking. Internal and external rotation become equal, and the hips extend.

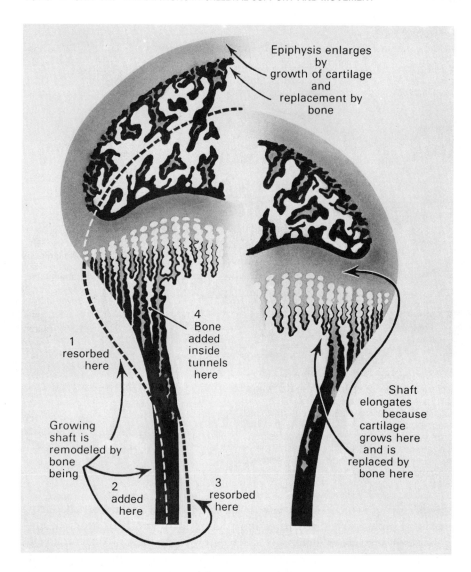

Figure 56-2 Diagram illustrating the surfaces where bone is deposited or resorbed during remodeling at the ends of growing long bones with flared extremities. (*Cormack DH: Ham's Histology, 9th ed, p 303. Philadelphia, JB Lippincott, 1987*)

Flexion contractures of the shoulders, elbows, and knees are also commonly seen in newborns, but they should disappear by 3 months of age.[2]

All infants and toddlers have lax ligaments that become tighter with age and assumption of the weight-bearing posture. The hypermobility that accompanies joint laxity along with torsional, or twisting, forces exerted on the limbs during growth are responsible for a number of variants seen in young children. Torsional forces caused by intrauterine positions or sleeping and sitting patterns twist the growing bones and can produce the deformities seen with growth and development.

Femoral anteversion

Femoral anteversion (internal femoral torsion) is a normal variant commonly seen during the first 6 years of life, especially in 3- and 4-year-old girls. Hip rotation in both flexion and extension can be measured with computed tomography. Internal rotation of the hips exceeds external rotation by 30 degrees or more. It is related to the increased ligamentous laxity of the anterior capsule of the hip: this joint does not provide the stable pressure needed to correct the approximately 50 degrees of anteversion present at birth. Children are most comfortable sitting in the "M" position, with the hips between the heels. When the child stands, the knees turn in while the feet appear to point straight ahead; and when the child walks, both knees and toes point in. Children with this problem are encouraged to sit in the so-called Indian chief, or "W," position. If left untreated, the tibiae compensate by becoming externally rotated so that by 8 to 12 years of age the knees may turn in but the feet no longer do. A derotational osteotomy is done in severe cases.

Toeing-out

Toeing-out is a common problem in children caused by external femoral torsion. This occurs when the femur can be externally rotated to about 90 degrees but internally rotated only to a neutral position or slightly beyond. When a child habitually sleeps in the prone position, the femoral torsion will persist and an external tibial torsion may also develop. If external tibial torsion is present, the feet point lateral to the midline of the medial plane. External tibial torsion rarely causes toeing-out: it only intensifies the condition. Toeing-out usually corrects itself as the child becomes proficient in walking. Occasionally a night splint is used.

Toeing-in

Toeing-in (pigeon toe) can be caused by torsion in the feet, lower legs, or entire leg. Toeing-in due to adduction of the forefoot (congenital metatarsus adductus) is usually the result of the fetal position maintained *in utero*. It may occur in one foot or bilaterally. A supple deformity can be passively manipulated into a straight position and requires no treatment. Treatment consisting of serial casting or an orthosis that pushes the metatarsals (not the hindfoot) into abduction is usually required in a fixed deformity (*i.e.,* one in which the forefoot cannot be passively manipulated into a straight position).

Internal tibial torsion

Internal tibial torsion (bowing of the tibia) is a rotation of the tibia that makes the feet appear to turn inward. It is present at birth and fails to correct itself if children either sleep on their knees with the feet turned in or sit on inturned feet. In 80% of cases, it will resolve itself by the time the child is 18 months of age.[3] In the other 20% of cases, the Denis Browne splint (a bar to which shoes are attached) may be used to put the feet into mild external rotation while the child is sleeping. This treatment stimulates the proximal growth plate of the tibia to grow in a spiral fashion and correct the defect. Surgery may be necessary if tibial torsion persists beyond age 3, but only if the condition is severe and significantly interferes with walking and running.

Genu varum and genu valgum

Genu varum (bowlegs) is an outward bowing of the knees when the medial malleoli of the ankles are touching. Most infants and toddlers have some bowing of their legs up to age 2. If there is a large separation between the knees (*i.e.,* greater than 15 degrees) after age 2, the child may require bracing. The child should also be evaluated for diseases such as rickets or tibia vara (Blount's disease).

Genu valgum (knock-knees) is a deformity in which there is decreased space between the knees. The medial malleoli in the ankles cannot be brought in contact with each other when the knees are touching. It is seen most frequently in children between the ages of 2 and 6 years. The condition is usually the result of lax medial collateral ligaments of the knee and may be exacerbated by sitting in the "M" position. Genu valgum can be ignored up to age 7, unless it is more than 15 degrees, unilateral, or associated with short stature. It usually resolves spontaneously and rarely requires treatment.

Flatfoot

Flatfoot is a deformity characterized by the absence of the longitudinal arch of the foot. Infants normally have a wider and fatter foot than adults. The fat pads that are normally accentuated by pliable muscles create an illusion of fullness often mistaken for flatfeet. Until the longitudinal arch develops at age 2 to 3 years, all children have flatfeet. The true criterion for flatfoot (pes planus) is that the head of the talus points medially and downward, so that the heel is everted and the forefoot must be inverted (toed in) in order for the metatarsal heads to be planted equally on the ground. Weight bearing may cause pain in the longitudinal arch and up the leg.

There are two types of flatfeet—supple and rigid. Supple flatfeet are always bilateral, occur more often in black people, and tend to be familial.[3] In supple flatfeet, the arch disappears only with weight bearing. The rigid flatfoot is fixed with no apparent arch in any position. It is seen in conjunction with neuromuscular diseases and juvenile rheumatoid arthritis.

In the adult, treatment of flatfeet is conservative and aimed at relieving fatigue, pain, and tenderness. Supportive well-fitting shoes with arch supports may be helpful and prevent prevent ligaments from becoming overstretched. Women may complain of pain in the forefoot when wearing poorly fitting high heels. Surgery may be done in cases of severe and persistant symptoms.

Juvenile osteochondroses

The term *juvenile osteochondroses* is used to describe a group of children's diseases in which one or more growth ossification centers undergo a period of degeneration, necrosis, or inactivity that is followed by regeneration and usually deformity. The osteochondroses are separated into two groups according to their etiologies. The first group consists of the *true osteonecrotic osteochondroses,* so called because the diseases are caused by localized osteonecrosis of an apophyseal or epiphyseal center (Legg–Calvé–Perthes disease, Freiberg's infarction, Panner's disease, and Kienbock's disease). The second group of juvenile osteochondroses are caused by abnormalities of endochondral ossification, due either to a genetically determined normal variation or to trauma (Osgood–Schlatter disease, Blount's disease, Sever's disease, and Scheuermann's disease). The discussion in this section focuses on Legge–Calvé–Perthes disease from the first group and Osgood–Schlatter disease from the second group.

Legg–Calvé–Perthes disease

Legg–Calvé–Perthes disease (coxa plana) is an osteonecrotic disease of the proximal femoral (capital) epiphysis, which is the growth center for the head of the femur. It occurs in 1 out of 1200 children, affecting primarily those between ages 3 and 12 years with a peak age of 6 years.[4] It occurs primarily in boys and is much more common in whites than blacks. Although no definite genetic pattern has been established, it occasionally affects more than one family member. The incidence for siblings developing the disease is 1 in 25.[5]

The cause of Legg-Calvé-Perthes disease is unknown. The disorder is usually insidious in onset and occurs in otherwise healthy children. It may, however, be associated with acute trauma. The children usually affected have a shorter stature. Undernutrition has been suggested as a causative factor. When girls are affected, they usually have a poorer prognosis than boys because they are skeletally more mature. This means that they would have a shorter period for growth and remodeling than boys of the same age. Although both legs can be affected, in 85% of the cases only one leg is involved.[5]

The primary pathologic feature of Legg–Calvé-Perthes disease is an avascular necrosis of the bone and marrow involving the epiphyseal growth center in the femoral head. The disorder may be confined to part of the epiphysis, or it may involve the entire epiphysis. In severe cases, there is a disturbance in the growth pattern that leads to a broad, short femoral neck. The necrosis is followed by slow absorption of the dead bone over a 2- to 3-year period. Although the necrotic trabeculae are eventually replaced by healthy new bone, the epiphysis rarely regains its normal shape. The process occurs in four predictable stages, each with its distinctive radiologic characteristics:

1. The incipient or synovitis stage, which is characterized by synovial inflammation and increased joint fluid. This stage usually lasts from 1 to 3 weeks.
2. The aseptic or avascular stage, during which the ossification center becomes necrotic. This stage may last from several months to a year. Damage to the femoral head is determined by the degree of necrosis that occurs during this stage. This stage lasts 3 to 6 months.
3. The regenerative or revascularization stage, which involves the resorption of the necrotic bone. This stage lasts for 1 to 3 years, during which time the necrotic bone is gradually re-

placed by new immature bone cells and the contour of the bone is remodeled.
4. The healed or residual stage, characterized by the formation and replacement of immature bone cells by normal bone cells. Remodeling of the femoral head continues throughout the growing years but is ultimately determined by the amount of collapse that has occurred during the avascular stage.

Legg–Calvé–Perthes disease has an insidious onset with a prolonged course. The main symptoms are pain in the groin, thigh, or knee and difficulty in walking. The child may have a painless limp with limited abduction and internal rotation, and a flexion contracture of the affected hip. The age of onset is important because young children have a greater capability for remodeling of the femoral head and acetabulum, and thus less flattening of the femoral head will occur. More than 50% of the cases occur between ages 5 and 7 years. Early diagnosis is important and is based on correlating physical symptoms with x-ray findings that are related to the stage of the disease.

The goal of treatment is to reduce deformity and preserve the integrity of the femoral head. Both conservative and surgical interventions are used in the treatment of Legg–Calvé–Perthes disease. Children under 4 years of age with little or no involvement of the femoral head may require only periodic observation. In all other children, some intervention is needed to relieve the force of weight bearing, the muscular tension, and subluxation of the femoral head. It is important to maintain the femur in a well-seated position in the concave acetabulum in order to prevent deformity. This is done by keeping the hip in abduction and mild internal rotation.

The initial treatment usually involves bed rest with Russell or Buck's traction (see Chapter 55) or with a device to keep the legs separated in abduction with mild internal rotation (e.g., hip spica cast or abduction brace). Once the inflammatory stage has subsided (usually several weeks), the child is allowed up but is not permitted to bear weight on the femoral head. The child walks with crutches and may be required to wear a brace, splint, or walking cast.

Surgery may be done to contain the femoral head within the acetabulum. This treatment is usually reserved for children older than 6 years who at the time of diagnosis have more serious involvement of the femoral head. Several sources indicate that the best surgical results are obtained when surgery is done early, before the epiphysis becomes necrotic.[6,7]

Osgood–Schlatter disease

Osgood–Schlatter disease is a partial separation of the tibial tuberosity caused by sudden or continued strain on the patellar tendon during growth. It occurs most frequently in boys between the ages of 10 and 16 years.[8] The disorder is characterized by pain in the front of the knee associated with inflammation and thickening of the patellar tendon. The disorder is not a true osteochondrosis. Instead, it probably represents a partial avulsion or tearing away of the tibial tubercle as the result of extraordinary stress placed on the knee during a critical growth period.[8] Follow-up studies have indicated that the disorder may really be a mechanical tendonitis with partial avulsion of the tibial tubercle.[8]

With Osgood–Schlatter disease, pain is usually associated with specific activities such as kneeling, running, bicycle riding, or stair climbing. The symptoms are self-limiting; although they may recur during adolescence, they usually resolve after closure of the tibial growth plate. In some cases, limitations on activity, braces, and even a plaster cast to immobilize the knee may be necessary to relieve the pain. Occasionally minor symptoms or an increased prominence of the tibial tubercle may continue into adulthood. Surgery may be indicated to excise painful bony fragments from the patellar tendon.

Slipped capital femoral epiphysis

Normally, the proximal femoral epiphysis unites with the neck of the femur between ages 16 and 19 years. Prior to this time (10 to 17 years in girls and 13 to 16 years in boys) the femoral head may slip from its normal position directly at the head of the femur and become displaced medially and posteriorly.[8] This produces an adduction, lateral rotation, and extension deformity. About 1 in 50,000 children suffer a slipped capital femoral epiphysis.[5]

The etiology of slipped capital femoral epiphysis is obscure, but it may be related to the child's susceptibility to stress on the femoral neck as a result of genetics or abnormal structure. Boys are affected twice as often as girls, and in 50% of cases the condition is bilateral.[8] Affected children are often overweight with poorly developed secondary sex characteristics or, in some instances, are extremely tall and thin. In many cases there is a history of rapid skeletal growth preceding displacement of the epiphysis.

There are often complaints of referred knee pain in children with the condition, accompanied by reports of difficulty walking, fatigue, and stiffness. The diagnosis is confirmed by x-ray studies in which the degree of slipping can be determined on a lateral view. Early treatment is imperative to prevent lifelong crippling. Avoidance of weight bearing on the femur and bed rest are essential parts of the treatment. Traction or gentle manipulation under anesthesia is used to reduce the slip. Surgical insertion of pins to keep the femoral neck and head of the femur aligned is a common method of treatment for children with moderate or severe slips. Crutches are used for several months following surgical correction to prevent full weight bearing until the growth plate is sealed by the bony union.

Scoliosis

Scoliosis is a lateral deviation of the spinal column that may or may not include rotation or deformity of the vertebrae. It has been estimated that over 1 million Americans have a significant degree of scoliosis.[9] It is most commonly seen during adolescence and is 8 times more frequent in girls than boys. An increase in joint laxity, which causes excessive joint motion and is more common in girls, has been associated with development of idiopathic scoliosis.[10]

Scoliosis can develop as the result of another disease condition or it can occur without known cause. Idiopathic scoliosis, or scoliosis of unknown cause, accounts for 75% to 80% of the total number of cases of the disorder and affects between 2% and 8% of the population in the United States.[11] The other 20% to 25% of cases are caused by over 50 different etiologies, including poliomyelitis, congenital hemivertebrae, neurofibromatosis and cerebral palsy. Family history is positive for scoliosis in about 30% of the cases.[12]

Scoliosis is classified as either postural or structural. With postural scoliosis there is a small curve that corrects with bending. It can be corrected with passive and active exercises. Structural scoliosis does not correct with bending. It is a fixed deformity classified into three categories based on etiology: (1) idiopathic, (2) congenital, and (3) neuromuscular.

Idiopathic scoliosis is a structural spinal curvature for which no etiology has been established. It occurs primarily in infants of the United Kingdom and Europe during the first 3 years of life. Its usual effect on males is a curve in the thoracic area that is convex and to the left. Juvenile idiopathic scoliosis occurs in children between 5 and 6 years of age and is quite rare. Adolescent idiopathic scoliosis is the most common type of scoliosis and usually appears in girls beginning at about age 10.[13]

Congenital scoliosis is caused by disturbances in vertebral development during the third to fifth week of embryologic development.[14] There are structural anomalies in the vertebrae that can cause a severe curvature. The child may have other anomalies and neurologic complications if the spine is involved.

Neuromuscular scoliosis develops from neuropathic or myopathic diseases. Neuropathic scoliosis is seen with cerebral palsy and poliomyelitis. There is often a long C-shaped curve from the cervical to the sacral region. In cerebral palsy there may be severe deformity that makes treatment quite difficult. Myopathic neuromuscular scoliosis develops with muscular dystrophy and is usually not severe.

Scoliosis is usually first noted because of the deformity it causes. A high shoulder, prominent hip, or projecting scapula may be noticed by a parent or in a school screening program. In girls, difficulty in hemming or fitting a dress may call attention to the deformity. Pain is present in severe cases, usually in the lumbar region. The pain may be caused by pressure on the ribs or the crest of the ilium. There may be shortness of breath as a result of diminished chest expansion and gastrointestinal disturbances from crowding of the abdominal organs. Adults with less severe deformity may experience mild backache. If scoliosis is left untreated, the curve may progress to a point where cardiopulmonary function is compromised and there is a risk of neurologic complications. New surgical techniques are available to successfully treat adults with undetected or progressive scoliosis.[15,16]

Early diagnosis of scoliosis is important in prevention of severe spinal deformity. School screening programs are an excellent method for early detection of scoliosis in adolescents. Screening should be done yearly in the fifth through tenth grades. School nurses and physical education teachers can be specially trained to carry out the examination, which takes about 30 seconds to complete. Both boys and girls should be screened. Students are examined from the front, back, and sides while standing and bending with arms both at the sides and out in front with palms

Table 56–1. Treatment parameters for scoliosis

Treatment	Indicators
I. Periodic assessment and exercise	Curvature of less than 20 degrees; resolving infantile curve; and curve in adults
II. External bracing: Milwaukee brace Orthoplast jacket Body cast	Curvature of 15 degrees to 25 degrees; skeletally immature curvature of 20 degrees to 40 degrees
III. Surgery: Harrington rod instrumentation Dwyer cable instrumentation Segmental (Luque) spinal instrumentation	Some curvatures of 20 degrees to 40 degrees; most curvatures of greater than 40 degrees

touching. The cardinal signs of scoliosis are: (1) uneven shoulders or iliac crest, (2) prominent scapula on the convex side of the curve, (3) malalignment of spinous processes, (4) asymmetry of the flanks, (5) asymmetry of the thoracic cage, and (6) rib hump or paraspinal muscle prominence when bending forward (Figure 56-3).

Diagnosis is made by physical examination and confirmed by radiography. The curve is measured by determining the amount of lateral deviation present on x-ray films and is labeled right or left for the convex portion of the curve. Several different methods are used.

The treatment of scoliosis depends on the severity of the deformity (Table 56-1). A conservative approach includes periodic assessment and either an exercise program or some form of external bracing. An exercise program is designed to promote the maximum degree of correction possible based on the degree of flexibility present at the time of diagnosis. The pelvic tilt exercise is an example of an exercise done both with and without a brace.

A brace is used to control the progression of the curvature during growth and also provides some correction. The most commonly used brace is the Milwaukee brace, which was developed by Blount and Schmitt in 1945 (Figure 56-4). This was the first brace to provide some degree of active correction. It is the treatment of choice for curvatures of 40 degrees or less in adolescents with idiopathic scoliosis. The decision to use the brace has to be an individual one, with consideration being given to the likelihood of progression to 40 degrees or more and the cosmetic impact on the individual. Lateral pads apply pressure to the apex of the curve (i.e., the point most deviated from the vertical axis) on the convex side. The brace is usually

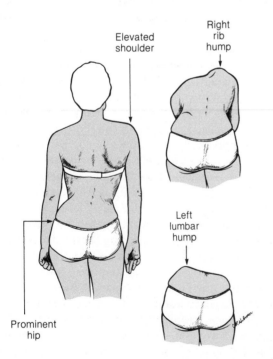

Elevated shoulder
Right rib hump
Left lumbar hump
Prominent hip

Figure 56-3 Scoliosis. Abnormalities to be determined at initial screening examination. (*Gore DR, Passehl R, Sepic S, Dalton A: Scoliosis screening: Results of a community project. Pediatrics 67[2], 1981. Copyright © 1981 by the American Academy of Pediatrics.*)

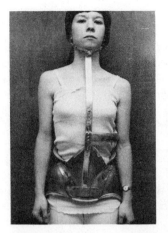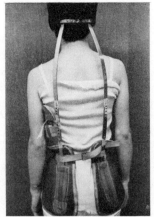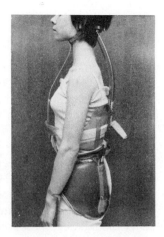

Figure 56-4 The Milwaukee brace as seen from front, back, and side. (*Farrell J: Illustrated Guide to Orthopedic Nursing, 2nd ed, p 172. Philadelphia, JB Lippincott, 1982*)

prescribed for 23 hours per day, with removal permitted only for hygienic purposes. In reality, however, few adolescents comply with this program. Compliance is higher in younger children, with most high-school-age children wearing their braces only 9 to 12 hours per day. Because of the high noncompliance in the full-time programs, part-time programs have been initiated with 16 hours or less of prescribed brace-wear for curvatures of less than 35 degrees.[17] In this program, the adolescent does not have to wear the brace to school.

Exercises are done during the time out of the brace and when the brace is on. Good skin care is essential in order to prevent breakdown under the brace. It is important for health care professionals to work with the adolescent in order to ensure their compliance with the treatment program. This is particularly important because the brace may present an additional stress to an already threatened body image.

Surgical intervention with instrumentation and spinal fusion is done in severe cases—when the curvature has progressed to 40 degrees or beyond at the time of diagnosis or when curves of a lesser degree are compounded with imbalance or rotation of the vertebrae. Three methods of instrumentation are used: (1) Harrington rod and posterior spinal fusion, (2) Dwyer (or Zielke) instrumentation and anterior spinal fusion, (3) segmental (Luque) spinal instrumentation and posterior spinal fusion, or (4) Cortrel-Dubousset bilateral segmental fixation. With the Harrington rod instrumentation and posterior spinal fusion, a distraction rod is attached to the posterior aspect of the spinal column on the concave side of the curvature. A second, more flexible rod, may be used to compress the convex side. The Drummond or Wisconsin technique includes wires placed through the base of the spinous process and around the Harring-

ton rod to provide multiple points of fixation. With the anterior instrumentation method, a wire cable (Dwyer) or steel rod (Zielke) is threaded through screw and staple units inserted directly into the vertebral body as a means of exerting tension on the convex side of the curve. The spine is then fused anteriorly. This is usually followed several weeks later by a posterior fusion done for added correction and stability. A Dwyer or Zielke instrumentation procedure is difficult because the anterior fusion requires a transthoracic and retroperitoneal approach (through the rib cage and pulmonary cavity). With the segmental instrumentation method a posterior fusion is used along with the Luque instrumentation. Wire loops are attached to the laminae as a means of securing rods to both sides of the spine. This provides a rigid internal fixation at the level of each vertebra. Cortrel-Dubousset instrumentation consists of two gnarled rods linked together with various hooks and transverse fixation rods that provide a three-dimensional correction of the curve and rotational stability. The system is used to treat a variety of spinal problems, including scoliosis, kyphosis, fractures, and tumors.

Patients who have had a Harrington rod inserted or a Dwyer procedure performed are immobilized in a body cast or Milwaukee brace. Traction may be used initially, applied directly to the Milwaukee brace. A CircOlectric bed, Stryker frame, or Foster frame may be used to assist with turning. Patients with a Harrington rod or Dwyer instrumentation require a longer period of postoperative bed rest than those who had the segmental (Luque) spinal instrumentation procedure. The Cortrel-Dubousset instrumentation system necessitates a shorter period of immobilization after surgery. A brace is not required except for adults or adolescents with neuromuscular disease.

Hereditary and congenital deformities

Congenital deformities are abnormalities that are present at birth. They can be caused by hereditary influences or by disturbances in embryonic development. They range in severity from mild limb deformities, which are relatively common, to major limb malformations, which are relatively rare. There may be a simple webbing of the fingers or toes (syndactyly) or the presence of an extra digit (polydactyly). Joint contractures and dislocations produce more severe deformity, as does the absence of entire bones, joints, or limbs. An epidemic of limb deformities occurred from 1957 to 1962 as a result of maternal ingestion of thalidomide. This drug was withdrawn from the market in 1961.

Congenital deformities are caused by many factors, some as yet unknown. These factors include genetic influences, external agents that injure the fetus (e.g., radiation, alcohol, medications, and viruses), and in utero environmental factors. As discussed in Chapter 4, the fourth to the seventh week of gestation is the most vulnerable period for development of limb deformities.

Congenital dislocation of the hip

Congenital dislocation of the hip is seen in 1.6 out of every 1000 live births. It occurs most frequently in first-born children and is six times more common in female than in male infants.[14] It is thought that the instability of the hip is a consequence of laxity of the ligaments, which is genetically determined, and displacement is the result of environmental factors such as fetal position or breech delivery.[14]

In a child with congenital dislocation of the hip, the head of the femur is located outside of the acetabulum. In less severe cases, the hip joint may be either unstable or subluxed, so that the joint surfaces are separated and there is a partial dislocation. Hip dislocation may be associated with ligamentous laxity and environmental influences such as intrauterine positioning or breech presentation during delivery.

Normal development of the hip requires that a normal positional relationship should exist between the femoral head and the acetabulum. If this relationship is not maintained, there may be a delay in the maturation, size, and development of both the femoral head and the acetabulum. Early diagnosis of congenital hip dislocation is important because treatment is easiest and most effective if begun during the first 6 months of life. Repeated dislocation causes damage to both the femoral head and the acetabulum. Clinical examinations to detect dislocation of the hip should be done at birth and every several months during the first

year of life. If the femoral head can be displaced by the examiner, it is considered dislocatable.

Several examination techniques are used to screen for congenital hip dislocation. In infants, signs of dislocation include asymmetry of the hip or gluteal folds, shortening of the thigh so that one knee (on the affected side) is higher than the other, and limited abduction of the affected hip (Figure 56-5). The asymmetry of gluteal folds is not definitive but indicates the need for further evaluation. A specific examination involves an attempt to manually dislocate and then reduce the abnormal hip while the infant is in the supine position with both knees flexed. With gentle downward pressure being applied to the knees, the knee and thigh is manually abducted as an upward and medial pressure is applied to the proximal thigh. In infants with the disorder, the initial downward pressure on the knee produces a dislocation of the hip, which is followed by a palpable or audible click (Ortolani sign) as the hip is reduced and moves back into the acetabulum. In an older child, instability of the hip may produce a delay in standing or walking and even-

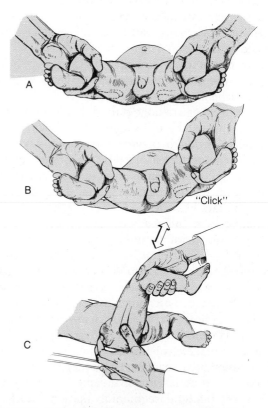

Figure 56-5 Congenital dislocation of the hip. (**A**) In the newborn, both hips can be equally flexed, abducted, and externally rotated without producing a "click." (**B**) A diagnosis of a congenital dislocation of the hip may be confirmed by the Ortolani "click" test. The involved hip cannot be abducted as far as the opposite one, and there is a "click" as the hip reduces. (**C**) Telescoping of the femur to aid in the diagnosis of a congenitally dislocated hip. (*Hoppenfeld's Physical Examination of the Spine and Extremities. New York, Appleton-Century-Croft, 1976*)

tually a characteristic waddling gait. When the thumbs are placed over the anterior iliac crest and the hands over the lateral pelvis in examination, the levels of the thumbs are not even; in addition, the child is unable to elevate the opposite side of the pelvis (positive Trendelenburg's test). Diagnosis is confirmed by radiography.

The treatment of congenital hip dislocation is begun as soon as the diagnosis has been made. The best results are obtained if the treatment is begun before there is weight bearing on the hip and the hip is reduced by 1 year of age. Treatment at any age includes reduction of the dislocation and immobilization of the legs in an abducted position. The most serious complication of any treatment is avascular necrosis of the femoral head as a result of the forced abduction. With children under 3 years of age, gentle traction is used when reduction cannot be easily obtained. This treatment is followed by several months of immobilization in a hip spica cast, plaster splints, or an abduction splint such as a Frejka pillow or Pavlik harness. The harness allows the child more mobility as the leg is slowly and gently brought into abduction. Failure to use the harness correctly can result in a need for surgery. Adults with unreduced congenital dislocation of the hip require a total hip replacement because of damage to the articulating surface of the joint. These individuals have considerable problems after surgery because of their soft tissue contractures.

Congenital clubfoot

Congenital clubfoot can affect one or both feet. Like congenital dislocation of hip, its occurrence follows a multifactorial inheritance pattern. The condition has an incidence of 1 per every 1,000 live births and occurs twice as often in males as in females.[18] The chance that a sibling will have the defect is 3% and that the offspring of an affected person will have the disorder, 8% to 11%.

In the most common form of clubfoot (95% of cases) the foot is plantar flexed and inverted.[18] This is the so-called *equinovarus* type where the foot resembles a horse's hoof (Figure 56-6). The other 5% of cases are of the *calcaneovalgus* type (reverse clubfoot), in which the foot is dorsiflexed and everted. The reverse clubfoot can occur as an isolated condition or in association with multiple congenital defects.

At birth, the feet of many infants assume one of these two positions, but they can be passively overcorrected or brought back into the opposite position. If the foot cannot be overcorrected, some type of correction may be necessary. Although the exact cause of clubfoot is unknown, there are three theories that are generally accepted: (1) an anomalous development occurs during the first trimester of pregnancy, (2) the

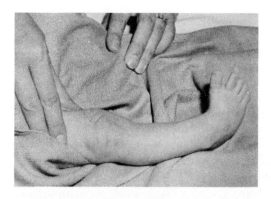

Figure 56-6 Talipes equinovarus deformity. Note the internal tibial torsion. (*Turek SL: Orthopaedics: Principles and Their Application, 4th ed. Philadelphia, JB Lippincott, 1984*)

leg fails to rotate inward and move from the equinovarus position at about the third month, or (3) the soft tissues in the foot do not mature and lengthen.

Clubfoot varies in severity from a mild deformity to one in which the foot is completely inverted. The treatment is begun as soon as the diagnosis is made. When treatment is initiated during the first few weeks of life, a nonoperative procedure is effective within a short period. Serial manipulations and casting is used to gently correct each component in the forefoot varus, the hindfoot varus, and the equinus. The treatment is continued until the foot is in a normal position with full correction evident clinically and on x-ray studies. Surgery may be required for severe deformities or when nonoperative treatment methods are unsuccessful. An external distractor, like the Ilizarov external fixator, is being used in Asia and Europe to correct the deformity of a relapsed or neglected clubfoot.[19]

Osteogenesis imperfecta

Osteogenesis imperfecta is a hereditary disease that is characterized by defective synthesis of connective tissue, including bone matrix. It is perhaps the most common hereditary bone disease, with an occurrence rate of approximately 1 in 40,000 births.[20] Although it is usually transmitted as an autosomal dominant trait, a distinct form of the disorder with multiple lethal defects is thought to be inherited as an autosomal recessive trait. In the latter case, as many as 25% of the offspring of carrier (asymptomatic) parents may be affected.[21]

The disorder is characterized by thin and poorly developed bones that are prone to multiple fractures. These children have short limbs and a soft, thin cranium with bifrontal prominences that give a triangular appearance to the face. Other problems associated with defective connective tissue synthesis include short stature, thin skin, blue sclera, loose-jointedness, scoliosis, and a tendency for hernia formation. Hearing loss is common in adults with this disorder because of otosclerosis of the middle and inner ear.

The most serious defects occur when the disorder is inherited as a recessive trait. Severely affected fetuses have multiple intrauterine fractures, and bowing and shortening of the extremities. Many of these babies are stillborn or die during infancy. Less severe affliction occurs when the disorder is inherited as a dominant trait. The skeletal system is not so weakened, and fractures often do not appear until the child becomes active and starts to walk, or even later in childhood. These fractures heal rapidly, but with a poor-quality callus. In some cases, parents may be suspected of child abuse when the child is admitted to the health care facility with multiple fractures.

At present there is no known medical treatment for correction of the defective collagen synthesis that is characteristic of osteogenesis imperfecta. Instead, current treatment modalities focus on preventing and treating fractures. Nonunion is common, especially with repeated fractures at a progressively deforming site. Surgical intervention is often needed to correct deformities, stabilize fractures, remove hardware devices after a nonunion, and occasionally amputate the site of a failed bone graft.

In summary, skeletal disorders can be due to congenital or hereditary influences or to factors that occur during normal periods of skeletal growth and development. Newborn infants undergo normal changes in muscle tone and joint motion, causing conditions such as femoral anteversion and toeing-in. Many of these conditions are corrected as skeletal growth and development take place. Other childhood skeletal disorders, such as the osteochondroses, slipped capital femoral epiphysis, and scoliosis, are not corrected by the growth process. These disorders are progressive, can cause permanent disability, and require treatment. Disorders such as congenital dislocation of the hip and congenital clubfoot are present at birth. Both of these disorders are best treated during infancy. Regular examinations during the first year of life are recommended as a means of achieving early diagnosis of such disorders. Osteogenesis imperfecta is a rare autosomal hereditary disorder that is characterized by defective synthesis of connective tissue, including bone matrix. It results in poorly developed bones that fracture easily.

Metabolic bone disease

The process of bone resorption and formation is continuous throughout life. This process is called

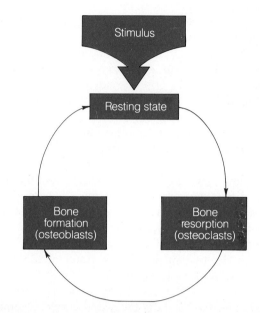

Figure 56-7 Coupled sequence of bone resorption and formation.

bone remodeling. There are two types of bone remodeling: structural and internal remodeling.[22] Structural remodeling involves deposition of new bone on the outer aspect of the shaft at the same time that bone is resorbed from the inner aspect of the shaft. It occurs during growth and results in a bone having adult form and shape. Internal remodeling involves the replacement of bone. In the adult skeleton, remodeling involves formation of new packets of bone on trabecular surfaces and is important in replacing existing bone. Internal remodeling involves a coupled sequence of bone cell activity (Figure 56-7). The sequence is activated by one of many stimuli, including the actions of parathyroid hormone. It begins with osteoclastic resorption of existing bone, during which both the organic and the inorganic components are removed. The sequence then proceeds to the formation of new bone by osteoblasts. In the adult, the length of one sequence (bone resorption and formation) is about 4 months.[22] Ideally, the replaced bone should equal the absorbed bone. If it does not, there is a net loss of bone. In the elderly, for example, bone resorption and formation are no longer perfectly coupled, and bone mass is lost.

The three major influences on the equilibrium of bone tissue are: (1) mechanical stress, which helps stimulate osteoblastic activity and formation of the organic matrix; (2) calcium and phosphate levels in the extracellular fluid; and (3) hormones and local factors, which influence bone resorption and formation. Mechanical stress stimulates osteoblastic activity and formation of organic matrix. It is important in preventing bone atrophy and in healing fractures. Bone serves as a storage site for extracellular calcium and phosphate ions. Consequently, alterations in the extracellular levels of these ions affect their deposition in bone (see Chapter 27).

Hormonal control of bone formation and metabolism

The process of bone formation and mineral metabolism is complex. It involves the interplay between the action of parathyroid hormone, calcitonin, and vitamin D. Other hormones, such as cortisol, growth hormone, thyroid hormone, and the sex hormones, also influence bone formation either directly or indirectly. The actions of parathyroid hormone, calcitonin, and vitamin D are summarized in Table 56-2.

Parathyroid hormone

Parathyroid hormone (PTH) is one of the important regulators of calcium and phosphate levels in the blood. The hormone is secreted by the parathyroid glands, which are located on the posterior outer surface of the thyroid gland.

PTH acts to prevent serum calcium levels from falling below and serum phosphate levels from rising above normal physiologic concentrations. The secretion of PTH is regulated by negative feedback according to serum calcium levels. PTH, which is released from the parathyroid gland in response to a decrease in plasma calcium, acts to restore the concentration of the calcium ion to just above the normal set point. This, in turn, inhibits further secretion of the hormone. Other factors, such as serum phosphate and arterial blood pH, indirectly influence parathyroid secretion by altering the amount of calcium that is complexed to phosphate or bound to albumin.

PTH functions to maintain serum calcium levels by initiating (1) release of calcium from bone, (2) conservation of calcium by the kidney, (3) enhanced intestinal absorption of calcium through activation of vitamin D, and (4) reduction of serum phosphate levels (Figure 56-8). PTH also increases the movement of calcium and phosphate from bone into the extracellular fluid. Calcium is immediately released from the canaliculi and bone cells; a more prolonged release of calcium and phosphate is mediated by increased osteoclast activity. In the kidney, PTH stimulates tubular reabsorption of calcium while reducing the reabsorption of phosphate. The latter effect ensures that increased release of phosphate from bone during mobilization of calcium does not produce an elevation in serum phosphate levels. PTH increases intestinal absorption of calcium because of its ability to stimulate production of 1,25-dihydroxy-vitamin D_3 by the kidney.

Calcitonin

Whereas PTH acts to increase blood calcium levels, the hormone calcitonin acts to lower blood calcium levels. Calcitonin (sometimes called thyrocalcitonin) is secreted by the parafollicular, or C, cells of the thyroid gland.

Calcitonin inhibits the release of calcium from bone into the extracellular fluid. It is thought to act by causing calcium to become sequestered in bone cells and by inhibiting osteoclast activity. Calcitonin also reduces the renal tubular reabsorption of calcium and phosphate; the decrease in serum calcium level that follows administration of pharmacologic doses of calcitonin may be related to this action.[23]

Table 56-2. Actions of parathyroid hormone, calcitonin, and vitamin D

Actions	Parathyroid hormone	Calcitonin	Vitamin D
Intestinal absorption of calcium	Increases indirectly through increased activation of vitamin D	Probably not affected	Increases
Intestinal absorption of phosphate	Increases	Probably not affected	Increases
Renal excretion of calcium	Decreases	Increases	Probably increases but less effect than PTH
Renal excretion of phosphate	Increases	Increases	Increases
Bone resorption	Increases	Decreases	$1,25(OH)_2D_3$ increases
Bone formation	Decreases	Uncertain	$24,25(OH)_2D_3$ increases(?)
Serum calcium levels	Produces a prompt increase	Decreases with pharmacologic doses	No effect
Serum phosphate levels	Prevents an increase	Decreases with pharmacologic doses	No effect

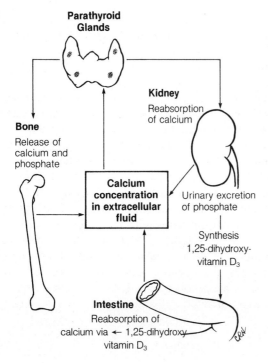

Figure 56-8 Regulation and actions of parathyroid hormone.

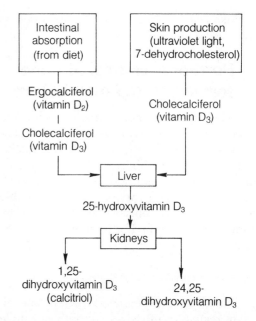

Figure 56-9 Sources and pathway for activation of vitamin D.

The major stimulus for calcitonin synthesis and release is a rise in serum calcium. The actual role of calcitonin in the overall mineral homeostasis is unclear. There are no clearly definable syndromes of calcitonin deficiency or excess, which suggests that calcitonin does not directly alter calcium metabolism. It has been suggested that the physiologic actions of calcitonin are related to the postprandial handling and processing of dietary calcium.[23] This theory proposes that after meals calcitonin maintains parathyroid secretion at a time when it normally would be reduced by calcium entering the blood from the digestive tract. Although excess or deficiency states associated with alterations in physiologic levels of calcitonin have not been observed, it has been shown that pharmacologic doses of the hormone reduce osteoclastic activity. Because of this action, calcitonin has proved effective in the treatment of Paget's disease. The hormone is also used to reduce serum calcium levels during hypercalcemic crises.

Vitamin D

It is now recognized that vitamin D and its metabolites are not vitamins but steroid hormones. There are two forms of vitamin D: vitamin D_2 (ergocalciferol) and vitamin D_3 (cholecalciferol). The two forms differ by the presence of a double bond, yet have identical biological activity. The term *vitamin D* is used to indicate both forms.

Vitamin D has little or no activity until it has been metabolized to compounds that mediate its activity. Figure 56-9 depicts sources of vitamin D and pathways for activation. The first step of the activation process occurs in the liver, where vitamin D is hydroxylated to form the metabolite 25-hydroxyvitamin D_3 (25-OH D_3). From the liver, 25-OH D_3 is transported to the kidneys, where it undergoes conversion to either 1,25-dihydroxyvitamin D_3 [1,25-$(OH)_2D_3$] or 24,25-dihydroxyvitamin D_3 [24,25-$(OH)_2D_3$]. Other metabolites of vitamin D have been and are still being discovered.

There are two sources of vitamin D: intestinal absorption and skin production. Intestinal absorption occurs mainly in the jejunum and includes both vitamin D_2 and vitamin D_3. The most important dietary sources of vitamin D are fish, liver, and irradiated milk. Because vitamin D is fat-soluble, its absorption is mediated by bile salts and occurs by means of the lymphatic vessels. In the skin, ultraviolet radiation from sunlight spontaneously converts 7-dehydrocholesterol previtamin D_3 to vitamin D_3. A circulating vitamin D–binding protein provides a mechanism to remove vitamin D from the skin and make it available to the rest of the body. With adequate exposure to sunlight, the amount of vitamin D that can be produced by the skin is usually sufficient to meet physiologic requirements. The importance of sunlight exposure is evidenced by population studies that report lower vitamin D levels in countries, such as England, that have less sunlight than the United States.[24] Elderly people who are either housebound or institutionalized frequently have low vitamin D levels.[25] The deficiency often goes undetected until there are problems such as psuedofractures or electrolyte imbalances. Seasonal variations in vitamin D levels probably reflect changes in sunlight exposure.

The most potent of the vitamin D metabolites is $1,25\text{-}(OH)_2D_3$. This metabolite increases intestinal absorption of calcium and resorption of calcium and phosphate from bone. Bone resorption by the osteoclasts is increased and bone formation by the osteoblasts is decreased; there is also an increase in acid phosphatase and a decrease in alkaline phosphatase. Both intestinal absorption and bone resorption increase the amount of calcium and phosphorus available to the mineralizing surface of the bone. The role of $24,25\text{-}(OH)_2D_3$ is less clear. There is increasing evidence that $24,25\text{-}(OH)_2D_3$, in conjunction with $1,25\text{-}(OH)_2D_3$, may be involved in normal bone mineralization.[26]

The regulation of vitamin D activity is influenced by several hormones. PTH and prolactin stimulate $1,25\text{-}(OH)_2D_3$ production by the kidney. States of hyperparathyroidism are associated with increased levels of $1,25\text{-}(OH)_2D_3$, whereas hypoparathyroidism leads to lowered levels of this metabolite. Prolactin may have an ancillary role in regulating vitamin D metabolism during pregnancy and lactation. Calcitonin inhibits $1,25\text{-}(OH)_2D_3$ production by the kidney. In addition to hormonal influences, changes in the concentration of ions such as calcium, phosphate, hydrogen, and potassium exert an effect on both $1,25\text{-}(OH)_2D_3$ and $24,25\text{-}(OH)_2D_3$ production. Under conditions of deprivation of phosphate and calcium, $1,25\text{-}(OH)_2D_3$ levels are increased, whereas hyperphosphatemia and hypercalcemia decrease the levels of metabolite.

—— Disorders of bone metabolism

—— Osteopenia

Osteopenia is a condition that is common to all metabolic bone diseases. It is characterized by a reduction in bone mass greater than expected for age, race, or sex, and it occurs because of a decrease in bone formation, inadequate bone mineralization, or excessive bone deossification. Osteopenia is not a diagnosis but a term used to describe an apparent lack of bone on x-ray studies. The major causes of osteopenia are osteoporosis, osteomalacia, malignancies such as multiple myeloma, and endocrine disorders such as hyperparathyroidism and hyperthyroidism.

—— Osteoporosis

Osteoporosis is a disorder in which the rate of bone resorption is greater than the rate of bone formation. There are parallel losses of both the organic matrix and mineral content of the bone. The total composition of bone remains the same: there is just too

little of it. Osteoporotic bone is brittle, fragile, and fractures easily. Osteoporosis can occur as the result of an endocrine disorder or malignancy but is most often associated with the aging process. Loss of bone mass begins at about age 25. After age 40, the rate of bone loss is approximately 0.5% per year, and it increases to about 1% per year or more in menopausal women.[27] It has been estimated that osteoporosis currently affects about 14 million women in the United States. Overall, up to 85% of the female population will develop osteoporosis.[28] Age-related bone losses in men are seen 15 to 20 years later than in women and occur at a slower rate.[29] It has also been shown that bone mass positively correlates with the amount of skin pigmentation; whites have the least amount of bone mass and blacks have the most.[29] Although osteoporosis is uncommon among black women, many cases are seen among postmenopausal women with brown and yellow skin. One of the reasons for the increased risk in postmenopausal women of white or Asian descent may be that their original bone mass is less and therefore the losses associated with aging affect them sooner.

With osteoporosis, changes occur in both the diaphysis and the metaphysis. The diameter of the bone enlarges with age, causing the outer supporting cortex to become thinner. In severe osteoporosis, the vertebrae and hip bones begin to resemble the fragile structure of a fine china vase. There is loss of trabeculae from cancellous bone and thinning of the cortex to such an extent that minimal stress causes fractures.

The development of osteoporosis involves many factors. It is related to hormone levels, physical fitness, and general nutrition. It is thought that an indirect action of estrogen is the suppression of bone resorption. This action is reduced after menopause. Exercise helps to prevent involutional bone loss and may serve to prevent or delay the progression of osteoporosis.[30,31] Poor nutrition or an age-related decrease in intestinal absorption of calcium because of deficient activation of vitamin D may contribute to osteoporosis, particularly in the elderly. Individuals with endocrine disorders such as hyperthyroidism, hyperparathyroidism, Cushing's syndrome, or diabetes mellitus are at high risk for developing osteoporosis. The prolonged use of certain drugs, such as corticosteroids, anticonvulsants, antacids, diuretics, or thyroid supplements, is also associated with bone loss.[32] Other factors found to be associated with osteoporosis are a diet high in protein, cigarette smoking, alcohol ingestion, and a family history of osteoporosis.[33]

Osteoporosis is rare in children. When it does occur, it is related to causes such as the excess corticosteroid levels associated with Cushing's syndrome, colon disease, prolonged immobility, or osteogenesis imperfecta. The cardinal features occur at the onset or just before puberty and may include pain in the back and extremities and multiple fractures. There is radiologic evidence of osteoporotic new bone. Idiopathic juvenile osteoporosis, which is more common in children, resembles rickets.

The true etiology of osteoporosis is unknown, but most data suggest that the primary problem is an acceleration of bone resorption. The serum alkaline phosphatase level, a measure of osteoblastic activity, is increased slightly.[29] There may also be a lower level of calcitonin and a decreased response to a calcium stimulus.[27] Decreases in sex hormone levels, which seem to act as an intermediate to prevent bone loss, in both men and women are somehow important in the pathogenesis of osteoporosis. In postmenopausal women, these changes can be reversed by estrogen therapy. There is some evidence that osteoporosis is caused, at least in part, by abnormalities in local factors, such as prostaglandins, interleukins, and growth factors, that influence bone cell function.[31] Further study is needed, particularly because local factors cannot be measured directly but have to be identified with *in vitro* organ-culture methods and tissues from laboratory animals.

The first clinical manifestations of osteoporosis are pain accompanied by skeletal fractures—a vertebral compression fracture or fractures of the hip, pelvis, humerus, or any other bone. Estimates are that 25% to 30% of all Caucasian women in the United States will experience an osteoposis-related fracture.[32] Unfortunately, fractures represent an end stage of the disease. Women who present with fractures are much more likely to suffer another fracture than are women of the same age without osteoporosis. Wedging and collapse of vertebrae causes a loss of height in the vertebral column and kyphosis, a condition commonly referred to as *dowager's hump*. Usually, there is no generalized bone tenderness. When pain occurs it is related to fractures.

The initial diagnosis of osteoporosis is usually made on the basis of standard x-ray studies when a woman presents with a fracture. However, radiologic evidence of decreased bone density is nonspecific. Bone loss is apparent on standard x-ray studies only when there is a 30% or greater loss in bone mass. A computed tomography (CT) scan is the most accurate indicator of early bone loss in the spine, but it is expensive and involves exposure to high radiation doses. Dual-photon absorptiometry of the spine and hip and single-photon absorptiometry of the wrist can detect bone losses of only 1% to 2%. The latter are used as an inexpensive diagnostic tool in osteoporosis screening programs.

In all cases of osteoporosis, clinical examination and x-ray findings must be considered in conjunction with various blood chemistry levels. Assays of calcium, phosphorus, and alkaline phosphatase levels and protein electrophoresis should be done before treatment is started. These levels may all be within the normal range in postmenopausal osteoporosis, with only a slight rise in serum calcium and phosphate reflecting the increased bone destruction. Unfortunately, the only measure of bone density and calcium level is through bone biopsy. This is usually reserved for people who do not respond to treatment.

Prevention and early detection of osteoporosis is essential to the prevention of the deformities and fractures associated with its presence. It is important to identify persons in high-risk groups so that treatment can be begun early. Postmenopausal women, women of small stature or lean body mass, those with sedentary life-styles, those whose calcium intake is poor, and those suffering from diseases that demineralize bone are at greatest risk. Regular exercise and adequate calcium intake are important factors in preventing osteoporosis. Recent studies have indicated that premenopausal women need over 1000 mg and postmenopausal women 1500 mg of calcium daily.[8] This means that adults should drink 3 to 4 glasses of milk daily or substitute other foods that are high in calcium. Unfortunately, the average American diet only provides about 600 mg.[8]

At present the efficacy of treatment methods for osteoporosis is questionable. A combination of fluoride, calcium, and vitamin D is most often used. A daily intake of 400 to 800 IU of vitamin D is recommended.[8] Administration of fluoride does lead to widespread formation of new bone, but the quality of the bone is still questionable. Because the new bone is laid down on existing bone, the treatment must be started while there is still adequate bone onto which the fluoride bone can be built. Calcitonin can be used to increase osteoblast activity. It has some effect on bone pain, but is only available by injection. There is evidence that deficient activation of vitamin D may be an important factor in the impaired intestinal absorption of calcium in the elderly. On the basis of this evidence, 1,25-dihydroxyvitamin D_3 is being studied as a treatment for osteoporosis.[34]

The use of estrogen therapy in postmenopausal women in the United States, while relatively common, is still controversial. Several studies have shown a reduction in postmenopausal bone loss in women using estrogen therapy, particularly those treated within the first 3 years of menopause.[31] Recent studies have indicated that administering estrogen to older women, at least up to age 74 years, may prevent hip fractures.[35] However, there is strong evidence that women who have not undergone a hysterectomy are at increased risk for developing endometrial cancer when taking estrogens.[31] This risk appears to be related to the length of treatment, dose, and concomitant use of progestins. Further research is needed to determine the ideal dose and duration of estrogen therapy needed to prevent loss of bone mass.

Persons with osteoporosis have many special needs. In treating fractures, it is important to minimize immobility. Bed rest is imposed only after recent fractures. The use of leg braces is avoided. Walking and swimming are encouraged. Unsafe conditions that predispose individuals to falls and fractures should be corrected or avoided.

Osteomalacia and rickets

In contrast to osteoporosis, which causes a loss of total bone mass and results in brittle bones, osteomalacia and rickets produce a softening of the bones and do not involve the loss of bone matrix. About 60% of bone is mineral content, about 30% is organic matrix, and the rest is living bone cells. Both the organic matrix and the inorganic mineral salts are needed for normal bone consistency. As an example, if the inorganic mineral salts are removed from fresh bone (dilute nitric acid will remove them), the organic matrix that remains will still resemble a bone, but it will be so flexible that it can be tied in a knot. On the other hand, when a bone is placed over a hot flame, the organic material is destroyed and the bone becomes very brittle.

Osteomalacia. Osteomalacia is a generalized bone condition in which inadequate mineralization of bone matrix results from a calcium or phosphate deficiency (or both). It is sometimes referred to as the adult form of rickets.

There are two main causes of osteomalacia: (1) insufficient calcium absorption from the intestine because of either a lack of calcium or resistance to the action of vitamin D and (2) increased renal phosphorus losses. As discussed previously, vitamin D is a fat-soluble vitamin that is either absorbed intact through the intestine or produced in the skin as a result of ultraviolet irradiation of 7-dehydrocholesterol. Vitamin D that is absorbed from the intestine or synthesized in the skin is inactive. Vitamin D is activated in a two-step process that begins in the liver and is completed in the kidney. Vitamin D deficiency is most commonly due to reduced vitamin D absorption as a result of biliary tract or intestinal diseases that impair fat and fat-soluble vitamin absorption. Lack of vitamin D in the diet is rare in the United States because many foods are fortified with the vitamin. Anticonvulsant medications, such as phenobarbital and phenytoin, induce hepatic hydroxylases that accelerate breakdown of the active forms of vitamin D. The long-term use of antacids, such as aluminum hydroxide, that bind dietary forms of phosphate and prevent their absorption is another cause of phosphate deficiency. Long-standing primary hyperparathyroid-

ism causes hypophosphatemia, which can lead to rickets in children and osteomalacia in adults. A form of osteomalacia called renal rickets occurs with chronic renal failure. It is caused by the inability of the kidney to activate vitamin D and excrete phosphate and is accompanied by hyperparathyroidism, increased bone turnover, and increased bone resorption. Another form of osteomalacia is due to renal tubular defects that cause excessive phosphorus loses. This form of osteomalacia is commonly referred to as vitamin D–resistant rickets and is often a familial disorder. It is inherited as an x-linked dominant gene, being passed by mothers to half of all their children and by fathers to their daughters only. This form of osteomalacia affects boys more severely than girls.

The incidence of osteomalacia is high among the elderly because of diets deficient in both calcium and vitamin D and is often compounded by intestinal malabsorption problems that accompany aging. Osteomalacia is often seen in cultures in which the diet is deficient in vitamin D, such as in northern China, Japan, and northern India. Women in these areas have a higher incidence of the disorder than men because of the combined effects of pregnancy, lactation, and more indoor confinement. Osteomalacia is occasionally seen in strict vegetarians; persons who have had a gastrectomy; and those on long-term anticonvulsant, tranquilizer, sedative, muscle relaxant, or diuretic drugs. There is also a greater incidence of osteomalacia in colder regions of the world, particularly during the winter months, probably because of lessened exposure to sunlight.

The clinical manifestations of osteomalacia are bone pain, tenderness, and fractures as the disease progresses. In severe cases, muscle weakness is often an early sign. The cause of muscle weakness is unclear, although experimental evidence suggests that vitamin D deficiency affects muscle metabolism.[21] The combined effects of gravity, muscle weakness, and bone softening contribute to the development of deformities. There may be a dorsal kyphosis in the spine, rib deformities, a heart-shaped pelvis, and marked bowing of the tibiae and femurs. Osteomalacia predisposes an individual to pathologic fractures in the weakened areas, especially in the distal radius and proximal femur. In contrast to osteoporosis, it is not a significant cause of hip fractures. There may be delayed healing and poor retention of internal fixation devices.

Osteomalacia is usually accompanied by a compensatory hyperparathyroidism stimulated by low serum calcium levels. Parathyroid hormone reduces renal absorption of phosphate and removes calcium from the bone. Thus, calcium levels are only slightly reduced in osteomalacia.

Diagnostic measures are directed toward

identifying osteomalacia and establishing its cause. Diagnostic methods include x-ray studies, laboratory workup, bone scan, and bone biopsy. X-ray findings typical of osteomalacia are the development of transverse lines or pseudofractures called Looser's zones. These are apparently caused by pulsations of the major arteries where they cross the bone.[21] A bone biopsy may be done to confirm the diagnosis of osteomalacia in a person with nonspecific osteopenia who shows no improvement after treatment with exercise, vitamin D, and calcium.

The treatment of osteomalacia is directed at the underlying cause. If the problem is nutritional, restoring adequate amounts of calcium and vitamin D to the diet may be sufficient. The elderly with intestinal malabsorption may also benefit from vitamin D. The least expensive and most effective long-term treatment is a diet rich in vitamin D (fish, dairy products, and margarine) along with careful exposure to the midday sun. Vitamin D is specific for adult osteomalacia and vitamin D–resistant rickets, but large doses are usually needed to overcome the resistance to its calcium absorption action and to prevent renal loss of phosphate. The biologically active form of vitamin D, calcitriol, is available for use in the treatment of osteomalacia resistant to vitamin D (*e.g.,* osteomalacia resulting from chronic liver disease and kidney failure). If osteomalacia is due to malabsorption, the treatment is directed toward correcting the primary disease condition. For example, adequate replacement of pancreatic enzymes is of paramount importance in pancreatic insufficiency. In renal tubular disorders, the treatment is directed at the altered renal physiology.

Rickets. Vitamin D deficiency rickets, seen in children, is called infantile or nutritional rickets. It is a disturbance in the formation of bone in the growing skeleton, characterized by softened and deformed bones caused by failure of the organic matrix of bone to calcify normally. Rickets occurs primarily in underdeveloped areas of the world and in urban areas where pigmented ethnic groups have migrated from sunny to cloudy climates. It is seen most often in infants from 6 to 24 months of age.

Nutritional rickets is caused by either a lack of vitamin D in the diet or malabsorption diseases. Inadequate amounts of calcium and phosphorus in the diet also play a part in the development of rickets. The bony changes are a result of inadequate absorption of calcium.

The pathology of rickets is the same as that of osteomalacia seen in adults. Because rickets affects children during periods of active growth, however, the structural changes are seen in the bone are somewhat different. Bones become deformed; ossification at epiphyseal plates is delayed and disordered. This results in widening of the epiphyseal cartilage plate. Any new bone that does grow is unmineralized.

The symptoms of rickets are usually noted between 6 months and 3 years. Early symptoms are lethargy and muscle weakness, which may be accompanied by convulsions or tetany related to hypocalcemia. Irritability is common. In severe cases, children lose their skin pigment, develop flabby subcutaneous tissue, and have poorly developed musculature. The ends of long bones and ribs are enlarged. The thorax may be abnormally shaped with prominent rib cartilage (rachitic rosary). The legs exhibit either bowlegged (varus) or knock-kneed (valgus) deformities. The skull is enlarged and soft, and closure of the fontanels is delayed. The child is slow to develop teeth and may have difficulty standing.

Rickets is treated with a balanced diet sufficient in calcium, phosphorus, and vitamin D. Exposure to sunshine is also important, especially for premature infants and those on artificial milk feedings. Supplemental vitamin D in excess of normal requirements is given for several months. Maintaining good posture, positioning, and bracing in older children are used to prevent deformities. Once the disease is controlled, deformities may have to be surgically corrected as the child grows.

Paget's disease (osteitis deformans)

Paget's disease is discussed separately because it is not a true metabolic disease. It is a progressive skeletal disorder that involves excessive bone destruction and repair and is characterized by increasing structural changes of the long bones, spine, pelvis, and cranium. The disease affects about 3% of the population over age 40 and 10% of those over age 70.[36] It is rarely diagnosed before age 40. In children, hyperostosis corticalis deformans juvenilis (a rare inherited disorder), hyperphosphatemia, and diseases that cause diaphyseal stenosis may mimic Paget's disease and are sometimes referred to as juvenile Paget's disease. The etiology of Paget's disease is unknown. Recent studies propose that it may be caused by a virus with osteoclastic capability.[37]

The disease usually begins insidiously and progresses slowly over many years. An initial osteolytic phase is followed by an osteoblastic sclerotic phase. During the initial osteolytic phase, abnormal osteoclasts proliferate. Bone resorption occurs so rapidly that new bone formation cannot keep up, and the bone is replaced by fibrous tissue. The bones actually increase in size and thickness because of accelerated bone resorption followed by abnormal regeneration. Irregular bone formation results in sclerotic and osteoblastic lesions. The result is a thick layer of coarse bone with a rough and pitted outer surface that has the appearance of pumice. Histologically, the Paget's lesions show increased vascularity and bone marrow fibrosis with intense cellular activity. The bone has a somewhat mosaic pattern caused by areas of density outlined by heavy blue lines, called cement lines.

The disease varies in severity and may be present long before it is clinically detected. The clinical manifestations of Paget's disease depend on the specific area involved. About 20% of those persons with the disorder are totally asymptomatic, and the disease is discovered accidentally.[37] Involvement of the skull causes headaches, intermittent tinnitus, vertigo, and eventual hearing loss. In the spine, collapse of the anterior vertebrae causes kyphosis of the thoracic spine. The femur and tibia become bowed. Softening of the femoral neck can cause coxa vara (reduced angle of the femoral neck). Coxa vara, in combination with softening of the sacral and iliac bones, causes a waddling gait. When the lesion affects only one bone, it may cause only mild pain and stiffness. Progressive deossification weakens and distorts the bone structure. The deossification process begins along the inner cortical surfaces and continues until the substance of the bone disappears. Pathologic fractures may occur, especially in the bones subjected to the greatest stress (e.g., the upper femur, lower spine, and pelvic bones). These fractures often heal poorly, with excessive and poorly distributed callus.

Other manifestations of Paget's disease include nerve palsy syndromes from lesions in the upper extremities, mental deterioration, and cardiovascular disease. Cardiovascular disease is the most serious complication and is listed as the most common cause of death in advanced generalized Paget's disease. It is caused by vasodilation of the vessels in the skin and subcutaneous tissues overlying the affected bones. When one-third to one-half of the skeleton is affected, the increased blood flow may lead to high-output cardiac failure.[37] Ventilatory capacity may be limited by rib and spine involvement.

Sarcoma occurs in about 7% of persons with Paget's disease, with a slight predominance in men.[38] One-fifth of all osteogenic sarcomas in persons 50 years or older originate in persons with Paget's disease.[39] The bones most often affected, in order of frequency, are the femur, pelvis, humerus, and tibia. There appears to be a close histopathogenic relationship between Paget's disease and the associated sarcoma.[40] The fact that the cellular activity seen in sarcoma (e.g., these tumors have a large number of osteoclasts and atypical osteoblasts) seems to be an exaggeration of the remodeling process of Paget's disease gives credence to the theory that both diseases have a viral origin.[38]

Diagnosis of Paget's disease is based on char-acteristic bone deformities and x-ray changes. Elevated levels of serum alkaline phosphatase and urinary hydroxyproline support the diagnosis, and continued surveillance of these levels may be used to monitor the effectiveness of treatment. Bone scans are used to detect the rapid bone turnover indicative of active disease and to monitor the response to treatment. The scan cannot identify bone activity due to malignant lesions. Bone biopsy may be done to differentiate the lesion from osteomyelitis or a primary or metastatic bone tumor.

The treatment of Paget's disease is based on the degree of pain and the extent of the disease. Pain can be reduced with either nonsteroidal or other anti-inflammatory agents. Suppressive agents such as calcitonin, mithramycin, and diphosphate compounds are used to manage pain and prevent further spread of the disease and neurologic defects. Calcitonin and etidronate disodium (a phosphate compound) decrease bone resorption. Mithramycin is a cytotoxic agent that causes osteoclasts to reduce their resorption of bone. Because this drug is very toxic, it is reserved for resistant cases. Decreases in serum alkaline phosphatase and urinary hydroxyproline levels and radiologically evident improvement indicate response to treatment. However, symptomatic improvement is usually considered the best measure of success.

In summary, metabolic bone diseases such as osteoporosis, osteomalacia, rickets, and Paget's disease are the result of a disruption in the equilibrium of bone formation and resorption. Osteoporosis, which is the most common of the metabolic bone diseases, occurs when the rate of resorption is greater than that of bone formation. It is seen frequently in postmenopausal women and is the major cause of fractures in people over 45 years of age. Osteomalacia and rickets are caused by inadequate mineralization of bone matrix, primarily because of a deficiency of vitamin D. Paget's disease results from excessive osteoclastic activity and is characterized by the formation of poor-quality bone. The success rate of the various drugs and hormones that are used to treat metabolic bone diseases varies. Further research is needed to clarify the etiology, pathology, and treatment of these diseases.

Neoplasms

Neoplasms in the skeletal system are usually referred to as bone tumors. Primary malignant tumors of the bone are uncommon, constituting about 1% of all cancers.[39] Metastatic disease of the bone, however, is relatively common. Primary bone tumors may arise from any of the skeletal components, including osseous bone tissue, cartilage, and bone marrow. The discussion in this section focuses on primary benign and malignant bone tumors of osseous or cartilaginous origin and metastatic bone disease. Tumors of bone marrow origin (leukemia and multiple myeloma) are discussed in Chapter 14.

Like other types of neoplasms, bone tumors may be either benign or malignant. The benign types, such as osteochondromas and giant cell tumors, tend to grow rather slowly and usually do not destroy the supporting or surrounding tissue or spread to other parts of the body. Malignant tumors, such as osteosarcoma and Ewing's sarcoma, grow rapidly and can spread to other parts of the body through the bloodstream or lymphatics.

Specific types of bone tumors affect different age groups. Adolescents have the highest incidence, with a rate of 3 cases per 100,000. In children less than 15 years of age, only 3.2% of all malignancies are primary bone tumors.[39] The two major forms of bone cancer in children and young adults are osteogenic sarcoma and Ewing's sarcoma. It is unusual for either condition to be seen after age 25. The incidence of bone tumors declines in young adults to a rate of 0.3 per 100,000 between the ages of 30 and 35 years and then slowly begins to rise until the incidence at age 60 equals that at adolescence.[39] The classification of benign and malignant bone tumors is described in Table 56-3.

Characteristics of bone tumors

There are three major symptoms of bone tumors: pain, presence of a mass, and impairment of function (Chart 56-1).[41] Pain is a feature common to almost all malignant tumors but may or may not be present in benign tumors. For example, a benign bone cyst is usually asymptomatic until a fracture occurs. Pain that persists at night and is not relieved by rest is suggestive of malignancy. A mass or hard lump may be the first sign of a bone tumor. A malignant tumor is suspected when a painful mass exists that is enlarging or eroding the cortex of the bone. The ease of discovery of a mass depends on the location of the tumor: A small lump arising on the surface of the tibia is easy to detect, whereas a tumor that is deep in the medial portion of the thigh may grow to a considerable size before it is noticed. Both benign and malignant tumors may cause the bone to erode to the point where it cannot withstand the strain of ordinary use. In such cases, even a small amount of bone stress or trauma precipitates a pathologic fracture. A tumor may produce pressure on a peripheral nerve causing decreased sensation, numbness, a limp, or limitation of movement.

Benign neoplasms

Benign bone tumors usually are found to be limited to the confines of the bone, have well-demarcated edges, and are surrounded by a thin rim of sclerotic bone. The four most common types of benign bone tumors are (1) osteoma, (2) chondroma, (3) osteochondroma, and (4) giant cell tumor.

An *osteoma* is a small bony tumor found on the surface of a long bone, flat bone, or the skull. It is usually composed of hard, compact (ivory osteoma) or spongy (cancellous) bone. It may be either excised or left alone.

A *chondroma* is a tumor composed of cartilage. It either grows outward from the bone (ecchondroma) or within the bone (enchondroma). These tumors

Table 56-3.	Classification of primary bone neoplasms	
Tissue type	**Benign neoplasm**	**Malignant neoplasm**

Bone	Osteoid osteoma
	Benign
	  osteoblastoma
	Osteoma
		Osteosarcoma
		Parosteal
		  osteogenic
		  sarcoma

Cartilage	Osteochondroma Chondroma Chondroblastoma Chondromyxoid fibroma	Chondrosarcoma

Bone marrow		Multiple
		  myeloma
		Reticulum cell
		  sarcoma

Uncertain	Giant cell tumor
	Fibrous
	  histiocytoma
		Ewing's sarcoma
		Malignant giant
		  cell tumor
		Malignant fibrous
		  histiocytoma
		Adamantinoma

Chart 56-1: Symptoms of bone cancer

Bone pain in an adult or child that lasts for as long as a week, is constant or intermittent, and is usually worse at night

Unexplained swelling over the knee, thigh, or other bone

Skin over the bone that feels considerably warmer than the rest of the body, or veins that are noticeably prominent

(Adapted from Facts on Bone Cancer. American Cancer Society, 1978. The American Cancer Society suggests that persons with these symptoms see their physician.)

may become large and are especially common in the hands and feet. At times a chondroma may persist for many years and then take on the attributes of a malignant chondrosarcoma. A chondroma is usually not treated unless it becomes unsightly or uncomfortable.

An *osteochondroma* is the most common form of benign tumor in the skeletal system. It grows only during periods of skeletal growth, originating in the epiphyseal cartilage plate and growing out of the bone like a mushroom. An osteochondroma is composed of both cartilage and bone and usually occurs singly but may affect several bones in a condition called multiple exostoses. Malignant changes are rare, and excision of the tumor is done only when necessary.

A *giant cell tumor,* or osteoclastoma, is an aggressive tumor of multinucleated cells that often behaves like a malignant tumor, metastasizing through the bloodstream and recurring locally following excision. It occurs most often in young adults, predominantly female, and is most commonly found in the knee, wrist, or shoulder. The tumor begins in the metaphyseal region, grows into the epiphysis, and may extend into the joint surface itself. Pathologic fractures are common because the tumor destroys the bone substance. Clinically pain may occur at the tumor site, with gradually increasing swelling. X-rays show destruction of the bone with expansion of the cortex.

The treatment of giant cell tumors depends on their location. If the affected bone can be eliminated without loss of function, such as the clavicle or fibula, the entire bone or part of it may be removed. When the tumor is near a major joint, such as the knee or shoulder, a local excision is done. Irradiation may be used in an attempt to prevent recurrence of the tumor.

Malignant bone tumors

In contrast to benign tumors, malignant tumors tend to be ill-defined, lack sharp borders, and extend beyond the confines of the bone, showing that it has destroyed the cortex. Although malignant bone tumors are rare, they have a high mortality rate. In addition, there is much morbidity and trauma from the often mutilating surgical excision. Surgery often leads to amputation or removal of a large part of the bone, which causes disability.

Methods used in the diagnosis of bone tumors include roentgenography (x-ray), computed tomography, radionuclide bone scanning, and biopsy of the tumor. Biopsy can be performed by means of a large needle or open surgical methods.

The treatment of malignant bone tumors primarily involves surgical removal of the tumor with either amputation of the limb or wide resection of the tumor and surrounding tissue. Radiation therapy is used as a definitive and adjuvant treatment to slow the progression of the cancer, decrease bone pain, and prevent pathologic fractures. A pathologic fracture spreads the tumor cells through formation of a hematoma. Because high-grade bone and soft tissue sarcomas produce clinically undetectable metastases called micrometastases, immunotherapy, irradiation, and chemotherapy are often used in combination as adjuvant therapy. Chemotherapy is the most effective modality for controlling metastases. Extremely aggressive drug combinations have been developed, particularly in the pediatric and young adult age groups. Many advances have been made in the limb salvage surgical procedures now being used as an alternative to limb amputation. They are most often used in younger individuals in an attempt to increase their functioning and mobility. The tumor must have minimal soft tissue involvement and no involvement of major blood vessels.

Osteogenic sarcoma

An osteogenic tumor is one arising from or having genesis within bone tissue. Osteogenic sarcoma involves proliferation of osteoid or immature bone.

Osteogenic sarcoma is the most common and most fatal primary malignant bone tumor, with the exception of multiple myeloma. It is a disease primarily of children and young adults between the ages of 10 and 20 years, with males being affected slightly more often than females. The tumor occurs most frequently during periods of peak skeletal growth, with the growth potential of each long bone determining the frequency of tumor occurrence. The most common sites of occurrence are the distal femur (41.5%), proximal tibia (16%), and proximal humerus (15%).[42] Occasionally, malignancies arise from the middle portion of the long bones. Persons affected with osteogenic sarcoma are usually tall and are found to have a high plasma level of somatomedin. Osteogenic sarcoma is an aggressive tumor that grows rapidly. The tumor moves from the metaphysis of the bone out to the periosteum, much like the process of acute hematogenous osteomyelitis. The causes of osteogenic sarcoma are unknown. It has been shown that viruses can induce sarcomas in laboratory animals. In addition, radiation from either an internal source, such as the radioactive pharmaceutical technetium used in bone scans, or an external source, such as x-rays, may also be a causative factor.

The primary clinical feature of osteosarcoma is severe pain in the affected bone, usually of sudden onset. There is a wide variation in the hardness of osteogenic tumors. Osteosarcoma usually begins as a firm white or reddish mass and later becomes softer with a viscous interior. Swelling is often present over the area. The skin overlying the tumor may be very shiny and stretched, with prominent superficial veins. The range of motion of the adjacent joint may be restricted. Even though this type of tumor extends through the medullary cavity, there is usually no evidence on x-ray images.

Sarcomas infrequently metastasize to the lymph nodes because the cells are unable to grow within the node. Nodal metastases usually occur only in the late course of disseminated disease. Most often the tumor cells exit the primary tumor through the venous end of the capillary, and early metastasis to the lung is common: In osteosarcoma, the cause of death in 60% to 80% of cases is metastatic lung disease.[39] Lung metastases, even if massive, are usually relatively asymptomatic. The prognosis in osteosarcoma depends on the aggressiveness of the disease, radiologic features, presence or absence of pathologic fracture, size of the tumor, rapidity of tumor growth, and sex of the individual. There is some suggestion that females have a better survival rate than males.[41]

Chemotherapy, using various drug combinations, is the most effective treatment for metastatic osteosarcoma. The treatment for sarcomas is a combination of surgery, chemotherapy and radiation therapy used preoperatively or postoperatively. In the past, treatment usually entailed amputation above the level of the tumor. Currently, limb salvage surgical procedures, using a metal prosthesis or cadaver allografts, are becoming a more viable alternative. The allografts, however, have a high rate of failure due to fracture.[44] Studies have shown that limb salvage surgery has no adverse effects on the long-term survival of people with osteosarcoma. The success of limb salvage appears to depend on the use of a wide surgical margin and use of adjuvant chemotherapy.[45] Microscopic examination has shown that tumor filaments may extend 1 to 3 inches or more beyond the cortical bone.[43] Advanced imaging techniques and the use of angiography assist the surgeon in determining the best type of definitive surgery. Successful limb conservation has been achieved in a limited population with a technique involving *en bloc resection* (removal of the tumor and a portion of uninvolved soft tissue), extracorporeal irradiation, and reimplantation of the irradiated bone.[46] When a tumor is inoperable or metastases are widespread, chemotherapy with or without irradiation may be used. Pulmonary irradiation is being used with increasing success to treat pulmonary metastases in children under age 12. The use of immunotherapy, including interferon, is still in the experimental stage, as it is with other types of cancers.

Chondrosarcoma

Chondrosarcoma, a malignant tumor of cartilage that can develop either within the medullary cavity or peripherally, is the second most common form of malignant bone tumor.[39] It is about one-half as common as osteosarcoma, accounting for about 13% of bone tumors, and it affects males slightly more often than females.[39] It is found in an older age group than osteogenic sarcoma, with the peak incidence occurring around 45 years of age. The tumor arises from points of muscle attachment to bone, particularly the knee, shoulder, hip, and pelvis. About 10% of all chondrosarcomas arise from underlying benign lesions.[40]

Chondrosarcomas are slow-growing, metastasize late, and are often painless. They can remain hidden in an area like the pelvis for a long time. This type of tumor, like many primary malignancies, tends to destroy bone and extend into the soft tissues beyond the confines of the bone of origin. Chondrosarcomas mainly affect the bones of the trunk, pelvis, or proximal femur and rarely develop in the distal portion of a bone. Often irregular flecks and ringlets of calcification are a prominent radiographic finding.

Early diagnosis is important because chondrosarcoma responds well to early radical surgical excision. It is generally resistant to radiation therapy and currently available chemotherapeutic agents.

Ewing's sarcoma

Ewing's sarcoma is the third most common type of primary bone tumor and is highly malignant, often with only a 3- to 5-year survival rate.[39] It is frequently seen in males under 30 years of age, with the incidence being highest in the second decade of life. Ewing's tumor arises from immature bone marrow cells and causes bone destruction from within. It can occur in any bone, with pelvic tumors having the worst prognosis.

Manifestations of Ewing's tumor include pain, tenderness, fever, and leukocytosis. Pathologic fractures are common because of bone destruction. The primary treatment of Ewing's sarcoma is irradiation along with combination chemotherapy. Ewing's sarcoma is more radiosensitive than other primary bone tumors. The use of central nervous system irradiation is being investigated. Wide resection of the tumor is considered if the nerves and blood vessels are free of disease. Radical amputation is often necessary because of the aggressiveness of the tumor.

Metastatic bone disease

Metastatic tumors are the most common malignancy of osseous tissue, accounting for 60% to 65% of all skeletal tumors.[47] Metastatic lesions are seen most often in the spine and pelvis and are less common in anatomic sites that are further removed from the trunk of the body. Tumors that frequently spread to the skeletal system are those of the breast, lung, prostate, kidney, and thyroid, although any cancer can ultimately involve the skeleton. More than 80% of bone metastases are due to primary lesions in the breast, lung, or prostate.[48] The incidence of metastatic bone disease is highest in persons over 40 years of age. In 90% of cases, there are several bony metastases, with or without metastatic spread to other organs.[47] Because of the effectiveness of current cancer treatment modalities, cancer patients are living longer, so that the incidence of clinically apparent skeletal involvement appears to be increasing in the long run. These skeletal metastases cause great pain, increase the risk of fractures, and increase the disability of the cancer patient.

Metastasis to the bone frequently occurs without involving other organs. This is because the blood flow in the veins of the skeletal system is sluggish. These are thin-walled valveless veins, and there are many storage sites along the way. The pattern of metastasis is often related to the specific vascular pathway involved: for example, metastases to the shoulder girdle and pelvis occur when prostatic cancers invade the vertebral vein system. If metastasis is limited to the skeletal system, without other major organ involvement, a person can live for many years. Death is usually a consequence of metastasis to vital organs rather than a consequence of the primary tumor itself.

The major symptom of bone metastasis is pain with evidence of an impending pathologic fracture. Pain is caused by either stretching of the periosteum of the involved bone or by nerve entrapment, as in the nerve roots of the spinal cord by the vertebral body. X-ray examinations are used along with computed tomography or bone scans to detect, diagnose, and localize metastatic bone lesions. About one-third of persons with skeletal metastases have positive bone scans without radiologic findings, and about 28% have metastatic lesions on x-ray studies with a negative bone scan.[49] Arteriography, using radiopaque contrast media, may be helpful in outlining the tumor margins. Serum levels of alkaline phosphatase and calcium are often elevated in persons with metastatic bone disease. A bone biopsy usually is done when there is a question regarding the diagnosis or treatment.

The primary goals in treatment of metastatic bone disease are to prevent pathologic fractures and to promote survival with maximum functioning in order to help the patient maintain as much mobility and pain control as possible. Treatment methods include surgery, chemotherapy, and irradiation. The discov-

ery of new and more effective drugs along with the use of combination protocols has increased the effectiveness of chemotherapy in treating metastatic bone disease secondary to tumors of the breast, prostate, and lung.[50] Radiation therapy is primarily used as a palliative treatment to alleviate pain and prevent pathologic fractures. Localized radiation therapy provides partial or complete pain relief and prevention of fractures in about 73% to 96% of people with metastases to weight-bearing bones.[48]

Pathologic fractures occur in about 10% to 15% of persons with metastatic bone disease. The affected bone appears to be eaten away on x-ray images, and in severe cases, crumbles on impact, much like dried toast. Many pathologic fractures occur in the femur, humerus, and vertebrae. In the femur, fractures occur because the proximal aspect of the bone is under great mechanical stress. Lesions may be treated prophylactically with surgery and radiation therapy to prevent pathologic fractures. Flexible intramedullary rods, such as an Enders rod, may be used to stabilize long bones when lytic lesions involve 30% or more of the bone or are longer than 3 cm and in nonweight-bearing bones (humerus, ulna, and radius) when lesions involve 50% or more of the bone or are longer than 5 cm.[48] When a pathologic fracture has occurred, traction, intramedullary nailing, casting, or bracing can be used. Because adequate fixation is often difficult in diseased bone, bone cement (methyl methacrylate) is often used with internal fixation devices in order to stabilize the bone. The selection of a treatment modality for either prevention or treatment of pathologic fractures depends on the severity of the lesion, the degree of pain, and the life expectancy of the patient. The goal is to give people flexibility, mobility, and pain relief. Surgeons employ a certain degree of aggressiveness in treating metastatic lesions so that patients can function as normally as possible.

In summary, bone tumors, like any other type of neoplasms, may be either benign or malignant. Benign bone tumors grow slowly and usually do not destroy the surrounding tissues. Malignant tumors can be either primary or metastatic. Primary bone tumors are relatively rare, grow rapidly, metastasize to the lungs and other parts of the body through the bloodstream, and have a high mortality rate. Metastatic bone tumors are usually multiple, originating primarily from cancers of the breast, lung, and prostate. The incidence of metastatic bone disease is probably increasing because the improved treatment methods enable people with cancer to live longer. Recent advances in chemotherapy, radiation therapy, and surgical procedures have substantially increased the survival and cure rates for many types of bone cancers. A primary goal in metastatic bone disease is the prevention of pathologic fractures.

References

1. Moore KL: Before We are Born, pp 2–3. Philadelphia, WB Saunders, 1983
2. Hopper WC: Genetics in orthopedics. Orthop Nurs 1:38, 1983
3. DeAngles C: Pediatric Primary Care, pp 289, 292. Boston, Little, Brown, 1984
4. Core Curriculum for Orthopedic Nursing, p 125. Pitman, NJ, National Association of Orthopedic Nurses, 1986
5. Renshaw TS: Pediatric Orthopedics, pp 77, 83. Philadelphia, WB Saunders, 1986
6. Axer A, Gershuni DH, Hendel D, Mirovski Y et al: Indications for femoral osteotomy in Legge Calvé Perthes disease. Clin Orthop 150(July–Aug):78, 1980
7. Jani LFH, Dick W: Results of three different types of therapeutic groups in Perthes disease. Clin Orthop 150(4):88, 1980
8. Rodman GP, Shumacker HR (ed): Primer on Rheumatic Disorders. 9th ed, pp 243, 245, 277. Atlanta, GA, Arthritis Foundation, 1988
9. Harrel J, Meehan PL: School screening in spinal deformity. ONAJ 6:201, 1977
10. Binns M: Joint laxity in idiopathic adolescent scoliosis. J Bone Joint Surg 70(B):420, 1988
11. Harrington PR: The etiology of idiopathic scoliosis. Clin Orthop 126(July–Aug):17, 1977
12. Bunnell WP: The natural history of idiopathic scoliosis. Clin Orthop 229(April):20, 1988
13. Segil C: Current concepts in management of scoliosis. Nurs Clin North Am 11:691, 1976
14. Holt deToledo C: The patient with scoliosis: The defect, the classification, and detection. Am J Nurs 79:1588, 1979
15. Rodts MF: Surgical intervention for adult scoliosis. Orthop Nurs 6(6):11, 1987
16. Bradford DS: Adult scoliosis: Current concepts of treatment. Clin Orthop 229:70, 1988
17. Kehl DK and Morrissy RT: Brace treatment in adolescent scoliosis: An update on concepts and techniques. Clin Orthop 229:34, 1988
18. Hooker CW, Greene WB: Congenital malformations. In Wilson FC (ed): The Musculoskeletal System, 2nd ed, p.27. Philadelphia, JB Lippincott, 1983
19. Grill F, Franke J: The Ilizarov distractor for correction of relapsed or neglected clubfoot. J Bone Joint Surg 69(B):593, 1987
20. Duncan C: Osteogenesis imperfecta. ONA 6:193, 1979
21. Robbins SL, Cotran RS: Pathologic Basis of Disease, pp 1480, 1491. Philadelphia, WB Saunders, 1979
22. Ham AW, Cormack DH: Histology, 8th ed, p 441. Philadelphia, JB Lippincott, 1979
23. Talmadge RV, Grubb SA, VanderWeil CJ: Physiologic processes in bone. In Wilson FC (ed): The Musculoskeletal System, 2nd ed. Philadelphia, JB Lippincott, 1983
24. Stamp TCB, Round JM: Seasonal changes in human plasma levels of 25-dihydroxyvitamin D. Nature 247:563, 1974
25. Anderson MEK, Conley DM: Let the sun shine in. Geriatric Nurs 8:174, 1987
26. Bickle DD: The vitamin D endocrine system. Ann Intern Med 27:45, 1982
27. Raisz LG: Osteoporosis. J Am Geriatr Soc 30:127, 1982
28. Gregory CA: Possible influence of physical activity on musculoskeletal symptoms of menopause and postmenopausal women. J Obstet Gynecol Nurs 11:103, 1982
29. Gordon GS, Vaughn C: Osteoporosis: Early detection, prevention, and treatment. Consultant 25:64, 1980
30. Aloia JF: Estrogen and exercise in prevention and treatment of osteoporosis. Geriatrics 37(6):81, 1982
31. Raisz LC: Local and systemic factors in the pathogenesis of osteoporosis. N Engl J Med 318:818, 1988
32. Notelovitz M, Ware M: Stand tall: The Informed Woman's Guide to Osteoporosis. Gainesville, FL, Triad Publishing, 1988
33. Spencer H: Osteoporosis: Goals of therapy. Hosp Pract 3:131, 1982
34. Slovik DM, Adams JS, Neer RM, et al: Deficient production of 1,25 dihydroxyvitamin D in elderly osteoporotic patients. N Engl J Med 305:372, 1981
35. Kiel DP, Felson DT, Anderson JJ, et al: Hip fracture and the use of estrogens in postmenopausal women: The Framingham Study. N Engl J Med 317:1169, 1987
36. Aroncheck JM, Haddad JG. Paget's disease. Orthop Clin North Am 14:3, 1983
37. Wallach S. Treatment of Paget's disease. Adv Intern Med 27:1,1982
38. Schajowicz F, Arauyo ES, Bernestein M: Sarcoma complicating Paget's disease of bone. J Bone Joint Surg 65(B):299,1983
39. Rubin R (ed): Clinical Oncology: A Multidisciplinary Approach, pp 296–306. New York, American Cancer Society, 1983
40. Dahlin DC: Bone Tumors: General Aspects and Data on 6,221 Cases, 3rd ed. Springfield, IL, Charles C Thomas, 1978
41. Facts on Bone Cancer. New York, American Cancer Society, 1978
42. Huvos AG: Bone Tumors: Diagnosis, Treatment and Prognosis. Philadelphia, WB Saunders, 1979
43. Brashear HR: Tumors and tumorlike conditions of bone. In Wilson FC (ed): The Musculoskeletal System, 2nd ed, p 158. Philadelphia, JB Lippincott, 1980
44. Nirenberg A: The adolescent with osteogenic sarcoma. Orthop Nurs 4(5):11, 1985
45. Simon MA: Limb salvage for osteosarcoma. J Bone Joint Surg 70(A):307, 1987
46. Uyttendaele D, DeSchyver A, Claessen H: Limb conservations in primary bone tumors by resection, extracorporeal irradiation and re-implantation. J Bone Joint Surg 70(B):348, 1988
47. Sherry HS, Levy RN, Siffert RS: Metastatic disease of bone in orthopedic surgery. Clin Orthop 169:44, 1982
48. Mauch PM, Drew MA: Treatment of metastatic cancer to bone. In DeVita VT, Hellman S, Rosenberg SA (eds): Cancer: Principles of Practice of Oncology, 2nd ed, pp 2132, 2135, 2133. Philadelphia, JB Lippincott, 1985
49. Bhardwaj S, Holland JF: Chemotherapy of metastatic cancer in bone. Clin Orthop 169:28, 1982
50. Schocker JD, Brady LW: Radiation therapy for bone metastasis. Clin Orthop 169:38, 1982

Bibliography

Abramowicz M (ed): Prevention and treatment of postmenopausal osteoporosis. Medical Letter 29, No 746:75, 1987

Albright JA: Management overview of osteogenesis imperfecta. Clin Orthop Rel Res 159:80, 1981

Aloia JF: Estrogen and exercise in prevention and treatment of osteoporosis. Geriatrics 37(6):81, 1982

Binder H, Hawks L, Graybill G, et al: Osteogenesis imperfecta: Rehabilitation approach with infants and young children. Arch Phys Med Rehabil 65:537, 1984

Birch JC, Herrig JH, Roach JW, et al: Cortrel-Dubousset instrumentation in idiopathic scoliosis. Clin Orthop Rel Res 228:25, 1988

Bowen JR, Foster BK, Hartzell CR: Legg–Calvé–Perthes disease. Clin Orthop Rel Res 185:97, 1984

Brewer V, Meyer BM, Keele MS, et al: Role of exercise in prevention of involutional bone loss. Med Sci Sports Exercise 15:445, 1983

Bridwell KH: Cortrel-Dubousset instrumentation. Orthop Nurs 7(1):11, 1988

Christodouloy AG, Prince HG, Webb JK, et al: Adolescent idiopathic thoracic scoliosis: A prospective trial with and without bracing during postoperative care. J Bone Joint Surg 69(1):13, 1987

Corbett D: Information needs of parents of a child with Pavlik harness. Orthop Nurs 7(2):20, 1988

Dalinka MK, Aronchick JM, Haddad JG: Paget's disease. Orthop Clin North Am 14:3, 1983

Dell DD, Regan R: Juvenile idiopathic scoliosis. Orthop Nurs 6(6):23, 1987

Gamble JG, Rinsky LA, Strudwick J, et al: Non-union of fractures in children who have osteogenesis imperfecta. J Bone Joint Surg 70(A):439, 1988

Gelberman RH, Cohen MS, Desai SS, et al: Femoral anteversion: A clinical assessment of idiopathic intoeing gait in children. J Bone Joint Surg 69(B):75, 1987

Gershuni DH: Preliminary evaluation and prognosis in Legg–Calvé–Perthes disease. Clin Orthop 150(4):16, 1980

Graham BA, Gleit CJ: Osteoporosis: A major health problem in postmenopausal women. Orthop Nurs 3(6):19, 1984

Ippolito E, Tudisco C, Farsetti P: The long-term prognosis of unilateral Perthes disease. J Bone Joint Surg 69(B):243, 1987

Jackson MA, Nelson D: Etiology and medical management of acute suppurative joint infections in pediatric patients. J Pediatr Orthop 2:313, 1982

Kaplan FS, Soffer SR, Fallon MD, et al: Osteomalacia as a very late manifestation of primary hyperparathyroidism. Clin Orthop 228:26, 1988

Lahde RE: Luque rod instrumentation. AORN 38:35, 1983

Lamphier PC: Primary bone tumors. Orthop Nurs 4(5):17, 1985

Li WK, Lane JM, Rosen G, et al: Pelvic Ewing's sarcoma: Advances in treatment. J Bone Joint Surg 65(A):737, 1983

McKibbin B, Freedman L, Howard C, et al: The management of congenital dislocation of the hip in the newborn. J Bone Joint Surg 70(B):423, 1988

Madigan RR, Wallace SL: What's new in scoliosis. J Tennessee Med Assoc 76:292, 1983

Mann RA: Acquired flatfoot in adults. Clin Orthop Rel Res 181:46, 1983

Pitt M: Osteopenic bone disease. Orthop Clin North Am 14:65, 1983

Renshaw TS: Screening school children for scoliosis. Clin Orthop 229:26, 1988

Sachs B, Bradford D, Winter R, et al: Scheuerman kyphosis: Followup of the Milwaukee brace treatment. J Bone Joint Surg 69(A): 50, 1987

Siris ES, Jacobs TP, Canfield RE: Paget's disease of bone. Bull N Y Acad Med 56:285, 1980

Slovik DM, Adams JS, Neer RM, et al: Deficient production of 1,25-dihydroxyvitamin D in elderly osteoporotic patients. N Engl J Med 305:372, 1981

Spencer H: Osteoporosis: Goals of therapy. Hosp Pract 17(3):131, 1982

Thomas IH, Cole WG, Waters KD: Function after partial pelvic resection of Ewing's sarcoma. J Bone Joint Surg 69(B):271, 1987

Victoria-Diaz A, Victoria-Diaz V: Pathogenesis of idiopathic club foot. Clin Orthop 185:14, 1984

Wallack S: Treatment of Paget's disease. Adv Intern Med 27:1, 1982

Weatherly CR, Draycott V, O'Brien JD: The rib deformity in adolescent idiopathic scoliosis: A prospective study to evaluate changes after Harrington distraction and posterior fusion. J Bone Joint Surg 69(B):179, 1987

Wilton TJ, Hosking DJ, Pawley E, et al: Osteomalacia and femoral neck fractures in the elderly patient. J Bone Joint Surg 69(B):388, 1987

Winter RB: Adolescent idiopathic scoliosis. N Engl J Med 314:1379, 1986

Wynne-Davies R: Some etiologic factors in Perthes disease. Clin Orthop 150(4):12, 1980

Wynne-Davies R, Gormley J: Clinical and genetic patterns in osteogenesis imperfecta. Clin Orthop Rel Res 159:26, 1981

Janice Smith Pigg

CHAPTER 57

Alterations in Skeletal Function: Rheumatic Disorders

Objectives

After you have studied this chapter, you should be able to meet the following objectives:

_____ Describe the pathologic changes that may be found in the joint of an individual with rheumatoid arthritis.

_____ List the extra-articular manifestations of rheumatoid arthritis.

_____ List the components of a basic treatment program for rheumatoid arthritis.

_____ Compare rheumatoid arthritis and osteoarthritis in terms of joint involvement, level of inflammation, and local and systemic manifestations.

_____ Describe the pathologic joint changes associated with osteoarthritis.

_____ Cite the primary features of ankylosing spondylitis.

_____ Describe how the site of inflammation differs in spondyloarthropathies from that in rheumatoid arthritis.

_____ Cite the common features in the management of rheumatoid arthritis, osteoarthritis, and ankylosing spondylitis.

_____ Differentiate between the type of crystals found in the joint in acute gout and pseudogout.

_____ Describe renal mechanisms for eliminating uric acid.

_____ State two mechanisms of hyperuricemia.

_____ List three drugs that are used in the treatment of gout and describe their mechanisms of action.

Arthritis, or inflammation of the joint, is a rheumatic disorder characterized by inflammatory and degenerative joint changes. More than 100 different types of arthritis exist, and one person in every seven is affected.[1] Arthritis affects people in all age groups and is the second leading cause of disability in the United States.[2] The disabling effects may be manifested in an individual's personal, professional, and social activities.

There is a wide spectrum of perceptions about arthritis. Some people perceive arthritis as a minor ache or pain; others envision being in a wheelchair within a matter of months. Because arthritis is not often perceived as life-threatening, sufferers frequently do not seek treatment until the disorder has significantly affected their life.

Some forms of arthritis may develop as a primary joint disorder, while other forms may occur as a secondary disorder resulting from another disease condition. Chart 57-1 provides a classification of rheumatic diseases. The discussion in this chapter is limited to rheumatoid arthritis, osteoarthritis, spondyloarthropathies, and crystal-induced arthropathies.

Rheumatoid arthritis

Rheumatoid arthritis is a systemic inflammatory disease that affects 0.3% to 1.5% of the population, women being affected two to three times more frequently than men.[3] Although rheumatoid arthritis occurs in all age groups, its prevalence increases with age. In women the peak incidence is between ages 40 and 60.

Although the cause of rheumatoid arthritis remains somewhat mysterious, there is evidence that immunologic events may play an important role. About 70% of those with the disease have the rheumatoid factor (RF), which is considered to be an antibody to an autologous (self-produced) immunoglobulin in their blood.[4]

Why the body would begin to produce antibodies against its own IgG cannot be answered as yet. It is possible that an infectious agent, such as a virus, could alter the immunoglobulin so that it is recognized as foreign. Another possibility is that genetic predisposition plays a role in the development of the response. A large number of persons with rheumatoid arthritis have been found to have the histocompatibility antigen, human lymphocyte antigen, HLA-DR4 (discussed in Chapter 11).[3]

The rheumatoid factor has been found not only in the blood, but also in the synovial fluid and synovial membrane of affected persons. In fact, it has been shown that much of the rheumatoid factor is produced by lymphocytes in the inflammatory infiltrate of the synovial tissue.[5] To partially explain the destructive changes that occur in rheumatoid arthritis, it has been suggested that the rheumatoid factor reacts with IgG or other types of antibodies to form immune complexes. These immune complexes activate the complement system, which, in turn, initiates the inflammatory reaction. Polymorphonuclear leukocytes, monocytes, and lymphocytes are attracted to the area. These cells phagocytize the immune complexes and, in the process, release lysosomal enzymes capable of causing destructive changes in the joint cartilage. The inflammatory response that follows attracts additional lymphocytes and plasma cells, setting into motion a chain of events that perpetuates the condition.

Pathologic changes

In rheumatoid arthritis the pathologic changes begin with inflammatory changes in the synovial membrane. The synovial cells and the subsynovial tissue undergo a reactive hyperplasia. Vasodilation and increased blood flow cause warmth and redness. Swelling results from the increased capillary permeability that accompanies the inflammatory process.

Characteristic of rheumatoid arthritis is the development of a destructive vascular granulation tissue called *pannus,* which extends from the synovium to involve the articular cartilage (Figure 57-1). The inflammatory cells found in the pannus have a destructive effect on the adjacent cartilage and bone. Eventually, the pannus develops between the joint margins, leading to reduced joint motion and the possibility of eventual ankylosis. With the progression of the disease, joint inflammation and the resulting structural changes can lead to joint instability, muscle atrophy from disuse, stretching of the ligaments, and involvement of the tendons and muscles. The effect of the pathologic changes in the joint is related to the disease activity, which can change at any time. The destructive changes are irreversible.

Clinical manifestations

Rheumatoid arthritis is often associated with extra-articular as well as articular manifestations. The disease, which is characterized by exacerbations and remissions, may involve only a few joints for brief durations or it may be relentlessly progressive and debilitating. About 3% of persons with the disease have a progressive, unremitting form of rheumatoid arthritis that does not respond to aggressive therapy.[6]

Joint manifestations

Rheumatoid arthritis usually has an insidious onset marked by systemic manifestations such as fatigue, anorexia, weight loss, and generalized aching and stiffness. Joint involvement is usually symmetrical and polyarticular. Any diarthrodial joint can be involved. The individual may complain of joint pain and swelling in addition to stiffness. Morning stiffness usually lasts 30 minutes and frequently lasts for several hours. The limitation of joint motion that occurs early in the disease is usually due to pain; later it is due to fibrosis. The most frequently affected joints initially are the fingers, hands, wrists, knees, and feet. Later, other diarthrodial joints may become involved. Spinal involvement is usually limited to the cervical region.

In the *hands* there is usually bilateral and symmetrical involvement of the proximal interphalangeal (PIP) and metacarpophalangeal (MCP) joints in the early stages of rheumatoid arthritis; the distal interphalangeal (DIP) joints are rarely affected. The fingers often take on a spindle-shaped appearance because of inflammation of the proximal interphalangeal joints (Figure 57-2).

Progressive joint destruction may lead to subluxation and instability as well as limitation in movement. Swelling and thickening of the synovium can result in stretching of the joint capsule and ligaments. When this occurs, muscle and tendon imbalance develop, and mechanical forces applied to the joints through daily activities produce joint deformities. In the metacarpophalangeal joints, the extensor tendons can slip to the ulnar side of the metacarpal head, causing ulnar deviation of the fingers. Subluxation of the metacarpophalangeal joints may develop when this deformity is present (Figure 57-3). Hyperextension of the proximal interphalangeal joint and partial flexion of the distal interphalangeal joint is called a *swan neck deformity* (Figure 57-4). Once this condition becomes fixed, severe loss of function occurs, because the person can no longer make a fist. When flexion of the proximal interphalangeal joint with hyperextension of the distal interphalangeal joint occurs it is called a *boutonnière deformity* (Figure 57-5).

In rheumatoid arthritis a condition called *carpal tunnel syndrome* can occur when the median nerve is compressed as a result of synovial hypertrophy and tenosynovitis on the volar aspect of the wrist. Carpal tunnel syndrome is an entrapment neuropathy and is a common cause of paresthesias of the hand in rheumatoid arthritis as well as other conditions. Burning pain and tingling of the hands occurs, often at night. Numbness of the middle or three radial fingers is common. Occasionally the pain spreads above the wrist into the arm. As the condition progresses, muscle weakness may develop and there may be difficulty in abducting the thumb or opposing the thumb to the index finger.

The knee is one of the most commonly affected joints and is responsible for much of the disability associated with the disease.[7] Active synovitis may be apparent as visible swelling that obliterates the normal contour over the medial and lateral aspects of the patella. The bulge sign, which involves milking fluid from the lateral to the medial side of the patella, may be used to determine the presence of excess fluid when it is not visible. Joint contractures, instability, and valgus deformity are further manifestations that can occur (Figure 57-6). There is often severe quadriceps atrophy, which contributes to disability. A Baker's cyst may occur behind the knee. This is caused by enlargement of the bursa and usually does not cause symptoms unless the cyst ruptures, in which case symptoms mimicking thrombophlebitis appear.

Disease activity can limit flexion and extension of the ankle, which can create difficulty in walking. Involvement of the metatarsophalangeal joints can cause subluxation, hallux valgus, and cock-up toe deformities (Figure 57-7).

Neck discomfort is common. In rare cases, longstanding disease can lead to neurologic complications. Dislocation of the first cervical vertebra or subluxation of the odontoid process of the second vertebra into the foramen magnum are uncommon but potentially fatal complications.

Extra-articular manifestations

Although characteristically a joint disease, rheumatoid arthritis can affect a number of other tissues. The extra-articular manifestations probably occur with a fair degree of frequency but are usually mild enough to cause few problems. They are most likely to be present in persons with a positive rheumatoid factor assay.

Because rheumatoid arthritis is a systemic disease, it may be accompanied by the previously mentioned complaints of fatigue, weakness, anorexia, weight loss, and low-grade fever when the disease is active. The erythrocyte sedimentation rate (ESR), which is commonly elevated during inflammatory processes, has been found to correlate with the amount of disease activity.[3] Anemia associated with a low serum iron level or low iron-binding capacity is common.[3] This anemia is generally resistant to iron therapy. The finding of rheumatoid factor is helpful but not diagnostic of rheumatoid arthritis.[3]

Rheumatoid nodules are granulomatous lesions that develop around small blood vessels. The nodules may be tender or nontender, movable or immovable. The size is variable. Typically they are found over pressure points such as the extensor surfaces of the ulna (Figure 57-8). The nodules may remain unless surgically removed, or they may resolve spontaneously.

Vasculitis is an uncommon manifestation of rheumatoid arthritis seen in persons with a long his-

Chart 57-1: Classification of the rheumatic diseases

I. Diffuse connective tissue diseases
   A. Rheumatoid arthritis
   B. Juvenile arthritis
      1. Systemic onset (Still's disease)
      2. Polyarticular onset
      3. Pauciarticular onset
   C. Systemic lupus erythematosus
   D. Systemic sclerosis
   E. Polymyositis/dermatomyositis
   F. Necrotizing vasculitis and other vasculopathies
      1. Polyarteritis nodosa group (includes hepatitis B–associated arteritis and Churg–Strauss allergic granulomatosis)
      2. Hypersensitivity vasculitis (includes Schönlein-Henoch purpura)
      3. Wegener's granulomatosis
      4. Giant cell arteritis (temporal arteritis, Takayasu's arteritis)
      5. Mucocutaneous lymph node syndrome (Kawasaki disease)
      6. Behcet's disease
      7. Cryoglobulinemia
      8. Juvenile dermatomyositis
   G. Sjögren's syndrome
   H. Overlap syndromes (includes undifferentiated and mixed connective tissue disease)
   I. Others (includes polymyalgia rheumatica, panniculitis (Weber–Christian disease), erythema nodosum, relapsing polychondritis, diffuse fasciitis with esosinophilia, adult onset Still's disease and others)

II. Arthritis associated with spondylitis
   A. Ankylosing spondylitis
   B. Reactive arthritis (Reiter's syndrome)
   C. Psoriatic arthritis
   D. Arthritis associated with chronic inflammatory bowel disease

III. Degenerative joint disease (osteoarthritis, osteoarthrosis)
   A. Primary (includes erosive osteoarthritis)
   B. Secondary

IV. Arthritis, tenosynovitis, and bursitis associated with infectious agents
   A. Direct
      1. Bacterial (staphylococci, gonococci, mycobacteria, spirochetes, and others)
      2. Viral, including hepatitis
      3. Fungal
      4. Parasitic
      5. Unknown, suspected (Whipple's disease)
   B. Indirect (reactive)
      1. Bacterial (includes acute rheumatic fever, intestinal bypass, postdysenteric—shigella, yersinia)
      2. Viral (hepatitis B)

V. Metabolic and endocrine diseases associated with rheumatic states
   A. Crystal-induced conditions
      1. Monosodium urate (gout)
      2. Calcium pyrophosphate dihydrate (pseudogout, chondrocalcinosis)
      3. Apatite and other basic calcium phosphates
      4. Oxalate

   B. Biochemical abnormalities
      1. Amyloidosis
      2. Vitamin C deficiency (scurvy)
      3. Specific enzyme deficiency states (includes Fabry's, Farber's, and others)
      4. Hyperlipoproteinemias (types II, IIa, IV, and others)
      5. Mucopolysaccharidoses
      6. Hemoglobinopathies (SS disease and others)
      7. True connective tissue disorders (Ehlers-Danlos, Marfan's, osteogenesis imperfecta, and pseudoxanthoma elasticum)
      8. Hemochromatosis
      9. Wilson's disease (hepatolenticular degeneration)
      10. Ochronosis (alkaptonuria)
      11. Gaucher's disease
      12. Others
   C. Endocrine diseases
      1. Diabetes mellitus
      2. Acromegaly
      3. Hyperparathyroidism
      4. Thyroid disease (hyperthyroidism, hypothyroidism, thyroiditis)
   D. Immunodeficiency diseases (primary immunodeficiency, acquired immunodeficiency syndrome (AIDS))
   E. Other hereditary disorders
      1. Arthrogryposis multiplex congenita
      2. Hypermobility syndromes
      3. Myositis ossificans progressiva

VI. Neoplasms
   A. Primary (*e.g.*, synovioma, synoviosarcoma)
   B. Metastasis
   C. Multiple myeloma
   D. Leukemia and lymphoma
   E. Villonodular synovitis
   F. Osteochondromatosis
   G. Others

VII. Neuropathic disorders
   A. Charcot's joints
   B. Compression neuropathies
      1. Peripheral entrapment (carpal tunnel syndrome and others)
      2. Radiculopathy
      3. Spinal stenosis
   C. Reflex sympathetic dystrophy
   D. Others

VIII. Bone, periosteal, and cartilage disorders associated with articular manifestations
   A. Osteoporosis
      1. Generalized
      2. Localized (regional and transient)
   B. Osteomalacia
   C. Hypertrophic osteoarthropathy
   D. Diffuse idiopathic skeletal hyperostosis (includes ankylosing vertebral hyperostosis—Forrestier's disease)
   E. Osteitis
      1. Generalized (osteitis deformans—Paget's disease of bone)
      2. Localized (osteitis condensans ilii; osteitis pubis)

(continued)

      F.   Osteonecrosis
      G.   Osteochondritis (osteochondritis dissecans)
      H.   Bone and joint dysplasias
      I.   Slipped capital femoral epiphysis
      J.   Costochondritis (includes Tietze's syndrome)
      K.   Osteolysis and chondrolysis
      L.   Osteomyelitis
  IX. Nonarticular rheumatism
      A.   Myofascial pain syndromes
            1.   Generalized (fibrositis, fibromyalgia)
            2.   Regional
      B.   Low back pain and intervertebral disc disorders
      C.   Tendinitis (tenosynovitis) and/or bursitis
            1.   Subacromial/subdeltoid bursitis
            2.   Bicipital tendinitis, tenosynovitis
            3.   Olecranon bursitis
            4.   Epicondylitis, medial or lateral humeral
            5.   DeQuervain tenosynovitis
            6.   Adhesive capsulitis of the shoulder (frozen shoulder)
            7.   Trigger finger
            8.   Others
      D.   Ganglion cysts
      E.   Faciitis
      F.   Chronic ligament and muscle strain
      G.   Vasomotor disorders
            1.   Erythromelalgia
            2.   Raynaud's disease or phenomenon

      H.   Miscellaneous pain syndromes (includes weather sensitivity, psychogenic rheumatism)
  X. Miscellaneous disorders
      A.   Disorders frequently associated with arthritis
            1.   Trauma (the result of direct trauma)
            2.   Internal derangement of joints
            3.   Pancreatic disease
            4.   Sarcoidosis
            5.   Palindromic rheumatism
            6.   Intermittent hydrarthrosis
            7.   Erythema nodosum
            8.   Hemophilia
      B.   Other conditions
            1.   Multicentric reticulohistiocytosis (nodular panniculitis)
            2.   Familial Mediterranean fever
            3.   Goodpasture's syndrome
            4.   Chronic active hepatitis
            5.   Drug-induced rheumatic syndromes
            6.   Dialysis-associated syndromes
            7.   Foreign body synovitis
            8.   Acne and hyradenitis suppurativa
            9.   Pustulosis palmaris et plantaris
         10.   Sweet's syndrome
         11.   Others

(Primer on the Rheumatic Diseases, 9th ed. Atlanta, Arthritis Foundation, 1988)

tory of active arthritis and high titers of rheumatoid factor. It is possible that some persons have vasculitis that remains silent. Vasculitis is caused by the inflammatory process affecting the small and medium-sized arterioles. Manifestations include ischemic areas in the nailfold and digital pulp that appear as brown spots. Ulcerations may occur in the lower extremities, particularly around the malleolar areas. In some cases, neuropathy may be the only symptom of vasculitis. The visceral organs, such as the heart, lungs, and gastrointestinal tract may also be affected.

Secondary Sjögren's syndrome is present in about 10% to 15% of persons with rheumatoid arthritis.[3] It may also be present with other connective tissue diseases or be a disorder without an accompanying disease process. The primary symptoms are reduced lacrimal and salivary gland secretion, frequently referred to as the *sicca complex*. The eyes may feel sandy or gritty, as if foreign bodies are in them. The mouth feels dry, and the sufferer usually feels thirsty. The person is more prone than normal to dental caries and halitosis because saliva is not present to reduce these problems. The dryness associated with Sjögren's syndrome can affect any of the mucous membranes. The treatment is generally symptomatic. Artificial tears, or 0.5% methylcellulose eye drops, provide temporary relief of dry eyes. Sugarless hard candy, artificial saliva

products, and the use of a home humidifier can help reduce mouth and throat dryness. The use of water-soluble lubricants during sexual activity can be helpful if vaginal dryness is a problem.[8]

Other extra-articular manifestations include eye lesions such as episcleritis and scleritis, hematologic abnormalities, pulmonary disease, cardiac complications, infection, and Felty's syndrome (leukopenia with or without splenomegaly).

Diagnosis and treatment

The diagnosis of rheumatoid arthritis is based on history, physical examination, and laboratory tests. The diagnostic criteria developed by the American Rheumatism Association are used in establishing the diagnosis (Chart 57-2). At least four of the criteria must be present to make a diagnosis of rheumatoid arthritis.

In the early stages, the disease is much more difficult to diagnose. On physical examination the affected joints show signs of inflammation, swelling, tenderness, and possibly warmth and reduced motion. The joints have a soft, spongy feeling because of the synovial thickening and inflammation. Body movements may be guarded to prevent pain. Changes in joint structure are usually not visible early in the dis-

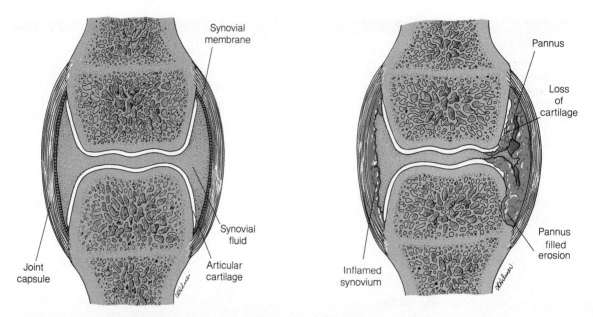

Figure 57-1 (**Left**) Normal joint structures; (**right**) joint changes in rheumatoid arthritis. The left side denotes early changes occurring within the synovium, and the right side shows progressive disease that leads to erosion and the formation of pannus.

ease. Information should be elicited regarding the duration of symptoms, systemic manifestations, stiffness, and family history.

The rheumatoid factor may be used as a diagnostic test, but is inconclusive, because 1% to 5% of healthy persons have rheumatoid factor.[3] The presence of rheumatoid factor seems to be more common with advancing age. It is important to note than an individual can have rheumatoid arthritis without the rheumatoid factor being present. X-ray findings are

not diagnostic in rheumatoid arthritis because joint erosions are not often seen on radiographic images in the early stages of the disorder.

Synovial fluid analysis can be helpful in the diagnostic process. The fluid has a cloudy appearance because the white blood cell count is elevated as a result of inflammation, while the complement components of the synovial fluid are depressed.

The treatment goals for a person with rheumatoid arthritis are to reduce pain, minimize stiffness

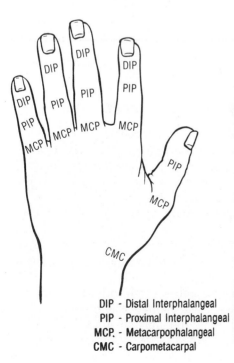

DIP - Distal Interphalangeal
PIP - Proximal Interphalangeal
MCP. - Metacarpophalangeal
CMC - Carpometacarpal

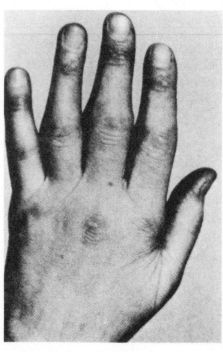

Figure 57-2 (**Left**) Diagram of the joints of the hand; (**right**) early rheumatoid arthritis—spindling of the fingers. (*Photograph reprinted from the Revised Clinical Slide Collection on the Rheumatic Diseases, © 1972. Used by permission of the Arthritis Foundation.*)

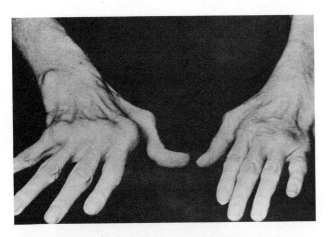

Figure 57-3 Swelling and atrophy of the metacarpophalangeal joints in both hands. Ulnar deviation and subluxation of the metacarpophalangeal joints in the right hand. (*Reprinted from the Arthritis Teaching Slide Collection, 2nd ed, © 1980. Used by permission of the Arthritis Foundation.*)

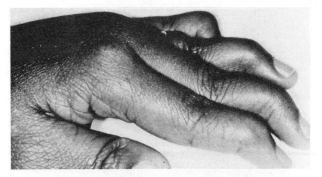

Figure 57-4 Swan neck deformity, in which the proximal interphalangeal (middle) joint is hyperextended and the distal interphalangeal joint is in flexion. (*Reprinted from the Arthritis Teaching Slide Collection, © 1980. Used by permission of the Arthritis Foundation.*)

and swelling, maintain mobility, and become an informed health care consumer. The treatment plan includes education about the disease and its treatment, rest, therapeutic exercises, and medications. Because of the chronicity of the disease and the need for continuous long-term adherence to the prescribed treatment modalities, it is important that the treatment be integrated with the individual's life-style.

Basic education is fundamental in removing misconceptions. Both the individual with arthritis and the general population need to know that although arthritis cannot be cured, much can be done to control its progress. Fear of being crippled is a major concern that should be addressed, so that the disease can be perceived realistically. All aspects of the treatment require that the individual with arthritis accept responsibility for the health care program. Family members should be included in education programs; their support in integrating prescribed treatment regimens is very important. Because many unproven remedies for arthritis are offered, patients need information on how to assess the validity of the available treatments. The Arthritis Foundation provides information and community services to people with arthritis and their families.

Both physical and emotional rest are important aspects of care. Physical rest reduces joint stress. Rest should include total body rest of 8 hours to 10 hours at night and one to two naps or rest periods during the day. Rest of specific joints is recommended to relieve pain. For example, sitting reduces the weight on an inflamed knee and the use of lightweight splints reduces undue movement of the hand or wrist. Emotional rest is also important. Some persons find that discomfort increases with emotional stress; with

emotional rest, muscles relax and discomfort is reduced.

Although rest is essential, therapeutic exercises are important in maintaining joint motion and muscle strength. Range of motion exercises involve the active and passive movement of joints. Isometric (muscle tensing) exercises may be used to strengthen muscles. These exercises are frequently taught by a physical therapist and then performed daily at home. There is also a need to emphasize the difference between normal activity and therapeutic exercise.

Instruction in the safe use of heat and cold modalities to relieve discomfort and in the use of relaxation techniques is also important. Proper posture, positioning, body mechanics, and the use of supportive shoes can provide further comfort. Patients often need information about the principles of joint protection and work simplification. Some need assistive devices to reduce pain and improve their ability to perform activities of daily living.

Strategies to aid in symptom control also in-

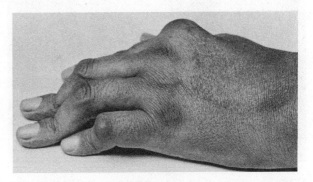

Figure 57-5 Boutonnière deformity, which is characterized by flexion of the proximal interphalangeal joint, hyperextension of the distal interphalangeal joint, and inability to straighten the joint. (*Reprinted from the Arthritis Teaching Slide Collection, 2nd ed, © 1980. Used by permission of the Arthritis Foundation.*)

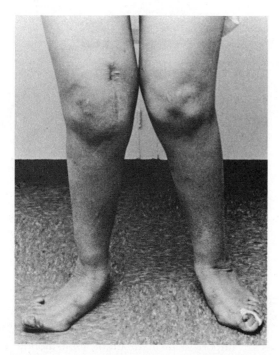

Figure 57-6 Genu valgum (knock knees). This abnormal position is the result of a gradual wearing of cartilage and weakened ligaments in the knee joint. (*Reprinted from the Arthritis Teaching Slide Collection, © 1980. Used by permission of the Arthritis Foundation.*)

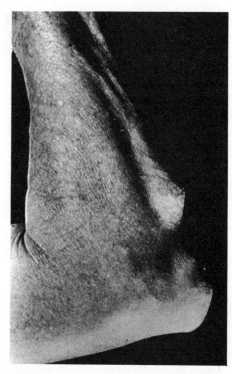

Figure 57-8 Rheumatoid nodules on the elbow. (*Reprinted from the Revised Clinical Slide Collection on the Rheumatic Diseases, © 1972. Used by permission of the Arthritis Foundation.*)

volve regulating activity by pacing, establishing priorities, and setting realistic goals. Support groups and group education experiences benefit some persons. The home and work environments should be assessed and interventions incorporated as the situation warrants.

Salicylates and their derivatives are often selected as the first medication of choice in treatment of rheumatoid arthritis. The dose required for treatment is within a range that will reduce inflammation. The analgesic dose of aspirin is often less than the dose required to suppress inflammation, and persons should be instructed that the anti-inflammatory dose needs to be maintained to control symptoms. The

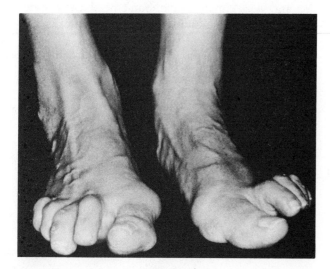

Figure 57-7 Hallus valgus and hammer toes. The "cock-up" toe deformities are associated with subluxation at the metatarsophalangeal joints. Painful corns and bunions are made worse by irritation caused by faulty shoes. (*Reprinted from the Arthritis Teaching Slide Collection, 2nd ed, © 1980. Used by permission of the Arthritis Foundation.*)

Chart 57-2: Proposed 1987 revised American Rheumatism Association criteria for rheumatoid arthritis

Four or more of the following conditions must be present to establish a diagnosis of rheumatoid arthritis

1. Morning stiffness for at least 1 hour and present for at least 6 weeks.
2. Swelling of three or more joints for at least 6 weeks.
3. Swelling of wrist, metacarpophalangeal or proximal interphalangeal joints for 6 or more weeks.
4. Symmetrical joint swelling.
5. Hand roentgenogram changes typical of rheumatoid arthritis that must include erosions or unequivocal bony decalcification.
6. Rheumatoid nodules.
7. Serum rheumatoid factor found present by a method that is positive in less than 5% of normals.

(Primer on the Rheumatic Diseases, 9th ed. Atlanta, Arthritis Foundation, © 1988. Used with the permission of the Arthritis Foundation.)

exact mechanism of aspirin's action is not completely understood, but it is known to inhibit prostaglandin synthesis. Enteric-coated and buffered forms of aspirin are available and are sometimes better tolerated in persons who are prone to gastrointestinal side effects. Tinnitus and decreased hearing are common side effects that resolve when the medication dosage is reduced or discontinued. Sometimes other aspirin preparations are better tolerated, such as salicylate, choline magnesium trisalicylate, and diflunisal.[3] If the individual cannot tolerate or does not receive benefit from aspirin, other nonsteroidal anti-inflammatory drugs (NSAID) from six major chemical classes may be tried. These include: (1) indoles—indomethacin, sulindac, and tolmetin; (2) propionic acid derivatives —ibuprofen, naproxen, fenoprofen, ketoprofen, suprofen; (3) anthranilic acids—meclofenamate sodium; (4) oxicams—piroxicam; (5) pyrazolons— phenylbutazone and oxyphenbutazone; and (6) phenylacetic acid. These medications have antipyretic and anti-inflammatory properties similar to aspirin. Persons with active peptic ulcers or blood coagulation problems should not be given these preparations, because, like aspirin, they have gastrointestinal side effects and impair platelet function.

A slow-acting drug may be added to the medication regimen to induce remission of the disease if it is not responding to the NSAIDs or other conservative therapy. The exact mechanism of action for the slow-acting medications such as gold compounds, hydroxychloroquine, or penicillamine is unknown. Their beneficial effects do not usually become evident until after 2 months of therapy. These drugs and their side effects are summarized in Table 57-1.

Corticosteroid drugs are used to reduce discomfort, but to avoid long-term side effects are only used in specific situations for short-term therapy at a low dose level. They may be used for unremitting disease with extra-articular manifestations. This medication does not modify the disease, so it is unable to prevent joint destruction. Intra-articular corticosteroid injections can provide rapid relief of acute or subacute inflammatory synovitis (after infection is ruled out) in a few joints. They should not be repeated more than a few times a year.

Immunosuppressant drugs, such as azathioprine, cyclophosphamide, chlorambucil, sulfasalazine, and levamisole have the potential for modifying the disease process in rheumatoid arthritis. Only azathioprine has FDA approval for treatment of arthritis. Plasmapheresis, leukopheresis, lymphapheresis thoracic-duct drainage, chemical or local radiation synovectomy, and total body irradiation are procedures which are currently considered experimental. These treatments may hold promise for the future.

Surgery may be indicated as part of the treatment of rheumatoid arthritis. Synovectomy may be indicated to reduce pain and joint damage when synovitis does not respond to medical treatment. The most common soft tissue surgery is tenosynovectomy (repair of damaged tendons) of the hand to release nerve entrapments. Total joint replacements may be indicated to reduce pain and increase motion.

Although the course of rheumatoid arthritis is unpredictable, the past 20 years have brought more effective treatment for the disease. Sufferers are now being diagnosed and treated earlier. Criteria have been developed for remission in rheumatoid arthritis (Chart 57-3).

Juvenile rheumatoid arthritis

Juvenile rheumatoid arthritis is a chronic disease that affects approximately 60,000 to 200,000 children in the United States.[3] It is characterized by synovitis and can influence epiphyseal growth by

Table 57-1. Slow-type medications used in the treatment of rheumatoid arthritis

Medication	Side effects
Gold compounds	
Intramuscular	Skin rash, pruritus
Sodium thiomalate (Myochrysine)	Stomatitis (may be preceded by metallic taste)
Aurothioglucose (Solganal)	Nephrotic syndrome
	Glomerulitis with hematuria
Oral	Albuminuria
Auranofin	Blood dyscrasias
	Granulocytopenia
	Thrombocytopenia
	Hypoplastic and aplastic anemia
	Reduction of hemoglobin
	Leukopenia
	Nitritoid reaction: flushing, dizziness, fainting, sweating
	Nausea, vomiting, diarrhea
	Hair loss
Antimalarial	
Hydroxychloroquine	Retinopathy, corneal changes
Chloroquine	Visual field defects
	Alopecia
	Skin rashes, pruritus
	Gastrointestinal disturbances
Penicillamine	Dermatitis, pruritus
	Fever, lymphadenopathy
	Gastrointestinal disturbances
	Loss of taste
	Stomatitis
	Bone marrow depression and blood dyscrasias
	Proteinuria and hematuria

Chart 57-3: Proposed criteria for clinical remission in rheumatoid arthritis

Five or more of the following requirements must be fulfilled for at least 2 consecutive months

1. Duration of morning stiffness not exceeding 15 minutes.
2. No fatigue.
3. No joint pain (by history).
4. No joint tenderness or pain on motion.
5. No soft tissue swelling in joints or tendon sheaths.
6. Erythrocyte sedimentation rate (Westergren method) less than 30 mm/hr for a female or 20 mm/hr for a male.

(Primer on Rheumatic Diseases, 9th ed. Atlanta, Arthritis Foundation, © 1988. Used with permission of the Arthritis Foundation.)

stimulating growth of the affected side. Generalized stunted growth may also occur.

Systemic onset (Still's disease) affects about 20% of children with juvenile rheumatoid arthritis.[3] The symptoms include a daily intermittent high fever, which is usually accompanied by a rash, generalized lymphadenopathy, hepatosplenomegaly, leukocytosis, and anemia. Most of these children also have joint involvement. Systemic symptoms usually subside in 6 to 12 months. This form of juvenile rheumatoid arthritis can also make an initial appearance in adulthood. Infections, heart disease, and adrenal insufficiency may cause death.

A second subgroup of juvenile rheumatoid arthritis, pauciarticular arthritis, affects no more than four joints. This subgroup affects 40% of children with juvenile rheumatoid arthritis.[3] The pauciarticular arthritis affects two distinct groups. The first group generally consists of females less than 6 years of age with chronic uveitis. Antinuclear antibody testing in this group is usually positive. The second group, in whom the arthritis is of late onset, is most commonly made up of males. The HLA-B27 tests are positive in over half of this group. Sacroiliitis is present and the arthritis is usually in the lower extremities.

The third subgroup of juvenile rheumatoid arthritis, accounting for about 40% of the total, is polyarticular onset disease. It affects more than four joints during the first 6 months of the disease. This form of arthritis more closely resembles the adult form of the disease than the other two subgroups. Rheumatoid factor is sometimes present and may indicate a more active disease process. Systemic features include a low-grade fever, weight loss, malaise, anemia, stunted growth, slight organomegaly (*e.g.,* hepatosplenomegaly), and adenopathy.[3]

The prognosis for most children with rheumatoid arthritis is good. Aspirin is the main medica-

tion used. Although some nonsteroidal anti-inflammatory drugs are available, not all have been approved by the FDA for use in children. Intramuscular gold therapy is often used when aspirin or nonsteroidal anti-inflammatory drugs have proven ineffective. Other aspects of treatment of children with juvenile rheumatoid arthritis are similar to those used for the adult with rheumatoid arthritis. Children are encouraged to lead as normal a life as possible.

In summary, rheumatoid arthritis is a systemic inflammatory disorder that affects 0.3% to 1.5% of the population. Women are affected more frequently than men. This form of arthritis, the cause of which is unknown, has a chronic course and is usually characterized by remissions and exacerbations. Joint involvement is symmetrical and begins with inflammatory changes in the synovial membrane. As joint inflammation progresses, structural changes can occur, leading to joint instability. Systemic manifestations include weakness, anorexia, weight loss, and low-grade fever. Some extra-articular features include rheumatoid nodules, vasculitis, and Sjögren's syndrome. The treatment goals include reducing pain, stiffness, and swelling, maintaining mobility, and assisting the individual to become an informed health care consumer.

Osteoarthritis

Osteoarthritis, also referred to as degenerative joint disease, is the most common form of arthritis. It is a chronic disease of unknown etiology that can lead to loss of mobility and chronic pain. It often causes significant disability, especially when the involved joints are critical to the performance of daily activities. The incidence of osteoarthritis increases with age until by age 60 years more than 60% of the population probably have some degree of cartilage abnormality in many of their major joints.[9]

The joint changes associated with osteoarthritis are progressive through the loss of articular cartilage and are characterized by development of joint pain, stiffness, limitation of motion, and possibly joint instability and deformity. The associated synovitis is secondary.[3] Although there may be periods when mild inflammation is present, it is not the severe type seen in the inflammatory forms of rheumatic diseases such as rheumatoid arthritis.

Osteoarthritis may occur as a primary idiopathic or a secondary disorder. Primary osteoarthritis occurs without an obvious reason and is the most common form. The secondary form of the disease develops because of some identifiable reason. For example, osteoarthritis can occur secondary to joint instability caused by injury to a knee ligament or a meniscus cartilage tear. Other joint disorders such as rheumatoid arthritis, damage from metabolic alterations of the cartilage, congenital abnormalities, childhood changes in joint structure, and crystal deposition may also cause secondary osteoarthritis.

Several additional factors warrant mention. The hypothesis that osteoarthritis is a result of aging has been fairly well discredited.[9] There is a genetic predisposition to some forms of osteoarthritis, as in Heberden's nodes, which affect the distal interphalangeal joints of the hand. The relationship between obesity and the development of osteoarthritis is still controversial, but obesity has been associated with osteoarthritis of the knee in women, probably as a result of additional mechanical stress.

Pathologic changes

Osteoarthritis affects the articular cartilage and subchondral bone (Figure 57-9). Normally, cartilage is a translucent, white, smooth material. In osteoarthritis, the cartilage softens and acquires a yellowish appearance early in the disease process; as the disease progresses, the joint becomes rough because of fissuring, pitting, and erosions followed by the development of focal and eventually diffuse ulcerations. Eventually erosion of the cartilage occurs, leading to thinning and destruction of cartilage down to the bone. Although this process is occurring in the cartilage, changes are also taking place in the subchondral

bone underlying the cartilage. Sclerosis, or formation of new bone and cysts, usually occurs in the juxta-articular bone—that is, the bone near the joint. Formation of new bone that occurs at the joint margins is called *osteophyte spur formation.*

Mild synovitis may also occur. This is more likely to be seen in advanced disease. In certain cases, the synovitis may be related to the release of calcium pyrophosphate dihydrate from the cartilage or calcium hydroxyapatite crystals from synovial tissues.

As a working hypothesis it has been suggested that the cellular events responsible for the development of osteoarthritis begin with some type of insult involving the chondrocytes that degrade matrix proteoglycans and collagen. Biochemical events such as collagen fatigue and fracture occur with less stress as cartilage ages. Attempts at repair by increased matrix synthesis and cellular proliferation maintain the integrity of the cartilage until failure of reparative processes allows the degenerative changes to progress. Inflammatory mediators (*e.g.,* prostaglandins) may increase the inflammatory and degenerative response. Recent studies also implicate immunologic factors in the perpetuation and acceleration of the osteoarthritic change.[3]

Clinical manifestations

The manifestations of osteoarthritis may occur suddenly or insidiously. Initially, pain may be described as aching and may be somewhat difficult to localize. Pain usually follows the use of the involved joints and is relieved by rest. As the disease advances, even minimal activity may cause pain. Pain usually increases throughout the day, causing most discomfort in the evening; overactivity can also increase pain.

The most frequently affected joints are the hips, knees, lumbar and cervical vertebrae, proximal and distal interphalangeal joints of the hand, the first carpometacarpal joint, and the first metatarsophalangeal joints of the feet. Stiffness is localized to the involved joints. It is usually present in the morning, on awakening, and lasts until the person can "work it out" by moving about. Usually, morning stiffness is reduced in about 30 minutes. Sitting also causes stiffness, and persons need to limit the duration of sitting to avoid prolonged stiffness. Pain may occur with passive motion of the involved joint. Crepitus and grinding may also be evident when the joint is moved.

Other clinical features are limitations of joint motion and joint instability. Joint enlargement is usually due to new bone formation, so that the joint feels hard, in contrast with the soft, spongy feeling characteristic of rheumatoid arthritis. Sometimes mild synovitis or increased synovial fluid are present, which can also cause joint enlargement.

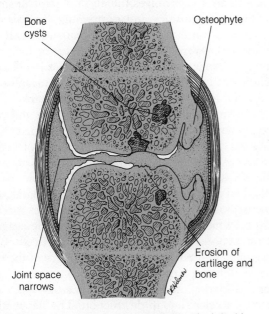

Figure 57-9 Joint changes in osteoarthritis. The left side denotes early changes, joint space narrowing with cartilage breakdown. The right side shows more severe disease progression with lost cartilage and osteophyte formation.

Bone cysts

Osteophyte

Joint space narrows

Erosion of cartilage and bone

——— Diagnosis and treatment

The diagnosis of osteoarthritis is usually determined by history and physical examination, x-ray studies, and laboratory findings that exclude other diseases. Table 57-2 identifies the joints that are commonly affected by osteoarthritis and the common clinical features correlated with the disease activity of each particular joint. Although pain and stiffness are common features of the disease, the impact of the disease will vary with each person.

Table 57–2. Clinical features of osteoarthritis

Joint	Clinical features
Distal interphalangeal joint (DIP) Heberden's nodes	Occurs more frequently in women; usually involves multiple DIPs, lateral flexor deviation of joint, spur formation at joint margins, pain and discomfort following joint use
Proximal interphalangeal joint (PIP) Bouchard's nodes	Same as for distal interphalangeal joint disease
First carpometacarpal joint (CMC)	Tenderness at base of thumb; squared appearance to joint
First metatarsal phalangeal joint (MTP)	Insidious onset; irregular joint contour; pain and swelling aggravated by tight shoes
Hip	Most common in older male adults; characterized by insidious onset of pain, localized to groin region or inner aspect of the thigh; may be referred to buttocks, sciatic region, or knee; reduced hip motion; leg may be held in external rotation with hip flexed and adducted; limp or shuffling gait; difficulty getting in and out of chairs
Knee	Localized discomfort with pain on motion; limitation of motion; crepitus; quadriceps atrophy due to lack of use; joint instability; genu varus or valgus; joint effusion
Cervical spine	Localized stiffness; radicular or nonradicular pain; posterior osteophyte formation may cause vascular compression*
Lumbar spine	Low back pain and stiffness; muscle spasm; decreased back motion; nerve root compression causing radicular pain*; spinal stenosis*

* Rare complication.

In osteoarthritis, the most beneficial method of diagnosis is radiography. If pathologic changes are mild, the x-ray images may be normal. Characteristic radiologic changes include joint space narrowing, osteophyte formation, subchondral bony sclerosis, and cyst formation. Laboratory studies are usually normal because the disorder is not a systemic disease. The sedimentation rate may be slightly elevated in generalized osteoarthritis or erosive inflammatory variations of the disease. If inflammation is present, there may be a slight increase in cell count. The synovial fluid is also usually normal. However, calcium pyrophosphate dihydrate or hydroxyapatite crystals may be seen in the synovial fluid.

The treatment of osteoarthritis is directed toward the relief of pain and the maintenance of mobility and is tailored to the needs of the individual. Specific treatments are determined by the extent of the disease, the joints involved, and the response to previous and current treatment regimens. Education about the disease and type of treatment methods is important. The treatment continuum may range from no treatment to very extensive forms of treatment. Excessive stress on the affected joints should be avoided. Pain and stiffness may be controlled by a balance of activity and rest of the affected joints. A cane or walker may be helpful for reducing the load on weight-bearing joints; control of body weight also reduces the stress placed on the weight-bearing joints. The work environment should be evaluated to reduce repetitive movements and allow for joint rest when possible. The patient should be instructed in activity pacing, planning, priority setting, and simplification of movement that involves the affected joint. Instruction in proper posture and positioning may also be warranted. Heat treatments and therapeutic exercises are directed toward improving and reducing pain and stiffness. Application of cold, provided it is not contraindicated by other medical conditions, may also be used if the individual finds heat uncomfortable.

Analgesics, such as acetaminophen and propoxyphene derivatives, may be used as needed. Narcotics are rarely used except in instances of severe disease exacerbation. Aspirin may be used as an analgesic or as an anti-inflammatory medication. If the individual cannot tolerate aspirin, a nonsteroidal anti-inflammatory drug may be used. The exact mechanism by which these medications act on the osteoarthritic process is unknown. Local corticosteroid injections are used during the acute stages of the disease to reduce pain. These injections are used only after considering other conservative measures, as their use may accelerate joint destruction. The destruction occurs because pain is reduced after the injection and then the joint may be overused. Corticosteroid injections are used infrequently, especially in weight-bearing joints.

Surgery is considered when the person is having severe pain and joint function is severely reduced. Procedures include bunion resections, osteotomies to change alignment of the knee and hip joints, and decompression of the spinal roots in osteoarthritic vertebral stenosis. Total hip replacements have provided effective relief of symptoms and improved range of motion for many persons, as have total knee replacements, although the latter procedure has produced less consistent results. Joint replacement is available for the first carpometacarpal joint. Arthrodesis is used in advanced disease to reduce pain; however this results in loss of motion.

In summary, osteoarthritis is the most common form of arthritis; it can occur as either a primary or a secondary disorder. It is a localized condition affecting primarily the weight-bearing joints. The disorder is characterized by degeneration of the articular cartilage and subchondral bone. Joint enlargement is usually due to new bone formation, which causes the joint to feel hard. Pain and stiffness are primary features of the disease. The treatment is directed toward the relief of pain and maintenance of mobility.

Spondyloarthropathies

Spondyloarthropathies are diseases of the axial skeleton, and particularly the joints of the spine. The seronegative (*rheumatoid-factor negative*) spondyloarthropathies include ankylosing spondylitis, juvenile ankylosing spondylitis, reactive arthritis, psoriatic arthritis, and enteropathic arthritis. These disorders are characterized by involvement of the sacroiliac joints, peripheral inflammatory arthropathy, and the absence of rheumatoid factor. Inflammation of the axial skeleton develops at sites where ligament inserts into bone (enthesis) rather than the synovium. Sometimes a person with spondyloarthropathy will also have inflammation and involvement of the peripheral joints in which case the signs and symptoms overlap with other inflammatory types of arthritis (*e.g.*, rheumatoid arthritis). There is also clinical evidence of overlap between the various seronegative spondylarthritides.

There is a familial tendency toward development of spondyloarthropathy. The reactive arthropathies are typically genetically-determined HLA-B27 antigen (see Chapter 11). Not all HLA-B27 antigen-positive persons develop one of the spondyloarthropathies. Although all HLA-B27 antigen-positive persons are presumed to have contact with environmental triggering agents, only 10%–20% actually develop a spondyloarthropathy. Some of the triggering events are known, as in the case of enteropathic arthritis after exposure to *Shigella*. In the case of ankylosing spondylitis, the precipitating cause is not known. Although the seronegative spondyloarthropathies are believed to be caused by HLA-associated immunologic mechanisms, their pathogenesis remains obscure.

Ankylosing spondylitis

Ankylosing spondylitis is an inflammatory disease of the axial skeleton, including the sacroiliac joints, intervertebral disk spaces, and the apophyseal and costovertebral articulations. Bilateral sacroiliitis is a primary feature of the disease. Occasionally large synovial joints may be involved, usually the hips, knees, and shoulders. Small peripheral joints are usually not affected. This disorder is more common than was once believed; it probably affects about 1% to 2% of the population, which is comparable to the prevalence of rheumatoid arthritis.[11] At one time the disease was thought to occur four to ten times more frequently in men than in women. It now appears that the prevalence in women is probably the same or only slightly less than in men, but the disease is not usually as severe in women.[3] Although ankylosing spondylitis can occur in persons of any age, it is usually diagnosed in the second or third decade of life. The disease is seen frequently in North American native Americans and is rarely seen in blacks and Orientals.[10] In children, HLA-B27 is a marker of spondyloarthropathy. Typically, juvenile ankylosing spondylitis affects boys in late childhood.

Ankylosing spondylitis may cause the development of fibrosis, calcification, and ossification of joints with progression to ankylosis. The disease generally brings to mind an image of an individual with a rigid bamboo-like spine. Fortunately, however, few persons develop a progressive disease pattern that leads to this outcome. The disease spectrum ranges from an asymptomatic sacroiliitis to a progressive disease that can affect many body systems. When a progressive disease pattern does develop, it is usually in men.

Clinical manifestations

The individual with ankylosing spondylitis will typically complain of low back pain, which may be persistent or intermittent. The pain may initially be blamed on muscle strain or spasm from physical activity. Lumbosacral pain may also be present, with discomfort in the buttocks and hip areas. Sometimes pain can radiate to the thigh in a manner similar to that of sciatic pain. Although the pain is usually in the lower back, some persons may complain of pain at a higher vertebral level as an initial symptom. In some persons, other problems, such as tendinitis and peripheral joint changes, may precede back pain. Prolonged stiffness is present in the morning and after periods of rest.

Mild activity helps reduce pain and stiffness. It is understandable that sleep patterns are frequently interrupted because of these manifestations. Walking or exercise may be needed to provide the comfort needed in order to return to sleep. Muscle spasm may also contribute to discomfort.

Loss of motion in the spinal column is characteristic of the disease. The severity and duration of disease activity influence the degree of mobility. Motion can be lost in anterior or lateral flexion, extension, and rotation of the spinal column. Loss of lumbar lordosis occurs as the disease progresses, and this is followed by kyphosis of the thoracic spine and extension of the neck.

Because ankylosing spondylitis affects the sites of enthesis, recurrent tendinitis may develop. This usually occurs at the Achilles tendon or the areas of intercostal muscle insertion, and as plantar fasciitis. Little residual damage is done in these situations.

Peripheral arthritis occurs in 20% to 30% of persons with ankylosing spondylitis.[10] Women seem to have peripheral joint disease more frequently than men.[3] Involvement is usually asymmetric and affects hip, shoulder, and knee joints. Hip pain can be a major cause of disability.

The lower the age at onset, the greater the likelihood of progression to total hip replacement.[3] Heel pain is commonly seen as a result of plantar fasciitis.

The disease process varies considerably among individuals. Exacerbations and remissions are common; their unpredictability can create uncertainty in planning daily activities as well as future goals and expectations. Fortunately, most of those affected are able to lead productive lives.

Systemic features of weight loss, fever, and fatigue may be apparent. Thoracic involvement including manubriosternal and sternoclavicular inflammation can create symptoms similar to those of conditions such as angina or esophageal dysfunctions. Uveitis develops in up to 25% of those affected by ankylosing spondylitis.[3] Osteoporosis can occur, especially in the spine, which contributes to the risk of spinal fracture. Fusion of the costovertebral joints can lead to reduced lung volume.

Complications of ankylosing spondylitis, although infrequent, include fractures in ankylosed areas of the spine, atlantoaxial subluxation (the atlas is the first cervical vertebra and articulates above with the occipital bone and below with the axis), spinal cord compression, aortic regurgitation, apical fibroses of the lung, amyloidosis, and cauda equina syndrome with bowel and bladder dysfunction. The complications are more likely in longstanding disease.

The prognosis in ankylosing spondylitis is generally good. The first decade of disease predicts the remainder. Severe disease usually occurs early and is marked by peripheral arthritis, especially of the hip. Mortality is low (6%) and significant disability occurs in less than 20% of persons with the disorder.

Diagnosis and treatment

The diagnosis of ankylosing spondylitis is based on history, physical examination, and x-ray examination. Several methods are available to assess mobility and detect sacroiliitis. Although these measures alone do not provide a diagnosis of ankylosing spondylitis or other spondyloarthropathies, they can provide useful measurements for monitoring the disease status. Sacroiliitis can be detected by having the individual lean forward over a table and pressing firmly on the sacroiliac joints. Pain or tenderness may be elicited and spinal muscle spasm may also be detected.

General fitness and hip mobility can be measured by having the individual flex forward from the waist with the knees straight and extend the arms to touch the floor. The distance from the fingertips to the floor is then measured.

The modified Schober's test is also used to determine lumbar spine involvement. With this test, an imaginary perpendicular line is drawn from a mark placed midpoint between the postiliac spines to 10 cm above this point. The individual is then asked to bend forward; the distance between the two points is noted. The distance increases to 15 cm or more with flexion in normal persons. To determine lateral flexion, the top point of the midaxillary line serves as one reference point, and a point 20 cm below is a second reference point. An increase in distance between these two points to 25 cm to 30 cm is normal with contralateral flexion.

Chest expansion may be used as an indirect indicator of thoracic involvement, which usually occurs late in the disease. Measurements are taken at the fourth intercostal space. Normally the chest expands by 4 cm to 5 cm with inspiration. This measurement is more difficult to obtain in women. Expansion may also be measured at the xyphoid process.

The measurement of the occiput to the wall is determined by having the individual stand erect with the back against the wall and measuring the distance from the occiput to the wall. This is most appropriate to provide the parameters for monitoring late disease, to show loss of normal vertebral structure, and to expose hip flexion contractures.

Laboratory findings frequently include an elevated erythrocyte sedimentation rate. A mild normocytic normochromic anemia may also be present. HLA typing is not diagnostic of the disease and should not be used as a routine screening procedure.

Radiologic evaluations will help differentiate

sacroiliitis from other diseases. Symmetric sacroiliitis is usually identified when the first radiographically visible changes are noted; however, in early disease x-ray images may be normal. Vertebrae are normally concave on the anterior border. In ankylosing spondylitis the vertebrae take on a squared appearance. This is caused by erosion of the upper and lower margins of the vertebrae at the site of insertion of the anulus fibrosus. Syndesmophyte formation occurs as a result of the inflammatory process in the outer layers of the anulus fibrosus. Progressive ossification can occur. Spinal changes usually follow a progressive ascending pattern up the spine.

Treatment is directed at controlling pain and maintaining mobility by suppressing inflammation. Patient education is essential because regimens require that the individual patient take responsibility for self-care activities. This requires understanding of the disease process and course as well as the rationale for the modalities of treatment. Instruction should address proper posture and positioning. This includes sleeping in a supine position on a firm mattress using one small pillow or no pillow. Sleeping in extension may reduce the possibility of flexion contractures. A bed board may be used to supply additional firmness. Some persons find the most comfort by sleeping on the floor. Therapeutic exercises are important to assist in maintaining motion in peripheral joints and in the spine. Muscle-strengthening exercises for extensor muscle groups are also prescribed. Heat applications or a shower or bath may be beneficial before exercise to improve ease of movement. These strategies can also be used in the morning or at bedtime to reduce stiffness and pain. Immobilizing joints is not recommended.

The patient should maintain good general health: maintaining ideal weight, for example, reduces the stress on weight-bearing joints. Smoking should be discouraged because it can exacerbate respiratory problems. Swimming is an excellent general conditioning exercise that avoids joint stress and enhances muscle tone. Occupational counseling or job evaluation may be warranted because of postural abnormalities.

Aspirin or nonsteroidal anti-inflammatory medications are used to reduce inflammation, which in turn helps to control pain and reduce muscle spasm. Phenylbutazone is highly effective but its use should be limited to persons with severe disease in whom other agents have failed because of potential bone marrow suppression in long term usage.[10,11]

Most peripheral joint pain and limitations of motion occur in the hip. Total hip replacement surgery has contributed to pain reduction. Anesthesia can be problematic for persons with cervical rigidity or with reduced chest expansion. These factors need to be weighed before surgery is considered.

Other types of spondyloarthropathies

Reactive arthritis, including Reiter's syndrome, is a seronegative arthritis in which an infective trigger (sexually-transmitted or enteric infection) is suspected. The reactive arthropathies may be defined as a sterile inflammatory arthropathy distant in time and place from the initial inciting infective process. It can occur following *Shigella-, Salmonella-, Camperobacter-,* or *Yersina*-associated diarrhea or sexually-transmitted ureaplasma or chlamydial infections (the gonococcus produces direct infection of the joint and is not a cause of reactive arthritis). More recently, reactive arthritis has been observed in persons with acquired immunodeficiency syndrome (AIDS).[11] Urethritis is ordinarily the first feature of the disease; conjunctivitis and arthritis, typically of the lower extremities, usually follow. Not all individuals exhibit this triad of features; some individuals may have only one or two of them. In addition to urethritis, other mucocutaneous manifestations may be present, including mouth ulcerations, balanitis circinata, and skin rashes. Low back pain is common. Spinal radiologic changes are similar to ankylosing spondylitis but may be more asymptomatic. Reactive arthritis may follow a self-limited course; it may involve recurrent episodes of arthritis, or in a small number of cases it may follow a continuous unremitting course. The treatment is largely symptomatic. The NSAIDS are used in treating the arthritic symptoms. Although the disease is precipitated by an infection, at present there is no evidence that antibiotic therapy will alter the course of the disease.

Psoriatic arthritis is a seronegative inflammatory arthropathy that affects 5% to 7% of persons with cutaneous psoriasis. Psoriatic arthritis tends to be slowly progressive. Asymmetric oligoarthritis occurs most commonly. When fingers or toes are involved, there is diffuse swelling or *sausaging*. Often, affected joints are surprisingly functional and only minimally symptomatic.

Spondyloarthritis is also associated with inflammatory bowel diseases such as Crohn's disease and ulcerative colitis. When arthritis is present, it has usually developed before the bowel disease, especially in Crohn's disease. Sacroiliitis occurs in approximately 10% of persons with inflammatory bowel disease. In this form of arthritis, the activity of the bowel disease is not related to the activity of the arthritis.[12]

In summary, spondyloarthropathies affect the axial skeleton. Inflammation develops at sites where ligaments insert into bone. Ankylosing spondylitis is considered a prototype of this classification category. Bilateral sacroiliitis is the primary feature of ankylosing spondylitis. The disease spectrum ranges from asymptomatic sacroiliitis to a progressive disorder affecting many body systems. The etiology remains unknown; however, a strong association between HLA-B27 antigen and ankylosing spondylitis has been identified. Loss of motion in the spinal column is characteristic of the disease. Peripheral arthritis may occur in some persons. Other forms of spondyloarthritis include reactive arthritis and spondyloarthritis associated with inflammatory bowel disease.

Crystal-induced arthropathies

Crystal deposition within joints has been shown to produce arthritis. In gout, monosodium urate or uric acid crystals, are found in the joint cavity; and in another condition called pseudogout, calcium pyrophosphate dihydrate (CPPD) crystals are found in the joints.

Gout

The manifestations of the heterogenous group of diseases known as the gout syndrome include: (1) acute gouty arthritis with recurrent attacks of severe articular and periarticular inflammation; (2) tophi or the accumulation of crystalline deposits in articular surfaces, bones, soft tissue, and cartilage; (3) gouty nephropathy or renal impairment; and (4) uric acid kidney stones. Primary gout is predominantly a disease of men with peak incidence in the fourth or sixth decade. Only 3% to 7% of cases occur in women, and most of these are in postmenopausal women.[13]

Uric acid metabolism and elimination

Uric acid is a metabolite of the purines, adenine and guanine, that serve as the nitrogenous bases for the biosynthesis of nucleotides. The nucleotides of a cell undergo continuous turnover and therefore require a continuous supply of purine bases for their renewal. Xanthine, an intermediate in the formation of uric acid, is produced when the purine bases are degraded. The conversion of xanthine to uric acid takes place in the liver where the enzyme xanthine oxidase, which is needed for conversion, is present in the greatest quantity.

Normally about two-thirds of the uric acid produced each day is excreted through the kidneys; the rest is eliminated through the gastrointestinal tract. Normal renal handling of uric acid involves three steps: (1) filtration, (2) reabsorption, and (3) secretion. Uric acid is freely filtered across the glomerulus, is completely reabsorbed in the proximal

tubule, and then is secreted back into the tubular fluid by another mechanism for the transport of organic acids in the distal end of the proximal tubule or distal tubule. It is the tubular secretion and postsecretory reabsorption that determines the final concentration of uric acid in the urine.

Most persons with gout have a reduced urate clearance. In these persons the serum urate level becomes elevated so that a normal amount of urate can be excreted and urate homeostasis achieved. Most persons with increased production of urate will have increased excretion of uric acid. However, if kidney damage is present, an increased amount of uric acid will be eliminated by the gastrointestinal tract.

Small doses of uricosuric agents may preferentially reduce secretion and increase uric acid retention, whereas therapeutic doses block reabsorption and increase uric acid elimination. The salicylates reduce secretion and cause net retention of uric acid when given at doses used for pain relief; very large doses are needed to block both reabsorption and secretion. Consequently aspirin and other salicylates are not recommended for use as an analgesic in persons with gout. Some of the diuretics, including the thiazides, which are weak acids, are secreted by the proximal tubular cells and can also interfere with the excretion of uric acid.

Mechanisms of hyperuricemia

Hyperuricemia reflects a metabolic derangement in extracellular fluids. Asymptomatic hyperuricemia is a laboratory finding and not a disease. Hyperuricemia is defined as a serum urate concentration greater than 7.0 mg/dl measured by the specific uricase method.[14] Monosodium urate crystal deposition develops when hyperuricemia is present. However, most persons with hyperuricemia do not develop gout. Attacks of gout seem to be related to sudden increases or decreases in serum uric acid levels. Hyperuricemia may occur because of overproduction of uric acid, underexcretion of uric acid, or a combination of the two. Primary and secondary forms of hyperuricemia exist. Primary causes are related to genetic defects in purine metabolism. Secondary forms of hyperuricemia are related to certain disease conditions and medications.

An attack of gout occurs when the monosodium urate crystals precipitate within the joint and initiate an inflammatory response. This may follow a sudden rise in the serum urate levels. The excess urate is not soluble and therefore precipitates. Gout can also occur with a sudden drop in the urate level. In either situation, crystals are released into the synovial fluid and an inflammatory response is initiated.

Phagocytosis of urate crystals by the polymorphonuclear leukocytes occurs and leads to cell death and release of lysosomal enzymes. As this process continues, the inflammation causes destruction of the cartilage and subchondral bone. Tophi are large, hard nodules that have an irregular surface and contain crystalline deposits of monosodium urate that incite an inflammatory response. They are most commonly found in the synovium, olecranon bursa, Achilles tendon, subchondral bone, and extensor surface of the forearm and may be mistaken for rheumatoid nodules. Tophi usually do not appear until an average of 10 years or more after the first gout attack. This stage of gout, called chronic tophaceous gout, is characterized by more frequent and prolonged attacks, which are often polyarticular. Crystal deposition usually occurs in peripheral areas of the body such as the great toe and the pinnae of the ear. Sodium urate is less soluble at temperatures below 37°C.[15] The peripheral tissues are cooler than other parts of the body, and this may at least partially explain why gout occurs most frequently in peripheral joints.[15]

The typical acute attack of gout is monoarticular and usually affects the first metatarsophalangeal joint. The tarsal joints, insteps, ankles, heels, knees, wrists, fingers, and elbows may also be initial sites of involvement.[13] Acute gout often begins at night following more than usual exercise. The onset of pain is typically abrupt with redness and swelling. The attack may last for days or weeks. Pain may be severe enough to be aggravated even by the weight of a bed sheet covering the affected area. Attacks of gout may be precipitated by certain medications, foods, or alcohol. After the first attack, it may be months or years before another attack. The attacks usually become more frequent, and as they do, more joints become affected.

In the early stages of gout after the initial attack has subsided, the individual is asymptomatic, and joint abnormalities are not evident. This is referred to as intercritical gout. As attacks recur with increased frequency, joint changes occur and become permanent.

—— Diagnosis and treatment

A definitive diagnosis of gout can be made only when monosodium urate crystals are present in the synovial fluid or in tissue sections of tophaceous deposits. Synovial fluid analysis is useful in ruling out other conditions, such as septic arthritis, pseudogout, and rheumatoid arthritis. The presence of hyperuricemia cannot be equated with gout, because many persons with this condition never develop gout.

Those in whom gout has been diagnosed are usually evaluated to determine if the disorder is related to overproduction or to underexcretion of uric acid. Blood is drawn to determine the uric acid levels

and a 24-hour urine sample is collected. Ideally the person should be on a purine-free diet during the time the urine specimen is being collected, in which case the normal urate values range from 264 to 588 mg/day, as compared to values close to 1000 mg/day when there are no dietary restrictions of purines. Values above these levels indicate an overproduction of uric acid.[13] The normal serum urate concentration is 5.1 ± 1.0 mg/dl in men and 4.0 + 1.0 mg/dl in women.

The objectives in the treatment of gout are: (1) termination and prevention of the acute attacks of gouty arthritis and (2) correction of hyperuricemia, with consequent inhibition of further precipitation of sodium urate and absorption of urate crystal deposits already in the tissues. Management of acute disease is directed toward reducing joint inflammation. Hyperuricemia and related problems of tophi, joint destruction, and renal problems are treated after the acute inflammatory process has subsided. Treatment with colchicine is used early in the acute stage. Although the drug is usually given orally, a more rapid response is obtained when colchicine is given intravenously. The fact that the drug causes nausea and diarrhea when large doses are given orally is often a limiting factor in oral therapy. However, these side effects are essentially eliminated when the drug is given intravenously. The acute symptoms of gout usually subside within 48 hours after treatment with oral colchicine has been instituted and after 12 hours following intravenous administration of the drug.

Nonsteroidal anti-inflammatory medications are effective during the acute stage when used at their maximum dosage and are sometimes preferred to colchicine because they have fewer toxic side effects. Phenylbutazone is usually very effective but is usually only used on a short-term basis because long-term use can cause bone marrow suppression. The corticosteroid drugs are not recommended for treatment of gout unless all other medications have proved unsuccessful. Intra-articular injections of corticosteroid agents may be used when only one joint is involved and the individual is unable to take colchicine or nonsteroidal drugs.

With the exception of phenylbutazone, the drugs used to treat acute gout have no effect on the serum urate level and thus are valueless in tophaceous gout and the control of hyperuricemia.[16] After the acute attack has been relieved, the hyperuricemia is treated. One method is to reduce hyperuricemia through the use of allopurinol or a uricosuric agent. These compounds are not used in the treatment of acute gouty arthritis, and if given, will only tend to exacerbate and prolong the inflammation.[16] These uricosuric medications prevent the tubular reabsorption of urate. The serum urate concentrations are monitored to determine efficacy and dosage. Urico-suric agents include probenecid or sulfinpyrazone, a phenylbutazone derivative. These drugs are usually started in small doses and gradually increased over 7 to 10 days. Aspirin should not be used with these medications because it decreases the urinary excretion of uric acid.

Hyperuricemia can also be treated with allo-purinol, which inhibits the production of uric acid. Allopurinol inhibits xanthine oxidase, an enzyme needed for the conversion of hypoxanthine to xan-thine and xanthine to uric acid. There is a slight possibility that xanthine kidney stones can develop if allopurinol is used for many years. It is usually re-served for the individual who does not have an ade-quate response or is unable to tolerate other forms of treatment.

Treatment of hyperuricemia is aimed at maintaining normal uric acid levels and requires life-long treatment. Prophylactic colchicine or nonsteroi-dal anti-inflammatory drugs may be used between gout attacks. If the uric acid level is normal and the person has not had recurrent attacks of gout, these medications may be discontinued.

Gout can be effectively controlled by medical management; however, it often is not, because many persons with gout have a limited understanding of the disease and therefore a low compliance with treat-ment.[17] Education about the disease and its manage-ment is fundamental to the treatment and manage-ment of gout. The sufferer should be made aware that the prognosis is very good and that the disease, al-though chronic, can be controlled in almost all cases. Some changes in life-style may be needed, such as maintenance of ideal weight, moderation in alcohol consumption, and avoidance of purine-rich foods. Ad-equate fluid intake of at least 2 liters per day may help to prevent the development of uric acid renal calculi (see Chapter 31). Adherence to the lifelong use of medications may be the only major life-style change for many persons.

Calcium crystal deposition disease

Calcium pyrophosphate dihydrate crystal de-position disease (CPPD), or pseudogout, is an acute, inflammatory arthritis caused by the deposition of cal-cium pyrophosphate dihydrate crystals within the joint. The inflammation can occur in one or several joints and lasts for several days. Because degenerative changes and inflammation are present, the disorder can mimic other forms of arthritis, leading to difficulty in establishing a diagnosis. Chondrocalcinosis is used to describe the radiologic appearance of calcified joint cartilage. The diagnosis is confirmed by x-ray studies,

synovial fluid analysis, or biopsy. The knee and wrist are the joints most commonly involved. As in gout, the individual with pseudogout may be asymptomatic be-tween attacks.

Pseudogout is four times more common in men than women. There may be an inherited ten-dency toward the disorder. It is commonly seen in metabolic disorders such as hyperparathyroidism. Nonsteroidal anti-inflammatory drugs are used to re-duce inflammation. Colchicine may be used to treat an acute attack. Unlike gout, there are no drugs that can remove the CPPD crystals from the joints. The degenerative changes associated with pseudogout are treated by supportive measures similar to those used in the treatment of osteoarthritis.

Other calcium phosphates, including hy-droxyapatite, and calcium oxalate cause extraskeletal calcific deposits. Articular and periarticular calcifica-tions are often of no consequence. However, crystal shedding can result in acute inflammation, and the crystals have been associated with osteoarthritis and destructive arthropathies. Calcium oxalates have been identified in connective tissue disease and may be a factor in some renal-dialysis arthropathies.[3]

In summary, crystal-induced arthropathies are characterized by crystal deposition within the joint. Gout is the prototype of this group. Acute at-tacks of arthritis occur with gout and are characterized by the presence of monosodium urate crystals in the joint. The disorder is accompanied by hyperuricemia, which results either from overproduction of uric acid or from the reduced ability of the kidney to rid the body of excess uric acid. Management of acute disease is first directed toward the reduction of joint inflam-mation; then the hyperuricemia is treated. Hyperuri-cemia is treated with uricosuric agents, which prevent the tubular reabsorption of urate, or with medication that inhibits the production of uric acid. Although gout is chronic, in most cases it can be controlled.

References

1. Meenan RF, Liang MH, Hadler NM, and the Disability Task Force of the Arthritis Foundation: Social security disability and the arthritis patient. Bull Rheumatic Dis 33, No 1, 1983
2. Harris ED. Rheumatoid arthritis: The clinical spectrum. In Kelley WN, Harris ED, Ruddy S et al (eds): Textbook of Rheumatology, 1st ed vol 1, p 930. Philadelphia, WB Saunders, 1981.
3. Schumacher HR (ed): Primer on the Rheumatic Dis-eases, 9th ed. Atlanta, GA, Arthritis Foundation, 1988
4. Carson DA: Rheumatoid factor. In Kelley WN, Harris ED, Ruddy S et al (eds): Textbook of Rheumatology, vol 1, 2nd ed, p 667. Philadelphia, WB Saunders, 1985

Environmental Chemistry

WHEN ASTRONOMERS SPECULATE about life elsewhere in the universe, they look for the possibility of planets within a size and temperature range that allows for liquid water and a gaseous atmosphere. Most of the other worlds in our solar system do not meet this criterion. Instead, they are either barren and airless, like Earth's moon and Mercury, or else have crushing atmospheres—as do Jupiter, Saturn, Uranus, and Neptune—exerting pressures thousands of times greater than the atmospheric pressure on Earth.

Life is intimately dependent on water because only water has the unique properties required to sustain life. The presence of large amounts of liquid water makes our planet unusual in the solar system: It is probably the only one capable of supporting higher forms of life. Scientists who look for life elsewhere in our solar system place their scant hope on the presence of water beneath the dry surface of Mars or the existence of liquid water beneath the frozen seas of Jupiter's moon Europa. If we should someday discover higher forms of life on distant planets of other suns, it will likely be on another watery planet similar to our own.

In this chapter, we look at the composition and properties of Earth's atmosphere and water supplies and at some of the ways in which human activities affect our air and water. Mostly, though, we focus on how knowledge of chemistry can illuminate environmental issues and how chemistry can often be used to alleviate environmental problems. Proper use of scientific knowledge is essential to protecting the only planet that we know to be hospitable to life.

Earth's Atmosphere

Let us look first at Earth's atmosphere. Is the air we breathe unique? A look at other worlds in our solar system gives us a clue. Astronauts have walked on the dry, dusty, airless surface of the moon. Scientists have sent robotic probes down through clouds of sulfuric acid and a thick blanket of carbon dioxide to land on the hot, inhospitable surface of Venus. Other space probes have descended through the sparse atmosphere

CONTENTS

◀ We inhabit the solid surface of planet Earth, but it is the liquid water on its surface and the gaseous atmosphere that makes it hospitable to higher forms of life. In this chapter, we examine Earth's atmosphere and waters and some of the effects of human activities on our environment. In doing so, we apply some of the chemistry we learned in preceding chapters. A knowledge of chemistry is essential to understanding environmental problems and to their solution.

of Mars and used a robot to analyze its rocks. Still other spacecraft have examined the crushing, turbulent, toxic atmospheres of Jupiter, Saturn, Uranus, and Neptune. We do not know much about the atmosphere of distant Pluto because it has not been examined except from vast distances.

Of all the worlds in the solar system, Earth's atmosphere is unique in its ability to support human life. In the sections that follow, we consider first the normal composition of the atmosphere and then some substances introduced into the atmosphere by human activities.

25.1 Atmospheric Composition, Structure, and Natural Cycles

Without food, we can live about a month; without water, a few days; but without air, we would die within minutes. Air is vital because it contains free oxygen (O_2), an element essential to the basic processes of respiration and metabolism. However, life as we know it could not exist in an atmosphere of pure oxygen, because oxidation processes would be greatly accelerated by the increased concentration of O_2. The oxygen in air is diluted with nitrogen, thus lessening the tendency for everything in contact with air to become oxidized. Carbon dioxide and water vapor are but minor components in air, and yet they are the primary raw materials of the plant kingdom; and plants produce the food on which we and all other animal life depend. Even ozone, a gas present only in trace quantities, plays vital roles in shielding Earth's surface from harmful ultraviolet radiation and in maintaining a proper energy balance in the atmosphere.

On a mole percent basis, dry air in the lower atmosphere consists of about 78% N_2, 21% O_2, and 1% Ar. Among the minor constituents of dry air, the most abundant is carbon dioxide. The concentration of CO_2 in air has increased from about 275 ppm in 1880 to 368 ppm in 2001. It continues to rise about 1.5 ppm per year and most likely will continue to rise as more and more fossil fuels (coal, oil, and natural gas) are burned. The composition of dry air is summarized in Table 25.1.

Altogether, the thin blanket of gases that makes up the atmosphere is spread over a surface area of 5.0×10^8 km² and has a mass of about 5.2×10^{15} metric tons (1 metric ton = 1000 kg). That is about 10 million metric tons of air over each square kilometer of surface, or 10 metric tons over each square meter, or about 1 metric ton (nearly the mass of one small automobile) over each square foot.

How deep is the atmosphere? It is hard to say because the atmosphere does not end abruptly. Instead, it gradually fades away with increasing distance from Earth's surface. At sea level, the density of air is about 1.3 g/L, but at an altitude of about 50 km, the density drops into the range of micrograms and even nanograms per liter.

Application Note

Even though the atmosphere has an extremely low density at high altitudes, there is still sufficient air present to cause significant drag on large objects. Between October 2000 and February 2001, atmospheric drag caused the International Space Station to drop from an altitude of 390 km to an altitude of 360 km. The drag will increase as more parts are added to the station.

Table 25.1 Composition of Dry Air (near sea level)	
Component	**Mole Percent**[a]
Nitrogen (N_2)	78.084
Oxygen (O_2)	20.946
Argon (Ar)	0.934
Carbon dioxide (CO_2)	0.0368
Neon (Ne)	0.001818
Helium (He)	0.000524
Methane (CH_4)	0.0002
Krypton (Kr)	0.000114
Hydrogen (H_2)	0.00005
Dinitrogen monoxide (N_2O)	0.00005
Xenon (Xe)	0.000009
	Plus traces of: ozone (O_3); sulfur dioxide (SO_2); nitrogen dioxide (NO_2); ammonia (NH_3); carbon monoxide (CO); iodine (I_2)

[a] The compositions of gaseous mixtures are often expressed in percent by volume. Volume percent and mole percent compositions have the same numeric values.

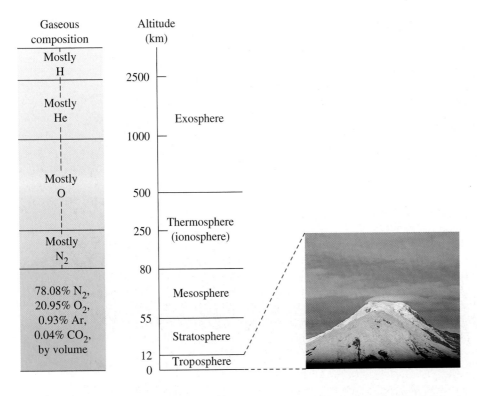

Atmospheric Layers activity

◀ **FIGURE 25.1   Layers of the atmosphere**

The altitudes of the several layers of the atmosphere are only approximate. For example, the height of the troposphere varies from about 8 km at the poles to 16 km at the equator. The approximate temperatures in these layers are cited in the text.

QUESTION: The troposphere, stratosphere, and mesosphere have the same percent composition by volume. How do these layers differ in absolute composition per unit volume?

However, 99% of the mass of the atmosphere lies within 30 km of Earth's surface—a thin layer of air indeed, akin to the peel of an apple, only relatively thinner.

Rather arbitrarily, we divide the atmosphere into the layers shown in Figure 25.1. The layer nearest Earth's surface, the *troposphere,* extends about 12 km above the surface and contains about 90% of the mass of the atmosphere. Weather and nearly all human activity occur in the troposphere. Temperatures generally decline as altitude increases in the troposphere, ranging from a maximum of about 320 K at Earth's surface to a minimum of about 220 K in the upper troposphere.

The next layer, the *stratosphere,* extends from about 12 km above Earth's surface to 55 km. The ozone layer that shields living creatures from deadly UV radiation lies in the stratosphere. Supersonic aircraft fly in the lower part of the stratosphere. Temperatures in the stratosphere are fairly constant at about 220 K from 12 to 25 km, then rise with increasing altitude to about 280 K at 50 km.

The layer above the stratosphere, ranging from about 55 to 80 km, is called the *mesosphere.* Here the temperature falls continuously to about 180 K as altitude increases.

The layer above the mesosphere is known as either the *thermosphere* or the *ionosphere.* In this region, molecules can absorb such highly energetic electromagnetic radiation from the Sun that they dissociate into atoms; some of the atoms are further broken down into positive and negative ions and free electrons. Temperatures in the thermosphere rise to about 1500 K as the altitude increases,* but high temperatures in this region do not have the same significance as on Earth's surface. The temperatures are high because the average kinetic energy of the gaseous particles is high. However, because there are relatively few of these particles per unit volume, little energy is transferred through collisions. A cold object brought into this region does not get hot, because there are far too few collisions to bring the object to temperature equilibrium with the gas molecules.

Water Vapor in the Atmosphere

Unless it has been specially dried, air invariably contains water vapor. Atmospheric water vapor plays one of the key roles in the **hydrologic (water) cycle**—the series of natural processes by which water is recycled through the environment (Figure 25.2).

Mt. Cayambe in Ecuador is almost on the equator, but its peak is snow-capped, illustrating the decrease in temperature with altitude in the troposphere. Mt. Cayambe's summit, at 5.79 km, is about halfway through the troposphere.

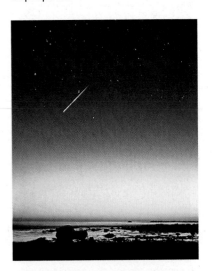

▲ This meteor seen against a starry sky at dusk is an extraterrestrial chunk of matter that has entered Earth's atmosphere. It emits light because it is heated to a high temperature. This heating occurs not from the high temperature in the thermosphere but through frictional resistance the object encounters as it passes through gases in the portion of the atmosphere that lies between about 80 to 100 km.

*The temperature in the thermosphere depends on the amount of solar radiation reaching this region. It varies with sunspot activity and is higher during the day than at night.

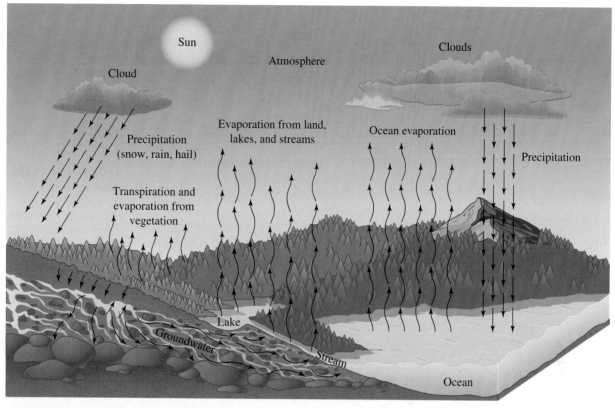

▲ **FIGURE 25.2** **The hydrologic (water) cycle**

The oceans on Earth are vast reservoirs of water. Water evaporates from the oceans, producing moist air masses that move over the land. When the moist air is cooled, the water vapor forms clouds and the clouds produce rain. Rainwater replenishes groundwater and forms lakes and streams, and this water eventually returns to the ocean. Water is also returned to the atmosphere by evaporation throughout the cycle.

 Hydrologic Cycle activity

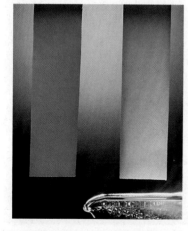

▲ **FIGURE 25.3** **An old-fashioned indicator of relative humidity**

The strips of filter paper were impregnated with an aqueous solution of cobalt(II) chloride and allowed to dry. Because it is in dry air, the strip on the left is blue, the color of anhydrous $CoCl_2$. In the more humid air above a beaker of water, a portion of the strip on the right is pink, the color of the hexahydrate, $CoCl_2 \cdot 6\,H_2O$. Test strips of this sort have been used in the past to signal large changes in the relative humidity of air.

The proportion of water vapor in air is quite variable, ranging from trace amounts to about 4% by volume. *Humidity* is a general term describing the water vapor content of air. The *absolute humidity* is the quantity of water vapor present in an air sample, usually expressed in g H_2O/m^3 air. The *relative humidity* of air is a measure of water vapor content as a percentage of the maximum possible; it compares the partial pressure of water vapor in an air sample to the maximum partial pressure possible at the given temperature—the vapor pressure of water:

$$\text{Relative humidity} = \frac{\text{partial pressure of water vapor}}{\text{vapor pressure of water}} \times 100\% \quad \textbf{(25.1)}$$

A number of experimental methods exist for determining the relative humidity of air. A crude but colorful method for estimating relative humidity is illustrated in Figure 25.3.

Example 25.1

The partial pressure of water vapor in a certain air sample at 20.0 °C is 12.8 mmHg. What is the relative humidity of this air?

STRATEGY

To determine the relative humidity using Equation (25.1), we need (1) the partial pressure of water vapor in the sample and (2) the vapor pressure of water at the given temperature. The first quantity is given (12.8 mmHg). For the second, we need the vapor pressure of water at 20.0 °C. We can find it in a tabulation such as Table 11.2.

SOLUTION

$$\text{Relative humidity} = \frac{12.8 \text{ mmHg}}{17.5 \text{ mmHg}} \times 100\% = 73.1\%$$

If an air sample at 20.0 °C has a relative humidity of 38.5%, what is the partial pressure of water vapor in this sample?

What mass of water vapor is contained in 10.0 L of air at 20.0 °C and 73.1% relative humidity?

If we warm the air sample described in Example 25.1, the relative humidity decreases because the vapor pressure of water increases sharply with temperature but the partial pressure of water vapor in the sample remains essentially unchanged. If we cool the air sample, we observe the opposite—the relative humidity increases. By consulting an extensive table of vapor-pressure data, we would find that the vapor pressure of water is 12.8 mmHg at 15.0 °C. When cooled to 15.0 °C, the air sample in Example 25.1 would be *saturated* with water vapor. At temperatures below 15.0 °C, the relative humidity would exceed 100%, and the air would be *supersaturated* with water vapor. This is an unstable situation that is not at equilibrium; it cannot persist. Some of the water vapor would condense as droplets of liquid water that we call *dew*.

The highest temperature at which condensation of water vapor from an air sample can occur is known as the *dew point*. When the dew point is below the freezing point of water (0 °C), the water condenses as *frost* without going through the liquid state.

The water vapor that condenses from air at the dew point is pure water. The liquid in Figure 25.4 also results from the condensation of atmospheric water vapor, but it is not pure water. Rather, it is a solution of calcium chloride, formed in this way: If the partial pressure of water vapor in the air exceeds the vapor pressure of a saturated solution of $CaCl_2 \cdot 6 H_2O$, water vapor condenses on the solid $CaCl_2 \cdot 6 H_2O$ and dissolves some of it, producing a saturated solution. This condensation of water vapor on a solid followed by solution formation is called **deliquescence;** it continues until all the solid has dissolved and the vapor pressure of the solution (now unsaturated) equals the partial pressure of water vapor in the air.

Nitrogen Fixation: The Nitrogen Cycle

Although it exists in large quantities in the atmosphere, nitrogen, an element essential to life, cannot be used directly by higher plants or animals. The N_2 molecules must first be converted to compounds that are more readily usable by living organisms. This conversion of atmospheric nitrogen into nitrogen compounds is called **nitrogen fixation**.

Certain bacteria, such as the cyanobacteria (blue-green algae) found in water and a variety of bacteria that live in root nodules of specific plants, are able to fix atmospheric nitrogen by converting it to ammonia. These nitrogen-fixing bacteria are concentrated in the roots of leguminous plants, such as clover, soybeans, and peas.

Other plants take up nitrogen atoms in the form of nitrate ions or ammonium ions from soil or water. Nitrogen atoms in plants combine with carbon compounds from photosynthesis to form amino acids, the building blocks of proteins. Thus the food chain for animals originates with plant life. The decay of plant and animal life returns nitrogen to the environment as nitrates and ammonia. Eventually the nitrogen in these compounds is returned to the atmosphere as N_2 when *denitrifying* bacteria act on the nitrates and ammonia.

Lightning also fixes some atmospheric nitrogen by creating a high-energy environment in which nitrogen and oxygen can combine. Nitrogen monoxide and nitrogen dioxide are formed in this way:

$$N_2(g) + O_2(g) \xrightarrow{\text{Lightning}} 2 NO(g)$$

$$2 NO(g) + O_2(g) \longrightarrow 2 NO_2(g)$$

The nitrogen dioxide then reacts with water to form nitric acid:

$$3 NO_2(g) + H_2O(l) \longrightarrow 2 HNO_3(aq) + NO(g)$$

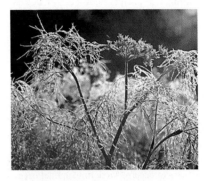

▲ Dill covered with morning dew. When the temperature drops to the point where the absolute humidity of the air is greater than the vapor pressure of water, water vapor condenses to the familiar liquid known as dew.

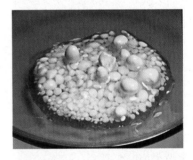

▲ **FIGURE 25.4** **Deliquescence of calcium chloride**

Water vapor from the air condenses onto the solid $CaCl_2 \cdot 6 H_2O$ and produces a solution of $CaCl_2(aq)$. Here the solution is saturated, but eventually all the solid will dissolve and the solution will become unsaturated. The deliquescence of $CaCl_2 \cdot 6 H_2O$ occurs only when the relative humidity exceeds 32%. Other water-soluble solids deliquesce under other conditions of relative humidity.

QUESTION: Why will calcium chloride not deliquesce if the relative humidity is less than 32%?

Alfalfa can fix 100 kg/acre or more of atmospheric nitrogen, the equivalent of almost 300 kg of ammonium nitrate fertilizer.

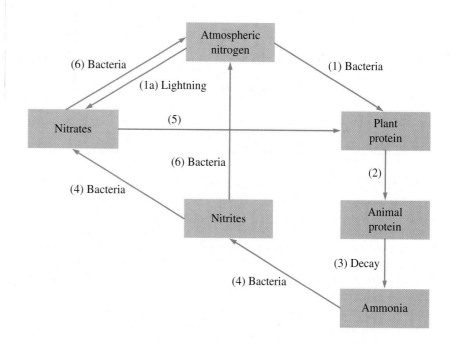

▶ **FIGURE 25.5** **The nitrogen cycle**
Bacteria fix atmospheric nitrogen by converting it to plant proteins (1). Nitrates are also converted to proteins by plants (5). Animals feed on plants and other animals (2). The decay of plant and animal proteins produces ammonia (3). Through a series of bacterial actions, ammonia is converted to nitrites and nitrates (4). Denitrifying bacteria decompose nitrites and nitrates, returning N_2O and N_2 to the atmosphere (6). Some atmospheric nitrogen is converted to nitrates during electrical storms (1a). A significant amount of nitrogen fixation and denitrification occurs in oceans. Modern manufacturing and agricultural processes also play important roles in the cycle.

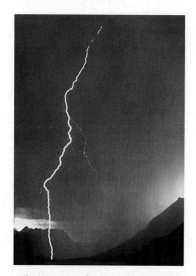

▲ The nitrogen fixation that occurs during electrical storms is an important part of the natural nitrogen cycle.

The nitric acid falls in rainwater, adding to the available nitrates in sea and soil. The net effect of all these natural activities is a constant recycling of nitrogen atoms in the environment in a **nitrogen cycle** (Figure 25.5).

Industrial fixation of nitrogen by the manufacture of inorganic nitrogen fertilizers has modified the nitrogen cycle. These fertilizers have greatly increased the world's food supply because the availability of fixed nitrogen is often the limiting factor in the production of food. Not all the consequences of this interference have been favorable, however. Excessive runoff of dissolved nitrogen fertilizers has led to serious water pollution in some areas, but modern methods of high-yield farming seem to demand synthetic fertilizers.

The Carbon Cycle

Carbon atoms are cycled throughout Earth's solid crust, oceans, and atmosphere by natural processes. In the process of photosynthesis, atmospheric CO_2 is converted to carbohydrates, the chief structural material of plants. For example, the photosynthesis of glucose, one of the simplest carbohydrates, occurs through dozens of sequential steps leading to the net change:

$$6 \, CO_2(g) + 6 \, H_2O(l) \longrightarrow C_6H_{12}O_6(s) + 6 \, O_2(g)$$

Animals acquire carbon compounds by consuming plants or other animals, and they return CO_2 to the atmosphere as a product of respiration. The decay of plant and animal matter also returns CO_2 to the air. Most photosynthesis occurs in the oceans, where algae and related plants convert CO_2 into organic compounds. Some of Earth's carbon is locked up in fossilized forms—in coal, petroleum, and natural gas produced eons ago from decaying organic matter and in limestone from the shells of decayed mollusks from ancient seas. Figure 25.6 shows a simplified **carbon cycle**.

Note in Figure 25.6 that human activities today play a key role in the carbon cycle by releasing carbon atoms as CO and CO_2 when we burn wood and fossil fuels.

25.2 Air Pollution

Human activities affect the atmosphere in many ways. In addition to the release of carbon dioxide into the atmosphere, the combustion of fossil fuels causes regional problems with high levels of carbon monoxide and particles of ash, dust, and soot, and with sulfur dioxide pollution and acid rain. Oxides of nitrogen, formed by high-temperature combustion in air, are involved in the production of photochemical smog. In general, we consider an **air pollutant** to be any substance that is found in air in greater abun-

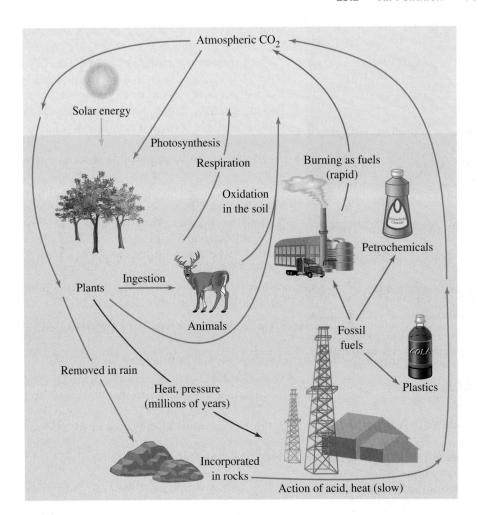

▲ **FIGURE 25.6   The carbon cycle**

The natural main cycle is indicated by blue arrows. Some carbon atoms are locked up by the formation of fossil fuels and limestone deposits, in what are called fossilization tributaries (red arrow). Disruption of the cycle by human activities is becoming increasingly important (purple arrows).

QUESTION: The carbon released when fossil fuels are burned is isotopically different from the carbon released when wood is burned. Why? (See Section 19.3.)

dance than normally occurs naturally and that has one or more harmful effects on human health or the environment.

Carbon Monoxide

It is estimated that, on a global basis, up to 80% of the carbon monoxide in the atmosphere comes from natural sources. Nature is able to prevent the buildup of CO in the atmosphere, however, because bacteria in soil convert it to CO_2. The other 20% comes from human activity, and this is the part that is the problem. Both carbon monoxide and carbon dioxide are formed in varying quantities when fossil fuels are burned. For instance, the combustion of methane, the major component of natural gas, yields both gases:

$$CH_4(g) + \tfrac{3}{2}O_2(g) \longrightarrow CO(g) + 2\,H_2O(l)$$

$$CH_4(g) + 2\,O_2(g) \longrightarrow CO_2(g) + 2\,H_2O(l)$$

With an excess of O_2, as is the case when air is readily available, the combustion products are almost exclusively $CO_2(g)$ and $H_2O(l)$. If the quantity of air is more limited, as in a dust- or dirt-clogged heater, $CO(g)$ is also formed.

The chief source of $CO(g)$ in polluted air is the incomplete combustion of hydrocarbons in automobile engines. Thus carbon monoxide is a local pollution problem,

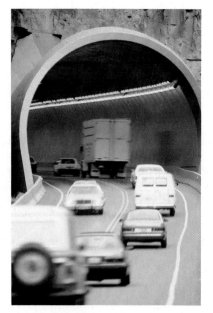

▲ Crowded parking garages and tunnels can have dangerously high levels of carbon monoxide gas.

Application Note

The Clean Air Act of 1990 instituted maximum limits for emission of CO and of other pollutants from new automobiles. In addition, to reduce local pollution, many large and moderate-sized cities now require periodic testing of emissions from individual automobiles. Some areas also mandate the use of oxygenated fuels to reduce carbon monoxide emissions.

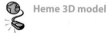 Heme 3D model

▶ **FIGURE 25.7   A molecular view of carbon monoxide poisoning**

The hemoglobin molecule consists of thousands of atoms, but key portions of the molecule are four heme groups, one of which is shown here. Each heme has an iron atom (shown in rust color here) in the center of a square formed by four nitrogen atoms (blue). The heme group is able to bind one small molecule to the iron atom. Ordinarily, it binds an O_2 molecule, but the heme group has a much higher affinity for CO (shown here pointing up from the iron atom) than for O_2. As a result, even when the CO(g) concentration is low, O_2 molecules are easily displaced by CO.

with the greatest threat being in urban areas with heavy vehicular traffic. Millions of tons of this invisible but deadly gas are poured into the atmosphere each year, about 75% of it from automobile exhausts. The U.S. government has set danger levels at 9 ppm CO averaged over an 8-hour period and 35 ppm averaged over a 1-hour period. Even in off-street urban areas, levels often reach 8 ppm or more. On streets and in parking garages, danger levels are exceeded much of the time. Such levels do not cause immediate death, but exposure over a long period can cause physical and mental impairment.

Because CO is an invisible, odorless, tasteless gas, we cannot tell when it is around without using test reagents or instruments. Drowsiness is usually the only symptom of carbon monoxide poisoning, and drowsiness is not always unpleasant. How many auto accidents are caused by drowsiness or sleep induced by CO(g) escaping into the car from a faulty exhaust system? No one knows for sure.

Carbon monoxide exerts its insidious effect by replacing O_2 molecules normally bonded to Fe atoms in hemoglobin in blood. We represented the heme units and polypeptide chains in hemoglobin in Figure 22.9. The form of hemoglobin carrying carbon monoxide is shown in Figure 25.7. In the reversible uptake of O_2 and CO by hemoglobin (Hb) to form HbO_2 and HbCO,

$$(1) \qquad Hb + O_2 \rightleftharpoons HbO_2$$
$$(2) \qquad Hb + CO \rightleftharpoons HbCO$$

The CO is highly effective in displacing O_2 from HbO_2 because reaction (2) proceeds much farther toward product than does reaction (1).

The symptoms of carbon monoxide poisoning are those of oxygen deprivation. All except the most severe cases of the poisoning are reversible, though the process may be very slow. The best antidote is the administration of pure oxygen. At high concentrations, the O_2 can cause the reaction

$$HbCO + O_2 \rightleftharpoons HbO_2 + CO$$

to proceed farther toward products. Artificial respiration may help if pure oxygen is not available.

Chronic exposure to CO, even to low levels, as through cigarette smoking, puts an added strain on the heart and increases the chances of a heart attack. Carbon monoxide impairs the blood's ability to transport oxygen, and consequently the heart has to work harder to supply oxygen to tissues.

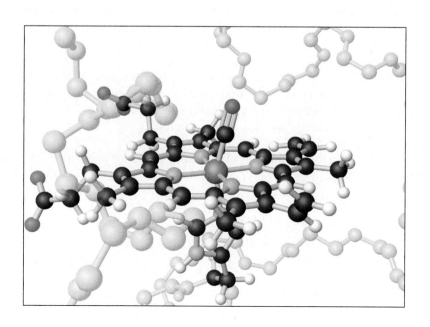

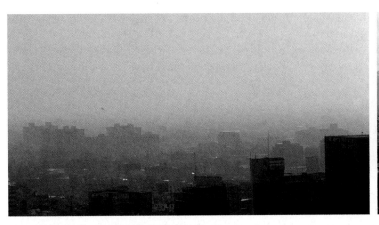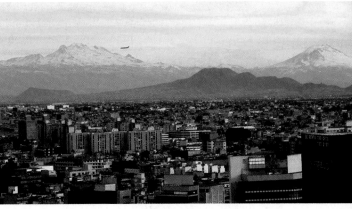

▲ **FIGURE 25.8   Photochemical smog**
(Left) Mexico City on January 9, 1996, when air pollution approached levels classified as "dangerous". (Right) A photograph taken one week earlier, from the same location, on a rare clear day.

Photochemical Smog

We usually think of sunlight as something pleasant. However, when sunlight falls on air containing a mixure of nitrogen oxides, hydrocarbons, and other substances, the light produces a mixture of pollutants called **photochemical smog** (Figure 25.8).

Photochemical smog production starts with the formation of nitrogen monoxide (NO). The reaction between $N_2(g)$ and $O_2(g)$ at ordinary temperatures is obviously extremely slow because these gases coexist in the atmosphere. However, at high temperatures, such as those attained by the combustion of a fuel in air, some NO is formed:

$$N_2(g) + O_2(g) \longrightarrow 2\,NO(g)$$

This reaction takes place in power plants that burn fossil fuels and in incinerators. The greatest source of NO, though, is in the exhaust fumes of automobile engines.

In sufficiently high concentrations, NO can react with hemoglobin in blood and rob it of its oxygen-carrying ability, just as CO does. However, such NO concentrations are rarely reached in polluted air. The main role of NO as an air pollutant is its participation in various reactions that yield several other pollutants.

Nitrogen dioxide, the gas that gives the amber color often seen in polluted air in major urban centers, is formed by the oxidation of NO. Nitrogen dioxide is an irritant to the eyes and respiratory system. Tests with laboratory animals indicate that chronic exposure to levels of NO_2 in the range of 10–25 ppm might lead to emphysema or other degenerative lung diseases. However, as with NO, we are concerned not so much with the direct effects of NO_2 but with its chemical reactions.

In the presence of sunlight, represented here as $h\nu$,* NO_2 decomposes:

$$NO_2(g) + h\nu \longrightarrow NO(g) + O(g)$$

Oxygen *atoms* produced by the photochemical (light-induced) decomposition of NO_2 are highly reactive. They react with many substances that are generally available in polluted air. For example, they react with O_2 molecules to form ozone (O_3):

$$O(g) + O_2(g) \longrightarrow O_3(g)$$

This reaction leads to an ozone concentration in photochemical smog that is considerably higher than normal. Ozone is the main cause of the breathing difficulties some

---

*The expression $h\nu$ is derived from the equation for the energy of a photon of light, $E = h\nu$ (Chapter 7). Here it represents a photon of sunlight. One photon of the proper energy can split one molecule of $NO_2(g)$ into a molecule of NO(g) and an oxygen atom, represented as O(g).

people experience during smog episodes. Another effect of ozone is that it causes rubber to crack and deteriorate.

In addition to ozone, nitrogen oxides, and hydrocarbons, photochemical smog contains *peroxyacetyl nitrate* (PAN), an organic compound formed by the combination of two free radicals:

$$CH_3\overset{\overset{\displaystyle O}{\|}}{C}{-}O{-}O\cdot \ + \ \cdot NO_2 \ \longrightarrow \ CH_3\overset{\overset{\displaystyle O}{\|}}{C}{-}O{-}ONO_2$$

(Recall from Chapter 9 that NO_2 is an odd-electron molecule; it has an unpaired electron and is therefore a free radical.) PAN is a powerful *lachrymator;* it makes the eyes form tears.

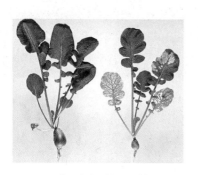

▲ A normal radish plant (left) and one damaged by air pollution (right).

In addition to their role in smog formation, NO and NO_2 (collectively called NO_x) contribute to the fading and discoloration of fabrics. By forming nitric acid, they contribute to the acidity of rainwater, which accelerates the corrosion of metals and building materials. They also produce crop damage, although specific effects of these gases are difficult to separate from those of other pollutants.

The reactions that form photochemical smog are exceedingly complex and are still not completely understood. We will point out only a few of the more important features of this reaction chemistry.

We have already noted two reactions: the photochemical decomposition of NO_2 and the production of ozone. If ozone formation is to continue, there must be a continuous source of NO_2. In Section 25.1, we noted one reaction for the formation of NO_2:

$$2\ NO(g) + O_2(g) \longrightarrow 2\ NO_2(g)$$

However, at the low concentrations of NO in a smoggy atmosphere and at normal air temperatures, this reaction is too slow to produce much NO_2. Instead, the NO appears to be converted to NO_2 in another—much faster—reaction that involves hydrocarbons, which come mostly from automotive exhaust. The process begins with a hydrocarbon molecule, RH, reacting with an oxygen atom to produce the free radicals R· and ·OH, followed by the ·OH radical's reaction with another hydrocarbon molecule:

$$RH + O \longrightarrow R\cdot + \cdot OH$$

$$RH + \cdot OH \longrightarrow R\cdot + H_2O$$

The hydrocarbon radicals, R·, can react with O_2 to produce new radicals called *peroxyl* radicals:

$$R\cdot + O_2 \longrightarrow RO_2\cdot$$

Then the peroxyl radicals can react with NO to form NO_2:

$$RO_2\cdot + NO \longrightarrow RO\cdot + NO_2$$

Automotive exhaust is a major contributor to the production of photochemical smog, but geographic factors are also important. Smog is especially likely to occur in a region like the Los Angeles basin, which is surrounded by mountains. In the absence of strong winds in the basin, the only direction in which mixing and dilution of air pollutants can occur is vertically into the atmosphere. However, at times, the region may also experience a temperature inversion—a mass of warm air overlaying a mass of colder air. The warmer top layer acts like a lid on a reaction vessel, keeping pollutants from moving upward and thereby being diluted, but it does let sunlight through. The sunlight acts on the pollutants to form smog, which is then trapped in the cooler stagnant layer of air. The most severe smog episodes usually occur during strong temperature inversions.

Control of Photochemical Smog

Most measures to reduce levels of photochemical smog focus on automobiles, but potential sources of smog precursors range from power plants to lawn mowers to charcoal lighter fluid. In many parts of the world, automobiles are now equipped with cat-

alytic converters. The first function of these converters is to catalyze the oxidation of carbon monoxide and unburned hydrocarbons to CO_2 and H_2O. The catalyst is usually palladium (Pd) or platinum (Pt) or a mixture of the two. To remove NO from automotive exhaust by reducing it to N_2 requires a reduction catalyst, which is different from the Pt/Pd oxidation catalyst. Some automobiles therefore use a dual catalyst system. Using a fuel–air mixture that is very rich in fuel can also lower the NO content of automotive exhaust because burning such a mixture results in some unburned hydrocarbons and CO(g). The CO can then reduce some of the NO in the exhaust stream to N_2:

$$2\,CO(g) + 2\,NO(g) \longrightarrow 2\,CO_2(g) + N_2(g)$$

Excess unburned hydrocarbons and CO(g) are then oxidized to CO_2 and H_2O in the catalytic converter.

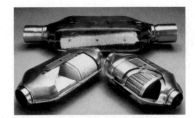

▲ A cutaway view of a dual-bed automobile catalytic converter.

Industrial Smog

Photochemical smog occurs mainly in warm, sunny weather and is characterized by high levels of hydrocarbons, nitrogen oxides, and ozone. The other major kind of smog is usually associated with industrial activities and is therefore called **industrial smog.** It occurs mainly in cool, damp weather and is usually characterized by high levels of sulfur oxides (SO_2 and SO_3, collectively called SO_x) and of particulate matter (dust, smoke, and so on).

A major source of SO_x in some areas is smelters, where sulfide ores are roasted as the first step in the production of copper, lead, and zinc. For example, the smelting of zinc ore to produce ZnO also yields SO_2:

$$2\,ZnS(s) + 3\,O_2(g) \longrightarrow 2\,ZnO(s) + 2\,SO_2(g)$$

Another source of SO_x is coal, especially soft coal from the eastern United States, which has a relatively high sulfur content. When this coal is burned, sulfur compounds in the coal also burn, forming SO_2. This choking, acrid gas is readily absorbed in the respiratory system. It is a powerful irritant and is known to aggravate the symptoms of people who suffer from asthma, bronchitis, emphysema, and other lung diseases.

Some of the sulfur dioxide reacts further with oxygen in air to form sulfur trioxide:

$$2\,SO_2(g) + O_2(g) \longrightarrow 2\,SO_3(g)$$

Sulfur trioxide then reacts with water to form sulfuric acid:

$$SO_3(g) + H_2O(l) \longrightarrow H_2SO_4(aq)$$

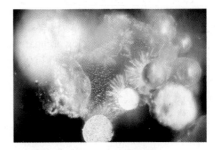

▲ This copper smelter emitted 900 tons of SO_2 daily before it ceased operation in January 1987.

Fine droplets of this acid form an aerosol mist that is even more irritating to the respiratory tract than sulfur dioxide.

Particulate matter consists of solid and liquid particles of greater than molecular size (Figure 25.9). The largest particles often are visible in air as dust and smoke. Smaller particles, 1 μm or less in diameter, are called *aerosols* and are often invisible to the naked eye.

Particulate matter consists in part of *soot* (unburned carbon). A larger portion is made up of the mineral matter that occurs in coal but does not burn. In the roaring fire of a huge boiler in a factory or power plant, some of this solid mineral matter is left behind as *bottom ash*. However, a lot of solid matter is carried aloft in the tremendous draft created by the fire. This *fly ash* settles over the surrounding area, covering everything with dust. It is also inhaled, contributing to respiratory problems.

Perhaps the most insidious form of particulate matter is the sulfates. Some of the sulfuric acid in smog reacts with ammonia to form solid ammonium sulfate:

$$2\,NH_3(g) + H_2SO_4(aq) \longrightarrow (NH_4)_2SO_4(s)$$

The solid ammonium sulfate and minute liquid droplets of sulfuric acid are trapped in the lungs, where they can cause considerable damage.

The harmful effects of sulfur dioxide and particulate matter may be magnified by their interaction. A certain level of sulfur dioxide, without the presence of particulate

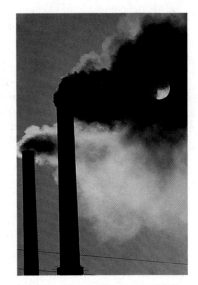

▲ FIGURE 25.9 **False-color scanning electron micrograph of fly ash from a coal-burning power plant**

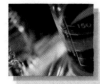

Natural Pollutants

Even before there were people, there was pollution. This pollution frequently came from erupting volcanoes, which spewed ash and poisonous gases into the atmosphere. And today, of course, they still do. Kilauea in Hawaii, for example, emits 200–300 tons of SO_2 per day. Acid rain downwind from this volcano has created a barren region called the Kau desert.

The 1991 eruption of Mt. Pinatubo in the Philippines injected such vast quantities of particulates into the stratosphere that the reflection of incoming solar radiation by these particles apparently produced a temporary reversal of the trend toward global warming. Earth's average surface temperature fell from 15.47 °C in 1990 to 15.13 °C in 1992.

Dust storms, especially in arid regions, can add massive amounts of particulate matter to the atmosphere. Smoke and dust from forest fires in Mexico and Central America drift across the United States and into Canada. Dust from the Sahara reaches the Caribbean area and South America. Swamps and marshes emit noxious gases such as hydrogen sulfide, a toxic gas with the odor of rotten eggs.

An important source of particulates in the atmosphere is the sea. Wave action causes seawater droplets to be suspended in the air, and when these droplets evaporate, salt particles are left behind in the air. Tropical thunderstorms carry chloride ions into the stratosphere, where they can be converted to chlorine atoms and perhaps contribute to the destruction of ozone. Thus, the greatest contributor to all the particulate matter in the atmosphere is ordinary salt from a perfectly natural source, reminding us yet again that nature is not always benign.

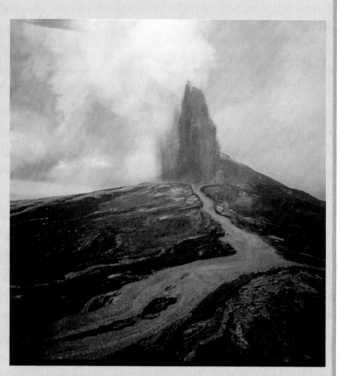

▲ An eruption at Kilauea volcano on the island of Hawaii.

According to the World Health Organization, Mexico City has the world's worst air pollution. Pollution levels are at least double those considered safe. One five-day episode in 1996 caused 400,000 pollution-related hospital and clinic contacts. The pollution originates from automobiles, industries, and propane used in home heating and cooking. The problem is compounded by location: Mexico City is in a valley surrounded by mountains.

matter, might be reasonably safe. A certain level of particulate matter, without sulfur dioxide around, might also be reasonably safe. Take these same levels of the two together, however, and the effect might be considerably exacerbated, aggravating respiratory problems such as bronchitis or triggering acute asthma attacks. *Synergistic effects* such as this are quite common whenever certain chemicals are brought together: The effect of the two together is much greater than the sum of their individual effects. For example, some forms of asbestos are carcinogenic, and about 35 or 40 of the chemicals in cigarette smoke are carcinogens. Asbestos workers who smoke develop cancer at a much greater rate than do people who are exposed to one of these carcinogens but not the other.

When inhaled deeply into the lungs, the pollutants in industrial smog break down the cells of the tiny air sacs, called alveoli, where oxygen and carbon dioxide exchange ordinarily occurs. The alveoli lose their resilience; as a result, it becomes difficult for them to expel carbon dioxide. Such lung damage contributes to pulmonary emphysema, a condition characterized by an increasing shortness of breath. Emphysema is one of the fastest-growing causes of death in the United States. Although the principal factor in the rise of emphysema is cigarette smoking, air pollution is also a factor.

Not only are the oxides of sulfur and the aerosol mists of sulfuric acid damaging to humans and other animals, they damage plants as well. Leaves become bleached and mottled when exposed to sulfur oxides. The yield and quality of farm crops can be severely affected. In addition, these compounds are also major contributors to acid rain.

Controlling Industrial Smog

Soot and fly ash can be removed from smokestack gases in several ways. One method, the use of electrostatic precipitators, is illustrated in Figure 25.10. The particles in the smokestack gases are given an electric charge, and the charged particles deposit on the oppositely charged collector plate. The energy requirement of this method is high. About 10% of the electricity produced in a power plant is required to operate the electrostatic precipitators. And the ash has to be put somewhere. Ash production in the United States is about 70 million metric tons per year. Some of the ash is used in making cement, and some is melted and formed into fibers called mineral wool, used for insulation. Most of the ash is simply stored on the ground or buried in landfills.

Emissions of SO_x can be reduced by removing sulfur-containing minerals before burning the coal. For example, FeS_2 (*pyrite*) can be concentrated and removed by flotation (Figure 24.1). Another way is to convert the coal to gaseous or liquid hydrocarbons by reaction with $H_2(g)$, leaving minerals such as pyrite behind. Both methods are expensive, however.

An alternative is to remove SO_2 from stack gases after the coal has been burned. In one method, powdered coal and limestone are burned together. The limestone decomposes to CaO and CO_2, and SO_2 reacts with the CaO:

$$CaCO_3(s) \longrightarrow CaO(s) + CO_2(g)$$
$$CaO(s) + SO_2(g) \longrightarrow CaSO_3(s)$$

Sulfur dioxide can also be reacted with hydrogen sulfide, producing elemental sulfur that is easily recovered:

$$2\,H_2S(g) + SO_2(g) \longrightarrow 3\,S(s) + 2\,H_2O(l)$$

Still another possibility is to convert sulfur dioxide to sulfuric acid. However, if all the SO_2 in smokestack gases were converted to sulfuric acid, the quantity produced would greatly exceed current demand. Then the sulfuric acid would present a disposal problem.

25.3 The Ozone Layer

The **ozone layer** is a band of the stratosphere about 20 km thick, centered at an altitude of about 25–30 km. This layer has a much higher ozone concentration than the rest of the atmosphere. Ozone absorbs harmful UV radiation, and the ozone layer thus protects life on Earth.

Ultraviolet radiation, invisible to human eyes, has profound effects on living matter. Proteins, nucleic acids, and other cell components are broken down by any UV radiation of wavelength shorter than about 290 nm. Wavelengths below 230 nm are filtered out by O_2 and other atmospheric components, but ozone alone absorbs in the wavelength range from 230 to 290 nm. In addition, radiation with wavelengths from 290 to 320 nm, called UV-B radiation, produces sunburn and can also cause eye damage and skin cancer; this radiation is only partially absorbed by ozone. Thus, the total amount of UV radiation reaching Earth's surface is critically dependent on the concentration of $O_3(g)$ in the ozone layer. Society therefore faces a challenge to maintain the appropriate concentration of ozone in the ozone layer.

When two opposing processes occur, one producing and the other consuming a substance, the result is a fairly constant concentration. Let us consider the processes that lead to a natural balanced concentration of about 8 ppm of ozone in the ozone layer. Ozone is produced in the upper atmosphere in a sequence of two reactions. First, an O_2 molecule absorbs UV radiation and dissociates into two O atoms:

$$O_2 + h\nu \longrightarrow O + O$$

Then atomic and molecular oxygen react to form ozone. The highly energetic O_3 thus formed would simply decompose back to O_2 and O except for the fact that some excess energy is dissipated when O_3 molecules collide with a third body, M, often a N_2 molecule. This dissipation of excess energy makes an accumulation of O_3 possible:

$$O_2 + O + (M) \longrightarrow O_3 + (M)$$

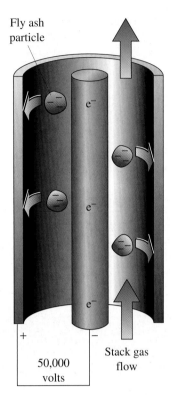

Fly ash particle

▲ **FIGURE 25.10 An electrostatic precipitator**
Electrons emitted from the negatively charged electrode in the center attach themselves to the particles of fly ash, giving them a negative charge. The negatively charged particles are attracted to the positively charged cylindrical collector plate and are deposited there.

 Statospheric Ozone animation

Catalytic Destruction of Stratospheric Ozone animation

CFCs and Stratospheric Ozone animation

Ozone is decomposed in a sequence of two reactions. First, an ozone molecule decomposes when it absorbs UV radiation:

$$O_3 + h\nu \longrightarrow O_2 + O$$

Then, an atom of oxygen reacts with another ozone molecule, forming two O_2 molecules and releasing heat to the environment:

$$O + O_3 \longrightarrow 2\,O_2 \qquad \Delta H = -391.9\;kJ$$

The heat released in this reaction accounts for the characteristic temperature increase with altitude in the stratosphere (page 1037).

Other naturally occurring species also contribute to the decomposition of ozone. Atmospheric NO, produced mainly from N_2O released by soil bacteria, decomposes ozone through this sequence of reactions:

$$
\begin{array}{rl}
(1) & \cancel{NO} + O_3 \longrightarrow \cancel{NO_2} + O_2 \\
(2) & \cancel{NO_2} + O \longrightarrow \cancel{NO} + O_2 \\
\hline
\textit{Overall reaction:} & O_3 + O \longrightarrow 2\,O_2
\end{array}
$$

Note that NO is consumed in the first reaction but regenerated in the second, which means that a little NO goes a long way. Moreover, we should expect that the injection of any additional NO into the stratosphere would increase the destruction of ozone and reduce its steady-state concentration. This additional NO can come, for example, from combustion processes in supersonic jets operating in the stratosphere. Perhaps the best evidence for the depletion of stratospheric ozone is that obtained from studies in Antarctica (Figure 25.11).

Of all human activities that affect the ozone layer, release of chlorofluorocarbons (CFCs) is thought to be the most significant. Because CFCs have a long lifetime in the atmosphere, some of the molecules eventually rise and appear in low concentrations in the stratosphere. There, they absorb UV radiation and decompose to produce atomic and molecular fragments (free radicals):

$$CCl_2F_2 + h\nu \longrightarrow \cdot CClF_2 + Cl\cdot$$

The ozone-destroying cycles set up beyond this point are quite complex, but a simplified representation is

$$
\begin{array}{rl}
(1) & \cancel{Cl\cdot} + O_3 \longrightarrow \cancel{ClO\cdot} + O_2 \\
(2) & \cancel{ClO\cdot} + O \longrightarrow \cancel{Cl\cdot} + O_2 \\
\hline
\textit{Overall reaction:} & O_3 + O \longrightarrow 2\,O_2
\end{array}
$$

The chlorine atom that reacts in step 1 is regenerated in step 2; one chlorine atom can therefore destroy thousands of ozone molecules. (As in polymerization, the reaction proceeds until ended by the combination of two radicals.)

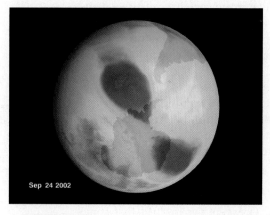 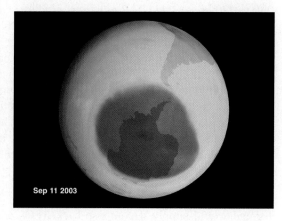

▲ **FIGURE 25.11**

The dark blue region indicates depletion of the ozone layer as measured by satellite on September 24, 2002 (left) and on September 11, 2003 (right). Notice the dramatic difference in area of the ozone hole.

QUESTION: What factors influence the size of the ozone hole over Antartica?

Currently, CFCs and other chlorine- or bromine-containing compounds that might diffuse into the stratosphere and contribute to ozone depletion are being replaced with more benign substances. Hydrofluorocarbons, such as CH_2FCH_3, have no Cl or Br to form radicals and are one kind of replacement. Another kind are hydrochlorofluoro-carbons (HCFCs), such as CH_3CCl_2F. These molecules break down more readily in the troposphere, and thus fewer ozone-destroying molecules reach the stratosphere.

25.4 Global Warming: Carbon Dioxide and the Greenhouse Effect

We all exhale carbon dioxide with every breath; it is a normal product of respiration. Consequently, we generally do not think of CO_2 as an air pollutant. Low levels of CO_2 are not toxic, and this gas is a minor component of Earth's atmosphere. However, CO_2 plays a role in determining Earth's climate. Small increases in the concentration of CO_2 could have a profound effect on the environment by producing a significant increase in the average global temperature, an effect called **global warming.**

When electromagnetic radiation from the Sun reaches Earth, some is reflected back into space, some is absorbed by substances in the atmosphere, and some reaches Earth's surface and is absorbed there. The surface then gets rid of some of this absorbed solar energy by emitting infrared radiation toward outer space. Certain atmospheric gases, principally $CO_2(g)$ and $H_2O(g)$, absorb some of this infrared radiation, and as a result, this radiant energy is retained in the atmosphere and warms it. The process, known as the **greenhouse effect** because it resembles the retention of heat in a greenhouse, is summarized in Figure 25.12. The greenhouse effect is natural, and it is crucial to maintaining the proper temperature for life on Earth. Without it, Earth would be an icehouse, permanently covered with snow and ice. Scientists are concerned, however, with the effects of continued increases in the concentrations of greenhouse-enhancing gases.

Increased levels of CO_2 and other greenhouse gases are readily measured. Computer models of the atmosphere indicate that a CO_2 buildup is likely to cause an increase in Earth's average temperature. There are still uncertainties because it is impossible to identify all the factors that should be included in computer models and to know how heavily to weight each factor. For example, warming of the atmosphere could lead to the increased evaporation of water and an accompanying increase in cloud cover. Because clouds reflect some incoming radiation back into space, this

Trees consume water vapor and carbon dioxide gas in the process of photosynthesis. The deforestation of tropical rain forests, as in "slash-and-burn" clearing for agriculture, is a contributing factor in the increase of atmospheric $CO_2(g)$ levels.

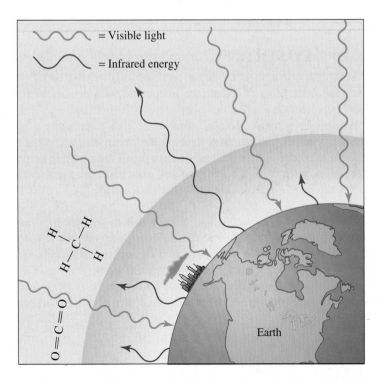

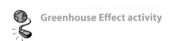 Greenhouse Effect activity

◀ **FIGURE 25.12   The greenhouse effect**

Electromagnetic radiation from the Sun, in the form of visible light, passes through the atmosphere and is absorbed by ground and ocean, warming Earth's surface. The warm surface then emits infrared radiation. Some of this infrared radiation is absorbed by CO_2, H_2O, and other gases and retained in the atmosphere as thermal energy.

QUESTION: By what mechanism do the greenhouse gases absorb infrared radiation? (See Section 23.12.)

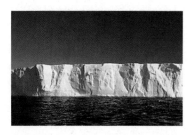

▲ The number of huge icebergs that break off the continental ice shelf in Antarctica may increase as a result of global warming.

Motion pictures such as *Deep Impact* and *Armageddon* feature a large comet or asteroid threatening Earth. In reality, if such a comet or asteroid landed in an ocean, it would blast vast quantities of water vapor into the atmosphere. Because water vapor is a powerful greenhouse gas, one result of such an impact could be severe global warming. Even before impact, the frictional heat generated by the object moving through Earth's atmosphere would cause nitrogen and oxygen in the atmosphere to form vast quantities of NO. The NO could lead to substantial destruction of the ozone layer.

could cause global cooling rather than global warming. However, the models are being steadily improved, and almost all predict warming.

In 2001, the United Nations–sponsored Intergovernmental Panel on Climate Change summarized the various forecasts, predicting a global temperature increase of from 1.4 to 5.8 °C by 2100. New evidence suggests that "most of the observed warming" in recent decades has come from gases released as a result of human activities. The panel of scientists predicted that rising temperatures could lead to drastic shifts in weather, with droughts striking farming areas. They expressed fears that melting glaciers could raise sea levels, flooding densely populated coastal areas of China, Egypt, Bangladesh, and other countries. These effects could be experienced as early as the middle of the twenty-first century.

Scientists are not limited to computer modeling to assess the likelihood of global warming. Direct experimental evidence also exists. For example, the ice in the Greenland and Antarctic icecaps is laid down in layers much like the annual growth rings of trees. Analyses of tiny air bubbles trapped in these layers show a strong correlation between atmospheric CO_2 content and estimated global temperatures over the past 160,000 years—lower CO_2 levels correlate with lower temperatures, and higher levels with higher temperatures. Thus it seems reasonable to expect that global temperatures will continue to rise as CO_2 levels increase.

Most atmospheric scientists think that global warming is already under way. Both the atmosphere and the oceans have warmed measurably in the last 50 years, and these changes have been firmly linked to human activities. A few scientists still question the reality of global warming, noting large swings in average temperatures over the years. The uncertainty arises from the fact that the measured increase in average temperature over the past 50 years has been only a few tenths of a degree Celsius, whereas annual variations in certain regions are often as much as 4 or 5 °C.

The main strategy for countering a possible global warming is to curtail the use of fossil fuels, but this may not be enough. For example, several gases—methane, ozone, nitrous oxide (N_2O), and CFCs—are even better absorbers of infrared radiation than is carbon dioxide. (The 1.3 billion cattle in the world alone produce about 20% of the atmospheric methane.) At an international meeting in Kyoto, Japan, in 1998, most of the world's industrial nations agreed to limit emissions of CO_2 over the next several decades. However, the agreement has not yet been implemented. The debate continues about the need for immediate action and how drastic our efforts should be. The debate may continue for years.

The Hydrosphere

Earth is a water world. Most of its surface is covered with oceans, seas, lakes, and streams—waters collectively called the *hydrosphere*. The human body is mostly water, too—about two-thirds by mass. The concentration of salts in the water in blood is similar to the concentration of salts in the water in the ocean. In fact, we are much like walking sacks of seawater. Although primitive life forms are found in some seemingly inhospitable places on Earth and could possibly exist elsewhere in the solar system, Earth alone has the large quantity of liquid water necessary for higher life forms as we know them.

Some of the properties of water that make it able to support life, however, also make it easy to pollute. Many chemical substances are soluble in water. In fact, much of the chemistry we have studied is that of aqueous solutions. Soluble substances are easily dispersed and eventually enter our water supplies. Once they are there, removing them is often quite difficult. A daily supply of clean drinking water is essential to life and good health because contaminated water can cause disease and, in some cases, death.

25.5 Earth's Natural Waters

We have noted the unusual properties of water in previous chapters. The following list provides a quick review of some of the properties and their consequences.

- Water commonly occurs as a liquid, the only prevalent naturally occurring liquid on Earth's surface.

- The solid form of water (ice) is less dense than the liquid form; therefore water expands when it freezes.

- Water has a higher density than most other familiar liquids; hydrocarbons and other organic compounds that are insoluble in water and less dense than water float on its surface.

- Water has a high heat capacity and a high heat of vaporization. Thus, a given quantity of heat produces a much greater temperature increase in a landmass than in a body of water covering the same area. Bodies of water tend to make daily and seasonal temperature variations more moderate along their shores.

Although three-fourths of Earth's surface is covered with water, nearly 98% is salty seawater, unfit for drinking and unsuitable for most industrial purposes. More than 1% of Earth's water is frozen in the polar icecaps, which leaves less than 1% available as fresh water. Fresh water falls on Earth in enormous amounts as rain and snow, but most of it falls into the sea or in areas that are otherwise inaccessible. Thus, available water is not always where the people are. Some areas with adequate rainfall are unsuitable for human habitation because of extremely cold climates or steep mountain slopes. Some areas have adequate *average* rainfall but have periods of drought and flooding. In some places with adequate freshwater supplies, the water is too polluted for many uses.

Natural waters such as rainwater and groundwater are not pure H_2O. Rainwater carries dust particles from the atmosphere and dissolves a little oxygen, nitrogen, and carbon dioxide as it falls through the atmosphere. During electrical storms, traces of nitric acid are found in rainwater as well. Groundwater dissolves minerals from rocks and soil as it moves along on or beneath Earth's surface. Groundwater also dissolves matter from decaying plants and animals. The principal cations in natural groundwater are Na^+, K^+, Ca^{2+}, Mg^{2+}, and sometimes Fe^{2+} or Fe^{3+}. The anions are usually SO_4^{2-}, HCO_3^-, and Cl^-. Table 25.2 provides a summary of substances found in natural waters.

Table 25.2 Some Substances Found in Natural Waters

Substance	Formula	Source
Carbon dioxide	CO_2	Atmosphere
Dust	—	Atmosphere
Nitrogen	N_2	Atmosphere
Oxygen	O_2	Atmosphere
Nitric acid (thunderstorms)	HNO_3	Atmosphere
Sand and soil particles	—	Soil and rock
Sodium ions	Na^+	Soil and rock
Potassium ions	K^+	Soil and rock
Calcium ions	Ca^{2+}	Limestone rock
Magnesium ions	Mg^{2+}	Dolomite rock
Iron(II) ions	Fe^{2+}	Soil and rock
Chloride ions	Cl^-	Soil and rock
Sulfate ions	SO_4^{2-}	Soil and rock
Bicarbonate ions	HCO_3^-	Soil and rock

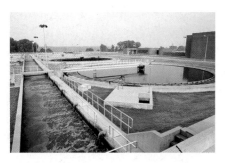

▲ Modern treatment procedures in the United States produce water that is clean and free of disease-causing organisms.

25.6   Water Pollution

Early people did little to pollute the water and the air, if only because their numbers were few. The Industrial Revolution and a concurrent large increase in population led to serious pollution of the environment. However, the pollution was mostly local and largely biological. Human wastes were dumped on the ground or into the nearest stream. Disease organisms were transmitted through food, water, and direct contact.

Contamination of water supplies by microorganisms from human wastes was a severe problem throughout the world until about 100 years ago. As population increased over the centuries, pollution became more and more of a problem. Then, starting in the 1830s, severe epidemics of cholera swept the Western world, and typhoid fever and dysentery were common decade after decade. In 1900, for example, there were more than 35,000 deaths from typhoid in the United States. It was at about this time that scientists began making the connection between disease and contaminated water. Today, as a result of chemical treatment, municipal water supplies in the more developed nations are generally safe. However, waterborne diseases are still quite common in much of Asia, Africa, and Latin America. Worldwide, an estimated 80% of all the world's sickness is caused by contaminated water. People with waterborne diseases fill half the world's hospital beds and die at a rate of 25,000 per day. Fewer than 10% of the people of the world have access to sufficient clean water, with the consequence that there are still epidemics of cholera, typhoid, and dysentery in many parts of the world.

How much water does one really need? Even though one person needs only about 1.5 L per day for drinking, the average U.S. resident uses about 7 L for drinking and cooking and overall consumes directly almost 400 L each day (Table 25.3). The combined residential, industrial, commercial, and agricultural use of water adds up to an average of 6900 L per person per day, and the rate of use is rapidly increasing. Much of this water is used indirectly in agriculture and industry to produce food and other materials. For example, it takes 800 L of water to produce 1 kg of vegetables and 13,000 L of water to produce a steak from beef cattle fed from irrigated croplands.

We also use water for recreation—for example, swimming, boating, and fishing. For most of these purposes, we need water that is free from bacteria, viruses, and parasitic organisms.

The threat of biological contamination has not been totally eliminated from developed nations. An estimated 30 million people in the United States are at risk because of bacterial contamination of drinking water, for example. Even in the most developed nations, hepatitis A, a viral disease spread through drinking water and contaminated food, at times threatens to reach epidemic proportions. Biological contamination also lessens the recreational value of water, leading to a ban of swimming in many areas.

Table 25.3 Average Daily Per-Person Use of Water in the United States	
Use	**Amount (L)**
Direct use	
Drinking and cooking	7
Flushing toilets	80
Supplying swimming pools and watering lawns	85
Dish washing	14
Bathing	70
Laundry	35
Miscellaneous	90
Total direct use	**381**
Indirect use	
Industrial	3800
Irrigation (agriculture)	2150
Municipal water (nonindustrial)	550
Total indirect use	**6500**
Total overall use	**6881**

Chemical Contamination: From Farm, Factory, and Home

In the past, factories often were built on the banks of streams, and wastes were dumped into the water to be carried away. Currently, fertilizers and pesticides used in agriculture and on lawns and recreational areas such as golf courses have found their way into the water system and have further contaminated it. Transportation of petroleum results in oil spills in oceans, estuaries, and rivers. Acids enter waterways from mines and factories and from acid precipitation. Household chemicals also contribute to water pollution when detergents, solvents, and other chemicals are dumped down drains.

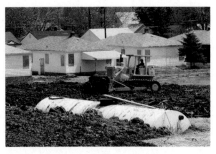

▲ Most of the homes in the Love Canal area near Niagara Falls, New York, have been abandoned because the ground on which they stand has been contaminated by industrial waste.

About half the people in the United States drink surface water (from streams and lakes). The other half get their drinking water from groundwater. Toxic chemicals from various sources have been found in both kinds of water supplies. For example, people living close to the Rocky Mountain Arsenal, near Denver, have found their wells contaminated by wastes from the production of pesticides. Wells near Minneapolis are contaminated with creosote, a chemical used as a wood preservative. Water wells in Wisconsin and on Long Island, New York, have been contaminated with aldicarb, a pesticide used on potato crops. Community water supplies in New Jersey have been shut down because of contamination with industrial wastes.

Chemicals buried in dumps—often years ago, before there was much awareness of environmental problems—have now infiltrated groundwater supplies. Often, as at the Love Canal site in Niagara Falls, New York, people built schools and houses on or near old dumpsites. Common contaminants are hydrocarbon solvents, such as benzene and toluene, and chlorinated hydrocarbons, such as carbon tetrachloride (CCl_4), chloroform ($CHCl_3$), and methylene chloride (CH_2Cl_2). Especially common is trichloroethylene (CCl_2CHCl), widely used as a dry-cleaning solvent and as a degreasing compound. These organic compounds dissolve in water only in trace quantities, often in the ppm or ppb range, and it is these tiny amounts that are found in groundwater. However, these chlorinated hydrocarbons are unwanted even in trace amounts, for most of them are suspected carcinogens. Unfortunately, the compounds are notably lacking in reactivity. They therefore decompose so slowly that they are likely to be around for a long time.

Another major source of groundwater contamination is leaking underground storage tanks. Gasoline at service stations has traditionally been stored in buried steel tanks. There are perhaps 2.5 million such tanks in the United States. The tanks last an average of about 15 years before they rust through and begin to leak. As many as 200,000 may now be leaking, many of them at stations that went out of business during the fuel shortages of the 1970s. In many areas of the country, gasoline is now found in water wells near these tanks. Laws now require replacement of old gasoline storage tanks and proper cleanup of any contaminated ground. Groundwater contamination is a serious long-term problem because, once contaminated, an underground aquifer may remain unusable for decades or longer. There is no easy way to remove the contaminants. Pumping out the water and purifying it could take years and cost billions of dollars.

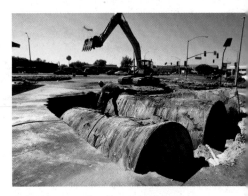

▲ Rusting gasoline storage tanks can leak gasoline and its additives into the environment. Methyl *tert*-butyl ether (MTBE) is one such additive that is now of environmental concern.

Although groundwater pollution can be a serious problem, it is often overdramatized by the media. The amounts of contaminants are often truly minute. For example, the U.S. Environmental Protection Agency (EPA) has set a safety limit of 10 ppb for aldicarb—that is 10 mg of aldicarb in 1000 L of water. You would have to drink 32,000 L of water to get as much aldicarb as there is aspirin in one tablet. Aldicarb is moderately toxic to mammals, but it breaks down rather quickly in the environment. Contamination of groundwater by toxic substances is serious, but biological contamination is much more widespread and often more deadly than chemical contamination.

Industries in the United States have eliminated a considerable proportion of the water pollution they once produced. Most industries are now in compliance with the Water Pollution Control Act, which requires that they use the best practicable technology. Let us consider a specific case in pollution control.

Waste chromium, in the form of chromate ions (CrO_4^{2-}), and cyanide ions (CN^-) are products of the chromium plating of steel. In the past, these toxic substances were often dumped into waterways. Nowadays, they may be removed to a large extent by

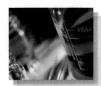

Ironing Out Pollutants

Contaminated groundwater from a leaking landfill often moves in a plume toward a nearby lake or stream. Is there an effective way to remove contaminants as the water moves through the ground? A relatively inexpensive and quite effective way of removing chlorinated compounds is to place a pit containing scrap-iron filings as a barrier in the path of the flow (Figure 25.13).

Recall that iron corrodes through a redox reaction in which dissolved oxygen is the oxidizing agent and iron is the reducing agent:

Oxidation half-reaction:

$$2\{Fe \longrightarrow Fe^{2+} + 2\,e^-\}$$

Reduction half-reaction:

$$O_2 + 4\,H^+ + 4\,e^- \longrightarrow 2\,H_2O$$

Overall reaction:

$$2\,Fe + O_2 + 4\,H^+ \longrightarrow 2\,Fe^{2+} + 2\,H_2O(l)$$

In a reaction with chlorinated compounds, Fe atoms give electrons to the chlorine atoms, converting them to chloride ions. In the reduction half-reaction, a chlorine-containing compound, designated RCl, is converted to a hydrocarbon, RH:

Reduction half-reaction: $RCl + H^+ + 2\,e^- \longrightarrow RH + Cl^-$

The overall reaction can be written

$$Fe + RCl + H^+ \longrightarrow Fe^{2+} + RH + Cl^-$$

The hydrocarbons formed are generally less toxic and more easily degraded by microorganisms than the chlorine-containing compounds.

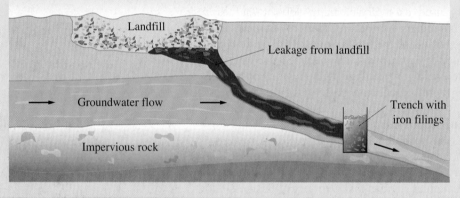

◀ **FIGURE 25.13   Using iron filings to remove chlorinated hydrocarbons from contaminated groundwater**

As contaminated groundwater from a leaking landfill moves toward a nearby lake or stream, it passes through a barrier of iron filings. The iron converts the chlorinated compound to a hydrocarbon plus chloride ions.

chemical treatment. Cyanide ions are removed by a reaction with chlorine in basic solution to form nitrogen gas, bicarbonate ions, and chloride ions:

$$10\,OH^-(aq) + 2\,CN^-(aq) + 5\,Cl_2(g) \longrightarrow N_2(g) + 2\,HCO_3^-(aq) + 10\,Cl^-(aq) + 4\,H_2O(l)$$

Bicarbonate and chloride ions are generally not considered toxic at the levels formed in this reaction.

Chromate ions are removed by reduction with sulfur dioxide, forming Cr^{3+} ion and sulfate ions:

$$2\,CrO_4^{2-}(aq) + 3\,SO_2(g) + 2\,H_2O(l) \longrightarrow 2\,Cr^{3+}(aq) + 3\,SO_4^{2-}(aq) + 4\,OH^-(aq)$$

The Cr^{3+} ions can be precipitated and removed as $Cr(OH)_3(s)$. However, proper control of the pH is essential because $Cr(OH)_3$ is amphoteric; it redissolves in a solution that is either too acidic or too basic. Sulfate ion is usually not a serious pollutant.

Many industries have contributed to water pollution. Wastes from the textile industries include conditioners, dyes, bleaches, oils, dirt, and other organic debris. Most of these can be removed by conventional sewage treatment. Wastes from meat-packing plants include blood and various animal parts. These and other food industry wastes are usually treated by sewage treatment plants.

Some Chemistry and Biology of Sewage

Dumping human sewage into waterways spreads *pathogenic* (disease-causing) microorganisms, but disease is not the only problem. The organic matter in sewage is decomposed by bacteria, and this process depletes dissolved oxygen [$O_2(aq)$] in the water and overfertilizes the water with plant nutrients. A flowing stream can handle a small amount of waste without difficulty, but large quantities of raw sewage cause undesirable changes.

Most organic material can be degraded (broken down) by microorganisms. This biodegradation can be either *aerobic* or *anaerobic*. **Aerobic oxidation** occurs in the presence of dissolved oxygen. The **biochemical oxygen demand (BOD)** measures the quantity of oxygen, in milligrams, needed for the aerobic oxidation of the organic compounds in 1 L of water. If the BOD is high enough, oxygen is depleted, and higher life forms, such as fish, can no longer survive in the water. However, rapidly flowing streams can regenerate themselves downstream as oxygen from the air enters the moving water and dissolves.

With adequate dissolved oxygen, aerobic bacteria (those that require oxygen) oxidize the organic matter to carbon dioxide, water, and a variety of inorganic ions (Table 25.4). The water is relatively clean, but the ions, particularly the nitrates and phosphates, may serve as nutrients for the growth of algae, which also cause problems. When the algae die, they become organic waste and increase the BOD through a process called **eutrophication.** Algal bloom and die-off are also stimulated by the runoff of fertilizers from farms and lawns and seepage from feedlots. This combination leads to dead and dying streams and lakes that nature cannot purify nearly as quickly as we can pollute them.

When the dissolved oxygen in a body of water is depleted by too much organic matter—whether from sewage, dying algae, or other sources—**anaerobic decay** processes take over. Instead of oxidizing the organic matter, anaerobic bacteria reduce it. Methane (CH_4) is formed. Sulfur is converted to hydrogen sulfide (H_2S) and other foul-smelling organic compounds. Nitrogen is reduced to ammonia and odorous amines. The foul odors indicate that the water is overloaded with organic wastes. No life, other than a few anaerobic organisms, can survive in such water.

Water Treatment: A Drop to Drink

Many cities use water that has been used by other cities upstream. Such water may be polluted with chemicals and pathogenic microorganisms. Making the water safe and palatable involves several steps of physical and chemical treatment (Figure 25.14). The water usually is placed in a settling basin, where it is treated with slaked lime [$Ca(OH)_2(aq)$] and a flocculating agent, such as aluminum sulfate. These materials react to form a gelatinous mass (called *flocs*) of aluminum hydroxide that carries down dirt particles and bacteria:

$$3\ Ca(OH)_2(aq)\ +\ Al_2(SO_4)_3(aq)\ \longrightarrow\ 2\ Al(OH)_3(s)\ +\ 3\ CaSO_4(s)$$

Slaked lime

The water is then filtered through sand and gravel.

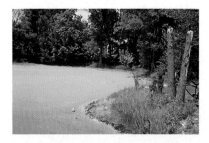

▲ An algal bloom leads to oxygen depletion in the water of this pond.

Table 25.4 Some Substances Added to Water by the Breakdown of Organic Matter

Substance	Formula
Aerobic conditions	
Carbon dioxide	CO_2
Nitrate ions	NO_3^-
Phosphate ions	PO_4^{3-}
Sulfate ions	SO_4^{2-}
Bicarbonate ions	HCO_3^-
Anaerobic conditions	
Methane	CH_4
Ammonia	NH_3
Amines	RNH_2
Hydrogen sulfide	H_2S
Methanethiol	CH_3SH

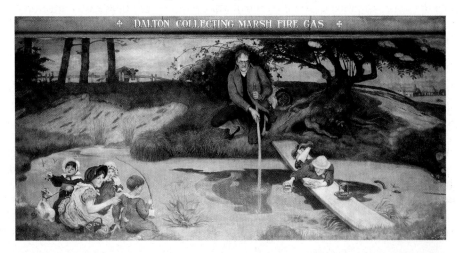

◀ Methane, sometimes called marsh gas, is formed by the anaerobic decay of organic matter. This painting, *Dalton Collecting Marsh Fire Gas,* shows John Dalton, developer of the atomic theory (Chapter 2). *Source:* Ford Madox Brown (1821–1893), "Dalton Collecting Marsh Fire Gas." © Manchester Art Gallery. Photo by John Ingram.

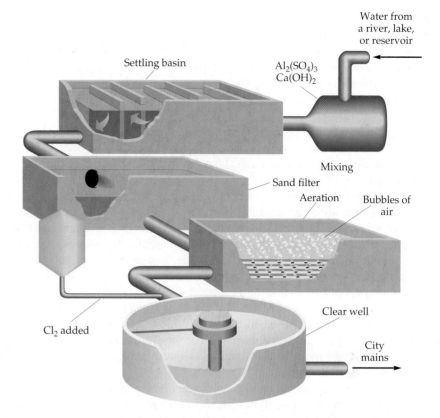

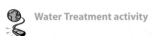
Water Treatment activity

▶ **FIGURE 25.14** **A diagram of a municipal water purification plant**

The next step is usually *aeration:* The water is sprayed into the air to remove odorous compounds and to improve its taste (water without dissolved air tastes flat). Sometimes the water is filtered through charcoal, which adsorbs colored and odorous compounds. In the final step, the water is *chlorinated:* Chlorine is added to kill any remaining bacteria. In some communities that use lake or river water, a lot of chlorine is needed to kill all the bacteria, and the residual chlorine imparts an unpleasant taste to the water.

Some pollutants are difficult to remove from water. For example, nitrates get in groundwater from fertilizers used on farms and lawns, from decomposition of organic wastes in sewage treatment, and from runoff from animal feedlots. Nitrate compounds are highly soluble, and only expensive treatment can remove them from water once they are there.

Many people drink bottled water to avoid real or perceived problems with public water supplies. Bottled water was largely unregulated until 1995, when the Food and Drug Administration set standards to ensure that its minimum quality was equal to that of public water supplies. Much bottled water comes from the same municipal supplies as tap water.

In addition to chlorination to kill bacteria, many communities add fluorides to drinking water to prevent dental caries (tooth decay). Tooth decay was once considered to be the leading chronic disease of childhood, but its incidence has decreased dramatically, thanks in part to fluoridation of drinking water. Only 29% of the nine-year-olds in the United States were cavity-free in 1971, but today more than two-thirds of that age group are cavity-free. Recall that tooth enamel is a complex calcium phosphate called hydroxyapatite (page 692). Fluoride ions replace some of the hydroxide ions, forming a harder mineral called fluorapatite:

$$Ca_5(PO_4)_3OH + F^- \longrightarrow Ca_5(PO_4)_3F + OH^-$$

Enough fluoride (usually as H_2SiF_6 or Na_2SiF_6) is added to the water to give concentrations of 0.7 to 1.1 ppm (by mass) of fluoride. Evidence indicates that such fluoridation results in a reduction in the incidence of dental caries by as much as two-thirds in some areas.

There is some concern about the cumulative effects of consuming fluorides in drinking water, in the diet, in toothpaste, and from other sources. Excessive fluoride

consumption during early childhood can cause mottling of the tooth enamel. The enamel becomes brittle in certain areas and gradually discolors. At concentrations higher than those found in drinking water, fluorides may interfere with calcium metabolism, with kidney action, with thyroid function, and with the actions of other glands and organs. In moderate to high concentrations, fluorides are acute poisons. Indeed, sodium fluoride is used as a poison for roaches and rats. However, there is little or no evidence that fluoridation at the levels now used causes any health problems.

Wastewater Treatment Plants

For many years, most communities simply held sewage in settling ponds for a while before discharging it into a stream, lake, or ocean. This constitutes what now is called **primary sewage treatment.** Primary treatment removes some of the solids as *sludge,* but the effluent still has a huge BOD. Often all the dissolved oxygen in the pond is used up, and anaerobic decomposition—with its resulting odors—takes over. Effluent from a primary treatment plant contains considerable dissolved and suspended organic matter. A **secondary sewage treatment** plant passes effluent from a settling tank through sand and gravel filters. There is some aeration in this step, and aerobic bacteria convert most of the organic matter to stable inorganic materials.

A combination of primary and secondary treatment methods, known as the **activated sludge method** (Figure 25.15), is frequently employed. The sewage is placed in tanks and aerated with large blowers. This causes the formation of large, porous flocs, which serve to filter and absorb contaminants. The aerobic bacteria further convert the organic material to sludge. A part of the sludge is recycled to keep the process going, but huge quantities must be removed for disposal. This sludge is stored on land (where it requires large areas), dumped at sea (where it pollutes the ocean), or burned in incinerators (where it requires energy—such as natural gas—and contributes to air pollution). Sometimes the sludge is processed for use as fertilizer.

In many areas, secondary treatment of wastewater is inadequate. **Advanced treatment,** sometimes called *tertiary treatment,* is increasingly required. Several advanced processes are now in use. One process that is becoming more important is charcoal filtration. Charcoal adsorbs organic molecules that are difficult to remove by other methods. There are federal mandates for more communities to treat their water with charcoal, but some cities have not yet complied because of the expense. Even more costly processes, such as reverse osmosis (page 513), may be needed in some cases. Table 25.5 provides a summary of wastewater treatment methods.

The effluent from sewage plants usually is treated with chlorine before being returned to a waterway. Chlorine is added in an attempt to kill any pathogenic microorganisms that might remain. Such treatment has been quite effective in preventing the spread of such waterborne infectious diseases as typhoid fever. Further, some chlorine remains in the water, providing residual protection against pathogenic bacteria. However, chlorination is not effective against viruses, such as those that cause hepatitis.

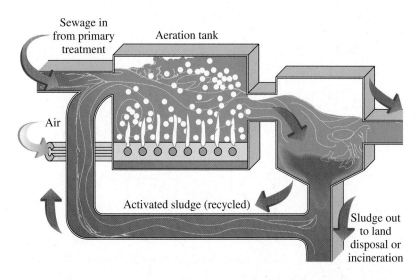

Sewage in from primary treatment

Aeration tank

Air

Activated sludge (recycled)

Sludge out to land disposal or incineration

◀ FIGURE 25.15   **A diagram of a secondary sewage treatment plant that uses the activated sludge method**

Table 25.5 Summary of Wastewater Treatment Methods

Method	Cost	Material Removed	Percent Removed
Primary			
Sedimentation	Low	Dissolved organics	25–40
		Suspended solids	40–70
Secondary			
Trickling filters	Moderate	Dissolved organics	80–95
		Suspended solids	70–92
Activated sludge	Moderate	Dissolved organics	85–95
		Suspended solids	85–95
Advanced (tertiary)			
Carbon bed with regeneration	Moderate	Dissolved organics	90–98
Ion exchange	High	Nitrates and phosphates	80–92
Chemical precipitation	Moderate	Phosphates	88–95
Filtration	Low	Suspended solids	50–90
Reverse osmosis	Very high	Dissolved solids	65–95
Electrodialysis	Very high	Dissolved solids	10–40
Distillation	Extremely high	Dissolved solids	90–98

25.7 Acid Rain and Acid Waters

We have seen how sulfur oxides are converted to sulfuric acid, and nitrogen oxides to nitric acid, in the atmosphere. These acids reach Earth as acid rain or acid snow, in the form of deposits from acid fog, or as adsorbents on particulate matter. When rainfall is more acidic than it would be if it contained just dissolved atmospheric $CO_2(g)$, it is called **acid rain.** Some rainfall has been reported that is even more acidic than vinegar or lemon juice.

Acid rain corrodes metals, limestone, and marble, and even ruins the finish on automobiles. It comes mainly from sulfur oxides emitted from power plants and smelters and from nitrogen oxides from automobiles. These acids may be carried for hundreds of kilometers before falling as rain or snow (Figure 25.16). (In addition to

Carbon Dioxide Behaves as an Acid in Water movie

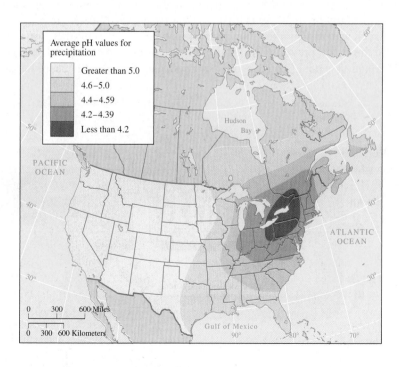

▶ **FIGURE 25.16   Acid rain**
Acids formed from sulfur oxides, mainly from coal-burning power plants, and nitrogen oxides from power plants and automobiles may fall in rain hundreds of kilometers from their sources. These acids cross oceans and international boundaries, causing political as well as environmental problems. This map shows that acid deposition is most severe over the northeastern United States and eastern Canada.

rainfall, another way surface waters are made acidic is from acids flowing into streams from abandoned mines.)

Acid Waters: Dead Lakes

Acid water is detrimental to life in lakes and streams. More than 1000 bodies of water in the eastern United States are acidified, and 11,000 others have only a limited ability to neutralize the acids that enter them. In the Canadian province of Ontario, 48,000 lakes are threatened, and more than 100 lakes in New York's Adirondack Mountains are so acidic that they are devoid of life. The acid rain falling on these areas is thought to originate mainly in the Ohio River Valley and Great Lakes regions.

Acid water has been linked to declining crop and forest yields, but its effects on living organisms are hard to pin down precisely. Probably the greatest effect of acidity is that it causes the release of toxic ions from rocks and soil. For example, aluminum ions, which are tightly bound in clays and other minerals, are released in acidic solution:

A clay   Sand

$$Al_2Si_2O_5(OH)_4(s) + 6\,H_3O^+(aq) \longrightarrow 2\,Al^{3+}(aq) + 2\,SiO_2(s) + 11\,H_2O(l)$$

Aluminum ions have low toxicity to humans, but they seem to be deadly to young fish. Many of the dying lakes have only mature fish; none of the young survive. Ironically, lakes destroyed by excess acidity are often quite beautiful. The water is clear and sparkling—quite a contrast to the water in lakes where fish are killed by oxygen depletion following algal blooms.

Acids are no threat to lakes and streams in areas where the rock is limestone, which can neutralize excess acid. Where rock is principally granite, however, no such neutralization occurs. Acidic waters can be neutralized by adding lime or pulverized limestone. A few such attempts have been carried out, but the process is costly and the results last only a few years. An obvious way to lessen the problem is to either remove the sulfur from coal before burning it or scrub the sulfur oxides from smokestack gases. Considerable progress has been made in this area, but these remedies are expensive, and they add to the cost of electricity.

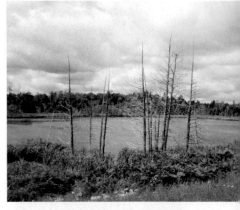

▲ The appearance of an acid lake can be quite deceiving. It can be quite beautiful, yet there is not a fish to be found in it. The lake is devoid of life. Acid rain has wiped out entire fish populations and other aquatic life in lakes that lack neutralizing limestone rocks in their watershed.

Toxic Substances in the Biosphere

In concluding this chemistry text, we briefly consider the most important "sphere" on Earth—the **biosphere,** that relatively thin film of air, water, and soil in which almost all life on Earth exists. Nearly all the processes in the biosphere are driven by energy from the Sun. About 23% of the solar energy that reaches Earth drives the water cycle. A tiny portion is absorbed by green plants, which use it to power photosynthesis, directly supplying the energy that sustains life. Let us now turn our attention to some toxic substances that sometimes seem to threaten living things.

One of the main concerns about certain pollutants is their toxicity. Toxic substances, often called poisons, have always been with us. Today our knowledge of poisons is greater than in times past, plus there are more of them than ever before. Industrial accidents, such as that at Bhopal, India, in 1984, which killed 2500 people and injured perhaps 100,000 others, have made the public acutely aware of problems with toxic substances. People are also concerned about long-term exposure to toxic substances in the air, in their drinking water, and in their food. Chemists can detect exceedingly tiny quantities of such substances. It is still quite difficult, however, to determine what effects these trace amounts of toxic materials have on human health. **Toxicology** is the study of the effects of poisons, their identification or detection, and the development and use of antidotes.

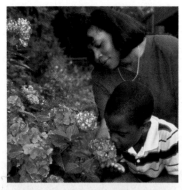

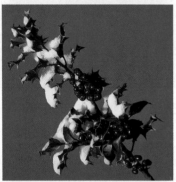

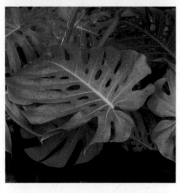

▲ Many common plants and plant parts are poisonous, including hydrangeas (top), holly berries (middle), and philodendron (bottom). Plants that produce toxic substances have evolved by the process of natural selection. The toxic substances serve as antifeedants that poison the animals that would otherwise eat the plants.

25.8 Poisons

What is a poison? Perhaps a better question would be, How much is a poison? A substance may be harmless—or even a necessary nutrient—in one amount but injurious or even deadly in another. Even a common substance such as table salt can be poisonous when eaten in abnormally large amounts; too much salt ingested at one time can induce vomiting. There have even been cases of fatal poisoning when salt was accidentally substituted for lactose (milk sugar) in formulas for infants. Some substances are obviously more toxic than others, however. It would take a massive dose of salt to kill the average healthy adult, whereas only a few micrograms of some of the nerve poisons can be fatal. Toxicity depends largely on the chemical nature of the substance.

People also respond differently to the same chemical. To cite an extreme case, 10–20 grams of sugar would cause no acute symptoms in most people but might be dangerous to a diabetic. Excessive amounts of sodium chloride would be especially serious to a person with edema (swelling due to excessive amounts of fluid in the tissues).

Still another complicating factor is that chemicals behave differently when administered in different ways. Nicotine is more than 50 times as toxic when applied intravenously as when taken orally. Good, fresh water is delightful when we drink it, but even water can be deadly when inhaled into the lungs in sufficient quantity. Further complications arise from the fact that even closely related animal species can react differently to a given chemical. Even individuals within a species may react to different degrees.

Poisons Around the House and in the Garden

Many household chemicals are poisonous. Drain cleaners, oven cleaners, and toilet bowl cleaners are highly corrosive to tissues. Some insecticides and rodenticides are quite toxic. Laundry bleach and ammonia are both toxic, and when they are mixed together, the combination can be deadly. Sodium hypochlorite in the bleach reacts with NH_3 to form highly toxic chloramines (NH_2Cl, $NHCl_2$, and NCl_3) and nitrosyl chloride ($NOCl$).

Even seemingly harmless products around the house can be dangerous to young children. A bottle of cough syrup can trigger an emergency visit to the hospital. Toxic substances are also used in home gardens. Herbicides and insecticides are not the only poisons you are likely to find in a garden. Sometimes the plants themselves are toxic. Irises are beautiful, and so are azaleas, hydrangeas, and oleander, but all of these popular perennials are poisonous. Holly berries, wisteria seeds, and the leaves and berries of privet hedges are also among the more poisonous products of the home garden. Some houseplants, such as the philodendron, are also toxic.

Corrosive Poisons

Strong acids and bases and strong oxidizing agents are highly corrosive to human tissue. These chemicals indiscriminately destroy living cells. Both acids and bases, even in dilute solutions, catalyze the hydrolysis of protein molecules in living cells. These reactions involve the breaking of the amide (peptide) linkages in the molecules. In cases of severe exposure, the fragmentation continues until the tissue is completely destroyed.

Acidic air pollutants, such as sulfuric acid aerosols and acids formed in the incineration of plastics and other wastes, are particularly destructive of lung tissue. Other air pollutants also damage living cells. Ozone, peroxyacetyl nitrate (PAN), and the other oxidizing components of photochemical smog probably do their main damage through the deactivation of enzymes. The active sites of enzymes often incorporate —SH groups, and ozone can oxidize these thiol groups to sulfonic acid groups ($—SO_3H$). This change renders an enzyme inactive and halts vital processes in the cell. No doubt, oxidizing agents can also break bonds in many of the chemical substances in a cell. Such powerful agents as ozone are more likely to make an indiscriminate attack than to react in a highly specific way.

Agents that Block Oxygen Transport and Use

Certain chemical substances block the transport of oxygen in the bloodstream and prevent the oxidation of metabolites by oxygen in the cells. All act on the iron atoms in complex protein molecules. Carbon monoxide binds tightly to the iron atom in hemo-

globin, blocking the transport of oxygen (Section 25.2). Nitrates also diminish the ability of hemoglobin to carry oxygen. They are reduced to nitrites by microorganisms in the digestive tract, and in turn the iron atoms in hemoglobin are oxidized from Fe^{2+} to Fe^{3+}. The resulting *methemoglobin* is incapable of carrying oxygen.

Cyanides are among the most notorious poisons in both fact and fiction. Sodium cyanide is used to extract gold and silver from ores and in electroplating baths, and cyanides can enter the environment from these processes. Hydrogen cyanide is used (with great care by specially trained experts) to exterminate insects and rodents in the holds of ships, in warehouses, in railway cars, and on citrus and other fruit trees. Hydrogen cyanide is generated easily enough by treating a cyanide salt with an acid:

$$CN^-(aq) + H_3O^+(aq) \longrightarrow HCN(g) + H_2O(l)$$

NaCN can be accidentally or deliberately ingested, and HCN can be inhaled. In either case, cyanides act almost instantaneously, and it takes only tiny quantities to kill. The average fatal dose for an adult is only 50–200 mg.

Cyanide blocks the oxidation of glucose inside the cell by forming a stable complex with iron- and copper-containing enzymes called *cytochrome oxidases*. The enzymes normally act by providing electrons for the reduction of oxygen in the cell. Cyanide ties up these mobile electrons, rendering them unavailable for the reduction process and bringing an abrupt end to cellular respiration.

Sodium thiosulfate ($Na_2S_2O_3$) is an antidote for cyanide poisoning, but it must be administered quickly. A sulfur atom is transferred from the thiosulfate ion to the cyanide ion, converting cyanide to relatively innocuous thiocyanate ions (SCN^-):

$$S_2O_3{}^{2-} + CN^- \longrightarrow SCN^- + SO_3{}^{2-}$$

Unfortunately, few victims of acute cyanide poisoning survive long enough to be treated.

Heavy Metal Poisons

Most metals and their compounds show some toxicity when ingested in large amounts. Even the essential mineral nutrients can be toxic when taken in excessive amounts. In many cases, too much of a metal nutrient (a toxic level) can be as dangerous as too little (deficiency). This concept is illustrated in Figure 25.17. For example, the average adult requires 10–18 mg of iron every day. If less is taken in, the person suffers from anemia. Yet an overdose can cause vomiting, diarrhea, shock, coma, and even death. As few as 10–15 tablets containing 325 mg each of iron (as $FeSO_4$) have been fatal to children.

We are not certain how iron poisoning works. However, the heavy metals—those near the bottom of the periodic table—exert their action primarily by inactivating enzymes (Section 13.11). Both mercury (as Hg^{2+}) and lead (as Pb^{2+}) act in this way. The symptoms of mercury poisoning, which include loss of equilibrium, sight, feeling, and hearing, often do not show up for several weeks. By the time the symptoms become recognizable, extensive damage has already been done to the brain and the rest of the nervous system. This damage is largely irreversible.

Lead poisoning can be treated if detected early enough. As we saw in Chapter 22, it usually is treated by intravenous administration of the calcium salt of EDTA. The Pb^{2+} ions are exchanged for the Ca^{2+} ions, and the lead–EDTA complex is excreted. As with mercury poisoning, the neurological damage done by lead compounds is essentially irreversible. Treatment must be performed early to be effective.

Cadmium (as Cd^{2+}) is also toxic (page 915). Its mode of action is different from that of lead and mercury. Cadmium poisoning leads to loss of calcium ions from the bones, leaving them brittle and easily broken. It also causes severe abdominal pain, vomiting, diarrhea, and a choking sensation.

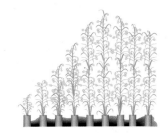

▲ **FIGURE 25.17** **The effect of copper ion on the height of oat seedlings**

From left to right, the concentrations of Cu^{2+} are 0, 3, 6, 10, 20, 100, 500, 2000, and 3000 mg/L. Plants on the left show varying degrees of deficiency; those on the right show copper ion toxicity. The optimum level of Cu^{2+} for oat seedlings is therefore about 100 mg/L.

Nerve Poisons

To understand how nerve poisons work, let us consider the action of acetylcholine as a neurotransmitter, with the help of the following equation:

$$CH_3COOCH_2CH_2N^+(CH_3)_3 + H_2O \underset{\text{Acetylase}}{\overset{\text{Cholinesterase}}{\rightleftharpoons}} CH_3COOH + HOCH_2CH_2N^+(CH_3)_3$$

Acetylcholine   Acetic Acid   Choline

Acetylcholine carries a signal from one nerve cell to another. After doing so, it hydrolyzes to acetic acid and choline through the action of the enzyme *cholinesterase.* Another enzyme, *acetylase,* converts acetic acid and choline back to acetylcholine, which is then ready to carry the next nerve impulse.

Nerve poisons can disrupt the acetylcholine cycle in three ways:

- Botulin, the deadly toxin given off by the anaerobic bacterium *Clostridium botulinum* found in improperly processed canned food, blocks the synthesis of acetylcholine. No messenger is formed, and no messages are carried between nerve cells. Paralysis sets in and death occurs, usually by respiratory failure.
- Curare, atropine, and some local anesthetics block the acetylcholine receptor sites. In this case, the message is sent but not received. In the case of local anesthetics, this can be good for pain relief in a limited area, but anesthetics, too, can be lethal in sufficient quantity.
- *Anticholinesterase poisons* inhibit the action of cholinesterase. This inhibition keeps the level of acetylcholine high; the message is turned on continuously, overstimulating the receptor cells. Anticholinesterase poisons include the organic phosphorus insecticides and chemical warfare compounds such as tabun, sarin, and soman.

The nerve poisons are among the most toxic synthetic chemicals known. They kill when they are inhaled or absorbed through the skin, resulting in the complete loss of muscular coordination and subsequent death by cessation of breathing. The usual antidote is atropine injection and artificial respiration. Without the antidote, death may occur in 2–10 minutes.

Chlorinated hydrocarbon pesticides, such as DDT, are relatively safe to mammals, but they are also nerve poisons. Acute DDT poisoning causes tremors, convulsions, and cardiac or respiratory failure. Chronic exposure to DDT leads to the degeneration of the central nervous system. Other chlorinated compounds, such as the PCBs, act in a similar manner.

Despite their tremendous potential for death and destruction, the nerve poisons have helped us gain an understanding of the chemistry of the nervous system. That knowledge enables scientists to design antidotes for the nerve poisons. In addition, our increased understanding should contribute to progress along more positive lines—in the control of pain, for example.

Detoxification and Potentiation of Poisons

The human body can handle moderate amounts of some poisons. The liver is able to detoxify some compounds by oxidation, reduction, or coupling with amino acids or other normal body chemicals. Perhaps the most common route is oxidation. Ethanol is detoxified by oxidation to acetaldehyde, which in turn is oxidized to acetic acid, a normal constituent of cells. The acetic acid is then oxidized to carbon dioxide and water.

Highly toxic nicotine from tobacco is detoxified by oxidation to cotinine:

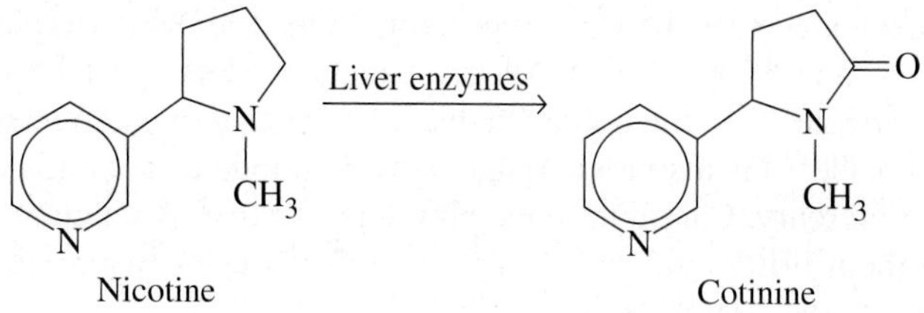

Nicotine   Cotinine

Cotinine is less toxic than nicotine. The added oxygen atom also makes cotinine more water-soluble than nicotine and thus more readily excreted in the urine.

The liver is equipped with a system of enzymes, called P-450, that oxidizes fat-soluble substances. The P-450 system converts these fat-soluble compounds, which are likely to be retained in the body, into water-soluble ones that are readily excreted. It can also join molecules to amino acids. For example, toluene is essentially insoluble in water. The P-450 enzymes oxidize toluene to more soluble benzoic acid. The latter

Application Note

Extremely small amounts of one type of botulism toxin have been found useful in treatment of certain muscle spasms. Injection of the toxin into the muscle blocks synthesis of acetylcholine and can relieve spasms for up to three months. The well-known BOTOX® cosmetic treatment is a form of botulism toxin.

is then coupled with the amino acid glycine to form hippuric acid, which is still more soluble and is readily excreted:

Toluene $\xrightarrow{\text{Oxidation}}$ Benzoic acid $\xrightarrow[\text{(Glycine)}]{\text{H}_2\text{N}-\text{CH}_2-\overset{\text{O}}{\overset{\|}{\text{C}}}-\text{OH}}$ Hippuric acid

The liver enzymes simply oxidize, reduce, or join molecules together. The end product is not necessarily less toxic. For example, methanol is oxidized to the more toxic substance formaldehyde. It is probably the reaction of formaldehyde with the protein in cells that causes the blindness, convulsions, respiratory failure, and death that are characteristic of methanol poisoning. Also, the same enzymes that oxidize alcohols deactivate the male hormone, testosterone. The buildup of these enzymes in a chronic alcoholic leads to a more rapid destruction of testosterone. This appears to be the mechanism for alcoholic impotence, a well-known characteristic of alcoholism.

Benzene, because of its general inertness in the body, is not acted on until it reaches the liver. There, it is slowly oxidized to an epoxide, which is a cyclic ether containing a three-membered ring:

$$\text{benzene} \xrightarrow[\text{the liver}]{\text{Oxidation in}} \text{epoxide}$$

This type of reaction, called *potentiation,* converts a relatively harmless chemical into a much more toxic one. In this benzene potentiation, the product epoxide is a highly reactive molecule that can attack certain key proteins, causing damage that sometimes results in leukemia.

Carbon tetrachloride, CCl_4, is also quite inert in the body. When it reaches the liver, however, it is converted to the reactive trichloromethyl free radical $Cl_3C\cdot$, which attacks unsaturated fatty acids in the body. This action can trigger cancer.

25.9 Carcinogens and Anticarcinogens

Tumors, abnormal growths of new tissue, may be either benign or malignant. Benign tumors are characterized by slow growth; they often regress spontaneously, and they do not invade neighboring tissues. Malignant tumors, often called *cancers,* may grow slowly or rapidly, but their growth is generally irreversible. Malignant growths invade and destroy neighboring tissues. Cancer is not a single disease, but rather a catchall term for more than 200 different afflictions. Many are not even closely related to one another.

What causes cancer? The answers to this seemingly simple question are quite varied and anything but simple. Some chemicals modify DNA, thus scrambling the code for replication and for the synthesis of proteins. For example, aflatoxin B is known to bind to guanine residues in DNA. Just how this initiates cancer, however, is not known for sure.

There is a genetic component to the development of many forms of cancer. Certain genes, called *oncogenes,* seem either to trigger or to sustain the processes that convert normal cells to cancerous ones. Oncogenes arise from ordinary genes that regulate cell growth and cell division and then can be activated by chemical carcinogens, radiation, or perhaps by some viruses. It seems that more than one oncogene must be turned on, perhaps at different stages of the process, before a cancer develops.

We also have suppressor genes that ordinarily prevent the development of cancers. These genes must be inactivated before a cancer develops. Suppressor gene inactivation can occur through mutation, alteration, or loss of the gene. In all, 10 or 15 mutations may be required in a cell before it turns cancerous. Thus, our bodies have some natural protection against cancer.

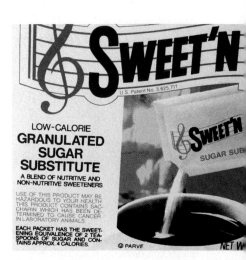

▲ A surprising number of consumer products warn us about containing suspected carcinogens, such as saccharine.

A **carcinogen** is a material that causes cancer. Many people seem to believe that chemicals are a major cause of cancer, but most cancers are caused by lifestyle factors. Nearly two-thirds of all cancer deaths in the United States are linked to tobacco, diet, and lack of exercise with resulting obesity. Even among the chemicals that are most suspect, such as pesticides, many have not been shown to be carcinogenic. Only about 30 chemical compounds have been identified as human carcinogens. Another 300 or so have been shown to cause cancer in laboratory animals, but it is often difficult to equate the results of tests on laboratory animals with risks to humans. Some of these 300 are widely used and are therefore a subject of some concern.

There are strong correlations between carcinogenicity and certain molecular sizes and shapes, and some of the more notorious carcinogens are polycyclic aromatic hydrocarbons, of which 3,4-benzpyrene is perhaps the best known:

3,4-Benzpyrene

Carcinogenic polycyclic hydrocarbons are formed during the incomplete burning of nearly any organic material. They have been found in charcoal-grilled meats, cigarette smoke, automobile exhausts, coffee, burnt sugar, and many other materials.

Another important class of carcinogens is the aromatic amines. Two prominent ones are β-naphthylamine and benzidine. These compounds once were used widely in the dye industry. They were responsible for a high incidence of bladder cancer among dye-industry workers.

Not all carcinogens are aromatic compounds. Prominent among the aliphatic carcinogens are dimethylnitrosamine [$(CH_3)_2NNO$] and vinyl chloride, the monomer from which the polymer polyvinyl chloride is made. Other aliphatic carcinogens include some epoxides, such as bis(epoxy)butane, and some other three- and four-membered heterocyclic rings containing oxygen or nitrogen.

Few of the known carcinogens are synthetic chemicals. Some, such as safrole in sassafras and the aflatoxins produced by molds on foods, occur naturally. Some researchers estimate that 99.99% of all carcinogens that we ingest are natural ones. Plants produce compounds to protect themselves from fungi, insects, and higher animals, including humans. Some carcinogenic compounds are found in mushrooms, basil, celery, figs, mustard, pepper, fennel, parsnips, and citrus oils—almost every place a curious chemist looks. Carcinogens are also produced during cooking and as products of normal metabolism.

With so many natural carcinogens in food, why do we not all get cancer? Part of the answer to this question is that some substances in food act as **anticarcinogens.** Fiber is believed to protect against colon cancer, for example; the food additive BHT (butylated hydroxytoluene) may protect against stomach cancer, and certain vitamins have anticarcinogenic effects.

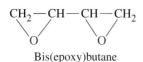

Bis(epoxy)butane

N-Laurylethyleneimine

β-Propiolactone

▲ Three small-ring heterocyclic carcinogens. The top molecule is an epoxide.

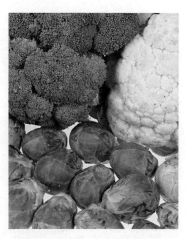

▲ Broccoli, cauliflower, and brussels sprouts are among the cruciferous vegetables that have been shown to reduce the incidence of cancer in humans.

BHT

A diet rich in cruciferous vegetables (cabbage, broccoli, brussels sprouts, kale, and cauliflower) has been shown to reduce the incidence of cancer in both animals and humans. We still do not know for sure what components of these foods protect against cancer. Perhaps it is a combination of substances rather than just one. The vitamins that are antioxidants (vitamin C, vitamin E, and β-carotene, a precursor to vitamin A)

How Cigarette Smoking Causes Cancer

The association between cigarette smoking and cancer has been known for decades, but the precise mechanism was not known until 1996. The research scientists who found the link focused on a tumor-suppressor gene called *P53*, a gene that is mutated in about 60% of all lung cancers. They also focused on a metabolite of benzpyrene, a carcinogen found in tobacco smoke.

In the body, benzpyrene is oxidized to an epoxide that is an active carcinogen and binds to specific nucleotides in the gene—sites called hot spots—where mutations frequently occur. It seems quite likely that the benzpyrene metabolite causes many of those mutations in the *P53* gene.

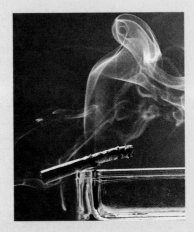

◄ Cigarette smoke contains at least 40 carcinogens, including 3,4-benzpyrene.

seem to exhibit the strongest anticancer properties. Some studies with vitamins A, C, and E, used separately or in combination, have confirmed that each of these vitamins has some ability to lower the incidence of cancer. There probably are many other anti-carcinogens in our food that have not yet been identified.

25.10 Hazardous Materials

Stories about toxic substances have caused increasing concern about hazardous materials in the environment. Problems with chemical dumps have made household words out of Love Canal in New York State and Valley of the Drums in Kentucky. Although often overblown in the news media, serious problems do exist.

The U.S. EPA categorizes **hazardous materials** on the basis of their properties:

- **Ignitable materials** are substances that catch fire readily, such as gasoline and other hydrocarbons.
- **Corrosive materials** are substances that corrode storage containers and other equipment, such as strong acids.
- **Reactive materials** are substances that react or decompose readily, possibly producing hazardous by-products. Examples include explosives and materials that react with water to produce toxic fumes, such as powdered bleach (calcium hypochlorite).
- **Toxic materials** are substances that are injurious when inhaled or ingested, such as chlorine, ammonia, formaldehyde, and pesticides.

From this list, we see that hazardous materials can cause fires or explosions, pollute the air, contaminate our food and water, and occasionally poison by direct contact. As long as we want the products our industries produce, however, we will have to deal with the problems of hazardous wastes (Table 25.6).

Many hazardous materials can be rendered less harmful by chemical treatment. For example, acid wastes can be neutralized with inexpensive bases, such as lime. However, the best way to handle hazardous wastes is not to produce them in the first place. Many industries have modified processes to minimize the amount of wastes produced, and some wastes that are produced can be reprocessed to recover energy or materials. Hydrocarbon solvents can be either purified and reused or else burned as fuels. Sometimes, one industry's waste can be a raw material for another industry. For example, waste nitric acid from the metals industry can be converted to fertilizer. Finally, if a hazardous waste cannot be used, incinerated, or treated to render it less

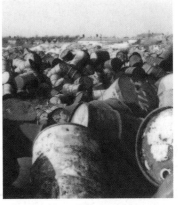

(a)

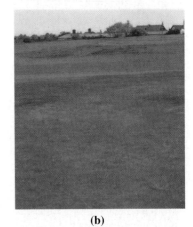

(b)

▲ (a) A waste dump in 1970 at Malkins Bank, Cheshire, England, with drums leaking chemical wastes. (b) The same site, cleaned up and restored, is now a municipal golf course.

Table 25.6 Industrial Products and Hazardous Waste By-products	
Product	**Associated Waste**
Plastics	Organic chlorine compounds
Pesticides	Organic chlorine compounds, organophosphate compounds
Medicines	Organic solvents and residues, heavy metals (for example, mercury and zinc)
Paints	Heavy metals, pigments, solvents, organic residues
Oil, gasoline	Oil, phenols and other organic compounds, heavy metals, ammonium salts, acids, caustics
Metals	Heavy metals, fluorides, cyanides, acidic and alkaline cleaners, solvents, pigments, abrasives, plating salts, oils, phenols
Leather	Heavy metals, organic solvents
Textiles	Heavy metals, dyes, organic chlorine compounds, solvents

hazardous, it must be stored in a secure landfill. Unfortunately, landfills often leak, contaminating groundwater. When this happens, we clean up one toxic waste dump and move the materials to another, playing a rather macabre shell game.

The best technology at present for treating organic wastes, including chlorinated compounds, appears to be incineration. For example, combustion at 1260 °C eliminates more than 99.9999% of chlorinated compounds, such as PCBs.

Perhaps *biodegradation* of wastes will be the way of the future. Some microorganisms can degrade hydrocarbons in gasoline, for example, and there are bacteria that, when provided with proper nutrients, can degrade chlorinated hydrocarbons.

Weighing Risks and Benefits

Increasingly, we have to decide whether the benefits we gain from hazardous substances are worth the risks we assume by using them. Many issues involving toxic chemicals are emotional, and most of the decisions regarding them are political. Nevertheless, possible solutions to problems posed by toxic chemicals often lie in the field

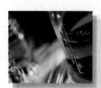

Phytoremediation

Many of the *d*-block elements and some of the lower *s*-block and *p*-block elements, such as lead and barium, are toxic. Sites of heavy contamination of toxic metals are major problems. A direct method of cleanup is to dig up the contaminated soil and move it elsewhere, but that is very expensive and merely moves a large contamination problem to a new location.

Phytoremediation is a technique that shows promise for ridding contaminated soil of heavy metals as well as petroleum products and other organic compounds. Certain plant species are *hyperaccumulators,* meaning they have a high affinity for various metal ions or other specific chemical species. These plants are cultivated in the problem area. The plants may be harvested and further processed by dehydration and/or ashing. The residue from the plants is far smaller than the mass of the contaminated soil, and disposal is much easier.

The efficacy of phytoremediation has been improved in some cases by watering the plants with a solution of a chelating agent such as EDTA (Section 22.12). Chelated metals are more easily accumulated in the plant. For example, chelation has been

found to increase phytoremediation of lead by a factor of 100 or more in some cases.

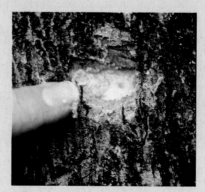

▲ The Italian serpentine plant *Alyssum bertolonii* can accumulate so much nickel(II) ion that its sap is green! It is thought that the ability to accumulate heavy metals may be related to the toxic effects of those elements on insects that might otherwise feast on these plants.

of chemistry. We hope the chemistry you have learned in this text will help you make intelligent decisions. Most of all, we hope you will continue to learn more about chemistry, because chemistry affects nearly everything you do. We wish you success and happiness, and may the joy of learning go with you always.

Cumulative Example

A large coal-fired electric plant burns 2500 tons of coal per day. **(a)** Determine the number of homes that this plant can supply with electricity, assuming that coal is nearly pure carbon, that the efficiency of the plant is 41%, and that one home consumes 85 kWh each day. **(b)** The coal that is burned contains 0.65% S by mass. Assume that all the sulfur is converted to SO_2 and that, because of a thermal inversion, the SO_2 remains trapped for one day in a parcel of air that is 45 km × 60 km × 0.40 km. Will the level of SO_2 in this air exceed the primary national air-quality standard of 365 μg SO_2/m^3 air?

STRATEGY

For part (a), we can determine the enthalpy change for the combustion of 2500 tons of solid carbon to carbon dioxide. Next, we must convert that enthalpy change first to kilowatt-hours (using the conversion factor, 1 kWh = 3600 kJ, from the inside back cover) and then to number of homes. In applying the plant efficiency factor, we use the unit kJ(electric)/kJ(thermal) to extract that portion of the energy of combustion of the coal that actually appears as electricity (the rest is waste heat). For part (b), we first calculate the mass of sulfur in the coal and then use simple stoichiometry to determine the mass of sulfur dioxide produced. Next, we convert that mass to micrograms and then divide the mass by the volume of air (in cubic meters).

SOLUTION

(a) First, we write the combustion equation and determine the enthalpy change. Because of our assumption that the coal is pure carbon, the enthalpy change is simply the standard enthalpy of formation of $CO_2(g)$.

$$C(graphite) + O_2(g) \longrightarrow CO_2(g) \qquad \Delta H° = -393.5 \text{ kJ/mol}$$

The next step is to convert 2500 tons of carbon to grams.

$$? \text{ g C} = 2500 \text{ tons C} \times \frac{2000 \text{ lb}}{1 \text{ ton}} \times \frac{453.6 \text{ g}}{1 \text{ lb}} = 2.3 \times 10^9 \text{ g C}$$

Now we can use the molar mass of carbon, the enthalpy change, the plant efficiency factor, and the conversion factors from kJ(thermal) to kWh and from kWh to homes.

$$? \text{ homes} = 2.3 \times 10^9 \text{ g C} \times \frac{1 \text{ mol C}}{12.011 \text{ g C}} \times \frac{393.5 \text{ kJ(thermal)}}{1 \text{ mol C}}$$

$$\times \frac{0.41 \text{ kJ(electric)}}{1 \text{ kJ(thermal)}} \times \frac{1 \text{ kWh}}{3600 \text{ kJ(electric)}} \times \frac{1 \text{ home}}{85 \text{ kWh}}$$

$$= 1.0 \times 10^5 \text{ homes}$$

(b) We begin with a balanced equation for combustion of sulfur.

$$S(s) + O_2(g) \longrightarrow SO_2(g)$$

Next, we use the percent sulfur to find the grams of sulfur associated with the calculated mass of carbon and then convert this mass stoichiometrically to grams of sulfur dioxide.

$$? \text{ g SO}_2 = 2.3 \times 10^9 \text{ g C} \times \frac{0.65 \text{ g S}}{100 \text{ g C}} \times \frac{1 \text{ mol S}}{32.07 \text{ g S}} \times \frac{1 \text{ mol SO}_2}{1 \text{ mol S}} \times \frac{64.06 \text{ g SO}_2}{1 \text{ mol SO}_2}$$

$$= 3.0 \times 10^7 \text{ g SO}_2$$

Finally, we express the concentration as grams of SO_2 per cubic kilometer and convert to the desired units of μg SO_2/m^3.

$$\frac{? \, \mu\text{g SO}_2}{\text{m}^3} = \frac{3.0 \times 10^7 \text{ g SO}_2}{(45 \times 60 \times 0.40) \text{ km}^3} \times \frac{10^6 \, \mu\text{g}}{1 \text{ g}} \times \left(\frac{1 \text{ km}}{1000 \text{ m}}\right)^3 = 28 \, \mu\text{g SO}_2/\text{m}^3$$

The $SO_2(g)$ content of the air does not exceed the primary air-quality standard.

ASSESSMENT

It appears that the SO_2 content of the air during the thermal inversion is well below the primary national air-quality standard. Indeed, ten times this concentration of SO_2 still would not exceed the standard. However, we have made a very questionable assumption: that the SO_2 is uniformly dispersed. In practice, it seems almost certain that regions closer to the plant would exhibit much higher levels of SO_2 than more distant regions of this large parcel of air.

Concept Review with Key Terms

25.1 Atmospheric Composition, Structure, and Natural Cycles—Starting at Earth's surface, the primary regions of the atmosphere are called the troposphere, stratosphere, mesosphere, and thermosphere (ionosphere). The chief components of dry air are N_2, O_2, and Ar. Water vapor is an important participant in the **hydrologic (water) cycle**. The humidity of air is a measure of its water vapor content. Dew and frost formation and **deliquescence** are phenomena related to relative humidity.

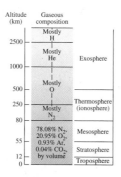

Nitrogen fixation describes the conversion of atmospheric nitrogen into nitrogen-containing compounds and is an important step in the **nitrogen cycle**. Chemical fixation of nitrogen to make fertilizers has greatly increased the world's food supply but has also altered the natural nitrogen cycle. Atmospheric CO_2 is the carbon source for carbohydrate synthesis in the **carbon cycle**. Some carbon is locked out of the cycle in fossil fuels (coal, natural gas, and petroleum), but the combustion of these fuels returns CO and CO_2 to the cycle.

25.2 Air Pollution—Carbon monoxide is an **air pollutant** commonly found in high concentrations in urban areas with heavy vehicular traffic. In the presence of unburned hydrocarbons and sunlight, oxides of nitrogen lead to **photochemical smog**. Temperature inversions also contribute to smog conditions. Smog-control measures focus on catalytic converters for use in automobiles and the control of combustion

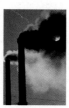

processes to reduce emissions. **Industrial smog** is associated with industrial processes and practices that produce high levels of sulfur oxides and **particulate matter**.

25.3 The Ozone Layer—Ozone, O_3, in the stratosphere protects living organisms by absorbing ultraviolet radiation. The integrity of the **ozone layer** is threatened by human activities, such as the release of chlorofluorocarbons (CFCs) into the atmosphere.

25.4 Global Warming: Carbon Dioxide and the Greenhouse Effect—The continuous buildup of CO_2 in the atmosphere may result in **global warming**. The **greenhouse effect** is a natural process in which infrared radiation emitted by Earth's surface is absorbed by atmospheric gases such as CO_2 and H_2O. In-

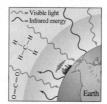

creased levels of these "greenhouse" gases may contribute to increased global warming.

25.5 Earth's Natural Waters—Water covers three-fourths of Earth's surface, but only about 1% of it is available as fresh water. Water has a higher density, specific heat, and heat of vaporization than most other liquids. Unlike most liquids, water expands when it freezes.

25.6 Water Pollution—Fresh water is easily contaminated by various chemicals and microorganisms, some coming from natural processes and others from human activities. Dumping sewage into water increases the amount of organic material in the water. The breakdown of this material by dissolved oxygen is known as **aerobic oxidation**. At high levels of organic material, aerobic oxidation can lead to an increase in **biochemical oxygen demand (BOD)** and eventually harm higher forms of aquatic life. Water pollutants that are nutrients for the growth of algae can lead to **eutrophication** of a lake or stream. When oxygen levels are depleted, **anaerobic decay**—the reduction of organic material to CH_4, H_2S, and NH_3—further harms aquatic life.

Groundwater and surface water each provide drinking water for about half the U.S. population. Municipal water supplies are treated in several physical and chemical steps: settling, filtration, aeration, and chlorination. Fluoridation appears to have greatly reduced the incidence of dental caries.

Wastewater treatment usually includes several processes. **Primary sewage treatment** uses settling ponds for sludge removal. **Secondary sewage treatment** entails sand and gravel filtration. A combination of these methods is known as the **activated sludge method**. **Advanced treatment** methods include charcoal filtration, ion exchange, and reverse osmosis.

25.7 Acid Rain and Acid Waters—Sulfur oxides and nitrogen oxides can react with water in the atmosphere to produce **acid rain**. This form of pollution causes lakes and streams to become so acidic that the acidic water damages fish and other aquatic life.

25.8 Poisons—A number of processes threaten forms of life in the Earth's **biosphere**. **Toxicology** is the study of the responses of living organisms to poisons. Strong acids and bases are corrosive poisons. Substances such as ozone are toxic because they are strong oxidizing agents. Carbon monoxide and nitrites are toxic because they interfere with the blood's ability to transport oxygen. Cyanides are poisons because they shut down cellular respiration. Heavy metal poisons, such as lead and mercury, inactivate enzymes by tying up their SH groups. Nerve poisons, such as organophosphates, interfere with the acetylcholine cycle.

25.9 Carcinogens and Anticarcinogens—Carcinogens are slow poisons that trigger the growth of malignant tumors. Some natural substances in foods act to inhibit cancerous growth and are known as **anticarcinogens**.

25.10 Hazardous Materials—**Hazardous materials** are industrial products and by-products that can cause illness or death. The four classes of hazardous materials are **ignitable materials**, **corrosive materials**, **reactive materials**, and **toxic materials**.

Assessment Goals

When you have mastered the material in this chapter, you will be able to:

- List the different layers of the atmosphere and their composition.
- Describe the three natural cycles of our biosphere involving water, nitrogen, and carbon.
- Distinguish between air pollutants, photochemical smog, and industrial smog.

- Describe approaches to controlling the different forms of air pollution.
- Describe the properties of ozone, the importance of the ozone layer, and the effect of human activities on the ozone layer.
- Explain the relationship between carbon dioxide and the greenhouse effect.
- List the sources of natural waters within the hydrosphere.

- Describe different forms of chemical contamination of water and the remediation steps used to address these, including treatment of municipal water, wastewater, and sewage.
- Describe the sources of acid rain and its impact on the environment.
- Describe poisons, their mechanisms of toxicity, their control, and their antidotes.
- Describe natural and synthetic carcinogens, their mechanism of action, and the activity of anticarcinogens.
- Distinguish between the four classes of hazardous materials in terms of their chemical identity and impact.

Self-Assessment Questions

1. Which layer of the atmosphere (a) lies nearest the surface of Earth? (b) Contains the ozone layer?

2. List the three major components of dry air, and give the approximate (nearest whole number) mole percent of each.

3. What is the nitrogen cycle? How has industrial fixation of nitrogen to make fertilizers affected the nitrogen cycle?

4. Briefly describe each of the following terms dealing with a natural phenomenon.

    (a) deliquescence   (b) the greenhouse effect

5. What specific materials are implied by these terms for atmospheric pollutant(s)?

    (a) PAN   (b) SO_x (c) fly ash

6. By name and/or formula, identify (a) two gases able to displace O_2 in blood hemoglobin; (b) two "greenhouse" gases, in addition to CO_2 and H_2O; and (c) a constituent of acid rain.

7. List two uses of chlorofluorocarbons (CFCs), and describe how CFCs are implicated in the depletion of the ozone layer.

8. What is photochemical smog? What is the role of sunlight in its formation?

9. What is industrial smog? How is it formed?

10. What conditions favor the formation of carbon monoxide during the combustion of gasoline in an automobile engine? How does carbon monoxide exert its poisonous effect?

11. What is synergism? Indicate one specific example of a synergistic effect concerning air pollution.

12. What are the health effects associated with ozone in the stratosphere and at ground level? Why are they not the same?

13. How is each of the following used to reduce air pollution?

    (a) electrostatic precipitator

    (b) catalytic converter

14. Which of the following are important contributors to the formation of photochemical smog, and which are not? Explain.

    (a) NO   (c) hydrocarbon vapors

    (b) CO   (d) SO_2

15. What is a temperature inversion? How does a temperature inversion contribute to air pollution problems?

16. How are the following terms related to one another regarding air pollution: aerosol, fly ash, and particulate matter?

17. Describe measures that can be used to control the emission of nitrogen oxides in automotive exhaust, and explain why these are not the same measures used to control emissions of hydrocarbons and carbon monoxide.

18. What proportion of Earth's water is seawater? Why are the seas salty?

19. List some waterborne diseases. Why are these diseases no longer common in developed countries?

20. What impurities are present in rainwater?

21. List four cations and three anions present in groundwater.

22. What is BOD? Why is a high BOD undesirable?

23. What are the products of the breakdown in water of organic matter by aerobic bacteria? By anaerobic bacteria?

24. List some ways in which groundwater is contaminated. What are some common industrial contaminants of groundwater?

25. Why do chlorinated hydrocarbons remain in groundwater for such a long time?

26. List two ways by which lakes and streams have become acidic. Why is acidic water especially hazardous to fish?

27. List several ways by which the acidity of rain can be reduced. What kind of rocks tend to neutralize acidic waters? How can we restore (at least temporarily) lakes that are too acidic?

28. List two toxic compounds found in wastes from the chromium plating process. How is each removed?

29. Describe (a) a primary sewage treatment plant and (b) a secondary sewage treatment plant. What impurities are removed by each? What impurities remain in wastewater after each form of treatment?

30. Describe the activated sludge method of sewage treatment. Why is wastewater chlorinated before it is returned to a waterway?

31. What is meant by advanced treatment of wastewater? What kinds of substances are removed from wastewater by charcoal filtration? Why is it so difficult to remove nitrate ions from water?

32. Why are municipal water supplies (a) treated with aluminum sulfate and slaked lime, (b) aerated, and (c) chlorinated?

33. Give an example that shows how the toxicity of a substance depends on the route of administration.

34. List three corrosive poisons. How do dilute solutions of acids and bases damage living cells? How does ozone damage living cells?

35. How do cyanides exert their toxic effect? How does sodium thiosulfate act as an antidote for cyanide poisoning?

36. Iron (as Fe^{2+}) is a necessary nutrient. What are the effects of too little Fe^{2+}? Of too much?

37. What is acetylcholine? Describe its action.

38. How do (a) botulin, (b) sarin, and (c) organophosphorus compounds affect the acetylcholine cycle?

39. What is the P-450 system? What is its function? Does it always detoxify foreign substances?

40. List two ways that the conversion of nicotine to cotinine in the liver lessens the risk of nicotine poisoning.

41. List two steps in the detoxification of ingested toluene. What is the effect of these steps?

42. What is a tumor? How are benign and malignant tumors different?

43. What are (a) oncogenes and (b) suppressor genes? How is each involved in the development of cancer?

44. List some conditions under which polycyclic hydrocarbons are formed.

45. What is a hazardous material?

46. Define and give an example of (a) a reactive material, (b) an ignitable material, and (c) a corrosive material.

Problems

Earth's Atmosphere

47. The text states that 99% of the mass of the atmosphere lies within 30 km of the surface of Earth. Which of the following values is a reasonable estimate of air pressure at an altitude of 30 km: **(a)** 0.1 mmHg, **(b)** 1 mmHg, **(c)** 10 mmHg, or **(d)** 100 mmHg? Explain your reasoning. (*Hint:* Recall the basic ideas relating to pressure from Section 5.3.)

48. When present in a very small proportion in air, the concentration of a gas is customarily indicated in parts per million (ppm) rather than in mole percent or volume percent. Use data in Table 25.1 to determine the parts per million in air of the noble gases that are listed there.

49. Suggest a likely reason for the observed change in composition with altitude—from N_2 to O to He to H—shown in Figure 25.1.

50. Part of the design criteria for the International Space Station included a requirement that parts of the station exposed to space be as chemically nonreactive as possible. Suggest a likely reason for this requirement. (*Hint:* Refer to Figure 25.1 and the note on page 1036.)

Water Vapor in the Atmosphere

51. What are the mole percent and ppm of H_2O in an air sample at STP in which the partial pressure of water vapor is 2.00 mmHg?

52. What should be the relative humidity of a sample of air at 25 °C in which the partial pressure of water vapor is 10.5 mmHg? (*Hint:* Use data from Table 11.2.)

53. What is the partial pressure of water vapor in a sample of air having a relative humidity of 75.5% at 20 °C? (*Hint:* Use data from Table 11.2.)

54. A parcel of air has an absolute humidity, expressed as a partial pressure of water vapor, of 18.0 mmHg. At which of the following temperatures does the air have the greatest relative humidity: 25 °C, 30 °C, or 40 °C? Explain.

55. What is the dew point of the parcel of air described in Problem 54? (*Hint:* Use data from Table 11.2.)

56. Why is it that condensed water vapor can be seen above a kettle of boiling water even in a hot kitchen, whereas you can see your breath only on a cold day?

Carbon, CO, and CO₂

57. The combustion of a hydrocarbon, especially if the quantity of oxygen is limited, produces a mixture of carbon dioxide and carbon monoxide. The decomposition of a metal carbonate by an acid produces only carbon dioxide, even if the quantity of acid is limited. Explain this difference in behavior.

58. Indicate a natural process or processes by which carbon atoms are **(a)** removed from the atmosphere, **(b)** returned to the atmosphere, **(c)** effectively withdrawn from the carbon cycle.

59. Write an equation that represents the complete combustion of the hydrocarbon hexane, $C_6H_{14}(l)$. Explain why it is not possible to write a unique equation to represent its incomplete combustion.

60. Carbon monoxide is a poisonous gas, even in low concentrations, whereas carbon dioxide is not. Yet, except in some local situations, there is less environmental concern over carbon monoxide than over carbon dioxide. Explain why this is so.

61. The United States leads the world in per capita emissions of $CO_2(g)$, amounting to 19.8 metric tons (t) per person per year (1 t = 1000 kg). What mass, in metric tons, of each of the following fuels would yield this quantity of CO_2?
(a) CH_4 **(b)** C_8H_{18} **(c)** coal (94.1% C by mass)

62. Tabulations on carbon dioxide emissions often list cement manufacture as one of the sources. Describe two ways in which the manufacture of Portland cement injects carbon dioxide into the atmosphere.

Air Pollution

63. Although alternative automotive fuels can reduce some types of air pollution, they still produce other types of pollution, such as nitrogen oxides. Explain why.

64. Per ton of material consumed, which of the following would you expect to produce the greatest quantity of $SO_2(g)$: **(a)** smelting zinc sulfide, **(b)** smelting lead sulfide, **(c)** burning coal, or **(d)** burning natural gas? Explain.

65. Write equations for the following reactions.
(a) Sulfur burns in air, forming sulfur dioxide.
(b) Zinc sulfide, heated in air, yields zinc oxide and sulfur dioxide.
(c) Sulfur dioxide reacts with oxygen, forming sulfur trioxide.
(d) Sulfur trioxide reacts with water, forming sulfuric acid.
(e) Sulfuric acid is completely neutralized by aqueous ammonia.

66. Identify each species, NO, NO_2, Cl, and ClO, as a catalyst or a reactive intermediate in the chemical reactions involved in the ozone layer.

67. Describe how the following particulate matter may be produced.
(a) sodium chloride from seawater
(b) sulfate particles in an industrial smog

68. The average person takes 15 breaths per minute, inhaling 0.50 L of air with each breath. What mass of particulates, in milligrams, would the person breathe in a day if the particulate level in air were 75 $\mu g/m^3$?

Water and Water Pollution

69. Give the equation that shows the neutralization of acidic water by limestone.

70. Wastewater disinfected with chlorine must be dechlorinated before it is returned to sensitive bodies of water. The dechlorinating agent often is sulfur dioxide. Write the equation for the reaction. Is the chlorine oxidized or reduced? Identify the oxidizing agent and reducing agent in the reaction.

71. How many kilograms of $Ca(OH)_2$ are needed to neutralize a lake that has been made 2.0×10^{-4} M in sulfuric acid by acid rain and is 300×200 m, with an average depth of 5.0 m?

72. Suggest a reason for the "extremely high" cost of distillation as compared to other methods of tertiary wastewater treatment (Table 25.5).

Additional Problems

Problems marked with an * may be more challenging than others.

73. Assume that typical urban air contains 100 μg of suspended particles per m^3 of air. Assume that the average particle is spherical in shape, with a diameter of 1 μm and a density of 1 g/cm^3. Estimate the number of particles per cm^3 of the air.

* 74. The text states that 5.2×10^{15} metric tons of atmospheric gases are spread over a surface area of 5.0×10^8 km^2. Use these facts, together with data from Appendix B, to estimate a value of standard atmospheric pressure.

75. At 20 °C, the vapor pressure observed for a saturated solution of $CaCl_2 \cdot 6\,H_2O$ is 5.67 mmHg. If a quantity of this solution is placed in a large sealed container at 20 °C and the solution is kept saturated by the presence of excess solid, what relative humidity will be maintained in the air in the container? How effective is $CaCl_2 \cdot 6\,H_2O$ in dehumidifying air?

* 76. A 12.012-L sample of air becomes saturated with water vapor at 25.0 °C. The air is then cooled to 20.0 °C. What mass of water (dew) will deposit on the walls of the container?

77. There are different ways to assess how much the combustion of various fuels contributes to the buildup of CO_2 in the atmosphere. One relates the mass of CO_2 formed to the mass of fuel burned; another relates the mass of CO_2 to the quantity of heat evolved in the combustion. Which of the three fuels C(graphite), $CH_4(g)$, or $C_4H_{10}(g)$ produces the smallest mass of CO_2 (a) per gram of fuel, (b) per kJ of heat evolved? (Hint: Use data from Appendix C, and assume that all the products of each combustion are gases.)

* 78. It has been estimated that if all the ozone in the atmosphere were brought to sea level at STP, the gas would form a layer 0.3 cm thick. (a) Estimate the number of O_3 molecules in Earth's atmosphere. (b) Comment on the feasibility of a caller's suggestion to a radio science program that depleted ozone in the stratosphere be replaced by transporting unwanted ozone from low altitudes into the stratosphere.

* 79. A small gasoline-powered engine with a 1-L storage tank is inadvertently left running overnight in a large warehouse, 95 m $\times$ 38 m $\times$ 16 m. When workers arrive in the morning, are they likely to enter an environment in which the level of CO exceeds the danger level of 35 ppm? (Hint: Use C_8H_{18} as a representative formula of gasoline, and make other reasonable assumptions.)

80. To prevent tooth decay, drinking water is usually treated to contain 1.00 ppm of F^- ion. A cylindrical water tank has a diameter of 5.00 m and a depth of 12.0 m. What mass of NaF(s) is needed to establish a F^- ion concentration of 1.00 ppm in a tankful of water? What volume of 0.150 M NaF would be needed to achieve 1.00 ppm of F^-?

81. The workplace standard for $SO_2(g)$ in air is 5 ppm. Approximately what mass of sulfur could be burned in an enclosed workplace, 10.5 m $\times$ 5.4 m $\times$ 3.6 m, before this limit is exceeded?

82. The decomposition of ozone by chlorine atoms can be described by the rate law: rate = $k[Cl][O_3]$.

$$Cl(g) + O_3(g) \longrightarrow ClO(g) + O_2(g)$$
$$k = 7.2 \times 10^9 \text{ M}^{-1}\text{ s}^{-1} \text{ at 298 K}$$

How would the rate of ozone destruction be affected by doubling the concentration of chlorine atoms?

* 83. A newspaper article states the following: "Never dump oil down a sewer or water main. One quart of motor oil can make 250,000 gallons of water undrinkable. That is more water than 30 people drink in a lifetime." Estimate the concentration of the oil in the contaminated water, assuming thorough mixing. What other assumptions must you make?

84. The concentration of trichloroethane, CH_3CCl_3, in a sample of groundwater is 34 ppb. What is the concentration in nanomoles per liter?

* 85. A leaking tank spills 875 kg of 2-propanol into a lake with a volume of 1.8×10^8 L. How much is the BOD (in mg/L) increased by the spill? Assume that the 2-propanol is oxidized to CO_2.

86. Chlorine, even at very low concentrations, can be quite toxic to aquatic organisms. It also reacts with organic substances in the water to form toxic chlorinated organic compounds such as chloroform and chlorinated phenols. Wastewater that contains chlorine is therefore often dechlorinated before it is discharged. At low pH (below pH 1), chlorine exists principally as $Cl_2(aq)$. At high pH (above pH 8.5), the chlorine largely disproportionates to OCl^- and Cl^-. Two principal reagents are used to dechlorinate wastewater: sulfur dioxide (or salts that release SO_2, such as $NaHSO_3$) and hydrogen peroxide. Write equations for the reaction of OCl^- in wastewater with a pH of 12.3 with (a) $NaHSO_3$ and (b) H_2O_2.

87. Various regulations often require the reduction of phosphate levels before wastewater can be discharged to waterways. This can be done with any of several different precipitating agents such as (a) iron(III) chloride, (b) aluminum sulfate, or (c) CaO. Write the equation for the precipitation reaction that occurs with each of the reagents. In each case, calculate the cation concentration that must be present if the concentration of PO_4^{3-} is to be reduced to 10 ppm.

88. In investigating an old dump, a student finds a metal container filled with 12 oz of liquid. The label indicates that the can contains a substance that a reference book lists as a carcinogen. The concentration of the substance is given as 8.2 mg/fluid oz. On

further investigation, he finds that 20 billion such containers were once filled and distributed in the United States each year. **(a)** How many milligrams of the carcinogen are in each can? **(b)** How many metric tons of the carcinogen were distributed in this manner each year?

* **89.** If the average relative humidity on Earth's surface is 70% at the average Earth temperature of 14 °C, estimate the mass of water vapor in the lowest 1.0 km of the atmosphere. Earth has a land surface area of 1.5×10^6 km^2 and an area of 3.6×10^6 km^2 covered by water. Seawater is about 0.44 M in NaCl and 0.051 M in MgCl$_2$.

* **90.** An air conditioner takes outside air at 1.0 atm, 30 °C, and relative humidity of 85%, and cools it to 10 °C air that is saturated with water vapor. That cool air is exhausted into a room, which maintains the room at 21 °C. The vapor pressure of water at 10 °C is 9.2 Torr. **(a)** If the only source of water vapor is from the cooled air, what is the relative humidity in the room? **(b)** If 100 cubic feet of air is processed each minute, what mass of water vapor is condensed by the air conditioner over 8.0 hours of operation? **(c)** How much energy, in kilojoules, is released by the condensation described in (b)?

Apply Your Knowledge

* **91.** **[Collaborative]** Many industrial wastewater streams are contaminated with metal ions. Many of these ions can be effectively removed by precipitation as insoluble salts. As^{3+}, Cd^{2+}, Cr^{3+}, Cu^{2+}, Fe^{2+}, Mn^{2+}, Ni^{2+}, Pb^{2+}, and Zn^{2+} can be precipitated as hydroxides. Cd^{2+}, Co^{2+}, Cu^{2+}, Fe^{2+}, Hg^{2+}, Mn^{2+}, Ni^{2+}, Ag$^+$, Sn^{2+}, and Zn^{2+} can be precipitated as sulfides. Cd^{2+}, Ni^{2+}, and Pb^{2+} can be precipitated as carbonates. All these reactions are sensitive to the pH of the solution. For each group, write an equation for a representative reaction and state whether the reaction should be carried out at high pH or low pH. Explain.

* **92.** **[Environmental]** For the complete combustion of gasoline, the mass ratio of air to fuel should be about 14.5 to 1. Use ideas from this chapter and elsewhere in the text to show that this is about the ratio that you would predict. (*Hint:* Assume that C$_8$H$_{18}$ is a representative formula of gasoline, and use the composition of air given in Table 25.1.)

93. **[Environmental]** Propose a disposal method for each of the following wastes. Be as specific as possible, and justify your choice.

(a) hydrochloric acid contaminated with iron salts

(b) picric acid (an explosive)

(c) pentane contaminated with residues from penicillin production

* **94.** **[Environmental]** Use the following and other data from the text to show that if all the sulfur in coal used in electric power plants were converted to sulfuric acid, the quantity of acid produced would exceed current demand. (1) Annual U.S. coal consumption by electric power plants: approximately 8.7×10^8 ton. (2) Average SO$_2$ formation in the combustion of coal: 2 mg SO$_2$/kJ heat evolved. (3) Typical annual U.S. production of sulfuric acid: approximately 8.0×10^{10} lb. [*Hint:* You need to estimate the heat of combustion of coal. To do this, assume that coal is 100% C(graphite) and use data from Appendix C.]

* **95.** **[Environmental]** The world's termite population is estimated to be 2.4×10^{17}. Annually, these termites produce an estimated 4.6×10^{16} g CO$_2$. The atmosphere contains 5.2×10^{15} metric tons of air (1 metric ton = 1000 kg). On a number basis, the current CO$_2$ level in the atmosphere is 368 ppm. What fraction of this CO$_2$ level could be attributed to termites if none of the termite-produced CO$_2$ were removed by natural processes?

* **96.** **[Environmental]** An important variable in the combustion of gasoline in an internal combustion engine is the air : fuel ratio. The figure that follows shows how the emission of pollutants is related to the air : fuel ratio. Provide a plausible interpretation of

this figure. (*Hint:* Refer to Problem 92. Also, recall that RH represents hydrocarbons.)

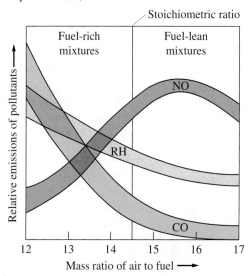

* **97.** **[Environmental]** To grow properly, common species of algae need carbon, nitrogen, and phosphorus atoms in the approximate ratio 106 C : 16 N : 1 P.

(a) Which is the limiting nutrient in a lake that has the following concentrations: C, 505 mg/L; N, 92 mg/L; and P, 14 mg/L?

(b) A scientific team wants to study algal growth in an experimental pond having the following atom ratio of nutrients: 44 C : 7 N : 1 P. They plan to achieve the appropriate nutrient mix by using a particular combination of *three* of the following chemicals: CO(NH$_2$)$_2$, CH$_3$CHOHCOOH, NH$_4$NO$_3$, NH$_4$H$_2$PO$_4$, (NH$_4$)$_2$HPO$_4$. Which three chemicals should they use if they wish to keep the total mass of chemicals *to a minimum*? What is the required *mass* ratio of these three chemicals?

* **98.** **[Environmental]** The herbicide dichlobenil (2,6-dichlorobenzonitrile, C$_7$H$_3$Cl$_2$N) has a solubility of 18 mg/L in water at 20 °C. The herbicide disintegrates with a half-life (first order) of 1.00 year. Suppose that 5.00×10^2 kg of dichlobenil is applied in the fields surrounding a 7.91-acre pond having an average depth of 5.25 ft. Suppose further that half of the dichlobenil permeates into the pond and that this happens within a few days.

(a) After a few days, what will be the concentration of dichlobenil in the pond, in ppm by mass and in molecules of dichlobenil per liter of pond water?

(b) How long would it take for the dichlobenil concentration in the pond to drop to 1.00 ppm following this single application?

(c) Suppose that the fields are treated with the dichlobenil in six-month intervals (fall and spring) each year for a number of years. What will be the concentration of dichlobenil in the pond just before the sixth application of the herbicide is made?

(d) Will the pond water eventually become saturated in dichlobenil? If so, when?

99. [Biochemical] A television mystery story indicated that a corpse contained 12 mg of chloroform. No liquid chloroform was found in the victim's stomach. This quantity supposedly could not have been self-administered as a vapor because the person would have become unconscious before achieving that quantity in her system. The quantity also was said to be less than a lethal dose. The *Merck Index* gives two values for the LD_{50} of chloroform: 2.18 mL/kg of body weight (14 day, orally in rats) and 0.9 mL/kg (organism and duration unspecified). The term LD_{50} refers to the dose that is lethal to half the administered population. Assuming that the corpse weighs 135 lb, how does the quantity of chloroform in her body compare to the lethal dose? What are some of the limitations of these calculations?

100. [Collaborative] The following quotations relating to hydrogen as a fuel are from "Letters to the Editor" in *Chemical and Engineering News*. How is it possible for scientists to have such divergent views on a seemingly straightforward matter?

April 1, 2002, D. C. MacWilliams, Alamo, CA: "The hydrogen fuel cell just shifts the pollution from the vehicle to the manufacturing facility. I believe that methane (or another hydrocarbon) fuel cell should be the focus."

April 1, 2002, George R. Lester, Salem, VA: "'Abundant, pollution-free hydrogen fuel' is a misleading myth unless it has been produced from nonfossil fuels such as solar, nuclear, wind (indirect solar), hydroelectric (very indirect solar), or the like."

April 29, 2002, Jerald A. Cole and Henry Wedaa, California Hydrogen Business Council, Long Beach, CA: "Furthermore, Lester's statement that "'Abundant, pollution-free hydrogen fuel' is a misleading myth" is absolutely untrue. Pollution-free hydrogen is even now being safely manufactured daily in factories around the world by the electrolysis of water—with an impeccable safety record."

June 3, 2002, Jason R. Guth, Chandler, AZ: "Converting fossil fuels to hydrogen can in no way reduce reliance on fossil fuels."

e-Media Problems

The activities described in these problems can be found in the Interactive student Tutorial (IST) module of the Companion Website, *http://chem.prenhall.com/hillpetrucci*.

101. View the **Heme** 3-D model (*Section 25-2*). By using the pop-up menu (right-click for Windows, click and hold for MacIntosh), change the representation of the model from ball-and-stick to space-filling. Why is the heme structure capable of bonding only to small molecules?

102. Consider the chemical reaction $3\ O_2(g) \longrightarrow 2\ O_3(g)$ described in detail in the **Stratospheric Ozone** animation (*Section 25-3*). **(a)** What is (are) the intermediate(s) of the reaction converting oxygen to ozone? **(b)** Construct an energy level diagram of the three elementary reactions leading to the production of ozone in an "energy-stabilized" state.

103. Compare the two sets of reactions seen in the **Catalytic Destruction of Stratospheric Ozone** animation and the **CFCs and Stratospheric Ozone** animation (*Section 25-3*). **(a)** What feature(s) is (are) common to the reaction mechanisms involving NO and Cl? **(b)** What extra energetic step is required to initiate the process described in the second animation?

104. View the **Carbon Dioxide Behaves as an Acid in Water** movie (*Section 25-7*). Review the properties of polyprotic acids in Section 15.5. **(a)** For the process seen in the movie, what species are present at equilibrium following the addition of dry ice to water? Write equations describing the corresponding reactions of **(b)** $SO_2(g)$ and **(c)** $SO_3(g)$.

Some Mathematical Operations

A.1 Exponential Notation

A number is in exponential form when it is written as the product of a coefficient—usually with a value between 1 and 10—and a power of ten. Following are two examples of *exponential notation*, a form usually employed by scientists and sometimes called *scientific notation*.

$$4.18 \times 10^3 \quad \text{and} \quad 6.57 \times 10^{-4}$$

Numbers are expressed in exponential form for two reasons: (1) We can write very large or very small numbers in a minimum of printed space and with a reduced chance of typographical error. (2) Numbers in exponential form convey explicit information about the precision of measurements: The number of significant figures in a measured quantity is stated unambiguously.

In the expression 10^n, n is the exponent of ten, and we say that the number ten is raised to the nth power. If n is a *positive* quantity, 10^n has a value *greater than 1*. If n is a *negative* quantity, 10^n has a value *less than 1*. We are particularly interested in cases where n is an integer, as in the following examples.

Positive Powers of 10
$10^0 = 1$
$10^1 = 10$
$10^2 = 10 \times 10 = 100$
$10^3 = 10 \times 10 \times 10 = 1000$
  and so on

The power of ten determines the number of zeros that follow the digit *1*.

Negative Powers of 10
$10^0 = 1$
$10^{-1} = 1/10 = 0.1$
$10^{-2} = 1/(10 \times 10) = 0.01$
$10^{-3} = 1/(10 \times 10 \times 10) = 0.001$
  and so on

The power of ten determines the number of places to the right of the decimal point where the digit *1* appears.

We express (a) 612,000 and (b) 0.000505 in exponential form as follows.

(a) $\quad 612{,}000 = 6.12 \times 100{,}000 = 6.12 \times 10^5$

(b) $\quad 0.000505 = 5.05 \times 0.0001 = 5.05 \times 10^{-4}$

The following approach provides a more direct method for converting numbers to the exponential form.

- Count the number of places a decimal point must be moved to produce a coefficient having a value between 1 and 10.
- The number of places counted then becomes the power of ten.
- The power of ten is *positive* if the decimal point is moved to the *left*.

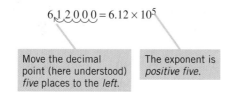

Move the decimal point (here understood) *five* places to the *left*.

The exponent is *positive five*.

One of the most common questions instructors encounter is "How do I use my calculator to do this?" You may find it a useful exercise to go through the calculations shown in this Appendix, using your calculator, to insure that you understand its use.

• The power of ten is *negative* if the decimal point is moved to the *right*.

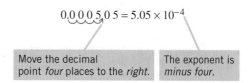

$$0.0\,0\,0\,5.0\,5 = 5.05 \times 10^{-4}$$

| Move the decimal point *four* places to the *right*. | The exponent is *minus four*. |

To convert a number from exponential form to the conventional form, move the decimal point in the opposite direction.

$$3.75 \times 10^6 = 3.7\,5\,0\,0\,0\,0. = 3{,}750{,}000$$

| The exponent is *six*. | Move the decimal point six places to the *right*. |

$$7.91 \times 10^{-7} = 0\,0\,0\,0\,0\,0\,0\,7\,.\,9\,1 = 0.000000791$$

| The exponent is *minus seven*. | Move the decimal point seven places to the *left*. |

Your calculator may require different keystrokes than those shown here. Check the specific instructions in the manual supplied with the calculator. Some two-line and graphing calculators may display the entire result, that is, 2.85×10^7 or 1.67×10^{-5}.

It is easy to handle exponential numbers on most calculators. A typical procedure is to enter the number, followed by the key EXP and then the exponent. To enter the number 2.85×10^7, the keystrokes required are [2] [.] [8] [5] [EXP] [7], and the result is displayed as 2.85^{07}. For the number 1.67×10^{-5}, the keystrokes are [1] [.] [6] [7] [EXP] [5] [±], and the result is displayed as 1.67^{-05}.

Many calculators can be set to convert all numbers and calculated results to the exponential form, regardless of the form in which the numbers are entered. Generally, the calculator can also be set to display a fixed number of significant figures in results.

Addition and Subtraction

With modern calculators it is rarely necessary to carry out operations such as addition and subtraction of exponential numbers by hand. However, it is quite important that you understand how such operations are carried out, so that you can correctly evaluate a calculator answer.

To add or subtract numbers in exponential notation with pencil and paper only, we must express each quantity as the same power of ten. This treats the power of ten in the same way as a unit—it is simply "carried along" in the calculation. In the following, each quantity is expressed to the power 10^{-3}.

$$(3.22 \times 10^{-3}) + (7.3 \times 10^{-4}) - (4.8 \times 10^{-4})$$
$$= (3.22 \times 10^{-3}) + (0.73 \times 10^{-3}) - (0.48 \times 10^{-3})$$
$$= (3.22 + 0.73 - 0.48) \times 10^{-3}$$
$$= 3.47 \times 10^{-3}$$

In contrast, most calculators perform these operations automatically, and you generally will not need to convert the numbers to the same power of ten when using a calculator.

Multiplication and Division

To multiply numbers expressed in exponential form, *multiply* all coefficients to obtain the coefficient of the result and *add* all exponents to obtain the power of ten in the result.

$$0.0803 \times 0.0077 \times 455 = (8.03 \times 10^{-2}) \times (7.7 \times 10^{-3}) \times (4.55 \times 10^2)$$
$$= (8.03 \times 7.7 \times 4.55) \times 10^{(-2-3+2)}$$
$$= (2.8 \times 10^2) \times 10^{-3} = 2.8 \times 10^{-1}$$

To divide two numbers in exponential form, *divide* the coefficients to obtain the coefficient of the result and *subtract* the exponent in the denominator from the exponent in the numerator to obtain the power of ten. The following example combines

multiplication and division. First, we apply the rule for multiplication separately to the numerator and to the denominator, and then we use the rule for division.

$$\frac{0.015 \times 0.0088 \times 822}{0.092 \times 0.48} = \frac{(1.5 \times 10^{-2})(8.8 \times 10^{-3})(8.22 \times 10^2)}{(9.2 \times 10^{-2})(4.8 \times 10^{-1})}$$

$$\frac{1.1 \times 10^{-1}}{4.4 \times 10^{-2}} = 0.25 \times 10^{-1-(-2)} = 0.25 \times 10^1$$

$$= 2.5 \times 10^{-1} \times 10^1 = 2.5$$

As with addition and subtraction, most calculators perform multiplication, division, and combinations of the two with no need to record intermediate results.

Raising a Number to a Power and Extracting the Root of an Exponential Number

To raise an exponential number to a given power, raise the coefficient to that power, and multiply the exponent by that power. For example, we can *cube* a number (raise it to the *third* power) in the following manner:

$$(0.0066)^3 = (6.6 \times 10^{-3})^3 = (6.6)^3 \times 10^{(-3) \times 3}$$

| Rewrite in exponential form. | Cube the coefficient. | Multiply the exponent by 3. |

$$= (2.9 \times 10^2) \times 10^{-9} = 2.9 \times 10^{-7}$$

To extract the root of an exponential number, we raise the number to a *fractional* power: one-half power for a square root, one-third power for a cube root, and so on. Most calculators have keys designed for extracting square roots and cube roots. Thus, to extract the square root of 1.57×10^{-5}, enter the number 1.57×10^{-5} into the calculator and use the $\left(\sqrt{} \right)$ key.

$$\sqrt{1.57 \times 10^{-5}} = 3.96 \times 10^{-3}$$

To extract the cube root of 3.18×10^{10}, enter the number 3.18×10^{10} and use the $\left(\sqrt[3]{} \right)$ key.

$$\sqrt[3]{3.18 \times 10^{10}} = 3.17 \times 10^3$$

Some calculators allow you to extract roots by keying in the root as a fractional exponent.

$$(2.75 \times 10^{-9})^{1/5} = 1.94 \times 10^{-2}$$

We can also extract the roots of numbers by using logarithms.

A.2 Logarithms

The common logarithm (log) of a number (N) is the exponent (x) to which the base 10 must be raised to yield the number.

$$\log N = x$$
$$N = 10^x$$
$$N = 10^{\log N}$$

Equivalent expressions

In the following expressions, the numbers N are printed in blue and their logarithms ($\log N$) are printed in red.

$$\log 1 = \log 10^0 = 0 \qquad\qquad \log 1 = \log 10^0 = 0$$
$$\log 10 = \log 10^1 = 1 \qquad\qquad \log 0.1 = \log 10^{-1} = -1$$
$$\log 100 = \log 10^2 = 2 \qquad\qquad \log 0.01 = \log 10^{-2} = -2$$
$$\log 1000 = \log 10^3 = 3 \qquad\qquad \log 0.001 = \log 10^{-3} = -3$$

Most of the numbers that we commonly encounter are not integral powers of ten, and their logarithms are not integral numbers. However, the preceding pattern gives us a general idea of what their logarithms might be. Consider, for example, the numbers 655 and 0.0078.

$$100 < 655 < 1000 \qquad 0.001 < 0.0078 < 0.01$$
$$2 < \log 655 < 3 \qquad -3 < \log 0.0078 < -2$$

Note that log 655 is between 2 and 3 and that log 0.0078 is between -3 and -2. To get a more exact value, however, we must use a table of logarithms or the [LOG] key on a calculator.

$$\log 655 = 2.816 \qquad \log 0.0078 = -2.11$$

In working with logarithms, we often need to find the *antilogarithm*, the number that has a certain value for its logarithm. We can think of the antilogarithm in the following terms.

$$\text{If } \log N = 3.576, \text{ then } N = 10^{3.576} = 3.77 \times 10^3.$$
$$\text{If } \log N = -4.57, \text{ then } N = 10^{-4.57} = 2.7 \times 10^{-5}.$$

With a calculator, we simply enter the value of the logarithm (3.576 or -4.57) and then use the $\left[10^x\right]$ key.

On some calculators, antilogarithms are found by entering the number, pressing a "second function" ([2nd]) key, then the [LOG] key.

Significant Figures in Logarithms

As they are written, $\log N = 3.576$ appears to have four significant figures and $N = 3.77 \times 10^3$ to have only three, but in reality both values have only *three*. Digits to the *left* of the decimal point in a logarithm simply relate to the power of ten in the exponential form of a number. The only significant digits in a logarithm are those to the *right* of the decimal point. The coefficient of the exponential form of the number should have this same number of digits. Thus, to express the logarithm of 2.5×10^{-12} to two significant figures, we would write $\log 2.5 \times 10^{-12} = -11.60$.

Some Relationships Involving Logarithms

We can use the definition of logarithms to write $M = 10^{\log M}$ and $N = 10^{\log N}$. For the product $(M \times N)$, we can write either of the following:

$$(M \times N) = 10^{\log M} \times 10^{\log N} = 10^{(\log M + \log N)}$$
$$(M \times N) = 10^{\log(M \times N)}$$

This means that the logarithm of the product of several terms is equal to the sum of the logarithms of the individual terms. Thus,

$$\log(M \times N) = (\log M + \log N) \qquad \textbf{(A.1)}$$

We can establish two other relationships in a similar manner.

$$\log \frac{M}{N} = (\log M - \log N) \qquad \textbf{(A.2)}$$

$$\log N^a = a \log N \qquad \textbf{(A.3)}$$

Equation (A.3) affords a simple method of extracting the roots of numbers. For example, to determine $(2.75 \times 10^{-9})^{1/5}$, write

$$\log(2.75 \times 10^{-9})^{1/5} = 1/5 \times \log(2.75 \times 10^{-9})$$
$$= 1/5 \times (-8.561) = -1.712$$
$$(2.75 \times 10^{-9})^{1/5} = 10^{-1.712} = 0.0194$$

Most scientific calculators have x^y and $\sqrt[y]{x}$ keys to determine powers and roots.

Natural Logarithms

Choosing *10* as the base for common logarithms is arbitrary. Other choices can be made as well. For example, to the base 2, $\log_2 8 = 3$. This simply means that $2^3 = 8$. And $\log_2 10 = 3.322$ means that $2^{3.322} = 10$.

Several of the relationships in this text involve *natural logarithms*. The base for natural logarithms (ln) is the quantity e, which has the value $e = 2.71828\cdots$. We

encounter the ln function in circumstances in which the rate of change of a variable is proportional to the value of that variable at the time the rate is measured. Such circumstances are common in physical science, including, for example, the rate of decay of a radioactive material (Section 19.3).

Generally we can work entirely within the natural logarithm system by using the calculator keys [ln] and $[e^x]$ rather than [LOG] and $[10^x]$. However, if we need to convert between natural and common logarithms, we can use the following conversion factor based on the relationship $\log_e 10 = 2.303$:

$$\ln N = 2.303 \log N \qquad \textbf{(A.4)}$$

A.3   Algebraic Operations

To solve an algebraic equation requires that we isolate one quantity—the unknown—on one side of the equation and the known quantities on the other side. This generally requires rearranging terms in the equation, and in these rearrangements, the guiding principle is that *whatever we do to one side of the equation, we must do to the other side as well*. Consider the equation

$$\frac{(5x^2 - 12)}{(x^2 + 4)} = 3$$

1. Multiply both sides of the equation by $(x^2 + 4)$.

$$\cancel{(x^2+4)}\frac{(5x^2 - 12)}{\cancel{(x^2+4)}} = 3 \times (x^2 + 4)$$

$$5x^2 - 12 = 3x^2 + 12$$

2. Subtract $3x^2$ from each side of the equation.

$$5x^2 - 3x^2 - 12 = \cancel{3x^2} - \cancel{3x^2} + 12$$

$$2x^2 - 12 = 12$$

3. Add 12 to each side of the equation.

$$2x^2 - \cancel{12} + \cancel{12} = 12 + 12 = 24$$

4. Divide each side of the equation by 2.

$$\frac{\cancel{2}x^2}{\cancel{2}} = \frac{24}{2} = 12$$

5. Extract the square root of each side of the equation.

$$\sqrt{x^2} = \pm\sqrt{12} = \pm\sqrt{4} \times \sqrt{3}$$

$$x = \pm 2\sqrt{3}$$

$$x = \pm 3.464$$

Quadratic Equations

A quadratic equation has *2* as the highest power of the unknown *x*. At times, quadratic equations are of the form

$$(x + n)^2 = m^2$$

To solve for *x*, extract the square root of each side.

$$(x + n) = \sqrt{m^2} = \pm m$$

and

$$x = m - n \quad \text{or} \quad x = -m - n$$

You will find a quadratic equation of this type in Example 14.12.

More often, however, the quadratic equation will be of the form

$$ax^2 + bx + c = 0$$

where a, b, and c are constants. To solve this equation for x, we can use the *quadratic formula*.

$$x = \frac{-b \pm \sqrt{b^2 - 4ac}}{2a} \qquad \text{(A.5)}$$

Consider the solution of the following quadratic equation.

$$50.3x^2 - 13.4x + 0.787 = 0$$

$$x = \frac{-(-13.4) \pm \sqrt{(-13.4)^2 - (4 \times 50.3 \times 0.787)}}{2 \times 50.3}$$

$$x = \frac{13.4 \times \sqrt{21.22}}{100.6} = \frac{13.4 \pm 4.61}{100.6}$$

$$x = \frac{13.4 + 4.61}{100.6} = 0.179 \quad \text{and} \quad x = \frac{13.4 - 4.61}{100.6} = 0.0874$$

We encounter this particular quadratic equation in Example 14.13, where we find that the only physically significant answer is $x = 0.0874$.

Solving Equations by Approximation

If an equation is of higher degree than quadratic, the most direct solution is often one of successive approximations. We gather the terms involving the unknown on one side of the equation and a constant term on the other side of the equation. Then we apply trial and error with a little reasoning. For example, consider the following equation:

$$\frac{4x^3}{(0.492 - 2x)^2} = 0.023$$

Suppose, based on the physical situation, that x must be a positive quantity smaller than 0.246. Then, let's guess at a possible value of x and see how close the result is to 0.023 when we substitute this value of x into the equation.

Try $x = 0.100$:

$$\frac{4x^3}{(0.492 - 2x)^2} = \frac{4 \times (0.100)^3}{[0.492 - (2 \times 0.100)]^2} = \frac{4 \times 10^{-3}}{[0.492 - 0.200]^2} = 0.0469$$

Because $0.0469 > 0.023$, our guess is not good enough. Now let's make a second approximation.

Try $x = 0.050$:

$$\frac{4x^3}{(0.492 - 2x)^2} = \frac{4 \times (0.050)^3}{[0.492 - (2 \times 0.050)]^2} = \frac{5.0 \times 10^{-4}}{[0.492 - 0.100]^2} = 0.0033$$

Now our result $0.0033 < 0.023$. We seem to be on the other side of the desired answer. We need to try a value $0.050 < x < 0.100$. We need a third approximation.

Try $x = 0.080$:

$$\frac{4x^3}{(0.492 - 2x)^2} = \frac{4 \times (0.080)^3}{[0.492 - (2 \times 0.080)]^2} = \frac{2.0 \times 10^{-3}}{[0.492 - 0.160]^2} = 0.018$$

In this third approximation, we have $0.018 < 0.023$. We are now much closer to an acceptable value of x. In some cases, this might be close enough, but suppose we try one more approximation, with $0.080 < x < 0.10$.

Try $x = 0.085$:

$$\frac{4x^3}{(0.492 - 2x)^2} = \frac{4 \times (0.085)^3}{[0.492 - (2 \times 0.085)]^2} = \frac{2.5 \times 10^{-3}}{[0.492 - 0.170]^2} = 0.024$$

Now we are very close to the correct answer, since $0.024 \approx 0.023$. (A further approximation would show that $0.084 < x < 0.085$.)

This method may seem laborious, but usually it is not. Once the format of the approximations is set up, the calculations can be quickly performed with a calculator.

Many graphing calculators will solve such equations very easily. Likewise, a computer spreadsheet such as Excel™ or Quattro Pro™ can be used to perform the successive approximations much more readily than can be done with a calculator.

A.4 Graphs

Suppose we obtain the following data for the quantities x and y as a result of laboratory measurements:

$$x = 0, y = 2 \qquad x = 2, y = 6 \qquad x = 4, y = 10$$
$$x = 1, y = 4 \qquad x = 3, y = 8 \qquad \ldots$$

Just by inspecting these data, you can probably see that they fit the equation

$$y = 2x + 2$$

Sometimes an exact equation cannot be written from the experimental data, or the form of the equation may not be immediately obvious from the data themselves. In these cases, it often proves helpful to graph the data. The data points listed above are plotted in the graph, in which the x values are placed along the horizontal axis (abscissa) and the y values along the vertical axis (ordinate). For each point in the figure, the x and y values are listed in the order (x, y).

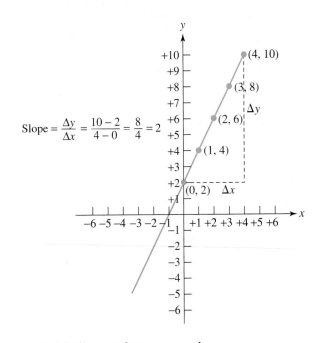

A straight-line graph: $y = mx + b$

We see that the data fall on a straight line. The equation for a straight-line graph is

$$y = mx + b$$

To obtain a value of the *intercept*, b, we set $x = 0$ and obtain the value of y. From the graph, we see that $y = 2$ when $x = 0$. To obtain the slope of the line, we can work with two points on the graph, denoted as points 1 and 2 below.

$$y_2 = mx_2 + b \quad \text{and} \quad y_1 = mx_1 + b$$

The *difference* between these two equations is

$$y_2 - y_1 = m(x_2 - x_1) + b - b$$

If the points do not fall exactly on the line, we draw the "best" straight line represented by the points, and select two points on it. Alternately, a computer spreadsheet will plot the data and determine the slope and intercept automatically. It is well worth your time to learn to use such tools.

The value of m is

$$m = \frac{y_2 - y_1}{x_2 - x_1} = \frac{\Delta y}{\Delta x}$$

The slope is evaluated in the figure; it is 2. Thus, the equation of the straight line is

$$y = mx + b = 2x + 2$$

A.5 Some Key Equations

On several occasions in the text, we refer to this appendix for details on the derivations of key equations or their manipulation into more useful forms. Abbreviated treatments follow. The first two require some prior knowledge of calculus.

Integrated Rate Equation for First-Order Reaction (Equation (13.7))

For the reaction

$$A \longrightarrow products$$

having the rate law

$$Rate\ of\ reaction = -(rate\ of\ disappearance\ of\ A) = k[A]$$

1. Replace the rate of disappearance of A by the derivative $d[A]/dt$.

$$-\frac{d[A]}{dt} = k[A]$$

2. Rearrange this expression to the form

$$\frac{d[A]}{[A]} = -kdt$$

3. Integrate between the limits A_0 at time $t = 0$ and A_t at time t.

$$\int_{[A]_0}^{[A]_t} \frac{d[A]}{[A]} = -k \int_0^t dt$$

4. The result obtained is

$$\ln\frac{[A]_t}{[A]_0} = -kt$$

Integrated Rate Equation for Second-Order Reaction (Equation (13.11))

For the reaction

$$A \longrightarrow products$$

having the rate law

$$Rate\ of\ reaction = -(rate\ of\ disappearance\ of\ A) = k[A]^2$$

1. Replace the rate of disappearance of A by the derivative $d[A]/dt$.

$$-\frac{d[A]}{dt} = k[A]^2$$

2. Rearrange this expression to the form

$$\frac{d[A]}{[A]^2} = -kdt$$

3. Integrate between the limits A_0 at time $t = 0$ and A_t at time t.

$$\int_{[A]_0}^{[A]_t} \frac{d[A]}{[A]^2} = -k \int_0^t dt$$

4. The result obtained is

$$-\frac{1}{[A]_t} + \frac{1}{[A]_0} = -kt \quad \text{or} \quad \frac{1}{[A]_t} = kt + \frac{1}{[A]_0}$$

The Arrhenius Equation (Equation (13.16))

Our goal is to convert the equation for the straight-line graph of Figure 13.15,

$$\ln k = \frac{-E_a}{RT} + \ln A$$

into an equation that eliminates the constant term, $\ln A$.

1. Write the equation for two different temperatures, T_1 and T_2, at which the rate constants are k_1 and k_2. (E_a and R are constants.)

$$\ln k_2 = \frac{-E_a}{RT_2} + \ln A \qquad \ln k_1 = \frac{-E_a}{RT_1} + \ln A$$

2. Subtract $\ln k_1$ from $\ln k_2$

$$\ln k_2 - \ln k_1 = \frac{-E_a}{RT_2} + \ln A - \left(\frac{-E_a}{RT_1} + \ln A\right)$$

3. Replace $\ln k_2 - \ln k_1$ by $\ln \frac{k_2}{k_1}$, and eliminate $\ln A$.

$$\ln \frac{k_2}{k_1} = \frac{E_a}{RT_1} - \frac{E_a}{RT_2} + \ln A - \ln A$$

4. Rearrange the equation to the final form.

$$\ln \frac{k_2}{k_1} = \frac{E_a}{R}\left(\frac{1}{T_1} - \frac{1}{T_2}\right)$$

The van't Hoff Equation (Equation (17.14))

Our goal is to convert the equation for the straight-line graph of Figure 17.13,

$$\ln K_{eq} = \frac{-\Delta H^\circ}{RT} + \text{constant}$$

into an equation that eliminates the term "constant," represented below as A.

1. Write the equation for two different temperatures, T_1 and T_2, at which the equilibrium constants are K_1 and K_2. (ΔH° and R are constants.)

$$\ln K_2 = \frac{-\Delta H^\circ}{RT_2} + \ln A \qquad \ln K_1 = \frac{-\Delta H^\circ}{RT_1} + \ln A$$

2. Subtract $\ln K_1$ from $\ln K_2$.

$$\ln K_2 - \ln K_1 = \frac{-\Delta H^\circ}{RT_2} + \ln A - \left(\frac{-\Delta H^\circ}{RT_1} + \ln A\right)$$

3. Replace $\ln K_2 - \ln K_1$ by $\ln \frac{K_2}{K_1}$, and eliminate $\ln A$.

$$\ln \frac{K_2}{K_1} = \frac{\Delta H^\circ}{RT_1} - \frac{\Delta H^\circ}{RT_2} + \ln A - \ln A$$

4. Rearrange the equation to the final form.

$$\ln \frac{K_2}{K_1} = \frac{\Delta H^\circ}{R}\left(\frac{1}{T_1} - \frac{1}{T_2}\right)$$

Some Basic Physical Concepts

B.1 Velocity and Acceleration

The speed of an object is the distance it travels per unit time. An automobile with a speedometer that reads 105 km/h will, if it continues at this constant speed for exactly one hour, travel a distance of 105 km. For scientific work, *velocity* is a more appropriate term. Velocity has two components: a *magnitude* (speed) and a *direction* (up, down, east, southwest, and so on). The SI units of velocity are distance $\times$ time^{-1}(m s^{-1}).

The velocity of an object changes if its speed or direction of motion changes. The rate of change of velocity is called *acceleration*, which has the units of velocity $\times$ time^{-1}(m s^{-1} $\times$ s^{-1} = m s^{-2}). For an object under a constant acceleration (a), its velocity (v) as a function of time (t) is

$$v = at \tag{B.1}$$

The distance (d) traveled is given by the following equation, which can be established by the methods of calculus.

$$d = \tfrac{1}{2}at^2 \tag{B.2}$$

The *constant acceleration due to gravity* (g) experienced by a freely falling body is 9.0866 m s^{-2}.

B.2 Force and Work

According to Newton's *first law* of motion, an object has a natural tendency—called *inertia*—to remain in motion at a constant velocity if it is moving or to remain at rest if it is not moving. A *force* is required to overcome the inertia of an object—that is, to give motion to an object at rest or to change the velocity of a moving object. Because a change in velocity is an acceleration, we can say that *a force is required to provide acceleration to an object*.

Newton's *second law* of motion describes the force (F) required to produce an acceleration (a) in an object of mass (m).

$$F = ma \tag{B.3}$$

The SI unit of force is the *newton* (N). It is the force required to produce an acceleration of 1 m s^{-2} in a 1-kg mass.

$$1 \text{ N} = 1 \text{ kg} \times 1 \text{ m s}^{-2} = 1 \text{ kg m s}^{-2} \tag{B.4}$$

The weight (W) of an object is the force of gravity on the object. It is the mass of the object multiplied by the acceleration due to gravity.

$$W = F = mg$$

Work is done when a force acts through a distance.

$$\text{Work}(w) = \text{force}(F) \times \text{distance}(d)$$

A joule (J) is the work done when a force of one newton acts through a distance of one meter. When we combine this definition and the SI units of the newton from Equation (B.4), we obtain the SI units of the joule.

$$1 \text{ J} = 1 \text{ N} \times 1 \text{ m} = 1 \text{ N m}$$

$$1 \text{ J} = 1 \text{ kg} \times 1 \text{ m s}^{-2} \times 1 \text{ m} = 1 \text{ kg m}^2 \text{ s}^{-2}$$

B.3   Energy

Energy is the capacity to do work. A moving object has *kinetic* energy as a result of its motion. The work associated with the moving object is given by the previous expressions (page A10).

$$w = F \times d = ma \times d$$

From Equation (B.2), we can substitute the expression for the distance, d, that is, $d = \frac{1}{2}at^2$.

$$w = ma \times \tfrac{1}{2}at^2 = \tfrac{1}{2} \times m(at)^2$$

Now, from Equation (B.1), we can substitute velocity (v) for the term at.

$$w = \tfrac{1}{2} \times m \times v^2$$

This is the work required to provide an object of mass m with a velocity v. This quantity of work appears as the kinetic energy (E_k) of the moving object.

$$E_k = \tfrac{1}{2}mv^2$$

In addition to kinetic energy associated with motion, an object may possess *potential energy*. Potential energy is stored energy that can be released under appropriate circumstances. Think of it as energy that stems from the condition, position, or composition of an object. In principle, equations can be written for the various ways in which potential energy is stored in an object, but we do not specifically use such equations in the text.

B.4   Magnetism

Attractive and repulsive forces associated with magnets are centered in regions of the magnets called *poles*. A magnet has a north pole and a south pole. If two magnets are arranged so that the north pole of one magnet is brought near the south pole of another magnet, there is an attractive force between the magnets. If like poles are brought close together—either both north poles or both south poles—there is a repulsive force. *Unlike poles attract, and like poles repel.*

A magnetic field exists in the region surrounding a magnet in which the influence of the magnet can be felt. For example, a magnetic field can be detected through deflections of a compass needle, or the field can be visualized through the attractive forces that cause a characteristic alignment of iron filings.

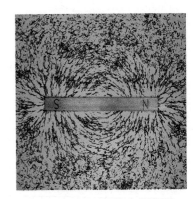

▲ **Visualizing a magnetic field of a bar magnet**

The sprinkling of iron filings outlines the magnetic field of a bar magnet.

B.5   Electricity

Electricity is a phenomenon closely related to magnetism. Ultimately, all bulk matter contains electrically charged particles: protons and electrons. However, an object displays a net electric charge—positive or negative—only when the numbers of electrons and protons in the object are unequal. The basic expression dealing with stationary electrically charged particles—static electricity—is Coulomb's law: The magnitude of the force (F) between electrically charged objects is directly proportional to the magnitudes of the charges (Q) and inversely proportional to the *square* of the distance (r) between them.

$$F \propto \frac{Q_1 \times Q_2}{r^2}$$

- *Like charges repel.* Whether both charges are positive or both are negative, their product is a positive quantity. A *positive* force is a *repulsive force.*
- *Unlike charges attract.* If one charge is positive and the other negative, their product is a negative quantity. A *negative* force is an *attractive* force.

An *electric field* exists in the region surrounding an electrically charged object in which the influence of the electric charge is felt. If an uncharged object is brought into

the field of a charged object, an electric charge of the opposite sign may be *induced* in the previously uncharged object. This leads to a force of attraction between the two. (See Figure 11.17.)

Electric current is a flow of charged particles—electrons in metallic conductors and positive and negative ions in molten salts and in aqueous salt solutions. The unit of electric charge is the *coulomb* (C). The unit of electric current is the *ampere* (A). A current of one ampere is the flow of one coulomb of electric charge per second.

$$1 \text{ A} = 1 \text{ C}/1 \text{ s} = 1 \text{ C s}^{-1}$$

Electric potential, or voltage, is the energy per unit of charge in an electric current. With coulomb as the unit of charge and joule as the unit of energy, the unit of electrical potential, 1 *volt* (V), is

$$1 \text{ V} = \frac{1 \text{ J}}{1 \text{ C}}$$

Electric *power* is the rate of production (or consumption) of electric energy. The electric power unit, the *watt* (W), signifies the production (or consumption) of one joule of energy per second.

$$1 \text{ W} = 1 \text{ J s}^{-1}$$

Because electric energy in joules is the product (volts × coulombs) and because coulombs per second (C s^{-1}) represents a current in amperes (A), we can also write the following expressions.

$$1 \text{ W} = 1 \text{ V C s}^{-1} = 1 \text{ V} \times 1 \text{ A}$$

As an example, the electric power associated with the passage of 10.0 amp through a 110-volt electric circuit is

$$110 \text{ V} \times 10.0 \text{ A} = 1100 \text{ W}$$

B.6   Electromagnetism

A variety of relationships between electricity and magnetism, collectively called *electromagnetism*, underlie some important practical applications: (1) Magnetic fields are associated with the flow of electrons, as in *electromagnets* (demonstrated in the photograph below). (2) Forces are experienced by current-carrying conductors in a magnetic field, as in *electric motors*. (3) Electric currents are induced when electric conductors are moved through a magnetic field, as in *electric generators*. Several phenomena described in this text are electromagnetic effects.

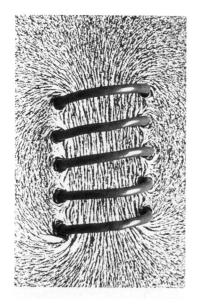

▲ **Visualizing a magnetic field of an electromagnet**

An electric current flowing through a coil of wire produces a magnetic field, outlined here by a sprinkling of iron filings.

▶ **An electromagnet**

Electric current from the battery passes through the coil of wire wrapped around an iron bar. The electric current induces a magnetic field and causes the bar to act as a magnet, attracting small iron objects. When the electric current is cut off, the magnetic field dissipates and the bar loses its magnetism.

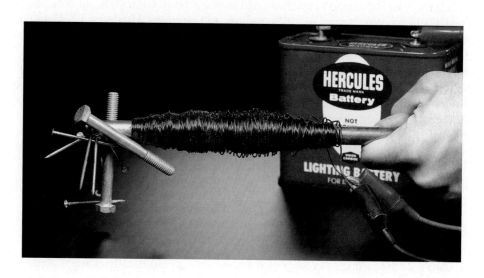

Data Tables

C.1 Thermodynamic Properties of Substances at 298.15 K*

Inorganic Substances

	ΔH_f°, kJ mol^{-1}	ΔG_f°, kJ mol^{-1}	S°, J mol^{-1}K^{-1}		ΔH_f°, kJ mol^{-1}	ΔG_f°, kJ mol^{-1}	S°, J mol^{-1}K^{-1}
Aluminum				BrCl(g)	14.6	−0.96	240.0
Al(s)	0	0	28.3	BrF$_3$(g)	−255.6	−229.5	292.4
Al^{3+}(aq)	−531	−485	−321.7	BrF$_3$(l)	−300.8	−240.6	178.2
AlCl$_3$(s)	−705.6	−630.1	109.3				
Al$_2$Cl$_6$(g)	−1291	−1221	490	**Cadmium**			
AlF$_3$(s)	−1504	−1425	66.48	Cd(s)	0	0	51.76
Al$_2$O$_3$(α, s)	−1676	−1582	50.92	Cd^{2+}(aq)	−75.90	−77.61	−73.2
Al(OH)$_3$(s)	−1276	—	—	CdCl$_2$(s)	−391.5	−344.0	115.3
Al$_2$(SO$_4$)$_3$(s)	−3441	−3100	239	CdO(s)	−258	−228	54.8
Barium				**Calcium**			
Ba(s)	0	0	62.3	Ca(s)	0	0	41.4
Ba^{2+}(aq)	−537.6	−560.8	9.6	Ca^{2+}(aq)	−542.8	−553.6	−53.1
BaCO$_3$(s)	−1216	−1138	112	CaBr$_2$(s)	−682.8	−663.6	130
BaCl$_2$(s)	−858.1	−810.4	123.7	CaCO$_3$(s)	−1207	−1128	88.70
BaF$_2$(s)	−1209	−1159	96.40	CaCl$_2$(s)	−795.8	−748.1	105
BaO(s)	−548.1	−520.4	72.09	CaF$_2$(s)	−1220	−1167	68.87
Ba(OH)$_2$(s)	−946.0	−859.4	107	CaH$_2$(s)	−186	−147	42
Ba(OH)$_2 \cdot$ 8 H$_2$O(s)	−3342	−2793	427	Ca(NO$_3$)$_2$(s)	−938.4	−743.2	193
BaSO$_4$(s)	−1473	−1362	132	CaO(s)	−635.1	−604.0	39.75
Beryllium				Ca(OH)$_2$(s)	−986.1	−898.6	83.39
Be(s)	0	0	9.54	Ca$_3$(PO$_4$)$_2$(s)	−4121	−3885	236
BeCl$_2$(s)	−496.2	−449.5	75.81	CaSO$_4$(s)	−1434	−1322	106.7
BeF$_2$(s)	−1027	−979.5	53.35	**Carbon** (See also the table of organic substances.)			
BeO(s)	−608.4	−579.1	13.77	C(g)	716.7	671.3	158.0
Bismuth				C (diamond)	1.90	2.90	2.38
Bi(s)	0	0	56.74	C (graphite)	0	0	5.74
BiCl$_3$(s)	−379	−315	177	CCl$_4$(g)	−102.9	−60.63	309.7
Bi$_2$O$_3$(s)	−573.9	−493.7	151	CCl$_4$(l)	−135.4	−65.27	216.2
Boron				C$_2$N$_2$(g)	308.9	297.2	242.3
B(s)	0	0	5.86	CO(g)	−110.5	−137.2	197.6
BCl$_3$(l)	−427.2	−387	206	CO$_2$(g)	−393.5	−394.4	213.6
BF$_3$(g)	−1137	−1120.3	254.0	CO$_3^{2-}$(aq)	−677.1	−527.8	−56.9
B$_2$H$_6$(g)	36	86.6	232.0	C$_3$O$_2$(g)	−93.72	−109.8	276.4
B$_2$O$_3$(s)	−1273	−1194	53.97	C$_3$O$_2$(l)	−117.3	−105.0	181.1
Bromine				COCl$_2$(g)	−220.9	−206.8	283.8
Br(g)	111.9	82.43	174.9	COS(g)	−138.4	−165.6	231.5
Br$^-$(aq)	−121.6	−104.0	82.4	CS$_2$(l)	89.70	65.27	151.3
Br$_2$(g)	30.91	3.14	245.4	**Chlorine**			
Br$_2$(l)	0	0	152.2	Cl(g)	121.7	105.7	165.1
				Cl$^-$(aq)	−167.2	−131.2	56.5

* Substances are at 1 atm pressure, and solutes in aqueous solutions are at unit activity ($\approx$1 M). Differences between these data and those based on the IUPAC recommended standard-state pressure of 1 bar, where they exist, are very small.

Inorganic Substances (continued)

	ΔH_f°, kJ mol^{-1}	ΔG_f°, kJ mol^{-1}	S°, J mol^{-1}K^{-1}		ΔH_f°, kJ mol^{-1}	ΔG_f°, kJ mol^{-1}	S°, J mol^{-1}K^{-1}
$Cl_2(g)$	0	0	223.0	$ICl(l)$	−23.89	−13.60	135.1
$ClF_3(g)$	−163.2	−123.0	281.5	**Iron**			
$ClO_2(g)$	102.5	120.5	256.7	$Fe(s)$	0	0	27.28
$Cl_2O(g)$	80.33	97.49	267.9	$Fe^{2+}(aq)$	−89.1	−78.90	−137.7
Chromium				$Fe^{3+}(aq)$	−48.5	−4.7	−315.9
$Cr(s)$	0	0	23.66	$FeCO_3(s)$	−740.6	−666.7	92.88
$Cr_2O_3(s)$	−1135	−1053	81.17	$FeCl_3(s)$	−399.5	−334.1	142.3
$CrO_4^{2-}(aq)$	−881.2	−727.8	50.21	$FeO(s)$	−272	−251.5	60.75
$Cr_2O_7^{2-}(aq)$	−1490	−1301	261.9	$Fe_2O_3(s)$	−824.2	−742.2	87.40
Cobalt				$Fe_3O_4(s)$	−1118	−1015	146
$Co(s)$	0	0	30.0	$Fe(OH)_3(s)$	−823.0	−696.6	107
$CoO(s)$	−237.9	−214.2	52.97	**Lead**			
$Co(OH)_2$ (pink, s)	−539.7	−454.4	79	$Pb(s)$	0	0	64.81
Copper				$Pb^{2+}(aq)$	−1.7	−24.43	10.5
$Cu(s)$	0	0	33.15	$PbI_2(s)$	−175.5	−173.6	174.8
$Cu^{2+}(aq)$	64.77	65.49	−99.6	$PbO_2(s)$	−277	−217.4	68.6
$CuCO_3 \cdot Cu(OH)_2(s)$	−1051	−893.7	186	$PbSO_4(s)$	−919.9	−813.2	148.6
$Cu_2O(s)$	−168.6	−146.0	93.14	**Lithium**			
$CuO(s)$	−157.3	−129.7	42.63	$Li(s)$	0	0	29.12
$Cu(OH)_2(s)$	−450.2	−373	108	$Li^+(aq)$	−278.5	−293.3	13.4
$CuSO_4 \cdot 5\,H_2O(s)$	−2279.6	−1880.1	300.4	$LiCl(s)$	−408.6	−384.4	59.33
Fluorine				$Li_2O(s)$	−597.94	−561.18	37.57
$F(g)$	78.99	61.92	158.7	$LiOH(s)$	−484.9	−439.0	42.80
$F^-(aq)$	−332.6	−278.8	−13.8	$LiNO_3(s)$	−483.1	−381.1	90.0
$F_2(g)$	0	0	202.7	**Magnesium**			
Helium				$Mg(s)$	0	0	32.69
$He(g)$	0	0	126.0	$Mg^{2+}(aq)$	−466.9	−454.8	−138.1
Hydrogen				$MgCl_2(s)$	−641.3	−591.8	89.62
$H(g)$	218.0	203.3	114.6	$MgCO_3(s)$	−1096	−1012	65.7
$H^+(aq)$	0	0	0	$MgF_2(s)$	−1124	−1071	57.24
$H_2(g)$	0	0	130.6	$MgO(s)$	−601.7	−569.4	26.94
$HBr(g)$	−36.40	−53.43	198.6	$Mg(OH)_2(s)$	−924.7	−833.9	63.18
$HCl(g)$	−92.31	−95.30	186.8	$MgSO_4(s)$	−1285	−1171	91.6
$HCl(aq)$	−167.2	−131.3	56.48	**Manganese**			
$HCN(g)$	135	125	201.7	$Mn(s)$	0	0	32.0
$HF(g)$	−271.1	−273.2	173.7	$Mn^{2+}(aq)$	−220.8	−228.1	−73.6
$HI(g)$	26.48	1.72	206.5	$MnO_2(s)$	−520	−465.2	53.05
$HNO_3(l)$	−173.2	−79.91	155.6	$MnO_4^-(aq)$	−541.4	−447.2	191.2
$HNO_3(aq)$	−207.4	−113.3	146.4	**Mercury**			
$H_2O(g)$	−241.8	−228.6	188.7	$Hg(g)$	61.32	31.85	174.9
$H_2O(l)$	−285.8	−237.2	69.91	$Hg(l)$	0	0	76.02
$H_2O_2(g)$	−136.1	−105.5	232.9	$HgO(s)$	−90.83	−58.56	70.29
$H_2O_2(l)$	−187.8	−120.4	110	**Nitrogen**			
$H_2S(g)$	−20.63	−33.56	205.7	$N(g)$	472.7	455.6	153.2
$H_2SO_4(l)$	−814.0	−690.1	156.9	$N_2(g)$	0	0	191.5
$H_2SO_4(aq)$	−909.3	−744.6	20.08	$NF_3(g)$	−124.7	−83.2	260.7
Iodine				$NH_3(g)$	−46.11	−16.48	192.3
$I(g)$	106.8	70.28	180.7	$NH_3(aq)$	−80.29	−26.57	111.3
$I^-(aq)$	−55.19	−51.57	111.3	$NH_4^+(aq)$	−132.5	−79.31	113.4
$I_2(g)$	62.44	19.36	260.6	$NH_4Br(s)$	−270.8	−175	113.0
$I_2(s)$	0	0	116.1	$NH_4Cl(s)$	−314.4	−203.0	94.56
$IBr(g)$	40.84	3.72	258.7	$NH_4F(s)$	−464.0	−348.8	71.96
$ICl(g)$	17.78	−5.44	247.4	$NH_4HCO_3(s)$	−849.4	−666.1	121

Inorganic Substances (continued)

	ΔH_f°, kJ mol^{-1}	ΔG_f°, kJ mol^{-1}	S°, J mol^{-1}K^{-1}		ΔH_f°, kJ mol^{-1}	ΔG_f°, kJ mol^{-1}	S°, J mol^{-1}K^{-1}
$NH_4I(s)$	−201.4	−113	117	**Silver**			
$NH_4NO_3(s)$	−365.6	−184.0	151.1	$Ag(s)$	0	0	42.55
$NH_4NO_3(aq)$	−339.9	−190.7	259.8	$Ag^+(aq)$	105.6	77.11	72.68
$(NH_4)_2SO_4(s)$	−1181	−901.9	220.1	$AgBr(s)$	−100.4	−96.90	107
$N_2H_4(g)$	95.40	159.3	238.4	$AgCl(s)$	−127.1	−109.8	96.2
$N_2H_4(l)$	50.63	149.2	121.2	$AgI(s)$	−61.84	−66.19	115
$NO(g)$	90.25	86.57	210.6	$AgNO_3(s)$	−124.4	−33.5	140.9
$N_2O(g)$	82.05	104.2	219.7	$Ag_2O(s)$	−31.0	−11.2	121
$NO_2(g)$	33.18	51.30	240.0	$Ag_2SO_4(s)$	−715.9	−618.5	200.4
$N_2O_4(g)$	9.16	97.82	304.2	**Sodium**			
$N_2O_4(l)$	−19.6	97.40	209.2				
$N_2O_5(g)$	11.3	115.1	355.7	$Na(g)$	107.3	76.78	153.6
$NO_3^-(aq)$	−205.0	−108.7	146.4	$Na(l)$	2.41	0.50	57.86
$NOBr(g)$	82.17	82.4	273.5	$Na(s)$	0	0	51.21
$NOCl(g)$	51.71	66.07	261.6	$Na^+(aq)$	−240.1	−261.9	59.0
				$Na_2(g)$	142.0	104.0	230.1
Oxygen				$NaBr(s)$	−361.1	−349.0	86.82
$O(g)$	249.2	231.7	160.9	$Na_2CO_3(s)$	−1131	−1044	135.0
$O_2(g)$	0	0	205.0	$NaHCO_3(s)$	−950.8	−851.0	102
$O_3(g)$	142.7	163.2	238.8	$NaCl(s)$	−411.1	−384.0	72.13
$OH^-(aq)$	−230.0	−157.2	−10.75	$NaCl(aq)$	−407.3	−393.1	115.5
$OF_2(g)$	24.5	41.8	247.3	$NaClO_3(s)$	−365.8	−262.3	123
				$NaClO_4(s)$	−383.3	−254.9	142.3
Phosphorus				$NaF(s)$	−573.7	−543.5	51.46
$P(\alpha, white)$	0	0	41.1	$NaH(s)$	−56.27	−33.5	40.02
$P(red)$	−17.6	−12.1	22.8	$NaI(s)$	−287.8	−286.1	98.53
$P_4(g)$	58.9	24.5	279.9	$NaNO_3(s)$	−467.9	−367.1	116.5
$PCl_3(g)$	−287.0	−267.8	311.7	$NaNO_3(aq)$	−447.4	−373.2	205.4
$PCl_3(l)$	−319.7	−272.3	217.1	$Na_2O_2(s)$	−510.9	−447.7	94.98
$PCl_5(g)$	−374.9	−305.0	364.5	$NaOH(s)$	−425.6	−379.5	64.48
$PCl_5(s)$	−443.5	—	—	$NaOH(aq)$	−469.2	−419.2	48.1
$PH_3(g)$	5.4	13.4	210.1	$NaH_2PO_4(s)$	−1537	−1386	127.5
$P_4O_{10}(s)$	−2984	−2698	228.9	$Na_2HPO_4(s)$	−1748	−1608	150.5
$PO_4^{3-}(aq)$	−1277	−1019	−222	$Na_3PO_4(s)$	−1917	−1789	173.8
				$NaHSO_4(s)$	−1125	−992.9	113
Potassium				$Na_2SO_4(s)$	−1387	−1270	149.6
$K(g)$	89.24	60.63	160.2	$Na_2SO_4(aq)$	−1390	−1268	138.1
$K(l)$	2.28	0.26	71.46	$Na_2SO_4 \cdot 10\,H_2O(s)$	−4327	−3647	592.0
$K(s)$	0	0	64.18	$Na_2S_2O_3(s)$	−1123	−1028	155
$K^+(aq)$	−252.4	−283.3	102.5	**Sulfur**			
$KBr(s)$	−393.8	−380.7	95.90				
$KCN(s)$	−113	−101.9	128.5	$S(rhombic)$	0	0	31.8
$KCl(s)$	−436.7	−409.2	82.59	$S_8(g)$	102.3	49.16	430.2
$KClO_3(s)$	−397.7	−296.3	143	$S_2Cl_2(g)$	−18.4	−31.8	331.5
$KClO_4(s)$	−432.8	−303.2	151.0	$SF_6(g)$	−1209	−1105	291.7
$KF(s)$	−567.3	−537.8	66.57	$SO_2(g)$	−296.8	−300.2	248.1
$KI(s)$	−327.9	−324.9	106.3	$SO_3(g)$	−395.7	−371.1	256.6
$KNO_3(s)$	−494.6	−394.9	133.1	$SO_4^{2-}(aq)$	−909.3	−744.5	20.1
$KOH(s)$	−424.8	−379.1	78.87	$S_2O_3^{2-}(aq)$	−648.5	−522.5	67
$KOH(aq)$	−482.4	−440.5	91.63	$SO_2Cl_2(g)$	−364.0	−320.0	311.8
$K_2SO_4(s)$	−1438	−1321	175.6	$SO_2Cl_2(l)$	−394.1	−314	207
				Tin			
Silicon							
$Si(s)$	0	0	18.8	$Sn(white)$	0	0	51.55
$SiH_4(g)$	34	56.9	204.5	$Sn(gray)$	−2.1	0.1	44.14
$Si_2H_6(g)$	80.3	127	272.5	$SnCl_4(l)$	−511.3	−440.2	259
$SiO_2(quartz)$	−910.9	−856.7	41.84	$SnO(s)$	−286	−257	56.5
				$SnO_2(s)$	−580.7	−519.7	52.3

Inorganic Substances (continued)

	ΔH_f°, kJ mol^{-1}	ΔG_f°, kJ mol^{-1}	S°, J mol^{-1}K^{-1}		ΔH_f°, kJ mol^{-1}	ΔG_f°, kJ mol^{-1}	S°, J mol^{-1}K^{-1}
Titanium				$UF_6(s)$	−2197	−2069	228
Ti(s)	0	0	30.6	$UO_2(s)$	−1085	−1032	77.03
$TiCl_4(g)$	−763.2	−726.8	355	**Zinc**			
$TiCl_4(l)$	−804.2	−737.2	252.3	Zn(s)	0	0	41.6
$TiO_2(s)$	−944.7	−889.5	50.33	$Zn^{2+}(aq)$	−153.9	−147.1	−112.1
Uranium				$ZnCl_2(s)$	−415.1	−369.4	111.5
U(s)	0	0	50.21	ZnO(s)	−348.3	−318.3	43.64
$UF_6(g)$	−2147	−2064	378				

Organic Substances

Formula	Name	ΔH_f°, kJ mol^{-1}	ΔG_f°, kJ mol^{-1}	S°, J mol^{-1}K^{-1}
$CH_4(g)$	Methane(g)	−74.81	−50.75	186.2
$C_2H_2(g)$	Acetylene(g)	226.7	209.2	200.8
$C_2H_4(g)$	Ethylene(g)	52.26	68.12	219.4
$C_2H_6(g)$	Ethane(g)	−84.68	−32.89	229.5
$C_3H_8(g)$	Propane(g)	−103.8	−23.56	270.2
$C_4H_{10}(g)$	Butane(g)	−125.7	−17.15	310.1
$C_6H_6(g)$	Benzene(g)	82.93	129.7	269.2
$C_6H_6(l)$	Benzene(l)	48.99	124.4	173.3
$C_6H_{12}(g)$	Cyclohexane(g)	−123.1	31.8	298.2
$C_6H_{12}(l)$	Cyclohexane(l)	−156.2	26.7	204.3
$C_{10}H_8(g)$	Naphthalene(g)	149	223.6	335.6
$C_{10}H_8(s)$	Naphthalene(s)	75.3	201.0	166.9
$CH_2O(g)$	Formaldehyde(g)	−117.0	−110.0	218.7
$CH_3OH(g)$	Methanol(g)	−200.7	−162.0	239.7
$CH_3OH(l)$	Methanol(l)	−238.7	−166.4	126.8
$CH_3CHO(g)$	Acetaldehyde(g)	−166.1	−133.4	246.4
$CH_3CHO(l)$	Acetaldehyde(l)	−191.8	−128.3	160.4
$CH_3CH_2OH(g)$	Ethanol(g)	−234.4	−167.9	282.6
$CH_3CH_2OH(l)$	Ethanol(l)	−277.7	−174.9	160.7
$C_6H_5OH(s)$	Phenol(s)	−165.0	−50.42	144.0
$(CH_3)_2CO(g)$	Acetone(g)	−216.6	−153.1	294.9
$(CH_3)_2CO(l)$	Acetone(l)	−247.6	−155.7	200.4
$CH_3COOH(g)$	Acetic acid(g)	−432.3	−374.0	282.5
$CH_3COOH(l)$	Acetic acid(l)	−484.1	−389.9	159.8
$CH_3COOH(aq)$	Acetic acid(aq)	−488.3	−396.6	178.7
$C_6H_5COOH(s)$	Benzoic acid(s)	−385.1	−245.3	167.6
$CH_3NH_2(g)$	Methylamine(g)	−23.0	32.3	242.6
$C_6H_5NH_2(g)$	Aniline(g)	86.86	166.7	319.2
$C_6H_5NH_2(l)$	Aniline(l)	31.6	149.1	191.3
$C_6H_{12}O_6(s)$	Glucose(s)	−1273.3	−910.4	212.1

C.2   Equilibrium Constants

A. Ionization Constants of Weak Acids at 25 °C

Name of Acid	Formula	K_a	Name of Acid	Formula	K_a
Acetic	$HC_2H_3O_2$	1.8×10^{-5}	Hyponitrous	HONNOH	8.9×10^{-8}
Acrylic	$HC_3H_3O_2$	5.5×10^{-5}		$HONNO^-$	4×10^{-12}
Arsenic	H_3AsO_4	6.0×10^{-3}	Iodic	HIO_3	1.6×10^{-1}
	$H_2AsO_4^-$	1.0×10^{-7}	Lactic	$HC_3H_5O_2$	1.4×10^{-4}
	$HAsO_4^{2-}$	3.2×10^{-12}	Malonic	$H_2C_3H_2O_4$	1.5×10^{-3}
Arsenous	H_3AsO_3	6.6×10^{-10}		$HC_3H_2O_4^-$	2.0×10^{-6}
Benzoic	$HC_7H_5O_2$	6.3×10^{-5}	Nitrous	HNO_2	7.2×10^{-4}
Bromoacetic	$HC_2H_2BrO_2$	1.3×10^{-3}	Oxalic	$H_2C_2O_4$	5.4×10^{-2}
Butyric	$HC_4H_7O_2$	1.5×10^{-5}		$HC_2O_4^-$	5.3×10^{-5}
Carbonic	H_2CO_3	4.4×10^{-7}	Phenol	HOC_6H_5	1.0×10^{-10}
	HCO_3^-	4.7×10^{-11}	Phenylacetic	$HC_8H_7O_2$	4.9×10^{-5}
Chloroacetic	$HC_2H_2ClO_2$	1.4×10^{-3}	Phosphoric	H_3PO_4	7.1×10^{-3}
Chlorous	$HClO_2$	1.1×10^{-2}		$H_2PO_4^-$	6.3×10^{-8}
Citric	$H_3C_6H_5O_7$	7.4×10^{-4}		HPO_4^{2-}	4.2×10^{-13}
	$H_2C_6H_5O_7^-$	1.7×10^{-5}	Phosphorus	H_3PO_3	3.7×10^{-2}
	$HC_6H_5O_7^{2-}$	4.0×10^{-7}		$H_2PO_3^-$	2.1×10^{-7}
Cyanic	HOCN	3.5×10^{-4}	Propionic	$HC_3H_5O_2$	1.3×10^{-5}
Dichloroacetic	$HC_2HCl_2O_2$	5.5×10^{-2}	Pyrophosphoric	$H_4P_2O_7$	3.0×10^{-2}
Fluoroacetic	$HC_2H_2FO_2$	2.6×10^{-3}		$H_3P_2O_7^-$	4.4×10^{-3}
Formic	$HCHO_2$	1.8×10^{-4}		$H_2P_2O_7^{2-}$	2.5×10^{-7}
Hydrazoic	HN_3	1.9×10^{-5}		$HP_2O_7^{3-}$	5.6×10^{-10}
Hydrocyanic	HCN	6.2×10^{-10}	Selenic	H_2SeO_4	strong acid
Hydrofluoric	HF	6.6×10^{-4}		$HSeO_4^-$	2.2×10^{-2}
Hydrogen peroxide	H_2O_2	2.2×10^{-12}	Selenous	H_2SeO_3	2.3×10^{-3}
Hydroselenic	H_2Se	1.3×10^{-4}		$HSeO_3^-$	5.4×10^{-9}
	HSe^-	1×10^{-11}	Succinic	$H_2C_4H_4O_4$	6.2×10^{-5}
Hydrosulfuric	H_2S	1.0×10^{-7}		$HC_4H_4O_4^-$	2.3×10^{-6}
	HS^-	1×10^{-19}	Sulfuric	H_2SO_4	strong acid
Hydrotelluric	H_2Te	2.3×10^{-3}		HSO_4^-	1.1×10^{-2}
	HTe^-	1.6×10^{-11}	Sulfurous	H_2SO_3	1.3×10^{-2}
Hypobromous	HOBr	2.5×10^{-9}		HSO_3^-	6.2×10^{-8}
Hypochlorous	HOCl	2.9×10^{-8}	Thiophenol	HSC_6H_5	3.2×10^{-7}
Hypoiodous	HOI	2.3×10^{-11}	Trichloroacetic	$HC_2Cl_3O_2$	3.0×10^{-1}

B. Ionization Constants of Weak Bases at 25 °C

Name of Base	Formula	K_b
Ammonia	NH_3	1.8×10^{-5}
Aniline	$C_6H_5NH_2$	7.4×10^{-10}
Codeine	$C_{18}H_{21}O_3N$	8.9×10^{-7}
Diethylamine	$(C_2H_5)_2NH$	6.9×10^{-4}
Dimethylamine	$(CH_3)_2NH$	5.9×10^{-4}
Ethylamine	$C_2H_5NH_2$	4.3×10^{-4}
Hydrazine	NH_2NH_2	8.5×10^{-7}
	$NH_2NH_3^+$	8.9×10^{-16}
Hydroxylamine	NH_2OH	9.1×10^{-9}
Isoquinoline	C_9H_7N	2.5×10^{-9}
Methylamine	CH_3NH_2	4.2×10^{-4}
Morphine	$C_{17}H_{19}O_3N$	7.4×10^{-7}
Piperidine	$C_5H_{11}N$	1.3×10^{-3}
Pyridine	C_5H_5N	1.5×10^{-9}
Quinoline	C_9H_7N	6.3×10^{-10}
Triethanolamine	$C_6H_{15}O_3N$	5.8×10^{-7}
Triethylamine	$(C_2H_5)_3N$	5.2×10^{-4}
Trimethylamine	$(CH_3)_3N$	6.3×10^{-5}

C. Solubility Product Constants[a]

Name of Solute	Formula	K_{sp}	Name of Solute	Formula	K_{sp}
Aluminum hydroxide	$Al(OH)_3$	1.3×10^{-33}	Copper(II) carbonate	$CuCO_3$	1.4×10^{-10}
Aluminum phosphate	$AlPO_4$	6.3×10^{-19}	Copper(II) chromate	$CuCrO_4$	3.6×10^{-6}
Barium carbonate	$BaCO_3$	5.1×10^{-9}	Copper(II) ferrocyanide	$Cu_2[Fe(CN)_6]$	1.3×10^{-16}
Barium chromate	$BaCrO_4$	1.2×10^{-10}	Copper(II) hydroxide	$Cu(OH)_2$	2.2×10^{-20}
Barium fluoride	BaF_2	1.0×10^{-6}	Copper(II) sulfide[b]	CuS	6×10^{-37}
Barium hydroxide	$Ba(OH)_2$	5×10^{-3}	Iron(II) carbonate	$FeCO_3$	3.2×10^{-11}
Barium sulfate	$BaSO_4$	1.1×10^{-10}	Iron(II) hydroxide	$Fe(OH)_2$	8.0×10^{-16}
Barium sulfite	$BaSO_3$	8×10^{-7}	Iron(II) sulfide[b]	FeS	6×10^{-19}
Barium thiosulfate	BaS_2O_3	1.6×10^{-5}	Iron(III) arsenate	$FeAsO_4$	5.7×10^{-21}
Bismuthyl chloride	$BiOCl$	1.8×10^{-31}	Iron(III) ferrocyanide	$Fe_4[Fe(CN)_6]_3$	3.3×10^{-41}
Bismuthyl hydroxide	$BiOOH$	4×10^{-10}	Iron(III) hydroxide	$Fe(OH)_3$	4×10^{-38}
Cadmium carbonate	$CdCO_3$	5.2×10^{-12}	Iron(III) phosphate	$FePO_4$	1.3×10^{-22}
Cadmium hydroxide	$Cd(OH)_2$	2.5×10^{-14}	Lead(II) arsenate	$Pb_3(AsO_4)_2$	4.0×10^{-36}
Cadmium sulfide[b]	CdS	8×10^{-28}	Lead(II) azide	$Pb(N_3)_2$	2.5×10^{-9}
Calcium carbonate	$CaCO_3$	2.8×10^{-9}	Lead(II) bromide	$PbBr_2$	4.0×10^{-5}
Calcium chromate	$CaCrO_4$	7.1×10^{-4}	Lead(II) carbonate	$PbCO_3$	7.4×10^{-14}
Calcium fluoride	CaF_2	5.3×10^{-9}	Lead(II) chloride	$PbCl_2$	1.6×10^{-5}
Calcium hydrogen phosphate	$CaHPO_4$	1×10^{-7}	Lead(II) chromate	$PbCrO_4$	2.8×10^{-13}
Calcium hydroxide	$Ca(OH)_2$	5.5×10^{-6}	Lead(II) fluoride	PbF_2	2.7×10^{-8}
Calcium oxalate	CaC_2O_4	2.7×10^{-9}	Lead(II) hydroxide	$Pb(OH)_2$	1.2×10^{-15}
Calcium phosphate	$Ca_3(PO_4)_2$	2.0×10^{-29}	Lead(II) iodide	PbI_2	7.1×10^{-9}
Calcium sulfate	$CaSO_4$	9.1×10^{-6}	Lead(II) sulfate	$PbSO_4$	1.6×10^{-8}
Calcium sulfite	$CaSO_3$	6.8×10^{-8}	Lead(II) sulfide[b]	PbS	3×10^{-28}
Chromium(II) hydroxide	$Cr(OH)_2$	2×10^{-16}	Lead(II) thiosulfate	PbS_2O_3	4.0×10^{-7}
Chromium(III) hydroxide	$Cr(OH)_3$	6.3×10^{-31}	Lithium fluoride	LiF	3.8×10^{-3}
Cobalt(II) carbonate	$CoCO_3$	1.4×10^{-13}	Lithium phosphate	Li_3PO_4	3.2×10^{-9}
Cobalt(II) hydroxide	$Co(OH)_2$	1.6×10^{-15}	Magnesium ammonium phosphate	$MgNH_4PO_4$	2.5×10^{-13}
Cobalt(III) hydroxide	$Co(OH)_3$	1.6×10^{-44}	Magnesium carbonate	$MgCO_3$	3.5×10^{-8}
Copper(I) chloride	$CuCl$	1.2×10^{-6}	Magnesium fluoride	MgF_2	3.7×10^{-8}
Copper(I) cyanide	$CuCN$	3.2×10^{-20}	Magnesium hydroxide	$Mg(OH)_2$	1.8×10^{-11}
Copper(I) iodide	CuI	1.1×10^{-12}	Magnesium phosphate	$Mg_3(PO_4)_2$	1×10^{-25}
Copper(II) arsenate	$Cu_3(AsO_4)_2$	7.6×10^{-36}			

[a] Data are at various temperatures around room temperature, from 18 to 25 °C.

[b] For a solubility equilibrium of the type $MS(s) + H_2O \rightleftharpoons M^{2+}(aq) + HS^-(aq) + OH^-(aq)$.

C. Solubility Product Constants (continued)

Name of Solute	Formula	K_{sp}	Name of Solute	Formula	K_{sp}
Manganese(II) carbonate	$MnCO_3$	1.8×10^{-11}	Silver nitrite	$AgNO_2$	6.0×10^{-4}
Manganese(II) hydroxide	$Mn(OH)_2$	1.9×10^{-13}	Silver sulfate	Ag_2SO_4	1.4×10^{-5}
Manganese(II) sulfide[b]	MnS	3×10^{-14}	Silver sulfide[b]	Ag_2S	6×10^{-51}
Mercury(I) bromide	Hg_2Br_2	5.6×10^{-23}	Silver sulfite	Ag_2SO_3	1.5×10^{-14}
Mercury(I) chloride	Hg_2Cl_2	1.3×10^{-18}	Silver thiocyanate	$AgSCN$	1.0×10^{-12}
Mercury(I) iodide	Hg_2I_2	4.5×10^{-29}	Strontium carbonate	$SrCO_3$	1.1×10^{-10}
Mercury(II) sulfide[b]	HgS	2×10^{-53}	Strontium chromate	$SrCrO_4$	2.2×10^{-5}
Nickel(II) carbonate	$NiCO_3$	6.6×10^{-9}	Strontium fluoride	SrF_2	2.5×10^{-9}
Nickel(II) hydroxide	$Ni(OH)_2$	2.0×10^{-15}	Strontium sulfate	$SrSO_4$	3.2×10^{-7}
Scandium fluoride	ScF_3	4.2×10^{-18}	Thallium(I) bromide	$TlBr$	3.4×10^{-6}
Scandium hydroxide	$Sc(OH)_3$	8.0×10^{-31}	Thallium(I) chloride	$TlCl$	1.7×10^{-4}
Silver arsenate	Ag_3AsO_4	1.0×10^{-22}	Thallium(I) iodide	TlI	6.5×10^{-8}
Silver azide	AgN_3	2.8×10^{-9}	Thallium(III) hydroxide	$Tl(OH)_3$	6.3×10^{-46}
Silver bromide	$AgBr$	5.0×10^{-13}	Tin(II) hydroxide	$Sn(OH)_2$	1.4×10^{-28}
Silver carbonate	Ag_2CO_3	8.5×10^{-12}	Tin(II) sulfide[b]	SnS	1×10^{-26}
Silver chloride	$AgCl$	1.8×10^{-10}	Zinc carbonate	$ZnCO_3$	1.4×10^{-11}
Silver chromate	Ag_2CrO_4	1.1×10^{-12}	Zinc hydroxide	$Zn(OH)_2$	1.2×10^{-17}
Silver cyanide	$AgCN$	1.2×10^{-16}	Zinc oxalate	ZnC_2O_4	2.7×10^{-8}
Silver iodate	$AgIO_3$	3.0×10^{-8}	Zinc phosphate	$Zn_3(PO_4)_2$	9.0×10^{-33}
Silver iodide	AgI	8.5×10^{-17}	Zinc sulfide[b]	ZnS	2×10^{-25}

D. Complex Ion Formation Constants[a]

Formula	K_f	Formula	K_f
$[Ag(CN)_2]^-$	5.6×10^{18}	$[Fe(en)_3]^{2+}$	5.0×10^9
$[Ag(EDTA)]^{3-}$	2.1×10^7	$[Fe(ox)_3]^{4-}$	1.7×10^5
$[Ag(en)_2]^+$	5.0×10^7	$[Fe(CN)_6]^{3-}$	10^{42}
$[Ag(NH_3)_2]^+$	1.6×10^7	$[Fe(EDTA)]^-$	1.7×10^{24}
$[Ag(SCN)_4]^{3-}$	1.2×10^{10}	$[Fe(ox)_3]^{3-}$	2×10^{20}
$[Ag(S_2O_3)_2]^{3-}$	1.7×10^{13}	$[Fe(SCN)]^{2+}$	8.9×10^2
$[Al(EDTA)]^-$	1.3×10^{16}	$[HgCl_4]^{2-}$	1.2×10^{15}
$[Al(OH)_4]^-$	1.1×10^{33}	$[Hg(CN)_4]^{2-}$	3×10^{41}
$[Al(ox)_3]^{3-}$	2×10^{16}	$[Hg(EDTA)]^{2-}$	6.3×10^{21}
$[Cd(CN)_4]^{2-}$	6.0×10^{18}	$[Hg(en)_2]^{2+}$	2×10^{23}
$[Cd(en)_3]^{2+}$	1.2×10^{12}	$[HgI_4]^{2-}$	6.8×10^{29}
$[Cd(NH_3)_4]^{2+}$	1.3×10^7	$[Hg(ox)_2]^{2-}$	9.5×10^6
$[Co(EDTA)]^{2-}$	2.0×10^{16}	$[Ni(CN)_4]^{2-}$	2×10^{31}
$[Co(en)_3]^{2+}$	8.7×10^{13}	$[Ni(EDTA)]^{2-}$	3.6×10^{18}
$[Co(NH_3)_6]^{2+}$	1.3×10^5	$[Ni(en)_3]^{2+}$	2.1×10^{18}
$[Co(ox)_3]^{4-}$	5×10^9	$[Ni(NH_3)_6]^{2+}$	5.5×10^8
$[Co(SCN)_4]^{2-}$	1.0×10^3	$[Ni(ox)_3]^{4-}$	3×10^8
$[Co(EDTA)]^-$	10^{36}	$[PbCl_3]^-$	2.4×10^1
$[Co(en)_3]^{3+}$	4.9×10^{48}	$[Pb(EDTA)]^{2-}$	2×10^{18}
$[Co(NH_3)_6]^{3+}$	4.5×10^{33}	$[PbI_4]^{2-}$	3.0×10^4
$[Co(ox)_3]^{3-}$	10^{20}	$[Pb(OH)_3]^-$	3.8×10^{14}
$[Cr(EDTA)]^-$	10^{23}	$[Pb(ox)_2]^{2-}$	3.5×10^6
$[Cr(OH)_4]^-$	8×10^{29}	$[Pb(S_2O_3)_3]^{4-}$	2.2×10^6
$[CuCl_3]^{2-}$	5×10^5	$[PtCl_4]^{2-}$	1×10^{16}
$[Cu(CN)_4]^{3-}$	2.0×10^{30}	$[Pt(NH_3)_6]^{2+}$	2×10^{35}
$[Cu(EDTA)]^{2-}$	5×10^{18}	$[Zn(CN)_4]^{2-}$	1×10^{18}
$[Cu(en)_2]^{2+}$	1×10^{20}	$[Zn(EDTA)]^{2-}$	3×10^{16}
$[Cu(NH_3)_4]^{2+}$	1.1×10^{13}	$[Zn(en)_3]^{2+}$	1.3×10^{14}
$[Cu(ox)_2]^{2-}$	3×10^8	$[Zn(NH_3)_4]^{2+}$	4.1×10^8
$[Fe(CN)_6]^{4-}$	10^{37}	$[Zn(OH)_4]^{2-}$	4.6×10^{17}
$[Fe(EDTA)]^{2-}$	2.1×10^{14}	$[Zn(ox)_3]^{4-}$	1.4×10^8

[a] The ligands referred to in this table are monodentate: Cl^-, CN^-, I^-, NH_3, OH^-, SCN^-, $S_2O_3^{2-}$; bidentate: ethylenediamine, en; oxalate ion, ox ($C_2O_4^{2-}$); tetradentate: ethylenediaminetetraacetato ion, $EDTA^{4-}$.

C.3 Standard Electrode (Reduction) Potentials at 25 °C

Reduction Half-Reaction	$E°$, V
$F_2(g) + 2\,e^- \longrightarrow 2\,F^-(aq)$	+2.866
$OF_2(g) + 2\,H^+(aq) + 4\,e^- \longrightarrow H_2O(l) + 2\,F^-(aq)$	+2.1
$O_3(g) + 2\,H^+(aq) + 2\,e^- \longrightarrow O_2(g) + H_2O(l)$	+2.075
$S_2O_8^{2-}(aq) + 2\,e^- \longrightarrow 2\,SO_4^{2-}(aq)$	+2.01
$Ag^{2+}(aq) + e^- \longrightarrow Ag^+(aq)$	+1.98
$H_2O_2(aq) + 2\,H^+(aq) + 2\,e^- \longrightarrow 2\,H_2O(l)$	+1.763
$MnO_4^-(aq) + 4\,H^+(aq) + 3\,e^- \longrightarrow MnO_2(s) + 2\,H_2O(l)$	+1.70
$PbO_2(s) + SO_4^{2-}(aq) + 4\,H^+(aq) + 2\,e^- \longrightarrow PbSO_4(s) + 2\,H_2O(l)$	+1.69
$Au^{3+}(aq) + 3\,e^- \longrightarrow Au(s)$	+1.52
$MnO_4^-(aq) + 8\,H^+(aq) + 5\,e^- \longrightarrow Mn^{2+}(aq) + 4\,H_2O(l)$	+1.51
$2\,BrO_3^-(aq) + 12\,H^+(aq) + 10\,e^- \longrightarrow Br_2(l) + 6\,H_2O(l)$	+1.478
$PbO_2(s) + 4\,H^+(aq) + 2\,e^- \longrightarrow Pb^{2+}(aq) + 2\,H_2O(l)$	+1.455
$ClO_3^-(aq) + 6\,H^+(aq) + 6\,e^- \longrightarrow Cl^-(aq) + 3\,H_2O(l)$	+1.450
$Au^{3+}(aq) + 2\,e^- \longrightarrow Au^+(aq)$	+1.36
$Cl_2(g) + 2\,e^- \longrightarrow 2\,Cl^-(aq)$	+1.358
$Cr_2O_7^{2-}(aq) + 14\,H^+(aq) + 6\,e^- \longrightarrow 2\,Cr^{3+}(aq) + 7\,H_2O(l)$	+1.33
$MnO_2(s) + 4\,H^+(aq) + 2\,e^- \longrightarrow Mn^{2+}(aq) + 2\,H_2O(l)$	+1.23
$O_2(g) + 4\,H^+(aq) + 4\,e^- \longrightarrow 2\,H_2O(l)$	+1.229
$2\,IO_3^-(aq) + 12\,H^+(aq) + 10\,e^- \longrightarrow I_2(s) + 6\,H_2O(l)$	+1.20
$ClO_4^-(aq) + 2\,H^+(aq) + 2\,e^- \longrightarrow ClO_3^-(aq) + H_2O(l)$	+1.19
$ClO_3^-(aq) + 2\,H^+(aq) + e^- \longrightarrow ClO_2(g) + H_2O(l)$	+1.175
$NO_2(g) + H^+(aq) + e^- \longrightarrow HNO_2(aq)$	+1.07
$Br_2(l) + 2\,e^- \longrightarrow 2\,Br^-(aq)$	+1.065
$NO_2(g) + 2\,H^+(aq) + 2\,e^- \longrightarrow NO(g) + H_2O(l)$	+1.03
$[AuCl_4]^-(aq) + 3\,e^- \longrightarrow Au(s) + 4\,Cl^-(aq)$	+1.002
$VO_2^+(aq) + 2\,H^+(aq) + e^- \longrightarrow VO^{2+}(aq) + H_2O(l)$	+1.000
$NO_3^-(aq) + 4\,H^+(aq) + 3\,e^- \longrightarrow NO(g) + 2\,H_2O(l)$	+0.956
$Hg^{2+}(aq) + 2\,e^- \longrightarrow Hg(l)$	+0.854
$Ag^+(aq) + e^- \longrightarrow Ag(s)$	+0.800
$Fe^{3+}(aq) + e^- \longrightarrow Fe^{2+}(aq)$	+0.771
$O_2(g) + 2\,H^+(aq) + 2\,e^- \longrightarrow H_2O_2(aq)$	+0.695
$2\,HgCl_2(aq) + 2\,e^- \longrightarrow Hg_2Cl_2(s) + 2\,Cl^-(aq)$	+0.63
$MnO_4^-(aq) + e^- \longrightarrow MnO_4^{2-}(aq)$	+0.56
$I_2(s) + 2\,e^- \longrightarrow 2\,I^-(aq)$	+0.535
$Cu^+(aq) + e^- \longrightarrow Cu(s)$	+0.520
$H_2SO_3(aq) + 4\,H^+(aq) + 4\,e^- \longrightarrow S(s) + 3\,H_2O(l)$	+0.449
$C_2N_2(g) + 2\,H^+(aq) + 2\,e^- \longrightarrow 2\,HCN(aq)$	+0.37
$[Fe(CN)_6]^{3-}(aq) + e^- \longrightarrow [Fe(CN)_6]^{4-}(aq)$	+0.361
$Cu^{2+}(aq) + 2\,e^- \longrightarrow Cu(s)$	+0.340
$VO^{2+}(aq) + 2\,H^+(aq) + e^- \longrightarrow V^{3+}(aq) + H_2O(l)$	+0.337
$PbO_2(s) + 2\,H^+(aq) + 2\,e^- \longrightarrow PbO(s) + H_2O(l)$	+0.28
$Hg_2Cl_2(s) + 2\,e^- \longrightarrow 2\,Hg(l) + 2\,Cl^-(aq)$	+0.2676
$HAsO_2(aq) + 3\,H^+(aq) + 3\,e^- \longrightarrow As(s) + 2\,H_2O(l)$	+0.240
$AgCl(s) + e^- \longrightarrow Ag(s) + Cl^-(aq)$	+0.2223
$SO_4^{2-}(aq) + 4\,H^+(aq) + 2\,e^- \longrightarrow 2\,H_2O(l) + SO_2(g)$	+0.17
$Cu^{2+}(aq) + e^- \longrightarrow Cu^+(aq)$	+0.159
$Sn^{4+}(aq) + 2\,e^- \longrightarrow Sn^{2+}(aq)$	+0.154
$S(s) + 2\,H^+(aq) + 2\,e^- \longrightarrow H_2S(g)$	+0.14
$AgBr(s) + e^- \longrightarrow Ag(s) + Br^-(aq)$	+0.071
$2\,H^+(aq) + 2\,e^- \longrightarrow H_2(g)$	0
$Pb^{2+}(aq) + 2\,e^- \longrightarrow Pb(s)$	−0.125
$Sn^{2+}(aq) + 2\,e^- \longrightarrow Sn(s)$	−0.137
$AgI(s) + e^- \longrightarrow Ag(s) + I^-(aq)$	−0.152

Reduction Half-Reaction (continued)	$E°$, V
$V^{3+}(aq) + e^- \longrightarrow V^{2+}(aq)$	-0.255
$Ni^{2+}(aq) + 2\,e^- \longrightarrow Ni(s)$	-0.257
$H_3PO_4(aq) + 2\,H^+(aq) + 2\,e^- \longrightarrow H_3PO_3(aq) + H_2O(l)$	-0.276
$Co^{2+}(aq) + 2\,e^- \longrightarrow Co(s)$	-0.277
$PbSO_4(s) + 2\,e^- \longrightarrow Pb(s) + SO_4^{2-}(aq)$	-0.356
$Cd^{2+}(aq) + 2\,e^- \longrightarrow Cd(s)$	-0.403
$Cr^{3+}(aq) + e^- \longrightarrow Cr^{2+}(aq)$	-0.424
$Fe^{2+}(aq) + 2\,e^- \longrightarrow Fe(s)$	-0.440
$2\,CO_2(g) + 2\,H^+(aq) + 2\,e^- \longrightarrow H_2C_2O_4(aq)$	-0.49
$Zn^{2+}(aq) + 2\,e^- \longrightarrow Zn(s)$	-0.763
$Cr^{2+}(aq) + 2\,e^- \longrightarrow Cr(s)$	-0.90
$Mn^{2+}(aq) + 2\,e^- \longrightarrow Mn(s)$	-1.18
$Ti^{2+}(aq) + 2\,e^- \longrightarrow Ti(s)$	-1.63
$U^{3+}(aq) + 3\,e^- \longrightarrow U(s)$	-1.66
$Al^{3+}(aq) + 3\,e^- \longrightarrow Al(s)$	-1.676
$Mg^{2+}(aq) + 2\,e^- \longrightarrow Mg(s)$	-2.356
$Na^+(aq) + e^- \longrightarrow Na(s)$	-2.713
$Ca^{2+}(aq) + 2\,e^- \longrightarrow Ca(s)$	-2.84
$Sr^{2+}(aq) + 2\,e^- \longrightarrow Sr(s)$	-2.89
$Ba^{2+}(aq) + 2\,e^- \longrightarrow Ba(s)$	-2.92
$Cs^+(aq) + e^- \longrightarrow Cs(s)$	-2.923
$K^+(aq) + e^- \longrightarrow K(s)$	-2.924
$Rb^+(aq) + e^- \longrightarrow Rb(s)$	-2.924
$Li^+(aq) + e^- \longrightarrow Li(s)$	-3.040

Basic Solution

$O_3(g) + H_2O(l) + 2\,e^- \longrightarrow O_2(g) + 2\,OH^-(aq)$	$+1.246$
$ClO^-(aq) + H_2O(l) + 2\,e^- \longrightarrow Cl^-(g) + 2\,OH^-(aq)$	$+0.890$
$HO_2^-(aq) + H_2O(l) + 2\,e^- \longrightarrow 3\,OH^-(aq)$	$+0.88$
$BrO^-(aq) + H_2O(l) + 2\,e^- \longrightarrow Br^-(aq) + 2\,OH^-(aq)$	$+0.766$
$ClO_3^-(aq) + 3\,H_2O(l) + 6\,e^- \longrightarrow Cl^-(aq) + 6\,OH^-(aq)$	$+0.622$
$2\,AgO(s) + H_2O(l) + 2\,e^- \longrightarrow Ag_2O(s) + 2\,OH^-(aq)$	$+0.604$
$MnO_4^-(aq) + 2\,H_2O(l) + 3\,e^- \longrightarrow MnO_2(s) + 4\,OH^-(aq)$	$+0.60$
$BrO_3^-(aq) + 3\,H_2O(l) + 6\,e^- \longrightarrow Br^-(aq) + 6\,OH^-(aq)$	$+0.584$
$Ni(OH)_3(s) + e^- \longrightarrow Ni(OH)_2(s) + OH^-(aq)$	$+0.48$
$2\,BrO^-(aq) + 2\,H_2O(l) + 2\,e^- \longrightarrow Br_2(l) + 4\,OH^-(aq)$	$+0.455$
$2\,IO^-(aq) + 2\,H_2O(l) + 2\,e^- \longrightarrow I_2(s) + 4\,OH^-(aq)$	$+0.42$
$O_2(g) + 2\,H_2O(l) + 4\,e^- \longrightarrow 4\,OH^-(aq)$	$+0.401$
$Ag_2O(s) + H_2O(l) + 2\,e^- \longrightarrow 2\,Ag(s) + 2\,OH^-(aq)$	$+0.342$
$Co(OH)_3(s) + e^- \longrightarrow Co(OH)_2(s) + OH^-(aq)$	$+0.17$
$NO_3^-(aq) + H_2O(l) + 2\,e^- \longrightarrow NO_2^-(aq) + 2\,OH^-(aq)$	$+0.01$
$CrO_4^{2-}(aq) + 4\,H_2O(l) + 3\,e^- \longrightarrow [Cr(OH)_4]^-(aq) + 4\,OH^-(aq)$	-0.13
$HPbO_2^-(aq) + H_2O(l) + 2\,e^- \longrightarrow Pb(s) + 3\,OH^-(aq)$	-0.54
$HCHO(aq) + 2\,H_2O(l) + 2\,e^- \longrightarrow CH_3OH(aq) + 2\,OH^-(aq)$	-0.59
$SO_3^{2-}(aq) + 3\,H_2O(l) + 4\,e^- \longrightarrow S(s) + 6\,OH^-(aq)$	-0.66
$AsO_4^{3-}(aq) + 2\,H_2O(l) + 2\,e^- \longrightarrow AsO_2^-(aq) + 4\,OH^-(aq)$	-0.67
$AsO_2^-(aq) + 2\,H_2O(l) + 3\,e^- \longrightarrow As(s) + 4\,OH^-(aq)$	-0.68
$2\,H_2O(l) + 2\,e^- \longrightarrow H_2(g) + 2\,OH^-(aq)$	-0.828
$OCN^-(aq) + H_2O(l) + 2\,e^- \longrightarrow CN^-(aq) + 2\,OH^-(aq)$	-0.97
$As(s) + 3\,H_2O(l) + 3\,e^- \longrightarrow AsH_3(g) + 3\,OH^-(aq)$	-1.21
$[Zn(OH)_4]^{2-}(aq) + 2\,e^- \longrightarrow Zn(s) + 4\,OH^-(aq)$	-1.285
$Sb(s) + 3\,H_2O(l) + 3\,e^- \longrightarrow SbH_3(g) + 3\,OH^-(aq)$	-1.338
$Al(OH)_4^-(aq) + 3\,e^- \longrightarrow Al(s) + 4\,OH^-(aq)$	-2.310
$Mg(OH)_2(s) + 2\,e^- \longrightarrow Mg(s) + 2\,OH^-(aq)$	-2.687

Organic Nomenclature

In the early days of organic chemistry, compounds were given common names, often based on natural sources. For example, butyric acid ($CH_3CH_2CH_2COOH$) was so named from the Latin *butyrum*, meaning butter. (The *but-* part of the name survives in the systematic names of compounds with four carbon atoms per molecule: $CH_3CH_2CH_2CH_3$, butane; $CH_3CH_2CH_2CH_2OH$, 1-butanol; and so on.) Today, there are millions of organic compounds, and we could no more memorize individual names for all of them than we could memorize all the listings in the New York City telephone directory. To bring some order to the haphazard naming of the rapidly increasing roster of organic compounds, an international assembly of chemists met in 1892 for the first of many meetings on nomenclature—a system for assigning names. This organization exists today as the International Union of Pure and Applied Chemistry (IUPAC). Here, we will examine some simple rules for naming a few families of organic compounds.

D.1 Alkanes

An IUPAC name of an organic compound often consists of three basic parts: one or more prefixes, a stem, and an ending. The following rules will enable us to name most alkanes.

1. Use the ending *-ane* to indicate that the compound is an alkane.
2. The longest continuous chain (LCC) of carbon atoms is the *parent chain;* it provides the *stem* name. For example, the following alkane is named as a derivative of hexane because there are six carbon atoms in the LCC:

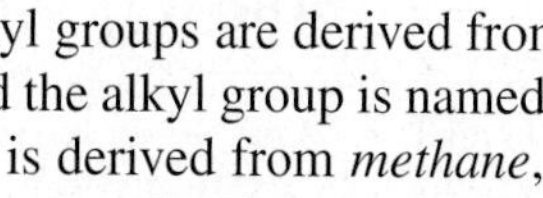

$$CH_3CH_2CHCH_2CH_2CH_3$$
$$|$$
$$CH_3$$

   The stem *hex-* and ending *-ane* combine to give *hexane.* (Recall that the names of the stems for chains with up to 10 carbon atoms were given in Table 2.6.)

3. The prefixes in a name indicate the groups attached to the parent chain. If the group contains only carbon and hydrogen with no double or triple bonds, it is called an *alkyl* group. Alkyl groups are derived from the corresponding alkane by removing one H atom, and the alkyl group is named after the alkane. For example, the *methyl* group $—CH_3$ is derived from *methane*, CH_4. There is only one alkyl group derived from methane and only one from ethane. For the general alkane C_nH_{2n+2} with $n = 3$ (propane) or higher, different alkyl groups are formed depending on which H atom is removed. For example, removal of an end H atom from propane gives a *propyl* group, whereas removal of a H atom from the middle carbon atom of propane yields an *isopropyl* group. The names and formulas of the four simplest alkyl groups are as follows:

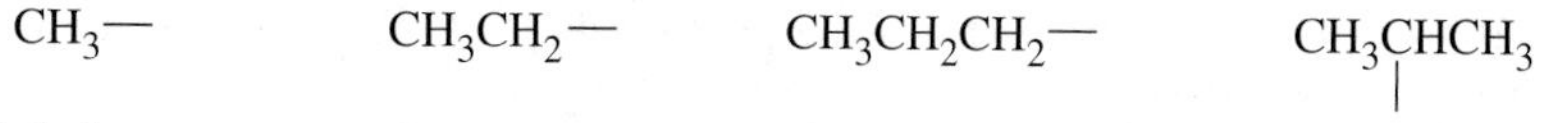

$$CH_3— \qquad CH_3CH_2— \qquad CH_3CH_2CH_2— \qquad CH_3CHCH_3$$
$$|$$

   Methyl group   Ethyl group   Propyl group   Isopropyl group

4. The smallest possible Arabic numerals are used to indicate the position(s) on the longest carbon chain at which the substituents (alkyl groups, in this case) are

attached. Thus, to complete the name of the alkane in item 2, we again identify the LCC (red):

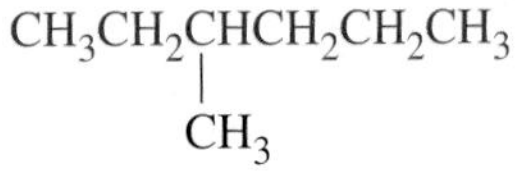

$$CH_3CH_2CHCH_2CH_2CH_3$$
$$|$$
$$CH_3$$

Next, we note that the methyl group —CH_3 is attached to the third carbon atom from the left end. Thus, the compound is *3-methylhexane*. Notice that if we number the carbon atoms from the right end, the methyl group is on the *fourth* carbon atom. The name "4-methylhexane" is incorrect, however, because we must use the *lowest* possible numbers for constituent groups.

5. We use the prefixes *di-* for two, *tri-* for three, and *tetra-* for four to denote two, three, or four identical groups attached to the parent chain. If two identical groups are bonded to the same carbon atom, we must repeat the position number for each group:

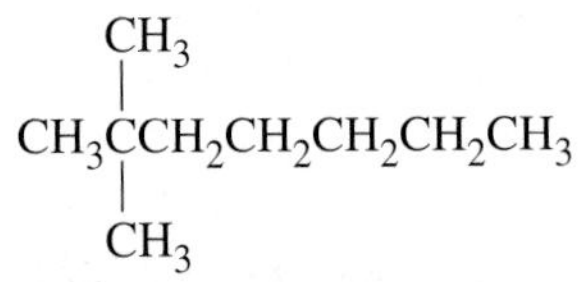

$$CH_3$$
$$|$$
$$CH_3CCH_2CH_2CH_2CH_3$$
$$|$$
$$CH_3$$
2,2-Dimethylheptane

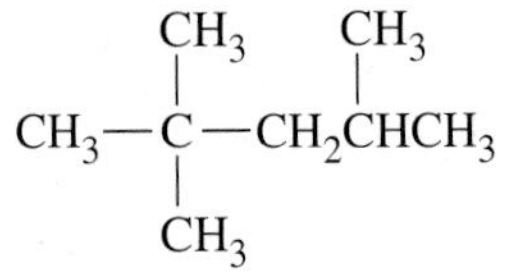

$$CH_3 \quad CH_3$$
$$| \quad \quad |$$
$$CH_3—C—CH_2CHCH_3$$
$$|$$
$$CH_3$$
2,2,4-Trimethylpentane

Commas are used to separate numbers from each other, and hyphens to separate numbers from words.

6. Groups are listed in alphabetical order. Thus, the proper name for the compound

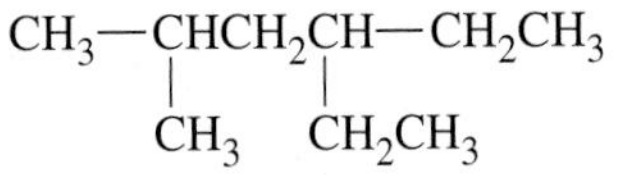

$$CH_3—CHCH_2CH—CH_2CH_3$$
$$| \quad \quad |$$
$$CH_3 \quad CH_2CH_3$$

is 4-ethyl-2-methylhexane, not "2-methyl-4-ethylhexane."

As a final example, let's name the following compound:

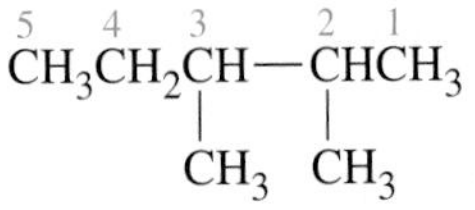

$$\overset{5}{C}H_3\overset{4}{C}H_2\overset{3}{C}H—\overset{2}{C}H\overset{1}{C}H_3$$
$$| \quad \quad |$$
$$CH_3 \quad CH_3$$

The LCC has five carbon atoms; the compound is named as a derivative of pentane. There are methyl groups attached to the second and third carbon atoms. The correct name is 2,3-dimethylpentane. Note that we numbered the carbon atoms so that the substituent groups would have the lowest numbers possible.

Example D.1

Give an appropriate IUPAC name for this compound:

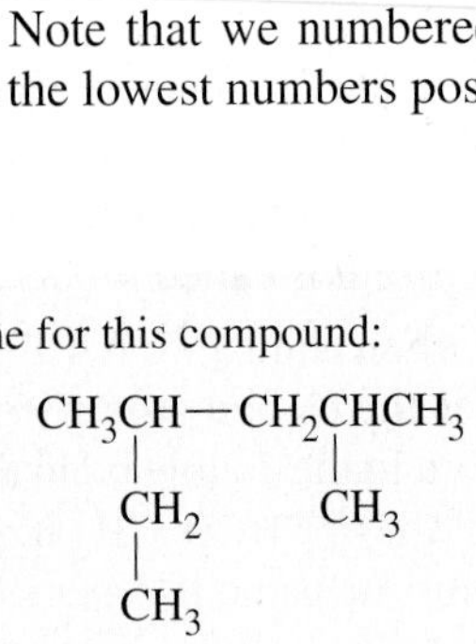

$$CH_3CH—CH_2CHCH_3$$
$$| \quad \quad |$$
$$CH_2 \quad CH_3$$
$$|$$
$$CH_3$$

SOLUTION

Let's begin by identifying the LCC. This one is a little tricky. The parent compound is the longest continuous chain, not necessarily the chain drawn straight across the page. The LCC (red) contains *six* carbon atoms.

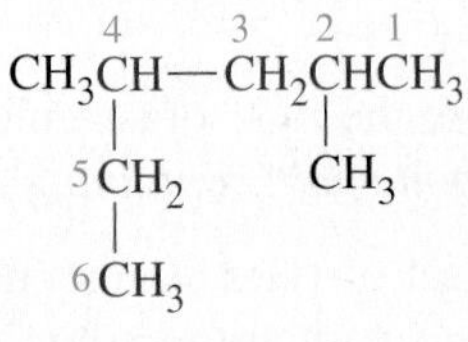

$$\overset{4}{C}H_3\overset{3}{C}H—\overset{2}{C}H_2\overset{1}{C}HCH_3$$
$$| \quad \quad |$$
$$^5CH_2 \quad CH_3$$
$$|$$
$$^6CH_3$$

The substituents (black) are two methyl groups, one on the second carbon atom of the LCC and one on the fourth. Again, we use the lowest combination of numbers, in this case requiring that we count from the left end. The correct name is 2,4-dimethylhexane, not "2-ethyl-4-methylpentane."

Example D.2

Give the structural formula for 5-isopropyl-2-methyloctane.

SOLUTION

The compound is derived from octane, so we start with a chain of eight carbon atoms.

$$-C-C-C-C-C-C-C-C-$$

Next, starting on the left, we attach a methyl group to the second C atom.

$$\begin{array}{c} CH_3 \\ | \\ -C-C-C-C-C-C-C-C- \\ 12345678 \end{array}$$

Then, continuing to count from the left, we add an isopropyl group to the fifth C atom. (Remember that an isopropyl group is a three-carbon chain attached by the *middle* carbon atom.)

$$\begin{array}{c} CH_3 \quad\quad CH_3CHCH_3 \\ | \quad\quad\quad\quad | \\ -C-C-C-C-C-C-C-C- \\ 12345678 \end{array}$$

Finally, we add enough H atoms to give each C atom four bonds. The structural formula is

$$\begin{array}{c} CH_3 \quad\quad CH_3CHCH_3 \\ | \quad\quad\quad\quad | \\ CH_3CHCH_2CH_2CHCH_2CH_2CH_3 \end{array}$$

D.2 Alkenes and Alkynes

A few simple alkenes are best known by common names (Section 9.11), but we need systematic names for the many isomers of higher alkenes. Some of the IUPAC rules for alkenes are as follows.

1. All alkenes have names ending in *-ene*.

2. The longest chain of carbon atoms *containing the double bond* is the parent chain. The stem name is the same as that of the alkane with the same number of carbon atoms. The compound $CH_2{=}CH_2$ has the same number of C atoms as ethane, CH_3CH_3; it is called *ethene*. Similarly, $CH_3CH{=}CH_2$ has the same number of C atoms as propane, $CH_3CH_2CH_3$; it is called *propene*.

3. For chains of four or more carbon atoms, we must indicate the location of the double bond. To do this, number the carbon atoms from the end of the parent chain that gives the first carbon atom in the double bond the lowest possible number. For example, the compound $CH_3CH{=}CHCH_2CH_3$ has the double bond between the second and third carbon atoms. Its name is *2-pentene*.

4. Substituent groups are named as in alkanes, and their positions are indicated by a number. Thus, the following alkene is 2-ethyl-5-methyl-1-hexene:

$$\begin{array}{c} \overset{1}{}\quad\overset{2}{}\overset{3}{}\quad\overset{4}{}\quad\overset{5}{}\quad\overset{6}{} \\ CH_2{=}CCH_2CH_2CHCH_3 \\ | \quad\quad\quad\quad | \\ CH_2CH_3 \;\; CH_3 \end{array}$$

Notice that we did not choose the LCC of seven carbon atoms (red) as the parent chain. We chose the *six-carbon chain containing the double bond*.

To name *alkynes*, we use a set of rules almost identical to those for the alkenes. Alkynes differ in that they have a carbon-to-carbon triple bond instead of a double

bond, and we use the ending *-yne* rather than the *-ene* ending for alkenes. The IUPAC name of $CH_2\!=\!CH_2$ is *ethyne*, and that of $CH_3C\!\equiv\!CH$ is *propyne*. The compounds $CH_3CH_2C\!\equiv\!CH$ and $CH_3C\!\equiv\!CCH_3$ are *1-butyne* and *2-butyne*, respectively.

Example D.3

Name the following compound:

$$CH_3C\!\equiv\!CCH_2CH\!-\!CHCH_3$$
$$\overset{|}{CH_3}\ \ \overset{|}{CH_3}$$

SOLUTION

The LCC containing the triple bond has seven carbon atoms; the seven-carbon alkyne is heptyne. We give the lowest position number to the triple bond, not to the substituent groups. To do this, we number the C atoms as shown here:

$$\overset{1}{C}H_3\overset{2}{C}\!\equiv\!\overset{3}{C}\overset{4}{C}H_2\overset{5}{C}H\!-\!\overset{6}{C}\overset{7}{H}CH_3$$
$$\overset{|}{CH_3}\ \ \overset{|}{CH_3}$$

The parent compound is 2-heptyne. There are methyl substituents on the fifth and sixth carbon atoms. The name of the compound is 5,6-dimethyl-2-heptyne.

Example D.4

Give the structural formula for **(a)** 2-methyl-2-pentene and **(b)** 4-methyl-2-hexyne.

SOLUTION

(a) The stem *pent* and ending *-ene* tell us that the LCC containing the double bond has five carbon atoms. The *2* indicates that the double bond is between the second and third carbon atoms.

$$C\!-\!C\!=\!C\!-\!C\!-\!C$$

The *2-methyl* locates the $-CH_3$ substituent on the second carbon atom.

$$C\!-\!C\!=\!C\!-\!C\!-\!C$$
$$\overset{|}{CH_3}$$

Adding enough hydrogen atoms to provide four bonds to each carbon atom gives us the structural formula.

$$CH_3\!-\!C\!=\!CH\!-\!CH_2\!-\!CH_3$$
$$\overset{|}{CH_3}$$

(b) The stem *hex-* and ending *-yne* tell us that the LCC containing a *triple* bond has six carbon atoms. The 2 tells us that the triple bond is between the second and third carbon atoms, and the *4-methyl* locates the $-CH_3$ substituent on the fourth carbon atom. Adding hydrogen atoms gives the structural formula.

$$CH_3C\!\equiv\!CCHCH_2CH_3$$
$$\overset{|}{CH_3}$$

D.3   Alcohols

In Section 2.9, we introduced alcohols as compounds with the general formula ROH, indicating a hydroxyl group (OH) bonded to a carbon atom of an alkyl group (R). The OH group is a substituent on the LCC, but we generally don't name it as a substituent. Rather, we indicate its presence by an ending:

- The presence of the OH functional group is denoted by an *-ol* ending on an alkane stem name (not through the prefix, hydroxyl).
- In numbering the carbon atoms of the LCC, the position of the OH group is given first priority; that is, it is given the lowest number possible.

The two simplest alcohols are known by the common names methyl alcohol and ethyl alcohol. The IUPAC name of CH_3OH is based on the alkane methane, CH_4. We drop the *-e* of methane and add the ending *-ol*; its name is *methanol*. Similarly, the name of CH_3CH_2OH is based on the alkane ethane, CH_3CH_3; its name is *ethanol*. There are two propyl alcohols. Their structures and names are given below.

$$CH_3CH_2CH_2OH$$

1-Propanol

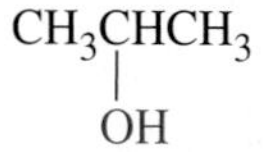

$$CH_3CHCH_3$$
$$|$$
$$OH$$

2-Propanol

Recall that their common names are propyl alcohol and isopropyl alcohol, respectively.

Example D.5

The compound commonly known as *tert*-butyl alcohol, $(CH_3)_3COH$, and its methyl ether, $(CH_3)_3COCH_3$, are used as octane boosters in gasoline. What is the IUPAC name of the alcohol?

SOLUTION

Let's begin by converting the condensed formula to a more complete structural formula. There are three methyl groups and a hydroxyl group, all attached to a single C atom.

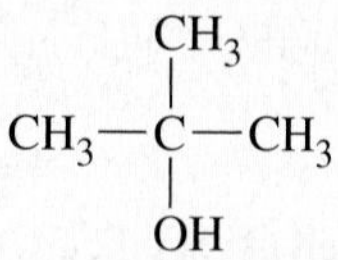

$$\begin{array}{c} CH_3 \\ | \\ CH_3-C-CH_3 \\ | \\ OH \end{array}$$

The LCC is three carbon atoms long, and the hydroxyl group is on the second carbon of this chain, yielding, for the moment, 2-propanol. There is also a methyl group attached to the second carbon of the parent chain, giving the IUPAC name *2-methyl-2-propanol*.

D.4 Carboxylic Acids

The simplest carboxylic acids are widely known by their common names. For example, HCOOH is called formic acid and CH_3COOH is called acetic acid. The IUPAC names are based on alkanes with the same number of carbon atoms. The *-e* ending of the alkane name is replaced by *-oic acid*. Thus, HCOOH is methanoic acid, and CH_3COOH is ethanoic acid. The carboxylic acid with an LCC of eight carbon atoms is octanoic acid. For locating substituents, numbering begins with the carboxylic carbon atom as number 1, as illustrated in Example D.6.

Example D.6

Give the structural formula for 4-ethyl-6-methyloctanoic acid.

SOLUTION

Octanoic tells us that the compound has an LCC of eight carbon atoms, with an end C atom as part of a carboxyl group.

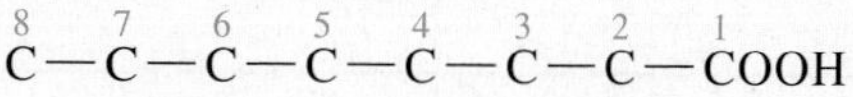

$$\overset{8}{C}-\overset{7}{C}-\overset{6}{C}-\overset{5}{C}-\overset{4}{C}-\overset{3}{C}-\overset{2}{C}-\overset{1}{COOH}$$

The substituents are an ethyl group on the fourth carbon atom (counting *from the carboxyl end*) and a methyl group on the sixth carbon atom. Adding these substituents and enough H atoms to give each C atom four bonds, we get

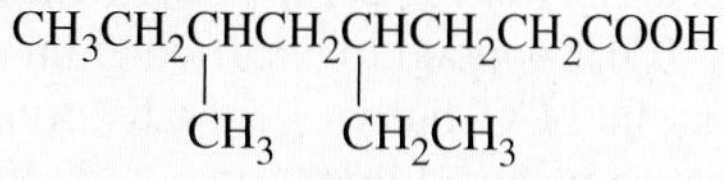

$$\begin{array}{c} CH_3CH_2CHCH_2CHCH_2CH_2COOH \\ | | \\ CH_3 CH_2CH_3 \end{array}$$

There are many other families of organic compounds. Table D.1 lists several of the most common functional groups and examples of compounds that contain them. With what we have presented here and in Chapters 2 and 23, you should be able to relate the names and formulas of many types of organic compounds.

Table D.1 Some Classes of Organic Compounds and Their Functional Groups

Class	General Structural Formula[a]	Example	Name of Example	Cross Reference
Alkane	R—H	$CH_3CH_2CH_2CH_2CH_2CH_3$	hexane	Sections 2.9, 6.8, Chap. 23
Alkene	$\diagdown C = C \diagdown$	$CH_2 = CHCH_2CH_2CH_3$	1-pentene	Section 9.11, Chap. 23
Alkyne	$-C \equiv C-$	$CH_3C \equiv CCH_2CH_2CH_2CH_2CH_3$	2-octyne	Section 9.11, Chap. 23
Alcohol	R—OH	$CH_3CH_2CH_2CH_2OH$	1-butanol	Section 2.9, Chap. 23
Alkyl halide	R—X[b]	$CH_3CH_2CH_2CH_2CH_2CH_2Br$	1-bromohexane	Chap. 23
Ether	R—O—R	$CH_3—O—CH_2CH_2CH_3$	1-methoxypropane (methyl propyl ether)[c]	Chap. 23
Amine	$R—NH_2$	$CH_3CH_2CH_2—NH_2$	1-aminopropane (propylamine)[c]	Section 4.2, Chap. 15
Aldehyde	$R—\overset{\overset{\displaystyle O}{\|\|}}{C}—H$	$CH_3CH_2CH_2\overset{\overset{\displaystyle O}{\|\|}}{C}—H$	butanal (butyraldehyde)[c]	Section 4.5, Chap. 23
Ketone	$R—\overset{\overset{\displaystyle O}{\|\|}}{C}—R$	$CH_3CH_2\overset{\overset{\displaystyle O}{\|\|}}{C}CH_2CH_2CH_3$	3-hexanone (ethyl propyl ketone)[c]	Section 4.5, Chap. 23
Carboxylic acid	$R—\overset{\overset{\displaystyle O}{\|\|}}{C}—OH$	$CH_3CH_2CH_2\overset{\overset{\displaystyle O}{\|\|}}{C}—OH$	butanoic acid (butyric acid)[c]	Sections 2.9, 4.2, Chap. 15, 23
Ester	$R—\overset{\overset{\displaystyle O}{\|\|}}{C}—OR$	$CH_3CH_2CH_2\overset{\overset{\displaystyle O}{\|\|}}{C}—OCH_3$	methyl butanoate (methyl butyrate)[c]	Section 6.8, Chap. 23, Chap. 24 (polymers)
Amide	$R—\overset{\overset{\displaystyle O}{\|\|}}{C}—NH_2$	$CH_3CH_2CH_2\overset{\overset{\displaystyle O}{\|\|}}{C}—NH_2$	butanamide (butyramide)[c]	Chap. 23, Chap. 24 (polymers)
Arene	Ar—H[d]	⬡—CH_2CH_3	ethylbenzene	Section 10.8, Chap. 23
Aryl halide	Ar—X[b]	⬡—Br	bromobenzene	Chap. 23
Phenol	Ar—OH	Cl—⬡—OH	4-chlorophenol (p-chlorophenol)[c]	Section 10.9, Chap. 23

[a] The functional group is shown in red. R stands for an alkyl group.
[b] X stands for a halogen atom—F, Cl, Br, or I.
[c] Common name.
[d] Ar— stands for an aromatic (aryl) group such as the benzene ring.

Glossary

Absolute configuration is the three-dimensional arrangement of groups about a chiral center in a molecule.

Absolute zero is the lowest possible temperature: $-273.15\ °C = 0\ K$.

The **accuracy** of a set of measurements refers to the closeness of the average of the set to the most probable value.

An **acid** is (1) a hydrogen-containing compound that can produce hydrogen ions, H^+, in aqueous solution (Arrhenius theory); (2) a proton donor (Brønsted–Lowry theory); (3) an atom, ion, or molecule that can accept a pair of electrons to form a covalent bond (Lewis theory).

An **acid–base indicator** is a substance added to the reaction mixture in a titration that changes color at or near the equivalence point.

An **acidic oxide** is a nonmetal oxide whose reaction with water produces a ternary acid as its sole product.

The **acid ionization constant** (K_a) is the equilibrium constant for the reversible ionization of a weak acid.

Acid rain is rainfall that is more acidic than is water in equilibrium with atmospheric carbon dioxide.

The **actinide** elements constitute the portion of the f-block of the periodic table in which the $5f$ subshell fills in the aufbau process.

An **activated complex** is an aggregate of atoms in the transition state of a reaction formed by a favorable collision. (*See also* **transition state**.)

The **activated sludge method** of sewage treatment is a process in which sludge from the secondary stage is put into aeration tanks to facilitate decomposition by aerobic microorganisms.

The **activation energy** (E_a) of a reaction refers to the minimum total kinetic energy that molecules must bring into their collisions so that a chemical reaction may occur.

The **active site** on an enzyme is the region of the enzyme molecule where the substrate attaches and a chemical reaction occurs. (*See also* **enzyme** and **substrate**.)

Activity is the effective concentration of a species, and in dilute solutions is often approximated by molar concentration.

The **activity series of the metals** is a listing of the metals in order of their ability to displace one another from solutions of their ions or to displace H^+ as $H_2(g)$ from acidic solutions. (See also Figure 4.13.)

The **actual yield** is the measured quantity of a desired product obtained in a chemical reaction. (*See also* **theoretical yield** and **percent yield**.)

Addition polymerization is a type of polymerization reaction in which monomers add to one another to produce a polymeric product that contains all the atoms of the starting monomers.

In an **addition reaction**, substituent groups join to hydrocarbon molecules at points of unsaturation—double or triple bonds.

An **adduct** is a compound that results from the addition, through a coordinate covalent bond, of one structure to another.

Adhesive forces are intermolecular forces between unlike molecules, for example, between those in a liquid and those in a surface over which the liquid is spread.

Advanced treatment (*tertiary treatment*) is a third stage of sewage treatment in which nitrates, phosphates, and (sometimes) dissolved organic substances are removed from the effluent of a secondary treatment process.

Aerobic oxidation is an oxidation process that occurs in the presence of oxygen.

An **air pollutant** is a substance that is found in air in greater abundance than normally occurs naturally and that has some harmful effect(s) on the environment.

An **alcohol (ROH)** is an organic substance whose molecules contain the hydroxyl group, OH, attached to an alkyl group.

An **aldehyde (RCHO)** is an organic compound whose molecules have a carbonyl functional group with a hydrogen atom attached to the carbonyl carbon.

Aliphatic compounds are those organic compounds with open chains of carbon atoms, or rings of carbon atoms that are similar in structure and properties to the open-chain compounds. (*See also* **aromatic compounds**.)

An **alkane** is a saturated hydrocarbon having the general formula C_nH_{2n+2}. (*See also* **saturated hydrocarbon**.)

An **alkene** is a hydrocarbon whose molecules contain at least one carbon-to-carbon double bond.

An **alkyl group (R)** is a substituent group in organic molecules derived from an alkane molecule by removal of one hydrogen atom.

An **alkyne** is a hydrocarbon whose molecules contain at least one carbon-to-carbon triple bond.

An **allotrope** is one of two or more forms of an element that differ in their basic molecular structure.

An **alloy** is a metallic material consisting of two or more elements.

An **alpha** (α) **particle** consists of two protons and two neutrons. It is identical to a doubly ionized helium ion, He^{2+}.

An **amide (RCONH₂)** is an organic compound in which a nitrogen atom is bonded to the carbon atom of a carbonyl group.

An **amine** is an organic substance in which one or more H atoms of an ammonia molecule are replaced by a hydrocarbon residue.

The **ampere (A)** is the basic unit of electric current. One ampere is a current of 1 coulomb per second: $1\ A = 1\ C/s$.

An **amphiprotic** substance can ionize either as a Brønsted–Lowry acid or base, depending on the acid–base properties of other species in the solution.

An **amphoteric** substance (usually an oxide or hydroxide) can react either with an acid or a base. The central element of the oxide or hydroxide appears in a cation in acidic solutions and in an anion in basic solutions.

Anaerobic decay is decomposition in the absence of oxygen.

The **analyte** is the sought-for substance in an analysis such as a titration.

Analytical chemistry is the branch of chemistry that deals with determination of the composition and properties of substances and mixtures.

An **anion** is a negatively charged ion.

An **anode** is an electrode at which an oxidation half-reaction occurs. It is the negative electrode in a voltaic cell and the positive electrode in an electrolytic cell.

An **antibonding molecular orbital** places a high electron charge density (electron probability) away from the region between bonded atoms. (*See also* **bonding molecular orbital** and **molecular orbital**.)

An **anticarcinogen** is a substance that opposes the action of a carcinogen; it prevents or retards the development of cancer.

An **aqueous solution** is a solution in which water is the solvent.

Aromatic compounds are organic compounds with benzene-like structures. To describe their electronic structures (Lewis structures), resonance theory is used.

The **atmosphere (atm)** is a unit used to measure gas pressure. It is equal to the pressure of a column of mercury having a height of exactly 760 mm. That is, 1 atm = 760 mmHg.

The **atomic mass** of an element is the weighted average of the masses of the atoms of the naturally occurring isotopes of the element.

An **atomic mass unit (u)** is exactly one-twelfth the mass of an atom of carbon-12.

The **atomic number (Z)** of an atom is the number of protons in the atomic nucleus.

An **atomic orbital** is a wave function for an electron corresponding to the assignment of specific values to the n, l, and m_l quantum numbers in a wave equation.

The **atomic radius** is a measure of the size of an atom based on the measurement of internuclear distances. (*See also* **covalent radius**, **ionic radius**, and **metallic radius**.)

Atoms are the smallest distinctive units of a sample of matter. Atoms of one element differ from atoms of all other elements. (*See also* **element**.)

The **aufbau principle** is a hypothetical process for building up an atom from the atom of the preceding atomic number by adding a proton and the requisite number of neutrons to the nucleus and one electron to the appropriate atomic orbital.

Average bond energy is the average of the bond-dissociation energies for a number of different molecular species containing the particular bond. (*See also* **bond-dissociation energy**.)

Avogadro's hypothesis states that equal numbers of molecules of different gases, when compared at the same temperature and pressure, occupy equal volumes.

Avogadro's law states that at a fixed temperature and pressure, the volume of a gas is directly proportional to the amount of gas.

Avogadro's number (N_A) is the number of elementary units in a mole—$6.02214199 \times 10^{23}$ mol^{-1}.

A **band**, in describing bonding in metals and semiconductors, is a collection of a large number of closely spaced molecular orbitals, obtained by combining atomic orbitals of many atoms.

A **barometer** is a device used to measure the pressure exerted by the atmosphere.

A **base** is (1) a compound that produces hydroxide ions, OH^-, in aqueous solution (Arrhenius theory); (2) a proton acceptor (Brønsted–Lowry theory); (3) an atom, ion, or molecule that donates a pair of electrons to form a covalent bond (Lewis theory).

The **base ionization constant (K_b)** is the equilibrium constant for the reversible ionization of a weak base.

A **basic oxide** is a metal oxide whose reaction with water produces a base.

A **beta (β^-) particle** is identical to an electron and is emitted by the nuclei of certain radioactive atoms as they undergo decay. In the decaying nucleus, the atomic number increases by one unit and the mass number remains unchanged.

A **bidentate** ligand has two points of attachment to a metal center in a complex.

A **bimolecular reaction** is an elementary reaction in a reaction mechanism that involves the collision of two molecules.

Biochemical oxygen demand (BOD) measures the amount of oxygen needed by aerobic microorganisms to metabolize the organic wastes in water.

The **biosphere** is the part of Earth occupied by living organisms.

A **body-centered cubic (bcc)** crystal structure has as its unit cell a cube with a structural unit at each corner and one in the center of the cell. (*See also* **unit cell**.)

The **boiling point** of a liquid is the temperature at which the liquid boils—the temperature at which the vapor pressure of the liquid is equal to the prevailing atmospheric pressure.

The **bond-dissociation energy (D)** of a particular covalent bond between two atoms is the quantity of energy required to break one mole of bonds of that type in a gaseous species.

A **bonding molecular orbital** places a high electron charge density (electron probability) in the region between two bonded atoms. (*See also* **antibonding molecular orbital** and **molecular orbital**.)

A **bonding pair** is a pair of electrons shared between two atoms in a molecule.

The **bond length** of a particular covalent bond is the distance between the nuclei of two atoms joined by that type of bond.

A **bond moment** describes the extent to which a separation of positive ($\delta+$) and negative ($\delta-$) charges exists in a covalent bond between two atoms.

Bond order refers to the number of electron pairs in a covalent bond—that is, whether a single pair (bond order = 1), two pairs (bond order = 2), or three pairs (bond order = 3). In molecular orbital theory, it is one-half the difference between the number of electrons in bonding molecular orbitals and in antibonding molecular orbitals.

Boyle's law states that for a given amount of gas at a constant temperature, the volume of a gas varies inversely with its pressure. That is, $V \propto 1/P$ or PV = constant.

A **buffer solution** is a solution containing a weak acid and its conjugate base or a weak base and its conjugate acid. Small quantities of added acid are neutralized by one buffer component and small quantities of added base by the other. As a result, the solution pH is maintained nearly constant.

A **buret** is a long graduated tube constructed to deliver precise volumes of a liquid solution through a stopcock valve.

A **calorie (cal)** is the energy needed to raise the temperature of 1 g of water by 1 °C (more precisely, from 14.5 to 15.5 °C). 1 cal = 4.184 J.

A **calorimeter** is a device in which quantities of heat are measured.

A **carbocation** is an intermediate species in certain reactions of organic compounds in which a positive charge is centered on a carbon atom in the species.

A **carbohydrate** is a compound consisting of carbon, hydrogen, and oxygen, generally with twice as many hydrogen atoms as oxygen atoms; a starch, sugar, or cellulose.

The **carbon cycle** refers to the totality of activities in which carbon atoms are cycled through the environment.

A **carboxylic acid (RCOOH)** is an organic substance whose molecules contain the carboxyl group, COOH.

A **carcinogen** is an agent that causes cancer.

Cast iron is a carbon–iron alloy that is cast into shape and contains 1.8–4.5% C.

A **catalyst** is a substance that increases the rate of a reaction without itself being consumed in the reaction. A catalyst changes a reaction mechanism to one with a lower activation energy.

A **cathode** is an electrode at which a reduction half-reaction occurs. It is the positive electrode in a voltaic cell and the negative electrode in an electrolytic cell.

A **cathode ray** is a beam of electrons that travels from the cathode to the anode when an electric discharge is passed through an evacuated tube.

A **cation** is a positively charged ion.

A **cell diagram** is a schematic representation of an electrochemical cell.

Cell potential (E_{cell}) (cell voltage) refers to the potential difference between the electrodes in an electrochemical cell.

A **central atom** in a molecule or polyatomic ion is an atom bonded to two or more other atoms.

A **ceramic** is an inorganic solid generally produced at high temperature, and often containing silica or silicates. Most ceramics are hard, brittle, and stable at high temperatures.

Charles's law states that the volume of a fixed amount of a gas at a constant pressure is directly proportional to its Kelvin temperature. That is, $V \propto T$, or $V = $ constant $\times T$.

A **chelate** is a five- or six-membered ring structure produced in a complex through the attachment of one or more polydentate ligands to a metal center.

A **chemical bond** is a force that holds atoms together in molecules or ions together in crystals.

Chemical change. *See* **chemical reaction**.

A **chemical equation** is a description of a chemical reaction that uses symbols and formulas to represent the elements and compounds involved in the reaction. Numerical coefficients preceding each symbol or formula and indicating molar proportions may be needed to balance a chemical equation.

A **chemical formula** indicates the composition of a compound through symbols of the elements present and subscripts to indicate the relative numbers of atoms of each element.

Chemical kinetics is the study of the rates of chemical reactions, the factors that affect rates, and reaction mechanisms.

Chemical nomenclature is a systematic way of relating the names and formulas of chemical compounds.

A **chemical property** is a characteristic that matter displays as it undergoes a change in composition.

A **chemical reaction** is a process in which a sample of matter undergoes a change in composition and/or structure of its molecules. One or more original substances (reactants) are changed into one or more new substances (products).

Chemical shift is a term used in nuclear magnetic resonance (NMR) spectroscopy to indicate the location of an absorption peak relative to a standard. The magnitudes of the chemical shifts can be used to determine structural features of a molecule.

A **chemical symbol** is a representation of an element made up of one or two letters derived from the English name of the element (or sometimes from the Latin name of the element or one of its compounds).

Chemistry is a study of the composition, structure, and properties of matter and of the changes that occur in matter.

A **chiral carbon** is a carbon atom that is attached to four different groups.

Cis isomers have two substituent groups attached to the two atoms on the same side of a double bond in an organic molecule, or along the same edge of a square planar or octahedral complex ion. (*See also* **geometric isomers**.)

Cohesive forces are intermolecular forces between like molecules.

A **colligative property** is a physical property—such as vapor pressure lowering, freezing point depression, boiling point elevation, and osmotic pressure—that depends on the concentration of solute in the solution but not on the identity of the solute.

A **colloid** is a dispersion in which the dispersed matter has one or more dimensions (length, width, or thickness) in the range from about 1 nm to 1000 nm.

The **combined gas law** combines Boyle's, Charles's, and Avogadro's laws into a single relationship, written as $\dfrac{P_1 V_1}{n_1 T_1} = \dfrac{P_2 V_2}{n_2 T_2}$.

The **common ion effect** refers to the ability of an ion X to (a) suppress the ionization of a weak acid or weak base that produces X, or (b) reduce the solubility of a slightly soluble ionic compound that produces X.

A **complex** consists of a central atom, which is usually a metal ion, and coordinately covalently bonded groups called ligands.

A **complex ion** is a complex that carries a net electric charge, either positive (a complex cation) or negative (a complex anion).

A **composite** is composed of two or more physically distinct materials that, when combined, exploit the desired structural and mechanical properties of the individual components.

Composition refers to the types of atoms and their relative proportions in a sample of matter.

A **compound** is a substance made up of atoms of two or more elements, with the different atoms joined in fixed proportions.

A **concentration cell** is a voltaic cell having identical electrodes in contact with solutions of different concentrations.

A **concentration equilibrium constant** (K_c) is the numerical value of an equilibrium constant expression in which molarities of products and reactants are used.

Condensation is the conversion of a gas (vapor) to a liquid.

In **condensation polymerization**, monomers with at least two functional groups link together by eliminating small-molecule by-products.

A **conduction band** is a partially filled band of very closely spaced energy levels.

A **conjugate acid** is formed when a Brønsted–Lowry base accepts a proton. Every base has a conjugate acid.

A **conjugate base** is formed when a Brønsted–Lowry acid donates a proton. Every acid has a conjugate base.

A **conjugated bonding system** refers to a molecular structure having a series of alternate single and double bonds. Substances having this feature can absorb UV and/or visible light.

A **continuous spectrum** exhibits a broad range of wavelengths emitted or absorbed without a significant break or gap. (*See also* **emission spectrum** and **line spectrum**.)

Contributing structure. *See* **resonance structure**.

A **conversion factor** is a ratio of terms—equivalent to the number 1—that is used to change the unit(s) in which a quantity is expressed.

A **cooling curve** is a graph of temperature as a function of time, obtained as a substance is cooled. Constant-temperature segments of the curve correspond to phase changes, for example, condensation and freezing.

A **coordinate covalent bond** is a linkage between two atoms in which one atom provides both of the electrons of the shared pair.

A **coordination compound** is a substance made up of one or more complexes.

The **coordination number** of the metal center in a complex is the total number of points around this central atom at which bonding to ligands can occur.

Core electrons are electrons found in the inner electronic shells of atoms. (*See also* **valence electrons**.)

A **corrosive material** is one that degrades a metal or alloy by a chemical reaction. A corrosive material requires a special container because it corrodes conventional container materials.

The **coulomb** (**C**) is the SI unit of electric charge. The electric charge on an electron, for example, is -1.602×10^{-19} C.

A **coupled reaction** is one that involves two separate processes that can be combined to give a single reaction. In most cases, a thermodynamically unfavorable reaction is combined with another reaction to give an overall reaction that is thermodynamically favorable.

A **covalent bond** is a bond formed by a pair of electrons shared between atoms.

The **covalent radius** of an atom is one-half the distance between the nuclei of two like atoms joined in a molecule.

Critical mass is the minimum mass of a fissionable element that must be present to sustain a chain reaction. This is the mass required to produce an explosion of a nuclear bomb.

The **critical point** refers to the condition at which the liquid and gaseous (vapor) states of a substance become identical. It is the highest temperature point on a vapor pressure curve.

The **critical pressure** of a substance is the pressure at its critical point.

The **critical temperature** of a substance is the temperature at its critical point.

A **crystal** is a structure having plane surfaces, sharp edges, and a regular geometric shape. The fundamental units—atoms, ions, or molecules—are assembled in a regular, repeating manner extending in three dimensions through the crystal.

Crystal field theory is a theory of bonding in complexes that focuses on the abilities of ligands to produce a splitting of a d-subshell energy level of the metal center in a complex.

A **cubic close-packed (ccp)** structure has units (atoms, ions, or molecules) arranged in one of the two ways that minimize the voids between the units. The layers are stacked in the arrangement ABCABC. (*See also* **hexagonal close-packed**.)

Dalton's law of partial pressures states that in a mixture of gases, each gas expands to fill the container and exerts its own pressure, called a partial pressure. The total pressure of the mixture is the sum of the partial pressures exerted by the separate gases.

Data are the facts collected by careful observations and measurements made during experiments.

The **d-block** is the portion of the periodic table in which the $(n - 1)d$ subshell (the d subshell of the next-to-outermost shell) fills in the aufbau process. The d-block comprises the B-group elements in the periodic table.

The **debye (D)** is the unit used to express the dipole moments of polar molecules. One debye is equal to 3.34×10^{-30} C m.

Degenerate orbitals are two or more orbitals that are at the same energy level.

Deionized water is water that has been freed of ions through ion-exchange processes.

Deliquescence is the condensation of water vapor on a solid followed by solution formation.

Delocalized electrons are bonding electrons that are spread out over several atoms, rather than being in a fixed location between two atoms.

The **density (d)** of a sample of matter is its mass per unit volume, that is, the mass of the sample divided by its volume: $d = m/V$.

Deoxyribonucleic acid (DNA) is a polymer of nucleotides. The nucleotides consist of the sugar deoxyribose, a phosphate ester, and a cyclic amine base (adenine, guanine, thymine, or cytosine).

A **dextrorotatory** (+) substance rotates the plane of polarized light to the right.

A **diagonal relationship** refers to the similarity of certain second-period elements in one group of the periodic table with third-period elements of the next group to the right.

Diamagnetism is the weak repulsion by a magnetic field of a substance in which all electrons are paired.

Diffusion is the process by which one substance mixes with one or more other substances as a result of the random motion of molecules.

Dilution is a process of producing a solution of lower concentration from a more concentrated one by the addition of an appropriate quantity of solvent.

The **dipole moment (μ)** of a polar molecule is the product of the magnitude of the charges (δ) and the distance that separates them.

A **disaccharide** is a carbohydrate with molecules that can be hydrolyzed to two monosaccharide units.

A **dispersion force** is an attractive force between an instantaneous dipole and an induced dipole.

A **disproportionation reaction** is an oxidation–reduction reaction in which the same substance is both oxidized and reduced.

Doping refers to the addition of trace amounts of certain elements to a semiconductor to change the semiconducting properties. (*See also **n-type semiconductor** and **p-type semiconductor**.*)

A **double bond** is a covalent linkage in which two atoms share two pairs of electrons between them.

Dynamic equilibrium occurs when two opposing processes occur at exactly the same rate, with the result that no net change occurs.

The **effective nuclear charge (Z_{eff})** acting on an electron in an atom is the actual nuclear charge less the screening effect of other electrons in the atom.

Effusion is a process in which a gas escapes from its container through a tiny hole (an orifice). (*See also **Graham's law of effusion**.*)

An **elastomer** is a polymeric material that can be stretched significantly by a relatively low stress and upon release of the stress will return substantially to its original length.

An **electrochemical cell** is a combination of two half-cells in which metal electrodes are joined by a wire and the solutions are brought into contact through a salt bridge or by other means. (*See also **electrolytic cell**, **half-cell**, and **voltaic cell**.*)

Electrochemistry is a study of the relationships between electrical energy and chemical reactions.

An **electrode** is a conductive solid dipped into a solution or molten electrolyte to carry electricity to or from the liquid. (*See also **anode** and **cathode**.*)

Electrode potential is a property related to the tendency of a species to be reduced at an electrode.

Electrolysis is the decomposition of compounds by passing electricity through an ionic solution or a molten salt. A nonspontaneous chemical change occurs.

An **electrolyte** is a compound that conducts electricity when molten or in a liquid solution.

An **electrolytic cell** is an electrochemical cell in which electrolysis occurs.

The **electromagnetic spectrum** is the range of wavelengths and frequencies found for electromagnetic waves, extending from very long wavelength radio waves to the shortest gamma rays.

An **electromagnetic wave** originates in the vibrations of electrically charged objects and is propagated through oscillations of electric and magnetic fields.

An **electron** is a particle carrying the fundamental unit of negative electric charge. Electrons have a mass of 0.0005486 u and are found outside the nuclei of atoms.

Electron affinity is the energy change that occurs when an electron is added to an atom in the gaseous state.

Electron capture (EC) is a type of radioactive decay in which a nucleus absorbs an electron from the first or second electronic shell.

The **electron configuration** of an atom describes the distribution of electrons among atomic orbitals in the atom.

The **electronegativity (EN)** of an element is a measure of the tendency of its atoms in molecules to attract bonding electrons to themselves.

An **electron group** is a collection of valence electrons localized in a region around a central atom that exerts repulsions on other groups of valence electrons. It may be a bonding pair of electrons in a single bond, two pairs of electrons in a double bond, three pairs of electrons in a triple bond, a lone pair of electrons, or even an unpaired electron.

The **electron-group geometry** of a molecule or ion is the arrangement of all the electron groups—both bonding and nonbonding—about a central atom.

The **electron spin quantum number** (m_s) is a fourth quantum number (in addition to the three required by the Schrödinger wave equation) needed to complete the orbital designation of an electron. The two possible values of the spin quantum number are $+\frac{1}{2}$ and $-\frac{1}{2}$.

The **electron-Volt** is a unit of energy equal to that acquired by an electron as it passes through a potential difference of 1 V in a vacuum.

Electrophilic aromatic substitution is a reaction type in which an electrophile attaches to an aromatic ring such as benzene, replacing a hydrogen atom on the ring.

An **electrophilic reagent** is an electron-deficient molecule or ion that accepts an electron pair from a molecule, forming a covalent bond.

An **element** is a substance that cannot be broken down into simpler substances by chemical reactions. All atoms of a given element have the same atomic number.

An **elementary reaction** represents, at the molecular level, a single stage in the overall mechanism by which a chemical reaction occurs. (*See also* **bimolecular**, **termolecular**, and **unimolecular reaction**.)

An **emission (line) spectrum** is a dispersion of electromagnetic radiation into a discrete set of wavelength components. These components can be rendered as images of a slit (lines) in light from a spectroscope.

An **empirical formula** is the *simplest* formula describing the elements in a compound and the smallest integral (whole number) ratio in which their atoms are combined.

Enantiomers are pairs of mirror-image isomers that differ only in the direction in which they rotate the plane of polarized light. One isomer rotates the plane to the right, and the other rotates the plane to the same degree, but to the left.

An **endothermic reaction** is a reaction in which thermal energy is converted to chemical energy. In an endothermic process, a temperature decrease occurs in an isolated system, or in a nonisolated system, heat is absorbed from the surroundings.

The **endpoint** is the point in a titration at which an added indicator changes color. An indicator is chosen so that its endpoint matches the equivalence point of the reaction. (*See also* **equivalence point**.)

An **energy gap** (E_g) is the energy separation between a valence band and a conduction band that lies above it. In a semiconductor, the gap is relatively small, and in an insulator it is very large. (*See also* **conduction band**) and **valence band**.

An **energy level (shell)** is the state of an atom determined by the location of its electrons among the various principal shells and subshells.

Enthalpy (H) is a thermodynamic function defined as the sum of the internal energy and the pressure–volume product: $H = E + PV$.

The **enthalpy change** (ΔH) in a chemical reaction is equal to the heat of reaction at constant temperature and pressure, q_P.

An **enthalpy diagram** is a graphical representation of the change in enthalpy that occurs in a chemical reaction.

The **enthalpy (heat) of fusion** (ΔH_{fusion}) is the quantity of heat required to melt a given quantity of a solid.

The **enthalpy (heat) of sublimation** (ΔH_{subl}) is the quantity of heat required to vaporize a given quantity of solid at a constant temperature. It is equal to the sum of the enthalpies of fusion and vaporization.

The **enthalpy (heat) of vaporization** (ΔH_{vapn}) is the quantity of heat required to vaporize a given quantity of liquid at a constant temperature.

Entropy (S) is a property related to the distribution of the energy of a system among the available energy levels.

Entropy change (ΔS) is the difference in entropy between two states of a system, as between the products and reactants of a chemical reaction.

An **enzyme** is a protein that catalyzes reactions occurring in living organisms.

Equilibrium is a condition that is reached when two opposing processes occur at equal rates. As a result, the concentrations (or partial pressures) of the reacting species remain constant with time.

An **equilibrium constant expression** is a particular ratio of concentrations (or partial pressures) of products to reactants in a chemical reaction at equilibrium. The expression has a constant value that is independent of the manner in which equilibrium is reached. (*See also* K_c and K_p.)

The **equilibrium constant** (K_{eq}) is the form of the equilibrium constant based on activities and used in thermodynamic relationships. In the K_{eq} expression, species in solution are usually represented by their molarities and in gases by their partial pressures in atm.

The **equivalence point** of a titration is the point at which two reactants have been introduced into a reaction mixture in their stoichiometric proportions.

An **essential amino acid** is an amino acid that cannot be synthesized in the body and must therefore be included in the diet.

An **ester** $(R'COOR)$ is a compound derived from a carboxylic acid and an alcohol. The OH of the acid is replaced by an OR group.

An **ether** $(R'OR)$ is a compound having two hydrocarbon groups joined through an oxygen atom.

Eutrophication describes a process in which an overabundance of nutrients leads to an overgrowth of algae in a body of water. The algae then die, and their decay depletes the dissolved oxygen in the water.

An **excited state** of an atom is one in which one or more electrons has been promoted to a higher energy level than in the ground state. (*See also* **ground state**.)

An **exothermic reaction** is a reaction in which chemical energy is converted to thermal energy. In an exothermic process, a temperature increase occurs in an isolated system, or in a nonisolated system, heat is given off to the surroundings.

An **expanded valence shell** of a central atom in a Lewis structure is one that can accommodate more than the usual octet (8) of electrons.

An **experiment** is a carefully controlled procedure devised to test a hypothesis.

An **extensive property** is a physical property, such as mass or volume, that depends on the size or quantity of the sample of matter being considered.

A **face-centered cubic (fcc)** crystal structure has as its unit cell a cube with a structural unit at each of the corners and in the center of each face of the cube. (*See also* **unit cell**.)

The **Faraday constant** (F) is the electric charge, in coulombs, per mole of electrons—96,485 C/mol.

The **f-block** is the portion of the periodic table in which the $(n - 2)f$ subshell (the f subshell of the second-from-outermost shell) fills in the aufbau process. The f-block consists of the lanthanides and actinides.

Ferromagnetism is a magnetic effect much stronger than paramagnetism and associated with iron, cobalt, nickel, and certain alloys. It requires that atoms be both paramagnetic and of the right size to be able to form magnetic domains.

The **first law of thermodynamics** states that the internal energy of an isolated system is constant, or if a system interacts with its surroundings by exchanging heat and/or work, the exchange must occur in such a way that no energy is created or destroyed. (*See also* **law of conservation of energy**.)

A **first-order reaction** has a rate equation in which the sum of the exponents, $m + n + \cdots = 1$.

Flotation is a metallurgical method by which an ore is separated from waste rock, based on selective wetting of the ore by a surface-active agent.

Formal charge, a concept used in writing Lewis structures, is the number of valence electrons in an isolated atom minus the number of electrons assigned to that atom in a Lewis structure.

The **formation constant** (K_f) describes equilibrium between a complex ion and the cation and ligands from which it is formed.

Formula mass is the mass of a formula unit relative to that of a carbon-12 atom; it is the sum of the masses of the atoms or ions represented by the formula.

A **formula unit** is the simplest combination of atoms or ions consistent with the formula of a compound. In an ionic compound, it is the smallest possible electrically neutral collection of ions.

Fractional crystallization is a method of purifying a solid by dissolving it in a suitable solvent and changing the solution temperature to a value where the solute solubility is lower (usually a lower temperature). Excess solute crystallizes as pure solid, and soluble impurities remain in solution.

Fractional distillation is a method of separating the volatile components of a solution having different vapor pressure and boiling points. It involves repeated vaporizations and condensations occurring continuously in a distillation column.

The **free electron model** of metals considers the metal to be composed of positive ions surrounded by a "sea" of mobile electrons.

The **free energy change** (ΔG) is the difference in free energy between two states of a system, as between the free energies of the products and reactants of a chemical reaction. It is given by the equation $\Delta G = \Delta H - T\Delta S$.

A **free radical** is a highly reactive atom or molecular fragment characterized by having one or more unpaired electrons. Free radicals are encountered as intermediates in some chemical reactions.

Freezing point is the temperature at which a liquid freezes—that is, the liquid comes into equilibrium with solid. For a pure substance, the freezing point and melting point are the same.

The **frequency** (ν) of a wave is the number of cycles of the wave (the number of wavelengths) that pass through a point in a unit of time.

A **functional group** is an atom or grouping of atoms attached to or within a hydrocarbon chain or ring that confers characteristic properties to the molecule as a whole.

Fusion (melting) is the process of changing a solid to a liquid.

Galvanic cell *See* **voltaic cell**.

A **gamma** (γ) **ray** is a highly penetrating form of electromagnetic radiation emitted by the nuclei of certain radioactive atoms as they undergo decay.

The **gas constant** (R) is a proportionality constant used in the ideal gas law and in other relationships, and has a value of 0.082057 L atm/(mol K) or 8.314 J/(mol K).

A **gene** is a section of a DNA molecule found in the chromosomes of cells; genes are the basic units of heredity.

Geometric isomers in organic compounds are isomers (cis, trans) that differ in the positions of attachment of substituent groups at a double bond. In complexes, the isomers differ in the positions of attachment of ligands to the central metal ion.

Gibbs free energy (G), a thermodynamic function used in establishing criteria for equilibrium and for spontaneous change, is defined as $G = H - TS$, where H is the enthalpy, T is the Kelvin temperature, and S is the entropy of a system.

Global warming refers to the anticipated increase in Earth's average temperature resulting from the accumulation of CO_2 and other infrared-absorbing gases in the atmosphere.

Graham's law of effusion states that the rates of effusion of gas molecules are inversely proportional to the square roots of their molar masses.

The **greenhouse effect** refers to the ability of $CO_2(g)$ and certain other gases to absorb and trap energy radiated by Earth's surface as infrared radiation.

The **ground state** of an atom is the atom at its lowest energy level. (*See also* **excited state**.)

Groups of the periodic table are the vertical columns of elements having similar properties.

A **half-cell** is an electrode in a solution of ions; the reaction in the half-cell is either an oxidation or a reduction. (*See also* **electrochemical cell**.)

The **half-life** ($t_{1/2}$) of a chemical reaction is the time required to consume one-half of the initial quantity of a reactant. For radioactive decay, it is the time in which one-half of the atoms of a radioactive nuclide disintegrate.

A **half-reaction** is that portion of an oxidation–reduction reaction that represents either the oxidation process or the reduction process.

Hard water is groundwater containing significant concentrations of doubly charged cations derived from natural sources, such as Ca^{2+}, Mg^{2+}, Fe^{2+}, and associated anions.

A **hazardous material** is one that, when improperly managed, can cause or contribute to death or illness or threaten human health or the environment.

Heat (q) is an energy transfer into or out of a system caused by a difference in temperature between a system and its surroundings.

Heat capacity (C) of a system is the quantity of heat needed to raise the temperature of a system by 1 °C or 1 K.

A **heating curve** is a graph of temperature as a function of time obtained by gradually heating a substance. Constant-temperature segments of the curve correspond to phase changes. (*See also* **cooling curve**.)

The **heat of reaction** (q_{rxn}) is the quantity of heat exchanged between a system and its surroundings when a chemical reaction occurs at a constant temperature and pressure.

The **Henderson–Hasselbalch equation** is used to relate the pH of a solution of a weak acid and its conjugate base to the pK_a of the weak acid and to the ratio of the stoichiometric concentration of the conjugate base to that of the weak acid: pH = pK_a + log ([conjugate base]/[weak acid]).

Henry's law states that the solubility of a gas is directly proportional to the partial pressure of the gas in equilibrium with the solution.

Hess's law states that the enthalpy change of a reaction is constant, whether the reaction is carried out directly in one step or indirectly through a number of steps.

A **heterogeneous mixture** is a mixture in which the composition and/or properties vary from one region to another within the mixture.

A **hexagonal close-packed (hcp)** structure is one of the two crystal arrangements in which the structural units are close-packed. The layers are stacked in the arrangement ABABAB. (*See also* **cubic close-packed**.)

A **homogeneous mixture** is a mixture having the same composition and properties throughout the given mixture.

A **homologous series** is a series of organic compounds whose formulas and structures vary in a regular manner and whose properties are predictable based on this regularity.

Humidity is a measure of the water vapor content of air. The *absolute humidity* is the actual quantity of water vapor present in an air sample, and the *relative humidity* of air is a measure of water vapor content as a percentage of the maximum possible quantity.

Hund's rule states that electrons occupy atomic orbitals of identical energy singly before any pairing of electrons occurs. Furthermore, the electrons in the singly occupied orbitals have parallel spins.

Hybridization is a hypothetical process in which pure atomic orbitals are combined to produce a set of new orbitals called hybrid orbitals to describe covalent bonding by the valence bond method. (*See also* sp, sp^2, sp^3, sp^3d, sp^3d^2 hybridization.)

Hybrid orbitals are formed by a combination of atomic orbitals to produce a set of new orbitals.

A **hydrate** is a compound that incorporates water molecules into its basic solid structure. The formula unit of a hydrate includes a fixed number of water molecules.

A **hydrocarbon** is a compound containing only hydrogen and carbon atoms.

In a **hydrogenation reaction**, $H_2(g)$ is a reactant and H atoms are added to C atoms at a carbon-to-carbon double or triple bond.

A **hydrogen bond** is a type of intermolecular force in which a hydrogen atom covalently bonded in one molecule is simultaneously attracted to a nonmetal atom in a neighboring molecule. In most cases, both the atom to which the hydrogen atom is bonded and the one to which it is attracted must be small atoms of high electronegativity, usually N, O, or F.

The **hydrologic (water) cycle** is the series of natural processes by which water is recycled through the environment—Earth's solid crust, oceans and freshwater bodies, and the atmosphere.

In a general sense, **hydrolysis** is the reaction of a substance with water in which both the substance and the water molecules split apart. In a more limited sense, it is an acid–base reaction between an ion and water.

Hydrometallurgy is the extraction of a metal from its ores by processes that involve water and aqueous solutions.

A **hypertonic** solution is a solution having an osmotic pressure greater than that of body fluids (blood, tears). A hypertonic solution has a greater osmotic pressure than does an isotonic solution.

A **hypothesis** is a tentative explanation or prediction concerning some phenomenon.

A **hypotonic** solution is a solution having an osmotic pressure less than that of body fluids (blood, tears). A hypotonic solution has a lower osmotic pressure than does an isotonic solution.

An **ideal gas** is a hypothetical gas that strictly obeys the simple gas laws and the ideal gas law.

The **ideal gas law** or **ideal gas equation** states that the volume of a gas is directly proportional to the amount of a gas and its Kelvin temperature and is inversely proportional to its pressure: $PV = nRT$.

An **ideal solution** is one for which the heat of solution is zero and the volume of solution is the total of the volumes of the solution components. In general, the physical properties of an ideal solution can be predicted from the properties of its components.

An **ignitable material** is one that burns readily on ignition, presenting a fire hazard.

An **indicator** is a substance added to the reaction mixture in a titration that changes color at or near the equivalence point.

Industrial smog is polluted air associated with industrial activities. The principal pollutants are oxides of sulfur and particulate matter.

An **inert pair** refers to the ns^2 electrons in the valence shell of the posttransition elements of groups 3A, 4A, and 5A. These electrons may remain in the valence shell following the loss of the np electrons, as in Tl^+, Sn^{2+}, Pb^{2+}, and Bi^{3+}.

The **initial rate of reaction** is the rate of a reaction immediately after the reactants are brought together. The rate is generally expressed in terms of the rate of change with time of the concentration of one of the reactants or one of the products.

An **instantaneous rate of reaction** is the rate of a reaction at some particular time in the course of a reaction. It is established through a tangent line to a concentration versus time graph at the time in question.

An **integrated rate law** is an equation derived from the rate law for a reaction that expresses the concentration of a reactant as a function of time. (*See also* **rate law**.)

An **intensive property** is a property of a sample of matter, such as temperature or density, that is independent of the quantity of matter being considered.

An **interhalogen compound** is a compound of two (sometimes three) halogen elements.

An **intermediate** is a substance that is produced in one elementary step in a reaction mechanism and consumed in another. The intermediate does not appear in the chemical equation for the overall reaction.

An **intermolecular force** is a force *between* molecules.

The **internal energy** (**U**) is the total amount of energy contained in a thermodynamic system. The components of internal energy are energy associated with random molecular motion (thermal energy) and that associated with chemical bonds and intermolecular forces (chemical energy).

An **ion** is an electrically charged particle comprised of one or more atoms.

Ion exchange is the replacement in solution of ions of one type for ions of another type, using an ion-exchange resin or zeolite.

Ionic bonds are attractive forces between positive and negative ions, holding them together in solid crystals.

An **ionic compound** is a compound that consists of oppositely charged ions held together by electrostatic attractions.

Ionic radius is a measure of the size of a cation or anion based on the distance between the centers of ions in an ionic compound.

Ionization energy is the energy required to remove the least tightly bound electron from a ground-state atom (or ion) in the gaseous state.

The **ion product of water** (K_w) is the equilibrium constant for autoionization of water into H_3O^+ and OH^-. At 25 °C, its value is 1.0×10^{-14}.

The **isoelectric point (pI)** is the pH value at which an amino acid exists as a zwitterion.

Isoelectronic species (atoms, ions, molecules) have the same number of electrons.

Isomers are compounds having the same molecular formula but different structural formulas.

An **isotonic** solution is one that has the same osmotic pressure as body fluids (blood, tears).

Isotopes are atoms that have the same number of protons in their nuclei—the same atomic number—but different numbers of neutrons and, therefore, different mass numbers.

The **joule (J)** is the basic unit of energy in SI. It is the work done by a force of 1 newton (N) acting over a distance of 1 meter. That is, $1 \text{ J} = 1 \text{ N m} = 1 \text{ kg m}^2 \text{ s}^{-2}$.

K_c is the numerical value of an equilibrium constant expression in which molarities of products and reactants are used.

K_p is the numerical value of an equilibrium constant expression in which the partial pressures (usually in atm) of gaseous products and reactants are used.

A **kelvin (K)** is the SI base unit of temperature. An interval of 1 kelvin on the Kelvin scale is the same as one degree on the Celsius scale.

The **Kelvin scale** is an absolute temperature scale with its zero at −273.15 °C; its relationship to the Celsius scale is $T(K) = T(°C) + 273.15$.

A **ketone** is an organic substance whose molecules have a carbonyl group between two other C atoms.

The **kilogram (kg)** is the SI base unit of mass.

A **kilopascal (kPa)** is 1000 pascals (Pa). (*See also* **pascal**.)

Kinetic energy (E_k) is energy of motion, given by the expression $E_k = \frac{1}{2}mv^2$.

The **kinetic-molecular theory of gases** is a theory based on a small number of postulates concerning gas molecules from which simple gas laws, the ideal gas law, and equations dealing with temperature and molecular speeds can be derived.

The **lanthanide** elements constitute the portion of the f-block of the periodic table in which the $4f$ subshell fills in the aufbau process.

The **lanthanide contraction** describes the general downward trend in the radii of lanthanide atoms and ions with increasing atomic number.

Lattice energy is the enthalpy change that accompanies the formation of one mole of an ionic solid from its gaseous ions.

The **law of combining volumes** states that when gases measured at the same temperature and pressure are allowed to react, the volumes of gaseous reactants and products are in small whole-number ratios.

The **law of conservation of energy** states that in a physical or chemical change, energy can be neither created nor destroyed.

The **law of conservation of mass** states that the total mass remains constant during a reaction. That is, the mass of the products of a reaction is always equal to the total mass of the reactants consumed.

The **law of constant composition** or **law of definite proportions** states that all samples of a particular compound have the same composition. That is, all samples have the same proportions by mass of the elements present.

The **law of multiple proportions** states that when two or more different compounds of the same two elements are compared, the masses of one element that combine with a fixed mass of the second element are in the ratio of small whole numbers.

Le Châtelier's principle is a statement that permits qualitative predictions about the effects produced by changes (amounts of reactants or products, reaction volume, temperature, etc.) imposed on a system at equilibrium. (*See* page 589 for a statement of the principle.)

A **levorotatory** (−) substance rotates the plane of polarized light to the left.

Lewis acid. *See* **acid.**

Lewis base. *See* **base.**

A **Lewis structure** is a representation of covalent bonding through Lewis symbols, shared electron pairs, and lone-pair electrons.

A **Lewis symbol** is a representation of an element in which the chemical symbol stands for the core of the atom and dots placed around the symbol represent its valence electrons.

A **ligand** is a species (atom, molecule, anion, or, rarely, cation) that is bonded to a metal center in a complex by a coordinate covalent bond.

The **limiting reactant** (reagent) is the reactant that is completely consumed in a chemical reaction, thereby limiting the amounts of products formed.

The **line spectrum** of an element reflects the discrete wavelengths of light emitted by the element. (*See also* **emission spectrum.**)

A **liquid crystal** is a physical form of a substance that has the fluid properties of a liquid and the optical properties of a crystalline solid.

A **lipid** is a cellular component that is insoluble in water but soluble in solvents of low polarity such as hexane, diethyl ether, and benzene.

A **liter (L)** is a metric unit of volume equal to 1 cubic decimeter or 1000 cubic centimeters: $1\ L = 1\ dm^3 = 1000\ cm^3$.

Lone pairs are electron pairs assigned exclusively to one of the atoms in a Lewis structure. They are not shared and hence are not involved in the chemical bonding.

Macromolecules are giant molecules (polymers) having small molecules (monomers) as their building blocks.

Magic numbers are numbers of protons and neutrons in stable nucleon shells that make up especially stable atomic nuclei.

The **magnetic quantum number** (m_l) is the last of three parameters that must be assigned a specific value to achieve a solution of Schrödinger's wave equation for the hydrogen atom: m_l is an integer between $-l$ and $+l$ (including 0). (*See also* **orbital angular momentum quantum number** and **principal quantum number.**)

A **main-group element** is an element in which the subshell being filled in the aufbau process is either an s or a p subshell of the principal shell of highest principal quantum number (the outermost shell). Main-group elements are located in the s- and p-blocks of the periodic table.

A **manometer** is a device used to measure pressure of a confined gas.

Mass is the quantity of matter in an object. It is related to the force required to move the object or to change its velocity if the object is already in motion.

The **mass percent composition** of a substance is the proportion, by mass, of each element in the substance expressed as a percentage.

The **mass number** (A) is the sum of the number of protons and neutrons in the nucleus of an atom. It is also called the *nucleon number*.

A **mass spectrometer** is a device that separates ions according to their mass-to-charge ratios.

Matter is anything that occupies space and has mass.

The **melting point** of a solid is the temperature at which it melts, that is, the temperature at which it comes into equilibrium with the liquid phase.

A **meniscus** is the interface between a liquid and the air above it.

A **meta director** is a substituent already on a benzene ring, such as —COOH or —NO$_2$, that causes an incoming electrophile to substitute mainly in the meta position.

A **metal** is an element having a distinctive set of properties: luster, good heat and electrical conductivity, malleability, and ductility. Metal atoms generally have small numbers of valence electrons and a tendency to form cations. Metals are found to the left of the stepped diagonal line in the periodic table.

The **metallic radius** is one-half the distance between the nuclei of adjacent atoms in a solid metal.

A **metalloid** is an element that has the physical appearance of a metal but some nonmetallic properties as well. Metalloids are located along the stepped diagonal line in the periodic table.

The **meter (m)** is the SI base unit of length.

The **method of initial rates** is an experimental method of establishing the rate law of a reaction. To establish the order of the reaction with respect to one of the reactants, the initial rates are compared for two different concentrations of that reactant, with the concentrations of all other reactants held constant. (*See also* **initial rate of reaction**, **rate law**, and **order of a reaction.**)

A **millimeter of mercury (mmHg)** is a unit used to express gas pressure: 1 mmHg = 1/760 atm (exactly). (*See also* **atmosphere.**)

A **mixture** is a type of matter with composition and properties that may vary from one sample to another. (*See also* **heterogeneous mixture** and **homogeneous mixture.**)

The **molality (m)** of a solution is the amount of solute, in moles, per kilogram of solvent (not of solution).

Molar concentration. *See* **molarity.**

Molar heat capacity is the quantity of heat required to change the temperature of one mole of a substance by 1 °C (or 1 K); it is the heat capacity of one mole of substance.

The **molarity (M)** of a solution is the amount of solute, in moles, per liter of solution.

The **molar mass** of a substance is the mass of one mole of that substance. It is numerically equal to the atomic mass, molecular mass, or formula mass, and expressed as g/mol.

The **molar volume of a gas** refers to the volume occupied by one mole of gas at a fixed temperature and pressure; it is essentially independent of the identity of the gas. At standard temperature and pressure, the molar volume of an ideal gas is 22.4141 L.

A **mole (mol)** is an amount of substance that contains as many elementary units (atoms, molecules, formula units) as there are atoms in exactly 12 g of the isotope carbon-12.

A **molecular compound** has molecules as its smallest characteristic entities, and these molecules determine the properties of the compound.

A **molecular formula** gives the symbol and *exact* number of each kind of atom found in a molecule.

Molecular geometry describes the geometric figure formed when appropriate atomic nuclei in a molecule or polyatomic ion are joined by straight lines. Molecular geometry refers to the geometric shape of a molecule or polyatomic ion.

The **molecularity** of a reaction is the number of molecules (or ions) that come together to form the activated complex.

Molecular mass is the average mass of a molecule of a substance relative to that of a carbon-12 atom; it is the sum of the masses of the atoms represented in the molecular formula.

A **molecular orbital** is a region in a molecule where there is a high electron charge density or a high probability of finding an electron. (*See also* **antibonding molecular orbital** and **bonding molecular orbital**.)

A **molecule** is a group of two or more atoms held together in a definite arrangement by forces called covalent bonds.

The **mole fraction (*x*)** of a component in a homogeneous mixture (a solution) is the fraction of all the molecules in the mixture contributed by that component.

The **mole percent** of a component in a homogeneous mixture (a solution) is the percentage of all the molecules in the mixture contributed by that component.

Mole ratio. *See* **stoichiometric factor**.

A **monodentate ligand** attaches to the metal center in a complex through one pair of electrons on a donor atom.

Monomers are small molecules that are capable of independent existence, but which under appropriate conditions can join together to form a giant molecule called a polymer. (*See also* **polymerization**.)

A **monoprotic acid** has one ionizable hydrogen atom per molecule.

A **monosaccharide** is a carbohydrate that cannot be hydrolyzed into simpler sugars.

A **multiple bond** is a covalent linkage in which two atoms share either two pairs (double bond) or three pairs (triple bond) of electrons between them.

Nanomaterials are materials possessing unique and desirable properties when the length scale of the sample is reduced to a nanometer scale.

The **Nernst equation** relates a cell voltage under nonstandard conditions, E_{cell}, to the standard cell potential, E°_{cell}, and the concentrations of reactants and products of a redox reaction. Its form at 25 °C is $E_{cell} = E^{\circ}_{cell} - (0.0592/n) \log Q$, where n is the number of moles of electrons transferred in the oxidation and reduction half-reactions of a redox reaction and Q is the reaction quotient.

A **net ionic equation** is an equation that represents the actual molecules or ions that participate in a chemical reaction, eliminating all nonparticipating species (so-called spectator ions).

In a **network covalent solid**, covalent bonds extend throughout the crystalline solid.

A **neutralization** reaction is one in which an acid and a base react in such a manner that there is neither excess acid nor base in the final solution. The products of the reaction are water and a salt.

The **neutron** is a fundamental particle of matter found in the nuclei of atoms. Neutrons have a mass of 1.0087 u and no electric charge.

A **newton (N)** is the basic unit of force in SI. It is the force required to give a 1-kg mass an acceleration of 1 m/s^2. That is, 1 N = 1 kg m s^{-2}.

The **nitrogen cycle** refers to the totality of activities in which nitrogen atoms are cycled through the environment.

Nitrogen fixation refers to the conversion of atmospheric nitrogen (N_2) into nitrogen compounds. This occurs naturally in the nitrogen cycle and artificially in the synthesis of ammonia. (*See also* **nitrogen cycle**.)

A **noble gas** is an element in group 8A of the periodic table. Noble gases have the valence-shell electron configuration ns^2np^6 (except helium, $1s^2$).

A **nonelectrolyte** is a substance that exists exclusively or almost exclusively in molecular form, whether in the pure state or in solution.

A **nonmetal** is an element that lacks metallic properties. Nonmetals are generally poor conductors of heat and electricity and brittle when in the solid state. Nonmetal atoms generally have larger numbers of valence electrons than do metals and they tend to form anions. Nonmetal atoms are confined to the *p*-block of the periodic table (plus hydrogen and helium).

In a **nonpolar covalent bond**, there is an equal sharing of the electrons between the bonded atoms. The electrons are no closer to one atom than to the other, so there is no charge separation.

A **nonspontaneous process** will not occur in a system left to itself. It can be made to occur only through intervention from outside the thermodynamic system.

The **normal boiling point** of a liquid is the temperature at which the liquid boils at 1 atm pressure.

The **normal melting point** of a solid is the temperature at which the solid melts at 1 atm pressure.

An ***n*-type semiconductor** is a semiconductor doped with donor atoms that can lose electrons to the conduction band. Electric current in this type of semiconductor is carried primarily by these donor electrons. (*See also* **doping**.)

Nuclear binding energy is the energy released when the nucleons are bound together into the nucleus of an atom. It is the energy equivalent of the mass lost in creating a nucleus from its individual protons and neutrons.

Nuclear fission is the splitting of a large unstable nucleus into two lighter fragments and two or more neutrons. In this process, mass is converted to an equivalent quantity of energy, which is released.

Nuclear fusion is the joining together, or fusing, of lighter nuclei into a heavier one. In the process, some matter is converted to energy, which is released.

Nucleon is the general term for the nuclear particles protons and neutrons.

A **nucleophile** is a molecule or ion that donates a lone pair of electrons to another molecule, forming a covalent bond.

Nucleotides are the structural units, consisting of a sugar, a phosphate ester group, and a cyclic amine base, that make up deoxyribonucleic acid (DNA) and ribonucleic acid (RNA).

The **nucleus** of an atom is the densely packed, positively charged core of an atom, containing the protons, the neutrons, and most of the atom's mass.

Nuclide is a term used to signify an atomic species having a particular atomic number and mass number, such as $^{12}_{6}C$. (*See also* **isotopes**.)

The **octet rule** states that most covalently bonded atoms represented in a Lewis structure have eight electrons in their outermost (valence) shells. In the formation of ionic compounds, the ions of the main-group elements also tend to follow the octet rule.

Optical isomers are molecules or species that are nonsuperimposable mirror images; they differ only in the way they rotate the plane of polarized light. (*See also* **enantiomers**.)

The **orbital angular momentum quantum number (*l*)** is the second of three parameters that must be assigned a specific value to achieve a solution of Schrödinger's wave equation for the hydrogen atom: $l = 0, 1, 2, 3, \ldots, n - 1$. The value of l establishes a particular sublevel or subshell within a principal energy level.

An **orbital diagram** is a method of denoting an electron configuration in which parentheses or boxes are used to represent orbitals within

subshells and arrows are used to represent electrons in the orbitals.

The **order of a reaction** is determined by the exponents of the concentration terms in the rate law for the reaction: Rate of reaction $= k[A]^m[B]^n \ldots$. The order of the reaction with respect to A is m; with respect to B, it is n; and so on. The overall order of the reaction is $m + n + \ldots$.

An **ore** is a naturally occurring mineral containing a metal in a form and concentration that makes extraction of the metal feasible.

Osmosis is the net flow of a solvent through a semipermeable membrane, from pure solvent into a solution or from a solution of a lower concentration into one of a higher concentration.

The **osmotic pressure** of a solution is the pressure that must be applied to a solution to prevent the flow of solvent molecules into the solution when the solution and pure solvent are separated by a semipermeable membrane.

The **overvoltage** of an electrode reaction is the excess voltage above that calculated from $E°$ values required to bring about the reaction.

Oxidation is a process in which the oxidation number of an element increases. It is the half-reaction of an oxidation–reduction reaction in which electrons are given up.

The **oxidation number** of an element in a compound is a means of designating the number of electrons that its atoms have lost, gained, or shared in forming that compound.

An **oxidizing agent** (oxidant) is a substance that makes possible the oxidation that occurs in an oxidation–reduction reaction. The oxidizing agent itself is reduced.

The **ozone layer** is a band of the stratosphere, about 20 km thick and centered at an altitude of about 25 to 30 km, that has a much higher concentration of ozone than the rest of the atmosphere.

Paramagnetism is the attraction into an external magnetic field of substances that have unpaired electrons.

Partial pressure. *See* **Dalton's law of partial pressure**.

A **partial pressure equilibrium constant** (K_p) is the numerical value of an equilibrium constant expression in which the partial pressures (usually in atm) of gaseous products and reactants are used.

Particulate matter is an air pollutant consisting of solid and liquid particles of greater than molecular size but small enough to remain suspended in air.

Parts per billion (ppb) expresses the composition of a mixture as the number of parts of one component per billion parts of the mixture as a whole, usually on a mass basis for liquid solutions and a mole basis for gaseous mixtures.

Parts per million (ppm) expresses the composition of a mixture as the number of parts of one component per million parts of the mixture as a whole, usually on a mass basis for liquid solutions and a mole basis for gaseous mixtures.

Parts per trillion (ppt) expresses the composition of a mixture as the number of parts of one component per trillion parts of the mixture as a whole, usually on a mass basis for liquid solutions and a mole basis for gaseous mixtures.

A **pascal (Pa)** is the basic unit of pressure in SI. It is a pressure of 1 newton per square meter, 1 N m^{-2}.

The **Pauli exclusion principle** states that no two electrons in an atom may have all four quantum numbers alike. Consequences of this principle are that there may be no more than two electrons in an orbital and that the two electrons must have opposing spins.

The **p-block** is the portion of the periodic table in which the np subshell (the p subshell of the outer shell) fills in the aufbau process. The p-block elements are all main-group elements.

A **peptide** is composed of a chain of two or more amino acids joined through peptide (amide) linkages in chains of peptides, polypeptides, and proteins.

The **percent yield** is the ratio of the actual yield to the theoretical yield of a chemical reaction, expressed as a percentage.

The **periodic law** states that certain sets of physical and chemical properties recur at regular intervals (periodically) when the elements are arranged according to increasing atomic number.

A **periodic table** is a tabular arrangement of the elements according to increasing atomic number that places elements having similar properties into the same vertical columns. (Mendeleev's original periodic table was arranged according to atomic weights, not atomic numbers.)

Permanent hardness in water is the condition in which the predominant anions are other than HCO_3^-. (*See also* **hard water**.)

The **pH** is the negative of the logarithm of the hydronium ion concentration in a solution: $pH = -\log[H_3O^+]$.

A **phase change** is a change from one phase to another, as in solid to liquid or liquid to gas.

A **phase diagram** is a pressure–temperature plot indicating the conditions under which a substance exists as a solid phase, a liquid, a gas, or some combination of these in equilibrium.

Photochemical smog is air that is polluted with oxides of nitrogen and unburned hydrocarbons, together with ozone and several other components produced by the action of sunlight.

The **photoelectric effect** refers to the emission of electrons from the surface of certain materials when they absorb light of the appropriate frequency.

A **photon** is a quantum of energy in the form of light. The energy of the photon is given by the expression $E = h\nu$.

A **photovoltaic cell** is a device that uses semiconductors to convert solar energy (light) into electricity.

In a **physical change**, a sample of matter undergoes a change in phase or state or other property that is observable but does not involve a change in composition.

A **physical property** is a characteristic that a sample of matter displays without undergoing a change in composition.

A **pi (π) bond** forms by the overlap in a parallel or side-by-side fashion of p orbitals of the bonded atoms. A double bond consists of one σ and one π bond; a triple bond, of one σ and two π bonds.

Pig iron is crude, high-carbon iron produced by reduction of iron ore in a blast furnace.

pK_a is the negative of the logarithm of the ionization constant of an acid: $pK_a = -\log K_a$.

pK_b is the negative of the logarithm of the ionization constant of a base: $pK_b = -\log K_b$.

pK_w is the negative of the logarithm of the ion product of water: $pK_w = -\log K_w = -\log(1.0 \times 10^{-14}) = 14.00$ (at 25 °C). (*See also* **ion product of water**.)

Planck's constant (h) is the numerical constant relating the energy of a photon of light and its frequency: $E = h\nu$. Its value is $6.62606876 \times 10^{-34}$ J s.

pOH is the negative of the logarithm of the hydroxide concentration in an aqueous solution: $pOH = -\log[OH^-]$.

In a **polar** bond between two atoms, electrons are drawn closer to the more electronegative atom, creating a separation of charge. One end of the bond has a small negative charge, $\delta-$, and the other end, a small positive charge, $\delta+$.

Polarizability is a measure of the ease with which electron charge density in an atom or molecule is distorted by an external electric field. It measures the ease with which a dipole can be induced in an atom or molecule.

In a **polar molecule**, a small separation of positive ($\delta+$) and negative ($\delta-$) charge exists, caused by electronegativity differences and molecular geometry.

A **polyatomic ion** is a charged particle containing two or more covalently bonded atoms.

A **polydentate** ligand attaches to a metal center in a complex at more than one point.

A **polymer** is a giant molecule formed by the combination of smaller molecules (monomers) in a repeating manner.

Polymerization is a type of reaction in which small repeating units (monomers) combine to form giant molecules (polymers).

Polymorphism is the property of a substance crystallizing in two or more forms, such as sulfur in its rhombic and monoclinic forms.

A **polypeptide** is a polymer of amino acids; it is usually of lower molecular mass than a protein.

A **polyprotic acid** has more than one ionizable H atom per molecule. The ionization of a polyprotic acid occurs in discrete steps.

A **polysaccharide** is a carbohydrate, each molecule of which can be hydrolyzed into many monosaccharide units.

A **positive hole** is a "missing electron" in a semiconductor; the vacancy acts like a positive ion.

A **positron** (β^+) is a positively charged particle having the same mass as a β^- particle.

The **potential difference**, measured in volts, is the difference in electric potential between two points in an electric circuit, for example, between the electrodes in an electrochemical cell.

Potential energy is energy that is due to position or arrangement. It is the energy associated with forces of attraction and repulsion between objects.

A **precipitate** is an insoluble compound formed by a reaction in solution.

A **precipitation reaction** is a chemical reaction between ions in solution that produces an insoluble solid—a precipitate.

The **precision** of a set of measurements refers to how closely members of a set of measurements agree with one another. It reflects the degree of reproducibility of the measurements.

Pressure (P) is a force per unit area—that is, $P = F/A$.

Primary sewage treatment involves treatment of sewage in a holding pond intended to remove some of the sewage solids as sludge by simple sedimentation (settling).

The **primary structure** is the amino acid sequence in a protein or of nucleotides in a nucleic acid.

The **principal quantum number** (n) is the first of three quantum numbers that must be assigned a specific numerical value to achieve a solution to Schrödinger's wave equation for the hydrogen atom: $n = 1, 2, 3, \ldots$. Its value designates the principal energy level of an electron in an atom.

A **principal shell** (level) refers to the collection of orbitals having the same principal quantum number.

A **product** is a substance that is produced in a chemical reaction. The formulas of products appear on the right side of a chemical equation.

A **protein** is a high-molecular-mass polymer of amino acids.

A **proton** is a nuclear particle carrying the fundamental unit of positive charge and having a mass of 1.0073 u.

A **proton acceptor** is a Brønsted–Lowry base. (*See also* **base**.)

A **proton donor** is a Brønsted–Lowry acid. (*See also* **acid**.)

Pseudohalogens are certain groupings of atoms, such as CN and OCN, that mimic the characteristics of a halogen atom.

A **p-type semiconductor** is a semiconductor that has been doped with acceptor atoms that extract electrons from chemical bonds in the semiconductor, producing positive holes in the valence band. Electric current in these semiconductors is carried primarily by positive holes. (*See also* **doping**.)

Pyrometallurgy includes metallurgical methods based on high-temperature reactions involving solids.

A **quantum** is the smallest quantity of energy that can be emitted or absorbed in a process, as given by the expression $E = h\nu$.

Quantum (wave) **mechanics** is the mathematical description of atomic structure based on the wave properties of subatomic properties.

Quantum numbers are certain integral values assigned to three parameters in a wave equation to obtain acceptable solutions to the equation.

The **quaternary structure** of a protein is the arrangement of protein subunits in geometric shapes.

A **rad** (radiation absorbed dose) corresponds to the absorption of 1×10^{-2} J of energy per kilogram of matter.

The **radioactive decay law** states that the rate of disintegration of a radioactive isotope, called the decay rate or activity, is directly proportional to the number of atoms present.

A **radioactive decay series** is a sequence of nuclear processes involving α and β emissions by which an initial long-lived radioactive nucleus is eventually converted to a stable nonradioactive nucleus.

A **radioactive tracer** is a radionuclide that can be used to follow a physical or chemical process through the ionizing radiation that it emits.

Radioactivity (radioactive decay) is the spontaneous emission of ionizing radiation by the atomic nuclei of certain isotopes.

Raoult's law states that the addition of a solute lowers the vapor pressure of the solvent and that the fractional lowering of the vapor pressure is equal to the mole fraction of the solute.

The **rate constant** (k) of a reaction is a numerical constant that relates the rate of the reaction to the concentrations of the reactants. Rate constants are functions of temperature. (*See also* **rate law**.)

The **rate-determining step** in a reaction mechanism is the step (usually the slowest) that is crucial in establishing the rate of an overall reaction.

The **rate law** (rate equation) of a chemical reaction is an expression relating the rate of the reaction to the concentrations of the reactants.

Rate of a reaction is the increase in concentration of a product per unit of time or the decrease in concentration of a reactant per unit of time, usually expressed as M s^{-1}.

A **reactant** is a starting material or substance consumed in a chemical reaction. The formulas of reactants appear on the left side of a chemical equation.

A **reaction mechanism** is a detailed representation of a chemical reaction consisting of a series of elementary reactions. A plausible mechanism must be consistent with the stoichiometry and the rate law of the net reaction.

A **reaction profile** is a schematic representation of changes in energy during the course of a reaction. The profile shows activation energies and enthalpies of reaction and identifies the energies of reactants, transition state(s), and products.

A **reaction quotient** (Q_c) or (Q_p) has the same format as an equilibrium constant (K) but uses initial concentrations rather than equilibrium concentrations.

A **reactive material** is one that tends to react spontaneously or to react vigorously with air or water.

A **reducing agent** (reductant) is a substance that makes possible the reduction that occurs in an oxidation–reduction reaction. The reducing agent itself is oxidized.

Reduction is a process in which the oxidation number of an element decreases. It is the half-reaction of an oxidation–reduction reaction in which electrons are "gained."

Refining is the process of removing impurities from a metal by any of a variety of chemical or physical means.

A **rem** (roentgen equivalent for man) is a *rad* multiplied by a factor that takes into account the fact that different types of radiation of the same energy have different effects on people.

Resonance is a term used to describe a situation in which several plausible Lewis structures can be written to represent a species but

in which the true structure cannot be written. The plausible structures are called contributing structures or resonance structures; the true structure, which is a composite of the contributing structures, is called the resonance hybrid.

A **resonance hybrid** is a composite of two or more plausible contributing Lewis structures. The resonance hybrid represents the true structure of a molecule or ion.

A **resonance structure** is one of two or more plausible Lewis structures that can be written to represent a molecule or ion.

The **resultant dipole moment** is the dipole moment of a molecule as a whole based on an assessment of bond moments and the molecular geometry. (*See also* **bond moment** and **dipole moment**.)

Reverse osmosis refers to the net flow of solvent through a semipermeable membrane in the opposite direction from that expected for osmosis. It is produced by applying pressure to a solution in excess of its osmotic pressure. (*See also* **osmosis**.)

Ribonucleic acid (RNA) is a polymer of nucleotides. The nucleotide consists of the sugar ribose, a phosphate ester, and a cyclic amine base (adenine, guanine, uracil, or cytosine).

The **root-mean-square speed** (u_{rms}) of the molecules of a gas is the square root of the average of the squares of the molecular speeds.

A **salt** is an ionic compound in which hydrogen atoms of an acid are replaced by metal ions. Salts are produced in the reaction of an acid and a base.

A **salt bridge** is a salt solution used to connect the two solutions in a voltaic cell. It permits ions to migrate without mixing of the solutions.

Saponification is the alkaline hydrolysis of a fat or other ester.

A **saturated hydrocarbon** has molecules that contain the maximum number of hydrogen atoms for the carbon atoms present. All bonds in the molecules are single covalent bonds.

A **saturated solution** is one in which dynamic equilibrium exists between undissolved solute and the solution. The solution contains the maximum amount of solute that can be dissolved in a particular quantity of solvent at the given temperature.

The **s-block** is the portion of the periodic table in which the ns subshell (the s subshell of the outer shell) fills in the aufbau process.

A **scientific law** is a brief statement, sometimes in mathematical terms, used to summarize and describe patterns in large collections of scientific data.

The **second (s)** is the SI base unit of time.

Secondary sewage treatment consists of passing the effluent from a primary treatment plant through gravel and sand filters to aerate the water and remove finer suspended solids.

The **secondary structure** of a protein is the arrangement of the protein chains with respect to the nearest neighbor amino acid units, for example, a helix or a pleated sheet.

One statement of the **second law of thermodynamics** is that all natural or spontaneous processes are accompanied by an increase in entropy of the universe. That is, $\Delta S_{univ} = \Delta S_{system} + \Delta S_{surroundings} > 0$.

A **second-order reaction** has a rate equation in which the sum of the exponents $m + n + \cdots = 2$.

A **semiconductor** is a substance in which there is only a small energy gap between the valence and conduction band. The electrical conductivity of a semiconductor is not nearly as good as that of a metal, but still much better than that of an insulator.

A **semipermeable membrane** is a material that permits the flow of solvent molecules but severely restricts the flow of solute molecules of a solution.

A **sigma (σ) bond** results from the end-to-end overlap of pure or hybridized atomic orbitals between the bonded atoms. A σ bond exists along a line joining the nuclei of the bonded atoms.

The **significant figures** in a measured quantity are all the digits known with certainty plus the first uncertain digit.

A **simple cubic cell** has an atom, molecule, or ion at each corner of a cube.

A **single bond** is a covalent linkage in which two atoms share one pair of electrons between them.

The **skeletal structure** of a polyatomic species (molecule, ion) indicates the order in which atoms are attached to one another.

Slag is a metallurgical term for a relatively low-melting-point product of the reaction of an acidic oxide and a basic oxide.

Soaps are salts of long-chain carboxylic acids called fatty acids (because they are derived from fats).

The **solubility** of a solute in a particular solvent refers to the concentration of the solute in a saturated solution.

The **solubility product constant** (K_{sp}) describes the equilibrium that exists between a slightly soluble ionic solute and its ions in a saturated aqueous solution.

Solubility rules are a set of generalizations used to classify substances as soluble or insoluble in water.

A **solute** is a solution component that is dissolved in a solvent. A solution may have several solutes, which are generally present in lesser amounts than is the solvent.

A **solution** is a homogeneous mixture of two or more substances. The composition and properties are uniform throughout a solution.

A **solvent** is the solution component (usually present in greatest amount) in which one or more solutes are dissolved to form the solution.

sp **hybridization** describes a scheme in the valence bond method in which one s and one p orbital are combined into two sp hybrid orbitals oriented in a linear fashion.

spdf **notation** uses numbers to designate a principal shell and the letters s, p, d, and f to identify a subshell.

sp^2 **hybridization** describes a scheme in the valence bond method in which one s and two p orbitals are combined into three sp^2 hybrid orbitals oriented in a trigonal planar fashion.

sp^3 **hybridization** describes a scheme in the valence bond method in which one s and three p orbitals are combined into four sp^3 hybrid orbitals oriented in a tetrahedral fashion.

sp^3d **hybridization** describes a scheme in the valence bond method in which one s, three p, and one d orbital are combined into five sp^3d hybrid orbitals oriented in a trigonal bipyramidal fashion.

sp^3d^2 **hybridization** describes a scheme in the valence bond method in which one s, three p, and two d orbitals are combined into six sp^3d^2 hybrid orbitals oriented in an octahedral fashion.

The **specific heat** of a substance is the quantity of heat required to raise the temperature of 1 gram of substance by 1 °C (or 1 K).

Spectator ions do not participate in an acid–base, precipitation, or redox reaction, but serve only to maintain electrical neutrality. (*See also* **net ionic equation**.)

The **spectrochemical series** is a listing of ligands in order of their abilities to produce a splitting of a d-subshell energy level in a complex. Ligands in the series are referred to as strong field, intermediate field, or weak field, depending on the degree of splitting they produce. (*See also* **crystal field theory**.)

Spectroscopy is a study, using various instrumental methods, of atomic and molecular properties through the absorption or emission of electromagnetic radiation by a substance.

A **spontaneous process** is one that occurs in a system left to itself. Once started, no action from outside the system is required to keep the process going.

A **standard cell potential** (E°_{cell}) (standard cell voltage) is the potential difference (in volts) between the electrodes in a voltaic cell

when all species are present in their standard states.

The **standard electrode potential** ($E°$) measures the tendency of a reduction process to occur when all species in a half-cell are present in their standard states. This tendency is measured in volts, relative to an assigned value of zero for the standard hydrogen electrode.

The **standard enthalpy of formation** (ΔH_f°) of a substance is the enthalpy change that occurs in the formation of 1 mol of the substance in its standard state from the reference forms of its elements in their standard states. The reference forms of the elements are generally their most stable forms at the given temperature and 1 atm pressure.

The **standard enthalpy of reaction** ($\Delta H°$) is the enthalpy change for a reaction in which all reactants and products are in their standard states.

The **standard free energy change** ($\Delta G°$) is the free energy change of a process in which the reactants and products are all in their standard states.

The **standard free energy of formation** (ΔG_f°) of a substance is the free energy change that occurs in the formation of one mole of the substance in its standard state from the reference forms of its elements in their standard states. The reference forms of the elements are generally their most stable forms at the given temperature and 1 atm pressure.

A **standard hydrogen electrode (SHE)** has hydrogen gas at 1 atm pressure and hydronium ion at unit activity (about 1 M) in oxidation–reduction equilibrium on an inert platinum electrode. The potential arbitrarily assigned to this electrode is exactly 0 V.

The **standard molar entropy** ($S°$) of a substance is its entropy at standard pressure and a specified temperature.

The **standard state** of a solid or liquid substance is the pure element or compound at 1 atm pressure and at the temperature of interest. For a gaseous substance, the standard state is the (hypothetical) pure gas behaving as an ideal gas at 1 atm pressure and the temperature of interest.

Standard temperature and pressure (STP) for a gas are 273.15 K (0 °C) and 1 atm (760 mmHg).

A **state** of a system is its exact condition, determined by the kinds and amounts of matter present; the structure of this matter at the molecular level; and the prevailing temperature and pressure.

A **state function** is a property that has a unique value that depends only on the present state of a system and not on how that state was reached.

The **states of matter** are the three fundamental conditions in which samples of matter may be obtained: solid, liquid, and gas.

Steel is an alloy of iron containing small amounts of carbon and usually containing other metals such as manganese, nickel, and chromium.

Stereoisomers are isomers that have the same molecular formulas but differ in the arrangement of atoms in three-dimensional space.

A **stoichiometric coefficient** is a coefficient placed in front of a formula in a chemical equation to balance the equation.

A **stoichiometric factor** or mole ratio is a conversion factor relating molar amounts of two species involved in a chemical reaction (that is, a reactant to a product, one reactant to another, and so on). The numerical values used in formulating the factor are the stoichiometric coefficients.

Stoichiometric proportions refer to relative amounts of reactants that are in the mole ratios corresponding to the coefficients in a balanced equation; no reactants are in excess.

Stoichiometry refers to quantitative measurements and relationships involving substances and mixtures of chemical interest.

A **strong acid** is an acid that is essentially completely ionized in solution, that is, an acid that is a strong electrolyte. (*See also* **acid**.)

A **strong base** is a base that is essentially completely ionized in solution, that is, a base that is a strong electrolyte. (*See also* **base**.)

A **strong electrolyte** is a substance that exists almost exclusively in ionic form in solution.

A **structural formula** is a chemical formula that shows how the atoms in a molecule are attached to one another.

Sublimation is the direct passage of molecules from the solid state to the vapor state.

A **sublimation curve** is a graph of the vapor pressure (sublimation pressure) of a solid as a function of temperature. It is analogous to the vapor pressure curve of a liquid.

A **subshell (sublevel)** is the collection of orbitals of a given type (specified by n and l) present in a principal shell. For example, the three $2p$ orbitals constitute the $2p$ subshell.

Subshell (sublevel) notation is a method of denoting an electron configuration that uses numbers to represent the principal shells and the letters s, p, d, and f for subshells. A superscript number following the letter indicates the number of electrons in the subshell.

A **substance** is a type of matter having a definite, or fixed, composition and fixed properties that do not vary from one sample to another. All substances are either elements or compounds.

In a **substitution reaction**, a substituent group replaces a hydrogen atom in a hydrocarbon molecule. This type of reaction is characteristic of alkanes and aromatic hydrocarbons.

The **substrate** in an enzyme-catalyzed reaction is the reactant species that attaches to the active site on an enzyme molecule and undergoes chemical reaction.

A **superconductor** is a metal, alloy, or ceramic material whose resistance to the flow of electricity vanishes at a sufficiently low temperature.

Supercooling is a condition in which a liquid is cooled below its freezing point without the appearance of any solid.

A **supercritical fluid** is a fluid at a temperature above its critical temperature and at a pressure above its critical pressure.

A **supersaturated** solution contains more solute than is present in a saturated solution in equilibrium with undissolved solute.

Surface tension is the amount of work required to extend a liquid surface, usually expressed in joules per square meter, $J\,m^{-2}$.

The **surroundings** refer to that part of the universe with which a system interacts by exchanging heat and/or work and/or matter.

A **system** is that part of the universe chosen for a thermochemical or thermodynamic study. (*See also* **surroundings**.)

Temperature is a physical property, related to the mean kinetic energies of the atoms or molecules in a substance, that indicates the direction of heat flow. Kinetic energy, as heat, is transferred from more energetic (higher temperature) to less energetic (lower temperature) atoms or molecules.

Temporary hardness is present in hard water that has HCO_3^- as its primary anion. (*See also* **hard water**.)

A **terminal atom** in a polyatomic species (molecule, ion) is bonded to just one other atom.

A **termolecular reaction** in a reaction mechanism involves the simultaneous collision of three molecules.

The **tertiary structure** refers to the folds, bends, and twists in a protein or nucleic acid structure.

The **theoretical yield** is the calculated quantity of a product expected in a chemical reaction.

A **theory** provides explanations of observed phenomena and predictions that can be tested by experimentation. It is the intellectual frame-

work for explaining scientific data and scientific laws.

Thermochemistry is the study of energy changes associated with chemical reactions or physical processes, especially energy changes that appear as heat.

Thermodynamics is the science dealing with the relationship between heat and motion (work) and with transformations of energy from one form to another. Thermochemistry is a subfield within thermodynamics.

A **thermoplastic polymer** is one that can be softened by heating and formed into desired shapes by applying pressure.

A **thermosetting polymer** becomes permanently hard at elevated temperatures and pressures.

The **third law of thermodynamics** states that the entropy of a pure, perfect crystal at 0 K is zero. This is the starting point for the experimental determination of absolute molar entropies.

The **titrant** in a titration is the solution, usually of accurately known concentration, that is added to the analyte through a buret.

Titration is a laboratory procedure in which the amount or concentration of one reactant is found by adding a known solution of a second reactant in stoichiometric proportions.

A **titration curve** in a neutralization reaction is a graph of pH versus volume of titrant added from a buret.

A **torr** is a unit used to express gas pressure: 1 Torr = 1 mmHg. (*See also* **millimeter of mercury**.)

A **toxic material** is one that contains or releases poisonous substances in amounts large enough to threaten human health or the environment.

Toxicology is a study of the effects of poisons on the body, their identification and detection, and remedies against them.

Trans isomers have two groups attached to opposite sides of a double bond in an organic molecule, at opposite corners of a square in a square planar complex, or above and below the central plane in an octahedral complex.

Transcription is the process by which DNA directs the synthesis of an mRNA molecule during protein synthesis.

A **transition element** is one in which the subshell being filled in the aufbau process is in a principal shell of less than the highest quantum number (an inner shell). Transition elements are located in the *d*- and *f*-blocks of the periodic table.

A **transition state** is a state that lies between the reactants and products of a chemical reaction. It is produced as a result of collisions between especially energetic molecules.

Translation is the process by which the information contained in a base triplet of an mRNA molecule is converted to a protein structure.

The **transuranium elements** are those with atomic number (Z) greater than 92.

A **triglyceride** is an ester formed by the chemical combination of glycerol with three fatty acids. It is also called a *triacylglycerol*.

A **triple bond** is a covalent linkage in which two atoms share three pairs of electrons between them.

A **triple point** is a particular temperature and pressure at which three phases of a pure substance are at equilibrium—solid, liquid, and vapor; or two solid phases and the liquid; or two solid phases and the vapor.

Trouton's rule states that the entropy of vaporization of a nonpolar liquid at its normal boiling point is approximately 87 J K^{-1} mol^{-1}.

The **Tyndall effect** is the scattering of light by colloidal particles, which makes a colloidal dispersion distinguishable from a true solution.

Heisenberg's **uncertainty principle** states that the product of the uncertainty in the position of an object and the uncertainty in its momentum (mass, m, times speed, u) cannot be less than $h/4\pi$. Thus, it is not possible to know with certainty both the position of a subatomic particle and details of its motion.

A **unimolecular reaction** in a reaction mechanism is one in which a single molecule undergoes rearrangement or decomposition.

The **unit cell** of a crystal structure is the simplest parallelepiped that can be used to generate the entire crystalline lattice through straight-line displacements in all three dimensions.

In the **unit-conversion method**, a given quantity is multiplied by a conversion factor to change the unit of the quantity to a different, desired unit.

The **universal gas constant (R)** is the numerical constant required to relate pressure, volume, amount, and temperature of a gas in the ideal gas equation, $PV = nRT$. Its numerical value is 0.082057 L atm mol^{-1} K^{-1} or 8.3145 J mol^{-1} K^{-1}.

An **unsaturated hydrocarbon** is a carbon–hydrogen compound having one or more multiple bonds (double, triple) between carbon atoms.

An **unsaturated** solution contains less of a solute in a given quantity of solution than is present in a saturated solution. It is a solution having a concentration less than the solubility limit.

A **valence band** is formed by combining atomic orbitals of the valence electrons of a large number of atoms into a set of molecular orbitals very closely spaced in energy. If the band is only partially filled with electrons, it is also a conduction band. (*See also* **band** and **conduction band**.)

The **valence bond theory** describes a covalent bond as a region of high electron charge density that results from the overlap of atomic orbitals between the bonded atoms.

Valence electrons are electrons with the highest principal quantum number. They are found in the outermost electronic shells of atoms. (*See also* **core electrons**.)

The **valence shell** is the outer shell of electrons of an atom, the electrons with the highest principal quantum number.

The **valence-shell electron-pair repulsion (VSEPR) method** is an approach to describing the geometric shapes of molecules and polyatomic ions in terms of the geometrical distribution of electron groups in the valence shell(s) of central atom(s).

van der Waals forces are short-range attractive forces between molecules that include dispersion forces, dipole-dipole forces, and dipole-induced dipole forces.

The **van't Hoff factor (i)** is a correction factor that must be incorporated into equations for colligative properties so that the equations may be applied to solutions of strong or weak electrolytes.

A **vapor** is a gas at a temperature below its critical temperature. A vapor can be liquefied by application of pressure without lowering the temperature.

Vaporization, or evaporation, is the process of conversion of a liquid to a gas (vapor).

The **vapor pressure** of a liquid is the pressure exerted by the vapor in dynamic equilibrium with the liquid at a constant temperature.

A **vapor pressure curve** is a graph of the vapor pressure of a liquid as a function of temperature. The curve is the boundary between the liquid and vapor areas in a phase diagram.

The **viscosity** of a liquid substance is a measure of its resistance to flow.

Volt (V) is the unit used to measure electrode potentials and electrical potential differences.

A **voltaic cell** is an electrochemical cell that produces electricity through an oxidation–reduction reaction.

A **wave** is a progressive, repeating disturbance propagated from a point of origin to a more distant point.

The **wavelength** is the distance between any two identical points in consecutive cycles of a wave, for example, the distance between the peaks or crests of the wave.

The **wavenumber** ($\widetilde{\nu}$) of radiation expresses the frequency of radiation as the number of cycles per centimeter of the wave.

A **weak acid** is an acid that exists partly in ionic form and partly in molecular form in solution, that is, an acid that is a weak electrolyte. (*See also* **acid**.)

A **weak base** is a base that exists partly in ionic form and partly in molecular form in solution, that is, a base that is a weak electrolyte. (*See also* **base**.)

A **weak electrolyte** is a substance that is present partly in molecular form and partly in ionic form in its solutions.

Work is (1) the result of a force acting through a distance, for example, $1\ J = 1\ N \times 1\ m$, or (2) an energy transfer into or out of a thermodynamic system that can be expressed as the product of a force and a distance.

An **X ray** is high-energy electromagnetic radiation produced by the impact of cathode rays (electrons) on a solid, such as on a dense metal anode (a target) in a cathode-ray tube.

A **zero-order reaction** has a rate that is independent of the concentration of reactant(s). The sum of the exponents in its rate equation, $m + n + \cdots = 0$.

Zone refining is a process of purification in which a rod of material is subjected to repeated cycles of melting and freezing. This sweeps impurities in a molten zone to the end of the rod, which is then cut off.

Answers to Selected Problems

These answers are for in-text Exercises and selected end-of-chapter problems. *Note:* Some of your answers may differ slightly from those given here, depending on the number of digits used in expressing atomic masses and other precisely known quantities and whether intermediate results were rounded off.

Chapter 1

Exercises: 1.1A (a) 2.05 μm; (b) 4.03 kg; (c) 7.06 ns; (d) 5.15 cm. **1.1B** (a) 6.217 $\times$ 10^3 g; (b) 1.6 $\times$ 10^{-3} s; (c) 7.17 $\times$ 10^{-2} g; (d) 3.87 $\times$ 10^2 m. **1.2A** (a) 3.55 $\times$ 10^{-4} s; (b) 1.885 $\times$ 10^6 m; (c) 1.350 $\times$ 10^1 m; (d) 4.25 $\times$ 10^{-7} m. **1.2B** (a) 2.28 $\times$ 10^2 kg; (b) 8.3 $\times$ 10^{-4} m; (c) 4.05 $\times$ 10^{-4} m; (d) 1.215 $\times$ 10^3 s. **1.3A** (a) 185 °F; (b) 10.0 °F; (c) 168 °C; (d) $-$29.3 °C. **1.3B** $-$459.67 °F. **1.4A** 8.9 $\times$ 10^{-3} m^3. **1.4B** 8.9 $\times$ 10^3 cm^3. **1.5A** 925 g zinc. **1.5B** 5.1 cm^2. **1.6A** (a) 100.5 m; (b) 1.50 $\times$ 10^2 g; (c) 415 g; (d) 6.3 L. **1.6B** (a) 1.80 $\times$ 10^3 m^2; (b) 2.33 g/mL; (c) 72 kg/m^3; (d) 0.63 g/cm^3. No differences between rounding of intermediate results and a final rounding only. **1.7A** (a) 7.63 $\times$ 10^{-2} m; (b) 8.56 $\times$ 10^4 mg; (c) 1.82 $\times$ 10^3 ft. **1.7B** (a) 5.53 $\times$ 10^4 μg; (b) 448 fl oz; (c) 23.6 km. **1.8A** (a) 73.8 in.^{2}; (b) 0.256 m^3. **1.8B** 1.00 $\times$ 10^3 g/L. **1.9A** 1.034 $\times$ 10^4 kg/m^2. **1.9B** 177 lb. **1.10A** 7.80 g/cm^3. **1.10B** 7.40 g/cm^3. **1.11A** 3.34 gal. **1.11B** 17.2 kg. **1.12A** 20 kg. **1.12B** (a). **1.13A** Although the mass is the same at 21 °C and 25 °C, volume varies with temperature, and so does density. We are given the density at 25 °C and not 21 °C. **1.13B** 0.69 g/cm^3. **1.14A** Remove the ebony wood and replace it by the block of plastic floating about $\frac{3}{4}$ submerged in the chloroform. **1.14B** The observations: (a) 75.0 g; (b) plastic rests at the bottom of the beaker filled with ethyl alcohol; (c) plastic is about 80% submerged in chloroform; (d) plastic weighs 13.5 g when submerged in water. **Self-Assessment Questions: 1.** (d), (f). **8.** (c). **9.** (c). **10.** (a), (c), (e) are elements; the rest are compounds, each made of two elements. **11.** (a). **16.** (b). **20.** (d). **22.** (b). **Problems: 23.** (a), (b), and (d). **25.** (a), (b), (d) are physical, (c) is chemical. **27.** (a) is a substance; (b), (c), (d) are mixtures. **29.** Both mass and weight have changed; body fat has been removed, which has mass (and weight). **31.** Yes, if all the results have the same amount and direction of error. Yes, if the positive and negative errors cancel. **33.** Mass is probably more consistent. Volume varies with particle size, sifting, settling, type of flour, etc. **35.** (a) 8.01 μg; (b) 7.9 mL; (c) 1.05 km. **37.** (a) 209 °F; (b) 576.1 °C; (c) $-$62 °F. **39.** Yes. **41.** (a) 0.0374 L; (b) 1.55 $\times$ 10^5 m; (c) 0.198 g; (d) 1.19 $\times$ 10^4 cm^2; (e) 0.078 ms; (f) 24.4 m/s. **43.** (a) 6.68 kg; (b) 3.8 $\times$ 8.9 $\times$ 235 cm; (c) 0.26 m^3. **45.** (4) < (3) < (1) < (2). **47.** 7.92 in. **49.** (a) 3; (b) 3; (c) 4; (d) 4; (e) 3; (f) 3. **51.** (a) 2.804 $\times$ 10^3 m; (b) 9.01 $\times$ 10^2 s; (c) 9.0 $\times$ 10^{-4} cm; (d) 2.210 $\times$ 10^2 s. **53.** (a) 505.5 m; (b) 2120 s, 3 SF; (c) 0.00610, 3 SF; (d) 40,000 L, 3 SF (last two zeroes are not significant). **55.** (a) 45.8 cm; (b) 167 cm; (c) 44.5 g; (d) 10.1 L. **57.** (a) 2.32 $\times$ 10^3 mm^3; (b) 4.80 $\times$ 10^3 cm^2/g; (c) 4.6 $\times$ 10^4 mm^2/mg; (d) 1.92 $\times$ 10^{-4} g/mL. **59.** 1.14 g/mL.

61. 5.23 g/cm^3. **63.** 5.4 $\times$ 10^2 g. **65.** 6.73 $\times$ 10^{-6} cm. **67.** 0.0042 g/cm^3. **69.** (b). **71.** 7.1 g/cm^3. **Additional Problems: 74.** Yes, both are linear relationships, and the lines cross at $-$40 °C. **76.** 0.02 m^2. **79.** 116.18 mph. **83.** 2.36 $\times$ 10^5 nails/roll. **86.** 4.9 mg/m^2. **88.** The second (cork). The cork floats and will displace its mass, 8.8 g or 8.8 mL, of water. The brass sinks and will displace its volume, 8.0 mL. **92.** (a) 4.8 $\times$ 10^{-5} cm; (b) 0.60 g/cm^3. **93.** (a) Volume is about 30 $\times$ 13 $\times$ 11 or 4300 cm^3, so $d >$ 1 g/cm^3 and the object will not float; (b) new $d =$ 1.16 g/cm^3; (c) 3 more holes. **96.** 66.8 mL chloroform and 33.2 mL bromoform **98.** Floating ice displaces its mass of water, not its volume. No effect on the level. **Apply Your Knowledge: 101.** 10 mg/10 L $=$ 10^2 μg/dL, not 10 μg/dL. **102.** (a) 0.8790 g/mL; (b) 7.135 g/cm^3.

Chapter 2

Exercises: 2.1A 45.07 g. The mass of magnesium oxide (the product) is equal to the sum of the masses magnesium and oxygen consumed. The masses of material not involved in the reaction are unchanged. **2.1B** The principal products of the combustion—carbon dioxide gas and water vapor—escape into the air. The mass of the match residue will be less than the original mass. **2.2A** 3.779 g magnesium oxide. **2.2B** 2.361 g magnesium burned; 3.915 g magnesium oxide formed. **2.3A** $^{116}_{50}$Sn. **2.3B** $^{116}_{48}$Cd; 48 p, 48 e, 68 n. **2.4A** 20.18 u. **2.4B** 69.16% copper-63; 30.84% copper-65. **2.5A** Magnesium-24 is most abundant; its mass is closest to 24.305 u. To determine the second-most abundant, at least one of the actual percent abundances would have to be known. **2.5B** (a) No. (b) Assuming only a trace of magnesium-26, the weighted-average atomic mass of ^{24}Mg and ^{25}Mg would be 24.305 u if the percent ^{24}Mg were 68.03%. If the amount of ^{26}Mg is more than a trace, the percent ^{24}Mg would have to be larger. **2.6A** N$_2$F$_4$; dinitrogen tetrafluoride. **2.6B** S$_8$O; octasulfur monoxide. **2.7A** (a) P$_4$O$_{10}$; (b) heptasulfur dioxide. **2.7B** SO$_2$F$_2$ is a plausible formula based on Figure 2.9 and the nomenclature rules for binary molecular compounds, but this is a ternary molecular compound. **2.8A** (a) K$_2$S; (b) Li$_2$O; (c) AlF$_3$. **2.8B** (a) Cr$_2$O$_3$; (b) FeS; (c) Li$_3$N. **2.9A** (a) calcium bromide; (b) lithium sulfide; (c) iron(II) bromide; (d) copper(I) iodide. **2.9B** (a) Cu$_2$S; (b) Co$_2$O$_3$; (c) Mg$_3$N$_2$. **2.10A** (a) (NH$_4$)$_2$CO$_3$; (b) Ca(ClO)$_2$; (c) Cr$_2$(SO$_4$)$_3$. **2.10B** (a) KAl(SO$_4$)$_2$; (b) MgNH$_4$PO$_4$. **2.11A** (a) potassium hydrogen carbonate; (b) iron(III) phosphate; (c) magnesium dihydrogen phosphate. **2.11B** (a) sodium selenate; (b) iron(III) arsenide; (c) disodium hydrogen phosphite. **Self-Assessment Questions: 1.** (c). **3.** No, Cl atoms must form something; they are not in water or carbon dioxide. **7.** (b) are isotopes;

(a) are isobars. **8. (a)** ^8_5B; **(b)** $^{14}_6C$; **(c)** $^{235}_{92}U$; **(d)** $^{60}_{27}Co$. **12.** (a), (d), (f). **19.** molecular formula (a), (b), (d); structural formula (c) and (e). **Problems: 21.** Yes; mass of product & unreacted reactant in excess equals sum of reactant masses. **23. (a)** 104.3 g; **(b)** 40.3 g MgO; **(c)** conservation of mass and definite proportions; **(d)** 80.6 g MgO. **25.** Yes. **27.** 2.61 g. **29.** (a) and (c). **31. (a)** 30p, 34n, 30e; **(b)** 47p, 62n, 47e; **(c)** 6p, 8n, 6e; **(d)** 95p, 148n, 95e. **33.** #2, $^{40}_{20}Ca$; #6, $^{48}_{22}Ti$; #7, $^{48}_{20}Ca$; #2 and #7 are isotopes. **35.** Bromine must consist of isotopes of significant abundance both above and below mass number 80 (in nature, almost equal abundances of isotopes 79 and 81). **37.** 69.7 u. **39.** 28.09 u. **41.** 72.163% Rb-85, 27.387% Rb-87. **43.** group, period, class are: **(a)** 3A, 4, metal; **(b)** 5A, 3, nonmetal; **(c)** 7A, 5, nonmetal; **(d)** 2A, 7, metal; **(e)** 1A, 2, metal; **(f)** 3B, 6, metal; **(g)** 8A, 5, nonmetal. **45. (a)** N_2; **(b)** H_2; **(c)** I_2; **(d)** P_4. **47.** (a), (c), and (d); (b) is ionic, (e) contains three elements. **49. (a)** $SiCl_4$; **(b)** SF_6; **(c)** CS_2; **(d)** Cl_2O_3; **(e)** dinitrogen monoxide; **(f)** diiodine pentoxide; **(g)** phosphorus pentachloride; **(h)** diphosphorus trioxide. **51. (a)** Mg^{2+}; **(b)** Br^-; **(c)** Ti^{4+}; **(d)** iodide ion; **(e)** sulfide ion; **(f)** chromium(II) ion. **53. (a)** ammonium ion; **(b)** hypochlorite ion; **(c)** phosphate ion; **(d)** hydrogen sulfate ion; **(e)** OH^-; **(f)** SO_3^{2-}; **(g)** CH_3COO^-; **(h)** CO_3^{2-}. **55. (a)** potassium iodide; **(b)** magnesium fluoride; **(c)** nickel(II) sulfate; **(d)** titanium(IV) bromide; **(e)** ammonium hydrogen sulfate; **(f)** aluminum oxide; **(g)** barium chloride dihydrate; **(h)** lithium oxalate; **(i)** sodium sulfate decahydrate. **57. (a)** KCl; **(b)** $CaCO_3$; **(c)** Cr_2O_3 **(d)** $KClO_4$; **(e)** $NaClO_3$; **(f)** $FeSO_4 \cdot 7 H_2O$. **59. (a)** Na_2O; **(b)** CuOH; **(c)** BaI_2; **(d)** $Al_2(SO_4)_3$; **(e)** sodium bromate; **(f)** lithium hydrogen sulfate; **(g)** ammonium dichromate; **(h)** nickel(II) oxalate. **61. (a)** Cl is not chlorate, NH_4ClO_3; **(b)** nitrate has three O atoms, KNO_3; **(c)** SO_4^{2-} needs two sodium ions, Na_2SO_4; **(d)** Ba^{2+} needs two OH^- ions; $Ba(OH)_2$; **(e)** O is oxide, ZnC_2O_4; **(f)** IV signifies 4+ charge, MnO_2; **(g)** Sr and CrO_4 are both divalent, $SrCrO_4$; **(h)** II signifies 2+ charge, $Cu_3(PO_4)_2$. **63. (a)** hydrobromic acid; **(b)** nitrous acid; **(c)** phosphorous acid; **(d)** $HClO_2$; **(e)** KOH; **(f)** H_2SO_3; **(g)** barium hydroxide; **(h)** HI. **65.** IO_3^-, HIO_3, iodic acid.

67. (a) H—C—C—C—C—C—H, $CH_3(CH_2)_3CH_3$; (with H atoms on each C)

(b) H—C—C—C—C—O—H, $CH_3(CH_2)_2COOH$;

(c) H—O—C—C—C—H
HOCH$_2$CH$_2$CH$_3$

(d) H—C—C—H, H—C—C—H, CH_2—CH_2 CH_2—CH_2;

(e) H—C—C—C—H, $CH(CH_3)_3$;

(f) H—C—C—C—O—H, CH_3CH_2COOH.

69. (a) H—C—C—C—C—O—H   H—C—C—C—O—H (with H—C—H branch)

(b) $CH_3(CH_2)_2COOH$; $(CH_3)_2CHCOOH$

(c) (two structures with O and OH groups)

(d) isomers **71. (a)** straight chain alkane; **(b)** alcohol; **(c)** cyclic alkane; **(d)** hydrocarbon; **(e)** carboxylic acid; **(f)** inorganic; **(g)** carboxylic acid; **(h)** inorganic. **73.** (b). **75. (a)** dimethyl ether, methanol; **(b)** ethyl methyl ether, ethanol and methanol; **(c)** diethyl ether, ethanol. **77.** $CH_3CH_2OCH_2CH_3$, $CH_3CH_2CH_2OCH_3$, $(CH_3)_2CHOCH_3$.

79. (a) (structure) **(b)** (structure) **(c)** (structure)

Additional Problems: 82. (c). **86.** H_2, HD, D_2 (least abundant); 10. **89.** No, although the %C and %H are constant, we do not know about %N and %O, only that their sum is constant. **92.** The composition of N_2O_5 is different from those of the other three oxides, while N_2O_4 has the same composition as NO_2. **94.** $^{25}Mg = 10.00\%$; $^{26}Mg = 11.01\%$. **98. (a)** $C_nH_{2n+1}OH$; **(b)** $C_nH_{2n}O_2$; **(c)** $C_nH_{2n}O_2$. **103.** empirical formula C_2H_6N; molecular formula $C_4H_{12}N_2$. **105. (a)** $CH_3(CH_2)_{10}COONH_4$; **(b)** $Ca[CH_3(CH_2)_{16}COO]_2$; **(c)** $CH_3(CH_2)_7CH=CH(CH_2)_7COOK$.

107. (a) methyl acetate; methyl alcohol and acetic acid; **(b)** propyl acetate; propyl alcohol and acetic acid; **(c)** isopropyl formate; isopropyl alcohol and formic acid.

110. $CH_3(CH_2)_4CH_3$, hexane; $(CH_3)_2CH(CH_2)_2CH_3$, 2-methylpentane; $CH_3CH_2CH(CH_3)CH_2CH_3$, 3-methylpentane; $(CH_3)_3CCH_2CH_3$, 2,2-dimethylbutane; $(CH_3)_2CHCH(CH_3)_2$, 2,3-dimethylbutane. **111. (a)** $^{40}_{20}Ca$; **(b)** $^{234}_{90}Th$; **(c)** $^{120}_{48}Cd$; **(d)** $^{64}_{30}Zn^{2+}$. **114. (a)** propyl bromide; **(b)** isobutyl chloride; **(c)** ethyl iodide; **(d)** *t*-butyl fluoride **Apply Your Knowledge: 116. (a)** Physicist's scale, the mixture with heavier isotopes is heavier than O-16 alone, so physicist ratios are slightly larger; **(b)** Atomic mass of C-12 is divisible by 4, and the new atomic mass of O is 15.9994 which is a change of 0.0006/16 = 4/100,000. **120.** Atomic masses are (mostly) averages of several isotopes rather than single isotopes. Fractional masses can arise

from integral masses and different abundances; i.e., Cl = 35.5 can arise from three Cl-37 and one Cl-35.

Chapter 3

Exercises: 3.1A (a) 124 u, **(b)** 92.0 u, **(c)** 98.1 u, **(d)** 74.1 u. **3.1B (a)** 208.24 u, **(b)** 108.01 u, **(c)** 88.106 u, **(d)** 100.161 u. **3.2A (a)** 29.9 u; **(b)** 148 u; **(c)** 234 u; **(d)** 295 u. **3.2B (a)** 104.06 u; **(b)** 117.49 u; **(c)** 392.18 u; **(d)** 249.69 u. **3.3A (a)** 14.5 mg Ag; **(b)** 2.47×10^{25} O atoms. **3.3B (a)** 17 mol Al; **(b)** 173 mL liquid bromine. **3.4A (a)** 3.11×10^{24} Cl atoms; **(b)** 90.5 g sucrose. **3.4B** 555 mL solution. **3.5A (d)**; the sample is about 1/6 mol Mg (about 4 g). **3.5B (b)**. C accounts for less than 1/3 the mass of CO_2 (compound a). In propane (compound b), C accounts for the bulk of the mass. Acetic acid (compound c) has the same number of C atoms per molecule as propane, but also two more massive O atoms. Diethyl ether (compound d) has 4 C atoms per molecule, but this is offset by an additional O and 4 H atoms. **3.6A (a)** 6.102% H, 21.20% N, 48.43% O, 24.27% S; **(b)** 20.00% C, 6.713% H, 46.65% N, 26.64% O; urea has the greatest percent nitrogen. **3.6B (a)** 9.388% N, **(b)** 10.77% O, **(c)** 36.08% H_2O **3.7A** 1.37×10^3 mg Na^+. **3.7B** 1.40×10^2 g N. **3.8A** LiH_2PO_4 has the smallest mass of cation (7 g Li^+) per mol P when compared with $Ca(H_2PO_4)_2$ (20 g Ca^{2+}) and $(NH_4)_2HPO_4$ (36 g NH_4^+). Thus, it has the highest %P. **3.8B** Hydrocarbons should have higher percentages of C than the oxygen-containing methanol and acetic acid. The hydrocarbon octane, C_8H_{18}, has a higher proportion of C to H than does butane, C_4H_{10} (equivalent to C_8H_{20}). C_8H_{18} has the highest %C. **3.9A** $C_6H_{12}O$. **3.9B** $C_5H_{10}NO_2$. **3.10A** C_7H_5. **3.10B (a)** Fe_3O_4; **(b)** CCl_2F_2; **(c)** $C_7H_5N_3O_6$. **3.11A** ethylene, C_2H_4; cyclohexane, C_6H_{12}; 1-pentene, C_5H_{10}. **3.11B (a)** P_2O_3; **(b)** C_2H_3; **(c)** $C_3H_4O_3$; **(d)** $C_2H_4O_3$; **(e)** CH_3O; **(f)** $CuCO_3$. **3.12A (a)** 60.0% C, 13.4% H, 26.6% O; **(b)** C_3H_8O or C_3H_7OH. **3.12B (a)** 80.24% C; 9.62% H, 10.14% O; **(b)** $C_{21}H_{30}O_2$. **3.13A (a)** $SiCl_4 + 2 H_2O \longrightarrow$ $SiO_2 + 4 HCl$; **(b)** $PCl_5 + 4 H_2O \longrightarrow H_3PO_4 + 5 HCl$; **(c)** $6 CaO + P_4O_{10} \longrightarrow 2 Ca_3(PO_4)_2$. **3.13B (a)** $Pb(NO_3)_2(aq)$ $+ 2 KI(aq) \longrightarrow 2 KNO_3(aq) + PbI_2(s)$; **(b)** $4 HCl(g) + O_2(g)$ $\longrightarrow 2 H_2O(g) + 2 Cl_2(g)$. **3.14A (a)** $2 C_4H_{10} + 13 O_2 \longrightarrow$ $8 CO_2 + 10 H_2O$; **(b)** $CH_3CH_2CH_2CHOHCH_2OH + 7 O_2$ $\longrightarrow 5 CO_2 + 6 H_2O$. **3.14B** $2 C_5H_{12}O + 15 O_2 \longrightarrow$ $10 CO_2 + 12 H_2O$. **3.15A (a)** $FeCl_3 + 3 NaOH \longrightarrow Fe(OH)_3$ $+ 3 NaCl$; **(b)** $3 Ba(NO_3)_2 + Al_2(SO_4)_3 \longrightarrow 3 BaSO_4 +$ $2 Al(NO_3)_3$. **3.15B** $3 Ca(OH)_2(s) + 2 H_3PO_4(aq) \longrightarrow$ $Ca_3(PO_4)_2(s) + 6 H_2O(l)$. **3.16A** $2 C_6H_{14}O_4 + 15 O_2 \longrightarrow$ $12 CO_2 + 14 H_2O$. **3.16B** $2 Pb(NO_3)_2(s) \longrightarrow 2 PbO(s) +$ $4 NO_2(g) + O_2(g)$. **3.17A (a)** 1.59 mol CO_2; **(b)** 305 mol H_2O; **(c)** 0.6060 mol CO_2. **3.17B (a)** 3.83 mol CO_2; **(b)** 6.22 mol O_2. **3.18A** 21.4 g Mg. **3.18B** 26.4 g N_2 and 15.1 g O_2. **3.19A** 774 ml H_2O. **3.19B** 28.9 mL H_2O. **3.20A** 4.77 g H_2S; 0.9 g FeS in excess. **3.20B** 1.40 g H_2. **3.21A** 26.8 g. **3.21B** 374 g. **3.22A** 1.35 kg $(NH_4)_2HPO_4$. **3.22B** aluminum. **3.23A (a)** 1.26 M; **(b)** 0.0242 M; 0.0349 M. **3.23B (a)** 6.99×10^{-3} M; **(b)** 7.19 M; **(c)** 0.34 M. **3.24A (a)** 673 g KOH; **(b)** 0.0561 g KOH; **(c)** 4.91 g KOH. **3.24B** 23.2 mL. **3.25A** 23.5 M HCOOH. **3.25B** 70.4% $HClO_4$. **3.26A** 466 mL. **3.26B** 17.0 mL. **3.27A** 375 mL. **3.27B (a)** 11.9 g CO_2; **(b)** 0.662 M NaCl. **Self-Assessment Questions: 2.** 6.02×10^{23} molecules O_2, 1.20×10^{24} atoms O. **3.** (c). **4. (a)** 6.02×10^{23} Ca^{2+} ions, 1.20×10^{24} NO_3^- ions; **(b)** 1.20×10^{24} N atoms, 3.61×10^{24} O atoms. **5. (a)** HO;

(b) CH_2; **(c)** C_5H_4; **(d)** C_3H_6O. **8.** (b). **9. (a)** $Hg(NO_3)_2(s) \xrightarrow{\Delta}$ $Hg(l) + 2 NO_2(g) + O_2(g)$ **(b)** $Na_2CO_3(aq) + 2 HCl(aq) \longrightarrow$ $H_2O(l) + CO_2(g) + 2 NaCl(aq)$ **(c)** $C_3H_4O_4(s) + 2 O_2(g) \longrightarrow$ $3 CO_2(g) + 2 H_2O(l)$ **10.** (c). **11.** (a). **14.** They are equal. To change g/L to mg/mL, numerator and denominator are both divided by 1000. **Problems: 17. (a)** 122.99 u (molecular); **(b)** 146.35 u; **(c)** 325.33 u; **(d)** 404.02 u; **(e)** 383.97 u; **(f)** 135.04 u (molecular); **(g)** 102.18 u (molecular); **(h)** 114.22 u (molecular). **19. (a)** 324.36 u; **(b)** 152.15 u. **21. (a)** 43.4 g; **(b)** 42.5 g; **(c)** 44.5 g; **(d)** 0.0345 g. **23. (a)** 3.78 mol; **(b)** 0.204 mol; **(c)** 0.139 mol; **(d)** 3.51×10^{-3} mol; **(e)** 3.78×10^5 mol. **25.** 1.81×10^{24} oxide ions, 1.20×10^{24} iron(III) ions. **27. (a)** 2.82×10^{24} molecules; **(b)** 2.22×10^{23} ions; **(c)** 2.119×10^{-22} g; **(d)** 1.651×10^{-22} g. **29.** mol of atoms: Al (<1 mol) $<$ U (just over 1 mol) $<$ HCl ($\sim$1.5 mol) $< O_2$ ($\sim$2 mol). **31. (a)** 45.94% K; 16.46% N; 37.60% O; **(b)** 64.81% C; 13.60% H; 21.59% O; **(c)** 10.22% Al; 35.21% P; 54.57% O; **(d)** 19.05% C; 4.80% H; 76.15% O. **33. (a)** 48.44% O; **(b)** 13.85% N; **(c)** 5.03% Be. **35. (a)** N_2O_5; **(b)** C_5H_{11}. **37. (a)** $C_6H_4Cl_2$; **(b)** $C_6H_{12}O_6$. **39. (a)** $C_{18}H_{21}NO_3$; **(b)** $Mg_2P_2O_7$. **41.** $C_6H_6O_2$. **43.** $LiClO_4 \cdot 3 H_2O$. **45.** NH_4NO_2. **47.** CH_3S, $C_2H_6S_2$. **49.** C_4H_4S. **51. (a)** MTBE $<$ ethanol $<$ methanol; **(b)** yes; **(c)** 15% MTBE. **53. (a)** $Cl_2O_5 + H_2O \longrightarrow 2 HClO_3$; **(b)** $V_2O_5 + 2 H_2 \longrightarrow$ $V_2O_3 + 2 H_2O$; **(c)** $4 Al + 3 O_2 \longrightarrow 2 Al_2O_3$; **(d)** $TiCl_4 +$ $2 H_2O \longrightarrow TiO_2 + 4 HCl$; **(e)** $Sn + 2 NaOH \longrightarrow Na_2SnO_2$ $+ H_2$; **(f)** $PCl_5 + 4 H_2O \longrightarrow 5 HCl + H_3PO_4$; **(g)** $CH_3SH +$ $3 O_2 \longrightarrow CO_2 + SO_2 + 2 H_2O$; **(h)** $3 Zn(OH)_2 + 2 H_3PO_4$ $\longrightarrow Zn_3(PO_4)_2 + 6 H_2O$; **(i)** $3 CH_3CH_2OH + PCl_3 \longrightarrow$ $3 CH_3CH_2Cl + H_3PO_3$. **55.** $2 Mg(s) + O_2(g) \longrightarrow$ $2 MgO(s)$; 1 mol $O_2 \backsimeq$ 2 mol Mg; 1 mol $O_2 \backsimeq$ 2 mol MgO. **57. (a)** $2 HCl(aq) + Zn(s) \longrightarrow H_2(g) + ZnCl_2(aq)$; **(b)** $C_2H_6(g)$ $+ 2 H_2O(g) \longrightarrow 2 CO(g) + 5 H_2(g)$; **(c)** $P_4O_{10}(s) + 6 H_2O(l)$ $\longrightarrow 4 H_3PO_4(l)$; **(d)** $Pb(s) + PbO_2(s) + 2 H_2SO_4(aq) \longrightarrow$ $2 PbSO_4(s) + 2 H_2O(l)$. **59.** $3 Fe_2O_3(s) + H_2(g) \longrightarrow H_2O(g) +$ $2 Fe_3O_4(s)$. **61.** $4 NH_3 + 5 O_2 \longrightarrow 4 NO + 6 H_2O$. **63. (a)** 3.61×10^3 mol CO_2; **(b)** 7.31×10^3 mol O_2; **(c)** 1.69×10^3 mol H_2O; **(d)** 1.8×10^3 mol C_8H_{18}. **65.** $CaCN_2$. **67.** 1.78×10^4 g CO_2. **69. (a)** 3.77 g CO_2; **(b)** 68.0% $CaCO_3$. **71.** The reactant that is consumed completely and determines the amount of product formed; when the two reactants are in stoichiometric proportions. **73.** LiOH is limiting; 2.20 mol Li_2CO_3. **75.** (d); 4.00 g is about 1/8 or 0.125 mol O_2, Hg is limiting and produces 0.200 mol HgO, leaving a small excess of O_2. **77. (a)** 516 g KI; **(b)** $KHCO_3$, 6.7 g. **79.** Yes. **81.** 0.727 g ZnS, 83.4% **83.** 51.3 g NH_4HCO_3. **85. (a)** 2.26 M; **(b)** 0.0700 M; **(c)** 0.7802 M; **(d)** 0.963 M; **(e)** 0.9462 M; **(f)** 1.83 M. **87. (a)** 0.0294 mol; **(b)** 7.66 g; **(c)** 206 g; **(d)** 87.9 mL. **89. (a)** 403 mL; **(b)** 2.49×10^3 mL; **(c)** 104 mL. **91.** 14.6 M. **93.** 0.0291 M. **95. (a)** 165.2 mL; **(b)** 16.20 mL. **97.** The final molarity cannot be the simple average (0.15 M) of the two because a greater volume is used of the 0.20 M solution. The answer is (c), 0.17 M. **99.** Pipet 3×25 mL and 2×10 mL into a 100 mL volumetric flask. Add 1.05 g $AgNO_3$, mix to dissolve, dilute to the mark. Other approaches possible. **101.** 46.5 g $BaSO_4$. **103.** 2.19 M. **105.** 1.91 g CO_2. **107. (a)** 0.2 cm²; **(b)** 13 drops. **Additional Problems: 110.** 5 tablets. **113.** $BrCl_3$. **115.** 55.85 u, Fe. **118.** 70.1%. **120.** Empirical CHF; molecular $C_3H_3F_3$; $4 C_3H_3F_3 +$ $12 O_2 \longrightarrow 3 CF_4 + 6 H_2O + 9 CO_2$. **123. (a)** 48.4 g; **(b)** 45.9 g; **(c)** 9.4 g MgO, 40.5 g Mg_3N_2. **124.** $3 C_2H_4O_2 + PCl_3$ $\longrightarrow H_3PO_3 + 3 C_2H_3OCl$. **Apply Your Knowledge:**

128. (a) 4% P, 4% K; (b) 35-0-0; (c) KH_2PO_4 and $(NH_4)_2HPO_4$; (d) 20 g K_2O requires 42.9 g KNO_3 and contains 5.9 g N, 20 g P_2O_5 requires 33.8 g NaH_2PO_4. Additional 14.1 g N requires 40.2 g NH_4NO_3, total = 116.9 g > 100 g, not possible. **130.** 70.58%. **132.** 1.81 g Na. **133.** 0.4065 g $MgCl_2$, 0.2053 g NaCl.

Chapter 4

Exercises: 4.1A $[Na^+]$ = 0.438 M; $[Mg^{2+}]$ = 0.0512 M; $[Cl^-]$ = 0.540 M. **4.1B** $[Na^+]$ = 0.093 M; $[K^+]$ = 0.020 M; $[Cl^-]$ = 0.080 M; $[C_6H_5O_7^{3-}]$ = 0.011 M; $[C_6H_{12}O_6]$ = 0.111 M. **4.2A** (a) $Ca(OH)_2(aq) + 2 HCl(aq) \longrightarrow CaCl_2(aq) + 2 H_2O(l)$; (b) $Ca^{2+}(aq) + 2 OH^-(aq) + 2 H^+(aq) + 2 Cl^-(aq) \longrightarrow Ca^{2+}(aq) + 2 Cl^-(aq) + 2 H_2O(l)$; (c) $OH^-(aq) + H^+(aq) \longrightarrow H_2O(l)$. **4.2B** (a) $2 KHSO_4(aq) + 2 NaOH(aq) \longrightarrow K_2SO_4(aq) + Na_2SO_4(aq) + 2 H_2O(l)$; (b) $K^+(aq) + HSO_4^-(aq) + Na^+(aq) + OH^-(aq) \longrightarrow K^+(aq) + Na^+(aq) + SO_4^{2-}(aq) + H_2O(l)$; (c) $HSO_4^-(aq) + OH^-(aq) \longrightarrow SO_4^{2-}(aq) + H_2O(l)$. **4.3A** The bulb will be dimly lit with CH_3NH_2 (weak base) and brightly lit with HNO_3 (strong acid). When the solutions are mixed, the $CH_3NH_3^+NO_3^-$ (salt) formed maintains the brightly lit bulb. **4.3B** $Mg(OH)_2(s)$ is essentially insoluble, and the very low ion concentration in $Mg(OH)_2(aq)$ produces only a dim glow in the bulb. The bulb grows brighter as $Mg(CH_3COO)_2(aq)$ forms, and brightest when the $Mg(OH)_2(aq)$ is completely neutralized. Beyond this point, additional $CH_3COOH(aq)$ produces little change because $CH_3COOH(aq)$ is a weak acid. **4.4A** (a) $Mg^{2+}(aq) + 2 OH^-(aq) \longrightarrow Mg(OH)_2(s)$; (b) $2 Fe^{3+}(aq) + 3 S^{2-}(aq) \longrightarrow Fe_2S_3(s)$; (c) $Sr^{2+}(aq) + SO_4^{2-}(aq) \longrightarrow SrSO_4(s)$. **4.4B** (a) $Zn^{2+}(aq) + SO_4^{2-}(aq) + Ba^{2+}(aq) + S^{2-}(aq) \longrightarrow ZnS(s) + BaSO_4(s)$; (b) no reaction; (c) $2 HCO_3^-(aq) + Ca^{2+}(aq) + 2 OH^-(aq) \longrightarrow CaCO_3(s) + CO_3^{2-}(aq) + 2 H_2O(l)$. **4.5A** H^+ from the acid combines with OH^- from $Fe(OH)_3$ to form $H_2O(l)$: $Fe(OH)_3(s) + 3 H^+(aq) \longrightarrow Fe^{3+}(aq) + 3 H_2O(l)$. **4.5B** The likely precipitate is calcium palmitate, $Ca[CH_3(CH_2)_{14}COO]_2(s)$. Ionic equation: $2 K^+(aq) + 2 CH_3(CH_2)_{14}COO^-(aq) + Ca^{2+} + 2 Cl^-(aq) \longrightarrow 2 K^+(aq) + 2 Cl^-(aq) + Ca[CH_3(CH_2)_{14}COO]_2(s)$; net ionic equation: $Ca^{2+}(aq) + 2 CH_3(CH_2)_{14}COO^-(aq) \longrightarrow Ca[CH_3(CH_2)_{14}COO]_2(s)$. **4.6A** 42.20% NaCl. **4.6B** 17.4 g AgCl(s); 14.9 g $Mg(OH)_2(s)$. **4.7A** (a) Al, +3, O, −2; (b) P, 0; (c) C, −2, H, +1, F, −1; (d) H, +1, As, +5, O, −2; (e) Na, +1, Mn, +7, O, −2; (f) Cl, +3, O, −2; (g) Cs, +1, O, −1/2. **4.7B** (a) +5; (b) +2; (c) +5; (d) +5/2; (e) +4/3; (f) +5; (g) +3. **4.8A** $Cr_2O_7^{2-}(aq)$ and $HNO_3(aq)$ are oxidizing agents and do not react with each other. HCl(aq) is a reducing agent; $Cl^-(aq)$ is oxidized, probably to $Cl_2(g)$. The $Cr_2O_7^{2-}$ is reduced to Cr^{3+}, accounting for the green color. **4.8B** The solution would be $ZnCl_2(aq)$ in HCl(aq) instead of unreacted HCl(aq), as in (a), or $Cu^{2+}(aq)$ and $Zn^{2+}(aq)$ in $HNO_3(aq)$, as in (b). **4.9A** 74.53 mL. **4.9B** 1.10×10^2 mL. **4.10A** 12.6 mL. **4.10B** 31.7% H_2SO_4. **4.11A** 0.009815 M. **4.11B** 23.42 mL **4.12A** 22.04 mL. **4.12B** 14.23 mL. **Self-Assessment Questions: 1.** (a). **2.** (a) weak acid; (b) strong acid; (c) strong base; (d) weak base; (e) salt; (f) weak acid. **3.** (c) highest, (b) lowest. **4.** (c). **5.** (a), it is a strong electrolyte and is completely ionized; while (b) and (c) have a higher concentration and are only slightly ionized. **6.** (a). **9.** (c). **11.** (d), most sulfates are soluble but lead is an exception. **12.** (c), $MgCl_2(aq) + Na_2CO_3 \longrightarrow 2 NaCl(aq) + MgCO_3(s)$. **17.** (d). **18.** (a) 0; (b) +3; (c) −2; (d) +6; (e) −3; (f) +4; (g) +4; (h) +5;

(i) +5/2; (j) −1. **19.** (a) −3; (b) +2; (c) +1; (d) −2; (e) +3. **24.** (b) **Problems: 25.** (a), (b), (c), (e), (f) are strong electrolytes; (d) is weak. **27.** All; they are all soluble and are strong electrolytes. **29.** (a) $[Li^+]$ = $[NO_3^-]$ = 0.647 M; (b) $[Ca^{2+}]$ = 0.035 M, $[I^-]$ = 0.070 M; (c) $[Al^{3+}]$ = 2.14 M, $[SO_4^{2-}]$ = 3.21 M. **31.** $[Na^+]$ = 0.0844 M, $[Cl^-]$ = 0.0554 M, $[SO_4^{2-}]$ = 0.0145 M. **33.** 3.384 L. **35.** 0.040 M $Al(NO_3)_3$ > 0.1 M KNO_3 > 0.047 M $Ca(NO_3)_2$. **37.** 0.261 M. **39.** 1.92×10^3 mg Cl/L. **41.** 67.5 mL. **43.** (a) < (d) < (c) < (b). **45.** (a) $HBr(aq) \longrightarrow H^+(aq) + Br^-(aq)$; (b) $LiOH(aq) \longrightarrow Li^+(aq) + OH^-(aq)$; (c) $HF(aq) \rightleftharpoons H^+(aq) + F^-(aq)$. (d) $HIO_3(aq) \rightleftharpoons H^+(aq) + IO_3^-(aq)$; (e) $(CH_3)_2NH(aq) + H_2O(l) \rightleftharpoons (CH_3)_2NH_2^+(aq) + OH^-(aq)$; (f) $HCOOH(aq) \rightleftharpoons H^+(aq) + HCOO^-(aq)$. **47.** (d) < (c) < (a) < (b). **49.** (b); for (a) no reaction; (b) $H^+(aq) + OH^-(aq) \longrightarrow H_2O(l)$; (c) $NH_3(aq) + H^+(aq) \longrightarrow NH_4^+(aq)$. **51.** $CaCO_3(s) + 2 H^+(aq) \longrightarrow Ca^{2+}(aq) + H_2O(l) + CO_2(g)$. **53.** (a) $2 I^-(aq) + Pb^{2+}(aq) \longrightarrow PbI_2(s)$; (b) no reaction; (c) $Cr^{3+}(aq) + 3 OH^-(aq) \longrightarrow Cr(OH)_3(s)$; (d) no reaction; (e) $OH^-(aq) + H^+(aq) \longrightarrow H_2O(l)$; (f) $HSO_4^-(aq) + OH^-(aq) \longrightarrow H_2O(l) + SO_4^{2-}(aq)$. **55.** (a) $Mg(OH)_2(s) + 2 H^+(aq) \longrightarrow Mg^{2+}(aq) + 2 H_2O(l)$; (b) $HCOOH(aq) + NH_3(aq) \longrightarrow NH_4^+(aq) + HCOO^-(aq)$; (c) no reaction; (d) $Cu^{2+}(aq) + CO_3^{2-}(aq) \longrightarrow CuCO_3(s)$; (e) no reaction. **57.** (a), (b), (c) soluble; (d) insoluble. **59.** No; $MgSO_4$ is soluble in H_2O and $Mg(OH)_2$ reacts with acid to dissolve. Add water to the powder; if it dissolves it is $MgSO_4$. **61.** $Cu^{2+}(aq) + CO_3^{2-}(aq) \longrightarrow CuCO_3(s)$. **63.** Add $Ba^{2+}(aq)$ to each, Na_2SO_4 precipitates $BaSO_4$; add H_2SO_4 to each, $Ba(NO_3)_2$ precipitates $BaSO_4$; the nonreacting solution is NH_3. **65.** (a) oxidation, Cr^{2+} to Cr^{3+}; (b) neither, no atom changes oxidation number; (c) neither, no atom changes oxidation number. **67.** (a) $4 HCl + O_2 \longrightarrow 2 H_2O + 2 Cl_2$; (b) $2 NO + 5 H_2 \longrightarrow 2 H_2O + 2 NH_3$; (c) $CH_4 + 4 NO \longrightarrow 2 N_2 + 2 H_2O + CO_2$; (d) $3 Ag + 4 H^+ + NO_3^- \longrightarrow NO + 2 H_2O + 3 Ag^+$; (e) $IO_4^- + 7 I^- + 8 H^+ \longrightarrow 4 I_2 + 4 H_2O$. **69.** Oxidizing agent and reducing agent, respectively: (a) O_2, HCl; (b) NO, H_2; (c) NO, CH_4; (d) NO_3^-, Ag; (e) IO_4^-, I^-. **71.** (a) both Pb^{2+} and V^{3+} are being oxidized, but nothing is reduced; (b) only S^{2-} is being reduced, nothing is oxidized. **73.** (a) $Zn + 2 H^+ \longrightarrow Zn^{2+} + H_2$; (b) no reaction; (c) $Fe + 2 Ag^+ \longrightarrow Fe^{2+} + 2 Ag$; (d) no reaction. **75.** (a) 46.8 ml; (b) 11.9 mL; (c) 23.1 mL. **77.** 0.8051 M. **79.** (a) 487 mg $CaCO_3$; (b) 195 mg Ca^{2+}. **81.** Tums. **83.** (d); 22.00 mL is about 10% excess OH^-, and the CH_3COOH has been consumed. **85.** (a) 147.7 mL; (b) 111.6 mL; (c) 29.1 mL. **87.** $Ba^{2+}(aq) + SO_4^{2-}(aq) \longrightarrow BaSO_4(s)$; 0.04329 M. **89.** (a) 12.39 mL; (b) 47.67 mL. **91.** 0.1226 M. **93.** 0.235 M Cl^-. **Additional Problems: 96.** 6.4 mL. **99.** 1.5×10^3 kg. **101.** 1.2 M OH^-. **104.** 9.26 g. **107.** +5. **110.** 86.2 mL. **113.** KCl; 3.43 g. **115.** 0.0345% S. **Apply Your Knowledge: 116.** 49.0% protein. **118.** $Ag^+ + SCN^- \longrightarrow AgSCN(s)$; 93.71% Ag **122.** No.

Chapter 5

Exercises: 5.1A (a) 720 mmHg; (b) 737 Torr; (c) 760.7 Torr; (d) 1.01 atm. **5.1B** 2.00×10^2 kPa; 1.97 atm. **5.2A** 6.50 m. **5.2B** 2.90 atm due to the water; 3.90 atm total. **5.3A** 735 mmHg < 745 mmHg < 750 mmHg < 101 kPa < "above 762 mmHg"; but because 103 kPa = 773 mmHg, we are uncertain how to compares it with "above 762 mmHg." That is, we don't know which of the two comes last in the series. **5.3B** (a) When air is sucked through the straw, the pressure of the remaining air drops. Air pres-

sure outside the straw exceeds that within the straw and pushes liquid up the straw. **(b)** The hand-operated water pump acts in the same way as the soda straw. The height limitation arises because of the maximum height of a water column that can be sustained by atmospheric pressure (see Example 5.2). **5.4A** 503 Torr. **5.4B** 17.8 mL. **5.5A** 400 mmHg. **5.5B** (d). The PV product is constant in Exercise 5.5A. Both (a) and (b) use the wrong volume in the PV product, and (c) is not a PV product. Response (d) is a PV product equivalent to 1.2×10^4 Torr L, when properly converted. **5.6A** 234 L. **5.6B** 338 K (65 °C). **5.7A** 7.5 L. **5.7B** (b). The final pressure must be larger than the initial pressure, but not three times as great. Responses (a), (c) and (d) must all be incorrect. Note that the correct answer is roughly 4/3 of the initial pressure (the temperature ratio is 423 K/323 K ∼ 4/3). **5.8A** 98.4 g C_3H_8. **5.8B** 3.75×10^3 L CO_2. **5.9A** Greater than 6.7×10^2 °C. **5.9B** $P_2 = (n_2/n_1) \times P_1$. Pressure is directly proportional to amount of gas. With more molecules in the same volume, the frequency of molecular collisions, and hence the pressure, increases. **5.10A** 1.58 mol N_2. **5.10B** 0.93 mol N_2. **5.11A** -139 °C. **5.11B** 21.6 g N_2. **5.12A** 74.3 g/mol. **5.12B** 2.0 atm. **5.13A** 126 u. **5.13B** $C_4H_6O_2$. **5.14A** 1.25 g/L. **5.14B** C_4H_{10}. **5.15A** 94 °C. **5.15B** 92 °C. **5.16A** 2.78 L $O_2(g)$. **5.16B** 207 L $O_2(g)$. **5.17A** 4.16×10^4 L $CO_2(g)$. **5.17B** 746 L $C_5H_{10}(l)$. **5.18A** Partial pressures: O_2, 0.209 atm; Ar, 0.00932 atm; CO_2, 0.0005 atm; total pressure: 0.999 atm. **5.18B** 12.9 atm. **5.19A** Partial pressures: N_2, 0.741 atm; O_2, 0.150 atm; H_2O, 0.060 atm; Ar, 0.009 atm; CO_2, 0.040 atm. **5.19B** Mole fractions: CH_4, 0.636; C_2H_6, 0.253; C_3H_8, 0.054; C_4H_{10}, 0.0562. **5.20A** If only H_2 were added, its partial pressure would be 2.50 atm instead of 2.00 atm. A gas other than H_2 is needed at a partial pressure of 0.50 atm; it can be additional He, but does not have to be. **5.20B** The pressure increases by the factor 673 K/273 K ≈ 2.5, even if no N_2 is added. Responses (a) and (b) are incorrect. N_2 must be removed. However, since the amount of N_2 initially is slightly less than 0.10 mol, response (c) is incorrect. The correct response is (d). **5.21A** Total mass of wet gas: 0.0235 g; mass of H_2: 0.0197 g. **5.21B** 0.502 g $KClO_3$. **5.22A** Estimate the value of $\sqrt{T/M}$ for each of the four responses. Choose the one with the largest value. It is (d). **5.22B** The temperature must exceed 273 K multiplied by the ratio of the molar mass of O_2 to H_2. Only response (d), 5000 K, does. **5.23A** N_2 effuses faster by the factor $(39.95/28.01)^{1/2} = 1.194$. **5.23B** NO effuses faster by the factor $(46.07/30.01)^{1/2} = 1.239$, or 23.9% faster. **5.24A** 59 g/mol. **5.24B** 166 s. **Self-Assessment Questions: 3.** (b). **5.** **(a)** 0.7326 atm; **(b)** 0.762 atm; **(c)** 0.691 atm; **(d)** 1.17 atm. **6.** **(a)** V decreases; **(b)** V decreases; **(c)** indeterminate; **(d)** V increases. **7.** **(a)** P increases; **(b)** P increases; **(c)** P increases; **(d)** indeterminate. **9.** (b), (c), (d). **10.** (d). **11.** (a). **12.** (c). **13.** **(a)** A more dense; **(b)** same density; **(c)** B more dense. **14.** (a). **15.** (b). **16.** (d). **17.** (c). **18.** (a). **19.** (b). **20.** (b). **Problems: 21.** **(a)** 7.10×10^2 Torr; **(b)** 1.01 atm; **(c)** 93.1 kPa; **(d)** 1.73×10^3 mmHg **23.** 121 atm **25.** 0.958 m **27.** 756 mmHg **29.** The height in mm must be greater than the pressure in mmHg, since 1 mm of height = 1 mmHg pressure. **31.** **(a)** 922 mL; **(b)** 632 mL; **(c)** 707 mL. **33.** 46.4 m³. **35.** **(a)** 6.54×10^3 L; **(b)** 817 min. **37.** 478 mL. **39.** 150 K. **41.** 3.26 kg CH_4. **43.** 575 mL. **45.** (d). **47.** 2.49×10^3 Torr. **49.** 24.5 L. **51.** 0.489 m³. **53.** **(a)** 46.9 L; **(b)** 26.9 atm; **(c)** 8.64 mg H_2; **(d)** 248 kPa. **55.** 7.48 L. **57.** 71.5 L. **59.** 178 u. **61.** C_7H_8. **63.** **(a)** 0.901 g/L; **(b)** 0.968 g/L. **65.** 0.803 atm. **67.** S_8. **69.** (c). **71.** 18.8 L. **73.** 4.50 L. **75.** 28.1 mg Mg. **77.** 122 L. **79.** 123 mL. **81.** 585 mmHg

N_2, 153 mmHg O_2, 24 mmHg CO_2. **83.** **(a)** $x_{He} = 0.205$, $x_{O_2} = 0.795$; **(b)** $P_{He} = 2.40$ atm; $P_{O_2} = 9.30$ atm; **(c)** $P_{total} = 11.70$ atm. **85.** $P_{O_2} = 736$ mmHg, $x_{O_2} = 0.974$. **87.** 0.154 g O_2, 0.145 g glucose. **89.** (b). **91.** A mixture expands to fill the entire container and so all the gases have the same volume. If the gases of the mixture were at different temperatures, they would quickly equilibrate to the same temperature. Since P_{gas} is directly related to the number of moles of the gas, pressures may be different if the number of moles differ. **93.** **(a)** 81 u; **(b)** 26 u. **Additional Problems: 95.** 80 g air, 36 lb/in² **97.** 0.181 g He. **100.** 661 mL. **102.** 54.09 u. **105.** No. **107.** 5.75×10^{15} tons. **110.** 44.5% Li, 55.5% Mg. **113.** 1.26×10^4 L air; 1.47×10^3 L CO_2. **117.** **(a)** 9.78 atm; **(b)** 9.38 atm; **(c)** The a-term, intermolecular attraction, is more important than the b-term, molecular volume, so the real pressure is lower than the ideal pressure. **119.** 2-methylpentane and 3-methylpentane, $(CH_3)_2CHCH_2CH_2CH_3$ and $CH_3CH_2CH(CH_3)CH_2CH_3$. **Apply Your Knowledge: 121.** 144 u. **123.** Slightly over 30 km. **124.** Atomic mass of X = 16.0 u; number of X atoms = 2, 1, 1, 2, respectively; X = oxygen.

Chapter 6

Exercises: 6.1A $\Delta U = -478$ J. **6.1B** The system absorbs heat; $q = +122.6$ J. **6.2A** **(a)** gas does work $(w < 0)$; **(b)** internal energy decreases $(\Delta U < 0)$; **(c)** temperature decreases $(\Delta T < 0)$. **6.2B** The process can occur. The values of w are different for the expansion and the compression because w is path-dependent. However, because the gas is returned to the identical starting condition, $\Delta U = 0$. **6.3A** $\Delta H = +142.7$ kJ. **6.3B** $\Delta H = -148.9$ kJ. **6.4A** $H_2O(s) \longrightarrow H_2O(l)$ $\Delta H = +6.02$ kJ. **6.4B** $N_2O_3(g) \longrightarrow NO(g) + NO_2(g)$ $\Delta H = +40.5$ kJ. **6.5A** $\Delta H = -1.17 \times 10^3$ kJ. **6.5B** 2.80×10^4 L $CH_4(g)$. **6.6A** 11 J/°C. **6.6B** $q = -153$ kJ. **6.7A** $q = 6.67 \times 10^4$ cal = 66.7 kcal. **6.7B** 4.39×10^5 kg H_2O. **6.8A** 95.1 °C. **6.8B** 1.57×10^3 g Cu. **6.9A** 0.13 J g⁻¹ °C⁻¹. **6.9B** 1.64 J g⁻¹ °C⁻¹. **6.10A** 60 °C. **6.10B** 27.8 °C. **6.11A** $q_{rxn} = 2.81$ kJ. **6.11B** The result should be substantially the same. The net ionic reactions are the same in the two neutralizations, $H^+(aq) + OH^-(aq) \longrightarrow H_2O(l)$. **6.12A** $\Delta H = -56.2$ kJ **6.12B** 29.9 °C. **6.13A** $\Delta H = -395$ kJ. **6.13B** 5.99 kJ/°C. **6.14A** $\Delta H = -1215$ kJ. **6.14B** $\Delta H = -137.0$ kJ. **6.15A** $\Delta H° = -44.2$ kJ. **6.15B** $2 C_4H_{10}(g) + 13 O_2(g) \longrightarrow 8 CO_2(g) + 10 H_2O(l)$, $\Delta H° = -5755$ kJ. **6.16A** $\Delta H_f° = -52$ kJ/mol $C_2Cl_4(l)$. **6.16B** $\Delta H_f° = +81$ kJ/mol $C_4H_4S(l)$. **6.17A** $\Delta H_f°$ of CH_3CH_2OH and CH_3OH differ only by 39 kJ/mol. In contrast, the enthalpies of the combustion products are much lower for CH_3CH_2OH than for CH_3OH [by 1 mol each of $CO_2(g)$ and $H_2O(l)$]. Per mole, combustion of CH_3CH_2OH gives off the greater amount of heat. **6.17B** The complete combustion of 1 mol $CH_3COOH(l)$ yields 2 mol each of $CO_2(g)$ and $H_2O(l)$. This final state is at a higher enthalpy than the 2 mol $CO_2(g)$ + 3 mol $H_2O(l)$ formed in the combustion of 1 mol of $CH_3CH_2OH(l)$. At the same time, the initial state of 1 mol $CH_3COOH(l)$ is at a lower enthalpy than the initial states of 1 mol $C_2H_6(g)$ and 1 mol $CH_3CH_2OH(l)$. The magnitudes of the enthalpies of combustion are: $CH_3COOH(l) < CH_3CH_2OH < C_2H_6$. **6.18A** $\Delta H_f°$ [$BaSO_4$] $= -1473$ kJ/mol. **6.18B** $\Delta H° = +2.4$ kJ [per mole of $Mg(OH)_2(s)$ formed]. **Self-Assessment Questions: 3.** (c). **6.** (a). **8.** (d). **9.** (a). **10.** (b). **12.** (d). **13.** (a). **14.** $2 Fe(s) + 3/2 O_2(g) \longrightarrow Fe_2O_3(s)$. **18.** 53 kcal, 17%. **Problems: 19.** $+442$ J. **21.** 515 J absorbed. **23.** Yes, yes.

25. Endothermic, $+241$ kJ, ΔH because the system is at constant pressure. **27.** $CaO(s) + H_2O(l) \longrightarrow Ca(OH)_2(s)$, $\Delta H = -65.2$ kJ. **29. (a)** -31 kJ; **(b)** $+138$ kJ. **31.** $1/4\ P_4(s) + 3/2\ Cl_2(g) \longrightarrow PCl_3(g)$, $\Delta H = -287$ kJ. **33.** 1591 kJ evolved. **35.** 416 kJ evolved. **37.** 447 L. **39.** Yes. **41.** 757 g CaO. **43.** 13 J/°C. **45. (a)** 108 kJ; **(b)** 14.8 kJ. **47.** 52.0 °C. **49.** 0.485 J/(g°C). **51.** No. **53.** Cu. **55.** -53.7 kJ/mol. **57.** $+27$ kJ/mol. **59.** 28.6 kJ evolved per g coal. **61.** 9.32 kJ/°C. **63.** -5.64×10^3 kJ/mol. **65.** -221.0 kJ. **67.** -818.2 kJ. **69.** -1155.4 kJ. **71. (a)** -19 kJ; **(b)** -1095.9 kJ; **(c)** $+168.0$ kJ; **(d)** -1084.3 kJ. **73.** -206 kJ/mol. **75.** -628 kJ/mol. **77.** $+30.6$ kJ. **79.**

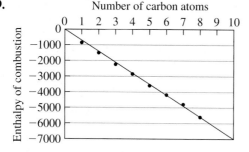

Number of carbon atoms

Slope $= -650.7$ kJ/C atom, intercept $= -260.4$ kJ, so for $C_{10}H_{22}$, $\Delta H_{comb} = -6767$ kJ/mol; for $C_{12}H_{24}$, $\Delta H_{comb} = -8069$ kJ/mol. **81.** 14%. **Additional Problems: 83.** (c). **85.** 27.8 °C. **88.** The aluminum foil; we need only calculate the product (mass $\times$ specific heat). **90.** 1.28×10^3 kJ. **93.** About 69 °C. **95.** 33.54 °C. **98. (a)** ΔH is a state function and depends on the concentration of solute; **(b)** For dilution, Equation (6.21) becomes $\Delta H_f^{\circ}(\text{dilute}) - \Delta H_f^{\circ}(\text{concd})$; since ΔH_f° becomes more negative with dilution, the dilution is exothermic. **99.** $C_2H_6O(g) + 3\ O_2(g) \longrightarrow 2\ CO_2(g) + 3\ H_2O(l)$; $\Delta H^{\circ} = -1.45 \times 10^3$ kJ. **102.** $\Delta H_f^{\circ} = -156$ kJ/mol. **Apply Your Knowledge: 104. (a)** $2\ C_6H_{14}(l) + 19\ O_2(g) \longrightarrow 12\ CO_2(g) + 14\ H_2O(l)$; $\Delta H^{\circ} = -8314.0$ kJ; **(b)** $(CH_3)_2CHCH_2CH_2CH_3$ or $CH_3CH_2CH(CH_3)CH_2CH_3$; **(c)** 12.1 gal. **107. (a)** 25.2; **(b)** Plot specific heat vs. 1/(molar mass); **(c)** 59.4 g/mol; **(d)** about 83 mL. **109.** -74.9 kJ (lab), -82 kJ (theor); Reasons for error: assumption of specific heat of solutions; heat absorbed by calorimeter; solutions not at 1 M concentration; and so on.

Chapter 7

Exercises: 7.1A 2.80×10^{11} Hz. **7.1B** 3.07×10^3 nm. **7.2A** Microwave radiation has longer wavelengths than visible light. **7.2B** (b); comparisons can be made with the information in Figure 7.11. **7.3A** 1.91×10^{-23} J/photon. **7.3B** 8.46×10^{-19} J/photon. **7.4A** 299 kJ/mol photons. **7.4B** infrared (≈ 1200 nm). **7.5A** $E_6 = -6.053 \times 10^{-20}$ J. **7.5B** No. The allowable energy levels are $n = (-2.179 \times 10^{-18}/E_n)^{1/2}$, where n must be an integer; $(1 \times 10^1)^{1/2} = 3.16$—not an integer. **7.6A** $\Delta E_{level} = 4.086 \times 10^{-19}$ J. **7.6B** Yes. Find a pair of integers such that $(4.269 \times 10^{-20}\ \text{J}/2.179 \times 10^{-18}\ \text{J}) = (1/n_1^2 - 1/n_2^2)$. The pair must be larger than $n_1 = 5$ and $n_2 = 3$, because the energy difference, 4.269×10^{-20} J, is smaller than the 1.550×10^{-19} J found in Example 7.6. Try combinations such as 5,4; 6,5; 6,4; 7,6; 7,5; and 7,4. The combination 7,5 works. **7.7A** $\nu = 3.083 \times 10^{15}$ s^{-1}. **7.7B** $\lambda = 434.1$ nm (visible region). **7.8A (a)** ΔE_{level} between $n = 1$ and $n = 2$ is $3/4\ B$. The only transitions that would require more energy are from $n = 1$ to $n \geq 3$. **7.8B** No. The energy cited is less than the minimum energy for an emission from the level

$n = 4$, that is, less than $E = 2.179 \times 10^{-18}$ J $\times (1/3^2 - 1/4^2) = 1.2 \times 10^{-19}$ J. **7.9A** $\lambda = 0.105$ nm. **7.9B** $\nu = 1.50 \times 10^3$ m/s. **7.10A** (b), (c) are possible; (a), (d) are not possible because m_l cannot be less than $-l$ nor greater than $+l$. **7.10B (a)** $m_l = -1, 0, 1$; **(b)** $l = 2$ or 3; **(c)** $n \geq 4$, $m_l = -3, -2, -1, 0, 1, 2, 3$. **7.11A (a)** three; **(b)** the f subshells of $n \geq 4$. **7.11B (a)** Sixteen orbitals in $n = 4$ (one $4s$, three $4p$, five $4d$, seven $4f$); **(b)** total number of orbitals $= n^2$. **Self-Assessment Questions: 1.** (b). **5.** (d). **6.** (b). **7.** (a). **9.** (b). **10.** At the microscopic level, energy changes are very small, and the discontinuities due to quantization are very important. At the macroscopic level, energy changes are much larger and energy transfer appears to be continuous. **12.** The negative sign indicates attractive force. The smaller the value of n, the closer the electron is to the nucleus, and the stronger should be that attractive force. The incorrect expression $E_n = -B \times n^2$ predicts an increase in E as n increases. **13.** (a). **17. (a)** $3d$; **(b)** $2s$; **(c)** $4p$; **(d)** $4f$. **18.** (d). **19. (a)** 3; **(b)** 2; **(c)** 4. **21.** (d). **Problems: 23.** Charge 1.602×10^{-19} C, mass 1.672×10^{-27} kg. **25.** 1.6×10^{-19} C, the common factor. **27. (a)** 8.3×10^{-7} kg/C; **(b)** 9.3×10^{-8} kg/C; **(c)** 4.1×10^{-7} kg/C; without knowledge of actual isotope masses, we must use mass numbers. **29.** 72.5 u. **31. (a)** 414 m, AM radio; **(b)** 0.541 m, radio; **(c)** 2.86×10^{-11} m, X ray. **33.** $\lambda = 700$ nm, $\nu = 4.29 \times 10^{14}$ s^{-1}. **35.** 1.5×10^4 s. **37.** 4.92×10^{-19} J; greater, because 655 nm falls in the red region of the spectrum, and violet light has a shorter wavelength and higher energy. **39.** 2.55×10^{-19} J/photon; 154 kJ/mol photons. **41.** 427 nm. **43.** 246 nm, UV region. **45. (a)** 2.118×10^{-18} J; **(b)** 7.566×10^{-20} J. **47. (a)** 6.906×10^{14} s^{-1}; **(b)** 2.923×10^{15} s^{-1}. **49.** No; $n^2 = -B/E = 0.2179$, and there is no integer, squared, that gives 0.2179. **51.** 1312 kJ/mol. **53.** 0.00204 nm. **55.** 1.43×10^8 m/s. **57. (a)** $n = 2$; **(b)** $n = 4$. **59.** For $n = 4$, $l = 0, 1, 2,$ or 3; for $l = 1$, $m_l = 1, 0,$ or -1. **61. (a)** Magnitude of m_l cannot exceed l; **(b)** allowed; **(c)** allowed; **(d)** n must be 1 or greater. **63. (a)** $n = 4$, $l = 1$, $m_l = 1, 0,$ or -1; **(b)** $n = 4$, $l = 3$, $m_l = 3, 2, 1, 0, -1, -2,$ or -3; **(c)** $3d$. **65. (a)** $n = 2$ or greater, $m_s = +\frac{1}{2}$ or $-\frac{1}{2}$; **(b)** $l = 1$ or 2; **(c)** $l = 2, 3,$ or 4, $m_s = +\frac{1}{2}$ or $-\frac{1}{2}$; **(d)** $n = 1$ or greater, $m_l = 0$. **67.** $n = 3$, $l = 2$, $m_l = 0$, $m_s = -\frac{1}{2}$; any set for which $n = 3$, $l = 2$, $m_l = 2, 1, -1,$ or -2, and $m_s = +\frac{1}{2}$ or $-\frac{1}{2}$. **Additional Problems: 69.** 200.6 u, abundances are precisely known but masses are not (mass numbers). **71.** 0.017 s; period $= 1/\nu$. **74.** 2.37×10^{15} Hz; yes, the transition in H from $n = 2$ to $n = 1$ has slightly more energy than is needed, and the additional energy would be converted to kinetic energy of the two N atoms. **77.** maximum $= 121.6$ nm, minimum 91.2 nm. **79.** $n = 4$ to $n = 2$. **82.** Pfund transitions are to $n = 5$, 7400 nm is $n = 6$ to $n = 5$. **84.** 2.41×10^{-34} m. **87.** 7.65×10^3 m/s. **89.** About 700 photons/s. **93.** 0.00251 nm, ten times smaller than observed. **97. (a)** 5.16×10^{14} s^{-1}; **(b)** no, 1000 nm $= 3 \times 10^{14}$ s^{-1}; **(c)** 5.25×10^5 m/s. **Apply Your Knowledge: 101. (a)** 7.3×10^5 m/s; **(b)** 2.4×10^{14} rev/s. **103.** Note that sig. fig. convention is not followed, for clarity. **(a)** 6.6×10^{-34}%, 100%; **(b)** 0.02%, 99.98%; **(c)** 0.003%, 99.997%; **(d)** Decreasing flame temperature by 500 K decreases the number of emitting atoms, and the emission intensity, by a factor of 12; **(e)** number of ground-state atoms is virtually the same in (b) and (c).

Chapter 8

Exercises: 8.1A (a) $1s^2 2s^2 2p^6 3s^2 3p^5$; **(b)** $[Ne]3s^2 3p^5$;

(c)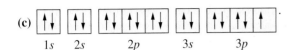
1s   2s   2p   3s   3p

8.1B Only (b) and (c) are valid electron configurations (for oxygen). Response (a) violates Hund's rule; (d) has unpaired electrons with opposing, rather than parallel, spins. **8.2A (a)** Mo: $1s^2 2s^2 2p^6 3s^2 3p^6 3d^{10} 4s^2 4p^6 4d^5 5s^1$; [Kr]$4d^5 5s^1$; **(b)** Bi: $1s^2 2s^2 2p^6 3s^2 3p^6 3d^{10} 4s^2 4p^6 4d^{10} 4f^{14} 5s^2 5p^6 5d^{10} 6s^2 6p^3$; [Xe]$4f^{14} 5d^{10} 6s^2 6p^3$. **8.2B (a)** Sn: [Kr]$4d^{10} 5s^2 5p^2$;

(b) Zr: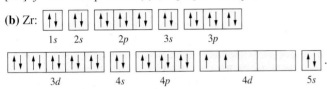
1s   2s   2p   3s   3p

3d   4s   4p   4d   5s

8.3A Se^{2-}, [Ar]$3d^{10} 4s^2 4p^6$; Pb^{2+}: [Xe]$4f^{14} 5d^{10} 6s^2$.

8.3B I$^-$: [Kr]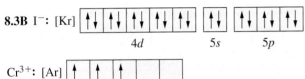
4d   5s   5p

Cr^{3+}: [Ar]
3d

8.4A (a) 2; **(b)** 4; **(c)** 0; **(d)** 0; **(e)** 0; **(f)** 4. **8.4B** The paramagnetic species and odd number of electrons are (a), 1; (d), 3; (f), 2; (g), 1. **8.5A (a)** F < N < Be; **(b)** Be < Ca < Ba; **(c)** F < Cl < S; **(d)** Mg < Ca < K. **8.5B** Based on trends noted in the text: P < Ge < Sn < Pb < Cs. The case of Ca is uncertain. Ca, in the fourth period, is a larger atom than P and Ge, in the third and fourth periods. The Ca atom, far to the left in its period, is probably larger than Sn and Pb, rather far to the right. The Cs atom in the lower left of the periodic table is largest. Probable order: P < Ge < Sn < Pb < Ca < Cs. **8.6A** Y^{3+} < Sr^{2+} < Rb$^+$ < Br$^-$ < Se^{2-}. **8.6B** Cr^{3+} < Cr^{2+} < Ca^{2+} < K$^+$ < Cs$^+$. **8.7A (a)** Be < N < F; **(b)** Ba < Ca < Be; **(c)** S < P < F; **(d)** K < Ca < Mg. **8.7B** I_1 for Al < I_1 for S < I_1 for H < I_2 for Mg < I_1 for Ar < I_2 for K. [I_1 for H (1312) can be calculated from the value of B in the Bohr H atom; other values can be found in the text.]. **8.8A** +400 kJ/mol; Se^{2-} is larger than S^{2-}, for which EA$_2 \approx$ 450 kJ/mol. **8.8B (a)** Adding one electron to Si would produce a half-filled p subshell. Adding one electron to Al results in only two electrons in the subshell. **(b)** Adding one electron to P would be adding to a half-filled subshell but adding one electron to Si would produce a half-filled subshell. **8.9A** More nonmetallic: **(a)** O; **(b)** S; **(c)** F. **8.9B** Na (alkali metal) ≈ Ba (alkaline earth metal) > Fe = Co(transition metals) > Sb(metalloid) > Se (nonmetal) > S(nonmetal). In general, group 1A elements are somewhat more metallic than group 2A. However, Na (third period) and Ba (sixth period) are comparable in metallic character. Fe and Co are very similar in atomic radius and ionization energy. The placement of Sb, Se, and S is based on their relative positions in the periodic table. **8.10A (a)** $Z = 52$ (Te); **(b)** $Z = 21$ (Sc); **(c)** lowest I_1, $Z = 39$ (Y); highest I_1, $Z = 48$ (Cd); **(d)** N. **8.10B (a)** Lowest I_1 value: In ($Z = 49$), highest I_1 value: Xe ($Z = 54$); **(b)** K ($Z = 19$), Cr ($Z = 24$), Cu ($Z = 29$); **(c)** Mg ($Z = 12$), Ar ($Z = 18$). **Self-Assessment Questions: 1.** (b), (c). **2.** (c). **3.** The second response. **4. (a)** F; **(b)** Ca; **(c)** N; **(d)** Na; **(e)** Fe. **5. (a)** ns; **(b)** np; **(c)** (n − 1)d; **(d)** (n − 2)f. **7. (a)** 4 valence, 2 core; **(b)** 8, 2; **(c)** 7, 2; **(d)** 3, 10; **(e)** 2, 10. **11.** (c), (e).

12. (d). Yes, odd number of electrons means at least one unpaired electron; No, electrons may be unpaired in degenerate orbitals in a subshell. **15.** (d). **16.** (b). **17.** (a). **19.** (c). **Problems: 21. (a)** Parallel spins in one $2p$ orbital; **(b)** Three electrons in one $2p$ orbital; **(c)** Non-parallel spins in three degenerate orbitals. **23. (a)** $3s$ subshell must fill before $3p$; **(b)** $4s$ subshell not occupied, $3d$ is occupied; **(c)** $2d$ subshell does not exist. **25. (a)** Pauli exclusion principle; **(b)** Pauli exclusion and aufbau; **(c)** Rules for quantum numbers n and l. **27. (a)** $1s^2 2s^2 2p^6 3s^2$; **(b)** $1s^2 2s^2 2p^5$; **(c)** $1s^2 2s^2 2p^4$; **(d)** $1s^2 2s^2$; **(e)** $1s^2 2s^2 2p^6 3s^2 3p^3$; **(f)** $1s^2 2s^2 2p^6 3s^2 3p^2$; **(g)** $1s^2 2s^2 2p^2$; **(h)** $1s^2 2s^2 2p^6 3s^2 3p^6 4s^1$; **(i)** $1s^2 2s^2 2p^6 3s^2 3p^6 3d^1 4s^2$. **29. (a)** [Xe] $6s^1$; **(b)** [Kr] $5s^2$; **(c)** [Ar] $3d^2 4s^2$; **(d)** [Kr] $4d^{10} 5s^2 5p^3$; **(e)** [Ar] $3d^{10} 4s^2 4p^5$; **(f)** [Xe] $5d^{10} 6s^2 6p^2$.

31. (a)
1s   2s   2p

(b)
1s   2s   2p

(c) [Ne]
3s   3p

(d) [Ar]
4s

(e) [Ne]
3s   3p

(f) [Ar]
4s   3d

33.
4f   5d   6s

as the fifth element in the d-block of the sixth period, Re has filled $4f$ and $6s$ subshells and a half-filled $5d$ subshell.

35. (a) [Ar];

(b) [Ar]
3d

(c) [Xe]
4f   5d   6s

(d) [Ne].

37. None; the configuration has $3d$ but no $4s$ electrons, and must therefore be a cation, but Co^{3+} would have a $3d^6$ configuration, Ni^{2+} would have $3d^8$, Cu^{2+} would have $3d^9$. **39.** 3+ (loss of $4p$ electrons) and 5+ (further loss of $4s$ electrons). **41. (a)** 2, 6A; **(b)** 3, 4A; **(c)** 3, 1A; **(d)** 2, 2A; **(e)** 2, 5A; **(f)** 3, 3A. **43. (a)** 5; **(b)** 32; **(c)** 5; **(d)** 2; **(e)** 10. **45. (a)** diamagnetic, valence $4s$ electrons paired; **(b)** paramagnetic, unpaired $2p$ electron;

(c) diamagnetic, [Ar] configuration; **(d)** paramagnetic, unpaired $3p$ electron; **(e)** diamagnetic, pseudo-noble gas configuration. **47.** Ca, Zn, Kr. **49. (a)** Al, lower Z_{eff}; **(b)** Cl^-, isoelectronic but with fewer protons; **(c)** Ba, higher period number (n); **(d)** K (higher n) is larger than Na, which is larger than Na^+ (cation from the atom). **51. (a)** B < Al < Mg < K; B has lowest n, Al has Z_{eff} greater than Mg, K has higher n and lower Z_{eff} than Mg; **(b)** Cl < P < Br < Br^-; Cl slightly higher Z_{eff} than P, Br has higher n than P, Br^- anion larger than Br atom. **53.** At the lower left; highest value of n, lowest Z_{eff}. **55. (a)** Yes, using general trends in size; **(b)** Yes, the species are isoelectronic and F^- has fewer protons, and so is larger. **57. (a)** Ba < Ca < Mg, I decreases with n; **(b)** Al < P < Cl, I increases with Z_{eff}; **(c)** Na < Fe < Cl < F < Ne; both F < Ne and Na < Fe due to Z_{eff}, and F > Cl due to size. **59.** $I_1 < I_2 < I_3 < I_4$ because each successive electron comes from an increasingly positive ion; at I_4 a core electron is removed. **61.** The halogens (7A), because each needs only one electron for a filled shell. **63.** Adding an electron to P produces a pair in one $3p$ orbital, and these electrons repel one another.

65.

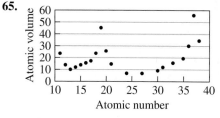

67. Atomic radius (metallic character increases with increase) and ionization energy (metallic character decreases with increase); P < Ge < Bi < Al < Ca < K < Rb. **69.** Tl < Ge < Se < S < Ne. **71. (a)** $Cl_2(g) + 2\ Br^-(aq) \longrightarrow 2\ Cl^-(aq) + Br_2(aq)$; **(b)** no reaction; **(c)** $Br_2(l) + 2\ I^-(aq) \longrightarrow 2\ Br^-(aq) + I_2(aq)$ **73. (a)** $N_2O_5(s) + H_2O(l) \longrightarrow 2\ HNO_3(aq)$; **(b)** $MgO(s) + 2\ CH_3COOH(aq) \longrightarrow Mg(CH_3COO)_2(aq) + H_2O(l)$; **(c)** $Li_2O(s) + H_2O(l) \longrightarrow 2\ LiOH\ (aq)$. **Additional Problems:**

75.

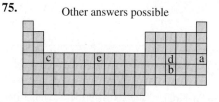

Other answers possible

78. $I_1(Cs) < I_1(B) < I_2(Sr) < I_2(In) < I_2(Xe) < I_3(Ca)$; Cs is larger than B; for Sr, In, Xe, I_2 increases from left to right; for Ca, I_3 involves removal of a core electron. **81. (a)** $1s^3 2s^3 2p^9 3s^3 3p^9 3d^7 4s^3$; **(b)** $1s^2 1p^6 2s^2 2p^6 2d^{10} 3s^2 3p^6 3d^{14} 4s^2$; No, in (a) Rb would be a transition metal and Na = $1s^3 2s^3 2p^5$, a late p-block element; in (b) Rb would be a transition metal and Na = $1s^2 1p^6 2s^2 2p^1$, an early p-block element. **82.** More protons in He attract the electrons more strongly; -5.23×10^3 kJ/mol for the (one) electron in the He^+ ion, which will have a different energy than that of the (two) electrons in a He atom. **85.** 1312 kJ/mol for (a) and (b), because the Balmer line involves the energy difference between E_∞ and E_2, and the Lyman line involves the energy difference between E_2 and E_1. Ionization energy involves E_∞ and E_1, the sum. **87.** $2\ Cl(g) + 2\ e^- \longrightarrow 2\ Cl^-(g)$, $\Delta H = 2 \times$ electron affinity = -698 kJ; $\Delta H_{overall} = -455$ kJ/mol Cl_2; exothermic. **Apply Your Knowledge: 92. (a)** where Sr is; In_2O_3; where it is now; **(b)** Dulong & Petit atomic mass is 232 u; which gives a formula of $UCl_{3.90}$ which

is about UCl_4; assuming U atomic mass of 240 u gives $UCl_{4.04}$ which is about UCl_4. **94. (a)** A = 2.5×10^{15}, b = 1.18; **(b)** A = 2.5×10^{15}, b = 1.16; they are essentially the same; **(c)** 6.85×10^{-9} cm.

Chapter 9

Exercises: 9.1A (a) :Är: **(b)** :Ḃr: **(c)** K·

9.1B (a) :Äs· **(b)** Rb· **(c)** :Ṫe·

9.2A Ba^{2+} + $2\left[:\ddot{I}:\right]^-$ **9.2B** $2\ Al^{3+}$ + $3\left[:\ddot{O}:\right]^{2-}$

9.3A $\Delta H_f^\circ = -617$ kJ/mol LiF(s). **9.3B** Lattice energy = -861 kJ/mol LiCl(s). **9.4A (a)** Ba < Ca < Be; **(b)** Ga < Ge < Se; **(c)** Te < S < Cl. **9.4B** Cl > S > B > Fe > Sc > Na > Rb. **9.5A** C—S < C—H < C—Cl < C—O < C—Mg. **9.5B (a)** Si—F; **(b)** S—Se.

9.6A H—N—N—H (with H atoms attached to each N) **9.6B** H—C—C—Cl: (with H atoms attached) **(d)**

9.7A :S̈=C=Ö: **9.7B** :Ö=N̈—C̈l:.

9.8A $\left[:\ddot{O}-\overset{\overset{\displaystyle :\ddot{O}:}{|}}{\underset{\underset{\displaystyle :\ddot{O}:}{|}}{Cl}}-\ddot{O}:\right]^-$ **9.8B** $\left[:\ddot{O}=N=\ddot{O}:\right]^+$

9.9A H—N̈—Ö—H (with H on N); the second structure has formal charges of +1 (O) and −1 (N), so the first structure with all formal charges of zero is better. **9.9B** H—C—C—Ö—C—H (with O double bond and H atoms attached).

9.10A $\left[:\ddot{O}-N=\ddot{O}:\right]^- \longleftrightarrow \left[:\ddot{O}-N-\ddot{O}:\right]^- \longleftrightarrow \left[:\ddot{O}=N-\ddot{O}:\right]^-$; the resonance hybrid involves equal contributions from the three structures. **9.10B (a)** Two resonance structures for HCO_3^-; **(b)** a single Lewis structure for HOClO; **(c)** a single Lewis structure for CN^-; **(d)** a single Lewis structure for C_2^{2-}; and **(e)** two resonance structures for $HCOO^-$.

9.11A :C̈l—P̈—C̈l: (with Cl above) **9.11B (a)** :F̈—C̈l—F̈: **(b)** :F̈—S̈—F̈: (with F atoms above and below)

9.12A (a) Incorrect. ClO_2 has 19 valence electrons, but the Lewis structure has 20. **(b)** Correct. **(c)** Incorrect. The structure has 26 electrons rather than the 24 available. **9.12B (1)** One structure limits the valence shell of the central S atom to eight, producing formal charges of +2 on the S atom and −1 on the two terminal O atoms bonded to it. The two central O atoms bonded to the S atom, and the two H atoms bonded to them, have formal charges of zero. **(2)** A set of resonance structures has a valence shell expansion of central S atom to 12 electrons and all formal charges = 0. The two terminal O atoms are doubly bonded to the S atom and the two

central O atoms are joined to the S and two H atoms by single bonds. (3) Another set of resonance structures has a valence shell expansion to 10 electrons, one sulfur-to-oxygen double bond, and formal charges of +1 and −1. **9.13A** 144 pm. **9.13B** 145 pm. **9.14A** $\Delta H = -113$ kJ. **9.14B** Bond energy, N—F = 278 kJ/mol.

Self-Assessment Questions: 3. (a) Na·   **(b)** $:\overset{\bullet}{\underset{\bullet\bullet}{O}}:$

(c) ·Si·   **(d)** $:\overset{\bullet\bullet}{\underset{\bullet\bullet}{Br}}·$ **(e)** ·Ca·   **(f)** $·\overset{\bullet\bullet}{As}·$

5. (a) Ca· + 2 $:\overset{\bullet\bullet}{\underset{\bullet\bullet}{Br}}:$ ⟶ Ca^{2+} + 2 $\left[:\overset{\bullet\bullet}{\underset{\bullet\bullet}{Br}}:\right]^-$

(b) Ba· + $·\overset{\bullet\bullet}{\underset{\bullet\bullet}{O}}:$ ⟶ Ba^{2+} + $\left[:\overset{\bullet\bullet}{\underset{\bullet\bullet}{O}}:\right]^{2-}$

(c) 2 ·Al· + 3 $·\overset{\bullet\bullet}{\underset{\bullet\bullet}{S}}:$ ⟶ 2 Al^{3+} + 3 $\left[:\overset{\bullet\bullet}{\underset{\bullet\bullet}{S}}:\right]^{2-}$

6. $:\overset{\bullet\bullet}{\underset{\bullet\bullet}{I}}—\overset{\bullet\bullet}{\underset{\bullet\bullet}{I}}:$; one bonding pair (dash), six unshared pairs (double dots). **7.** $H—\overset{\bullet\bullet}{\underset{\bullet\bullet}{F}}:$ with $\overset{\delta+}{H}\overset{\delta-}{F}$. **9. (a)** N; **(b)** Cl; **(c)** F; **(d)** O. **10. (a)** F; **(b)** Br; **(c)** Cl; **(d)** N. **11. (a)** ionic; **(b)** polar covalent; **(c)** ionic; **(d)** polar covalent; **(e)** ionic; **(f)** ionic; **(g)** nonpolar covalent; **(h)** nonpolar covalent; **(i)** polar covalent. **12. (a)** 1; **(b)** 4; **(c)** 2; **(d)** 1; **(e)** 3; **(f)** 1. **13.** (a); compact structure, low EN atom in center. **14.** (c).

15. (a) $:\overset{\bullet\bullet}{\underset{\bullet\bullet}{F}}—P\overset{\overset{\textstyle:\overset{\bullet\bullet}{F}:}{|}}{\underset{\underset{\textstyle:\overset{\bullet\bullet}{F}:}{|}}{\diagup}}\overset{\bullet\bullet}{\underset{\bullet\bullet}{F}}:$ **(c)** $:N=\overset{\bullet\bullet}{O}:$ **(e)** $:\overset{\bullet\bullet}{\underset{\bullet\bullet}{O}}—\overset{\bullet\bullet}{Br}—\overset{\bullet\bullet}{\underset{\bullet\bullet}{O}}:$

16. (a), (b), (d). **17.** (c). **18.** (b) < (a) < (d) < (c). **19.** (b). **20.** 759 kJ/mol. **21. (a)** alkyne; **(b)** alkene; **(c)** alkyne; **(d)** saturated hydrocarbon. **Problems: 23.** (a), (b), (c), (e).

25. (a) $Li^+\left[:\overset{\bullet\bullet}{\underset{\bullet\bullet}{Br}}:\right]^-$; **(b)** 2 Cs^+ + $\left[:\overset{\bullet\bullet}{\underset{\bullet\bullet}{S}}:\right]^{2-}$;

(c) 3 Na^+ + $\left[:\overset{\bullet\bullet}{\underset{\bullet\bullet}{N}}:\right]^{3-}$; **(d)** 2 Y^{3+} + 3 $\left[:\overset{\bullet\bullet}{\underset{\bullet\bullet}{S}}:\right]^{2-}$.

27. −420 kJ/mol; Appendix C = −436.7 kJ/mol. **29.** −703 kJ/mol. **31.** −1965 kJ/mol.

33. (a) $H—\overset{\overset{\textstyle H}{|}}{\underset{\underset{\textstyle H}{|}}{Si}}—H$ **(b)** $:\overset{\bullet\bullet}{\underset{\bullet\bullet}{Cl}}—\overset{\bullet}{\underset{\underset{\textstyle :\overset{\bullet\bullet}{Cl}:}{|}}{N}}—\overset{\bullet\bullet}{\underset{\bullet\bullet}{Cl}}:$

37. Structure (a) should display an ionic bond not a covalent bond, (b) should have covalent bonds not ionic bonds, (c) shows 17 electrons but only has 16 available, (d) has 16 available but only shows 14. **39. (a)** K < As < Br; **(b)** Cs < Ca < Be; **(c)** Pb < Sb < Cl.

41. (a) $\overset{\delta+\ \delta-}{H—H}$ < $\overset{\delta+\ \delta-}{H—C}$ < $\overset{\delta+\ \delta-}{H—N}$ < $\overset{\delta+\ \delta-}{H—O}$ < $\overset{\delta+\ \delta-}{H—F}$

(b) C—C ≈ $\overset{\delta+\ \delta-}{C—I}$ < $\overset{\delta+\ \delta-}{C—Br}$ < $\overset{\delta+\ \delta-}{C—Cl}$ < $\overset{\delta+\ \delta-}{C—F}$

43. (a) periodic table; **(b)** periodic table; **(c)** values of EN needed; **(d)** periodic table. **45.** From left to right: **(a)** −1, +1; **(b)** 0, 0, 0; **(c)** −1, +1, −1; **(d)** 0, 0, −1. **47.** From left to right: **(a)** −1, +1, 0; **(b)** 0, +1, −1; (b) is preferred.

49. $\left[H—\overset{\bullet\bullet}{\underset{\bullet\bullet}{O}}—\overset{\overset{\textstyle}{}}{\underset{\underset{\textstyle:\overset{\bullet\bullet}{O}:}{||}}{C}}—\overset{\bullet\bullet}{\underset{\bullet\bullet}{O}}:\right]^-$ ⟷ $\left[H—\overset{\bullet\bullet}{\underset{\bullet\bullet}{O}}—\overset{\overset{\textstyle}{}}{\underset{\underset{\textstyle:\overset{\bullet\bullet}{O}:}{|}}{C}}=\overset{\bullet\bullet}{O}:\right]^-$; the resonance structure is a hybrid of the two structures–the bonds to the terminal oxygen atoms are intermediate between single and double bonds.

51. (a) $H—\overset{\bullet\bullet}{\underset{\bullet\bullet}{O}}—N=\overset{\bullet\bullet}{O}:$ **(b)** Resonance structures are important only in nitric acid, which has two terminal oxygen atoms rather than the single one seen in nitrous acid.

53. (a) ·$\overset{\bullet}{N}=\overset{\bullet\bullet}{O}:$ $:\overset{\bullet\bullet}{\underset{\bullet\bullet}{F}}—\overset{\bullet}{\underset{\underset{\textstyle:\overset{\bullet\bullet}{F}:}{|}}{Cl}}—\overset{\bullet\bullet}{\underset{\bullet\bullet}{F}}:$ $:\overset{\bullet\bullet}{\underset{\bullet\bullet}{Cl}}—\overset{\underset{\textstyle:\overset{\bullet\bullet}{Cl}:}{|}}{B}—\overset{\bullet\bullet}{\underset{\bullet\bullet}{Cl}}:$ $:\overset{\bullet\bullet}{\underset{\bullet\bullet}{F}}—\overset{\overset{\textstyle:\overset{\bullet\bullet}{F}:}{|}}{\underset{\underset{\textstyle:\overset{\bullet\bullet}{F}:}{|}}{Se}}—\overset{\bullet\bullet}{\underset{\bullet\bullet}{F}}:$;

        (b)   **(c)**   **(d)**

NO is a free radical, the B in BCl_3 has an incomplete octet; ClF_3 and SeF_4 both have expanded valence shells.

55. (a) $:\overset{\bullet\bullet}{S}=\overset{\bullet}{\underset{\underset{\textstyle:\overset{\bullet\bullet}{\underset{\bullet\bullet}{F}}:}{|}}{S}}—\overset{\bullet\bullet}{\underset{\bullet\bullet}{F}}:$ **(b)** $\left[:\overset{\bullet\bullet}{\underset{\bullet\bullet}{I}}—\overset{\bullet\bullet}{\underset{\bullet\bullet}{I}}—\overset{\bullet\bullet}{\underset{\bullet\bullet}{I}}:\right]^-$

(c) $H—\overset{\bullet\bullet}{\underset{\bullet\bullet}{O}}—\overset{\underset{\underset{\textstyle:O:}{||}}{}}{C}—\overset{\bullet\bullet}{\underset{\bullet\bullet}{O}}—H$ **(d)** $[:C\equiv N:]^-$

(e) $\left[\overset{\overset{\textstyle:\overset{\bullet\bullet}{F}:\ :\overset{\bullet\bullet}{F}:}{}}{:\overset{\bullet\bullet}{\underset{\bullet\bullet}{F}}—\overset{\underset{\textstyle:\overset{\bullet\bullet}{F}:}{}}{S}—\overset{\bullet\bullet}{\underset{\bullet\bullet}{F}}:}\right]^-$ **(f)** $\left[:\overset{\bullet\bullet}{\underset{\bullet\bullet}{O}}—\overset{\overset{\textstyle:\overset{\bullet\bullet}{O}:}{}}{Br}—\overset{\bullet\bullet}{\underset{\bullet\bullet}{O}}:\right]^-$

57. (a) $H—\overset{\overset{\textstyle H}{|}}{\underset{\underset{\textstyle H}{|}}{C}}—\overset{\overset{\textstyle H}{|}}{\underset{\underset{\textstyle :\overset{\bullet\bullet}{\underset{\textstyle H}{O}}:}{|}}{C}}—\overset{\overset{\textstyle H}{|}}{\underset{\underset{\textstyle H}{|}}{C}}—H$ **(c)** $H—\overset{\overset{\textstyle H}{|}}{\underset{\underset{\textstyle H}{|}}{C}}—\overset{\bullet\bullet}{\underset{\bullet\bullet}{O}}—\overset{\overset{\textstyle H}{|}}{\underset{\underset{\textstyle H}{|}}{C}}—H$

(b) $H—\overset{\overset{\textstyle:O:}{||}}{C}—\overset{\bullet\bullet}{\underset{\bullet\bullet}{O}}—H$

59. In (a) the N is electron deficient, in (b) N cannot have an expanded shell, in (c) there is a negative formal charge on N and positive on O. Better structures are

(a) $\left[\overset{\overset{\textstyle:\overset{\bullet\bullet}{O}:}{|}}{\overset{\bullet\bullet}{\underset{\bullet\bullet}{O}}=N—\overset{\bullet\bullet}{\underset{\bullet\bullet}{O}}:}\right]^-$ **(b)** $H—\overset{\overset{\textstyle H}{|}}{\underset{\bullet}{N}}—C\equiv N:$

(c) $H—\overset{\bullet}{N}=C=\overset{\bullet\bullet}{O}:$

61. The empirical formula C_2H_5O has an odd number of electrons; several unsatisfactory structures can be drawn (below). Doubling the empirical formula to give $C_4H_{10}O_2$ gives many possible structures

$·\overset{\overset{\textstyle H\ \ H}{|\ \ \ |}}{\underset{\underset{\textstyle H\ \ H}{|\ \ \ |}}{C—C}}—\overset{\bullet\bullet}{\underset{\bullet\bullet}{O}}—H$ $H—\overset{\bullet\bullet}{\underset{\bullet\bullet}{O}}—\overset{\overset{\textstyle H}{|}}{\underset{\underset{\textstyle H}{|}}{C}}—\overset{\overset{\textstyle H}{|}}{\underset{\underset{\textstyle H}{|}}{C}}—\overset{\overset{\textstyle H}{|}}{\underset{\underset{\textstyle H}{|}}{C}}—\overset{\overset{\textstyle H}{|}}{\underset{\underset{\textstyle H}{|}}{C}}—\overset{\bullet\bullet}{\underset{\bullet\bullet}{O}}—H$

    Unsatisfactory   Satisfactory

63. (a) 233 pm; **(b)** 149 pm—likely to be high; very polar bond. **65.** HI, with the lowest ΔEN. **67.** $:\ddot{F}\!—\!\ddot{N}\!=\!\ddot{N}\!—\!\ddot{F}:$. **69.** -535 kJ. **71.** exothermic, breaking a CH bond and Cl_2 bond, forming a CCl bond and a HCl bond. **73.** 302 kJ/mol bonds. **75.** 416 kJ/mol (experimental) vs. 414 kJ/mol (table). **77. (a)** $H_2C\!=\!CHCH_3$; **(b)** $HC\!\equiv\!CCH_2CH_3$; **(c)** $H_2C\!=\!CHCH_2CH_2CH_3$; **(d)** $CH_3CH_2C\!\equiv\!CCH_2CH_3$ **79. (a)** $H_2C\!=\!CH_2 + H_2 \longrightarrow H_3CCH_3$; **(b)** $HC\!\equiv\!CH + 2H_2 \longrightarrow H_3CCH_3$. **81. (a)** -128 kJ; **(b)** -136.94 kJ. **83. (a)** $\dashv CH_2CH_2CH_2\ CH_2CH_2CH_2CH_2CH_2 \vdash$ **(b)** $\dashv CHClCH_2\!—\!CHClCH_2\!—\!CHClCH_2\!—\!CHClCH_2\vdash$ **(c)** $\dashv CH(CH_3)CH_2\!—\!CH(CH_3)CH_2\!—\!CH(CH_3)CH_2\!—\!CH(CH_3)CH_2\vdash$ **Additional Problems: 85.** In an alkane all of the carbon atoms have as many bonds as possible (4), so there are no lone pairs, and the skeletal structure completes the Lewis structure. Organic compounds containing O, N, S, Cl, etc., have lone-pair electrons that do not appear in the structural formula.

87.

$$
\begin{array}{ccc}
& \text{H} & \text{H} \\
& | & | \\
\text{H}—\text{C}—\ddot{\text{O}}—\text{C}—\text{H} \\
& | & | \\
& \text{H} & \text{H}
\end{array}
\qquad
\begin{array}{ccc}
& \text{H} & \text{H} \\
& | & | \\
\text{H}—\text{C}—\text{C}—\ddot{\text{O}}—\text{H} \\
& | & | \\
& \text{H} & \text{H}
\end{array}
$$

91. $H\!—\!\ddot{N}\!—\!N\!\equiv\!N: \longleftrightarrow H\!—\!\ddot{N}\!=\!N\!=\!\ddot{N}:$

93. $+111$ kJ/mol. **95.** -616 kJ/mol; Mg^+ does not have an octet of electrons. **96.** -65 kJ/mol. **98.** Both NO_2 and NO_2^- have resonance structures (two each) with a single and a double NO bond. **102.** 632 kJ/mol (calculated) vs. 590 kJ/mol (table). **Apply Your Knowledge: 104. (a)** 3500 cm; **(b)** 290 pages. **105.** $+97$ kJ/mol. **106. (a)** 106 kJ; **(b)** 0.91; **(c)** 2.96.

Chapter 10

Exercises: 10.1A (a) $SiCl_4$: VSEPR notation, AX_4: electron-group geometry and molecular geometry both tetrahedral. **(b)** $SbCl_5$: VSEPR notation, AX_5: electron-group geometry and molecular geometry both trigonal bipyramidal. **10.1B (a)** BF_4^-: VSEPR notation, AX_4: electron-group geometry and molecular geometry both tetrahedral (Lewis structure on page 362). **(b)** N_3^-: Lewis structure, $\left[\ddot{N}\!=\!N\!=\!\ddot{N}\right]^-$, VSEPR notation, AX_2; electron-group geometry and molecular geometry both linear. **10.2A** SF_4: VSEPR notation, AX_4E. Electron-group geometry is trigonal bipyramidal. In the seesaw structure (Table 10.1), two LP-BP repulsions at $90°$; and two at $120°$; in the pyramidal structure given, three LP-BP at $90°$ and one at $180°$. Because $90°$ LP-BP interactions are especially unfavorable, the seesaw structure is adopted. **10.2B** ClF_3: VSEPR notation AX_3E_2: Electron-group geometry is trigonal bipyramidal. In the T-shaped structure (Table 10.1), four LP-BP repulsions at $90°$; in the trigonal planar structure, six LP-BP repulsions at $90°$. The T-shaped structure is observed. **10.3A** For Lewis structure of $(CH_3)_2O$, see answer to Chapter 9, Problem 57(c). Each C atom bonded to four atoms in tetrahedral fashion (AX_4). The O atom (AX_2E_2) has tetrahedral electron-group geometry, and the $C\!—\!O\!—\!C$ linkage is angular or bent (bond angle $\approx 109°$). **10.3B** The three H atoms in the CH_3 group and the two H atoms in the CH_2 group are in a tetrahedral arrangement about the C atom. The $C\!—\!C\!—\!C$ bond angle is tetrahedral. The $—CHO$ end of the molecule is trigonal planar, with $H\!—\!C\!—\!O$, $H\!—\!C\!—\!C$, and $C\!—\!C\!—\!O$ bond angles of $120°$. **10.4A** Polar: SO_2, angular or bent (AX_2E); BrCl, linear but with a small ΔEN between atoms. Nonpolar: BF_3, symmetrical,

trigonal planar (AX_3); N_2, linear, no polarity in bond. **10.4B** SO_3, symmetrical, trigonal planar (AX_3)—nonpolar; SO_2Cl_2, symmetrical, tetrahedral (AX_4), but with different EN for terminal O and Cl atoms—polar; ClF_3 nonsymmetric, T-shaped (AX_3E_2)—polar; BrF_5, nonsymmetric, square pyramidal shape (AX_5E)—polar. **10.5A** NOF, $110°$; NO_2F, $118°$. LP-BP repulsions from lone-pair electrons on the N atom force O and F atoms closer together in NOF than in NO_2F, with no lone-pair electrons on N atom. **10.5B** COF_2. CS_2 is a symmetrical, linear molecule and SO_3, symmetrical trigonal planar. Neither has a resultant dipole moment. NO should have only a small dipole moment because of the EN difference between N and O is small. NO_2F has $\mu = 0.47$ D, as indicated in Example 10.5. COF_2 should have $\mu > 0.47$ D because its geometrical shape is like that of NOF_2, but the EN of C is less than that of N. **10.6A** $SiCl_4$ is a tetrahedral molecule (AX_4); hybridization scheme for Si: sp^3. **10.6B** I_3^-, a linear ion with trigonal bipyramidal electron group geometry; sp^3d hybridization for central I atom. **10.7A (a)** Tetrahedral molecular geometry around C atom and angular or bent around O atom. **(b)** Hybridization: sp^3 for both C and O. **(c)** $3\ \sigma\ C(sp^3)\!—\!H(1s)$; $\sigma\ C(sp^3)\!—\!O(sp^3)$; $\sigma\ O(sp^3)\!—\!H(1s)$. **10.7B (a)** $:N\!\equiv\!C\!—\!C\!\equiv\!N:$ Linear molecule, **(b)** Hybridization: sp for both C and N. **(c)** $\sigma\ C(sp)\!—\!C(sp)$; $2\ \sigma\ C(sp)\!—\!N(sp) + 4\pi C(2p)\!—\!N(2p)$. **10.8A** The third isomer is 1,1-dichloroethene, $Cl_2C\!=\!CH_2$; it is a polar molecule. **10.8B (a)** Planar $H_2C\!=\!CH_2$ is nonpolar, but replacing one H with F makes $H_2C\!=\!CHF$ polar. **(b)** Because of the very small ΔEN between C and H and the symmetrical shape of *trans*-2-butene (see page 415), the molecule is *nonpolar*. **(c)** Acetylene, $H\!—\!C\!\equiv\!C\!—\!H$, is a symmetrical, linear *nonpolar* molecule. **(d)** Substitute Cl atoms for the two H atoms at the double bond in *cis*-2-butene, and EN differences make the resulting nonsymmetric molecule *polar*. **10.9A** H_2^- should be somewhat stable; two electrons in bonding MO and one, in antibonding MO; bond order is $1/2$. **10.9B** The molecule He_2, has two electrons in a bonding MO and two in an antibonding MO. Its bond order is zero and the molecule is not stable. In the ion, He_2^+, there are two electrons in the bonding MO and one in the antibonding MO. The diatomic ion has a bond order of $\frac{1}{2}$ and should be stable. Presumably, He_2 ions with $2+$ or $3+$ charges would also be stable. **10.10A** No effect for Li_2 and Be_2 because the σ_{2p} and π_{2p} molecular orbitals are empty. No effect for N_2 because the σ_{2p} and π_{2p} molecular orbitals are filled. No effect for O_2, F_2 and Ne_2 because the σ_{2p} and π_{2p} molecular orbitals are filled, and the highest energy orbitals with electrons are the π_{2p}^* orbitals (σ_{2s}^* in Ne_2). In B_2, reversal of the σ_{2p} and π_{2p} orbitals would replace the two unpaired electrons in the π_{2p} orbitals by a pair of electrons in the σ_{2p}; the bond order would be unchanged, but the molecule would be diamagnetic instead of paramagnetic. In C_2, the bond order would be unchanged, but the species would be paramagnetic instead of diamagnetic. **10.10B** The 11 valence electrons are distributed in the MO diagram of either N_2 or O_2. In either case, bond order $= (8 - 3)/2 = 2.5$. **Self-Assessment Questions: 3.** (c). **4.** (a). **5.** sp^2, sp^2, sp^3. **6. (a)** $180°$; **(b)** $120°$; **(c)** $109.5°$. **7.** (b). **10.** (a). **14.** (c). **15.** Five σ, one π. **17.** (b). **Problems: 21. (a)** AX_2E_2; **(b)** AX_4; **(c)** AX_3E. **23. (a)** angular; **(b)** tetrahedral; **(c)** trigonal pyramidal. **25. (a)** linear; **(b)** linear; **(c)** tetrahedral; **(d)** trigonal planar. **27. (a)** angular; **(b)** trigonal pyramidal; **(c)** square planar; **(d)** trigonal pyramidal. **29. (a)** Tetrahedral around CH_3 carbon, C-C-N is linear; **(b)** trigonal planar around both nitrogen atoms; **(c)** tetrahedral

around CH_3 carbon, C-S-H is angular (109°). **31.** B has 3 electron groups, all bonded, while Cl has 5 electron groups, 3 bonded; AX_3 vs. AX_3E_2. **33.** In CH_4 all four bonds are identical; in $COCl_2$ there are two C—Cl single bonds and one C=O double bond. The difference in bonds is more likely to cause $COCl_2$ to deviate from the predicted angles. **35.** The angle of an angular molecule depends on the electron-group geometry. Tetrahedral EG geometry produces a bond angle of about 109° (in H_2O), and trigonal planar EG geometry produces a bond angle of about 120° (in SO_2). **37.** (a) polar; (b) polar; (c) polar; (d) nonpolar. **39.** Both have the same angular geometry, based on AX_2E_2, with similar bond angles. However, ΔEN for each O—H bond is greater than that for each O—F bond, so water should have the greater dipole moment.

41.

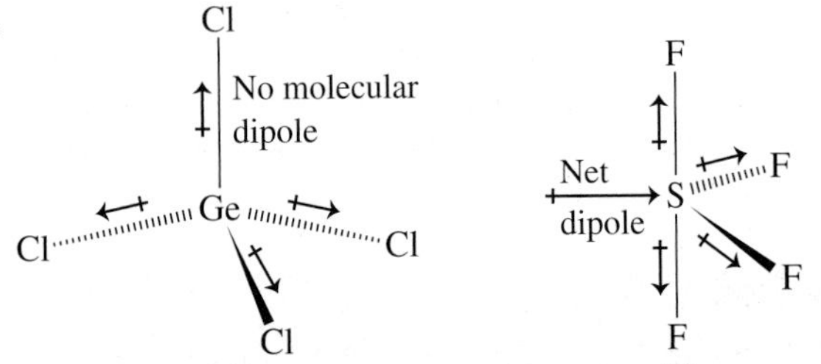

(a)   (b)

43. Li_2 is formed by overlap of two $2s$ orbitals, F_2 is formed by overlap of two $2p$ orbitals. The lobes of $2p$ orbitals can overlap more than the spherical $2s$ orbitals, so the F_2 bond should be stronger. **45.** (a) sp^2; (b) sp; (c) sp^3; (d) sp^3d^2. **47.** (a) N is sp^2, C is sp; (b) CH_3 carbon is sp^3, CN carbon is sp; (c) two CH_3 carbon atoms are sp^3, the two inner carbon atoms are sp; (d) Both C and N are sp^3. **49.** (a) Trigonal planar around N, H—O—N bond is about 109°; (b) Octahedral; (c) Tetrahedral around CH_3 carbon, and H—C≡C—C is linear;

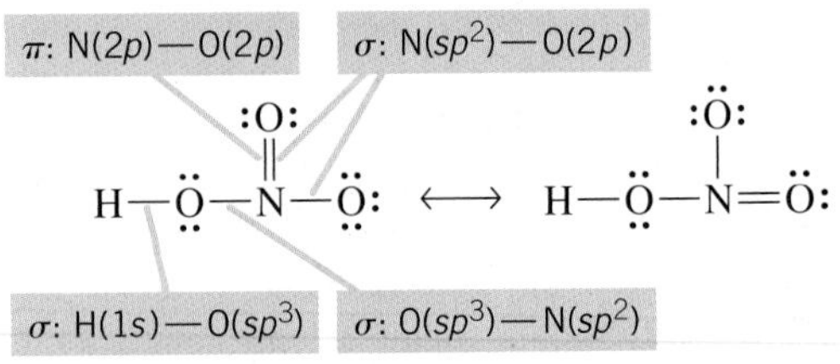

(a)

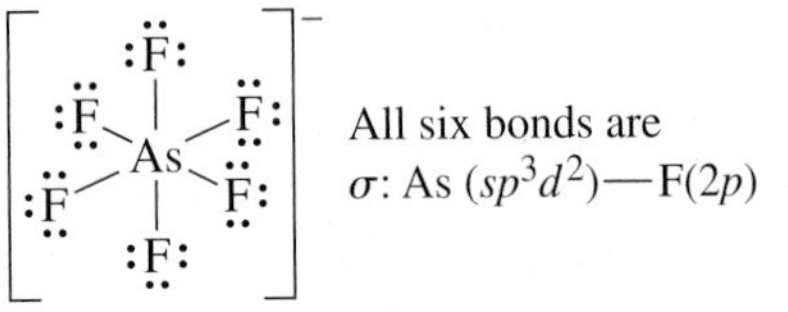

(b)

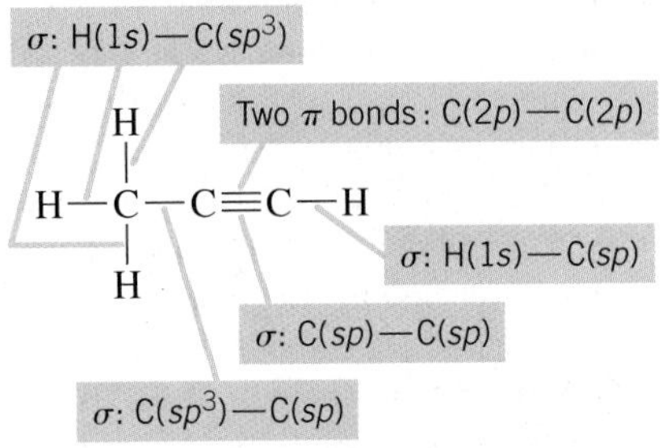

(c)

51. No. There are different numbers of electrons in the two species. Adding two electrons adds an additional lone pair on the central

atom, changing the geometry. **53.** There are four resonance structures, so the two π bonds are delocalized over all four C—O bonds, making the four C—O bonds all the same length and strength. Both carbon atoms are sp^2 hybridized. Selecting one resonance structure for the bonding scheme:

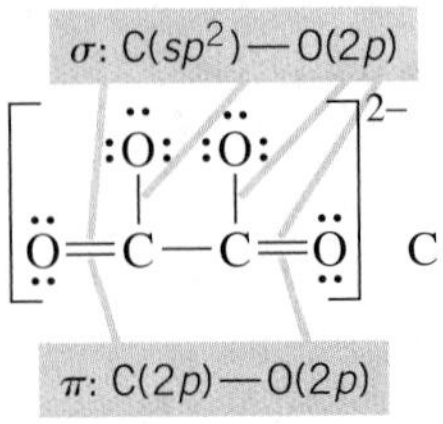

55.

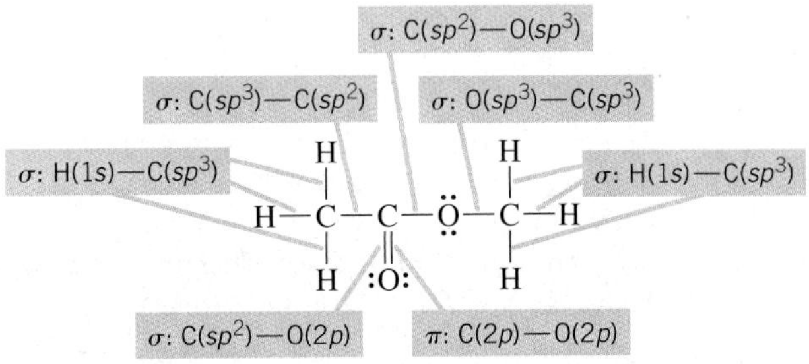

(a)

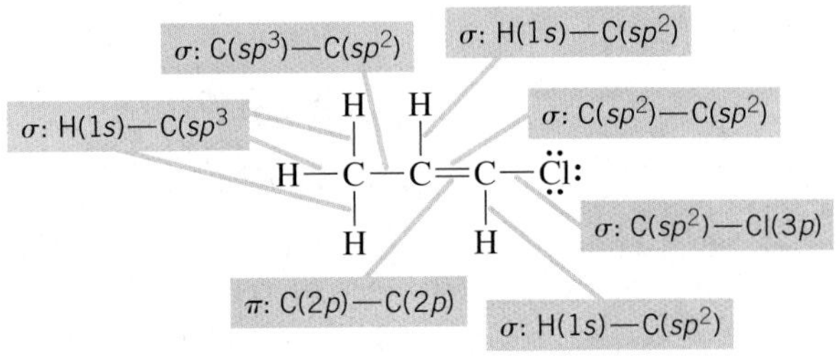

(b)

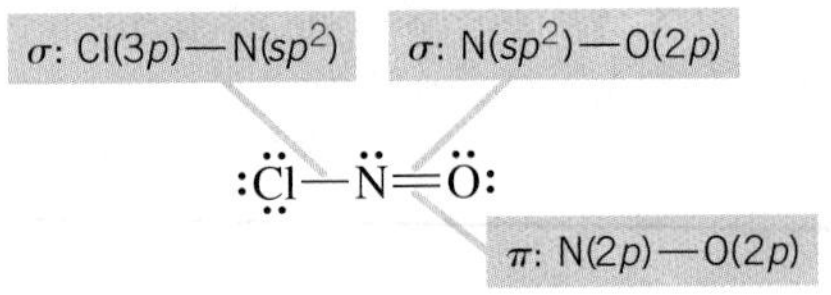

(c)

57. (a), (c). Each side of the double bond must have two different groups or atoms attached. **59.** No, there are two hydrogen atoms on the one side of the double bond. Yes, substituting a chlorine atom as described gives two different groups attached to each side of the double bond. **61.** F_2^+ has greater bond energy because it has fewer antibonding electrons. **63.** Bond order from Lewis structure is 4, and it is 2 from molecular orbital theory. Lewis bonding theory does not account for antibonding electrons. **65.** (a) CN^- (isoelectronic with N_2) has the stronger bond, with a bond order of 3; the bond order of CN^+ (isoelectronic with C_2) is 2; (b) All electrons are paired, so neither is paramagnetic. **67.** O_2^{2-} has a bond order of 1 and is diamagnetic; O_2^- has a bond order of 1.5 and is paramagnetic.

69.

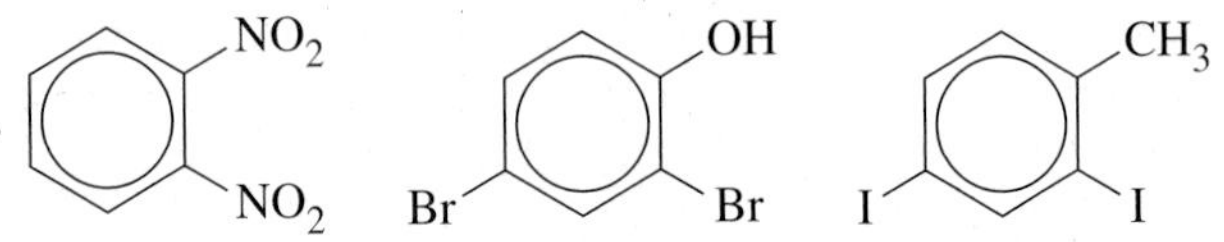

(a)   (b)   (c)

71. **(a)** 2,5-diiodoaniline; **(b)** 1,2,4-trifluorobenzene; **(c)** 3,4,5-tribromotoluene.

73.

$$\ddot{N}=\ddot{N} \qquad \ddot{N}=N$$

(a)

(b) All C and N atoms are sp^2 hybridized; **(c)** All bond angles (H—C—C, C—C—C, C—C—N, C—N=N) are about 120°, though the C—N—N bond angles are slightly less due to LP-BP repulsion. **Additional Problems: 75.** Not necessarily; bond dipoles may cancel depending on the shape of the molecule. **77.** The electronegativity of fluorine is greater than that of oxygen, resulting in a small shift in electron density toward the fluorine atom. **79.** **(a)** seesaw (AX_4E); **(b)** square pyramidal (AX_5E). **82.** ethane < methylamine < methanol < fluoromethane; the C and H atoms have little effect on dipole moment since their electronegativities are about the same. Ethane is nonpolar, and polarity of the other three is dictated by increasing electronegativity from N to O to F. **84.** Linear molecule;

σ: C(sp)—O(2p)

σ: C(sp)—C(sp)

$$\ddot{O}=C=C=C=\ddot{O}$$

π: C(2p)—C(2p)

π: C(2p)—O(2p)

87. The central carbon atom is sp hybridized, and the other two carbon atoms are sp^2 hybridized. **90.** 6.09 D, 17.6% ionic character. **92.** We can draw a right triangle for which the hypotenuse is the magnitude of the O-H dipole, the adjacent side is half the net dipole moment (there are two O—H bonds and both contribute to the net dipole), and the included angle ϕ is half the bond angle of 104.5°, and solve for the adjacent side

(a) $\cos\phi = \dfrac{a}{h}$

$$\cos\frac{104.5°}{2} = \frac{(1.84\ D/2)}{h}$$

$$h = 1.50\ D$$

(b) Substitute S for O:

$$\cos\phi = \frac{a}{h}$$

$$\cos\phi = \frac{(0.93\ D/2)}{0.67\ D} = 0.69$$

$$\phi = 46° \quad 2\phi = \text{bond angle} = 92°$$

Apply Your Knowledge: 95. (a)

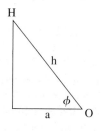 Cyclopentane

(b) Propene

(d) No. **96.** **(a)** $Li_2 \longrightarrow Li_2^+ + e^-$; $Be_2 \longrightarrow Be_2^+ + e^-$; $B_2 \longrightarrow B_2^+ + e^-$; $C_2 \longrightarrow C_2^+ + e^-$; $N_2 \longrightarrow N_2^+ + e^-$; $O_2 \longrightarrow O_2^+ + e^-$; $F_2 \longrightarrow F_2^+ + e^-$; $Ne_2 \longrightarrow Ne_2^+ + e^-$; **(b)** Yes, Ne_2^+ has more bonding electrons than antibonding electrons; BO = 0.5; **(c)** An energy diagram similar to Figure 10.25 for F_2 shows that the electron comes from the π^* antibonding orbital of F_2, which is at a higher energy level than the p orbital in F; **(d)** The electron comes from the π^* antibonding orbital of O_2, which is at a higher energy level than the p orbital in O, so O_2 has a lower first ionization energy than O; **(e)** The electron comes from the σ *bonding* orbital of N_2, which is at a *lower* energy level than the p orbital in N, so N_2 has a *higher* first ionization energy than N; **(f)** The first ionization energy increases as $O_2 < O < N < N_2$, so N_2 has a much higher ionization energy than does O_2 and is thereby better suited for plasma spectrometry than is O_2. Helium, having an even higher ionization energy because of its smaller size and the fact that it is a noble gas, is also a good candidate.

Chapter 11

Exercises: 11.1A $\Delta H_{vapn} = 34.0\ kJ/mol\ C_6H_6$. **11.1B** $\Delta H_{total} = 92.0\ kJ$. **11.2A** CCl_4. A relatively low ΔH_{vapn} and a relatively high molar mass lead to the smallest heat requirement per kilogram. **11.2B** Approximately 97 g. **11.3A** 4.00×10^2 mmHg. **11.3B** 5.33×10^{-3} g H_2O. **11.4A** Room temperature is far above T_c of methane; the methane is present as a gas of relatively low mass, and a pressure gauge is better used to measure its amount. **11.4B** What is observed depends on the initial volume of liquid. To see the disappearance of the meniscus, both liquid and vapor must be present as T_c is reached. Because the densities of the liquid and vapor are equal at T_c, the required mass of substance for the critical phenomena to be observed is the product of the volume of the tube and the critical density. Thus, for example, if the initial mass of liquid is less than this calculated mass, all of the liquid will have vaporized before T_c is reached. **11.5A** If only gas were present, the pressure would be 10 atm—far in excess of the vapor pressure of H_2O at 30.0 °C. Most of the H_2O condenses to liquid. (It cannot all be liquid, because the liquid volume is only about 20 mL and the system volume is 2.61 L.) The final condition is a point on the vapor pressure curve at 30.0 °C. **11.5B** The very cold, solid dry ice (-78.5°C) absorbs heat from the much warmer water. The $CO_2(s)$ sublimes, producing a large volume of cold $CO_2(g)$, which escapes as large bubbles. Water vapor in contact with the cold $CO_2(g)$ condenses to droplets of $H_2O(l)$ ("fog"). This fog of $H_2O(l)$ is carried off by the invisible $CO_2(g)$ and down the walls of the beaker. The $CO_2(g)$ is more dense than air. **11.6A** IBr and BrCl have about the same polarity, but IBr has a greater molar mass. IBr has stronger intermolecular forces and is the solid. BrCl is the gas. **11.6B (a)** The molar masses are comparable, but aniline is somewhat polar and toluene is nonpolar. Toluene has the lower boiling point. **(b)** The lower boiling point is that of nonpolar trans-1,2-dichloroethene; the cis isomer is polar. **(c)** The symmetrical placement of Cl atoms in para-dichlorobenzene makes it nonpolar and gives it a lower boiling point; the ortho isomer is polar. **11.7A** The boiling point of butane should be about 36 °C below the boiling point of pentane, that is, about 0 °C. **11.7B** $C_{11}H_{24}$ to about $C_{15}H_{32}$. **11.8A** Hydrogen bonding is an important intermolecular force in NH_3, C_6H_5OH, CH_3COOH, H_2O_2. **11.8B** (d) < (b) < (a) < (c). Isobutane (d) and carbon disulfide (b) are both nonpolar molecules with intermolecular forces limited to dispersion forces.

For these two the order is (d) < (b). Isopropanol (a) and ethylene glycol (c) are both polar and both undergo hydrogen bonding. This suggests that both should have boiling points above that of carbon disulfide, despite their somewhat smaller molar masses. Ethylene glycol has two —OH groups whereas isopropanol has only one —OH group, so we should expect the ethylene glycol to have the highest boiling point. The actual boiling points are (d) isobutane, $-11.7°C$, (b) carbon disulfide, 46.6 °C, (a) 2-propanol, 82.4 °C, (c) ethylene glycol, 197.3 °C. **11.9A** $CsBr < KI < KCl < MgF_2$. **11.9B** MgF_2 is water insoluble. We expect that the interionic forces of attraction in MgF_2 should be considerably greater than in the other three compounds, because of the smaller size and higher charge of Mg^{2+} compared to K^+ and Cs^+, and because of the smaller size of F^- relative to Cl^-, Br^-, and I^-. **11.10A** 286.6 pm. **11.10B** $V = (286.6)^3$ pm$^3 = 2.354 \times 10^{-23}$ cm^3; number Fe atoms/unit cell $= 2$. **11.11A** $N_A = 6.05 \times 10^{23}$. **11.11B** void fraction $= [(2r)^3 - 4/3 \times \pi r^3]/(2r^3) = [(8 - 4\pi/3)/8] = 0.4764$; % voids $= 0.4764 \times 100\% = 47.64\%$. **Self-Assessment Questions: 3.** (a). **5.** (d). **7.** (a). **8.** (d). **10.** (c). **13.** (b). **14.** (c). **16.** (b). **Problems: 17.** 1280 kJ. **19.** 199 kJ **21.** 328 g. **23.** When holding your hand in the oven, you are feeling the slow transfer of heat from air to your hand; the air remains in the gas phase. Above the boiling water, steam condenses to liquid water on the skin, with evolution of the very large heat of condensation onto the skin. **25.** (a) ~40 mmHg; **(b)** ~62 °C. **27.** 1.57 L. **29.** 214 mmHg. **31.** The sample cannot be liquid only; 1.82 g $H_2O(l)$ occupies less than 2 mL volume and the container holds 2.55 L. It cannot be vapor only because the $H_2O(g)$ would exert a pressure (749 mmHg) far in excess of the vapor pressure at 30.0 °C. It is a mixture of liquid and gas. **33.** Heat goes into vaporizing water—the water boils at a constant temperature. Because its ignition temperature is greater than 100 °C, the paper does not burn. **35.** A gas cannot be liquefied above T_c, regardless of the pressure applied. A gas can be either liquefied or solidified by a sufficient lowering of the temperature, regardless of its pressure. A gas can always be liquefied by an appropriate combination of pressure and temperature changes. **37.** 7.8 kJ. **39.** 8.4 °C. **41.** (c).

43. (a)

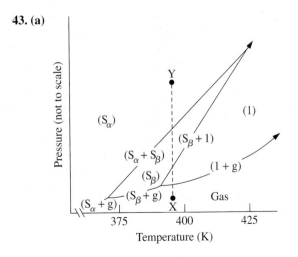

(b) The 2 triple points at the bottom have S_α, S_β and gas present. The triple point at the top has S_α, S_β and liquid present. **(c)** The sulfur gas becomes liquid, then monoclinic sulfur and finally rhombic sulfur as pressure increases.

45.

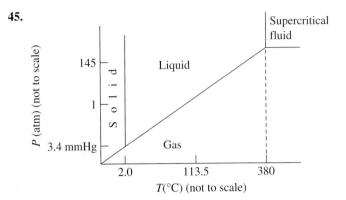

47.

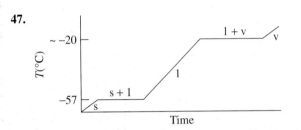

The solid CO_2 becomes a liquid slightly above -56.7 °C (the triple point is 5.1 atm and -56.7 °C). The liquid then converts to a gas at a temperature that is probably below room temperature (the critical point is at 72.9 atm and 304.2 K). **49.** Both are nonpolar, CF_4 has fewer electrons and weaker dispersion forces than PBr_5, so CF_4 is lower boiling. **51.** The substances have similar molar mass, but 1-pentanol molecules can form intermolecular hydrogen bonds and 3,3-dimethylpentane molecules cannot. Further, 3,3-dimethylpentane molecules are more compact, have less intermolecular contact and therefore weaker dispersion forces than 1-pentanol. 1-Pentanol has the higher melting point. **53.** BF_3 is the gas. It has small, non-polar molecules; NI_3 is a solid; it has large molecules, large dispersion forces, and is slightly polar; PCl_3 is a liquid with an intermediate molecular mass; CH_3COOH is a liquid–similar mass to BF_3, but it undergoes hydrogen bonding. **55.** $CH_4 < CH_3CH_3 < NH_3 < H_2O$; first two are nonpolar and CH_4 molecules are smaller and thus lower boiling. Both NH_3 and H_2O have hydrogen bonding, but oxygen is more electronegative than nitrogen, so water is higher boiling. **57.** $CH_3OH < C_6H_5OH < NaOH < LiOH$; first two undergo hydrogen bonding, with methanol molecules being smaller (weaker dispersion forces). The other two are ionic with strong interionic forces. The melting point of LiOH is higher than that of NaOH due to the high charge density of the Li^+ ion. **59.** 1-Octanol undergoes hydrogen bonding while octane has only dispersion forces, so 1-octanol has stronger intermolecular forces and a higher surface tension. **61.** Water "wets" glass because the adhesive forces between water molecules and glass exceed the cohesive forces in liquid water (glass surface is polar due to lone pairs on the oxygen atoms in SiO_2). The reverse is true with substances that water does not wet, for example, Teflon® or wax paper. Additives can make water "wetter" if they either reduce cohesive forces or increase adhesive forces (wetting agents usually do the latter). **63. (a)** The larger unit is a unit cell, but not the smaller one. The larger cell can be shifted left, right, up, and down by one unit cell (four symbols) and will coincide with the original pattern. In contrast, when a second small square is stacked on top of the first, the two sides of the interface show different symbols. **(b)** There are 3 hearts, 3 diamonds, and

3 clubs in a unit cell. **65.** (a) 501 pm; (b) 1.26×10^{-22} cm^3; (c) 3.62 g/cm^3. **Additional Problems: 67.** (a) 404 pm; (b) 6.4×10^{23} formula unit/mol. **69.** For Ti^{4+}, $8 \times (1/8) + 1 = 2$; for O^{2-}, $4 \times (1/2) + 2 = 4$. The formula Ti$_2$O$_4$ reduces to TiO$_2$. Ti^{4+} coordination number is 6; that of O^{2-} is 3. No, because there are twice as many O^{2-} as Ti^{4+}, the coordination number of Ti^{4+} should be twice that of O^{2-}. **71.** 1.2×10^{-3}. **73.** (a) 0.213 kJ; (b) 28.7 L; (c) only gas. **76.** (a) Hydrogen bonding is most important. There are also dipole-dipole and dispersion forces. (b) Dipole-dipole forces are most important. There are also dispersion forces. (c) Ionic bonding is the most important. There are also dispersion forces. **78.** The density of H$_2$O(l) rises from its value at the melting point to a maximum at 3.98 °C. Above this temperature its density falls with temperature as with most substances. Thus, for every density in the temperature range from 0 °C to 3.98 °C, there is another temperature in a range extending a bit above 3.98 °C at which the same density is observed. **80.** (a) 56.9 mmHg; (b) −33.36 °C; (c) 108.9 atm. **81.** The Group 4A hydrides show the expected trend: dispersion forces and boiling points increase with increasing molar mass. For the Group 5A, 6A, and 7A hydrides of periods 3, 4, and 5, boiling points also increase with molar mass. Three anomalies are seen for NH$_3$, H$_2$O, HF. The unusually high boiling points for NH$_3$, H$_2$O, and HF result from hydrogen bonding in these liquids. **83.** 4.0×10^2 mmHg. **85.** 27 °C. **90.** 3.516 g/mL. **94.** 1.41×10^3 g. **98.** (a) 599 mmHg; (b) 93 °C. **100.** 9.5 mmHg at −101.65 °C. **Apply Your Knowledge: 102.** 0.021 J/m^2. **104.** 22 times.

Chapter 12

Exercises: 12.1A 17.8% glucose, by mass; only the mass ratio of glucose to solution enters into the calculation, not the formula of glucose. **12.1B** 6.98% sucrose, by mass. **12.2A** 34.8% toluene, by volume. **12.2B** (a) 34.4% toluene, by mass; (b) $d = 0.874$ g/mL. **12.3A** (a) 0.1 ppb; (b) 100 ppt. **12.3B** 69.9 ppm Na$^+$. **12.4A** 0.317 m C$_6$H$_{12}$O$_6$ **12.4B** 3.56 m. **12.5A** 0.418 mL CH$_3$CH$_2$OH. **12.5B** 253 mL H$_2$O. **12.6A** (a) 2.53 m CH$_3$OH; (b) 1.86 mol% CO(NH$_2$)$_2$. **12.6B** (a) 8.50% CH$_3$OH, by mass; (b) 2.61 M CH$_3$OH; (c) 4.97 mol% CH$_3$OH. **12.7A** (b). The solutions are all rather dilute and have densities of approximately 1.0 g/mL. The mole percents of CH$_3$CH$_2$OH are not large, and we expect the largest to be in the solution having the greatest quantity of CH$_3$CH$_2$OH per liter or kilogram of solution. Solution (a) has 0.5 mol CH$_3$CH$_2$OH per liter; (b) has slightly more than 1 mol CH$_3$CH$_2$OH per kilogram of solution; (c) has slightly less than 0.5 mol CH$_3$CH$_2$OH per kilogram of solution; (d) has somewhat less than 1 mol CH$_3$CH$_2$OH per liter. **12.7B** (d). Compare 1.0 kg of each of the four solutions, keeping in mind that 1000 mL H$_2$O ≈ 1000 g H$_2$O ≈ 55 mol H$_2$O. All the solutions are rather dilute and have H$_2$O as the preponderant component. Solution (a) has about 0.01 mol Na$^+$, whereas solution (b) has about 0.02 mol Na$^+$ (for dilute aqueous solutions molality and molarity are very nearly the same). Solution (c) has 10 g NaNO$_3$ per kg solution, making it about 10/85 m NaNO$_3$ and containing slightly more than 0.10 mol Na$^+$. In solution (d), for every 1000 g H$_2$O present there would be about 55 mol H$_2$O and about 0.55 mol Na$^+$. Solution (d) has the greatest concentration of Na$^+$, whether expressed on a mol or ppm basis. **12.8A** Because of the similarity of its structure to that of benzene, nitrobenzene is more soluble in benzene

than in water. **12.8B** The molecular models: (a) acetic acid, (b) 1-hexanol, (c) hexane, (d) butanoic acid; the order of increasing solubility in water: c < b < d < a. **12.9A** 5.5×10^{-2} mg CO$_2$/100 g H$_2$O. **12.9B** 2.1×10^2 mg. **12.10A** 93.9 mmHg. **12.10B** 8.03 g C$_{10}$H$_8$ **12.11A** Partial and total pressures: $P_{\text{benz}} = 51.4$ mmHg; $P_{\text{tol}} = 13.0$ mmHg; $P_{\text{total}} = 64.4$ mmHg. **12.11B** Mole fractions: 0.230 for benzene and 0.770 for toluene. **12.12A** The solution with equal masses has a greater mole fraction of the more volatile benzene (78 g/mol) than of toluene (92 g/mol); it produces vapor with the greater x_{benzene}. **12.12B** $P_{\text{benzene}} = 73.2$ mmHg, $P_{\text{toluene}} = 6.53$ mmHg. **12.13A** No. Water vapor passes from the more dilute (B) to the more concentrated solution (A) until the two solutions have the same concentration. Then, there is no further net transfer of water between the solutions. **12.13B** There are several possibilities as to what might happen. If the second liquid is miscible with water in all proportions and is also volatile (e.g., methanol, ethanol), vapor escaping from each pure liquid will dissolve into the other liquid; given enough time the two solutions would attain the same mole fraction composition. If the second liquid is miscible with water in all proportions but is essentially nonvolatile (e.g., glycerol), only water vapor will be transferred, and in time all the water would be transferred from beaker A to B. If the second liquid is immiscible with water or nearly so, very little, if any, substance will be transferred through the vapor phase. **12.14A** −2.46 °C. **12.14B** 18 g sucrose. **12.15A** C$_6$H$_6$O$_4$. **12.15B** No. The greatest freezing point depression would occur if the solid were pure glucose (the substance with the smaller molar mass). The molality of the glucose solution would be 0.555 m; the freezing point of the solution would be −1.03 °C. The freezing point of the solution could not be as low as −1.25 °C. **12.16A** 6.86×10^4 g/mol. **12.16B** 9.33 mm H$_2$O. **12.17A** Lowest fp: 0.0080 M HCl; highest fp: 0.010 m C$_6$H$_{12}$O$_6$. **12.17B** They are the results expected for the expression: $\Delta T_f = -i\, K_f\, m$, with $i = 1$ for HCl dissolved in C$_6$H$_6$, and $i = 2$, in H$_2$O. **Self-Assessment Questions: 2.** Molarity involves a volume, which varies with T. Molality does not involve a volume and is therefore independent of T. Mole fraction and mass percent do not involve a volume and are therefore independent of T. Volume percent varies with T. **5.** (c), (e); (Each involves two nonpolar substances.). **6.** (c). **7.** (a). **9.** (b). **10.** Usually not. If only the solvent is volatile, the vapor cannot have the same composition as the solution because the vapor is pure solvent. If all components are volatile, the vapor and solution compositions are likely to differ because of differences in the volatilities of the components. **13.** (a) **17.** No. Osmotic flow is of *solvent* molecules from a *dilute* solution, which has a higher vapor pressure, into a more concentrated one. The concentration of solvent is greater in the dilute solution, so the situation is similar to gases diffusing from higher to lower pressure. **20.** (a) 0.1 M NaHCO$_3$; (b) 1 M NaCl; (c) 1 M CaCl$_2$; (d) 3 M glucose. **Problems: 21.** Mix 112 g NaNO$_3$ and 2.19 kg water. **23.** (a) 17.5% by mass; (b) 17.9% by mass; (c) 42.7% by mass. **25.** a) 9.28% by volume; (b) 11.7% by volume; (c) 29.3% by volume. **27.** 12 g. **29.** (a) 5 ppb trichloroethylene; (b) 2.5 ppm KI; (c) 3.9×10^{-4} M SO$_4$$^{2-}$. **31.** ppt < ppb < ppm < 1 mg/dL < 1%. **33.** 5.38 m. **35.** 0.598 M; 0.624 m. **37.** 10.7 mol. **39.** (a) 0.0434; (b) 0.0192. **41.** The solution with the greatest amount of solute per unit mass of solvent—(b) in this case—has the greatest mole fraction of solute. Solution (a) has exactly 1 mol solute per 1000 g H$_2$O. (b) has slightly more than 1 mol solute in 950 g H$_2$O. Solution (c) has about 0.3 mol solute per 900 g H$_2$O.

43. (a) $CHCl_3$, insoluble; **(b)** C_6H_5COOH, slightly soluble; **(c)** $CH_3CHOHCH_2OH$, highly soluble. **45.** Unsaturated. **47. (a)** 21 g water; **(b)** about 44 °C. **49.** Yes. Allow solvent to evaporate. When the solution becomes saturated, crystallization begins to occur. **51. (a)** 1.38×10^{-3} M; **(b)** 7.2 atm. **53. (a)** Partial pressures: pentane, 88.2 mmHg; hexane, 96.8 mmHg; **(b)** Vapor composition: $x_{pent} = 0.477$; $x_{hex} = 0.523$. **55.** 17.4 mmHg. **57. (a)** -0.47 °C; **(b)** 3.70 °C. **59.** 1.28 m. **61.** $K_f = 4.27$ °C m^{-1}. **63.** $C_6H_3O_6N_3$. **65.** The salt solution has the higher osmotic pressure. As it shrinks into a pickle, the cucumber loses water to NaCl(aq). **67.** 9.94 atm. The solution is hypertonic. **69.** To the right (from A to B). **71. (a)** $i = 1$; $T_f = -0.19$ °C; **(b)** $i \approx 3$; $T_f \approx -0.57$ °C; **(c)** i is slightly greater than 1; T_f is slightly less than -0.19 °C; **(d)** $i \approx 2$; $T_f \approx -0.38$ °C. Answer (a) is most precise, since glucose has i of precisely 1. The others are electrolytes and dissociate; i depends on concentration and is less precisely known. **73.** 3; CaO will form $Ca(OH)_2$ in solution, which is partially soluble in water. **75.** Order of decreasing freezing points: (b) > (a) > (e)>(c) > (d). **77.** 2.4×10^2 g NaCl. **79.** The charge on the particles is negative. Al^{3+} is the most highly charged cation of the three, making $AlCl_3$(aq) the most effective coagulant. **Additional Problems: 81. (a)** 15.1% by volume; **(b)** 12.2% by mass; **(c)** 11.9% mass/volume; **(d)** 7.25 mole %. **84.** 27.0% H_2O by mass. **86.** 486 g sucrose. **88.** 11.7% nitrobenzene by mass; 95% nitrobenzene by mass; They will not have the same boiling points, because the constants are different and the initial boiling points are different. **91. (a)** 0.20 m $(CH_3)_2CO$ has the highest total vapor pressure because x_{water} is as great as in the other solutions and $(CH_3)_2CO$ is volatile; **(b)** NaCl(satd. aq) has the highest concentration of solute particles and the lowest freezing point. **(c)** The vapor pressure of NaCl(satd. aq) remains constant because its concentration does not change as H_2O(g) is lost. The concentrations and vapor pressures of the other solutions do change. **93. (a)** $x_{benzene} = 0.256$; $x_{toluene} = 0.744$; **(b)** $x_{benzene} = 0.455$; $x_{toluene} = 0.545$. **96.** At equilibrium, each solution has a mass fraction of urea of 0.230 and a mole fraction of 0.0822. **100.** 48.6% by mass sucrose, 51.3% by mass glucose. **102.** The liquid is $CaCl_2$(aq). Water from the air condenses on the solid and dissolves it to form saturated $CaCl_2$(aq). A solid will not act this way if the vapor pressure of the saturated solution exceeds the partial pressure of water in the atmosphere. **104. (a)** 14 divisions; **(b)** total volume = 1 cm^3; total surface area = 9.82×10^4 cm^2; The smaller the particle, the larger the surface area to volume ratio. **Apply Your Knowledge: 105.** 9×10^9 Zn atoms **107. (a)** The weight molarity only depends on mass, so it is not dependent on temperature. **(b)** 0.3473 $M_{(wt)}$; 32.40% by mass sulfuric acid **109.** 0.36 L

Chapter 13

Exercises: 13.1A (a) 0.0259 M min^{-1}; **(b)** 8.63×10^{-4} M s^{-1}. **13.1B (a)** 1.05×10^{-5} M s^{-1}; **(b)** 3.15×10^{-5} M s^{-1}. **13.2A (a)** 1.11×10^{-3} M s^{-1}; **(b)** $[H_2O_2]_{310s} = 0.287$ M. **13.2B** about 270 s. **13.3A** 0.0912 M s^{-1}. **13.3B** 3/2 order. **13.4A (a)** $t = 255$ min; **(b)** $[NH_2NO_2] = 0.0139$ M. **13.4B** 3.46×10^{-4} M min^{-1}. **13.5A (a)** $t \approx 480$ s; **(b)** 0.150 g N_2O_5. **13.5B** $P_{tot} = 1850$ mmHg. **13.6A** Slightly above 50 mmHg, perhaps 52 mmHg. **13.6B** 640 mmHg. **13.7A** $k = 0.023$ M^{-1} s^{-1}. **13.7B** The half-life doubles for each succeeding half-life period—55 s for the first $t_{1/2}$, 110 s for the

second $t_{1/2}$, 220 s for the third $t_{1/2}$, and so on. To two significant figures (corresponding to "55 s"), $[A] = 0.20$ M at $t = (55 + 110) = 1.7 \times 10^2$ s, and $[A] = 0.10$ M at $t = (55 + 110 + 220)$ s $= 3.9 \times 10^2$ s. **13.8A** $Rate_2 = 3.2 \times 10^{-3}$ M s^{-1}, $rate_1 = 8.0 \times 10^{-4}$ M s^{-1}, $rate_2/rate_1 = 2^n = 4$, and $n = 2$. For straight-line graphs, plot $1/[A]$ versus t with data from the graphs given. **13.8B** The $[A]_t$ vs. t graph for the first-order reaction starts at $t = 0$ and 2.00 M, above the graph for the second-order reaction having $[A]_0 = 1.00$ M. After 693 s, $[A]_t$ in the first-order reaction has fallen to 1.00 M, and at 2×693 s $= 1386$ s, to $[A]_t = 0.50$ M. For the second-order graph. $[A]_t = 0.50$ M at 1000 s. At 1386 s, the first-order graph still lies above the second-order graph. After $t = 3 \times 693$ s $= 2079$ s, $[A]_t$ in the first-order reaction has fallen to 0.25 M. In the second-order reaction, $[A]_t$ does not reach 0.25 M until $t = 1000$ s $+ 2000$ s $= 3000$ s. The first-order graph falls below the second-order graph some time between 1386 s and 2079 s. The two graphs share one point in common. The time at this intersection of the two graphs can be estimated by trial and error. Substitute different times into the integrated rate equations for the two reaction orders to obtain values of $[A]_t$. Find the time (about 1700 s) at which the $[A]_t$ values of the two graphs are the same. **13.9A** $T = 288$ K (15 °C). **13.9B** $E_a = 163$ kJ/mol. **13.10A** First step: (slow, rate-determining), $NOCl \longrightarrow NO + Cl$; second step (fast), $NOCl + Cl \longrightarrow NO + Cl_2$. Rate of reaction $= k[NOCl]$. **13.10B** The mechanism consists of a fast, reversible first

step: $NO + O_2 \underset{k_{-1}}{\overset{k_1}{\rightleftharpoons}} NO_3$ followed by a slow, rate-determining

step: $NO_3 + NO \overset{k_2}{\longrightarrow} 2 NO_2$. Overall reaction is $2 NO + O_2 \longrightarrow 2 NO_2$. Assume rapid equilibrium in the first step to establish the rate law: rate $= k[NO]^2[O_2]$. **Self-Assessment Questions: 3.** The *average* rate is the rate (change in concentration of reactant or product/change in time) over a finite time period. The *instantaneous* rate is the slope of a tangent line to a plot of concentration of reactant or product vs. time, corresponding to the rate at a specific instant. The *initial* rate is the instantaneous rate at time $= 0$. The average rate approaches the instantaneous rate as the change in time interval decreases. The initial rate is an instantaneous rate, but the reverse is not necessarily true. **6.** (c). **7.** (d). **8.** (a). **9.** (b). **12.** (c). **15.** (c). **Problems: 23.** 0.222 M. **25. (a)** 3.1×10^{-4} M/s; **(b)** 9.3×10^{-4} M/s; **(c)** rate of reaction of A $= 3.1 \times 10^{-4}$ M/s. **27.** It is not zero order. **29. (a)** False, this would be true only for a second-order reaction, which has not been established. **(b)** True, A is consumed twice as fast as B is produced. **31. (a)** First order in $S_2O_8^{2-}$, first order in I^-, second order overall; **(b)** 6.1×10^{-3} M^{-1} s^{-1}; **(c)** 5.8×10^{-5} M/s. **33.** Zero order–rate is independent of concentration. **35.** 7.5×10^{-3} M/s. **37. (a)** 0.325 M; **(b)** 84 min. **39. (a)** 2.2×10^{-5} s^{-1}; **(b)** 569 mmHg; **(c)** 22.1 h. **41.** 1.4×10^{14} molecules/L. **43. (a)** 0.096 M; **(b)** 25 min. **45.** For a zero-order reaction, half-life is directly proportional to concentration, so the half-life is longest initially, when the concentration is highest. For a second-order reaction the half-life is inversely proportional to concentration, so the half-life is shortest initially. **47.** Rate $= k[A]^2$; $k = 9.77 \times 10^{-4}$ M^{-1} s^{-1}. **49.** 84 ms. **51.** The calculation involves the frequency of *effective* collisions, which depends on orientation of colliding molecules and is very difficult to determine accurately. **53.** No. Looking at Figure 13.14 for an endothermic process, it is obvious that the activation energy must be greater

than the enthalpy change, since the energy barrier must be at least equal to the energy (enthalpy change) required to reach the products. Looking at Figure 13.13 for an exothermic reaction, it is clear that the activation energy "hill" can be virtually zero, but cannot be defined in relation to the enthalpy change. **55.** 91 kJ/mol. **57. (a)** 7.14×10^{-7} min^{-1}; **(b)** 649 K. **59.** A unimolecular step may occur when a molecule acquires enough energy from collisions with other molecules to dissociate. **61. (a)** A + 2 B $\longrightarrow$ C + D; **(b)** Rate = k[A][B]. **63.** 2 NO$_2$ $\longrightarrow$ NO$_3$ + NO (slow); NO$_3$ + CO $\longrightarrow$ NO$_2$ + CO$_2$ (fast). **65.** The rate law derived from this slow equilibrium/fast step mechanism is Rate = $k_2 (k_1/k_{-1})$([NO]^2[Cl$_2$]/[NOCl]), which does not match the observed rate law. **67.** rate = k_2 [Hg][Tl^{3+}] k_1/k_{-1} = [Hg][Hg^{2+}]/[Hg$_2^{2+}$] or [Hg] = (k_1/k_{-1})[Hg$_2^{2+}$]/[Hg^{2+}] so rate = $k_2 (k_1/k_{-1})$[Hg$_2^{2+}$][Tl^{3+}]/[Hg^{2+}] **69.** Since I$^-$ is a catalyst, [I$^-$] remains unchanged, and the rate law simplifies to rate = k' [H$_2$O$_2$], where k' depends on the initial [I$^-$]. **71.** An inhibitor may block the active site of the enzyme or it may react with the enzyme to change the shape of the active site. **73.** Both require that reactions occur at active sites. The kinetics of each type of reaction is governed by the availability of these sites. **Additional Problems: 75.** 2.6×10^{-3} M/s. **76.** 0 s, 35.3 mL; 60 s, 27.9 mL; 120 s, 22.6 mL; 180 s, 18.3 mL; 240 s, 14.9 mL; 300 s, 11.9 mL; 360 s, 9.44 mL; 420 s, 7.52 mL; 480 s, 6.08 mL; 540 s, 4.80 mL; 600 s, 3.76 mL. **79. (a)** 1.06 atm; **(b)** 2.12 atm; **(c)** 2.46 atm. **82.** 35.9 min. **85. (a)** 1, 1, −1, 1; **(b)** rate = k[OCl$^-$][I$^-$]/[OH$^-$], k = 60 s^{-1}; **(c)** second step is rate-determining; rate = k_2[I$^-$][HOCl]; the first step is a fast reversible reaction where [HOCl] = (k_1/k_{-1})[OCl$^-$][H$_2$O]/[OH$^-$]; note that [H$_2$O] is constant, so rate = k_{total}[OCl$^-$][I$^-$]/[OH$^-$]; **(d)** No; OH$^-$ is formed in the first step and consumed in the third step, so it is an intermediate. **86.** O$_3$ $\rightleftharpoons$ O + O$_2$ (fast); O + O$_3$ $\longrightarrow$ 2 O$_2$ (slow). **89.** Second order, k = 0.066 g^{-1} h^{-1}. **90.** 173.2 h. **Apply Your Knowledge: 92.** As the solution becomes more acidic, NH$_2$ groups become NH$_3^+$ groups and COOH groups retain their protons. The groups that are necessary for the reaction to occur are NH$_2$ and COO$^-$. **94. (a)** 51.3 kJ/mol; **(b)** 126 chirps/min; **(c)** 71 °F versus 68 °F, so it is close, but not exact. **95. (a)** Rate = $(\Delta[I_3^-]/\Delta t)$ and $\Delta[I_3^-]$ = the constant amount of S$_2$O$_3^{2-}$ initially added, so an increase in Δt means a decrease in rate; **(b)** first, first, second; **(c)** 3.7×10^{-5} M/s; **(d)** 0.0062 M^{-1} s^{-1}; **(e)** S$_2$O$_3^{2-}$ + 3 I$^-$ $\longrightarrow$ 2 SO$_4^{2-}$ + 3 I$_3^-$, rate = k[S$_2$O$_3^{2-}$][I$^-$]; The first step should be slow because the species colliding are negatively charged (repulsive forces). Step 2 (fast) involves unimolecular decomposition of an unstable, highly charged species. Step 3 (fast) involves collision of species that have opposite charges (attractive forces). Steps 2 and 3 should be largely independent of orientation (2 is unimolecular, and 3 involves monatomic ions).

Chapter 14

Exercises: 14.1A No. [COCl]$_2$ = K_c[CO]^2, but there are many possible values for [CO] = [Cl$_2$], and thus for [COCl$_2$]. **14.1B** [SO$_2$] and [SO$_3$] do not have unique values, but the following ratios do: [SO$_3$]^2/[SO$_2$]^2, [SO$_2$]^2/[SO$_3$]^2, [SO$_3$]/[SO$_2$], [SO$_2$]/[SO$_3$]. If [O$_2$] = 1.00 M, [SO$_3$] = 10.0[SO$_2$]. **14.2A** K_c = 2.5×10^{-3}. **14.2B** K_c = 6.64×10^{78}. **14.3A** K_P = 4.6×10^3. **14.3B** K_c = 3.0×10^{60}. **14.4A** K_P = $P_{CO}P_{H_2}/P_{H_2O}$. **14.4B** K_c = [H$_2$]^4/[H$_2$O]^4; K_P = $P_{H_2}^4/P_{H_2O}^4$. **14.5A** Reaction probably does not go to completion.

K_c = 1.2×10^3 is not a particularly large value. **14.5B** K_P = 10.0. For the two smallest values of K_P, the pressure of H$_2$O could be significant, but not those of CO and H$_2$. For the two largest values, the reaction goes essentially to completion. For the value K_P = 10.0, all the gas partial pressures are most likely to be significant. **14.6A** Net reaction goes to the right. **14.6B** Compared to initial values, at equilibrium: P_{H_2S} increases, P_{HI} decreases, amount of I$_2$(s) increases, amount of S(s) decreases. **14.7A** Compared to the original equilibrium, there will be **(a)** more NH$_3$ and H$_2$, less N$_2$ (equilibrium shifts to the right); **(b)** less NH$_3$ and N$_2$, more H$_2$ (to the left); **(c)** less NH$_3$, N$_2$, and H$_2$ (to the right). **14.7B** Addition of CH$_3$COOH(aq) represents adding both a reactant and a product. If the acetic acid is nearly pure, equilibrium should shift to the right—formation of more products. If the acetic acid is very dilute, equilibrium should shift to the left—formation of more reactants. For intermediate concentrations, the result depends on the exact concentration of the CH$_3$COOH(aq). **14.8A** There is no change because no. mol gaseous products = no. mol gaseous reactants. **14.8B** Both changes shift equilibrium to the left. The amounts of NO and O$_2$ increase as well as the amount of NO$_2$. **14.9A** At low temperatures, because the forward reaction is exothermic. **14.9B** Using data from the problem and Appendix C, we find that the formation of N$_2$O$_3$(g) is an exothermic reaction. Thus, its formation is favored at the lower temperature—the freezing point of water. **14.10A (a)** More CO, H$_2$O, and H$_2$ and less CO$_2$ (equilibrium shifts to the left). **(b)** Prediction not possible. Added H$_2$ favors the reverse reaction; added H$_2$O, the forward reaction. **(c)** Both changes shift equilibrium to the right. There will be more CO$_2$ and H$_2$, and less CO. Whether the amount of H$_2$O increases or decreases depends on the original equilibrium condition. **14.10B** The reaction is CH$_4$(g) + 2 H$_2$O(g) $\rightleftharpoons$ CO$_2$(g) + 4 H$_2$(g). Formation of H$_2$(g) is favored at (a) higher temperatures (the reaction is endothermic); and (b) lower pressures (the number of moles of products is greater than the number of moles of reactants). **14.11A** K_c = 25. **14.11B** K_P = 0.429. **14.12A** 0.0828 mol H$_2$, and P_{H_2} = 0.815 atm. **14.12B** If the equilibrium concentrations are written with the unit mol/L, the unit L will cancel if it appears as many times in the numerator as in the denominator. This occurs only if the same total number of moles of gas appears on each side of the reaction equation. **14.13A** 0.085 mol COCl$_2$. **14.13B** x_{NO} = 0.018. **14.14A** 1.76×10^{-2} mol H$_2$, 7.6×10^{-3} mol I$_2$, 0.085 mol HI. **14.14B** 0.0128 mol H$_2$; 0.0128 mol I$_2$; 0.094 mol HI. **14.15A** P_{CO} = P_{Cl_2} = 0.19 atm; P_{COCl_2} = 0.81 atm; P_{total} = 1.19 atm. **14.15B** P_{total} = 0.658 atm. **Self-Assessment Questions: 2.** (d). **3.** (b). **4.** (c). **5.** (d). **7.** (d), (f). **9.** (c). **10. (a)** K_p = $P_{CO_2}P_{H_2}/P_{CO}P_{H_2O}$; **(b)** K_p = $P_{NH_3}^2/P_{H_2}^3 P_{N_2}$; **(c)** K_p = $P_{NH_3}P_{H_2S}$. **11. (a)** K_p = $P_{NO}/P_{N_2}^{1/2}P_{O_2}^{1/2}$; **(b)** K_p = $P_{NH_3}/P_{H_2}^{3/2}P_{N_2}^{1/2}$; **(c)** K_p = $P_{NOCl}/P_{N_2}^{1/2}P_{O_2}^{1/2}P_{Cl_2}^{1/2}$. **12. (a)** K_c = [CO$_2$]^2[N$_2$]/[CO]^2[NO]^2; **(b)** K_c = [H$_2$O]^6[NO]^4/[O$_2$]^5[NH$_3$]^4; **(c)** K_c = [H$_2$O][CO$_2$]. **14.** (a), (c). **17.** (b). **18.** (d). **Problems: 19. (a)** 1.2×10^{-3}; **(b)** 4.79×10^{-3}; **(c)** 1.23×10^3. **21.** 3.59×10^{-3}. **23.** 6.35. **25.** 1.13×10^{-10}. **27.** 3.0×10^{66}. **29.** No, it depends on the value of K_c; if K_c < 1, then K_c' > K_c. **31.** 2.3×10^3. **33.** 0.0126 M. **35.** 0.134 atm. **37.** 9. **39.** (b), (e). **41.** (c). **43. (a)** increase; **(b)** none; **(c)** increase; **(d)** decrease; **(e)** none; **(f)** increase; **(g)** none. **45.** All of the reactions are endothermic, because energy must be expended to break stable bonds. Dissociation is favored by increasing the temperature. **47.** (b), (d) greater. **49.** Q_c = 8.88 < K_c, shifts to the right.

51. $Q_P = 97.4 < K_p$, shifts to the right. **53.** $K_p = 1.80 \times 10^{-6}$; $K_p = 6.78 \times 10^{-5}$. **55.** $NH_2COONH_4(s) \rightleftharpoons 2\,NH_3(g) + CO_2(g)$; $K_p = 6.7 \times 10^{-4}$. **57.** 1.49×10^{-3}. **59.** 12.5 g. **61.** 0.0436 mol. **63.** 48.2 g. **65.** $PCl_3 = Cl_2 = 0.082$ mol; $PCl_5 = 0.028$ mol. **67.** 46%. **69. (a)** 0.0271 atm; **(b)** 0.179 atm. **71.** 3.65 atm. **73.** 1 atm. **Additional Problems: 75. (a)** shift to the left; **(b)** left; **(c)** right; **(c)** right; **(d)** right; **(e)** right; **(f)** right. **77. (a)** Left; **(b)** 0.164 mol H_2; 0.164 mol CO_2; 0.036 mol CO; 0.136 mol H_2O. **79.** 5.60. **80.** 3.9; high P and low T. **82.** 8.32×10^{-3} atm. **85.** 78.3%. **88.** 0.92 mol; increase. **Apply Your Knowledge: 90.** 3.9. **92.** 0.0149.

Chapter 15

Exercises: 15.1A (a) base: NH_3, conjugate acid, NH_4^+; acid: HCO_3^-, conjugate base, CO_3^{2-}; **(b)** acid: H_3PO_4, conjugate base, $H_2PO_4^-$; base: H_2O, conjugate acid, H_3O^+. **15.1B** Amphiprotic species in 15.1A: HCO_3^- acts as an acid in (a), and as a base in $HCO_3^- + H_3O^+ \rightleftharpoons H_2CO_3 + H_2O$; H_2O acts as a base in (b), and as an acid in $H_2O + NH_3 \rightleftharpoons OH^- + NH_4^+$. As we will discover later in the chapter, $H_2PO_4^-$ is also amphoteric. In reaction (b) it acts as a base in the reverse reaction, but it is an acid in the reaction $H_2PO_4^- + NH_3 \rightleftharpoons NH_4^+ + HPO_4^{2-}$. **15.2A (a)** H_2Te. The Te atom is larger than S, and the H—Te bonds are weaker. **(b)** $CH_3CH_2CH_2CHBrCOOH$. Although Cl is somewhat more electronegative than Br, it is located much farther from the —COOH group, thereby weakening its electron-withdrawing ability. **15.2B** a < d < b < c. The Cl and Br atoms are electron-withdrawing. The effect is weakest with Br opposite the —COOH group, but stronger with Cl adjacent to the group, and stronger still with two Cl atoms adjacent. **15.3A** d < a < c < b. Aromatic amines are much weaker than aliphatic ones. Cl atoms weaken amine bases because they are electron-withdrawing, and more so with more Cl atoms closer to the —NH_2 group. **15.3B (a)** —$CH_2CH_2CH_3$, no electron-withdrawing groups; **(b)** The $C_6H_3Br_2$ group produces an aromatic amine with two electron-withdrawing bromine atoms near the —NH_2 group. **15.4A** pH = 1.331. **15.4B** pH = 12.624. **15.5A** Basic. OH^- from the NaOH raises $[OH^-]$ above the 1.0×10^{-7} M found in water. **15.5B** The pure water has a pH = 7.00. The pH of each solution is also very close to 7.00, one slightly acidic and the other slightly basic. Because equal amounts of excess H_3O^+ and OH^- are present, complete neutralization occurs and the final mixture is pH neutral. **15.6A** pH = 2.74. **15.6B** pH = 4.52. **15.7A** pH = 2.20. **15.7B** The two relationships that must be simultaneously satisfied are $x^2/M = 1.4 \times 10^{-3}$ and $x/M = 0.050$. The minimum molarity is 0.56 M. **15.8A** pH = 11.96. **15.8B** pH = 9.35. **15.9A** $K_a = 6.2 \times 10^{-5}$; $pK_a = 4.21$. **15.9B** $[NH_3] = 6.56$ M. **15.10A** Methylamine. A larger K_b and higher molarity make $[OH^-]$ and pH of CH_3NH_2 greater than those of NH_3(aq). **15.10B** 0.0010 M HCl(aq). In 0.0010 M HCl(aq), a strong acid, $[H_3O^+] = 0.0010$ M, and pH = 3. In 0.10 M CH_3COOH(aq), a weak acid, $[H_3O^+] = \sqrt{K_a \times 0.10} = \sqrt{1.8 \times 10^{-6}} > 1.0 \times 10^{-3}$ M, and pH < 3. **15.11A** pH = 1.48. **15.11B** The molarity of H_3PO_4 in the cola is between about 4.4×10^{-3} M and 6.4×10^{-3} M. The corresponding pH values are 2.52 and 2.39, respectively, and they correlate well the pH ≈ 2.5 stated in the problem. **15.12A** Assume complete ionization: pH = 2.77. **15.12B (b)**—complete ionization in the first step and limited in the second. Response (a) has no ionization in the second step and (c), nearly complete ionization. In (d), $[H_3O^+]$ cannot exceed 0.040 M.

15.13A (a) Neutral—salt of strong acid and strong base; **(b)** basic—salt of weak acid and strong base. **15.13B** HCl(aq) < NH_4Br(aq) < NaCl(aq) < KNO_2(aq) < NaOH(aq). **15.14A** pH = 5.27. **15.14B** Neutralization produces 0.0873 M CH_3COONa; pH = 8.84. **15.15A** 0.29 M CH_3COONa(aq). **15.15B** 0.10 M NH_4CN. HCN is a much weaker acid than HNO_2 —the weaker the acid, the stronger the anion as a base. **15.16A** pH = 8.89. **15.16B** H_3O^+ is the common ion; $[H_3O^+] = 0.10$ M, $[CH_3COO^-] = 1.8 \times 10^{-5}$ M. **15.17A** pH = 9.10. **15.17B** 0.020 mol NaOH. **15.18A** $[CH_3COOH] = 0.43$ M. **15.18B** 3.2 g NH_4Cl. **15.19A** The pH ≈ 5. This eliminates (b)—a basic buffer—and (c)—strongly acidic. Add a small quantity of acid or base. If there is a color change, the solution is (a); if not, it is the buffer (d). **15.19B** 0.0200 mol NaOH converts all the CH_3COOH to CH_3COO^-. The pH is approximately 9, about the pH at which thymol blue changes color. **15.20A (a)** pH = 2.90; **(b)** pH = 3.90; **(c)** pH = 10.10; **(d)** pH = 11.10. **15.20B** pH = 13.02. **15.21A (a)** pH = 4.96; **(b)** pH = 11.10. **15.21B (a)** pH = 13.22; **(b)** pH = 9.07; **(c)** pH = 5.04; **(d)** pH = 4.74. The titration curve starts at a high pH; has a pH > 7 at the equivalence point; and progresses through a buffer region in a weakly acidic solution beyond the equivalence point. **15.22A** $K_b \approx 1 \times 10^{-5}$; pH at the equiv. point: ≈5 (estimated from graph); 4.7 (calculated, assuming $K_b = 1 \times 10^{-5}$). **15.22B** This would not be a satisfactory titration. The change in slope of the titration curve would be too gradual. For instance, the initial pH would be about 11; the pH at the equivalence point would be about 7; and the final pH, about 4. **Self-Assessment Questions: 1.** Arrhenius: $HI(aq) \longrightarrow H^+ + I^-$; Brønsted-Lowry: $HI(aq) + H_2O \longrightarrow H_3O^+ + I^-$. **3.** (c). **4.** (b), (d). **5. (a)** $HClO_2 + H_2O \rightleftharpoons H_3O^+ + ClO_2^-$;

$$K_a = \frac{[H_3O^+][ClO_2^-]}{[HClO_2]}$$

(b) $CH_3CH_2COOH + H_2O \rightleftharpoons H_3O^+ + CH_3CH_2COO^-$;

$$K_a = \frac{[H_3O^+][CH_3CH_2COO^-]}{[CH_3CH_2COOH]};$$

(c) $HCN + H_2O \rightleftharpoons H_3O^+ + CN^-$; $K_a = \frac{[H_3O^+][CN^-]}{[HCN]}$;

(d) $C_6H_5OH + H_2O \rightleftharpoons H_3O^+ + C_6H_5O^-$

$$K_a = \frac{[H_3O^+][C_6H_5O^-]}{[C_6H_5OH]}.$$

6. (d). **9.** (a). **12.** (d). **13.** $K_a \times K_b = 10^{-14}$ **16.** Equivalence point: the point at which acid and base are in the exact stoichiometric proportions. Endpoint: the point at which the indicator changes color. The indicator ordinarily is selected so that the endpoint occurs at the equivalence point. **17.** (b). **18.** The pH is highest initially (basic solution), it is lowest when the last of the acid has been added. **19. (a)** above 7; **(b)** below 7; **(c)** at 7. **Problems: 21. (a)** $HIO_4 + NH_3 \rightleftharpoons IO_4^- + NH_4^+$; **(b)** $H_2O + NH_2OH \rightleftharpoons OH^- + NH_2OH_2^+$; **(c)** $H_3BO_3 + NH_2^- \rightleftharpoons H_2BO_3^- + NH_3$.

23. (a) $\underset{\text{acid 1}}{HOClO_2} + \underset{\text{base 2}}{H_2O} \rightleftharpoons \underset{\text{acid 2}}{H_3O^+} + \underset{\text{base 1}}{ClO_2^-}$;

(b) $\underset{\text{acid 1}}{HSeO_4^-} + \underset{\text{base 2}}{NH_3} \rightleftharpoons \underset{\text{acid 2}}{NH_4^+} + \underset{\text{base 1}}{SeO_4^{2-}}$;

(c) $HCO_3^- + OH^- \rightleftharpoons CO_3^{2-} + H_2O$
   acid 1   base 2   base 1   acid 2 ;

(d) $C_5H_5NH^+ + H_2O \rightleftharpoons C_5H_5N + H_3O^+$
   acid 1   base 2   base 1   acid 2 .

25. $H_2PO_4^- + H_2O \rightleftharpoons H_3PO_4 + OH^-$; $H_2PO_4^- + H_2O \rightleftharpoons HPO_4^{2-} + H_3O^+$. **27.** HCl is the strongest acid, so the reaction with HCl will proceed farthest to the right. **29.** CH_3COOH is a stronger acid than is H_2O, and so aniline accepts a proton more readily from CH_3COOH than from H_2O. **31. (a)** H_2Se is stronger, because Se is larger than S and H_2Se has a lower bond dissociation energy; **(b)** $HClO_3$ is stronger because Cl is more electronegative than I and withdraws more electron density from the H—O bond; **(c)** H_3AsO_4 is stronger because As is larger than P, and because the H^+ is being removed from a neutral molecule, not a 1– ion; **(d)** HBr is stronger because of the greater electronegativity difference; **(e)** HN_3 is stronger because three electronegative nitrogen atoms withdraw electron density more than does one N; **(f)** HNO_3 is stronger because the H^+ is being removed from a neutral molecule and not from a 1– ion. **33.** See p. 623; **(a)** About 4×10^{-3}; less than that of 2,2-dichloropropanoic acid but more than that of 2-chloropropanoic acid; **(b)** About 5×10^{-5}; less than that of 3-chloropropanoic acid but slightly more than that of 1-pentanoic acid or acetic acid; the Cl atom is some distance from the —COOH group and has little effect. **35.** phenol < (d) < (a) < (b) < (c). **37. (a)** 0.0012 M; **(b)** 5.5×10^{-10} M; **(c)** 4.5×10^{-5} M; **(d)** 0.00011 M. **39. (a)** 1.41; **(b)** 12.85; **(c)** 0.19; **(d)** 10.70. **41. (a)** 1.14; **(b)** −0.24; **(c)** 1.05; **(d)** 12.95. **43.** Dilute 10.0 mL of 0.250 M NaOH to 5.00 L. **45.** The $Ba(OH)_2$; its $[OH^-] = 2 \times 0.0062 = 0.0124$ M, pOH = 1.91, pH = 12.09. **47. (a)** 2.48; **(b)** 1.95. **49.** 1.6 M. **51.** 3.6×10^{-4}. **53.** 1.08. **55.** 0.016 M. **57.** 0.0045 M H_2SO_4. **59. (a)** pH = 0.70; **(b)** 5.3×10^{-5} M. **61. (a)** 1.53; **(b)** 0.12 M; **(c)** 0.029 M; **(d)** 6.3×10^{-8} M; **(e)** 9.3×10^{-19} M. **63. (a)** neutral; **(b)** acidic, $CH_3CH_2NH_3^+ + H_2O \rightleftharpoons H_3O^+ + CH_3CH_2NH_2$; **(c)** acidic; both $HCOO^- + H_2O \rightleftharpoons HCOOH + OH^-$ and $NH_4^+ + H_2O \rightleftharpoons H_3O^+ + NH_3$ occur, but $K_a(NH_4^+) > K_b(HCOO^-)$. **65.** (c). **67. (a)** $OCl^- + H_2O \rightleftharpoons HOCl + OH^-$; **(b)** $K_b = 3.4 \times 10^{-7}$; **(c)** pH = 10.22. **69.** 0.23 M. **71.** (c) supplies H_3O^+, and (d) supplies $HCOO^-$. **73.** 1.8×10^{-4} M. **75.** 4.24. **77. (a)** pH < 7; **(b)** pH > 7; **(c)** pH < 7; **(d)** pH < 7; **(e)** pH > 7; **(f)** pH > 7. **79.** $HPO_4^{2-} + H_2O \rightleftharpoons PO_4^{3-} + H_3O^+$, $HPO_4^{2-} + H_2O \rightleftharpoons H_2PO_4^- + OH^-$; basic. **81.** 3.65. **83.** 0.37 g. **85.** 3.63. **87.** No, the components must be a conjugate (weak) acid-base pair. **89.** Suitable endpoints for a strong acid-strong base titration occur over a much wider pH range than for a weak acid-strong base titration (Figures 15.15, 15.16). **91. (a)** yellow; **(b)** blue; **(c)** red; **(d)** violet. **93.** Yellow. **95.** The pH is high at the beginning of the titration; the pH drops slowly until just before the equivalence point; just before the equivalence point the pH drops sharply; at the equivalence point the pH is 7.00; just past equivalence the pH continues its sharp drop; further beyond equivalence the pH continues to drop but much more slowly. The same indicators may be used for both titrations because the steep change in pH occurs over the same span in pH. **97.** 4.52. **99. (a)** 16.0 mL; **(b)** 11.28; **(c)** 9.60; **(d)** 9.26; **(e)** 9.03; **(f)** 5.05; **(g)** 1.48. **101.** Lewis acid and base are, respectively: **(a)** $Al(OH)_3$ and OH^-; **(b)** Cu^{2+} and NH_3; **(c)** CO_2 and OH^-. **Additional Problems: 103. (a)** 7.7 g; **(b)** 3.0 g acetic acid, 0.21 g NaOH. **106.** 5.36. **108.** Yes; yes; no the solutions will not be the same. **110.** 0.026 M. **113.** 2.8 %NaCl; an indicator that produces an endpoint very near pH = 7. **116. (a)** pH = 11.23; **(b)** 34 mg NaOH. **117. (a)** Strong base titrated with weak acid; **(b)** $pK_a \approx 3.8$; **(c)** pH = 8.75. **120.** $pK_{a_1} = 3.16$; $pK_{a_2} = 5.22$. **122. (a)** 2 mol acetic acid per 1 mol sodium acetate; **(b)** 3 mol acetic acid per 1 mol NaOH; **(c)** 3 mol sodium acetate per 2 mol HCl. Solution (c) forms 2 mol NaCl from the HCl and has a high ionic strength, which will affect activity and pH. **125.** pH = 2.25. **Apply Your Knowledge: 127.** pH = 4.3. Distilled water with even a tiny amount of acidic or basic contaminant will have a pH significantly different from 7.00. One suitable buffer would have $[HPO_4^{2-}]/[H_2PO_4^-] = 0.63$. **129.** 1.8×10^2 g CaO. **130.** $K_a = 1.4 \times 10^{-4}$. **133.** pH = 5.68.

Chapter 16

Exercises: 16.1A (a) $MgF_2(s) \rightleftharpoons Mg^{2+}(aq) + 2 F^-(aq)$, $K_{sp} = [Mg^{2+}][F^-]^2$; **(b)** $Li_2CO_3(s) \rightleftharpoons 2 Li^+(aq) + CO_3^{2-}(aq)$, $K_{sp} = [Li^+]^2[CO_3^{2-}]$; **(c)** $Cu_3(AsO_4)_2(s) \rightleftharpoons 3 Cu^{2+}(aq) + 2 AsO_4^{3-}(aq)$, $K_{sp} = [Cu^{2+}]^3[AsO_4^{3-}]^2$. **16.1B (a)** $MgF_2(s) \rightleftharpoons Mg^{2+}(aq) + 2 F^-(aq)$, $K_{sp} = [Mg^{2+}][F^-]^2$; **(b)** $Li_2CO_3(s) \rightleftharpoons 2 Li^+(aq) + CO_3^{2-}(aq)$, $K_{sp} = [Li^+]^2[CO_3^{2-}]$; **(c)** $Cu_3(AsO_4)_2(s) \rightleftharpoons 3 Cu^{2+}(aq) + 2 AsO_4^{3-}(aq)$, $K_{sp} = [Cu^{2+}]^3[AsO_4^{3-}]^2$. **16.2A** $K_{sp} = 2.0 \times 10^{-11}$. **16.2B** $K_{sp} = 1.1 \times 10^{-12}$ M. **16.3A** 1.4×10^{-6} M. **16.3B** 3.1×10^2 ppm of I^-. **16.4A** The trend in molar solubilities is the same as that of K_{sp} values because all four formulas are of the form MX_2: $CaF_2(K_{sp} = 5.3 \times 10^{-9}) < PbI_2(7.1 \times 10^{-9}) < MgF_2(3.7 \times 10^{-8}) < PbCl_2(1.6 \times 10^{-5})$. **16.4B** For $BaSO_4$, the solubility, $s = \sqrt{K_{sp}} \approx 1 \times 10^{-5}$ M. For CaF_2 and PbI_2, $s = (K_{sp})^{1/3}/4 \approx (K_{sp})^{1/3}$. Both K_{sp} values are to the power 10^{-9}, so $s \approx 10^{-3}$ M. The coefficient in the K_{sp} of PbI_2 is larger than in the K_{sp} of CaF_2, so PbI_2 is most soluble. **16.5A** 1.4×10^{-5} M. **16.5B** 4.9 g $AgNO_3$. **16.6A** Yes, $Q_{ip}(4.6 \times 10^{-8}) > K_{sp}$. **16.6B** No, $Q_{ip}(1.3 \times 10^{-12}) < K_{sp}$. **16.7A** Add KI(aq) dropwise from a buret to a known volume of solution of known $[Pb^{2+}]$. Stir after each drop is added, observing first the appearance and then disappearance of PbI_2(s). Continue until a single drop produces a lasting precipitate. Now, $Q_{ip} = K_{sp}$. Calculate K_{sp} from the $[Pb^{2+}]$ and $[I^-]$. **16.7B (a)** The observations should be similar. At the point of impact of the first droplet K_{sp} of PbI_2 is exceeded and precipitate should first form and then disappear as complete mixing occurs. **(b)** No precipitate should form because the ion product cannot exceed $[Pb^{2+}][I^-]^2 = (0.10)(1 \times 10^{-4})^2 < K_{sp} = 7.1 \times 10^{-9}$. **16.8A** Yes, $Q_{ip}(5 \times 10^{-8}) > K_{sp}$. **16.8B** 3.3 g KI. **16.9A** Yes, only $\approx 0.01\%$ of Ca^{2+} remains in solution. **16.9B** (c) < (a) < (b) < (d). (c) No precipitation of cation occurs; $MgSO_4$ is water-soluble. (a) The mixture becomes $CaSO_4$(s) with excess $[Ca^{2+}] = 0.020$ M. Slightly less than 0.090/0.110 of the Ca^{2+} precipitates; about 20% of the Ca^{2+} remains in solution. (c) The mixture becomes $PbCl_2$(s) with excess $[Cl^-] = 0.01$ M. The solubility in this case is slightly less than $S = (K_{sp}/4)^{1/3} \approx 0.016$ M. The fraction of Pb^{2+} precipitating is about $(0.120 - 0.016)/0.120$, and about 13% of the Pb^{2+} remains in solution. (d) The mixture becomes AgCl(s) with excess $[Cl^-] = 0.005$ M. The solubility is slightly less than $S = \sqrt{K_{sp}} \approx 1 \times 10^{-5}$ M. Precipitation of the Ag^+ is essentially complete. **16.10A (a)** Br^- precipitates first; **(b)** $[Br^-] = 2.8 \times 10^{-5}$ M when Cl^- begins to precipitate; **(c)** precipitation of Br^- is not quite complete. **16.10B** I^- and Br^- can be separated. K_{sp} for AgI and AgBr differ by nearly 6000-fold, much greater

than 360-fold between AgBr and AgCl. **16.11A** 0.80 M. **16.11B** No, $Q_{ip}(7 \times 10^{-33}) > K_{sp}$. **16.12A** $Mg(OH)_2(s) + 2 NH_4^+(aq) \longrightarrow Mg^{2+}(aq) + 2 H_2O(l) + 2 NH_3(aq)$. **16.12B** Most soluble in 1.00 M $NH_4NO_3(aq)$. Solubility is reduced in 1.00 M $Na_2SO_3(aq)$ due to the common ion effect, and in 1.00 M $NH_3(aq)$ due to the high pH. $NH_4NO_3(aq)$ is slightly acidic and will increase the solubility of $SrSO_3$ over its solubility in pure water, by reacting to form the weak acid HSO_3^-. **16.13A** $[Ag^+] = 9.2 \times 10^{-15}$ M. **16.13B** $[NH_3]_{total} = 0.66$ M. **16.14A** No, $Q_{ip}(5.5 \times 10^{-17}) < K_{sp}$ of AgI. **16.14B** 4.8×10^{-3} g KBr. **16.15A** 0.22 M. **16.15B** $NaCN(aq)$. K_f of $[Ag(CN)_2]^-$ is much larger than that of $[Ag(S_2O_3)_2]^{3-}$ or $[Ag(NH_3)_2]^+$. **16.16A** No; NH_4^+ does not react with NO_3^-. The complex ion is not destroyed and the concentration of free Ag^+ remains too low for $AgCl(s)$ to precipitate. **16.16B** (a) $Zn^{2+}(aq) + 2 NH_3(aq) + 2 H_2O(l) \longrightarrow Zn(OH)_2(s) + 2 NH_4^+(aq)$; (b) $Zn(OH)_2(s) + 4 NH_3(aq) \longrightarrow [Zn(NH_3)_4]^{2+}(aq) + 2 OH^-(aq)$; (c) $[Zn(NH_3)_4]^{2+}(aq) + 2 OH^-(aq) + 6 CH_3COOH(aq) \longrightarrow Zn^{2+}(aq) + 6 CH_3COO^-(aq) + 4 NH_4^+(aq) + 2 H_2O(l)$ **Self-Assessment Questions: 1.** (a) $K_{sp} = [Fe^{3+}][OH^-]^3$; (b) $K_{sp} = [Au^{3+}]^2[C_2O_4^{2-}]^3$ **4.** (a) The compounds are of the same type (MX); $PbSO_4$ has the larger K_{sp} and is the more soluble. (b) The compounds are of the same type (MX_2); PbI_2 has the larger K_{sp} and is the more soluble. **5.** (a). **6.** (c). **9.** HCl and CH_3COOH react with OH^-, increasing $[Fe^{3+}]$. The other solutions reduce $[Fe^{3+}]$ by supplying the common ion OH^-. **11.** (a) $K_f = [[Ag(NH_3)_2]^+]/[Ag^+][NH_3]^2$; (b) $K_f = [[Zn(NH_3)_4]^{2+}]/[Zn^{2+}][NH_3]^4$; (c) $K_f = [[Ag(S_2O_3)_2]^{3-}]/[Ag^+][S_2O_3^{2-}]^2$. **12.** $Pb(NO_3)_2(aq)$ reduces the solubility of $PbCl_2$ through the common-ion effect; $HCl(aq)$ increases it through the formation of the complex ion $[PbCl_3]^-$. **13.** (a). **14.** (b). **15.** $[Al(H_2O)_6]^{3+} + H_2O \rightleftharpoons H_3O^+ + [AlOH(H_2O)_5]^{2+}$. **Problems: 19.** $Hg_2(CN)_2(s) \rightleftharpoons Hg_2^{2+}(aq) + 2 CN^-(aq)$, $K_{sp} = [Hg_2^{2+}][CN^-]^2 = 5 \times 10^{-40}$; **21.** $Ag_3AsO_4(s) \rightleftharpoons 3 Ag^+(aq) + AsO_4^{3-}(aq)$, $K_{sp} = [Ag^+]^3[AsO_4^{3-}] = 1.0 \times 10^{-22}$. **23.** Molar solubility and K_{sp} cannot have the same value. Molar solubility is equal to an ion concentration or some fraction of it; K_{sp} is a *product* of two ion concentrations raised to powers. Molar solubilities are generally larger than K_{sp} because the roots of a number <1 are larger than the number. **25.** (a) $K_{sp} = 1.46 \times 10^{-10}$; (b) $K_{sp} = 1.2 \times 10^{-33}$; (c) $K_{sp} = 3.7 \times 10^{-8}$. **27.** (a) Ag_2CrO_4; (b) $MgCO_3$. **29.** $K_{sp} = 1.6 \times 10^{-5}$. **31.** $CaSO_4$ is more soluble than $CaCO_3$; it has a larger K_{sp}. $[Ca^{2+}]$ is greater in $CaSO_4$(satd aq) than in CaF_2(satd aq), because $(9.1 \times 10^{-6})^{1/2}$ is larger than $[(5.3/4) \times 10^{-9}]^{1/3}$. **33.** Yes. **35.** Yes, 22 mg $PbCl_2$ should precipitate. **37.** Pure water. The other two solutions contain common ions and reduce the solubility. **39.** (a) $s = 6.7 \times 10^{-6}$ M; (b) $s = 1.6 \times 10^{-6}$ M. **41.** $[Pb^{2+}] = 4.4 \times 10^{-8}$ M; $[I^-] = 0.400$ M. **43.** (a) $[Ag^+] = 3.0 \times 10^{-2}$ M; (b) 62 g Na_2SO_4. **45.** 2.7×10^{-3} M. **47.** $[CrO_4^{2-}] = 1.0 \times 10^{-6}$ M. **49.** (a) No; (b) Yes, $Pb_3(AsO_4)_2$ will form. **51.** No, $Q_{ip}(5.5 \times 10^{-12}) < K_{sp}$ of CaF_2. **53.** $CaCO_3$, 3.1×10^{-6} M. **55.** (a) $[Mg^{2+}] = 4.5 \times 10^{-6}$ M; (b) Yes, only 0.0076% of Mg^{2+} remains in solution. **57.** pH = 10.85. **59.** (a) $CaF_2(s)$; (b) $[F^-] = 1.9 \times 10^{-3}$ M; (c) No, 15% of the Ca^{2+} remains in solution when $MgF_2(s)$ begins to precipitate. **61.** (a) Essentially complete precipitation of 1.0×10^{-3} mol $AgCl(s)$ occurs. (b) Because $[Ag^+]$ is too low following precipitation of $AgCl(s)$, Ag_2SO_4 does not precipitate. **63.** $NaHSO_4$. The reaction, $HSO_4^- + CO_3^{2-} \longrightarrow HCO_3^- + SO_4^{2-}$, replaces insoluble $CaCO_3$ by the more soluble

$Ca(HCO_3)_2$. **65.** 2.5×10^{-16} M **67.** $CaCO_3(s) + 2 H_3O^+(aq) \longrightarrow Ca^{2+}(aq) + 3 H_2O(l) + CO_2(g)$; $CaCO_3(s) + 2 CH_3COOH(aq) \longrightarrow Ca^{2+}(aq) + 2 CH_3COO^-(aq) + H_2O(l) + CO_2(g)$. **69.** $[CrCl_2(NH_3)_4]^+$. **71.** Both H_3O^+ from HCl (d) and HSO_4^- from $NaHSO_4$ (b) can donate protons to NH_3 in the complex ion, causing the complex ion to dissociate and the concentration of free Zn^{2+} to increase. **73.** $2 Ag^+(aq) + SO_4^{2-}(aq) \longrightarrow Ag_2SO_4(s)$; $Ag_2SO_4(s) + 4 NH_3(aq) \longrightarrow 2[Ag(NH_3)_2]^+(aq) + SO_4^{2-}(aq)$; $[Ag(NH_3)_2]^+(aq) + 2 H_3O^+(aq) \longrightarrow Ag^+(aq) + 2 NH_4^+(aq) + 2 H_2O(l)$. **75.** (a) $Fe(OH)_3(s) + 3 H^+(aq) \longrightarrow Fe^{3+}(aq) + 3 H_2O(l)$; (b) NR; (c) $Cr^{3+}(aq) + 4 OH^-(aq) \longrightarrow [Cr(OH)_4]^-(aq)$. **77.** $[Zn^{2+}] = 1.2 \times 10^{-10}$ M. **79.** A trace of $PbI_2(s)$ should precipitate; $Q_{sp}(2.1 \times 10^{-8})$ is slightly larger than K_{sp}. **81.** 4.0 mg KBr. **83.** 0.043 M. **85.** $K_{sp}(PbS) \ll K_{sp}(PbCl_2)$. Enough Pb^{2+} remains from cation group 1 that K_{sp} of PbS is exceeded. $[Ag^+]$ in equilibrium with $AgCl(s)$ is so low that Ag^+ does not later precipitate as Ag_2S. **87.** Hg_2^{2+} is definitely present; the presence of Ag^+ and Pb^{2+} is uncertain—no tests were performed. **Additional Problems: 91.** Yes. **92.** $K_{sp} = 1.62 \times 10^{-7}$. **94.** $Pb(N_3)_2(s) + 2 H_3O^+(aq) \rightleftharpoons Pb^{2+}(aq) + 2 HN_3(aq) + 2 H_2O(l)$; $K_c = 6.9$. Solubility at pH 2.85 is 0.015 mol $Pb(N_3)_2/L$. **98.** 0.10 mL 0.0050 M NaBr. **101.** 6.5×10^{-4} M. **103.** (a) Yes; (b) 2.3 g calcium palmitate. **Apply Your Knowledge: 104.** (a) 34.32% Ca; (b) 0.6231 g $CaCO_3$, 34.22% Ca. **105.** (a) $[Ba^{2+}]$ in saturated $BaSO_4(aq)$ is too low to be hazardous. (b) 1.4 mg Ba^{2+}/L. (c) SO_4^{2-} from $MgSO_4$ reduces the solubility of $BaSO_4$. **108.** (a) 29-30 drops; (b) In (a) the $[Pb^{2+}]$ is essentially fixed at 0.020 M and the $[I^-]$ is increased until K_{sp} is reached. In (b) the $[I^-]$ is fixed at 0.020 M and the $[Pb^{2+}]$ is gradually increased. Since $[I^-]$ is squared but $[Pb^{2+}]$ is taken to the first power in the expression for K_{sp}, the amount of the second ion needed will differ. **110.** (a) $s = 1.2 \times 10^{-2}$ M; (b) $s = 6.0 \times 10^{-2}$ M.

Chapter 17

Exercises: 17.1A (a) Spontaneous. Cellulose decomposes into simpler molecules, such as CO_2 and H_2O, through the action of microorganisms. (b) Nonspontaneous. A compound cannot be decomposed through a physical change. (c) Spontaneous. $HCl(g)$ dissociates completely simply by dissolving in water. **17.1B** (a) Spontaneous; the liquids are miscible in all proportions at all temperatures at which the liquids exist. (b) Uncertain. All compounds decompose at very high temperatures, but it is uncertain whether this decomposition will produce $CO_2(g)$ at 1 atm at 600 °C. (c) Uncertain. Whether the condensation is spontaneous depends on the temperature; that is, spontaneous at all temperatures below that at which the sublimation pressure of $CO_2(s) = 0.50$ atm. (d) Nonspontaneous. $Cu(s)$ lies below $H_2(g)$ in the activity series (Figure 4.13) and will not displace $H_2(g)$ from acidic solution. **17.2A** (a) Decrease. Two moles of gas are converted to one of solid. (b) Increase. Two moles of solid are converted to two moles of solid and three moles of gas. (c) Uncertain. Two moles of gaseous reactants produce two moles of gaseous products. **17.2B** Vaporization produces an increase in entropy (disorder), but enthalpy also increases. In condensation, entropy and enthalpy both decrease. At equilibrium vaporization and condensation occur at equal rates. **17.3A** $\Delta S° = -42.1$ J/K. **17.3B** $\Delta S° = 131.0$ J/K. **17.4A** (a) $\Delta S < 0$, $\Delta H < 0$, case 2; (b) $\Delta S > 0$, $\Delta H > 0$, case 3. **17.4B** $\Delta S > 0$, $\Delta H° = -56.9$ kJ, case 1. **17.5A** -78.5 °C(See Figure 11.12). **17.5B** Both dissociation

reactions have $\Delta S° > 0$, but only the dissociation of $NO_2(g)$ has $\Delta H° < 0$, making it spontaneous at all temperatures. For the dissociation of $NH_3(g)$, $\Delta H° > 0$, and so the dissociation is spontaneous only at higher temperatures. **17.6A (a)** $\Delta G° = -70.5$ kJ; **(b)** $\Delta G° = 447.5$ kJ. **17.6B (a)** $\Delta G° = -66.9$ kJ; **(b)** $\Delta G° = -1305.7$ kJ. **17.7A** $\Delta H°_{vap} = 36$ kJ mol^{-1}. **17.7B** Because of extensive hydrogen bonding in $CH_3OH(l)$, $\Delta S°_{vap} > 87$ J mol^{-1} K^{-1}. $\Delta S° = 112.9$ J mol^{-1} K^{-1} is based on $S°$ values in Appendix C; it is 112.5 J mol^{-1} K^{-1} based on $\Delta H°_f$ values and $\Delta S° = \Delta H°/T_{bp}$. **17.8A** $K_{eq} = [Al^{3+}](P_{H_2})^3/[H^+]^6$. **17.8B** $Mg(OH)_2(s) + 2 H_3O^+(aq) \rightleftharpoons Mg^{2+}(aq) + 4 H_2O(l)$; $K_{eq} = [Mg^{2+}]/[H_3O^+]^2$. **17.9A** $K_{eq} = 3.02 \times 10^{-21}$. **17.9B** $K_{eq} = 27$; $P_{NO} = 0.16$ atm, $P_{NOBr} = 0.84$ atm. **17.10A** $K_{eq} = 0.45$. **17.10B** With the Clausius-Clapeyron equation, $P_{H_2O} = 55.7$ mmHg; from Table 11.2, $P_{H_2O} = 55.3$ mmHg. **Self-Assessment Questions: 1.** (a), (c). **2.** (c). **3. (a)** Decrease (liquid $\longrightarrow$ solid); **(b)** increase (solid $\longrightarrow$ gas); **(c)** increase (liquid + oxygen gas $\longrightarrow$ large volume of gaseous products). **9.** NOF_3 has a greater number of atoms and vibrational modes, and hence a greater entropy, than NO_2F. **10.** (b). **11.** Low temperatures. The ΔH term dominates in the Gibbs equation, offsetting a positive value of $-T\Delta S$ and making $\Delta G < 0$. **13.** (d). **14.** (c). **18.** (d). **Problems: 19. (a)** Increase—system energy dispersed over more levels in gas than in liquid. **(b)** Increase—process produces increased number of molecules of gas. **(c)** Indeterminate—same number of moles of gas on each side of equation. **(d)** Increase—large amount of gas produced from a solid. **(e)** Decrease—system energy is spread among fewer levels in solid than in liquid. **(f)** Indeterminate—The gases are all diatomic and the same number of moles of gas appear on each side of the equation. **(g)** Increase—A liquid decomposes to produce a large amount of gas. **(h)** Entropy decreases when a large volume of gas dissolves in water. **21.** The final state: heterogeneous mixture of octane floating on water. Solution formation would require $\Delta H > 0$ to break hydrogen bonds in the water. The increase in entropy would not be sufficient to overcome the large ΔH. **23.** Correct: For a process to occur spontaneously, the total entropy—S_{univ}—must increase. Errors in other statements: (a) Entropy of the system may increase in some cases and decrease in others; (b) Entropy of the surroundings may also increase or decrease; (c) Entropy of the system and surroundings need not both increase, as long as the increase in one exceeds the decrease in the other. **25.** Rather than two vertical sections, the graph has one vertical section at 194.5 K corresponding to sublimation. **27.** No. The disintegration of an aluminum can is spontaneous, but because a protective coating of Al_2O_3 forms on the surface, complete disintegration takes a very long time. "Spontaneous" does not mean "fast." **29.** A criterion based on ΔS requires assessing both ΔS_{syst} and ΔS_{surr}; the free energy change requires only measurements in the system: $\Delta G = \Delta H - T\Delta S$.

The $T\Delta S$ line does not cross the ΔH line, so ΔG is always negative and the reaction is spontaneous at all temperatures. **33. (a)** The change in *enthalpy* indicates whether the reaction is endothermic or exothermic; **(b)** The *entropy change* indicates whether the reaction involves an increase or decrease in available energy levels; **(c)** The *relative values of ΔH and $T\Delta S$* indicate whether equilibrium in the reaction is favored at high or low temperatures. **35. (a)** Melting of a solid is nonspontaneous below its melting point and spontaneous above its melting point—0 °C for water. **(b)** The condensation of a vapor at 1 atm pressure to liquid is spontaneous below the normal boiling point and nonspontaneous above the normal boiling point. For water, this temperature is 100 °C. **37.** High temperature, since $\Delta S < 0$ and $\Delta G = \Delta H - T\Delta S$ **39. (a)** $\Delta G° = +22.9$ kJ; **(b)** $\Delta G° = -163$ kJ. **41.** $\Delta H° = -1076.8$ kJ; $\Delta S° = -56.5$ J/K; $\Delta G° = -1060.1$ kJ. **43.** With $\Delta G°$, we can evaluate K_{eq}: $\Delta G° = -RT \ln K_{eq}$. With K_{eq}, we can determine an equilibrium condition. To evaluate ΔG for nonstandard conditions we use $\Delta G = \Delta G° + RT \ln Q$ (where Q is reaction quotient). However, we cannot obtain ΔG without knowing $\Delta G°$. **45.** 364 K (91 °C). **47.** $\Delta H°_{vap} = +29.8$ kJ/mol (Trouton's rule); +30.1 kJ/mol (Appendix C). **49. (a)** $\Delta G = 0$ kJ; **(b)** $K_p = 171$. **51. (a)** $K_{eq} = P_{H_2O}P_{SO_2} = K_p$; **(b)** $K_{eq} = [Mg^{2+}][OH^-]^2 = K_{sp}$; **(c)** $K_{eq} = [CH_3COOH][OH^-]/[CH_3COO^-] = K_b$. **53. (a)** $K_p = 7.2 \times 10^{24}$; **(b)** $K_p = 1.3 \times 10^{-20}$. **55.** $P_{C_{10}H_8} = 0.063$ mmHg. **57. (a)** $\Delta G° = -15.9$ kJ. **(b)** Direction of net reaction: $\longrightarrow$. **(c)** 0.037 mol CO, 0.064 mol H_2O, 0.193 mol CO_2, 0.274 mol H_2. **59.** The reaction to be coupled with the given reaction must have $\Delta G° < -237.9$ kJ. Only (c) will work; it has $\Delta G° = -257.2$ kJ. **61.** $K_{eq} = 3.5 \times 10^{10}$. **63.** 390.4 K. **65.** $K_p = 2.0 \times 10^6$. **67.** Estimated boiling point: 348 K. Use $\Delta H°_{298}$ and $\Delta G°_{298}$ from Appendix C; calculate K_p at 298 K; use the van't Hoff equation to determine T at which $K_p = 1.00$ atm. **69.** 424 K. **Additional Problems: 71.** The expansion in Figure 6.8 is not reversible because the process cannot be reversed by an infinitesimal change. The weights are too large, the change occurs too quickly. **74.** In Chapter 14, we saw that an endothermic reaction would be forced to the right by an increase in temperature. The effect of being forced to the right increases the K_{eq}. From the van't Hoff equation, for positive ΔH (endothermic) an increase in temperature increases the K_{eq}. That is, for $\Delta H > 0$ and $T_2 > T_1$, $K_2 > K_1$. **75.** 393 K. **77. (a)** 3.47 kJ; **(b)** to the left; **(c)** 0.0554 mol CO_2, 0.0754 mol H_2, 0.0346 mol CO, 0.0796 mol H_2O. **81.** Sublimation pressure of Hg(s) at -78.5 °C: $\approx 10^{-9}$ mmHg. **83.** $T = 631$ K. **87. (a)** true from definition of $\Delta G°$, so (c) is false; (d) is true, nonspontaneous process so (b) is false. **89.** $P_{PCl_5} = 1.79$ atm, $P_{PCl_3} = P_{Cl_2} = 0.95$ atm, $P_{total} = 3.69$ atm. **Apply Your Knowledge: 92. (a)** Using van't Hoff's equation, $T = 523$ °C; **(b)** H_2, graphite, CO, Cu_2O, SO_2, and Al. **94.** At body temperature (37 °C), a concentration of glucose-6-phosphate 627 times the glucose concentration. **97.** $\Delta G = -26.3$ kJ. **98. (a)** $T = 491$ K; the temperature is probably higher because some heat is lost to the surroundings; **(b)** 22 atm; **(c)** "You can't win" because you can't get more work out of the engine than the energy put into the engine; "you can't break even" because you can't even get 100% efficiency; the engine always operates "at a loss."

31.

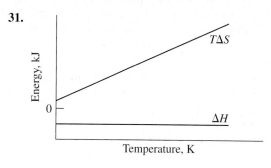

Chapter 18

Exercises: 18.1A $4 Zn(s) + 2 NO_3^-(aq) + 10 H^+(aq) \longrightarrow 4 Zn^{2+}(aq) + N_2O(g) + 5 H_2O(l)$. **18.1B** $3 P_4(s) + 20 NO_3^-(aq)$

$+ 8 H_2O(l) + 8 H^+(aq) \longrightarrow 12 H_2PO_4^-(aq) + 20 NO(g)$.
18.2A $2 OCN^-(aq) + 3 OCl^-(aq) + 2 OH^-(aq) \longrightarrow$
$2 CO_3^{2-}(aq) + N_2(g) + H_2O(l) + 3 Cl^-(aq)$. **18.2B** $4 MnO_4^-(aq)$
$+ 3 CH_3CH_2OH(aq) \longrightarrow 4 MnO_2(s) + 3 CH_3COO^-(aq) +$
$OH^-(aq) + 4 H_2O(l)$. **18.3A** $2 Al(s) + 6 H^+(aq) \longrightarrow$
$2 Al^{3+}(aq) + 3 H_2(g)$. **18.3B** $Cu(s)|Cu^{2+}(aq)||Ag^+(aq)|Ag(s)$.
18.4A $E^\circ_{Sm^{2+}/Sm} = -2.67$ V. **18.4B** $E^\circ_{ClO_4^-/Cl_2} = 1.392$ V.
18.5A **(a)** $E^\circ_{cell} = 2.016$ V; **(b)** $E^\circ_{cell} = -0.499$ V.
18.5B $2 Mn^{2+}(aq) + 5 S_2O_8^{2-}(aq) + 8 H_2O(l) \longrightarrow$
$2 MnO_4^-(aq) + 10 SO_4^{2-}(aq) + 16 H^+(aq)$, $E^\circ_{cell} = 0.50$ V.
18.6A No, $E^\circ_{cell} = -0.431$ V. **18.6B** The reverse reaction is spontaneous; for the forward reaction, $E^\circ_{cell} = -0.31$ V. **18.7A** Similar
to Example 18.7, Zn is oxidized, and electrons pass through the
voltmeter to the Cu electrode, where H^+ (from lemon juice) is
reduced to $H_2(g)$. **18.7B (a)** Result should be similar to what is
seen in Figure 18.10, but the gas evolution would probably be less
vigorous because $[H^+]$ is lower in $CH_3COOH(aq)$, a weak acid,
than in HCl(aq), a strong acid. **(b)** $NO_3^-(aq)$ is a stronger oxidizing agent in acidic solutions than is $H^+(aq)$, and the reduction
product should be mostly NO(g) or $NO_2(g)$, rather than $H_2(g)$.
Moreover, the copper strip would react as well as the zinc, producing a blue solution characteristic of $Cu^{2+}(aq)$ (recall Figure 4.14).
(c) Result should be similar to Figure 18.10, but with the copious
collection of $H_2(g)$ bubbles on the surface of the pool of mercury
and a smaller amount on the zinc strip. **18.8A** $\Delta G^\circ = -394$ kJ;
$K_{eq} = 1 \times 10^{69}$. **18.8B** For the reaction: $3 Ag(s) + 4 H^+(aq) +$
$NO_3^-(aq) \longrightarrow 3 Ag^+(aq) + NO(g) + 2 H_2O(l)$,
$E^\circ_{cell} = 0.156$ V; $K_{eq} = 8.0 \times 10^7$. **18.9A (a)** $E_{cell} = 1.056$ V;
(b) $E_{cell} = 1.150$ V. **18.9B** $E_{cell} = 1.045$ V. **18.10A** The bend,
like the head and tip, is strained and more energetic than the body
of the nail. It is an anodic area (blue precipitate). **18.10B** The same
half-reactions occur even if the early indicators of those half-
reactions, the phenolphthalein and potassium ferricyanide, are
missing. Over time, in the presence of dissolved $O_2(g)$, the
$Fe^{2+}(aq)$ produced in the oxidation will be converted to red-brown
$Fe_2O_3(s)$, as outlined in Figure 18.18. The first appearance of this
"rust" should be at the same points where the blue precipitate is
seen in Figure 18.19. **18.11A** $2 Br^-(aq) + 2 H_2O(l) \longrightarrow Br_2(l)$
$+ 2 OH^-(aq) + H_2(g)$; $E^\circ_{cell} = -1.893$ V. **18.11B** To force the
electrolysis, Ag(s, anode) $\longrightarrow$ Ag(s, cathode), the external
voltage > 0.460 V. Otherwise, this reaction can occur: Cu(s) $+$
$2 Ag^+(aq) \longrightarrow Cu^{2+}(aq) + 2 Ag(s)$, $E^\circ_{cell} = 0.460$ V.
18.12A Cell A: $Cu(s) + Zn^{2+}(1.0$ M$) \longrightarrow Cu^{2+}(0.10$ M$) +$
Zn(s); cell B: $Zn(s) + Cu^{2+}(1.0$ M$) \longrightarrow Zn^{2+}(0.10$ M$) + Cu(s)$.
18.12B As current flows, $[Zn^{2+}]$ and $[Cu^{2+}]$ change in both cells;
when concentrations in the two cells are the same, current stops.
18.13A 22.5 min. **18.13B (a)** 1945 C; **(b)** 1.529 A.
18.14A NaCl(aq). The oxidation $H_2O \longrightarrow O_2$ produces
0.25 mol O_2 per mol e^-; $Cl^- \longrightarrow Cl_2$ produces 0.5 mol Cl_2 per
mol e^-. Oxidation of I^- produces solid I_2. **18.14B** Choice (a) produces $H_2(g)$ rather than metallic sodium. The answer will be the
solution requiring the smallest number of moles of electrons transferred in the electrolysis. In solution (b) the number of moles of Cu
in 1.00 g is 1.00/63.55 = 0.0157 mol Cu; the electrolysis requires
2 mol e^- per mol Cu or a total of about 0.03 mol electrons. By contrast, in solution (c) 1.00 g of metal corresponds to about
1.00/107.87 = 0.009 mol Ag, requiring 0.009 mol e^- for its elec-
trodeposition. The situation with solution (d) is roughly the same
as with solution (b). Solution (c) is the answer we seek, provided
that there is sufficient Ag^+ in the solution to yield at least 1.00 g

Ag(s). There is, since 0.150 L $\times 0.25$ mol Ag^+/L > 0.009 mol
Ag^+. Note that we did not have to determine whether solutions (b)
and (d) have enough solute to yield 1.00 g of the solid metal, nor
did we have to use the magnitude of the current since it was the
same in all cases. **Self-Assessment Questions: 5.** (c). **6.** (d). **8.** If
the reduction most easily achieved is assigned $E^\circ = 0$, all others
will have $E^\circ < 0$. If the reduction most difficult to achieve is
assigned $E^\circ = 0$, all others will have $E^\circ > 0$. **9.** (d). **11.** Ag, Au.
12. E°_{cell} values are based on E° values and related to ΔG° values
for *redox* reactions. Predictions based on E°_{cell} are the same as if
based on ΔG°. They apply regardless of how redox reactions are
carried out. **13.** $E^\circ_{cell} < 0$ means that a reaction is nonspontaneous
when reactants and products are in their standard states. The reaction may be spontaneous for specific nonstandard conditions.
21. E° data are used to determine E°_{cell} for the nonspontaneous
reaction occurring in electrolysis; the applied voltage must exceed
this E°_{cell}. **22.** (a). **23.** An object to be electroplated is the cathode,
and the metal to be plated out, in solution as cations. **24.** (d).
Problems: 25. (a) $HNO_2(aq) \longrightarrow NO_2(g) + H^+(aq) + e^-$;
(b) $PbO_2(s) + 2 H^+(aq) + 2 e^- \longrightarrow PbO(s) + H_2O(l)$;
(c) $12 OH^-(aq) + CH_3CH_2OH(aq) \longrightarrow 2 CO_2(g) + 9 H_2O(l)$
$+ 12 e^-$. **27. (a)** $6 Fe^{2+} + Cr_2O_7^{2-} + 14 H^+ \longrightarrow 6 Fe^{3+} +$
$2 Cr^{3+} + 7 H_2O$; **(b)** $S_8 + 12 O_2 + 8 H_2O \longrightarrow 8 SO_4^{2-} +$
$16 H^+$; **(c)** $4 Fe^{3+} + 2 NH_2OH_2^+ \longrightarrow 4 Fe^{2+} + H_2O + N_2O +$
$6 H^+$. **29. (a)** $4 Fe(OH)_2(s) + O_2(g) + 2 H_2O(l) \longrightarrow$
$4 Fe(OH)_3(s)$; **(b)** $S_8(s) + 12 OH^-(aq) \longrightarrow 2 S_2O_3^{2-}(aq) +$
$4 S^{2-}(aq) + 6 H_2O(l)$; **(c)** $2 CrI_3(s) + 27 H_2O_2(aq) + 10 OH^-(aq)$
$\longrightarrow 2 CrO_4^{2-}(aq) + 6 IO_4^-(aq) + 32 H_2O(l)$.
31. (a) $5 H_2C_2O_4(aq) + 2 MnO_4^-(aq) + 6 H^+(aq) \longrightarrow$
$2 Mn^{2+}(aq) + 10 CO_2(g) + 8 H_2O(l)$; **(b)** $Cr_2O_7^{2-}(aq) +$
$3 UO^{2+}(aq) + 8 H^+(aq) \longrightarrow 2 Cr^{3+}(aq) + 3 UO_2^{2+}(aq) +$
$4 H_2O(l)$; **(c)** $4 Zn(s) + NO_3^-(aq) + 6 H_2O(l) \longrightarrow 4 Zn^{2+}(aq)$
$+ NH_3(g) + 9 OH^-(aq)$. **33. (a)** 0.118 V; **(b)** -0.508 V;
(c) 0.595 V. **35.** $E^\circ_{cathode} = 0.20$ V. **37.** $E^\circ_{V^{2+}/V} = -1.13$ V.
39. (a) $Fe^{2+} \longrightarrow Fe^{3+} + e^-$, $Cr_2O_7^{2-} + 14 H^+ + 6 e^- \longrightarrow$
$2 Cr^{3+} + 7 H_2O$, $6 Fe^{2+} + Cr_2O_7^{2-} + 14 H^+ \longrightarrow 6 Fe^{3+} +$
$2 Cr^{3+} + 7 H_2O$; $E^\circ_{cell} = 0.56$ V; **(b)** $NO + 2 H_2O \longrightarrow NO_3^-$
$+ 4 H^+ + 3 e^-$, $H_2O_2 + 2 H^+ + 2 e^- \longrightarrow 2 H_2O$, $2 NO +$
$3 H_2O_2 \longrightarrow 2 NO_3^- + 2 H^+ + 2 H_2O$; $E^\circ_{cell} = 2.619$ V.
41. (a) $Fe^{3+} + e^- \longrightarrow Fe^{2+}$, $Sn^{2+} \longrightarrow Sn^{4+} + 2 e^-$,
$2 Fe^{3+} + Sn^{2+} \longrightarrow Sn^{4+} + 2 Fe^{2+}$, $Pt|Sn^{2+}, Sn^{4+}||Fe^{2+}, Fe^{3+}|Pt$,
$E^\circ_{cell} = 0.617$ V; **(b)** $Cu(s) \longrightarrow Cu^{2+} + 2 e^-$, $4 H^+ + NO_3^- +$
$3 e^- \longrightarrow 2 H_2O + NO(g)$, $3 Cu(s) + 8 H^+ + 2 NO_3^- \longrightarrow$
$3 Cu^{2+} + 4 H_2O + 2 NO(g)$, $Cu|Cu^{2+}(aq)||H^+(aq), NO_3^-(aq)$,
$NO(g)|Pt$; $E^\circ_{cell} = 0.616$ V. **43. (a)** No; **(b)** Yes. **45. (a)** No;
(b) Yes; **(c)** Yes. **47. (a)** H^+ is not a good enough oxidizing agent to
oxidize Ag(s) to Ag^+; $2 Ag(s) + 2 H^+(aq) \longrightarrow 2 Ag^+(aq) +$
$H_2(g)$, $E^\circ_{cell} = -0.800$ V. **(b)** $NO_3^-(aq)$ oxidizes Ag(s) to Ag^+,
$3 Ag(s) + 4 H^+(aq) + NO_3^-(aq) \longrightarrow 3 Ag^+(aq) + NO(g) +$
$2 H_2O(l)$, $E^\circ_{cell} = 0.156$ V. **49.** 0.800 V $< E^\circ_{Pd^{2+}/Pd} < 0.956$ V.
51. (a) $E^\circ_{cell} = 0.694$ V, $\Delta G^\circ = -268$ kJ; **(b)** $E^\circ_{cell} = 0.99$ V,
$\Delta G^\circ = -5.7 \times 10^2$ kJ. **53. (a)** $K_{eq} = [Pb^{2+}]P_{Cl_2}/([H^+]^4[Cl^-]^2)$
$= 3.6 \times 10^6$; **(b)** $K_{eq} = [BrO_3^-]^2/([Br^-]^2 P_{O_2}^3) = 8.1 \times 10^{-38}$.
55. $Cu(s) + 2 Ag^+(aq) \longrightarrow Cu^{2+}(aq) + 2 Ag(s)$ at equilibrium
$[Ag^+] = 1.2 \times 10^{-8}$ M, $[Cu^{2+}] = 0.50$ M. **57. (a)** $E_{cell} =$
-0.026 V; **(b)** $E_{cell} = 0.19$ V. **59.** $E_{cell} = -0.15$ V.
61. pH = 1.82. **63.** The cell reaction is $Cu(s) + 2 Ag^+(aq) \longrightarrow$
$Cu^{2+}(aq) + 2 Ag(s)$. Cell (b) has a higher E_{cell} because it has a
lower ratio of $[Cu^{2+}]/[Ag^+]^2$. **65.** $2 Mg(s) + O_2(g) + 2 H_2O(l)$
$\longrightarrow 2 Mg(OH)_2(s)$, $E^\circ_{cell} = 2.757$ V. **67.** Anode:

$Zn(s) + 2\,OH^-(aq) \longrightarrow ZnO(s) + H_2O(l) + 2\,e^-$; cathode: $Ag_2O(s) + H_2O(l) + 2\,e^- \longrightarrow 2\,Ag(s) + 2\,OH^-(aq)$; cell reaction: $Zn(s) + Ag_2O(s) \longrightarrow ZnO(s) + 2\,Ag(s)$. **69.** Oxygen oxidizes $Fe(s)$ to $Fe^{2+}(aq)$ and $Fe^{3+}(aq)$. Water is involved in the reduction half-reaction and in the conversion of $Fe(OH)_2$ to $Fe(OH)_3$. The electrolyte completes the electric circuit between anodic and cathodic regions. **71.** The sacrificial anode is oxidized. Its sacrifice protects from oxidation the metal to which it is attached. **73.** Zinc is oxidized instead of iron (it is a sacrificial anode). There is a white precipitate of zinc ferricyanide but no Turnbull's blue. **75.** (a) $Cu(s, \text{anode}) \longrightarrow Cu(s, \text{cathode})$; (b) $2\,H_2O(l) + 2\,Cu^{2+}(aq) \longrightarrow 4\,H^+(aq) + O_2(g) + 2\,Cu(s)$; (c) $2\,H_2O(l) + 2\,Cu^{2+}(aq) \longrightarrow 4\,H^+(aq) + O_2(g) + 2\,Cu(s)$. **77.** (a) $BaCl_2(l) \longrightarrow Ba(l) + Cl_2(g)$, required voltage > 4.28 V; (b) $2\,HBr(aq) \longrightarrow H_2(g) + Br_2(l)$, required voltage > 1.065 V; (c) $2\,H_2O(l) \longrightarrow 2\,H_2(g) + O_2(g)$, required voltage > 2.057 V. **79.** 14.3 g Ag. **81.** 7.59×10^4 C. **83.** $AgNO_3$. $Ag^+(aq)$ yields 1 mol Ag/mol e^-, and $Cu^{2+}(aq)$ and $Zn^{2+}(aq)$ each yield 0.5 mol/mol e^-. Also, the molar mass of Ag exceeds that of Cu and Zn. **Additional Problems: 86.** $CN^- + 2\,OH^- + Cl_2 \longrightarrow OCN^- + 2\,Cl^- + H_2O$; $2\,OCN^- + 6\,OH^- + 3\,Cl_2 \longrightarrow 2\,HCO_3^- + N_2 + 6\,Cl^- + 2\,H_2O$. **88.** $2\,NO(g) + 5\,H_2(g) \longrightarrow 2\,NH_3(g) + 2\,H_2O(g)$; the method works because the ionic species that are introduced by employing aqueous solutions cancel out. **91.** 58.1 mL $O_2(g)$. **92.** 0.513 M $AgNO_3$. **96.** $E_{cell} = -0.457$ V. **99.** E_{cell} decreases as $[Cu^{2+}]$ increases at the anode and decreases at the cathode. When $[Cu^{2+}] = 0.76$ M in each half-cell, $E_{cell} = 0$ and the current stops. **102.** $Ag(s)|AgI(satd)| |Ag^+(0.100\text{ M})|Ag(s)$, $K_{sp} = 8.2 \times 10^{-17}$. **104.** The blue color will be seen. The Cu^{2+} is converted to $[Cu(NH_3)_4]^{2+}$, $[Cu(NH_3)_4]^{2+} = 4 \times 10^{-4}$ M. **106.** $[Hg^{2+}] = 0.177$ M; $[Fe^{2+}] = 0.034$ M; $[Fe^{3+}] = 0.356$ M. **109.** 3×10^3 ions. **112.** (a) cathode $O_2(g) + 2\,H_2O(l) + 4\,e^- \longrightarrow 4\,OH^-$, anode $H_2(g) + 2\,OH^- \longrightarrow 2\,H_2O(l) + 2\,e^-$, overall $2\,H_2(g) + O_2 \longrightarrow 2\,H_2O$; (b) $E_{cell} = 1.256$ V; (c) 7.50×10^5 kJ; (d) 868 watts; (e) Ideal gas behavior assumed; cell is nonstandard. **Apply Your Knowledge: 115.** 9.65×10^{-4} g. **116.** (a) $C_3H_5(NO_3)_3 + H^+ + 2\,e^- \longrightarrow C_3H_5OH(NO_3)_2 + NO_2^-$; $NO_2^- + 2\,H^+ + e^- \longrightarrow NO + H_2O$; (b) $C_3H_5(NO_3)_3 + NADH \longrightarrow C_3H_5OH(NO_3)_2 + NO_2^- + NAD^+$; $2\,NO_2^- + 3\,H^+ + NADH \longrightarrow 2\,NO + 2\,H_2O + NAD^+$.

Chapter 19

Exercises: 19.1A (a) $^{212}_{86}Rn \longrightarrow ^{208}_{84}Po + ^{4}_{2}He$; (b) $^{37}_{18}Ar + ^{0}_{-1}e \longrightarrow ^{37}_{17}Cl$; (c) $^{60}_{27}Co^* \longrightarrow ^{60}_{27}Co + \gamma$. **19.1B** (a) $^{218}_{84}Po \longrightarrow ^{214}_{82}Pb + ^{4}_{2}He$; (b) $^{36}_{17}Cl \longrightarrow ^{36}_{16}S + ^{0}_{1}e$. **19.2A** 5.20×10^2 atoms s^{-1}. **19.2B** $t = 1.60 \times 10^5$ y. **19.3A** Fraction remaining $= 1/2^{30} = 9.3 \times 10^{-10}$; time required, 30×8.040 days $= 241.2$ days. **19.3B** (b). There are about 10 times more ^{24}Na atoms than ^{11}C, but ^{11}C atoms disintegrate about 50 times as fast. There are about $10^4 - 10^5$ times as many ^{238}U atoms as ^{11}C, but $t_{1/2}$ of ^{238}U exceeds that of ^{11}C by a factor of more than 10^9. **19.4A** 6.0 dis min^{-1} per g carbon. **19.4B** The activity falls to one-half its initial value in 12.26 y ($t_{1/2}$ for tritium). The brandy is only about 12 years old, not 25. **19.5A** $^{35}_{17}Cl + ^{1}_{0}n \longrightarrow ^{35}_{16}S + ^{1}_{1}H$. **19.5B** $^{249}_{98}Cf + ^{15}_{7}N \longrightarrow ^{260}_{105}Db + 4\,^{1}_{0}n$. **19.6A** $^{74}_{30}Zn$ lies above the belt of stability and is radioactive. **19.6B** "Magic numbers" of protons and neutrons in ^{40}Ca and ^{48}Ca make them stable. (Isotopes with $Z = 20$ and $A = 42, 44$, and 46 are also stable.) ^{39}Ca is below the belt of stability in Figure 19.5 and is radioactive.

19.7A ^{84}Y has 39 protons and 45 neutrons and lies outside the belt of stability (Figure 19.5). It should decay by electron capture or positron emission to yield ^{84}Sr, which is within the belt of stability and could be stable. **19.7B** $^{17}_{9}F \longrightarrow ^{17}_{8}O + ^{0}_{1}e$ and $^{22}_{9}F \longrightarrow ^{22}_{10}Ne + ^{0}_{-1}e$. **19.8A** $\Delta E = -5.0$ MeV. **19.8B** Energy requirement $= \Delta E = 2.7$ MeV. To convert from atomic to nuclear masses subtract the mass of 15 electrons from each side of the equation. The same result is obtained by using either atomic or nuclear masses. **Self-Assessment Questions: 2.** (b). **3.** (c). **5.** (d). **7.** 74 days. **10.** (d). **11.** (a). **13.** (c). **15.** The minimum mass of a fissionable isotope that must be brought into a small volume for a self-sustaining nuclear fission reaction to occur. **Problems: 21.** (a) 86, ^{215}Po; (b) Tm, ^{167}Er; (c) ^{90}Y; (d) ^{79}Br. **23.** (a) Cd-123; (b) Rh-103; (c) Bi-209. **25.** (a) ^{7}Be; (b) ^{242}Pu.

27.

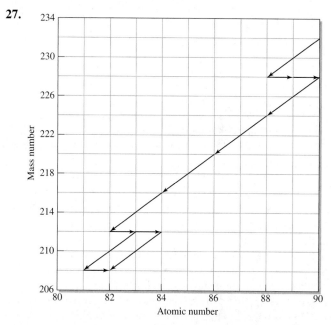

29. Chemical reactions occur as a result of collisions, and their rates depend on the reaction mechanism. Different mechanisms lead to different overall reaction orders. The rate at which the nuclei of a particular nuclide decay depends on how many of them are present. Thus, the process is first order. **31.** (a) ^{15}O has the shortest half-life and the greatest activity. (b) A 75% reduction represents two half-life periods. The required $t_{1/2}$ is one day, and the nuclide having about this half-life is ^{28}Mg. **33.** For equal masses, the number of atoms (N) is about four times as great for ^{32}P as for ^{131}I. The decay constant (λ) of ^{32}P is about one-half that of ^{131}I. Because A is proportional to both λ and N, A of ^{32}P is about twice that of $^{131}I(4 \times 1/2 = 2)$. **35.** (a) 6.03×10^4 atoms/h; (b) 2.04×10^6 atoms/h. **37.** $t_{1/2} = 88.5$ d. **39.** (a) Not quite 3 half-lives elapse, so the activity should be about 1/8 the original activity or 110 dis/min; (b) 119 dis/min. **41.** 11 dis min^{-1} per g carbon. **43.** (a) $^{1}_{0}n$; (b) $^{2}_{1}H$; (c) $^{4}_{2}He$. **45.** (a) $2\,^{2}_{1}H \longrightarrow ^{3}_{2}He + ^{1}_{0}n$; (b) $^{241}_{95}Am + ^{4}_{2}He \longrightarrow ^{243}_{97}Bk + 2\,^{1}_{0}n$; (c) $^{238}_{92}U + ^{4}_{2}He \longrightarrow ^{239}_{94}Pu + 3\,^{1}_{0}n$. **47.** $^{99}_{43}Tc + ^{1}_{0}n \longrightarrow ^{100}_{43}Tc \longrightarrow ^{100}_{44}Ru + ^{0}_{-1}e$. **49.** 0.5301 u. **51.** 8.520 MeV/nucleon. **53.** -1.8 MeV. **55.** (a) 227.9793 u; (b) 228.0287 u. **57.** 11.0 MeV. **59.** (a) is radioactive because there are fewer neutrons than protons; (d) should be radioactive with an odd number of neutrons and of protons; (b) and (c) have a neutron-to-proton ratio near 1 but greater than 1, and should be stable. **61.** ^{36}Cl (17p, 19n) and ^{64}Cu (29p, 35n) do not occur naturally, even though their atomic masses

are close to the weighted average atomic mass of the element (35.4527 u for Cl and 63.546 u for Cu). They are "odd-odd" nuclides and are radioactive. **63.** ^{40}Ca is a "doubly magic" nuclide (20p, 20n) with a neutron:proton ratio of 1 : 1. These factors contribute to the stability of a nuclide of relatively low atomic number. **65.** $\Delta E = -183.6$ MeV. **67.** A nuclide with a very short half-life decays so quickly that it is not a significant hazard, whereas one with a very long half-life has a very low activity and is less hazardous for that reason. **69.** 320 g $<$ mass of ^{131}I $<$ 400 g. **71.** A few micrometers at most. A positron will annihilate an electron upon encountering one, and there are a lot of electrons in matter, even gaseous matter. **73.** Inject a small amount of ^{3}H into the stream, or add an inert radioactive gaseous element such as ^{41}Ar($t_{1/2}$, 1.83 h) or ^{37}Ar($t_{1/2}$, 35 d) and look for radioactivity around the pipes. **Additional Problems: 78.** -4.3 MeV. **79.** 25 pm. **80.** (a) $4n + 2$; (b) $4n$; (c) $4n + 3$; (d) $4n + 3$. **81.** 4.01 MeV, 1.39×10^7 m/s. **82.** 3.65×10^{-7} g. **86.** 238 dis/s. **89.** 2.1×10^3 L. **92.** cobalt-57: $1s^12s^22p^63s^23p^64s^23d^7$, cobalt-57: $1s^22s^12p^63s^23p^64s^23d^7$, 6.70×10^5 kJ/mol. **93.** The stable isotopes of Cu are ^{63}Cu and ^{65}Cu. Unstable ^{64}Cu lies between the two in Figure 19.4, rather than above or below the stable isotopes. Thus, it attains stability by beta emission to form ^{64}Zn (stable) or by either positron emission or electron capture to form ^{64}Ni. **Apply Your Knowledge: 94.** Uranium I = ^{238}U; Uranium X$_1$ = ^{234}Th; Uranium X$_2$ = ^{234}Pa; Uranium II = ^{234}U; Ionium = ^{230}Th; Radium = ^{226}Ra **95.** $\sim 1.1 \times 10^{-5}$%, by calculating each element separately. **99.** Plot ln A versus time in minutes. The slope is -0.305 min^{-1}, the half-life = $-0.693/(-0.305$ min$^{-1}) = 2.27$ min.

Chapter 20

Exercises: 20.1A (a) 2 NaCl(l) $\xrightarrow{\text{electrolysis}}$ 2 Na(l) + Cl$_2$(g), followed by 2 Na(s) + H$_2$(g) $\longrightarrow$ 2 NaH(s); (b) 2 NaCl(aq) + 2 H$_2$O(l) $\xrightarrow{\text{electrolysis}}$ 2 NaOH(aq) + Cl$_2$(g) + H$_2$(g), followed by 2 NaOH(aq) + Cl$_2$(g) $\longrightarrow$ NaCl(aq) + NaOCl(aq) + H$_2$O(l). **20.1B** 2 Na(s) + 2 H$_2$O(l) $\longrightarrow$ 2 NaOH(aq) + H$_2$(g), NaOH(aq) + SO$_2$(g) $\longrightarrow$ Na$_2$SO$_3$(aq) **20.2A** Maximum mass: 1.658 g (exclusively MgO); minimum mass: 1.384 g (exclusively Mg$_3$N$_2$). **20.2B** Most of the product was MgO. Since N$_2$ is much more abundant in the atmosphere than is O$_2$, it would appear that the rate of reaction of Mg with O$_2$ is much greater than with N$_2$. **Self-Assessment Questions: 1.** Sodium, calcium; some common naturally occurring compounds: NaCl, Na$_2$CO$_3$; CaCl$_2$, CaCO$_3$, CaSO$_4$. **4.** There is no change in amount of H$_2$SO$_4$ because only H$_2$O(l) is electrolyzed. If significant amounts of water are electrolyzed, the concentration of H$_2$SO$_4$ increases. **5.** Because its filled 1s shell gives it properties similar to that of the noble gases. **7.** (c). **13.** (c). **Problems: 21.** Order of increasing solubility: MgCO$_3$ < Li$_2$CO$_3$ < Na$_2$CO$_3$. Interionic attractions are strongest between the small, highly charged Mg^{2+} and CO$_3$$^{2-}$, and are greater for Li$_2CO_3$ than Na$_2$CO$_3$ because Li$^+$ is a smaller ion than Na$^+$. **23.** Density, electrode potential, electrical conductivity, and hardness; these properties depend on two or more factors that vary down the periodic table. **25.** (a) potassium peroxide; (b) calcium hydrogen carbonate; (c) Ba$_3$(PO$_4$)$_2$; (d) Sr(NO$_3$)$_2 \cdot$ 4 H$_2$O. **27.** (a) CaO, calcium oxide; (b) Na$_2$SO$_4 \cdot$ 10 H$_2$O, sodium sulfate decahydrate; (c) CaSO$_4 \cdot$ 2 H$_2$O, calcium sulfate dihydrate; (d) CaCO$_3 \cdot$ MgCO$_3$, calcium magnesium carbonate. **29.** MgCO$_3$(s) + 2 HCl(aq) $\longrightarrow$ H$_2$O(l) + CO$_2$(g) + MgCl$_2$(aq)

$\xrightarrow{\text{evaporation}}$ MgCl$_2$(s) $\xrightarrow{\Delta,\text{ electrolysis}}$ Mg(l) + Cl$_2$(g). **31.** H$_2$SO$_4$(conc aq) + 2 NaCl(s) $\xrightarrow{\Delta}$ Na$_2$SO$_4$(s) + 2 HCl(g); Na$_2$SO$_4$(s) + 10 H$_2$O(l) $\longrightarrow$ Na$_2$SO$_4 \cdot$ 10 H$_2$O(s) (Glauber's salt). Heating the salt of a volatile acid with a nonvolatile acid drives off the volatile acid. **33.** NaOH(s) has to be prepared from NaCl(aq) by electrolysis. To obtain Na from NaOH requires an additional electrolysis. This is a more expensive route than to electrolyze NaCl(l), despite the requirement of a higher temperature.

35.

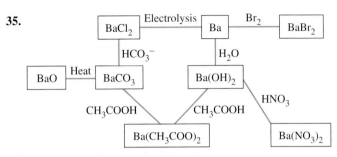

37. Electrolysis of MgCl$_2$(aq) will produce hydrogen gas rather than magnesium metal. **39.** (a) Ca(s) + 2 HCl(aq) $\longrightarrow$ H$_2$(g) + CaCl$_2$(aq); (b) KHCO$_3$(s) + HCl(aq) $\longrightarrow$ KCl(aq) + H$_2$O(l) + CO$_2$(g); (c) 2 NaF(s) + H$_2$SO$_4$(concd aq) $\xrightarrow{\Delta}$ Na$_2$SO$_4$(s) + 2 HF(g). **41.** (a) 2 Li(s) + Cl$_2$(g) $\longrightarrow$ 2 LiCl(s); (b) 2 K(s) + 2 H$_2$O(l) $\longrightarrow$ 2 KOH(aq) + H$_2$(g); (c) 2 Cs(s) + Br$_2$(l) $\longrightarrow$ 2 CsBr(s); (d) K(s) + O$_2$(g) $\longrightarrow$ KO$_2$(s). **43.** (a) BeF$_2$(s) + 2 Na(l) $\xrightarrow{\Delta}$ Be(s) + 2 NaF(s); (b) Ca(s) + 2 CH$_3$COOH(aq) $\longrightarrow$ Ca(CH$_3$COO)$_2$(aq) + H$_2$(g); (c) PuO$_2$(s) + 2 Ca(s) $\xrightarrow{\Delta}$ Pu(s) + 2 CaO(s); (d) CaCO$_3 \cdot$ MgCO$_3$(s) $\xrightarrow{\Delta}$ CaO(s) + MgO(s) + 2 CO$_2$(g). **45.** (a) MgCO$_3$(s) + 2 HCl(aq) $\longrightarrow$ MgCl$_2$(aq) + H$_2$O(l) + CO$_2$(g); (b) CO$_2$(g) + 2 KOH(aq) $\longrightarrow$ K$_2$CO$_3$(aq) + H$_2$O(l); (c) 2 KCl(s) + H$_2$SO$_4$(conc aq) $\xrightarrow{\Delta}$ K$_2$SO$_4$(s) + 2 HCl(g). **47.** (a) 2 NaCl(s) + H$_2$SO$_4$(conc aq) $\xrightarrow{\Delta}$ Na$_2$SO$_4$(s) + 2 HCl(g); (b) Mg(HCO$_3$)$_2$(aq) $\xrightarrow{\Delta}$ MgCO$_3$(s) + H$_2$O(l) + CO$_2$(g), followed by MgCO$_3$(s) $\xrightarrow{\Delta}$ MgO(s) + CO$_2$(g). **49.** 594 g CaH$_2$. **51.** 267 m^3 CO$_2$. **53.** 694 L seawater. **55.** (c). **57.** NH$_3$ (a base) reacts with HCO$_3$$^-$ (an acid): NH$_3$(aq) + HCO$_3$$^-$(aq) $\longrightarrow$ NH$_4$$^+$(aq) + CO$_3$$^{2-}$(aq). This is followed by M^{2+}(aq) + CO$_3$$^{2-}$(aq) $\longrightarrow$ MCO$_3$(s), where M^{2+} = Mg^{2+}, Ca^{2+}, or Fe^{2+}. **59.** 68.4-mg boiler scale (CaCO$_3$). **61.** A limestone cave and hard water both form through the forward direction of the reaction: CaCO$_3$(s) + H$_2$O(l) + CO$_2$(g) $\rightleftharpoons$ Ca(HCO$_3$)$_2$(aq). Stalactites and stalagmites form in the reverse of this reaction, as does boiler scale when hard water is boiled. **63.** In a cation exchange, all cations are replaced by H$^+$. Then, in an anion exchange, all anions are replaced by OH$^-$. The H$^+$ and OH$^-$ combine to form H$_2$O, and the water is essentially free of all ions. **Additional Problems: 65.** (a) 4 Li(s) + O$_2$(g) $\longrightarrow$ 2 Li$_2$O(s); (b) 6 Li(s) + N$_2$(g) $\longrightarrow$ 2 Li$_3$N(s); (c) Li$_2$CO$_3$ $\xrightarrow{\Delta}$ Li$_2$O(s) + CO$_2$(g). **66.** 2 Na$_2$O$_2$(s) + 2 CO$_2$(g) $\longrightarrow$ 2 Na$_2$CO$_3$(s) + O$_2$(g). **67.** The CaO(s) is converted to CaCO$_3$(s) by one or both of these routes: CaO(s) + CO$_2$(g) $\longrightarrow$ CaCO$_3$(s), or CaO(s) + H$_2$O(l) $\longrightarrow$ Ca(OH)$_2$(s), followed by Ca(OH)$_2$(s) + CO$_2$(g) $\longrightarrow$ CaCO$_3$(s) + H$_2$O(g). **71.** 60.2% MgO(s). **74.** (a) Ca^{2+}(aq) + Na$_2$CO$_3$(aq) $\longrightarrow$ CaCO$_3$(s) + 2 Na$^+$(aq); (b) 21 g. **80.** (a) 1.7 g sodium dodecyl sulfate; (b) 3.1×10^{-12} C; (c) The surfactant is a salt and does not dissolve well in oil-based (nonpolar solvent) paint. In

latex paint the surfactant dissolves readily and can easily be carried to the particles. **83.** Spectroscopic methods should reveal whether the emitted radiation is that of hydrogen or of other elements. **Apply Your Knowledge: 84.** 80.56 ppm Ca^{2+}. **85.** The battery operates for 34 years and consumes 0.13 g $Li(s)$. **89.** About $300,000. **91.** 246 kg/day.

Chapter 21

Exercises: 21.1A $2 BCl_3(g) + 3 H_2(g) \longrightarrow 2 B(s) + 6 HCl(g)$. **21.1B** $[B_2O_4(OH)_4]^{2-}(aq) + 4 H_2O(l) \longrightarrow 2 H_2O_2(aq) + 2[B(OH)_4]^-(aq)$ **21.2A** The reaction is nonspontaneous for standard-state conditions: $E°_{cell} = -0.90$ V and $\Delta G° = 174$ kJ. The $\Delta G°$ differs from Example 21.2 because of different standard states, such as 1 M $Br^-(aq)$ instead of $NaBr(s)$ and 1 M $H^+(aq)$ and 1 M $SO_4^{2-}(aq)$ instead of $H_2SO_4(l)$. **21.2B** The reaction in question differs from that in Example 21.2 only in that 2 $NaI(s)$ is substituted for 2 $NaBr(s)$ on the left and $I_2(g)$ for $Br_2(g)$ on the right. Instead of redoing the complete calculation of Example 21.2, replace 3.14 by 19.36 on the right and $2 \times (-349.0)$ by $2 \times (-286)$ on the left. Thus to the numerical answer for Example 21.2 (54), *add* $(19.36 - 3.14) = 16.22$; and *subtract* $[(-2 \times 286) - (-2 \times 349)] = 126$. The new answer is 54 kJ + 16.22 kJ − 126 kJ = −56 kJ. The oxidation of sodium iodide to $I_2(g)$ is spontaneous at 25 °C, and so it must become spontaneous at a lower temperature than does the oxidation of sodium bromide to $Br_2(g)$. **Self-Assessment Questions: 3.** Oxygen, silicon, aluminum. **4.** Most active *p*-block metal: Al; nonmetal, F. **8.** Even though a larger cable of Al is required to carry the same amount of current, the mass of the cable is less because of the considerably lower density of Al compared to Cu. **15.** Water has extensive hydrogen bonding between molecules, resulting in a higher boiling point than H_2S, for which hydrogen bonding is unimportant. **21. (a)** silver azide; **(b)** potassium thiocyanate; **(c)** astatine oxide, **(d)** telluric acid. **22. (a)** H_2SeO_4; **(b)** H_2Te; **(c)** $Pb(N_3)_2$; **(d)** $AgAt$. **23.** bauxite, Al_2O_3; boric oxide, B_2O_3; corundum, Al_2O_3; cyanogen, $(CN)_2$; hydrazine, N_2H_4; silica, SiO_2. **Problems: 25.** $3 Mg(s) + B_2O_3 \xrightarrow{\Delta} 2 B(s) + 3 MgO(s)$. **27.** H_3BO_3 is an acid because it accepts OH^- from water, forming H_3O^+. The $B(OH)_3$ molecule is able to accept only one OH^- through the lone pair of electrons on the boron atom, and is therefore monoprotic. H_3PO_4 donates protons and can lose three H^+ ions from the molecule. **29.** $Na_2B_4O_7 \cdot 10 H_2O + H_2SO_4 \longrightarrow$
$4 B(OH)_3 + Na_2SO_4 + 5 H_2O; 2 B(OH)_3 \xrightarrow{\Delta} B_2O_3 + 3 H_2O; B_2O_3 + 3 Cl_2 + 3 C \longrightarrow 3 CO + 2 BCl_3; 2 BCl_3 + 3 H_2 \longrightarrow 6 HCl + 2 B.$ **31.** $2 BCl_3 + 6 LiAlH_4 \longrightarrow B_2H_6 + 6 AlH_3 + 6 LiCl.$ **33.** $12 NaHCO_3 + 4 KAl(SO_4)_2 \xrightarrow{\Delta} 6 Na_2SO_4 + 2 K_2SO_4 + 4 Al(OH)_3 + 12 CO_2.$ **35.** Both iron and aluminum oxidize in air, but unlike iron(III) oxide, aluminum's oxide coating is thin and strongly adherent, and protects the underlying metal from further corrosion, so the metal appears not to "rust". **37.** $2 Al(s) + Fe_2O_3(s) \longrightarrow Al_2O_3(s) + 2 Fe(l); \Delta H \approx -852$ kJ. The ΔH value is only an estimate because it is based on data at 298 K, and because it assumes the product $Fe(s)$ rather than $Fe(l)$. **39.** Because the precipitate of $Al(OH)_3$ is amphoteric and will dissolve.

41. $\ddot{S}{=}C{=}\ddot{O}:$ $[:C{\equiv}N:]^-$ $[:\ddot{O}{-}C{\equiv}N:]^-$

43. $Al_4C_3(s) + 12 H_2O(l) \longrightarrow 3 CH_4 + 4 Al(OH)_3.$ **45.** Geometric structure: two tetrahedra sharing a corner. **47.** $KAl_2(AlSi_3O_{10})(OH)_2$. Oxidation numbers $[1 \times 1](K) + [3 \times 3](Al) + [3 \times 4](Si) + [12 \times (-2)](O) + [2 \times 1](H) = 0$. **49. (a)** $Si(CH_3)_4$; **(b)** $SiCl_2(CH_3)_2$; **(c)** $SiH(CH_2CH_3)_3$. **51. (a)** Yes; **(b)** No; **(c)** Yes; **(d)** No. **53. (a)** $Sn(s) + 2 HCl(aq) \longrightarrow SnCl_2(aq) + H_2(g)$; **(b)** $SnCl_2 + Cl_2(g) \longrightarrow SnCl_4$; **(c)** $SnCl_4(aq) + 4 NH_3(aq) + 2 H_2O(l) \longrightarrow SnO_2(s) + 4 NH_4^+(aq) + 4 Cl^-(aq)$. **55.** $f < d < c < a < b < e$. **57. (a)** $3 NO_2(g) + H_2O(l) \longrightarrow 2 HNO_3(l) + NO(g)$; **(b)** $4 NH_3(g) + 5 O_2(g) \longrightarrow 4 NO(g) + 6 H_2O(g)$; **(c)** $NH_4NO_3(s) \xrightarrow{200 °C} N_2O(g) + 2 H_2O(g)$. **59.** Oxidation: $NH_2NH_3^+(aq) \longrightarrow N_2(g) + 5 H^+(aq) + 4 e^-$; reduction: $Fe^{3+}(aq) + e^- \longrightarrow Fe^{2+}(aq)$; redox reaction: $4 Fe^{3+}(aq) + NH_2NH_3^+(aq) \longrightarrow 4 Fe^{2+}(aq) + N_2(g) + 5 H^+(aq)$; $E°_{N_2/NH_2NH_3^+} = -0.23$ V. **61.** Principal allotropes: white P and red P; structures: white P consists of individual P_4 tetrahedra and red P consists of P_4 units joined together into long chains. **63.** $P_4(s) + 3 KOH(aq) + 3 H_2O(l) \longrightarrow 3 KH_2PO_2(aq) + PH_3(g)$.

65. (a) $4 Al(s) + 3 O_2(g) \longrightarrow 2 Al_2O_3(s)$; **(b)** $2 KClO_3(s) \xrightarrow{\Delta} 2 KCl(s) + 3 O_2(g)$; **(c)** $2 Na_2O_2(s) + 2 H_2O(l) \longrightarrow 4 NaOH(aq) + O_2(g)$; **(d)** $Pb^{2+}(aq) + H_2O(l) + O_3(g) \longrightarrow PbO_2(s) + 2 H^+(aq) + O_2(g)$. **67.** Because of its low melting point (119 °C) S_8 is melted by superheated water. The water and $S_8(l)$ do not form a solution or react, and the mixture can be brought to the surface with compressed air. The $S_8(s)$ is in a pure state. **69.** Oxidation: $2 S(s) + 6 OH^- \longrightarrow S_2O_3^{2-} + 3 H_2O + 4 e^-$; reduction: $2 SO_3^{2-} + 3 H_2O + 4 e^- \longrightarrow S_2O_3^{2-} + 6 OH^-$; overall: $SO_3^{2-}(aq) + S(s) \longrightarrow S_2O_3^{2-}(aq)$. **71.** Only $Cl_2(g)$ will oxidize $Br^-(aq)$ to $Br_2(l)$. $I_2(s)$ is too poor an oxidizing agent for this, and I^-, Cl^-, and F^- can only act as reducing agents. **73.** $I^-(aq) + 3 Cl_2(g) + 3 H_2O(l) \longrightarrow IO_3^-(aq) + 6 Cl^-(aq) + 6 H^+(aq)$; $2 Br^-(aq) + Cl_2(g) \longrightarrow 2 Cl^-(aq) + Br_2(l)$; When the mixture, $IO_3^-(aq) + Cl^-(aq) + Br_2(l)$, is extracted with $CS_2(l)$, only the $Br_2(l)$ dissolves in the $CS_2(l)$. **75.** $MgBr_2$ is a halide, $NaClO_3$ is a halate (chlorate) salt, BrF_3 is neither. **77. (a)** $2 KI(s) + 2 H_2SO_4(concd aq) \longrightarrow I_2(s) + K_2SO_4(aq) + 2 H_2O(l) + SO_2(g)$; **(b)** $KI(s) + H_3PO_4(concd aq) \longrightarrow HI(g) + KH_2PO_4(s)$. **79. (a)** Square planar; **(b)** square pyramidal. **81.** Argon is produced only by the decay of potassium-40, whereas helium is derived from alpha particles. Alpha particles are emitted by many radioactive isotopes, particularly those of high atomic and mass numbers. **Additional Problems: 83. (a)** BrF_3: 28 valence electrons; VSEPR notation AX_3E_2; electron-group geometry, trigonal bipyramidal; molecular shape, T-shaped; **(b)** IF_5: 42 valence electrons; VSEPR notation AX_5E; electron-group geometry, octahedral; molecular shape, square pyramidal. **86.** $2 Al(s) + 2 KOH(aq) + 6 H_2O(l) \longrightarrow 2 KAl(OH)_4(aq) + 3 H_2(g)$; $KAl(OH)_4(aq) + 2 H_2SO_4(aq) + 8 H_2O(l) \longrightarrow KAl(SO_4)_2 \cdot 12 H_2O(s)$ **91.** 1.4×10^4 L air. **92.** 334 kg C, 1.89×10^3 kg Al_2O_3, 1.07×10^{10} coulombs. **95.** $[NO_3^-] = 0.1716$ M. **98. (a)** $\Delta H°_f[ClF] \approx -50$ kJ/mol; **(b)** $\Delta H°_f[OF_2] \approx 34$ kJ/mol; **(c)** $\Delta H°_f[Cl_2O] \approx 82$ kJ/mol; **(d)** $\Delta H°_f[NF_3] \approx -129$ kJ/mol. **Apply Your Knowledge: 105.** 5×10^{37} O_3 molecules.

Chapter 22

Exercises: 22.1A Essentially nothing. The match used in an attempt to ignite the dichromate salt might flare a bit initially, with

the dichromate, an oxidizing agent, promoting the oxidation of the match. However, a reaction could not be sustained, because there is no reducing agent in the solid. **22.1B** $4 \text{FeCr}_2\text{O}_4 + 16 \text{NaOH} + 7 \text{O}_2 \xrightarrow{\Delta} 8 \text{Na}_2\text{CrO}_4 + 4 \text{Fe(OH)}_3 + 2 \text{H}_2\text{O}$. **22.2A** $\text{MnO}_4^- (\text{aq}) + 2 \text{H}_2\text{O}(\text{l}) + 3 e^- \longrightarrow \text{MnO}_2(\text{s}) + 4 \text{OH}^-(\text{aq})$; $E° = 0.60$ V. In basic solution, MnO_4^- will oxidize any species having $E° < 0.60$ V, including $\text{Br}^-(\text{aq})$ to $\text{BrO}_3^-(\text{aq})$, $\text{Br}_2(\text{l})$ to $\text{BrO}^-(\text{aq})$, Ag(s) to $\text{Ag}_2\text{O}(\text{s})$, and $\text{NO}_2^-(\text{aq})$ to $\text{NO}_3^-(\text{aq})$. **22.2B (a)** *red*. $\text{BiO}_3^- + 4 \text{H}^+ + 2 e^- \longrightarrow \text{BiO}^+ + 2 \text{H}_2\text{O}$; *oxid*. $\text{Mn}^{2+} + 4 \text{H}_2\text{O} \longrightarrow \text{MnO}_4^- + 8 \text{H}^+ + 5 e^-$; *overall*: $2 \text{Mn}^{2+} + 5 \text{BiO}_3^- + 4 \text{H}^+ \longrightarrow 5 \text{BiO}^+ + 2 \text{MnO}_4^- + 2 \text{H}_2\text{O}$; **(b)** The standard electrode potential for the BiO_3^- reduction to BiO^+ must exceed that of the reduction of MnO_4^- to Mn^{2+}, which is 1.51 V. **22.3A** The coordination and oxidation numbers are **(a)** 6 and $+3$; **(b)** 6 and $+2$. **22.3B** $[\text{CrCl}_2(\text{H}_2\text{O})_4]\text{Cl}$. **22.4A (a)** hexaamminecobalt(II) ion; **(b)** pentaamminebromocobalt(III) bromide. **22.4B (a)** tetrachloroaurate(III) ion; **(b)** triamminediaquabromocobalt(III) tetracyanonickelate(II). **22.5A (a)** $[\text{Co(en)}_3]^{3+}$; **(b)** $[\text{CrCl}_4(\text{NH}_3)_2]^-$. **22.5B (a)** $[\text{Cr(NH}_3)_6][\text{Co(CN)}_6]$; **(b)** $[\text{PtCl}_2(\text{en})_2]\text{SO}_4$. **22.6A (a)** Isomers. NCS^- is bonded to Fe^{3+} through the S atom in one structure and the N atom in the other. **(b)** Isomers. The ligands, NH_3, are bonded to Zn^{2+} in one structure and Cu^{2+} in the other, similarly with Cl^-. **(c)** Not isomers. One compound has two NH_3 ligands and the other has four. **22.6B (a)** No isomerism. The H_2O molecule can take up any one of four equivalent positions, and the NH_3 molecules, the other three. **(b)** Yes, ligands can be interchanged between the complex cation and complex anion, as in $[\text{Pt(NH}_3)_4][\text{CuCl}_4]$. **22.7A** Assuming en ligands attach only at adjacent points on the hexagonal ring, all structures are identical to the following:

22.7B In $[\text{PtCl}_2(\text{NH}_3)_2]$, substitution at adjacent corners of the square (*cis*) is different from substitution at the ends of a diagonal (*trans*). In $[\text{ZnCl}_2(\text{NH}_3)_2]$, all four vertices of a tetrahedron are equivalent and there can be no isomerism. **22.8A** CN^- is a strong field ligand, and the energy separation (Δ) is large. The six d electrons of $[\text{Ar}]3d^6$ are found as three pairs in the lower-energy set of $3d$ orbitals. **22.8B** In a tetrahedral field, the eight $3d$ electrons of $[\text{Ar}]3d^8$ fill the two lower-level and one of the upper-level d orbitals. The other two upper level d orbitals have single electrons. There are two unpaired electrons. **Self-Assessment Questions: 2.** $[\text{Kr}]4d^{10}5s^25p^1$ is the electron configuration of indium, a fifth-period, p-block, main-group element; $[\text{Ar}]3d^74s^2$ is that of cobalt, a fourth-period, d-block, transition element. **5.** (c). **6.** (a). **7.** Co, Ni, and Fe each lose two $4s$ electrons to form 2+ ions, but when iron also loses a $3d$ electron, it obtains a half-filled $3d$ subshell which is especially stable. **8. (a)** scandium chloride; **(b)** iron(II) silicate; **(c)** sodium manganate; **(d)** chromium(VI) oxide. **12.** (c). **13.** (d). **18.** The central atom is part of a complex anion. **20.** (b). **Problems: 23.** To acquire the argon electron configuration, a Ca atom loses two electrons ($4s^2$), whereas Sc loses three ($3d^14s^2$). **25.** The +1 oxidation state might be expected because chromium has a $4s^13d^5$ configuration, and should be capable of losing a single valence electron. **27. (a)** Ca < K because $Z_{\text{eff}} \approx 2$ for Ca and ≈ 1 for K. The nucleus attracts the valence electrons more strongly in Ca.

(b) Mn < Ca because it has a larger nuclear charge but the same number of valence electrons as Ca. **(c)** The Mn and Fe atoms are the same size because they have the same Z_{eff} and the same number of valence electrons. **29. (a)** $2 \text{Sc}(\text{s}) + 6 \text{HCl}(\text{aq}) \longrightarrow 2 \text{ScCl}_3(\text{aq}) + 3 \text{H}_2(\text{g})$; **(b)** $\text{Sc(OH)}_3(\text{s}) + 3 \text{HCl}(\text{aq}) \longrightarrow \text{ScCl}_3(\text{aq}) + 3 \text{H}_2\text{O}(\text{l})$; **(c)** $\text{Sc(OH)}_3(\text{s}) + 3 \text{Na}^+(\text{aq}) + 3 \text{OH}^-(\text{aq}) \longrightarrow 3 \text{Na}^+(\text{aq}) + [\text{Sc(OH)}_6]^{3-}(\text{aq})$. **31. (a)** $\text{K}_2\text{Cr}_2\text{O}_7(\text{aq}) + 14 \text{HCl}(\text{aq}) \longrightarrow 3 \text{Cl}_2(\text{g}) + 2 \text{CrCl}_3(\text{aq}) + 2 \text{KCl}(\text{aq}) + 7 \text{H}_2\text{O}(\text{l})$, separate CrCl_3 and KCl by fractional crystallization; **(b)** $2 \text{MnO}_4^-(\text{aq}) + 5 \text{C}_2\text{O}_4^{2-}(\text{aq}) + 16 \text{H}^+(\text{aq}) \longrightarrow 10 \text{CO}_2(\text{g}) + 2 \text{Mn}^{2+}(\text{aq}) + 8 \text{H}_2\text{O}(\text{l})$, then $\text{Mn}^{2+}(\text{aq}) + \text{Na}_2\text{CO}_3(\text{aq}) \longrightarrow \text{MnCO}_3(\text{s}) + 2 \text{Na}^+(\text{aq})$. **33.** $3 \text{MnO}_2 + \text{KClO}_3 + 6 \text{KOH} \longrightarrow 3 \text{K}_2\text{MnO}_4 + \text{KCl} + 3 \text{H}_2\text{O}$, then $2 \text{K}_2\text{MnO}_4 + \text{Cl}_2 \longrightarrow 2 \text{KMnO}_4 + 2 \text{KCl}$ **35.** CrO_4^{2-} in equilibrium with $\text{Cr}_2\text{O}_7^{2-}$ combines with Pb^{2+} to form $\text{PbCrO}_4(\text{s})$; the net reaction goes to completion. **37.** Fe(s); it is most easily oxidized. That is, $\text{Fe}^{2+}(\text{aq}) + 2 e^- \longrightarrow \text{Fe}(\text{s})$ has the lowest value of $E°$ (-0.440 V). **39.** The reaction $4 \text{Co}^{3+}(\text{aq}) + 2 \text{H}_2\text{O}(\text{l}) \longrightarrow \text{O}_2(\text{g}) + 4 \text{H}^+(\text{aq}) + 4 \text{Co}^{2+}(\text{aq})$ is spontaneous with $E°_{\text{cell}} = 0.69$ V. **41. (a)** $2 \text{Ag}(\text{s}) + 2 \text{H}_2\text{SO}_4(\text{concd aq}) \longrightarrow \text{SO}_2(\text{g}) + 2 \text{H}_2\text{O}(\text{l}) + \text{Ag}_2\text{SO}_4(\text{s})$; **(b)** $3 \text{Ag}(\text{s}) + 4 \text{HNO}_3(\text{concd aq}) \longrightarrow \text{NO}(\text{g}) + 2 \text{H}_2\text{O}(\text{l}) + 3 \text{AgNO}_3(\text{aq})$. **43.** Compare three reduction half-reactions: (1) $\text{NO}_3^- + 4 \text{H}^+ + 3 e^- \longrightarrow \text{NO}(\text{g}) + 2 \text{H}_2\text{O}$, $E° = 0.956$ V; (2) $\text{Ag}^+ + e^- \longrightarrow \text{Ag}(\text{s})$, $E° = 0.800$ V; (3) $\text{Au}^{3+} + 3 e^- \longrightarrow \text{Au}(\text{s})$, $E° = 1.52$ V. The combination of (1) and the reverse of (2) has $E°_{\text{cell}} > 0$; (1) and the reverse of (3) has $E°_{\text{cell}} < 0$. **45.** Compared to Group 2A, the 2B elements form many complex ions and have smaller atomic radii, higher ionization energies, and $E°$ values that are less negative. **47.** No; although $E°$ for Cd^{2+}/Cd is -0.403 V, that potential is less negative than that of the Fe^{2+}/Fe reduction, and so the iron metal will be oxidized while the cadmium remains unchanged. **49. (a)** $3 \text{Hg}(\text{l}) + 2 \text{NO}_3^-(\text{aq}) + 8 \text{H}^+(\text{aq}) \longrightarrow 3 \text{Hg}^{2+}(\text{aq}) + 2 \text{NO}(\text{g}) + 4 \text{H}_2\text{O}(\text{l})$; **(b)** $\text{ZnO}(\text{s}) + 2 \text{CH}_3\text{COOH}(\text{aq}) \longrightarrow \text{Zn}^{2+}(\text{aq}) + 2 \text{CH}_3\text{COO}^-(\text{aq}) + \text{H}_2\text{O}(\text{l})$. **51. (a)** 6; **(b)** 2; **(c)** 4. **53. (a)** 6; **(b)** 3; **(c)** 3; **(d)** 1. **55. (a)** $+2$; **(b)** $+3$; **(c)** $+4$; **(d)** 0. **57. (a)** hexamminezinc(II); **(b)** tetrachloroferrate(II); **(c)** tetramminedichloroplatinum(IV); **(d)** tris(ethylenediamine)cobalt(III). **59. (a)** $[\text{CoF}_6]^{3-}$; **(b)** $[\text{CrCl}_2(\text{H}_2\text{O})_4]^+$; **(c)** $[\text{CoBr}_2(\text{en})_2]^+$. **61. (a)** potassium hexacyanochromate(II); **(b)** potassium tris(oxalato)chromate(III). **63. (a)** $[\text{Cu(NH}_3)_4]\text{Cl}_2$; **(b)** $[\text{Cr(en)}_3][\text{Co(CN)}_6]$; **(c)** $[\text{Pt(NH}_3)_4][\text{PtCl}_4]$. **65. (a)** It is a cation, so the name ends with "copper(II)": tetraaquacopper(II) ion; **(b)** The oxidation state is not given. The correct name could be a neutral complex, pentaamminesulfatocobalt(II), but is more likely a complex ion, pentaamminesulfatocobalt(III) ion. **67. (a)** Yes, these are structural isomers. The NCS^- ion is bonded through the N atom in one and through the S atom in the other; **(b)** Yes, these are isomers. Both have the formula $\text{Pt}_3\text{Cl}_6\text{N}_6\text{H}_{18}$, but the cations and anions differ in composition; **(c)** No, these are different compounds since they have different numbers of K atoms; **(d)** Yes, these are structural isomers, they differ in the ligands on the central metal ion. **69.** The sketch should have Cr^{3+} as the central ion in an octahedron. No matter which pair of adjacent vertices is chosen for linkage of the en ligand, the remaining four vertices for linkage of Cl^- are equivalent. **71.** Yes. Refer to Figure 22.15. Replace any two en ligands by ox, both in the structure on the left and in its mirror image. The resulting structures are still nonsuperimposable mirror images. **73.** Four different groups can be arranged in just two

different ways in a tetrahedral complex, and those two ways are mirror images of one another. **75.** (a) $Cr^{3+}[Ar]3d^3$;

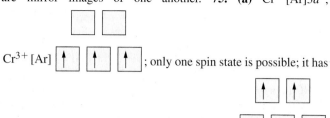

; only one spin state is possible; it has three unpaired e^-. (b) $Fe^{3+}[Ar]3d^5$; Fe^{3+} [Ar] because Cl^- is a weak-field ligand, we expect the high-spin state with all five e^- unpaired. (c) $Mn^{3+}[Ar]3d^4$;

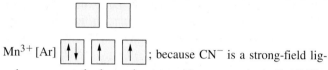

; because CN^- is a strong-field ligand, we expect the low-spin state with two unpaired e^-. (d) The d-orbital sets in a tetrahedral field are reversed from (a)–(c).

$Co^{2+}[Ar]3d^7$; Co^{2+} [Ar] ; only one spin state is possible, with three unpaired $3d$ e^-. **77.** NH_3 is a stronger field ligand than H_2O. Light of shorter wavelength (higher frequency) is absorbed, and light of longer wavelength is transmitted by the ammine complex than by the aqua complex. **Additional Problems: 80.** $2\,Cu(s) + O_2(g) + H_2O(l) + CO_2(g) \longrightarrow Cu_2(OH)_2CO_3(s)$. **81.** One or both of the following reactions should occur: (1) $5\,MnO_4^{2-} + 8\,H^+ \longrightarrow Mn^{2+} + 4\,MnO_4^- + 4\,H_2O$; (2) $3\,MnO_4^{2-} + 4\,H^+ \longrightarrow MnO_2(s) + 2\,MnO_4^- + 2\,H_2O$. **85.** 2.70 g Cr. **89.** In the complex $[Cr(L)_6]^{3+}$, the three d electrons of $Cr^{3+}([Ar]3d^3)$ remain unpaired regardless of the ligand (see also, answer to Problem 75a). **93.** (a) and (c) are identical, (a) and (b) [or (a) and (d)] are geometric isomers, and (b) and (d) are optical isomers. **Apply Your Knowledge: 97.** 61%. **99.** $K[PtCl_3(C_2H_4)]$. **105.** 0.0154 M. The results would have been the same with iron(III) because EDTA reacts with all metal ions in a one-to-one ratio regardless of charge.

Chapter 23

Exercises: 23.1A (a) Aliphatic. The conjugated system is incomplete, and the π-bonding system does not fit the $4n + 2$ rule. (b) Aliphatic. The structure fits the $4n + 2$ rule, but the conjugated system is incomplete. (c) Aliphatic. The conjugated system is complete, but the structure does not fit the $4n + 2$ rule. (d) Aromatic. The conjugated system extends throughout the structure, and 14 π electrons conform to the $4n + 2$ rule (where $n = 3$). **23.1B** The nitrogen atom is sp^2 hybridized, leaving an unshared pair of electrons in an unhybridized p-orbital to contribute to pi-bonding. Pyrrole therefore has six pi-electrons, which fits the $4n + 2$ rule, and the pi-electrons extend around the entire ring. **23.2A** The sign of the optical rotation cannot be predicted from the formulas alone. (a) Gulose is an L-aldohexose; (b) erythrulose is an L-ketoterose. **23.2B** No. The name D-(−)-fructose below the Fischer projection on the previous page establishes that the D-configuration of fructose has been found to be levorotatory. The dextrorotatory or (−) configuration must therefore be the L-configuration. **Self-Assessment Questions: 3.** (c). **6.** (a) aromatic; (b) aliphatic; (c) aliphatic; (d) both. **8.** (a). **13.** (c).

15. (b). **18.** A conjugated system has alternating double and single bonds. Examples: 1,3-butadiene, 1,3,5-hexatriene, lycopene. **19.** IR radiation induces various vibrations of bonds; UV and visible radiation causes electronic transitions. **20.** UV; NMR. **21.** $\tilde{\nu} = \nu/c$. **25.** Penicillin molecules have a β lactam, a four-membered ring with one nitrogen atom and three carbon atoms, one an amide. The amide carbon in penicillin attaches to the enzyme that catalyzes the synthesis of bacterial cell walls, deactivating the enzyme. Human cells do not have cell walls and are not harmed. **32.** When the urine has a lower pH (after a meal, after drinking alcohol, or during periods of stress), more nicotine (a base) is excreted because the conjugate acid (ionic) of nicotine is more soluble in urine. The more nicotine excreted, the more quickly the person craves another cigarette. **Problems:**

33. (a) $CH_2{=}CCH_2CH_3$
          CH_2CH_3

(b) $CH_3CHCH_2CHCH_2CH_3$
      CH_3 CH_2CH_3

(c) $CH_3C{=}CHCHCH_2CCH_3$ with CH_3 groups
      CH_3 CH_3 CH_3

(d) $CH_3CH_2CH{-}CHCH_2CH_2CH_2CH_3$
     $CH_3{-}CH$ CH_2CH_3
          CH_3

(e) $H_2C{-}CHCH_2CH_3$
    $H_2C{-}CH_2$

(f) $CH_3CH{=}CCH_2CH_3$
         CH_2CH_3

35. (a) 2-methyl-2-butene; (b) 1,1,6-trichloro-3-heptyne; (c) 2,2,4-trimethyl-3-hexene; (d) 2-methyl-1-pentene.

37. (a) 2,2-dimethyl-3-pentanol; (b) 2-methyl-1-propanol; (c) 2-chloro-4-iodobenzoic acid; (d) 4-chloro-2-nitroaniline.

39. (a) $CH_3CH_2CH(OH)CH_2CH_2CH_3$; (b) $CH_3CH(OH)C(CH_3)_3$; (c) $CH_3CH_2CH(OH)CH(CH_3)CH(CH_3)CH_2CH_3$; (d) $CH_3CH_2CH(CH_2CH_3)CH_2OH$;

(e) Br, Br ring —COOH   (f) CH_3CHCH_3 ring —COOH

41. (a) carboxylic acid, halide; (b) alkene; (c) carboxylic acid, aromatic ring, halide.

43. (a) $CH_3CH_2CHClCH_2COOH$ 3-chloropentanoic acid

(b) $CH_2{=}CCH_2CH_2CH_3$ 2-ethyl-1-pentene
    CH_2CH_3

(c) Br—ring(Br)—COOH 2,4-dibromobenzoic acid

45. (a) oxidation; (b) hydration. **47.** (a) $CH_3CH_2CH_2CH_3$; (b) $(CH_3)_2C(OH)CH(CH_3)_2$. **49.** (a) $CH_3CH_2CH_2OH$ $\xrightarrow{H_2SO_4, \Delta}$ $CH_3CH=CH_2$; (b) $2 CH_3CH_2CH_2OH$ $\xrightarrow{H_2SO_4}$ $(CH_3CH_2CH_2)_2O$. **51.** (a) $CH_3CH=CH_2$; (b) $CH_2=C(CH_3)_2$. **53.** (a) $CH_3CH_2CH_2COOH + NaHCO_3(aq)$ $\longrightarrow$ $CH_3CH_2CH_2COONa(aq) + CO_2(g) + H_2O(l)$; (b) $CH_3COOCH_2CH_3 + H_2O$ $\xrightarrow{H_2SO_4}$ $CH_3COOH + CH_3CH_2OH$. **55.** (a) Saturated, 8 carbon atoms; (b) unsaturated, 10 carbon atoms; (c) unsaturated, 18 carbon atoms.

57.

$CH_3(CH_2)_{16}COOH$
(a)

$CH_3(CH_2)_{12}COO^-K^+$
(b)

$CH_2OCO(CH_2)_7CH=CH(CH_2)_7CH_3$
$|$
$CHOCO(CH_2)_7CH=CH(CH_2)_7CH_3$
$|$
$CH_2OCO(CH_2)_7CH=CH(CH_2)_7CH_3$
(c)

$CH_2OCO(CH_2)_{14}CH_3$
$|$
$CHOCO(CH_2)_{14}CH_3$
$|$
$CH_2OCO(CH_2)_{14}CH_3$
(d)

59. (a) aldose, triose; (b) aldose, pentose; (c) aldose, pentose; (d) ketose, hexose; (e) aldose, hexose. **61.** (a) D-sugar; (b) L-sugar; (c) D-sugar.

63.

(a)

(b)

65. (a) β; (b) α. **67.** (a) $-CH_2COOH$; (b) $-CH_2SH$; (c) $-CH(CH_3)_2$; (d) $-CH_2OH$; (e) $-CH_2C_6H_5$ (CH_2 on phenyl ring). **69.** Lysine, $NH_2(CH_2)_4CH(NH_2)COOH$, also arginine or histidine (Table 23.2). **71.**

73. (a) pH < pI; (b) pH > pI; (c) pH = pI. **75.** The sugar is ribose; the heterocyclic base is the pyrimidine cytosine. **77.** The molecule is not a nucleotide (no phosphate unit). The base is a pyrimidine (thymine). The compound is incorporated in DNA. **79.** CTAATGT **81.** CUAAUGU **83.** AGGCTA **85.** (a) AAA; (b) GUA; (c) UCG; (d) GGC. **87.** CH_3COOH would show a broad OH peak around $3200-3600$ cm^{-1} while CH_3COOCH_3 would not. **89.** 2-butanol has an $-OH$ band between $3250-3450$ cm^{-1}, 2-butanone has a $C=O$ peak around 1700 cm^{-1}. Either of the two features would be sufficient to distinguish between the compounds. **91.** Yes. It is likely to have one or more of the structural features noted in Table 23.6. **93.** Yellow substances absorb blue-violet light. **Additional Problems: 96.** (a) $CH_3CH_2CH_2OH$; (b) $HOCH_2CH_2OH$; (c) CH_3OH; (d) $(CH_3)_2CHCH_2CH_2OH$.

99.

102. The conjugated system of azobenzene [first structure, $(C_6H_5N)_2$] extends over 14 atoms and should produce a colored compound, while p-hydroxyphenol (second structure) is colorless; its conjugated system is no more extensive than that of benzene. **103.** (a) The second compound has a $C-O$ stretch and CH_3 stretch; the first does not. (b) The first compound has an $O-H$ stretch, but not the second. The second has a $C-O$ stretch, but not the first. **113.** There are four isomers: $ClCH_2CH(CH_3)CH_2CH_3$ (31.1%), $CH_3CH(CH_3)CH_2CHCl$ (15.5%), $CH_3CCl(CH_3)$ CH_2CH_3 (22.3%), and $CH_3CH(CH_3)CHClCH_3$ (31.1%). **114.** (a) $CH_3CH_2CH_2COOCOCH_2CH_2CH_3 + H_2O \longrightarrow$ $2 CH_3CH_2CH_2COOH$, $CH_3CH_2CH_2COOCOCH_2CH_2CH_3 +$ $H_2O + 2 NH_3 \longrightarrow 2 CH_3CH_2CH_2COO^-NH_4^+$; (b) The product of the reaction with $NH_3(aq)$; it is ionic; (c) $CH_3CH_2CH_2CONH_2$. **Apply Your Knowledge: 115.** The molar mass is 5.10 g/0.0500 mol = 102 g/mol. Possible formulas have one COOH group and the molecular formula $C_5H_{10}O_2$: $CH_3CH_2CH_2CH_2COOH$; $CH_3CH_2CH(CH_3)COOH$; $(CH_3)_2CHCH_2COOH$; $(CH_3)_3CCOOH$. **117.** Carbon disulfide and carbon tetrachloride are nonpolar and most useful for infrared spectrometry. They are also useful for NMR because they have no hydrogen atoms to produce an interfering signal. Ionic compounds such as NaCl, AgCl, and KBr have no covalent bonds and no significant vibrational frequencies of absorbance.

Chapter 24

Exercises: 24.1A A metal more active than Zn (for example, Al) would displace some Zn(s), together with the less active metals. This would reduce the yield of Zn in the subsequent electrolysis. Also, a new cation (for example, Al^{3+}) would be introduced, which might deposit with the Zn during electrolysis. **24.1B** $Ag_2S(s) + 4 CN^-(aq) + 2 O_2(g) \longrightarrow 2 Ag(CN)_2^-(aq) + SO_4^{2-}(aq)$ **24.2A** The $-CH_3$ groups are side-chains of the polymer chain; they are not part of the main chain. Also, the repeating unit shown has one C atom with only three bonds in the $-CH-$ portion and one with five bonds in the $-CH_3-$ portion. **24.2B** Since the central carbon atom has no hydrogen atoms, a branched structure, in which the end of one or two propadiene molecules attaches to that central carbon, would be expected. **24.3A** $-[OCH_2CH_2(C=O)]_n$ **24.3B** Serine, threonine, tyrosine have $-OH$ groups in addition to the amino and carboxyl groups. These three could form polyesters as well as polyamides. Tryptophan, asparagine, glutamine, praline, lysine, arginine, and histidine have at least two basic nitrogen atoms in different locations and could form different polyamides. Aspartic and glutamic acid have two (different) carboxyl groups each, and either group could attach to the amino group. **Self-Assessment Questions: 1.** (c). **2.** (b). **5.** Reduction converts a metal oxide to the free metal. The most common reducing agent is carbon. In a few cases, such as HgO, the oxide decomposes to the free metal; a reducing agent is not needed. **7.** (b). **13.** One model of metallic bonding states that the valence electrons are free to move around the remaining atomic cores. It is this electron gas (comprised of valence electrons, not all electrons) in the metal crystal that bonds metal atoms together. **16.** A semiconductor that contains a carefully controlled trace of a specific impurity. A positive hole, characteristic of p-type semiconductor, is a vacancy in the valence band. When a potential is applied to the p-type semiconductor, an adjacent electron "jumps" into the hole, leaving another hole. **17.** (c). **20.** (d). **23.** (b). **Problems 25.** The metal has to be obtainable in a pure form in an economically feasible process. The ore richest in the metal may be

scarce, or it may be in a chemical form that is difficult to reduce. **27.** Cd occurs in Zn ores because of the chemical similarity of Zn and Cd. Cd(l) can be separated from Zn(l) by fractional distillation, or the less active Cd(s) can be displaced from a solution of Zn^{2+} and Cd^{2+} by Zn(s). **29.** Any HgO produced by roasting HgS immediately decomposes to Hg(l) and $O_2(g)$ in the overall reaction $HgS(s) + O_2(g) \longrightarrow Hg(l) + SO_2(g)$. **31.** $2[Ag(CN)_2]^-(aq) + Zn(s) \longrightarrow 2\,Ag(s) + [Zn(CN)_4]^{2-}(aq)$. **33.** (1) $ZnO(s) + H_2SO_4(aq) \longrightarrow ZnSO_4(aq) + H_2O(l)$; (2) $Zn(s) + Cd^{2+}(aq) + SO_4^{2-}(aq) \longrightarrow Cd(s) + Zn^{2+}(aq) + SO_4^{2-}(aq)$; (3) $2\,Zn^{2+}(aq) + 2\,SO_4^{2-}(aq) + 2\,H_2O(l) \xrightarrow{\text{electrolysis}} 2\,Zn(s) + 4\,H^+(aq) + 2\,SO_4^{2-}(aq) + O_2(g)$. Note that sulfuric acid produced in reaction (3) can be recycled into reaction (1). **35.** (1) $Sn(s) + 2\,Cl_2(g) \longrightarrow SnCl_4(l)$; (2) $SnCl_4(l) + (2 + x)H_2O \longrightarrow SnO_2 \cdot x\,H_2O + 4\,HCl(aq)$; (3) $SnO_2 \cdot x\,H_2O \xrightarrow{\Delta} SnO_2(s) + x\,H_2O(g)$; (4) $SnO_2(s) + 2\,C(s) \xrightarrow{\Delta} Sn(s) + 2\,CO(g)$. **37.** 1.7×10^7 kg ore. **39.** $2\,PbS(s) + 3\,O_2(g) \longrightarrow 2\,PbO(s) + 2\,SO_2(g)$; $PbO(s) + C(s) \longrightarrow Pb(l) + CO(g)$; $PbO(s) + CO(g) \longrightarrow Pb(l) + CO_2(g)$ **41.** The $4p$ band of Ca overlaps with the $4s$ band. The numbers of valence e^- and energy levels are greater in the two partly filled overlapping bands of Ca than in the half-filled $4s$ band in K. **43.** All electron transitions in the visible spectrum are possible between appropriate levels in an electron band. Because most of the incident light is reflected, metals have a luster. If certain wavelength components are reflected more strongly than others, the metal is colored. **45.** 1.37×10^{21} energy levels, 2.74×10^{21} electrons. **47.** In a semiconductor, there is an energy gap between the valence and conduction bands. In a metal, either the valence band is itself a conduction band or it overlaps one; there is no energy gap. **49.** (a) n-type; (b) p-type. **51.** See Figure 24.12. In n-type, electrons in the donor level are readily promoted. Positive holes left in the donor level are immobilized. Electrons predominate as charge carriers. In p-type, electrons are promoted to and immobilized in the low-lying acceptor level. Positive holes predominate as charge carriers. **53.** No, the number of electrons that jump the gap *decreases* as the temperature is lowered. **55.** ZnSe and GaP. **57.** (a) Cellophane is regenerated cellulose, the same material as rayon. It is made by treating cellulose with sodium hydroxide and carbon disulfide, and forcing the viscous solution through a narrow slit to form a film. (b) LDPE, low-density polyethylene, has the formula $-(CH_2CH_2)_n-$. It is made by the free-radical polymerization of ethylene, $CH_2{=}CH_2$. Its chains are branched and pack together poorly. **59.** Rubber is elastic because its coiled polymer chains are straightened out during stretching but return to their coiled state when relaxed. Vulcanization forms crosslinks between chains which pull the chains back into their original shape after stretching.

61.

63.

(a)

(b)

65.

(a)

(b)

67. (b) Terephthalic acid, $HO{-}\overset{\displaystyle O}{\overset{\|}{C}}{-}\bigcirc{-}\overset{\displaystyle O}{\overset{\|}{C}}{-}OH$,

and 1,4 phenylenediamine, $H_2N{-}\bigcirc{-}NH_2$

69. Tempered iron is more dense because fcc has a greater packing efficiency than bcc. All tempered metals need not follow this pattern. For example, if a metal underwent transition from fcc to bcc as the temperature was increased, a decrease in density would be seen. **71.** The rate should increase 200 times; the surface area of the finer catalyst is 2.3×10^2 m^2/g **Additional Problems: 73.** 55 g. **75.** In its "nonconducting" mode, the diode will actually conduct a tiny amount of current. The unintended impurity makes the p-type semiconductor behave as n-type to a very limited extent, and vice versa. **77.** Minimum wavelength is 1.09 μm, in the infrared region, so silicon should have sufficient energy levels in its conduction band so that it absorbs all visible light. **81.** 1,2-ethanediol has two $-OH$ groups, whereas 1,2,3-propanetriol has three. The polymer of 1,2,3-propanetriol and 1,2-benzenedicarboxylic acid has extensive crosslinking of polymer chains and is much more rigid than the polymer with 1,2-ethanediol. **84.** 760 u. **Apply Your Knowledge: 88.** 12.8% Mn. **91.** 3.60% Ni.

Chapter 25

Exercises: 25.1A 6.74 mmHg. **25.1B** 0.126 g water vapor. **Self-Assessment Questions: 1. (a)** troposphere; **(b)** stratosphere. **6. (a)** carbon monoxide, CO, and nitrogen oxide, NO; **(b)** CH_4 and CCl_2F_2; **(c)** HNO_3 and/or H_2SO_4. **10.** A combustion mixture that is rich in fuel and lean in $O_2(g)$ promotes the formation of CO(g). Carbon monoxide ties up the iron atoms in hemoglobin, preventing the transport of oxygen to the cells of the body. **13. (a)** The electrostatic precipitator applies a charge to particulates, collecting the particulates out of flue gases. **(b)** A catalytic converter dramatically increases the rate of conversion of hydrocarbons and carbon monoxide to water and carbon dioxide; it also speeds the breakdown of nitrogen oxides to nitrogen and oxygen gases. **19.** Cholera, typhoid fever, dysentery. Industrialized nations destroy disease organisms using Cl_2, O_3, or other oxidizing agents. **22.** BOD = biochemical oxygen demand; the amount of oxygen needed to decompose aerobically the organic matter in water. A high BOD means that there is a lot of organic material in the water, which usually means that the oxygen in the water is used up and living organisms will die. **25.** Because chlorinated hydrocarbons are chemically stable and do not react readily with other compounds. **Problems 47.** (c). Air pressure at 30 km is produced by the 1% of air that is at altitudes beyond 30 km. $P_{bar} \approx 0.01 \times 760$ mmHg ≈ 7.6 mmHg ≈ 10 mmHg. **49.** Lower-molecular-mass species predominate at higher altitudes due to their higher root-mean-square velocities. **51.** 0.263 mol% H_2O; 2.36×10^3 ppm H_2O. **53.** 13.2 mmHg. **55.** The dew point is about 20.4 °C, the temperature at which $P_{H_2O(g)} = 18.0$ mmHg. **57.** Combustion is a redox reaction. The oxidation numbers of the C atoms in fuel can be increased to either +4 (CO_2) or +2 (CO). The reaction of an acid and a carbonate is an acid-base reaction.

The oxidation number of C in carbonates is +4. Only CO_2 can form. **59.** $2 C_6H_{14}(l) + 19 O_2(g) \longrightarrow 12 CO_2(g) + 14 H_2O(l)$. If combustion is incomplete, some C atoms combine with two O atoms (CO_2), some with only one (CO), and some with none (C); we cannot write a unique equation. **61.** Masses in metric tons: **(a)** 7.22 t CH_4; **(b)** 6.42 t C_8H_{18}; **(c)** 5.74 t coal. **63.** At high temperatures, some NO (from N_2 and O_2) is formed in a combustion chamber that contains air, regardless of the fuel. **65. (a)** $S_8(s) + 8 O_2(g) \longrightarrow 8 SO_2(g)$; **(b)** $2 ZnS(s) + 3 O_2(g) \longrightarrow 2 ZnO(s) + 2 SO_2(g)$; **(c)** $2 SO_2(g) + O_2(g) \longrightarrow 2 SO_3(g)$; **(d)** $SO_3(g) + H_2O(l) \longrightarrow H_2SO_4(aq)$; **(e)** $H_2SO_4(aq) + 2 NH_3(aq) \longrightarrow (NH_4)_2SO_4(aq)$. **67. (a)** Water evaporates from sea spray and leaves particles of NaCl(s) suspended in the air. **(b)** Sulfur dioxide emissions are converted to $SO_3(g)$, which reacts with water vapor to form $H_2SO_4(aq)$. Droplets of $H_2SO_4(aq)$ are neutralized by a basic substance (e.g., NH_3) to form solid sulfate particles. **69.** $2 H_3O^+(aq) + CaCO_3(s) \longrightarrow Ca^{2+}(aq) + 3 H_2O(l) + CO_2(g)$. **71.** 4.4×10^3 kg. **Additional Problems: 78. (a)** 4×10^{37} molecules O_3; **(b)** It would be difficult to separate and store the ozone; ozone spontaneously breaks down into O_2 gas; the mass of ozone that would need to be transported is extremely large, on the order of millions of tons. **79.** If *all* the C_8H_{18} were converted to CO—an unlikely happening—the CO level would be about 24 ppm CO, well below the danger level of 35 ppm. **85.** 12 mg O_2/L. **90.** 4.5×10^{13} kg. **Apply Your Knowledge 94.** If all the S in coal were converted to H_2SO_4, about 1.8×10^{11} lb H_2SO_4 would be produced, about twice the current annual U.S. production. **97. (a)** C is limiting. **(b)** $CH_3CHOHCOOH$, $CO(NH_2)_2$, and $NH_4H_2PO_4$ in the mass ratio of 10.70 : 1.566 : 1.000. **98. (a)** 4.9 ppm, 1.40×10^{19} molecules/L; **(b)** 2.29 y; **(c)** 9.7 ppm; **(d)** No.

Photo Credits

Jim Zuckerman/Corbis/Bettmann. Page 460M: Carey B. Van Loon. Page 460T: Herman Eisenbeiss/Photo Researchers, Inc. Page 460BL: Reprinted with permission from Journal Langmuir, 2003, vol. 19., Cover. © 2003 American Chemical Society. Page 460BR, 475(11.7): Richard Megna/Fundamental Photographs. Page 461T: Carey B. Van Loon. Page 461B: Kristen Brochmann/Fundamental Photographs. Page 464: Michael J. Bronikowski, California Institute of Technology/Jet Propulsion Laboratory, Pasadena, CA. Page 467, 475(11.10): Richard Megna/Fundamental Photographs. Page 468a–b: Carey B. Van Loon. Page 469a–b: Carey B. Van Loon. Page 477: Carey B. Van Loon. Page 481: Richard Megna/Fundamental Photographs.

Chapter 12 Page 482: © Chris Newbert/Minden Pictures. Page 484: Photo © copyright Alliance Pharmaceutical Corp. Page 485R: Draeger Safety, Inc. Page 485L: DWI-Safe, Inc. Page 487: Richard Megna/Fundamental Photographs. Page 488a–b: Richard Megna/Fundamental Photographs. Page 492: Susanna Price/Dorling Kindersley Media Library. Page 493T: Richard Megna/Fundamental Photographs. Page 493B: Michael Baytoff/Black Star. Page 494: Richard Megna/Fundamental Photographs. Page 497T: Richard Megna/Fundamental Photographs. Page 497B a–c: Richard Megna/Fundamental Photographs. Page 498: Jens Gunelson. Page 499: Charles D. Winters/Photo Researchers, Inc. Page 501: F. Stuart Westmorland/Photo Researchers, Inc. Page 507: Randy Ury/Corbis/Stock Market. Page 509: Wayne County Government. Page 510: Rod Planck/Photo Researchers, Inc. Page 511: Tom J. Ulrich/Getty Images Inc. - Stone Allstock. Page 512a–c: © Dr. David Phillips/Visuals Unlimited. Page 513: Science Photo Library/Photo Researchers, Inc. Page 515T: Omikron/Science Source/Photo Researchers, Inc. Page 515B, 518(12.10): Stephen Frisch/Stock Boston. Page 516T: Richard Megna/Fundamental Photographs. Page 516B a–b: Carey B. Van Loon. Page 523: Richard Megna/Fundamental Photographs. Page 524a–c: © 2001 Richard Megna/Fundamental Photographs, NYC.

Chapter 13 Page 526: Dr. James E. Lloyd, University of Florida. Page 528T: Loren M. Winters/© Scott Butson, Stuart Pratt and Robert Watts. Page 528M: James Prince/Photo Researchers, Inc. Page 528B: AP/Wide World Photos. Page 530: © Phil Degginger/Color Pic, Inc. Page 554T: Charles D. Winters/Photo Researchers, Inc. Page 554B: Serco International Fire Training Centre, Teesside College. Teesside Airport, Darlington, U.K. Page 559: Richard Megna/Fundamental Photographs. Page 560a–b: Fundamental Photographs. Page 562: Phil Degginger/Color-Pic, Inc. Page 572: James H. Robinson/Photo Researchers, Inc.

Chapter 14 Page 574: Richard Megna/Fundamental Photographs. Page 589: Stock Boston. Page 590: Stamp from the private collection of Professor C.M. Lang, photography by Gary J. Shulfer, University of Wisconsin, Stevens Point. Scott Standard Postage Stamp Catalogue, Scott Pub. Co., Sidney, Ohio. Page 612: Carey B. Van Loon.

Chapter 15 Page 614: © 2003 Richard Megna/Fundamental Photographs. Page 616: Carey B. Van Loon. Page 629: Richard Megna/Fundamental Photographs. Page 631: Richard Megna/Fundamental Photographs. Page 639: Carey B. Van Loon. Page 641T: Carey B. Van Loon. Page 641a–d: Richard Megna/Fundamental Photographs. Page 645: Carey B. Van Loon. Page 649L: © David Papazian/CORBIS. Page 649R: Tom Pantages. Page 651: Dan McCoy/Rainbow. Page 653: Carey B. Van

Loon. Page 654: Richard Megna/Fundamental Photographs. Page 655: Richard Megna/Fundamental Photographs.

Chapter 16 Page 676: AP/Wide World Photos. Page 678: Science Source/Photo Researchers, Inc. Page 682a–b: Richard Megna/Fundamental Photographs. Page 684T: Dr. Terry McCreary. Page 684B: Richard Megna/Fundamental Photographs. Page 686a–b: Carey B. Van Loon. Page 687: Manfred Kage/Peter Arnold, Inc. Page 689a–b: Richard Megna/Fundamental Photographs. Page 691: Carey B. Van Loon. Page 692: Max Listgarten/Visuals Unlimited. Page 694: Richard Megna/Fundamental Photographs. Page 695: Richard Megna/Fundamental Photographs. Page 697: © Joel Gordon 2004. Page 698: Richard Megna/Fundamental Photographs. Page 700a: Richard Megna/Fundamental Photographs. Page 700b: Carey B. Van Loon. Page 702: Carey B. Van Loon. Page 709: Richard Megna/Fundamental Photographs. Page 711R: Kristen Brochmann/Fundamental Photographs. Page 711L: NYC Parks Photo Archive/Fundamental Photographs.

Chapter 17 Page 712: AP/Wide World Photos. Page 714: AP/Wide World Photos. Page 717: Corbis/Bettmann. Page 719: Carey B. Van Loon. Page 721: AP/Wide World Photos. Page 726: Library of Congress. Page 746T: Carey B. Van Loon. Page 746L: JPL/NASA Headquarters. Page 746R: Tom Bochsler/Pearson Education/PH College.

Chapter 18 Page 748: AP/Wide World Photos. Page 750a–b: Carey B. Van Loon. Page 751: Phil Degginger/Color-Pic, Inc. Page 755T: Carey B. Van Loon. Page 755B: Richard Megna/Fundamental Photographs. Page 758: Photograph courtesy of Virginia Tech/Rick Griffiths. Page 764: Carey B. Van Loon. Page 767: Carey B. Van Loon. Page 770: Science Photo Library/Photo Researchers, Inc. Page 774: Carey B. Van Loon. Page 777: Yardney Technical Products, Inc./Alupower, Inc. Page 778: Courtesy of Mercedes-Benz USA/H. Mock/Dr. R. Krauss. Page 779: John Mead/Science Photo Library/Photo Researchers, Inc. Page 780T: Phil Degginger/Color-Pic, Inc. Page 780B: Robert Erlbacher/Missouri Dry Dock and Repair Company, Inc. Page 781: Carey B. Van Loon. Page 785: Library of Congress. Page 788: PPG Industries Inc. Page 794: Carey B. Van Loon. Page 796: New York Convention & Visitors Bureau.

Chapter 19 Page 798: Bruce E. Zuckerman © West Semitic Research/Dead Sea Scrolls. CORBIS. Page 804: Science VU/National Library of Medicine/Visuals Unlimited. Page 807: Gianni Tortoli/Science Source/Photo Researchers, Inc. Page 809: Corbis/Bettmann. Page 810: AP/Wide World Photos. Page 816T: © Royalty-Free/CORBIS. Page 816B: © Y. Arthus-Bertrand/Peter Arnold, Inc. Page 818: U.S. Department of Energy/Photo Researchers, Inc. Page 819: Yoav Levy/Phototake NYC. Page 823: Runk/Schoenberger/Grant Heilman Photography, Inc.

Chapter 20 Page 832: H. Ford/JHU, and NASA. Page 834: Royal Observatory, Edinburgh, Scotland/Anglo-Australian Telescope Board/Science Photo Library/Photo Researchers, Inc. Page 835T: Ed Degginger/Color-Pic, Inc. Page 835B: © Reuters NewMedia Inc./CORBIS/Joe Polimeni. Page 836T: Richard Megna/Fundamental Photographs. Page 836B: Photo courtesy of Jonathan Slack, Lawrence Berkeley National Laboratory. Page 837a–c: Richard Megna/Fundamental Photographs Page 837d–e: Ed Degginger/Color-Pic, Inc. Page 838: H. Mock/Dr. R. Krauss/Mercedes-Benz USA, Photo Library. Page 839: Richard Megna/Fundamental Photographs. Page 840T: Mark E. Gibson/Visuals Unlimited. Page

840B: Photo Courtesy Mine Safety Appliances Company (MSA) www.msanet.com. Page 841T: Phil Degginger/Color-Pic, Inc. Page 841M: Department of Clinical Radiology, Salisbury District Hospital/Science Photo Library/Photo Researchers, Inc. Page 841B: NASA/Johnson Space Center. Page 843: Tom Pantages. Page 844, 856(20.7): David Cavagnaro/Peter Arnold, Inc. Page 845: Steve Gorton/Dorling Kindersley Media Library. Page 847T, 856(20.9): E. Nagele/Getty Images, Inc. - Taxi. Page 847M: © Jeff Scovil. Page 847B: Robert "Bob" Burns. Page 848: Richard Megna/Fundamental Photographs. Page 849T: Portland Cement Association. Page 849M: James L. Almos/Peter Arnold, Inc. Page 849B: Tom Pantages. Page 850: Michael Collier. Page 851T: Howard Sochurek/Corbis/Stock Market. Page 851B: Richard Megna/Fundamental Photographs. Page 852T, 856(20.12): Francoise Sauze/Science Photo Library/Photo Researchers, Inc. Page 852B: George Kelvin/Phototake NYC. Page 853: Dr. Terry McCreary. Page 854B: Richard Megna/Fundamental Photographs. Page 854T: Richard Megna/Fundamental Photographs.

Chapter 21 Page 862: Anderson, Theodore/Getty Images Inc. - Image Bank. Page 864: Richard Megna/Fundamental Photographs. Page 866T: © E. R. Degginger/Color Pic, Inc. Page 866B: Photo courtesy of U.S. Borax Inc. Page 867T: UPI/Corbis/Bettmann. Page 867B: Corbis/Bettmann. Page 869: Ed Degginger/Color-Pic, Inc. Page 870T: Carey B. Van Loon. Page 870a: Vaughan Fleming/Science Photo Library/Photo Researchers, Inc. Page 871T: Chatham Created Gems, Inc. Page 871B: Paul Silverman/Fundamental Photographs. Page 872T: Russell Munson/Corbis/Stock Market. Page 872B: J. and L. Weber/Peter Arnold, Inc. Page 873: Courtesy Inner Mountain Outfitters (www.caves.org/imo). Page 874T: L. Lefkowitz/Getty Images, Inc. - Taxi. Page 874B: Robert Essel/Corbis/Stock Market. Page 875: Paul Silverman/Fundamental Photographs. Page 876: M. Angelo/Corbis/Bettmann. Page 877B: Carey B. Van Loon. Page 877T: Water container. Lead, Roman, 1st-3rd century C.E. Museo Archeologico Nazionale, Naples, Italy. Photograph © Erich Lessing/Art Resource. Page 879T: Hank Morgan/Rainbow. Page 879B: Grant Heilman/Grant Heilman Photography, Inc. Page 880: Johnson Matthey Plc. Page 881: Jessica Wecker/Photo Researchers, Inc. Page 882T: NASA Headquarters. Page 882B: Ed Degginger/Color-Pic, Inc. Page 885T: Novosti/Sovfoto/Eastfoto. Page 885B: Tom Pantages. Page 886: Space Telescope Science Institute/NASA/Science Photo Library/Photo Researchers, Inc. Page 887a: Jeffrey A. Scovil. Page 887b: Tom Bochsler/Pearson Education/PH College. Page 887c: Carey B. Van Loon. Page 887d: Stephen Frisch/Stock Boston. Page 888T: Bill Pierce/Rainbow. Page 888B: Carey B. Van Loon. Page 889: Tom Pantages. Page 890T: Richard Megna/Fundamental Photographs. Page 890B: Ed Degginger/Color-Pic, Inc. Page 893T: Tom Pantages. Page 893B: Argonne National Laboratory. Page 894: © Carl & Ann Purcell/CORBIS.

Chapter 22 Page 902: © 2001 Richard Megna, Fundamental Photographs. Page 907T: Phil Degginger/Color-Pic, Inc. Page 907B: Richard Megna/Fundamental Photographs. Page 908T: Carey B. Van Loon. Page 908B: Carey B. Van Loon. Page 909T: Carey B. Van Loon. Page 909B: Tom Pantages. Page 910a–c: Carey B. Van Loon. Page 911: Steve Gorton/Dorling Kindersley Media Library. Page 912: Reprinted with permission from M. Seul, L.R. Monar, L. O'Gorman and R. Wolfe, Morphology and local structure in labyrinthine stripe domain phase, Science 254:1616-1618, Fig. 3 (1991). Copyright

Index